Hgb	hemoglobin	🔊 O.D.	right eye
HIT	heparin-induced thrombo-cytopenia	🔊 OJ	orange juice
		🔊 O.S.	left eye
HIV	human immunodeficiency virus	OTC	over the counter
		🔊 O.U.	each eye
HMG-CoA	3-hydroxy-3-methylglutaryl coenzyme A	oz	ounce
		p.c.	after meals
HR	heart rate	PCA	patient-controlled analgesia
🔊 h.s.	at bedtime		...gh, by ...th
🔊 H.S.	half-strength		
🔊 I.J.	injection		
I.M.	intramuscular		
🔊 I.N.	intranasal		
INR	International Normalized Ratio		...mbin time
IPPB	interm... press...		...al thromboplastin time
🔊 IU	international...		premature ventricular contraction
I.V.	intravenous		every
K	potassium	🔊 Q.D.	every day
kg	kilogram	🔊 q.h.s.	at bedtime
KVO	keep vein open	q.i.d.	four times daily
L	liter	🔊 Q.O.D.	every other day
LD	lactate dehydrogenase	RBC	red blood cell
LDL	low-density lipoprotein	RDA	recommended dietary allowance
LMW	low-molecular-weight		
m	meter	RNA	ribonucleic acid
m^2	square meters	RSV	respiratory syncytial virus
🔊 µg	microgram	SA	sinoatrial
MAO	monoamine oxidase	🔊 S.C.	subcutaneous
mcg	microgram	SI	International System of Units
MDI	metered-dose inhaler		
mEq	milliequivalent	SIADH	syndrome of inappropriate antidiuretic hormone secretion
mg	milligram		
🔊 $MgSO_4$	magnesium sulfate		
ml	milliliter	S.L.	sublingual
mm	millimeter	🔊 S.Q.	subcutaneous
mm^3	cubic millimeters	SSRI	selective serotonin reuptake inhibitor
mm Hg	millimeters of mercury		
mmol	millimole	T_3	triiodothyronine
🔊 MS	morphine sulfate	T_4	thyroxine
🔊 MSO_4	morphine sulfate	TCA	tricyclic antidepressant
Na	sodium	t.i.d.	three times daily
NA	not applicable	🔊 T.I.W.	three times a week
NaCl	sodium chloride	tRNA	transfer ribonucleic acid
ng	nanogram	tsp	teaspoon
NG	nasogastric	🔊 U	unit
N.P.O.	nothing by mouth	USP	United States Pharmacopeia
NSAID	nonsteroidal anti-inflam-matory drug	VMA	vanillylmandelic acid
		WBC	white blood cell

🔊 Clinical alert. **Do not use.**

McGraw-Hill

NURSE'S
DRUG
Handbook

McGraw-Hill

NURSE'S DRUG Handbook

SEVENTH EDITION

Patricia Dwyer Schull

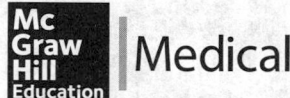

New York   Chicago   San Francisco   Lisbon   London   Madrid   Mexico City
Milan   New Delhi   San Juan   Seoul   Singapore   Sydney   Toronto

McGraw-Hill Nurse's Drug Handbook, Seventh Edition

6 7 8 9 0   LCR   21 20

ISBN 978-0-07-179942-3
MHID 0-07-179942-7
ISSN 1550-0543

This book was set in Minion by Cenveo® Publisher Services; project management was provided by Anupriya Tyagi, Cenveo Publisher Services.

The editors were Catherine A. Johnson and Robert Pancotti; and the production supervisor was Jeffrey Herzich.

This book was developed by MedVantage Publishing, LLC; the President was Patricia Dwyer Schull; the Clinical Manager was Minnie Bowen Rose; the Editorial and Copyedit Project Manager was Karen Comerford; the Designers were Stephanie Peters and Joseph John Clark; and the Editorial Supervisor was Julia S. Knipe.

LSC Communications was printer and binder.

This book is printed on acid-free paper.

McGraw-Hill books are available at special quantity discounts to use as premiums and sales promotions, or for use in corporate training programs.
To contact a representative, please e-mail us at bulksales@mcgraw-hill.com.

Contents

Part 3
Appendices

Foreword

Errors can and do occur at all phases of the medication delivery process, but more than 60% of them occur during drug administration, which is primarily the responsibility of nurses. That means nurses are the last line of defense against patient harm, and have a real opportunity to make medication delivery significantly safer.

To prevent errors, nurses must follow current and sanctioned safety guidelines, including the five rights of medication administration. But today nurses are doing more than that. They are spearheading efforts to prevent errors by improving the medication management process, using safety practices associated with fewer medication errors. These safety practices include questioning a patient's medication orders, clarifying unclear orders, reconciling patient medications from admission to discharge, and avoiding interruptions during administration.

Despite the implementation of these error-reduction strategies, protecting patients from medication errors continues to be a formidable task and a daily challenge. Nurses must stay on guard, especially as high-risk drugs appear on the market and are often prescribed for the sickest patients. And many newly approved drugs are being marketed directly to consumers.

To meet these challenges and protect patients, nurses need to use their skills and their smarts, and they need a clear nursing drug guide that focuses on patient safety from cover to cover. Since the first edition, the *McGraw-Hill Nurse's Drug Handbook* has done just that.

This handbook promotes safety by providing detailed administration guidelines and vital information for each drug, including adverse reactions, patient monitoring with a special emphasis on elderly and pediatric patients, patient education, clinical alerts, and Food and Drug Administration Boxed Warnings. Plus, the hallmark of the handbook, the special section called "Safe Drug Administration" (now 36 pages), is packed with invaluable information, such as drug compatibilities, drug names that look or sound alike, Tall Man letters, conversions and calculations, and much more.

In this seventh edition, the "Safe Drug Administration" section has a new feature, Guidelines for Timely Medication Administration, which addresses the most common violation of the five rights, the wrong time. This new feature provides the most current and authoritative guidelines for *defining* the right time for drug administration based on the nature of each prescribed drug and the relevant patient and clinical considerations. Because national regulations now require medication reconciliation to reduce errors and ensure patients understand their medications at discharge, the "Safe Drug Administration" section now also includes an updated algorithm on the steps nurses can take to reconcile patient medications.

Called the safest drug handbook for nurses by its users, this guide will help you meet the ongoing challenge of avoiding medication errors in today's complex clinical environment. With its emphasis on safe, effective drug administration in both the A-to-Z drug monographs and the full-color "Safe Drug Administration" section, the *McGraw-Hill Nurse's Drug Handbook* stands alone in the crowded, look alike, sound alike world of drug guides for nurses.

Peggy Kalowes, RN, PhD, CNS, FAHA
Director, Nursing Research and Evidence Based Practice
Long Beach Memorial and Miller Children's Hospital
Long Beach, CA

About the author

Patricia Dwyer Schull has more than 20 years' experience in nursing publishing. She is the editor and author of popular nursing journals, books, websites, and other publications and the President of MedVantage Publishing. She has held executive management positions with the top nursing publishers in the world. Before entering the publishing industry, she practiced as a professional nurse and held nursing positions in direct patient care, staff education, and hospital management. She has a Master of Science degree in Nursing, a Bachelor of Science degree, and a Registered Nurse Diploma in Nursing.

Advisors

Vicki L. Buchda, RN, MS, NEA-BC
Director of Patient Care Services
Straub Clinic and Hospital
Honolulu, HI

Pamela R. Dellinger, RN, PhD, CHCR
Director of Education
Carolinas Medical Center-Lincoln
Lincolnton, NC

**Maureen Duff, RGN, RM, RNT,
Pg Dip APS, BSc, MSc, NIP,
FFNMRCSI**
Programme Director, Nonmedical
Prescribing
School of Nursing, Midwifery and
Health
University of Stirling
Scotland, UK

Harriet R. Feldman, RN, PhD, FAAN
Dean and Professor
College of Health Professions and
Lienhard School of Nursing
Pace University
Pleasantville, NY

David Hawkins, PharmD
Vice President for Academic Affairs
and Dean of Pharmacy
California Health Sciences University
Fresno, CA

**Joyce E. Johnson, RN, PhD, NEA-BC,
FAAN**
Associate Dean, Clinical
Excellence/Clinical Professor
Rutgers University College of Nursing
New Brunswick, NJ

Peggy Kalowes, RN, PhD, CNS, FAHA
Director, Nursing Research and
Evidence Based Practice
Long Beach Memorial and Miller
Children's Hospital
Long Beach, CA

Terris Kennedy, RN, PhD
Chief Nursing Officer and Senior
Vice President
Riverside Health System
Newport News, VA

James A. Koestner, BS, PharmD
Program Director-Formulary
Management
Vanderbilt University Medical Center
Nashville, TN

Contributors and reviewers

Nancy Balkon, PhD, ANP-C, NPP, FAANP
Clinical Associate Professor
Stony Brook University School of Nursing
Stony Brook, NY

Cathy L. Bartels, PharmD
Clinical Pharmacist Educator
Children's Hospital & Medical Center
Pharmacy Department
Omaha, NE

Melanie Boock, RN, BSN, CEN, CPEN, CCRN
Emergency Department Nurse
Vail Valley Medical Center
Vail, CO

Vicky Borders-Hemphill, PharmD
Safety Evaluator
U.S. Food and Drug Administration
Silver Spring, MD

Jason Buckway, RN, BSN, MBA
Director, Cardiovascular/GI/Respiratory/Hospitalists Services
McKay-Dee Hospital Center
Intermountain Health Care
Ogden, UT

Melinda S. Carter, RPh, PharmD
Clinical Pharmacist
Coram Specialty Infusion Services
Wallingford, CT

Linda C. Copel, RN, PhD, PMHCNS, BC, CNE, NCC, FAPA
Professor, College of Nursing
Villanova University
Villanova, PA

Julie M. Gerhart, RPh, MS
Associate Director, Pharmacy Affairs
Merck & Co., Inc.
North Wales, PA

Franklin Grollman, PharmD, BCOP
Clinical Pharmacy Specialist, Hematology/Oncology Pharmacy
Walter Reed National Military Medical Center
Bethesda, MD

Delilah Hall-Towarnicke, RN, MSN, CNS, CRRN, CMSRN
Clinical Nurse Specialist Acute Rehabilitation
Cleveland Clinic Foundation
Cleveland, OH

Kathleen E. Jones, RN, CPN
Freelance Author
Centerburg, OH

Sandy Keefe, RN, MSN
Associate Director and Health Care Manager
Via West Campus
Cupertino, CA

Mary Jo Lombardo, RN, DNP, CEN
Clinical Education Program Manager, Emergency Department
Howard County General Hospital
Columbia, MD

Mary Jane McDevitt, RN, BSN, CDE
Program Director, Center for Diabetes
Springfield Hospital
Springfield, PA

Keith M. Olsen, PharmD, FCCP, FCCM
Professor and Chair, Department of Pharmacy Practice
College of Pharmacy
University of Nebraska Medical Center
Omaha, NE

Joanna Maudlin Pangilinan, PharmD, BCOP
Pharmacist
Comprehensive Cancer Center
University of Michigan Health System
Ann Arbor, MI

Lois A. Piano, RN, MSN, EdD
Research Consultant
Curtis Analytic Partners
Philadelphia, PA

Martha Polovich, RN, MN, AOCN
Oncology Clinical Nurse Specialist
Duke Oncology Network
Durham, NC

Christine Price, PharmD
Clinical Coordinator and PGY1
 Residency Director
Morton Plant Mease Health Care
Clearwater, FL

Barbara Putrycus, RN, MSN
Director of Quality, Infection Control
 Surgical Services
Oakwood Hospital & Medical Center
Dearborn, MI

Michele Riccardi, PharmD, BCPS
Pharmacy Clinical Coordinator
Midstate Medical Center
Meriden, CT

Minnie Bowen Rose, RN, BSN, MEd
Clinical Consultant
Philadelphia, PA

Cynthia Saver, RN, MS
President
CLS Development, Inc.
Columbia, MD

Ann Schlaffer, RN, PNP
Pediatric Nurse Practitioner
Eastern Shore Rural Health
Atlantic, VA

AnnMarie Smith, RN, BSN, MA
Clinical Instructor, Nursing Education
 and Professional Practice
 Development
Zielony Nursing Institute
Cleveland Clinic Foundation
Cleveland, OH

Mary E. Stassi, RN-BC
Health Occupations Coordinator
St. Charles Community College
Cottleville, MO

Jeannette Yeznach Wick, RPh, MBA, FASCP
Visiting Professor
University of Connecticut School of
 Pharmacy
Storrs, CT

Preface and user's guide

Despite ongoing and carefully considered efforts to curtail medication administration errors, medication errors continue to occur in all areas of health care—errors that affect all patient populations, resulting in increased attention by both health care professionals and consumers. Awareness of errors committed by nurses continues to increase due to numerous reports on their frequency. Consumer awareness of medication errors has also increased due to unfortunate and very publicized events at hospitals across the country, especially several cases of heparin overdose, causing deaths in infants.

The national attention focused on these upsetting events has shed light on the urgent need to develop new strategies to prevent medication errors. In response, many initiatives have been introduced to reduce the number of medication errors, and nurses are spearheading many of these endeavors.

At the same time, pharmaceutical companies continue to create powerful medications whose advanced pharmacologic features offer the promise of faster and more effective cures. Not only are many patients receiving these more powerful drugs but they're also receiving more drugs than ever before. Frequently, these patients are the sickest patients, and the patients most vulnerable to adverse drug reactions, interactions, and the life-threatening consequences of a medication error.

Further, public opinion polls consistently portray nursing as the most trusted profession, and patients look to us for guidance about their medications. Consequently, patient protection and advocacy related to drug therapy have become major challenges for nurses.

With all these challenges, nurses will always have an ongoing need to obtain more knowledge about current and newly approved medications, as well as a duty to use evidence-based best practices when giving drugs. To meet this challenge, you need a current, reliable, and practical source of drug information written especially for nurses. *McGraw-Hill Nurse's Drug Handbook,* Seventh edition, fits the bill precisely.

From its first edition, this book has focused on safe medication use. With each subsequent edition, we've added new safety-centered components and features to address newly introduced drugs, new uses for existing drugs, new drug concerns, and new evidence about the best medication administration practices. Over the past few years, as studies have shed more light on the causes of medication errors, as new drugs have been introduced, and as postmarketing ADE reports have been collected and analyzed, *McGraw-Hill Nurse's Drug Handbook* has been refined, updated, and augmented accordingly.

Targeting excellence

The quality, relevance, and success of any book for nurses hinge on whether it meets its audience's needs. To help us refine and update the book for this seventh edition, we took the same approach as with past editions, asking many practicing nurses, student nurses, nursing school deans, nursing executives, and pharmacists to review the previous edition. We also took to heart the valuable comments submitted by nurses who purchased the book. Most importantly, we've continually monitored the literature for pharmacotherapeutic research advances and innovations and emerging safety concerns.

Outstanding features

McGraw Hill Nurse's Drug Handbook, seventh edition continues to offer the outstanding features of previous editions while introducing new features reflecting recent research, readers' and reviewers' feedback, and the Joint Commission's patient safety goals and other mandates. You'll find alphabetically arranged drug monographs for approximately 1,000 generic drugs and 3,000 trade drugs. The information in these monographs has been reviewed and updated by dozens of practicing nurses and pharmacists, and then edited by our team of clinical and editorial experts. Features of this edition include:

• new monographs for newly approved drugs and certain other medications
• new indications, dosages, off-label uses, and safety warnings for preexisting drugs
• generic and trade-name drugs available in Canada (marked by a maple leaf) and the United Kingdom (UK), which are marked with a special icon (⊕)
• red "Clinical Alert" logos (◀€), which call attention to critical administration and safety considerations (especially for high-alert drugs)
• a scored tablet icon **⊘** to instantly guide your eye to the "Indications and dosages" section
• Food and Drug Administration (FDA) boxed warnings in the monographs of all drugs that have such warnings
• special icons in the monographs of every hazardous drug (⊛) or high-alert drug (⊗)
• detailed administration guidelines for each drug, with specific instructions on oral, I.M., I.V., subcutaneous, and other routes when applicable
• life-threatening adverse reactions shown in boldface
• interactions with other drugs, diagnostic tests, foods, herbs and nutritional supplements, and behaviors

• patient monitoring guidelines, including ongoing assessment, follow-up laboratory test results that indicate adverse reactions, and warning signs of an untoward event
• crucial information to consider when giving the drug to elderly or pediatric patients
• drug-altering laboratory values
• an enhanced version of our popular full-color "Safe drug administration" insert, which includes the FDA's list of recommended "tall man" names to distinguish drugs with look-alike or sound-alike names, along with guidelines for managing, preparing, and administering hazardous drugs, and a new algorithm on the steps nurses can take to reconcile patient medications and new sanctioned guidelines for timely administration of scheduled drugs
• updated and new appendices, including one on current drug shortages
• a comprehensive index so you can look up a drug by its generic name, trade name, or indications.

Drug administration guidelines

From the time a prescriber orders a drug to the time the patient receives it, the process of drug administration may involve anywhere from 80 to 200 individual steps. Missteps can happen at any point in this process—but you can help prevent some of these errors long before the dose is prepared.

Evidence-based best practices of drug administration

Best practices for preventing and detecting medication errors always starts with patient assessment at the time of admission and should be performed whenever the patient's symptoms change or a new symptom develops. During the initial patient evaluation, review the patient's current drug regimen, obtain drug allergy information, measure height and weight, and check the diagnosis and other baseline data to help determine the patient's risk of an adverse reaction. Also, make sure you're familiar with the drug's action, expected benefits, adverse reactions, and interaction potential in light of such patient factors as diagnosis and medical condition.

To further gauge your patient's risk of an ADE, ask yourself these questions:
• Is the patient elderly? Advanced age increases the risk of an ADE.
• Is the drug you're administering a high-alert or hazardous one? If so, find out what precautions you can take to reduce the chance of an ADE.
• Is the drug appropriate for the patient's diagnosis? Is it the drug of choice for this diagnosis—or just the prescriber's preference for reasons other than evidence, contraindications to alternative drugs, or a positive outcome?
• Is the patient receiving multiple drugs? Polypharmacy is extremely common, especially among older patients. The addition of each new drug increases the chance of an ADE by 10%. The more daily drugs, daily doses, and different prescribers and pharmacies involved in a patient's regimen, the greater the risk of ADEs.
• Is the patient especially vulnerable to a harmful interaction, such as a drug-drug, drug-food, drug-herb, drug-alcohol, or drug-behavior interaction?
• Has the drug been prescribed based on an altered laboratory value caused by another drug?
• Is the patient a child? Pediatric patients are at increased risk for ADEs. Drug formulations and labeling generally are geared to adults; to administer a drug to a child, you may need to calculate the pediatric dosage or mix the drug in a certain way, which increases the risk of error. Also, a child's body isn't completely developed and thus less able to overcome the effects of an overdose or interaction.

The "five rights" of drug administration

Nurses are legally responsible for applying and ensuring the "five rights" of drug administration. To help achieve these goals, use the following strategies:
• **Right patient.** Always confirm the patient's identity before administering a drug. Check his ID bracelet and ask him to state his name; then confirm his name, age, and allergies. The Joint Commission requires the use of two identifiers, such as the patient number, his telephone number, or his Social Security number. Ideally, match the ordered treatment to the patient using his name bracelet and ID number, comparing it to the drug order transcribed in the medication administration record (MAR). Be especially cautious if your patient is confused, because he may answer to the wrong name.
• **Right drug.** Giving the wrong drug is the most common type of medication error. It typically results from such factors as look-alike and sound-alike drug names, similar drug labels and packaging, and poor communication. Never try to decipher an illegible drug order, and never give a drug if you're not sure why it was prescribed.

To make sure you give the right drug, match the drug label against the order in the MAR *three times*—once when you remove the container from the patient's drug drawer, again before you remove the dose from the container and, finally, before you return the container to the drawer or discard it. Never give a drug from a container that is unlabeled or has an unreadable label, and never borrow a drug from another patient.

In an effort to reduce "wrong-drug" and other medication errors, many hospitals have adopted newer technologies, such as bar-code point-of-care drug administration systems. When using such a system, keep in mind that it must be monitored regularly for problems and that staff members must receive adequate training in its use.

• **Right dosage.** Check the dosage against the order in the MAR. Determine if it's appropriate based on the patient's age, size, vital signs, and condition. If the dose needs to be measured, use appropriate equipment—for instance, an oral syringe rather than a parenteral syringe to measure an oral liquid drug. Be on the lookout for misinterpretation of orders, incorrect calculation of volumes and infusion rates, misreading of decimal points, and labeling errors.

When administering a drug that can cause serious harm if given incorrectly (such as I.V. insulin or heparin) or when giving an infusion to a pediatric patient, always double-check the dosage and pump settings; then verify these with a colleague.

• **Right time.** The most common violation of the five rights of drug administration is giving a drug at the wrong time. For as long as many nurses can remember, the *right time* has been defined as up to 30 minutes before or after the scheduled administration time. In 2008, the Centers for Medicare & Medicaid Services (CMS) made this 30-minute rule part of their *Regulations and Interpretive Guidance for Hospitals,* which spells out the conditions of participation for receiving Medicare and Medicaid payments. In a 2010 survey by the Institute for Safe Medication Practices (ISMP), nurses described the CMS rule as unsafe, impossible to follow, and largely unnecessary.

The shortcuts and workarounds nurses used in their attempts to comply were eye-opening, and in November of 2011, recognizing the rule was no longer the standard of practice, the CMS removed it. The CMS now requires hospitals to develop their own drug administration policies and procedures based on established standards of practice and directs hospitals to consider the nature of each prescribed drug and the relevant patient and clinical considerations. In response to this new direction, we have included *Guidelines for Timely Administration of Medication* in the "Safe Drug Administration" insert, page S-8.

• **Right route.** Many drugs can be given by multiple routes. The prescriber chooses the route based on such factors as the patient's condition and the desired onset of action. In turn, the prescribed dosage is based on the administration route. Generally, oral dosages of a given drug are greater than injected dosages, so a serious overdose may occur if a dose intended for oral administration is given by injection instead.

Also, keep in mind that most serious error outcomes occur when the I.V. route is used. (Only a few high-risk drugs, such as warfarin, some chemotherapy drugs, and a few sedatives, are given orally.)

Finally, be aware that some drugs or drug forms (for instance, sustained-release tablets or capsules) should never be crushed. Crushing can alter the dosage delivered, causing the patient to receive a bolus of a drug that's meant to be released slowly over several hours.

Additional nursing responsibilities

Of course, nursing responsibilities don't stop with these five rights. Documentation, monitoring, and patient teaching are also crucial.

After giving the drug, always document that it was administered. Document the dose as soon as it is given—never before. When documenting, use only accepted abbreviations and avoid those that are used rarely or that could be misread or misinterpreted. (See *Avoiding dangerous abbreviations,*

Avoiding dangerous abbreviations

To help reduce medication errors, all health care team members must use abbreviations correctly. The Joint Commission mandates that health care organizations standardize a list of abbreviations, acronyms, and symbols that should not be used. A minimum required list of prohibited abbreviations, which includes the first five items shown below. The Joint Commission also advises organizations to consider adding the remaining items to their "Do not use" list.

Abbreviation	Potential problem	Solution
U (for "unit")	Mistaken as "0," "4," or "cc"	Write "unit."
IU (for "international unit")	Mistaken as "IV" ("intravenous") or 10 ("ten")	Write "international unit."
Q.D., Q.O.D. (for "once daily," "every other day")	Mistaken for each other. Period after "Q" may be mistaken for "I"; "O" may be mistaken for "I."	Write "daily" or "every other day."
Trailing zero (X.0 mg) (prohibited only for drug-related notations); lack of leading zero (.X mg)	Decimal point is missed.	Never write a zero by itself after decimal point (X mg); always use a zero before decimal point (0.X mg).
MS MSO$_4$ MgSO$_4$	Confused for one another. May mean "morphine sulfate" or "magnesium sulfate."	Write "morphine sulfate" or "magnesium sulfate."
> (greater than) or < (less than)	Misinterpreted as the number "7" or the letter "L"	Write "greater than" or "less than"
@	Mistaken for the number "2"	Write "at"
µg (for "microgram")	Mistaken for "mg" (milligrams), resulting in 1,000-fold overdose	Write "mcg."
H.S. (for "half-strength" or "at bedtime")	Mistaken for "half-strength" or "hour of sleep" ("at bedtime")	Write "half-strength" or "at bedtime."
q.H.S. (for "at bedtime")	Mistaken for "every hour"	Write "at bedtime."
T.I.W. (for "3 times a week")	Mistaken for "3 times a day" or "twice weekly"	Write "3 times weekly" or "three times weekly."
S.C. or S.Q. (for "subcutaneous")	Mistaken for "S.L." (sublingual) or "5 every"	Write "Sub-Q," "subQ," or "subcutaneously."
D/C (for "discharge")	Misinterpreted as "discontinue"	Write "discharge."
cc (for "cubic centimeters")	Mistaken for "U" (units) if poorly written	Write "ml" for milliliters.

Understanding pregnancy risk categories

Whenever possible, pregnant women should avoid drug therapy. The risks of taking drugs during pregnancy range from relatively minor fetal defects (such as ear tags or extra digits) to fetal death.

When drug therapy is considered, the drug's benefits to the mother must be weighed against the risk to the fetus. Ideally, the drug should provide clear benefits to the mother without harming the fetus. To help prescribers and pregnant patients assess a drug's risk-to-benefit ratio, the Food and Drug Administration assigns one of five pregnancy risk categories to each drug. In addition, certain drugs are not rated.

Category A: No evidence of risk exists. Adequate, well-controlled studies in pregnant women don't show an increased risk of fetal abnormalities during any trimester.

Category B: The risk of fetal harm is possible but remote. Animal studies show no fetal risk; however, controlled studies haven't been done in humans. Or animal studies do show a risk to the fetus, but adequate studies in pregnant women haven't shown such a risk.

Category C: Fetal risk can't be ruled out. Although animal studies show risks, adequate, well-controlled human studies are lacking. Despite the potential fetal risks, use of the drug may be acceptable because of benefits to the mother.

Category D: Positive evidence of fetal risk exists. Nevertheless, potential benefits from the drug may outweigh the risk. For example, the drug may be acceptable in a life-threatening situation or serious disease if safer drugs can't be used or are ineffective.

Category X: Contraindicated during pregnancy. Studies in animals or humans or reports of adverse reactions show evidence of fetal risk that clearly outweighs any possible benefit to the patient.

Category NR: Not rated.

page xvi, and the inside front cover, *Common abbreviations.*)

If the patient refuses a medication, report this to the prescriber immediately. Then record his refusal on both the MAR and the patient's record; include your initials, full name, and credentials on both records.

During the course of drug therapy, monitor the patient to determine drug efficacy and detect signs and symptoms of an adverse reaction or interaction. Teach the patient the name of the prescribed drug, its dosage, administration route, dosing frequency and times, and duration of therapy. Make sure he knows how to recognize the drug's therapeutic effects, adverse reactions, and interactions with other drugs, foods, herbs, and behaviors.

Be aware that the Joint Commission's 2009 National Patient Safety Goals mandate that health care facilities (and by extension, nurses) implement applicable practices that will improve or bring about the following:

- better communication among caregivers
- creation of a standardized list of abbreviations, symbols, and dose designations *not* to be used
- improved safety of drug use
- verification of all labels both verbally and visually by two qualified individuals, if the person preparing the drug is not the same person who will administer it
- accurate and complete medication reconciliation across the continuum of care
- reduction of the risk of patient harm stemming from falls caused by medications
- active involvement of patients in their own care (including teaching them about their drugs).

User's guide to *McGraw-Hill Nurse's Drug Handbook*

This book is organized in three main parts.

Part 1: A to Z drug monographs

Part 1 presents individual drug monographs in alphabetical order by generic name.

Where applicable, the top banner of the monograph includes an icon or logo denoting that the drug is a high-alert drug (⊗) or a hazardous drug (⊛). As defined by the Institute of Safe Medication Practices, *high-alert* drugs are those that can cause an increased risk of significant patient harm when used in error, and deserve special attention, caution, and safeguards.

Drugs designated as *hazardous* by the National Institute for Occupational Safety and Health, American Society of Health-System Pharmacists, and the Centers for Disease Control and Prevention include cancer chemotherapy agents, some antivirals, certain hormones, some bioengineered drugs, and selected miscellaneous drugs. These agents meet one or more of the following criteria: carcinogenicity, teratogenicity or other developmental toxicity, reproductive toxicity, organ toxicity at low doses, genotoxicity, or structure and toxicity profiles that mimic existing drugs determined to be hazardous by the above criteria. These drugs must be handled within an established safety program (see "Guidelines for preparing, handling, and administering hazardous drugs," in the "Safe drug administration" insert).

Below the banner, each monograph is presented in the following order:
Generic name. A drug's generic name is the nonproprietary name, typically assigned by the manufacturer. When more than one therapeutic form of the drug is available, generic names of these forms are listed alphabetically.

Schedules of controlled substances

The Controlled Substances Act of 1970 regulates the production and distribution of stimulants, narcotics, depressants, hallucinogens, and anabolic steroids. Drugs regulated by this law fall into five categories, or schedules, based on their abuse potential, medicinal value, and harmfulness. Schedule I drugs are the most hazardous; schedule V drugs, the least hazardous.

Schedule I: High potential for abuse; no currently accepted medical use in the United States. Using the drug even under medical supervision is thought to be unsafe.

Schedule II: High potential for abuse; currently accepted medical use in the United States (or currently accepted medical use with severe restrictions). Abuse may lead to severe psychological or physical dependence. Emergency telephone orders for limited quantities may be authorized, but the prescriber must provide a written, signed prescription order.

Schedule III: Lower abuse potential than schedule I and II drugs; currently accepted medical use in the United States. Abuse may lead to a moderate or low degree of physical dependence or high psychological dependence. Telephone orders are permitted.

Schedule IV: Lower abuse potential than schedule I, II, or III drugs; currently accepted medical use in the United States. Abuse may lead to limited physical dependence or psychological dependence. Telephone orders are permitted.

Schedule V: Low abuse potential compared to drugs in other schedules; currently accepted medical use in the United States. Abuse may lead to limited physical dependence or to psychological dependence. Some schedule V drugs may be available in limited quantities without a prescription (if state law permits).

High-alert drugs

SAFETY
GUIDELINES

Certain drugs expose patients to an increased risk of significant harm when used in error. In 2008, the Institute for Safe Medication Practices (ISMP) updated its list of high-alert drugs based on voluntary medication error reports, harmful medication errors described in the literature, practitioner feedback, and expert reviews. The ISMP has identified both high-alert drug classes (or categories) and specific high-alert drugs.

High-alert drug classes and categories

- adrenergic agonists, I.V.
- adrenergic antagonists, I.V.
- anesthetic agents, general, inhaled and I.V.
- antiarrhythmics, I.V.
- antithrombotic agents, including anticoagulants, Factor Xa inhibitors, direct thrombin inhibitors, thrombolytics, and glycoprotein IIb/IIIa inhibitors
- cardioplegic solutions
- chemotherapeutic agents
- dextrose (20% or greater)
- dialysis solutions
- epidural and intrathecal drugs
- hypoglycemics, oral
- inotropic drugs, I.V.
- liposomal drug forms
- moderate sedation agents, I.V. (or oral agents for children)
- narcotics and opioids
- neuromuscular blocking agents
- radiocontrast agents, I.V.
- total parenteral nutrition preparations

Specific high-alert drugs

- epoprostenol
- insulin, subcutaneous and I.V.
- magnesium sulfate injection
- methotrexate, oral nononcologic use
- opium tincture
- oxytocin
- potassium chloride for injection
- potassium phosphates injection
- promethazine, I.V.
- sodium chloride injection
- sodium nitroprusside for injection
- sterile water for injection, inhalation, and irrigation in containers of 100 ml or more
- Vasopressin, I.V. or intraosseous

Trade names. A drug's common trade, or brand, name is the proprietary, trademarked name under which it's marketed. Trade-name and generic drugs are therapeutically equivalent in strength, quality, performance, and use; when interchanged, they have the same effects and no differences. However, they may vary in preservatives, color, shape, labeling and, possibly, scoring. In the monographs, trade-name drugs available in Canada are marked with a maple leaf, and those available in the UK are marked with a ⊕ for easy identification.

Pharmacologic and therapeutic classes. This section specifies the drug's pharmacologic class (based on its pharmacologic properties and action—for example, sulfonamide or corticosteroid) and therapeutic class (based on approved therapeutic uses of the drug—for instance, antineoplastic or antihypertensive). Many drugs fall into multiple therapeutic classes.
Pregnancy risk category. This section lists the category assigned by the FDA to indicate the drug's potential danger to the fetus when taken during

pregnancy. (See *Understanding pregnancy risk categories,* page xvii.)

Controlled substance schedule. Narcotics, stimulants, and certain other drugs fall under the Controlled Substances Act. The Drug Enforcement Agency assigns each of these drugs a category, or schedule, based on its abuse potential and other factors. (See *Schedules of controlled substances,* page xviii.) When applicable, this section lists the drug's assigned schedule.

FDA boxed warning. The FDA assigns a boxed warning if:

• the drug may cause an adverse reaction so serious (relative to the drug's potential benefit) that prescribers must carefully weigh risk against benefit

• a serious adverse reaction can be prevented or reduced through careful patient selection, rigorous monitoring, avoiding certain concomitant therapy, adding another drug, managing the patient in a specific way, or avoiding use in a specific clinical situation

• the FDA approved the drug with restrictions to assure its safe use because it concluded that the drug can be used safely only if its distribution or use is restricted.

In this book, boxed warnings have been condensed and edited for space reasons. Be sure to review the complete package insert before administering the drug in question.

Action. This section summarizes how the drug achieves its therapeutic effect—the action that takes place when it reaches its target site and combines with cellular drug receptors to cause certain physiologic responses. When a drug's action isn't known or when researchers have proposed theories for the action but haven't clarified it definitively, we state this fact.

Availability. This section lists the physical forms in which the drug is produced and dispensed, plus available strengths (the amount of active ingredient present) for each form.

Indications and dosages. Marked with a red scored tablet icon **⊘** for quick identification, this section details the drug's FDA-approved indications for adults, children, infants, and neonates (when appropriate), along with recommended dosages, administration routes, and dosing frequency for each indication. The indications and dosages shown reflect current clinical trends, not unequivocal standards, and must be considered in light of the patient's condition and diagnosis. (Although we've made every effort to ensure the accuracy of all dosages, we urge you to become familiar with the official package insert for each drug you administer.)

Dosage adjustment. This section tells which patient groups (such as children or elderly patients), diseases, or disorders (such as renal or hepatic dysfunction) may necessitate dosage adjustment.

Off-label uses. Here you'll find a list of off-label (unlabeled or unapproved) uses of the drug, when applicable. Off-label drug use has become increasingly common as clinical research moves ahead of the FDA's approval process. In some cases, off-label use has become the standard of care.

Contraindications. This section lists conditions that contraindicate use of the drug, such as preexisting diseases. As a rule, never give a drug to a patient who has a history of hypersensitivity to that drug.

Drugs commonly implicated in hypersensitivity reactions include antibiotics, histamines, iodides, phenothiazines, tranquilizers, anesthetics, diagnostic agents (such as iodinated contrast media), and biologic agents (such as insulin, vaccines, and antitoxins).

Precautions. For some patients, a specific drug may pose an increased risk of untoward effects—yet the physician prescribes it because, in his judgment, the potential benefits outweigh the risks. For instance, many drugs can be dangerous for elderly patients, pregnant or breastfeeding women, young children, and patients with renal or hepatic dysfunction. This section tells you which patients to whom you must administer the drug cautiously. Precautions can be especially important if you're administering a high-alert drug. (See *High-alert drugs,* page xix.)

Administration. Here you'll find information to help you prepare the drug and administer it correctly and safely, regardless of the route—including whether to give it with or without food, how to mix it for I.V. or I.M. use, and what flow rate to use.

Route, onset, peak, and duration. Presented in table form, this section provides a pharmacokinetic profile—onset of action, peak blood level, and duration of action—for each route by which the drug is administered.

Adverse reactions. Occurring in roughly 30% of hospital patients, reactions can range from mild to life-threatening. They may arise immediately and suddenly, or take weeks or even months to develop.

Adverse reactions can be especially dangerous if a medication error occurs in a patient who's receiving a high-alert drug. The sickest patients—those in intensive care—typically receive anywhere from 20 to 40 different drugs. These patients are the most vulnerable to adverse reactions, drug interactions, and life-threatening consequences of a medication error. In this section, we list the most commonly reported adverse reactions by body system. Life-threatening reactions appear in **boldface.**

Interactions. With Americans taking more prescription and nonprescription drugs than ever, you're likely to encounter patients experiencing the effects of drug interactions. Many people also take herbs and nutritional supplements that can interact with drugs to cause dangerous effects or to impede a drug's intended effect. This section presents documented and clinically significant interactions that may occur if the drug is used concurrently with other drugs, specific foods, and certain herbs or supplements, or if it's combined with certain behaviors (for instance, smoking or alcohol use). It also describes the drug's effects on diagnostic test results, which can be especially important for hospital patients.

Patient monitoring. Close patient monitoring is essential during drug therapy (and in some cases, even after therapy ends) to help gauge whether the drug is effective and to detect untoward reactions or interactions. Early detection of troublesome side effects or drug inefficacy allows timely adjustments in therapy and may prevent patient injury or avoid a treatment delay.

To monitor your patient effectively, you must be familiar with the drug you're administering and its intended outcome. You must also determine whether this drug might interact with other drugs that your patient is receiving, and determine whether his medical condition, vital signs, or recent laboratory findings make him more vulnerable to interactions or adverse effects. This section discusses important nursing assessments and interventions to perform, such as monitoring blood drug levels to help determine the correct dosage and to prevent toxicity.

Patient teaching. The nurse's responsibility for teaching patients about their care has never been greater. What's more, patients are now demanding more information about their treatment. This section describes key teaching points you should cover with a patient who's receiving the drug, including essential information needed to create a patient teaching plan and protect your patient even after discharge.

Part 2: Drug classes, vitamins and minerals, herbs and supplements

Part 2 presents collective monographs on therapeutic drug classes and abbreviated monographs on vitamins, minerals, herbs, and nutritional supplements. Monographs on therapeutic drug classes familiarize you with the overall attributes of an entire drug class. These monographs also tell you which drugs the prescriber may order if a particular drug in the same class is unsuitable for your patient.

The use of herbal remedies and supplements is soaring—yet many users and health care practitioners are in the dark about these products' adverse effects and potential interactions with prescription and over-the-counter drugs. This section gives basic information that may help your patients use herbs more safely.

Part 3: Appendices, references, and index

Appendices serve as handy references on important drug topics and related issues—everything from normal laboratory values for monitoring and detecting drug levels to the top 200 most commonly prescribed drugs.

This seventh edition of *McGraw-Hill Nurse's Drug Handbook* includes a new appendix on Current Drug Shortages. In recent years, drug shortages in the United States have reached critical levels, adversely affecting drug therapy, delaying medical procedures and treatment, and contributing to medication errors. Nurses should keep informed about current drug shortages. By knowing which drugs are expected to be in short supply and discussing workable alternatives with physicians and pharmacists, nurses can ease the adverse effects of ongoing drug shortages.

Author Acknowledgments

A project of this scope and intensity demands incredible effort, hard work, and the expertise of a dedicated team. I'm indeed fortunate to work with such a group, the MedVantage Publishing team. I want to thank them all; in particular, Minnie Rose, our clinical manager, whose patience, knowledge, and attention to detail add so much to the success of this project; also Karen Comerford, editorial and copyedit project manager; Joseph John Clark, design manager; and Julia Knipe, administrator and editorial supervisor.

The entire McGraw-Hill team deserve a heartfelt thank you. Their continued support is, as always much appreciated.

I also wish to thank our advisors, contributors, and reviewers for continuing to share their expertise—and their valuable time. A project like this wouldn't be possible without them.

And a most-important thank you to all you wonderful nurses who give unselfishly of yourselves to ensure the best care and protection of your patients. I'm especially grateful to those of you who've written or e-mailed me with kind words. I appreciate your enthusiastic support.

I'm certain *McGraw-Hill Nurse's Drug Handbook* will continue to enhance your practice and help you continue to make drug therapy safer and more effective for your patients.

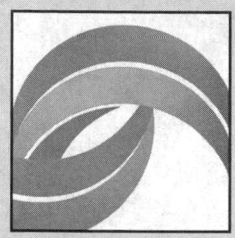

Part 1

Drug monographs A to Z
Safe drug administration

a

abacavir sulfate
Ziagen

Pharmacologic class: Carbocyclic nucleoside reverse transcriptase
Therapeutic class: Antiretroviral
Pregnancy risk category C

FDA | **BOXED WARNING**

• Drug may cause serious and potentially fatal hypersensitivity reactions, including multi-organ syndrome marked by fever, rash, GI distress, malaise, fatigue, achiness, dyspnea, cough, and pharyngitis. Discontinue immediately if you suspect such a reaction. If hypersensitivity can't be ruled out, discontinue permanently, even if other diagnoses are possible.
• After hypersensitivity reaction, never restart drug or other agents containing it, because more severe symptoms (including severe hypotension and death) may arise within hours.

Action
Converts via intracellular enzymes to active metabolite carbovir triphosphate, which inhibits activity of human immunodeficiency virus-1 (HIV-1) reverse transcriptase. Inhibits viral reproduction by interfering with DNA and RNA synthesis.

Availability
Oral solution: 20 mg/ml
Tablets: 300 mg

◑ Indications and dosages
➤ HIV-1 infection
Adults: 300 mg P.O. b.i.d. or 600 mg P.O. daily

Children ages 3 months to 16 years: 8 mg/kg P.O. b.i.d., to a maximum dosage of 300 mg b.i.d.

Contraindications
• Hypersensitivity to drug
• Hepatic disease, lactic acidosis
• Breastfeeding
• Children younger than age 3 months

Precautions
Use cautiously in:
• impaired renal function, bone marrow suppression
• risk factors for hepatic disease
• elderly patients
• pregnant patients.

Administration
• Always give in combination with other antiretrovirals.
◀≶ Be aware that drug may cause fatal hypersensitivity reactions.
• Give with food if GI upset occurs.

Route	Onset	Peak	Duration
P.O.	Unknown	0.5-1.7 hr	Unknown

Adverse reactions
CNS: headache, weakness, insomnia
GI: nausea, vomiting, diarrhea, poor appetite, pancreatitis
Hematologic: neutropenia, severe anemia
Hepatic: hepatic failure
Metabolic: mild hyperglycemia, **lactic acidosis**
Skin: rash, **erythema multiforme, toxic epidermal necrolysis**
Other: body fat redistribution, **Stevens-Johnson syndrome, fatal hypersensitivity reaction, immune reconstitution syndrome**

Interactions
Drug-drug. *Methadone:* Increased oral methadone clearance
Drug-diagnostic tests. *Alanine aminotransferase, aspartate aminotransferase, creatine phosphokinase, gammaglutamyltransferase, glucose, triglycerides:* increased levels

---

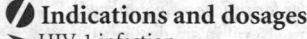

Reactions in **bold** are life-threatening.   ◀≶ Clinical alert

Drug-herbs. *St. John's wort:* decreased drug blood level and reduced drug effect

Drug-behaviors. *Alcohol use:* increased drug half-life and concentration

Patient monitoring

◄€ Assess for severe lactic acidosis, especially in women and obese patients.

◄€ Evaluate closely for signs and symptoms of hypersensitivity reaction, which can be fatal. These include fever, rash, fatigue, nausea, vomiting, diarrhea, abdominal pain, dyspnea, cough, and pharyngitis.

◄€ Be aware that immune reconstitution syndrome may occur in patients receiving combination antiretroviral therapy. During initial phase of therapy, patient whose immune system responds may develop inflammatory response to indolent or residual opportunistic infections (such as *Mycobacterium avium* complex, cytomegalovirus, *Pneumocystis jiroveci* pneumonia, and tuberculosis), which may necessitate further evaluation and treatment.

◄€ Never restart therapy if patient has experienced a previous hypersensitivity reaction to this drug.

• Check for liver enlargement.

• Monitor CBC, serum electrolytes, and liver and kidney function test results.

Patient teaching

• Advise patient to take drug with food to minimize GI upset.

• Instruct patient to refrigerate drug but not to freeze it.

◄€ Teach patient how to recognize hypersensitivity reaction. Instruct him to stop taking drug and contact prescriber immediately if signs or symptoms of such a reaction occur.

◄€ Tell patient to contact prescriber if he develops a rash (possible sign of Stevens-Johnson syndrome).

◄€ Instruct patient to immediately report signs and symptoms of immune reconstitution syndrome (such as new signs and symptoms of a previously subclinical infection, worsening or progression of a known infection despite treatment, a new infection or illness, or failure of antiretroviral therapy).

• Inform patient that drug doesn't cure HIV but lowers viral count.

• Instruct patient to obtain medication guide and warning card with each refill.

• Tell patient he'll undergo frequent blood and urine testing during therapy.

• Advise patient to consult prescriber before drinking alcohol or using herbs.

• As appropriate, review all other significant and life-threatening adverse reactions and interactions, especially those related to the drugs, tests, herbs, and behaviors mentioned above.

abatacept
Orencia

Pharmacologic class: Selective costimulation modulator

Therapeutic class: Antirheumatic

Pregnancy risk category C

Action

Inhibits T-cell activation by binding to CD80 and CD86, blocking interaction with CD28. (This interaction triggers costimulatory signal necessary for full activation of T cells, which are implicated in rheumatoid arthritis pathogenesis.)

Availability

Injection: 125 mg/ml in prefilled syringes

Powder for infusion (lyophilized): 250 mg/15 ml in single-use vial

Indications and dosages
➤ Moderate to severe adult rheumatoid arthritis as monotherapy or concomitantly with disease-modifying antirheumatic drugs other than tumor necrosis factor (TNF) antagonists

Adults weighing less than 60 kg (132 lb): 500 mg I.V. given over 30 minutes at weeks 0, 2, and 4; thereafter, give every 4 weeks. Or, 500 mg I.V. as a loading dose followed by 125 mg subcutaneously within a day, followed by 125 mg subcutaneously once weekly. For patients unable to receive an infusion, initiate weekly injections subcutaneously without an I.V. loading dose.

Adults weighing 60 to 100 kg (132 to 220 lb): 750 mg I.V. given over 30 minutes at weeks 0, 2, and 4; thereafter, give every 4 weeks. Or 750 mg I.V. as a loading dose followed by 125 mg subcutaneously within a day, followed by 125 mg subcutaneously once weekly. For patients unable to receive an infusion, may initiate weekly injections subcutaneously without an I.V. loading dose.

Adults weighing more than 100 kg: 1 g I.V. given over 30 minutes at weeks 0, 2, and 4; thereafter, give every 4 weeks. Or 1 g I.V. as a loading dose followed by 125 mg subcutaneously within a day, followed by 125 mg subcutaneously once weekly. For patients unable to receive an infusion, may initiate weekly injections subcutaneously without an I.V. loading dose.

➤ Moderately to severely active polyarticular juvenile idiopathic arthritis as monotherapy or concomitantly with methotrexate

Children age 6 and older weighing less than 75 kg: 10 mg/kg I.V. at weeks 0, 2, and 4; thereafter give every 4 weeks. Not to exceed a maximum dosage of 1 g.

Contraindications
• Hypersensitivity to drug or its components

Precautions
Use cautiously in:
• increased risk of infection or history of recurrent infections, immunocompromised state, chronic obstructive pulmonary disease (COPD)
• concurrent use of concomitant TNF antagonists
• patients older than age 65
• pregnant or breastfeeding patients
• children (safety and efficacy not established).

Administration
◀⧉ Reconstitute each vial with 10 ml sterile water for injection, using only silicone-free disposable syringe included with product.
◀⧉ During reconstitution, rotate vial by swirling gently. Avoid prolonged or vigorous agitation. Don't shake.
• Further dilute reconstituted solution to volume of 100 ml with normal saline solution.
• Use silicone-free syringe to add drug to infusion bag or bottle, and mix gently. Resulting drug concentration should be 5 mg/ml for two vials, 7.5 mg/ml for three vials, or 10 mg/ml for four vials, respectively.
• Administer infusion over 30 minutes using infusion set and nonpyrogenic, low protein-binding filter.
• Complete infusion within 24 hours of vial reconstitution.
• Don't infuse other drugs concurrently through same I.V. line.
• Watch for infusion-related reactions (hypotension or hypertension, dyspnea, nausea, dizziness, headache, flushing, urticaria, pruritus, rash, cough, or wheezing), which usually occur within 1 hour of administration. Be prepared to intervene appropriately.

Route	Onset	Peak	Duration
I.V.	Unknown	Unknown	Unknown

Adverse reactions
CNS: headache, dizziness
CV: hypertension, hypotension
EENT: nasopharyngitis
GI: nausea, dyspepsia, diverticulitis
GU: urinary tract infection, acute pyelonephritis
Musculoskeletal: back pain, extremity pain
Respiratory: cough, upper respiratory tract infection, pneumonia, wheezing, bronchitis, dyspnea
Skin: rash, flushing, urticaria, pruritus
Other: herpes zoster, pain, injection-site reactions, **malignancies**, infusion-related reactions, hypersensitivity reaction

Interactions
Drug-drug. *Immunizations:* possible decrease in immunization efficacy

Patient monitoring
• Continue to monitor patient for infusion-related events.
• Assess patient's overall health at each visit to evaluate infection status.
• Closely monitor COPD patient because of increased likelihood of adverse events.

Patient teaching
• If patient will self-administer drug, tell him to follow exact directions for injection and proper disposal of needles and syringes.
• Instruct patient to report signs and symptoms of infection.
• Caution patient to avoid immunizations during or within 3 months of stopping drug.
• Tell female with childbearing potential that pregnancy and breast-feeding aren't recommended during therapy.
• As appropriate, review all other significant adverse reactions and interactions, especially those related to the drugs mentioned above.

abciximab
ReoPro✲

Pharmacologic class: Platelet aggregation inhibitor
Therapeutic class: Antithrombotic, antiplatelet drug
Pregnancy risk category C

Action
Inhibits fibrinogen binding and platelet-platelet interaction by impeding fibrinogen binding to platelet receptor sites, thereby prolonging bleeding time

Availability
Injection: 2 mg/ml (5-ml vials containing 10 mg)

🕭 Indications and dosages
➤ Adjunct to aspirin and heparin to prevent acute cardiac ischemic complications in patients undergoing percutaneous coronary intervention (PCI)
Adults: 0.25 mg/kg I.V. bolus given 10 to 60 minutes before start of PCI, followed by infusion of 0.125 mcg/kg/minute for 12 hours. Maximum dosage is 10 mcg/minute.
➤ Adjunct to aspirin and heparin in patients with unstable angina who haven't responded to conventional medical therapy and will undergo PCI within 24 hours
Adults: 0.25 mg/kg I.V. bolus, followed by 18- to 24-hour infusion of 10 mcg/minute, ending 1 hour after PCI

Contraindications
• Hypersensitivity to drug or murine proteins
• Active internal bleeding
• Bleeding diathesis
• Severe, uncontrolled hypertension

- Thrombocytopenia (< 100,000 cells/mm³)
- Neutropenia
- Aneurysm
- Arteriovenous malformation
- History of cerebrovascular accident
- Oral anticoagulant therapy within past 7 days (unless prothrombin time is < 1.2 times control)

Precautions
Use cautiously in:
- patients receiving drugs that affect hemostasis (such as thrombolytics, anticoagulants, or antiplatelet drugs)
- pregnant or breastfeeding patients.

Administration
- I.V. bolus dose may be given undiluted. For I.V. infusion, further dilute the desired dose with normal saline or D_5W.
- Give through separate I.V. line with no other drugs.
- Avoid noncompressible I.V. sites, such as subclavian or jugular vein.
- ◄⏫ Stop continuous infusion after failed PCI.
- Restrict patient to bed rest for 6 to 8 hours after drug withdrawal or 4 hours after heparin withdrawal (whichever occurs first).
- After catheter removal, apply pressure to femoral artery for at least 30 minutes.

Route	Onset	Peak	Duration
I.V.	Rapid	30 min	48 hr

Adverse reactions
CNS: dizziness, anxiety, agitation, abnormal thinking, hypoesthesia, difficulty speaking, confusion, weakness, **cerebral ischemia, coma**
CV: pseudoaneurysm, palpitations, vascular disorders, arteriovenous fistula, hypotension, peripheral edema, weak pulse, intermittent claudication, bradycardia, **ventricular or supraventricular tachycardia, atrial fibrillation or flutter, atrioventricular block, nodal arrhythmias, pericardial effusion, embolism, thrombophlebitis**
EENT: abnormal or double vision
GI: nausea, vomiting, diarrhea, constipation, dyspepsia, ileus, gastroesophageal reflux, enlarged abdomen, dry mouth
GU: urinary tract infection, urine retention or urinary incontinence, painful or frequent urination, abnormal renal function, cystalgia, prostatitis
Hematologic: anemia, **leukocytosis, thrombocytopenia, bleeding**
Metabolic: diabetes mellitus, **hyperkalemia**
Musculoskeletal: myopathy, myalgia, increased muscle tension, reduced muscle stretching ability
Respiratory: pneumonia, crackles, rhonchi, bronchitis, pleurisy, **pleural effusion, bronchospasm, pulmonary edema, pulmonary embolism**
Skin: pallor, cellulitis, petechiae, pruritus, bullous eruptions, diaphoresis
Other: abscess, peripheral coldness, development of human antichimeric antibodies

Interactions
Drug-drug. *Drugs that affect hemostasis (such as aspirin, dextran, dipyridamole, heparin, nonsteroidal antiinflammatory drugs, oral anticoagulants, thrombolytics, and ticlopidine):* increased bleeding risk
Drug-diagnostic tests. *Activated partial thromboplastin time (APTT), clotting time, prothrombin time (PT):* increased values
Platelets: decreased count

Patient monitoring
- Assess platelet count before, during, and after therapy.
- ◄⏫ Monitor catheter insertion site frequently for bleeding.
- ◄⏫ During catheter insertion and for 6 hours after catheter removal, frequently

monitor digital pulse in leg where catheter was inserted.
• Monitor CBC, PT, APTT, and International Normalized Ratio.
• Minimize arterial or venous punctures, automatic blood pressure cuff use, I.M. injections, nasotracheal or nasogastric intubation, and urinary catheterization.
• Use indwelling venipuncture device, such as heparin lock, to draw blood.

Patient teaching
• Tell patient what to expect during and after drug administration.
• Advise patient to minimize GI upset by eating small, frequent servings of food and drinking plenty of fluids.
◀€ Instruct patient to immediately report unusual bleeding or bruising.
• Caution patient to avoid activities that may cause injury. Advise him to use soft toothbrush and electric razor to avoid gum and skin injury.
• Inform patient that he'll undergo regular blood testing during therapy.
• As appropriate, review all other significant and life-threatening adverse reactions and interactions, especially those related to the drugs and tests mentioned above.

abiraterone acetate
Zytiga

Pharmacologic class: CYP17 inhibitor
Therapeutic class: Antineoplastic
Pregnancy risk category X

Action
Converts from abiraterone acetate in vivo to abiraterone, an androgen biosynthesis inhibitor that inhibits 17α-hydroxylase/C17,20-lyase (CYP17), an enzyme that's expressed in testicular, adrenal, and prostatic tumor tissues and is required for androgen biosynthesis, thereby causing androgen-sensitive prostatic carcinoma to respond to such treatment that decreases androgen levels

Availability
Tablets: 250 mg

Indications and dosages
➤ Metastatic castration-resistant prostate cancer in combination with prednisone in patients who have received prior chemotherapy containing docetaxel
Adults: 1,000 mg P.O. daily in combination with prednisone 5 mg P.O. b.i.d.

Dosage adjustment
• Baseline moderate hepatic impairment (Child-Pugh Class B)

Contraindications
• Pregnancy
• Women of childbearing age

Precautions
Use cautiously in:
• mild to moderate hepatic disease, mineralocorticoid excess, adrenocortical insufficiency, CV disease
• co-administration of CYP2D6 substrates with a narrow therapeutic index (avoid use or if alternative treatments can't be used, consider a dosage reduction of the concomitant CYP2D6 substrate)
• co-administration of strong inhibitors and inducers of CYP3A4 (avoid or use with caution)
• breastfeeding women
• children (safety and efficacy not established).

Administration
◀€ Be aware that pregnant women and women of childbearing age shouldn't handle drug without wearing gloves.
• Control hypertension and correct hypokalemia before starting drug.

- Give tablets whole and be aware that patient shouldn't eat for at least 2 hours before drug is administered and for at least 1 hour after drug is administered.

🔊 Don't use in patients with baseline severe hepatic impairment (Child-Pugh Class C).

- Withhold drug in patients who develop hepatotoxicity during treatment until recovery. May restart drug at a reduced dosage.

🔊 Discontinue drug if patient develops severe hepatotoxicity.

- Be aware that safety isn't established in patients with left ventricular ejection fraction less than 50% or New York Heart Association Class III or IV heart failure.

Route	Onset	Peak	Duration
P.O.	Unknown	Unknown	Unknown

Adverse reactions

CV: hypertension, arrhythmia, **heart failure**
GI: diarrhea, dyspepsia
GU: urinary tract infection, urinary frequency, nocturia
Hepatic: hepatotoxicity
Metabolic: hypokalemia, mineralocorticoid excess with fluid retention, adrenocortical insufficiency, **hyperosmolar coma or death**
Musculoskeletal: joint swelling or discomfort, muscle discomfort, fractures, musculoskeletal and connective tissue disorders
Respiratory: cough, upper respiratory tract infection
Other: fluid retention, edema, hot flushes, chest pain or discomfort

Interactions

Drug-drug. *CYP2D6 substrates with a narrow therapeutic index (such as thioridazine):* increased CYP2D6 substrate C_{max} and area under the curve (AUC)
CYP3A4 inducers (such as carbamazepine, phenobarbital, phenytoin, rifabutin, rifapentine, rifampin): unknown effects
Strong CYP3A4 inhibitors (such as atazanavir, clarithromycin, indinavir, itraconazole, ketoconazole, nefazodone, nelfinavir, ritonavir, saquinavir, telithromycin, voriconazole): unknown effects
Drug-diagnostic tests. *ALT, AST, triglycerides, total bilirubin):* increased levels
Potassium: reduced level
Drug-food. *Any food:* increased abiraterone AUC

Patient monitoring

- Monitor hepatic function tests closely and modify, interrupt, or discontinue dosing as prescribed.
- Monitor blood pressure, serum potassium level, and signs and symptoms of fluid retention at least monthly.
- Monitor patient for signs and symptoms of adrenocortical insufficiency (such as hypoglycemia, hypotension, orthostatic hypotension, dehydration, weight loss, and nausea and vomiting); be aware that increased dosage of corticosteroids may be indicated before, during, and after stressful situations.

Patient teaching

- Tell patient to swallow tablets whole with water on an empty stomach (don't eat for at least 2 hours before taking drug and for at least 1 hour after taking drug).
- Instruct patient to take drug with prednisone as prescribed and not to interrupt or stop either drug without consulting prescriber.
- Instruct patient to report joint or muscle discomfort, urinary or respiratory tract infection, urinating more frequently or during the night, dizziness on standing, extreme thirst, or weight loss.

Reactions in **bold** are life-threatening. 🔊 Clinical alert

◀€ Advise pregnant women and women of childbearing age not to handle drug without wearing gloves.
• Advise male patient of child-producing age to use a condom and another effective contraceptive during therapy if having sex with a woman of childbearing potential.
• As appropriate, review all other significant and life-threatening adverse reactions and interactions, especially those related to the drugs, tests, and food mentioned above.

acamprosate calcium
Campral

Pharmacologic class: Gamma-aminobutyric acid (GABA) analogue
Therapeutic class: Detoxification agent
Pregnancy risk category C

Action
Unclear. May interact with glutamate and GABA neurotransmitter systems centrally, restoring balance between neuronal excitation and inhibition (which is altered by chronic alcoholism).

Availability
Tablets (enteric-coated): 333 mg

🕖 Indications and dosages
➤ To maintain abstinence from alcohol in patients with alcohol dependence who are abstinent when treatment begins
Adults: 2 tablets P.O. t.i.d.

Dosage adjustment
• Moderate renal impairment

Contraindications
• Hypersensitivity to drug
• Severe renal impairment

Precautions
Use cautiously in:
• mild to moderate renal impairment
• suicidal ideation or behavior
• elderly patients
• breastfeeding patients
• children.

Administration
• Give without regard to meals.
• Don't crush or break enteric-coated tablet.
• Know that drug helps maintain alcohol abstinence only when used as part of treatment program that includes counseling and support.

Route	Onset	Peak	Duration
P.O.	Unknown	3-8 hr	Unknown

Adverse reactions
CNS: apathy, confusion, agitation, neurosis, malaise, somnolence, abnormal thinking, vertigo, asthenia, anxiety, depression, dizziness, insomnia, paresthesia, tremor, withdrawal syndrome headache, migraine, abnormal dreams, hallucinations, **seizures, suicidal ideation or suicide attempt**
CV: chest pain, palpitations, syncope, hypotension, angina pectoris, varicose veins, phlebitis, peripheral edema, orthostatic hypotension, vasodilation, tachycardia, hypertension, **myocardial infarction**
EENT: abnormal vision, amblyopia, hearing loss, tinnitus, rhinitis, pharyngitis
GI: nausea, vomiting, diarrhea, constipation, abdominal pain, dyspepsia, flatulence, belching, gastroenteritis, gastritis, esophagitis, hematemesis, dry mouth, anorexia, pancreatitis, **rectal hemorrhage, GI hemorrhage**
GU: urinary frequency, urinary tract infection, urinary incontinence, erectile dysfunction, increased or decreased libido, metrorrhagia, vaginitis
Hematologic: anemia, ecchymosis, eosinophilia, lymphocytosis, **thrombocytopenia**
Hepatic: hepatic cirrhosis

Metabolic: hyperglycemia, diabetes mellitus, hyperuricemia, gout, avitaminosis
Musculoskeletal: joint, muscle, neck, or back pain
Respiratory: cough, dyspnea, bronchitis, epistaxis, pneumonia, **asthma**
Skin: pruritus, sweating
Other: abnormal taste, increased thirst, increased appetite, weight gain or loss, pain, infection, flulike symptoms, chills, abscess, hernia, allergic reaction, accidental or intentional injury, **intentional overdose**

Interactions
Drug-drug. *Naltrexone:* increased acamprosate blood level
Drug-diagnostic tests. *Bilirubin, eosinophils, lymphocytes:* increased levels
Liver function tests: abnormal results
Red blood cells: decreased count

Patient monitoring
◀€ Monitor patient for depression or expressed suicidal ideation.
• Monitor creatinine clearance during therapy.

Patient teaching
• Instruct patient to swallow tablet whole, with or without food.
• Advise patient to keep taking drug exactly as prescribed, even if he has a relapse. Encourage him to discuss any renewed alcohol consumption with prescriber.
◀€ Instruct patient to contact prescriber immediately if he experiences seizure, chest pain, suicidal thoughts, or symptoms of liver problems (such as unusual tiredness or yellowing of skin or eyes).
• Caution patient to move slowly to a sitting or standing position, to avoid dizziness or light-headedness from a sudden blood pressure decrease.
• Advise patient to avoid driving and other hazardous activities until he knows how drug affects concentration, alertness, vision, coordination, and physical dexterity.
• Instruct female patient to notify prescriber if she becomes or intends to become pregnant or to breastfeed during therapy.
• Inform patient that drug helps maintain abstinence from alcohol only when used as part of treatment program that includes counseling and support.
• Emphasize that drug doesn't eliminate or diminish alcohol withdrawal symptoms.
• As appropriate, review all other significant and life-threatening adverse reactions and interactions, especially those related to the drugs and tests mentioned above.

acarbose
Glucobay ⊕, Prandase ✤, Precose

Pharmacologic class: Alphaglucosidase inhibitor
Therapeutic class: Hypoglycemic
Pregnancy risk category B

Action
Improves blood glucose control by slowing carbohydrate digestion in intestine and prolonging conversion of carbohydrates to glucose

Availability
Tablets: 25 mg, 50 mg, 100 mg

⊘ Indications and dosages
➤ Treatment of type 2 (non-insulin-dependent) diabetes mellitus when diet alone doesn't control blood glucose
Adults: Initially, 25 mg P.O. t.i.d. Increase q 4 to 8 weeks as needed until maintenance dosage is reached. Maximum dosage is 100 mg P.O. t.i.d. for

---

adults weighing more than 60 kg (132 lb); 50 mg P.O. t.i.d. for adults weighing 60 kg or less.

Contraindications
- Hypersensitivity to drug
- Renal dysfunction
- Type 1 diabetes mellitus, diabetic ketoacidosis
- GI disease
- Cirrhosis
- Colonic ulcers
- Inflammatory bowel disease
- Intestinal obstruction
- Pregnancy or breastfeeding

Precautions
Use cautiously in:
- patients receiving concurrent hypoglycemic drugs
- children.

Administration
- Give with first bite of patient's three main meals.
- Know that drug prevents breakdown of table sugar (sucrose). Thus, mild hypoglycemia must be corrected with oral glucose (such as D-glucose or dextrose), and severe hypoglycemia may warrant I.V. glucose or glucagon injection.
- Be aware that drug may be used alone or in combination with insulin, metformin, or sulfonylureas (such as glipizide, glyburide, or glimepiride).

Route	Onset	Peak	Duration
P.O.	Rapid	1 hr	Unknown

Adverse reactions
GI: diarrhea, abdominal pain, flatulence
Metabolic: hypoglycemia (when used with insulin or sulfonylureas)
Other: edema, hypersensitivity reaction (rash)

Interactions
Drug-drug. *Activated charcoal, calcium channel blockers, corticosteroids, digestive enzymes, diuretics, estrogen, hormonal contraceptives, isoniazid,* *nicotinic acid, phenothiazines, phenytoin, sympathomimetics, thyroid products:* decreased therapeutic effect of acarbose
Digoxin: decreased digoxin blood level and reduced therapeutic effect
Insulin, sulfonylureas: hypoglycemia
Drug-diagnostic tests. *Alanine aminotransferase, aspartate aminotransferase:* increased levels
Calcium, vitamin B_6: decreased levels
Hematocrit: decreased

Patient monitoring
- Monitor patient for hypoglycemia if he's taking drug concurrently with insulin or sulfonylureas.
- Stay alert for hyperglycemia during periods of increased stress.
- Assess GI signs and symptoms to differentiate drug effects from those caused by paralytic ileus.
- Check 1-hour postprandial glucose level to gauge drug's efficacy.
- Monitor liver function test results. Report abnormalities so that dosage adjustments may be made as needed.

Patient teaching
- Inform patient that drug may cause serious interactions with many common medications, so he should tell all prescribers he's taking it.
- Teach patient about other ways to control blood glucose level, such as recommendations regarding diet, exercise, weight reduction, and stress management.
- Stress importance of testing urine and blood glucose regularly.
- Teach patient about signs and symptoms of hypoglycemia. Tell him that although this drug doesn't cause hypoglycemia when used alone, hypoglycemic symptoms may arise if he takes it with other hypoglycemics.
- Urge patient to keep oral glucose on hand to correct mild hypoglycemia; inform him that sugar in candy won't correct hypoglycemia.

♣ Canada   ✛ UK   ☣ Hazardous drug   ⊗ High-alert drug

- Inform patient that GI symptoms such as flatulence may result from delayed carbohydrate digestion in intestine.
- Advise patient to obtain medical alert identification and to carry or wear it at all times.
- As appropriate, review all other significant and life-threatening adverse reactions and interactions, especially those related to the drugs and tests mentioned above.

acetaminophen

Abenol✢, Acephen, Anadin Paracetamol❋, Apo-Acetaminophen✢, Aspirin Free Anacin, Atasol✢, Calpol❋, Cetaphen, Children's Tylenol Soft Chews, Disprol❋, Feverall, Galpamol❋, Genapap, Little Fevers, Mandanol❋, Mapap, Nortemp, Nortemp Children's, Novo-Gesic✢, Pain Eze, Panadol❋, Pediatrix✢, Silapap, Tempra✢, Tycolene, Tylenol 8 Hour, Tylenol, Tylenol Arthritis, Tylenol Extra Strength, Valorin

Pharmacologic class: Synthetic non-opioid *p*-aminophenol derivative
Therapeutic class: Analgesic, antipyretic
Pregnancy risk category B

Action
Unclear. Pain relief may result from inhibition of prostaglandin synthesis in CNS, with subsequent blockage of pain impulses. Fever reduction may result from vasodilation and increased peripheral blood flow in hypothalamus, which dissipates heat and lowers body temperature.

Availability
Caplets (extra-strength): 500 mg
Caplets, capsules: 160 mg, 500 mg, 650 mg (extended-release)
Drops: 100 mg/ml
Elixir: 80 mg/2.5 ml, 80 mg/5 ml, 120 mg/5 ml, 160 mg/5 ml
Gelcaps: 500 mg
Liquid: 160 mg/5 ml, 500 mg/15 ml
Solution: 80 mg/1.66 ml, 100 mg/1 ml, 120 mg/2.5 ml, 160 mg/5 ml, 167 mg/5 ml
Suppositories: 80 mg, 120 mg, 125 mg, 300 mg, 325 mg, 650 mg
Suspension: 32 mg/ml, 160 mg/5 ml
Syrup: 160 mg/5 ml
Tablets (chewable): 80 mg, 160 mg
Tablets (extended-release): 160 mg, 325 mg, 500 mg, 650 mg
Tablets (film-coated): 160 mg, 325 mg, 500 mg

💊 Indications and dosages
➤ Mild to moderate pain caused by headache, muscle ache, backache, minor arthritis, common cold, toothache, or menstrual cramps or fever
Adults and children age 12 and older: 325 to 650 mg P.O. q 4 to 6 hours, or 1,000 mg three or four times daily. Or two extended-release caplets or tablets P.O. q 8 hours, to a maximum dosage of 4,000 mg/day. Or 650 mg P.R. q 4 to 6 hours, to a maximum dosage of 4,000 mg/day. Or, two extra-strength caplets q 6 hours, to a maximum dosage of six caplets/day.
Children: 10 to 15 mg/kg, or as indicated below:

Oral use

Age	Usual dosage	Maximum dosage
11-12 years	480 mg q 4 hr	5 doses in 24 hr
9-10 years	400 mg q 4 hr	5 doses in 24 hr
6-8 years	320 mg q 4 hr	5 doses in 24 hr
4-5 years	240 mg q 4 hr	5 doses in 24 hr
2-3 years	160 mg q 4 hr	5 doses in 24 hr
1 year	120 mg q 4 hr	5 doses in 24 hr
4-11 months	80 mg q 4 hr	5 doses in 24 hr
0-3 months	40 mg q 4 hr	5 doses in 24 hr

Rectal use

Age	Usual dosage	Maximum dosage
12 years and older	325-650 mg q 4 hr	4,000 mg/day
11-12 years	320-480 mg q 4 hr	2,880 mg/day
6-11 years	325 mg q 4 hr	2,600 mg/day
3-6 years	120-125 mg q 6 hr	720 mg/day
1-3 years	80 mg q 4 hr	
3-11 months	80 mg q 6 hr	

Dosage adjustment
• Renal or hepatic impairment

Contraindications
• Hypersensitivity to drug

Precautions
Use cautiously in:
• anemia, hepatic or renal disease
• elderly patients
• pregnant or breastfeeding patients
• children younger than age 2.

Administration
• Be aware that although most patients tolerate drug well, toxicity can occur with a single dose.
• Know that acetylcysteine may be ordered to treat acetaminophen toxicity, depending on patient's blood drug level. Activated charcoal is used to treat acute, recent acetaminophen overdose (within 1 hour of ingestion).
• Determine overdose severity by measuring acetaminophen blood level no sooner than 4 hours after overdose ingestion (to ensure that peak concentration has been reached).

Route	Onset	Peak	Duration
P.O.	0.5-1 hr	10-60 min	3-8 hr (dose dependent)
P.R.	0.5-1 hr	10-60 min	3-4 hr

Adverse reactions
Hematologic: thrombocytopenia, hemolytic anemia, neutropenia, leukopenia, pancytopenia
Hepatic: jaundice, **hepatotoxicity**
Metabolic: hypoglycemic coma
Skin: rash, urticaria
Other: hypersensitivity reactions (such as fever)

Interactions
Drug-drug. *Activated charcoal, cholestyramine, colestipol:* decreased acetaminophen absorption
Barbiturates, carbamazepine, diflunisal, hydantoins, isoniazid, rifabutin, rifampin, sulfinpyrazone: increased risk of hepatotoxicity
Hormonal contraceptives: decreased acetaminophen efficacy
Oral anticoagulants: increased anti-coagulant effect
Phenothiazines (such as chlorproma-zine, fluphenazine, thioridazine): severe hypothermia
Zidovudine: increased risk of granulocytopenia
Drug-diagnostic tests. *Home glucose measurement systems:* altered results
Urine 5-hydroxyindole acetic acid: false-positive result
Drug-behaviors. *Alcohol use:* increased risk of hepatotoxicity

Patient monitoring
◀€ Observe for acute toxicity and overdose. Signs and symptoms of acute toxicity are as follows—*Phase 1:* Nausea, vomiting, anorexia, malaise, diaphoresis. *Phase 2:* Right upper quadrant pain or tenderness, liver enlargement, elevated bilirubin and hepatic enzyme levels, prolonged prothrombin time, oliguria (occasional). *Phase 3:* Recurrent anorexia, nausea, vomiting, and malaise; jaundice; hypoglycemia; coagulopathy; encephalopathy; possible renal failure and cardiomyopathy. *Phase 4:* Either recovery or progression to fatal complete hepatic failure.

❀ Canada   ⊕ UK   ☙ Hazardous drug   ⊗ High-alert drug

Patient teaching

- Caution parents or other caregivers not to give acetaminophen to children younger than age 2 without consulting prescriber first.
- Tell patient, parents, or other caregivers not to use drug concurrently with other acetaminophen-containing products or to use more than 4,000 mg of regular-strength acetaminophen in 24 hours.
- Inform patient, parents, or other caregivers not to use extra-strength caplets in dosages above 3,000 mg (six caplets) in 24 hours because of risk of severe liver damage.
- Advise patient, parents, or other caregivers to contact prescriber if fever or other symptoms persist despite taking recommended amount of drug.
- Inform patients with chronic alcoholism that drug may increase risk of severe liver damage.
- As appropriate, review all other significant and life-threatening adverse reactions and interactions, especially those related to the drugs, tests, and behaviors mentioned above.

acetazolamide

Acetazolam✱, AK-Zol, Apo-Acetazolamide✱, Diamox✱, Diamox Sequels

Pharmacologic class: Carbonic anhydrase inhibitor
Therapeutic class: Diuretic, antiglaucoma drug, anticonvulsant, altitude agent, urinary alkalinizer
Pregnancy risk category C

Action

Inhibits carbonic anhydrase in kidney, decreasing water reabsorption and increasing excretion of sodium, potassium, and bicarbonate. Lowers intraocular pressure by decreasing aqueous humor production. May raise seizure threshold by reducing carbonic anhydrase in CNS, thereby decreasing neuronal conduction.

Availability

Capsules (sustained-release): 500 mg
Injection: 500 mg/vial
Tablets: 125 mg, 250 mg

⬛ Indications and dosages

➤ Open-angle (chronic simple) glaucoma (given with miotics)
Adults: 250 mg P.O. one to four times daily, or 500-mg sustained-release capsule P.O. once or twice daily. Don't exceed total daily dosage of 1 g.
➤ Preoperative treatment of closed-angle (secondary) glaucoma
Adults: 250 mg P.O. q 4 hours or 250 mg P.O. b.i.d.; in acute cases only, 500 mg P.O. followed by 125 to 250 mg P.O. q 4 hours. For rapid relief of increased intraocular pressure, 500 mg I.V., repeated in 2 to 4 hours; then 125 to 250 mg P.O. q 4 to 6 hours.
Children: 10 to 15 mg/kg/day P.O. in divided doses q 6 to 8 hours, or 5 to 10 mg/kg I.V. q 6 hours
➤ Seizure disorder (given with other anticonvulsants)
Adults and children: 250 mg P.O. daily when given with another anticonvulsant, or 8 to 30 mg/kg daily P.O. in one to four divided doses. Usual dosage range is 375 mg to 1 g daily.
➤ Drug-induced edema or edema secondary to heart failure
Adults: Initially, 250 to 375 mg P.O. daily. If diuresis fails, give dose on alternate days, or give for 2 days alternating with day of rest.
Children: 5 mg/kg P.O. daily, or 150 mg/m² P.O. or I.V. once daily in morning
➤ Acute high-altitude (mountain) sickness
Adults: 500 mg to 1 g P.O. daily in divided doses, or sustained-release

capsule q 12 to 24 hours. Dosing should begin 24 to 48 hours before ascent and continue during ascent and for 48 hours after reaching desired altitude. For rapid ascent, 1-g P.O. dose is recommended.

Dosage adjustment
• Mild renal failure

Off-label uses
• Acute pancreatitis
• Alkalosis after open-heart surgery
• Hereditary ataxia
• Peptic ulcer
• Periodic paralysis
• Renal calculi
• Phenobarbital or lithium overdose
• Hydrocephalus in infants

Contraindications
• Hypersensitivity to drug or sulfonamides
• Adrenocortical insufficiency
• Closed-angle glaucoma
• Severe pulmonary obstruction
• Severe renal disease, hypokalemia, hyponatremia
• Hepatic disease

Precautions
Use cautiously in:
• respiratory, renal, or hepatic disease; diabetes mellitus, hypercalcemia, gout, adrenocortical insufficiency
• pregnant or breastfeeding patients.

Administration
◀€ Before giving, ask if patient is pregnant. Drug may cause fetal toxicity.
• Direct I.V. administration is preferred. When giving by direct I.V. route, reconstitute 500-mg vial with more than 5 ml of sterile water for injection; administer over 1 minute.
• When giving drug intermittently by I.V. infusion, further dilute with normal saline solution or dextrose solution and infuse over 4 to 8 hours.

• Be aware that I.M. administration is painful because solution is alkaline.
• If necessary, crush tablets and mix in nonsweet, nonalcoholic syrup or non-glycerin solution.

Route	Onset	Peak	Duration
P.O.	1 hr	2-4 hr	8-12 hr
P.O. (sustained)	2 hr	8-12 hr	18-24 hr
I.V., I.M.	1-2 min	15-18 min	4-5 hr

Adverse reactions
CNS: weakness, nervousness, irritability, drowsiness, confusion, dizziness, depression, tremor, headache, paresthesia, flaccid paralysis, **seizures**
EENT: transient myopia, tinnitus, hearing dysfunction, sensation of lump in throat
GI: nausea, vomiting, diarrhea, constipation, melena, abdominal distention, dry mouth, anorexia
GU: dysuria, hematuria, glycosuria, polyuria, crystalluria, renal colic, renal calculi, **uremia, sulfonamide-like renal lesions, renal failure**
Hematologic: thrombocytopenia, leukopenia, agranulocytosis, hemolytic anemia, thrombocytopenic purpura, pancytopenia, bone marrow depression with aplastic anemia
Hepatic: hepatic insufficiency
Metabolic: hypokalemia, hyperglycemia and glycosuria, hyperuricemia and gout, **metabolic acidosis, hyperchloremic acidosis**
Respiratory: hyperpnea
Skin: rash, pruritus, urticaria, photosensitivity, hirsutism, cyanosis
Other: altered taste and smell, weight loss, fever, excessive thirst, pain at I.M. injection site, hypersensitivity reaction, **Stevens-Johnson syndrome**

Interactions
Drug-drug. *Amphetamines, procainamide, quinidine, tricyclic antidepressants:* decreased excretion and

enhanced or prolonged effect of these drugs, leading to toxicity

Amphotericin B, corticosteroids, cortico-trophin, other diuretics: increased risk of hypokalemia

Lithium, phenobarbital, salicylates: increased excretion of these drugs, possibly reducing their efficacy

Methenamine compounds: inactivation of these drugs

Phenytoin, primidone: severe osteomalacia

Salicylates: increased risk of salicylate toxicity

Drug-diagnostic tests. *Ammonia, bili-rubin, calcium, chloride, glucose, uric acid:* increased levels

Thyroid iodine uptake: decreased in patients with hyperthyroidism or normal thyroid function

Urinary protein (with some reagents): false-positive result

Drug-behaviors. *Sun exposure:* increased risk of photosensitivity

Patient monitoring

◀≋ Evaluate for signs and symptoms of sulfonamide sensitivity; drug can cause fatal hypersensitivity.

◀≋ Monitor laboratory test results for hematologic changes; blood glucose, potassium, bicarbonate, and chloride levels; and liver and kidney function changes.

• Observe for signs and symptoms of bleeding tendency.

• Monitor fluid intake and output.

Patient teaching

• Advise patient to take drug with food if GI upset occurs.

• Caution patient to avoid driving and other hazardous activities until he knows how drug affects concentration and alertness.

• Tell patient to eat potassium-rich foods (such as seafood, bananas, and oranges) if taking drug long term or receiving other potassium-depleting drugs.

• Advise patient to avoid activities that can cause injury. Advise him to use soft toothbrush and electric razor to avoid gum and skin injury.

• Tell patient to report significant numbness or tingling.

• Inform patient that he'll undergo regular blood testing during therapy.

• As appropriate, review all other significant and life-threatening adverse reactions and interactions, especially those related to the drugs, tests, and behaviors mentioned above.

acetylcysteine (*N*-acetylcysteine)
Acetadote, Mucomyst✽, Mucosil-10, Mucosil-20, Parovelex✽⊕

Pharmacologic class: N-acetyl derivative of naturally occurring amino acid (L-cysteine)

Therapeutic class: Mucolytic, acetaminophen antidote

Pregnancy risk category B

Action
Decreases viscosity of secretions, promoting secretion removal through coughing, postural drainage, and mechanical means. In acetaminophen overdose, maintains and restores hepatic glutathione, needed to inactivate toxic metabolites.

Availability
Injection: 200 mg/ml
Solution: 10%, 20%

⑦ Indications and dosages
➤ Mucolytic agent in adjunctive treatment of acute and chronic bronchopulmonary disease (bronchitis, bronchiectasis, chronic asthmatic

---

bronchitis, emphysema, pneumonia, primary amyloidism of lungs, tuberculosis, tracheobronchitis), pulmonary complications of cystic fibrosis, atelectasis, or pulmonary complications related to surgery, posttraumatic chest conditions, tracheostomy care, or use during anesthesia

Adults and children: *Nebulization (face mask, mouthpiece, tracheostomy)*— 6 to 10 ml of 10% solution or 3 to 5 ml of 20% solution three or four times daily. Dosage range is 2 to 20 ml of 10% solution or 1 to 10 ml of 20% solution q 2 to 6 hours.

Nebulization (tent or croupette)—Volume of 10% or 20% solution that will maintain heavy mist for desired period

Instillation (direct)—1 to 2 ml of 10% to 20% solution q 1 hour p.r.n.

Instillation via syringe attached to percutaneous intratracheal catheter—2 to 4 ml of 10% solution or 1 to 2 ml of 20% solution q 1 to 4 hours

➤ Diagnostic bronchial studies

Adults and children: Two to three doses of 2 to 4 ml of 10% solution or 1 to 2 ml of 20% solution by nebulization or intratracheal instillation before procedure

➤ Acetaminophen overdose

Adults, elderly patients, children: Give immediately if 24 hours or less have elapsed since acetaminophen ingestion. Use the following protocol: empty stomach by lavage or emesis induction, and then have patient drink copious amounts of water. If activated charcoal has been given, perform lavage before giving acetylcysteine. Draw blood for acetaminophen plasma assay and baseline aspartate aminotransferase (AST), alanine aminotransferase (ALT), prothrombin time, bilirubin, blood glucose, blood urea nitrogen, electrolyte, and creatinine clearance levels. If ingested acetaminophen dose is in toxic range, give acetylcysteine 140 mg/kg P.O. as loading dose from 20% solution. Administer

17 maintenance doses of 70 mg/kg P.O. q 4 hours, starting 4 hours after loading dose. Repeat procedure until acetaminophen blood level is safe. If patient vomits loading dose or any maintenance dose within 1 hour of administration, repeat that dose.

Off-label uses
• Unstable angina

Contraindications
• Hypersensitivity to drug (except with antidotal use)
• Status asthmaticus (except with antidotal use)

Precautions
Use cautiously in:
• renal or hepatic disease, Addison's disease, alcoholism, brain tumor, bronchial asthma, seizure disorder, hypothyroidism, respiratory insufficiency, psychosis
• elderly patients
• pregnant or breastfeeding patients.

Administration
• Separate administration times of this drug and antibiotics.
• Use plastic, glass, or stainless steel container when giving by nebulizer, because solution discolors on contact with rubber and some metals.
• Once solution is exposed to air, use within 96 hours.
• Dilute solution before administering for acetaminophen overdose, to reduce risk of vomiting, drug's unpleasant odor, and irritating or sclerosing properties.
• Chill solution and have patient sip through straw, or, if necessary, give by nasogastric tube when administering for acetaminophen overdose.

Route	Onset	Peak	Duration
P.O.	30-60 min	1-2 hr	Unknown
Instillation, inhalation	1 min	5-10 min	2-3 hr

Adverse reactions

CNS: dizziness, drowsiness, headache
CV: hypotension, hypertension, tachycardia
EENT: severe rhinorrhea
GI: nausea, vomiting, stomatitis, constipation, anorexia
Hepatic: hepatotoxicity
Respiratory: hemoptysis, tracheal and bronchial irritation, increased secretions, wheezing, chest tightness, **bronchospasm**
Skin: urticaria, rash, clamminess, **angioedema**
Other: tooth damage, chills, fever, hypersensitivity including anaphylaxis

Interactions

Drug-drug. *Activated charcoal:* increased absorption and decreased efficacy of acetylcysteine
Nitroglycerin: increased nitroglycerin effects, causing hypotension and headache
Drug-diagnostic tests. *Liver function tests:* abnormal results

Patient monitoring

• Monitor respirations, cough, and character of secretions.

Patient teaching

• Instruct patient to report worsening cough and other respiratory symptoms.
• Advise patient to mix oral form with juice or cola to mask bad taste and odor.
• As appropriate, review all other significant and life-threatening adverse reactions and interactions, especially those related to the drugs and tests mentioned above.

a

acetylsalicylic acid (aspirin)

Alka⊕, Angettes⊕, Apo-Asa✦, Apo–ASEN✦, Arthrinol✦, Arthrisin✦, Artria S.R.✦, ASA, Aspercin, Aspergum, Aspir-Low, Aspirtab, Astrin✦, Bayer, Caprin⊕, Coryphen✦, Dispirin⊕, Easprin, Ecotrin, Enpirin⊕, Entrophen✦, Halfprin, Headache Tablet✦, Micoprin⊕, Novasen✦, Nu-Seals⊕, PMS-ASA✦, PostMI⊕, Sal-Adult✦, Sal-Infant✦, St. Joseph, Supasa✦, ZORprin

Pharmacologic class: Nonsteroidal anti-inflammatory drug (NSAID)
Therapeutic class: Nonopioid analgesic, antipyretic, antiplatelet drug
Pregnancy risk category C (with full dose in third trimester: *D*)

Action

Reduces pain and inflammation by inhibiting prostaglandin production. Fever reduction mechanism unknown; may be linked to decrease in endogenous pyrogens in hypothalamus resulting from prostaglandin inhibition. Exerts antiplatelet effect by inhibiting synthesis of prostacyclin and thromboxane A_2.

Availability

Gum (chewable): 227 mg
Suppositories: 60 mg, 120 mg, 200 mg, 300 mg, 325 mg, 600 mg, 650 mg
Tablets: 81 mg, 325 mg, 500 mg
Tablets (chewable): 81 mg
Tablets (enteric-coated, delayed-release): 81 mg, 162 mg, 325 mg, 500 mg, 650 mg, 975 mg
Tablets (extended-release): 650 mg, 800 mg
Tablets (film-coated): 325 mg, 500 mg

⬭ Indications and dosages

➤ Mild pain or fever
Adults: 325 to 500 mg P.O. q 3 hours, or 325 to 650 mg P.O. q 4 hours, or 650 to 1,000 mg P.O. q 6 hours, to a maximum dosage of 4,000 mg/day. *Extended-release tablets*—650 mg to 1,300 mg q 8 hours, not to exceed 3,900 mg/day; or 800 mg q 12 hours.
Children: 10 to 15 mg/kg P.O. or P.R. q 4 hours, not to exceed total daily dosage of 3.6 g, or up to 60 to 80 mg/kg/day. See chart below.

Age (years)	Dosage (q 4 hr)
12-14	648 mg
11-12	486 mg
9-10	405 mg
6-8	324 mg
4-5	243 mg
2-3	162 mg

➤ Mild to moderate pain caused by inflammation (as in rheumatoid arthritis or osteoarthritis)
Adults: Initially, 2,400 to 3,600 mg P.O. daily in divided doses. Dosage may be increased by 325 to 1,200 mg daily at intervals of at least 1 week. Usual maintenance dosage is 3.6 to 5.4 g/day P.O. in divided doses, to a maximum dosage of 6 g/day.
➤ Juvenile rheumatoid arthritis
Children: 60 to 130 mg/kg/day P.O. in children weighing 25 kg (55 lb) or less, or 2,400 to 3,600 mg P.O. daily in children weighing more than 25 kg P.O.; give in divided doses q 6 to 8 hours.
➤ Acute rheumatic fever
Adults: 5 to 8 g/day P.O. in divided doses
Children: Initially, 100 mg/kg/day P.O. in individual doses for first 2 weeks; then maintenance dosage of 75 mg/kg/day P.O. in divided doses for next 4 to 6 weeks
➤ To reduce the risk of transient ischemic attacks (TIAs) or cerebrovascular accident in men with a history of TIAs caused by emboli
Adults: 650 mg P.O. b.i.d. or 325 mg P.O. q.i.d.
➤ To reduce the risk of myocardial infarction (MI) in patients with a history of MI or unstable angina
Adults: 75 to 325 mg/day P.O.
➤ Kawasaki disease
Children: Initially during acute febrile period, 80 to 180 mg/kg/day P.O. in four divided doses. Maintenance dosage is 3 to 10 mg/kg/day given as a single dose for up to 8 weeks or until platelet count and erythrocyte sedimentation rate return to normal.
➤ Thromboembolic disorders
Adults: 325 to 650 mg P.O. once or twice daily

Contraindications

• Hypersensitivity to salicylates, other NSAIDs, or tartrazine
• Renal impairment
• Severe hepatic impairment
• Hemorrhagic states or blood coagulation defects
• Vitamin K deficiency caused by dehydration
• Concurrent anticoagulant use
• Pregnancy (third trimester) or breastfeeding

Precautions

Use with extreme caution, if at all, in:
• hepatic disorders, anemia, asthma, gastritis, Hodgkin's disease
• heart failure or other conditions in which high sodium content is harmful (buffered aspirin)
• patients receiving other salicylates or NSAIDs concurrently
• elderly patients
• children and adolescents.

Administration

◀᎑ Never administer to child or adolescent who has signs or symptoms of chickenpox or flulike illness.

◀🔊 Don't give within 6 weeks after administration of live varicella virus vaccine, because of risk of Reye's syndrome.
• Give with food or large amounts of water or milk to minimize GI irritation.
• Know that extended-release and enteric-coated forms are best for long-term therapy.
• Be aware that aspirin should be discontinued at least 1 week before surgery because it may inhibit platelet aggregation.

Route	Onset	Peak	Duration
P.O. (tablets)	15-30 min	1-2 hr	4-6 hr
P.O. (chewable)	Rapid	Unknown	1-4 hr
P.O. (enteric-coated)	5-30 min	2-4 hr	8-12 hr
P.O. (extended)	5-30 min	1-4 hr	3-6 hr
P.R.	5-30 min	3-4 hr	1-4 hr

Adverse reactions
EENT: hearing loss, tinnitus, ototoxicity
GI: nausea, vomiting, abdominal pain, dyspepsia, epigastric distress, heartburn, anorexia, **GI bleeding**
Hematologic: thrombocytopenia, hemolytic anemia, leukopenia, agranulocytosis, shortened red blood cell life span
Hepatic: hepatotoxicity
Metabolic: hyponatremia, hypokalemia, **hypoglycemia**
Respiratory: wheezing, hyperpnea, **pulmonary edema with toxicity**
Skin: rash, urticaria, bruising, angioedema
Other: hypersensitivity reactions, **salicylism or acute toxicity**

Interactions
Drug-drug. *Acidifying drugs (such as ammonium chloride):* increased salicylate blood level
Activated charcoal: decreased salicylate absorption

Alkalinizing drugs (such as antacids): decreased salicylate blood level
Angiotensin-converting enzyme (ACE) inhibitors: decreased antihypertensive effect
Anticoagulants, NSAIDs, thrombolytics: increased bleeding risk
Carbonic anhydrase inhibitors (such as acetazolamide): salicylism
Corticosteroids: increased salicylate excretion and decreased blood level
Furosemide: increased diuretic effect
Live varicella virus vaccine: increased risk of Reye's syndrome
Methotrexate: decreased methotrexate excretion and increased blood level, causing greater risk of toxicity
Nizatidine: increased salicylate blood level
Spironolactone: decreased spironolactone effect
Sulfonylureas (such as chlorpropamide, tolbutamide): enhanced sulfonylurea effects
Tetracycline (oral): decreased absorption of tetracycline (with buffered aspirin)
Drug-diagnostic tests. *Alanine aminotransferase, alkaline phosphatase, amylase, aspartate aminotransferase, coagulation studies, Paco_2, uric acid:* increased values
Cholesterol, glucose, potassium, protein-bound iodine, sodium, thyroxine, triiodothyronine: decreased levels
Pregnancy test, protirelin-induced thyroid stimulating hormone, radionuclide thyroid imaging, serum theophylline (Schack and Waxler method), urine catecholamines, urine glucose, urine hydroxyindoleacetic acid, urine ketones (ferric chloride method), urine vanillylmandelic acid: test interference
Tests using phenosulfonphthalein as diagnostic agent: decreased urinary excretion of phenosulfonphthalein
Urine protein: increased level
Drug-food. *Urine-acidifying foods:* increased salicylate blood level

---

Reactions in **bold** are life-threatening. ◀🔊 Clinical alert

Drug-herbs. *Anise, arnica, cayenne, chamomile, clove, fenugreek, feverfew, garlic, ginger, ginkgo biloba, ginseng, horse chestnut, kelpware, licorice:* increased bleeding risk

Drug-behaviors. *Alcohol use:* increased bleeding risk

Patient monitoring

🔊 Watch for signs and symptoms of hypersensitivity and other adverse reactions, especially bleeding tendency.

• Stay alert for signs and symptoms of acute toxicity, such as diplopia, ECG abnormalities, generalized seizures, hallucinations, hyperthermia, oliguria, acute renal failure, incoherent speech, irritability, restlessness, tremor, vertigo, confusion, disorientation, mania, lethargy, laryngeal edema, anaphylaxis, and coma.

• Monitor elderly patients carefully because they're at greater risk for salicylate toxicity.

• With prolonged therapy, frequently assess hemoglobin, hematocrit, International Normalized Ratio, and kidney function test results.

• Check salicylate blood levels frequently.

• Evaluate patient for signs and symptoms of ototoxicity (hearing loss, tinnitus, ataxia, and vertigo).

Patient teaching

• Tell patient to report ototoxicity symptoms, unusual bleeding, and bruising.

• Caution patient to avoid activities that may cause injury. Advise him to use soft toothbrush and electric razor to avoid gum and skin injury.

• Instruct patient to tell all prescribers he's taking the drug, because it may cause serious interactions with many common medications.

• Tell patient not to take other over-the-counter preparations containing aspirin.

• Inform patient that he may need to undergo regular blood testing during therapy.

• As appropriate, review all other significant and life-threatening adverse reactions and interactions, especially those related to the drugs, tests, foods, herbs, and behaviors mentioned above.

acitretin
Neotigason ✦ , Soriatane

Pharmacologic class: Second-generation retinoid
Therapeutic class: Antipsoriatic
Pregnancy risk category X

FDA | BOXED WARNING

• Drug may harm fetus and must not be used by pregnant patients, those who intend to become pregnant, or those who may not use reliable contraception during therapy and for at least 3 years afterward.

• Patient must commit to using two effective contraceptive forms simultaneously. At least one form must be primary, unless patient chooses absolute abstinence, has had a hysterectomy, or is postmenopausal.

• Drug should be prescribed only by clinicians with special competence in diagnosing and treating severe psoriasis, experience using systemic retinoids, and understanding of teratogenicity risk.

• Consider drug only for women with severe psoriasis unresponsive to other therapies or whose clinical condition contraindicates other therapies.

• Instruct patient not to donate blood during therapy and for at least 3 years afterward.

Action
Unclear. Promotes normal growth cycle of skin cells, possibly by targeting retinoid receptors in these cells and adjusting factors that affect epidermal proliferation and synthesis of RNA and DNA.

Availability
Capsules: 10 mg, 17.5 mg, 25 mg

✐ Indications and dosages
➢ Severe psoriasis
Adults and elderly patients: Initially, 25 to 50 mg/day P.O. as a single dose with main meal. If initial response is satisfactory, give maintenance dosage of 25 to 50 mg/day P.O.

Off-label uses
• Darier's disease (keratosis follicularis)
• Lamellar ichthyosis (in children)
• Lichen planus
• Nonbullous and bullous ichthyosiform erythroderma
• Palmoplantar pustulosis
• Sjögren-Larsson syndrome

Contraindications
• Hypersensitivity to drug or paraben (used as preservative in gelatin capsule)
• Pregnancy or anticipated pregnancy within 3 years after drug discontinuation (drug has teratogenic and embryotoxic effects)
• Women of childbearing age who may not use reliable contraception during therapy and for at least 3 years after drug discontinuation
• Breastfeeding

Precautions
Use cautiously in:
• hepatic or renal impairment, diabetes mellitus, obesity
• elevated cholesterol or triglyceride levels
• elderly patients.

Administration
◀﹦ Verify that patient isn't pregnant before giving drug.
• Give as a single dose with main meal.

Route	Onset	Peak	Duration
P.O.	Unknown	Unknown	Unknown

Adverse reactions
CNS: headache, depression, insomnia, drowsiness, fatigue, migraine, rigors, abnormal gait, nerve inflammation, hyperesthesia, paresthesia, **pseudotumor cerebri**
EENT: abnormal or blurred vision, dry eyes, eye irritation, eyebrow and eyelash loss, eyelid inflammation, cataract, conjunctivitis, corneal epithelial abnormality, reduced night vision, photophobia, recurrent styes, earache, tinnitus, hearing loss, epistaxis, rhinitis, sinusitis, **papilledema**
GI: nausea, vomiting, diarrhea, constipation, abdominal pain, gastritis, stomatitis, esophagitis, melena, painful straining at stool, pancreatitis, lip inflammation and cracking, dry mouth, anorexia
GU: abnormal urine, dysuria, atrophic vaginitis, leukorrhea
Hepatic: abnormal hepatic function, jaundice, **hepatitis**
Metabolic: poor blood glucose control
Musculoskeletal: joint, muscle, back, and bone pain; arthritis; bone disorders; spinal bone overgrowth; increased muscle tone or rigidity; tendinitis
Respiratory: coughing, increased sputum, laryngitis
Skin: dry skin, pruritus, skin atrophy, skin peeling, abnormal skin odor, sticky skin, seborrhea, dermatitis, diaphoresis, cold clammy skin, skin infection, rash, pyrogenic granuloma, skin ulcers, skin fissures, sunburn, flushing, purpura, nail disorder, inflammation of tissue surrounding nails, abnormal hair texture, alopecia

---

Reactions in **bold** are life-threatening. ◀﹦ Clinical alert

Other: abnormal taste, glossitis, tongue ulcers, gingival bleeding, gingivitis, edema, thirst, hot flashes

Interactions
Drug-drug. *Glyburide:* increased blood glucose clearance
Methotrexate: increased risk of hepatotoxicity
Oral contraceptives ("minipill"): decreased contraceptive efficacy
Drug-diagnostic tests. *Alanine aminotransferase, aspartate aminotransferase, triglycerides:* increased levels
Low-density lipoproteins: decreased level
Drug-behaviors. *Alcohol use:* interference with acitretin elimination, possible drug toxicity

Patient monitoring
• Monitor patient who has early signs or symptoms of pseudotumor cerebri, such as headache, nausea, vomiting, and visual disturbances. Discontinue drug immediately if papilledema occurs.
• Check blood lipid levels before therapy begins and every 1 to 2 weeks during therapy.
• Monitor blood glucose levels and kidney and liver function test results.
• If drug causes open skin lesions resulting from dermatitis or blisters, watch for signs and symptoms of infection.
• Assess for pain, stinging, and itching. Apply cool compresses as needed for relief.
◀€ Be aware that women taking this drug must avoid alcohol-containing foods, beverages, medications, and over-the-counter products during therapy and for 2 months afterward.

Patient teaching
• Instruct patient to take drug with main meal to minimize GI upset.
• Tell patient to avoid driving and other hazardous activities until he knows how drug affects concentration, alertness, and vision.
• Caution patient not to drink alcohol during therapy.
◀€ Advise females to use effective contraception for at least 1 month before starting drug, throughout entire course of therapy, and for 3 years after discontinuing drug.
• Explain that disease may seem to worsen at start of therapy.
• Tell contact lens wearers that lens intolerance may develop.
• As appropriate, review all other significant and life-threatening adverse reactions and interactions, especially those related to the drugs, tests, and behaviors mentioned above.

activated charcoal
Actidose, Actidose-Aqua, Bragg's Medicinal Charcoal ⊕, Carbomix ⊕, Charcadote ♣, Char-Caps, Charco Caps, EZ-Char

Pharmacologic class: Carbon residue
Therapeutic class: Antiflatulent, antidote
Pregnancy risk category C

Action
Binds to poisons, toxins, irritants, and drugs, forming a barrier between particulate material and GI mucosa that inhibits absorption of this material in GI tract. As an antiflatulent, reduces intestinal gas volume and relieves related discomfort.

Availability
Capsules: 260 mg
Granules: 15 g/120 ml
Liquid: 15 g/120 ml, 50 g/240 ml, 208 mg/1 ml

Oral suspension: 12.5 g/60 ml, 15 g/75 ml, 25 g/120 ml, 30 g/120 ml, 50 g/240 ml
Powder: 15, 30, 40, 130, 240 g/container

⬤ Indications and dosages
➤ Poisoning
Adults: 25 to 100 g P.O. (or 1 g/kg, or about 10 times the amount of poison ingested) as a suspension in 120 to 240 ml (4 to 8 oz) of water
Children: Initially, 1 to 2 g/kg P.O. (or 10 times the amount of poison ingested) as a suspension in 120 to 240 ml (4 to 8 oz) of water
➤ Flatulence
Adults: 600 mg to 5 g P.O. as a single dose, or 975 mg to 3.9 g in divided doses

Off-label uses
• Diarrhea
• GI distress
• Hypercholesterolemia

Contraindications
None

Precautions
Use cautiously in:
• patients who have aspirated corrosives or hydrocarbons and are vomiting.

Administration
◀€ Don't try to give activated charcoal to semiconscious patient.
◀€ If signs of aspiration occur, stop giving drug immediately to avoid fatal airway obstruction or infection.
• Administer by large-bore nasogastric tube after gastric lavage, as needed.
• Give within 30 minutes of poison ingestion when possible.
• Mix powder with tap water to form thick syrup. Add fruit juice or flavoring to improve taste.
• Be aware that drug inactivates ipecac syrup.
• Know that drug is ineffective in poisoning from ethanol, methanol, and iron salts.

• Don't give children more than one dose of drug product containing sorbitol (sweetener).
• When used for indications other than as antidote, give drug at least 2 hours before or 1 hour after other drugs.

Route	Onset	Peak	Duration
P.O.	Immediate	Unknown	Unknown

Adverse reactions
GI: nausea, vomiting, diarrhea, constipation, black stools, **intestinal obstruction**

Interactions
Drug-drug. *Acetaminophen, barbiturates, carbamazepine, digitoxin, digoxin, furosemide, glutethimide, hydantoins, methotrexate, nizatidine, phenothiazines, phenylbutazones, propoxyphene, salicylates, sulfonamides, sulfonylurea, tetracycline, theophyllines, tricyclic antidepressants, valproic acid:* decreased absorption of these drugs
Ipecac syrup: ipecac absorption and inactivation
Drug-food. *Milk, ice cream, sherbet:* decreased absorptive activity of drug

Patient monitoring
• Monitor patient for constipation.
• If patient vomits soon after receiving dose, ask prescriber if dose should be repeated.

Patient teaching
• Instruct patient to drink six to eight glasses of fluid daily to prevent constipation.
• Tell patient that stools will be black as charcoal is excreted from body.
• As appropriate, review all other significant and life-threatening adverse reactions and interactions, especially those related to the drugs and foods mentioned above.

acyclovir

acyclovir sodium
Zovirax

Pharmacologic class: Acyclic purine nucleoside analogue
Therapeutic class: Antiviral
Pregnancy risk category B

Action
Inhibits viral DNA polymerase, thereby inhibiting replication of viral DNA. Specific for herpes simplex types 1 (HSV-1) and 2 (HSV-2), varicella-zoster virus, Epstein-Barr virus, and cytomegalovirus (CMV).

Availability
Capsules: 200 mg
Cream: 5% in 2-g tube
Injection: 50 mg/ml
Ointment: 5% in 15-g tube
Powder for injection: 500 mg/vial, 1,000 mg/vial
Suspension: 200 mg/5 ml
Tablets: 400 mg, 800 mg

🖉 Indications and dosages
➤ Acute treatment of herpes zoster (shingles)
Adults: 800 mg P.O. q 4 hours while awake (five times/day) for 7 to 10 days
➤ Initial episode of genital herpes
Adults: 200 mg P.O. q 4 hours while awake (1,000 mg/day) for 10 days
➤ Chronic suppressive therapy for recurrent genital herpes episodes
Adults: 400 mg P.O. b.i.d., or 200 mg P.O. three to five times daily for up to 12 months
➤ Intermittent therapy for recurrent genital herpes episodes
Adults: 200 mg P.O. q 4 hours while awake (five times/day) for 5 days, initiated at first sign or symptom of recurrence
➤ Management of initial episodes of genital herpes and limited, non-life-threatening mucocutaneous herpes simplex virus infections in immuno-compromised patients
Adults: Apply approximately ½" ribbon of ointment per 4 square inches of surface area to sufficiently cover all lesions q 3 hours, six times daily for 7 days.
➤ Treatment of recurrent herpes labialis (cold sores)
Adults and adolescents ages 12 and older: Apply cream to infected area five times daily for 4 days.
➤ Varicella (chickenpox)
Adults and children weighing more than 40 kg (88 lb): 800 mg P.O. q.i.d. for 5 days
Children older than age 2: 20 mg/kg P.O. q.i.d. for 5 days
➤ Mucosal and cutaneous HSV-1 and HSV-2 in immunocompromised patients
Adults and children older than age 12: 5 mg/kg I.V. infusion over 1 hour given q 8 hours for 7 days
Children younger than age 12: 10 mg/kg I.V. infusion over 1 hour given q 8 hours for 7 days
➤ Herpes simplex encephalitis
Adults and children older than age 12: 10 mg/kg I.V. over 1 hour given q 8 hours for 10 days
Children ages 3 months to 12 years: 20 mg/kg I.V. over 1 hour given q 8 hours for 10 days
Children from birth to 3 months: 10 mg/kg I.V. over 1 hour given q 8 hours for 10 days
➤ Varicella zoster infections in immunocompromised patients
Adults and adolescents older than age 12: 10 mg/kg I.V. over 1 hour given q 8 hours for 7 days
Children younger than age 12: 20 mg/kg I.V. over 1 hour given q 8 hours for 7 days

Dosage adjustment
- Renal impairment
- Obesity (adult dosage based on ideal weight)
- Elderly patients

Off-label uses
- Herpes zoster encephalitis
- CMV and HSV infection after bone marrow or kidney transplantation
- Infectious mononucleosis
- Varicella pneumonia

Contraindications
- Hypersensitivity to drug or valacyclovir

Precautions
Use cautiously in:
- preexisting serious neurologic, hepatic, pulmonary, or fluid or electrolyte abnormalities
- renal impairment
- obesity
- pregnant or breastfeeding patients.

Administration
- Make sure patient is adequately hydrated before starting therapy.
- Give single I.V. dose by infusion over at least 1 hour to minimize renal damage.
- Don't give by I.V. bolus or by I.M. or subcutaneous route.
- Be aware that absorption of topical acyclovir is minimal.

Route	Onset	Peak	Duration
P.O.	Variable	1.5-2 hr	4 hr
I.V.	Immediate	1 hr	8 hr
Topical	Unknown	Unknown	Unknown

Adverse reactions
CNS: aggressive behavior, dizziness, malaise, weakness, paresthesia, headache; with I.V. use—**encephalopathic changes** (lethargy, tremors, obtundation, confusion, hallucinations, agitation, seizures, coma)
CV: peripheral edema

EENT: vision abnormalities
GI: nausea, vomiting, diarrhea
GU: proteinuria, hematuria, crystalluria, vaginitis, candidiasis, changes in menses, vulvitis, oliguria, renal pain, **renal failure, glomerulonephritis**
Hematologic: anemia, lymphadenopathy, **thrombocytopenia, thrombotic thrombocytopenic purpura/hemolytic uremic syndrome** (in immunocompromised patients), **disseminated intravascular coagulation, hemolysis, leukopenia, leukoclastic vasculitis**
Hepatic: jaundice, **hepatitis**
Musculoskeletal: myalgia
Skin: photosensitivity rash, pruritus, angioedema, alopecia, urticaria, severe local inflammatory reactions (with I.V. extravasation), **toxic epidermal necrolysis, erythema multiforme**
Other: gingival hyperplasia, fever, excessive thirst, pain at injection site, **anaphylaxis, Stevens-Johnson syndrome**

Interactions
Drug-drug. *Interferon:* additive effect
Nephrotoxic drugs: increased risk of nephrotoxicity
Probenecid: increased acyclovir blood level
Zidovudine: increased CNS effects, especially drowsiness
Drug-diagnostic tests. *Alanine aminotransferase, aspartate aminotransferase, bilirubin, blood urea nitrogen:* increased levels

Patient monitoring
- Monitor fluid intake and output.
- Assess for signs and symptoms of encephalopathy.
- Evaluate patient frequently for adverse reactions, especially bleeding tendency.
- Monitor CBC with white cell differential and kidney function test results.

Patient teaching

- Instruct patient to keep taking drug exactly as prescribed, even after symptoms improve.
- Advise patient to drink enough fluids to ensure adequate urinary output.
- Tell patient to monitor urine output and report significant changes.
- ◀ Instruct patient to immediately report unusual bleeding or bruising.
- Caution patient to avoid driving and other hazardous activities until he knows how drug affects concentration and alertness.
- Advise patient to minimize GI upset by eating small, frequent servings of food and drinking plenty of fluids.
- Tell patient to use soft toothbrush and electric razor to avoid injury to gums and skin.
- Advise patient to avoid sexual intercourse when visible herpes lesions are present.
- Inform patient that he may need to undergo regular blood testing during therapy.
- As appropriate, review all other significant and life-threatening adverse reactions and interactions, especially those related to the drugs and tests mentioned above.

adalimumab

Humira

Pharmacologic class: Biological modifier
Therapeutic class: Antirheumatic (disease-modifying), immunomodulator
Pregnancy risk category B

FDA BOXED WARNING

- There is increased risk of serious infections with drug use (including tuberculosis [TB], bacterial sepsis, invasive fungal infections [such as histoplasmosis], and infections due to other opportunistic pathogens) leading to hospitalization or death.
- Discontinue adalimumab if a serious infection or sepsis develops during treatment.
- Perform test for latent TB; if positive, start treatment for TB before starting adalimumab.
- Monitor all patients for active TB during treatment, even if initial latent TB test is negative.
- Lymphoma and other malignancies, some fatal, have been reported in children and adolescents treated with tumor necrosis factor (TNF) blockers, including adalimumab.
- Postmarketing cases of hepatosplenic T-cell lymphoma (HSTCL), a rare type of T-cell lymphoma, have been reported in patients treated with TNF blockers, including adalimumab. These cases have had a very aggressive disease course and have been fatal. The majority of reported TNF blocker cases have occurred in patients with Crohn's disease or ulcerative colitis, and the majority were in adolescent and young adult males. Almost all these patients had received azathioprine or 6-mercaptopurine concomitantly with a TNF blocker at or before diagnosis. It's uncertain whether the occurrence of HSTCL is related to use of a TNF blocker or a TNF blocker in combination with these other immunosuppressants.

Action

Human immunoglobulin (Ig) G1 monoclonal antibody that binds to human tumor necrosis factor (TNF), which plays a role in inflammation and immune responses. Also modulates biological responses induced or modulated by TNF.

Availability
Injection (preservative-free): 20 mg/0.4 ml in single-use prefilled glass syringe, 40 mg/0.8 ml in a single-use prefilled pen or single-use prefilled glass syringe

🞂 Indications and dosages
➤ To reduce signs and symptoms, slow disease progression, and improve physical function of moderately to severely active rheumatoid arthritis and to reduce signs and symptoms of psoriatic arthritis
Adults: 40 mg subcutaneously every other week alone or in combination with methotrexate or other disease-modifying antirheumatic drugs
➤ Moderate to severe chronic plaque psoriasis in patients who are candidates for systemic therapy or phototherapy and when other systemic therapies are medically less appropriate
Adults: Initially, 80 mg subcutaneously followed by 40 mg every other week starting 1 week after initial dose
➤ To reduce signs and symptoms of ankylosing spondylitis
Adults: 40 mg subcutaneously every other week
➤ Crohn's disease
Adults: Initially, 160 mg subcutaneously (four 40-mg injections in one day or two 40-mg injections per day for two consecutive days), followed by 80 mg subcutaneously 2 weeks later (day 15). Two weeks later (day 29), begin a maintenance dose of 40 mg subcutaneously every other week.
➤ Moderately to severely active polyarticular juvenile idiopathic arthritis as monotherapy or concomitantly with methotrexate
Children age 4 and older weighing 15 kg (33 lb) to less than 30 kg (66 lb): 20 mg subcutaneously every other week
Children age 4 and older weighing 30 kg (66 lb) or more: 40 mg subcutaneously every other week

Contraindications
• Hypersensitivity to drug
• Active infection, including chronic or localized infection

Precautions
Use cautiously in:
• preexisting or recent onset of demyelinating disorders, immunosuppression, or lymphoma
• elderly patients
• pregnant or breastfeeding patients
• children.

Administration
• Give subcutaneously; rotate injection sites.
• Be aware that patients not receiving methotrexate concurrently may benefit from dosage increase to 40 mg weekly.
• Store in refrigerator and protect from light.

Route	Onset	Peak	Duration
Subcut.	Slow	75-187 hr	Unknown

Adverse reactions
CNS: headache, **demyelinating disease**
CV: hypertension, **arrhythmias**
EENT: sinusitis
GI: nausea, vomiting, abdominal pain
GU: urinary tract infection, hematuria
Metabolic: hyperlipidemia, hypercholesterolemia
Musculoskeletal: back pain
Respiratory: upper respiratory tract infection
Skin: rash
Other: accidental injury, pain and swelling at injection site, flulike symptoms, lupuslike syndrome, fungal infection, allergic reactions, **tuberculosis reactivation, malignancies**

Interactions
Drug-drug. *Immunosuppressants (including corticosteroids):* serious infection
Live-virus vaccines: serious illness
Drug-diagnostic tests. *Alkaline phosphatase:* elevated level

---

Patient monitoring

📢 Monitor for signs and symptoms of infection if patient is receiving concurrent corticosteroids or other immunosuppressants (because of risk that infection may progress).

• Monitor CBC.

Patient teaching

• Teach patient how to recognize and report signs and symptoms of allergic response and other adverse reactions.

• Inform patient that drug lowers resistance to infection. Instruct him to immediately report fever, cough, breathing problems, and other infection symptoms.

• Instruct patient to minimize GI upset by eating small, frequent servings of healthy food and drinking plenty of fluids.

• As appropriate, review all other significant and life-threatening adverse reactions and interactions, especially those related to the drugs and tests mentioned above.

adefovir dipivoxil

Hepsera

Pharmacologic class: Nucleotide reverse transcriptase inhibitor

Therapeutic class: Antiviral

Pregnancy risk category C

FDA | BOXED WARNING

• Severe acute hepatitis exacerbations have occurred after drug withdrawal. Monitor hepatic function closely for at least several months in patients who discontinue drug or other anti–hepatitis B therapy; if appropriate, resume such therapy.

• Long-term therapy may cause nephrotoxicity in patients with or at risk for underlying renal dysfunction. Monitor renal function closely and adjust dosage as needed.

• Human immunodeficiency virus (HIV) resistance may occur during therapy in patients with chronic hepatitis B infection who have unrecognized or untreated HIV infection.

• Lactic acidosis and severe hepatomegaly with steatosis (including fatal cases) may occur with use of drug alone or combined with other antiretrovirals.

Action

Inhibits hepatitis B virus (HBV) DNA polymerase and suppresses HBV replication

Availability

Tablets: 10 mg

🖊 Indications and dosages

➤ Chronic HBV with active viral replication plus persistent elevations in alanine aminotransferase (ALT) or aspartate aminotransferase (AST) or histologically active disease

Adults: 10 mg P.O. daily

Dosage adjustment

• Renal impairment

Contraindications

• Hypersensitivity to drug

Precautions

Use cautiously in:

• lactic acidosis, renal or hepatic impairment

• elderly patients

• pregnant or breastfeeding patients

• children.

Administration

• Offer HIV testing before starting therapy. (Drug may increase resistance to antiretrovirals in HIV patients.)

• Give with or without food.

Route	Onset	Peak	Duration
P.O.	Rapid	0.6-4 hr	Unknown

Adverse reactions

CNS: headache
GI: nausea, vomiting, diarrhea, abdominal pain, flatulence, dyspepsia, anorexia, pancreatitis
GU: renal dysfunction
Hepatic: severe hepatomegaly with steatosis, hepatitis exacerbation (if therapy is withdrawn)
Metabolic: lactic acidosis
Respiratory: pneumonia
Other: fever, infection, pain, antiretroviral resistance in patients with unrecognized HIV

Interactions

Drug-drug. *Acetaminophen, aspirin, indomethacin:* granulocytopenia
Acyclovir, adriamycin, amphotericin B, benzodiazepines, cimetidine, dapsone, doxorubicin, experimental nucleotide analogue, fluconazole, flucytosine, ganciclovir, indomethacin, interferon, morphine, phenytoin, probenecid, sulfonamide, trimethoprim, vinblastine, vincristine: increased risk of nephrotoxicity
Drug-diagnostic tests. *Amylase, blood glucose, blood urea nitrogen, creatine kinase, hepatic enzymes, lipase:* elevated levels

Patient monitoring

• Monitor fluid intake and output.
• Watch for hematuria.
• Assess for signs and symptoms of lactic acidosis, especially in women and overweight patients.
• Check for liver enlargement.
• Monitor liver and kidney function test results.
• After therapy ends, monitor patient for evidence of serious hepatitis exacerbation.

Patient teaching

• Advise patient to take drug with or without food.
• Instruct patient to drink plenty of fluids to ensure adequate urine output.
• Advise patient to monitor urine output and color and to report significant changes.
• Tell patient that drug may cause weakness. Discuss appropriate lifestyle adjustments.
• Caution patient not to take over-the-counter analgesics without prescriber's approval.
• Inform patient that he'll undergo regular blood testing during therapy.
• As appropriate, review all other significant and life-threatening adverse reactions and interactions, especially those related to the drugs and tests mentioned above.

adenosine

Adenacor ⊕ , Adenocard, Adenoscan

Pharmacologic class: Endogenous nucleoside
Therapeutic class: Antiarrhythmic
Pregnancy risk category C

Action

Converts paroxysmal supraventricular tachycardia (PSVT) to normal sinus rhythm by slowing conduction through atrioventricular (AV) node and interrupting reentry pathway. Also used as a diagnostic agent in thallium scanning.

Availability

Injection: 3 mg/ml

Indications and dosages

Adenocard—
➤ PSVT, including that associated with Wolff-Parkinson-White syndrome (after attempting vagal maneuvers, when appropriate)
Adults and children weighing more than 50 kg (110 lb): Initially, 6 mg by rapid I.V. bolus over 1 to 2 seconds.

If desired effect isn't achieved within 1 to 2 minutes, give 12 mg by rapid I.V. bolus; may repeat 12-mg I.V. bolus dose as needed. Maximum single dosage is 12 mg.

Children weighing less than 50 kg (110 lb): 0.05 to 0.1 mg/kg by rapid I.V. bolus. If this dosage proves ineffective, increase in 1 to 2 minutes by 0.05 mg/kg q 2 minutes, to a maximum single dosage of 0.3 mg/kg. Maximum single dosage is 12 mg.

Adenoscan—

➤ Diagnosis of coronary artery disease in conjunction with thallium-201 myocardial perfusion scintigraphy in patients unable to exercise adequately during testing

Adults: 140 mcg/kg/minute by I.V. infusion over 6 minutes, for a total dosage of 0.84 mg/kg. Required dose of thallium-201 is injected at midpoint (after first 3 minutes) of Adenoscan infusion.

Off-label uses

- Diagnosis of supraventricular arrhythmias
- Pulmonary hypertension

Contraindications

- Hypersensitivity to drug
- Second- or third-degree AV block
- Sinus node disease
- Bronchoconstrictive lung disease

Precautions

Use cautiously in:
- asthma, angina
- elderly patients
- pregnant patients
- children.

Administration

- Don't administer through central line (may cause asystole).
- Don't give more than 12 mg Adenocard as a single dose.
- Don't dilute Adenocard. Administer Adenocard by I.V. injection as a rapid bolus directly into vein whenever possible during cardiac monitoring.
- After administering Adenocard, flush I.V. line immediately and rapidly with normal saline solution to drive drug into bloodstream.
- Dilute a single dose of Adenoscan in sufficient normal saline solution to be given by continuous infusion over 6 minutes.

Route	Onset	Peak	Duration
I.V.	Immediate	10 sec	20-30 sec

Adverse reactions

CNS: light-headedness, dizziness, apprehension, headache, tingling in arms, numbness

CV: chest pain, palpitations, hypotension, ST-segment depression, **first- or second-degree AV block, atrial tachyarrhythmias, other arrhythmias**

EENT: blurred vision, tightness in throat

GI: nausea, pressure in groin

Musculoskeletal: discomfort in neck, jaw, and arms

Respiratory: chest pressure, dyspnea and urge to breathe deeply, hyperventilation

Skin: burning sensation, facial flushing, sweating

Other: metallic taste

Interactions

Drug-drug. *Carbamazepine:* worsening of progressive heart block

Digoxin, verapamil: increased risk of ventricular fibrillation

Dipyridamole: increased adenosine effect

Theophylline: decreased adenosine effect

Drug-food. *Caffeine:* decreased adenosine effect

Drug-herbs. *Aloe, buckthorn bark or berry, cascara sagrada, rhubarb root, senna leaf or fruits:* increased adenosine effect

Guarana: decreased adenosine effect

Drug-behaviors. *Smoking:* increased risk of tachycardia

Patient monitoring

- Monitor heart rhythm for new arrhythmias after administering dose.
- Check vital signs. Assess for chest pain or pressure, dyspnea, and sweating.
- ◄€ Watch for bronchoconstriction in patients with asthma, emphysema, or bronchitis.
- Ask patient if he has recently used aloe, buckthorn, cascara sagrada, guarana, rhubarb root, or senna. If response is positive, notify prescriber.

Patient teaching

- Advise patient to report problems at infusion site.
- Tell patient he may experience 1 to 2 minutes of flushing, chest pain and pressure, and breathing difficulty during administration. Assure him that these effects will subside quickly.
- Advise patient to minimize GI upset by eating small, frequent servings of healthy food and drinking plenty of fluids.
- As appropriate, review all other significant and life-threatening adverse reactions and interactions, especially those related to the drugs, foods, herbs, and behaviors mentioned above.

---

aflibercept
Eylea

Pharmacologic class: Vascular endothelial growth factor (VEGF) inhibitor
Therapeutic class: Ophthalmic agent
Pregnancy risk category C

Action

VEGF-A and placental growth factor (PlGF) are members of the VEGF family of angiogenic factors that can act as mitogenic, chemotactic, and vascular permeability factors for endothelial cells. VEGF acts via two receptor tyrosine kinases, VEGFR-1 and VEGFR-2, present on the surface of endothelial cells. PlGF binds only to VEGFR-1, which is also present on the surface of leucocytes. Activation of these receptors by VEGF-A can result in neovascularization and vascular permeability. Aflibercept acts as a soluble decoy receptor that binds VEGF-A and PlGF, and thereby can inhibit the binding and activation of these cognate VEGF receptors.

Availability

Solution for ophthalmic injection: 40 mg/ml in 3-ml (0.278-ml fill) single-use vials

Ø Indications and dosages

➤ Neovascular (wet) age-related macular degeneration
Adults: 2 mg (0.05 ml) by intravitreal injection into affected eye q 4 weeks for the first 3 months, followed by 2 mg (0.05 ml) once q 8 weeks

Contraindications

- Hypersensitivity to drug or its components
- Ocular or periocular infection
- Active intraocular inflammation

Precautions

Use cautiously in:
- pregnant or breastfeeding patients
- children (safety and efficacy not established).

Administration

- Be aware that drug should be administered by ophthalmic intravitreal injection only under controlled aseptic conditions by a qualified health care professional.
- Provide adequate anesthesia and a topical broad-spectrum anti-infective before the injection, as prescribed.
- Inspect drug for particulate matter and discoloration before administering.

Reactions in **bold** are life-threatening.   ◄€ Clinical alert

- Use a filter needle to draw up the prescribed dose; remove the filter needle from syringe, and attach a 30G, $1/_2$-inch injection needle for the intravitreal injection. Discard unused drug after injection.
- Be aware that each vial should only be used for the treatment of a single eye. If the contralateral eye requires treatment, use a new vial and change all equipment.
- Immediately following the intravitreal injection, assess patient for increased intraocular pressure (IOC).

Route	Onset	Peak	Duration
Intravitreous	Unknown	1-3 days	Unknown

Adverse reactions
CNS: nonfatal stroke
CV: nonfatal MI, vascular death
EENT: conjunctival hyperemia, conjunctival hemorrhage, eye pain, cataract, vitreous detachment, vitreous floaters, increased IOC, endophthalmitis, corneal erosion, corneal edema, retinal detachment, retinal tear, retinal pigment epithelium tear, injection-site pain, injection-site hemorrhage, foreign body sensation in eye, increased lacrimation, blurred vision, eyelid edema
Other: hypersensitivity

Interactions
None

Patient monitoring
- Continue to monitor patient for increased IOP, endophthalmitis, retinal detachment, and arterial thromboembolic events and be prepared to treat appropriately.

Patient teaching
◀€ Instruct patient to contact ophthalmologist immediately if treated eye becomes red, light sensitive, or painful, or if vision change occurs.

◀€ Instruct patient to immediately report signs and symptoms of stroke (such as weakness on one side of body or slurred speech), chest pain, or other new signs and symptoms.
- Caution patient to avoid driving and other hazardous activities until visual function has recovered sufficiently.
- As appropriate, review all other significant and life-threatening adverse reactions mentioned above.

agalsidase beta
Fabrazyme, Fibrazyme

Pharmacologic class: Homodimeric glycoprotein
Therapeutic class: Recombinant human alpha-galactosidase enzyme
Pregnancy risk category B

Action
Provides exogenous source of alpha-galactosidase A (which is deficient in Fabry disease) and reduces deposits of globotriaosylceramide in kidney and other body tissues

Availability
Powder for reconstitution: for injection, lyophilized: 5 mg, 35 mg

⬤ Indications and dosages
➤ Fabry disease
Adults: 1 mg/kg I.V. q 2 weeks. Infuse no faster than 0.25 mg/minute; if tolerated, increase rate by 0.05 to 0.08 mg/minute in subsequent infusions.

Contraindications
None

Precautions
Use cautiously in:
- advanced Fabry disease, cardiac dysfunction

- pregnant or breastfeeding patients
- children.

Administration

- Premedicate with antipyretics, as prescribed.
- To reconstitute, slowly inject 7.2 ml of sterile water for injection into vial; then roll and tilt vial gently to mix drug.
- Don't shake drug, and don't use filter needles.
- Dilute reconstituted solution with normal saline injection to a final volume of 500 ml.
- Infuse through separate I.V. line; don't mix with other drugs.

Route	Onset	Peak	Duration
I.V.	End of infusion	90 min	Up to 5 hr

Adverse reactions

CNS: anxiety, depression, dizziness, paresthesias
CV: dependent edema, chest pain, **cardiomegaly**
EENT: rhinitis, sinusitis, laryngitis, pharyngitis
GI: nausea, dyspepsia
GU: testicular pain
Musculoskeletal: arthrosis, bone pain
Respiratory: bronchitis, **bronchospasm**
Skin: pallor
Other: pain, allergic reactions, **infusion reactions** (hypertension, chest tightness, dyspnea, fever, rigors, hypotension, abdominal pain, pruritus, myalgia, headache, urticaria)

Interactions

Drug-drug. *Amiodarone, chloroquine, gentamicin, monobenzone:* inhibition of intracellular agalsidase activity

Patient monitoring

- Watch closely for signs and symptoms of allergic or infusion reaction.
- Monitor vital signs and fluid intake and output. Stay alert for dependent edema, blood pressure changes, and chest pain.

- Measure temperature. Watch for signs and symptoms of infection (particularly EENT and respiratory infections).
- Evaluate patient's mood. Report significant anxiety or depression.

Patient teaching

◀€ Teach patient to recognize and immediately report signs and symptoms of allergic or infusion reaction.

- Caution patient to avoid driving and other hazardous activities until he knows how drug affects mood, balance, and blood pressure.
- Advise patient to report signs and symptoms of infection (particularly EENT and respiratory infections).
- Inform patient that drug can cause depression and anxiety. Instruct him to notify prescriber if these effects occur.
- As appropriate, review all other significant and life-threatening adverse reactions and interactions, especially those related to the drugs mentioned above.

albuterol (salbutamol)
Proventil

albuterol sulfate (salbutamol sulfate)
AccuNeb, Gen-Salbutamol✦, Nu-Salbutamol✦, ProAir HFA, Proventil HFA, Ventolin HFA, Vospire-ER

Pharmacologic class: Sympathomimetic (beta$_2$-adrenergic agonist)
Therapeutic class: Bronchodilator, antiasthmatic
Pregnancy risk category C

Action

Relaxes smooth muscles by stimulating beta$_2$-receptors, thereby causing bronchodilation and vasodilation

---

Reactions in **bold** are life-threatening.　　　　　◀€ Clinical alert

Availability

Aerosol: 90 mcg/actuation,
108 mcg/inhalation
Oral solution: 2 mg/5 ml
Solution for inhalation: 0.083% (3 ml),
0.5% (0.5 and 20 ml), 0.63 mg/3 ml,
1.25 mg/3 ml
Syrup: 2 mg/5 ml
Tablets: 2 mg, 4 mg
Tablets (extended-release): 4 mg, 8 mg

⬮ Indications and dosages

➤ To prevent and relieve bronchospasm in patients with reversible
obstructive airway disease
Adults and children ages 12 and older:
Tablets—2 to 4 mg P.O. three or four
times daily, not to exceed 32 mg daily.
Extended-release tablets—4 to 8 mg P.O.
q 12 hours, not to exceed 32 mg daily in
divided doses. *Syrup*—2 to 4 mg (1 to
2 tsp or 5 to 10 ml) three or four times
daily, not to exceed 8 mg q.i.d.
Aerosol—one to two inhalations q 4
to 6 hours to relieve bronchospasm;
two inhalations q.i.d. to prevent
bronchospasm. *Solution for
inhalation*—2.5 mg three to four times
daily by nebulization, delivered over 5 to
15 minutes.
Children ages 6 to 12: *Tablets*—2 mg
P.O. three or four times daily; maximum daily dosage is 24 mg, given in
divided doses. *Extended-release
tablets*—4 mg q 12 hours; maximum
daily dosage is 24 mg/kg given in
divided doses. *Syrup*—2 mg (1 tsp or
5 ml) three or four times daily, not to
exceed 24 mg.
**Adults and children age 4 and older
(with ProAir HFA):** Two inhalations q
4 to 6 hours to treat acute bronchospasm
**Children ages 2 to 12 weighing more
than 15 kg (33 lb):** *Solution for
inhalation*—2.5 mg three to four
times/day by nebulization
Children ages 2 to 6: *Syrup*—Initially,
0.1 mg/kg P.O. t.i.d., not to exceed

2 mg (1 tsp) t.i.d. Maximum dosage is
4 mg (2 tsp) t.i.d.
➤ To prevent exercise-induced
bronchospasm
**Adults and children older than age 4
(older than age 12 with Proventil):**
Two inhalations 15 minutes before
exercise
**Adults and children age 4 and older
(with ProAir HFA):** Two inhalations q
15 to 30 minutes before exercise

Dosage adjustment

• Sensitivity to beta-adrenergic
stimulants
• Elderly patients

Off-label uses

• Chronic obstructive pulmonary
disease
• Hyperkalemia with renal failure
• Preterm labor management

Contraindications

• Hypersensitivity to drug

Precautions

Use cautiously in:
• cardiac disease, hypertension, diabetes mellitus, glaucoma, seizure disorder, hyperthyroidism, exercise-induced
bronchospasm, prostatic hypertrophy
• elderly patients
• pregnant or breastfeeding patients
• children.

Administration

• Give extended-release tablets whole;
don't crush or mix with food.
• Administer solution for inhalation by
nebulization over 5 to 15 minutes, after
diluting 0.5 ml of 0.5% solution with
2.5 ml of sterile normal saline solution.
• Know that children weighing less
than 15 kg (33 lb) who require less
than 2.5 mg/dose should receive 0.5%
inhalation solution.

Route	Onset	Peak	Duration
P.O.	15-30 min	2-3 hr	6-12 hr
P.O. (extended)	30 min	2-3 hr	12 hr
Aerosol	6-10 min	30 min-1 hr	2-4 hr
Inhalation	5 min	30 min-1 hr	2-4 hr

Adverse reactions

CNS: dizziness, excitement, headache, hyperactivity, insomnia
CV: hypertension, palpitations, tachycardia, chest pain
EENT: conjunctivitis, dry and irritated throat, pharyngitis
GI: nausea, vomiting, anorexia, heartburn, GI distress, dry mouth
Metabolic: hypokalemia
Musculoskeletal: muscle cramps
Respiratory: cough, dyspnea, wheezing, **paradoxical bronchospasm**
Skin: pallor, urticaria, rash, angioedema, flushing, sweating
Other: tooth discoloration, increased appetite, **hypersensitivity reaction**

Interactions

Drug-drug. *Beta-adrenergic blockers:* inhibited albuterol action, possibly causing severe bronchospasm in asthmatic patients
Digoxin: decreased digoxin blood level
MAO inhibitors: increased cardiovascular adverse effects
Oxytoxics: severe hypotension
Potassium-wasting diuretics: ECG changes, hypokalemia
Theophylline: increased risk of theophylline toxicity
Drug-food. *Caffeine-containing foods and beverages (such as coffee, tea, chocolate):* increased stimulant effect
Drug-herbs. *Cola nut, ephedra (ma huang), guarana, yerba maté:* increased stimulant effect

Patient monitoring

◀€ Stay alert for hypersensitivity reactions and paradoxical bronchospasm. Stop drug immediately if these occur.

• Monitor serum electrolyte levels.

Patient teaching

• Tell patient to swallow extended-release tablets whole and not to mix them with food.
• Follow manufacturer's directions supplied with inhalation drugs.
◀€ Teach patient signs and symptoms of hypersensitivity reaction and paradoxical bronchospasm. Tell him to stop taking drug immediately and contact prescriber if these occur.
◀€ Instruct patient to notify prescriber immediately if prescribed dosage fails to provide usual relief, because this may indicate seriously worsening asthma.
• Advise patient to limit intake of caffeine-containing foods and beverages and to avoid herbs unless prescriber approves.
• Caution patient to avoid driving and other hazardous activities until he knows how drug affects concentration and alertness.
• Advise patient to establish effective bedtime routine and to take drug well before bedtime to minimize insomnia.
• As appropriate, review all other significant and life-threatening adverse reactions and interactions, especially those related to the drugs, foods, and herbs mentioned above.

aldesleukin (interleukin-2, IL-2)

Proleukin

Pharmacologic class: Interleukin-2 (IL-2), human recombinant (cytokine)
Therapeutic class: Antineoplastic (miscellaneous)
Pregnancy risk category C

FDA | BOXED WARNING

• Give only to patients with normal cardiac and pulmonary function, as shown by thallium stress testing and pulmonary function testing. Use extreme caution when giving to patients with normal thallium stress test and normal pulmonary function tests who have a history of cardiac or pulmonary disease.

• Give under supervision of physician experienced in cancer chemotherapy, in setting where intensive care facilities and cardiopulmonary or intensive care specialists are available.

• Drug is linked to capillary leak syndrome, which causes hypotension and reduced organ perfusion (possibly severe and resulting in death).

• Before starting drug, preexisting bacterial infections must be treated, because drug may impair neutrophil function and increase disseminated infection risk. Patients with indwelling central lines are at special risk for infection with gram-positive microorganisms. Prophylactic antibiotics can help prevent staphylococcal infections.

• Withhold drug in patients who develop moderate to severe lethargy or somnolence; continued administration may cause coma.

Action

Activates cellular immunity and inhibits tumor growth by increasing lymphocytes and cytokines, which lyse tumor cells

Availability

Injection: 22 million international units/vial

🚺 Indications and dosages

➤ Metastatic renal cell carcinoma and metastatic melanoma

Adults older than age 18: 600,000 international units/kg I.V. given over 15 minutes q 8 hours for a maximum of 14 doses, followed by 9 days of rest. Repeat for another 14 doses, for a maximum of 28 doses per course.

Off-label uses

• Colorectal cancer
• Kaposi's sarcoma
• Non-Hodgkin's lymphoma

Contraindications

• Hypersensitivity to drug
• Arrhythmias, cardiac tamponade, seizures, severe GI bleeding, coma or toxic psychosis lasting more than 48 hours
• Organ allograft
• Abnormal thallium stress test or pulmonary function test results

Precautions

Use cautiously in:

• anemia, bacterial infections, heart disease, CNS metastases, hepatic disease, pulmonary disease, renal disease, thrombocytopenia
• pregnant or breastfeeding patients
• children.

Administration

• Make sure patient's thallium stress test and pulmonary function test results are normal before giving.

◀≀ Don't give if patient is drowsy or severely lethargic; contact prescriber immediately.

• Reconstitute drug according to label directions with 1.2 ml of sterile water for injection by injecting diluent against side of vial (to prevent excessive foaming).

• Further dilute reconstituted dose with 50 ml of 5% dextrose injection.

• Administer I.V. infusion over 15 minutes.

• Don't use in-line filter.

Route	Onset	Peak	Duration
I.V.	5 min	13 min	3-4 hr

Adverse reactions

CNS: dizziness, mental status changes, syncope, sensory or motor dysfunction, headache, fatigue, rigors, weakness, malaise, poor memory, depression, sleep disturbances, hallucinations

CV: bradycardia, sinus tachycardia, premature atrial complexes, premature ventricular contractions, **arrhythmias, myocardial ischemia, cardiac arrest, capillary leak syndrome and severe hypotension, myocardial infarction**

EENT: reversible vision changes, conjunctivitis

GI: nausea, vomiting, diarrhea, constipation, dyspepsia, abdominal pain, stomatitis, anorexia, **intestinal perforation, ileus, GI bleeding**

GU: hematuria, proteinuria, dysuria, **renal failure, oliguria or anuria**

Hematologic: anemia, purpura, eosinophilia, **thrombocytopenia, coagulation disorders, leukopenia, leukocytosis**

Hepatic: jaundice, ascites

Metabolic: hyperglycemia, **hypoglycemia, acidosis, alkalosis**

Musculoskeletal: joint and back pain, myalgia

Respiratory: cough, chest pain, tachypnea, wheezing, dyspnea, pulmonary congestion, **pulmonary edema, respiratory failure, apnea, pleural effusion**

Skin: erythema, pruritus, rash, dry skin, petechiae, urticaria, exfoliative dermatitis

Other: weight gain or loss, fever, chills, edema, infection, pain or reaction at injection site, hypersensitivity reaction

Interactions

Drug-drug. *Aminoglycosides, asparaginase, cytotoxic chemotherapy agents, doxorubicin, indomethacin, methotrexate:* increased toxicity

Antihypertensives: increased hypotensive effect

Glucocorticoids: reduced antitumor effects

Drug-diagnostic tests. *Alkaline phosphatase, bilirubin, glucose, blood urea nitrogen, creatinine, potassium, transaminases:* increased levels

Calcium, glucose, magnesium, phosphorus, potassium, protein sodium, uric acid: decreased levels

Patient monitoring

- Monitor heart rate and rhythm, vital signs, and fluid intake and output.
- Assess for signs and symptoms of hypersensitivity reaction and infection.
- Monitor for adverse CNS effects. Report these immediately.
- Evaluate chest X-rays.
- Monitor CBC, electrolyte levels, and liver and kidney function test results.

Patient teaching

◄€ Tell patient that drug lowers resistance to infections. Advise him to immediately report fever, cough, breathing problems, and other signs or symptoms of infection.

◄€ Advise patient to immediately report chest pain, irregular or fast heart beats, easy bruising or bleeding, or abdominal pain.

- Instruct patient to minimize GI upset by eating small, frequent servings of food and drinking plenty of fluids.
- Provide dietary counseling. Refer patient to dietitian if adverse GI effects significantly limit food intake.
- Notify patient that he'll undergo blood testing and have chest X-rays taken during therapy.
- As appropriate, review all other significant and life-threatening adverse reactions and interactions, especially those related to the drugs and tests mentioned above.

alendronate sodium

Apo-Alendronate✤, Co Alendronate✤,
Dom-Alendronate✤ Fosamax,
Gen-Alendronate✤, Ratio-
Alendronate✤, Sandoz Alendronate

Pharmacologic class: Bisphosphonate
Therapeutic class: Bone-resorption
inhibitor
Pregnancy risk category C

Action
Impedes bone resorption by inhibiting
osteoclast activity, absorbing calcium
phosphate crystal in bone, and directly
blocking dissolution of hydroxyapatite
crystal of bone

Availability
Tablets: 5 mg, 10 mg, 35 mg, 40 mg, 70 mg

⊘ Indications and dosages
➤ Paget's disease of bone (men and
women)
Adults: 40 mg P.O. daily for 6 months
➤ Prevention of osteoporosis in postmenopausal women
Adults: 5 mg P.O. daily or 35 mg P.O.
once weekly for up to 7 years
➤ Glucocorticoid-induced osteoporosis in men and women
Adults: 5 mg P.O. daily. For postmenopausal women not receiving estrogen,
recommended dosage is 10 mg P.O.
once daily.
➤ Treatment of osteoporosis in
postmenopausal women; treatment to
increase bone mass in men with
osteoporosis
Adults: 70-mg tablet or 70 mg oral solution P.O. weekly or 10-mg tablet P.O. daily

Contraindications
• Hypersensitivity to drug or its com-
ponents
• Hypocalcemia

• Esophageal abnormalities such as
stricture or achalasia that delay
esophageal emptying
• Inability to stand or sit upright for
30 minutes
• Increased risk of aspiration (oral
solution)

Precautions
Use cautiously in:
• Severe renal insufficiency (creatinine
clearance less than 35 ml/minute),
esophageal disease, GI ulcers, gastritis,
osteonecrosis of jaw
• pregnant or breastfeeding patients
• children.

Administration
• Give with 6 to 8 oz of water 30 minutes before first food, beverage, or
medication of day.
• Don't give at bedtime or before
patient arises for the day.
• Don't give food, other beverages, or
oral drugs for at least 30 minutes after
giving tablets.
• Keep patient upright for at least 30
minutes after giving dose to avoid serious esophageal irritation.
• Follow oral solution with at least
60 ml (2 oz) of water to facilitate
gastric emptying.
• Be aware that patients should receive
supplemental calcium and vitamin D if
dietary intake is inadequate.
• Be aware that aspirin and nonsteroidal
anti-inflammatory drugs (NSAIDs) may
worsen GI upset. Discuss alternative
analgesics with prescriber.

Route	Onset	Peak	Duration
P.O.	1 mo	3-6 mo	3 wk-7 mo

Adverse reactions
CNS: headache
CV: hypertension
GI: nausea, vomiting, diarrhea, constipa-
tion, abdominal pain, acid regurgitation,
esophageal ulcer, flatulence, dyspepsia,
abdominal distention, dysphagia
GU: urinary tract infection

Hematologic: anemia
Metabolic: hypomagnesemia, hypo-phosphatemia, hypokalemia, **fluid overload**
Musculoskeletal: bone or muscle pain
Skin: rash, redness, photosensitivity
Other: abnormal taste

Interactions

Drug-drug. *Antacids, calcium supplements:* decreased alendronate absorption
NSAIDs, salicylates: increased risk of GI upset
Ranitidine: increased alendronate effect
Drug-diagnostic tests. *Calcium, phosphate:* decreased levels
Drug-food. *Any food, caffeine (as in coffee, tea, cocoa), mineral water, orange juice:* decreased drug absorption

Patient monitoring

• Monitor for signs and symptoms of GI irritation, including ulcers.
• Monitor blood pressure.
• Evaluate blood calcium and phosphate levels.

Patient teaching

◀€ Tell patient to immediately report serious vomiting, severe chest or abdominal pain, difficulty swallowing, or abdominal swelling.
• Instruct patient to take tablets first thing in the morning on an empty stomach, with 6 to 8 oz of water only.
• Instruct patient to follow oral solution with at least 60 ml (2 oz) of water.
• Tell patient not to lie down, eat, drink, or take other oral medications for 30 minutes after taking dose.
• Advise patient to take only those pain relievers suggested by prescriber. Inform him that some over-the-counter pain medications (such as aspirin and NSAIDs) may worsen drug's adverse effects.
• As appropriate, review all other significant and life-threatening adverse reactions and interactions, especially those related to the drugs, tests, and foods mentioned above.

alfuzosin

Besavar ⊕, Uroxatral, Xatral ✿ ⊕

Pharmacologic class: Alpha$_1$-adrenergic receptor blocker
Therapeutic class: Benign prostatic hyperplasia agent
Pregnancy risk category B

Action

Selectively inhibits alpha$_1$-adrenergic receptors in lower urinary tract, relaxing smooth muscle in bladder neck and prostate

Availability

Tablets (extended-release): 10 mg

⊘ Indications and dosages

➤ Signs and symptoms of benign prostatic hyperplasia
Adults: 10 mg P.O. once daily with food, given at same meal each day

Contraindications

• Hypersensitivity to drug or its components
• Moderate or severe hepatic impairment
• Concomitant use of potent CYP-4503A4 inhibitors (such as itraconazole, ketoconazole, or ritonavir)

Precautions

Use cautiously until prostate cancer is ruled out. Also use cautiously in:
• severe renal impairment
• mild hepatic impairment
• angina pectoris, orthostatic hypotension, syncope, or concomitant treatment with phosphodiesterase-5 (PDE-5) inhibitors, antihypertensives or nitrates

---

• concomitant use of other alpha blockers (use not recommended)
• QT prolongation, concomitant use of drugs that prolong QT interval
• cataract surgery.

Administration
• Administer with food.
• Don't crush or break tablet.
• Be aware that prostate carcinoma should be ruled out before starting therapy.

Route	Onset	Peak	Duration
P.O.	Unknown	8 hr	Unknown

Adverse reactions
CNS: dizziness, headache, fatigue
EENT: sinusitis, pharyngitis
GI: nausea, constipation, abdominal pain, dyspepsia
GU: priapism
Respiratory: upper respiratory tract infection, bronchitis
Other: pain

Interactions
Drug-drug. *Alpha adrenergic antagonists, antihypertensives, PDE-5 inhibitors:* increased risk of symptomatic hypotension, orthostatic hypotension, or syncope *CYP3A4 inhibitors (such as itraconazole, ketoconazole, ritonavir):* increased alfuzosin blood level
Other alpha adrenergic antagonists: increased antagonistic effect
Drug-food. *Any food:* increased alfuzosin absorption

Patient monitoring
◀€ Discontinue drug if signs or symptoms of angina pectoris appear or worsen.

Patient teaching
• Instruct patient to take drug with food at same time each day.
• Tell patient not to break, chew, or crush tablet.

• Caution patient to avoid driving and other hazardous activities until he knows if drug makes him dizzy.
• As appropriate, review all other significant adverse reactions and interactions, especially those related to the drugs and foods mentioned above.

aliskiren
Tekturna

Pharmacologic class: Direct renin inhibitor
Therapeutic class: Antihypertensive
Pregnancy risk category C (first trimester), *D* (second and third trimesters)

FDA | BOXED WARNING
• Drugs that act directly on the renin-angiotensin system can cause injury and death to a developing fetus.
• Discontinue drug as soon as possible when pregnancy is detected.

Action
Decreases plasma renin activity and inhibits conversion of angiotensinogen to angiotensin

Availability
Tablets: 150 mg, 300 mg

Indications and dosages
➤ Hypertension (alone or in combination with other antihypertensives)
Adults: Initially, 150 mg P.O. once daily; may increase to 300 mg if blood pressure isn't adequately controlled

Contraindications
• Concurrent use of angiotensin receptor blockers (ARBs) or ACE inhibitors in patients with diabetes

---

Precautions

Use cautiously in:
- patients with severe renal dysfunction, nephrotic syndrome, renovascular hypertension, or history of dialysis
- angioedema (laryngeal edema)
- concurrent use of ACE inhibitors or ARBs in patients with renal impairment (GFR less than 60 ml/minute; avoid use)
- concurrent use of NSAIDs including selective COX-2 inhibitors, potassium-sparing diuretics, potassium supplements, salt substitutes containing potassium, or other drugs that increase potassium levels
- females of childbearing age
- pregnant or breastfeeding patients
- children (safety and efficacy not established).

Administration

- Give consistently with or without food, but not with high-fat foods.

Route	Onset	Peak	Duration
P.O.	Unknown	1-3 hr	Unknown

Adverse reactions

CNS: headache, fatigue
CV: dizziness, hypotension
EENT: nasopharyngitis
GI: diarrhea, gastroesophageal reflux
Musculoskeletal: back pain
Respiratory: upper respiratory tract infection, cough
Skin: rash
Other: edema, angioedema

Interactions

Drug-drug. *ACE inhibitors, ARBs:* increased risk of renal impairment, hypotension, and hyperkalemia
Cyclosporine, itraconazole: significantly increased aliskiren level
NSAIDs (including selective COX-2 inhibitors): increased risk of deterioration of renal function, including possible acute renal failure, and increased aliskiren antihypertensive effect

Drug-diagnostic tests. *BUN, creatine kinase, potassium, serum creatinine, serum uric acid:* increased values
Hematocrit, hemoglobin: decreased values
Drug-food. *High-fat meals:* decreased drug absorption

Patient monitoring

- Stay alert for signs and symptoms of renal dysfunction, especially in patients receiving NSAIDs.
- ◀ Monitor patient for signs and symptoms of angioedema; discontinue drug if signs and symptoms are present.

Patient teaching

- Instruct patient to take drug consistently with or without food, but not with high-fat foods.
- Instruct patient not to stop drug suddenly because doing so could result in uncontrolled high blood pressure.
- Advise female to tell prescriber if she's pregnant or breastfeeding before taking drug.
- As appropriate, review all other significant adverse reactions and interactions, especially those related to the drugs, tests, and foods mentioned above.

alitretinoin
Panretin

Pharmacologic class: Second-generation retinoid
Therapeutic class: Topical antineoplastic
Pregnancy risk category D

Action

Binds to and activates intracellular retinoid receptor subtypes, regulating expression of genes that control cellular differentiation and proliferation

Availability

Topical gel: 0.1%

🖊 Indications and dosages

➤ Treatment of cutaneous lesions in patients with AIDS-related Kaposi's sarcoma

Adults: Apply to lesions b.i.d., gradually increasing to t.i.d. or q.i.d. according to individual lesion tolerance

Contraindications

• Hypersensitivity to retinoids or other drug components

Precautions

Use cautiously in:
• photosensitivity
• concomitant use of insecticides containing diethyltoluamide (DEET)
• elderly patients
• pregnant or breastfeeding patients
• children.

Administration

• Apply generous amount of gel to affected area. Let it dry for 3 to 5 minutes before covering with clothing.

Route	Onset	Peak	Duration
Topical	Unknown	Unknown	Unknown

Adverse reactions

CNS: paresthesia
Skin: rash, pruritus, exfoliative dermatitis, skin disorder at application site (such as abrasion, burning, blisters, excoriation, scab, cracking, crusting, drainage, eschar, fissure, oozing, peeling, redness, or swelling), edema
Other: pain, increased sensitivity to sunlight or sun lamps

Interactions

Drug-behaviors. *DEET-containing insect repellents:* increased adverse reactions to DEET

Patient monitoring

• Monitor patient for serious adverse effects, especially burns caused by exposure to sunlight or sun lamps.

Patient teaching

• Instruct patient to apply generous amount of gel to affected skin area and let dry for 3 to 5 minutes before covering area with clothing.
• Caution patient to avoid applying gel to mucous membranes or to normal skin surrounding lesions.
🔊 Inform patient that drug increases sensitivity to sunlight and that exposure to sunlight or sun lamps (even through window glass or on a cloudy day) may cause serious burn of treated areas. Caution him to avoid such exposure.
• Tell patient to avoid insect repellents containing DEET during therapy.
• Emphasize importance of keeping all medical appointments so prescriber can check progress and monitor for unwanted drug effects.
• Advise females of childbearing potential to avoid becoming pregnant while using this drug.
• As appropriate, review all other significant adverse reactions and interactions, especially those related to the behaviors mentioned above.

allopurinol

Apo-Allopurinol🍁, Caplenol⊕, Cosuric⊕, Nu-purol🍁, Rimapurinol ⊕, Zyloprim, Zyloprim🍁

allopurinol sodium

Aloprim

Pharmacologic class: Xanthine oxidase inhibitor
Therapeutic class: Antigout drug
Pregnancy risk category C

Action

Inhibits conversion of xanthine to uric acid and increases reutilization of hypoxanthine and xanthine for nucleic acid synthesis, thereby decreasing uric acid levels in both serum and urine

Availability
Powder for injection: 500-mg vial
Tablets: 100 mg, 300 mg

⬤ Indications and dosages
➤ Gout in patients with frequent disabling attacks; gout resulting from hyperuricemia, acute or chronic leukemia, psoriasis, or multiple myeloma
Adults: 200 to 300 mg P.O. daily in mild cases or 400 to 600 mg P.O. daily in severe cases, to a maximum dosage of 800 mg/day; or 200 to 400 mg/m²/day I.V. as a single infusion or in equally divided doses q 6, 8, or 12 hours to a maximum dosage of 600 mg/day
Children ages 6 to 10: 300 mg P.O. daily
Children younger than age 6: 150 mg P.O. daily
➤ To prevent acute gout attacks
Adults: 100 mg P.O. daily; increase by 100 mg at weekly intervals without exceeding maximum dosage of 800 mg, until uric acid level falls to 6 mg/dl or less
➤ Recurrent calcium oxalate calculi
Adults: 200 to 300 mg P.O. daily in single dose or divided doses
➤ To prevent uric acid nephropathy during cancer chemotherapy
Adults: 600 to 800 mg P.O. daily for 2 to 3 days, accompanied by high fluid intake

Dosage adjustment
• Renal impairment

Off-label uses
• Hematemesis caused by gastritis induced by nonsteroidal anti-inflammatory drugs
• Pain from acute pancreatitis
• Seizures refractory to standard therapy

Contraindications
• Hypersensitivity to drug

Precautions
Use cautiously in:
• acute gout attack, renal insufficiency, dehydration
• pregnant or breastfeeding patients.

Administration
• Reconstitute single-dose vial with 25 ml sterile water for injection. Further dilute with normal saline solution or D₅W to a concentration of 6 mg/ml or less.
• Infuse over 30 to 60 minutes.
• Don't mix I.V. form with other drugs or give through same I.V. port as drugs that may be incompatible.
• Divide oral doses larger than 300 mg.
• Give oral form with or right after meals.
• Don't give oral form with mineral water, orange juice, or caffeinated beverages.

Route	Onset	Peak	Duration
P.O.	2-3 days	0.5-2 hr	1-2 wk
I.V.	Unknown	0.5 hr	Unknown

Adverse reactions
CNS: drowsiness, dizziness, headache, peripheral neuropathy, neuritis, paresthesia
CV: hypersensitivity vasculitis, **necrotizing vasculitis**
EENT: retinopathy, cataract, epistaxis
GI: nausea, vomiting, diarrhea, abdominal pain, dyspepsia, gastritis
GU: exacerbation of gout and renal calculi, **uremia, renal failure**
Hematologic: eosinophilia, anemia, **thrombocytopenia, bone marrow depression, agranulocytosis, leukocytosis, aplastic anemia, leukopenia**
Hepatic: cholestatic jaundice, **hepatomegaly, hepatitis, hepatic necrosis**
Musculoskeletal: myopathy, joint pain
Skin: rash; alopecia; maculopapular, urticarial, or purpuric lesions; severe furunculosis of nose; ichthyosis; bruising; **scaly or exfoliative erythema multiforme; toxic epidermal necrolysis**

Other: abnormal taste, loss of taste, fever, chills

Interactions

Drug-drug. *Amoxicillin, ampicillin, bacampicillin:* increased risk of rash
Anticoagulants (except warfarin): increased anticoagulant effect
Antineoplastics: increased risk of myelosuppression
Azathioprine, mercaptopurine: inhibition of allopurinol metabolism
Chlorpropamide: increased hypoglycemic effects
Diazoxide, diuretics, mecamylamine, pyrazinamide: increased uric acid levels
Ethacrynic acid, thiazide diuretics: increased risk of allopurinol toxicity
Uricosurics: increased uric acid excretion
Urine-acidifying drugs (ammonium chloride, ascorbic acid, potassium or sodium phosphate): increased risk of renal calculi
Xanthines: increased theophylline levels
Drug-diagnostic tests. *Alanine aminotransferase, alanine phosphatase, aspartate aminotransferase, bilirubin, eosinophils:* increased levels
Granulocytes, hemoglobin, platelets, white blood cells: decreased levels
Drug-food. *Caffeine-containing beverages and foods, mineral water, orange juice:* decreased drug absorption, increased uric acid level
Drug-behaviors. *Alcohol use:* increased uric acid level

Patient monitoring

• Assess fluid intake and output. Intake should be sufficient to yield daily output of at least 2 L of slightly alkaline urine.
• Monitor uric acid level to help evaluate drug efficacy.

Patient teaching

◀€ Instruct patient to promptly report painful urination, bloody urine, rash, eye irritation, or swelling of lips and mouth.

• Tell patient to take drug with food or milk, exactly as prescribed.
• Explain that gout attacks may not ease significantly until 2 to 6 weeks of therapy.
• Caution patient to avoid driving and other hazardous tasks until he knows how drug affects concentration and alertness.
• Advise patient to avoid alcohol, caffeine-containing beverages and foods, mineral water, and orange juice during therapy.
• As appropriate, review all other significant and life-threatening adverse reactions and interactions, especially those related to the drugs, tests, foods, and behaviors mentioned above.

almotriptan malate

Axert

Pharmacologic class: Serotonin (5-hydroxytryptamine [5-HT]) receptor agonist

Therapeutic class: Vascular headache suppressant, antimigraine drug

Pregnancy risk category C

Action

Promotes vascular constriction and relieves migraine by stimulating specific 5-HT receptors in intracranial blood vessels and sensory trigeminal nerves

Availability

Tablets: 6.25 mg, 12.5 mg

⚠ Indications and dosages

➢ Acute migraine

Adults: Single dose of 6.25 to 12.5 mg P.O. at first sign or symptom of migraine; may be repeated after 2 hours. Don't exceed two doses in a 24-hour period.

Dosage adjustment
• Severe renal or hepatic impairment

Contraindications
• Hypersensitivity to drug
• Ischemic heart disease, history of myocardial infarction (MI), documented silent ischemia, symptoms or findings consistent with ischemic heart disease, cerebrovascular accident, uncontrolled hypertension, coronary artery vasospasm
• Ischemic bowel disease
• Basilar or hemiplegic migraine
• MAO inhibitor use in past 14 days
• Use of other 5-HT agonists or ergotamine-containing or ergot-type drugs within past 24 hours

Precautions
Use cautiously in:
• impaired renal or hepatic function
• cardiovascular risk factors
• pregnant or breastfeeding patients
• children younger than age 18 (use not recommended).

Administration
• Give with or without food.
• Wait at least 2 hours after initial dose before giving repeat dose.
• Don't exceed two doses in 24 hours.
◀ Don't give within 14 days of MAO inhibitors or within 24 hours of other 5-HT agonists or ergotamine-containing or ergot-type drugs.

Route	Onset	Peak	Duration
P.O.	Variable	1-3 hr	Unknown

Adverse reactions
CNS: headache, anxiety, dizziness, fatigue, malaise, weakness, cold or hot sensations, sedation, numbness, burning or tingling sensations
CV: blood pressure changes, palpitations, tachycardia, **coronary artery vasospasm, MI, ventricular fibrillation, ventricular tachycardia**

EENT: vision changes; nasal, throat, and mouth discomfort
GI: nausea, abdominal distress, dysphagia, dry mouth
Musculoskeletal: weakness, stiff neck, muscle pain
Respiratory: chest tightness or pressure
Skin: sweating, flushing

Interactions
Drug-drug. *CYP2D6 inhibitors (erythromycin, itraconazole, ritonavir):* increased almotriptan effect
Ergot derivatives, other 5-HT agonists: prolonged vasoactive action
Ketoconazole and other CYP3A inhibitors: increased almotriptan blood level, leading to toxicity
MAO inhibitors: decreased almotriptan absorption
Selective serotonin reuptake inhibitors: weakness, hyperreflexia, poor coordination

Patient monitoring
• Assess patient's cardiovascular status, noting chest tightness or pressure.
• Monitor vital signs.

Patient teaching
◀ Tell patient to immediately report chest tightness or pressure.
• Inform patient that he may take drug with or without food.
• If second dose is needed, tell patient to take it at least 2 hours after first.
• Caution patient not to take more than two doses in 24 hours.
• Instruct patient to avoid driving and other hazardous activities until he knows how drug affects concentration and alertness.
• As appropriate, review all other significant and life-threatening adverse reactions and interactions, especially those related to the drugs mentioned above.

---

alosetron hydrochloride
Lotronex

Pharmacologic class: Serotonin receptor antagonist
Therapeutic class: Agent for irritable bowel syndrome
Pregnancy risk category B

FDA | BOXED WARNING

- Infrequent but serious GI problems have occurred, resulting in hospitalization and, rarely, blood transfusions, surgery, and death.
- Only physicians enrolled in Glaxo-SmithKline's Prescribing Program for Lotronex should prescribe Lotronex.
- Drug is indicated only for women with severe, diarrhea-predominant irritable bowel syndrome who don't respond adequately to conventional therapy. Patient must read and sign agreement before receiving initial prescription.
- Discontinue immediately if patient develops constipation or ischemic colitis symptoms. Don't resume therapy in patients who developed ischemic colitis. Patients with resolved constipation should resume only on advice of physician.

Action
Inhibits activation of nonselective cation channels, resulting in modulation of enteric nervous system

Availability
Tablets: 0.5 mg, 1 mg

ⓘ Indications and dosages
➤ Women with severe, diarrhea-predominant irritable bowel syndrome (IBS) who have chronic symptoms not caused by anatomic or biochemical abnormalities and who are unresponsive to conventional therapy
Adult women: Initially, 0.5 mg P.O. b.i.d. If after 4 weeks dose is well tolerated but doesn't adequately control IBS, may increase to 1 mg P.O. b.i.d.; therapy should be discontinued in patients not responding to 1 mg P.O. b.i.d. after 4 weeks.

Contraindications
- Concurrent use of fluvoxamine
- Severe hepatic impairment
- Current constipation or history of chronic or severe constipation
- History of complications related to constipation
- History of intestinal obstruction, stricture, toxic megacolon, GI perforation, or adhesion
- History of ischemic colitis, impaired intestinal circulation, thrombophlebitis, or hypercoagulable state
- Current Crohn's disease or ulcerative colitis, active diverticulitis, or history of these disorders
- Inability to understand or comply with patient-physician agreement for drug

Precautions
Use cautiously in:
- hepatic insufficiency
- moderate CYP/A2 inhibitors, such as quinolone antibiotics and cimetidine (avoid use)
- elderly patients
- pregnant or breastfeeding patients
- children.

Administration
◀℈ Before administering, know that drug is approved with the following marketing restrictions: Ensure that patient understands that drug has serious risks, patient reads and signs patient-physician agreement, and patient follows directions in accompanying medication guide.

♣ Canada   ✚ UK   ☣ Hazardous drug   ⊗ High-alert drug

- Know that anatomical and biochemical abnormalities of GI tract should be ruled out before drug therapy starts.
- Give with or without food.
- ◀≹ Don't administer drug if patient is constipated.
- ◀≹ Stop therapy immediately if patient develops constipation or signs or symptoms of ischemic colitis.

Route	Onset	Peak	Duration
P.O.	Rapid	1 hr	Unknown

Adverse reactions
CNS: anxiety, malaise
CV: increased blood pressure, extrasystoles, tachyarrhythmias, **arrhythmias**
GI: nausea; constipation; GI pain, discomfort, or spasms; abdominal distention; regurgitation or gastroesophageal reflux; hemorrhoids; decreased salivation; dyspepsia; **ischemic colitis; GI perforation; small-bowel mesenteric ischemia**
GU: urinary frequency
Hematologic: hemorrhage
Respiratory: breathing disorders
Skin: sweating, urticaria
Other: fatigue, cramps, disturbed temperature regulation

Interactions
Drug-drug. *CYP450 inducers or inhibitors:* altered alosetron clearance
Fluvoxamine: increased alosetron concentration and half-life
Drug-diagnostic tests. *Blood glucose, calcium, phosphate:* increased or decreased level

Patient monitoring
◀≹ Monitor patient closely for adverse reactions, especially such GI reactions as constipation and signs or symptoms of ischemic colitis.

Patient teaching
◀≹ Make sure patient knows about drug's marketing restrictions, which stipulate that she understands drug has serious risks, that she reads and signs patient-physician agreement, and that she follows directions in accompanying medication guide.

- Tell patient to take drug exactly as prescribed, with or without food.
- ◀≹ Instruct patient to contact prescriber immediately if she develops constipation or symptoms of insufficient blood flow to bowel (such as new or worsening pain in bowels or bloody bowel movements).
- As appropriate, review all other significant and life-threatening adverse reactions and interactions, especially those related to the drugs and tests mentioned above.

alprazolam
Apo-Alpraz✳, Niravam, Novo-Alprazol✳, Nu-Alpraz✳, Xanax, Xanax TS✳, Xanax XR

Pharmacologic class: Benzodiazepine
Therapeutic class: Anxiolytic
Controlled substance schedule IV
Pregnancy risk category D

Action
Unclear. Thought to act at limbic, thalamic, and hypothalamic levels of CNS to produce sedative, anxiolytic, skeletal muscle relaxant, and anticonvulsant effects.

Availability
Solution: 1 mg/ml
Tablets (extended-release): 0.5 mg, 1 mg, 2 mg, 3 mg
Tablets (immediate-release): 0.25 mg, 0.5 mg, 1 mg, 2 mg
Tablets (orally disintegrating): 0.25 mg, 0.5 mg, 1 mg, 2 mg

🖊 Indications and dosages

➤ Anxiety disorders

Adults: Initially, 0.25 to 0.5 mg P.O. t.i.d. Maximum dosage is 4 mg daily in divided doses.

Elderly patients: Initially, 0.25 mg P.O. two or three times daily. Maximum dosage is 4 mg daily in divided doses.

➤ Panic disorders

Adults: *Immediate-release or orally disintegrating tablets*—Initially, 0.5 mg P.O. t.i.d. *Extended-release tablets*—Initially, 0.5 to 1 mg P.O. daily. Usual dosage is 3 to 6 mg daily, with a maximum dosage of 10 mg daily. For all dosage forms, increase by a maximum of 1 mg daily at intervals of 3 to 4 days, with a maximum of 10 mg daily in divided doses.

Dosage adjustment

- Hepatic impairment

Off-label uses

- Agoraphobia
- Depression
- Premenstrual syndrome

Contraindications

- Hypersensitivity to benzodiazepines
- Narrow-angle glaucoma
- Labor and delivery
- Pregnancy or breastfeeding

Precautions

Use cautiously in:
- hepatic dysfunction
- history of attempted suicide or drug dependence
- elderly patients.

Administration

- Don't give with grapefruit juice.
- Make sure patient swallows extended-release tablets whole without chewing or crushing.
- Mix oral solution with liquids or semisolid foods and instruct patient to consume entire amount immediately.
- Administer orally disintegrating tablets by placing tablet on patient's tongue. If only one-half of scored tablet is used, discard unused portion immediately.

🔊 Don't withdraw drug suddenly. Seizures and other withdrawal symptoms may occur unless dosage is tapered carefully.

Route	Onset	Peak	Duration
P.O.	30 min	1-2 hr	4-6 hr

Adverse reactions

CNS: dizziness, drowsiness, depression, fatigue, light-headedness, disorientation, anger, hostility, euphoria, hypomanic episodes, restlessness, confusion, crying, delirium, headache, stupor, rigidity, tremor, paresthesia, vivid dreams, extrapyramidal symptoms

CV: bradycardia, tachycardia, hypertension, hypotension, palpitations, **CV collapse**

EENT: blurred or double vision, nystagmus, nasal congestion

GI: gastric disorders, dysphagia, anorexia, increased salivation, dry mouth

GU: menstrual irregularities, urinary retention, urinary incontinence, libido changes, gynecomastia

Hematologic: blood dyscrasias such as eosinophilia, **agranulocytosis, leukopenia, and thrombocytopenia**

Hepatic: hepatic dysfunction (including **hepatitis**)

Musculoskeletal: muscle rigidity, joint pain

Skin: dermatitis, rash, pruritus, urticaria, increased sweating

Other: weight loss or gain, hiccups, fever, edema, psychological drug dependence, drug tolerance

Interactions

Drug-drug. *Antidepressants, antihistamines, opioids, other benzodiazepines:* increased CNS depression

Barbiturates, rifampin: increased metabolism and decreased efficacy of alprazolam

---

🍁 Canada   ⊕ UK   ☠ Hazardous drug   ⊗ High-alert drug

Cimetidine, disulfiram, erythromycin, fluoxetine, hormonal contraceptives, isoniazid, ketoconazole, metoprolol, propoxyphene, propranolol, valproic acid: decreased metabolism and increased action of alprazolam
Digoxin: increased risk of digoxin toxicity
Levodopa: decreased antiparkinsonian effect
Theophylline: increased sedative effect
Tricyclic antidepressants (TCAs): increased TCA blood levels
Drug-diagnostic tests. *Itraconazole, ketoconazole:* increased alprazolam plasma level
Drug-food. *Grapefruit juice:* decreased drug metabolism and increased blood level
Drug-herbs. *Chamomile, hops, kava, skullcap, valerian:* increased CNS depression
Drug-behaviors. *Alcohol use:* increased CNS depression
Smoking: decreased alprazolam efficacy

Patient monitoring
• Watch for excessive CNS depression if patient is concurrently taking antidepressants, other benzodiazepines, antihistamines, or opioids.
• If patient is taking TCAs concurrently, watch for increase in adverse TCA effects.
• Monitor CBC and liver and kidney function test results.
• Monitor vital signs and weight.
• Report signs of drug abuse, including frequent requests for early refills.

Patient teaching
• Instruct patient to swallow extended-release tablets whole without crushing or chewing.
◀€ Tell patient that drug may make him more depressed, angry, or hostile. Urge him to contact prescriber immediately if he thinks he's dangerous to himself or others.

• Inform patient that drug may cause tremors, muscle rigidity, and other movement problems. Advise him to report these effects to prescriber.
◀€ Caution patient not to stop taking drug suddenly. Withdrawal symptoms, including seizures, may occur unless drug is tapered carefully.
• Advise patient to avoid driving and other hazardous activities until he knows how drug affects concentration and alertness.
• As appropriate, review all other significant and life-threatening adverse reactions and interactions, especially those related to the drugs, tests, foods, herbs, and behaviors mentioned above.

alteplase (tissue plasminogen activator, recombinant)
Actilyse ⊕, Activase, Activase rt-PA ✿, Cathflo Activase

Pharmacologic class: Plasminogen activator
Therapeutic class: Thrombolytic
Pregnancy risk category C

Action
Converts plasminogen to plasmin, which in turn breaks down fibrin and fibrinogen, thereby dissolving thrombus

Availability
Injection: 2-mg single-patient vials; 50-mg, 100-mg vials

⁄ Indications and dosages
➤ Lysis of thrombi obstructing coronary arteries in acute myocardial infarction (MI)

3-hour infusion—
Adults: 100 mg I.V. over 3 hours as follows: 60 mg over first hour (give 6 to 10 mg as bolus over first 1 to 2 minutes), then 20 mg I.V. over second hour, then 20 mg I.V. over third hour
Adults weighing less than 65 kg (143 lb): 1.25 mg/kg I.V. in divided doses over 3 hours, not to exceed 100 mg
Accelerated infusion—
Adults weighing more than 67 kg (147 lb): Give total dosage of 100 mg as follows: 15 mg I.V. bolus over 1 to 2 minutes, then 50 mg I.V. over next 30 minutes, then 35 mg I.V. over next 60 minutes.
Adults weighing 67 kg (147 lb) or less: 15 mg I.V. bolus over 1 to 2 minutes, followed by 0.75 mg/kg I.V. over next 30 minutes (not to exceed 50 mg), followed by 0.5 mg/kg I.V. over next hour, not to exceed 35 mg
➤ Acute ischemic cerebrovascular accident (CVA)
Adults: 0.9 mg/kg I.V. over 1 hour, to a maximum dosage of 90 mg, with 10% of total dosage given as I.V. bolus within first minute
➤ Acute massive pulmonary embolism
Adults: 100 mg I.V. over 2 hours, followed by heparin
➤ Restoration of function of central venous access device
Adults weighing 30 kg (66 lb) or more: *Cathflo Activase*—2 mg/2-ml concentration instilled in dysfunctional catheter. If catheter function isn't restored in 120 minutes after first dose, may give second dose.
Adults weighing 10 kg (22 lb) to less than 30 kg: *Cathflo Activase*—Use 110% of catheter lumen volume not to exceed 2 mg/2-ml concentration instilled in dysfunctional catheter. If catheter function isn't restored in 120 minutes after first dose, may give second dose.

Off-label uses
• Small-vessel occlusion by microthrombi
• Peripheral arterial thromboembolism

Contraindications
• Hypersensitivity to drug or its components (Cathflo Activase)
• Seizures, stroke, aneurysm, intracranial neoplasm, bleeding diathesis

Precautions
Use cautiously in:
• hypersensitivity to anistreplase or streptokinase
• GI or genitourinary bleeding, ophthalmic hemorrhage, organ biopsy, severe hepatic or renal disease
• elderly patients
• pregnant or breastfeeding patients
• children.

Administration
◀ Be aware that intracranial hemorrhage must be ruled out before therapy begins.
◀ To treat acute ischemic CVA, give within 3 hours of initial signs or symptoms.
◀ If uncontrolled bleeding occurs, stop infusion and notify prescriber immediately.
• Give I.V. only, using controlled-infusion pump.
• Reconstitute with unpreserved sterile water for injection. May be further diluted with normal saline solution or D_5W.

Route	Onset	Peak	Duration
I.V.	Unknown	Unknown	Unknown

Adverse reactions
CNS: cerebral hemorrhage, cerebral edema, CVA (with accelerated infusion)
CV: hypotension, bradycardia, recurrent ischemia, **pericardial effusion, pericarditis, mitral regurgitation, electromechanical dissociation,**

arrhythmias, cardiogenic shock, heart failure, cardiac arrest, cardiac tamponade, myocardial rupture, embolization, venous thrombosis
GI: nausea, vomiting, **GI bleeding**
GU: GU tract bleeding
Hematologic: spontaneous bleeding, bone marrow depression
Musculoskeletal: musculoskeletal pain
Respiratory: pulmonary edema
Skin: bruising, flushing
Other: fever, edema, phlebitis or bleeding at I.V. site, hypersensitivity reaction (including rash, **anaphylactic reaction, laryngeal edema**), **sepsis**

Interactions

Drug-drug. *Aspirin, drugs affecting platelet activity (such as abciximab, heparin, dipyridamole, oral anticoagulants, vitamin K antagonists):* increased risk of bleeding
Drug-diagnostic tests. *Blood urea nitrogen:* elevated level

Patient monitoring

• Monitor vital signs, ECG, and neurologic status.
• Maintain strict bed rest.
• Watch for signs and symptoms of bleeding tendency and hemorrhage.
• Monitor patient on Cathflo Activase for GI bleeding, venous thrombosis, and sepsis.
• Evaluate results of clotting studies.

Patient teaching

• As appropriate, explain therapy and monitoring to patient and family.

aluminum hydroxide
AlternaGEL, Alu-Cap, Alu-Tab

Pharmacologic class: Inorganic salt
Therapeutic class: Antacid
Pregnancy risk category NR

Action
Dissolves in acidic gastric secretions, releasing anions that partially neutralize gastric hydrochloric acid. Also elevates gastric pH, inhibiting the action of pepsin (an effect important in peptic ulcer disease).

Availability
Capsules: 400 mg, 475 mg, 500 mg
Oral suspension: 320 mg/5 ml, 450 mg/5 ml, 600 mg/5 ml, 675 mg/5 ml
Tablets: 300 mg, 500 mg, 600 mg

Indications and dosages
➤ Hyperacidity
Adults: 500 to 1,500 mg (tablet or capsule) P.O. 1 hour after meals and at bedtime; or 5 to 30 ml (oral suspension) between meals and at bedtime, as needed or directed

Off-label uses
• Bleeding from stress ulcers
• Gastroesophageal reflux disease

Contraindications
• Signs or symptoms of appendicitis or inflamed bowel

Precautions
Use cautiously in:
• gastric outlet obstruction, hypercalcemia, hypophosphatemia, massive upper GI hemorrhage
• patients using other aluminum products concurrently
• patients on dialysis
• pregnant or breastfeeding patients.

Administration
• Administer with water or fruit juice.
• Give 1 hour after meals and at bedtime.
• In reflux esophagitis, administer 20 to 40 minutes after meals and at bedtime.
• Don't give within 1 to 2 hours of antibiotics, histamine$_2$ (H$_2$) blockers, iron preparations, corticosteroids, or enteric-coated drugs.

Reactions in **bold** are life-threatening.   🔊 Clinical alert

• Provide care as appropriate if patient becomes constipated.

Route	Onset	Peak	Duration
P.O.	15-30 min	30 min	30 min-3 hr

Adverse reactions

CNS: malaise (with prolonged use), **neurotoxicity, encephalopathy**
GI: constipation, anorexia (with prolonged use), **intestinal obstruction**
Metabolic: hypophosphatemia (with prolonged use)
Musculoskeletal: osteomalacia and chronic phosphate deficiency with bone pain, malaise, muscle weakness (with prolonged use)
Other: aluminum toxicity

Interactions

Drug-drug. *Allopurinol, anti-infectives (including quinolones, tetracyclines), corticosteroids, diflunisal, digoxin, ethambutol, H$_2$ blockers, hydantoins, iron salts, isoniazid, penicillamine, phenothiazines, salicylates, thyroid hormone, ticlopidine:* decreased effects of these drugs
Enteric-coated drugs: premature release of these drugs in stomach
Drug-diagnostic tests. *Gastrin:* increased level
Phosphate: decreased level
Some imaging studies: test interference
Drug-food. *Milk, other foods high in vitamin D:* milk-alkali syndrome (nausea, vomiting, distaste for food, headache, confusion, hypercalcemia, hypercalciuria)

Patient monitoring

• Monitor long-term use of high doses if patient is on sodium-restricted diet. (Drug contains sodium.)
• Assess for GI bleeding.
• Watch for constipation.
• With long-term use, monitor blood phosphate level and assess for signs and symptoms of hypophosphatemia (anorexia, malaise, muscle weakness). Also monitor bone density.

Patient teaching

• Tell patient to take drug 1 hour after meals and at bedtime.
• Caution patient not to take drug within 1 to 2 hours of anti-infectives, H$_2$ blockers, iron, corticosteroids, or enteric-coated drugs.
• Advise patient to take drug with water or fruit juice.
• Instruct patient to report signs and symptoms of GI bleeding and hypophosphatemia (appetite loss, malaise, muscle weakness).
• Recommend increased fiber and fluid intake and regular physical activity to help ease constipation.
• Inform patient that drug contains sodium, so he should discuss drug therapy with health care providers if he's later told to consume a low-sodium diet.
• Advise patient that he'll need to undergo periodic blood testing and bone mineral density tests if he's receiving long-term therapy.
• As appropriate, review all other significant and life-threatening adverse reactions and interactions, especially those related to the drugs, tests, and foods mentioned above.

amantadine hydrochloride
Dom-Amantadine✤, Gen-Amantadine✤, Lysovir⊕, PMS-Amantadine✤

Pharmacologic class: Anticholinergic-like agent

Therapeutic class: Antiviral, antiparkinsonian

Pregnancy risk category C

Action
Antiviral action unclear; may prevent penetration of influenza A virus into host cell. Antiparkinsonian action unknown; may ease parkinsonian symptoms by increasing dopamine release, preventing dopamine reuptake into presynaptic neurons, stimulating dopamine receptors, or enhancing dopamine sensitivity.

Availability
Capsules (liquid-filled): 100 mg
Syrup: 50 mg/5 ml
Tablets: 100 mg

𝟋 Indications and dosages
➤ Symptomatic treatment or prophylaxis of influenza type A virus in patients with respiratory conditions
Adults older than age 65 with normal renal function: 100 mg P.O. once daily
Adults to age 64 with normal renal function: 200 mg (tablets) or 4 tsp of syrup P.O. daily in a single dose, or 100 mg tablet or 2 tsp of syrup P.O. b.i.d.
Children ages 9 to 12: 100 mg P.O. q 12 hours
Children ages 1 to 9 or weighing less than 45 kg (99 lb): 4.4 to 8.8 mg/kg/day of syrup P.O. q 12 hours, not to exceed 150 mg daily
➤ Parkinson's disease
Adults: Initially, 100 mg P.O. daily, increased to 100 mg b.i.d. if needed. If patient doesn't respond adequately, give 200 mg b.i.d., up to 400 mg/day.
➤ Drug-induced extrapyramidal reactions
Adults: 100 mg P.O. b.i.d.; may increase dosage to maximum of 300 mg daily in divided doses

Dosage adjustment
• Renal impairment

Contraindications
• Hypersensitivity to drug

Precautions
Use cautiously in:
• cardiac disease, hepatic disease, renal impairment, seizure disorder, psychiatric problems
• untreated closed-angle glaucoma (use not recommended)
• elderly patients
• pregnant or breastfeeding patients.

Administration
• For antiviral use, start therapy within 24 to 48 hours of symptom onset and continue for 24 to 48 hours after symptoms resolve.
• When giving as prophylactic antiviral, start therapy as soon as possible and continue for at least 10 days after exposure to virus.
• When giving with influenza vaccine, continue drug for 2 to 3 weeks while patient develops antibody response to vaccine.

Route	Onset	Peak	Duration
P.O.	48 hr	2 wk	Unknown

Adverse reactions
CNS: depression, dizziness, drowsiness, insomnia, light-headedness, anxiety, irritability, hallucinations, confusion, ataxia, headache, nervousness, abnormal dreams, agitation, fatigue, delusions, aggressive behavior, manic reaction, psychosis, slurred speech, euphoria, abnormal thinking, amnesia, increased or decreased motor activity, paresthesia, tremor, abnormal gait, delirium, stupor, **coma**
CV: orthostatic hypotension, tachycardia, peripheral edema, **heart failure, cardiac arrest, arrhythmias**
EENT: blurred vision, mydriasis, keratitis, photosensitivity, optic nerve palsy, nasal congestion
GI: nausea, vomiting, diarrhea, constipation, dry mouth, dysphagia, anorexia
GU: urine retention, decreased libido
Hematologic: leukocytosis

Reactions in **bold** are life-threatening.　　　◀€ Clinical alert

Musculoskeletal: involuntary muscle contractions
Respiratory: tachypnea, **acute respiratory failure, pulmonary edema**
Skin: purplish skin discoloration, rash, pruritus, diaphoresis
Other: edema, fever, allergic reactions including **anaphylaxis**

Interactions

Drug-drug. *Anticholinergics, antihistamines, phenothiazines, quinidine, tricyclic antidepressants:* increased atropine-like adverse effects
CNS stimulants: increased CNS stimulation
Hydrochlorothiazide, triamterene: increased amantadine effects
Drug-diagnostic tests. *Alanine aminotransferase, alkaline phosphatase, aspartate aminotransferase, bilirubin, blood urea nitrogen, creatine kinase, creatinine, gamma-glutamyltransferase, lactate dehydrogenase:* increased levels
Drug-herbs. *Angel's trumpet, jimsonweed, scopolia:* increased cardiac and anticholinergic-like effects
Drug-behaviors. *Alcohol use:* increased CNS adverse reactions

Patient monitoring

◀€ Monitor patient for depression and suicidal ideation.
• Watch for mental status changes, especially in elderly patients.
• Stay alert for worsening of psychiatric problems if patient has a history of such problems or substance abuse.
• Monitor for orthostatic hypotension.
• Evaluate for signs and symptoms of fluid overload.
• Monitor kidney and liver function test results.

Patient teaching

◀€ Caution patient that taking more than prescribed dosage may lead to serious adverse reactions or even death.

• Advise patient to establish effective bedtime routine and to take drug several hours before bedtime to minimize insomnia.
• Caution patient to avoid driving and other hazardous activities until he knows how drug affects concentration and alertness.
• Advise patient to minimize GI upset by eating small, frequent servings of foods and drinking plenty of fluids.
• Instruct patient to contact prescriber if he develops signs or symptoms of depression.
• As appropriate, review all other significant and life-threatening adverse reactions and interactions, especially those related to the drugs, tests, herbs, and behaviors mentioned above.

amifostine
Ethyol

Pharmacologic class: Organic thiophosphate cytoprotective drug
Therapeutic class: Cytoprotectant
Pregnancy risk category C

Action

Undergoes conversion to free thiol, an active metabolite that reduces toxic effects of cisplatin on renal tissue

Availability

Powder for injection: 500-mg anhydrous base and 500 mg mannitol in 10-ml vials

⑦ Indications and dosages

➢ To reduce cumulative renal toxicity of cisplatin therapy in patients with ovarian cancer or non-small-cell lung cancer

Adults: 910 mg/m² I.V. daily as a 15-minute infusion, starting 30 minutes before chemotherapy

➤ To reduce moderate to severe xerostomia in patients undergoing postoperative radiation treatment for head or neck cancer

Adults: 200 mg/m² I.V. daily as a 3-minute infusion, starting 15 to 30 minutes before standard fraction radiation therapy

Off-label uses
• Protection against cisplatin- and paclitaxel-induced neurotoxicity

Contraindications
• Hypersensitivity to drug
• Hypotension

Precautions
Use cautiously in:
• arrhythmias, heart failure, ischemic heart disease, renal impairment, hearing impairment, hypocalcemia, myasthenia gravis, nausea, vomiting, hypotension, obesity
• history of cerebrovascular accident or transient ischemic attacks
• concurrent antihypertensive therapy that can't be discontinued for 24 hours before amifostine therapy (not recommended)
• definitive radiotherapy (not recommended)
• elderly patients
• pregnant patients (safety and efficacy not established)
• breastfeeding patients
• children (safety and efficacy not established).

Administration
• Ensure that patient is adequately hydrated before starting drug.
• Give antiemetics before and during therapy.
• Reconstitute single-dose vial with 9.7 ml of sterile normal saline injection. May be further diluted with normal saline solution up to a concentration of 40 mg/ml.
• Don't mix with other drugs or solutions.
• Know that drug also can be prepared in polyvinyl chloride bags.
• Don't infuse longer than 15 minutes; doing so increases risk of adverse reactions.
◀€ Keep patient supine during administration.

Route	Onset	Peak	Duration
I.V.	5-8 min	Unknown	Unknown

Adverse reactions
CNS: dizziness, drowsiness, rigors
CV: hypotension
GI: nausea, vomiting
Metabolic: hypocalcemia
Respiratory: dyspnea, sneezing
Skin: flushing, rash, urticaria, **erythema multiforme**
Other: chills, warm sensation, hiccups, allergic reactions

Interactions
Drug-drug. *Antihypertensives:* increased risk of hypotension
Drug-diagnostic tests. *Calcium:* decreased level

Patient monitoring
• Monitor blood pressure every 5 minutes during infusion and immediately after infusion as clinically indicated.
• Assess for severe nausea and vomiting.
• Monitor fluid intake and output.
• Monitor blood calcium level. Give calcium supplements as ordered.

Patient teaching
• Emphasize importance of remaining supine during drug administration to prevent hypotension.
• Caution patient to avoid driving and other hazardous activities until he knows how drug affects concentration and alertness.

Reactions in **bold** are life-threatening.   ◀€ Clinical alert

- Advise patient to minimize GI upset by eating small, frequent servings of food and drinking plenty of fluids.
- Provide dietary counseling. Refer patient to dietitian if adverse GI effects significantly limit food intake.
- Inform patient that sneezing is a normal effect of drug.
- As appropriate, review all other significant and life-threatening adverse reactions and interactions, especially those related to the drugs and tests mentioned above.

amikacin sulfate

Pharmacologic class: Aminoglycoside
Therapeutic class: Anti-infective
Pregnancy risk category D

FDA | BOXED WARNING

- Observe patient closely because of potential ototoxicity and nephrotoxicity. Safety isn't established for treatment exceeding 14 days.
- Neuromuscular blockade and respiratory paralysis have occurred after parenteral injection, topical use (as in orthopedic and abdominal irrigation), and oral use.
- Monitor renal function and eighth-nerve function closely, especially in patients with known or suspected renal impairment at onset of therapy, as well as those with initially normal renal function who develop signs of renal dysfunction during therapy.
- Avoid concurrent use with potent diuretics (such as furosemide and ethacrynic acid) because diuretics may cause ototoxicity. Also, I.V. diuretics may increase aminoglycoside toxicity by altering antibiotic serum and tissue levels.
- Avoid concurrent and sequential systemic, oral, or topical use of other neurotoxic or nephrotoxic products and other aminoglycosides. Advanced age and dehydration also may increase toxicity risk.

Action
Interferes with protein synthesis in bacterial cells by binding to 30S ribosomal subunit, leading to bacterial cell death

Availability
Injection: 50 mg/ml, 250 mg/ml

Indications and dosages
➤ Severe systemic infections caused by sensitive strains of *Pseudomonas aeruginosa, Escherichia coli,* or *Proteus, Klebsiella, Serratia, Enterobacter, Actinobacter, Providencia, Citrobacter,* or *Staphylococcus* species
Adults, children, and older infants: 15 mg/kg/day I.V. or I.M. in two to three divided doses q 8 to 12 hours in 100 to 200 ml of dextrose 5% in water (D_5W) over 30 to 60 minutes. Maximum dosage is 1.5 g/day.
Neonates: Initially, 10 mg/kg I.M., then 7.5 mg/kg I.M. q 12 hours
➤ Uncomplicated urinary tract infections caused by susceptible organisms
Adults, children, and older infants: 250 mg I.M. or I.V. twice daily

Dosage adjustment
- Renal impairment (adults)
- Patients undergoing hemodialysis

Off-label uses
- *Mycobacterium avium-intracellulare* infection

Contraindications
- Hypersensitivity to aminoglycosides
- Breastfeeding

Precautions
Use cautiously in:
- decreased renal function, neuromuscular disorders
- parkinsonism, myasthenia gravis

- concurrent or serial use of other nephrotoxic and ototoxic drugs
- elderly patients
- pregnant patients.

Administration

- Don't physically mix amikacin with other drugs. Administer separately.
- For I.V. use, dilute in 100 to 200 ml of normal saline solution or D_5W and give over 30 to 60 minutes.
- Ensure adequate fluid intake to avoid dehydration.
- Draw peak blood level 1 hour after I.M. infusion or 30 to 60 minutes after I.V. infusion.
- Draw trough blood level just before next dose.

Route	Onset	Peak	Duration
I.V.	Immediate	30 min	8-12 hr
I.M.	Variable	1 hr	8-12 hr

Adverse reactions

CNS: dizziness, vertigo, tremor, numbness, depression, confusion, lethargy, headache, paresthesia, ataxia, **neuromuscular blockade, seizures, neurotoxicity**

CV: hypotension, hypertension, palpitations

EENT: nystagmus and other visual disturbances, ototoxicity, hearing loss, tinnitus

GI: nausea, vomiting, splenomegaly, stomatitis, increased salivation, anorexia

GU: azotemia, increased urinary excretion of casts, polyuria, painful urination, impotence, **nephrotoxicity**

Hematologic: purpura, eosinophilia, **leukemoid reaction, aplastic anemia, neutropenia, agranulocytosis, leukopenia, thrombocytopenia, pancytopenia, hemolytic anemia**

Hepatic: hepatomegaly, hepatic necrosis, hepatotoxicity

Musculoskeletal: joint pain, muscle twitching

Respiratory: apnea

Skin: rash, alopecia, urticaria, itching, exfoliative dermatitis

Other: weight loss, superinfection, pain and irritation at I.M. site

Interactions

Drug-drug. *Acyclovir, amphotericin B, cephalosporin, cisplatin, diuretics, vancomycin:* increased risk of ototoxicity and nephrotoxicity

Depolarizing and nondepolarizing neuromuscular junction blockers, general anesthetics: increased amikacin effect, possibly leading to respiratory depression

Dimenhydrinate: masking of ototoxicity signs and symptoms

Indomethacin: increased trough and peak amikacin levels

Parenteral penicillin: amikacin inactivation

Drug-diagnostic tests. *Alanine aminotransferase, alkaline phosphatase, aspartate aminotransferase, bilirubin, blood urea nitrogen, creatinine, lactate dehydrogenase, nonprotein nitrogen, nitrogen compounds (such as urea):* increased levels

Calcium, potassium, magnesium, sodium: decreased levels

Reticulocytes: increased or decreased count

Patient monitoring

- Monitor kidney function test results and urine cultures, output, protein, and specific gravity.
- Monitor results of peak and trough drug blood levels.
- Evaluate for signs and symptoms of ototoxicity (hearing loss, tinnitus, ataxia, and vertigo).
- Assess for secondary superinfections, particularly upper respiratory tract infections.

Patient teaching

◀€ Inform patient that drug may cause hearing loss, seizures, and other neurologic problems. Tell him to report these symptoms immediately.

Reactions in **bold** are life-threatening.   ◀€ Clinical alert

• Instruct patient to immediately report fever, cough, breathing problems, sore throat, and other signs and symptoms of infection.
• Caution patient to avoid driving and other hazardous activities until he knows how drug affects concentration and alertness.
• Instruct patient to notify prescriber if he's urinating much more or much less than normal.
• Advise patient to minimize GI upset by eating small, frequent servings of food, and drinking plenty of fluids.
• Inform patient that he'll undergo regular blood and urine testing during therapy.
• As appropriate, review all other significant and life-threatening adverse reactions and interactions, especially those related to the drugs and tests mentioned above.

aminocaproic acid
Amicar

Pharmacologic class: Carboxylic acid derivative
Therapeutic class: Antihemorrhagic, antifibrinolytic
Pregnancy risk category C

Action
Interferes with plasminogen activator substances and blocks action of fibrinolysin (plasmin)

Availability
Injection: 250 mg/ml
Syrup: 250 mg/ml
Tablets: 500 mg, 1,000 mg

Indications and dosages
➤ Excessive bleeding caused by fibrinolysis

Adults: 5 g P.O. during first hour; then 1 to 1.25 g/hour until drug blood level of 0.13 mg/ml is reached and sustained and bleeding is controlled. Or 4 to 5 g in 250 ml of compatible diluent I.V. over 1 hour, followed by continuous infusion of 1 g/hour in 50 ml of diluent. Continue for 8 hours or until bleeding stops. Maximum daily dosage is 30 g.

Off-label uses
• Dental extractions
• Hemorrhage

Contraindications
• Hypersensitivity to drug
• Disseminated intravascular coagulation
• Neonates (injectable form)

Precautions
Use cautiously in:
• heart, hepatic, or renal failure
• upper urinary tract bleeding.

Administration
• Dilute I.V. form in normal saline solution, dextrose 5% in water, or Ringer's solution for injection. Give at prescribed rate.
• Know that oral and I.V. doses are the same.

Route	Onset	Peak	Duration
P.O.	1 hr	2 hr	Unknown
I.V.	1 hr	Unknown	3 hr

Adverse reactions
CNS: dizziness, malaise, headache, delirium, hallucinations, weakness, **seizures**
CV: hypotension, ischemia, **thrombophlebitis, cardiomyopathy, bradycardia, arrhythmias**
EENT: conjunctival suffusion, tinnitus, nasal congestion
GI: nausea, vomiting, diarrhea, abdominal pain, dyspepsia

 Canada   ⊕ UK   ☒ Hazardous drug   ⊗ High-alert drug

GU: intrarenal obstruction, renal failure
Hematologic: bleeding tendency, generalized thrombosis, agranulocytosis, leukopenia, thrombocytopenia
Musculoskeletal: myopathy, rhabdomyolysis
Respiratory: dyspnea, pulmonary embolism
Skin: rash, pruritus

Interactions

Drug-drug. *Estrogens, hormonal contraceptives:* increased risk of hypercoagulation
Activated prothrombin, prothrombin complex concentrates: increased signs of active intravascular clotting
Drug-diagnostic tests. *Alanine aminotransferase, aldolase, aspartate aminotransferase, blood urea nitrogen, creatinine, creatine kinase, potassium:* increased levels
Drug-herbs. *Alfalfa, anise, arnica, astragalus, bilberry, black currant seed oil, capsaicin, cat's claw, celery, chaparral, clove oil, dandelion, dong quai, evening primrose oil, feverfew, garlic, ginger, ginkgo, papaya extract, rhubarb, safflower oil, skullcap:* increased anticoagulant effect
Coenzyme Q10, St. John's wort: reduced anticoagulant effect

Patient monitoring

• Monitor vital signs, fluid intake and output, and ECG.
◀≋ Assess for signs and symptoms of thrombophlebitis and pulmonary embolism.
◀≋ Monitor neurologic status, especially for signs of impending seizure.
• Monitor kidney and liver function test results, serum electrolyte levels, and CBC with white cell differential.
• Evaluate for blood dyscrasias, particularly bleeding tendencies.

Patient teaching

• Tell patient that drug may significantly affect many body systems. Assure him that he'll be monitored closely.
◀≋ Instruct patient to immediately report signs and symptoms of thrombophlebitis, pulmonary embolism, or unusual bleeding.
• Tell patient he'll undergo frequent blood testing during therapy.
• As appropriate, review all other significant and life-threatening adverse reactions and interactions, especially those related to the drugs, tests, and herbs mentioned above.

aminophylline (theophylline, ethylenediamine)

Amnivent✸, Phyllocontin✢

Pharmacologic class: Xanthine
Therapeutic class: Bronchodilator
Pregnancy risk category C

Action

Unclear. Thought to directly relax smooth muscle of bronchial airways and increase pulmonary blood flow by inhibiting phosphodiesterase.

Availability

Injection: 250 mg/10 ml
Oral liquid: 105 mg/5 ml
Tablets: 100 mg, 200 mg

🕗 Indications and dosages

➤ Symptomatic relief of bronchospasm in patients with acute symptoms who require rapid theophyllinization
Adults (nonsmokers): 0.7 mg/kg/hour I.V. for first 12 hours. Maintenance dosage is 0.5 mg/kg/hour I.V.

Children ages 9 to 16: 1 mg/kg/hour I.V. for first 12 hours. Maintenance dosage is 0.8 mg/kg/hour I.V.
Children ages 6 months to 9 years: 1.2 mg/kg/hour I.V. for first 12 hours. Maintenance dosage is 1 mg/kg/hour I.V.
➤ Chronic bronchial asthma
Adults and children: Dosage is highly individualized. Common initial dosage is 16 mg/kg/24 hours I.V. or 400 mg/24 hours I.V. in divided doses at 6- or 8-hour intervals. If needed, dosage may be increased 25% at 3-day intervals.

Dosage adjustment
- Heart failure
- Hepatic disease
- Elderly patients
- Smokers

Off-label uses
- Dyspnea in patients with chronic obstructive pulmonary disease (COPD)

Contraindications
- Hypersensitivity to xanthine compounds or ethylenediamine
- Seizure disorders

Precautions
Use cautiously in:
- COPD, diabetes mellitus, glaucoma, renal or hepatic disease, heart failure or other cardiac or circulatory impairment, hypertension, hyperthyroidism, peptic ulcer, severe hypoxemia
- active peptic ulcer disease
- elderly patients
- neonates, infants, and young children.

Administration
- For I.V. use, dilute according to label directions and infuse at a rate no faster than 25 mg/minute.
- Don't give in I.V. solutions containing invert sugar, fructose, or fat emulsions.

- Give oral form at meals with 8 oz of water.

Route	Onset	Peak	Duration
P.O. (extended)	Variable	Variable	Variable
P.O. (liquid)	15-60 min	1-7 hr	Variable
I.V.	Immediate	Immediate	6-8 hr

Adverse reactions
CNS: irritability, dizziness, nervousness, restlessness, headache, insomnia, stammering speech, abnormal behavior, mutism, unresponsiveness alternating with hyperactivity, **seizures**
CV: palpitations, sinus tachycardia, extrasystoles, **marked hypotension, arrhythmias, circulatory failure**
GI: nausea, vomiting, diarrhea, epigastric pain, hematemesis, gastroesophageal reflux, anorexia
GU: urine retention (in men with enlarged prostate), diuresis, increased excretion of renal tubular cells and red blood cells, proteinuria
Metabolic: hyperglycemia
Musculoskeletal: muscle twitching
Respiratory: tachypnea, **respiratory arrest**
Skin: flushing
Other: fever, hypersensitivity reactions (including exfoliative dermatitis and urticaria)

Interactions
Drug-drug. *Adenosine:* decreased antiarrhythmic effect of adenosine
Barbiturates, nicotine, phenytoin, rifampin: decreased aminophylline blood level
Beta-adrenergic blockers: antagonism of aminophylline effects
Calcium channel blockers, cimetidine, ciprofloxacin, disulfiram, erythromycin, hormonal contraceptives, influenza vaccine, interferon, methotrexate: elevated aminophylline blood level

Carbamazepine, isoniazid, loop diuretics (such as furosemide): increased or decreased aminophylline blood level

Ephedrine, other sympathomimetics: toxicity, arrhythmias

Lithium: increased lithium excretion

Drug-diagnostic tests. *Aspartate aminotransferase, glucose:* increased levels

Drug-herbs. *Cayenne:* increased risk of aminophylline toxicity

Drug-behaviors. *Smoking:* increased aminophylline elimination

Patient monitoring

◀€ Monitor aminophylline blood level. Adjust dosage if patient has signs or symptoms of toxicity (tachycardia, headache, anorexia, nausea, vomiting, diarrhea, restlessness, and irritability).

• Assess for arrhythmias, especially after giving loading dose.

• Check vital signs and fluid intake and output.

• Monitor patient's response to drug, and assess pulmonary function test results.

Patient teaching

• Advise patient to take oral doses at meals with 8 oz of water.

• Caution patient to avoid driving and other hazardous activities until he knows how drug affects concentration and alertness.

• Tell patient to minimize GI upset by eating small, frequent servings of food and drinking plenty of fluids.

• Advise patient to establish effective bedtime routine to minimize insomnia.

• Caution patient not to change aminophylline brands.

• If patient smokes, tell him to notify prescriber if he stops smoking; dosage may need to be adjusted.

• As appropriate, review all other significant and life-threatening adverse reactions and interactions, especially those related to the drugs, tests, herbs, and behaviors mentioned above.

amiodarone hydrochloride
Amyben✚, Cordarone, Cordarone X✚, Nexterone, Pacerone

Pharmacologic class: Benzofuran derivative
Therapeutic class: Antiarrhythmic (class III)
Pregnancy risk category D

FDA BOXED WARNING

Oral products

• Because of substantial toxicity, drug is indicated only in patients with life-threatening arrhythmias.

• Drug may cause potentially fatal pulmonary toxicities, including hypersensitivity pneumonitis and interstitial/alveolar pneumonitis. Pulmonary toxicity is fatal about 10% of time.

• Hepatic injury is common but usually mild, manifesting only as abnormal liver enzyme levels. However, overt hepatic disease can occur and, in rare cases, is fatal.

• Drug may exacerbate arrhythmias by reducing tolerance for them or making them harder to reverse. Arrhythmias and significant heart block or sinus bradycardia occur in 2% to 5% of patients.

• Even in patients at high risk for arrhythmic death in whom toxicity is an acceptable risk, drug poses major management problems. Therefore, other agents should be tried first whenever possible.

• Difficulty of using drug effectively and safely poses significant risk. Patients with indicated arrhythmias

---

must be hospitalized to receive loading dose; response generally takes at least 1 week, but usually 2 or more.

Action
Prolongs duration and refractory period of action potential. Slows electrical conduction, electrical impulse generation from sinoatrial node, and conduction through accessory pathways. Also dilates blood vessels.

Availability
Injection: 50 mg/ml in 3-ml ampules
Injection, premixed in dextrose:
1.5 mg/ml (150 mg/100 ml), 1.8 mg/ml (360 mg/200 ml) in single-use plastic containers
Tablets: 100 mg, 200 mg, 400 mg

⃠ Indications and dosages
➤ Life-threatening ventricular arrhythmias
Adults: 150 mg in 100 ml of dextrose 5% in water (D_5W) by rapid I.V. infusion over 10 minutes; then dilute 900 mg in 500 ml of D_5W and administer 360 mg by slow I.V. infusion over next 6 hours; then 540-mg I.V. maintenance infusion over next 18 hours. Or 800 to 1,600 mg P.O. daily in one to two doses for 1 to 3 weeks; then 600 to 800 mg P.O. daily in one to two doses for 1 month; then 400-mg P.O. daily as maintenance dosage. All dosages are titrated to individual patient's clinical needs.
➤ Frequently recurring ventricular fibrillation (VF), hemodynamically unstable ventricular tachycardia (VT)
Adults: Initially, 1,000 mg I.V. infusion over first 24 hours, by following infusion regimen: 150 mg/100 ml (1.5 mg/ml) rapid I.V. infusion over 10 minutes, followed by 360 mg (1 mg/minute) by slow I.V. infusion over 6 hours; then 540 mg (0.5 mg/minute) by slow I.V. infusion over remaining 18 hours as maintenance infusion. For breakthrough

episodes of VF or hemodynamically unstable VT, repeat initial loading dose of 150 mg/100 ml I.V. infusion over 10 minutes as needed. After first 24 hours, continue maintenance infusion of 720 mg/24 hours (0.5 mg/minute) for up to 3 weeks. Increase maintenance infusion rate to achieve effective arrhythmia suppression as needed.

Off-label uses
• Atrioventricular (AV) nodal reentry tachycardia (with parenteral use)
• Conversion of atrial fibrillation to normal sinus rhythm

Contraindications
• Hypersensitivity to drug or its components, including iodine
• Cardiogenic shock
• Second- or third-degree AV block
• Marked sinus bradycardia
• Breastfeeding
• Neonates

Precautions
Use cautiously in:
• electrolyte imbalances, severe pulmonary or hepatic disease, thyroid disorders
• history of heart failure
• elderly patients
• pregnant patients
• children.

Administration
◀⃛ Know that I.V. amiodarone is a high-alert drug.
◀⃛ Give loading dose only in hospital setting with continuous ECG monitoring.
• Administer oral loading dose in two equal doses with meals. Give maintenance dose daily or in two divided doses to minimize GI upset.
• Don't give I.V. unless patient is on continuous ECG monitoring.
• Dilute I.V. drug (except premixed drug) with dextrose 5% in water and use an in-line filter. Drug isn't compatible with normal saline solution.

• Don't combine premixed drug with any other product in the same I.V. line or premixed container.

◀◈ Don't use plastic containers in series connections because of risk of air embolism.

• Use central venous catheter when giving repeated doses. If possible, use dedicated catheter for drug.

Route	Onset	Peak	Duration
P.O.	Variable	3-7 hr	Wks-mos
I.V.	Hrs	Unknown	Variable

Adverse reactions

CNS: dizziness, fatigue, headache, insomnia, paresthesia, peripheral neuropathy, poor coordination, involuntary movements, tremor, sleep disturbances

CV: hypotension, **heart failure, worsening arrhythmia, AV block, sinoatrial node dysfunction, bradycardia, asystole, cardiac arrest, cardiogenic shock, electromechanical dissociation, ventricular tachycardia**

EENT: corneal microdeposits, corneal or macular degeneration, visual disturbances, dry eyes, eye discomfort, optic neuritis or neuropathy, scotoma, lens opacities, photophobia, visual halos, **papilledema**

GI: nausea, vomiting, constipation, abdominal pain, abnormal salivation, anorexia

GU: decreased libido

Hematologic: coagulation abnormalities, thrombocytopenia

Hepatic: nonspecific hepatic disorders, **hepatic dysfunction**

Metabolic: hypothyroidism, hyperthyroidism

Respiratory: cough, **adult respiratory distress syndrome, pulmonary inflammation or fibrosis, pulmonary edema**

Skin: flushing, photosensitivity, toxic epidermal necrolysis

Other: abnormal taste and smell, edema, fever, **Stevens-Johnson syndrome**

Interactions

Drug-drug. *Anticoagulants:* increased prothrombin time (PT)

Azole antifungals, fluoroquinolones, loratadine, macrolide antibiotics, trazodone: increased risk of life-threatening arrhythmias

Beta-adrenergic blockers: increased risk of bradycardia and hypotension

Calcium channel blockers: increased risk of AV block (with verapamil, diltiazem) or hypotension (with any calcium channel blocker)

Cholestyramine: decreased amiodarone blood level

Cimetidine, ritonavir: increased amiodarone blood level

Class I antiarrhythmics (disopyramide, flecainide, lidocaine, mexiletine, procainamide, quinidine): increased blood levels of these drugs, leading to toxicity

Cyclosporine: elevated cyclosporine and creatinine blood levels

Dextromethorphan: impaired dextromethorphan metabolism (with amiodarone therapy of 2 weeks or longer)

Digoxin: increased digoxin blood level, leading to toxicity

Fentanyl: increased bradycardia, hypotension

Methotrexate: impaired methotrexate metabolism, possibly causing toxicity (with amiodarone use longer than 2 weeks)

Phenytoin: decreased amiodarone blood level or increased phenytoin blood level (with amiodarone use longer than 2 weeks)

Protease inhibitors (atazanavir, indinavir, nelfinavir): possible increased amiodarone concentration

Rifampin: decreased amiodarone concentration

Theophylline: increased theophylline blood level (with amiodarone use longer than 1 week)

Drug-diagnostic tests. *Kidney function tests:* abnormal results

Drug-food. *Grapefruit juice:* increased drug concentration

Reactions in **bold** are life-threatening.　　　　　　◀◈ Clinical alert

Drug-herb. *St. John's wort:* decreased drug blood level

Patient monitoring

◀≋ Monitor patient closely. Drug may cause serious or life-threatening adverse reactions.

◀≋ Watch for slow onset of life-threatening arrhythmias, especially after giving loading dose.

◀≋ Monitor ECG continuously during loading dose and when dosage is changed.

• Check patient's blood pressure, pulse, and heart rhythm regularly.

• Assess for signs and symptoms of lung inflammation.

• Monitor baseline and subsequent chest X-rays, as well as pulmonary, liver, and thyroid function test results.

• Closely monitor patient who's receiving other drugs concurrently because amiodarone can interact with many drugs. Check digoxin blood level if patient is receiving digoxin; monitor PT or International Normalized Ratio if patient is receiving anticoagulants.

Patient teaching

◀≋ Inform patient that drug may cause serious adverse reactions. Instruct him to report these immediately.

• Tell patient to take oral doses with meals. Advise him to divide daily dose into two doses if drug causes GI upset.

• Tell patient that adverse reactions are most common with high doses and may become more frequent after 6 months of therapy.

• Inform patient that he'll undergo regular blood testing, eye examinations, chest X-rays, and pulmonary function tests during therapy.

• As appropriate, review all other significant and life-threatening adverse reactions and interactions, especially those related to the drugs and tests mentioned above.

amitriptyline hydrochloride
Apo-Amitriptyline, Levate✤, Novotriptyn✤

Pharmacologic class: Tricyclic compound
Therapeutic class: Antidepressant
Pregnancy risk category D

FDA | **BOXED WARNING**

• Drug may increase risk of suicidal thinking and behavior in children and adolescents with major depressive disorder and other psychiatric disorders. Risk is greater during first few months of treatment, and must be balanced with clinical need, as depression itself increases suicide risk. With patient of any age, observe closely for clinical worsening, suicidality, and unusual behavior changes when therapy begins. Advise family to observe patient closely and communicate with prescriber as needed.

• Drug isn't approved for use in pediatric patients.

Action

Unclear. Inhibits norepinephrine and serotonin reuptake at presynaptic neuron, increasing levels of these neurotransmitters in brain. Also has sedative, anticholinergic, and mild peripheral vasodilating effects.

Availability

Tablets: 10 mg, 25 mg, 50 mg, 75 mg, 100 mg, 150 mg

🖊 Indications and dosages

➢ Depression (often given in conjunction with psychotherapy)
Adults: 75 mg P.O. daily in divided doses; may increase gradually to 150 mg/day. Or start with 50 to 100 mg P.O. at bedtime and increase by 25 to

50 mg as needed, to a total dosage of 150 mg. Hospitalized patients initially may receive 100 mg P.O. daily, with gradual increases as needed to a total dosage of 300 mg P.O.

Dosage adjustment

- Elderly patients
- Adolescents
- Outpatients

Off-label uses

- Analgesic adjunct for phantom limb pain or chronic pain

Contraindications

- Hypersensitivity to drug or other tricyclic antidepressants (TCAs)
- Acute recovery phase after myocardial infarction
- MAO inhibitor use within past 14 days
- Children younger than age 12

Precautions

Use cautiously in:

- seizures, cardiovascular disease, renal or hepatic impairment, urinary retention, hyperthyroidism, increased intraocular pressure, closed-angle glaucoma, prostatic hypertrophy, bipolar disorder, schizophrenia, paranoia
- elderly patients
- pregnant or breastfeeding patients.

Administration

- Administer full dose at bedtime to minimize orthostatic hypotension.
- Don't withdraw drug suddenly. Instead, taper dosage gradually.
- If patient is scheduled for surgery, discuss dosage tapering with prescriber.
- Be aware that drug is often used in conjunction with psychotherapy.

Route	Onset	Peak	Duration
P.O.	2-4 wk	2-6 wk	Unknown

Adverse reactions

CNS: headache, fatigue, agitation, numbness, paresthesia, peripheral neuropathy, weakness, restlessness, panic, anxiety, dizziness, drowsiness, difficulty speaking, excitement, hypomania, psychosis exacerbation, extrapyramidal effects, poor coordination, hallucinations, insomnia, nightmares, **seizures, coma, suicidal behavior or ideation (especially in children and adolescents)**

CV: ECG changes, tachycardia, hypertension, orthostatic hypotension, **arrhythmias, heart block, myocardial infarction**

EENT: blurred vision, dry eyes, mydriasis, abnormal visual accommodation, increased intraocular pressure, tinnitus

GI: nausea, vomiting, constipation, dry mouth, epigastric pain, anorexia, **paralytic ileus**

GU: urinary retention, delayed voiding, urinary tract dilation, gynecomastia

Hematologic: agranulocytosis, thrombocytopenia, thrombocytopenic purpura, leukopenia

Metabolic: changes in blood glucose level

Skin: photosensitivity rash, urticaria, flushing, diaphoresis

Other: increased appetite, weight gain, high fever, edema, hypersensitivity reaction

Interactions

Drug-drug. *Activated charcoal:* decreased amitriptyline absorption

Adrenergics, anticholinergics, anticholinergic-like drugs: increased anticholinergic effects

Amiodarone, cimetidine, quinidine, ritonavir: increased amitriptyline effects

Barbiturates: decreased amitriptyline blood level, increased CNS and respiratory effects

Clonidine: hypertensive crisis

CNS depressants (including antihistamines, opioids, sedative-hypnotics): increased CNS depression

Drugs metabolized by CYP-4502D6 (such as other antidepressants,

phenothiazines, carbamazepine, class 1C antiarrhythmics): decreased amitriptyline clearance, possibly causing toxicity
Guanethidine: antagonism of antihypertensive action
Levodopa: delayed or decreased levodopa absorption, hypertension
MAO inhibitors: hypotension, tachycardia, potentially fatal reactions
Rifabutin, rifampin, rifapentine: decreased amitriptyline blood level and effects
Selective serotonin reuptake inhibitors: increased risk of toxicity
Sympathomimetics: increased pressor effect of direct-acting sympathomimetics (epinephrine, norepinephrine), possibly causing arrhythmias; decreased pressor effect of indirect-acting sympathomimetics (ephedrine, metaraminol)
Drug-diagnostic tests. *Eosinophils, liver function tests:* increased values
Glucose, granulocytes, platelets, white blood cells: increased or decreased levels
Drug-herbs. *Angel's trumpet, jimsonweed, scopolia:* increased anticholinergic effects
Chamomile, hops, kava, skullcap, valerian: increased CNS depression
St. John's wort: decreased drug blood level and reduced efficacy
Drug-behaviors. *Alcohol use:* increased CNS sedation
Smoking: increased drug metabolism and altered effects
Sun exposure: increased risk of photosensitivity reaction

Patient monitoring
• Evaluate for signs and symptoms of psychosis. If present, discuss possible dosage change with prescriber.
• Assess for changes in patient's mood or mental status.
 Monitor for signs and symptoms of depression and assess for suicidal ideation (especially in child or adolescent).

• Check blood pressure for orthostatic hypertension.
• Monitor CBC with white cell differential, glucose levels, and liver function test results.

Patient teaching
 Instruct patient, parent, or caregiver to contact prescriber if severe mood changes or suicidal thoughts occur (especially if patient is child or adolescent).
• Tell patient that drug may cause temporary blood pressure decrease if he stands up suddenly. Advise him to rise slowly and carefully.
• Caution patient to avoid driving and other hazardous activities until he knows how drug affects concentration and alertness.
• Advise patient to minimize GI upset by eating small, frequent servings of food and drinking plenty of fluids.
• Inform patient that he'll undergo frequent blood testing during therapy.
• As appropriate, review all other significant and life-threatening adverse reactions and interactions, especially those related to the drugs, tests, herbs, and behaviors mentioned above.

amlodipine besylate
Norvasc

Pharmacologic class: Calcium channel blocker
Therapeutic class: Antihypertensive
Pregnancy risk category C

Action
Inhibits influx of extracellular calcium ions, thereby decreasing myocardial contractility, relaxing coronary and vascular muscles, and decreasing peripheral resistance

---

Availability
Tablets: 2.5 mg, 5 mg, 10 mg

⚠️ Indications and dosages
➤ Essential hypertension, chronic stable angina pectoris, and vasospastic angina (Prinzmetal's angina)
Adults: 5 to 10 mg P.O. once daily

Dosage adjustment
• Hepatic impairment
• Elderly patients

Off-label uses
• Pulmonary hypertension
• Raynaud's disease

Contraindications
• Hypersensitivity to drug

Precautions
Use cautiously in:
• aortic stenosis, severe hepatic impairment, heart failure
• elderly patients
• pregnant or breastfeeding patients
• children.

Administration
• Be aware that this drug may be given alone or with other drugs to relieve hypertension or angina.

Route	Onset	Peak	Duration
P.O.	Unknown	6-9 hr	24 hr

Adverse reactions
CNS: headache, dizziness, drowsiness, light-headedness, fatigue, weakness, lethargy
CV: peripheral edema, angina, bradycardia, hypotension, palpitations
GI: nausea, abdominal discomfort
Musculoskeletal: muscle cramps, muscle pain or inflammation
Respiratory: shortness of breath, dyspnea, wheezing
Skin: rash, pruritus, urticaria, flushing

Interactions
Drug-drug. *Beta-adrenergic blockers:* increased risk of adverse effects
Fentanyl, nitrates, other antihypertensives, quinidine: additive hypotension
Drug-behaviors. *Acute alcohol ingestion:* additive hypotension

Patient monitoring
◀€ Monitor patient for worsening angina.
• Monitor heart rate and rhythm and blood pressure, especially at start of therapy.
◀€ Assess for heart failure; report signs and symptoms (peripheral edema, dyspnea) to prescriber promptly.
◀€ Give sublingual nitroglycerin, as prescribed, if patient has signs or symptoms of acute myocardial infarction (especially when dosage is increased).

Patient teaching
• If patient also uses sublingual nitroglycerin, tell him he can take nitroglycerin as needed for acute angina.
• Caution patient to avoid driving and other hazardous activities until he knows how drug affects concentration and alertness.
• As appropriate, review all other significant adverse reactions, especially those related to the drugs and behaviors mentioned above.

amoxicillin

amoxicillin trihydrate
Amix❖, Amox♣, Amoxident❖, Amoxil, Apo-Amoxil♣, Moxatag♣, Novamoxin♣, Nu-Amoxil♣, Trimox

Pharmacologic class: Aminopenicillin
Therapeutic class: Anti-infective
Pregnancy risk category B

Action

Inhibits cell-wall synthesis during bacterial multiplication, leading to cell death. Shows enhanced activity toward gram-negative bacteria compared to natural and penicillinase-resistant penicillins.

Availability

Capsules: 250 mg, 500 mg
Powder for oral suspension: 50 mg/ml and 125 mg/5 ml (pediatric), 200 mg/5 ml, 250 mg/5 ml, 400 mg/5 ml
Tablets: 500 mg, 875 mg
Tablets for oral suspension: 200 mg, 400 mg
Tablets (chewable): 125 mg, 200 mg, 250 mg, 400 mg

💋 Indications and dosages

➤ Uncomplicated gonorrhea
Adults and children weighing at least 40 kg (88 lb): 3 g P.O. as a single dose
Children ages 2 and older weighing less than 40 kg (88 lb): 50 mg/kg P.O. given with probenecid 25 mg/kg P.O. as a single dose
➤ Bacterial endocarditis prophylaxis for dental, GI, and GU procedures
Adults: 2 g P.O. 1 hour before procedure
Children: 50 mg/kg P.O. 1 hour before procedure
➤ Lower respiratory tract infections caused by streptococci, pneumococci, non-penicillinase-producing staphylococci, and *Haemophilus influenzae*
Adults and children weighing more than 20 kg (44 lb): 875 mg P.O. q 12 hours or 500 mg P.O. q 8 hours
Children weighing less than 20 kg (44 lb): 45 mg/kg/day P.O. in divided doses q 12 hours or 40 mg/kg/day P.O. in divided doses q 8 hours
➤ Ear, nose, and throat infections caused by streptococci, pneumococci, non-penicillinase-producing staphylococci, and *H. influenzae;* GU infections caused by *Escherichia coli, Proteus mirabilis,* and *Streptococcus faecalis*
Adults and children weighing more than 20 kg (44 lb): 500 mg P.O. q 12 hours or 250 mg P.O. q 8 hours
Children weighing less than 20 kg (44 lb): 45 mg/kg/day P.O. in divided doses q 12 hours or 20 to 40 mg/kg P.O. in divided doses q 8 hours
➤ Eradication of *Helicobacter pylori* to reduce risk of duodenal ulcer recurrence
Adults: 1 g P.O. q 12 hours for 14 days in combination with clarithromycin and lansoprazole, or in combination with lansoprazole alone as 1 g t.i.d. for 14 days
➤ Postexposure anthrax prophylaxis
Adults: 500 mg P.O. t.i.d. for 60 days
Children: 80 mg/kg/day P.O. t.i.d. for 60 days
➤ Skin and skin-structure infections caused by streptococci (alpha- and beta-hemolytic strains), staphylococci, and *E. coli*
Adults: 500 mg P.O. q 12 hours to 250 mg P.O. q 8 hours. For severe infections, 875 mg P.O. q 12 hours or 500 mg P.O. q 8 hours.
Children older than age 3 months: 25 mg/kg/day P.O. in divided doses q 12 hours or 20 mg/kg/day P.O. in divided doses every 8 hours. For severe infections, 45 mg/kg/day P.O. in divided doses q 12 hours or 40 mg/kg/day P.O. in divided doses every 8 hours.

Dosage adjustment

• Renal impairment
• Hemodialysis
• Infants ages 3 months and younger

Off-label uses

• *Chlamydia trachomatis* infection in pregnant patients

Contraindications

• Hypersensitivity to drug or any penicillin

Precautions
Use cautiously in:
- severe renal insufficiency, infectious mononucleosis, hepatic dysfunction
- pregnant patients.

Administration
◀≋ Ask about history of penicillin allergy before giving.
- Give with or without food.
- Store liquid form in refrigerator when possible.
- Know that maximum dosage for infants ages 3 months and younger is 30 mg/kg/day divided q 12 hours.

Route	Onset	Peak	Duration
P.O.	30 min	1-2 hr	8-12 hr

Adverse reactions
CNS: lethargy, hallucinations, anxiety, confusion, agitation, depression, dizziness, fatigue, hyperactivity, insomnia, behavioral changes, **seizures** (with high doses)
GI: nausea, vomiting, diarrhea, bloody diarrhea, abdominal pain, gastritis, stomatitis, glossitis, black "hairy" tongue, furry tongue, enterocolitis, **pseudomembranous colitis**
GU: vaginitis, nephropathy, **interstitial nephritis**
Hematologic: eosinophilia, anemia, **thrombocytopenia, thrombocytopenic purpura, leukopenia, hemolytic anemia, agranulocytosis, bone marrow depression**
Hepatic: cholestatic jaundice, hepatic cholestasis, **cholestatic hepatitis, nonspecific hepatitis**
Respiratory: wheezing
Skin: rash
Other: superinfections (oral and rectal candidiasis), fever, **anaphylaxis**

Interactions
Drug-drug. *Allopurinol:* increased risk of rash

Chloramphenicol, macrolides, sulfonamides, tetracycline: decreased amoxicillin efficacy
Hormonal contraceptives: decreased contraceptive efficacy
Probenecid: decreased renal excretion
Drug-diagnostic tests. *Alanine aminotransferase, alkaline phosphatase, eosinophils, lactate dehydrogenase:* increased levels
Granulocytes, hemoglobin, platelets, white blood cells: decreased values
Direct Coombs' test, urine glucose, urine protein: false-positive results
Drug-food. *Any food:* delayed or reduced drug absorption
Drug-herbs. *Khat:* decreased antimicrobial efficacy

Patient monitoring
- Monitor for signs and symptoms of hypersensitivity reaction.
◀≋ Evaluate for seizures when giving high doses.
- Monitor patient's temperature and watch for other signs and symptoms of superinfection (especially oral or rectal candidiasis).

Patient teaching
◀≋ Instruct patient to immediately report signs and symptoms of hypersensitivity reactions, such as rash, fever, or chills.
- Tell patient he may take drug with or without food.
- Tell patient not to chew or swallow tablets for suspension, because they're not meant to be dissolved in mouth.
- Advise patient to minimize GI upset by eating small, frequent servings of food and drinking plenty of fluids.
- Tell patient taking hormonal contraceptives that drug may reduce contraceptive efficacy. Suggest she use alternative birth control method.
- Inform patient that drug lowers resistance to other types of infections. Instruct him to report new signs and symptoms of infection, especially in mouth or rectum.

- Tell parents they may give liquid form of drug directly to child or may mix it with foods or beverages.
- As appropriate, review all other significant and life-threatening adverse reactions and interactions, especially those related to the drugs, tests, foods, and herbs mentioned above.

amoxicillin and clavulanate potassium

Apo-Amoxi-Clav✣, Augmentin, Augmentin-Duo✤, Augmentin XR, Clavulin✣, Novo-Clavamoxin✣

Pharmacologic class: Aminopenicillin
Therapeutic class: Anti-infective
Pregnancy risk category B

Action
Amoxicillin inhibits transpeptidase, preventing cross-linking of bacterial cell wall and leading to cell death. Addition of clavulanate (a beta-lactam) increases drug's resistance to beta-lactamase (an enzyme produced by bacteria that may inactivate amoxicillin).

Availability
Oral suspension: 125 mg amoxicillin with 31.25 mg clavulanic acid/5 ml, 200 mg amoxicillin with 28.5 mg clavulanic acid/5 ml, 250 mg amoxicillin with 62.5 mg clavulanic acid/ 5 ml, 400 mg amoxicillin with 57 mg clavulanic acid/5 ml, 600 mg amoxicillin with 42.9 mg clavulanic acid/5 ml
Tablets (chewable): 200 mg amoxicillin with 28.5 mg clavulanate, 400 mg amoxicillin with 57 mg clavulanate
Tablets (extended-release): 1,000 mg amoxicillin with 62.5 mg clavulanate
Tablets (film-coated): 250 mg amoxicillin with 125 mg clavulanate, 500 mg amoxicillin with 125 mg clavulanate, 875 mg amoxicillin with 125 mg clavulanate

⏀ Indications and dosages
➤ Lower respiratory tract infections, otitis media, sinusitis, skin and skin-structure infections, and urinary tract infections (UTIs) caused by susceptible strains of gram-negative and gram-positive organisms
Adults and children weighing more than 40 kg (88 lb): 500 mg q 12 hours or 250 mg P.O. q 8 hours (based on amoxicillin component). For severe infections, 875 mg P.O. q 12 hours or 500 mg P.O. q 8 hours.
➤ Serious infections and community-acquired pneumonia
Adults and children weighing more than 40 kg (88 lb): 875 mg P.O. q 12 hours or 500 mg P.O. q 8 hours
Infants and children ages 3 months and older weighing less than 40 kg (88 lb): 20 to 45 mg/kg/day P.O. in divided doses q 12 hours or 20 or 25 to 40 mg/kg/day in divided doses q 8 hours, based on severity of infection and amoxicillin component (125 mg/5 ml or 250 mg/5 ml suspension)
Infants younger than 3 months: 30 mg/kg/day P.O. (based on amoxicillin component) divided q 12 hours. (125 mg/ 5 ml oral suspension is recommended.)
➤ Recurrent or persistent acute otitis media caused by *Streptococcus pneumoniae, Haemophilus influenzae,* or *Moraxella catarrhalis* in children ages 2 and younger and in children who have received antibiotic therapy within last 3 months
Children ages 3 months to 12 years: 90 mg/kg/day of Augmentin ES-600 P.O. q 12 hours for 10 days

Dosage adjustment
- Severe renal impairment
- Hemodialysis
- Infants ages 3 months and younger

Contraindications
- Hypersensitivity to drug or any penicillin
- Phenylketonuria (some products)

---

a

• History of cholestatic jaundice or hepatic dysfunction associated with this drug

Precautions
Use cautiously in:
• severe renal insufficiency, infectious mononucleosis
• pregnant patients.

Administration
◀ Ask about history of penicillin allergy before giving.
• Give with or without food.
• Know that maximum dosage for infants ages 3 months and younger is 30 mg/kg/day divided q 12 hours.
• Be aware that 12-hour dosing is recommended to reduce diarrhea.

Route	Onset	Peak	Duration
P.O.	Unknown	1-2.5 hr	6-8 hr
P.O. (extended)	Unknown	1-4 hr	Unknown

Adverse reactions
CNS: lethargy, hallucinations, anxiety, confusion, agitation, depression, dizziness, fatigue, hyperactivity, insomnia, behavioral changes, **seizures** (with high doses)
GI: nausea, vomiting, diarrhea, abdominal pain, stomatitis, glossitis, gastritis, black "hairy" tongue, furry tongue, enterocolitis, **pseudomembranous colitis**
GU: vaginitis, nephropathy, **interstitial nephritis**
Hematologic: anemia, **thrombocytopenia, thrombocytopenic purpura, leukopenia, hemolytic anemia, agranulocytosis, bone narrow depression,** eosinophilia
Hepatic: cholestatic hepatitis
Respiratory: wheezing
Skin: rash
Other: superinfections (oral and rectal candidiasis), fever, **anaphylaxis**

Interactions
Drug-drug. *Any food:* enhanced clavulanate absorption
Chloramphenicol, macrolides, sulfonamides, tetracycline: decreased amoxicillin efficacy
Hormonal contraceptives: decreased contraceptive efficacy
Probenecid: decreased renal excretion and increased blood level of amoxicillin
Drug-food. *Any food:* enhanced clavulanate absorption
Drug-herbs. *Khat:* decreased antimicrobial effect

Patient monitoring
• Monitor patient carefully for signs and symptoms of hypersensitivity reaction.
◀ Monitor for seizures when giving high doses.
• Check patient's temperature and watch for other signs and symptoms of superinfection, especially oral or rectal candidiasis.

Patient teaching
◀ Instruct patient to immediately report signs or symptoms of hypersensitivity reaction, such as rash, fever, or chills.
• Tell patient he may take drug with or without food.
• Inform patient that drug lowers resistance to some types of infections. Instruct him to report new signs or symptoms of infection (especially of mouth or rectum).
• Advise patient to minimize GI upset by eating small, frequent servings of food and drinking plenty of fluids.
• Tell patient taking hormonal contraceptives that drug may reduce contraceptive efficacy. Suggest she use alternative birth control method.
• Inform parents that they may give liquid form of drug directly to child or may mix it with foods or beverages.
• As appropriate, review all other significant and life-threatening adverse

---

◀ Clinical alert

reactions and interactions, especially those related to the drugs, foods, and herbs mentioned above.

amphotericin B cholesteryl sulfate
Amphocil✴, Amphotec

amphotericin B desoxycholate
Fungilin✴, Fungizone Intravenous

amphotericin B lipid complex
Abelcet

amphotericin B liposome⊗
AmBisome

Pharmacologic class: Systemic polyene antifungal
Therapeutic class: Antifungal
Pregnancy risk category B

FDA | BOXED WARNING

• Amphotericin B desoxycholate should be used mainly to treat progressive and potentially life-threatening fungal infections. It shouldn't be used to treat noninvasive forms of fungal disease (such as oral thrush, vaginal candidiasis, or esophageal candidiasis) in patients with normal neutrophil counts.

Action
Binds to sterols in fungal cell membrane, increasing permeability. This allows potassium to exit the cell, causing fungal impairment or death.

Availability
Amphotericin B cholesteryl sulfate—
Injection: 50 mg, 100 mg
Amphotericin B desoxycholate—
Injection: 50-mg vial
Oral suspension: 100 mg/ml in 24-ml bottles
Amphotericin B lipid complex—
Suspension for injection: 100 mg/20-ml vials
Amphotericin B liposome—
Injection: 50 mg

🖊 Indications and dosages
➤ Invasive aspergillosis
Adults: *Amphotericin B desoxycholate*—For patients with good cardiorenal function who tolerate test dose, give 0.25 to 0.3 mg/kg daily by slow I.V. infusion (0.1 mg/ml over 2 to 6 hours). Gradually increase to 0.5 to 0.6 mg/kg daily. Patients with neutropenia or rapidly progressing, potentially fatal infections may require higher dosages (1 to 1.5 mg/kg daily).
Adults and children ages 1 month and older: *Amphotericin B liposome*—3 to 5 mg/kg I.V. daily
➤ Invasive aspergillosis in patients with renal impairment or unacceptable toxicity who can't tolerate or don't respond to amphotericin B desoxycholate in effective doses
Adults and children: *Amphotericin B cholesteryl sulfate*—3 to 4 mg/kg daily reconstituted in sterile water for injection and diluted in dextrose 5% in water (D_5W) and give by continuous infusion at 1 mg/kg/hour. *Amphotericin B lipid complex*—5 mg/kg daily I.V. prepared as 1-mg/ml infusion and delivered at a rate of 2.5 mg/kg/hour.
➤ Systemic histoplasmosis
Adults: *Amphotericin B desoxycholate*—If patient tolerates test dose, gradually increase from initial recommended dosage of 0.25 to 0.3 mg/kg daily by slow I.V. infusion (0.1 mg/ml over 2 to 6 hours) to usual dosage of

0.5 to 0.6 mg/kg daily I.V. for 4 to 8 weeks; higher dosages (0.7 to 1 mg) may be necessary for rapidly progressing, potentially fatal infections.

➤ Systemic coccidioidomycosis and blastomycosis

Adults: *Amphotericin B desoxycholate*— If patient tolerates test dose, gradually increase from initial recommended dosage of 0.25 to 0.3 mg/kg daily by slow I.V. infusion (0.1 mg/ml over 2 to 6 hours) to usual dosage of 0.5 to 1 mg/kg daily I.V. for 4 to 12 weeks.

➤ Systemic cryptococcosis

Adults: *Amphotericin B desoxycholate*—If patient tolerates test dose, gradually increase from initial recommended dosage of 0.25 to 0.3 mg/kg daily by slow I.V. infusion (0.1 mg/ml over 2 to 6 hours) to usual dosage of 0.3 to 1 mg/kg daily I.V. (with or without flucytosine) for 2 weeks to several months. For patients with human immunodeficiency virus (HIV) infection, usual dosage is 0.7 mg/kg daily I.V. for 4 weeks, followed by 0.7 mg/kg I.V. given on alternate days for 4 additional weeks. If patient can't tolerate or doesn't respond to amphotericin B desoxycholate, give amphotericin B cholesteryl sulfate at a dosage of 3 to 6 mg/kg daily I.V.

Adults and children ages 1 month and older: *Amphotericin B liposome*—3 to 5 mg/kg daily I.V.

➤ Cryptococcal meningitis in HIV-infected patients

Adults: *Amphotericin B desoxycholate*—If patient tolerates test dose, gradually increase from initial recommended dosage of 0.25 to 0.3 mg/kg daily by slow I.V. infusion (0.1 mg/ml over 2 to 6 hours) to usual dosage of 0.3 to 1 mg/kg daily I.V. (with or without flucytosine) for 2 weeks to several months. *Amphotericin B lipid complex*—5 mg/kg I.V. infusion daily for 6 weeks, followed by 12 weeks of oral fluconazole therapy. *Amphotericin B liposome*—6 mg/kg I.V. infusion daily.

➤ Disseminated candidiasis

Adults: *Amphotericin B desoxycholate*—If patient tolerates test dose, gradually increase from initial recommended dosage of 0.25 to 0.3 mg/kg daily by slow I.V. infusion (0.1 mg/ml over 2 to 6 hours) to usual dosage of 0.4 to 0.6 mg/kg daily by slow I.V. infusion for 7 to 14 days (low-risk patients) or for 6 weeks (high-risk patients). For hepatosplenic candidiasis, 1 mg/kg daily I.V. given with oral flucytosine; for severe or refractory esophageal candidiasis in HIV-infected patients, 0.3 mg/kg daily I.V. for at least 5 to 7 days; for candiduria, 0.3 mg/kg daily I.V. for 3 to 5 days.

Adults and children ages 1 month and older: *Amphotericin B liposome*—3 to 5 mg/kg/day I.V. for 5 to 7 days

➤ Systemic zygomycosis, including mucormycosis

Adults: *Amphotericin B desoxycholate*—If patient tolerates test dose, gradually increase from initial recommended dosage of 0.25 to 0.3 mg/kg daily by slow I.V. infusion (0.1 mg/ml over 2 to 6 hours) to usual dosage of 1 to 1.5 mg/kg daily I.V. for 2 to 3 months. For rhinocerebral phycomycosis form, total dosage is 3 g I.V.

➤ Systemic disseminated sporotrichosis

Adults: *Amphotericin B desoxycholate*—If patient tolerates test dose, gradually increase from initial recommended dosage of 0.25 to 0.3 mg/kg daily by slow I.V. infusion (0.1 mg/ml over 2 to 6 hours) to usual dosage of 0.4 to 0.5 mg/kg daily I.V. for 2 to 3 months.

➤ Cutaneous leishmaniasis

Adults and children: *Amphotericin B desoxycholate*—If patient tolerates test dose, gradually increase from initial recommended dosage of 0.25 to 0.5 mg/kg/day given by slow I.V. infusion (0.1 mg/ml over 2 to 6 hours) until 0.5 to 1 mg/kg/day is reached; then give every other day. Usual duration is 3 to 12 weeks.

➤ Visceral leishmaniasis in immuno-competent patients

Adults and children ages 1 month and older: *Amphotericin B liposome*—3 mg/kg given I.V. over 2 hours on days 1 through 5, 14, and 21. Repeat course if initial treatment fails to clear parasites.

➤ Visceral leishmaniasis in immuno-compromised patients

Adults and children ages 1 month and older: *Amphotericin B liposome*—4 mg/kg given I.V. over 2 hours on days 1 through 5, 10, 17, 24, 31, and 38

➤ Empiric therapy for presumed fungal infection in febrile, neutropenic patients

Adults: *Amphotericin B desoxycholate*—If patient tolerates test dose, gradually increase from initial recommended dosage of 0.25 to 0.3 mg/kg daily by slow I.V. infusion (0.1 mg/ml over 2 to 6 hours) to usual dosage of 0.25 to 1 mg/kg daily I.V. *Amphotericin B liposome*—3 mg/kg daily given I.V. over 120 minutes for 2 weeks.

Off-label uses

• Chemoprophylaxis in immunocompromised patients
• Coccidioidal arthritis
• Prophylaxis of fungal infections in bone-marrow transplant recipients, patients with primary amoebic meningoencephalitis caused by *Naegleria fowleri*, and patients with ocular aspergillosis

Contraindications

• Hypersensitivity to drug and its components
• Severe respiratory distress

Precautions

Use cautiously in:
• renal impairment, electrolyte abnormalities
• pregnant or breastfeeding patients
• children.

Administration

• Know that amphotericin B should be given only by health care professionals thoroughly familiar with drug, its administration, and adverse reactions.

🔊 Before giving first dose of conventional amphotericin B (desoxycholate form), test dose may be ordered (due to widely varying tolerance and clinical status) as follows: 1 mg in 20 ml of D_5W over 20 to 30 minutes; monitor vital signs every 30 minutes for next 2 hours.

• Know that if desoxycholate form is discontinued for 1 week or longer, drug should be restarted at 0.25 mg/kg daily, with dosage then increased gradually.

• Pretreat with antihistamines, antipyretics, or corticosteroids, as prescribed.

• Give through separate I.V. line, using infusion pump and in-line filter with pores larger than 1 micron.

• Choose distal vein for I.V. site. Alternate sites regularly.

• Mix with sterile water to reconstitute. Don't mix with sodium chloride, other electrolytes, or bacteriostatic products.

• Flush I.V. line with 5% dextrose injection before and after infusion.

• Keep dry form of drug away from light. Once mixed with fluid, solution can be kept in light for up to 8 hours.

🔊 Know that total daily dosage of amphotericin B desoxycholate form should never exceed 1.5 mg/kg.

Route	Onset	Peak	Duration
P.O.	Unknown	Unknown	Unknown
I.V.	Rapid	End of infusion	24 hr

Adverse reactions

CNS: anxiety, confusion, headache, insomnia, weakness, depression, dizziness, drowsiness, hallucinations, speech difficulty, ataxia, vertigo, stupor, psychosis, **seizures**

CV: hypotension, hypertension, tachycardia, phlebitis, chest pain, orthostatic hypotension, vasodilation, **asystole, atrial fibrillation, bradycardia, cardiac arrest, shock, supraventricular tachycardia**

EENT: double or blurred vision, amblyopia, eye hemorrhage, hearing loss, tinnitus, epistaxis, rhinitis, sinusitis, pharyngitis

GI: nausea, vomiting, diarrhea, melena, abdominal pain, abdominal distention, dry mouth, oral inflammation, oral candidiasis, anorexia, **GI hemorrhage**

GU: painful urination, hematuria, albuminuria, glycosuria, excessive urea buildup, urine of low specific gravity, nephrocalcinosis, **renal failure, renal tubular acidosis, oliguria, anuria**

Hematologic: eosinophilia; normochromic, normocytic, or hypochromic anemia; **leukocytosis; thrombocytopenia; leukopenia; agranulocytosis; coagulation disorders**

Hepatic: jaundice, **acute hepatic failure, hepatitis**

Metabolic: hypomagnesemia, hypokalemia, hypocalcemia, hypernatremia, hyperglycemia, dehydration, hypoproteinemia, hypervolemia, hyperlipidemia, **acidosis**

Musculoskeletal: muscle, joint, neck, or back pain

Respiratory: increased cough, hypoxia, lung disorders, hyperventilation, wheezing, dyspnea, hemoptysis, tachypnea, **asthma, bronchospasm, respiratory failure, pulmonary edema, pleural effusion**

Skin: discoloration, bruising, flushing, pruritus, urticaria, acne, rash, sweating, nodules, skin ulcers, alopecia, maculopapular rash

Other: gingivitis, fever, infection, peripheral or facial edema, weight changes, pain or reaction at injection site, tissue damage with extravasation, hypersensitivity reactions including **anaphylaxis**

Interactions

Drug-drug. *Antineoplastics (such as mechlorethamine):* renal toxicity, bronchospasm, hypotension

Cardiac glycosides: increased risk of digitalis toxicity (in potassium-depleted patients)

Corticosteroids: increased potassium depletion

Cyclosporine, tacrolimus: increased creatinine levels

Flucytosine: increased flucytosine toxicity

Imidazoles (clotrimazole, fluconazole, ketoconazole, miconazole): antagonism of amphotericin B effects

Leukocyte transfusion: pulmonary reactions

Nephrotoxic drugs (such as antibiotics, pentamidine): increased risk of renal toxicity

Thiazides: increased electrolyte depletion

Skeletal muscle relaxants: increased skeletal muscle relaxation

Zidovudine: increased myelotoxicity and nephrotoxicity

Drug-diagnostic tests. *Alanine aminotransferase, alkaline phosphatase, aspartate aminotransferase, bilirubin, blood urea nitrogen, creatinine, gamma-glutamyltransferase, lactate dehydrogenase, nitrogenous compounds (urea), uric acid:* increased levels

Calcium, hemoglobin, magnesium, platelets, potassium, protein: decreased levels

Eosinophils, glucose, white blood cells: increased or decreased levels

Liver function tests: abnormal results

Prothrombin time: prolonged

Drug-herbs. *Gossypol:* increased risk of renal toxicity

Patient monitoring

◀€ Monitor for infusion-related reactions (fever, chills, hypotension, GI symptoms, breathing difficulties, and headache). Stop infusion and notify prescriber immediately if reaction occurs.

Reactions in **bold** are life-threatening.   ◀€ Clinical alert

◀€ After giving test dose, monitor vital signs and temperature every 30 minutes for 2 to 4 hours, as ordered.
• Assess fluid intake and output.
• Monitor kidney and liver function test results and serum electrolyte levels.
• Assess for signs and symptoms of ototoxicity (hearing loss, tinnitus, ataxia, and vertigo).

Patient teaching
◀€ Advise patient to contact prescriber immediately if he has fever, chills, headache, vomiting, diarrhea, cough, or breathing problems.
• Instruct patient to report hearing loss, dizziness, or unsteady gait.
• Caution patient to avoid driving and other hazardous activities until he knows how drug affects concentration, alertness, and vision.
• Instruct patient to drink plenty of fluids.
• Tell patient to monitor urine output and report significant changes.
• Advise patient to minimize GI upset by eating small, frequent servings of food and drinking plenty of fluids.
• As appropriate, review all other significant and life-threatening adverse reactions and interactions, especially those related to the drugs, tests, and herbs mentioned above.

ampicillin sodium
Apo-Ampi✤, Novo-Ampicillin✤, Nu-Ampi✤, Penbritin✤⊕, Rimacillin⊕

Pharmacologic class: Aminopenicillin
Therapeutic class: Anti-infective
Pregnancy risk category B

Action
Destroys bacteria by inhibiting bacterial cell-wall synthesis during microbial multiplication

Availability
Capsules: 250 mg, 500 mg
Oral suspension: 125 mg/5 ml, 250 mg/5 ml
Powder for injection: 125 mg, 250 mg, 500 mg, 1 g, 2 g, 10 g

⏺ Indications and dosages
➣ Respiratory tract, skin, and soft-tissue infections caused by *Haemophilus influenzae*, staphylococci, and streptococci
Adults and children weighing 40 kg (88 lb) or more: 250 to 500 mg I.V. or I.M. q 6 hours
Adults and children weighing less than 40 kg (88 lb): 25 to 50 mg/kg/day I.M. or I.V. in divided doses q 6 to 8 hours
Adults and children weighing more than 20 kg (44 lb): 250 mg P.O. q 6 hours
Children weighing 20 kg (44 lb) or less: 50 mg/kg/day P.O. in divided doses q 6 to 8 hours
➣ Bacterial meningitis caused by *Neisseria meningitidis, Escherichia coli,* group B streptococci, or *Listeria monocytogenes*; septicemia caused by *Streptococcus* species, penicillin G–susceptible staphylococci, enterococci, *E. coli, Proteus mirabilis,* or *Salmonella* species
Adults: 150 to 200 mg/kg/day by continuous I.V. infusion or I.M. injection in equally divided doses q 3 to 4 hours, to a maximum dosage of 14 g
Children: 100 to 200 mg/kg/day I.V. in divided doses q 3 to 4 hours
➣ GI or urinary tract infections, including *Neisseria gonorrhoeae* infection in women
Adults and children weighing more than 40 kg (88 lb): 500 mg I.M. or I.V. q 6 hours

Adults and children weighing 40 kg (88 lb) or less: 50 to 100 mg/kg/day I.M. or I.V. in equally divided doses q 6 to 8 hours

➤ Endocarditis prophylaxis for dental, oral, or upper respiratory tract procedures

Adults: 2 g I.M. or I.V. within 30 minutes before procedure

Children: 50 mg/kg I.V. or I.M. within 30 minutes before procedure

➤ Prevention of bacterial endocarditis before GI or GU surgery or instrumentation

High-risk adults: 2 g I.M. or I.V. with gentamicin 1.5 mg/kg I.M. or I.V. within 30 minutes before procedure. Six hours later, give ampicillin 1 g I.M. or I.V., or amoxicillin 1 g P.O.

High-risk children: 50 mg/kg I.M. or I.V. with 1.5 mg/kg of gentamicin I.M. or I.V. within 30 minutes before procedure; 6 hours later, give ampicillin 25 mg/kg I.M. or I.V. or ampicillin 25 mg/kg P.O.

Moderate-risk adults: 2 g I.M. or I.V. within 30 minutes before procedure

Moderate-risk children: 50 mg/kg I.M. or I.V. within 30 minutes before procedure

➤ Prophylaxis for neonatal group B streptococcal disease

Adult women: During labor, loading dose of 2 g I.V.; then 1 g I.V. q 4 hours until delivery

➤ *N. gonorrhoeae* infections

Adults: Single dose of 3.5 g P.O. given with 1 g probenecid

Children weighing 40 kg (88 lb) or more: 500 mg I.M. or I.V. q 6 hours

Children weighing less than 40 kg (88 lb): 50 mg/kg/day in divided doses q 6 to 8 hours

➤ Urethritis caused by *N. gonorrhoeae* (in males)

Adults and children weighing 40 kg (88 lb) or more: 500 mg I.V. or I.M., repeated 8 to 12 hours later

➤ Prophylaxis against sexually transmitted diseases in adult rape victims

Adults: 3.5 g P.O. with 1 g probenecid as a single dose

Dosage adjustment
• Renal impairment

Contraindications
• Hypersensitivity to penicillins, cephalosporins, imipenem, or other beta-lactamase inhibitors

Precautions
Use cautiously in:
• severe renal insufficiency, infectious mononucleosis
• pregnant or breastfeeding patients.

Administration
• Ask patient about history of penicillin allergy before giving.
• For I.V. use, mix powder with bacteriostatic water for injection in amount listed on label.
• For direct I.V. injection, give over 10 to 15 minutes. Don't exceed 100 mg/minute.
• For intermittent I.V. infusion, mix with 50 to 100 ml of normal saline solution and give over 15 to 30 minutes.
• Change I.V. site every 48 hours.
• Give oral doses 1 hour before or 2 hours after meals.

Route	Onset	Peak	Duration
P.O.	30 min	2 hr	6-8 hr
I.V.	Immediate	5 min	6-8 hr
I.M.	15 min	1 hr	6-8 hr

Adverse reactions
CNS: lethargy, hallucinations, anxiety, confusion, agitation, depression, fatigue, dizziness, **seizures**
CV: vein irritation, **thrombophlebitis, heart failure**
EENT: blurred vision, itchy eyes
GI: nausea, vomiting, diarrhea, abdominal pain, enterocolitis, gastritis, stomatitis, glossitis, black "hairy" tongue, furry tongue, oral or rectal candidiasis, **pseudomembranous colitis**

Reactions in **bold** are life-threatening.   🔊 Clinical alert

GU: vaginitis, nephropathy, **interstitial nephritis**
Hematologic: anemia, eosinophilia, **agranulocytosis, hemolytic anemia, leukopenia, thrombocytopenic purpura, thrombocytopenia, neutropenia**
Hepatic: nonspecific hepatitis
Musculoskeletal: arthritis exacerbation
Respiratory: wheezing, dyspnea, hypoxia, **apnea**
Skin: rash, urticaria, fever, diaphoresis
Other: pain at injection site, superinfections, hyperthermia, hypersensitivity reaction, **anaphylaxis, serum sickness**

Interactions

Drug-drug. *Allopurinol:* increased risk of rash
Chloramphenicol: synergistic or antagonistic effects
Hormonal contraceptives: decreased contraceptive effect, increased risk of breakthrough bleeding
Probenecid: decreased renal excretion of ampicillin, increased ampicillin blood level
Tetracyclines: reduced bactericidal effect
Drug-diagnostic tests. *Conjugated estrone, estradiol, estriol-glucuronide, total conjugated estriols:* increased levels in pregnant patients
Granulocytes, hemoglobin, platelets, white blood cells: decreased levels
Coombs' test, urine glucose: false-positive results
Eosinophils: increased count
Drug-food. *Any food:* reduced ampicillin efficacy

Patient monitoring

• Watch for signs and symptoms of hypersensitivity reaction.
◀€ Monitor for seizures when giving high doses.
• Frequently measure patient's temperature and check for signs and symptoms of superinfection, especially oral or rectal candidiasis.
• Monitor for bleeding tendency or hemorrhage.

Patient teaching

• Tell patient to take oral dose with 8 oz of water 1 hour before or 2 hours after a meal.
◀€ Instruct patient to immediately report signs and symptoms of hypersensitivity reaction, such as rash, fever, or chills.
• Inform patient that drug lowers resistance to certain other infections. Tell him to report new signs or symptoms of infection, especially in mouth or rectum.
• Advise patient to minimize GI upset by eating small, frequent servings of food and drinking plenty of fluids.
◀€ Instruct patient to promptly report unusual bleeding or bruising.
• Tell patient to avoid activities that can cause injury. Advise him to use soft toothbrush and electric razor to avoid gum and skin injury.
• Inform patient taking hormonal contraceptives that drug may reduce contraceptive efficacy. Advise her to use alternative birth control method.
• As appropriate, review all other significant and life-threatening adverse reactions and interactions, especially those related to the drugs, tests, and foods mentioned above.

ampicillin sodium and sulbactam sodium
Unasyn

Pharmacologic class: Aminopenicillin/beta-lactamase inhibitor
Therapeutic class: Anti-infective
Pregnancy risk category B

Action
Destroys bacteria by inhibiting bacterial cell-wall synthesis during microbial multiplication. Addition of sulbactam enhances drug's resistance to beta-lactamase, an enzyme that can inactivate ampicillin.

Availability
Injection: Vials; piggyback vials containing 1.5 g (1 g ampicillin sodium and 0.5 g sulbactam sodium), 3 g (2 g ampicillin sodium and 1 g sulbactam sodium), and 15 g (10 g ampicillin sodium and 5 g sulbactam sodium)

🚫 Indications and dosages
➤ Intra-abdominal, gynecologic, and skin-structure infections caused by susceptible beta-lactamase-producing strains
Adults and children weighing 40 kg (88 lb) or more: 1.5 to 3 g (1 g ampicillin and 0.5 g sulbactam to 2 g ampicillin and 1 g sulbactam) I.M. or I.V. q 6 hours. Maximum dosage is 4 g sulbactam daily.
Children ages 1 year and older: 300 mg/kg/day (200 mg ampicillin/100 mg sulbactam) by I.V. infusion q 6 hours in equally divided doses

Dosage adjustment
• Renal impairment

Contraindications
• Hypersensitivity to penicillins, cephalosporins, imipenem, or other beta-lactamase inhibitors

Precautions
Use cautiously in:
• severe renal insufficiency, infectious mononucleosis
• pregnant or breastfeeding patients.

Administration
• Ask patient about history of penicillin allergy before giving.

• Let vial stand several minutes until foam has evaporated before administering drug.
• Don't mix I.V. form with other I.V. drugs.
• Give direct I.V. dose over 10 to 15 minutes.
• Give intermittent infusion in 50 to 100 ml of compatible solution over 15 to 30 minutes.
• Change I.V. site every 48 hours.
• Don't give I.M. to children.

Route	Onset	Peak	Duration
I.V.	Immediate	End of infusion	6-8 hr
I.M.	Rapid	1 hr	6-8 hr

Adverse reactions
CNS: lethargy, hallucinations, anxiety, confusion, agitation, depression, fatigue, dizziness, **seizures**
CV: vein irritation, **thrombophlebitis, heart failure**
EENT: blurred vision, itchy eyes
GI: nausea, vomiting, diarrhea, abdominal pain, enterocolitis, gastritis, stomatitis, glossitis, black "hairy" tongue, furry tongue, oral and rectal candidiasis, **pseudomembranous colitis**
GU: hematuria, hyaline casts in urine, vaginitis, nephropathy, **interstitial nephritis**
Hematologic: anemia, eosinophilia, **agranulocytosis, hemolytic anemia, leukopenia, thrombocytopenic purpura, thrombocytopenia, neutropenia**
Hepatic: nonspecific hepatitis
Musculoskeletal: arthritis exacerbation
Respiratory: wheezing, dyspnea, hypoxia, **apnea**
Skin: rash, urticaria, diaphoresis
Other: pain at injection site, fever, hyperthermia, superinfections, hypersensitivity reactions, **anaphylaxis, serum sickness**

Interactions

Drug-drug. *Allopurinol:* increased risk of rash

Chloramphenicol: synergistic or antagonistic effects

Hormonal contraceptives: decreased contraceptive efficacy, increased risk of breakthrough bleeding

Probenecid: decreased renal excretion and increased blood level of ampicillin

Tetracyclines: reduced bactericidal effect

Drug-diagnostic tests. *Alanine aminotransferase, alkaline phosphatase, aspartate aminotransferase, bilirubin, blood urea nitrogen, creatine kinase, creatinine, gamma-glutamyltransferase, eosinophils, lactate dehydrogenase:* increased levels

Estradiol, estriol-glucuronide, granulocytes, hemoglobin, lymphocytes, neutrophils, platelets, white blood cells: decreased levels

Coombs' test: false-positive result

Urinalysis: red blood cells, hyaline casts

Patient monitoring

• Monitor for signs and symptoms of hypersensitivity reaction.

• Check for signs and symptoms of infection at injection site.

◀≋ Monitor for seizures when giving high doses.

• Watch for bleeding tendency and hemorrhage.

• Check patient's temperature and watch for other signs and symptoms of superinfection, especially oral or rectal candidiasis.

• Monitor CBC and liver function test results.

Patient teaching

◀≋ Instruct patient to immediately report signs and symptoms of hypersensitivity reaction, such as rash, fever, or chills.

• Tell patient to report signs and symptoms of infection or other problems at injection site.

• Advise patient to minimize GI upset by eating small, frequent servings of food and drinking plenty of fluids.

• Inform patient that drug lowers resistance to certain infections. Instruct him to report new signs or symptoms of infection, especially in mouth or rectum.

◀≋ Tell patient to promptly report unusual bleeding or bruising.

• Inform patient taking hormonal contraceptives that drug may reduce contraceptive efficacy. Advise her to use alternative birth control method.

• Instruct patient to avoid activities that can cause injury. Advise him to use soft toothbrush and electric razor to avoid gum and skin injury.

• Inform patient that he may need to undergo regular blood testing during therapy.

• As appropriate, review all other significant and life-threatening adverse reactions and interactions, especially those related to the drugs and tests mentioned above.

amyl nitrite
Amyl Nitrite

Pharmacologic class: Coronary vasodilator

Therapeutic class: Antianginal

Pregnancy risk category C

Action

Relaxes vascular smooth muscle, thereby dilating large coronary vessels, decreasing systemic vascular resistance, reducing afterload, decreasing cardiac output, and relieving angina

Availability

Ampules: 0.3 ml

⊘ Indications and dosages

➣ Acute angina attack
Adults: 0.18 to 0.3 ml by inhalation, repeated in 3 to 5 minutes if needed
➣ Antidote for cyanide poisoning
Adults and children: 0.3 ml by inhalation for 15 to 30 seconds q 5 minutes until sodium nitrite infusion is available

Contraindications

• Hypersensitivity to drug

Precautions

Use cautiously in:
• glaucoma, hypotension, hyperthyroidism, severe anemia, early myocardial infarction
• elderly patients
• pregnant or breastfeeding patients.

Administration

• Crush ampule and wave under patient's nose one to six times. If needed, repeat in 3 to 5 minutes.

Route	Onset	Peak	Duration
Inhalation	30 sec	Unknown	3-5 min

Adverse reactions

CNS: headache, dizziness, weakness, syncope, restlessness
CV: orthostatic hypotension, flushing, palpitations, **tachycardia**
EENT: increased intraocular pressure
GI: nausea, vomiting, fecal incontinence
GU: urinary incontinence
Hematologic: hemolytic anemia, methemoglobinemia
Skin: cutaneous vasodilation, rash, pallor, facial and neck flushing

Interactions

Drug-drug. *Aspirin:* increased amyl nitrite blood level and action
Calcium channel blockers: increased risk of symptomatic orthostatic hypotension
Sildenafil: increased risk of hypotension
Sympathomimetics: decreased antianginal effects, hypotension, tachycardia
Drug-behaviors. *Alcohol use:* severe hypotension, cardiovascular collapse

Patient monitoring

• Monitor vital signs. Stay alert for tachycardia and orthostatic hypotension.
• Assess for bowel and bladder incontinence.
• Monitor neurologic response. Watch closely for dizziness and syncope.
• Assess level of headache pain.
• In long-term therapy, monitor CBC.

Patient teaching

• Teach patient to crush capsule and wave it under his nose until angina is relieved (usually after one to six inhalations).
• Tell patient that drug often causes dizziness, orthostatic hypotension, and syncope. Advise him to sit or lie down until these effects subside.
• Inform patient that drug often causes headache. Instruct him to follow prescriber's recommendations for pain relief.
• Tell patient that drug may cause fecal or urinary incontinence. Encourage him to use bathroom frequently to avoid accidents.
• As appropriate, review all other significant and life-threatening adverse reactions and interactions, especially those related to the drugs and behaviors mentioned above.

anagrelide hydrochloride
Agrylin, Xagrid ✙

Pharmacologic class: Hematologic drug
Therapeutic class: Antiplatelet drug
Pregnancy risk category C

Action
Unclear. May reduce platelet production by decreasing megakaryocytic hypermaturation, thereby decreasing platelet count and inhibiting platelet aggregation (at higher doses).

Availability
Capsules: 0.5 mg, 1 mg

Indications and dosages
➤ Essential thrombocythemia
Adults: 0.5 mg P.O. q.i.d. or 1 mg P.O. b.i.d. for 1 week. Adjust as needed to lowest effective dosage that maintains platelet count below 600,000/mm³. Maximum dosage is 10 mg daily or 2.5 mg as a single dose.

Dosage adjustment
• Hepatic or renal disease

Contraindications
• Prolonged exposure to sunlight
• Women who are or may become pregnant

Precautions
Use cautiously in:
• renal, hepatic, or cardiac dysfunction
• pregnant or breastfeeding patients
• children younger than age 16.

Administration
• Give 1 hour before or 2 hours after meals.

Route	Onset	Peak	Duration
P.O.	Immediate	1 hr	48 hr

Adverse reactions
CNS: amnesia, confusion, depression, dizziness, drowsiness, weakness, headache, syncope, insomnia, migraine, nervousness, pain, paresthesia, malaise, **seizures, cerebrovascular accident**
CV: angina, chest pain, hypertension, palpitations, orthostatic hypotension, peripheral edema, vasodilation, **arrhythmias, tachycardia, heart failure, hemorrhage, myocardial infarction, cardiomyopathy, cardiomegaly, atrial fibrillation, complete heart block, pericarditis**
EENT: amblyopia, abnormal or double vision, visual field abnormalities, tinnitus, epistaxis, rhinitis, sinusitis
GI: nausea, vomiting, diarrhea, constipation, abdominal pain, melena, gastric or duodenal ulcers, dyspepsia, aphthous stomatitis, anorexia, flatulence, gastritis, pancreatitis, **GI hemorrhage**
GU: painful urination, hematuria
Hematologic: lymphadenoma, **bleeding tendency, anemia, thrombocytopenia**
Metabolic: dehydration
Musculoskeletal: leg cramps; joint, back, muscle, neck pain
Respiratory: bronchitis, dyspnea, pneumonia, respiratory disease, **asthma, pulmonary infiltrates, pulmonary fibrosis, pulmonary hypertension**
Skin: bruising, pruritus, rash, alopecia, urticaria, skin disease, photosensitivity reaction
Other: chills, fever, flulike symptoms, edema

Interactions
Drug-drug. *Sucralfate:* interference with anagrelide absorption
Drug-diagnostic tests. *Hemoglobin, platelets:* decreased values
Hepatic enzymes: elevated values
Drug-food. *Any food:* decreased drug bioavailability
Drug-herbs. *Evening primrose oil, feverfew, garlic, ginger, ginkgo biloba, ginseng, grapeseed:* increased antiplatelet effect

Patient monitoring
◀€ Watch for signs and symptoms of vasodilation, heart failure, and arrhythmias in patients with cardiovascular disease.
• For first 2 weeks, monitor CBC and liver and kidney function test results.

- Monitor platelet count regularly until maintenance dosage is established.
- Check regularly for adverse reactions, especially bleeding tendency.
- Monitor blood pressure for orthostatic hypertension.

Patient teaching
- Instruct patient to take drug 1 hour before or 2 hours after meals.
- Tell patient that drug may cause a temporary blood pressure decrease if he sits or stands up suddenly. Tell him to rise slowly and carefully.
- ◀€ Instruct patient to report unusual bleeding or bruising or difficulty breathing.
- ◀€ Tell patient to avoid prolonged exposure to sunlight.
- Caution patient to avoid driving and other hazardous activities until he knows how drug affects concentration, alertness, and vision.
- Inform patient using hormonal contraceptives that drug may interfere with contraceptive efficacy. Advise her to use alternative birth control method.
- Tell patient to avoid activities that may cause injury. Tell him to use soft toothbrush and electric razor to avoid gum and skin injury.
- Advise patient to minimize GI upset by eating small, frequent servings of food and drinking plenty of fluids.
- Notify patient that he'll undergo regular blood testing during therapy.
- As appropriate, review all other significant and life-threatening adverse reactions and interactions, especially those related to the drugs, tests, foods, and herbs mentioned above.

anakinra
Kineret

Pharmacologic class: Interleukin-1 (IL-1) blocker
Therapeutic class: Immunomodulator, antirheumatic
Pregnancy risk category B

Action
Inhibits binding of IL-1 with IL type I receptors, thereby mediating immunologic, inflammatory, and other physiologic responses

Availability
Prefilled glass syringes: 100 mg/0.67 ml

⟁ Indications and dosages
➣ Moderately to severely active rheumatoid arthritis in patients ages 18 and older who don't respond to disease-modifying antirheumatics alone
Adults: 100 mg/day subcutaneously, given at same time each day

Contraindications
- Hypersensitivity to drug or *Escherichia coli*–derived protein
- Serious infections

Precautions
Use cautiously in:
- immunosuppression, active infection, chronic illness, renal impairment
- elderly patients
- pregnant or breastfeeding patients
- children.

Administration
◀€ Withhold drug and notify prescriber if patient shows signs or symptoms of active infection.

◀€ Use extreme caution if patient is concurrently receiving drugs that block tumor necrosis factor (TNF), because of increased risk of serious infection.

• Give entire dose from prefilled syringe.

• Don't freeze or shake syringe.

Route	Onset	Peak	Duration
Subcut.	Slow	3-7 hr	Unknown

Adverse reactions

CNS: headache

EENT: sinusitis

GI: nausea, diarrhea, abdominal pain

Hematologic: thrombocytopenia, neutropenia

Respiratory: upper respiratory tract infection

Skin: rash, pruritus, injection site reaction or bruising, rash, erythema, inflammation

Other: flulike symptoms, infections

Interactions

Drug-drug. *Etanercept, infliximab, other drugs that block TNF:* increased risk of serious infection

Live-virus vaccines: vaccine inefficacy

Drug-diagnostic tests. *Neutrophils:* decreased count

Patient monitoring

• Monitor CBC with white cell differential.

• Assess injection site for reactions.

Patient teaching

◀€ Tell patient to immediately report signs or symptoms of infection.

• Advise patient to report signs and symptoms of allergic response.

• Instruct patient to take drug at same time each day for best response.

• Teach patient about proper drug disposal (in puncture-resistant container). Also caution him against reusing needles, syringes, and drug product.

• Tell patient not to freeze or shake drug.

• As appropriate, review all other significant and life-threatening adverse reactions and interactions, especially those related to the drugs and tests mentioned above.

anastrozole
Arimidex

Pharmacologic class: Nonsteroidal aromatase inhibitor

Therapeutic class: Antineoplastic

Pregnancy risk category D

Action

Reduces serum estradiol levels with no significant effect on adrenocorticoid or aldosterone level; decreases stimulating effect of estrogen on tumor growth

Availability

Tablets: 1 mg

⍟ Indications and dosages

➤ Postmenopausal women with hormone receptor-unknown or hormone receptor-positive advanced breast cancer or with advanced breast cancer after tamoxifen therapy; adjuvant treatment for hormone receptor-positive breast cancer

Adults: 1 mg P.O. daily

Contraindications

• Hypersensitivity to drug or its components

• Women of childbearing age

Precautions

Use cautiously in:

• ischemic heart disease

• breastfeeding patients

• children (safety and efficacy not established).

Administration
• Verify that patient isn't pregnant before giving drug.

Route	Onset	Peak	Duration
P.O.	>24 hr	Unknown	<6 days

Adverse reactions
CNS: headache, weakness, dizziness, depression, paresthesia, lethargy
CV: chest pain, peripheral edema, vasodilation, hypertension, **thromboembolic disease**
EENT: pharyngitis
GI: nausea, vomiting, diarrhea, constipation, abdominal pain, anorexia, dry mouth
GU: vaginal bleeding, leukorrhea, vaginal dryness, pelvic pain
Musculoskeletal: decreased bone mineral density, fractures, bone or back pain, muscle weakness
Respiratory: dyspnea, cough
Skin: rash
Other: food distaste, weight gain, swelling, hot flashes, flulike symptoms, tumor flare **hypersensitivity reactions** (including **anaphylaxis, angioedema, urticaria**)

Interactions
Drug-diagnostic tests. *Hepatic enzymes, low-density lipoproteins, total cholesterol:* increased levels

Patient monitoring
◀≲ Monitor patient closely for hypersensitivity reactions.
• Check regularly for signs and symptoms of thromboembolic disease, especially dyspnea and chest pain.
• Monitor for circulatory overload (suggested by peripheral edema, cough, and dyspnea).
• Assess for signs and symptoms of depression. Evaluate patient for suicidal ideation.
• Monitor liver function test results.

Patient teaching
◀≲ Instruct patient to immediately notify prescriber if signs and symptoms of hypersensitivity occur (such as itching or swelling of face, lips, or throat).
◀≲ Advise patient to immediately report signs and symptoms of thromboembolic disease and circulatory overload.
• Emphasize importance of preventing pregnancy during therapy.
• Tell patient to contact prescriber if she develops signs or symptoms of depression.
• Caution patient to avoid driving and other hazardous activities until she knows how drug affects concentration and alertness.
• Advise patient to minimize GI upset by eating small, frequent servings of food and drinking plenty of fluids.
• Inform patient that she'll undergo regular blood testing during therapy.
• As appropriate, review all other significant and life-threatening adverse reactions and interactions, especially those related to the tests mentioned above.

anidulafungin
Eraxis

Pharmacologic class: Semisynthetic echinocandin
Therapeutic class: Antifungal
Pregnancy risk category C

Action
Inhibits glucan synthase, an enzyme present in fungal (but not mammalian) cells; this action inhibits formation of 1,3-beta-D-glucan, an essential component of fungal cell wall.

Availability
Powder for injection (lyophilized): 50-mg single-use vial

◀≲ Clinical alert

⏀ Indications and dosages

➤ Candidemia and other *Candida* infections (intra-abdominal abscess, peritonitis)

Adults: Single 200-mg loading dose by I.V. infusion on day 1, followed by 100 mg I.V. daily thereafter. Duration depends on clinical response; generally, therapy continues at least 14 days after last positive culture.

➤ Esophageal candidiasis

Adults: Single 100-mg loading dose by I.V. infusion on day 1, followed by 50 mg I.V. daily thereafter. Treatment should continue for at least 14 days, and for at least 7 days after symptoms resolve; duration depends on clinical response. Due to risk of esophageal candidiasis relapse in patients with human immunodeficiency virus, suppressive antifungal therapy may be considered after treatment ends.

Contraindications

• Hypersensitivity to drug, its components, or other echinocandins

Precautions

Use cautiously in:
• hepatic impairment
• pregnant or breastfeeding patients
• children (safety and efficacy not established).

Administration

◀︎≣ Don't give by I.V. bolus.
• Reconstitute only with supplied diluent (20% dehydrated alcohol in water for injection).
• Further dilute only with 5% dextrose injection or normal saline solution, to yield infusion solution concentration of 0.5 mg/ml.
• Give by I.V. infusion within 24 hours of reconstitution.
◀︎≣ Don't infuse at a rate exceeding 1.1 mg/minute.

• Don't dilute with other solutions or infuse through same I.V. line with other drugs or electrolytes.

Route	Onset	Peak	Duration
I.V.	Unknown	Unknown	Unknown

Adverse reactions

CNS: headache
CV: hypotension, phlebitis
GI: aggravated dyspepsia, nausea, vomiting
Hematologic: neutropenia, leukopenia
Respiratory: dyspnea
Skin: rash, urticaria, pruritus, flushing
Other: fever

Interactions

Drug-diagnostic tests. *Alanine aminotransferase, aspartate aminotransferase, gamma glutamyltransferase:* increased

Patient monitoring

• If patient has abnormal liver function tests during therapy, monitor for evidence of worsening hepatic function and weigh risks and benefits of continuing therapy.
• Monitor for rash, urticaria, flushing, dyspnea, and hypotension. (However, these are rare when drug is administered slowly.)

Patient teaching

◀︎≣ Instruct patient to report rash, itching, unusual bruising or bleeding, unusual tiredness, or yellowing of skin or eyes.
• Advise patient to report troublesome side effects such as GI upset.
• As appropriate, review all other significant adverse reactions and interactions, especially those related to the tests mentioned above.

antihemophilic factor
(AHF, factor VIII)
Advate, Alphanate, Hemofil M, Koate-DVI, Kogenate FS, Monarc-M, Monoclate-P, Recombinate, ReFacto

Pharmacologic class: Hemostatic
Therapeutic class: Antihemophilic
Pregnancy risk category C

FDA | BOXED WARNING

• Drug is made from human plasma and may contain infectious agents. Plasma donor screening, testing, and inactivation or removal methods reduce this risk.

Action
Promotes conversion of prothrombin to thrombin (necessary for hemostasis and blood clotting). Also replaces missing or deficient clotting factors, thereby controlling or preventing bleeding.

Availability
I.V. injection: 250, 500, 1,000, or 1,500 international units/vial in numerous preparations

🕖 Indications and dosages
➤ Spontaneous hemorrhage in patients with hemophilia A (factor VIII deficiency)
Adults and children: Dosage is highly individualized, calculated as follows: AHF required (international units) equals weight (kg) multiplied by desired factor VIII increase (% of normal) multiplied by 0.5.

To control bleeding, desired factor VIII level is 20% to 40% of normal for minor hemorrhage; 30% to 60% of normal for moderate hemorrhage; or 60% to 100% of normal for severe hemorrhage. To prevent spontaneous hemorrhage, desired factor VIII level is 5% of normal.

Contraindications
• Hypersensitivity to drug or to mouse, hamster, or bovine protein

Precautions
Use cautiously in:
• hepatic disease
• blood types A, B, and AB
• patients receiving factor VIII inhibitors
• pregnant patients
• neonates and infants.

Administration
• Before giving, verify that patient has no history of hypersensitivity to drug or to mouse, hamster, or bovine protein.
• Follow prescriber's instructions regarding hepatitis B prophylaxis before starting therapy.
• Refrigerate concentrate until ready to reconstitute drug; then warm to room temperature before mixing.
• Roll bottle gently between hands until drug is well-mixed.
• Give a single dose over 5 to 10 minutes at rate of 2 to 10 ml/minute, as appropriate.
• After drug is reconstituted, don't refrigerate, shake, or store near heat.
• Don't mix with other I.V. solutions.
• Use plastic (not glass) syringe and filter.

Route	Onset	Peak	Duration
I.V.	Immediate	1-2 hr	Unknown

Adverse reactions
CNS: headache; lethargy; fatigue; dizziness; jitteriness; drowsiness; depersonalization; tingling in arms, ears, and face
CV: chest tightness, angina pectoris, tachycardia, slight hypotension, **thrombosis**

Reactions in **bold** are life-threatening.   ◀€ Clinical alert

EENT: blurred or abnormal vision, eye disorder, otitis media, epistaxis, rhinitis, sore throat
GI: nausea, vomiting, diarrhea, constipation, stomachache, abdominal pain, gastroenteritis, anorexia,
Hematologic: forehead bruises, **increased bleeding tendency, thrombocytopenia, hemolytic anemia, intravascular hemolysis, hyperfibrinogenemia**
Hepatic: hepatitis B transmission
Musculoskeletal: myalgia, muscle weakness, bone pain, finger pain
Respiratory: dyspnea, coughing, wheezing, **bronchospasm**
Skin: rash, acne, flushing, diaphoresis, urticaria
Other: taste changes, allergic reaction, fever, chills, cold feet, cold sensations, infected hematoma, stinging at injection site, **anaphylaxis, human immunodeficiency virus transmission**

Interactions
Drug-diagnostic tests. *Bilirubin, creatine kinase:* increased levels
Hemoglobin, platelets: decreased values

Patient monitoring
◀┊ Monitor for signs and symptoms of anaphylaxis and hemolysis.
◀┊ Watch for bleeding tendency and hemorrhaging.
• Check vital signs regularly.
• Monitor CBC and coagulation studies.
◀┊ Assess for severe headache (may indicate intracranial hemorrhage).

Patient teaching
◀┊ Tell patient to immediately report signs and symptoms of allergic response or bleeding tendency.
• Caution patient not to use aspirin during therapy.
• Instruct patient to contact prescriber if drug becomes less effective.

• Tell patient to report signs or symptoms of hepatitis B.
• Caution patient to avoid driving and other hazardous activities until he knows how drug affects concentration, alertness, and vision.
• Advise patient to minimize GI upset by eating small, frequent servings of food and drinking plenty of fluids.
• Notify patient that he'll undergo regular blood testing during therapy.
• As appropriate, review all other significant and life-threatening adverse reactions and interactions, especially those related to the tests mentioned above.

antithrombin III, human (AT-III, heparin cofactor 1)
Thrombate III

Pharmacologic class: Blood derivative, coagulation inhibitor
Therapeutic class: Antithrombin
Pregnancy risk category B

Action
Inactivates thrombin and activated forms of factors IXa, Xa, XIa, and XIIa, thereby inhibiting coagulation and thromboembolism formation

Availability
Injection: 500 international units, 1,000 international units

🕖 Indications and dosages
➤ Thromboembolism related to AT-III deficiency
Adults: Initial dosage is individualized to amount required to increase AT-III activity to 120% of normal (determined 20 minutes after administration). Usual infusion rate is 50 to

a maximum of 100 international units/minute I.V. Dosage calculation is based on anticipated 1.4% increase in plasma AT-III activity produced by 1 international unit/kg of body weight.

Use this formula to calculate dosage: Required dosage (international units) equals desired activity (%) minus baseline AT-III activity (%) multiplied by weight (kg) divided by 1.4 (international units/kg).

Maintenance dosage is individualized to amount required to maintain AT-III activity at 80% of normal.

Contraindications
None

Precautions
Use cautiously in:
• pregnant or breastfeeding patients
• children (safety and efficacy not established).

Administration
• Reconstitute drug concentrate with 10 ml of sterile water, normal saline solution, or dextrose 5% in water.
• Use filter needle provided by manufacturer to draw up solution.
• Don't shake vial.
• Know that drug may be diluted further in same solution if desired.
• Don't mix with other solutions.
• Infuse over 10 to 20 minutes.
• Administer within 3 hours of reconstitution.
◀€ If adverse reactions occur, decrease infusion rate or, if indicated, stop infusion until symptoms disappear.

Route	Onset	Peak	Duration
I.V.	Immediate	Unknown	4 days

Adverse reactions
CNS: dizziness, light-headedness, headache

CV: vasodilation, reduced blood pressure, chest pain
EENT: perception of "film" over eyes
GI: nausea, sensation of intestinal fullness
GU: diuresis
Musculoskeletal: muscle cramps
Respiratory: dyspnea, shortness of breath
Skin: urticaria, oozing lesions, hives, hematoma
Other: foul taste, chills, fever

Interactions
Drug-drug. *Heparin:* increased anticoagulant effect

Patient monitoring
• Monitor AT-III activity levels regularly.
◀€ Watch for signs and symptoms of too-rapid infusion, such as dyspnea and hypertension.
• Monitor vital signs and temperature.
• Assess fluid intake and output to detect dehydration.

Patient teaching
◀€ Instruct patient to immediately report chest tightness, dizziness, and fever.
• Caution patient to avoid driving and other hazardous activities until he knows how drug affects concentration and alertness.
• Advise patient to minimize GI upset and unpleasant taste by eating small, frequent servings of healthy food and drinking plenty of fluids.
• Tell patient that he'll undergo regular blood testing during therapy.
• As appropriate, review all other significant adverse reactions and interactions, especially those related to the drugs mentioned above.

apomorphine hydrochloride
APO-go ⊕, Apokyn

Pharmacologic class: Dopaminergic, dopamine-receptor agonist
Therapeutic class: Antiparkinsonian
Pregnancy risk category C

Action
Unclear. May stimulate postsynaptic dopamine D_2-type receptors in caudate-putamen of brain.

Availability
Ampules: 10 mg/ml in 2- and 3-ml cartridges

𝟎 Indications and dosages
➣ Acute intermittent treatment of hypomobility and "off" ("end-of-dose wearing off" and unpredictable "on/off") episodes associated with Parkinson's disease
Adults: 0.2-ml (2-mg) test dose injected subcutaneously during "off" state in setting where medical personnel can monitor blood pressure. If patient tolerates test dose, give 0.2 ml subcutaneously p.r.n. to treat "off" episodes no sooner than 2 hours after previous dose. Establish dosage based on tolerance and efficacy; increase in 0.1-ml (1 mg) increments, usually to 0.3 to 0.4 ml. Maximum dosage, 0.6 ml up to five times daily.

Patient who tolerates but doesn't respond to test dose may receive 0.4 ml (4 mg) at next observed "off" period, but no sooner than 2 hours after initial 0.2-ml test dose. If patient tolerates 0.4-ml test dose, give starting dosage of 0.3 ml (3 mg) p.r.n. to treat "off" episodes. If needed, increase in increments of 0.1 ml every few days on outpatient basis.

If patient doesn't tolerate 0.4-ml test dose, 0.3-ml test dose may be given during separate "off" period no sooner than 2 hours after 0.4-ml test dose.

If patient tolerates 0.3-ml test dose, starting dosage should be 0.2 ml p.r.n. to treat existing "off" episodes. If needed and if patient tolerates 0.2-ml dose, dosage can be increased to 0.3 ml after several days; in this case, it ordinarily shouldn't be increased to 0.4 ml on outpatient basis.

Dosage adjustment
• Mild or moderate renal impairment

Contraindications
• Hypersensitivity to drug or its components
• Concurrent use of 5-hydroxytryptamine$_3$ (5-HT$_3$) antagonists (such as alosetron, dolasetron, granisetron, ondansetron, palonosetron)

Precautions
Use cautiously in:
• renal or hepatic impairment
• pregnant or breastfeeding patients
• children (safety and efficacy not established).

Administration
• If prescribed, give trimethobenzamide (antiemetic) for 3 days before starting apomorphine and continuing throughout therapy.
• Give only by subcutaneous injection.
◀€ Don't give I.V. because this may cause serious adverse events, such as I.V. crystallization of apomorphine, leading to thrombus formation and pulmonary embolism.
• Titrate dosage based on efficacy and patient tolerance.
• Check supine and standing blood pressure before giving test dose and 20, 40, and 60 minutes after. If patient experiences clinically significant

orthostatic hypotension in response to test dose, don't give drug.

Route	Onset	Peak	Duration
Subcut.	Unknown	10-60 min	Unknown

Adverse reactions

CNS: drowsiness, somnolence, dizziness, hallucinations, confusion, syncope, dyskinesias
CV: orthostatic hypotension, chest pain, chest pressure, angina, cardiac valvulopathy
EENT: rhinorrhea
GI: nausea, vomiting, retroperitoneal fibrosis
GU: priapism
Respiratory: pulmonary infiltrates, pleural effusion, pleural thickening
Other: yawning, edema of extremities, injection site reactions, abuse potential, allergic reactions

Interactions

Drug-drug. *Antihypertensive agents, vasodilators:* increased incidence of hypotension, myocardial infarction, serious pneumonia, serious falls, bone and joint injuries
Dopamine antagonists: decreased apomorphine efficacy
5-HT$_3$ antagonists: profound hypotension
Drug-behaviors. *Alcohol use:* additive drowsiness and somnolence

Patient monitoring

• Monitor for serious cardiovascular and respiratory adverse reactions.
• Monitor for unexpected somnolence, which may interfere with daily activities.

Patient teaching

• Instruct patient to take drug as described in patient instruction leaflet.
• Make sure patient knows that dosages are in milliliters, not milligrams.
• Instruct patient to rotate injection site.

• Inform patient that drug may cause hallucinations and unexpected sleepiness.
• Tell patient that drug may cause blood pressure to drop. Caution him to rise slowly from sitting or lying position.
• Urge patient to consult prescriber before taking other drugs.
• Caution patient not to use alcohol during therapy.
• Advise patient to avoid driving and other hazardous activities until drug effects are known.
• As appropriate, review all other significant adverse reactions and interactions, especially those related to the drugs mentioned above.

aprepitant fosaprepitant dimeglumine
Emend, Emend for Injection

Pharmacologic class: Substance P and neurokinin-1 antagonist
Therapeutic class: Adjunctive antiemetic
Pregnancy risk category B

Action

Augments antiemetic activity of ondansetron (a 5-hydroxytryptamine$_3$-receptor antagonist) and dexamethasone. Also inhibits cisplatin-induced emesis.

Availability

Capsules: 40 mg, 80 mg, 125 mg
Powder for injection, lyophilized: 115 mg, 150 mg in single-dose vials

Indications and dosages

➤ To prevent acute and delayed nausea and vomiting caused by highly emetogenic cancer chemotherapy

---

Reactions in **bold** are life-threatening.   ◀€ Clinical alert

Adults: 125 mg P.O. 1 hour before chemotherapy on day 1; then 80 mg P.O. once daily in morning on days 2 and 3. Give with 12 mg dexamethasone P.O. and 32 mg ondansetron I.V. on day 1, and with 8 mg dexamethasone P.O. on days 2 to 4.

Adults: Single-dose regimen: 150 mg (fosaprepitant dimeglumine) by I.V. infusion over 20 to 30 minutes starting 30 minutes before chemotherapy, with 12 mg dexamethasone P.O. once daily and 32 mg ondansetron I.V. 30 minutes before chemotherapy once daily on day 1. On day 2, give dexamethasone 8 mg P.O. once daily in the morning. On days 3 and 4, give dexamethasone 8 mg P.O. b.i.d.

Adults: Three-day dosing regimen; 115 mg (fosaprepitant dimeglumine) by I.V. infusion over 15 minutes starting 30 minutes before chemotherapy, with 12 mg dexamethasone P.O. 30 minutes before chemotherapy once daily and 32 mg ondansetron I.V. once daily on day 1. On days 2 and 3, give 80 mg (aprepitant) capsules P.O. once daily and dexamethasone 8 mg P.O. once daily. On day 4, give dexamethasone 8 mg P.O. once daily.

➤ To prevent nausea and vomiting caused by moderately emetogenic cancer chemotherapy

Adults: Three-day dosing regimen; 115 mg (fosaprepitant dimeglumine) by I.V. infusion over 15 minutes starting 30 minutes before chemotherapy, with 12 mg dexamethasone P.O. 30 minutes before chemotherapy once daily and 8 mg ondansetron P.O. b.i.d. (one capsule 30 to 60 minutes before chemotherapy and one capsule 8 hours after first dose) on day 1. Give 80 mg (aprepitant) capsules P.O. once daily on days 2 and 3.

➤ Prevention of postoperative nausea and vomiting

Adults: 40 mg P.O. once within 3 hours before induction anesthesia

Contraindications
- Hypersensitivity to drug
- Concurrent pimozide, terfenadine, astemizole, or cisapride therapy
- Breastfeeding

Precautions
Use cautiously in:
- patients receiving concurrent warfarin or CYP3A4 inhibitors
- pregnant patients.

Administration
- Give with other antiemetics as prescribed.
- For the 115-mg and 150-mg I.V. dose, reconstitute powder with 5 ml normal saline solution in vial and inject in infusion bag containing 110 ml and 145 ml normal saline solution, respectively, to yield a final concentration of 1 mg/ml. Then gently invert I.V. bag two or three times. Don't mix with other solutions, including lactated Ringer's and Hartmann's solutions.

Route	Onset	Peak	Duration
P.O.	Unknown	Unknown	Unknown

Adverse reactions
CNS: dizziness, neuropathy, headache, insomnia, asthenia, fatigue
EENT: tinnitus
GI: nausea, vomiting, constipation, diarrhea, epigastric discomfort, gastritis, heartburn, abdominal pain, anorexia
Hematologic: neutropenia
Other: fever, dehydration, hiccups

Interactions
Drug-drug. *CYP3A4 inducers (carbamazepine, phenytoin, rifampin):* decreased aprepitant blood level
CYP3A4 inhibitors (azole antifungals, clarithromycin, nefazodone, ritonavir): increased aprepitant blood level
Dexamethasone, methylprednisolone: increased steroid exposure

Docetaxel, etoposide, ifosfamide, imatinib, irinotecan, paclitaxel, vinblastine, vincristine, vinorelbine: increased blood levels of these drugs

Hormonal contraceptives: decreased contraceptive efficacy

Paroxetine: decreased efficacy of either drug

Pimozide: increased blood level and toxic effects of aprepitant

Tolbutamide, warfarin: CYP2C9 induction, decreased efficacy of these drugs

Patient monitoring

• Monitor neurologic status. Institute measures to prevent injury as needed.

• Assess nutritional and hydration status.

• Monitor CBC.

Patient teaching

• Tell patient that drug may cause CNS effects. Explain that he'll be monitored to ensure his safety.

• Advise patient to minimize GI upset by eating small, frequent servings of food and drinking plenty of fluids.

• Caution patient to avoid driving and other hazardous activities until he knows how drug affects concentration, hearing, strength, balance, and alertness.

• As appropriate, review all other significant and life-threatening adverse reactions and interactions, especially those related to the drugs mentioned above.

argatroban

Acova

Pharmacologic class: L-arginine–derived thrombin inhibitor

Therapeutic class: Anticoagulant

Pregnancy risk category B

Action

Binds rapidly to site of thrombi, neutralizing conversion of fibrinogen to fibrin, activation of coagulation factors, and platelet aggregation (processes required for thrombus formation)

Availability

Injection: 100 mg/ml in 2.5-ml vials

Indications and dosages

➤ Treatment or prophylaxis of thrombosis in patients with heparin-induced thrombocytopenia

Adults: 2 mcg/kg/minute as a continuous I.V. infusion, to a maximum dosage of 10 mcg/kg/minute. Adjust dosage as needed to maintain activated partial thromboplastin time (APTT) at 1.5 to 3 times initial baseline value (not to exceed 100 seconds).

➤ Anticoagulation during percutaneous coronary intervention in patients who have or are at risk for heparin-induced thrombocytopenia

Adults: Start continuous I.V. infusion at 25 mcg/kg/minute and give loading dose of 350 mcg/kg by I.V. bolus over 3 to 5 minutes. Check activated clotting time (ACT) 5 to 10 minutes after bolus dose is given; adjust dosage until ACT is between 300 and 450 seconds. If ACT is below 300 seconds, give additional I.V. bolus dose of 150 mcg/kg; then increase infusion rate to 30 mcg/kg/minute, and check ACT after 5 to 10 minutes. If ACT exceeds 450 seconds, decrease infusion rate to 15 mcg/kg/minute, and check ACT after 5 to 10 minutes. Maintain adjusted infusion dosage once therapeutic ACT has been reached.

Dosage adjustment

• Hepatic impairment

Contraindications

• Hypersensitivity to drug

• Overt major bleeding

Precautions

Use cautiously in:
- hepatic impairment or disease, intracranial bleeding
- pregnant or breastfeeding patients
- children younger than age 18.

Administration

- Stop all parenteral anticoagulants before starting argatroban.
- Dilute in normal saline solution, dextrose 5% in water, or lactated Ringer's solution to a concentration of 1 mg/ml.
- Inject contents of 2.5-ml vial into 250-ml bag of diluent.
- Protect solution from direct sunlight.

Route	Onset	Peak	Duration
I.V.	Rapid	1-3 hr	Duration of infusion

Adverse reactions

CNS: headache
CV: hypotension, unstable angina, **atrial fibrillation, cardiac arrest, ventricular tachycardia, cerebrovascular disorders**
GI: nausea, vomiting, diarrhea, abdominal pain, anorexia, **GI bleeding**
GU: urinary tract infection, minor GU tract bleeding and hematuria, **renal dysfunction**
Hematologic: groin bleeding, brachial bleeding, **hypoprothrombinemia, thrombocytopenia, bleeding or hemorrhage**
Respiratory: cough, dyspnea, pneumonia, hemoptysis
Skin: rash, bleeding at puncture site
Other: allergic reaction, pain, infection, fever, **sepsis, anaphylaxis**

Interactions

Drug-drug. *Oral anticoagulants:* prolonged prothrombin time, increased International Normalized Ratio, increased risk of bleeding
Thrombolytics: increased risk of intracranial bleeding

Drug-diagnostic tests. *Hematocrit, hemoglobin:* decreased values

Patient monitoring

◀€ Monitor patient for signs and symptoms of anaphylaxis.
◀€ Evaluate patient for bleeding tendency and hemorrhage.
- Assess neurologic status and vital signs frequently.
- Monitor CBC and coagulation studies, especially partial thromboplastin time.
◀€ Check for signs and symptoms of serious arrhythmias and hypotension.

Patient teaching

◀€ Instruct patient to immediately report allergic reaction and unusual bleeding or bruising.
- Tell patient to avoid activities that can cause injury. Advise him to use a soft toothbrush and electric razor to avoid gum and skin injury.
- Advise patient to minimize GI upset by eating small, frequent servings of food and drinking plenty of fluids.
- Tell patient that he'll undergo regular blood testing during therapy.
- As appropriate, review all other significant and life-threatening adverse reactions and interactions, especially those related to the drugs and tests mentioned above.

aripiprazole
Abilify

Pharmacologic class: Quinolone-derived atypical antipsychotic agent

Therapeutic class: Antipsychotic, neuroleptic

Pregnancy risk category C

FDA | BOXED WARNING

- Drug increased mortality in elderly patients with dementia-related psychosis. Although causes of death were varied, most appeared to be cardiovascular or infectious. Drug isn't approved to treat dementia-related psychosis.
- Children, adolescents, and young adults taking antidepressants for major depressive disorder and other psychiatric disorders are at increased risk for suicidal thinking and behavior.
- Drug isn't approved for use in children with depression.

Action

Unclear. Thought to exert partial agonist activity at central dopamine D_2 and type 1A serotonin (5-HT_{1A}) receptors and antagonistic activity at serotonin 5-HT_{2A} receptors. Also has alpha-adrenergic and histamine$_1$-blocking properties.

Availability

Injection: 9.75 mg/1.3 ml (7.5 mg/ml)
Oral solution: 1 mg/ml
Tablets: 2 mg, 5 mg, 10 mg, 15 mg, 20 mg, 30 mg
Tablets (orally disintegrating): 10 mg, 15 mg

✪ Indications and dosages

➤ Schizophrenia
Adults: 10 to 15 mg P.O. daily. If needed, increase to 30 mg daily after 2 weeks.
Adolescents ages 13 to 17: Initially, 2 mg P.O. daily; increase to 5 mg P.O. after 2 days. Then increase to 10 mg P.O. after 2 additional days. Subsequent dosage intervals should occur in increments no greater than 5 mg, up to a maximum of 30 mg.
➤ To maintain stability in schizophrenic patients

Adults: 15 mg P.O. daily. Therapy may continue for up to 26 weeks with periodic evaluations.
Adolescents ages 13 to 17: General recommendation, continue responding patients beyond the acute response but at the lowest dosage needed to maintain remission.
➤ Acute manic and mixed episodes associated with bipolar disorder
Adults: 30 mg P.O. daily for up to 3 weeks
➤ Agitation associated with schizophrenia or bipolar mania
Adults: Usual dosage, 5.25 to 15 mg I.M. as single dose. Recommended dosage is 9.75 mg I.M. as single dose. No additional benefit was demonstrated for 15 mg compared to 9.75 mg. Lower dosage of 5.25 mg may be considered when clinical factors warrant. If agitation warranting second dose persists following initial dose, cumulative dosages up to total of 30 mg/day may be given. However, efficacy of repeated doses in agitated patients hasn't been systematically evaluated in controlled clinical trials. Also, safety of total daily doses greater than 30 mg or injections given more frequently than every 2 hours hasn't been adequately evaluated in clinical trials. If ongoing aripiprazole therapy is clinically indicated, oral aripiprazole ranging from 10 to 30 mg/day P.O. should replace aripiprazole injection as soon as possible.
➤ Adjunctive treatment of major depressive disorder
Adults: Initially, 2 to 5 mg P.O. daily. May increase up to 15 mg daily at increments of up to 5 mg/day at intervals of no less than 1 week.

Dosage adjustment

- Concurrent use of potent CYP3A4 inhibitors (such as ketoconazole), CYP2D6 inhibitors (such as fluoxetine, paroxetine, quinidine), or CYP3A4 inducers (such as carbamazepine)

Reactions in **bold** are life-threatening.   ◀€ Clinical alert

Contraindications
• Hypersensitivity to drug

Precautions
Use cautiously in:
• cerebrovascular disease, hypotension, seizure disorder, suicidal ideation
• high risk for aspiration pneumonia
• neuroleptic malignant syndrome, tardive dyskinesia, diabetes mellitus
• leukopenia, neutropenia, agranulocytosis
• pregnant or breastfeeding patients
• elderly patients (with dementia-related psychosis)
• children, adolescents, and young adults with major depressive disorder

Administration
• Give with or without food.
• Don't administer with grapefruit juice.
• Be aware that oral solution may be substituted for tablets on a mg-to-mg basis up to 25-mg dose. Patients receiving 30 mg of tablets should receive 25 mg of oral solution.

Route	Onset	Peak	Duration
I.M.	Unknown	1-3 hr	Unknown
P.O.	Slow	3-5 hr	Unknown

Adverse reactions
CNS: dizziness, insomnia, akathisia, agitation, anxiety, headache, light-headedness, drowsiness, tremor, tardive dyskinesia, **seizures, neuroleptic malignant syndrome, increased suicide risk**
CV: orthostatic hypotension, hypertension, peripheral edema, chest pain, **bradycardia, tachycardia**
EENT: rhinitis
GI: nausea, vomiting, diarrhea, constipation, jaundice, abdominal pain, esophageal motility disorders, dysphagia
GU: urinary incontinence
Respiratory: cough

Skin: rash
Other: fever, **hypersensitivity reactions** (including **anaphylaxis**)

Interactions
Drug-drug. *CNS depressants:* increased sedation
Drugs that induce CYP3A4: decreased aripiprazole effect
Drugs that inhibit CYP3A4 or CYP2D6: serious toxic effects
Other antipsychotic agents: increased extrapyramidal effects
Drug-diagnostic tests. *Granulocytes, leukocytes, neutrophils:* decreased values
Serum glucose: increased level
Drug-herbs. *Kava:* increased CNS depression
Drug-behaviors. *Alcohol use:* increased sedation

Patient monitoring
◄€ Watch for signs and symptoms of depression, and evaluate patient for suicidal ideation.
• Monitor neurologic status closely. Watch for tardive dyskinesia.
◄€ Evaluate patient for neuroleptic malignant syndrome (fever, altered mental status, rigid muscles, arrhythmia, tachycardia, sweating). Stop drug and notify prescriber if these signs and symptoms occur.
• Monitor blood pressure, pulse, CBC with differential, and weight.
◄€ Monitor blood glucose level closely; be aware that in patients with diabetes mellitus or risk factors for diabetes, serious hyperglycemia possibly associated with coma or death may occur.

Patient teaching
◄€ Instruct patient to immediately contact prescriber if he experiences depression or has suicidal thoughts, altered mental status, rigid muscles, irregular heart beat, excessive sweating,

---

rash, itching, difficulty breathing, or excessive thirst or urination.
- Inform patient that symptoms will subside slowly over several weeks.
- Tell patient he may take drug with or without food.
- Caution patient to avoid driving and other hazardous activities until he knows how drug affects concentration and alertness.
- Tell patient that drug may cause urinary incontinence.
- Caution patient to avoid strenuous exercise and hot environments whenever possible.
- Instruct patient to move slowly when rising to avoid dizziness from sudden blood pressure decrease.
- As appropriate, review all other significant and life-threatening adverse reactions and interactions, especially those related to the drugs, herbs, and behaviors mentioned above.

arsenic trioxide
Trisenox

Pharmacologic class: Nonmetallic element, white arsenic
Therapeutic class: Antineoplastic
Pregnancy risk category D

FDA | BOXED WARNING

- Give under supervision of physician experienced in managing patients with acute leukemia.
- Some patients with acute promyelocytic leukemia (APL) treated with drug have had symptoms similar to retinoic-acid–acute promyelocytic leukemia (RA-APL) or APL differentiation syndrome, marked by fever, dyspnea, weight gain, pulmonary infiltrates, and pleural or pericardial effusions. Syndrome can be fatal; at first sign, give

high-dose steroids immediately, regardless of patient's white blood cell count; continue steroids for at least 3 days or longer until signs and symptoms abate. Most patients don't require arsenic trioxide termination during treatment of APL differentiation syndrome.
- Drug may prolong QT interval and cause complete atrioventricular block. QT prolongation can lead to torsades de pointes–type ventricular arrhythmia, which can be fatal.
- Before starting therapy, obtain 12-lead ECG and assess serum electrolyte (potassium, calcium, and magnesium) and creatinine levels. Correct electrolyte abnormalities and, if possible, discontinue drugs known to cause QT prolongation. During therapy, maintain potassium level above 4 mEq/L and magnesium level above 1.8 mg/dL. If patient reaches absolute QT interval value above 500 msec, reassess and take immediate action to correct concomitant risk factors.

Action
Unclear. May cause morphologic changes and DNA fragmentation in promyelocytic leukemia cells, causing cell death and degradation of or damage to PML/RAR alpha (a fusion protein).

Availability
Injection: 1 mg/ml

✔ Indications and dosages
➤ APL in patients who have relapsed or are refractory to retinoid and anthracycline chemotherapy
Adults and children ages 5 and older:
Induction phase—0.15 mg/kg I.V. daily until bone marrow remission occurs, to a maximum of 60 doses. *Consolidation phase*—0.15 mg/kg I.V. daily for 25 doses over 5 weeks, starting 3 to 6 weeks after completion of induction phase.

Reactions in **bold** are life-threatening.   ◀€ Clinical alert

Contraindications
- Hypersensitivity to drug
- Pregnancy

Precautions
Use cautiously in:
- renal impairment, cardiac abnormalities
- elderly patients
- breastfeeding patients
- children.

Administration
◀≋ Know that drug is carcinogenic. Follow facility policy for preparing and handling antineoplastics.
- Dilute in 100 to 250 ml of dextrose 5% in water or normal saline solution.
- Don't mix with other drugs.
- Infuse over 1 to 2 hours (may infuse over 4 hours if patient has vasomotor reaction).

Route	Onset	Peak	Duration
I.V.	Unknown	Unknown	Unknown

Adverse reactions
CNS: headache, insomnia, paresthesia, dizziness, tremor, drowsiness, anxiety, confusion, agitation, rigors, weakness, **seizures, coma**
CV: ECG abnormalities, palpitations, chest pain, hypotension, hypertension, tachycardia, **prolonged QT interval, torsades de pointes**
EENT: blurred vision, painful red eye, dry eyes, eye irritation, swollen eyelids, tinnitus, earache, nasopharyngitis, postnasal drip, epistaxis, sinusitis, sore throat
GI: nausea, vomiting, constipation, diarrhea, abdominal pain, fecal incontinence, dyspepsia, dry mouth, mouth blisters, oral candidiasis, anorexia, **GI hemorrhage**
GU: urinary incontinence, intermenstrual bleeding, renal impairment, **oliguria, renal failure, vaginal hemorrhage**

Hematologic: anemia, lymphadenopathy, **leukocytosis, thrombocytopenia, neutropenia, disseminated intravascular coagulation, hemorrhage**
Metabolic: hypokalemia, hypomagnesemia, hyperglycemia, acidosis, **hypoglycemia, hyperkalemia**
Musculoskeletal: joint, muscle, bone, back, neck, or limb pain
Respiratory: dyspnea, cough, hypoxia, wheezing, crackles, tachypnea, decreased breath sounds, crepitation, hemoptysis, rhonchi, upper respiratory tract infection, **pleural effusion**
Skin: flushing, erythema, pallor, bruising, petechiae, pruritus, dermatitis, dry skin, hyperpigmentation, urticaria, skin lesions, herpes simplex infection, local exfoliation, diaphoresis, night sweats
Other: fever, facial edema, weight gain or loss, bacterial infection, pain and edema at injection site, **hypersensitivity reaction, sepsis**

Interactions
Drug-drug. *Drugs that can cause electrolyte abnormalities (such as amphotericin B, diuretics):* increased risk of electrolyte abnormalities
Drugs that can prolong QT interval (antiarrhythmics, thioridazines, some quinolones): increased QT-interval prolongation
Drug-diagnostic tests. *Alanine aminotransferase, aspartate aminotransferase, calcium, magnesium, white blood cells:* increased levels
Glucose, potassium: altered levels
Hemoglobin, neutrophils, platelets: decreased values

Patient monitoring
◀≋ Watch for signs and symptoms of APL differentiation syndrome (fever, dyspnea, weight gain, pulmonary infiltrates, and pleural or pericardial effusions).
- Evaluate vital signs and neurologic status.

◀≽ Obtain baseline ECG; monitor ECG at least weekly.

• Assess for arrhythmias and conduction disorders.

◀≽ Discontinue drug and notify prescriber if patient develops syncope, tachycardia, or arrhythmias.

• Monitor serum electrolyte levels, CBC, and coagulation studies.

• Assess for hypoglycemia and hyperglycemia if patient is diabetic.

Patient teaching

◀≽ Watch for signs and symptoms of APL differentiation syndrome.

• Tell patient that drug increases risk of serious infection. Instruct him to report signs or symptoms of infection.

◀≽ Emphasize importance of avoiding pregnancy during therapy.

• Caution patient to avoid driving and other hazardous activities until he knows how drug affects concentration and alertness.

• Tell patient to minimize GI upset by eating small, frequent servings of food and drinking plenty of fluids.

• Advise patient to establish effective bedtime routine to minimize insomnia.

• Notify patient that he'll undergo regular blood testing during therapy.

• As appropriate, review all other significant and life-threatening adverse reactions and interactions, especially those related to the drugs and tests mentioned above.

asenapine
Saphris

Pharmacologic class: Dibenzo-oxepino pyrrole
Therapeutic class: Atypical antipsychotic
Pregnancy risk category C

| FDA | BOXED WARNING | a |

• Elderly patients with dementia-related psychosis treated with antipsychotics are at increased risk for death. Analyses of 17 placebo-controlled trials (modal duration of 10 weeks), largely in patients taking atypical antipsychotics, revealed a risk of death in the drug-treated patients of between 1.6 and 1.7 times that seen in placebo-treated patients. Over the course of a typical 10-week controlled trial, the rate of death in drug-treated patients was about 4.5%, compared to a rate of about 2.6% in the placebo group. Although causes of death were varied, most deaths appeared to be either cardiovascular (for example, heart failure, sudden death) or infectious (for example, pneumonia) in nature.

• Observational studies suggest that, similar to atypical antipsychotics, treatment with conventional antipsychotics may increase mortality.

• The extent to which findings of increased mortality in observational studies may be attributed to the antipsychotic as opposed to some characteristic(s) of the patients isn't clear.

• Asenapine isn't approved for treatment of patients with dementia-related psychosis.

Action

Unknown. May be mediated through a combination of antagonistic activity at D_2 and 5-HT_{2A} receptors.

Availability

Tablet (sublingual): 5 mg, 10 mg

🖊 Indications and dosages

➢ Acute treatment of schizophrenia in adults
Adults: 5 mg S.L. b.i.d.

➤ Acute treatment of manic or mixed episodes associated with bipolar I disorder in adults

Adults: Initially, 10 mg S.L. b.i.d.; may be decreased to 5 mg S.L. b.i.d. if adverse reactions occur

Dosage adjustment
• Hypotension
• Severe neutropenia

Contraindications
None

Precautions
Use cautiously in:
• severe hepatic impairment (use not recommended)
• neuroleptic malignant syndrome, tardive dyskinesia, history of seizures or conditions that potentially lower seizure threshold (such as Alzheimer's dementia)
• diabetes mellitus
• dysphagia, patients at risk for aspiration pneumonia (avoid use)
• leukopenia, neutropenia
• antipsychotic-naïve patients
• cerebrovascular or cardiovascular disease; patients with risk factors for prolonged QT interval; concomitant use of drugs known to prolong QT interval, including Class 1A and Class III antiarrhythmics, other antipsychotics, and some antibiotics (avoid use)
• concomitant use of fluvoxamine (a CYP1A2 inhibitor), drugs that are both substrates and inhibitors of CYP2D6 (such as paroxetine), other centrally acting drugs, certain antihypertensives, alcohol
• patients who experience conditions that may contribute to core body temperature elevation (such as strenuous exercise, exposure to extreme heat, concomitant medication with anticholinergic activity, dehydration)

• elderly patients with dementia-related psychosis
• pregnant or breastfeeding patients
• children (safety and efficacy not established).

Administration
• Don't give within 10 minutes of a meal.
• Don't give water for at least 10 minutes following sublingual dose.

Route	Onset	Peak	Duration
S.L.	Rapid	0.5-1.5 hr	Unknown

Adverse reactions
CNS: headache, somnolence, insomnia, fatigue, anxiety, depression, irritability, dizziness, syncope, akathisia, extrapyramidal symptoms other than akathisia (including dystonia, oculogyration, dyskinesia, tardive dyskinesia, muscle rigidity, parkinsonism, tremor), **neuroleptic malignant syndrome, seizures**
CV: hypertension, orthostatic hypotension, **QT-interval prolongation**
GI: constipation, dry mouth, oral hypoesthesia, dysphagia, salivary hypersecretion, vomiting, increased appetite, dyspepsia
Hematologic: leukopenia, neutropenia, **agranulocytosis**
Metabolic: hyperglycemia, hyperprolactinemia
Musculoskeletal: arthralgia, extremity pain
Other: weight gain, toothache, dysgeusia

Interactions
Drug-drug. *Antibiotics (such as gatifloxacin, moxifloxacin), antipsychotics (such as chlorpromazine, thioridazine, ziprasidone), Class 1A antiarrhythmics (such as procainamide, quinidine), Class III antiarrhythmics (such as amiodarone, sotalol):* increased risk of QT-interval prolongation

Antihypertensives: possible enhanced effects of these agents

CYP1A2 inhibitors (such as fluvoxamine), other centrally acting drugs: possible increased asenapine plasma concentration

CYP2D6 substrates and inhibitors (such as paroxetine): possible enhanced inhibitory effects of paroxetine on its own metabolism

Drug-food. *Any food:* decreased asenapine effect

Drug-behaviors. *Alcohol:* possible enhanced alcohol effects

Patient monitoring

◀▧ Immediately discontinue drug and closely monitor patient if signs and symptoms of neuroleptic malignant syndrome occur, such as hyperpyrexia, muscle rigidity, altered mental status, and evidence of autonomic instability (irregular pulse or blood pressure, tachycardia, diaphoresis, and cardiac arrhythmia). Additional signs and symptoms may include elevated creatine kinase level, myoglobinuria (rhabdomyolysis), and acute renal failure.

◀▧ Discontinue drug if signs and symptoms of tardive dyskinesia occur (syndrome of potentially irreversible, involuntary, dyskinetic movement).

◀▧ Watch closely for suicide attempt in patients with inherent psychotic illnesses and bipolar disorder.

• Monitor blood glucose level closely in patient with or at risk for diabetes mellitus.

• Carefully monitor CBC with differential for neutropenia (fever or other signs and symptoms of infection) and treat promptly if such signs or symptoms occur. Discontinue drug immediately if WBC count decreases in absence of other causative factors or if severe neutropenia occurs (absolute neutrophil count less than 1,000/mm³).

• Carefully evaluate patient for history of drug abuse; if history exists, observe patient for signs and symptoms of misuse or abuse (such as drug-seeking behavior and increases in dosage).

• Monitor liver function tests closely.

Patient teaching

• Instruct patient not to remove tablet from packet until ready to take.

• Instruct patient to gently remove medication from packaging by peeling back tab with dry hands and not to push tablet through packaging.

• Tell patient to place tablet under the tongue and allow it to dissolve completely; caution patient not to chew, crush, or swallow tablet whole.

• Instruct patient not to eat or drink anything for 10 minutes after taking this medication.

◀▧ Instruct patient to immediately discontinue drug and notify prescriber if the following signs or symptoms occur: overheating, muscle rigidity, altered mental status, irregular pulse or blood pressure, rapid or irregular heart beat, excessive sweating, or involuntary muscle movements.

◀▧ Advise patient or caregiver to immediately notify prescriber if suicidal thoughts or behavior develops.

• Advise patient to avoid alcoholic beverages.

• Caution patient to avoid driving and other hazardous activities until drug's effects on concentration and alertness are known.

• Inform patient that drug may elevate body temperature and to avoid activities that may cause overheating and dehydration (such as strenuous work or exercise in hot weather, using hot tubs) and to seek immediate medical attention if fever, mental or mood change, headache, or dizziness occurs.

• Inform patient to move slowly when rising to avoid dizziness from sudden blood pressure decrease.

Reactions in **bold** are life-threatening.   ◀▧ Clinical alert

- As appropriate, review all other significant and life-threatening adverse reactions and interactions, especially those related to the drugs, foods, and behaviors mentioned above.

asparaginase
Elspar, Kidrolase✤

Pharmacologic class: Enzyme
Therapeutic class: Antineoplastic (miscellaneous)
Pregnancy risk category C

Action
Hydrolyzes asparagine (an amino acid needed for malignant cell growth in acute lymphocytic leukemia), resulting in leukemic cell death

Availability
Injection: 10,000 international units/vial (with mannitol)

⏀ Indications and dosages
➤ Acute lymphocytic leukemia (given with other drugs, such as prednisone or vincristine, as part of antineoplastic regimen)
Children: 1,000 international units/kg I.V. daily for 10 successive days, with asparaginase initiated on day 22 of regimen, or 6,000 international units/m² I.M. on days 4, 7, 10, 13, 16, 19, 22, 25, and 28
➤ Sole agent used to induce remission of acute lymphocytic leukemia
Adults and children: 200 international units/kg I.V. daily for 28 days
➤ Drug desensitization regimen
Adults and children: Initially, 1 international unit I.V. Then double the dosage q 10 minutes until total planned daily dosage has been given.

Contraindications
- Hypersensitivity to drug
- Pancreatitis or history of pancreatitis

Precautions
Use cautiously in:
- bone marrow depression, hepatic or renal disease, CNS depression, clotting abnormalities, infection
- pregnant or breastfeeding patients
- women of childbearing age.

Administration
◀ Administer intradermal skin test as ordered at start of therapy and when drug hasn't been given for 1 week or more.
- Follow prescriber's orders for drug desensitization when indicated (usually before therapy starts and again during retreatment).
◀ Know that drug may be carcinogenic, mutagenic, or teratogenic. Follow appropriate facility policy for handling and preparing.
- Before starting drug, give allopurinol as prescribed to lower risk of neuropathy.
- Add sterile water or normal saline solution (5 ml for I.V. dose, 2 ml for I.M. dose) to powdered drug in vial.
- Filter through 5-micron filter.
- For I.V. use, inject into normal saline solution or dextrose 5% in water and infuse over 30 minutes.
- For I.M. use, give a maximum of 2 ml at any one site.
- Don't use solution unless it's clear.
◀ If drug touches skin or mucous membranes, rinse with copious amounts of water for at least 15 minutes.
- Provide adequate fluid intake to prevent tumor lysis.

Route	Onset	Peak	Duration
I.V.	Immediate	Immediate	23-33 days
I.M.	Immediate	14-24 hr	23-33 days

Adverse reactions
CNS: confusion, drowsiness, depression, hallucinations, fatigue, agitation, headache, lethargy, irritability, **seizures, coma, intracranial hemorrhage and fatal bleeding**
GI: nausea, vomiting, anorexia, abdominal cramps, stomatitis, **hemorrhagic pancreatitis, fulminant pancreatitis**
GU: glycosuria, polyuria, uric acid nephropathy, **uremia, renal failure**
Hematologic: anemia, **leukopenia, hypofibrinogenemia, depression of clotting factor synthesis, bone marrow depression**
Hepatic: fatty liver changes, **hepatotoxicity**
Metabolic: hyperglycemia, hyperuricemia, hypocalcemia, hyperammonemia, **hypoglycemia**
Musculoskeletal: joint pain
Skin: rash, urticaria
Other: chills, fever, weight loss, hypersensitivity reactions, **anaphylaxis, fatal hyperthermia**

Interactions
Drug-drug. *Methotrexate:* decreased methotrexate efficacy
Prednisone: hyperglycemia, increased drug toxicity
Vincristine: hyperglycemia, increased drug toxicity, increased risk of neuropathy
Drug-diagnostic tests. *Alanine aminotransferase, ammonia, aspartate aminotransferase, blood urea nitrogen, glucose, uric acid:* increased levels
Calcium, hemoglobin, white blood cells: decreased levels
Thyroid function tests: interference with test interpretation

Patient monitoring
◀€ Observe for signs and symptoms of anaphylaxis.
◀€ Monitor for bleeding and hemorrhage. Watch closely for signs and symptoms of intracranial hemorrhage.

• Assess vital signs, temperature, and neurologic status.
• Monitor CBC, blood and urine glucose levels, and liver, kidney, and bone marrow function test results.
• Monitor fluid intake and output.

Patient teaching
◀€ Instruct patient to immediately report allergic response, severe abdominal pain, and unusual bleeding or bruising.
• Caution patient to avoid driving and other hazardous activities until he knows how drug affects concentration and alertness.
• Advise patient to drink plenty of fluids to ensure adequate urine output.
• Tell patient to monitor urine output and report significant changes.
• Instruct patient to avoid activities that can cause injury. Tell him to use soft toothbrush and electric razor to avoid injury to gums and skin.
• Advise patient to minimize GI upset by eating small, frequent servings of food and drinking plenty of fluids.
• Tell patient that he'll undergo regular blood testing during therapy.
• As appropriate, review all other significant and life-threatening adverse reactions and interactions, especially those related to the drugs and tests mentioned above.

atazanavir
Reyataz

Pharmacologic class: HIV-1 protease azapeptide inhibitor
Therapeutic class: Antiretroviral
Pregnancy risk category B

Action
Selectively inhibits the virus-specific processing of viral Gag and Gag-Pol

◀€ Clinical alert

polyproteins in human immunodeficiency virus (HIV)-1 infected cells, preventing formation of mature virions

Availability
Capsules: 100 mg, 150 mg, 200 mg, 300 mg

⟋ Indications and dosages
➤ Treatment-naïve patients with HIV-1 infection in combination with ritonavir

Adults: 300 mg with ritonavir 100 mg P.O. daily. When administered with tenofovir, H2-receptor antagonists, or proton pump inhibitors, give 300 mg with ritonavir 100 mg P.O. daily. When administered with efavirenz, give 400 mg with ritonavir 100 mg P.O. daily. Give 400 mg P.O. daily if patient is unable to tolerate ritonavir.

Adults and children at least age 13 weighing at least 40 kg (88 lb) who are unable to tolerate ritonavir: 400 mg (without ritonavir) P.O. daily (For patients at least age 13 and at least 40 kg receiving concomitant tenofovir, H_2-receptor antagonists, or proton pump inhibitors, atazanavir should not be administered without ritonavir.)

➤ Treatment-experienced patients with HIV-1 infection in combination with other antiretrovirals

Adults: 300 mg with ritonavir 100 mg P.O. daily. When administered with an H_2-receptor antagonist, give 300 mg with ritonavir 100 mg P.O. daily. When administered with tenofovir and an H_2-receptor antagonist, give 400 mg with ritonavir 100 mg P.O. daily.

➤ HIV-1 infection

Children ages 6 to younger than 18 weighing at least 40 kg (88 lb): 300 mg with ritonavir 100 mg P.O. daily

Children ages 6 to younger than 18 weighing at least 20 kg (44 lb) to less than 40 kg: 200 mg with ritonavir 100 mg P.O. daily

Children ages 6 to younger than 18 weighing at least 15 kg (33 lb) to less than 20 kg: 150 mg with ritonavir 100 mg P.O. daily

Dosage adjustment
• Hepatic impairment
• Administration with sildenafil citrate, tadalafil, or vardenafil
• Treatment-experienced pregnant women during second or third trimester, when administered with either an H_2-receptor antagonist or tenofovir

Contraindications
• Hypersensitivity to drug or its components
• Administration with alfuzosin, triazolam, oral midazolam, ergot derivatives, rifampin, irinotecan, lovastatin, simvastatin, indinavir, cisapride, pimozide, sildenafil (Revatio), or St. John's wort

Precautions
Use cautiously in:
• hepatic impairment (use not recommended)
• renal impairment (drug shouldn't be administered to HIV treatment-experienced patients with end-stage renal disease managed with hemodialysis)
• conduction abnormalities and coadministration of drugs that may prolong PR interval, especially those metabolized by CYP3A (such as verapamil)
• concomitant use of antiarrhythmics (such as amiodarone, bepridil, systemic lidocaine, quinidine); antidepressants (such as trazodone, tricyclic antidepressants); high doses of ketoconazole and itraconazole (above 200 mg/day); calcium channel blockers; hormonal contraceptives
• concomitant use of endothelin-receptor antagonist (such as bosentan) without ritonavir (use not recommended)

Safe drug administration

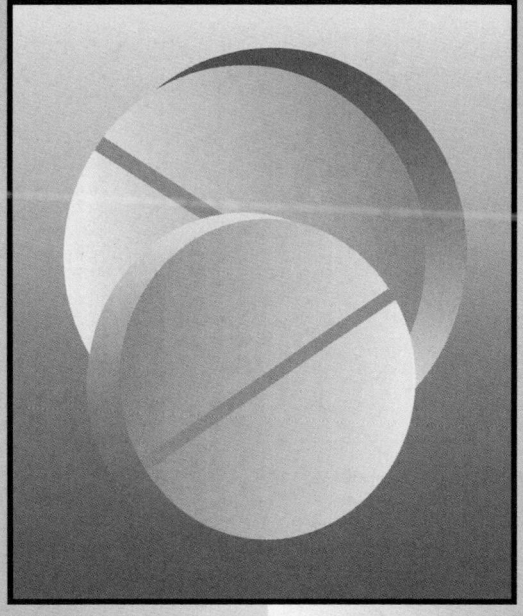

The following guidelines on preparing, administering, and monitoring drug therapy will help you ensure patient safety and drug effectiveness.

Drug compatibilities

Use the table below to determine if you can safely mix two drugs together in the same syringe or administer them together through the same I.V. line.

KEY
C: compatible
I: incompatible
∗: conflicting data exist
Blank space: no data available

	acyclovir sodium	amikacin	amiodarone	amphotericin B	aztreonam	calcium chloride	calcium gluconate	cefazolin	cefepime	ceftazidime	clindamycin	cyclosporine	dexamethasone	digoxin	diltiazem	diphenhydramine	dobutamine	dopamine	enalaprilat
acyclovir sodium															I		I	I	
amikacin			C	I	C	C	C	C	C	I	C	C	C	C	C	C			C
amiodarone		C		C		C	C	I			I	C		I			C	C	
amphotericin B		I	C		I										C	∗	I	I	I
aztreonam		C		I		C	C	C		C	C		C		C	C	C	C	C
calcium chloride		C	C		C								C				∗	C	
calcium gluconate		C	C		C			I			I		C			C	∗		C
cefazolin		C	I		C		I				∗	C	C		C				C
cefepime		C									C		C						
ceftazidime		I	I		C						C				C				C
clindamycin		C	I		C		I	∗	C	C		C	C						C
cyclosporine		C						C			C							∗	
dexamethasone		C			C	C	C	C	C		C					∗			
digoxin		C	I													I	I		
diltiazem	I	C		C	C			C		C	C						C	C	
diphenhydramine		C		∗	C		C						∗	I					
dobutamine	I		C	I	C	∗	∗							I	C			C	C
dopamine	I		C	I	C	C						∗			C		C		C
enalaprilat		C		I	C		C	C		C	C						C	C	
epinephrine		C	C			∗	∗								C				
esmolol		C	C			C		C		C	C				C		C	C	C
famotidine	C		C	C			C	C		C			C	C		C	C	C	C
fluconazole		C		C				C		C	C	C							
furosemide		∗	∗												I		I	I	

epinephrine	esmolol	famotidine	fluconazole	furosemide	heparin	hydrocortisone	hydromorphone hydrochloride	imipenem and cilastatin sodium	insulin	labetalol	levofloxacin	lorazepam	magnesium	methylprednisolone	metoclopramide hydrochloride	metoprolol	metronidazole	midazolam	milrinone	morphine	nitroglycerin	nitroprusside	norepinephrine	ondansetron	phenylephrine	potassium chloride	prochlorperazine	sodium bicarbonate	tobramycin	vancomycin
		C																												
C	C			C	*	I	C			C	C	C	C			C	C	C	C				C		C			C		C
C	C	C	C	C	*				C	C		C	*	C			C	C	C	C	C	*			C	C			I	C
		C			I	I	I						*	C			I												I	I
				C	C			C	C				I	C	C		I			C					C			C	C	*
*	C				C								I					C	C	C						I				
*		C	C		C	C				C			*	C				C	C						C	C	I	I	C	C
	C	C			*					C	C					*	C	C	C	C					C			C	C	*
						C											C								C				I	C
	C	C	C		*						C						C	I			C				C			I	*	*
	C		C		C	C				C	C			I	C		C		C	C	C	C			C				*	
													*				C						*					C	C
	C			C	C				C	*			C			I	C	C			C				C		C	C	I	I
	C	C				C						I						C	C	C						C				
	C	C			C	C						I	C	C			C						C		C			C	C	C
	C	C			C	C			C		C	I	C	C	C			C			C		C	C	C	C	C	C		C
C	C				I	C				C	C	C		C	C	C			C			C			C	C			I	
	C				I	C	C			C	C					C			C	C				C	C	C			C	C
C	C			*	C	C			C	C	C		C	C	C			C			C		C	C	C	C	C			C
		C			C								C				C						C					C		
C	I	*			C	C				I	I	C		I		I	I	I	C	C			I		C	*			C	*

Drug compatibilities (continued)

KEY
C: compatible
I: incompatible
∗: conflicting data exist
Blank space: no data available

	acyclovir sodium	amikacin	amiodarone	amphotericin B	aztreonam	calcium chloride	calcium gluconate	cefazolin	cefepime	ceftazidime	clindamycin	cyclosporine	dexamethasone	digoxin	diltiazem	diphenhydramine	dobutamine	dopamine	enalaprilat
heparin		I		I	C		C	∗	C	∗	C		C	C	∗	∗	∗	C	C
hydrocortisone		C		I	C	C	C				C		C		∗	C		C	C
hydromorphone hydrochloride																			
imipenem and cilastatin sodium			I		C										C				
insulin			C		C			C						I	∗		∗	I	
labetalol		C	C				C	C		C	C						C	C	C
levofloxacin		C									C		C				C	C	
lorazepam		C	C		I								C		C	I			
magnesium		C	∗	∗		C	I	∗	C		I	C					∗		C
methylprednisolone			C	C	C			C			C				∗	I		C	C
metoclopramide hydrochloride													C						
metoprolol																			
metronidazole		C	C		I			∗	C	C	C	C						∗	C
midazolam		C	C				C	C			I	C		∗	C		∗	C	
milrinone		C	C			C	C	C		C	C		C	C	C		C	C	
morphine		C	C		C	C		C		C	C		C	C		C	C	C	C
nitroglycerin			C												C		C	C	
nitroprusside			∗		C												C	C	C
norepinephrine			C												C		C	C	
ondansetron		C		I	C			C		C	C	∗	∗			C		C	
phenylephrine			C				C										C	C	
potassium chloride		C	C		C		C	C	C	C				C	C		∗	∗	C
prochlorperazine				I			I							I					
sodium bicarbonate		C	I		C	I	I			I					∗		I	I	
tobramycin			C		C		C	C	I	∗	∗	C			C				C
vancomycin		C	C		∗		C	∗	C	∗			I		C	C			C

	epinephrine	esmolol	famotidine	fluconazole	furosemide	heparin	hydrocortisone	hydromorphone hydrochloride	imipenem and cilastatin sodium	insulin	labetalol	levofloxacin	lorazepam	magnesium	methylprednisolone	metoclopramide hydrochloride	metoprolol	metronidazole	midazolam	milrinone	morphine	nitroglycerin	nitroprusside	norepinephrine	ondansetron	phenylephrine	potassium chloride	prochlorperazine	sodium bicarbonate	tobramycin	vancomycin
heparin	C	C	C	C	C	■	*			C	I	*	I	C	C	*			C	C	C	I	*	C			C	C	C	I	*
hydrocortisone	C	C	C		C	*	■			C			C	*		C		C		I			C				C			I	C
hydromorphone hydrochloride					C			■			C				C			I				C		C	C	I					
imipenem and cilastatin sodium			C		C				■	C			I				I	I			C						C				
insulin		C	C			I	C		C	■	I	I		C			C	C	C	C	C	I		C			C		*	C	C
labetalol		C	C		I	*				I	■			C			C	C		C	C	C	C				C		*	C	C
levofloxacin	C				I	I				I		■	C				C	I	I				C			C			C		C
lorazepam			C		C	C	C	C	I			C	■			C		C			*		C								C
magnesium		C	C			C	*			C	C			■			C		C	C			*		C		C		I	C	C
methylprednisolone			C			*									■	C	*	C	C				*		I						
metoclopramide hydrochloride					I		C									■	C		C						I						
metoprolol																	■											C			
metronidazole		C		C		C	C				C		C	C	C			■	C	C	C									C	
midazolam		C	C		I	C	I	C	I	C	C				*	C		C	■	C	C	C	C	C	C		C	I	I	C	C
milrinone	C				I	C			I	C			C	C	C			C	C	■	C	C	C	C	C		C		C	C	C
morphine	C	C	C	C	I	I	C			C	C	C		C	C	C	C	C	C		■	C	C	C		C	C	C	I	C	C
nitroglycerin		C	C		C	*				C	C	I				C	C			C	C	■	C				C				
nitroprusside	C	C	C		C	C				C	C	I		C			C			C	C	C	■	C		C			C		
norepinephrine			C							I	C			C	C	C			C	C	C		C	■		C					C
ondansetron			C		I	C	C	C	C				*		*			C		C					■			C	I		C
phenylephrine		C				C					C							C	C	C	C					■					C
potassium chloride	C	C	C	C	I	C			C	C		C	C		C	C				C	C	C		C		C	■		C		
prochlorperazine						I	I	I	C										I		C							■			
sodium bicarbonate			C	C	C	I				*	*	C		I					I	C	I						I		■		I
tobramycin		C			*	I			C	C			C			C			I	C	C	C	C							■	
vancomycin		C	C		*	I			C	C	C	C	C	C				C	C	C					C	C			I		■

Conversions and calculations

SAFETY GUIDELINES

Accurate conversions and calculations are crucial to ensuring safe drug administration. Use the tables below when you need to convert one unit to another, find equivalent measures, convert temperatures between Celsius and Fahrenheit, or calculate dosages or administration rates.

Metric measures

Solids
1 milligram (mg) = 1,000 micrograms (mcg)
1 gram (g) = 1,000 mg
1 kilogram (kg) = 1,000 g

Liquids
1 milliliter (ml) = 1 cubic centimeter (cc)
1 ml = 1,000 microliters (mcl)
1 cc = 1,000 mcl
1 liter (L) = 1,000 ml
1 L = 1,000 cc

Household to metric equivalents
1 teaspoon (tsp) = 5 ml
1 tablespoon (tbs) = 15 ml
1 ounce (oz) = 30 ml
2 tbs = 30 ml
1 oz = 30 g
1 pound (lb) = 454 g
2.2 lb = 1 kg
1 inch = 2.54 centimeters (cm)

Temperature conversions

To convert Celsius (°C) to Fahrenheit (°F)
Use the following equation:
$(°C \times 9/5) + 32 = °F$
Example: 38 °C times 9/5 is 68.4; 68.4 plus 32 equals 100.4 °F.

To convert °F to °C
$(°F - 32) \times 5/9 = °C$
Example: 98.6 °F minus 32 is 66.8; 66.8 times 5/9 equals 37 °C.

Calculating dosages and administration rates

Concentration of solution in mg/ml $= \dfrac{\text{mg of drug}}{\text{ml of solution}}$

Infusion rate in mg/minute $= \dfrac{\text{mg of drug}}{\text{ml of solution}} \times \text{flow rate (ml/hour)} \div 60 \text{ minutes}$

Concentration of solution in mcg/ml $= \dfrac{\text{mg of drug} \times 1,000}{\text{ml of solution}}$

Infusion rate in mcg/minute =
$\dfrac{\text{mg of drug} \times 1,000}{\text{ml of solution}} \times \text{flow rate (ml/hour)} \div 60 \text{ minutes}$

Infusion rate in mcg/kg/minute =
$\dfrac{\text{mg of drug} \times 1,000}{\text{ml of solution}} \times \text{flow rate (ml/hour)} \div 60 \text{ minutes} \div \text{weight in kg}$

Infusion rate in ml/hour = ml of solution $\div$ 60 minutes

Infusion rate in gtt/minutes $= \dfrac{\text{ml of solution}}{\text{time in minutes}} \times \text{drip factor (gtt/ml)}$

Medication Reconciliation

SAFETY
GUIDELINES

Changes to patients' medication regimens make inadvertent duplication, omission, and other unintended inconsistencies possible during admission, transfer, and discharge handoffs. To correct this problem, the Joint Commission made medication reconciliation across the care continuum a National Patient Safety Goal in 2005. Medication reconciliation helps avoid potentially dangerous inconsistencies through review and comparison of the complete medication regimen on admission, transfer, and discharge. To conduct a patient medication interview and verify, clarify, and reconcile any inconsistencies, use the algorithm below.

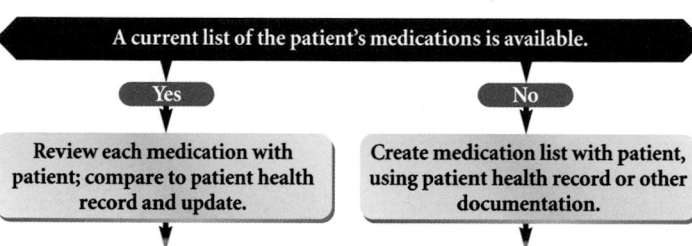

A current list of the patient's medications is available.

Yes → Review each medication with patient; compare to patient health record and update.

No → Create medication list with patient, using patient health record or other documentation.

Use the following questions to verify, update, or create list.
- What medications are you currently taking? When are you taking them? What dose/form are you taking? Who prescribed your medications?
- Do you have any allergies?
- Are you taking any new medications or have there been any changes to your existing medications?
- What over-the-counter drugs are you taking? Vitamins? Herbals? Supplements?
- Incorporate probing questions to trigger memory, such as: What medications do you take for your blood pressure? For your diabetes? For pain? For sleep?

Update and record list at end of interview; identify new or discontinued medications and changes made to existing medications.

Compare current medications, identifying vulnerabilities for error (such as omissions, duplications, incorrect dosing or timing, or adverse reactions or interactions). Discuss concerns or discrepancies with patient's physician or prescriber.

Give list to patient and family/caregiver. Counsel patient on any changes to regimen.

Record current medication regimen in patient health record, and communicate updated regimen to next care provider.

Repeat this process at each transition along the continuum of care.

Guidelines for timely administration of scheduled drugs

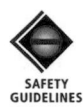

SAFETY
GUIDELINES

The most common violation of the five rights of drug administration is giving a drug at the wrong time. For as long as many nurses can remember, the *right time* has been defined as up to 30 minutes before or after the scheduled administration time. In 2008, the Centers for Medicare & Medicaid Services (CMS) made this 30-minute rule part of their *Regulations and Interpretive Guidance for Hospitals,* which spells out the conditions of participation for receiving Medicare and Medicaid payments.

In a 2010 survey by the Institute for Safe Medication Practices (ISMP), nurses described the CMS rule as unsafe, impossible to follow, and largely unnecessary. Of 17,500 responding nurses, 70% said their organizations mandated the 30-minute rule. Only 5% said they were able to comply with it. The shortcuts and workarounds nurses used in their attempts to comply were eye-opening, and in November of 2011, recognizing the rule was no longer the standard of practice, the CMS removed it.

The CMS now requires hospitals to develop their own drug administration policies and procedures based on established standards of practice and directs hospitals to consider the nature of each prescribed drug and the relevant patient and clinical considerations. In response to this new direction, ISMP formed an interdisciplinary advisory group and developed the *Acute Care Guidelines for Timely Administration of Medication.* The following guidelines are based on and adapted from the ISMP Acute Care Guidelines.

How to use the guidelines

In acute-care organizations, an inter-disciplinary team that includes nurses should translate these general guidelines into policies and procedures based on specific patient populations and drug systems, including available technology.

Definitions

Scheduled drugs include all drugs prescribed in maintenance doses and given according to a standard, repeated cycle of frequency, such as q 4 hours, q.i.d., t.i.d., b.i.d., daily, weekly, monthly, and annually. Scheduled drugs, as defined here, do not include the following types of drugs or drugs given in the following doses:

- STAT and now doses
- p.r.n. drugs
- First doses and loading doses
- One-time doses

- Specifically timed doses (for example, a preoperative antibiotic dose given a specified amount of time before incision and drug desensitization protocols)
- On-call doses (for example, preprocedure sedation)
- Time-sequenced or concomitant drugs (for example, chemotherapy and rescue agents or *n*-acetylcysteine and iodinated contrast media)
- Drugs given at specific times to ensure accurate peak or trough serum drug levels
- Investigational drugs in clinical trials.

Time-critical scheduled drugs are drugs that may result in harm or substantially suboptimal therapy or pharmacologic effect when given more than 30 minutes early or late.

Non–time-critical scheduled drugs are drugs that should not result in harm or substantially suboptimal therapy or pharmacologic effect when given more than 30 minutes early or late.

Time-critical scheduled drugs

As a member of the interdisciplinary team, you will participate in creating a list of time-critical scheduled drugs and establishing appropriate guidelines.

1. Create a list

Based on the patient population of a unit or an entire hospital, create a list of time-critical scheduled drugs.

For all hospitals, include these drugs:
• All prescribed drugs given more than every 4 hours
• Scheduled (not prn) opioids for chronic pain or palliative care
• Immunosuppressants for preventing solid-organ transplant rejection or treating myasthenia gravis
• Drugs that must be administered at different times, such as antacids and fluoroquinolones
• Drugs given with meals or within a certain period before or after meals—for example, rapid-, short-, or ultra-short-acting insulins; certain oral antidiabetics, such as acarbose, nateglinide, repaglinide, and glimepiride; alendronate; and pancrelipase.

Administration times of drugs given around meals require nursing judgment because they vary based on meal delivery, meal consumption, and patient condition.

Be sure to include drugs that are time-critical for a specific diagnosis or indication—for example, parenteral anti-infectives for patients with worsening sepsis. Also, allow prescribers, pharmacists, and nurses to include the designation of "time-critical" with the medication order or medication administration record

(MAR) entry for any scheduled drug.

2. Establish guidelines

Create guidelines that promote timely administration of time-critical drugs and exact-time administration of drugs such as rapid-, short-, and ultra-short-acting insulins. Ensure that MAR entries remind staff members of the need for timely or exact-time administration.

Non–time-critical scheduled drugs

As a member of the interdisciplinary team, you will participate in creating guidelines for all drugs given less than every 4 hours.

1. Establish guidelines for daily, weekly, and monthly drugs

Create guidelines that allow staff members to give these drugs up to 2 hours before or after the scheduled time. Though exceeding this 4-hour window may be safe, it may also increase the risk of failing to give a dose at all.

2. Establish guidelines for drugs given between 4 and 24 hours

Create guidelines that allow staff members to give these drugs up to 1 hour before or after the scheduled time.

First doses and subsequent doses

Define the time limits for giving a first dose or loading dose of critically needed drugs, such as I.V. anti-infectives, I.V. anticoagulants, and I.V. antiepileptics. Also, define the time limits for giving subsequent, less urgent doses. Include procedures that help achieve the administration time goals.

Technologic challenges

Be aware that your hospital's bar-coding software may need an update to trigger an alert for delayed and early doses when a dosage has more than one time interval. Software for electronic medication administration records (eMARs) also may require updates to change the appearance of a medication entry for delayed doses and to set different time limits for removing scheduled drugs from automated dispensing cabinets. Highlighting time-critical scheduled drugs on eMARs and differentiating between first and subsequent doses also present technologic challenges.

Approval

After establishing new policies and procedures based on the patient population, and current drug systems, the interdisciplinary team must obtain the approval of the medical staff.

Operational support guidelines

To enhance safe, timely drug administration, follow these operational support guidelines:

- Base staffing levels in the pharmacy and patient-care units on workload and patient acuity.
- When assigning nurses, consider the total number of drugs given daily, the types of drugs prescribed, the number of time-critical drugs, the complexity and frequency of drug administration, and the ability of patients to swallow oral drugs.
- Ensure that the number of automated dispensing cabinets on patient-care units facilitates safe and timely drug administration.
- Define acceptable reasons for administering doses early or late.

- Require staff members to document the exact time they administer drug doses. Ensure MARs provide sufficient space and prompts.
- Require staff members to check the MAR for the time of the last dose before giving the next dose.
- Create eMAR alerts indicating that a dose will soon be overdue or is overdue.
- Adhere to standard drug administration schedules based on the prescribed dosing frequency whenever possible.
- Establish a procedure for staff members who will administer or have administered a time-critical scheduled drug early or late. Include prescriber notification when an adverse outcome is anticipated or has occurred, documentation of the reason for untimely administration, and evaluation of the need to change the timing of future doses.
- Establish a streamlined process for reporting untimely administration of time-critical scheduled drugs, even if the reason is documented and justifiable. Use these reports to learn the causes of untimely administration and make improvements
- Review data from event reports, end-of-shift reports, and aggregate data collection to identify the causes of early or late drug administration, revise the list of time-critical drugs, and make system-based changes.

Adapted with permission from the Institute of Safe Medical Practices. ISMP Acute Care Guidelines for Timely Administration of Scheduled Medications. www.ismp.org/tools/guidelines/acutecare/tasm.pdf.

Drug names that look or sound alike

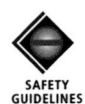

SAFETY
GUIDELINES

The drug names below can easily be confused, either verbally or in writing, because they either sound alike or have similar spellings. Generic names of these drugs appear in regular type; trade names are capitalized and in **boldface**.

Accupril, Accutane
Accutane, Anturane
acetazolamide, acetohexamide
acetylcholine, acetylcysteine
Aciphex, Aricept
Adderall, Inderal
albuterol, atenolol
Aldactazide, Aldactone
Aldomet, Aldoril
Aldoril, Elavil
alfentanil, fentanyl, **Sufenta, sufentanil**
Allegra, Viagra
alprazolam, diazepam, lorazepam,
    midazolam
Altace, alteplase
Alupent, Atrovent
amantadine, rimantadine
Ambien, Amen
Amicar, Amikin
amiloride, amiodarone, amlodipine
amitriptyline, nortriptyline
amoxicillin, **Augmentin**
Anafranil, enalapril
Apresazide, Apresoline
ASA, 5-ASA
Asacol, Os-Cal
Asacol, Os-Cal, Oxytrol
Atarax, Ativan
atenolol, timolol
avanafil, **Avandia, Avandryl**
Avinza, Invanz
azithromycin, erythromycin
baclofen, **Bactroban**
Benadryl, Bentyl, Benylin, Betalin
bepridil, **Prepidil**
Betagan, BetaGen
Bumex, Buprenex
bupivacaine, ropivacaine
bupropion, buspirone

Calan, Colace
calcifediol, calcitriol
Capitrol, captopril
carboplatin, cisplatin
Cardene, Cardizem
Cardene, codeine
cefazolin, cefprozil
cefotaxime, ceftizoxime
cefuroximine, deferoxamine
Cefzil, Kefzol
Celexa, Cerebyx
chlorpromazine, promethazine
ciprofloxacin, ofloxacin
Clinoril, Clozaril
clofazimine, clonidine, clozapine
clomiphene, clomipramine
clonazepam, clorazepate
clonidine, quinidine
clotrimazole, co-trimoxazole
codeine, **Lodine**
Coreg, Zomig
Cozaar, Zocor
cyclobenzaprine, cyproheptadine
cycloserine, cyclosporine
dacarbazine, procarbazine
dactinomycin, daunorubicin
Dantrium
Darvon, Diovan
daunorubicin, idarubicin
Decadron, Percodan
desipramine, imipramine
Desogen, desonide
desoximetasone, dexamethasone
Desoxyn, digitoxin, digoxin
Diabeta, Zebeta
diazepam, **Ditropan**
dimenhydrinate, diphenhydramine

Drug names that look or sound alike (continued)

Diprivan, Ditropan
dipyridamole, disopyramide
dobutamine, dopamine
doxapram, doxazosin, doxepin,
    doxycycline
Doxil, Paxil, Plavix
dronabinol, droperidol
dyclonine, dicyclomine
Dynacin, DynaCirc
Echogen, Epogen
Elavil, Equanil, Mellaril
Eldepryl, enalapril
Elmiron, Imuran
eloxatin, Exelon
enalapril, ramipril
Entex, Tenex, Xanax
ephedrine, epinephrine
esmolol, Osmitrol
Estraderm, Estratab, Estratest
Estraderm, Testoderm
ethosuximide, methsuximide
etidronate, etretinate
Eurax, Urex
Evista, E-vista
Femara, FemHRT
fenoprofen, flurbiprofen
fentanyl, sulfentanil
Fioricet, Fiorinal
Flaxedil, Flexeril
Flomax, Fosamax
flunisolide, fluocinonide
fluoxetine, fluvastatin, fluvoxamine,
    paroxetine
flurazepam, temazepam
Folotyn, folic acid, folinic acid
Foradil, Toradol
fosinopril, lisinopril, Risperdal
fosphenytoin, phenytoin
furosemide, torsemide
glimepiride, glipizide, glyburide
Granulex, Regranex
guaifenesin, guanfacine
Haldol, Stadol
heparin, Hepsera, Hespan

Hycodan, Vicodin
hydralazine, hydroxyzine
hydromorphone, morphine
Hyperstat, Nitrostat
imipenem, Omnipen
imipramine, Norpramin
Inderal, Inderide, Isordil
Intropin, Isoptin
Keflex, Ketek
Klonopin, Clonidine
Lamasil, Lomotil
Lamictal, Lamisil
lamivudine, lamotrigine
Lanoxin, Lasix, Lonox
Levatol, Lipitor
Levbid, Lithobid
Levitra, Raptiva
Librax, Librium
Loniten, Lotensin, lovastatin
Lorabid, Slo-bid
losartan, valsartan
Mandol, nadolol
Maxidex, Maxzide
Mazicon, Mevacor, Mivacron
methimazole
meclizine, memantine
melphalan, Mephyton
meperidine, meprobamate
Mesantoin, Mestinon
methicillin, mezlocillin
methotrexate, metolazone
metoprolol, misoprostol
minoxidil, Monopril
mithramycin, mitomycin
nadolol, nevivolol
naloxone, naltrexone
Naprelan, Naprosyn
Navane, Nubain
nelfinavir, nevirapine
Neurontin, Noroxin
niacinamide, nicardipine
nicardipine, nifedipine, nimodipine
Norpace, Norpramin
Ocufen, Ocuflox

(continued)

olanzapine, olsalazine
Orinase, Ornade
oxaprozin, oxazepam
oxycodone, **OxyContin**
paclitaxel, paclitaxel protein-bound
   particles
paclitaxel, paroxetine
Panadol, pindolol, **Plendil**
pancuronium, pipecuronium
Parlodel, pindolol
paroxetine, pralidoxime, pyridoxine
pentobarbital, phenobarbital
pentosan, pentostatin
Percocet, Percodan, Procet
Phenaphen, Phenergan
phenelzine, **Phenylzin**
phentermine, phentolamine
pioglitazone, rosiglitazone
Pitocin, Pitressin
Pravachol, Prevacid
Pravachol, propranolol
prednisolone, prednisone, primidone
Premarin, Primaxin
Prilosec, Prinivil, Proventil
Prilosec, Prozac
ProAmatine, protamine
probenecid, **Procanbid**
promazine, promethazine
Proscar, Provenge, Provera, Prozac
protamine, **Protopam, Protropin**
Quarzan, Questran
quinidine, quinine
ranitidine, rimantadine
Relpax, Revex, Revia
Reminyl, Robinul
reserpine, **Risperdal**
Restoril, Vistaril
Retrovir, ritonavir
ribavirin, riboflavin
rifabutin, rifampin
Rifadin, Rifamate, Rifater
Rifadin, Ritalin, ritodrine
Roxanol, Roxicet
Salbutamol, salmeterol
saquinavir, **Sinequan**
selegiline, **Stelazine**
Serentil, Serevent

Seroquel, Serzone
Solu-Cortef, Solu-Medrol
somatropin, sumatriptan
Spiriva, Stalevo
Sufenta, Survanta
sumatriptan, zolmitriptan
Tambocor, tamoxifen
Tequin, Ticlid
terbinafine, terbutaline, terfenadine
terbutaline, tolbutamide
terconazole, tioconazole
testolactone, testosterone
thiamine, **Thorazine**
tiagabine, tizanidine
Timoptic, Viroptic
Tobradex, Tobrex
tolazamide, tolbutamide
tolnaftate, **Tornalate**
tramadol, trazodone
Trandate, Tridate
Trendar, Trental
tretinoin, trientine
triamcinolone, **Triaminicin,**
   Triaminicol
triaminic, **Triaminicin**
triamterene, trimipramine
trifluoperazine, triflupromazine
Ultracef, Ultracet
Ultrase, Ultresa
Urised, Urispas
valacyclovir, valganciclovir
Vancenase, Vanceril
Vanceril, Vansil
VePesid, Versed
verapamil, **Verelan**
Verelan, Virilon
vinblastine, vincristine, vindesine,
   vinorelbine
Voltaren, Voltarol, Votrient
Wellbutrin, Wellcovorin, Wellferon
Xanax, Zantac
Zantac, Zyrtec
Zestril, Zostrix
Zocor, Zoloft
Zofran, Zosyn
Zymar, Zyprexa, Zyrtec

Identifying injection sites

SAFETY
GUIDELINES

Injection sites vary with administration route. The instructions below describe proper identification sites for I.M., subcutaneous, and I.V. drugs.

To begin, wash your hands, put on gloves, and locate the appropriate site. Clean the site with an alcohol pad, and administer the injection as described here.

I.M. injections

You can administer an I.M. injection into the muscles shown below. In these illustrations, specific injection sites are shaded.

Deltoid site
- Locate the lower edge of the acromial process.
- Insert the needle 1" to 2" below the acromial process at a 90-degree angle.

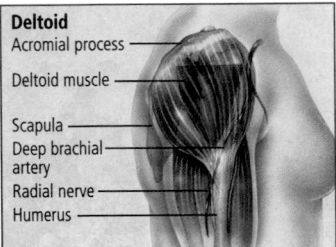

Deltoid
Acromial process
Deltoid muscle
Scapula
Deep brachial artery
Radial nerve
Humerus

Dorsogluteal site
- Draw an imaginary line from the posterior superior iliac spine to the greater trochanter.
- Insert the needle at a 90-degree angle above and outside the drawn line.
- You can administer a Z-track injection through this site. After drawing up the drug, change the needle, displace the skin lateral to the injection site, withdraw the needle, and then release the skin.

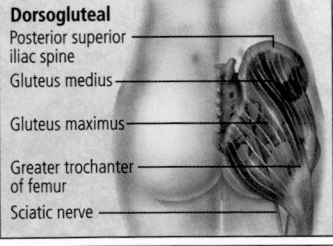

Dorsogluteal
Posterior superior iliac spine
Gluteus medius
Gluteus maximus
Greater trochanter of femur
Sciatic nerve

Ventrogluteal site
- With the palm of your hand, locate the greater trochanter of the femur.
- Spread your index and middle fingers posteriorly from the anterior superior iliac spine to the furthest area possible. This is the correct injection site.
- Remove your fingers and insert the needle at a 90-degree angle.

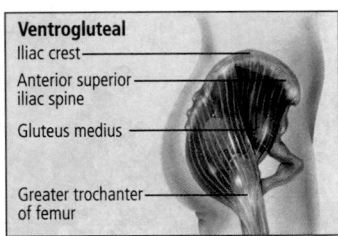

Ventrogluteal
Iliac crest
Anterior superior iliac spine
Gluteus medius
Greater trochanter of femur

Vastus lateralis and rectus femoris sites
- Find the lateral quadriceps muscle for the vastus lateralis, or the anterior thigh for the rectus femoris.
- Insert the needle at a 90-degree angle into the middle third of the muscle, parallel to the skin surface.

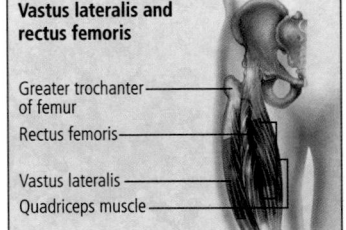

Vastus lateralis and rectus femoris
Greater trochanter of femur
Rectus femoris
Vastus lateralis
Quadriceps muscle

Subcutaneous injections

Subcutaneous drugs can be injected into the fat pads on the abdomen, buttocks, upper back, and lateral upper arms and thighs (shaded in the illustrations below). If your patient requires frequent subcutaneous injections, make sure to rotate injection sites.

• Gently gather and elevate or spread subcutaneous tissue.
• Insert the needle at a 45- or 90-degree angle, depending on the drug or the amount of subcutaneous tissue at the site.

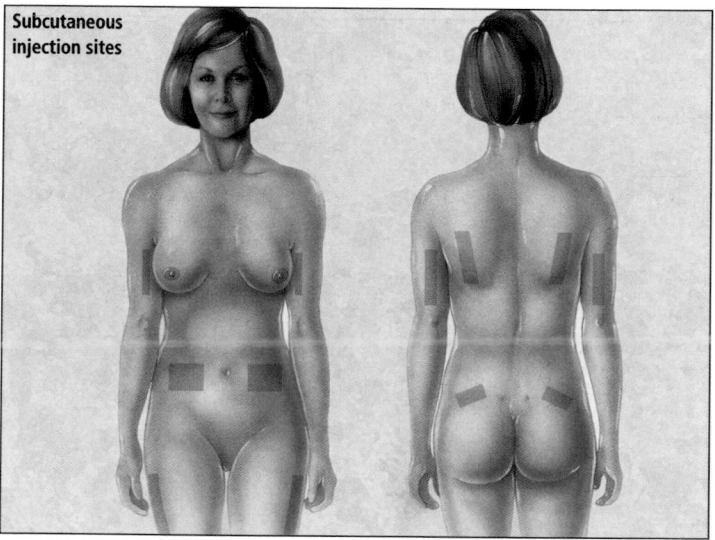

Subcutaneous injection sites

I.V. injections

I.V. drugs can be injected into the veins of the arms and hands. The illustration on the right shows commonly used sites.

• Locate the vein using a tourniquet.
• Insert the catheter at a slight angle (about 10 degrees).
• Release the tourniquet when blood appears in the syringe or tubing.
• Slowly inject the drug into the vein.

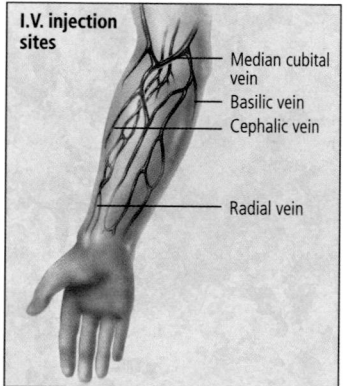

I.V. injection sites

Median cubital vein
Basilic vein
Cephalic vein

Radial vein

Illustrator: Kevin A. Somerville

Tall Man letters

SAFETY
GUIDELINES

In 2001, the Office of Generic Drugs requested manufacturers of some look-alike name pairs to voluntarily differentiate the drug names by using "Tall Man" letters to minimize medication errors. The list below shows the revisions that highlight dissimilar letters by using upper and lower case for drugs that have similar letters.

Established name	Recommended name
acetazolamide	acetaZOLAMIDE
acetohexamide	acetaHEXAMIDE
bupropion	buPROPion
buspirone	busPIRone
chlorpromazine	chlorproMAZINE
chlorpropamide	chlorproPAMIDE
clomiphene	clomiPHENE
clomipramine	clomiPRAMINE
cycloserine	cycloSERINE
cyclosporine	cycloSPORINE
daunorubicin	DAUNOrubicin
doxorubicin	DOXOrubicin
dimenhydrinate	dimenhyDRINATE
diphenhydramine	diphenhydrAMINE
dobutamine	DOBUTamine
dopamine	DOPamine
glipizide	glipiZIDE
glyburide	glyBURIDE
hydralazine	hydrALAZINE
hydromorphone	HYDROmorphone
hydroxyzine	hydrOXYzine
medroxyprogesterone	medroxyPROGESTERone
methylprednisolone	methylPREDNISolone
methyltestosterone	methylTESTOSTERone
mitoxantrone	mitoXANTRONE
nicardipine	NiCARDipine
nifedipine	NIFEdipine
prednisolone	prednisoLONE
prednisone	predniSONE
risperidone	risperiDONE
ropinirole	rOPINIRole
solu-medrol	solu-medrol
sulfadiazine	sulfaDIAZINE
sulfisoxazole	sulfiSOXAZOLE
tolazamide	TOLAZamide
tolbutamide	TOLBUTamide
vinblastine	vinBLAStine
vincristine	vinCRIStine

Tablets and capsules *not* to crush

Crushing extended-release or other long-acting oral drug forms can cause the ingredients to be released all at once instead of gradually. Similarly, crushing can break the coating of enteric-coated drugs, leading to GI irritation. Other drugs may taste bad or have carcinogenic or teratogenic potential when crushed. Never crush the trade-name drugs listed below.

Aciphex
Actiq
Actonel
Adalat CC
Adderall XR
Afeditab CR
Afinitor
Aggrenox
Allegra D
Alprazolam ER
Altoprev
Ambien CR
Amibid DM
Amitiza
Ampyra
Amrix
Aplenzin
Apriso
Aptivus
Aricept 23 mg
Arthrotec
Asacol
Aspirin EC
Atelvia
Augmentin XR
Avinza
Avodart
Azulfidine EN
Biaxin XL
Bisacodyl
Boniva
Bromfed PD
Budeprion SR
Calan SR
Carbatrol
Cardene SR
Cardizem CD, LA, SR
Carvedilol
Cefaclor ER
Ceftin

Cefuroxime
CellCept
Charcoal Plus
Chlor-Trimeton
Cipro XR
Claritin-D
Claritin-D 24 Hour
Colace
Colestid
Concerta
Cotazym-S
Covera-HS
Creon
Crixivan
Cymbalta
Cytovene
Cytoxan
Depakene
Depakote, Depakote ER, Depakote Sprinkles
Detrol LA
Dexilant
Dilacor XR
Dilatrate-SR
Dilt CD
Diltia XT
Ditropan XL
Divalproex ER
Doxidan
Drisdol
Droxia
Dulcolax
DynaCirc CR
EC-Naprosyn
Ecotrin
E.E.S. 400
Effer K
Effervescent Potassium
Effexor XR
Embeda

E-Mycin
Enablex
Entocort EC
Equetro
Ergomar
Erivedge
Ery-Tab
Erythromycin Base
Erythromycin stearate
Erythromycin Delayed-Release
Evista
Exalgo
Extendryl
Factive
Feen-a-mint
Feldene
FentaNYL
Fentora
Feosol
Feratab
Fergon
Ferro-Grad 500
Ferro-Sequel
Flagyl ER
Fleet Laxative
Flomax
Focalin XR
Fosamax
Gleevec
Glucophage XR
Glucotrol XL
Glumetza
Gralise
Guaifed, Guaifed PD
Guaifenesin and pseudoephedrine
Guaifenex DM, GP, PSE
Guaimax D
Halprin 81
Horizant
Hista-Vent DA
Hydrea
Imdur
Inderal LA
Indocin SR
Indomethacin SR
InnoPran XL
Intelence
Intermezzo
Intuniv
Invega

Isoptin SR
Isordil Sublingual
Isosorbide Dinitrate Sublingual
Isosorbide SR
ISOtretinoin
Jakafi
Jalyn
Janumet XR
Kadian
Kaletra
Kapidex
Kapvay
K-Dur
Keppra
Keppra XL
Ketex
Klor-Con, Klor-Con M
K-Lyte, K-Lyte CL, DS
Kombiglyze XR
K-Tab
LaMICtal XR
Lescol XL
Letairis
Levbid
Levsinex
Lialda
Liquibid
Lithobid
Lodrane 24, 24D
LoHIST 12 Hour
Lovaza
Luvox CR
Maxifed DM, DMX
Maxifen DM
Mestinon ER
Metadate CD, ER
Methylin ER
Metoprolol ER
Micro-K Extencaps
Mirapex ER
Morphine sulfate extended release
Motrin
Moxatag
MS Contin
Mucinex, Mucinex DM
Myfortic
Namenda XR
Naprelan
Nexium
Niaspan

Nicotinic Acid
Nifediac CC
Nifedical XL
Nitrostat
Norflex ER
Norpace CR
Norvir
Nucynta ER
Oleptro
Opana ER
Oracea
Oramorph SR
Orphenadrine citrate ER
OxyContin
Oxymorphone ER
Pancrease Delayed-Release
Pancrecarb
Pancrelipase
Paxil CR
Pentasa
Plendil
Pradaxa
Pre-Hist-D
Prevacid
Prevacid SoluTab
Prilosec
Pristiq
Procardia XL
Propecia
Proquin XR
Proscar
Protonix
Prozac Weekly
Qdall, Qdall AR
Ranexa
Rapamune
Rayos
Razadyne ER
Renagel
Renvela
Requip XL
Rescon, Rescon JR, MX
Respahist
Respaire SR
Revlimid
Ritalin LA, Ritalin-SR
R-Tanna
Rythmol SR
Ryzolt
Sensipar

Seroquel XR
Sinemet CR
Sinuvent PE
Slo-Niacin
Solodyn
Somnote
Sprycel
Strattera
Sudafed 12 Hour
Sular
Symax Duotab, Symax XR
Tasigna
Taztia XT
Tegretol-XR
Temodar
Tessalon Perles
Theochron
Theo-24
Tiazac
Topamax
Toprol XL
Touro CC-LD, Touro LA-LD
Toviaz
Tracleer
Trental
Treximet
Trilpix
Tylenol Arthritis
Ultram ER
Ultrase
Uniphyl
Urocit-K
Uroxatral
Valcyte
Verapamil SR
Verelan, Verelan PM
Videx EC
Vimovo
Viramune XR
VolSpire ER
Voltaren, XR
Voltrient
Wellbutrin SR, XL
Xanax-XR
Zegerid OTC
Zenpep
Zolinza
Zortress
Zyban
Zyflo CR

Monitoring blood levels

SAFETY
GUIDELINES

The table below shows therapeutic and toxic blood levels for selected drugs. Keep in mind that such levels may vary slightly among laboratories.

Drug	Therapeutic blood level	Toxic blood level
acetaminophen	10 to 20 mcg/ml	> 150 mcg/ml
alprazolam	0.025 to 0.102 mcg/ml	Not defined
amikacin	Peak: 25 to 35 mcg/ml	> 35 mcg/ml
	Trough: 5 to 10 mcg/ml	> 10 mcg/ml
aminophylline	10 to 20 mcg/ml	> 20 mcg/ml
amiodarone	1 to 2.5 mcg/ml	> 2.5 mcg/ml
amitriptyline	120 to 250 ng/ml	> 500 ng/ml
amobarbital	1 to 5 mcg/ml	> 10 mcg/ml
atenolol	0.2 to 0.7 mcg/ml	35 mcg/ml
bepridil	1 to 2 ng/ml	> 2 ng/ml
calcium	9 to 10.5 mg/dl	> 12 mg/dl
carbamazepine	4 to 14 mcg/ml	> 15 mcg/ml
clonazepam	10 to 80 ng/ml	> 100 ng/ml
creatinine	0.6 to 1.2 mg/dl	> 4 mg/dl
cyclosporine	50 to 300 ng/ml	> 400 ng/ml
desipramine	115 to 300 ng/ml	> 400 ng/ml
diazepam	0.5 to 2 mcg/ml	> 3 mcg/ml
digoxin	0.8 to 2 ng/ml	Adults: > 2.5 ng/ml
	Trough (> 12 hours after dose):	Children: > 3 ng/ml
	Heart failure: 0.8 to 1.5 ng/ml	
	Arrhythmias: 1.5 to 2 ng/ml	
diltiazem	0.05 to .40 mcg/ml	3.7 to 6.1 mcg/ml
diphenylhydantoin	10 to 20 mcg/ml	20 to 50 mcg/ml
disopyramide	2 to 8 mcg/ml	> 8 mcg/ml
ethosuximide	40 to 100 mcg/ml	> 100 mcg/ml
flecainide	0.2 to 1 mcg/ml	> 1 mcg/ml
fluconazole	5 to 15 mcg/ml	Not defined
fluoxetine	0.09 to 0.40 mcg/ml	Not defined
gentamicin	Peak: 4 to 12 mcg/ml	> 12 mcg/ml
	Trough: 1 to 2 mcg/ml	> 2 mcg/ml
glucose	70 to 110 mg/dl	> 300 mg/dl
glutethimide	2 to 6 mcg/ml	> 5 mcg/ml
haloperidol	5 to 20 ng/ml	> 20 ng/ml
hydromorphone	0.008 to 0.049 mcg/ml	Not defined

Drug	Therapeutic blood level	Toxic blood level
imipramine	225 to 300 ng/ml	> 500 ng/ml
lidocaine	1.5 to 6 mcg/ml	> 6 mcg/ml
lithium	0.6 to 1.2 mEq/L	> 1.5 mEq/L
lorazepam	50 to 240 ng/ml	300 to 600 ng/ml
magnesium	12 to 32 mcg/ml	80 to 120 mcg/ml
meperidine	100 to 550 ng/ml	> 1,000 ng/ml
meprobamate	6 to 12 mcg/ml	> 60 mcg/ml
methotrexate	> 0.01 mcmol	> 10 mcmol/24 hr
methsuximide	10 to 40 mcg/ml	> 44 mcg/ml
methylphenidate	0.01 to 0.06 mcg/ml	0.8 mcg/ml
metoprolol	0.03 to 0.27 mcg/ml	Not defined
mezlocillin	35 to 45 mcg/ml	> 45 mcg/ml
milrinone	150 to 250 ng/ml	> 250 ng/ml
nifedipine	0.025 to 0.1 mcg/ml	> 0.1 mcg/ml
nortriptyline	50 to 140 ng/ml	> 300 ng/ml
oxazepam	0.2 to 1.4 mcg/ml	> 2 mcg/ml
paroxetine	0.031 to 0.062 mcg/ml	Not defined
phenobarbital	10 to 40 mcg/ml	> 40 mcg/ml
phenytoin	10 to 20 mcg/ml	> 20 mcg/ml
potassium	3.5 to 5.0 mEq/L	> 6 mEq/L
primidone	4 to 12 mcg/ml	> 12 mcg/ml
procainamide	4 to 8 mcg/ml	> 10 mcg/ml
propranolol	50 to 200 ng/ml	> 200 ng/ml
quinidine	2 to 5 mcg/ml	> 5 mcg/ml
salicylates	100 to 300 mcg/ml	> 300 mcg/ml
sertraline	0.055 to 0.25 mcg/ml	Not defined
sodium	135 to 145 mEq/L	> 160 mEq/L
streptomycin	25 mcg/ml	> 25 mcg/ml
tacrolimus	0.005 to 0.02 mcg/ml	> 0.03 mcg/ml
theophylline	10 to 20 mcg/ml	> 20 mcg/ml
tobramycin	Peak: 4 to 12 mcg/ml	> 12 mcg/ml
	Trough: 1 to 2 mcg/ml	> 2 mcg/ml
tocainide	4 to 10 mcg/ml	Not defined
valproic acid	50 to 100 mcg/ml	> 100 mcg/ml
vancomycin	Peak: 20 to 40 mcg/ml	> 40 mcg/ml
	Trough: 5 to 15 mcg/ml	> 15 mcg/ml
verapamil	0.08 to 0.3 mcg/ml	Not defined
zolpidem	0.003 to 0.018 mcg/ml	Not defined

Effects of dialysis on drug therapy

SAFETY
GUIDELINES

A patient receiving a drug that's removed by hemodialysis (HD) or peritoneal dialysis (PD) will need supplemental doses of that drug. The chart below shows which drugs are removed by dialysis and therefore will necessitate supplemental dosing during or after dialysis. Drugs listed as "unlikely" haven't been studied; however, because of their chemical properties, dialysis is unlikely to remove them.

Generic drug	Removed by HD	Removed by PD
acetaminophen	Yes	No
acyclovir	Yes	No
adenosine	Unlikely	Unlikely
albumin	Unlikely	Unlikely
alendronate	No	No data
allopurinol	Yes	No data
alprazolam	No	Unlikely
amikacin	Yes	Yes
amiodarone	No	No
amitriptyline	No	No
amlodipine	No	No
amoxicillin	Yes	No
amphotericin B	No	No
ampicillin	Yes	No
ascorbic acid	Yes	Yes
aspirin	Yes	Yes
atenolol	Yes	No
atorvastatin	No	Unlikely
aztreonam	Yes	No
bleomycin	No	No
bumetanide	No	Unlikely
bupropion	No	No
buspirone	No	No data
candesartan	No	No data
captopril	Yes	No
carbamazepine	No	No
carbenicillin	Yes	No
carboplatin	Yes	No data
carisoprodol	Yes	Yes
carmustine	No	No data
cefaclor	Yes	Yes
cefadroxil	Yes	No
cefazolin	Yes	No
cefepime	Yes	Yes
cefoperazone	No	No
cefotaxime	Yes	No

Generic drug	Removed by HD	Removed by PD
cefotetan	Yes	Yes
cefoxitin	Yes	No
cefpodoxime	Yes	No
ceftazidime	Yes	Yes
ceftriaxone	No	No
cefuroxime	Yes	No
cephalexin	Yes	No
chlorpheniramine	Yes	No
cimetidine	No	No
ciprofloxacin	No	No
citalopram	No	Unlikely
clindamycin	No	No
clofibrate	No	No
clonazepam	No	Unlikely
clonidine	No	No
codeine	No	Unlikely
colchicine	No	No
cyclophospha-mide	Yes	No data
cyclosporine	No	No
dapsone	Yes	No data
desipramine	No	No
dexamethasone	No	No
diazepam	No	Unlikely
dicloxacillin	No	No
digoxin	No	No
diltiazem	No	No
diphenhydramine	Unlikely	Unlikely
divalproex	No	No
dobutamine	No	No
dopamine	No	Unlikely
doxazosin	No	No
doxepin	No	No
doxycycline	No	No
edetate calcium	Yes	Yes

Generic drug	Removed by HD	Removed by PD
enalapril	Yes	Yes
epinephrine	No data	No data
epoetin alfa	No	No
ertapenem	Yes	No data
erythromycin	No	No
esmolol	Yes	Yes
estradiol	No	No data
ethacrynic acid	No	Unlikely
etoposide	No	No
enoxaparin	No	Unlikely
famciclovir	Yes	No data
famotidine	No	No
felodipine	No	Unlikely
fenofibrate	No	Unlikely
filgrastim	No	Unlikely
flecainide	No	Unlikely
fluconazole	Yes	Yes
flucytosine	Yes	Yes
fluoxetine	No	No
folic acid	Yes	No data
foscarnet	Yes	No data
furosemide	No	Unlikely
gabapentin	Yes	No data
ganciclovir	Yes	No data
gemfibrozil	No	No
gentamicin	Yes	Yes
glyburide	No	Unlikely
haloperidol	No	No
heparin	No	No
hydralazine	No	No
hydrochloro- thiazide	No	Unlikely
hydrocodone	No data	No data
hydromorphone	No data	No data
hydroxyzine	No	No
ibuprofen	No	Unlikely
ibutilide	No data	No data
imipenem	Yes	Yes
imipramine	No	No
indomethacin	No	Unlikely
insulin	No	No
irbesartan	No	No data
isoniazid	No	No
isosorbide dinitrate	No	No
isosorbide mono- nitrate	Yes	No
isradipine	No	No
itraconazole	No	Unlikely
ketoconazole	No	No
ketoprofen	Unlikely	Unlikely
labetalol	No	No
lansoprazole	No	Unlikely
levetiracetam	Yes	No data
levofloxacin	Unlikely	Unlikely
lidocaine	No	Unlikely
linezolid	Yes	No data
lisinopril	Yes	No data
lithium	Yes	Yes
loracarbef	Yes	No data
loratadine	No	No
lorazepam	No	Unlikely
losartan	No	No
lovastatin	Unlikely	Unlikely
loxapine	No data	No data
mannitol	Yes	Yes
maprotiline	No	Unlikely
melphalan	No	No data
meperidine	No	Unlikely
mercaptopurine	Yes	No data
meropenem	Yes	No data
mesalamine	Yes	Unlikely
mesna	No data	No data
metformin	Yes	No data
methadone	No	No
methicillin	No	No
methotrexate	Yes	No
methyldopa	Yes	Yes
methylprednisolone	Yes	No data
metoclopramide	No	No
metoprolol	Yes	No data
metronidazole	Yes	No
miconazole	No	No
midazolam	No	Unlikely
minoxidil	Yes	Yes
morphine	No data	No
nadolol	Yes	No data
nalbuphine	No data	No data
naloxone	No data	No data
naltrexone	No data	No data

(continued)

Generic drug	Removed by HD	Removed by PD	Generic drug	Removed by HD	Removed by PD
naproxen	No	Unlikely	ranitidine	No	No
neomycin	Yes	yes	reserpine	No	No
nicardipine	No	Unlikely	reteplase	No data	No data
nifedipine	No	No	rifampin	No	No
nilutamide	No data	No data	risperidone	No data	No data
nimodipine	No	No	ritodrine	Yes	Yes
nitrofurantoin	Yes	No data	ritonavir	Unlikely	No
nitroglycerin	No	No	rosiglitazone	No	Unlikely
nitroprusside	Yes	Yes	rosuvastatin	No	No data
nortriptyline	No	No	sertraline	No	Unlikely
octreotide	Yes	No data	simvastatin	Unlikely	Unlikely
ofloxacin	Yes	No	sotalol	Yes	No data
olanzapine	No	No	stavudine	Yes	No data
omeprazole	Unlikely	Unlikely	streptomycin	Yes	Yes
ondansetron	Unlikely	Unlikely	sulfamethoxazole	Yes	No
oxazepam	No	Unlikely	tamoxifen	No data	No data
oxycodone	No data	No data	temazepam	No	Unlikely
paclitaxel	No	Unlikely	terazosin	No	No
pancuronium	No data	No data	tetracycline	No	No
pantoprazole	No	No data	theophylline	Yes	No
paricalcitol	Yes	Yes	thiamine	No	Unlikely
paroxetine	No	Unlikely	ticarcillin	Yes	No
penicillin	Yes	No	timolol	No	No
phenobarbital	Yes	Yes	tirofiban	Yes	No data
phenytoin	No	No	tobramycin	Yes	Yes
piperacillin	Yes	No	torsemide	No	Unlikely
pravastatin	No	No data	tramadol	No	No data
prednisone	No	No	trimethoprim	Yes	No
primidone	Yes	No data	valacyclovir	Yes	No
procainamide	Yes	No	valproic acid	No	No
promethazine	No	No data	valsartan	No	Unlikely
propafenone	No	No	vancomycin	No	No
propoxyphene	No	No	venlafaxine	No	Unlikely
propranolol	No	No	verapamil	No	No
propylthiouracil	No	No data	vinblastine	Unlikely	Unlikely
pseudoephedrine	No	Unlikely	vincristine	Unlikely	Unlikely
quinapril	No	No	voriconazole	Yes	Unlikely
quinidine	No; removed by hemoperfusion	No	warfarin	No	No
			zalcitabine	No data	No data
quinine	No	No	ziprasidone	No	Unlikely
ramipril	No	No data	zolpidem	No	Unlikely

Anaphylaxis: Treatment guidelines

SAFETY GUIDELINES

A hypersensitivity reaction may occur when a patient comes in contact with a certain agent, such as a drug, food, or other foreign protein. In some patients, this reaction progresses to life-threatening anaphylaxis, marked by sudden development of urticaria and respiratory distress. If this reaction continues, it may precipitate vascular collapse, leading to shock and, occasionally, death.

Hypersensitivity reaction

Adults: Epinephrine 0.2 to 0.5 ml of 1:1,000 solution subcutaneously or intramuscularly; repeat q 10 to 15 minutes to maximum dosage of 1 mg.
Children: Epinephrine 10 mcg/kg of 1:1,000 solution subcutaneously or intramuscularly, to maximum of 500 mcg/dose; may repeat q 15 minutes for 2 doses, then q 4 hours p.r.n.

↓

Adults or children: Diphenhydramine 1 to 2 mg/kg I.V. or I.M.

↓

Adults: Hydrocortisone 100 mg I.V. initially; then administer as indicated.
Children: Hydrocortisone 0.16 to 1 mg/kg I.V. given once or twice daily.

↓

If poor response, use anaphylaxis algorithm.

KEY
CPR: cardiopulmonary resuscitation

Anaphylaxis

Administer CPR if patient loses circulation or breathing; follow Advanced Cardiac Life Support guidelines.

↓

If hypotension occurs, give vasopressors (such as dopamine, norepinephrine, or neosynephrine). Provide fluid resuscitation with large volumes of normal saline or lactated Ringer's solution.

↓

Adults and children: If bronchospasm occurs, give 1 to 2 nebulized treatments of inhaled bronchodilator and consider loading dose of 6 mg/kg theophylline I.V., followed by maintenance dose as indicated.

↓

Adults: Epinephrine 0.2 to 0.5 ml of 1:1,000 solution subcutaneously or intramuscularly; repeat q 10 to 15 minutes to maximum dosage of 1 mg.
Children: Epinephrine 10 mcg/kg of 1:1,000 solution subcutaneously or intramuscularly; to maximum of 500 mcg/dose; may repeat dose q 15 minutes for 2 doses, then q 4 hours as needed.

↓

If patient doesn't respond, dilute epinephrine to yield 1:10,000 solution. For adults, infuse at 1 mcg/minute; may titrate to 2 to 10 mcg/minute. For children, infuse at 0.1 mcg/kg/minute.

Adult cardiac arrest: Treatment guidelines

SAFETY GUIDELINES

If you suspect your patient is in cardiac arrest, take appropriate steps, as described below.

↓

Assess responsiveness.

↓

Unresponsive
Begin chest compressions, at least 100/minute, (5 cycles of 30 compressions to 2 breaths). Activate emergency response system. Call for defibrillator. Assess breathing (open airway). Consider Advanced Airway (quantitative waveform capnography).

↓

Not breathing
Continue chest compressions. Give two breaths. Assess pulse. Continue CPR for 2 minutes (5 cycles of 30 compressions to 2 breaths). Assess pulse and cardiac rhythm. Attach monitor or defibrillator.

↓

No pulse
Initiate CPR (5 cycles of 30 compressions to 2 breaths) for 2 minutes. Assess cardiac rhythm.

VF or VT on monitor
Administer CPR until defibrillator charged: give 1 shock (360j for monophasic defibrillator; 200j for biphasic defibrillator). Immediately restart CPR for 2 minutes. After 2 minutes, check cardiac rhythm and pulse; if VF or VT, give 1 shock (360j for monophasic defibrillator or 200 to 300j for biphasic defibrillator). Start CPR immediately after the shock is delivered. Continue CPR for 2 minutes. Assess pulse and cardiac rhythm.

Asystole or PEA on monitor

Administer CPR for 2 minutes. After 2 minutes of CPR, check cardiac rhythm and pulse, then immediately restart CPR if PEA and asystole persist. Always verify asystole in 2 leads.

Conduct secondary survey

Breathing: Continue chest compressions at 100/minute.

Airway: Once an advanced airway device is in place, give 8 to 10 breaths/minute; provide ventilation and oxygenation.

Circulation: Obtain I.V. or I.O. access, administer adrenergic drug, and consider pacing. For asystole or PEA, give epinephrine 1 mg I.V.; repeat every 3 to 5 minutes. Give vasopressin 40 units to replace the first or second dose of epinephrine. For VF/VT, give epinephrine 1 mg I.V. or I.O.; repeat every 3 to 5 minutes. May use vasopressin 40 units to replace the first or second dose of epinephrine. For refractory VF/VT, give amiodarone 300 mg bolus for first dose, then 150 mg bolus for second dose, as directed.

Differential diagnosis: Search for and treat reversible causes.

KEY   CPR: cardiopulmonary resuscitation   VF: ventricular fibrillation
       I.O.: intraosseous   VT: ventricular tachycardia
       PEA: pulseless electrical activity

Pediatric cardiac arrest: Treatment guidelines

SAFETY GUIDELINES

For a pediatric patient in suspected cardiac arrest, take the following steps.

↓

Assess responsiveness.

↓

Unresponsive
Begin chest compressions, at least 100/minute, (5 cycles of 30 compressions to 2 breaths). Activate emergency response system. Attach monitor/defibrillator as soon as possible. Assess breathing (open airway).

↓

Not breathing
Continue chest compressions. Give two breaths that make the chest rise. Assess pulse.
Assess pulse. Start chest compressions (5 cycles of 30 compressions to 2 breaths) if patient is pulseless.

↓

No pulse
Continue CPR. Assess heart rhythm.

VF or VT on monitor
Attempt defibrillation
Deliver 1 shock at 2 J/kg. Resume CPR immediately for 2 minutes.
After 2 minutes, if VF or pulseless VT continues, deliver 1 shock at 4 J/kg. Give epinephrine I.V. or I.O. at 0.01 mg/kg. Resume CPR immediately for 2 minutes. After 2 minutes, if VF or pulseless VT continues. Deliver 1 shock at 4 J/kg.

Asystole or PEA on monitor
Give epinephrine 0.01 mg/kg I.V. or I.O. Continue CPR for 2 minutes then reassess; pulse and cardiac rythm. Always verify asystole in 2 leads.

↓

Conduct secondary survey
Airway and Breathing: Insert, confirm, and secure airway device; ventilate and oxygenate.
Circulation: Obtain I.V. access; defibrillate and give drugs as appropriate.
  *For VF/VT, give epinephrine 0.01 mg/kg (0.1 ml/kg of 1:10,000 solution)
  I.V. or I.O.; repeat q 3 to 5 minutes; then consider amiodarone.
  For asystole, give epinephrine 0.01 mg/kg (0.1 ml/kg of 1:10,000 solution)
  I.V. or I.O.; repeat q 3 to 5 minutes.
Differential diagnosis: Search for and treat reversible causes, including hypoxemia, hypovolemia, metabolic disorders, and thromboembolism.

KEY   CPR: cardiopulmonary resuscitation   PEA: pulseless electrical activity
      I.O.: intraosseus   VF: ventricular fibrillation
      J: joules   VT: ventricular tachycardia

Acute coronary syndrome: Treatment guidelines

Chest pain suggestive of ischemia

Immediate assessment (within 10 minutes):
- Measure vital signs and oxygen saturation.
- Obtain I.V. access, 12-lead ECG, and initial serum cardiac marker levels.
- Perform brief history and physical exam; review/complete fibrinolytic eligibility and contraindications.
- Obtain initial electrolyte and coagulation studies and cardiac marker levels.
- Request and review portable chest x-ray within 30 minutes.

Assess initial 12-lead ECG.

- ST elevation or new LBBB (strongly suggests injury) • ST-elevation AMI

Start adjunctive treatments
(as indicated; do not delay reperfusion therapy)
- Beta-adrenergic blockers I.V.
- Nitroglycerin I.V., heparin I.V.
- Clopidogrel, GPIIb/IIIa inhibitors, heparin (UFH or LMWH)

Time from symptom onset?   **> 12 hours**

< 12 hours

Choose reperfusion strategy based on local resources.
- Angiography
- PCI (angioplasty +/− stent)

- If signs of cardiogenic shock, PCI is treatment of choice.
- If PCI not available, use fibrinolytics (if no contraindications).

Fibrinolytic therapy chosen:
- alteplase or
- reteplase or
- tenecteplase
Goal: Door-to-drug within 30 minutes

Primary PCI chosen:
- Door-to-balloon inflation within 90 minutes
- Experienced operators
- High-volume medical center
- Cardiac surgical capability

KEY
ACE: angiotensin-converting enzyme
AMI: acute myocardial infarction

APSAC: anisoylated plasminogen streptokinase activator complex
LBBB: left bundle-branch block; O_2: Oxygen
PCI: percutaneous coronary intervention

SAFETY GUIDELINES

Immediate general treatment:
- O_2 not needed if oxyhemoglobin saturation is ≥ 94% in absence of respiratory distress
- Aspirin 160 to 325 mg (may be given by EMS).
- Nitroglycerin S.L. or by spray or I.V.
- Morphine I.V. (if nitroglycerin does not relieve pain).

Use MONA as memory aid: Morphine, Oxygen, Nitroglycerin, Aspirin.

EMS personnel can perform immediate assessment and treatment, including 12-lead ECG and review for fibrinolytic eligibility and administering aspirin, nitroglycerin and morphine.

- ST depression or dynamic T-wave inversion (strongly suggests ischemia)
- High-risk unstable angina/non-ST-elevation AMI

- Non-diagnostic ECG: no ST segment or T-wave changes
- Intermediate- or low-risk unstable angina

Start adjunctive treatments (as indicated, no contraindications):
- Heparin (UFH or LMWH)
- Clopidogrel
- Glycoprotein IIb/IIIa inhibitors
- Nitroglycerin I.V.
- Beta-adrenergic receptor blockers

← **Yes** — **Meets criteria for unstable or new-onset angina? Or troponin positive?**

No

Assess clinical status.

High-risk patient, defined by:
- persistent symptoms
- recurrent ischemia
- depressed left ventricular function
- widespread ECG changes
- previous AMI, PCI, or CABG

Admit to monitored bed.
- Obtain serial serum markers (including troponin).
- Repeat ECG/continuous ST monitoring.
- Consider imaging study.

Perform cardiac catheterization. Anatomy suitable for revascularization?

Clinically stable?

No → **Yes**

Evidence of ischemia or infarction?

Yes

Revascularization:
- PCI
- CABG

Admit to critical care unit.
- Continue or start treatment.
- Obtain serial cardiac markers and ECG.
- Consider imaging study.

No

Discharge acceptable
- Arrange follow-up

Preventing and treating extravasation

SAFETY GUIDELINES

Extravasation—escape of a vesicant drug into surrounding tissues—can result from a damaged vein or from leakage around a venipuncture site. Vesicant drugs (such as daunorubicin and vincristine) can cause severe tissue damage if extravasation occurs.

To help prevent extravasation, make sure the existing I.V. line is patent before you administer a drug by the I.V. route. Check patency by:
- inspecting the site for edema or pain
- flushing the I.V. line with 0.9% sodium chloride solution
- gently aspirating blood from the catheter.

Alternatively, you may insert a new I.V. catheter to ensure correct catheter placement. For vesicant drugs, consider using a central venous catheter.

If extravasation occurs, stop the infusion at once. Notify the physician to obtain treatment orders. Administer the antidote as ordered. Aspirate the remaining drug from the catheter before removing the I.V. line (unless you need the catheter to administer an antidote). *If you're unable to aspirate from the catheter, don't instill the antidote through the existing I.V.* If the extravasated drug was daunorubicin or doxorubicin, apply a cold compress to the area for 24 to 48 hours; if it was vinblastine or vincristine, apply a warm compress. Then elevate the affected extremity.

Administering antidotes
Antidotes for extravasation typically are either given through the existing I.V. line or injected subcutaneously around the infiltrated site using a 1-ml tuberculin syringe. Be sure to use a new needle for each antidote injection.

Extravasated drug	Antidote and dosage
• aminophylline • calcium solutions • contrast media • dextrose solutions (concentrations of 10% or more) • etoposide • nafcillin • potassium solutions • teniposide • total parenteral nutrition solutions • vinblastine • vincristine	**hyaluronidase:** 15 units/ml, as 0.2 ml subcutaneous injection near extravasation site
• dactinomycin	**ascorbic acid injection:** 50 mg
• daunorubicin • doxorubicin	**hydrocortisone sodium succinate:** 100 mg/ml: 50 to 200 mg
• dopamine • epinephrine • metaraminol • norepinephrine	**phentolamine:** 5 to 10 mg diluted in 10 to 15 ml of normal saline solution, administered within 12 hours of extravasation
• mechlorethamine	**sodium thiosulfate 10%:** 10 ml

Guidelines for handling, preparing, and administering hazardous drugs

SAFETY GUIDELINES

Health care professionals who work with or near hazardous drugs may be exposed to these agents in the air; on work surfaces, clothing, or medical equipment; or through contact with patient urine or feces. Hazardous drugs include many cancer chemotherapy agents, antivirals, hormones, and certain miscellaneous drugs. (Follow these hazardous drug guidelines for handling, preparation, and administration of all drugs with the special "hazardous drug" icon [☣] at the top of the monograph.)

The safety of health care workers who handle hazardous drugs is an ongoing concern. More than 5 million health care workers, including nurses, pharmacists, and physicians, are thought to be at risk. The greatest exposure occurs during preparation, administration, and disposal of these agents. In 2004, the National Institute for Occupational Safety and Health (NIOSH) issued an alert to inform workers of the possible risks of hazardous drugs. The alert included the following:

Warning! Working with or near hazardous drugs in health care settings may cause skin rashes, infertility, miscarriage, birth defects, and possibly leukemia or other cancers.

In 2006, the American Society of Health-System Pharmacists (ASHP) published revised guidelines on handling hazardous drugs. The following guidelines reflect the latest recommendations of ASHP, NIOSH, and the Centers for Disease Control and Prevention.

General preparation

• Read all material safety data sheets for each hazardous drug you handle.
• Prepare hazardous drugs in a controlled area designated for that purpose alone and restricted to authorized personnel. Identify these areas clearly with warning signs.
• Prepare hazardous drugs inside a ventilated cabinet with negative air pressure, to avoid spread of airborne drug contaminants and protect drugs that require sterile handling.
• Always work below eye level, within easy reach of a spill kit and a hazardous drug waste container.
• Wash hands with soap and water immediately before and after preparation.
• Use stringent sterile technique during any procedure in which sterile dosage forms are manipulated with needles and syringes.
• Whenever possible, use luer-lock syringes, I.V. administration sets, and connections, as these are less likely to separate during preparation.
• When supplemental protection is needed, use closed-system drug-transfer devices, glove bags, and needleless systems inside the ventilated cabinet.
• Know that hazardous drugs must be clearly labeled. Preparation and cleaning areas also need to be identified with warning signs or labels that are clear to non-English readers.

Personal protective equipment

Always wear personal protective equipment (PPE) during any activity involving hazardous drugs, including:

- reconstituting or admixing these drugs
- handling vials or finished products
- opening drug packaging
- assembling the delivery system
- administering these drugs
- labeling hazardous containers
- disposing of drug-related waste
- handling excretions from patients who have received hazardous drugs.

Gloves

- Wear two pairs of powder-free gloves. Make sure the inner pair is beneath the cuff of your gown and the outer pair covers the outside cuff.
- Before donning gloves, inspect them for defects.
- Remove the outer gloves after wiping down the final drug preparation but before labeling or removing it from the designated area. Place these gloves in a containment bag.
- Use clean gloves (the inner pair) to wipe the surface of the container, put the label on the final preparation, and place the drug container into the pass-through.
- Don fresh gloves to complete the final check and place the container for transport.
- Change gloves every 30 minutes during compounding, or immediately if damaged or contaminated.

Gown

Wear a disposable, nonabsorbent gown made of polypropylene material with a closed front, long sleeves, and elastic cuffs.

Face and eye shield

Wear a face or eye shield (as appropriate) if splashes, sprays, or aerosolizations to the eyes, nose, or mouth are possible during drug handling or administration.

Proper sequence for donning PPE

After washing your hands, don the first pair of gloves, then the gown and face shield (as appropriate), and then the second pair of gloves (which should extend beyond the cuff of your gown).

Dose reconstitution

- Avoid pressurizing vial contents, as this may cause the drug to spray out around or through the needle. To avoid pressurization, draw air into the syringe to create negative pressure in the vial.
- Transfer small amounts of diluent slowly as equal volumes of air are removed.
- Keeping the needle in the vial, swirl contents slowly until they dissolve.
- Make sure the syringe is no more than three-quarters full when it holds the final drug dosage.

Dose withdrawal and transfer

- Keeping the vial inverted, withdraw only the proper amount of drug solution.
- Remove the needle with the vial upright, making sure the needle hub is clear.
- To withdraw a dose from an ampule, gently tap the neck of the ampule. Then wipe the neck with alcohol and attach a 5-micron filter needle to a syringe. Draw the solution through the needle, clearing it from the needle and hub.
- If the drug will be dispensed in the syringe, draw back the plunger to clear fluid from the needle and hub. Replace the needle with a locking cap, and then wipe and lock the syringe.
- When using a needleless system, use gauze pads at connection points to contain leaks.
- If the drug will be transferred to an I.V. bag or bottle, prime the I.V. set before adding the drug. Puncture only the septum of the injection port. After injecting the drug solution into the bag, wipe the port, container, and I.V. set (if attached).
- Once drug preparation is complete, seal the final product in a plastic bag or other sealable container for transport

before taking it out of the ventilated cabinet; then label it with a unique identifier. Seal and wipe all waste containers inside the ventilated cabinet before removal. Finally, remove your outer gloves and sleeve covers (if used) and bag them while still inside the ventilated cabinet.

Administration

• Wash your hands and don gloves and gown. If spraying, splashing, or aerosolization is anticipated, wear a face shield or goggles.
• Visually examine the drug dose while it's still in the transport bag. If it appears intact, remove it from the bag.
• Place an absorbent pad on the work or administration area to contain spills or contamination.

Oral (noninjectable or nonparenteral) administration
• Oral hazardous drugs should be dispensed in the final dosage and form whenever possible.
• Avoid crushing tablets or opening capsules; instead, use liquid forms whenever possible.
• Never crush or compound an oral drug in an unprotected environment.
• Be aware that liquid hazardous drugs should be dispensed and maintained in sealable plastic bags.

I.M. or subcutaneous administration
• Remove the syringe cap and connect the appropriate safety needle.
• Don't expel air from the syringe or prime the safety needle.
• After administering the dose, discard the syringe (with safety needle attached) directly into an appropriate waste container.

I.V. administration
• If priming is necessary at the administration site, prime the I.V. tubing with an I.V. solution that doesn't contain a hazardous drug, or by using the backflow method.

• Place gauze pads under the connections at injection ports to catch leaks during administration.
• Use the transport bag as a containment bag for contaminated materials. Discard hazardous drug bags and bottles with their administration sets attached.

Disposal and clean-up

• Handle hazardous wastes and contaminated materials separately from other trash.
• Wash surfaces contaminated with hazardous drugs with detergent, hypochlorite solution, and neutralizer, as appropriate.
• Clean and decontaminate work areas before and after each hazardous drug-handling activity and at the end of each shift. Clean up small spills immediately.
• Dispose of drug-contaminated syringes and needles in puncture-proof containers labeled "Chemotherapy waste" or "Hazardous waste."
• Never push or force materials contaminated with hazardous drugs into waste containers.

After exposure to a hazardous drug

• In case of skin contact with a cytotoxic drug, immediately remove contaminated clothing and wash the affected area with soap and water. Don't scrub, because this will abrade the skin. Rinse the area thoroughly, and consult a physician for further treatment and monitoring.
• In case of eye contact, flush the affected eye with water or normal saline solution continuously for 15 minutes. Consult a physician for further treatment and monitoring.
• Document the exposure incident in your employee record and your facility's medical surveillance log.

Managing poisonings and overdoses

**SAFETY
GUIDELINES**

This chart serves as a quick reference for managing poisonings and drug overdoses. For more detailed instructions, consult your local poison control center. To find your local center, call the American Association of Poison Control Centers at 1-800-222-1222 or visit http://www.aapcc.org/findyour.htm.

Poison or drug	Antidote and dosage
acetaminophen	**acetylcysteine (Acetadote, Mucomyst)** Give P.O. as 5% solution by diluting with carbonated beverage or fruit juice. Loading dose: 140 mg/kg followed by 17 additional doses of 70 mg/kg q 4 hours. Repeat dose if patient vomits within 1 hour of administration. I.V. dose: 150 mg/kg over 15 minutes. Maintenance dose: 50 mg/kg infused over 4 hours, followed by 100 mg/kg infused over 16 hours.
anticholinergic agents antihistamines atropine	**physostigmine (Antilirium)** *Adults:* 0.5 to 2 mg slow I.V. injection (not to exceed 1 mg/minute). May repeat q 20 minutes until response or adverse effects occur. If initial dose is effective, additional doses of 1 to 4 mg may be given q 30 to 60 minutes as life-threatening signs (arrythmias, seizures, deep coma) recur. *Children:* 0.02 mg/kg I.M. or slow I.V. injection (not to exceed 0.5 mg/minute). May repeat q 5 to 10 minutes until therapeutic response occurs or maximum dosage of 2 mg is given.
arsenic trioxide	**dimercaprol (BAL)** *Adults:* 3 mg/kg I.M. q 4 hours until immediate life-threatening toxicity has subsided. Thereafter, give penicillamine 250 mg P.O. up to maximum frequency of four times daily (maximum: 1 g/day).
benzodiazepines	**flumazenil (Romazicon)** *Adults:* Initially, 0.2 mg I.V. injected over 30 seconds; follow with 0.3 mg if desired level of consciousness isn't reached. May give further doses of 0.5 mg at 60-second intervals until therapeutic response occurs or cumulative dosage of 3 mg is given. If partial response is achieved at 3 mg, patients may rarely need additional doses up to a total of 5 mg. If sedation recurs, repeat dose at 20-minute intervals. Maximum dosage is 3 mg/hour. *Children:* Initially 0.01 mg/kg (maximum dosage 0.2 mg) with repeat doses of 0.01 mg/kg (maximum dosage 0.2 mg) given q minute to maximum cumulative dosage of 1 mg.
calcium channel blockers	**activated charcoal** Consider prehospital administration of activated charcoal as a slurry in patient with potentially toxic ingestion who is awake and able to protect airway. Use minimum of 240 ml water/30 g charcoal. *Adults and adolescents:* Usual dosage, 25 to 100 g P.O. *Children ages 1 to 12:* 25 to 50 g P.O. (or 0.5 to 1 g/kg) *Children < age 1:* 0.5 to 1 g/kg P.O.

Poison or drug	Antidote and dosage
	calcium chloride *Adults:* If massive overdose occurs with hypotension remaining unresponsive to supportive measures, administer vasopressors (such as phenylephrine) as prescribed. Calcium gluconate 2 g/hour I.V. titrated to maintain blood pressure has been used successfully.
cholinergic agonists	**activated charcoal** Administer charcoal as a slurry (240 ml water/30 g charcoal). *Adults and adolescents:* Usual dosage, 25 to 100 g P.O. *Children ages 1 to 12:* 25 to 50 g P.O. *Children < age 1:* 1 g/kg P.O. **atropine sulfate** Atropine is the drug of choice for significant muscarinic symptoms. *Adults:* 2 to 4 mg I.V., repeated q 3 to 60 minutes as needed to control symptoms, then p.r.n. for 24 to 48 hours *Children:* 0.04 to 0.08 mg/kg I.V. (up to 4 mg), repeated q 5 to 60 minutes as needed **epinephrine** Epinephrine may help overcome severe cardiovascular or bronchoconstrictor responses. *Adults:* 0.1 to 1 mg subcutaneously
digoxin	**digoxin immune Fab (Digibind, DigiFab)** Calculate dosage as number of 38-mg vials, using this formula: Digoxin level (in ng) × patient's weight (in kg) divided by 100. Usual dosage range is four to six vials. If ingested amount of digoxin is unknown, give 10 to 20 vials (380 to 800 mg) I.V. over 30 minutes through a 0.22-micron filter. May give bolus dose if cardiac arrest is imminent.
ethylene glycol	**fomepizole (Antizol)** Loading dose: 15 mg/kg I.V. over 30 minutes, followed by 10 mg/kg I.V. over 30 minutes q 12 hours for four doses Maintenance dose: 15 mg/kg I.V. over 30 minutes q 12 hours until ethylene glycol level falls below 20 mg/dl
heparin	**protamine sulfate** Dosage is based on partial thromboplastin time; usually, 1 mg for each 100 units of heparin. Give I.V. over 10 minutes (maximum rate of 5 mg/minute) in doses not exceeding 50 mg. Patients allergic to fish, vasectomized or infertile men, and patients taking protamine-insulin products are at increased risk for protamine hypersensitivity.
hypercalcemic emergency	**edetate disodium (Endrate)** *Adults:* 50 mg/kg/day by slow I.V. infusion over at least 3 hours, up to a maximum of 3 g/day. *Children:* 40 mg/kg/day by slow I.V. infusion over at least 3 hours, up to a maximum of 70 mg/kg/day. Dilute with normal saline solution or dextrose 5% in water; don't infuse rapidly. Keep patient in bed for 15 minutes after infusion to avoid orthostatic hypotension. Keep I.V. calcium readily available, because drug may cause profound hypocalcemia, leading to tetany, seizures, arrhythmias, and respiratory arrest. Alternate I.V. sites daily to decrease risk of thrombophlebitis. **Alert:** Do not confuse drug with edetate calcium disodium, used as lead poisoning antidote.

(continued)

Managing poisonings and overdoses (continued)

Poison or drug	Antidote and dosage
iron	**deferoxamine (Desferal)** *Acute iron intoxication:* Initially, 1 g I.M., followed by 500 mg q 4 hours for two doses depending on clinical response, and then 500 mg q 4 to 12 hours, up to 6 g/day. May give I.V. infusion of 10 to 15 mg/kg/hour for first 1 g. Subsequent doses shouldn't exceed 125 mg/hour. Maximum dosage is 6 g in 24 hours. *Chronic iron intoxication:* In adults, 1 to 2 g/day subcutaneously. In children, maximum dosage of 2 g/day subcutaneously.
opioid overdose and dependence	**naloxone hydrochloride (Narcan)** *Opioid overdose* *Adults:* 0.4 to 2 mg I.V., I.M., or subcutaneously; repeat q 2 to 3 minutes, p.r.n., up to 10 mg If ordered, give initial adult dose of 0.1 mg I.V. to assess patient's response. Give subsequent doses of 0.4 mg or less (undiluted) by direct injection over 15 seconds, or titrate based on response. As needed, give continuous I.V. infusion, diluting 2 mg of naloxone with 500 ml of normal saline solution or dextrose 5% in water for a final concentration of 4 mcg/ml; titrate based on patient's response. *Children > age 5 or ≥ 20 kg:* 2 mg/dose; repeat q 2 to 3 minutes. *Children < age 5 or < 20 kg:* 0.1 mg/kg; repeat q 2 to 3 minutes. *Postoperative opioid-induced respiratory depression* *Adults:* 0.1 to 0.2 mg I.V. q 2 to 3 minutes, p.r.n. *Children:* 0.005 to 0.01 mg/kg q 2 to 3 minutes. *Opioid dependence* **naltrexone (Depade, ReVia)** *Adults:* Initially, 25 mg P.O.; give an additional dose of 25 mg if no withdrawal symptoms occur within 1 hour. When patient is receiving 50 mg q 24 hours, a maintenance schedule of 50 to 150 mg/day P.O. may be used. Don't initiate therapy until patient has been opiate-free for 7 to 10 days; do not begin for opioid dependence until a naloxone challenge test has been given. **Alert:** Do not confuse naltrexone with naloxone.
organophosphate insecticides	**pralidoxime (Protopam)** *Adults:* 1 to 2 g I.V. in 100 ml of normal saline solution infused over 15 to 30 minutes. If pulmonary edema occurs, may give as 5% solution I.V. over 5 minutes. May repeat dose in 1 hour if muscle weakness persists; may give additional doses at 10- to 12-hour intervals cautiously if muscle weakness continues. *Children:* 20 to 50 mg/kg (up to 1 g) in 250 ml normal saline solution I.V. over 30 minutes
warfarin	**phytonadione (Vitamin K)** *Adults:* 2.5 to 10 mg subcutaneously based on prothrombin time/International Normalized Ratio; may repeat in 6 to 8 hours as needed. In emergency, 2.5 to 25 mg slow I.V. (no faster than 1 mg/minute); may repeat 6 to 8 hours after first dose.
miscellaneous drug overdose	**activated charcoal** *Adults:* 1 to 2 g/kg with at least a 10:1 ratio of activated charcoal to intoxicant (usual dose is 25 to 100 g charcoal in water or sorbitol) and administered P.O. or by nasogastric tube. Do not give doses greater than 100 g. *Children:* 1 to 2 g/kg or 25 to 50 g charcoal. The use of repeated oral charcoal with sorbitol doses is not recommended.

- children younger than age 3 months (avoid use).

Administration
- Perform liver function tests before starting therapy.
- Administer drug with food.

⚡ Be aware that drug isn't recommended for treatment-experienced patients with prior virologic failure.

⚡ Don't administer to patient with severe hepatic impairment or treatment-experienced patient who is receiving dialysis for end-stage renal disease.

Route	Onset	Peak	Duration
P.O.	Unknown	Unknown	Unknown

Adverse reactions
CNS: headache, insomnia, dizziness, peripheral neurologic symptoms, depression.
CV: cardiac conduction abnormalities
EENT: scleral icterus
GI: nausea, vomiting, diarrhea, abdominal pain
GU: nephrolithiasis
Hematologic: neutropenia, thrombocytopenia, leukopenia, increased bleeding (in patients with hemophilia A and B)
Hepatic: jaundice, hepatotoxicity
Metabolic: hyperbilirubinemia, hyperglycemia, possible exacerbation of or new-onset diabetes mellitus
Musculoskeletal: myalgia
Respiratory: cough
Skin: rash, erythema multiforme, toxic skin eruptions, Stevens-Johnson syndrome
Other: fever, body fat redistribution or accumulation, immune reconstitution syndrome

Interactions
Drug-drug. Antacids, buffered drugs, H₂-receptor antagonists, proton pump inhibitors: decreased atazanavir plasma concentration

- concomitant use of inhaled nasal steroid (such as fluticasone propionate) and atazanavir without ritonavir
- concomitant use of inhaled nasal steroid (such as fluticasone propionate) and atazanavir with ritonavir (use not recommended unless potential benefit to patient outweighs risk of systemic corticosteroid adverse effects)
- concomitant use of proton pump inhibitors (such as omeprazole) (shouldn't be used in treatment-experienced patients receiving atazanavir)
- concomitant use of opioid (such as buprenorphine) and atazanavir with ritonavir (shouldn't be coadministered)
- administration of drugs highly dependent on CYP2C8 with narrow indices (such as paclitaxel, repaglinide) when atazanavir is administered without ritonavir
- concomitant use of antifungal (such as voriconazole) (shouldn't be administered with atazanavir/ritonavir unless benefit/risk assessment justifies use of voriconazole)
- concomitant use of antigout agent (such as colchicine) (shouldn't be administered with atazanavir to patients with hepatic or renal impairment)
- concomitant use of atazanavir with efavirenz in treatment-experienced patients (don't coadminister)
- concomitant use of inhaled beta agonist (such as salmeterol) (use not recommended)
- pregnant (avoid use without ritonavir) or breastfeeding patients
- patients less than 40 kg (88 lb) receiving concomitant tenofovir, H₂-receptor antagonists, or proton-pump inhibitors (not recommended)
- children younger than age 13 (avoid use without ritonavir)
- children ages 3 months to 6 years (safety and efficacy not established)

Antiarrhythmics (such as amiodarone, bepridil, systemic lidocaine, quinidine), tricyclic antidepressants): increased risk of serious or life-threatening adverse reactions

Atorvastatin, rosuvastatin: increased risk of myopathy including rhabdomyolysis

Bosentan: decreased atazanavir level, increased bosentan level

Buprenorphine: increased buprenorphine and its active metabolite norbuprenorphine plasma concentrations, decreased atazanavir level

Calcium channel blockers (such as diltiazem, felodipine, nifedipine, nicardipine, verapamil): increased calcium channel blocker effect

Clarithromycin: increased atazanavir and clarithromycin levels resulting in prolonged QTc interval; significantly reduced active clarithromycin metabolite level

Colchicine: increased colchicine effect

Cyclosporine, sirolimus, tacrolimus: increased immunosuppressant levels

Didanosine (buffered tablets): marked decrease in atazanavir exposure

Drugs primarily metabolized by CYP3A, UGT1A1, other drugs (such as alfuzosin, cisapride, ergot derivatives, indinavir, irinotecan, lovastatin, oral midazolam, pimozide, rifampin, sildenafil [Revatio], simvastatin, triazolam): increased plasma concentration of these drugs resulting in serious or life-threatening adverse reactions

Drugs that prolong PR interval (beta blockers other than atenolol, digoxin, verapamil): expected additive effect of atazanavir

Efavirenz: decreased atazanavir exposure

Ethinyl estradiol with norgestimate: decreased ethinyl estradiol level, increased norgestimate level

Ethinyl estradiol with norethindrone: increased ethinyl estradiol and norethindrone levels

Fluticasone: increased fluticasone plasma concentration

Fluticasone and atazanavir/ritonavir: increased fluticasone plasma concentration resulting in significantly reduced cortisol levels

H_2-receptor antagonists: decreased atazanavir plasma concentration resulting in loss of therapeutic effect and development of resistance

Itraconazole, ketoconazole: increased atazanavir area under the curve (AUC) and C_{max}, increased itraconazole and ketoconazole effects

Midazolam (parenteral): increased midazolam plasma concentrations, risk of respiratory depression and prolonged sedation

Nevirapine: markedly decreased atazanavir effect; increased nevirapine effect with risk of nevirapine-associated toxicity

Other protease inhibitors: expected increased effect of these drugs

Rifabutin: increased risk of rifabutin-associated adverse reactions

Ritonavir: increased atazanavir effect

Salmeterol: increased risk of cardiovascular adverse reactions including prolonged QT interval, palpitations, and sinus tachycardia

Sildenafil, tadalafil, vardenafil: possible increased phosphodiesterase inhibitor–associated adverse reactions (hypotension, syncope, visual disturbances, priapism)

Tenofovir: decreased atazanavir AUC and C_{min}, increased tenofovir level

Trazodone: increased trazodone plasma level

Warfarin: increased risk of serious or life-threatening bleeding

Drug-diagnostic tests. Alanine aminotransferase, aspartate aminotransferase, amylase, blood glucose, creatine kinase, high-density lipoproteins, lipase, low-density lipoproteins, total bilirubin, total cholesterol, triglycerides: increased levels

Hemoglobin, neutrophils, platelets: decreased levels

Drug-food. *Any food:* enhanced bioavailability and reduced pharmacokinetic variability

Drug-herbs. *St. John's wort:* decreased atazanavir plasma concentrations

Patient monitoring

◀€ Monitor patient closely and discontinue drug if severe rash occurs (possible sign of Stevens-Johnson syndrome).

◀€ Be aware that immune reconstitution syndrome may occur in patients receiving combination antiretroviral therapy. During initial phase of therapy, patient whose immune system responds may develop inflammatory response to indolent or residual opportunistic infections (such as Mycobacterium avium complex, cytomegalovirus, Pneumocystis jiroveci pneumonia, tuberculosis), which may necessitate further evaluation and treatment.

◀€ Temporarily interrupt or discontinue drug if signs or symptoms of nephrolithiasis occur.

• Monitor blood glucose level during therapy; watch for signs or symptoms of new-onset or exacerbation of diabetes mellitus and redistribution or accumulation of body fat.

• Monitor CBC with differential and liver and kidney function tests closely.

Patient teaching

• Instruct patient to take drug by mouth with food, to swallow capsules whole, and not to crush or chew them.

• Instruct patient to take drug 2 hours before or 1 hour after taking antacids or a buffered form of drugs.

◀€ Instruct patient to immediately report severe rash, changes in pulse or heart beat, signs or symptoms of kidney stones (pain in the side, blood in urine, or pain when urinating), yellowing of eyes, or signs and symptoms of immune reconstitution syndrome (such as new signs or symptoms of a previously subclinical infection, worsening or progression of a known infection despite treatment, a new infection or illness, or failure of antiretroviral therapy).

• Inform patient that drug may cause increase in blood glucose level and redistribution or accumulation of body fat.

• Advise patient to consult prescriber before using other prescription or over-the-counter drugs or herbs.

• Advise male patient taking sildenafil, tadalafil, or vardenafil to promptly report hypotension, visual changes, or prolonged penile erection to prescriber.

• As appropriate, review all other significant and life-threatening adverse reactions and interactions, especially those related to the drugs, tests, foods, and herbs mentioned above.

atenolol

Antipressan ⊕, Atenix ⊕, Novo-Atenol ✽, Tenormin

Pharmacologic class: Beta-adrenergic blocker (selective)

Therapeutic class: Antianginal, antihypertensive

Pregnancy risk category D

FDA | **BOXED WARNING**

• Caution patients with coronary artery disease (CAD) not to discontinue drug abruptly, because this may cause severe angina exacerbation, myocardial infarction, and ventricular arrhythmias. (The last two complications may occur with or without preceding angina exacerbation.) With planned drug discontinuation, observe patients carefully and advise them to minimize physical activity; if angina worsens or acute coronary insufficiency develops, drug should be reinstituted promptly, at least temporarily. Because CAD is common and may go unrecognized, abrupt withdrawal may pose a risk even in patients treated only for hypertension.

Action

Selectively blocks beta$_1$-adrenergic (myocardial) receptors; decreases cardiac output, peripheral resistance, and myocardial oxygen consumption. Also depresses renin secretion without affecting beta$_2$-adrenergic (pulmonary, vascular, uterine) receptors.

Availability

Tablets: 25 mg, 50 mg, 100 mg

🚺 Indications and dosages

➤ Hypertension
Adults: Initially, 50 mg P.O. once daily, increased to 100 mg after 7 to 14 days if needed
➤ Angina pectoris
Adults: Initially, 50 mg P.O. once daily, increased to 100 mg after 7 days if needed. Some patients may require up to 200 mg daily.
➤ Acute myocardial infarction
Adults: 50 mg tablet P.O., then give 50 mg P.O. in 12 hours. Maintenance dosage is 100 mg P.O. daily or 50 mg b.i.d. for 6 to 9 days.

Dosage adjustment

• Renal impairment
• Elderly patients

Contraindications

• Cardiogenic shock
• Sinus bradycardia
• Greater than first-degree heart block
• Heart failure (unless secondary to tachyarrhythmia treatable with beta-adrenergic blockers)

Precautions

Use cautiously in:
• renal failure, hepatic impairment, pulmonary disease, diabetes mellitus, thyrotoxicosis
• pregnant or breastfeeding patients
• children.

Administration

◀€ Adjust initial and subsequent dosages downward depending on clinical observations, including pulse rate and blood pressure.
◀€ Don't discontinue drug suddenly. Instead, taper dosage over 2 weeks.

Route	Onset	Peak	Duration
P.O.	1 hr	2 hr	24 hr

Adverse reactions

CNS: fatigue, lethargy, vertigo, drowsiness, dizziness, depression, disorientation, short-term memory loss
CV: hypertension, intermittent claudication, cold arms and legs, orthostatic hypotension, **bradycardia, arrhythmias, heart failure, cardiogenic shock, myocardial reinfarction**
EENT: blurred vision, dry eyes, eye irritation, conjunctivitis, stuffy nose, rhinitis, pharyngitis, **laryngospasm**
GI: nausea, vomiting, diarrhea, constipation, gastric pain, flatulence, anorexia, **ischemic colitis, retroperitoneal fibrosis, acute pancreatitis, mesenteric arterial thrombosis**
GU: impotence, decreased libido, dysuria, nocturia, Peyronie's disease, **renal failure**
Hematologic: agranulocytosis
Hepatic: hepatomegaly
Metabolic: hypoglycemia
Musculoskeletal: muscle cramps, back and joint pain
Respiratory: dyspnea, wheezing, respiratory distress, **bronchospasm, bronchial obstruction, pulmonary emboli**
Other: decreased exercise tolerance, allergic reaction, fever, development of antinuclear antibodies, hypersensitivity reaction

Interactions

Drug-drug. *Amiodarone, cardiac glycosides, diltiazem, verapamil:* increased myocardial depression, causing excessive bradycardia and heart block

Amphetamines, cocaine, ephedrine, norepinephrine, phenylephrine, pseudoephedrine: excessive hypertension, bradycardia

Ampicillin, calcium salts: decreased antihypertensive and antianginal effects

Aspirin, bismuth subsalicylate, magnesium salicylate, nonsteroidal anti-inflammatory drugs: decreased antihypertensive effect

Clonidine: life-threatening blood pressure increase after clonidine withdrawal or simultaneous withdrawal of both drugs

Dobutamine, dopamine: decrease in beneficial beta-cardiovascular effects

Lidocaine: increased lidocaine levels, greater risk of toxicity

MAO inhibitors: bradycardia

Prazosin: increased risk of orthostatic hypotension

Reserpine: increased hypotension, marked bradycardia

Theophylline: decreased theophylline elimination

Drug-diagnostic tests. *Alanine aminotransferase, alkaline phosphatase, aspartate aminotransferase, antinuclear antibody titer, blood urea nitrogen, creatinine, lactate dehydrogenase, platelets, potassium, uric acid:* increased levels

Glucose: increased or decreased level

Insulin tolerance test: false result

Drug-behaviors. *Alcohol use:* increased hypotension

Patient monitoring

• Watch for signs and symptoms of hypersensitivity reaction.

• Monitor vital signs (especially blood pressure), ECG, and exercise tolerance.

• Check closely for hypotension in hemodialysis patients.

• Monitor blood glucose level regularly if patient is diabetic; drug may mask signs and symptoms of hypoglycemia.

Patient teaching

◀€ Instruct patient to immediately report signs and symptoms of allergic response, breathing problems, and chest pain.

• Advise patient to take drug at same time every day.

◀€ Inform patient that he may experience serious reactions if he stops taking drug suddenly. Advise him to consult prescriber before discontinuing.

• Caution patient to avoid driving and other hazardous activities until he knows how drug affects concentration and alertness.

• Tell patient that drug may cause a temporary blood pressure decrease if he stands or sits up suddenly. Instruct him to rise slowly and carefully.

• Inform women that drug shouldn't be taken during pregnancy. Urge them to report planned or suspected pregnancy.

• Tell men that drug may cause erectile dysfunction. Advise them to discuss this issue with prescriber.

• As appropriate, review all other significant and life-threatening adverse reactions and interactions, especially those related to the drugs, tests, and behaviors mentioned above.

atomoxetine hydrochloride
Strattera

Pharmacologic class: Selective norepinephrine reuptake inhibitor

Therapeutic class: Central nervous system agent

Pregnancy risk category C

- Drug may increase risk of suicidal ideation in children or adolescents with attention deficit hyperactivity disorder (ADHD). Risk must be balanced with clinical need. Observe patient closely for clinical worsening, suicidality, and unusual behavior changes when therapy begins. Advise family to observe patient closely and communicate with prescriber as needed.
- Drug is approved for ADHD in pediatric and adult patients. It's not approved for major depressive disorder.

Action

Unclear. May block norepinephrine reuptake at neuronal synapse.

Availability

Capsules: 10 mg, 18 mg, 25 mg, 40 mg, 60 mg, 80 mg, 100 mg

🚫 Indications and dosages

➤ Acute treatment of ADHD

Children and adolescents weighing 70 kg (154 lb) or less: Initially, total daily dose of approximately 0.5 mg/kg P.O.; increase after minimum of 3 days to target total daily dose of approximately 1.2 mg/kg given either as single daily dose in morning or as evenly divided doses in morning and late afternoon or early evening. Total daily dosage in children and adolescents shouldn't exceed 1.4 mg/kg or 100 mg, whichever is less.

Children, adolescents, and adults weighing more than 70 kg (154 lb): Initially, total daily dose of 40 mg P.O.; increase after minimum of 3 days to target total daily dose of approximately 80 mg given either as single daily dose in morning or as evenly divided doses in morning and late afternoon or early evening. After 2 to 4 additional weeks, dosage may be increased to maximum of 100 mg in patients who haven't achieved optimal response. Maximum recommended total daily dosage is 100 mg.

➤ Maintenance and extended treatment of ADHD

Children ages 6 to 15: In general, continue dosage at which patient experienced continuous response.

Dosage adjustment

- Hepatic impairment
- Concurrent use of potent CYP2D6 inhibitors (such as fluoxetine, paroxetine, quinidine) in children weighing less than 70 kg (154 lb)

Contraindications

- Hypersensitivity to drug
- Closed-angle glaucoma, pheochromocytoma or history of pheochromocytoma, severe CV disorders
- MAO inhibitor use within past 14 days

Precautions

Use cautiously in:

- hypotension; impaired renal, cerebrovascular, hepatic, or endocrine function
- serious cardiac structural or heart rhythm abnormalities, cardiomyopathy (use not recommended)
- patients whose underlying medical conditions could be worsened by increased heart rate or blood pressure
- pregnant or breastfeeding patients
- children younger than age 6.

Administration

- Give as a single dose in morning, or give half of total daily dose in morning and other half in late afternoon or early evening.
- Check patient's baseline pulse and blood pressure.

🔊 Don't give to patient who has taken MAO inhibitors within past 14 days.

Route	Onset	Peak	Duration
P.O.	Rapid	1-2 hr	Unknown

Adverse reactions

CNS: aggression, insomnia, dizziness, drowsiness, headache, irritability, crying, mood swings, fatigue, rigors, **cerebrovascular accident, suicidal ideation**

CV: orthostatic hypotension, palpitations, tachycardia, Raynaud's phenomenon, **MI, sudden death**

EENT: rhinorrhea, sinusitis

GI: nausea, vomiting, constipation, upper abdominal pain, flatulence, dyspepsia, dry mouth

GU: urinary retention, urinary hesitancy, dysmenorrhea, erectile problems, ejaculation failure, impotence, prostatitis, priapism

Hepatic: severe liver injury

Musculoskeletal: muscle pain

Respiratory: cough

Skin: dermatitis, sweating

Other: fever, hot flashes, growth retardation (in children), decreased appetite, weight loss, **hypersensitivity reactions (including angioedema)**

Interactions

Drug-drug. *Albuterol:* increased cardiovascular effects

MAO inhibitors: hyperthermia, myoclonus, rapid changes in vital signs

Potent CYP2D6 inhibitors: increased atomoxetine effects in children weighing less than 70 kg (154 lb)

Vasopressors: hypertensive crisis

Drug-diagnostic tests. *Liver enzymes:* elevated levels

Patient monitoring

◀€ Monitor liver function tests closely; discontinue drug, and don't restart if liver enzymes are elevated or jaundice occurs.

• Monitor growth in children.

• Assess for weight loss.

• Check blood pressure and pulse, especially after dosage changes.

◀€ Monitor for changes in mood, sleep patterns, and behavior (especially aggressive behavior or hostility) and consider discontinuing drug if psychotic or manic symptoms occur.

• Evaluate for urinary hesitancy or urinary retention and sexual dysfunction.

• Provide dietary counseling. Refer patient to dietitian if adverse GI effects significantly limit food intake.

Patient teaching

◀€ Instruct patient to immediately report difficulty breathing, swelling of lips or throat, itching, dark urine, yellowing of skin or eyes, right upper quadrant tenderness, or flulike symptoms.

◀€ Instruct patient or caregiver to immediately report depression or suicidal thoughts.

• To minimize insomnia, advise patient to establish effective bedtime routine and to take drug in single morning dose or in divided half-doses in morning and late afternoon or early evening.

• Caution patient to avoid driving and other hazardous activities until he knows how drug affects concentration and alertness.

• Advise patient to minimize GI upset by eating small, frequent servings of food and drinking plenty of fluids.

• As appropriate, review all other significant adverse reactions and interactions, especially those related to the drugs mentioned above.

atorvastatin calcium
Lipitor

Pharmacologic class: HMG-CoA reductase inhibitor

Therapeutic class: Lipid-lowering agent

Pregnancy risk category X

Action

Inhibits HMG-CoA reductase, which catalyzes first step in cholesterol synthesis; this action reduces concentrations of serum cholesterol and low-density lipoproteins (LDLs), linked to increased risk of coronary artery disease (CAD). Also moderately increases concentration of high-density lipoproteins (HDLs), associated with decreased risk of CAD.

Availability
Tablets: 10 mg, 20 mg, 40 mg, 80 mg

🖊 Indications and dosages
➤ Adjunct to diet for controlling LDL, total cholesterol, apo-lipoprotein B, and triglyceride levels and to increase HDL levels in patients with primary hypercholesterolemia and mixed dyslipidemia; primary dysbetalipoproteinemia in patients unresponsive to diet alone; adjunct to diet to reduce elevated triglyceride levels
Adults: Initially, 10 mg P.O. daily; increase to 80 mg P.O. daily if needed. Adjust dosage according to patient's cholesterol level.
➤ Adjunct to other lipid-lowering treatments in patients with homozygous familial hypercholesterolemia
Adults: 10 to 80 mg P.O. daily
➤ Adjunct to diet to decrease total cholesterol, LDL, and apo-lipoprotein B levels in boys and postmenarchal girls ages 10 to 17 with familial and nonfamilial heterozygous hypercholesterolemia
Boys and girls: Initially, 10 mg P.O. daily; adjust dosage upward or downward based on lipid levels. Maximum dosage is 20 mg daily.
➤ Prevention of cardiovascular disease in patients without clinically evident coronary heart disease (CHD) but with multiple CHD risk factors
Adults: 10 mg P.O. daily
➤ Prevention of stroke and myocardial infarction in patients with type 2 diabetes who have multiple risk factors for CHD but without clinically evident CHD

Adults: Dosage individualized according to patient characteristics, such as goal of therapy and response according to National Cholesterol Education Program guidelines

Contraindications
• Hypersensitivity to drug or its components
• Active hepatic disease or unexplained, persistent serum transaminase elevations
• Pregnancy or breastfeeding

Precautions
Use cautiously in:
• hypotension, uncontrolled seizures, myopathy, alcoholism
• severe metabolic, endocrine, or electrolyte disorders
• concurrent use of cyclosporine, HIV protease inhibitors tipranavir or lopinavir plus ritonavir, hepatitis C protease inhibitor telaprevir, HMG-CoA reductase inhibitor gemfibrozil (avoid use)
• concurrent use of colchicine, fibric acid products, lipid-modifying doses (1 g/day or more) of niacin, clarithromycin and itraconazole (with atorvastatin dose above 20 mg), or grapefruit juice (more than 1.2 L/day)
• women of childbearing age
• children younger than age 18.

Administration
• Give with or without food.
• Don't give with grapefruit juice or antacids.
• If patient is also taking a CYP450 3A4 inducer (such as efavirenz or rifampin), give simultaneously with atorvastatin because delayed atorvastatin administration after rifampin administration has been associated with a significant reduction in atorvastatin plasma concentration.

Route	Onset	Peak	Duration
P.O.	Unknown	1-2 hr	Unknown

Adverse reactions
CNS: amnesia, abnormal dreams, emotional lability, headache, hyperactivity, poor coordination, malaise, paresthesia, peripheral neuropathy, drowsiness, syncope, weakness
CV: orthostatic hypotension, palpitations, phlebitis, vasodilation, **arrhythmias**
EENT: amblyopia, altered refraction, glaucoma, eye hemorrhage, dry eyes, hearing loss, tinnitus, epistaxis, sinusitis, pharyngitis
GI: nausea, vomiting, diarrhea, constipation, abdominal cramps, abdominal or biliary pain, colitis, indigestion, dyspepsia, flatulence, stomach ulcers, gastroenteritis, melena, tenesmus, glossitis, mouth sores, dry mouth, dysphagia, esophagitis, pancreatitis, **rectal hemorrhage**
GU: hematuria, nocturia, dysuria, urinary frequency or urgency, urinary retention, cystitis, nephritis, renal calculi, abnormal ejaculation, decreased libido, erectile dysfunction, epididymitis
Hematologic: anemia, **thrombocytopenia**
Hepatic: jaundice, **hepatic failure, hepatitis**
Metabolic: hyperglycemia, **hypoglycemia**
Musculoskeletal: bursitis, joint pain, back pain, leg cramps, gout, muscle pain or aches, myositis, myasthenia gravis, neck rigidity, torticollis, **rhabdomyolysis**
Respiratory: dyspnea, pneumonia, bronchitis
Skin: alopecia, acne, contact dermatitis, eczema, dry skin, pruritus, rash, urticaria, skin ulcers, seborrhea, photosensitivity, diaphoresis, **toxic epidermal necrolysis**
Other: taste loss, gingival bleeding, fever, facial paralysis, facial or generalized edema, flulike symptoms, infection, appetite changes, weight gain, allergic reaction, **Stevens-Johnson syndrome**

Interactions
Drug-drug. *Antacids, colestipol, CYP450 3A4 (such as efavirenz, rifampin):* decreased atorvastatin blood level
Azole antifungals, colchicine, cyclosporine, erythromycin, fibric acid derivatives, HIV protease inhibitors, lipid-modifying doses of niacin, other HMG-CoA reductase inhibitors, strong CYP3A4 inhibitors (such as clarithromycin, itraconazole): protease inhibitors: increased risk of myopathy or rhabdomyolysis
Digoxin: increased digoxin level, greater risk of toxicity
Hormonal contraceptives: increased levels of these drugs
Drug-diagnostic tests. *Alanine aminotransferase, aspartate aminotransferase, creatine kinase:* increased levels
Drug-food. *Grapefruit juice:* increased drug blood level, greater risk of adverse effects

Patient monitoring
• Monitor patient for signs and symptoms of allergic response.
◀€ Evaluate for muscle weakness (a symptom of myositis and possibly rhabdomyolysis).
• Be aware that reduction in dosage and periodic monitoring of creatine kinase level may be considered for patients taking drugs that may increase atorvastatin level.
• Monitor liver function test results and blood lipid levels.

Patient teaching
• Tell patient he may take drug with or without food.
◀€ Advise patient to immediately report allergic response, irregular heart beats, unusual bruising or bleeding, unusual tiredness, yellowing of skin or eyes, or muscle weakness.

Reactions in **bold** are life-threatening.   ◀€ Clinical alert

- Caution patient to avoid driving and other hazardous activities until he knows how drug affects concentration, alertness, and vision.
- Inform patient taking hormonal contraceptives that drug increases estrogen levels. Instruct her to tell all prescribers she's taking drug.
- Tell men that drug may cause erectile dysfunction and abnormal ejaculation. Encourage them to discuss these issues with prescriber.
- Tell patient he'll undergo regular blood testing during therapy.
- As appropriate, review all other significant and life-threatening adverse reactions and interactions, especially those related to the drugs, tests, foods, and herbs mentioned above.

atropine sulfate
AtroPen

atropine sulfate ophthalmic

Pharmacologic class: Anticholinergic (antimuscarinic)
Therapeutic class: Antiarrhythmic
Pregnancy risk category C

Action
Inhibits acetylcholine at parasympathetic neuroeffector junction of smooth muscle and cardiac muscle, blocking sinoatrial (SA) and atrioventricular (AV) nodes. These actions increase impulse conduction and raise heart rate. In ophthalmic use, blocks cholinergic stimulation to iris and ciliary bodies, causing pupillary dilation and accommodation paralysis.

Availability
Injection: 0.05 mg/ml, 0.1 mg/ml, 0.3 mg/ml, 0.4 mg/ml, 0.5 mg/ml, 0.8 mg/ml, 1 mg/ml

Ophthalmic solution: 0.5%, 1%, 2%
Tablets: 0.4 mg

🕖 Indications and dosages
➤ Bradyarrhythmias, symptomatic bradycardia
Adults: 0.5 to 1 mg by I.V. push repeated q 3 to 5 minutes as needed, to a maximum dosage of 2 mg
Children: 0.01 mg/kg I.V. to a maximum dosage of 0.4 mg or 0.3 mg/m². May repeat I.V. dose q 4 to 6 hours.
➤ Antidote for anticholinesterase insecticide poisoning
Adults: 2 to 3 mg I.V. repeated q 5 to 10 minutes until symptoms disappear or a toxic level is reached. For severe poisoning, 6 mg q hour.
Children: 0.05 mg/kg I.M. or I.V. repeated q every 10 to 30 minutes until symptoms disappear or a toxic level is reached
➤ Preoperatively to diminish secretions and block cardiac vagal reflexes
Adults and children weighing more than 40.8 kg (90 lb): 0.4 to 0.5 mg I.M., I.V., or subcutaneously 30 to 60 minutes before anesthesia
Children weighing 29.5 to 40.8 kg (65 to 90 lb): 0.4 mg I.M., I.V., or subcutaneously 30 to 60 minutes before anesthesia
Children weighing 18.1 to 29.5 kg (40 to 65 lb): 0.3 mg I.M., I.V., or subcutaneously 30 to 60 minutes before anesthesia
Children weighing 10.9 to 18.1 kg (24 to 40 lb): 0.2 mg I.M., I.V., or subcutaneously 30 to 60 minutes before anesthesia
Children weighing 7.3 to 10.9 kg (16 to 24 lb): 0.15 mg I.M., I.V., or subcutaneously 30 to 60 minutes before anesthesia
Children weighing 3.2 to 7.3 kg (7 to 16 lb): 0.1 mg I.M., I.V., or subcutaneously 30 to 60 minutes before anesthesia
➤ Peptic ulcer disease, functional GI disorders (such as hypersecretory states)
Adults: 0.4 to 0.6 mg P.O. q 4 to 6 hours

Children: 0.01 mg/kg or 0.3/m² P.O. q 4 to 6 hours
➤ Parkinsonism
Adults: 0.1 to 0.25 mg P.O. q.i.d.
➤ Antidote for muscarine-induced mushroom toxicity
Adults: 1 to 2 mg/hour I.M. or I.V. until respiratory function improves
➤ Pupillary dilation in acute inflammatory conditions of iris and uveal tract
Adults: Instill one or two drops of 0.5% or 1% solution into eye(s) up to q.i.d.
Children: Instill one or two drops of 0.5% solution into eye(s) up to t.i.d.
➤ To produce mydriasis and cycloplegia for refraction
Adults: Instill one or two drops of 1% solution into eye(s) 1 hour before refraction.
Children: Instill one or two drops of 0.5% solution into eye(s) b.i.d. for 1 to 3 days before examination.

Off-label uses
• Cholinergic-mediated bronchial asthma

Contraindications
• Hypersensitivity to drug or other belladonna alkaloids
• Acute narrow-angle glaucoma
• Adhesions between iris and lens (ophthalmic form)
• Obstructive GI tract disease
• Unstable cardiovascular status
• Asthma
• Myasthenia gravis
• Thyrotoxicosis
• Infants ages 3 months and younger

Precautions
Use cautiously in:
• chronic renal, hepatic, pulmonary, or cardiac disease
• intra-abdominal infection, prostatic hypertrophy
• elderly patients
• pregnant or breastfeeding patients
• children.

Administration
• For I.V. dose, infuse directly into large vein or I.V. tubing over at least 1 minute.
• Be aware that doses of 0.5 mg may cause paradoxical bradycardia because of central or peripheral parasympathomimetic effects of low doses in adults.
• Don't administer oral dose within 1 hour of giving antacids.
• Be aware that patients with Down syndrome may be unusually sensitive to drug.

Route	Onset	Peak	Duration
P.O.	0.5-2 hr	1-2 hr	4-6 hr
I.V.	Immediate	2-4 min	4-6 hr
I.M., subcut.	Rapid	15-50 min	4-6 hr

Adverse effects
CNS: headache, restlessness, ataxia, disorientation, delirium, insomnia, dizziness, drowsiness, agitation, nervousness, confusion, excitement
CV: palpitations, **bradycardia, tachycardia**
EENT: photophobia, blurred vision, increased intraocular pressure, mydriasis, cycloplegia, nasal congestion
GI: nausea, vomiting, constipation, bloating, dyspepsia, ileus, abdominal distention (in infants), dysphagia, dry mouth
GU: urinary retention, urinary hesitancy, impotence
Skin: decreased sweating, flushing, urticaria, dry skin
Other: thirst, **anaphylaxis**

Interactions
Drug-drug. *Amantadine, antiarrhythmics, anticholinergics, antihistamines, antiparkinsonian drugs, glutethimide, meperidine, muscle relaxants, phenothiazines, tricyclic antidepressants:* increased atropine effects
Antacids, antidiarrheals: decreased atropine absorption

Antimyasthenics: decreased intestinal motility

Cyclopropane: ventricular arrhythmias

Ketoconazole, levodopa: decreased absorption of these drugs

Metoclopramide: decreased effect of atropine on GI motility

Potassium chloride wax-matrix tablets: increased severity of mucosal lesions

Drug-herbs. *Jaborandi tree, pill-bearing spurge:* decreased drug effect

Jimsonweed: changes in cardiovascular function

Squaw vine: reduced metabolic breakdown of drug

Drug-behaviors. *Sun exposure:* increased risk of photophobia

Patient monitoring

◀€ Watch closely for signs and symptoms of anaphylaxis.

• Monitor heart rate for bradycardia or tachycardia.

• Evaluate fluid intake and output.

• Assess for urine retention or urinary hesitancy.

• Monitor for signs and symptoms of glaucoma.

Patient teaching

◀€ Instruct patient to immediately report allergic response.

◀€ Inform patient that headache, eye pain, and blurred vision may signal glaucoma. Tell him to report these symptoms at once.

• Caution patient to avoid driving and other hazardous activities until he knows how drug affects concentration, alertness, and vision.

• Encourage patient to establish an effective bedtime routine to minimize insomnia.

• Tell patient to apply pressure to inside corner of eye during instillation of ophthalmic solution and for 1 to 2 minutes afterward.

• As appropriate, review all other significant and life-threatening adverse reactions and interactions, especially those related to the drugs, herbs, and behaviors mentioned above.

avanafil
Stendra

Pharmacologic class: Phosphodiesterase type 5 (PDE5) inhibitor

Therapeutic class: Erectile dysfunction agent

Pregnancy risk category C

Action

Enhances the effect of nitric oxide by inhibiting PDE5, which is responsible for degradation of cyclic guanosine monophosphate in the corpus cavernosum. Because sexual stimulation is required to initiate the local release of nitric oxide, the inhibition of PDE5 has no effect in the absence of sexual stimulation.

Availability

Tablets: 50 mg, 100 mg, 200 mg

🥼 Indications and dosages

➤ Erectile dysfunction

Adults: Initially, 100 mg P.O. approximately 30 minutes before sexual activity on an as-needed basis. May increase dosage to 200 mg or decrease to 50 mg based on efficacy or tolerability; use the lowest dosage that provides benefit. Not to exceed one dose daily.

Dosage adjustment

• Concurrent use of moderate CYP3A4 inhibitors

• Concurrent use of alpha blockers

Contraindications

• Hypersensitivity to drug or its components

- Concurrent use of any form of organic nitrates

Precautions

Use cautiously in:
- severe hepatic or renal impairment (avoid use)
- mild to moderate hepatic or renal impairment
- patients in whom sexual activity is inadvisable due to CV status (particularly those with left ventricular outflow obstruction, such as aortic stenosis or idiopathic hypertrophic subaortic stenosis, and those with severely impaired autonomic blood pressure control)
- patients who have suffered MI, stroke, life-threatening arrhythmia, or coronary revascularization within the last 6 months; patients with resting hypotension (blood pressure less than 90/50 mm Hg) or hypertension (blood pressure greater than 170/100 mm Hg); patients with unstable angina, angina with sexual intercourse, or New York Heart Association Class 2 or greater congestive heart failure; patients with known hereditary degenerative retinal disorders, including retinitis pigmentosa (use not recommended)
- patients with anatomical deformation of the penis (such as angulation, cavernosal fibrosis, or Peyronie's disease); patients who have conditions that may predispose them to priapism (such as sickle cell anemia, multiple myeloma, or leukemia); patients with bleeding disorders or active peptic ulceration
- concurrent use of strong CYP3A4 inhibitors, CYP 450 inducers, or other PDE5 inhibitors, or erectile dysfunction therapies (use not recommended)
- concurrent use of moderate CYP3A4 inhibitors
- concurrent use of CYP3A4 inducers (not recommended)

- concurrent use of alpha blockers or other antihypertensives or substantial amounts of alcohol
- elderly patients
- women (not indicated)
- children younger than age 18 (safety and efficacy not established).

Administration

◀€ Don't give concurrently with nitrates. In a patient who has taken this drug, where nitrate administration is deemed medically necessary in a life-threatening situation, allow at least 12 hours to elapse after the last dose of avanafil before considering nitrate administration. In such circumstances, administer nitrates under close medical supervision with appropriate hemodynamic monitoring.

Route	Onset	Peak	Duration
P.O.	Unknown	30-45 min	Unknown

Adverse reactions

CNS: headache, dizziness
CV: hypertension, ECG abnormality
EENT: sudden decrease or loss of hearing, tinnitus, nasal congestion, nasopharyngitis, sinusitis, sinus congestion
GI: dyspepsia, nausea, constipation, diarrhea
GU: priapism
Musculoskeletal: back pain, arthralgia
Respiratory: upper respiratory tract infection, bronchitis
Skin: flushing, rash, pruritus
Other: influenza, hypersensitivity

Interactions

Drug-drug. *Alpha blockers (such as alfuzosin, tamsulosin), antihypertensives, nitrates (such as isosorbide, nitroglycerin)*: increased risk of hypotension
Amlodipine: increased avanafil C_{max} and area under the curve (AUC)
CYP2C8 substrates (rosiglitazone): increased rosiglitazone AUC and decreased rosiglitazone C_{max}

Desipramine, omeprazole: increased AUC and C_{max} of these drugs
Moderate CYP3A4 inhibitors (such as amprenavir, aprepitant, diltiazem, erythromycin, fluconazole, fosamprenavir, verapamil), strong CYP3A4 inhibitors (such as atazanavir, clarithromycin, indinavir, itraconazole, ketoconazole, nefazodone, ritonavir, saquinavir, telithromycin): increased avanafil plasma concentration
Drug-food. Grapefruit juice: potentially increased avanafil exposure
High-fat diet: reduced drug absorption, decreased peak level
Drug-behaviors. *Alcohol use (substantial amounts):* increased risk of hypotension

Patient monitoring
• Monitor CV status carefully.
• Monitor patient's hearing.

Patient teaching
• Tell patient to take tablets with or without food but not to take with grapefruit juice.
• Tell patient that high-fat diet may interfere with drug efficacy.
• Advise patient to take drug 30 minutes before sexual activity.
• Tell patient not to exceed prescribed dosage or take more than one dose daily.
◀≋ Instruct patient to stop sexual activity and contact prescriber immediately if chest pain, dizziness, or nausea occurs.
◀≋ Teach patient to recognize and immediately report serious cardiac and vision problems, and sudden decrease in or loss of hearing.
◀≋ Caution patient never to take drug with nitrates, because of risk of significant hypotension.
• Advise patient to avoid or limit alcohol use, because substantial use may cause increase in heart rate, decrease in standing blood pressure, dizziness, and headache.

• Inform patient that this drug can cause serious interactions with many common drugs. Instruct him to tell all prescribers he's taking avanafil.
• Instruct patient not to take other erectile dysfunction drugs while taking this drug.
• Instruct patient to report priapism (persistent, painful erection) or erections lasting more than 4 hours.
• Caution patient to avoid driving and other hazardous activities until he knows how drug affects concentration and alertness.
• As appropriate, review all other significant adverse reactions and interactions, especially those related to the drugs, foods, and behaviors mentioned above.

axitinib
Inlyta

Pharmacologic class: Kinase inhibitor
Therapeutic class: Antineoplastic
Pregnancy risk category D

Action
Inhibits receptor tyrosine kinases, including vascular endothelial growth factor receptors (VEGFR)-1, VEGFR-2, and VEGFR-3 at therapeutic plasma concentrations that are implicated in pathologic angiogenesis, tumor growth, and cancer progression

Availability
Tablets: 1 mg, 5 mg

⏀ Indications and dosages
➤ Advanced renal cell carcinoma after failure of one prior systemic therapy
Adults: Initially, 5 mg P.O. b.i.d., with dosage adjustments based on individual safety and tolerability

Dosage adjustment
- Moderate hepatic impairment
- Moderate to severe proteinuria
- Concurrent use of strong CYP3A4/5 inhibitors

Contraindications
None

Precautions
Use cautiously in:
- moderate hepatic impairment, proteinuria, end-stage renal disease (creatinine clearance less than 15 ml/minute)
- severe hepatic impairment (safety and efficacy not established)
- persistent hypertension, hypothyroidism, reversible posterior leukoencephalopathy syndrome
- patient at increased risk for arterial and venous thrombotic events or GI perforation or fistula
- patient with untreated brain metastasis or recent active GI bleeding (avoid use)
- patient undergoing surgery
- concurrent use of moderate or strong CYP3A4/5 inducers or strong CYP3A4/5 inhibitors, grapefruit, grapefruit juice (avoid use)
- pregnant or breastfeeding patients
- children younger than age 18 (safety and efficacy not established).

Administration
- Administer tablets whole with a glass of water approximately 12 hours apart with or without food.
- Don't give with grapefruit juice.
- Ensure that blood pressure is well controlled and assess thyroid function before starting drug.
- Watch for proteinuria before starting drug; reduce dosage or temporarily interrupt treatment if moderate to severe proteinuria occurs during treatment.
- Evaluate patient for elevated ALT, AST, and bilirubin levels; decrease starting dosage as appropriate in patients with moderate hepatic impairment.
- ◀€ Permanently discontinue drug if signs or symptoms of posterior leukoencephalopathy syndrome occur (such as headache, seizures, lethargy, confusion, blindness, or other visual and neurologic disturbances).
- Stop drug at least 24 hours before scheduled surgery.

Route	Onset	Peak	Duration
P.O.	Unknown	2.5-4.1 hr	Unknown

Adverse reactions
CNS: headache, fatigue, asthenia, **posterior leukoencephalopathy syndrome**
CV: hypertension
GI: nausea, vomiting, diarrhea, constipation, stomatitis, abdominal pain, dyspepsia, **GI perforation or fistula**
GU: proteinuria
Hematologic: hemorrhagic events
Hepatic: increased ALT, AST, and bilirubin levels
Metabolic: hypothyroidism, hypocalcemia, hyperglycemia, hypoglycemia, hyperkalemia, hyponatremia, hypophosphatemia
Musculoskeletal: arthralgia, extremity pain
Respiratory: cough, dyspnea
Skin: rash, dry skin, pruritus, erythema, alopecia
Other: decreased appetite, dysphonia, dysgeusia, weight loss, mucosal inflammation, palmar-plantar erythrodysesthesia syndrome

Interactions
Drug-drug. *Antacids (such as rabeprazole):* decreased axitinib area under the curve and C_{max}
Moderate CYP3A4/5 inducers (such as bosentan, efavirenz, etravirine, modafinil, nafcillin): possibly decreased axitinib plasma exposure
Strong CYP3A4/5 inducers (such as carbamazepine, dexamethasone,

---

Reactions in **bold** are life-threatening.　　◀€ Clinical alert

phenobarbital, phenytoin, rifabutin, rifampin, rifapentin): decreased axitinib plasma exposure

Strong CYP3A4/5 inhibitors (such as ketoconazole): increased axitinib plasma exposure

Drug-diagnostic tests. *Albumin, bicarbonate, calcium, hemoglobin, lymphocytes, phosphorus, platelets, WBCs:* decreased levels

Alkaline phosphatase, ALT, amylase, AST, creatinine, lipase, potassium, sodium: increased levels

Serum glucose: increased or decreased level

Drug-food. *Grapefruit, grapefruit juice:* increased axitinib plasma exposure

Drug-herbs. *St. John's wort:* decreased axitinib plasma exposure

Patient monitoring

• Monitor CBC with differential and renal function (especially for proteinuria) and hepatic function tests closely.

• Continue to monitor thyroid function periodically throughout treatment.

◀≶ Closely monitor patient at risk for arterial and venous thrombotic events, hemorrhagic events, and GI perforation and fistula.

◀≶ Continue to monitor patient for posterior leukoencephalopathy syndrome.

Patient teaching

• Tell patient to take tablets whole with a glass of water approximately 12 hours apart with or without food.

• Tell patient not to take drug with grapefruit juice or grapefruit products.

• Advise patient that hypertension may develop during treatment and that blood pressure should be monitored regularly.

◀≶ Instruct patient to immediately report signs or symptoms of arterial and venous thromboembolic events (such as chest pain or pressure, shortness of breath, numbness or weakness on one side of body, difficulty speaking, or vision changes), bleeding, or persistent or severe abdominal pain.

• Advise patient to report signs and symptoms of decreased thyroid function (such as fatigue, weight gain, depression, sensitivity to cold, brittle hair and nails, and thinning hair).

• Instruct patient to report signs and symptoms of palmar-plantar erythrodysesthesia syndrome (such as redness, swelling, tingling or burning, tenderness, or skin tightness on palms of hands or soles of feet).

• Instruct patient to tell prescriber about all drugs he's taking, because some drugs have potential for serious drug interactions.

• Advise female patient of childbearing age to avoid pregnancy and breastfeeding while taking this drug.

• As appropriate, review all other significant and life-threatening adverse reactions and interactions, especially those related to the drugs, tests, foods, and herbs mentioned above.

azacitidine
Vidaza

Pharmacologic class: Pyrimidine antimetabolite
Therapeutic class: Antineoplastic
Pregnancy risk category D

Action

Unclear. Thought to exert antineoplastic effect by causing DNA hypomethylation and direct cytotoxicity on abnormal hematopoietic bone marrow cells. Cytotoxicity causes death of rapidly growing cells, including cancer cells no longer responsive to normal growth control mechanisms.

Availability

Powder for injection (lyophilized): 100-mg single-use vials

🚺 Indications and dosages

➤ Treatment of the following myelodysplastic syndrome subtypes: refractory anemia or refractory anemia with ringed sideroblasts (if accompanied by neutropenia or thrombocytopenia or requiring transfusion), refractory anemia with excess blasts, refractory anemia with excess blasts in transformation, and chronic myelomonocytic leukemia

Adults: For first treatment cycle: 75 mg/m^2 subcutaneously or I.V. daily for 7 days; for subsequent treatment cycles, repeat cycle every 4 weeks. Dosage may be increased to 100 mg/m^2 if beneficial effect doesn't occur after two cycles and no toxicity (other than nausea and vomiting) develops. Patient should be treated for at least four cycles. Continue therapy as long as patient benefits from it.

Dosage adjustment

• Based on hematologic response (after administration of recommended dosage for first cycle)
• Unexplained serum bicarbonate reduction below 20 mEq/L
• Unexplained blood urea nitrogen or serum creatinine elevation

Off-label uses

• Acute myeloid leukemia

Contraindications

• Hypersensitivity to drug or mannitol
• Advanced malignant hepatic tumor

Precautions

Use cautiously in:
• impaired renal or hepatic function, myelodysplastic syndrome
• pregnant or breastfeeding patients
• children (safety and efficacy not established).

Administration

• Obtain CBC, liver function tests, and serum creatinine level before starting drug.
• For subcutaneous administration, reconstitute with 4 ml sterile water for injection. Inject diluent slowly into vial; invert vial two or three times and rotate gently until uniform suspension appears. Resulting suspension (which will be cloudy) contains azacitidine 25 mg/ml.
• Invert syringe two to three times and gently roll between palms for 30 seconds immediately before administration.
• When giving subcutaneously, divide doses above 4 ml equally in two syringes, and inject subcutaneously in separate sites.
• Administer within 1 hour after reconstitution.
• When giving subcutaneously, rotate sites for each injection (thigh, abdomen, or upper arm). Give new injection at least 1″ from old site and never into tender, bruised, red, or hard area.
• For I.V. administration, reconstitute each vial with 10 ml sterile water for injection. Vigorously shake or roll bottle until all solids have dissolved.
• Prepare I.V. solution by adding reconstituted drug to 50- to 100-ml infusion bag of normal saline solution injection or lactated Ringer's injection.
• Administer I.V. solution over 10 to 40 minutes; administration must be completed within 1 hour of vial reconstitution.

Route	Onset	Peak	Duration
I.V.	Unknown	Unknown	Unknown
Subcut.	Unknown	30 min	Unknown

Adverse reactions

CNS: fatigue, headache, confusion, dizziness, anxiety, depression, insomnia,

---

Reactions in **bold** are life-threatening.   ◀╠ Clinical alert

lethargy, weakness, rigors, malaise, hypoesthesia, **cerebral hemorrhage**

CV: chest pain, cardiac murmur, tachycardia, hypotension, peripheral edema, syncope

EENT: rhinorrhea, epistaxis, sinusitis, nasopharyngitis, pharyngitis, postnasal drip, **eye hemorrhage**

GI: nausea, vomiting, diarrhea, constipation, anorexia, abdominal pain or tenderness, abdominal distention, dyspepsia, hemorrhoids, dysphagia, gingival bleeding, oral mucosal petechiae, stomatitis, tongue ulcers, **mouth hemorrhage**

GU: dysuria, urinary tract infection

Hematologic: anemia, thrombocytopenia, leukopenia, neutropenia, febrile neutropenia, lymphadenopathy, aggravated anemia, **postprocedural hemorrhage, pancytopenia, bone marrow failure**

Musculoskeletal: myalgia, muscle cramps, arthralgia, limb pain, back pain

Respiratory: cough (possibly productive), dyspnea, exertional or exacerbated dyspnea, upper respiratory tract infection, pneumonia, crackles, wheezing, decreased breath sounds, pleural effusion, rhonchi, atelectasis

Skin: lesion, rash, pruritus, herpes simplex, increased sweating, urticaria, dry skin, skin nodule, erythema, pallor, cellulitis

Other: decreased appetite, weight loss, fever, pitting edema, hematoma, night sweats, peripheral swelling, injection-site reactions, tumor lysis syndrome, Sweet's syndrome (acute febrile neutrophilic dermatosis) transfusion reaction, chest-wall pain, postprocedural or other pain, **neutropenic sepsis, septic shock**

Interactions

Drug-diagnostic tests. *Potassium:* decreased

Patient monitoring

• Monitor CBC during therapy.
• Monitor liver function tests and serum creatinine frequently.

• Watch for renal tubular acidosis (serum bicarbonate level below 20 mEq/L associated with alkaline urine and hypokalemia, and serum potassium level below 3 mEq/L).

• Monitor patient for signs and symptoms of tumor lysis syndrome (such as irregular heartbeat, shortness of breath, high potassium level, high uric acid level, impaired mental ability, kidney failure).

Patient teaching

🔊 Instruct patient to call prescriber immediately if shortness of breath, high potassium level, impaired mental ability, rash, easy bruising or bleeding, or respiratory symptoms develop.

• Advise male patient not to father a child during therapy.

• Caution female of childbearing potential to avoid pregnancy and breastfeeding during therapy.

• As appropriate, review all other significant and life-threatening adverse reactions, especially those related to the tests mentioned above.

azathioprine

Apo-Azathioprine✤, Azasan, Gen-Azathioprine✤, Immunoprin⊕, Imuran, Novo-Azathioprine✤

Pharmacologic class: Purine antagonist

Therapeutic class: Immunosuppressant

Pregnancy risk category D

FDA **BOXED WARNING**

• Drug may cause chronic immunosuppression, increasing neoplasia risk. Physicians using it should be familiar with this risk and with possible

---

hematologic toxicities and mutagenic potential in both sexes.

Action

Prevents proliferation and differentiation of activated B and T cells by interfering with synthesis of purine, DNA, and RNA

Availability

Injection: 100-mg vial
Tablets : 50 mg, 75 mg, 100 mg

❶ Indications and dosages

➤ To prevent rejection of kidney transplant

Adults and children: Initially, 3 to 5 mg/kg/day P.O. or I.V. as a single dose. Give on day of transplantation or 1 to 3 days before day of transplantation; then 3 to 5 mg/kg/day I.V. after surgery until patient can tolerate P.O. route. Maintenance dosage is 1 to 3 mg/kg/day P.O.

➤ Rheumatoid arthritis

Adults and children: Initially, 1 mg/kg P.O. or I.V. in one or two daily doses. Increase dosage in steps at 6 to 8 weeks and thereafter at 4-week intervals; use dosage increments of 0.5 mg/kg/day, to a maximum dosage of 2.5 mg/kg/day. Once patient stabilizes, decrease in decrements of 0.5 mg/kg/day to lowest effective dosage.

Dosage adjustment

• Renal disease
• Concurrent allopurinol therapy
• Elderly patients

Off-label uses

• Crohn's disease
• Myasthenia gravis
• Chronic ulcerative colitis

Contraindications

• Hypersensitivity to drug
• Pregnancy or breastfeeding

Precautions

Use cautiously in:
• chickenpox, herpes zoster, impaired hepatic or renal function, decreased bone marrow reserve
• previous therapy with alkylating agents (cyclophosphamide, chlorambucil, melphalan) for rheumatoid arthritis
• elderly patients
• women of childbearing age.

Administration

• Give after meals.
• Be aware that I.V. administration is intended for use only when patients can't tolerate oral medications.

Route	Onset	Peak	Duration
I.V.	Unknown	Unknown	Unknown
P.O.	6-8 wks	12 wks	Unknown

Adverse reactions

CNS: malaise
EENT: retinopathy
GI: nausea, vomiting, diarrhea, stomatitis, esophagitis, anorexia, mucositis, pancreatitis
Hematologic: anemia, **thrombocytopenia, leukopenia, pancytopenia**
Hepatic: jaundice, **hepatotoxicity**
Musculoskeletal: muscle wasting, joint and muscle pain
Skin: rash, alopecia
Other: chills, fever, **serum sickness, neoplasms, serious infection**

Interactions

Drug-drug. *Allopurinol:* increased therapeutic and adverse effects of azathioprine
Angiotensin-converting enzyme (ACE) inhibitors, co-trimoxazole: severe leukopenia
Anticoagulants, cyclosporine: decreased actions of these drugs
Atracurium, pancuronium, tubocurarine, vecuronium: reversal of these drugs' actions

---

Reactions in **bold** are life-threatening. ◀€ Clinical alert

Drugs affecting bone marrow and bone marrow cells (such as ACE inhibitors, co-trimoxazole): severe leukopenia
Drug-diagnostic tests. *Alanine aminotransferase, alkaline phosphatase, amylase, aspartate aminotransferase, bilirubin:* increased levels
Albumin, hemoglobin, uric acid: decreased levels
Urine uric acid: decreased level
Drug-herbs. *Astragalus, echinacea, melatonin:* interference with immunosuppressant action

Patient monitoring

◀≋ Monitor CBC, platelet level, and liver function test results.
• Assess for signs and symptoms of hepatotoxicity (clay-colored stools, pruritus, jaundice, and dark urine).
• Watch for signs and symptoms of infection.
• Monitor for bleeding tendency and hemorrhage.

Patient teaching

◀≋ Tell patient that drug lowers resistance to infection. Instruct him to immediately report fever, cough, breathing problems, chills, and other symptoms.
◀≋ Instruct patient to immediately report unusual bleeding or bruising.
• Tell patient that drug effects may not be obvious for up to 8 weeks in immunosuppression and up to 12 weeks for rheumatoid arthritis relief.
◀≋ Emphasize importance of avoiding pregnancy during therapy and for 4 months afterward.
• Caution patient to avoid activities that may cause injury. Tell him to use soft toothbrush and electric razor to avoid gum and skin injury.
• Advise patient to minimize GI upset by eating small, frequent servings of food and drinking plenty of fluids.
• Tell patient he'll undergo regular blood testing during therapy.

• As appropriate, review all other significant and life-threatening adverse reactions and interactions, especially those related to the drugs, tests, and herbs mentioned above.

azelastine

Astelin, Astepro, Optivar

Pharmacologic class: Histamine 1 (H_1)-receptor antagonist
Therapeutic class: Respiratory inhalant, ophthalmologic agent
Pregnancy risk category C

Action

Selectively antagonizes H_1 and inhibits release of histamine and other mediators from cells (such as mast cells) involved in allergic response. Based on in vitro studies using human cell lines, inhibition of other mediators involved in allergic reactions (such as leukotrienes and platelet-aggregating factor) has also been demonstrated. Decreased chemotaxis and activation of eosinophils has also been demonstrated.

Availability

Nasal spray (Astepro): 0.15% (205.5 mcg in each 0.137-ml spray)
Nasal spray, metered (Astelin): 137-mcg spray
Ophthalmic solution (Optivar): 0.05%

ⓘ Indications and dosages

➤ Seasonal and allergic rhinitis
Adults and children age 12 and older: 1 or 2 sprays (Astelin, Astepro) per nostril b.i.d. or 2 sprays (Astepro) per nostril once daily
Children ages 5 to 11: 1 spray (Astelin) per nostril b.i.d.
➤ Perennial allergic rhinitis, vasomotor rhinitis

Adults and adolescents age 12 and older: 2 sprays (Astelin) per nostril b.i.d.

➤Allergic conjunctivitis

Adults and adolescents age 3 and older: 1 drop (Optivar) in each eye b.i.d.

Contraindications

• Hypersensitivity to drug or its components (Astelin, Optivar)
• None (Astepro)

Precautions

Use cautiously in:

• concurrent use of alcohol and CNS depressants (avoid Astepro use)
• pregnant or breastfeeding patients
• children (safety and efficacy not established for those younger than age 3 [Optivar]; age 5 [Astelin]; age 12 [Astepro]).

Administration

• Follow manufacturer's directions and prime Astelin nasal spray before use.
• Prime Astepro nasal spray before initial use and when it hasn't been used for 3 or more days.
• Be aware that patient shouldn't wear contact lenses when the eyes are red and that Optivar shouldn't be used to treat redness caused by contact lenses.
• Wait 10 minutes before allowing patient to put soft contact lenses back in after Optivar administration, because the preservative benzalkonium chloride may be absorbed.

Route	Onset	Peak	Duration
Nasal	Unknown	2-3 hr	Unknown
Ophthalmic	Unknown	Unknown	Unknown

Adverse reactions

CNS: dizziness (with Astelin); headache, fatigue, somnolence (with Astelin, Astepro)
EENT: transient eye burning or stinging (with Optivar); nasal burning, nasal discomfort, sneezing (with Astepro); pharyngitis, paroxysmal sneezing, rhinitis, epistaxis (with Astelin)
GI: nausea, dry mouth (with Astelin); nasal discomfort (with Astepro); epistaxis (with Astelin, Astepro)
Other: weight increase (with Astelin); bitter taste

Interactions

Drug-drug. *Cimetidine:* increased mean C_{max} and area under the curve of orally administered azelastine
CNS depressants: additional decreased alertness and impairment of CNS performance (with Astelin, Astepro)
Drug-behaviors. *Alcohol use:* decreased alertness and impairment of CNS performance (with Astelin, Astepro)

Patient monitoring

• Monitor patient for bothersome adverse reactions.

Patient teaching

• Instruct patient on proper use of nasal spray and eyedrops.
• Advise patient to avoid other antihistamines, alcohol, and other CNS depressants such as sedatives while using nasal spray.
• Instruct patient to avoid spraying nasal spray into the eyes.
• Advise patient not to wear contact lenses if the eyes are red. Instruct the patient who wears soft contact lenses and whose eyes aren't red to wait at least 10 minutes after instilling eyedrops before inserting contact lenses.
• Caution patient to avoid driving and other hazardous activities until drug's effects on concentration and alertness are known.
• As appropriate, review all other significant adverse reactions and interactions, especially those related to the drugs and behaviors mentioned above.

Reactions in **bold** are life-threatening.   ◀€ Clinical alert

azilsartan medoxomil
Edarbi

Pharmacologic class: Angiotensin II receptor blocker
Therapeutic class: Antihypertensive
Pregnancy risk category D

• When pregnancy is detected, discontinue drug as soon as possible.
• Drugs that act directly on the renin angiotensin system can cause injury and death to a developing fetus.

Action
Inhibits the pressor effects of an angiotensin II infusion in a dose-related manner. Effects of angiotensin II, the principal pressor agent of the renin-angiotensin system, include vasoconstriction, aldosterone release, and sodium reabsorption from the kidneys.

Availability
Tablets: 40 mg, 80 mg

Indications and dosages
➤ Hypertension alone or in combination with other antihypertensives
Adults: 80 mg P.O. daily. Consider a starting dose of 40 mg for patients who are being treated with high-dose diuretics

Contraindications
None

Precautions
Use cautiously in
• renal impairment, renal artery stenosis

• hypotension in volume- or salt-depleted patients
• patients whose renal function may depend on activity of the renin-angiotensin system
• elderly patients
• pregnant or breastfeeding patients
• children younger than age 18 (safety and efficacy not established).

Administration
• Administer with or without food.
• Correct volume or salt depletion before starting drug.

Route	Onset	Peak	Duration
P.O.	Unknown	1.5-3 hr	Unknown

Adverse reactions
CV: hypotension, orthostatic hypotension
GI: diarrhea
GU: oliguria or progressive azotemia with acute renal failure (rare)
Other: death (rare)

Interactions
Drug-drug. NSAIDs, including selective COX inhibitors: deteriorated renal function, including possible acute renal failure in patients who are elderly, volume-depleted, or who have compromised renal function; attenuated azilsartan antihypertensive effect
Drug-diagnostic tests. Serum creatinine: small reversible increases

Patient monitoring
• Watch for hypotension in volume- or salt-depleted patients, such as those receiving high-dose diuretics.
• Observe for increasing serum creatinine level in patients with moderate to severe renal impairment and worsening renal function in elderly patients and those receiving NSAIDs, including COX-2 inhibitors.
◀ Watch for oliguria or progressive azotemia that could possibly lead to

acute renal failure and death in patients whose renal function depends on the activity of the renin-angiotensin system (such as patients with severe congestive heart failure, renal artery stenosis or volume depletion).

Patient teaching
• Tell patient to take drug with or without food.
◀€ Instruct patient to promptly report changes in urinary function.
• Advise female patient of childbearing age to immediately notify prescriber if she becomes pregnant.
• Because of the potential for adverse effects in the breastfeeding infant, a decision should be made whether to discontinue breastfeeding or discontinue drug, taking into account importance of drug to the mother.
• As appropriate, review all significant and life-threatening adverse reactions and interactions, especially those related to the drugs and tests mentioned above.

azithromycin, azithromycin dihydrate
Azasite, Zithromax, Zmax

Pharmacologic class: Macrolide
Therapeutic class: Anti-infective
Pregnancy risk category B

Action
Bactericidal and bacteriostatic; inhibits protein synthesis after binding with 50S ribosomal subunit of susceptible organisms. Demonstrates cross-resistance to erythromycin-resistant gram-positive strains and resistance to most strains of *Enterococcus faecalis* and methicillin-resistant *Staphylococcus aureus.*

Availability
Oral suspension: 100 mg/5 ml in 15-ml bottles; 200 mg/5 ml in 15-ml, 22.5-ml, and 30-ml bottles
Oral suspension (Zmax extended-release): 2-g bottle
Powder for injection: 500 mg in 10-ml vials
Powder for oral suspension: 100 mg/ 5 ml, 200 mg/5 ml, 1,000 mg/packet
Solution (ophthalmic): 1% in 5-ml bottle filled with 2.5 ml solution
Tablets: 250 mg, 500 mg, 600 mg
Tablets (Tri-Pak): three 500-mg tablets
Tablets (Z-Pak): six 250-mg tablets

Indications and dosages
➤ Bacterial conjunctivitis caused by CDC coryneform group G, *H. influenzae, S. aureus, Streptococcus mitis* group, and *S. pneumoniae*
Adults: Instill 1 drop in affected eye(s) b.i.d., 8 to 12 hours apart for first 2 days then instill 1 drop in affected eye(s) once daily for next 5 days
➤ Mild community-acquired pneumonia
Adults: 500 mg P.O. on first day, then 250 mg/day for next 4 days. Or, 2 g P.O. as single dose (extended-release oral suspension).
Children ages 6 months and older: 10 mg/kg P.O. (no more than 500 mg/dose) on day 1, then 5 mg/kg (no more than 25 mg/dose) for 4 more days
➤ Community-acquired pneumonia caused by *Chlamydia pneumoniae, Haemophilus influenzae, Mycoplasma pneumoniae, Streptococcus pneumoniae, Legionella pneumophila, Moraxella catarrhalis,* and *S. aureus*
Adults and adolescents ages 16 and older: 500 mg I.V. daily for at least two doses, then 500 mg P.O. daily for total of 7 to 10 days
Children ages 6 months to 16 years: 10 mg/kg P.O. as a single dose on day 1, then 5 mg/kg P.O. on day 2 through 5

➤ Pharyngitis and tonsillitis
Adults: 500 mg P.O. on day 1, then 250 mg/day for next 4 days, to a total dosage of 1.5 g
Children ages 2 and older: 12 mg/kg P.O. daily for 5 days. Maximum dosage is 500 mg.

➤ Skin and skin-structure infections
Adults: 500 mg P.O. on first day, then 250 mg/day for next 4 days, to total dosage of 1.5 g

➤ Acute bacterial sinusitis
Adults: 500 mg P.O. daily for 3 days; or, 2 g P.O. as single dose (extended-release oral suspension)
Children ages 6 months and older: 10 mg/kg (maximum, 500 mg) P.O. daily for 3 days

➤ Mild to moderate acute exacerbation of chronic obstructive pulmonary disease
Adults: 500 mg/day for 3 days or 500 mg P.O. on day 1, then 250 mg P.O. daily on days 2 through 5; or, 2 g P.O. (extended-release oral suspension) as single dose

➤ Pelvic inflammatory disease caused by *Chlamydia trachomatis*, *Neisseria gonorrhoeae*, or *Mycoplasma hominis*
Adults: 500 mg I.V. daily on days 1 and 2, then 250 mg P.O. daily for a total of 7 days. If anaerobes are suspected, give continually with appropriate anti-anaerobic antibiotic, as ordered.

➤ Nongonococcal urethritis or cervicitis caused by *C. trachomatis;* genital ulcers caused by *Haemophilus ducreyi* (chancroid)
Adults: 1 g P.O. as a single dose

➤ Urethritis and cervicitis caused by *N. gonorrhoeae*
Adults: 2 g P.O. as a single dose

➤ To prevent disseminated *Mycobacterium avium* complex disease in patients with advanced human immunodeficiency virus
Adults: 1.2 g P.O. once weekly (given alone or with rifabutin)

➤ Acute otitis media
Children ages 6 months and older: 30 mg/kg as a single dose or 10 mg/kg once daily for 3 days; or 10 mg/kg as a single dose on day 1, followed by 5 mg/kg on days 2 through 5

Off-label uses

• Uncomplicated gonococcal infections of cervix, urethra, rectum, and pharynx

Contraindications

• Hypersensitivity to drug, erythromycin, or other macrolide anti-infectives
• None (ophthalmic solution)

Precautions

Use cautiously in:
• severe hepatic impairment, severe renal insufficiency, prolonged QT interval
• breastfeeding patients.

Administration

• Obtain specimens for culture and sensitivity testing before starting therapy.
• Administer tablets and single-dose packets with or without food.
• Give oral suspension 1 hour before meals or 2 hours afterward. With 1-g packet, or single 2-g bottles, mix entire contents in 2 oz of water.
🔇 Don't administer as I.V. bolus or I.M. injection.
• For I.V. use, reconstitute 500-mg vial with 4.8 ml of sterile water for injection.
• As appropriate, dilute solution further using normal or half-normal saline solution, dextrose 5% in water, or lactated Ringer's solution.
• Infuse injection over no less than 60 minutes. Infuse 1 mg/ml over 3 hours or 2 mg/2 ml over 1 hour.
• Know that 1,000-mg packet and extended-release oral suspension aren't for pediatric use.

Route	Onset	Peak	Duration
P.O.	Rapid	2.5-3.2 hr	24 hr
I.V.	Rapid	End of infusion	24 hr

Adverse reactions

CNS: dizziness, drowsiness, fatigue, headache, vertigo
CV: chest pain, palpitations
EENT: eye irritation (with ophthalmic use)
GI: nausea, diarrhea, abdominal pain, cholestatic jaundice, dyspepsia, flatulence, melena, **pseudomembranous colitis**
GU: nephritis, vaginitis, candidiasis
Metabolic: hyperglycemia, **hyperkalemia**
Skin: photosensitivity, rashes, angioedema
Other: overgrowth of nonsusceptible organisms (with prolonged use)

Interactions

Drug-drug. *Antacids containing aluminum or magnesium:* decreased peak azithromycin blood level
Arrhythmias (such as amiodarone, quinidine): increased risk of life-threatening arrhythmias
Carbamazepine, cyclosporine, digoxin, dihydroergotamine, ergotamine, hexobarbital, phenytoin, theophylline, triazolam: increased blood levels of these drugs
HMG-CoA reductase inhibitors (such as atorvastatin, lovastatin): increased risk of myopathy or rhabdomyolysis
Pimozide: prolonged QT interval, ventricular tachycardia
Warfarin: increased International Normalized Ratio
Drug-food. *Any food:* decreased absorption of multidose oral suspension
Drug-behaviors. *Sun exposure:* photosensitivity

Patient monitoring

• Monitor temperature, white blood cell count, and culture and sensitivity results.

• Assess for signs and symptoms of infection.
• Monitor patients at risk for cardiac arrhythmia.

Patient teaching

• Tell patient he may take tablets with or without food.
• Advise patient to take suspension 1 hour before or 2 hours after meals.
• Remind patient to complete entire course of therapy as ordered, even after symptoms improve.
• Advise patient not to wear contact lenses if signs or symptoms of bacterial conjunctivitis exist.
• As appropriate, review all other significant and life-threatening adverse reactions and interactions, especially those related to the drugs, foods, and behaviors mentioned above.

aztreonam, aztreonam lysine
Azactam, Cayston

Pharmacologic class: Monobactam
Therapeutic class: Anti-infective
Pregnancy risk category B

Action

Inhibits bacterial cell-wall synthesis during active multiplication by binding with penicillin-binding protein 3, resulting in cell-wall destruction

Availability

Inhalation solution: 75-mg single-use vial
Powder for injection: 500-mg vial, 1-g vial, 2-g vial, 1 g/50-ml I.V. bag, 2 g/50-ml I.V. bag

---

Reactions in **bold** are life-threatening.   ◀€ Clinical alert

⊘ Indications and dosages

➤ Cystic fibrosis in patients with *Pseudomonas aeruginosa*

Adults and children age 7 and older: 75 mg t.i.d. at least 4 hours apart for 28-day course, followed by 28 days off

➤ Infections caused by susceptible gram-negative organisms

Adults: For urinary tract infections, 500 mg or 1 g I.M. or I.V. q 8 or 12 hours; for moderately severe systemic infections, 1 or 2 g I.M. or I.V. q 8 or 12 hours; for severe or life-threatening infections, 2 g I.M. or I.V. q 6 or 8 hours. Maximum dosage is 8 g/day.

Children: For mild to moderate infections, 30 mg/kg I.M. or I.V. q 8 hours; for moderate to severe infections, 30 mg/kg I.M. or I.V. q 6 or 8 hours. Maximum dosage is 120 mg/kg/day.

Dosage adjustment

- Severe renal failure

Contraindications

- Hypersensitivity ˅ drug or its components

Precautions

Use cautiously in:
- renal or hepatic impairment
- elderly patients
- pregnant or breastfeeding patients.

Administration

- Flush I.V. tubing with compatible solution before and after giving drug.
- Compatible solutions include 0.9% sodium chloride injection, 5% or 10% dextrose injection, Ringer's or lactated Ringer's injection, 5% dextrose and 0.9% sodium chloride injection, and 5% dextrose and 0.45% sodium chloride injection.
- After adding diluent to vial or infusion bottle, shake immediately and vigorously.
- For I.V. bolus injection, reconstitute powder for injection by adding 6 to 10 ml of sterile water for injection. Inject prescribed dosage into tubing of compatible I.V. solution slowly over 3 to 5 minutes.
- For intermittent I.V. infusion, reconstitute powder for injection by adding compatible I.V. solution to yield a concentration not exceeding 20 mg/ml. Administer prescribed dosage over 20 to 60 minutes.
- 🔊 Thaw commercially available frozen drug at room temperature and give by intermittent I.V. infusion only.
- For I.M. injection, reconstitute powder for injection by adding 3 ml of sterile water for injection or 0.9% sodium chloride injection.
- Give I.M. injection deep into large muscle mass.
- Reconstitute inhalation solution with 1 ml sterile diluent supplied and administer only with nebulizer supplied. Don't reconstitute until ready to administer.
- Know that patient should use a bronchodilator as prescribed before using inhalation solution.

Route	Onset	Peak	Duration
I.V., I.M.	Organism & dose dependent	1 hr	4-12 hr
Inhalation	Unknown	1 hr	Unknown

Adverse reactions

CNS: dizziness, confusion, **seizures**
CV: phlebitis, **thrombophlebitis**
EENT: diplopia, tinnitus
GI: nausea, vomiting, diarrhea (including diarrhea associated with *Clostridium difficile*), **pseudomembranous colitis**
Hematologic: neutropenia, **pancytopenia**
Hepatic: hepatitis
Respiratory: bronchospasm
Skin: rash, **toxic epidermal necrolysis**
Other: altered taste, angioedema, **anaphylaxis**

Interactions

Drug-drug. *Aminoglycosides:* increased risk of nephrotoxicity and ototoxicity
Beta-lactamase-inducing antibiotics (such as cefoxitin, imipenem): antagonism with aztreonam
Furosemide, probenecid: increased aztreonam levels
Drug-diagnostic tests. *Alanine aminotransferase (ALT), aspartate aminotransferase (AST), creatinine, eosinophils, platelets, prothrombin time (PT), partial thromboplastin time (PTT):* increased values
Coombs' test: positive result
Neutrophils: decreased count

Patient monitoring

◀€ Assess patient closely for signs and symptoms of pseudomembranous colitis.
◀€ Monitor patient carefully for hypersensitivity reaction, especially if he's allergic to penicillin, carbapenems or cephalosporins.
• Monitor CBC with differential, AST, ALT, PT, PTT, and serum creatinine values.
• Monitor renal and hepatic function.

Patient teaching

• Show patient how to reconstitute inhalation solution using diluent supplied and tell patient not to reconstitute until ready to use. Advise patient to use only the nebulizer supplied and to use a bronchodilator as prescribed before using inhalation solution.
◀€ Instruct patient to immediately report severe diarrhea or signs or symptoms of hypersensitivity reaction, such as rash or difficulty breathing.
• Tell female patient to notify prescriber if she is pregnant or breastfeeding.
• As appropriate, review all other significant and life-threatening adverse reactions and interactions, especially those related to the tests mentioned above.

baclofen

Apo-Baclofen✦, Baclofen, Gen-Baclofen✦, Kemstro, Lioresal, Lioresal Intrathecal, Liotec✦, Lyflex⊕, Nu-Baclo✦, PMS-Baclofen✦

Pharmacologic class: Skeletal muscle relaxant
Therapeutic class: Antispasmodic
Pregnancy risk category C

FDA | BOXED WARNING

• With intrathecal form, abrupt withdrawal may cause high fever, altered mental status, exaggerated rebound spasticity, and muscle rigidity; in rare cases, patient progresses to rhabdomyolysis, multisystem failure, and death. To prevent abrupt withdrawal, pay careful attention to programming and monitoring of infusion system, refill scheduling and procedures, and pump alarms. Advise patients and caregivers of importance of keeping scheduled refill visits, and teach about early drug withdrawal symptoms. Give special attention to patients at apparent risk (those with spinal cord injuries at T6 or above, communication problems, or history of withdrawal symptoms from oral or intrathecal baclofen).

Action

Relaxes muscles by acting specifically at spinal end of upper motor neurons

Availability

Intrathecal injection: 10 mg/20 ml (500 mcg/ml), 10 mg/5 ml (2,000 mcg/ml)
Tablets: 10 mg, 20 mg

Reactions in **bold** are life-threatening.   ◀€ Clinical alert

Ⓘ Indications and dosages

➤ Reversible spasticity associated with multiple sclerosis or spinal cord lesions

Adults: Initially, 5 mg P.O. t.i.d. May increase by 5 mg q 3 days to a maximum dosage of 80 mg/day.

Children ages 4 and older: 25 to 1,200 mcg/day by intrathecal infusion; (average is 275 mcg/day); dosage determined by response during screening phase.

➤ Severe spasticity in patients who don't respond to or can't tolerate oral baclofen

Adults: *Screening phase*—Before pump implantation and intrathecal infusion, give test dose to check responsiveness. Administer 1 ml of 50 mcg/ml dilution over 1 minute by barbotage into intrathecal space. Within 4 to 8 hours, muscle spasms should become less severe or frequent and muscle tone should decrease; if patient's response is inadequate, give second test dose of 75 mcg/1.5 ml 24 hours after first dose. If patient is still unresponsive, may give final test dose of 100 mcg/2 ml 24 hours later. Patients unresponsive to 100-mcg dose aren't candidates for intrathecal baclofen. Following appropriate responsiveness, adjust dosage to twice the screening dose and give over 24 hours. If screening dose efficacy is maintained for 12 hours, don't double the dosage. After 24 hours, increase dosage slowly as needed and tolerated by 10% to 30% daily.

Maintenance therapy—During prolonged maintenance therapy, adjust daily dosage by 10% to 40% as needed and tolerated to maintain adequate control of symptoms. Maintenance dosage ranges from 12 mcg to 2,000 mcg daily.

Dosage adjustment

• Renal impairment
• Seizure disorders
• Elderly patients

Off-label uses

• Cerebral palsy
• Tardive dyskinesia
• Trigeminal neuralgia

Contraindications

• Hypersensitivity to drug
• Rheumatic disorders

Precautions

Use cautiously in:
• renal impairment
• epilepsy
• patients who use spasticity to maintain posture and balance
• elderly patients
• pregnant or breastfeeding patients
• children.

Administration

• Give oral doses with food or milk.
• Dilute only with sterile, preservative-free sodium chloride for injection.
• Know that intrathecal infusion should be performed only by personnel who have been trained in the procedure.

Route	Onset	Peak	Duration
P.O.	Unknown	2-3 hr	Unknown
Intrathecal	0.5-1 hr	4 hr	4-8 hr

Adverse reactions

CNS: dizziness, drowsiness, fatigue, confusion, depression, headache, insomnia, hypotonia, difficulty speaking, **seizures**
CV: edema, hypotension, hypertension, palpitations
EENT: blurred vision, tinnitus, nasal congestion
GI: nausea, vomiting, constipation
GU: urinary frequency, dysuria, erectile dysfunction
Metabolic: hyperglycemia
Skin: pruritus, rash, sweating
Other: weight gain, hypersensitivity reactions

Interactions

Drug-drug. *CNS depressants:* increased baclofen effect

MAO inhibitors: increased CNS depression, hypotension

Tricyclic antidepressants, drugs causing CNS depression: hypotonia, increased CNS depression

Drug-diagnostic tests. *Alkaline phosphatase, aspartate aminotransferase, glucose:* increased levels

Drug-behaviors. *Alcohol use:* CNS depression

Patient monitoring

• During intrathecal infusion, check pump often for proper functioning and check catheter for patency.

• Monitor patient's response continually to determine appropriate dosage adjustment.

◀ Observe closely for signs and symptoms of overdose (drowsiness, light-headedness, dizziness, respiratory depression), especially during initial screening and titration. No specific antidote exists. Immediately remove any solution from pump; if patient has respiratory depression, intubate until drug is eliminated.

Patient teaching

• Advise patient to take oral dose with food or milk.

• Instruct patient to avoid driving and other hazardous activities until he knows how drug affects concentration and alertness.

• Caution patient not to discontinue drug therapy abruptly. Doing so may cause hallucinations and rebound spasticity.

• Advise patient to avoid alcohol and other depressants such as sedatives while taking drug.

• As appropriate, review all other significant and life-threatening adverse reactions and interactions, especially those related to the drugs, tests, and behaviors mentioned above.

balsalazide disodium

Colazal, Colazide ✙

b

Pharmacologic class: GI agent
Therapeutic class: Anti-inflammatory
Pregnancy risk category B

Action

Metabolized in colon to mesalamine and then to 5-aminosalicylic acid, both of which are thought to exert local anti-inflammatory effect by inhibiting prostaglandin and acid metabolites.

Availability

Capsules: 750 mg

Indications and dosages

➤ Mildly to moderately active ulcerative colitis

Adults: Usual dosage, three 750-mg capsules P.O. t.i.d. (6.75 g daily) for up to 8 weeks; some patients may require 12 weeks

Children ages 5 to 17: Usual dosage, either three 750-mg capsules P.O. t.i.d. (6.75 g daily) for up to 8 weeks, or one 750-mg capsule P.O. t.i.d. (2.25 g daily) for up to 8 weeks

Contraindications

• Hypersensitivity to balsalazide, salicylates, or mesalamine

Precautions

Use cautiously in:
• renal impairment
• pyloric stenosis
• breastfeeding patients
• children younger than age 5 (safety and efficacy not established).

Administration

• Advise patient to swallow capsules whole, either always with or always without food.

• For those patients who can't swallow capsules whole, carefully open capsules and sprinkle contents on applesauce and have patient swallow contents immediately without chewing.

Route	Onset	Peak	Duration
P.O.	Unknown	1-2 hr	Unknown

Adverse reactions

CNS: headache, insomnia, dizziness, anxiety, confusion, agitation, **coma**
EENT: blurred vision, eye irritation, tinnitus, earache, epistaxis, sinusitis, sore throat, nasopharyngitis
GI: nausea, vomiting, diarrhea, constipation, abdominal pain, dyspepsia, anorexia, oral blisters, oral candidiasis, **GI hemorrhage**
GU: urinary tract infection
Musculoskeletal: arthralgia; myalgia; bone, back, neck, or limb pain
Respiratory: cough, upper respiratory tract infection
Skin: erythema
Other: generalized pain

Interactions

Drug-drug. *Oral antibiotics:* interference with balsalazide action

Patient monitoring

• Assess character and frequency of stools.
• Monitor CBC and liver and kidney function test results.

Patient teaching

• Instruct patient to take drug only as directed.
• Instruct patient to carefully open capsules and sprinkle contents on applesauce and swallow contents immediately without chewing if patient can't swallow capsules whole.
• Tell patient that teeth and tongue staining may occur when drug is taken by sprinkling on applesauce.
• As appropriate, review all other significant and life-threatening adverse reactions and interactions, especially those related to the drugs mentioned above.

basiliximab
Simulect

Pharmacologic class: Monoclonal antibody
Therapeutic class: Immunosuppressant
Pregnancy risk category B

FDA BOXED WARNING

• Give under supervision of physician experienced in immunosuppressive therapy and management of organ transplant recipients, in facility with adequate diagnostic and treatment resources.

Action

Blocks specific interleukin-2 (IL-2) receptor sites on activated T lymphocytes. Specific binding competitively inhibits IL-2-mediated activation and differentiation of lymphocytes responsible for cell-mediated immunity. Also impairs immunologic response to antigenic challenges.

Availability

Powder for injection: 10 mg, 20 mg in single-use vials

Indications and dosages

➤ Prevention of acute organ rejection in kidney transplantation
Adults and children weighing 35 kg (77 lb) or more: 20 mg I.V. 2 hours before transplantation surgery, then 20 mg I.V. 4 days after surgery. Withhold second dose if complications, hypersensitivity reaction, or graft loss occurs.

Children weighing less than 35 kg (77 lb): 10 mg I.V. 2 hours before transplantation surgery, then 10 mg I.V. 4 days after surgery. Withhold second dose if complications, hypersensitivity reaction, or graft loss occurs.

Contraindications
- Hypersensitivity to drug
- Pregnancy or breastfeeding

Precautions
Use cautiously in:
- elderly patients
- females of childbearing age.

Administration
◀€ Give by central or peripheral I.V. route only.
- Reconstitute by adding 5 ml of sterile water for injection to vial for bolus injection, or dilute with normal saline solution or dextrose 5% in water to a volume of 50 ml and infuse over 20 to 30 minutes. Discard any remaining product after preparing each dose.
- Don't infuse other drugs simultaneously through same I.V. line.
- Know that drug should be used only as part of regimen that includes cyclosporine and corticosteroids.

Route	Onset	Peak	Duration
I.V.	2 hr	Unknown	36 days

Adverse reactions
CNS: headache, insomnia, paresthesia, dizziness, drowsiness, tremor, anxiety, confusion, **coma, seizures**
CV: palpitations, edema, chest pain, ECG abnormalities, hypotension, hypertension, **prolonged QT interval**
EENT: blurred vision, eye irritation, tinnitus, earache, epistaxis, nasopharyngitis, sinusitis
GI: nausea, vomiting, diarrhea, constipation, abdominal pain, dyspepsia, anorexia, oral blisters, oral candidiasis, **GI hemorrhage**

GU: urinary incontinence, intermenstrual bleeding, **oliguria, renal failure**
Hematologic: anemia, **disseminated intravascular coagulation, hemorrhage, neutropenia, thrombocytopenia**
Metabolic: hypokalemia, hypomagnesemia, hyperglycemia, **acidosis, hypoglycemia, hyperkalemia**
Musculoskeletal: bone, back, neck, or limb pain
Respiratory: dyspnea, cough, hypoxia, tachypnea, hemoptysis, upper respiratory tract infection, **pleural effusions**
Skin: bruising, pruritus, dermatitis, skin lesions, diaphoresis, night sweats, erythema, hyperpigmentation, urticaria
Other: fever, lymphadenopathy, facial edema, bacterial infection, herpes simplex infection, injection site erythema, hypersensitivity reaction, **sepsis**

Interactions
Drug-drug. *Immunosuppressants:* additive immunosuppression
Drug-diagnostic tests. *Calcium, glucose, potassium:* increased or decreased levels
Hemoglobin, neutrophils, platelets: decreased values
Triglycerides: increased levels
White blood cells: decreased levels
Drug-herbs. *Astragalus, echinacea, melatonin:* interference with immunosuppressant action

Patient monitoring
◀€ Watch for signs and symptoms of hypersensitivity reaction. Keep emergency drugs at hand in case these occur.
- Monitor vital signs and observe patient frequently during I.V. infusion.
- Monitor laboratory values and drug blood level.

Patient teaching
- Teach patient about purpose of therapy. Explain that drug decreases the risk of acute organ rejection.

Reactions in **bold** are life-threatening.   ◀€ Clinical alert

- Tell patient he may be more susceptible to infection because of drug's immunosuppressant effect.
- Inform patient that he'll need lifelong immunosuppressant drug therapy.
- Advise women of childbearing age to use reliable contraception before, during, and for 2 months after therapy.
- As appropriate, review all other significant and life-threatening adverse reactions and interactions, especially those related to the drugs, tests, and herbs mentioned above.

beclomethasone dipropionate

AeroBec⊕, Apo-Beclomethasone✦, Asmabec⊕, Beclodisk✦⊕, Becloforte✦⊕, Beconase AQ Nasal Spray, Filair⊕, Hayfever Relief⊕, Nasobec⊕, Pollenase Nasal⊕, QVAR, Rivanase✦

Pharmacologic class: Corticosteroid
Therapeutic class: Anti-inflammatory agent
Pregnancy risk category C

Action

Unclear. May decrease inflammation by stabilizing leukocytic lysosomal membrane, decreasing number and activity of inflammatory cells, inhibiting bronchoconstriction (leading to direct smooth muscle relaxation), and reducing airway hyperresponsiveness.

Availability

Inhalation aerosol: 40-mcg metered inhalation in 7.3-g canister; 80-mcg metered inhalation in 7.3-g canister
Inhalation capsules: 100 mcg, 200 mcg
Nasal spray: 0.042% (25-g bottle containing 180 metered inhalations)

⊘ Indications and dosages

➤ Maintenance treatment of asthma as prophylaxis; asthma patients who require systemic steroids for whom adding an inhaled steroid may reduce or eliminate the need for systemic steroids

Adults and children ages 12 and older: When previous therapy was bronchodilator alone, 40 to 80 mcg by oral inhalation (QVAR) b.i.d.; maximum of 320 mcg b.i.d. When previous therapy was inhaled steroid, 40 to 160 mcg by oral inhalation (QVAR) b.i.d.; maximum of 320 mcg b.i.d.

Children ages 5 to 11: When previous therapy was bronchodilator alone, 40 mcg by oral inhalation (QVAR) b.i.d.; maximum of 80 mcg b.i.d. When previous therapy was inhaled steroid, 40 mcg by oral inhalation (QVAR) b.i.d.; maximum of 80 mcg b.i.d.

➤ Seasonal or perennial rhinitis
Adults and children ages 12 and older: One or two inhalations (42 to 84 mcg Beconase AQ Nasal Spray) in each nostril b.i.d.

Children ages 6 to 12: One inhalation (42 mcg Beconase AQ Nasal Spray) in each nostril b.i.d.

Contraindications

- Hypersensitivity to drug
- Status asthmaticus

Precautions

Use cautiously in:
- active untreated infections, diabetes mellitus, glaucoma, underlying immunosuppression
- patients receiving concurrent systemic corticosteroids
- pregnant or breastfeeding patients
- children younger than age 6.

Administration

- Use spacer device to ensure proper delivery of dose and to help prevent candidiasis and hoarseness.

• After inhalation, tell patient to hold his breath for a few seconds before exhaling.
• For greater efficacy, wait 1 minute between inhalations.
• If patient is also receiving a bronchodilator, administer it at least 15 minutes before beclomethasone.
• Discontinue drug after 3 weeks if symptoms don't improve markedly.

Route	Onset	Peak	Duration
Inhalation (nasal)	5-7 days	3 wk	Unknown
Inhalation (oral)	1-4 wk	Unknown	Unknown

Adverse reactions
CNS: headache
EENT: cataracts, nasal irritation or congestion, epistaxis, perforated nasal septum, nasopharyngeal or oropharyngeal fungal infections, hoarseness, throat irritation
GI: esophageal candidiasis
Metabolic: adrenal suppression
Respiratory: cough, wheezing, **bronchospasm**
Skin: urticaria, **angioedema**
Other: anosmia, Churg-Strauss syndrome, hypersensitivity reactions

Interactions
None significant

Patient monitoring
• Assess patient's mouth daily for signs of fungal infection.
• Observe patient for proper inhaler use.

Patient teaching
• Instruct patient to hold inhaled drug in airway for several seconds before exhaling and to wait 1 minute between inhalations.
• Advise patient to rinse mouth after using inhaler and to wash and dry inhaler thoroughly to help prevent fungal infections and sore throat.

• Encourage patient to document use of drug and his response in a diary.
• If patient is also using a bronchodilator, teach him to use it at least 15 minutes before beclomethasone.
• As appropriate, review all other significant and life-threatening adverse reactions.

b

benazepril hydrochloride
Apo-Benazepril✲, Lotensin

Pharmacologic class: Angiotensin-converting enzyme (ACE) inhibitor
Therapeutic class: Antihypertensive
Pregnancy risk category C (first trimester), *D* (second and third trimesters)

FDA BOXED WARNING

• When used during second or third trimester of pregnancy, drug may cause fetal injury and death. Discontinue as soon as possible when pregnancy is detected.

Action
Inhibits conversion of angiotensin I to angiotensin II, a vasoconstrictor that stimulates adrenal glands and promotes aldosterone secretion, thereby reducing sodium and water reabsorption and ultimately decreasing blood pressure. Decreased angiotensin also causes increased potassium level and fluid loss.

Availability
Tablets: 5 mg, 10 mg, 20 mg, 40 mg

⟡ Indications and dosages
➤ Hypertension
Adults: Initially, 5 to 10 mg/day P.O. as a single dose. Increase gradually to a maintenance dosage of 20 to 40 mg/day

---

Reactions in **bold** are life-threatening. ◀€ Clinical alert

as a single dose or in two divided doses. (Start with 5 mg/day in patients receiving diuretics.)

Dosage adjustment

• Renal impairment

Off-label uses

• Myocardial infarction
• Nephropathy

Contraindications

• Hypersensitivity to drug or to other ACE inhibitors
• Angioedema with or without previous ACE inhibitor treatment

Precautions

Use cautiously in:
• renal or hepatic impairment, hypovolemia, hyponatremia, aortic stenosis, hypertrophic cardiomyopathy, cerebrovascular or cardiac insufficiency
• patients receiving concurrent diuretics
• black patients
• elderly patients
• pregnant patients (use not recommended, particularly in second and third trimesters)
• breastfeeding patients
• children.

Administration

◀᪶ Use extreme caution if patient has family history of angioedema.
• When giving concurrently with diuretics, know that drug may cause excessive hypotension. If possible, stop diuretic therapy 2 to 3 days before starting benazepril.
• Give with or without food.
• Know that drug may be used alone or in conjunction with other antihypertensives.

Route	Onset	Peak	Duration
P.O.	0.5-1 hr	3-4 hr	24 hr

Adverse reactions

CNS: dizziness, drowsiness, fatigue, syncope, light-headedness, headache, insomnia
CV: angina pectoris, hypotension, tachycardia
EENT: sinusitis
GI: diarrhea, nausea, anorexia
GU: proteinuria, erectile dysfunction, decreased libido, **renal failure**
Hematologic: agranulocytosis
Metabolic: hyperkalemia
Respiratory: cough, dyspnea, bronchitis, **asthma, eosinophilic pneumonitis**
Skin: rash, **angioedema**
Other: fever, altered taste

Interactions

Drug-drug. *Allopurinol:* increased risk of hypersensitivity reaction
Antacids: decreased benazepril absorption
Antihypertensives, diuretics, general anesthetics, nitrates, phenothiazines: excessive hypotension
Cyclosporine, indomethacin, potassium-sparing diuretics, potassium supplements: hyperkalemia
Lithium: increased lithium blood level, greater risk of lithium toxicity
Nonsteroidal anti-inflammatory drugs: blunting of antihypertensive response
Drug-diagnostic tests. *Alanine aminotransferase, alkaline phosphatase, aspartate aminotransferase, bilirubin, blood urea nitrogen, creatinine, potassium:* increased levels
Antinuclear antibodies: positive result
Sodium: decreased level
Drug-food. *Salt substitutes containing potassium:* hyperkalemia
Drug-herbs. *Capsaicin:* cough
Drug-behaviors. *Acute alcohol ingestion:* increased hypotension

Patient monitoring

◀᪶ Monitor for signs and symptoms of angioedema, including laryngeal edema and shock.
• Measure blood pressure regularly.

- Monitor CBC, electrolyte levels, kidney and liver function test results, and urinary protein level.

Patient teaching

◀ Tell patient to immediately report change in urination pattern, difficulty breathing, or swelling of throat or lips.
- Instruct patient to record blood pressure at various intervals daily.
- Tell patient to report dizziness, fainting, or light-headedness during initial therapy.
- Advise patient to increase fluid intake during exercise and in hot weather.
- Caution patient to avoid salt substitutes, which may cause hyperkalemia.
- As appropriate, review all other significant and life-threatening adverse reactions and interactions, especially those related to the drugs, tests, foods, herbs, and behaviors mentioned above.

bendamustine hydrochloride
Treanda

Pharmacologic class: Alkylating agent
Therapeutic class: Antineoplastic
Pregnancy risk category D

Action

Unclear. Dissociates into electrophilic alkyl groups, which form covalent bonds with electron-rich nucleophilic moieties; bifunctional covalent linkage may cause cell death via several pathways. Acts against both quiescent and dividing cells.

Availability

Lyophilized powder for injection:
100 mg in 20-ml single-use vials (with mannitol)

🖋 Indications and dosages

➤ Chronic lymphocytic leukemia
Adults: 100 mg/m² by I.V. infusion over 30 minutes on days 1 and 2 of 28-day cycle for up to six cycles

Dosage adjustment

- Grade 4 hematologic toxicity or clinically significant nonhemologic toxicity at above grade 2

Off-label uses

- Non-Hodgkin's lymphoma

Contraindications

- Hypersensitivity to drug or mannitol

Precautions

Use cautiously in:
- mild or moderate renal impairment (not recommended in creatinine clearance less than 40 ml/minute)
- mild hepatic impairment (not recommended in moderate or severe hepatic impairment)
- myelosuppression
- concurrent use of CYP1A2 inhibitors or inducers
- pregnant or breastfeeding patients
- children (safety and efficacy not established).

Administration

- Give drug by I.V. infusion only.
- Reconstitute with 20 ml sterile water for injection. Wait until powder dissolves completely (approximately 5 minutes).
- Immediately transfer (within 30 minutes of reconstitution) to 500-ml infusion bag of normal saline injection. After transferring, thoroughly mix infusion bag contents. Admixture should be clear and colorless to slightly yellow.
◀ Stay alert for infusion reactions. Signs and symptoms include fever, chills, pruritus, and rash. Rarely, severe anaphylactic and anaphylactoid

---

reactions have occurred. Monitor patient and discontinue drug if severe reaction arises. Consider measures to prevent severe reactions, including antihistamines, antipyretics, and corticosteroids in subsequent cycles if patient had previous infusion reaction.
• Check I.V. site frequently to avoid extravasation.

Route	Onset	Peak	Duration
I.V.	Unknown	End of infusion	Unknown

Adverse reactions

CNS: asthenia, fatigue, malaise, weakness, somnolence, headache
CV: worsening hypertension
EENT: nasopharyngitis
GI: nausea, vomiting, diarrhea, constipation, dry mouth, mucosal inflammation, stomatitis
Hematologic: myelosuppression (**anemia, leukopenia,** lymphopenia, **neutropenia, thrombocytopenia**)
Metabolic: hyperuricemia
Respiratory: cough, pneumonia
Skin: rash, pruritus, toxic skin reactions, bullous exanthema, **Stevens-Johnson syndrome, toxic epidermal necrolysis**
Other: fever, chills, infection, herpes simplex, weight loss, **other malignancies, tumor lysis syndrome, sepsis, infusion reactions and anaphylaxis, hypersensitivity reaction**

Interactions

Drug-drug. *Allopurinol:* possible increased risk of skin reactions
CYP1A2 inducers (such as omeprazole): potentially decreased bendamustine blood level and increased active metabolite levels
CYP1A2 inhibitors (such as ciprofloxacin, fluvoxamine): potentially increased bendamustine blood level and decreased active metabolite levels
Drug-diagnostic tests. *ALT, AST, bilirubin, uric acid:* increased levels
Creatinine: altered level

Hemoglobin, lymphocytes, neutrophils, platelets, white blood cells: decreased levels
Potassium, uric acid: increased levels
Drug-behaviors. *Smoking:* potentially decreased bendamustine blood level and increased active metabolite levels

Patient monitoring

• Closely monitor complete blood count with differential and renal and hepatic function test results.
◀€ Monitor for skin reactions, including rash, toxic reactions, and bullous exanthema. Such reactions may be progressive and worsen with further treatment. In severe or progressive skin reaction, withhold or discontinue drug.
◀€ Watch for tumor lysis syndrome, especially during first treatment cycle. Signs and symptoms include irregular heartbeat, shortness of breath, high potassium level, high uric acid level, and impaired mental ability. Without intervention, acute renal failure and death may occur. Take preventive measures, as ordered, including maintaining adequate volume status, close monitoring of blood chemistry, and allopurinol administration during first 2 weeks of therapy in high-risk patients. However, be aware that concomitant use of allopurinol may increase risk of severe skin toxicity.

Patient teaching

• Instruct patient to report unusual bleeding or bruising, fever, chills, and lip or mouth sores.
• Inform patient that drug may increase risk of infection. Advise patient to wash hands frequently, wear mask in public places, and avoid people with infections.
• Advise female that drug may harm fetus; caution her to avoid becoming pregnant. If patient is pregnant during therapy or becomes pregnant, inform her of risk to fetus.

• As appropriate, review all other significant and life-threatening adverse reactions and interactions, especially those related to the drugs, tests, and behaviors mentioned above.

benztropine mesylate
Apo-Benztropine✣, Cogentin, PMS Benztropine✣

Pharmacologic class: Anticholinergic
Therapeutic class: Antiparkinsonian
Pregnancy risk category C

Action
Inhibits cholinergic excitatory pathways and restores balance of dopamine and acetylcholine in CNS, thereby decreasing excess salivation, rigidity, and tremors (parkinsonian symptoms)

Availability
Injection: 1 mg/ml in 2-ml ampules
Tablets: 0.5 mg, 1 mg, 2 mg

⊘ Indications and dosages
➤ Parkinsonism
Adults: Initially, 1 to 2 mg/day P.O. or I.M. at bedtime or in two or four divided doses. Dosage range is 0.5 to 6 mg/day.
➤ Acute dystonic reactions
Adults: Initially, 1 to 2 mg I.M. or I.V., then 1 to 2 mg P.O. b.i.d.
➤ Drug-induced extrapyramidal reactions (except tardive dyskinesia)
Adults: 1 to 4 mg P.O. or I.M. once or twice daily

Dosage adjustment
• Elderly patients

Off-label uses
• Excessive salivation

Contraindications
• Hypersensitivity to drug
• Angle-closure glaucoma
• Tardive dyskinesia
• Children younger than age 3

Precautions
Use cautiously in:
• seizure disorders, arrhythmias, tachycardia, hypertension, hypotension, hepatic or renal dysfunction, alcoholism, prostatic hypertrophy
• elderly patients
• pregnant or breastfeeding patients.

Administration
• Give after meals to prevent GI upset.
• Crush tablets if patient has difficulty swallowing them.
• Know that I.V. route is seldom used.
• Be aware that entire dose may be given at bedtime. (Drug has long duration of action.)

Route	Onset	Peak	Duration
P.O.	1-2 hr	Unknown	24 hr
I.V., I.M.	15 min	Unknown	24 hr

Adverse reactions
CNS: confusion, depression, dizziness, hallucinations, headache, weakness, memory impairment, nervousness, delusions, euphoria, paresthesia, sensation of heaviness in limbs, **toxic psychosis**
CV: hypotension, palpitations, **tachycardia, arrhythmias**
EENT: blurred vision, diplopia, mydriasis, angle-closure glaucoma
GI: nausea, constipation, dry mouth, **ileus**
GU: urinary hesitancy or retention, dysuria, difficulty maintaining erection
Musculoskeletal: paratonia, muscle weakness and cramps
Skin: rash, urticaria, decreased sweating, dermatoses

Interactions
Drug-drug. *Antacids, antidiarrheals:* decreased benztropine absorption

---

Reactions in **bold** are life-threatening.   ◀€ Clinical alert

Antihistamines, bethanechol, disopyramide, phenothiazines, quinidine, tricyclic antidepressants: additive anticholinergic effects

Drug-herbs. *Angel's trumpet, jimsonweed, scopolia:* increased anticholinergic effects

Drug-behaviors. *Alcohol use:* increased sedation

Patient monitoring

• Monitor blood pressure closely, especially in elderly patients.

• Monitor fluid intake and output; check for urinary retention.

• Assess for signs and symptoms of ileus, including constipation and abdominal distention.

Patient teaching

• Advise patient to use caution during activities that require physical or mental alertness, because drug causes sedation.

• Tell patient to avoid increased heat exposure.

◄€ Caution patient not to stop therapy abruptly.

• As appropriate, review all other significant and life-threatening adverse reactions and interactions, especially those related to the drugs, herbs, and behaviors mentioned above.

betamethasone
Betnelan✤, Celestone

betamethasone acetate and sodium phosphate
Celestone Soluspan

Pharmacologic class: Glucocorticoid (inhalation)

Therapeutic class: Antiasthmatic, anti-inflammatory (steroidal)

Pregnancy risk category C

Action

Stabilizes lysosomal neutrophils and prevents their degranulation, inhibits synthesis of lipoxygenase products and prostaglandins, activates anti-inflammatory genes, and inhibits various cytokines

Availability

Solution for injection: 3 mg betamethasone sodium phosphate with 3 mg betamethasone acetate/ml

Suspension for injection (acetate, phosphate): 6 mg (total)/ml

Syrup: 0.6 mg/5 ml

Tablets: 0.6 mg

Tablets (effervescent): 0.5 mg

Tablets (extended-release): 1 mg

⚫ Indications and dosages

➤ Inflammatory, allergic, hematologic, neoplastic, autoimmune, and respiratory diseases; prevention of organ rejection after transplantation surgery

Adults: 0.6 to 7.2 mg/day P.O. as single daily dose or in divided doses; or up to 9 mg I.M. of betamethasone acetate and sodium phosphate suspension.

➤ Bursitis or tenosynovitis

Adults: 1 ml of suspension intrabursally

➤ Rheumatoid arthritis or osteoarthritis

Adults: 0.5 to 2 ml of suspension intra-articularly

Off-label uses

• Respiratory distress syndrome

Contraindications

• Hypersensitivity to drug
• Breastfeeding

Precautions

Use cautiously in:

• systemic infections, hypertension, osteoporosis, diabetes mellitus, glaucoma, renal disease, hypothyroidism, cirrhosis, diverticulitis, thromboembolic disorders, seizures, myasthenia

gravis, heart failure, ocular herpes simplex, emotional instability
• patients receiving systemic corticosteroids
• pregnant patients
• children younger than age 6.

Administration

• Give as a single daily dose before 9:00 A.M.
• Give oral dose with food or milk.
• Administer I.M. injection deep into gluteal muscle (may cause tissue atrophy).
◀€ Don't give betamethasone acetate I.V.
• Be aware that typical suspension dosage ranges from one-third to one-half of oral dosage given q 12 hours.
◀€ To avoid adrenal insufficiency, taper dosage slowly and under close supervision when discontinuing.
• Know that drug may be given with other immunosuppressants.

Route	Onset	Peak	Duration
P.O.	Unknown	1-2 hr	3-25 days
I.M. (acetate/ phosphate)	1-3 hr	Unknown	1 wk

Adverse reactions

CNS: headache, nervousness, depression, euphoria, psychoses, **increased intracranial pressure**
CV: hypertension, **thrombophlebitis, thromboembolism**
EENT: cataracts, burning and dryness of eyes, rebound nasal congestion, sneezing, epistaxis, nasal septum perforation, difficulty speaking, oropharyngeal or nasopharyngeal fungal infections
GI: nausea, vomiting, anorexia, dry mouth, esophageal candidiasis, peptic ulcers
Metabolic: decreased growth, hyperglycemia, cushingoid appearance, **adrenal insufficiency or suppression**

Musculoskeletal: muscle wasting, muscle pain, osteoporosis, aseptic joint necrosis
Respiratory: cough, wheezing, **bronchospasm**
Skin: facial edema, rash, contact dermatitis, acne, ecchymosis, hirsutism, petechiae, urticaria, **angioedema**
Other: loss of taste, bad taste, weight gain or loss, Churg-Strauss syndrome, increased susceptibility to infection, hypersensitivity reaction

Interactions

Drug-drug. *Amphotericin B, loop and thiazide diuretics, ticarcillin:* additive hypokalemia
Barbiturates, phenytoin, rifampin: stimulation of betamethasone metabolism, causing decreased drug effects
Digoxin: increased risk of digoxin toxicity
Fluoroquinolones (such as ciprofloxacin, norfloxacin): increased risk of tendon rupture
Hormonal contraceptives: blockage of betamethasone metabolism
Insulin, oral hypoglycemics: increased betamethasone dosage requirement, diminished hypoglycemic effects
Live-virus vaccines: decreased antibody response to vaccine, increased risk of neurologic complications
Nonsteroidal anti-inflammatory drugs: increased risk of adverse GI effects
Drug-diagnostic tests. *Calcium, potassium:* decreased levels
Cholesterol, glucose: increased levels
Nitroblue tetrazolium test for bacterial infection: false-negative result
Drug-herbs. *Echinacea:* increased immune-stimulating effects
Ginseng: increased immune-modulating effects
Drug-behaviors. *Alcohol use:* increased risk of gastric irritation and GI ulcers

Patient monitoring

• Monitor weight daily and report sudden increase, which suggests fluid retention.

Reactions in **bold** are life-threatening.   ◀€ Clinical alert

- Monitor blood glucose level for hyperglycemia.
- Assess serum electrolyte levels for sodium and potassium imbalances.
- Watch for signs and symptoms of infection (which drug may mask).

Patient teaching

- Advise patient to report signs and symptoms of infection.
- Tell patient to report visual disturbances (long-term drug use may cause cataracts).
- Instruct patient to eat low-sodium, high potassium diet.
- ◀≋ Advise patient to carry medical identification describing drug therapy.
- Inform female patients that drug may cause menstrual irregularities.
- ◀≋ Caution patient not to stop taking drug abruptly.
- As appropriate, review all other significant and life-threatening adverse reactions and interactions, especially those related to the drugs, tests, herbs, and behaviors mentioned above.

bethanechol chloride
Duvoid✤, Myotonachol✤, Myotonine✜, PMS-Bethanecol Chloride✤, Urecholine

Pharmacologic class: Cholinergic
Therapeutic class: Urinary and GI tract stimulant
Pregnancy risk category C

Action
Stimulates parasympathetic nervous system and cholinergic receptors, leading to increased muscle tone in bladder and increased frequency of ureteral peristaltic waves. Also stimulates gastric motility, increases gastric tone, and restores rhythmic GI peristalsis.

Availability
Tablets: 5 mg, 10 mg, 25 mg, 50 mg

🕭 Indications and dosages
➢ Postpartal and postoperative non-obstructive urinary retention; urinary retention caused by neurogenic bladder
Adults: 10 to 50 mg P.O. three to four times daily; dosage may be determined by giving 5 or 10 mg q hour until response occurs or a total of 50 mg has been given.

Contraindications
- Hypersensitivity to drug
- GI or GU tract obstruction
- Hyperthyroidism
- Active or latent asthma
- Bradycardia
- Hypotension
- Atrioventricular conduction defects
- Coronary artery disease
- Seizure disorders
- Parkinsonism
- Peptic ulcer disease

Precautions
Use cautiously in:
- sensitivity to cholinergics or their effects and tartrazine (some products)
- pregnant or breastfeeding patients
- children.

Administration
- Give drug on empty stomach 1 hour before or 2 hours after a meal to help prevent nausea and vomiting.

Route	Onset	Peak	Duration
P.O.	30-90 min	1 hr	6 hr

Adverse reactions
CNS: headache, malaise, seizures
CV: bradycardia, hypotension, **heart block, syncope with cardiac arrest**
EENT: excessive lacrimation, miosis
GI: nausea, vomiting, diarrhea, abdominal discomfort, belching
GU: urinary urgency

Respiratory: increased bronchial secretions, **bronchospasm**
Skin: diaphoresis, flushing
Other: hypothermia

Interactions

Drug-drug. *Anticholinergics:* decreased bethanechol efficacy
Cholinesterase inhibitors: additive cholinergic effects
Depolarizing neuromuscular blockers: decreased blood pressure
Ganglionic blockers: severe hypotension
Procainamide, quinidine: antagonism of cholinergic effects
Drug-herbs. *Angel's trumpet, jimsonweed, scopolia:* antagonism of cholinergic effects

Patient monitoring

• Monitor blood pressure. Be aware that hypertensive patients may experience sudden blood pressure drop.
• Stay alert for orthostatic hypotension, a common adverse effect.
• Monitor fluid intake and output and residual urine volume.

Patient teaching

• Tell patient that drug is usually effective within 90 minutes of administration.
• Advise patient to take drug on empty stomach 1 hour before or 2 hours after a meal to avoid GI upset.
• Instruct patient to move slowly when sitting up or standing, to avoid dizziness or light-headedness from blood pressure decrease.
• As appropriate, review all other significant and life-threatening adverse reactions and interactions, especially those related to the drugs, tests, and herbs mentioned above.

bevacizumab
Avastin

b

Pharmacologic class: Monoclonal antibody
Therapeutic class: Immunologic agent
Pregnancy risk category C

FDA BOXED WARNING

• Drug may cause GI perforation, in some cases leading to death. Include such perforation in differential diagnosis of patients who experience abdominal pain during therapy. Discontinue permanently in patients with GI perforation.
• Drug may lead to potentially fatal wound dehiscence. Discontinue permanently in patients with wound dehiscence requiring medical intervention.
• Serious and, in some cases fatal, hemoptysis has occurred in patients with non-small-cell lung cancer who received chemotherapy and bevacizumab. Don't give to patients with recent hemoptysis.

Action

Binds to vascular endothelial growth factor, preventing or reducing microvascular formation and growth and inhibiting metastatic disease progression

Availability

Solution for injection: 25 mg/ml in 4-ml and 16-ml vials

ⓘ Indications and dosages

➢ First-line treatment of metastatic cancer of colon or rectum (used in combination with 5-fluorouracil [5-FU]-based chemotherapy)

Adults: 5 mg/kg I.V. infusion q 14 days until disease progression occurs when used with 5-FU, irinotecan, and leucovorin or 10 mg/kg I.V. infusion q 14 days until disease progression occurs when used with 5-FU, oxaliplatin, and leucovorin

➤ Unresectable, locally advanced, recurrent or metastatic nonsquamous, non-small-cell lung cancer
Adults: 15 mg/kg I.V. infusion q 3 weeks

Contraindications
None

Precautions
Use cautiously in:
• hypersensitivity to drug
• cardiovascular disease
• development of immunogenicity
• patients sensitive to infusion reactions
• patients recovering from major surgery, nongastrointestinal fistula
• recent history of hemoptysis (Don't administer drug.)
• patients with proteinuria
• elderly patients
• pregnant or breastfeeding patients
• children.

Administration
• Withdraw necessary amount to obtain required dose, and dilute in 100 ml of 0.9% sodium chloride injection.
◀◊ Don't mix or administer drug with dextrose solutions.
◀◊ Don't deliver by I.V. push or bolus.
• Initially, infuse drug over 90 minutes. If patient tolerates infusion well, infuse over 60 minutes the second time; if he continues to tolerate it well, infuse each dose over 30 minutes thereafter.
◀◊ Withhold dose if hypertension occurs.
◀◊ Stop infusion if patient develops infusion reaction, hypertensive crisis, severe bleeding, abdominal pain (may signal intra-abdominal abscess or GI

perforation), wound dehiscence, or urinary problems.
• Be aware that drug shouldn't be given within 28 days after major surgery and that therapy should be suspended several weeks before elective surgery.

Route	Onset	Peak	Duration
I.V.	Unknown	Unknown	Unknown

Adverse reactions
CNS: asthenia, dizziness, headache, confusion, syncope, abnormal gait, transient ischemia attack, **reversible leukoencephalopathy syndrome, cerebral infarction**
CV: hypotension, hypertension, angina, **hypertensive crisis, heart failure, deep-vein thrombosis, intra-abdominal thrombosis, thromboembolism, MI**
EENT: excess lacrimation, visual disturbances, rhinitis, **severe epistaxis**
GI: nausea, vomiting, diarrhea, constipation, abdominal pain, stomatitis, dyspepsia, flatulence, colitis, dry mouth, anorexia, **GI perforation, intra-abdominal abscess, rectal hemorrhage**
GU: proteinuria, urinary frequency or urgency, **nephrotic syndrome**
Hematologic: leukopenia, neutropenia, hemorrhage
Hepatic: bilirubinemia
Metabolic: hypokalemia, hyponatremia
Musculoskeletal: myalgia, back pain
Respiratory: upper respiratory tract infection, dyspnea, **massive hemoptysis**
Skin: wound-healing complications, dry skin, **exfoliative dermatitis, wound dehiscence**
Other: abnormal taste, altered voice, pain, weight loss, **infusion reaction**

Interactions
Drug-drug. *Irinotecan:* increased concentration of irinotecan metabolite

Drug-diagnostic tests. *Leukocytes, potassium, sodium:* decreased levels
Urine protein: increased level

Patient monitoring

◀ Monitor patient closely and discontinue drug if signs and symptoms of thromboembolism and GI perforation (such as abdominal pain, vomiting, and constipation), serious bleeding, nephrotic syndrome, or hypertensive crisis develops.

◀ Stay alert for and discontinue drug if nongastrointestinal fistula formation, delayed wound healing, or wound dehiscence requiring medical intervention occurs.

◀ Stay alert for and discontinue drug if signs and symptoms of leukoencephalopathy occur (such as headache, seizures, lethargy, confusion, or blindness).

• Assess blood pressure frequently.
• Monitor CBC with differential and urine protein and serum electrolyte levels.

Patient teaching

◀ Tell patient to call prescriber immediately if he experiences dizziness, severe bleeding, stomach pain, or urinary problems or if a wound opens.

• Instruct patient to tell prescriber if he has been exposed to chickenpox or if he has gout, heart disease, viral infection, urinary problems, hepatic disease, or another form of cancer.

• Advise patient to tell prescriber if he has surgery planned; drug may delay wound healing.

• Caution patient not to get immunizations unless prescriber approves.

• Inform female patients of childbearing potential risk of ovarian failure before starting drug.

• Instruct female patient to tell prescriber if she is pregnant, plans to become pregnant, or is breast-feeding.

• As appropriate, review all other significant and life-threatening adverse reactions and interactions, especially those related to the drugs and tests mentioned above.

bicalutamide

Apo-Bicalutamide✦, Casodex, Dom-Bicalutamide✦, Gen-Bicalutamide✦, Novo-Bicalutamide✦, PHL-Bicalutamide✦, PMS-Bicalutamide✦, Ratio-Bicalutamide✦, Sandoz Bicalutamide✦

Pharmacologic class: Nonsteroidal antiandrogen
Therapeutic class: Antineoplastic
Pregnancy risk category X

Action

Antagonizes effects of androgen at cellular level by binding to androgen receptors on target tissues

Availability

Tablets: 50 mg

🕧 Indications and dosages

➤ Metastatic prostate cancer
Adults: 50 mg P.O. once daily

Contraindications

• Hypersensitivity to drug
• Women who are or may become pregnant

Precautions

Use cautiously in:
• previous hypersensitivity or serious adverse reaction to flutamide or nilutamide
• moderate to severe hepatic impairment
• children.

Administration

• Know that drug is given in combination with luteinizing hormone-releasing hormone (LHRH).
• Administer at same time each day.

Route	Onset	Peak	Duration
P.O.	Unknown	31 hr	Unknown

Adverse reactions

CNS: headache, weakness, dizziness, depression, hypertonia, paresthesia, lethargy

CV: chest pain, peripheral edema, vasodilation, hypertension, **thromboembolic disease**

EENT: pharyngitis, bronchitis

GI: nausea, vomiting, diarrhea, constipation, abdominal pain, anorexia, dry mouth

GU: urinary tract infection, impotence

Musculoskeletal: bone and back pain

Respiratory: dyspnea, cough

Skin: rash, alopecia

Other: food distaste, weight gain, edema, pain, hot flashes, flulike symptoms

Interactions

Drug-drug. *Warfarin:* increased bicalutamide effects

Drug-diagnostic tests. *Alanine aminotransferase, alkaline phosphatase, aspartate aminotransferase, bilirubin, cholesterol, BUN, creatinine:* increased levels

Hemoglobin, white blood cells: decreased values

Patient monitoring

• Monitor prostate-significant antigen levels, CBC, and liver and kidney function test results.

• If patient is receiving warfarin concurrently, evaluate prothrombin time and International Normalized Ratio.

Patient teaching

• Instruct patient to take drug at same time each day, along with prescribed LHRH analog.

• Tell patient that any drug-related hair loss should reverse once therapy ends.

• As appropriate, review all other significant and life-threatening adverse reactions and interactions, especially those related to the drugs and tests mentioned above.

bisacodyl

Alophen, Apo-bisacodyl✦, Biolax⊕, Bisac-Evac, Biscolax, Carter's Little Pills✦, Correctol, Dacodyl, Doxidan, Dulcolax, Ex-Lax Ultra, Femilax, Fleet Bisacodyl, Fleet Stimulant Laxative, Gentlax✦, Laxoberal⊕, Veracolate

Pharmacologic class: Stimulant laxative

Therapeutic class: Laxative

Pregnancy risk category B

Action

Unclear. Thought to stimulate colonic mucosa, producing parasympathetic reflexes that enhance peristalsis and increase water and electrolyte secretion, thereby causing evacuation of colon.

Availability

Enema: 0.33 mg/ml, 10 mg/ml

Powder for rectal solution: 1.5 mg bisacodyl and 2.5 g tannic acid

Suppositories (rectal): 5 mg, 10 mg

Tablets (enteric-coated): 5 mg

🖊 Indications and dosages

➢ Constipation; bowel cleansing for childbirth, surgery, and endoscopic examination

Adults and children ages 12 and older: 5 to 15 mg P.O. or 10 mg P.R. as a single dose

Children older than age 3: 5 to 10 mg or 0.3 mg/kg P.O. as a single dose

Children ages 2 and older: 5 to 10 mg P.R. as a single dose

Children younger than age 2: 5 mg P.R. as a single dose

Contraindications
- Hypersensitivity to drug
- Intestinal obstruction
- Gastroenteritis
- Appendicitis

Precautions
Use cautiously in:
- hypersensitivity to tannic acid
- severe cardiovascular disease, anal or rectal fissures
- pregnant or breastfeeding patients.

Administration
- Make sure patient swallows tablets whole without chewing.
- Don't give tablets within 1 hour of dairy products or antacids (may break down enteric coating).
- Know that drug should be used only for short periods.

Route	Onset	Peak	Duration
P.O.	6-12 hr	Variable	Variable
P.R.	15-60 min	Variable	Variable

Adverse reactions
CNS: dizziness, syncope
GI: nausea, vomiting, diarrhea (with high doses), abdominal pain, burning sensation in rectum (with suppositories), laxative dependence, protein-losing enteropathy
Metabolic: hypokalemia, fluid and electrolyte imbalances, **tetany, alkalosis**
Musculoskeletal: muscle weakness (with excessive use)

Interactions
Drug-drug. *Antacids:* gastric irritation, dyspepsia
Drug-diagnostic tests. *Calcium, magnesium, potassium:* decreased levels
Phosphate, sodium: increased levels
Drug-food. *Dairy products:* gastric irritation

Patient monitoring
- Assess stools for frequency and consistency.
- Monitor patient for electrolyte imbalances and dehydration.

Patient teaching
- Instruct patient to swallow (not chew) enteric-coated tablets no sooner than 1 hour before or after ingesting antacids or dairy products. Tell him not to chew tablets.
- Advise patient not to use bisacodyl or other laxatives habitually because this may lead to laxative dependence.
- Suggest other ways to prevent constipation, such as by eating more fruits, vegetables, and whole grains to increase dietary bulk and by drinking 8 to 10 glasses of water daily.
- As appropriate, review all other significant and life-threatening adverse reactions and interactions, especially those related to the drugs, tests, and foods mentioned above.

bismuth subsalicylate
Bismatrol, Bismatrol Maximum Strength, Diotame, Kao-Tin, Kaopectate, Kaopectate Extra Strength, Kapectolin, Maalox Total Stomach Relief, Pepto-Bismol, Pepto-Bismol Bismuth Maximum Strength, Pink Bismuth

Pharmacologic class: Adsorbent
Therapeutic class: Antidiarrheal, antibiotic, antiulcer drug
Pregnancy risk category C

Action
Promotes intestinal adsorption of fluids and electrolytes and decreases synthesis of intestinal prostaglandins.

Reactions in **bold** are life-threatening.　　　◀€ Clinical alert

Adsorbent action removes irritants from stomach and soothes irritated bowel lining. Also shows antibacterial activity to eradicate *Helicobacter pylori*.

Availability

Liquid: 130 mg/15 ml, 262 mg/15 ml, 525 mg/15 ml (maximum strength)
Tablets: 262 mg
Tablets (chewable): 262 mg, 300 mg

ⓘ Indications and dosages

➤ Adjunctive therapy for mild to moderate diarrhea, nausea, abdominal cramping, heartburn, and indigestion accompanying diarrheal illnesses

Adults: Two tablets or 30 ml P.O. (15 ml of maximum strength) q 30 minutes, or two tablets or 60 ml (30 ml of extra/maximum strength) q 60 minutes as needed. Don't exceed 4.2 g in 24 hours.

Children ages 9 to 12: One tablet or 15 ml P.O. (7.5 ml of maximum strength) q 30 to 60 minutes. Don't exceed 2.1 g in 24 hours.

Children ages 6 to 9: 10 ml (5 ml of maximum strength) P.O. q 30 to 60 minutes. Don't exceed 1.4 g in 24 hours.

Children ages 3 to 6: 5 ml (2.5 ml of maximum strength) P.O. q 30 to 60 minutes. Don't exceed 704 mg in 24 hours.

➤ Ulcer disease caused by *H. pylori*
Adults: Two tablets or 30 ml P.O. q.i.d. (15 ml of maximum strength)

Off-label uses

• Chronic infantile diarrhea
• Norwalk virus-induced gastroenteritis

Contraindications

• Hypersensitivity to aspirin
• Elderly patients with fecal impaction
• Children or adolescents during or after recovery from chickenpox or flu-like illness

Precautions

Use cautiously in:
• diabetes mellitus, gout

• patients taking concurrent aspirin
• elderly patients
• pregnant or breastfeeding patients
• infants.

Administration

• Know that tablets should be chewed or dissolved in mouth before swallowing.
• Be aware that drug is usually given with antibiotics (such as tetracycline or amoxicillin) when prescribed for ulcer disease.

Route	Onset	Peak	Duration
P.O.	1 hr	Unknown	Unknown

Adverse reactions

EENT: tinnitus, tongue discoloration
GI: nausea, vomiting, diarrhea, constipation, gray-black stools, fecal impaction
Respiratory: tachypnea
Other: salicylate toxicity

Interactions

Drug-drug. *Aspirin, other salicylates:* salicylate toxicity
Corticosteroids, probenecid (large doses), sulfinpyrazone: decreased bismuth efficacy
Enoxacin: decreased enoxacin bioavailability
Methotrexate: increased risk of bismuth toxicity
Tetracycline: decreased tetracycline absorption
Drug-diagnostic tests. *Radiologic GI tract examination:* test interference

Patient monitoring

• Monitor fluid intake and electrolyte levels.
• Monitor stool frequency and appearance.
• Assess infants and debilitated patients for fecal impaction.

Patient teaching
- Instruct patient to chew tablets or dissolve them in mouth before swallowing.
- Inform patient that drug may turn stools gray-black temporarily.
- Tell patient to notify prescriber if he has diarrhea with fever for more than 48 hours.
- As appropriate, review all other significant adverse reactions and interactions, especially those related to the drugs and tests mentioned above.

bisoprolol fumarate
Apo-Bisoprolol, Bisoprolol✤, Cardicor⊕, Emcor⊕, Emcor LS⊕, Monocor✤, Novo-Bisoprolol✤, PMS-Bisoprolol✤, Sandoz Bisoprolol✤, Zebeta

Pharmacologic class: Beta$_1$-adrenergic blocker
Therapeutic class: Antihypertensive
Pregnancy risk category C

Action
Blocks beta$_1$-adrenergic receptors of sympathetic nervous system in heart and kidney, thereby decreasing myocardial excitability, myocardial oxygen consumption, cardiac output, and renin release from kidney. Also lowers blood pressure without affecting beta$_2$-adrenergic (pulmonary, vascular, and uterine) receptor sites.

Availability
Tablets: 5 mg, 10 mg

⑦ Indications and dosages
➤ Hypertension
Adults: Initially, 2.5 to 5 mg P.O. daily. Dosages up to 20 mg P.O. daily have been used.

Dosage adjustment
- Renal or hepatic impairment

Contraindications
- Hypersensitivity to drug
- Sinus bradycardia
- Second- or third-degree heart block
- Cardiogenic shock
- Heart failure
- Children (safety and efficacy not established)

Precautions
Use cautiously in:
- renal or hepatic impairment, pulmonary disease, asthma, diabetes mellitus, thyrotoxicosis, peripheral vascular disease
- patients undergoing anesthesia or major surgery
- elderly patients
- pregnant or breastfeeding patients.

Administration
- Give with or without food, but be consistent to minimize variations in absorption.
- Be aware that drug may be given alone or added to diuretic therapy.

Route	Onset	Peak	Duration
P.O.	30-60 min	2 hr	12-15 hr

Adverse reactions
CNS: dizziness, depression, paresthesia, sleep disturbances, hallucinations, memory loss, slurred speech
CV: bradycardia, peripheral vascular insufficiency, claudication, hypotension, sinoatrial or atrioventricular (AV) node block, **second- or third-degree heart block, heart failure, pulmonary edema, cerebrovascular accident, arrhythmias**
EENT: blurred vision, dry eyes, conjunctivitis, tinnitus, rhinitis, pharyngitis
GI: nausea, vomiting, diarrhea, constipation, gastric pain, gastritis, flatulence, anorexia, **ischemic colitis, acute**

---

pancreatitis, renal and mesenteric arterial thrombosis
GU: dysuria, polyuria, nocturia, erectile dysfunction, Peyronie's disease, decreased libido
Hematologic: eosinophilia, **agranulocytosis, thrombocytopenia**
Hepatic: hepatomegaly
Metabolic: hyperglycemia, **hypoglycemia**
Musculoskeletal: arthralgia, muscle cramps
Respiratory: dyspnea, cough, **bronchial obstruction, bronchospasm**
Skin: rash, purpura, pruritus, dry skin, excessive sweating

Interactions

Drug-drug. *Amphetamines, ephedrine, epinephrine, norepinephrine, phenylephrine, pseudoephedrine:* unopposed alpha-adrenergic stimulation
Antihypertensives: increased hypotension
Digoxin: additive bradycardia
Dobutamine, dopamine: decrease in beneficial beta$_1$-adrenergic cardiovascular effects
General anesthetics, I.V. phenytoin, verapamil: additive myocardial depression
MAO inhibitors: hypertension (when taken within 14 days of bisoprolol)
Nonsteroidal anti-inflammatory drugs: decreased antihypertensive effect
Thyroid preparations: decreased bisoprolol efficacy
Drug-diagnostic tests. *Alanine aminotransferase, alkaline phosphatase, aspartate aminotransferase, blood urea nitrogen, glucose, low-density lipoproteins, potassium, uric acid:* increased levels
Antinuclear antibodies: increased titers
Insulin tolerance test: test interference
Drug-behaviors. *Acute alcohol ingestion:* additive hypotension
Cocaine use: unopposed alpha-adrenergic stimulation

Patient monitoring

• Closely monitor blood glucose levels in diabetic patients.

• Assess for signs and symptoms of heart failure, including weight gain.
• Stay alert for blood pressure variations. Low blood pressure may indicate overdose.

Patient teaching

• Tell patient to weigh himself daily at same time and to report gain of 3 to 4 lb/day.
• Instruct patient to move slowly when sitting up or standing, to avoid dizziness or light-headedness from blood pressure decrease.
• Caution patient to avoid driving and other hazardous activities until he knows how drug affects concentration and alertness.
• Advise patient to restrict salt intake to help avoid fluid retention.
• Caution patient not to discontinue drug abruptly unless prescriber approves.
• Tell patient to carry medical identification stating that he's taking a beta blocker.
• As appropriate, review all other significant and life-threatening adverse reactions and interactions, especially those related to the drugs, tests, and behaviors mentioned above.

bivalirudin
Angiomax, Angiox ✚

Pharmacologic class: Thrombin inhibitor
Therapeutic class: Anticoagulant
Pregnancy risk category B

Action

Selectively inhibits thrombin by binding to its receptor sites, causing inactivation of coagulation factors V, VIII, and XII and thus preventing conversion of fibrinogen to fibrin

Availability

Powder for injection: 250 mg/vial

⊘ Indications and dosages

➤ Patients with unstable angina who are undergoing percutaneous transluminal coronary angioplasty (PTCA); patients with or at risk for heparin-induced thrombocytopenia or heparin-induced thrombocytopenia and thrombosis syndrome undergoing percutaneous coronary intervention

Adults: 0.75 mg by I.V. bolus followed by 1.75 mg/kg/hour by I.V. infusion for duration of procedure. Five minutes after bolus is administered, an activated clotting time should be obtained and an additional bolus of 0.3 mg/kg should be given if needed. Continuation of infusion for up to 4 hours postprocedure is optional, and at discretion of treating physician. After 4 hours, an additional I.V. infusion may be initiated at rate of 0.2 mg/kg/hour for up to 20 hours if needed.

Dosage adjustment

• Renal impairment
• Dialysis patients

Off-label uses

• PCTA (regardless of history of unstable angina)
• Anticoagulation during orthopedic surgery

Contraindications

• Hypersensitivity to drug
• Active major bleeding

Precautions

Use cautiously in:
• renal impairment, severe hepatic dysfunction, bacterial endocarditis, cerebrovascular accident, severe hypertension, heparin-induced thrombocytopenia, thrombosis syndrome
• diseases associated with increased risk of bleeding

• concurrent use of other platelet aggregation inhibitors
• pregnant or breastfeeding patients
• children.

Administration

• For I.V. injection and infusion, add 5 ml of sterile water to each 250-mg vial; gently mix until dissolved. Further dilute in 50 ml of dextrose 5% in water or normal saline solution for injection to a final concentration of 5 mg/ml.
• Don't mix with other drugs.
• Don't give by I.M. route.
• Know that drug is intended for use with aspirin.

Route	Onset	Peak	Duration
I.V.	Immediate	Immediate	1-2 hr

Adverse reactions

CNS: headache, anxiety, nervousness, insomnia
CV: hypotension, hypertension, **bradycardia, ventricular fibrillation**
GI: nausea, vomiting, abdominal pain, dyspepsia, **severe spontaneous GI bleeding**
GU: urinary retention, **severe spontaneous GU bleeding**
Hematologic: severe spontaneous bleeding
Musculoskeletal: pelvic or back pain
Other: fever, pain at injection site

Interactions

Drug-drug. *Abciximab, anticoagulants (including heparin, low-molecular-weight heparins, and heparinoids), thrombolytics, ticlopidine, warfarin:* increased risk of bleeding
Drug-diagnostic tests. *Activated partial thromboplastin time, prothrombin time:* increased
Drug-herbs. *Ginkgo biloba:* increased risk of bleeding

Patient monitoring

◀€ Monitor blood pressure, hemoglobin, and hematocrit. Be aware that

---

decrease in blood pressure or hematocrit may signal hemorrhagic event.
• Monitor venipuncture site closely for bleeding.

Patient teaching

◀€ Instruct patient to immediately report bleeding, bruising, or tarry stools.
• Tell patient to avoid activities that can cause injury. Advise him to use soft toothbrush and electric razor to avoid gum and skin injury.

bleomycin sulfate
Blenoxane

Pharmacologic class: Antitumor antibiotic
Therapeutic class: Antineoplastic
Pregnancy risk category D

FDA | BOXED WARNING

• Give under supervision of physician in facility with adequate diagnostic and treatment resources.
• Pulmonary fibrosis is most severe toxicity, and most often presents as pneumonitis progressing to pulmonary fibrosis. Occurrence is highest in elderly patients and those receiving more than 400 units total dose.

Action
Unclear. Appears to inhibit DNA synthesis and, to a lesser degree, RNA and protein synthesis. Binds to DNA, causing severing of single DNA strands.

Availability
Injection: 15-unit vials, 30-unit vials

⟡ Indications and dosages
➤ Hodgkin's lymphoma

Adults: 10 to 20 units/m^2 I.V., I.M., or subcutaneously once or twice weekly. After 50% response, maintenance dosage is 1 unit/m^2 I.M. or I.V. daily or 5 units/m^2 I.M. or I.V. weekly.
➤ Malignant pleural effusion; prevention of recurrent pleural effusions
Adults: 60 units dissolved in 50 to 100 mg of normal saline solution, given through thoracostomy tube
➤ Squamous cell carcinoma of head, neck, skin, penis, cervix, or vulva; non-Hodgkin's lymphoma; testicular carcinoma
Adults and children ages 12 and older: 10 to 20 units/m^2 I.V., I.M., or subcutaneously once or twice weekly.

Dosage adjustment
• Renal impairment
• Elderly patients

Off-label uses
• Esophageal carcinoma
• Hemangioma
• AIDS-related Kaposi's sarcoma
• Osteosarcoma
• Verrucous carcinoma
• Warts

Contraindications
• Hypersensitivity to drug
• Pregnancy or breastfeeding

Precautions
Use cautiously in:
• renal or pulmonary impairment
• elderly patients
• females of childbearing age.

Administration
• Wash hands before and after preparing drug; wear gloves during handling and preparation.
• For I.M. or subcutaneous use, reconstitute 15-unit vial with 1 to 5 ml and 30-unit vial with 2 to 10 ml of sterile water for injection, normal saline solution for injection, or bacteriostatic water for injection.

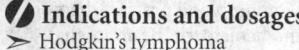

b

- For I.V. infusion, dissolve contents of 15- or 30-unit vial in 5 or 10 ml, respectively, of normal saline solution for injection.
- For intrapleural use, dissolve each 60 units in 50 to 100 ml of normal saline solution for injection, then administer through thoracostomy tube. Clamp tube after instilling drug. During next 4 hours, reposition patient from supine to right and left lateral positions several times. Then unclamp tube and restart suction.
- Premedicate patient with aspirin, as prescribed, to reduce risk of drug fever.

◀️≋ Know that cumulative dosages above 400 units should be given with extreme caution because of increased risk of pulmonary toxicity.

◀️≋ Know that in patients with lymphoma, anaphylactoid reaction may occur. Such patients should receive 2 units or less for the first two doses. If no reaction occurs, recommended doses may be given.

Route	Onset	Peak	Duration
I.V.	Immediate	10-20 min	Unknown
I.M., subcut.	15-20 min	30-60 min	Unknown

Adverse reactions

CNS: disorientation, weakness, aggressive behavior
CV: hypotension, peripheral vasoconstriction
GI: vomiting, diarrhea, anorexia, stomatitis
Hematologic: anemia, **leukopenia, thrombocytopenia**
Hepatic: hepatotoxicity
Metabolic: hyperuricemia
Respiratory: dyspnea, crackles, **pulmonary fibrosis, pneumonitis**
Skin: alopecia, erythema, rash, urticaria, vesicles, striae, hyperpigmentation, mucocutaneous toxicity
Other: fever, chills, weight loss, **anaphylactic reaction**

Interactions

Drug-drug. *Anesthestics:* increased oxygen requirement
Antineoplastics: increased risk of hematologic and pulmonary toxicity
Cardiac glycosides: decreased cardiac glycoside blood level
Cisplatin: decreased bleomycin elimination, increased risk of toxicity
Fosphenytoin, phenytoin: decreased blood levels of these drugs
Vinblastine: increased risk of Raynaud's syndrome
Drug-diagnostic tests. *Uric acid:* increased level

Patient monitoring

- Assess baseline pulmonary function status before initiating therapy; monitor throughout therapy.
- Monitor chest X-rays and assess breath sounds to detect signs of pulmonary toxicity.
- Assess oral cavity for sores, ulcers, pain, and bleeding.
- Monitor infusion site for irritation, burning, and signs of infection.
- Evaluate closely for signs and symptoms of drug fever.

Patient teaching

- Tell patient to avoid spicy, hot, or rough foods (may cause GI upset).
- Urge patient to use reliable contraceptive method during therapy.
- Tell patient not to receive vaccinations without consulting prescriber.

◀️≋ Instruct patient to immediately notify prescriber if breathing difficulties, fever, or chills occur.

- Tell patient to avoid activities that can cause injury. Advise him to use soft toothbrush and electric razor to avoid gum and skin injury.
- Inform patient that drug may cause hair loss but that hair will grow back after treatment ends.
- As appropriate, review all other significant and life-threatening adverse reactions and interactions, especially

---

Reactions in **bold** are life-threatening.   ◀️≋ Clinical alert

those related to the drugs and tests mentioned above.

boceprevir
Victrelis

Pharmacologic class: Hepatitis C NS3/4A protease inhibitor
Therapeutic class: Antiviral agent
Pregnancy risk category X

Action
Binds to the NS3 protease active site serine (S139) through an (alpha)-ketoamide functional group to inhibit viral replication in hepatitis C virus (HCV)-infected host cells

Availability
Capsules: 200 mg

🚫 Indications and dosages
➤ Chronic hepatitis C genotype 1 in patients with compensated hepatic disease (including cirrhosis) who are previously untreated or who have failed previous interferon and ribavirin therapy
Adults age 18 and older: 800 mg P.O. t.i.d. (q 7 to 9 hours) in combination with peginterferon alfa and ribavirin; in patients with compensated cirrhosis, give peginterferon alfa and ribavirin for 4 weeks followed by 44 weeks boceprevir 800 mg t.i.d. (q 7 to 9 hours) in combination with peginterferon alfa and ribavirin
➤ Chronic hepatitis C genotype 1 in patients with compensated hepatic disease (without cirrhosis) who are previously untreated or are partial responders or relapsers to interferon and ribavirin therapy
Adults age 18 and older: Initiate therapy with peginterferon alfa and ribavirin for 4 weeks (treatment weeks 1 to 4). Add boceprevir 800 mg P.O. t.i.d. (q 7 to 9 hours) to peginterferon alfa and ribavirin regimen after 4 weeks of treatment. Based on patient's HCV-RNA levels at treatment week 8, treatment week 12, and treatment week 24, use the following response-guided therapy guidelines below to determine duration of treatment.

Previously untreated patients

At treatment week 8	At treatment week 24
Undetectable	Undetectable

Complete three-drug regimen at treatment week 28.

At treatment week 8	At treatment week 24
Detectable	Undetectable

Continue all three drugs and finish through treatment week 36; then give peginterferon alfa and ribavirin and finish through treatment week 48.

Previous partial responders or relapsers

At treatment week 8	At treatment week 24
Undetectable	Undetectable

Complete three-drug regimen at treatment week 36.

At treatment week 8	At treatment week 24
Detectable	Undetectable

Continue all three drugs and finish through treatment week 36; then give peginterferon alfa and ribavirin and finish through treatment week 48.

Treatment futility
If the patient has HCV-RNA results of 100 international units/ml or greater at treatment week 12, discontinue three-drug regimen. If the patient has confirmed, detectable HCV-RNA at treatment week 24, discontinue three-drug regimen.

Contraindications

- Contraindications to peginterferon alfa and ribavirin (because boceprevir must be administered with these drugs)
- Concurrent use of drugs that are highly dependent on CYP3A4/5 for clearance, and for which elevated plasma concentrations are associated with serious or life-threatening events, including cisapride (not available in the United States), alfuzosin, dihydroergotamine, drospirenone, ergonovine, ergotamine, lovastatin, methylergonovine, oral midazolam, pimozide, sildenafil (Revatio) and tadalafil (Adcirca) when used for pulmonary arterial hypertension, simvastatin, and triazolam
- Concurrent use of potent CYP3A4/5 inducers when significantly reduced boceprevir plasma concentrations may be associated with reduced efficacy, including carbamazepine, phenobarbital, phenytoin, rifampin, and St. John's wort
- Pregnancy and in men whose female partners are pregnant

Precautions

Use cautiously in:
- patients with anemia or neutropenia
- patients with decompensated cirrhosis or organ transplant, co-infection with HCV and HIV, or hepatitis B virus
- patients with hepatic or renal impairment (avoid use)
- concurrent use of antidepressants such as trazodone, desipramine, or sedatives-hypnotics such as alprazolam and I.V. midazolam (requires close monitoring and consideration of dosage reduction of these drugs)
- concurrent use of antifungals (dosages of ketoconazole and itraconazole shouldn't exceed 200 mg/day if given with boceprevir)

- concurrent use of colchicine for gout flares, prophylaxis for gout flares, or familial Mediterranean fever (requires dosage reduction)
- concurrent use of rifabutin (not recommended)
- concurrent use of dihydropyridine calcium channel blockers, such as felodipine, nifedipine, and nicardipine (clinical monitoring recommended)
- concurrent use of dexamethasone (avoid use if possible or use with caution if use is necessary)
- concurrent use of inhaled corticosteroids budesonide, fluticasone (avoid use if possible, particularly for extended durations)
- concurrent use of bosentan (monitor patient closely)
- concurrent use of HIV non-nucleoside reverse transcriptase inhibitors such as efavirenz (avoid use)
- concurrent use of atazanavir/ritonavir, darunavir/ritonavir, or lopinavir/ritonavir combinations (not recommended)
- concurrent use of ritonavir
- concurrent use of atorvastatin (requires careful titration; atorvastatin dose not to exceed 20 mg daily)
- concurrent use of salmeterol (not recommended)
- concurrent use of methadone or buprenorphine (clinical monitoring recommended; may require altered methadone or buprenorphine dosage)
- concurrent use of sildenafil, tadalafil, or vardenafil when used for erectile dysfunction (don't exceed recommended reduced dosages of these drugs)
- elderly patients
- breastfeeding patients
- children (safety and efficacy not established).

Administration

- Administer with food (a meal or light snack).

◀€ Don't administer boceprevir without peginterferon alfa and ribavirin. Drug must not be used as monotherapy.

• Obtain CBC with WBC differential in all patients before starting drug. Be aware that decreased hemoglobin level or neutrophil count may require a decrease in dosage, interruption, or discontinuation of peginterferon alfa or ribavirin.

• Because this drug is given with ribavirin, ensure that a negative pregnancy test has been obtained immediately before starting therapy.

• Be aware that the Ribavirin Pregnancy Registry is available to monitor maternal-fetal outcomes of pregnancies in female patients and female partners of male patients exposed to ribavirin during treatment and for 6 months after treatment cessation.

• Be aware that boceprevir dosage reduction isn't recommended. If the patient has a serious adverse reaction potentially related to peginterferon alfa or ribavirin, the peginterferon alfa or ribavirin dosage should be reduced or discontinued.

Route	Onset	Peak	Duration
P.O.	Unknown	2 hr	Unknown

Adverse reactions

CNS: fatigue, headache, asthenia, dizziness, insomnia, irritability
GI: nausea, vomiting, diarrhea, dry mouth
Hematologic: anemia, neutropenia
Musculoskeletal: arthralgia
Respiratory: exertional dyspnea
Skin: alopecia, dry skin, rash
Other: chills, dysgeusia, decreased appetite

Interactions

Drug-drug. *Alpha₁-adrenoreceptors (alfuzosin):* increased alfuzosin concentration, resulting in hypotension

Antiarrhythmics (amiodarone, bepridil [not available in the United States], flecainide, propafenone, quinidine): increased antiarrhythmic concentration with risk of serious or life-threatening adverse events
Anticoagulants (warfarin): altered warfarin concentration
Anticonvulsants (carbamazepine, phenobarbital, phenytoin), antimycobacterials (rifampin): possible loss of virologic response to boceprevir
Antidepressants (desipramine, trazodone): increased trazodone and desipramine plasma concentrations, resulting in increased adverse reactions, such as dizziness, hypotension, and syncope
Antifungals (itraconazole, ketoconazole, posaconazole, voriconazole): increased plasma concentrations of these drugs
Antigout drugs (colchicine): significantly increased colchicine level, resulting in possible fatal toxicity
Anti-infectives (clarithromycin): increased clarithromycin concentration
Antimycobacterials (rifabutin): increased risk of rifabutin exposure and decreased risk of boceprevir exposure
Beta-agonists, inhaled (salmeterol): increased risk of salmeterol-associated CV events
Corticosteroids, inhaled (budesonide, fluticasone): increased budesonide and fluticasone plasma concentrations, resulting in significantly reduced serum cortisol concentration
Corticosteroids, systemic (dexamethasone): decreased boceprevir plasma concentration, with possible loss of boceprevir therapeutic effect
Digoxin: increased digoxin concentration, with risk of toxicity
Dihydropyridine calcium channel blockers (felodipine, nicardipine, nifedipine): increased dihydropyridine calcium channel blocker plasma concentration

Endothelin receptor antagonists (bosentan): increased bosentan concentration

Ergot derivatives (dihydroergotamine, ergonovine, ergotamine, methylergonovine): increased risk of acute ergot toxicity characterized by peripheral vasospasm and ischemia of extremities and other tissues

GI motility agents (cisapride, not available in the United States): increased risk of cardiac arrhythmias

HIV non-nucleoside reverse transcriptase inhibitors (efavirenz): decreased boceprevir plasma trough concentration, resulting in loss of boceprevir therapeutic effect

HIV protease inhibitor combinations (atazanavir/ritonavir): reduced steady-state exposure to atazanavir and ritonavir

HIV protease inhibitor combinations (darunavir/ritonavir, lopinavir/ ritonavir): reduced steady-state exposure to boceprevir, darunavir, lopinavir, and ritonavir

HIV protease inhibitors (ritonavir): decreased boceprevir concentration

HMG-CoA reductase inhibitors (atorvastatin): increased atorvastatin concentration

HMG-CoA reductase inhibitors (lovastatin, simvastatin): increased risk of myopathy, including rhabdomyolysis

Immunosuppressants (cyclosporine, sirolimus, tacrolimus): significantly increased cyclosporine, sirolimus, and tacrolimus plasma concentrations

Neuroleptics (pimozide): increased risk of cardiac arrhythmias

Opioid analgesics (buprenorphine, methadone): possible increased or decreased methadone or buprenorphine plasma concentration

Oral contraceptives (drospirenone): increased risk of hyperkalemia

Oral contraceptives (drospirenone, ethinyl estradiol): increased drospirenone and decreased ethinyl estradiol concentrations (effect on other progestins is unknown but increases in exposure are anticipated)

Phosphodiesterase type 5 enzyme inhibitors (sildenafil, tadalafil) when used for pulmonary arterial hypertension: increased risk of PDE5 inhibitor-associated adverse events, including visual abnormalities, hypotension, prolonged erection, and syncope

Phosphodiesterase type 5 enzyme inhibitors (sildenafil, tadalafil, vardenafil) when used for erectile dysfunction: increased sildenafil, tadalafil, and vardenafil levels, resulting in increased adverse reactions

Sedative-hypnotics (alprazolam, I.V. midazolam): increased concentrations of alprazolam and midazolam, with risk of respiratory depression or prolonged sedation

Sedative-hypnotics (triazolam, oral midazolam): prolonged or increased sedation or respiratory depression

Drug-diagnostic tests. *Hemoglobin, neutrophils, platelets:* decreased levels

Drug-food. *Any food:* enhanced boceprevir exposure

Drug-herbs. St. John's wort: possible loss of virologic response to boceprevir

Patient monitoring

• Continue to monitor CBC with WBC differential at treatment weeks 4, 8, and 12; closely monitor at other times as clinically appropriate.

• Monitor HCV-RNA levels at treatment weeks 4, 8, 12, and 24, at the end of treatment, during treatment follow-up, and at other times as clinically indicated. Be aware that discontinuation of therapy is recommended in all patients with HCV-RNA level of 100 international units/ml or greater at treatment week 12 or confirmed detectable HCV-RNA level at treatment week 24.

• If patient is also receiving antiarrhythmics, bosentan, calcium channel blockers, digoxin, immunosuppressants,

---

or opioid analgesics, monitor therapeutic levels of these drugs.

• Monitor INR closely if patient is receiving warfarin while taking this three-drug combination.

• Closely watch for adverse reactions in patients taking erectile dysfunction drugs while also taking this three-drug combination.

• Closely watch for respiratory depression or prolonged sedation in patients also taking sedatives or hypnotics with this three-drug combination.

Patient teaching

• Tell patient to take drug with food (a meal or light snack).

◀€ Advise patient that boceprevir must not be used alone, because of the high probability of resistance without combination anti-HCV therapies.

• Tell patient that if he misses a dose and it's less than 2 hours before the next dose is due, he should skip the missed dose. If he misses a dose and it's 2 or more hours before the next dose is due, he should take the missed dose and then resume the normal dosing schedule.

• Tell patient that laboratory evaluations are required before starting therapy and periodically thereafter.

• Inform female patient that she must have a negative pregnancy test before starting therapy and monthly thereafter during therapy.

• Advise female patient of childbearing age and female partners of male patients to avoid pregnancy during therapy with this three-drug combination by practicing effective contraception with at least two forms of contraceptives during therapy and for 6 months after therapy ends. Tell female patient not to rely on efficacy of systemic hormonal contraceptives during this treatment. Two alternative effective methods of contraception include intrauterine devices and barrier methods.

• Tell female patient of childbearing age that breastfeeding isn't recommended during therapy.

• Instruct patient to tell prescriber about all drugs and herbal products he's taking, because many drugs and some herbs have the potential for serious drug interactions and shouldn't be taken with boceprevir.

• Inform patient that it isn't known how treatment of hepatitis C virus infection affects transmission and that appropriate precautions to prevent transmission of hepatitis C virus should be taken.

• As appropriate, review all other significant adverse reactions and interactions, especially those related to the drugs, tests, food, and herbs mentioned above.

bortezomib
Velcade

Pharmacologic class: Proteasome inhibitor
Therapeutic class: Antineoplastic
Pregnancy risk category D

Action

Inhibits proteasomes (enzyme complexes that regulate protein homeostasis within cells). Reversibly inhibits chymotrypsin-like activity at 26S proteasome, leading to activation of signaling cascades, cell-cycle arrest, and apoptosis.

Availability

Powder for reconstitution (preservative-free): 3.5 mg (contains 35 mg of mannitol)

⚠ Indications and dosages

➤ Multiple myeloma, patients with mantle cell lymphoma who have received at least one prior therapy

Adults: 1.3 mg/m^2 I.V. or subcutaneously twice weekly for 2 weeks (days 1, 4, 8, and 11), followed by 10-day rest period (days 12 to 21). Allow at least 72 hours to elapse between doses. One treatment cycle equals 21 days (3 weeks).

Dosage adjustment

• Moderate or severe hepatic impairment
• Peripheral neuropathy
• Grade 3 nonhematologic events
• Grade 4 hematologic events

Contraindications

• Hypersensitivity to drug, mannitol, or boron

Precautions

Use cautiously in:
• peripheral neuropathy, dehydration, hepatic or renal impairment
• history of syncope or cardiovascular disorders
• pregnant or breastfeeding patients
• children.

Administration

• Be aware that drug is for I.V. or subcutaneous use only. Because each route of administration has a different reconstituted concentration, use caution when calculating volume to be administered.
• Reconstitute drug in vial with 3.5 ml of normal saline for injection to yield a concentration of 1 mg/ml for I.V. use.
• Reconstitute drug in vial with 1.4 ml of normal saline for injection to yield a concentration of 2.5 mg/ml for subcutaneous use.
• Give by I.V. push over 3 to 5 seconds or subcutaneously.
• Reconstituted solution must be used within 8 hours.

Route	Onset	Peak	Duration
I.V.	Unknown	Unknown	Unknown
Subcut.	Unknown	Unknown	Unknown

Adverse reactions

CNS: headache, insomnia, dizziness, anxiety, peripheral neuropathy, **reversible posterior leukoencephalopathy syndrome**
CV: tachycardia, hypotension
EENT: throat tightness
GI: nausea, vomiting, diarrhea, abdominal pain, dyspepsia
Hematologic: eosinophilia, anemia, **thrombocytopenia, neutropenia**
Hepatic: hyperbilirubinemia, **hepatitis, acute liver failure**
Metabolic: dehydration, pyrexia
Respiratory: cough, dyspnea, upper respiratory tract infection, **acute diffuse infiltrative pulmonary disease (pneumonitis, interstitial pneumonia, acute respiratory distress syndrome)**
Skin: rash, pruritus, urticaria
Other: altered taste, increased or decreased appetite, fever, chills, edema, **tumor lysis syndrome**

Interactions

Drug-drug. *CYP3A4 inducers (including amiodarone, carbamazepine, nevirapine, phenobarbital, phenytoin, and rifampin):* possible decrease in bortezomid serum level and efficacy
CYP3A4 inhibitors (including amiodarone, cimetidine, clarithromycin, delavirdine, diltiazem, disulfiram, erythromycin, fluoxetine, fluvoxamine, nefazodone, nevirapine, propoxyphene, quinupristin, verapamil, zafirlukast, and zileuton): possible increase in bortezomib serum level and efficacy
Drug-diagnostic tests. *Liver function tests:* increased levels
Drug-food. *Grapefruit juice:* increased bortezomib blood level, greater risk of toxicity

---

Reactions in **bold** are life-threatening.   🔊 Clinical alert

Patient monitoring

🔊 Monitor vital signs and temperature. Especially watch for tachycardia, fever, and hypotension.

🔊 Stay alert for and discontinue drug if posterior leukoencephalopathy (headache, seizures, lethargy, confusion, blindness) or tumor lysis syndrome occurs (irregular heartbeat, shortness of breath, high potassium level, high uric acid level, impairment of mental ability, kidney failure).

🔊 Closely monitor liver function tests and watch for signs and symptoms of hepatitis or liver failure.

• Monitor nutritional and hydration status for changes caused by GI adverse effects.

• Monitor CBC with white cell differential, and watch for signs and symptoms of blood dyscrasias.

🔊 Monitor respiratory status, watching for dyspnea, cough, and other signs and symptoms of upper respiratory tract infection.

Patient teaching

🔊 Inform patient that drug can cause serious blood dyscrasias. Teach him which signs and symptoms to report right away.

• Tell patient that drug may cause other significant adverse reactions. Reassure him he will be closely monitored.

• Instruct patient to move slowly when sitting or standing up to avoid dizziness or light-headedness from sudden blood pressure drop.

• Caution patient to avoid driving and other hazardous activities until he knows how drug affects concentration and alertness.

• Advise patient to minimize adverse GI effects by eating small frequent servings of healthy food and ensuring adequate fluid intake.

• Tell patient to immediately report signs and symptoms of upper respiratory tract infection.

• As appropriate, review all other significant and life-threatening adverse reactions and interactions, especially those related to the drugs and foods mentioned above.

bosentan
Tracleer

Pharmacologic class: Endothelin-receptor antagonist, vasodilator

Therapeutic class: Antihypertensive

Pregnancy risk category X

FDA | BOXED WARNING

• Drug causes at least 3 × ULN (upper limit of normal) of alanine aminotransferase and aspartate aminotransferase levels in about 11% of patients (along with elevated bilirubin in a few cases). These changes indicate potentially serious hepatic injury. Obtain serum transaminase levels before therapy begins and then monthly.

• Transaminase elevations warrant close attention. Avoid giving drug to patients with baseline transaminase levels more than 3 × ULN, because monitoring for hepatic injury may be more difficult. Stop therapy if transaminase elevations are accompanied by indications of hepatic injury or if bilirubin level is 2 × ULN or higher.

• Rare postmarketing cases of unexplained hepatic cirrhosis occurred after prolonged therapy in patients with multiple comorbidities and drug therapies.

• Drug is contraindicated in pregnancy because it's likely to cause major birth defects. Exclude pregnancy before therapy starts, and instruct patient to use reliable contraceptive method. Caution patient not to use hormonal contraceptives alone, because drug may

render these ineffective; instruct her to use additional forms of contraception. Obtain monthly pregnancy tests.
• Because of potential hepatic injury and to reduce risk of fetal exposure, drug may be prescribed only through Tracleer Access Program.

Action
Binds to and blocks receptor sites for endothelin A and B in endothelium and vascular smooth muscle. This action reduces elevated endothelin levels in patients with pulmonary arterial hypertension, and inhibits vasoconstriction resulting from endothelin-1 (ET-1).

Availability
Tablets: 62.5 mg, 125 mg

Indications and dosages
➤ Patients with pulmonary arterial hypertension (World Health Organization Group 1) to improve exercise ability and to decrease clinical worsening
Adults: Initially, 62.5 mg P.O. b.i.d. for 4 weeks; increase to maintenance dosage of 125 mg P.O. b.i.d. In patients older than age 12 who weigh less than 40 kg (88 lb), initial and maintenance dosages are 62.5 mg b.i.d.

Dosage adjustment
• Aminotransferase elevations more than 3 × upper limit of normal
• Concurrent use of lopinavir/ritonavir

Contraindications
• Hypersensitivity to drug
• Patients receiving concurrent cyclosporine or glyburide
• Pregnancy

Precautions
Use cautiously in:
• moderate to severe hepatic impairment (avoid use)

• mild hepatic impairment
• mitral stenosis, pulmonary veno-occlusive disease
• fluid retention, decreased sperm count, decreased hemoglobin level and hematocrit
• concurrent use of a CYP2C9 inhibitor and a strong or moderate CYP3A inhibitor (not recommended)
• concurrent use of tacrolimus
• elderly patients
• breastfeeding patients
• children younger than age 12 (safety and efficacy not established).

Administration
• Give tablets in morning and evening, with or without food.
• Consider gradual dosage reduction when discontinuing drug.

Route	Onset	Peak	Duration
P.O.	Variable	3-5 hr	Unknown

Adverse reactions
CNS: headache, fatigue
CV: edema, hypotension, palpitations
EENT: nasopharyngitis
GI: dyspepsia
Hepatic: hepatic dysfunction, hepatic injury, hepatotoxicity
Skin: pruritus, flushing

Interactions
Drug-drug. *Cyclosporine:* decreased cyclosporine blood level, increased bosentan blood level
CYP2C9 inhibitors (such as amiodarone, fluconazole), moderate CYP3A inhibitors (such as amprenavir, diltiazem, erythromycin, fluconazole), strong CYP3A inhibitors (such as itraconazole, ketoconazole): largely increased bosentan plasma concentration
Drugs metabolized by CYP2C9 and CYP3A: decreased plasma concentrations of these drugs

---

Glyburide: decreased blood levels of both drugs, increased risk of hepatic damage

Hormonal contraceptives: decreased bosentan efficacy

Lopinavir/ritonavir combination: increased bosentan trough concentration

Simvastatin and other statins: decreased effects of these drugs

Drug-diagnostic tests. *Hematocrit, hemoglobin:* decreased values

Transaminases: increased values

Patient monitoring

• Assess serum transaminase levels within first 3 days of therapy and then monthly.

• Evaluate hemoglobin level 1 month after therapy and then every 3 months.

◀€ If signs of pulmonary edema occur, consider the possibility of underlying pulmonary veno-occlusive disease and discontinue treatment if necessary.

• Assess female patient for pregnancy every month during therapy.

Patient teaching

• Tell patient to take drug with or without food in morning and evening.

• Caution female patient to avoid pregnancy, and discuss reliable contraceptive methods. Instruct her to contact prescriber immediately if she thinks she may be pregnant.

• Because of the potential for adverse effects in the breastfeeding infant, a decision should be made to discontinue breastfeeding or discontinue drug, taking into account the importance of drug to the mother.

• Inform patient that he'll undergo CBC measurement and liver function testing regularly during therapy.

• As appropriate, review all other significant and life-threatening adverse reactions and interactions, especially those related to the drugs and tests mentioned above.

brentuximab vedotin
Adcetris

Pharmacologic class: CD30-directed antibody-drug conjugate

Therapeutic class: Antineoplastic

Pregnancy risk category D

FDA | BOXED WARNING

• John Cunningham virus (JCV) infection resulting in progressive multifocal leukoencephalopathy (PML) and death has been reported in patients treated with brentuximab vedotin.

Action

Brentuximab vedotin antibody is a chimeric IgG1 directed against CD30. The small molecule MMAE is a microtubule-disrupting agent. MMAE is covalently attached to the antibody via a linker. Nonclinical data suggest that the anticancer activity of brentuximab vedotin is due to the binding of the antibody-drug conjugate (ADC) to CD30-expressing cells, followed by internalization of the ADC CD30 complex, and the release of MMAE via proteolytic cleavage. Binding of MMAE to tubulin disrupts the microtubule network within the cell, subsequently inducing cell-cycle arrest and apoptotic death of the cells.

Availability

Powder for reconstitution for injection, lyophilized: 50-mg single-use vial

⚠ Indications and dosages

➤ Hodgkin's lymphoma after failure of autologous stem cell transplant (ASCT) or after failure of at least two

---

prior multi-agent chemotherapy regimens in patients who aren't ASCT candidates; systemic anaplastic large cell lymphoma after failure of at least one prior multi-agent chemotherapy regimen

Adults: 1.8 mg/kg I.V. infusion over 30 minutes q 3 weeks; continue treatment until a maximum of 16 cycles, disease progression, or unacceptable toxicity occurs. Calculate dosage for patients weighing more than 100 kg (220 lb) based on a weight of 100 kg.

Dosage adjustment
• Neutropenia
• Peripheral neuropathy

Contraindications
• Concurrent use of bleomycin

Precautions
Use cautiously in:
• renal or hepatic impairment
• neutropenia, peripheral neuropathy, tumor lysis syndrome, Stevens-Johnson syndrome
• elderly patients (safety and efficacy not established)
• pregnant or breastfeeding patients
• children (safety and efficacy not established).

Administration
• Follow facility policy for handling, preparing, and administering carcinogenic, mutagenic, and teratogenic drugs.

◀≣ Don't administer by I.V. push or bolus.

◀≣ Obtain CBC with differential before each dose. Withhold drug for Grade 3 or 4 neutropenia until resolution to baseline or Grade 2 or lower. Be aware that growth factor support should be considered for subsequent cycles in patients who experience Grade 3 or 4 neutropenia. In patients with recurrent Grade 4 neutropenia despite the use of growth factors,

consider discontinuation or dosage reduction.

• Reconstitute each 50-mg vial with 10.5 ml sterile water for injection, to yield a single-use solution containing 5 mg/ml. Direct stream toward wall of vial and not directly at powder. Gently swirl vial to aid dissolution. Don't shake.

• Reconstituted solution should be clear to slightly opalescent, colorless, and free of visible particulates.

• Following reconstitution, dilute immediately into infusion bag, or store solution at 2° to 8° C (36° to 46° F) and use within 24 hours of reconstitution. Don't freeze. Discard unused portion.

• Immediately add reconstituted solution to infusion bag containing a minimum volume of 100 ml to achieve a final concentration of 0.4 to 1.8 mg/ml in 0.9% sodium chloride injection, 5% dextrose injection, or lactated Ringer's injection. Gently invert bag to mix solution. Following dilution, infuse solution immediately, or store solution at 2° to 8° C and use within 24 hours of reconstitution. Don't freeze.

• Don't mix drug with, or administer as an infusion with, other drug products.

◀≣ Manage neuropathy by using combination of dose delay and dosage reduction as prescribed. For new or worsening Grade 2 or 3 neuropathy, withhold dose until neuropathy improves to Grade 1 or baseline; then restart at dosage prescribed. For Grade 4 peripheral neuropathy, discontinue drug.

◀≣ If infusion reaction occurs, stop infusion and initiate appropriate medical management. If anaphylaxis occurs, discontinue infusion immediately and initiate appropriate medical management.

◀≣ If Stevens-Johnson syndrome occurs, discontinue drug and initiate appropriate medical therapy.

Reactions in **bold** are life-threatening.　　　　◀≣ Clinical alert

◀€ Consider the diagnosis of PML in any patient presenting with new-onset signs and symptoms of CNS abnormalities. Evaluation of PML includes, but isn't limited to, consultation with a neurologist, brain MRI, and lumbar puncture or brain biopsy. Withhold drug if PML is suspected; discontinue drug if PML is confirmed.

Route	Onset	Peak	Duration
I.V.	Unknown	End of infusion	Unknown

Adverse reactions

CNS: headache, dizziness, insomnia, anxiety, peripheral sensory neuropathy, peripheral motor neuropathy, fatigue
EENT: oropharyngeal pain
GI: nausea, vomiting, diarrhea, constipation, abdominal pain
Hematologic: neutropenia, anemia, thrombocytopenia
Musculoskeletal: arthralgia, myalgia, back pain, extremity pain, muscle spasms
Respiratory: upper respiratory tract infection, cough, dyspnea
Skin: rash, pruritus, alopecia, dry skin, **Stevens-Johnson syndrome**
Other: pyrexia, lymphadenopathy, chills, pain, peripheral edema, night sweats, decreased appetite, decreased weight, **tumor lysis syndrome, sepsis, infusion reactions and anaphylaxis**

Interactions

Drug-drug. *Strong CYP3A4 inducers (such as rifampin):* reduced MMAE exposure
Strong CYP3A4 inhibitors (such as ketoconazole): increased MMAE exposure and risk of adverse reactions

Patient monitoring

• Monitor renal and hepatic function tests closely.
• Monitor CBC with differential.
◀€ Continue to closely monitor patient for infusion reaction and take appropriate measures.

• Monitor patient for neuropathy and manage appropriately.
◀€ Be aware that concurrent use of bleomycin increases risk of pulmonary toxicity. Watch for cough, dyspnea, and other serious respiratory problems, such as interstitial infiltration or inflammation.
◀€ Be aware that patients with rapidly proliferating tumor and high tumor burden are at risk for tumor lysis syndrome; closely monitor these patients for hyperphosphatemia, hypocalcemia, hyperuricemia, hyperkalemia, and acute renal failure and take appropriate measures.
◀€ Continue to closely monitor neurologic function for signs and symptoms of PML (such as paresis, cognitive impairment, and problems with coordination).
◀€ Continue to closely monitor patients for signs and symptoms of Stevens-Johnson syndrome (such as hives, red or purple skin, rash, blisters).

Patient teaching

◀€ Instruct patient to immediately contact prescriber if signs and symptoms of infusion reactions (including fever, chills, rash, or breathing problems) occur within 24 hours of infusion.
◀€ Instruct patient to immediately contact prescriber if neurologic signs or symptoms of PML occur (such as problems with coordination, decreased strength or weakness, confusion, or problems thinking).
◀€ Instruct patient to immediately seek medical attention if hives, red or purple skin, rash, or blisters occur.
• Advise patient to report numbness or tingling of the hands or feet.
• Advise patient to contact prescriber if a fever (temperature of 38° C [100.5° F] or greater) or other evidence of potential infection (such as chills, cough, or pain on urination) develops.

• Counsel female patient of childbearing age to avoid pregnancy and breast-feeding while receiving this drug.
• As appropriate, review all other significant and life-threatening adverse reactions and interactions, especially those related to the drugs mentioned above.

bromocriptine mesylate
Apo-Bromocriptine✤, Cycloset,
Dom-Bromocriptine✤,
Parlodel, PMS-Bromocriptine✤

Pharmacologic class: Ergot-derivative dopamine agonist
Therapeutic class: Antiparkinsonian
Pregnancy risk category D

Action
Directly stimulates dopamine receptors in hypothalamus, causing release of prolactin-inhibitory factors and thereby relieving akinesia, rigidity, and tremors associated with Parkinson's disease. Also restores testicular or ovarian function and suppresses lactation. Cycloset's action in glycemic control is unknown.

Availability
Capsules: 5 mg
Tablets: 0.8 mg, 2.5 mg

ⓘ Indications and dosages
➤ Parkinson's disease
Adults: Initially, 1.25 mg P.O. b.i.d. Increase by 2.5 mg/day q 14 to 28 days depending on therapeutic response. Usual therapeutic dosage is 10 to 40 mg/day.
➤ Acromegaly
Adults: Initially, 1.25 to 2.5 mg/day P.O. for 3 days. Increase up to 1.25 to 2.5 mg/day q 3 to 7 days. Usual therapeutic dosage is 20 to 30 mg/day; not to exceed 100 mg/day.

➤ Hyperprolactinemia
Adults: Initially, 1.25 to 2.5 mg/day P.O. Increase gradually q 3 to 7 days up to 2.5 mg two to three times daily.
➤ Neuroleptic malignant syndrome
Adults: Initially, 5 mg P.O. once daily. Increase up to 20 mg/day.
➤ Pituitary tumors
Adults: Initially, 1.25 mg P.O. b.i.d. to t.i.d. Adjust dosage gradually over several weeks to a maintenance dosage of 10 to 20 mg/day given in divided doses.
➤ Type 2 diabetes mellitus
Adults: Initially, 0.8 mg P.O. daily within 2 hours of awakening; may increase by one tablet (0.8 mg) weekly until target range (1.6 to 4.8 mg) or maximal tolerance is reached.

Contraindications
• Hypersensitivity to drug, its components, or other ergot-related drugs
• Severe peripheral vascular disease
• Uncontrolled hypertension, syncopal migraines
• Breastfeeding

Precautions
Use cautiously in:
• impaired hepatic or cardiac function, renal disease, hypertension, pituitary tumor
• psychiatric disorders
• galactose intolerance, severe lactose deficiency, glucose-galactose malabsorption (use not recommended)
• Concomitant use with anti-hypertensives
• Concomitant use with dopamine antagonists such as neuroleptic agents (use not recommended)
• pregnant patients
• children younger than age 15.

Administration
• Give with meals or milk.
• If desired, give at bedtime to minimize dizziness and nausea.

- For Cycloset, administer within 2 hours of patient's waking in the morning and with food.

Route	Onset	Peak	Duration
P.O.	2 hr	8 hr	24 hr
P.O. (Cycloset)	Unknown	Unknown	Unknown

Adverse reactions

CNS: asthenia, confusion, headache, dizziness, fatigue, delusions, nervousness, mania, insomnia, nightmares, **seizures, cerebrovascular accident**
CV: hypotension, palpitations, extrasystoles, syncope, **arrhythmias, bradycardia, acute myocardial infarction**
EENT: blurred vision, diplopia, burning sensation in eyes, amblyopia, rhinitis, sinusitis, nasal congestion
GI: dyspepsia, nausea, vomiting, diarrhea, constipation, abdominal cramps, anorexia, dry mouth, **GI hemorrhage**
GU: urinary incontinence, polyuria, urinary retention
Musculoskeletal: leg cramps
Skin: urticaria, coolness and pallor of fingers and toes, rash on face and arms, alopecia
Other: metallic taste, digital vasospasm (in acromegaly use only), infection

Interactions

Drug-drug. *Amitriptyline, estrogens, haloperidol, hormonal contraceptives, imipramine, loxapine, MAO inhibitors, phenothiazines, progestins, reserpine:* interference with bromocriptine effects
Cyclosporine: inhibition of cyclosporine metabolism, leading to cyclosporine toxicity
Dopamine receptor antagonists (such as neuroleptics [including phenothiazines, butyrophenones, thioxanthenes]), metoclopramide: diminished effectiveness of Cycloset and these drugs

Ergot-related drugs: increased ergot-related adverse reactions, such as nausea, vomiting, and fatigue; decreased effectiveness of these drugs
Erythromycin: increased bromocriptine blood level and greater risk of adverse effects
Levodopa: additive effects of bromocriptine
Potent CYP3A4 inhibitors or inducers, substrates of CYP3A4 (such as azole antimycotics, HIV protease inhibitors): increased or decreased Cycloset circulating levels
Risperidone: increased prolactin blood level, interference with bromocriptine effects
Drug-diagnostic tests. *Alanine aminotransferase, alkaline phosphatase, aspartate aminotransferase, blood urea nitrogen, creatine kinase, growth hormone, uric acid:* increased levels
Drug-herbs. *Chaste tree fruit:* decreased bromocriptine effects
Drug-behaviors. *Alcohol use:* disulfiram-like reaction

Patient monitoring

- Monitor blood pressure to detect hypotension.
- When giving drug for hyperprolactinemia, monitor serum prolactin.
- When giving drug for acromegaly, monitor growth hormone levels to help guide dosage adjustment.
- When giving drug for diabetes mellitus, monitor blood glucose and hemoglobin A1C levels.
- In long-term use, monitor respiratory, hepatic, cardiovascular, and renal function.

Patient teaching

- Instruct patient to take Cycloset within 2 hours of waking in the morning and with food.
- 🔊 Caution patient not to drink alcohol because of risk of severe reaction.

• Advise patient to have regular dental exams. Drug causes dry mouth, possibly resulting in caries and periodontal disorders.

• To minimize constipation, instruct patient to exercise regularly, increase dietary fiber intake, and drink plenty of fluids (3,000 ml daily).

• Advise patient who doesn't desire pregnancy to use reliable contraceptive, because drug may restore fertility.

• Caution patient to avoid driving and other hazardous activities until he knows how drug affects concentration and alertness.

• As appropriate, review all other significant and life-threatening adverse reactions and interactions, especially those related to the drugs, tests, herbs, and behaviors mentioned above.

brompheniramine
Bromfenac, Dimetapp Allergy, Lodrane 24, LoHist 12D, Nasahist B, ND-Stat, TanaCof-XR, Vazol

Pharmacologic class: Histamine antagonist
Therapeutic class: Antihistamine
Pregnancy risk category C

Action
Antagonizes effects of histamine at histamine₁-receptor sites, but doesn't bind to or inactivate histamine. Also shows anticholinergic, antipruritic, and sedative activity.

Availability
Capsules (liquigels): 4 mg
Elixir: 2 mg/5 ml
Suspension: 12 mg/5 ml
Tablets: 4 mg, 8 mg, 12 mg
Tablets (extended-release): 8 mg, 12 mg

⟿ Indications and dosages
➤ Symptomatic relief of allergic symptoms caused by histamine release; severe allergic or hypersensitivity reactions

Adults and children ages 12 and older: 4 to 8 mg P.O. three to four times daily, or 8 to 12 mg extended-release tablets P.O. two or three times daily. Maximum dosage is 36 mg/day.

Children ages 6 to 12: 2 mg P.O. q 4 to 6 hours as needed, not to exceed 12 mg/day

Children ages 2 to 6: 1 mg P.O. q 4 to 6 hours p.r.n., not to exceed 6 mg/day

Contraindications
• Hypersensitivity to drug
• Coronary artery disease
• Urinary retention
• Pyloroduodenal obstruction
• Peptic ulcer
• MAO inhibitor use within past 14 days
• Breastfeeding

Precautions
Use cautiously in:
• angle-closure glaucoma, hepatic disease, hyperthyroidism, hypertension, bronchial asthma
• elderly patients
• pregnant patients.

Administration
• Give with food if GI upset occurs.
• Don't break or crush extended-release tablets.
• Shake oral suspension well before measuring dose.
◀╟ Check elixir and suspension doses carefully, because the mg/ml varies widely between the two liquids.

Route	Onset	Peak	Duration
P.O.	15-60 min	2-5 hr	3-24 hr

Adverse reactions

CNS: drowsiness, sedation, dizziness, excitation, irritability, syncope, tremor

CV: hypertension, hypotension, palpitations, tachycardia, extrasystole, **arrhythmias, bradycardia**

EENT: blurred vision, nasal congestion or dryness, dry or sore throat

GI: nausea, vomiting, constipation, dry mouth

GU: urinary retention or hesitancy, dysuria, early menses, decreased libido, impotence

Hematologic: hemolytic anemia, hypoplastic anemia, thrombocytopenia, agranulocytosis, leukopenia, pancytopenia

Respiratory: thickened bronchial secretions, chest tightness, wheezing

Skin: urticaria, rash

Other: increased or decreased appetite, weight gain

Interactions

Drug-drug. *CNS depressants (including opioids and sedative-hypnotics):* additive CNS depression

MAO inhibitors: intensified, prolonged anticholinergic effects

Drug-diagnostic tests. *Allergy tests:* false results

Granulocytes, platelets: decreased counts

Drug-behaviors. *Alcohol use:* increased CNS depression

Patient monitoring

• Monitor respiratory status.

• Stay alert for urinary retention, urinary frequency, and painful or difficult urination. Discontinue drug if these problems occur.

• With long-term use, monitor CBC.

• Monitor elderly patient for dizziness, sedation, and hypotension.

• If patient takes over-the-counter antihistamines, monitor him closely to avoid potential overdose.

Patient teaching

• Advise patient to take drug with meals if GI upset occurs.

• Instruct patient to avoid driving and other hazardous activities until he knows how drug affects concentration and alertness.

• Caution patient to avoid alcohol while taking drug.

• Urge patient to tell all prescribers which drugs and over-the-counter preparations he's taking.

• As appropriate, review all other significant and life-threatening adverse reactions and interactions, especially those related to the drugs, tests, and behaviors mentioned above.

budesonide

Budenofalk◈, Easyhaler Budesonide◈, Entocort CR◈, Entocort EC, Entocort Enema◈, Novolizer Budesonide◈, Pulmicort Flexhaler, Pulmicort Respules, Rhinocort Aqua

Pharmacologic class: Corticosteroid (inhalation)

Therapeutic class: Antiasthmatic, steroidal anti-inflammatory

Pregnancy risk category B (intranasal, inhalation); C (oral)

FDA | BOXED WARNING

• Pulmicort Respules is meant only for inhalation by compressed air-driven jet nebulizers (not ultrasonic devices). It must not be injected. Read patient instructions before using.

Action

Decreases inflammation by inhibiting migration of inflammatory mediators to injury site, where it reverses dilation and increases vessel permeability. Also decreases plasma exudation and mucus secretions within airway.

Availability

Capsules (extended-release): 3 mg
Inhalation powder: 90 mcg (Pulmicort Flexhaler), 180 mcg (Pulmicort Flexhaler)
Inhalation suspension (Respules): 0.25 mg/2 ml, 0.5 mg/2 ml, 1 mg/ml
Nasal spray: 32 mcg/metered spray (7-g canister)

Indications and dosages

➤ Maintenance treatment of asthma as prophylactic therapy
Adults: 360 mcg (powder for oral inhalation) inhaled b.i.d. For some patients, 180 mcg inhaled b.i.d. may be appropriate. Maximum dosage is 720 mcg b.i.d.
Children ages 6 to 17: 180 mcg (powder for oral inhalation) inhaled b.i.d. For some patients, dosage of 360 mcg inhaled b.i.d. may be appropriate. Maximum dosage is 360 mcg b.i.d.
➤ Seasonal or perennial allergic rhinitis
Adults and children ages 6 and older: Two sprays in each nostril in morning and evening, or four sprays in each nostril in morning. Maintenance dosage is fewest number of sprays needed to control symptoms.
➤ Mild to moderate active Crohn's disease involving ileum, ascending colon, or both
Adults: 9 mg P.O. daily for up to 8 weeks. For recurring episodes of active Crohn's disease, 8-week course can be repeated and tapered to 6 mg P.O. daily for 2 weeks before complete cessation.

Dosage adjustment

• Moderate to severe hepatic disease

Contraindications

• Hypersensitivity to drug
• Status asthmaticus

Precautions

Use cautiously in:
• renal disease, hepatic disease, heart failure, active untreated infections, systemic infections, hypertension, osteoporosis, diabetes mellitus, glaucoma, underlying immunosuppression, hypothyroidism, diverticulitis, nonspecific ulcerative colitis, recent intestinal anastomoses, thromboembolic disorders, seizures, myasthenia gravis, ocular herpes simplex infection
• patients receiving concurrent systemic corticosteroids
• pregnant or breastfeeding patients
• children younger than age 6.

Administration

• If patient also uses a bronchodilator, give that drug at least 15 minutes before budesonide.
• Know that using a spacer reduces risk of candidiasis and hoarseness.
• Make sure patient swallows capsules whole without crushing or chewing them.

Route	Onset	Peak	Duration
P.O.	Unknown	0.5-10 hr	Unknown
Inhalation (nasal)	Immediate	1-2 wk	Unknown

Adverse reactions

CNS: headache, nervousness, depression, euphoria, psychoses, **increased intracranial pressure**
CV: hypertension, Churg-Strauss syndrome, **thrombophlebitis, thromboembolism**
EENT: cataracts, nasal congestion, nasal burning or dryness, epistaxis, perforated nasal septum, hoarseness, nasopharyngeal and oropharyngeal fungal infections
GI: nausea, vomiting, peptic ulcers, anorexia, esophageal candidiasis, dry mouth
Metabolic: hyperglycemia, decreased growth (in children), cushingoid appearance (moon face, buffalo

---

hump), **adrenal suppression or insufficiency**

Musculoskeletal: muscle wasting, muscle pain, osteoporosis, aseptic joint necrosis

Respiratory: cough, wheezing, rebound congestion, **bronchospasm**

Skin: facial edema, rash, petechiae, contact dermatitis, acne, bruising, hirsutism, urticaria

Other: bad taste, anosmia, weight gain or loss, increased susceptibility to infection, **angioedema, hypersensitivity reaction**

Interactions

Drug-drug. *Amphotericin B, mezlocillin, piperacillin, thiazide and loop diuretics, ticarcillin:* additive hypokalemia

Digoxin: increased risk of digoxin toxicity

Erythromycin, indinavir, itraconazole, ketoconazole, ritonavir, saquinavir: increased blood level and effects of budesonide

Fluoroquinolones: increased risk of tendon rupture

Hormonal contraceptives: blockage of budesonide metabolism

Insulin, oral hypoglycemics: increased budesonide requirement

Live-virus vaccines: decreased antibody response to vaccine, increased risk of adverse effects from budesonide

Nonsteroidal anti-inflammatory drugs (including aspirin): increased risk of adverse GI effects

Phenobarbital, phenytoin, rifampin: decreased budesonide efficacy

Somatrem, somatropin: decreased response to budesonide

Drug-food. *Grapefruit, grapefruit juice:* increased blood level and effects of budesonide

High-fat meal: delayed peak budesonide concentration

Patient monitoring

• Monitor respiratory status to evaluate drug efficacy.

◀€ Stay alert for hypersensitivity reactions, especially angioedema.

• Evaluate liver function test results.

• Periodically observe patient for proper inhaler use.

• Assess oral cavity for infection.

Patient teaching

• Teach patient proper use of inhaler.

• Tell patient to swallow capsules whole without crushing or chewing them.

◀€ Instruct patient to contact prescriber immediately if he develops itching, rash, fever, swelling of face and neck, or difficulty breathing.

• Encourage patient to document medication use and his response in diary.

• Advise patient to report signs and symptoms of fungal infections of mouth.

• Tell female patient to inform prescriber if she is pregnant or plans to become pregnant.

• Caution patient to avoid exposure to chickenpox and measles, if possible.

• Emphasize importance of rinsing mouth after each inhaler treatment and washing and drying inhaler thoroughly after each use.

• Instruct patient to avoid high-fat meals, grapefruit, and grapefruit juice.

• As appropriate, review all other significant and life-threatening adverse reactions and interactions, especially those related to the drugs and foods mentioned above.

bumetanide
Bumetanide Injection

Pharmacologic class: Loop diuretic
Therapeutic class: Antihypertensive
Pregnancy risk category C

b

- Drug is a potent diuretic; excessive amounts may cause profound diuresis with fluid and electrolyte depletion. Give only under careful medical supervision; adjust dosage and dosing schedule to patient's needs.

Action
Inhibits reabsorption of sodium and chloride in distal renal tubules and ascending limb of loop of Henle; increases renal excretion of water, sodium, chloride, magnesium, hydrogen, and calcium. Also reduces increased fluid volume caused by renal vasodilation.

Availability
Injection: 0.25 mg/ml
Tablets: 0.5 mg, 1 mg, 2 mg

⏀ Indications and dosages
➣ Edema caused by heart failure or hepatic or renal disease; adult nocturia
Adults: 0.5 to 2 mg/day P.O. as a single dose; up to two additional doses may be given q 4 to 5 hours (up to 10 mg/day). Or 0.5 to 1 mg I.V. or I.M., repeated q 2 to 3 hours as needed, up to 10 mg/day.
➣ Hypertension
Adults: 0.5 mg/day P.O. Maximum dosage is 5 mg/day.

Dosage adjustment
- Renal impairment
- Elderly patients

Off-label uses
- Drug-related edema
- Hypercalcemia

Contraindications
- Hypersensitivity to drug or sulfonamides
- Uncorrected electrolyte imbalances
- Hepatic coma
- Anuria and oliguria

Precautions
Use cautiously in:
- severe hepatic disease, electrolyte depletion, diabetes mellitus, worsening azotemia
- elderly patients
- pregnant or breastfeeding patients
- children younger than age 18.

Administration
- Know that oral or I.V. route is preferred, because I.M. administration may cause pain at injection site.
- Be aware that drug may be given alone or with other antihypertensives.
- Dilute with dextrose 5% in water, normal saline solution, or lactated Ringer's injection.
- Give I.V. dose slowly over 2 minutes.
- Give P.O. form with food or milk.

Route	Onset	Peak	Duration
P.O.	30-60 min	1 hr	3-6 hr
I.V.	Within min	15-45 min	3-6 hr
I.M.	40 min	1-2 hr	4-6 hr

Adverse reactions
CNS: dizziness, headache, insomnia, nervousness, vertigo, weakness, paresthesia, confusion, fatigue, hand-flapping tremor, **encephalopathy**
CV: hypotension, ECG changes, chest pain, **thrombophlebitis, arrhythmias**
EENT: blurred vision, nystagmus, hearing loss, tinnitus
GI: nausea, vomiting, diarrhea, constipation, dyspepsia, gastric irritation, dry mouth, anorexia, **acute pancreatitis**
GU: polyuria, nocturia, glycosuria, premature ejaculation, difficulty maintaining erection, **oliguria, renal failure**
Hepatic: jaundice
Metabolic: dehydration, hyperglycemia, hyperuricemia, hypokalemia, hypomagnesemia, **hypochloremic alkalosis**
Musculoskeletal: arthralgia; muscle cramps, aching, or tenderness

---

Reactions in **bold** are life-threatening.

◀€ Clinical alert

Skin: photosensitivity, hives, rash, pruritus, urticaria, diaphoresis
Other: pain, nipple tenderness

Interactions

Drug-drug. *Aminoglycosides, cisplatin:* increased risk of ototoxicity
Amphotericin B, corticosteroids, mezlocillin, other diuretics, piperacillin, stimulant laxatives: additive hypokalemia
Anticoagulants, thrombolytics: increased bumetanide effects
Antihypertensives, nitrates: additive hypotension
Cardiac glycosides: increased risk of digoxin toxicity
Lithium: decreased lithium excretion, possible lithium toxicity
Neuromuscular blockers: prolonged neuromuscular blockade
Nonsteroidal anti-inflammatory drugs, probenecid: inhibition of diuretic response
Drug-diagnostic tests. *Blood urea nitrogen (BUN), cholesterol, creatinine, glucose, nitrogenous compounds:* increased levels
Calcium, magnesium, platelets, potassium, sodium: decreased levels
Drug-herbs. *Dandelion:* interference with diuretic activity
Ginseng: resistance to diuresis
Licorice: rapid potassium loss
Drug-behaviors. *Acute alcohol ingestion:* additive hypotension

Patient monitoring

• Weigh patient at start of therapy, and monitor weight throughout therapy.
• Monitor blood pressure regularly.
• Monitor serum electrolyte, uric acid, glucose, and BUN levels.
• Monitor elderly patients for extreme blood pressure changes, orthostatic hypotension, and dehydration.

Patient teaching

• Advise patient to take drug in morning to prevent nocturia, and to take second dose (if required) in late afternoon.
• Instruct patient to move slowly when sitting up or standing, to avoid dizziness or light-headedness from sudden blood pressure drop.
• Caution patient to avoid alcohol because of increased risk of hypotension.
• Advise patient to eat foods high in potassium. Provide other dietary counseling as appropriate to help prevent or minimize electrolyte imbalances.
• Instruct patient to weigh himself often to help detect fluid retention.
• As appropriate, review all other significant and life-threatening adverse reactions and interactions, especially those related to the drugs, tests, herbs, and behaviors mentioned above.

buprenorphine hydrochloride

Buprenex, Burinex✢, Subutex, Temgesic✢, Transtec✢

Pharmacologic class: Opioid agonist-antagonist
Therapeutic class: Opioid analgesic
Controlled substance schedule III
Pregnancy risk category C

Action

Unclear. May bind to opiate receptors in CNS, altering perception of and response to painful stimuli while causing generalized CNS depression. Also has partial antagonist properties, which may lead to opioid withdrawal effects in patients with physical drug dependence.

Availability

Injection: 300 mcg (0.3 mg)/ml
Tablets (sublingual): 2 mg, 8 mg

b

🚫 Indications and dosages
➤ Moderate to severe pain
Adults: 0.3 mg I.M. or slow I.V. q 6 hours as needed. Repeat initial dose after 30 to 60 minutes.
Children ages 2 to 12: 2 to 6 mcg (0.002 to 0.006 mg)/kg I.M. or slow I.V. q 4 to 6 hours
➤ Opioid dependence
Adults: 12 to 16 mg/day S.L.

Dosage adjustment
• Elderly patients

Contraindications
• Hypersensitivity to drug
• Elderly patients
• MAO inhibitor use within 14 days

Precautions
Use cautiously in:
• increased intracranial pressure (ICP); respiratory impairment; severe renal, hepatic, or pulmonary disease; hypothyroidism; adrenal insufficiency; undiagnosed abdominal pain; prostatic hypertrophy; systemic lupus erythematosus; gout; kyphoscoliosis; diabetes mellitus; alcoholism
• elderly patients
• pregnant or breastfeeding patients
• children younger than age 13.

Administration
• Mix with lactated Ringer's injection, dextrose 5% in water, or normal saline solution.
🔊 Give I.V. dose slowly over no less than 2 minutes. Drug may cause respiratory depression (especially initial dose).
• When giving I.M., rotate injection sites to prevent induration and abscess.
• If patient is immobilized, reposition him frequently and keep head of bed elevated.

Route	Onset	Peak	Duration
I.V.	Immediate	2 min	6 hr
I.M., S.L.	15 min	1 hr	6 hr

Adverse reactions
CNS: confusion, malaise, hallucinations, dizziness, euphoria, headache, unusual dreams, psychosis, slurred speech, paresthesia, depression, tremor, agitation, **seizures, coma, increased ICP**
CV: hypertension, hypotension, palpitations, tachycardia, Wenckebach (Mobitz Type 1) block, **bradycardia**
EENT: blurred vision, diplopia, amblyopia, miosis, conjunctivitis, tinnitus
GI: nausea, vomiting, constipation, flatulence, ileus, dry mouth
GU: urinary retention
Respiratory: hypoventilation, dyspnea, cyanosis, apnea, **respiratory depression**
Skin: diaphoresis, pruritus
Other: physical or psychological drug dependence, drug tolerance

Interactions
Drug-drug. *Antidepressants, antihistamines, sedative-hypnotics:* additive CNS depression
MAO inhibitors: increased CNS and respiratory depression, increased hypotension
Drug-herbs. *Chamomile, hops, kava, skullcap, valerian:* increased CNS depression
Drug-behaviors. *Alcohol use:* increased CNS depression

Patient monitoring
• Check hepatic function before and during therapy.
• Monitor respiratory status throughout therapy. Respiratory rate of 12 breaths/minute or less may warrant withholding dose or decreasing dosage.

Patient teaching
• Instruct patient to move slowly when sitting up or standing, to avoid dizziness or light-headedness from sudden blood pressure drop.
• Caution patient to avoid driving and other hazardous activities until he

knows how drug affects concentration and alertness.

• Advise patient to increase daily fluid intake to help prevent constipation.

• As appropriate, review all other significant and life-threatening adverse reactions and interactions, especially those related to the drugs, herbs, and behaviors mentioned above.

bupropion hydrobromide
Aplenzin

bupropion hydrochloride
Budeprion SR, Budeprion XL, Buproban, Wellbutrin, Wellbutrin SR, Wellbutrin XL, Zyban

Pharmacologic class: Aminoketone
Therapeutic class: Second-generation antidepressant, smoking-cessation aid
Pregnancy risk category C

FDA | BOXED WARNING

• Antidepressants increase risk of suicidal thinking and behavior in children, adolescents, and young adults with major depressive disorder and other psychiatric disorders. Risk must be balanced with clinical need, as depression itself increases suicide risk. With patient of any age, observe closely for clinical worsening, suicidality, or unusual behavior changes. Advise family or caregiver to observe patient closely and communicate with prescriber as needed.

• Bupropion hydrobromide (Aplenzin) and bupropion hydrochloride (Budeprion SR, Budeprion XL, Buproban, Wellbutrin, Wellbutrin SR, and Wellbutrin XL) aren't approved for smoking cessation treatment, but bupropion hydrochloride under the names of Buproban and Zyban is approved for this use. Serious neuropsychiatric events, including but not limited to depression, suicidal ideation, suicide attempt, and completed suicide, have been reported in patients taking Buproban and Zyban for smoking cessation. Some cases may have been complicated by the signs and symptoms of nicotine withdrawal in patients who stopped smoking. Risks should be weighed against benefits of their use in smoking cessation.

• Drug isn't approved for use in pediatric patients.

Action
Unclear. Thought to decrease neuronal reuptake of dopamine, serotonin, and norepinephrine in CNS. Action as smoking-cessation aid may result from noradrenergic or dopaminergic activity.

Availability
bupropion hydrobromide
Tablets (extended-release): 174 mg, 348 mg, 522 mg
bupropion hydrochloride
Tablets: 75 mg, 100 mg
Tablets (extended-release): 150 mg, 300 mg
Tablets (sustained-release): 100 mg, 150 mg, 200 mg

🖉 Indications and dosages
➤ Depression
Adults: Initially, 100 mg P.O. immediate-release tablet b.i.d. (morning and evening). After 3 days, may increase to 100 mg t.i.d. After 4 weeks, may increase to a maximum dosage of 450 mg/day in divided doses. No single dose should exceed 150 mg. With total daily dosage of 300 mg, wait at least 6 hours between doses; with total daily dosage of 450 mg, wait at least 4 hours between doses. Alternatively, give one 150-mg sustained-release tablet daily;

increase to 150-mg sustained-release tablet b.i.d. based on clinical response. Or initially, 174 mg P.O. extended-release tablet daily in the morning; if 174-mg dose is adequately tolerated, increase to 348 mg extended-release tablet daily as early as day 4. An increase in dosage to maximum of 522 mg extended-release tablet daily, given as a single dose, may be considered for patients in whom no clinical improvement is noted after several weeks of treatment at 348 mg/day. Don't exceed single dose of 150 mg for immediate-release tablets, 522 mg for extended-release tablets, or 200 mg for sustained-release tablets.

➤ Smoking cessation

Adults: 150 mg P.O. sustained-release tablet (Zyban) or 150 mg extended-release tablet (Buproban) once daily for 3 days, then 150-mg sustained-release tablet b.i.d. for 7 to 12 weeks. Space doses at least 8 hours apart. Don't exceed maximum dosage of 300 mg daily.

Contraindications

- Hypersensitivity to drug
- Seizures
- Anorexia nervosa or bulimia
- MAO inhibitor use within past 14 days
- Acute alcohol or sedative withdrawal
- Use of other bupropion products

Precautions

Use cautiously in:
- renal or hepatic impairment, unstable cardiovascular status
- patients with cranial trauma or other predispositions toward seizures, patients treated with other agents that lower seizure threshold (such as antipsychotics, other antidepressants, theophylline, systemic steroids)
- patients with recent history of myocardial infarction or unstable heart disease
- elderly patients

- pregnant or breastfeeding patients
- children.

Administration

- Be aware that patients should swallow extended- and sustained-release tablets whole and not crush or chew them.
- Be aware that treatment for smoking cessation should start while patient is still smoking, since approximately 1 week of treatment is required to achieve steady-state blood levels of bupropion.
- Avoid bedtime doses because they may worsen insomnia.

◀€ Know that drug shouldn't be withdrawn abruptly when used for depression.

Route	Onset	Peak	Duration
P.O.	Unknown	2 hr	Unknown
P.O. (extended, sustained)	Unknown	3 hr	Unknown

Adverse reactions

CNS: agitation, headache, insomnia, mania, psychoses, depression, dizziness, drowsiness, tremor, anxiety, nervousness, **seizures**

CV: hypertension, hypotension, tachycardia, palpitations, **severe hypertension, complete AV block**

EENT: blurred vision, amblyopia, auditory disturbances, epistaxis, rhinitis, pharyngitis

GI: nausea, vomiting, dyspepsia, abdominal pain, flatulence, mouth ulcers, dry mouth

GU: urinary retention, urinary frequency, nocturia, vaginal irritation, testicular swelling

Metabolic: hyperglycemia, changes in libido, **hypoglycemia, syndrome of inappropriate antidiuretic hormone secretion**

Musculoskeletal: arthralgia, myalgia, leg cramps, twitching, neck pain

---

Reactions in **bold** are life-threatening. ◀€ Clinical alert

Respiratory: bronchitis, increased cough, dyspnea

Skin: photosensitivity, dry skin, pruritus, rash, urticaria, diaphoresis, skin temperature changes, **erythema multiforme, Stevens-Johnson syndrome**

Other: altered taste, increased or decreased appetite, weight gain or loss, hot flashes, fever, allergic reaction, flu-like symptoms, **anaphylactoid reactions, anaphylaxis**

Interactions

Drug-drug. *Benzodiazepine withdrawal, corticosteroids, other antidepressants, over-the-counter stimulants, phenothiazines, theophylline:* increased risk of seizures

Cimetidine: inhibited bupropion metabolism

CYP2B6 substrates or inhibitors (such as clopidogrel, cyclophosphamide, orphenadrine, thiotepa, ticlopidine), efavirenz, fluvoxamine, nelfinavir, norfluoxetine, paroxetine, ritonavir, sertraline: increased bupropion activity

Despiramine, paroxetine, ritonavir, sertraline: possibly increased bupropion blood level

Levodopa, MAO inhibitors: increased risk of adverse reactions

Nicotine transdermal system: increased risk of severe hypertension

Drug-diagnostic tests. *Glucose:* increased level

Drug-behaviors. *Alcohol use or cessation:* increased risk of seizures

Sun exposure: increased risk of photosensitivity

Patient monitoring

• Monitor blood pressure, ECG, CBC, and renal and hepatic function. Monitor tricyclic antidepressant (TCA) blood level if patient's taking TCAs concurrently.

• Be aware that if patient is also on nicotine patch for smoking cessation, the combination may cause or increase risk of hypertension.

• Check for oral and dental problems.

Patient teaching

🔊 Instruct patient to seek immediate medical attention if itching, hives, swelling of the throat, or difficulty breathing occurs.

🔊 Instruct patient taking drug for smoking cessation to immediately notify prescriber if agitation, hostility, depressed mood, changes in thinking or behavior, suicidal ideation, or suicidal behavior occurs.

• Advise patient to set a "target quit date" within first 2 weeks of treatment for smoking cessation.

• Instruct patient to swallow extended- or sustained-release tablets without crushing or chewing.

🔊 Caution patient not to discontinue drug abruptly when taking drug for depression.

• Emphasize importance of frequent oral hygiene. (Dry mouth increases risk of caries and dental problems.)

• Caution patient to avoid alcohol, because it may increase risk of seizures.

• Advise patient to keep regular appointments for periodic blood tests and hepatic and renal studies.

• Advise breastfeeding patient that she should decide whether to discontinue breastfeeding or discontinue drug, taking into account the importance of drug for her treatment.

• As appropriate, review all other significant and life-threatening adverse reactions and interactions, especially those related to the drugs, tests, and behaviors mentioned above.

buspirone hydrochloride
BuSpar

Pharmacologic class: Azaspirodecanedione

Therapeutic class: Anxiolytic

Pregnancy risk category B

Action
Unclear. Thought to bind to serotonin and dopamine receptors in CNS, increasing dopamine metabolism and impulse formation. Also thought to inhibit neuronal firing and reduce serotonin turnover.

Availability
Tablets: 5 mg, 7.5 mg, 10 mg, 15 mg, 30 mg

⊘ Indications and dosages
➤ Anxiety disorders; anxiety symptoms

Adults: 7.5 mg P.O. b.i.d.; increase by 5 mg/day q 2 to 3 days as needed (not to exceed 60 mg/day). Common dosage is 20 to 30 mg/day in divided doses.

Off-label uses
• Parkinsonian syndrome
• Symptomatic relief of depression

Contraindications
• Hypersensitivity to drug
• Severe renal or hepatic impairment
• MAO inhibitor use within past 14 days

Precautions
Use cautiously in:
• patients receiving concurrent anxiolytics or psychotropics
• pregnant or breastfeeding patients
• children.

Administration
• Give with food to minimize GI upset.
• Know that full benefit of drug therapy may take up to 2 weeks.

Route	Onset	Peak	Duration
P.O.	7-10 days	3-4 wk	Unknown

Adverse reactions
CNS: dizziness, drowsiness, nervousness, headache, insomnia, weakness, personality changes, numbness, paresthesia, tremor, dream disturbances
CV: chest pain, palpitations, tachycardia, hypertension, hypotension
EENT: blurred vision, conjunctivitis, tinnitus, nasal congestion, sore throat
GI: nausea, vomiting, diarrhea, constipation, abdominal pain, dry mouth
GU: dysuria, urinary frequency or hesitancy, menstrual irregularities, menstrual spotting, libido changes
Musculoskeletal: myalgia
Respiratory: chest congestion, hyperventilation, dyspnea
Skin: rash, alopecia, blisters, pruritus, dry skin, easy bruising, edema, flushing, clammy skin, excessive sweating
Other: altered taste or smell, fever

Interactions
Drug-drug. *Erythromycin, itraconazole:* increased buspirone blood level
MAO inhibitors: hypertension
Trazodone: increased risk of adverse hepatic effects
Drug-food. *Grapefruit juice:* increased buspirone blood level and effects
Drug-herbs. *Hops, kava, skullcap, valerian:* increased CNS depression
Drug-behaviors. *Alcohol use:* increased CNS depression

Patient monitoring
• Monitor mental status closely.
• Assess hepatic and renal function regularly to detect drug toxicity.

Patient teaching
• Instruct patient to take drug with food.
• Advise patient not to use drug to manage everyday stress or tension.
• Instruct patient to avoid driving and other hazardous activities until he knows how drug affects concentration and alertness.
• Caution patient to avoid alcohol because it increases CNS depression.
• Emphasize importance of keeping follow-up appointments to check progress.
• As appropriate, review all other significant adverse reactions and interactions, especially those related to the

drugs, foods, herbs, and behaviors mentioned above.

busulfan
Busilvex✚, Busulfex, Myleran

Pharmacologic class: Alkylating agent
Therapeutic class: Antineoplastic
Pregnancy risk category D

FDA | BOXED WARNING

• Drug causes profound myelosuppression at recommended dosage. Give under supervision of physician experienced in allogeneic hematopoietic stem cell transplantation, cancer chemotherapy, and management of severe pancytopenia, in facility with adequate diagnostic and treatment resources.

Action
Unclear. Thought to interfere with bacterial cell-wall synthesis by cross-linking strands of DNA and disrupting RNA transcription, which causes cell to rupture and die. Exhibits minimal immunosuppressant activity.

Availability
Injection: 6 mg/ml in 10-ml ampules
Tablets: 2 mg

Indications and dosages
➤ Chronic myelogenous leukemia
Adults: 4 to 8 mg P.O. daily until white blood cell (WBC) count decreases to 15,000/mm³; then discontinue drug until WBC count rises to 50,000/mm³, and then resume as needed.
Children: 0.06 to 0.12 mg/kg/day P.O. or 1.8 to 4.6 mg/m²/day P.O. Adjust dosage to maintain WBC count at approximately 20,000/mm³. Drug should be withheld when WBC count

decreases to approximately 15,000/mm³.
➤ Allogenic hematopoietic stem cell transplantation
Adults: 0.8 mg/kg I.V. q 6 hours for 4 days. Starting 6 hours after 16th dose of busulfan injection, give cyclophosphamide 60 mg/kg/day I.V. over 1 hour for 2 days.

Off-label uses
• Adjunctive therapy in ovarian cancer
• Bone marrow transplantation

Contraindications
• Hypersensitivity to drug
• Patients not definitively diagnosed with chronic myelogenous leukemia
• Pregnancy or breastfeeding

Precautions
Use cautiously in:
• active infections, decreased bone marrow reserve, chronic debilitating disease, depressed neutrophil and platelet counts, seizure disorders, obesity
• patients receiving concurrent myelosuppressive or radiation therapy
• females of childbearing age.

Administration
• Give oral doses on empty stomach.
• When administering I.V., withdraw dose from ampule using 5-micron filter needle. Remove filter needle and use new needle to add busulfan to diluent.
• Dilute for injection using dextrose 5% in water or normal saline solution.
• Infuse I.V. dose over 2 hours, using an infusion pump.
• Flush I.V. catheter before and after each infusion with 5 ml D_5W or normal saline solution.
◀€ Be aware that drug is highly toxic and has a narrow therapeutic index.
• Maintain vigorous hydration to reduce risk of renal toxicity.
• Handle patient gently to avoid bruising.

Route	Onset	Peak	Duration
P.O.	1-2 wk	Wks	Up to 1 mo
I.V.	Unknown	Unknown	13 days

Adverse reactions

CNS: anxiety, confusion, depression, dizziness, headache, insomnia, weakness, **encephalopathy, seizures, cerebral hemorrhage, coma**

CV: chest pain, hypotension, hypertension, tachycardia, ECG changes, **heart block, left-sided heart failure, thrombosis, pericardial effusion, ventricular extrasystole, atrial fibrillation, arrhythmias, cardiac tamponade, cardiomegaly**

EENT: cataracts, ear disorders, epistaxis, pharyngitis

GI: nausea, vomiting, diarrhea, constipation, abdominal pain, dyspepsia, abdominal enlargement, pancreatitis, hematemesis, dry mouth, stomatitis, anorexia

GU: dysuria, hematuria, sterility, gynecomastia, **oliguria**

Hematologic: febrile neutropenia, thrombotic microangiopathy, profound myelosuppression

Hepatic: hepatitis, hepatomegaly

Metabolic: hypokalemia, hypomagnesemia, hypophosphatemia, hyperuricemia, hyperglycemia

Musculoskeletal: arthralgia, myalgia, back pain

Respiratory: hyperventilation, dyspnea, **pulmonary fibrosis**

Skin: pruritus, rash, acne, alopecia, erythema nodosum, exfoliative dermatitis, hyperpigmentation

Other: allergic reactions, chills, fever, injection site infection or inflammation; **severe bacterial, viral, fungal infections; sepsis; tumor lysis syndrome**

Interactions

Drug-drug. *Anticoagulants, aspirin, nonsteroidal anti-inflammatory drugs:* increased risk of bleeding

Live-virus vaccines: decreased antibody response to vaccine, increased risk of adverse reactions

Myelosuppressants: additive bone marrow depression

Nephrotoxic and ototoxic drugs (such as aminoglycosides, loop diuretics): additive nephrotoxicity and ototoxicity

Thioguanine: increased risk of hepatotoxicity

Drug-diagnostic tests. *Alkaline phosphatase, aspartate aminotransferase, bilirubin, nitrogenous compounds (urea):* increased levels

Hemoglobin, WBCs: decreased values

Patient monitoring

• Monitor patient closely for adequate hydration.

• Check for signs and symptoms of local or systemic infections.

• Assess for bleeding and excessive bruising.

• Evaluate oral hygiene regularly.

• Monitor CBC and WBC and platelet counts daily if patient is receiving I.V. busulfan.

• Monitor renal and hepatic function.

◀€ Know that diffuse pulmonary fibrosis ("busulfan lung") is a rare but potentially life-threatening complication, with symptom onset as late as 10 years after therapy.

Patient teaching

• Inform patient that drug doesn't cure leukemia but may induce remission.

• Advise patient to drink plenty of fluids to avoid dehydration.

◀€ Instruct patient to immediately report inability to eat or drink. Prescriber may add another drug to improve appetite.

• Inform patient that he's at increased risk for infection. Advise him to avoid contact with people with known infections and to avoid public transportation, if possible.

• Tell patient he's at increased risk for bleeding and bruising.

Reactions in **bold** are life-threatening.   ◀€ Clinical alert

- Advise patient to avoid activities that can cause injury and to use soft toothbrush and electric razor to avoid gum and skin injury.
- Inform patient that he'll undergo frequent blood testing to monitor drug effects.
- As appropriate, review all other significant and life-threatening adverse reactions and interactions, especially those related to the drugs and tests mentioned above.

butorphanol tartrate
APO-Butorphanol✦, PMS-Butorphanol✦, Stadol

Pharmacologic class: Opioid agonist-antagonist
Therapeutic class: Opioid analgesic
Controlled substance schedule IV
Pregnancy risk category C

Action
Alters perception of and emotional response to pain by binding with opioid receptors in brain, causing CNS depression. Also exerts antagonistic activity at opioid receptors, which reduces risk of toxicity, drug dependence, and respiratory depression.

Availability
Injection: 1 mg/ml, 2 mg/ml
Nasal spray: 10 mg/ml

🕖 Indications and dosages
➤ Moderate to severe pain
Adults: 1 to 4 mg I.M. q 3 to 4 hours as needed, not to exceed 4 mg/dose. Or 0.5 to 2 mg I.V. q 3 to 4 hours as needed. With nasal spray, 1 mg (one spray in one nostril) q 3 to 4 hours, repeated in 60 to 90 minutes if needed.
➤ Labor pains

Adults: 1 to 2 mg I.V. or I.M., repeated after 4 hours as needed
➤ Preoperative anesthesia
Adults: 2 mg I.M. 60 to 90 minutes before surgery
➤ Balanced anesthesia
Adults: 2 mg I.V. shortly before anesthesia induction, or 0.5 to 1 mg I.V. in increments during anesthesia

Dosage adjustment
- Renal or hepatic impairment
- Elderly patients

Off-label uses
- Headache
- Symptomatic relief of ureteral colic

Contraindications
- Hypersensitivity to drug

Precautions
Use cautiously in:
- head injury, ventricular dysfunction, coronary insufficiency, respiratory disease, renal or hepatic dysfunction
- history of drug abuse.

Administration
- Make sure solution is clear and free of particulates before giving.
- When using nasal spray, insert tip of the sprayer about ¼" into nostril, point tip backwards, and administer one spray.
- Be aware that I.V. route is preferred for severe pain.
🔊 Know that drug may cause infant respiratory distress in neonate of pregnant patient, especially if given within 2 hours of delivery.

Route	Onset	Peak	Duration
I.V.	2-3 min	30-60 min	3-4 hr
I.M.	10-15 min	30-60 min	3-4 hr
Intranasal	15 min	1-2 hr	4-5 hr

✦ Canada   ⊕ UK   ⚝ Hazardous drug   ⊗ High-alert drug

Adverse reactions

CNS: drowsiness, sedation, dizziness, tremor, irritability, syncope, stimulation

CV: hypertension, hypotension, palpitations, bradycardia, tachycardia, extrasystole, **arrhythmias**

EENT: blurred vision, nasal congestion or dryness, dry or sore throat

GI: nausea, vomiting, constipation, epigastric distress, dry mouth, **GI obstruction**

GU: urinary retention or hesitancy, dysuria, early menses, decreased libido, erectile dysfunction

Hematologic: hemolytic anemia, hypoplastic anemia, thrombocytopenia, agranulocytosis, leukopenia, pancytopenia

Respiratory: thickened bronchial secretions, chest tightness, wheezing

Skin: urticaria, rash, diaphoresis

Other: increased or decreased appetite, weight gain, local stinging, **anaphylactic shock, hypersensitivity reaction** (with I.V. use)

Interactions

Drug-drug. *CNS depressants:* additive CNS effects

Drugs-herbs. *Kava, St. John's wort, valerian:* increased CNS depression

Drug-behaviors. *Alcohol use:* additive CNS effects

Patient monitoring

• Monitor respiratory status closely, especially after I.V. administration.

• Watch for signs and symptoms of withdrawal in long-term use and in opioid-dependent patients.

• Assess elderly patient closely for sensitivity to drug.

Patient teaching

• Teach patient how to use nasal spray properly.

• Emphasize importance of using drug exactly as prescribed.

• Caution patient that drug may be habit-forming.

• Advise patient to avoid driving and other hazardous activities until he knows how drug affects concentration and alertness.

• As appropriate, review all other significant and life-threatening adverse reactions and interactions, especially those related to the drugs and behaviors mentioned above.

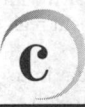

cabazitaxel
Jevtana

Pharmacologic class: Taxane
Therapeutic class: Antineoplastic
Pregnancy risk category D

FDA   BOXED WARNING

• Neutropenic deaths have been reported. Obtain frequent blood counts to monitor for neutropenia. Don't give drug if neutrophil count is 1,500 cells/mm³ or less.

• Severe hypersensitivity can occur and may include generalized rash, erythema, hypotension, and bronchospasm. Discontinue drug immediately if severe reactions occur and administer appropriate therapy.

• Drug is contraindicated in patients with history of severe hypersensitivity reactions to cabazitaxel or to drugs formulated with polysorbate 80.

Action

As a microtubule inhibitor, cabazitaxel binds to tubulin and promotes its assembly into microtubules while simultaneously inhibiting disassembly.

Reactions in **bold** are life-threatening.   ◀€ Clinical alert

This leads to the stabilization of microtubules, which results in the inhibition of mitotic and interphase cellular functions.

Availability

Injection: 60 mg/1.5 ml in single-use vial

🟡 Indications and dosages

➤ Metastatic hormone-refractory prostate cancer previously treated with a docetaxel-containing treatment regimen

Adults: 25 mg/m² I.V. by 1-hour infusion q 3 weeks in combination with prednisone 10 mg P.O. daily throughout treatment

Dosage adjustment

• Grade 3 or greater neutropenia for longer than 1 week despite appropriate treatment, including granulocyte-colony stimulating factor (G-CSF)
• Febrile neutropenia
• Grade 3 or greater diarrhea or persisting diarrhea despite appropriate treatment

Contraindications

• Hypersensitivity to drug or to other drugs formulated with polysorbate 80
• Patients with neutrophil counts of 1,500 cells/mm³ or less

Precautions

Use cautiously in:
• hepatic impairment with total bilirubin at or above the upper limit of normal (ULN), or AST or ALT levels 1.5 × ULN or greater (avoid use)
• severe renal impairment (creatinine clearance less than 30 mL/minute) and end-stage renal disease
• neutropenia
• GI symptoms
• infusion reactions
• concurrent use of strong CYP3A inducers or inhibitors (avoid use)
• elderly patients

• pregnant or breastfeeding patients
• children (safety and efficacy not established).

Administration

• Follow facility policy for handling, preparing, and administering carcinogenic, mutagenic, and teratogenic drugs.
◀€ Don't administer by I.V. push or bolus.
• Premedicate patient at least 30 minutes before each dose with the following I.V. drugs to reduce risk or severity of hypersensitivity: Antihistamine (dexchlorpheniramine 5 mg, or diphenhydramine 25 mg, or equivalent antihistamine), corticosteroid (dexamethasone 8 mg or equivalent steroid), H₂ antagonist (ranitidine 50 mg or equivalent H₂ antagonist).
• Give oral or I.V. antiemetic prophylaxis as needed.
• Don't use PVC infusion containers or polyurethane infusion sets for preparation or administration of drug.
• Be aware that drug requires two dilutions before administering.
• To reconstitute, use entire contents of accompanying diluent to achieve a concentration of 10 mg/ml. Withdraw only required amount of first dilution to prepare final infusion solution before administering. When transferring diluent, direct needle onto inside wall of vial and inject slowly to limit foaming. Remove syringe and needle and gently mix initial diluted solution by repeated inversions for at least 45 seconds to ensure full mixing of drug and diluent. Don't shake. Let solution stand for a few minutes to allow foam to dissipate; check that solution is homogeneous and contains no visible particulate matter.
• The second dilution should be done immediately (within 30 minutes) to obtain final infusion. Withdraw recommended dose from vial containing 10 mg/ml using calibrated syringe and

further dilute into sterile 250-ml PVC-free container of either normal saline solution or 5% dextrose solution for infusion. If dose greater than 65 mg is required, use larger volume of infusion vehicle so that a concentration of 0.26 mg/ml isn't exceeded. Concentration of final infusion solution should be between 0.10 and 0.26 mg/ml. Remove syringe and thoroughly mix final infusion solution by gently inverting bag or bottle. Final infusion solution in either normal saline solution or 5% dextrose solution should be used within 8 hours if kept at ambient temperature (including the 1-hour infusion) or within a total of 24 hours if refrigerated (including the 1-hour infusion).

• Inspect visually for particulate matter, crystals, and discoloration before administering. Discard unused portion.

• Discard first diluted solution or second (final) infusion solution if either isn't clear or appears to have precipitation.

• As final infusion solution is supersaturated, it may crystallize over time. If this occurs, don't use solution; discard it.

• Don't mix with other drugs.

• Use an in-line filter of 0.22-micrometer nominal pore size for administration.

◀≣ Reduce dosage as prescribed for Grade 3 or greater neutropenia lasting longer than 1 week despite appropriate treatment (including G-CSF), for febrile neutropenia, or for Grade 3 or greater diarrhea or persisting diarrhea despite appropriate treatment. Discontinue drug if patient continues to experience any of these reactions at prescribed lower dosage.

• Consider G-CSF and secondary prophylaxis in all patients considered to be at increased risk for neutropenia complications.

◀≣ Immediately discontinue infusion if severe hypersensitivity reactions

occur and initiate appropriate therapy. Be aware that patients with a history of severe hypersensitivity reactions shouldn't be rechallenged with this drug.

Route	Onset	Peak	Duration
I.V.	Unknown	End of infusion	Unknown

Adverse reactions

CNS: headache, dizziness, asthenia, fatigue, peripheral neuropathy
CV: hypotension, **arrhythmia**
GI: nausea, vomiting, diarrhea, constipation, abdominal pain, anorexia, dyspepsia, mucosal inflammation
GU: hematuria, urinary tract infection, dysuria, **renal failure**
Hematologic: neutropenia, anemia, leukopenia, thrombocytopenia
Musculoskeletal: back pain, arthralgia, muscle spasms
Respiratory: dyspnea, cough
Skin: alopecia
Other: pyrexia, dysgeusia, pain, weight loss, dehydration, peripheral edema, **hypersensitivity**

Interactions

Drug-drug. *Strong CYP3A inducers (such as carbamazepine, phenobarbital, phenytoin, rifabutin, rifampin, rifapentin):* decreased cabazitaxel concentration
Strong CYP3A inhibitors (such as atazanavir, clarithromycin, indinavir, itraconazole, ketoconazole, nefazodone, nelfinavir, ritonavir, saquinavir, telithromycin, voriconazole): increased cabazitaxel concentration
Drug-diagnostic tests. ALT, AST, bilirubin: increased levels
Drug-herbs. St. John's wort: decreased cabazitaxel concentration

Patient monitoring

• Monitor CBC with differential and renal and hepatic function tests closely.

• Be aware that the incidence of Grade 3 to 4 hematologic adverse reactions,

---

◀≣ Clinical alert

particularly neutropenia and febrile neutropenia, is higher in patients age 65 or older compared to younger patients.

◀ᣵ Be aware that cabazitaxel is extensively metabolized in the liver and hepatic impairment is likely to increase cabazitaxel concentration, with risk of severe and life-threatening complications in patients receiving other drugs belonging to same class.

◀ᣵ Continue to closely monitor patents for hypersensitivity reactions, especially during first and second infusions. Hypersensitivity reactions may occur within a few minutes after initiation of infusion; therefore, have facilities and equipment available for treatment of hypotension and bronchospasm. If severe hypersensitivity occurs that includes generalized rash, erythema, hypotension, and bronchospasm, immediately discontinue infusion and initiate appropriate therapy.

• Watch for dehydration if patient has nausea, vomiting, or severe diarrhea; be aware that intensive measures may be required for severe diarrhea and electrolyte imbalance. Initite appropriate measures, including rehydration and antidiarrheal or antiemetic medications, as needed. Delay or reduce dosage as necessary if patient has diarrhea at or above Grade 3.

◀ᣵ Be aware that renal failure may occur in association with sepsis, dehydration, or obstructive uropathy. Immediately take appropriate measures to identify causes of renal failure and treat aggressively.

Patient teaching

• Explain the importance of taking oral prednisone as prescribed.

• Explain the importance of routine blood cell counts and instruct patient to monitor temperature frequently.

◀ᣵ Instruct patient to immediately contact prescriber if signs and symptoms of hypersensitivity reactions occur, including rash or itching, skin redness, dizziness or faintness, chest or throat tightness, facial swelling, or breathing problems.

◀ᣵ Instruct patient to immediately contact prescriber if urinary tract problems, irregular heartbeat, significant vomiting or diarrhea, decreased urinary output, or blood in urine occurs.

• Advise patient to report numbness or tingling of the hands or feet or muscle problems.

• Advise patient to contact prescriber if a fever or other evidence of potential infection, such as cough or pain on urination, develops.

• Instruct patient to tell prescriber all drugs he's taking, because some drugs have potential for serious drug interactions and shouldn't be taken with cabazitaxel.

• Advise patient not to use St. John's wort without consulting prescriber.

• Advise female patient of childbearing age to avoid becoming pregnant while receiving this drug.

• Advise breastfeeding patient that she should decide whether to discontinue breastfeeding or discontinue drug, taking into account importance of drug for her treatment.

• As appropriate, review all other significant and life-threatening adverse reactions and interactions, especially those related to the drugs, tests, and herbs mentioned above.

calcitonin (salmon)
APO-Calcitonin, Calcimar, Caltine, Fortical, Miacalcic ✠, Miacalcin, Miacalcin Nasal Spray, Sandoz Calcitonin

Pharmacologic class: Hormone (calcium-lowering)
Therapeutic class: Hypocalcemic
Pregnancy risk category C

Action
Directly affects bone, kidney, and GI tract. Decreases osteoclastic osteolysis in bone; also reduces mineral release and collagen breakdown in bone and promotes renal excretion of calcium. In pain relief, acts through prostaglandin inhibition, pain threshold modification, or beta-endorphin stimulation.

Availability
Injection: 0.5 mg/ml (human), 1 mg/ml (human), 200 international units/ml in 2-ml vials (salmon)
Nasal spray (salmon): 200 international units/actuation, metered nasal spray in 3.7 ml-bottle

⑦ Indications and dosages
➤ Postmenopausal osteoporosis
Adults: *Calcitonin (salmon)*—100 international units/day I.M. or subcutaneously, or 200 international units/day intranasally with concurrent supplemental calcium and vitamin D
➤ Paget's disease of bone (osteitis deformans)
Adults: *Calcitonin (salmon)*—Initially, 100 international units/day I.M. or subcutaneously; after titration, maintenance dosage is 50 to 100 international units daily or every other day (three times weekly). *Calcitonin (human)*—0.5 mg I.M. or subcutaneously daily, reduced to 0.25 mg daily.

➤ Hypercalcemia
Adults: *Calcitonin (salmon)*—4 international units/kg I.M. or subcutaneously q 12 hours; after 1 or 2 days, may increase to 8 international units/kg q 12 hours; after 2 more days, may increase further, if needed, to 8 international units q 6 hours.

Contraindications
• Hypersensitivity to drug or salmon
• Pregnancy or breastfeeding

Precautions
Use cautiously in:
• renal insufficiency, pernicious anemia
• children.

Administration
◀⟨ Before salmon calcitonin therapy begins, perform skin test, if prescribed. Don't give drug if patient has positive reaction. Have epinephrine available.
• Bring nasal spray to room temperature before using.
• Give intranasal dose as one spray in one nostril daily; alternate nostrils every day.
• To minimize adverse effects, give at bedtime.
• Rotate injection sites to decrease inflammatory reactions.

Route	Onset	Peak	Duration
I.M., subcut.	15 min	4 hr	8-24 hr
Intranasal	Rapid	0.5 hr	1 hr

Adverse reactions
CNS: headache, weakness, dizziness, paresthesia
CV: chest pain
EENT: epistaxis, nasal irritation, rhinitis
GI: nausea, vomiting, diarrhea, epigastric pain or discomfort
GU: urinary frequency
Musculoskeletal: arthralgia, back pain
Respiratory: dyspnea
Skin: rash

Reactions in **bold** are life-threatening. ◀⟨ Clinical alert

Other: altered taste, allergic reactions including facial flushing, swelling, and **anaphylaxis**

Interactions
Drug-drug. *Previous use of bisphosphonates (alendronate, etidronate, pamidronate, risedronate):* decreased response to calcitonin

Patient monitoring
• Monitor for adverse reactions during first few days of therapy.
• Assess alkaline phosphatase level and 24-hour urinary excretion of hydroxyproline.
• Check urine for casts.
• Monitor serum electrolyte and calcium levels.

Patient teaching
• Instruct patient to take drug before bedtime to lessen GI upset. Tell him to call prescriber if he can't maintain his usual diet because of GI upset.
• Inform patient using nasal spray that runny nose, sneezing, and nasal irritation may occur during first several days as he adjusts to spray.
• Instruct patient to bring nasal spray to room temperature before using.
• Advise patient to blow nose before using spray, to take intranasal dose as one spray in one nostril daily, and to alternate nostrils with each dose.
• Tell patient to discard unrefrigerated bottles of calcitonin (salmon) nasal spray after 30 days.
• Encourage patient to consume a diet rich in calcium and vitamin D.
• As appropriate, review all other significant adverse reactions and interactions, especially those related to the drugs mentioned above.

calcium acetate
Phos-Ex⊕, PhosLo, PhosLo Gelcap

calcium carbonate
Adcal⊕, Alka-Mints, Cacit⊕, Calcarb 600, Calci-Chew, Calci-Mix, Caltrate 600, Children's Pepto Chooz, Florical, Maalox Regular Chewable, Mylanta Children's, Nephro-Calci, Nu-Cal✲, Os-Cal, Os-Cal 500, Oysco, Oyst-Cal 500, Oystercal 500, Rapeze⊕, Remegel⊕, Rennie Soft Chews⊕, Rolaids Calcium Rich, SeapCal⊕, Setlers⊕, Tums, Tums E-X, Tums Ultra

calcium chloride
Calciject✲, Cal-San✲, Cal-500✲, Calcarea✲, Calciforte✲, Cal Supp✲

calcium citrate
Cal-C-Caps, Cal-CEE

calcium gluconate

calcium lactate

tricalcium phosphate
Poster

Pharmacologic class: Mineral

Therapeutic class: Dietary supplement, electrolyte replacement agent

Pregnancy risk category C (calcium acetate, chloride, glubionate, gluceptate, phosphate), *NR* (calcium carbonate, citrate, gluconate, lactate)

Action
Increases serum calcium level through direct effects on bone, kidney, and GI tract. Decreases osteoclastic osteolysis by reducing mineral release and collagen breakdown in bone.

Availability

Calcium acetate—
Gelcaps: 667 mg
Tablets: 667 mg
Calcium carbonate—
Capsules: 1,250 mg
Lozenges: 600 mg
Oral suspension: 1,250 mg
Powder: 6.5 g
Tablets: 650 mg, 1,250 mg, 1,500 mg
Tablets (chewable): 750 mg, 1,000 mg, 1,250 mg
Tablets (gum): 300 mg, 450 mg, 500 mg
Calcium chloride—
Injection: 10% solution
Calcium citrate—
Tablets: 950 mg
Calcium gluceptate—
Injection: 22% solution
Calcium gluconate—
Injection: 10% solution
Tablets: 500 mg, 650 mg, 975 mg
Calcium lactate—
Tablets: 325 mg, 650 mg
Tricalcium phosphate—
Tablets: 600 mg

🅾 Indications and dosages

➤ Hypocalcemic emergency
Adults: 7 to 14 mEq I.V. of 10% calcium gluconate solution, 2% to 10% calcium chloride solution, or 22% calcium gluceptate solution
Children: 1 to 7 mEq calcium gluconate I.V.
Infants: Up to 1 mEq calcium gluconate I.V.
➤ Hypocalcemic tetany
Adults: 4.5 to 16 mEq calcium gluconate I.V., repeated as indicated until tetany is controlled
Children: 0.5 to 0.7 mEq/kg calcium gluconate I.V. three to four times daily as indicated until tetany is controlled
Neonates: 2.4 mEq/kg calcium gluconate I.V. daily in divided doses
➤ Cardiac arrest
Adults: 0.027 to 0.054 mEq/kg calcium chloride I.V., 4.5 to 6.3 mEq calcium

gluceptate I.V., or 2.3 to 3.7 mEq calcium gluconate I.V.
Children: 0.27 mEq/kg calcium chloride I.V., repeated in 10 minutes if needed. Check calcium level before giving additional doses.
➤ Magnesium intoxication
Adults: Initially, 7 mEq I.V.; subsequent dosages based on patient response
➤ Exchange transfusions
Adults: 1.35 mEq calcium gluconate I.V. with each 100 ml of citrated blood
➤ Hyperphosphatemia in patients with end-stage renal disease
Adults: Two tablets P.O. daily, given in divided doses t.i.d. with meals. May increase gradually to bring serum phosphate level below 6 mg/dl, provided hypercalcemia doesn't develop.
➤ Dietary supplement
Adults: 500 mg to 2 g P.O. daily

Off-label uses

• Osteoporosis

Contraindications

• Hypersensitivity to drug
• Ventricular fibrillation
• Hypercalcemia and hypophosphatemia
• Cancer
• Renal calculi
• Pregnancy or breastfeeding

Precautions

Use cautiously in:
• renal insufficiency, pernicious anemia, heart disease, sarcoidosis, hyperparathyroidism, hypoparathyroidism
• history of renal calculi
• children.

Administration

◀ᴇ When infusing I.V., don't exceed a rate of 200 mg/minute.
• Keep patient supine for 15 minutes after I.V. administration to prevent orthostatic hypotension.
• Administer P.O. doses 1 to 1½ hours after meals.

Reactions in **bold** are life-threatening.   ◀ᴇ Clinical alert

• Know that I.M. or subcutaneous administration is never recommended.
• Be aware that I.V. route is preferred in children.
• Be alert for extravasation, which causes tissue necrosis.

Route	Onset	Peak	Duration
P.O.	Unknown	Unknown	Unknown
I.V.	Immediate	Immediate	0.5-2 hr

Adverse reactions

CNS: headache, weakness, dizziness, syncope, paresthesia
CV: mild blood pressure decrease, **bradycardia, arrhythmias, cardiac arrest** (with rapid I.V. injection)
GI: nausea, vomiting, diarrhea, constipation, epigastric pain or discomfort
GU: urinary frequency, renal calculi
Metabolic: hypercalcemia
Musculoskeletal: joint pain, back pain
Respiratory: dyspnea
Skin: rash
Other: altered or chalky taste, excessive thirst, allergic reactions (including facial flushing, swelling, tingling, tenderness in hands, and **anaphylaxis**)

Interactions

Drug-drug. *Atenolol, fluoroquinolones, tetracycline:* decreased bioavailability of these drugs
Calcium channel blockers: decreased calcium effects
Cardiac glycosides: increased risk of cardiac glycoside toxicity
Iron salts: decreased iron absorption
Sodium polystyrene sulfonate: metabolic alkalosis
Verapamil: reversal of verapamil effects
Drug-diagnostic tests. *Calcium:* increased level
Drug-food. *Foods containing oxalic acid (such as spinach), phytic acid (such as whole grain cereal), or phosphorus (such as dairy products):* interference with calcium absorption

Patient monitoring

• Monitor calcium levels frequently, especially in elderly patients.

Patient teaching

• Instruct patient to consume plenty of milk and dairy products during therapy.
• Refer patient to dietitian for help in meal planning and preparation.
• As appropriate, review all other significant and life-threatening adverse reactions and interactions, especially those related to the drugs, tests, and foods mentioned above.

calcium polycarbophil

Equalactin, FiberCon, Fiber-Lax, Fiber-Tabs, Konsyl

Pharmacologic class: Bulk-forming agent
Therapeutic class: Laxative
Pregnancy risk category NR

Action

Absorbs water, thereby expanding and increasing bulk and moisture content of stool; increased bulk promotes peristalsis and bowel movement.

Availability

Tablets: 500 mg
Tablets (chewable): 500 mg, 1,250 mg

🖉 Indications and dosages

➤ Constipation
Adults and children ages 12 and older: 1 g P.O. q.i.d. as needed. Maximum dosage is 6 g daily.
Children ages 7 to 12: 500 mg P.O. one to three times daily as needed. Maximum dosage is 3 g daily.

Children ages 3 to 6: 500 mg P.O. b.i.d. as needed. Maximum dosage is 1.5 g daily.

➤ Diarrhea; irritable bowel syndrome
Adults and children ages 12 and older: 1 g P.O. q.i.d. as needed. Maximum dosage is 6 g daily.
Children ages 7 to 12: 500 mg P.O. one to three times daily as needed. Maximum dosage is 3 g in a 24-hour period.
Children ages 3 to 6: 500 mg P.O. b.i.d. as needed. Maximum dosage is 1.5 g daily.

Contraindications
• GI obstruction
• Difficulty swallowing

Precautions
Use cautiously in:
• pregnant or breastfeeding patients
• children.

Administration
• Give with at least 8 oz of water or other fluid.
• Administer at least 2 hours before or after other drugs.
• Make sure patient maintains adequate fluid intake.

Route	Onset	Peak	Duration
P.O.	12-24 hr	3 days	Variable

Adverse reactions
CV: chest pain
GI: nausea, vomiting, abdominal pain, flatulence, rectal bleeding, **intestinal obstruction**
Respiratory: difficulty breathing
Other: laxative dependence

Interactions
Drug-drug. *Tetracyclines:* impaired tetracycline absorption
Drug-herbs. *Lily of the valley, pheasant's eye, squill:* increased risk of adverse drug reactions

Patient monitoring
◀€ Monitor patient for difficulty breathing and signs and symptoms of intestinal obstruction.
• Assess for rectal bleeding and for failure to respond to drug.
• Monitor fluid intake and output, and assess hydration status regularly.

Patient teaching
• Instruct patient to take each dose with at least 8 oz of water or other fluid.
• Advise patient to space doses at least 2 hours apart from other drugs.
◀€ Urge patient to seek immediate medical attention if he experiences chest pain, vomiting, difficulty breathing, or rectal bleeding.
• Advise patient to tell prescriber if he's taking other drugs or if he has abdominal pain, nausea, vomiting, or a sudden change in bowel habits lasting 2 weeks or longer.
• As appropriate, review all other significant and life-threatening adverse reactions and interactions, especially those related to the drugs and herbs mentioned above.

calfactant
Infasurf

Pharmacologic class: Natural lung surfactant

Therapeutic class: Lung surfactant
Pregnancy risk category NR

Action
Adsorbs rapidly to air: liquid interface of lung alveoli, stabilizing and modifying surface tension. Restores adequate pressure volumes, gas exchange, and overall lung compliance.

Availability
Suspension for intratracheal injection: 6 ml in single-dose vials

⚠ Indications and dosages
➤ To prevent respiratory distress syndrome (RDS) in at-risk premature infants; treatment of infants who develop RDS
Premature infants: 3 ml/kg at birth intratracheally q 12 hours, up to three doses. Initial dose must be administered as two 1.5-ml/kg doses.

Contraindications
None

Precautions
Use cautiously in:
• altered ventilation requirements
• risk of cyanosis, bradycardia, or airway obstruction.

Administration
◀€ Know that drug is intended for intratracheal administration and should be given only by neonatologists or other clinicians experienced in neonatal intubation and ventilatory management in facilities with adequate personnel, equipment, and drugs.
◀€ Don't dilute drug or shake vial.
• Be aware that drug must be drawn into syringe through 20G or larger needle, taking care to avoid excessive foaming. Needle must be removed before drug is delivered through endotracheal tube.
◀€ Know that infant must receive continuous monitoring before, during, and after drug administration.

Route	Onset	Peak	Duration
Intratrach.	Rapid	Unknown	Unknown

Adverse reactions
CV: bradycardia
Respiratory: requirement for manual ventilation or reintubation, **airway** obstruction, reflux of drug into endotracheal tube, cyanosis

Interactions
None significant

Patient monitoring
◀€ Monitor infant's respiratory status continuously during and after drug administration.

Patient teaching
• Teach parents about treatment and assure them that infant will be monitored carefully.

candesartan cilexetil
Amias ⊕, Atacand

Pharmacologic class: Angiotensin II receptor antagonist
Therapeutic class: Antihypertensive
Pregnancy risk category D

FDA | BOXED WARNING
• When used during second or third trimester of pregnancy, drug may cause fetal injury and death. Discontinue as soon as possible when pregnancy is detected.

Action
Blocks aldosterone-producing and vasoconstrictive effects of angiotensin II at various receptor sites, including vascular smooth muscle and adrenal glands

Availability
Tablets: 4 mg, 8 mg, 16 mg, 32 mg

⚠ Indications and dosages
➤ Hypertension

Adults: 16 mg P.O. daily. Start at lower dosage if patient is receiving diuretics or is volume depleted. Range is 8 to 32 mg/day as a single dose or divided in two doses.

Children age 6 to younger than 17 weighing more than 50 kg (110 lb): 8 to 16 mg P.O. daily. Start at lower dosage if patient is receiving diuretics or is volume depleted. Range is 4 to 32 mg/day as a single dose or divided in two doses.

Children age 6 to younger than 17 weighing less than 50 kg: 4 to 8 mg P.O. daily. Start at lower dosage if patient is receiving diuretics or is volume depleted. Range is 4 to 16 mg/day as a single dose or divided in two doses.

Children age 1 to younger than 6: 0.20 mg/kg oral suspension P.O. daily. Start at lower dosage if patient is receiving diuretics or is volume depleted. Range is 0.05 to 0.4 mg/kg oral suspension P.O. daily as a single dose or divided in two doses.

➤Heart failure (New York Heart Association class II-IV)
Adults: 4-mg tablet P.O. daily. Increase to target maintenance dosage of 32 mg P.O. daily by doubling dose q 2 weeks, as tolerated.

Dosage adjustment
• Renal impairment
• Moderate hepatic insufficiency

Contraindications
• Hypersensitivity to drug or its components

Precautions
Use cautiously in:
• heart failure, renal or hepatic impairment
• volume- or salt-depleted patients receiving high doses of diuretics, hyperkalemia
• pregnant or breastfeeding patients
• children younger than age 1.

Administration
• Give with or without food.
• Be aware that pharmacist can prepare a suspension from tablets for children who can't swallow tablets.
🔊 Supervise patient closely if he is receiving concurrent diuretics or is otherwise at risk for intravascular volume depletion.
• Know that diuretic may be added to regimen if candesartan alone doesn't control blood pressure.

Route	Onset	Peak	Duration
P.O.	2-4 hr	6-8 hr	24 hr

Adverse reactions
CNS: dizziness, syncope, fatigue, headache
CV: hypotension, chest pain, peripheral edema, **mitral or aortic valve stenosis**
EENT: ear congestion or pain, sinus disorders, sore throat
GI: nausea, diarrhea, constipation, abdominal pain, dry mouth
GU: albuminuria, **renal failure**
Hepatic: hepatitis
Metabolic: gout, **hyperkalemia**
Musculoskeletal: arthralgia, back pain, muscle weakness
Respiratory: upper respiratory tract infection, cough, bronchitis
Other: dental pain, fever

Interactions
Drug-drug. *Diuretics, other antihypertensives:* increased risk of hypotension
Lithium: increased lithium blood level
Nonsteroidal anti-inflammatory drugs: decreased antihypertensive effect
Potassium-sparing diuretics, potassium supplements: increased risk of hyperkalemia
Drug-food. *Salt substitutes containing potassium:* increased risk of hyperkalemia
Drug-herbs. *Ephedra (ma huang), licorice, yohimbine:* decreased antihypertensive effect

---

Reactions in **bold** are life-threatening.　　　　🔊 Clinical alert

Patient monitoring
• Monitor electrolyte levels and kidney and liver function test results.
• Assess blood pressure regularly to gauge drug efficacy.
• Closely monitor patient with renal dysfunction who is receiving concurrent diuretics.

Patient teaching
• Tell patient to take drug with or without food.
• Inform caregiver that pharmacist will prepare a suspension for child who can't swallow tablets. Shake suspension well before each dose.
• Teach patient about lifestyle changes that help control blood pressure, such as proper diet, exercise, stress reduction, smoking cessation, and moderation of alcohol intake.
• Instruct patient to use reliable birth control method and to contact prescriber and discontinue drug if she suspects she's pregnant.
• Caution patient not to take herbs without consulting prescriber.
• As appropriate, review all other significant and life-threatening adverse reactions and interactions, especially those related to the drugs, foods, and herbs mentioned above.

---

capecitabine
Xeloda

Pharmacologic class: Fluoropyrimidine, antimetabolite (pyrimidine analog)

Therapeutic class: Antineoplastic

Pregnancy risk category D

FDA | BOXED WARNING

• In patients receiving concomitant oral coumarin-derivative anticoagulants (such as warfarin and phenprocoumon), monitor International Normalized Ratio (INR) or prothrombin time (PT) frequently to allow appropriate anticoagulant dosage adjustment. Altered coagulation parameters, bleeding, and death have occurred in patients taking this drug combination. Postmarketing reports show significant INR and PT increases in patients stabilized on anticoagulants when capecitabine therapy began. Age older than 60 and cancer diagnosis independently increase coagulopathy risk.

Action
Enzymatically converts to 5-fluorouracil, which injures cells by interfering with DNA synthesis, cell division, RNA processing, and protein synthesis

Availability
Tablets: 150 mg, 500 mg

Indications and dosages
➤ Metastatic breast cancer resistant to both paclitaxel and a chemotherapy regimen that includes anthracycline; metastatic colorectal cancer when treatment with fluoropyrimidine therapy alone is preferred
Adults: Initially, 2,500 mg/m²/day P.O. in two divided doses for 2 weeks, followed by a 1-week rest period; administered in 3-week cycles

Dosage adjustment
• Renal impairment
• Hepatic impairment
• Elderly patients

Contraindications
• Hypersensitivity to drug
• Severe renal impairment
• Pregnancy or breastfeeding

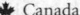

Precautions

Use cautiously in:

- mild to moderate renal impairment, hepatic impairment, severe diarrhea, coronary artery disease, intestinal disease, infection, coagulopathy
- children younger than age 18.

Administration

- Give with water within 30 minutes after a meal.
- If dosage must be lowered because of toxicity, don't increase dosage later.

Route	Onset	Peak	Duration
P.O.	Unknown	1.5-2 hr	Unknown

Adverse reactions

CNS: dizziness, fatigue, headache, insomnia, paresthesia
CV: edema
EENT: eye irritation
GI: nausea, vomiting, diarrhea, constipation, abdominal pain, dyspepsia, anorexia, stomatitis, **intestinal obstruction**
Hematologic: anemia, lymphopenia, **neutropenia, thrombocytopenia**
Metabolic: dehydration
Musculoskeletal: myalgia, limb pain
Skin: dermatitis, alopecia, nail disorder, hand and foot syndrome (palmar-plantar erythrodysesthesia)
Other: fever

Interactions

Drug-drug. *Antacids:* increased capecitabine blood level
Leucovorin: increased cytotoxicity
Live-virus vaccines: impaired ability to mount an immune response to vaccine
Phenytoin: increased phenytoin blood level
Warfarin: increased risk of bleeding
Drug-diagnostic tests. *Bilirubin:* increased level
Hemoglobin, neutrophils, platelets, white blood cells: decreased levels

Patient monitoring

- Monitor patient for signs and symptoms of toxicity. Be prepared to reduce dosage or withhold drug when indicated.
- Stay alert for signs and symptoms of infection.
- Carefully assess fluid and electrolyte status if patient has severe diarrhea.
- Monitor weight, CBC, International Normalized Ratio, prothrombin time, and kidney and liver function test results.
- Evaluate closely for adverse reactions in patients older than age 80.

Patient teaching

- Advise patient to take drug with water within 30 minutes after a meal.
- ◀ Instruct patient to immediately report nausea, vomiting, diarrhea, mouth ulcers, swollen joints, temperature above 100.5 °F (38 °C), and other signs or symptoms of infection.
- Tell patient to expect dosage adjustments during therapy.
- Urge patient to use reliable birth control method because drug may harm fetus if she becomes pregnant.
- Caution patient not to breastfeed during therapy.
- As appropriate, review all other significant and life-threatening adverse reactions and interactions, especially those related to the drugs and tests mentioned above.

captopril

Acepril ✚, Apo-Capto ✦, Dom-Captopril, Gen-Captopril ✦, Med-Captopril

Pharmacologic class: Angiotensin-converting enzyme (ACE) inhibitor

Therapeutic class: Antihypertensive

Pregnancy risk category C (first trimester), *D* (second and third trimesters)

• When used during second or third trimester of pregnancy, drug may cause fetal injury and death. Discontinue as soon as possible when pregnancy is detected.

Action
Prevents conversion of angiotensin I to angiotensin II, which leads to decreased vasoconstriction and, ultimately, to lower blood pressure. Also decreases blood pressure by increasing plasma renin secretion from kidney and reducing aldosterone secretion from adrenal cortex. Decreased aldosterone secretion prevents sodium and water retention.

Availability
Tablets: 12.5 mg, 25 mg, 50 mg, 100 mg

🍷 Indications and dosages
➤ Hypertension
Adults: 12.5 to 25 mg P.O. two to three times daily; may be increased up to 150/mg/day at 1- to 2-week intervals. Usual dosage is 50 mg t.i.d. If patient is receiving diuretics, start with 6.25 to 12.5 mg P.O. two to three times daily. If blood pressure isn't adequately controlled after 1 to 2 weeks, add diuretic, as prescribed. If further blood pressure decrease is needed, dosage may be raised to 150 mg P.O. t.i.d. while patient continues on diuretic. Maximum dosage is 450 mg/day.
➤ Heart failure
Adults: Usual initial dosage is 25 mg P.O. t.i.d. After increasing to 50 mg P.O. t.i.d. (if indicated), do not increase dosage further for 2 weeks, to determine satisfactory response. Don't exceed 450 mg/day.
➤ Left ventricular dysfunction after myocardial infarction

Adults: 6.25 mg P.O. as a test dose, followed by 12.5 mg t.i.d. May increase up to 50 mg t.i.d.
➤ Diabetic nephropathy
Adults: 25 mg P.O. t.i.d.

Dosage adjustment
• Renal impairment

Off-label uses
• Bartter's syndrome
• Hypertension associated with scleroderma
• Management of hypertensive crisis
• Raynaud's syndrome
• Rheumatoid arthritis
• Severe childhood hypertension

Contraindications
• Hypersensitivity to drug or other ACE inhibitors
• Angioedema (hereditary or idiopathic)
• Pregnancy

Precautions
Use cautiously in:
• renal or hepatic impairment, hypovolemia, hyponatremia, aortic stenosis and hypertrophic cardiomyopathy, cardiac or cerebrovascular insufficiency, systemic lupus erythematous
• family history of angioedema
• black patients with hypertension
• elderly patients
• breastfeeding patients
• children.

Administration
• Discontinue other antihypertensives 1 week before starting captopril, if possible.
• Give 1 hour before meals on empty stomach.

Route	Onset	Peak	Duration
P.O.	0.25-1 hr	1-1.5 hr	6-12 hr

Adverse reactions

CNS: headache, dizziness, drowsiness, fatigue, weakness, insomnia

CV: angina pectoris, tachycardia, **hypotension**

EENT: sinusitis

GI: nausea, diarrhea, anorexia

GU: proteinuria, erectile dysfunction, decreased libido, gynecomastia, **renal failure**

Hematologic: anemia, **agranulocytosis, leukopenia, pancytopenia, thrombocytopenia**

Metabolic: hyperkalemia

Respiratory: cough, asthma, bronchitis, dyspnea, **eosinophilic pneumonitis**

Skin: rash, **angioedema**

Other: altered taste, fever

Interactions

Drug-drug. *Allopurinol:* increased risk of hypersensitivity reaction

Antacids: decreased captopril absorption

Antihypertensives, general anesthetics that lower blood pressure, nitrates, phenothiazines: additive hypotension

Cyclosporine: hyperkalemia

Digoxin, lithium: increased blood levels of these drugs, increased risk of toxicity

Epoetin alfa: additive hyperkalemia

Indomethacin: reduced antihypertensive effect of captopril

Nonsteroidal anti-inflammatory drugs: decreased antihypertensive response

Potassium-sparing diuretics, potassium supplements: hyperkalemia

Probenecid: decreased elimination and increased blood level of captopril

Drug-diagnostic tests. *Alanine aminotransferase, alkaline phosphatase, aspartate aminotransferase, bilirubin, blood urea nitrogen, creatinine, potassium:* increased levels

Granulocytes, hemoglobin, platelets, red blood cells, sodium, white blood cells: decreased levels

Urine acetone: false-positive result

Drug-food. *Any food:* decreased captopril absorption

Salt substitutes containing potassium: hyperkalemia

Drug-herbs. *Capsaicin, yohimbine:* cough

Drug-behaviors. *Acute alcohol ingestion:* additive hypotension

Patient monitoring

◀€ Monitor for sudden blood pressure drop within 3 hours of initial dose if patient is receiving concurrent diuretics and on a low-sodium diet.

• Monitor hematologic, kidney, and liver function test results.

• Check for proteinuria monthly and after first 9 months of therapy.

Patient teaching

• Tell patient to take drug 1 hour before meals on empty stomach.

• Advise patient to report fever, rash, sore throat, mouth sores, fast or irregular heartbeat, chest pain, or cough.

• Inform patient that dizziness, fainting, and light-headedness usually disappear once his body adjusts to drug.

• Tell patient his ability to taste may decrease during first 2 to 3 months of therapy.

• Caution patient to avoid over-the-counter medications unless approved by prescriber.

• As appropriate, review all other significant and life-threatening adverse reactions and interactions, especially those related to the drugs, tests, foods, herbs, and behaviors mentioned above.

carbamazepine

Apo-Carbamazepine♣, Arbil⊕, Bio-Carbamazepine♣, Carbagen⊕, Carbamaz♣, Carbatrol, Dom-Carbamazepine♣, Epimaz⊕, Epitol, Equetro, Gen-Carbamazepine♣, Mazepine♣, Novo-Carbamazepine♣, Nu-Carbamazepine♣, PHL-Carbamazepine♣, PMS-Carbamazepine♣, Sandoz Carbamazepine♣, Tegretol, Tegretol-XR

Pharmacologic class: Iminostilbene derivative
Therapeutic class: Anticonvulsant
Pregnancy risk category D

FDA | BOXED WARNING

• Prescriber should be thoroughly familiar with prescribing information, particularly regarding use with other drugs (especially those that increase toxicity potential).
• Drug has been linked to aplastic anemia and agranulocytosis.
• Transient or persistent decreases in platelet or white blood cell (WBC) counts have occurred, but data aren't available to accurately estimate incidence or outcome. Rarely, leukopenia cases progressed to aplastic anemia or agranulocytosis.
• Obtain complete pretreatment hematologic tests as baseline. If WBC or platelet count drops during therapy, monitor closely. Consider withdrawing drug if evidence of significant bone marrow depression develops.

Action

Unclear. Chemically related to tricyclic antidepressants (TCAs). Anticonvulsant action may result from reduction in polysynaptic responses and blocking of post-tetanic potentiation.

Availability

Capsules (extended-release): 100 mg, 200 mg, 300 mg
Oral suspension: 100 mg/5 ml
Tablets: 200 mg
Tablets (chewable): 100 mg
Tablets (extended-release): 100 mg, 200 mg, 400 mg

🖊 Indications and dosages

➤ Prophylaxis of generalized tonic-clonic, mixed, and complex-partial seizures
Adults and children ages 12 and older: Initially, 200 mg P.O. b.i.d. (tablets) or 100 mg q.i.d. (oral suspension). Increase by up to 200 mg/day q 7 days until therapeutic blood levels are reached. Usual maintenance dosage is 600 to 1,200 mg/day in divided doses q 6 to 8 hours. In children ages 12 to 15, don't exceed 1 g/day. Give extended-release forms b.i.d.
Children ages 6 to 12: Initially, 100 mg P.O. b.i.d. (tablets) or 50 mg q.i.d. (oral suspension). Increase by up to 100 mg weekly until therapeutic levels are reached. Usual maintenance dosage is 400 to 800 mg/day. Don't exceed 1 g/ day. Give extended-release forms b.i.d.
Children younger than age 6: Initially, 10 to 20 mg/kg/day P.O. in two or three divided doses. May increase by up to 100 mg/day at weekly intervals. Usual maintenance dosage is 250 to 350 mg/day. Don't exceed 400 mg/day.
➤ Trigeminal neuralgia
Adults: Initially, 100 mg b.i.d. (tablets) or 50 mg q.i.d. (oral suspension). Increase by up to 200 mg/day until pain relief occurs; then give maintenance dosage of 200 to 1,200 mg/day in divided doses. Usual maintenance range is 400 to 800 mg/day.

♣ Canada   ⊕ UK   ⚘ Hazardous drug   ⊗ High-alert drug

Off-label uses
- Alcohol, cocaine, or benzodiazepine withdrawal
- Atypical psychoses
- Central diabetes insipidus
- Mood disorders
- Neurogenic pain

Contraindications
- Hypersensitivity to drug or TCAs
- MAO inhibitor use within past 14 days
- Bone marrow depression
- Pregnancy or breastfeeding

Precautions
Use cautiously in:
- cardiac disease, hepatic disease, increased intraocular pressure, mixed seizure disorders, glaucoma
- elderly males with prostatic hypertrophy
- psychiatric patients.

Administration
- Don't give within 14 days of MAO inhibitor.
- Give tablets with meals; may give extended-release capsules without regard to meals.
- Don't give with grapefruit juice.
- If desired, contents of extended-release capsules may be sprinkled over food; however, capsule and contents shouldn't be crushed or chewed.

Route	Onset	Peak	Duration
P.O.	Up to 1 mo	4-5 hr	6-12 hr
P.O. (extended)	Up to 1 mo	2-12 hr	12 hr

Adverse reactions
CNS: ataxia, drowsiness, fatigue, psychosis, syncope, vertigo, headache, **worsening of seizures**
CV: hypertension, hypotension, **arrhythmias, atrioventricular block, aggravation of coronary artery disease, heart failure**

EENT: blurred vision, diplopia, nystagmus, corneal opacities, conjunctivitis, pharyngeal dryness
GI: nausea, vomiting, diarrhea, abdominal pain, stomatitis, glossitis, dry mouth, anorexia
GU: urinary hesitancy, retention, or frequency; albuminuria; glycosuria; erectile dysfunction
Hematologic: eosinophilia, lymphadenopathy, **agranulocytosis, aplastic anemia, thrombocytopenia, leukopenia**
Hepatic: hepatitis
Metabolic: syndrome of inappropriate antidiuretic hormone secretion
Respiratory: pneumonitis
Skin: photosensitivity, rash, urticaria, diaphoresis, **erythema multiforme, Stevens-Johnson syndrome**
Other: weight gain, chills, fever

Interactions
Drug-drug. *Acetaminophen:* increased risk of acetaminophen-induced hepatotoxicity, decreased acetaminophen efficacy
Anticoagulants, bupropion: increased metabolism of these drugs, causing decreased efficacy
Barbiturates: decreased barbiturate blood level, increased carbamazepine blood level
Charcoal: decreased carbamazepine absorption
Cimetidine, danazol, diltiazem: increased carbamazepine blood level
Cyclosporine, felbamate, felodipine, haloperidol: decreased blood levels of these drugs
Doxycycline: shortened doxycycline half-life and reduced antimicrobial effect
Hormonal contraceptives: decreased contraceptive efficacy, possibly leading to pregnancy
Hydantoins: increased or decreased hydantoin blood level, decreased carbamazepine blood level

c

Isoniazid: increased risk of carbamazepine toxicity and isoniazid hepatotoxicity

Lithium: increased risk of CNS toxicity

Macrolide antibiotics (such as clarithromycin and erythromycin), propoxyphene, selective serotonin reuptake inhibitors (such as fluoxetine and fluvoxamine), verapamil: increased carbamazepine blood level, greater risk of toxicity

MAO inhibitors: high fever, hypertension, seizures, and possibly death

Nondepolarizing neuromuscular blockers: shortened carbamazepine duration of action

TCAs: increased carbamazepine blood level and greater risk of toxicity, decreased TCA blood level

Valproic acid: decreased valproic acid blood level with possible loss of seizure control, variable changes in carbamazepine blood level

Drug-diagnostic tests. *Blood urea nitrogen, eosinophils, liver function tests:* increased values

Granulocytes, hemoglobin, platelets, thyroid function tests, white blood cells: decreased values

Drug-food. *Grapefruit juice:* increased drug blood level and effects

Drug-herbs. *Plantain (psyllium seed):* inhibited GI absorption of drug

Patient monitoring

◀≶ Monitor patient closely. Institute seizure precautions if drug must be withdrawn suddenly.

• Assess for history of psychosis; drug may activate symptoms.

• Monitor baseline hematologic, kidney, and liver function test results.

• During dosage adjustments, monitor vital signs and fluid intake and output. Stay alert for fluid retention, renal failure, and cardiovascular complications.

• With high doses, monitor CBC weekly for first 3 months and then monthly to detect bone marrow depression.

Patient teaching

• Tell patient that he may sprinkle contents of extended-release capsules over food, but that he shouldn't crush or chew capsule or contents.

• Advise patient that coating on extended-release capsules may be visible in stools because it isn't absorbed.

• Tell patient to take drug with meals to minimize GI upset.

• Caution patient to avoid driving and other hazardous activities until he knows how drug affects concentration, alertness, and vision.

• Advise patient to avoid excessive sun exposure and to wear protective clothing and sunscreen.

• Inform female patient that drug may interfere with hormonal contraception. Advise her to use alternative birth-control method.

• As appropriate, review all other significant and life-threatening adverse reactions and interactions, especially those related to the drugs, tests, foods, and herbs mentioned above.

carbidopa-levodopa

Apo-Levocarb✦, Co-carledopa⊕, Dom-Levo-Carbidopa✦, Half Sinemet⊕, Novo-Levocarbidopa✦, Nu-Levocarb✦, Sinemet, Sinemet CR, Tilolec⊕

Pharmacologic class: Dopamine agonist

Therapeutic class: Antiparkinsonian

Pregnancy risk category C

Action

After conversion to dopamine in CNS, levodopa acts as a neurotransmitter, relieving symptoms of Parkinson's disease. Carbidopa prevents destruction of levodopa, making more levodopa available to be decarboxylated to dopamine in brain.

Availability

Tablets: 10 mg carbidopa/100 mg levodopa, 25 mg carbidopa/100 mg levodopa, 25 mg carbidopa/250 mg levodopa
Tablets (extended-release): 25 mg carbidopa/100 mg levodopa, 50 mg carbidopa/200 mg levodopa

⚠ Indications and dosages

➤ Idiopathic Parkinson's disease; parkinsonism; symptomatic parkinsonism
Conventional tablets—
Adults not currently receiving levodopa: Initially, 10 mg carbidopa/100 mg levodopa P.O. three to four times daily or 25 mg carbidopa/100 mg levodopa t.i.d.; may be increased q 1 to 2 days until desired effect occurs
Adults converting from levodopa alone (less than 1.5 g/day): Initially, 25 mg carbidopa/100 mg levodopa three to four times daily; may be increased q 1 to 2 days until desired effect occurs
Adults converting from levodopa alone (more than 1.5 g/day): Initially, 25 mg carbidopa/250 mg levodopa three to four times daily; may be increased q 1 to 2 days until desired effect occurs
Extended-release tablets—
Adults not currently receiving levodopa: Initially, 50 mg carbidopa/200 mg levodopa P.O. b.i.d., with doses spaced at least 6 hours apart
Adults converting from standard carbidopa-levodopa: Initiate therapy with at least 10% more levodopa content/day (may need up to 30% more) given at 4- to 8-hour intervals while awake; wait 3 days between dosage changes. Some patients may need higher dosages and shorter dosing intervals.

Contraindications

- Hypersensitivity to drug or tartrazine
- Angle-closure glaucoma
- MAO inhibitor use within past 14 days
- Malignant melanoma
- Breastfeeding

Precautions

Use cautiously in:
- cerebrovascular, renal, hepatic, or endocrine disease
- history of cardiac, psychiatric, or ulcer disease
- abrupt drug discontinuation or dosage
- pregnant patients
- children ages 18 and under (safety not established).

Administration

- Give dose as close as possible to time ordered to ensure stable drug blood level.
- Know that giving extended-release form with food increases drug bioavailability.
- If patient needs general anesthesia, continue drug therapy as appropriate (if he's allowed to have oral fluids and drugs).
◀ᣤ Be aware that drug shouldn't be withdrawn abruptly.

Route	Onset	Peak	Duration
P.O.	Unknown	40-120 min	Unknown

Adverse reactions

CNS: anxiety, dizziness, hallucinations, memory loss, headache, numbness, confusion, insomnia, nightmares, delusions, psychotic changes, depression, dementia, poor coordination, worsening hand tremor
CV: cardiac irregularities, palpitations, orthostatic hypotension
EENT: blurred vision, diplopia, mydriasis, eyelid twitching, difficulty swallowing

GI: nausea, vomiting, diarrhea, constipation, abdominal pain or discomfort, flatulence, excessive salivation, dry mouth, anorexia, **upper GI hemorrhage** (with history of peptic ulcer)
GU: urinary retention, urinary incontinence, dark urine
Hematologic: hemolytic anemia, leukopenia
Hepatic: hepatotoxicity
Musculoskeletal: muscle twitching, involuntary or spasmodic movements
Respiratory: hyperventilation
Skin: melanoma, flushing, rash, abnormally dark sweat
Other: altered or bitter taste, burning sensation of tongue, tooth grinding (especially at night), weight changes, hot flashes, hiccups

Interactions
Drug-drug. *Anticholinergics:* decreased carbidopa-levodopa absorption
Antihypertensives: additive hypotension
Haloperidol, papaverine, phenothiazines, phenytoin, reserpine: reversal of carbidopa-levodopa effects
Inhalation hydrocarbon anesthetics: increased risk of arrhythmias
MAO inhibitors: hypertensive reactions
Methyldopa: altered efficacy of carbidopa-levodopa, increased risk of adverse CNS reactions
Pyridoxine: antagonism of carbidopa-levodopa effects
Selegiline: increased risk of adverse reactions
Drug-diagnostic tests. *Alanine aminotransferase, alkaline phosphatase, aspartate aminotransferase, bilirubin, blood urea nitrogen, lactate dehydrogenase, low-density lipoproteins, protein-bound iodine, uric acid:* increased levels
Coombs' test: false-positive result
Granulocytes, hemoglobin, platelets, white blood cells: decreased values
Urine glucose, urine ketones: test interference

Drug-food. *Foods rich in pyridoxine (liver, yeast, cereals):* reversal of carbidopa-levodopa effects
Drug-herbs. *Kava:* decreased carbidopa-levodopa efficacy
Octacosanol: worsening of dyskinesia
Drug-behaviors. *Cocaine use:* increased risk of adverse reactions to carbidopa-levodopa

Patient monitoring
• Monitor patient for orthostatic hypotension.
• Assess patient's need for drug "holiday" if his response to drug decreases.

Patient teaching
◀€ Inform patient that muscle and eyelid twitching may indicate toxicity. Tell him to report these symptoms immediately.
◀€ Caution patient not to stop taking drug abruptly.
• Instruct patient to swallow extended-release tablets whole without crushing or chewing them.
• Advise patient to move slowly when sitting up or standing, to avoid dizziness or light-headedness caused by sudden blood pressure drop.
• Tell patient that drug may darken or discolor his urine and sweat.
• As appropriate, review all other significant and life-threatening adverse reactions and interactions, especially those related to the drugs, tests, foods, herbs, and behaviors mentioned above.

carboplatin
Pharmacologic class: Alkylating agent
Therapeutic class: Antineoplastic
Pregnancy risk category D

• Give under supervision of physician experienced in cancer chemotherapy, in facility with adequate diagnostic and treatment resources.
• Bone marrow suppression is dose-related and may be severe, resulting in infection and bleeding. Anemia may be cumulative and warrant transfusions.
• Vomiting is a common adverse effect.
• Anaphylactic-like reactions may occur within minutes of administration.

Action
Inhibits DNA synthesis by causing cross-linking of parent DNA strands; interferes with RNA transcription, causing growth imbalance that leads to cell death. Cell cycle phase nonspecific.

Availability
Injection: 50-mg, 150-mg, and 450-mg vials

📁 Indications and dosages
➤ Initial treatment of advanced ovarian cancer or palliative treatment of ovarian cancer unresponsive to other chemotherapeutic modalities
Adults: Initially, 300 mg/m^2 I.V. (given with cyclophosphamide) at 4-week intervals. For refractory tumors, 360 mg/m^2 I.V. as a single dose; may be repeated at 4-week intervals, depending on response. However, single dose shouldn't be repeated until neutrophil count is at least 2,000/mm^3 and platelet count at least 100,000/mm^3. Subsequent dosages are based on blood counts.

Dosage adjustment
• Renal impairment
• Reduced bone marrow reserve

Off-label uses
• Advanced endometrial cancer
• Advanced or recurrent squamous cell carcinoma of head and neck
• Relapsed and refractory acute leukemia
• Small-cell lung cancer
• Testicular cancer

Contraindications
• Hypersensitivity to drug, cisplatin, or mannitol
• Pregnancy or breastfeeding

Precautions
Use cautiously in:
• hearing loss, electrolyte imbalances, renal impairment, active infections, diminished bone marrow reserve
• females of childbearing age.

Administration
• Premedicate with antiemetics, as prescribed.
• When preparing and administering drug, follow facility protocol for handling cytotoxic drugs.
• Reconstitute powder for injection by adding sterile water for injection, 0.9% sodium chloride injection, or 5% dextrose injection, as appropriate, to provide 10-mg/ml solution. Drug may be further diluted to concentrations as low as 0.5 mg/ml.
• Don't use with needles or I.V. sets containing aluminum.
• Administer I.V. infusion over at least 15 minutes.
• Make sure patient maintains adequate fluid intake.
• Know that drug is given in combination with other agents.

Route	Onset	Peak	Duration
I.V.	Rapid	21 days	28 days

Adverse reactions
CNS: weakness, dizziness, confusion, peripheral neuropathy, **cerebrovascular accident**

CV: heart failure, embolism
EENT: visual disturbances, ototoxicity
GI: nausea, vomiting, constipation, diarrhea, abdominal pain, stomatitis
GU: gonadal suppression, **nephrotoxicity**
Hematologic: anemia, **leukopenia, thrombocytopenia, neutropenia**
Hepatic: hepatitis
Metabolic: hypocalcemia, hypokalemia, hypomagnesemia, hyponatremia
Respiratory: bronchospasm
Skin: alopecia, rash, urticaria, erythema, pruritus
Other: altered taste, hypersensitivity reactions, **anaphylaxis**

Interactions

Drug-drug. *Live-virus vaccines:* decreased antibody response to vaccine, increased risk of adverse reactions
Myelosuppressants: additive bone marrow depression
Nephrotoxic or ototoxic drugs (such as aminoglycosides, loop diuretics): additive nephrotoxicity or ototoxicity
Phenytoin: decreased phenytoin blood level

Drug-diagnostic tests. *Alkaline phosphatase (ALP), aspartate aminotransferase (AST), blood urea nitrogen, creatinine:* increased values
Electrolytes, hematocrit, hemoglobin. neutrophils, platelets, red blood cells, white blood cells: decreased values

Patient monitoring

• Assess for signs and symptoms of hypersensitivity reactions.
• Monitor CBC to help detect drug-induced anemia and other hematologic reactions.
• Monitor ALP, AST, and total bilirubin levels.
• Evaluate fluid and electrolyte balance.

Patient teaching

• Instruct patient to report signs and symptoms of allergic response and other adverse reactions, such as breathing problems, mouth sores, rash, itching, and reddened skin.
• Advise patient to report unusual bleeding or bruising.
• Caution patient to avoid driving and other hazardous activities until he knows how drug affects concentration and alertness.
• Urge patient to avoid activities that can cause injury. Advise him to use soft toothbrush and electric razor to avoid gum and skin injury.
• Instruct patient to drink plenty of fluids to ensure adequate urinary output.
• Provide dietary counseling and refer patient to dietitian as needed if GI adverse effects significantly limit food intake.
• As appropriate, review all other significant and life-threatening adverse reactions and interactions, especially those related to the drugs and tests mentioned above.

carisoprodol
Soma

Pharmacologic class: Carbamate derivative

Therapeutic class: Centrally acting skeletal muscle relaxant

Controlled substance schedule IV (in some states)

Pregnancy risk category C

Action

Unknown. May modify central perception of pain without modifying pain reflexes. Skeletal muscle relaxation may result from sedative properties or from inhibition of activity in descending reticular formation and spinal cord.

Availability
Tablets: 250 mg, 350 mg

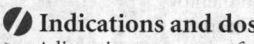 Indications and dosages
➤ Adjunctive treatment of muscle spasms associated with acute painful musculoskeletal conditions
Adults: 350 mg P.O. q.i.d.
➤ Relief of discomfort associated with acute painful musculoskeletal conditions
Adults: 250 to 350 mg P.O. t.i.d. and at bedtime

Contraindications
• Hypersensitivity to drug or meprobamate
• Porphyria or suspected porphyria

Precautions
Use cautiously in:
• severe hepatic or renal disease
• history of substance abuse
• pregnant or breastfeeding patients
• children ages 12 and younger.

Administration
• Give last daily dose at bedtime.
• Administer with food if GI upset occurs.
• If patient can't swallow tablets, mix with syrup, chocolate, or jelly.

Route	Onset	Peak	Duration
P.O.	30 min	1-2 hr	4-6 hr

Adverse reactions
CNS: dizziness, drowsiness, agitation, ataxia, depression, headache, insomnia, vertigo, tremor, depression
CV: hypotension, tachycardia
GI: nausea, vomiting, epigastric distress
Hematologic: eosinophilia, **leukopenia**
Respiratory: asthma attacks
Skin: flushing (especially of face), rash, pruritus, **erythema multiforme**
Other: hiccups, fever, psychological drug dependence, **anaphylactic shock**

Interactions
Drug-drug. *Antihistamines, opioids, sedative-hypnotics:* additive CNS depression
Drug-diagnostic tests. *Eosinophils:* increased count
Drug-herbs. *Chamomile, hops, kava, skullcap, valerian:* increased CNS depression
Drug-behaviors. *Alcohol use:* increased CNS depression

Patient monitoring
• When giving to breastfeeding patient, watch for signs of sedation and GI upset in infant.
• Monitor range of motion, stiffness, and discomfort level.
• Know that drug is metabolized to meprobamate. Monitor for drug dependence, especially in patients with history of substance abuse.

Patient teaching
• Tell patient that psychological drug dependence may occur.
• Instruct patient to avoid over-the-counter drugs and alcohol, because they may increase CNS depression.
• Caution patient to avoid driving and other hazardous activities until he knows how drug affects concentration and alertness.
• As appropriate, review all other significant and life-threatening adverse reactions and interactions, especially those related to the drugs, tests, herbs, and behaviors mentioned above.

carmustine
Gliadel Wafer

Pharmacologic class: Alkylating agent
Therapeutic class: Antineoplastic
Pregnancy risk category D

FDA | BOXED WARNING

- Give under supervision of physician experienced in cancer chemotherapy.
- Most common and severe toxic effect is bone marrow suppression—notably thrombocytopenia and leukopenia, which may contribute to bleeding and overwhelming infections in already compromised patient. Monitor blood counts weekly for at least 6 weeks after dose. Don't give courses more often than every 6 weeks.

Action

Unclear. Thought to interfere with bacterial cell-wall synthesis by cross-linking strands of DNA and disrupting RNA transcription, causing cell to rupture and die. Exhibits minimal immunosuppressant activity.

Availability

Intracavitary wafer implant: 7.7 mg (available in packages of eight wafers)
Powder for injection: 100-mg vials

🖊 Indications and dosages

➤ Brain tumor; multiple myeloma; Hodgkin's disease; other lymphomas
Adults and children: 150 to 200 mg/m^2 I.V. as a single dose q 6 to 8 weeks, or 75 to 100 mg/m^2/day for 2 days q 6 weeks, or 40 mg/m^2/day for 5 days q 6 weeks. Repeat dose q 6 weeks if platelet count exceeds 100,000/mm^3 and white blood cell (WBC) count exceeds 4,000/mm^3.
➤ Adjunct to brain surgery
Adults: Up to 61.6 mg (eight wafers) implanted in surgical cavity created during brain tumor resection

Dosage adjustment

- Based on WBC and platelet counts

Off-label uses

- Mycosis fungoides

Contraindications

- Hypersensitivity to drug
- Radiation therapy
- Chemotherapy
- Pregnancy or breastfeeding

Precautions

Use cautiously in:
- infection; depressed bone marrow reserve; respiratory, hepatic, or renal impairment
- females of childbearing age.

Administration

- Know that drug may be used alone or in conjunction with other treatments, such as surgery or radiation.
- Follow facility policy when preparing, administering, and handling drug.
- Reconstitute drug by dissolving vial of 100 mg with 3 ml of sterile dehydrated alcohol (provided with drug), followed by 27 ml of sterile water for injection; yields solution with concentration of 3.3 mg carmustine/ml. Solution may be further diluted with 5% dextrose injection and delivered by I.V. infusion over 1 to 2 hours.
- Know that infusion lasting less than 1 hour causes intense pain and burning at I.V. site.
- Infuse solution in glass containers only; drug is unstable in plastic I.V. bags.
- Know that skin contact with reconstituted drug may cause transient hyperpigmentation. If contact occurs, wash skin thoroughly with soap and water.
- Be aware that oxidized regenerated cellulose may be placed over wafers to secure them against surgical cavity surface.
- Know that resection cavity should be irrigated after wafer placement and that dura should be closed in watertight fashion.

Route	Onset	Peak	Duration
I.V.	Immediate	15 min	6 wk
Intra-cavitary	Unknown	Unknown	Unknown

Adverse reactions

CNS: ataxia, drowsiness
GI: nausea, vomiting, diarrhea, esophagitis, stomatitis, anorexia
GU: azotemia, **renal failure, nephrotoxicity**
Hematologic: anemia, **leukopenia, thrombocytopenia, cumulative bone marrow depression, bone marrow dysplasia**
Hepatic: hepatotoxicity
Respiratory: pulmonary fibrosis, pulmonary infiltrates
Skin: alopecia, hyperpigmentation, facial flushing, abnormal bruising
Other: I.V. site pain, **secondary malignancies**

Interactions

Drug-drug. *Anticoagulants, aspirin, nonsteroidal anti-inflammatory drugs:* increased risk of bleeding
Antineoplastics: additive bone marrow depression
Cimetidine: potentiation of bone marrow depression
Digoxin, phenytoin: decreased blood levels of these drugs
Live-virus vaccines: decreased antibody response to vaccines, increased risk of adverse reactions
Drug-diagnostic tests. *Alkaline phosphatase, aspartate aminotransferase, bilirubin, nitrogenous compounds (urea):* increased levels
Hemoglobin, WBCs: decreased values
Drug-behaviors. *Smoking:* increased risk of respiratory toxicity

Patient monitoring

• Assess baseline kidney and liver function tests.
• Monitor CBC for up to 6 weeks after giving dose to detect delayed bone marrow toxicity.
• Know that pulmonary function tests should be performed before therapy begins and regularly throughout therapy to assess for toxicity.

Patient teaching

• Instruct patient to report signs and symptoms of allergic response and other adverse reactions.
• Inform patient that severe flushing may follow I.V. dose but should subside in 2 to 4 hours.
• Tell patient to avoid activities that can cause injury. Advise him to use soft toothbrush and electric razor to avoid gum and skin injury.
• Advise patient to minimize GI upset by eating small, frequent servings of food and drinking plenty of fluids.
• Instruct patient to monitor urinary output and report significant changes.
• Inform patient that drug may cause hair loss.
• Advise patient that he'll undergo regular blood testing during therapy.
• As appropriate, review all other significant and life-threatening adverse reactions and interactions, especially those related to the drugs, tests, and behaviors mentioned above.

carteolol hydrochloride
Ocupress, Teoptic⊕

Pharmacologic class: Beta-adrenergic blocker (nonselective)
Therapeutic class: Antianginal, antihypertensive
Pregnancy risk category C

Action

Blocks stimulation of cardiac beta$_1$-adrenergic receptor sites and pulmonary beta$_2$-adrenergic receptor sites. Shows intrinsic sympathomimetic activity, causing slowing of heart rate, decreased myocardial excitability, reduced cardiac output, and decreased renin release from kidney. Also reduces intraocular pressure.

◀€ Clinical alert

Availability
Ophthalmic solution: 1%

⚕ Indications and dosages
➢ Open-angle glaucoma; ocular hypertension
Adults: One drop (1% solution) in affected eye(s) b.i.d.

Contraindications
• Hypersensitivity to drug or its components
• Other beta-adrenergic blockers
• Cardiogenic shock, bradycardia, second- or third-degree atrioventricular block
• Sinus bradycardia, bronchial asthma, severe obstructive pulmonary disease
• Overt heart failure

Precautions
Use cautiously in:
• pulmonary disease, diabetes mellitus, hypoglycemia, thyrotoxicosis, hypotension, respiratory depression, major surgery, history of bronchospasm
• angle-closure glaucoma
• pregnant or breastfeeding patients
• children.

Administration
• Be aware that if the patient's intraocular pressure isn't at a satisfactory level on prescribed regimen, concomitant therapy with pilocarpine and other miotics, or epinephrine or dipivefrin, or systemically administered carbonic anhydrase inhibitors such as acetazolamide may be instituted.

Route	Onset	Peak	Duration
Ophthalmic	Unknown	Unknown	Unknown

Adverse reactions
CNS: headache, fatigue, weakness, anxiety, depression, dizziness, insomnia, memory loss, nightmares, paresthesia, hallucinations, disorientation, slurred speech
CV: orthostatic hypotension, peripheral vasoconstriction, conduction disturbances, **bradycardia, heart failure**
EENT: decreased night vision and stinging, blurred vision, dry eyes, tinnitus, stuffy nose, nasal congestion, pharyngitis, **laryngospasm**
GI: nausea, vomiting, diarrhea, constipation, abdominal pain, dry mouth, anorexia
GU: dysuria, polyuria, nocturia, dark urine, erectile dysfunction, decreased libido, Peyronie's disease
Metabolic: hyperglycemia, **hypoglycemia**
Musculoskeletal: arthralgia, back or leg pain, muscle cramps
Respiratory: wheezing, **bronchospasm, respiratory distress, pulmonary edema**
Skin: pruritus, rash, sweating
Other: drug-induced lupuslike syndrome, **anaphylaxis**

Interactions
Drug-drug. *Adrenergics:* antagonism of carteolol effects
Allergen immunotherapy: increased risk of anaphylaxis
Amphetamines, ephedrine, epinephrine, norepinephrine, phenylephrine, pseudoephedrine: unopposed alpha-adrenergic stimulation, causing excessive hypertension and bradycardia
Antihypertensives, nitrates: additive hypotension
Clonidine: increased hypotension and bradycardia, exaggerated withdrawal phenomenon
Digoxin: additive bradycardia
Dobutamine, dopamine: decrease in beneficial cardiovascular effects
General anesthetics, I.V. phenytoin, verapamil: additive myocardial depression
Insulin, oral hypoglycemics: altered efficacy of these drugs
MAO inhibitors: hypertension

Nonsteroidal anti-inflammatory drugs: decreased antihypertensive effect
Thyroid preparations: decreased carteolol efficacy

Drug-diagnostic tests. *Blood urea nitrogen, lipoproteins, potassium, triglycerides, uric acid:* increased levels
Glucose or insulin tolerance test: test interference

Drug-behaviors. *Acute alcohol ingestion:* additive hypotension
Cocaine use: unopposed alpha-adrenergic stimulation, causing excessive hypertension and bradycardia
Sun exposure: photophobia

Patient monitoring

◀€ Monitor vital signs (especially blood pressure) and ECG. Drug may alter cardiac output and cause ineffective airway clearance. Discontinue drug at first sign of heart failure.

• Monitor for disorientation, agitation, visual disturbances, dizziness, ataxia and euphoria. Symptoms usually subside over several hours.

• Weigh patient daily and measure fluid intake and output to detect fluid retention.

• Assess blood glucose level regularly if patient has diabetes mellitus.

Patient teaching

• Instruct patient to take last dose at bedtime.

◀€ Instruct patient to report breathing problems immediately.

• Tell patient to report dizziness, confusion, depression, respiratory problems, or rash.

• Advise patient to move slowly when sitting up or standing to avoid dizziness or light-headedness from sudden blood pressure drop.

• Caution patient to avoid driving and other hazardous activities until he knows how drug affects concentration and alertness.

• Teach patient proper use of eyedrops. Tell him to wash hands first, not to

touch dropper tip to any surface, and not to use drops when contact lenses are in eyes.

• Inform patient that although eyedrops commonly cause stinging and blurred vision, he should notify prescriber if these symptoms are severe.

• As appropriate, review all other significant and life-threatening adverse reactions and interactions, especially those related to the drugs, tests, and behaviors mentioned above.

carvedilol
Apo-Carvedilol✤, Coreg, Dom-Carvedilol✤, Eucardic⊕

carvedilol phosphate
Coreg CR, Novo-Carvedilol✤, PHL-Carvedilol✤, PMS-Carvedilol✤

Pharmacologic class: Beta-adrenergic blocker (nonselective)
Therapeutic class: Antihypertensive
Pregnancy risk category C

Action
Blocks stimulation of cardiac beta$_1$-adrenergic receptor sites and pulmonary beta$_2$-adrenergic receptor sites. Shows intrinsic sympathomimetic activity, causing slowing of heart rate, decreased myocardial excitability, reduced cardiac output, and decreased renin release from kidney.

Availability
Capsules (extended-release): 10 mg, 20 mg, 40 mg, 80 mg
Tablets: 3.125 mg, 6.25 mg, 12.5 mg, 25 mg

⚫ Indications and dosages
➢ Hypertension

Adults: Initially, 6.25 mg P.O. b.i.d. (Coreg). May be increased q 7 to 14 days to a maximum dosage of 25 mg b.i.d. Or, 20 mg P.O. daily (Coreg CR). If tolerated, using standing systolic pressure about 1 hour after dosing, maintain dosage of Coreg CR for 7 to 14 days; then increase to 40 mg once daily if needed based on trough systolic standing blood pressure. Maintain this dosage for 7 to 14 days and adjust to 80 mg once daily if tolerated and needed. Total daily dose of Coreg CR shouldn't exceed 80 mg.

➤ Heart failure caused by ischemia or cardiomyopathy

Adults: Initially, 3.125 mg P.O. b.i.d. (Coreg) for 2 weeks. May increase to 6.25 mg b.i.d. Dosage may be doubled q 2 weeks as tolerated, not to exceed 25 mg b.i.d. in patients weighing less than 85 kg (187 lb) or 50 mg b.i.d. in patients weighing more than 85 kg. Or, 10 mg P.O. daily (Coreg CR) for 2 weeks. If tolerated, increase dosage to 20 mg, 40 mg, and 80 mg over successive intervals of at least 2 weeks.

➤ Left ventricular dysfunction following myocardial infarction

Adults: Initially, 6.25 mg P.O. b.i.d. (Coreg); increase after 3 to 10 days to 12.5 mg b.i.d. (based on tolerability), then increase to target dosage of 25 mg b.i.d. A lower starting dose (3.125 mg b.i.d.) or slower titration may be used if clinically indicated. Or, 20 mg P.O. once daily (Coreg CR); increase after 3 to 10 days to 40 mg daily (based on tolerability), then increase to target dose of 80 mg daily. A lower starting dose may be used (10 mg daily) or the rate of up titration may be slowed if clinically indicated.

Off-label uses

• Angina pectoris
• Idiopathic cardiomyopathy

Contraindications

• Hypersensitivity to drug
• Uncompensated heart failure
• Pulmonary edema
• Cardiogenic shock
• Bradycardia or heart block
• Severe hepatic impairment
• Bronchial asthma, bronchospasm

Precautions

Use cautiously in:

• renal or hepatic impairment, pulmonary disease, diabetes mellitus, hypoglycemia, thyrotoxicosis, peripheral vascular disease, hypotension, respiratory depression
• elderly patients
• pregnant or breastfeeding patients
• children.

Administration

• Ensure that patient is hemodynamically stable and fluid retention has been minimized before starting therapy.
• Give immediate-release form with food to slow absorption and minimize orthostatic hypotension.
• Give extended-release form in the morning with food and instruct patient to swallow capsule whole.
• For patients who can't swallow capsules whole, carefully open capsules and sprinkle contents on applesauce; have patient swallow contents immediately without chewing. Don't use warm applesauce; doing so could affect the modified-release properties of this formulation.
• When drug is used to treat heart failure, check apical pulse before administering. If it's below 60 beats/minute, withhold dosage and contact prescriber.
• When drug is used for hypertension, check standing systolic pressure about 1 hour after dosing for use as a guide for patient tolerance.
• Be aware that addition of diuretic may cause additive effects and may worsen orthostatic hypotension.

- Know that full antihypertensive effect takes 7 to 14 days.
- 🔊 Don't withdraw drug abruptly, because this may lead to withdrawal phenomenon (angina exacerbation, myocardial infarction, ventricular arrhythmias, and even death).

Route	Onset	Peak	Duration
P.O.	Within 1 hr	1-2 hr	12 hr

Adverse reactions

CNS: dizziness, fatigue, anxiety, depression, insomnia, memory loss, nightmares, headache, pain
CV: orthostatic hypotension, peripheral vasoconstriction, angina pectoris, chest pain, hypertension, **bradycardia, heart failure, atrioventricular block**
EENT: blurred or abnormal vision, dry eyes, stuffy nose, rhinitis, sinusitis, pharyngitis
GI: nausea, diarrhea, constipation
GU: urinary tract infection, hematuria, albuminuria, decreased libido, erectile dysfunction, **renal dysfunction**
Hematologic: bleeding, **purpura, thrombocytopenia**
Metabolic: hypovolemia, hypervolemia, hyperglycemia, hyponatremia, hyperuricemia, glycosuria, gout, **hypoglycemia**
Musculoskeletal: arthralgia, back pain, muscle cramps
Respiratory: wheezing, upper respiratory tract infection, dyspnea, bronchitis, **bronchospasm, pulmonary edema**
Skin: pruritus, rash
Other: weight gain, lupuslike syndrome, viral infection, **anaphylaxis**

Interactions

Drug-drug. *Antihypertensives:* additive hypotension
Calcium channel blockers, general anesthetics, I.V. phenytoin: additive myocardial depression
Cimetidine: increased carvedilol toxicity
Clonidine: increased hypotension and bradycardia, exaggerated withdrawal phenomenon

Digoxin: additive bradycardia
Dobutamine, dopamine: decrease in beneficial cardiovascular effects
Insulin, oral hypoglycemics: altered efficacy of these drugs
MAO inhibitors: hypertension
Nonsteroidal anti-inflammatory drugs: decreased antihypertensive action
Rifampin, thyroid preparations: decreased carvedilol efficacy
Theophyllines: reduced theophylline elimination, antagonistic effect that decreases theophylline or carteolol efficacy
Drug-diagnostic tests. *Antinuclear antibodies:* increased titers
Blood urea nitrogen, glucose, lipoproteins, potassium, triglycerides, uric acid: increased levels
Drug-food. *Any food:* delayed drug absorption
Drug-behaviors. *Acute alcohol ingestion:* additive hypotension

Patient monitoring

- Watch for signs and symptoms of hypersensitivity reaction.
- Assess baseline CBC and kidney and liver function test results.
- Monitor vital signs (especially blood pressure), ECG, and exercise tolerance. Drug may alter cardiac output and cause ineffective airway clearance.
- Weigh patient daily and measure fluid intake and output to detect fluid retention.
- Measure blood glucose regularly if patient has diabetes mellitus. Drug may mask signs and symptoms of hypoglycemia.

Patient teaching

- Instruct patient to take drug with food exactly as prescribed.
- Tell patient to take extended-release capsule in the morning with food, to swallow capsule whole, and not to chew, crush, or divide its contents.
- Instruct patient who can't swallow capsule whole to carefully open

---

Reactions in **bold** are life-threatening.　　　🔊 Clinical alert

capsule, sprinkle contents on cool or cold applesauce, and swallow contents immediately without chewing. Tell patient not to store mixture for future use.

◀€ Caution patient not to stop taking drug abruptly, because serious reactions may result.

• Advise patient to move slowly when sitting up or standing, to avoid dizziness or light-headedness from sudden blood pressure drop.

• Caution patient to avoid driving and other hazardous activities until he knows how drug affects concentration and alertness.

• Inform male patient that drug may cause erectile dysfunction. Advise him to discuss this issue with prescriber.

• Advise patient to use soft-bristled toothbrush and electric razor to avoid gum and skin injury.

• As appropriate, review all other significant and life-threatening adverse reactions and interactions, especially those related to the drugs, tests, foods, and behaviors mentioned above.

caspofungin acetate
Cancidas

Pharmacologic class: Echinocandin
Therapeutic class: Antifungal
Pregnancy risk category C

Action

Inhibits synthesis of beta (1, 3)-D-glucan, an important component of cell wall in *Aspergillus* and other fungal cells. This inhibition leads to cell rupture and death.

Availability

Lyophilized powder for injection:
50 mg and 70 mg in single-use vials

✔ Indications and dosages

➤ Invasive aspergillosis in patients - refractory to or intolerant of other therapies

Adults ages 18 and older: 70 mg I.V. as a single loading dose on first day, followed by 50 mg/day thereafter

Children ages 3 months to 17 years: 70 mg/m^2 I.V. as a single loading dose on first day, followed by 50 mg/m^2/day thereafter. Maximum loading dosage and daily maintenance dosage shouldn't exceed 70 mg, regardless of calculated dosage.

➤ Esophageal candidiasis

Adults ages 18 and older: 50 mg I.V. daily

Children ages 3 months to 17 years: 70 mg/m^2 I.V. as a single loading dose on first day, followed by 50 mg/m^2/day thereafter. Maximum loading dosage and daily maintenance dosage shouldn't exceed 70 mg, regardless of calculated dosage.

➤ Candidemia and other *Candida* infections (intra-abdominal abscesses, peritonitis, and pleural-space infections)

Adults ages 18 and older: 70 mg I.V. as a single loading dose on first day, followed by 50 mg/day thereafter. Continue therapy for at least 14 days after last positive culture. Consistently neutropenic patient may require longer course of therapy.

Children ages 3 months to 17 years: 70 mg/m^2 I.V. as a single loading dose on first day, followed by 50 mg/m^2/day thereafter. Maximum loading dosage and daily maintenance dosage shouldn't exceed 70 mg, regardless of calculated dosage.

➤ Empirical therapy for presumed fungal infections in febrile neutropenic patients

Adults ages 18 and older: 70 mg I.V. as a single loading dose on first day, followed by 50 mg/day thereafter. Continue therapy until neutropenia resolves, for at least 14 days in patients with fungal infections, or for at least 7 days after both neutropenia and symptoms resolve. If patient tolerates 50-mg dosage well but doesn't obtain adequate response, increase daily dosage to 70 mg.

Children ages 3 months to 17 years: 70 mg/m² I.V. as a single loading dose on first day, followed by 50 mg/m²/day thereafter. Maximum loading dosage and daily maintenance dosage shouldn't exceed 70 mg, regardless of calculated dosage.

Dosage adjustment
• Moderate hepatic insufficiency (adults)

Contraindications
• Hypersensitivity to drug or its components

Precautions
Use cautiously in:
• hepatic impairment
• renal insufficiency
• concurrent cyclosporine use
• pregnant or breastfeeding patients.

Administration
◀€ Don't mix with other drugs or with diluents containing dextrose.
• Reconstitute powder using 10.8 ml of normal saline solution for injection, sterile water for injection, or bacteriostatic water for injection. Mix gently until solution is clear. Add to I.V. bag or bottle containing 250 ml of normal, half-normal, or quarter-normal saline solution for injection or lactated Ringer's solution. Don't exceed concentration of 0.5 mg/ml.
◀€ Don't give by I.V. bolus.
• Administer by slow I.V. infusion over 1 hour.
• Know that in patients with human immunodeficiency virus, oral therapy may be given to help prevent oropharyngeal candidiasis relapse.

• Be aware that adults taking rifampin concurrently should receive 70-mg daily dosage.
• Know that dosage may need to be increased in patients receiving nevirapine, efavirenz, carbamazepine, dexamethasone, or phenytoin.

Route	Onset	Peak	Duration
I.V.	Immediate	9-11 hr	40-50 hr

Adverse reactions
CNS: headache
CV: tachycardia, phlebitis, hypotension, hypertension (children)
GI: nausea, vomiting, diarrhea, abdominal pain
GU: nephrotoxicity
Hematologic: anemia
Metabolic: hypokalemia, hyperkalemia
Musculoskeletal: pain, myalgia, back pain
Respiratory: tachypnea, cough, dyspnea, crackles, pneumonia, **respiratory distress (children), pleural effusion, respiratory failure**
Skin: erythema, pruritus (children), rash
Other: graft-versus-host disease, central line infection (children), chills, mucosal inflammation, peripheral edema, pyrexia, **infusion-related reactions,** septic shock

Interactions
Drug-drug. *Carbamazepine, dexamethasone, efavirenz, nelfinavir, nevirapine, phenytoin, rifampin:* reduced caspofungin blood level
Cyclosporine: markedly increased caspofungin blood level, transient ALT and AST increases
Tacrolimus: possible change in tacrolimus blood level
Drug-diagnostic tests. *Albumin, hematocrit, hemoglobin, magnesium, potassium, total protein (children), white blood cells:* decreased levels
ALP, ALT, AST, bilirubin, calcium, conjugated bilirubin, creatinine,

---

Reactions in **bold** are life-threatening. ◀€ Clinical alert

eosinophils, glucose, urea: increased levels
Potassium: decreased or increased level (children)
Urinary red blood cells: positive

Patient monitoring

◀€ Monitor closely for signs and symptoms of infusion-related reactions (pyrexia, chills, flushing, hypotension, hypertension, tachycardia, dyspnea, tachypnea, anaphylaxis). Be prepared to provide supportive care as needed.

• Monitor I.V. site carefully for phlebitis and other complications.

• Monitor complete blood count and serum electrolyte levels. Stay alert for signs and symptoms of hypokalemia.

• Monitor vital signs, especially for tachycardia and tachypnea.

• Closely monitor liver function tests; watch for evidence of worsening hepatic function.

Patient teaching

◀€ Instruct patient to immediately report signs or symptoms of infusion-related reaction, such as fever, chills, flushing, rapid heart beat, difficult or rapid breathing, or rash.

◀€ Tell patient drug may cause problems in vein used for infusion. Tell him to immediately report pain, swelling, or other symptoms.

• Instruct patient to report headache, nausea, or other unusual or troublesome symptoms.

• As appropriate, review all other significant and life-threatening adverse reactions and interactions, especially those related to the drugs and tests mentioned above.

cefaclor

Apo-Cefaclor✤, Distaclor⊕, PMS-Cefaclor✤, Raniclor

Pharmacologic class: Second-generation cephalosporin
Therapeutic class: Anti-infective
Pregnancy risk category B

Action

Interferes with bacterial cell-wall synthesis, causing cell to rupture and die

Availability

Capsules: 250 mg, 500 mg
Oral suspension: 125 mg/5 ml, 187 mg/5 ml, 250 mg/5 ml, 375 mg/5 ml
Tablets (extended-release): 500 mg

🖊 Indications and dosages

➤ Uncomplicated skin infections caused by *Staphylococcus aureus*
Adults and children ages 16 and older: 375 mg P.O. (extended-release tablet) q 12 hours for 7 to 10 days
➤ Pharyngitis and tonsillitis not caused by *Haemophilus influenzae*
Adults and children ages 16 and older: 375 mg P.O. (extended-release tablet) q 12 hours for 10 days
➤ Chronic bronchitis and acute bronchitis not caused by *H. influenzae*
Adults and children ages 16 and older: 500 mg P.O. (extended-release tablet) q 12 hours for 7 days
➤ Otitis media caused by staphylococci; lower respiratory tract infections caused by *H. influenzae, S. pyogenes,* and *S. pneumoniae;* pharyngitis and tonsillitis caused by *S. pyogenes;* urinary tract infections caused by *Klebsiella* species, *Escherichia coli, Proteus mirabilis,* and coagulase-negative staphylococci
Adults and children ages 13 to 17: 250 mg P.O. q 8 hours. For severe infections, 500 mg P.O. q 8 hours.

Children: 20 mg/kg/day P.O. in divided doses q 8 hours. For serious infections, 40 mg/kg/day P.O. in divided doses q 8 hours. Maximum dosage is 1 g/day.

Dosage adjustment
• Renal insufficiency
• Elderly patients

Contraindications
• Hypersensitivity to cephalosporins or penicillins

Precautions
Use cautiously in:
• renal impairment, phenylketonuria
• history of GI disease (especially colitis)
• emaciated patients
• elderly patients
• pregnant or breastfeeding patients
• children.

Administration
• Obtain specimens for culture and sensitivity testing as necessary before starting therapy.
• Be aware that cross-sensitivity to penicillins may occur.
• Give extended-release tablets with food to enhance absorption.
• Don't give antacids within 2 hours of extended-release form.

Route	Onset	Peak	Duration
P.O.	Rapid	30-60 min	6-12 hr
P.O. (extended)	Unknown	1.5-2.5 hr	12 hr

Adverse reactions
CNS: headache, lethargy, paresthesia, syncope, **seizures**
CV: hypotension, palpitations, chest pain, vasodilation
EENT: hearing loss
GI: nausea, vomiting, diarrhea, abdominal cramps, oral candidiasis, **pseudomembranous colitis**
GU: vaginal candidiasis, **nephrotoxicity**
Hematologic: lymphocytosis, eosinophilia, **bleeding tendency, hemolytic anemia, hypoprothrombinemia, neutropenia, thrombocytopenia, agranulocytosis, bone marrow depression**
Hepatic: hepatic failure, hepatomegaly
Musculoskeletal: arthralgia
Respiratory: dyspnea
Skin: urticaria, maculopapular or erythematous rash
Other: chills, fever, superinfection, **anaphylaxis, serum sickness**

Interactions
Drug-drug. *Aminoglycosides, loop diuretics:* increased risk of nephrotoxicity
Antacids: decreased absorption of extended-release cefaclor tablets
Chloramphenicol: antagonistic effect
Probenecid: decreased excretion and increased blood level of cefaclor
Drug-diagnostic tests. *Alanine aminotransferase, alkaline phosphatase, aspartate aminotransferase, bilirubin, blood urea nitrogen, creatinine, eosinophils, gamma-glutamyltransferase, lactate dehydrogenase:* increased levels
Coombs' test, urinary 17-ketosteroids, nonenzyme-based urine glucose tests (such as Clinitest): false-positive results
Hemoglobin, platelets, white blood cells: decreased values

Patient monitoring
• Assess CBC and kidney and liver function test results.
• With long-term therapy, obtain monthly Coombs' test.
• Monitor for signs and symptoms of superinfection and other serious adverse reactions.

Reactions in **bold** are life-threatening.   ◀€ Clinical alert

Patient teaching

- Instruct patient to take drug with food or milk to reduce GI upset.
- Advise patient to complete entire course of therapy even if he feels better.
- Tell patient to report signs and symptoms of allergic response and other adverse reactions, such as rash, easy bruising, bleeding, severe GI problems, or difficulty breathing.
- Instruct patient to avoid taking antacids within 2 hours of extended-release cefaclor.
- As appropriate, review all other significant and life-threatening adverse reactions and interactions, especially those related to the drugs and tests mentioned above.

cefadroxil

Baxan ✠, Novo-Cefadroxil ✦

Pharmacologic class: First-generation cephalosporin
Therapeutic class: Anti-infective
Pregnancy risk category B

Action

Interferes with bacterial cell-wall synthesis, causing cell to rupture and die

Availability

Capsules: 500 mg
Oral suspension: 250 mg/5 ml, 500 mg/5 ml
Tablets: 1 g

🕭 Indications and dosages

➤ Pharyngitis and tonsillitis caused by beta-hemolytic streptococci
Adults: 1 g/day P.O. or 500 mg P.O. b.i.d. for 10 days
Children: 30 mg/kg/day P.O. in divided doses q 12 hours for 10 days

➤ Skin infections caused by staphylococci and streptococci
Adults: 1 g/day P.O. or 500 mg P.O. q 12 hours
Children: 30 mg/kg/day P.O. in divided doses q 12 hours
➤ Urinary tract infections caused by *Proteus mirabilis, Escherichia coli,* and *Klebsiella* species
Adults: 1 to 2 g/day P.O. in divided doses q 12 hours
Children: 30 mg/kg/day P.O. in divided doses q 12 hours

Dosage adjustment

- Renal insufficiency
- Elderly patients

Off-label uses

- Bone and joint infections
- Unspecified respiratory infections

Contraindications

- Hypersensitivity to cephalosporins or penicillins

Precautions

Use cautiously in:
- renal impairment, phenylketonuria
- history of GI disease (especially colitis)
- elderly patients
- pregnant or breastfeeding patients
- children.

Administration

- Obtain specimens for culture and sensitivity testing as necessary before starting therapy.
- Give with or without food.

Route	Onset	Peak	Duration
P.O.	Rapid	1.5-2 hr	12-24 hr

Adverse reactions

CNS: headache, lethargy, paresthesia, syncope, **seizures**
CV: hypotension, palpitations, chest pain, vasodilation

EENT: hearing loss
GI: nausea, vomiting, diarrhea, cramps, oral candidiasis, **pseudomembranous colitis**
GU: vaginal candidiasis, **nephrotoxicity**
Hematologic: lymphocytosis, eosinophilia, **bleeding tendency, hemolytic anemia, hypoprothrombinemia, neutropenia, thrombocytopenia, agranulocytosis, bone marrow depression**
Hepatic: hepatic failure, hepatomegaly
Musculoskeletal: arthralgia
Respiratory: dyspnea
Skin: urticaria, maculopapular or erythematous rash
Other: chills, fever, superinfection, **anaphylaxis**

Interactions

Drug-drug. *Aminoglycosides, loop diuretics:* increased risk of nephrotoxicity
Probenecid: decreased excretion and increased blood level of cefadroxil
Drug-diagnostic tests. *Alanine aminotransferase, alkaline phosphatase, aspartate aminotransferase, bilirubin, blood urea nitrogen, creatinine, eosinophils, gamma-glutamyltransferase, lactate dehydrogenase:* increased levels
Coombs' test, urinary 17-ketosteroids, nonenzyme-based urine glucose tests (such as Clinitest): false-positive results
Hemoglobin, platelets, white blood cells: decreased values

Patient monitoring

• Assess baseline CBC and kidney and liver function test results.
• Monitor for signs and symptoms of superinfection and other serious adverse reactions.
• Be aware that cross-sensitivity to penicillins may occur.
• With long-term therapy, obtain monthly Coombs' test.

Patient teaching

• Advise patient to take drug with food or milk if GI upset occurs.

• Instruct patient to complete entire course of therapy even if he feels better.
• Tell patient to report signs and symptoms of allergic response and other adverse reactions, such as rash, easy bruising, bleeding, severe GI problems, wheezing, or difficulty breathing.
• As appropriate, review all other significant and life-threatening adverse reactions and interactions, especially those related to the drugs and tests mentioned above.

cefazolin sodium
Ancef

Pharmacologic class: First-generation cephalosporin
Therapeutic class: Anti-infective
Pregnancy risk category B

Action

Interferes with bacterial cell-wall synthesis, causing cell to rupture and die

Availability

Powder for injection: 500 mg, 1 g, 10 g, 20 g
Premixed containers: 500 mg/50 ml in dextrose 5% in water (D_5W), 1 g/50 ml in D_5W

Indications and dosages

➤ Respiratory tract infections caused by group A beta-hemolytic streptococci, *Klebsiella* species, *Haemophilus influenzae,* and *Staphylococcus aureus;* skin infections caused by *S. aureus* and beta-hemolytic streptococci; biliary tract infections caused by *Escherichia coli, Klebsiella* species, *Proteus mirabilis,* and *S. aureus;* bone and joint infections caused by *S. aureus;* genital infections caused by *E. coli, Klebsiella* species, *P. mirabilis,* and strains of enterococci; septicemia caused by *E.*

coli, Klebsiella species, *P. mirabilis, S. aureus,* and *S. pneumoniae;* endocarditis caused by *S. aureus* or beta-hemolytic streptococci

Adults: For mild infections, 250 to 500 mg q 8 hours I.V. or I.M. For moderate to severe infections, 500 to 1,000 mg I.V. or I.M. q 6 to 8 hours. For life-threatening infections, 1,000 to 1,500 mg I.M. or I.V. q 6 hours, to a maximum dosage of 6 g/day.

Children: For mild to moderate infections, 25 to 50 mg/kg/day I.V. or I.M. in divided doses t.i.d. or q.i.d. For severe infections, 100 mg/kg/day I.V. or I.M. in divided doses t.i.d. or q.i.d.

➤ Acute uncomplicated urinary tract infections (UTIs) caused by *E. coli, Klebsiella* species, *P. mirabilis,* and strains of *Enterococcus* and *Enterobacter* species

Adults: 1 g I.V. or I.M. q 12 hours

➤ Surgical prophylaxis

Adults: 1g I.V. or I.M. 30 to 60 minutes before surgery, then 0.5 to 1 g I.V. or I.M. q 6 to 8 hours for 24 hours. If surgery exceeds 2 hours, another 0.5- to 1-g dose I.M. or I.V. may be given intraoperatively.

➤ Pneumococcal pneumonia

Adults: 500 mg I.M. or I.V. infusion q 12 hours

Dosage adjustment
• Renal impairment
• Elderly patients

Contraindications
• Hypersensitivity to cephalosporins or penicillins

Precautions
Use cautiously in:
• renal impairment, phenylketonuria
• history of GI disease (especially colitis)
• emaciated patients
• elderly patients
• pregnant or breastfeeding patients
• children.

Administration
• Obtain specimens for culture and sensitivity testing as needed before starting therapy.
• For intermittent I.V. infusion, administer in volume-control set or in separate, secondary I.V. container over 30 to 60 minutes.
• For direct I.V. injection, dilute reconstituted dose in 5 ml of sterile water for injection and administer slowly over 3 to 5 minutes.
• Don't mix premixed solution with other drugs.
◀€ Don't use flexible container in series connections because of risk of air embolism.
• For I.M. use, reconstitute with sterile water for injection, bacteriostatic water, or normal saline solution for injection. Shake well until dissolved.
• Inject I.M. into large muscle mass.

Route	Onset	Peak	Duration
I.V.	Rapid	End of infusion	6-12 hr
I.M.	Rapid	1-2 hr	6-12 hr

Adverse reactions
CNS: headache, lethargy, confusion, hemiparesis, paresthesia, syncope, **seizures**
CV: hypotension, palpitations, chest pain, vasodilation
EENT: hearing loss
GI: nausea, vomiting, diarrhea, abdominal cramps, oral candidiasis, **pseudomembranous colitis**
GU: vaginal candidiasis, **nephrotoxicity**
Hematologic: lymphocytosis, eosinophilia, **bleeding tendency, hemolytic anemia, hypoprothrombinemia, neutropenia, thrombocytopenia, agranulocytosis, bone marrow depression**
Hepatic: hepatic failure, hepatomegaly
Musculoskeletal: arthralgia
Respiratory: dyspnea

Skin: urticaria, maculopapular or erythematous rash
Other: chills, fever, superinfection, **anaphylaxis, serum sickness**

Interactions
Drug-drug. *Aminoglycosides, loop diuretics:* increased risk of nephrotoxicity
Anticoagulants: increased anticoagulant effect
Chloramphenicol: antagonistic effect
Probenecid: decreased excretion and increased blood level of cefazolin
Drug-diagnostic tests. *Alanine aminotransferase, alkaline phosphatase, aspartate aminotransferase, bilirubin, blood urea nitrogen, creatinine, eosinophils, gamma-glutamyltransferase, lactate dehydrogenase:* increased levels
Coombs' test, urinary 17-ketosteroids, nonenzyme-based in the glucose tests (such as Clinitest): false-positive results
Hemoglobin, platelets, white blood cells: decreased values
Drug-behaviors. *Alcohol use:* acute alcohol intolerance (disulfiram-like reaction) if alcohol is consumed within 72 hours of drug administration

Patient monitoring
🔊 If patient is receiving high doses, monitor for extreme confusion, tonic-clonic seizures, and mild hemiparesis.
• Monitor CBC, prothrombin time, and kidney and liver function test results.
• Watch for signs and symptoms of superinfection and other serious adverse reactions.
• Be aware that cross-sensitivity to penicillins may occur.

Patient teaching
• Tell patient to report reduced urinary output, persistent diarrhea, bruising, or bleeding.
• Instruct patient to take drug exactly as prescribed and to complete full course of therapy even when he feels better.

• As appropriate, review all other significant and life-threatening adverse reactions and interactions, especially those related to the drugs, tests, and behaviors mentioned above.

cefdinir
Omnicef

Pharmacologic class: Third-generation cephalosporin
Therapeutic class: Anti-infective
Pregnancy risk category B

Action
Interferes with bacterial cell-wall synthesis and division by binding to cell wall, causing cell to die. Active against gram-negative and gram-positive bacteria, with expanded activity against gram-negative bacteria. Exhibits minimal immunosuppressant activity.

Availability
Capsules: 300 mg
Oral suspension: 125 mg/5 ml in 60- and 100-ml bottles

💊 Indications and dosages
➤ Acute bacterial otitis media caused by *Haemophilus influenzae, Streptococcus pneumoniae,* and *Moraxella catarrhalis*
Adults and children ages 13 and older: 300 mg P.O. q 12 hours or 600 mg P.O. q 24 hours for 10 days
Children ages 6 months to 12 years: 7 mg/kg P.O. q 12 hours for 5 to 10 days or 14 mg/kg P.O. q 24 hours for 10 days
➤ Uncomplicated skin and soft-tissue infections caused by *Staphylococcus aureus* and *Streptococcus pyogenes*
Adults and children ages 13 and older: 300 mg P.O. q 12 hours for 10 days. Maximum dosage is 600 mg/day.

Reactions in **bold** are life-threatening. 🔊 Clinical alert

➤ Acute maxillary sinusitis caused by
H. influenzae, S. pneumoniae, and *M.
catarrhalis*
Adults and children ages 13 and older:
300 mg P.O. q 12 hours or 600 mg P.O.
q 24 hours for 10 days. Maximum
dosage is 600 mg/day.
Children ages 6 months to 12 years:
7 mg/kg P.O. q 12 hours or 14 mg/kg
P.O. q 24 hours for 10 days
➤ Pharyngitis or tonsillitis caused by
S. pyogenes, chronic bronchitis caused
by *H. influenzae, S. pneumoniae,* and
M. catarrhalis
**Adults and children ages 13 and
older:** 300 mg P.O. q 12 hours for 5 to
10 days or 600 mg P.O. q 24 hours
for 10 days. Maximum dosage is
600 mg/day.
➤ Community-acquired pneumonia
caused by *H. influenzae, Haemophilus
parainfluenzae, S. pneumoniae,* and *M.
catarrhalis*
Adults and children ages 13 and older:
300 mg P.O. q 12 hours for 10 days.
Maximum dosage is 600 mg/day.

Dosage adjustment
• Renal impairment

Contraindications
• Hypersensitivity to cephalosporins
or penicillins

Precautions
Use cautiously in:
• renal impairment, phenylketonuria
• history of GI disease (especially
colitis)
• elderly patients
• pregnant or breastfeeding patients
• children.

Administration
• Obtain specimens for culture and
sensitivity tests as necessary before
starting therapy.
• Give with or without food.

• Administer 2 hours before or after
iron supplements or antacids containing aluminum or magnesium.
• Give capsules, if possible, to diabetic
patients (oral suspension contains
2.86 g of sucrose per teaspoon).

Route	Onset	Peak	Duration
P.O.	Rapid	2-4 hr	12-24 hr

Adverse reactions
CNS: headache, lethargy, paresthesia,
syncope, **seizures**
CV: hypotension, palpitations, chest
pain, vasodilation
EENT: hearing loss
GI: nausea, vomiting, diarrhea,
abdominal cramps, oral candidiasis,
pseudomembranous colitis
GU: vaginal candidiasis, **nephrotoxicity**
Hematologic: lymphocytosis, eosino-
philia, **bleeding tendency, hemolytic
anemia, hypoprothrombinemia, neu-
tropenia, thrombocytopenia, agranu-
locytosis, bone marrow depression**
Hepatic: hepatomegaly, hepatic failure
Musculoskeletal: arthralgia
Respiratory: dyspnea
Skin: chills, fever, urticaria, maculopapular or erythematous rash
Other: superinfection, **anaphylaxis,
serum sickness**

Interactions
Drug-drug. *Aminoglycosides, loop
diuretics:* increased risk of
nephrotoxicity
Antacids, iron-containing preparations:
decreased cefdinir absorption
Probenecid: decreased excretion and
increased blood level of cefdinir
Drug-diagnostic tests. *Alanine
aminotransferase, alkaline phosphatase,
aspartate aminotransferase, bilirubin,
blood urea nitrogen, creatinine, eosinophils, gamma-glutamyltransferase, lactate dehydrogenase:* increased levels
*Coombs' test, urinary 17-ketosteroids,
nonenzyme-based urine glucose tests
(such as Clinitest):* false-positive results

Hemoglobin, platelets, white blood cells: decreased values

Drug-herbs. *Angelica, anise, arnica, asafetida, bogbean, boldo, celery, chamomile, clove, danshen, fenugreek, feverfew, garlic, ginger, ginkgo, horse chestnut, horseradish, licorice, meadowsweet, onion, ginseng, papain, passionflower, poplar, prickly ash, quassia, red clover, turmeric, wild carrot, wild lettuce, willow:* increased risk of bleeding

Patient monitoring

• Monitor CBC and kidney and liver function test results.

• Monitor for signs and symptoms of superinfection and other serious adverse reactions.

Patient teaching

• Tell patient he may take drug with or without food.

• Instruct patient to report persistent diarrhea (more than four episodes daily) and other adverse effects.

• If patient uses antacids or iron-containing preparations (such as iron supplements), tell him to take these 2 hours before or after cefdinir.

• Inform patient that drug may temporarily discolor stools.

• As appropriate, review all other significant and life-threatening adverse reactions and interactions, especially those related to the drugs, tests, and herbs mentioned above.

cefepime hydrochloride
Maxipime

Pharmacologic class: Fourth-generation cephalosporin
Therapeutic class: Anti-infective
Pregnancy risk category B

Action

Interferes with bacterial cell-wall synthesis and division by binding to cell wall, causing cell to die. Active against gram-negative and gram-positive bacteria, with expanded activity against gram-negative bacteria. Exhibits minimal immunosuppressant activity.

Availability

Powder for injection: 500-mg vial, 1-g vial, 2-g vial; 1-g and 2-g piggyback bottles
Solution for injection (premixed): 1 g (50 ml in iso-osmotic dextrose), 2 g (100 ml in iso-osmotic dextrose)

⟐ Indications and dosages

➤ Urinary tract infections (UTIs) caused by *Escherichia coli, Klebsiella pneumoniae,* and *Proteus mirabilis*
Adults: 500 mg to 1g by I.V. infusion or I.M. q 12 hours for 7 to 10 days
➤ Severe UTIs caused by *E. coli* or *K. pneumoniae;* moderate to severe skin infections caused by *Staphylococcus aureus* or *Streptococcus pyogenes*
Adults: 2 g by I.V. infusion q 12 hours for 10 days
➤ Febrile neutropenia
Adults and children ages 2 months to 16 years: 2 g by I.V. infusion q 8 hours for 7 days
➤ Complicated intra-abdominal infections caused by alpha-hemolytic streptococci, *E. coli, K. pneumoniae, Pseudomonas aeruginosa, Enterobacter* species, *or Bacteroides fragilis*
Adults: 2 g by I.V. infusion q 12 hours for 7 to 10 days (given with metronidazole)
➤ Moderate to severe pneumonia caused by *K. pneumoniae, P. aeruginosa, Enterobacter* species, or *Streptococcus pneumoniae*
Adults: 1 to 2 g by I.V. infusion q 12 hours for 10 days

Dosage adjustment

• Renal impairment

Contraindications
- Hypersensitivity to cephalosporins or penicillins

Precautions
Use cautiously in:
- renal impairment, phenylketonuria
- history of GI disease
- elderly patients
- pregnant or breastfeeding patients
- children.

Administration
- Don't mix premixed solution with other drugs.
- 🔊 Don't use flexible container in series connections because of risk of air embolism.
- Obtain specimens for culture and sensitivity testing as needed before starting therapy.
- Don't mix with ampicillin (at concentrations above 40 mg/ml), metronidazole, aminoglycosides, or aminophylline if ordered concurrently. Give each drug separately.
- For I.V. infusion, use small I.V. needle and infuse into large vein over 30 to 60 minutes.
- For I.M. administration, inject deep into large muscle.

Route	Onset	Peak	Duration
I.V.	Rapid	End of infusion	12 hr
I.M.	Rapid	1-2 hr	12 hr

Adverse reactions
CNS: headache, lethargy, paresthesia, syncope, **seizures**
CV: phlebitis, hypotension, palpitations, chest pain, vasodilation, **thrombophlebitis**
EENT: hearing loss
GI: nausea, vomiting, diarrhea, abdominal cramps, oral candidiasis, **pseudomembranous colitis**
GU: vaginal candidiasis, **nephrotoxicity**
Hematologic: lymphocytosis, eosinophilia, **bleeding tendency, hemolytic anemia, hypoprothrombinemia, neutropenia, thrombocytopenia, agranulocytosis, bone marrow depression**
Hepatic: hepatic failure, hepatomegaly
Musculoskeletal: arthralgia
Respiratory: dyspnea
Skin: urticaria, maculopapular or erythematous rash, redness, swelling, induration
Other: chills, fever, superinfection, pain at I.M. site, phlebitis at I.V. site, **anaphylaxis, serum sickness**

Interactions
Drug-drug. *Aminoglycosides, loop diuretics:* increased risk of nephrotoxicity
Probenecid: decreased excretion and increased blood level of cefepime
Drug-diagnostic tests. *Alanine aminotransferase, alkaline phosphatase, aspartate aminotransferase, bilirubin, blood urea nitrogen, creatinine, eosinophils, gamma-glutamyltransferase, lactate dehydrogenase:* increased levels
Coombs' test, urinary 17-ketosteroids, nonenzyme-based urine glucose tests (such as Clinitest): false-positive results
Hemoglobin, platelets, white blood cells: decreased values
Drug-herbs. *Angelica, anise, arnica, asafetida, bogbean, boldo, celery, chamomile, clove, danshen, fenugreek, feverfew, garlic, ginger, ginkgo, ginseng, horse chestnut, horseradish, licorice, meadowsweet, onion, papain, passionflower, poplar, prickly ash, quassia, red clover, turmeric, wild carrot, wild lettuce, willow:* increased risk of bleeding

Patient monitoring
- Assess baseline CBC and kidney and liver function test results.
- Monitor for signs and symptoms of superinfection and other serious adverse reactions.
- Monitor for inflammation at infusion site.

• Be aware that cross-sensitivity to penicillins may occur.

Patient teaching
• Instruct patient to report reduced urinary output, persistent diarrhea, bruising, petechiae, or bleeding.
• Caution patient not to take herbs without consulting prescriber.
• As appropriate, review all other significant and life-threatening adverse reactions and interactions, especially those related to the drugs, tests, and herbs mentioned above.

cefixime
Suprax

Pharmacologic class: Third-generation cephalosporin
Therapeutic class: Anti-infective
Pregnancy risk category B

Action
Interferes with bacterial cell-wall synthesis and division by binding to cell wall, causing cell to die. Active against gram-negative and gram-positive bacteria, with expanded activity against gram-negative bacteria. Exhibits minimal immunosuppressant activity.

Availability
Oral suspension: 100 mg/5 ml
Tablets: 400 mg

⊘ Indications and dosages
➤ Uncomplicated gonorrhea caused by *Neisseria gonorrhoeae*
Adults and children weighing more than 50 kg (110 lb): 400 mg P.O. daily
➤ Uncomplicated urinary tract infections caused by *Escherichia coli* and *Proteus mirabilis;* otitis media caused by *Haemophilus influenzae, Moraxella catarrhalis,* and *Streptococcus pyogenes;*

pharyngitis and tonsillitis caused by *S. pyogenes;* acute bronchitis and acute exacerbation of chronic bronchitis caused by *H. influenzae* and *Streptococcus pneumoniae*
Adults and children older than age 12 or weighing more than 50 kg (110 lb): 400 mg P.O. daily or 200 mg P.O. q 12 hours
Children ages 12 and younger or weighing 50 kg (110 lb) or less: 8 mg/kg P.O. daily or 4 mg/kg P.O. q 12 hours

Dosage adjustment
• Renal impairment

Contraindications
• Hypersensitivity to cephalosporins or penicillins

Precautions
Use cautiously in:
• renal impairment, phenylketonuria
• history of GI disease
• elderly patients
• pregnant or breastfeeding patients
• children.

Administration
• Obtain specimens for culture and sensitivity testing as necessary before starting therapy.
• Know that drug may be taken with food.
• Be aware that suspension should be given for otitis media because it provides higher serum concentration.

Route	Onset	Peak	Duration
P.O.	Rapid	2-6 hr	24 hr

Adverse reactions
CNS: headache, lethargy, paresthesia, syncope, **seizures**
CV: hypotension, palpitations, chest pain, vasodilation
EENT: hearing loss
GI: nausea, vomiting, diarrhea, abdominal cramps, oral candidiasis, **pseudomembranous colitis**

GU: vaginal candidiasis, **nephrotoxicity**
Hematologic: lymphocytosis, eosinophilia, **bleeding tendency, hemolytic anemia, hypoprothrombinemia, neutropenia, thrombocytopenia, agranulocytosis, bone marrow depression**
Hepatic: hepatic failure, hepatomegaly
Musculoskeletal: arthralgia
Respiratory: dyspnea
Skin: urticaria, maculopapular or erythematous rash
Other: chills, fever, superinfection, **anaphylaxis, serum sickness**

Interactions

Drug-drug. *Aminoglycosides, loop diuretics:* increased risk of nephrotoxicity
Probenecid: decreased excretion and increased blood level of cefixime
Drug-diagnostic tests. *Alanine aminotransferase, alkaline phosphatase, aspartate aminotransferase, bilirubin, blood urea nitrogen, creatinine, eosinophils, gamma-glutamyltransferase, lactate dehydrogenase:* increased levels
Coombs' test, urinary 17-ketosteroids, nonenzyme-based urine glucose tests (such as Clinitest): false-positive results
Hemoglobin, platelets, white blood cells: decreased values
Drug-herbs. *Angelica, anise, arnica, asafetida, bogbean, boldo, celery, chamomile, clove, danshen, fenugreek, feverfew, garlic, ginger, ginkgo, ginseng, horse chestnut, horseradish, licorice, meadowsweet, onion, papain, passionflower, poplar, prickly ash, quassia, red clover, turmeric, wild carrot, wild lettuce, willow:* increased risk of bleeding

Patient monitoring

• Monitor baseline CBC and kidney and liver function test results.
• Monitor for signs and symptoms of superinfection and other serious adverse reactions.

• Be aware that cross-sensitivity to penicillins may occur.

Patient teaching

• Tell patient to take once-daily doses at same time each day.
• Advise patient to take drug exactly as prescribed and to continue to take full amount prescribed even when he feels better.
• Instruct patient to report signs and symptoms of allergic response and other adverse reactions, such as rash, easy bruising, bleeding, severe GI problems, or difficulty breathing.
• Caution patient not to take herbs without consulting prescriber.
• As appropriate, review all other significant and life-threatening adverse reactions and interactions, especially those related to the drugs, tests, and herbs mentioned above.

cefotaxime sodium
Claforan

Pharmacologic class: Third-generation cephalosporin
Therapeutic class: Anti-infective
Pregnancy risk category B

Action

Interferes with bacterial cell-wall synthesis and division by binding to cell wall, causing cell to die. Active against gram-negative and gram-positive bacteria, with expanded activity against gram-negative bacteria. Exhibits minimal immunosuppressant activity.

Availability

Powder for injection: 500 mg, 1 g, 2 g, 10 g
Premixed containers: 1 g/50 ml, 2 g/50 ml

🖊 Indications and dosages

➤ Perioperative prophylaxis

Adults and children weighing more than 50 kg (110 lb): 1 g I.V. or I.M. 30 to 90 minutes before surgery

➤ Prophylaxis in patients undergoing cesarean delivery

Adults: 1 g I.V. or I.M. as soon as umbilical cord is clamped

➤ Gonococcal urethritis and cervicitis

Adults weighing more than 50 kg (110 lb): 500 mg I.M. as a single dose

➤ Rectal gonorrhea (females)

Adults weighing more than 50 kg (110 lb): 500 mg I.M. as a single dose

➤ Rectal gonorrhea (males)

Adults weighing more than 50 kg (110 lb): 1 g I.M. as a single dose

➤ Disseminated gonorrhea

Adults and children weighing 50 kg (110 lb) or more: 1 g by I.V. infusion q 8 hours

➤ Uncomplicated infections caused by susceptible organisms

Adults and children weighing 50 kg (110 lb) or more: 1 g I.V. or I.M. q 12 hours

Children ages 1 month to 12 years weighing less than 50 kg (110 lb): 50 to 180 mg/kg/day I.V. or I.M. in four to six divided doses

➤ Moderate to severe infections caused by susceptible organisms

Adults and children weighing 50 kg (110 lb) or more: 1 to 2 g I.V. or I.M. q 8 hours

➤ Life-threatening infections caused by susceptible organisms

Adults and children weighing 50 kg (110 lb) or more: 2 g by I.V. infusion q 4 hours. Maximum dosage is 12 g/day.

➤ Septicemia and other infections that commonly require antibiotics in higher doses

Adults and children weighing 50 kg (110 lb) or more: 2 g by I.V. infusion q 6 to 8 hours

Dosage adjustment

- Renal impairment

Contraindications

- Hypersensitivity to cephalosporins or penicillins

Precautions

Use cautiously in:

- renal impairment, phenylketonuria
- history of GI disease
- elderly patients
- pregnant or breastfeeding patients
- children.

Administration

- Obtain specimens for culture and sensitivity testing as necessary before starting therapy.
- Reconstitute powder for I.V. injection with at least 10 ml of sterile water, and give over 3 to 5 minutes. For intermittent infusion, drug may be diluted further with 50 or 100 ml of normal saline solution or dextrose 5% in water (D_5W) and given over 30 minutes.
- Reconstituted drug may be diluted further for a continuous I.V. infusion of up to 1,000 ml with a compatible solution, such as normal saline solution, dextrose 5% or 10% in water, or D_5W and normal saline solution. Give over 6 to 24 hours, depending on concentration.
- Don't use diluents with pH above 7.5 (such as sodium bicarbonate).
- Rotate infusion sites.
- Inject I.M. deep into large muscle mass. Divide 2-g dose in half and inject into separate large muscle masses.

Route	Onset	Peak	Duration
I.V.	Rapid	End of infusion	4-12 hr
I.M.	Rapid	0.5 hr	4-12 hr

Adverse reactions

CNS: headache, lethargy, paresthesia, syncope, **seizures**

Reactions in **bold** are life-threatening. 🔊 Clinical alert

CV: hypotension, palpitations, chest pain, vasodilation
EENT: hearing loss
GI: nausea, vomiting, diarrhea, abdominal cramps, oral candidiasis, **pseudomembranous colitis**
GU: vaginal candidiasis, **nephrotoxicity**
Hematologic: lymphocytosis, eosinophilia, **bleeding tendency, hemolytic anemia, hypoprothrombinemia, neutropenia, thrombocytopenia, agranulocytosis, bone marrow depression**
Hepatic: hepatic failure, hepatomegaly
Musculoskeletal: arthralgia
Respiratory: dyspnea
Skin: urticaria, maculopapular or erythematous rash
Other: chills, fever, superinfection, pain at I.M. injection site, **anaphylaxis, serum sickness**

Interactions

Drug-drug. *Aminoglycosides, loop diuretics:* increased risk of nephrotoxicity
Probenecid: decreased excretion and increased blood level of cefotaxime
Drug-diagnostic tests. *Alanine aminotransferase, alkaline phosphatase, aspartate aminotransferase, bilirubin, blood urea nitrogen, creatinine, eosinophils, gamma-glutamyltransferase, lactate dehydrogenase:* increased levels
Coombs' test, urinary 17-ketosteroids, nonenzyme-based urine glucose tests (such as Clinitest): false-positive results
Hemoglobin, platelets, white blood cells: decreased values
Drug-herbs. *Angelica, anise, arnica, asafetida, bogbean, boldo, celery, chamomile, clove, danshen, fenugreek, feverfew, garlic, ginger, ginkgo, ginseng, horse chestnut, horseradish, licorice, meadowsweet, onion, papain, passionflower, poplar, prickly ash, quassia, red clover, turmeric, wild carrot, wild lettuce, willow:* increased risk of bleeding

Patient monitoring

• Monitor CBC and kidney and liver function test results.
• Monitor for signs and symptoms of superinfection and other serious adverse reactions.
• Be aware that cross-sensitivity to penicillins may occur.

Patient teaching

• Advise patient to report reduced urinary output, persistent diarrhea, bruising, and bleeding.
• As appropriate, review all other significant and life-threatening adverse reactions and interactions, especially those related to the drugs, tests, and herbs mentioned above.

cefoxitin sodium

Pharmacologic class: Second-generation cephalosporin
Therapeutic class: Anti-infective
Pregnancy risk category B

Action

Interferes with bacterial cell-wall synthesis and division by binding to cell wall, causing cell to die. Active against gram-negative and gram-positive bacteria, with expanded activity against gram-negative bacteria. Exhibits minimal immunosuppressant activity.

Availability

Powder for injection: 1 g, 2 g
Premixed containers: 1 g/50 ml in dextrose 5% in water (D_5W), 2 g/50 ml in D_5W

⦸ Indications and dosages

➤ Respiratory tract infections, skin infections, bone and joint infections, urinary tract infections, gynecologic infections, septicemia

Adults: For most infections, 1 g I.M. or I.V. q 6 to 8 hours. For severe infections, 1 g I.M. or I.V. q 4 hours or 2 g I.M. or I.V. q 6 to 8 hours. For life-threatening infections, 2 g I.V. q 4 hours or 3 g I.V. q 6 hours.

Children ages 3 months and older: For most infections, 13.3 to 26.7 mg/kg I.M. or I.V. q 4 hours or 20 to 40 mg/kg q 6 hours.

➤ Preoperative prophylaxis

Adults: 1 to 2 g I.V. within 60 minutes of incision, then q 6 hours for up to 24 hours

Dosage adjustment
• Renal failure

Contraindications
• Hypersensitivity to cephalosporins or penicillins

Precautions
Use cautiously in:
• renal impairment, hepatic disease, or biliary obstruction
• history of GI disease
• elderly patients
• children.

Administration
• Obtain specimens for culture and sensitivity testing as necessary before starting therapy.
• Reconstitute 1-g dose with 10 ml of sterile water; reconstitute 2-g dose with 10 to 20 ml.
• For direct I.V. injection, give 10 ml of sterile water with each gram of cefoxitin over 3 to 5 minutes. Inject into large vein and rotate sites, or give through existing I.V. tubing.
• For intermittent or continuous I.V. infusion, add reconstituted drug to compatible solution, such as D_5W, normal saline solution, or D_5W and normal saline solution.
• For I.M. injection, reconstitute each gram with 2 ml of sterile water or 2 ml

of 0.5% lidocaine hydrochloride (without epinephrine).
• Inject I.M. deep into large muscle mass; divide 2-g dose in half and inject into separate large muscle masses.
• Know that dry powder and solution may darken, but this does not alter drug efficacy.

Route	Onset	Peak	Duration
I.V.	Rapid	End of infusion	4-8 hr
I.M.	Rapid	30 min	4-8 hr

Adverse reactions
CNS: headache, lethargy, paresthesia, syncope, **seizures**
CV: hypotension, palpitations, chest pain, vasodilation, **thrombophlebitis**
EENT: hearing loss
GI: nausea, vomiting, diarrhea, abdominal cramps, oral candidiasis, **pseudomembranous colitis**
GU: vaginal candidiasis, **nephrotoxicity**
Hematologic: lymphocytosis, eosinophilia, **bleeding tendency, hemolytic anemia, hypoprothrombinemia, neutropenia, thrombocytopenia, agranulocytosis, bone marrow depression**
Hepatic: hepatic failure, hepatomegaly
Musculoskeletal: arthralgia
Respiratory: dyspnea
Skin: urticaria, maculopapular or erythematous rash
Other: chills, fever, superinfection, pain at I.M. site, **anaphylaxis, serum sickness**

Interactions
Drug-drug. *Aminoglycosides, loop diuretics:* increased risk of nephrotoxicity
Probenecid: decreased excretion and increased blood level of cefoxitin
Drug-diagnostic tests. *Alanine aminotransferase, alkaline phosphatase, aspartate aminotransferase, bilirubin, blood urea nitrogen, creatinine,*

---

eosinophils, gamma-glutamyltransferase, lactate dehydrogenase: increased levels
Coombs' test, urinary 17-ketosteroids, nonenzyme-based urine glucose tests (such as Clinitest): false-positive results
Hemoglobin, platelets, white blood cells: decreased values

Patient monitoring

• Assess CBC and kidney and liver function test results.
• Monitor fluid intake and output. Report significant decrease in output.
• Monitor for signs and symptoms of superinfection and other serious adverse reactions.
• Be aware that cross-sensitivity to penicillins may occur.

Patient teaching

• Instruct patient to report reduced urinary output, persistent diarrhea, bruising, and bleeding.
• As appropriate, review all other significant and life-threatening adverse reactions and interactions, especially those related to the drugs and tests mentioned above.

cefpodoxime proxetil
Orelox✦, Vantin

Pharmacologic class: Third-generation cephalosporin
Therapeutic class: Anti-infective
Pregnancy risk category B

Action

Interferes with bacterial cell-wall synthesis and division by binding to cell wall, causing cell to die. Active against gram-negative and gram-positive bacteria, with expanded activity against gram-negative bacteria. Exhibits minimal immunosuppressant activity.

Availability

Oral suspension: 50 mg/5 ml, 100 mg/5 ml
Tablets: 100 mg, 200 mg

⊘ Indications and dosages

➢ Acute community-acquired pneumonia caused by *Haemophilus influenzae* or *Streptococcus pneumoniae*
Adults and children ages 13 and older: 200 mg P.O. q 12 hours for 14 days
➢ Acute bacterial or chronic bronchitis
Adults and children ages 13 and older: 200 mg P.O. q 12 hours for 10 days
➢ Uncomplicated gonorrhea; rectal gonococcal infection caused by *Neisseria gonorrhoeae*
Adults: 200 mg P.O. as a single dose
➢ Uncomplicated urinary tract infections caused by *Escherichia coli, Klebsiella pneumoniae, Proteus mirabilis,* and *Staphylococcus saprophyticus*
Adults: 100 mg P.O. q 12 hours for 7 days
➢ Skin and soft-tissue infections caused by *Staphylococcus aureus* and *Streptococcus pyogenes*
Adults and children ages 13 and older: 400 mg P.O. q 12 hours for 7 to 14 days
➢ Acute otitis media caused by *H. influenzae, S. pneumoniae,* and *Moraxella catarrhalis*
Children ages 5 months to 12 years: 5 mg/kg P.O. q 12 hours (maximum of 200 mg/dose) or 10 mg/kg q 24 hours (maximum of 400 mg/dose) for 10 days
➢ Tonsillitis and pharyngitis caused by *S. pyogenes*
Adults and children ages 13 and older: 100 mg P.O. q 12 hours for 5 to 10 days
Children ages 2 months to 12 years: 5 mg/kg P.O. q 12 hours for 5 to 10 days

Dosage adjustment

• Renal impairment

Contraindications

- Hypersensitivity to cephalosporins or penicillins

Precautions

Use cautiously in:

- renal impairment, phenylketonuria
- history of GI disease
- elderly patients
- pregnant or breastfeeding patients
- children.

Administration

- Obtain specimens for culture and sensitivity testing as necessary before starting therapy.
- Give tablets with food to enhance absorption. Oral suspension may be given with or without food.
- Don't give antacids within 2 hours of cefpodoxime.

Route	Onset	Peak	Duration
P.O.	Unknown	2-3 hr	12 hr

Adverse reactions

CNS: headache, lethargy, paresthesia, syncope, **seizures**
CV: hypotension, palpitations, chest pain, vasodilation
EENT: hearing loss
GI: nausea, vomiting, diarrhea, abdominal cramps, oral candidiasis, **pseudomembranous colitis**
GU: vaginal candidiasis, **nephrotoxicity**
Hematologic: lymphocytosis, eosinophilia, **bleeding tendency, hemolytic anemia, hypoprothrombinemia, neutropenia, thrombocytopenia, agranulocytosis, bone marrow depression**
Hepatic: hepatic failure, hepatomegaly
Musculoskeletal: arthralgia
Respiratory: dyspnea
Skin: urticaria, maculopapular or erythematous rash
Other: chills, fever, superinfection, **anaphylaxis, serum sickness**

Interactions

Drug-drug. *Aminoglycosides, loop diuretics:* increased risk of nephrotoxicity
Antacids: decreased cefpodoxime absorption
Probenecid: decreased excretion and increased blood level of cefpodoxime
Drug-diagnostic tests. *Alanine aminotransferase, alkaline phosphatase, aspartate aminotransferase, bilirubin, blood urea nitrogen, creatinine, eosinophils, gamma-glutamyltransferase, lactate dehydrogenase:* increased levels
Coombs' test, urinary 17-ketosteroids, nonenzyme-based urine glucose tests (such as Clinitest): false-positive results
Hemoglobin, platelets, white blood cells: decreased values
Drug-herbs. *Angelica, anise, arnica, asafetida, bogbean, boldo, celery, chamomile, clove, danshen, fenugreek, feverfew, garlic, ginger, ginkgo, ginseng, horse chestnut, horseradish, licorice, meadowsweet, onion, papain, passionflower, poplar, prickly ash, quassia, red clover, turmeric, wild carrot, wild lettuce, willow:* increased risk of bleeding

Patient monitoring

- Assess CBC and kidney and liver function test results.
- Monitor for signs and symptoms of superinfection and other serious adverse reactions.
- Be aware that cross-sensitivity to penicillins may occur.

Patient teaching

- Instruct patient to take drug with food or milk to reduce GI distress and enhance absorption.
- Advise patient not to take antacids within 2 hours of drug.
- Tell patient to continue to take full amount prescribed even when he feels better.
- Instruct patient to report signs and symptoms of allergic response and other adverse reactions, such as rash,

---

easy bruising, bleeding, severe GI problems, or difficulty breathing.

• If patient is being treated for gonorrhea, instruct him to have partner tested and treated (as needed) and to use barrier contraception to prevent reinfection.

• As appropriate, review all other significant and life-threatening adverse reactions and interactions, especially those related to the drugs, tests, and herbs mentioned above.

cefprozil
Apo-Cefprozil✤, Cefzil, Ran-Cefprozil✤, Sandoz Cefprozil✤

Pharmacologic class: Second-generation cephalosporin
Therapeutic class: Anti-infective
Pregnancy risk category B

Action
Interferes with bacterial cell-wall synthesis and division by binding to cell wall, causing cell to die. Active against gram-negative and gram-positive bacteria, with expanded activity against gram-negative bacteria. Exhibits minimal immunosuppressant activity.

Availability
Powder for suspension: 125 mg/5 ml, 250 mg/5 ml
Tablets: 250 mg, 500 mg

❂ Indications and dosages
➤ Uncomplicated skin infections caused by *Staphylococcus aureus* and *Streptococcus pyogenes*
Adults and children ages 13 and older: 250 to 500 mg P.O. q 12 hours or 500 mg P.O. daily for 10 days
➤ Pharyngitis or tonsillitis caused by *S. pyogenes*

Adults and children ages 13 and older: 500 mg P.O. daily for at least 10 days
➤ Acute bronchitis; acute bacterial chronic bronchitis caused by *Streptococcus pneumoniae, Haemophilus influenzae,* and *Moraxella catarrhalis*
Adults and children ages 13 and older: 500 mg P.O. q 12 hours for 10 days
➤ Acute sinusitis caused by *S. pneumoniae, H. influenzae,* and *M. catarrhalis*
Adults and children ages 13 and older: 250 mg P.O. q 12 hours for 10 days; for moderate to severe infections, 500 mg P.O. q 12 hours for 10 days
Children ages 6 months to 12 years: 7.5 mg/kg P.O. q 12 hours for 10 days; for moderate to severe infections, 15 mg/kg P.O. q 12 hours for 10 days
➤ Otitis media caused by *S. pneumoniae, H. influenzae,* and *M. catarrhalis*
Children ages 6 months to 12 years: 15 mg/kg P.O. q 12 hours for 10 days

Dosage adjustment
• Renal impairment

Contraindications
• Hypersensitivity to cephalosporins or penicillins
• Renal failure

Precautions
Use cautiously in:
• renal or hepatic impairment
• pregnant or breastfeeding patients
• children.

Administration
• Obtain specimens for culture and sensitivity testing as necessary before starting therapy.
• Give drug with food.

Route	Onset	Peak	Duration
P.O.	Unknown	6-10 hr	24-28 hr

Adverse reactions

CNS: headache, dizziness, drowsiness, hyperactivity, hypotonia, insomnia, confusion, **seizures**

GI: nausea, vomiting, diarrhea, abdominal pain, dyspepsia, **pseudomembranous colitis**

GU: hematuria, vaginal candidiasis, genital pruritus, **renal dysfunction, toxic nephropathy**

Hematologic: eosinophilia, **aplastic anemia, hemolytic anemia, hemorrhage, bone marrow depression, hypoprothrombinemia**

Hepatic: hepatic dysfunction

Skin: toxic epidermal necrolysis, diaper rash, **erythema multiforme, Stevens-Johnson syndrome**

Other: allergic reactions, carnitine deficiency, drug fever, superinfection, **serum sickness–like reaction, anaphylaxis**

Interactions

Drug-drug. *Aminoglycosides:* increased risk of nephrotoxicity

Antacids containing aluminum or magnesium, histamine$_2$-receptor antagonists: increased cefprozil absorption

Probenecid: decreased excretion and increased blood level of cefprozil

Drug-diagnostic tests. *Alanine aminotransferase, alkaline phosphatase, aspartate aminotransferase, bilirubin, blood urea nitrogen, creatinine, eosinophils, gamma-glutamyltransferase, lactate dehydrogenase, white blood cells in urine:* increased levels

Blood glucose, Coombs' test, urine glucose tests using Benedict's solution: false-positive results

Platelets, white blood cells: decreased counts

Drug-food. *Moderate- or high-fat meal:* increased drug bioavailability

Patient monitoring

◀€ Stay alert for life-threatening reactions, including anaphylaxis, serum sickness–like reaction, Stevens-Johnson syndrome, and pseudomembranous colitis.

• Monitor neurologic status, particularly for signs and symptoms of impending seizures.

• Monitor kidney and liver function test results and assess fluid intake and output.

• Monitor CBC with white cell differential, prothrombin time, and bleeding time. Watch for signs and symptoms of blood dyscrasias, especially hypoprothrombinemia.

• Monitor temperature. Stay alert for signs and symptoms of superinfection.

Patient teaching

◀€ Advise patient to immediately report rash, bleeding tendency, or CNS changes.

• Teach patient to recognize signs and symptoms of superinfection, and instruct him to report these right away.

• Tell patient to take drug with food.

• As appropriate, review all other significant and life-threatening adverse reactions and interactions, especially those related to the drugs, tests, and foods mentioned above.

ceftazidime
Fortaz, Fortum ⊕, Tazicef

Pharmacologic class: Third-generation cephalosporin

Therapeutic class: Anti-infective

Pregnancy risk category B

Action

Interferes with bacterial cell-wall synthesis and division by binding to cell wall, causing cell to die. Active against gram-negative and gram-positive bacteria, with expanded activity against gram-negative bacteria. Exhibits minimal immuno-suppressant activity.

Availability

Powder for injection: 500 mg, 1 g, 2 g, 6 g

Premixed containers: 1 g/50 ml, 2 g/50 ml

⚕ Indications and dosages

➣ Skin infections; bone and joint infections; urinary tract and gynecologic infections, including gonorrhea; respiratory tract infections; intra-abdominal infections; septicemia

Adults and children ages 12 and older: For most infections, 500 mg to 2 g I.V. or I.M. q 8 to 12 hours. For pneumonia and skin infections, 0.5 to 1 g I.V. or I.M. q 8 to 12 hours. For bone and joint infections, 2 g I.V. or I.M. q 12 hours. For severe and life-threatening infections, 2 g I.V. q 8 hours. For complicated urinary tract infections (UTIs), 500 mg q 8 to 12 hours. For uncomplicated UTIs, 250 mg I.M. or I.V. q 12 hours.

Children ages 1 month to 12 years: 30 to 50 mg/kg I.V. q 8 hours

Neonates younger than 4 weeks: 30 mg/kg I.V. q 12 hours

Dosage adjustment

• Renal impairment

Off-label uses

• Febrile neutropenia
• Prophylaxis of perinatal infections

Contraindications

• Hypersensitivity to cephalosporins or penicillins

Precautions

Use cautiously in:

• renal impairment, hepatic disease, biliary obstruction, phenylketonuria
• history of GI disease
• elderly patients
• pregnant or breastfeeding patients
• children.

Administration

• Obtain specimens for culture and sensitivity testing as necessary before starting therapy.
• Reconstitute powder for injection with sterile water, following manufacturer's directions for amount of diluent to use.
• For I.V. injection, dilute in sterile water as directed, and give single dose over 3 to 5 minutes. Inject into large vein; rotate injection sites.
• For intermittent I.V. infusion, dilute further with 100 ml of sterile water or another compatible fluid, such as normal saline solution or dextrose 5% in water. Infuse over 30 minutes.
• Don't dilute with sodium bicarbonate.
• For I.M. injection, reconstitute with sterile water, bacteriostatic water, or 0.5% or 1% lidocaine hydrochloride.
• When giving I.M., inject deep into large muscle mass.

Route	Onset	Peak	Duration
I.V.	Rapid	End of infusion	6-12 hr
I.M.	Rapid	1 hr	6-12 hr

Adverse reactions

CNS: headache, confusion, hemiparesis, lethargy, paresthesia, syncope, asterixis, neuromuscular excitability (with increased drug blood levels in renally impaired patients), **seizures, encephalopathy**

CV: hypotension, palpitations, chest pain, vasodilation

EENT: hearing loss

GI: nausea, vomiting, diarrhea, abdominal cramps, oral candidiasis, **pseudomembranous colitis**

GU: vaginal candidiasis, **nephrotoxicity**

Hematologic: lymphocytosis, eosinophilia, **bleeding tendency, hemolytic anemia, hypoprothrombinemia, neutropenia, thrombocytopenia, agranulocytosis, bone marrow depression**

Hepatic: hepatic failure, hepatomegaly

Musculoskeletal: arthralgia
Respiratory: dyspnea
Skin: urticaria, maculopapular or erythematous rash
Other: chills, fever, superinfection, I.M. site pain, **anaphylaxis, serum sickness**

Interactions

Drug-drug. *Aminoglycosides, loop diuretics:* increased risk of nephrotoxicity
Chloramphenicol: antagonism of ceftazidime's effects
Probenecid: decreased excretion and increased blood level of ceftazidime
Drug-diagnostic tests. *Alanine aminotransferase, alkaline phosphatase, aspartate aminotransferase, bilirubin, blood urea nitrogen, creatinine, eosinophils, gamma-glutamyltransferase, lactate dehydrogenase:* Increased levels
Hemoglobin, platelets, white blood cells: decreased values
Coombs' test, urinary 17-ketosteroids, nonenzyme-based urine glucose tests (such as Clinitest): false-positive results
Drug-herbs. *Angelica, anise, arnica, asafetida, bogbean, boldo, celery, chamomile, clove, danshen, fenugreek, feverfew, garlic, ginger, ginkgo, ginseng, horse chestnut, horseradish, licorice, meadowsweet, onion, papain, passionflower, poplar, prickly ash, quassia, red clover, turmeric, wild carrot, wild lettuce, willow:* increased risk of bleeding

Patient monitoring

◀€ Monitor for extreme confusion, tonic-clonic seizures, and mild hemiparesis when giving high doses.
• Assess CBC and kidney and liver function test results.
• Monitor for signs and symptoms of superinfection and other serious adverse reactions.

• Be aware that cross-sensitivity to penicillins may occur.

Patient teaching

• Instruct patient to report reduced urine output, persistent diarrhea, bruising, and bleeding.
• As appropriate, review all other significant and life-threatening adverse reactions and interactions, especially those related to the drugs, tests, and herbs mentioned above.

ceftibuten
Cedax

Pharmacologic class: Third-generation cephalosporin
Therapeutic class: Anti-infective
Pregnancy risk category B

Action

Interferes with bacterial cell-wall synthesis and division by binding to cell wall, causing cell to die. Active against gram-negative and gram-positive bacteria, with expanded activity against gram-negative bacteria. Exhibits minimal immunosuppressant activity.

Availability

Capsules: 400 mg
Oral suspension: 90 mg/5 ml

⚠ Indications and dosages

➤ Acute bacterial exacerbations of chronic bronchitis caused by *Haemophilus influenzae, Moraxella catarrhalis,* and *Streptococcus pneumoniae;* pharyngitis and tonsillitis caused by *Streptococcus pyogenes;* acute bacterial otitis media caused by *H. influenzae, M. catarrhalis,* and *S. pyogenes*
Adults and children ages 12 and older: 400 mg P.O. q 24 hours for 10 days

---

Children ages 12 and younger: 9 mg/kg P.O. daily for 10 days. Maximum dosage shouldn't exceed 400 mg daily.

Dosage adjustment
• Renal impairment

Off-label uses
• Urinary tract infections

Contraindications
• Hypersensitivity to cephalosporins and penicillins

Precautions
Use cautiously in:
• renal impairment, hepatic disease, biliary obstruction, phenylketonuria
• history of GI disease
• elderly patients
• pregnant or breastfeeding patients
• children.

Administration
• Obtain specimens for culture and sensitivity testing as necessary before starting therapy.
• Give oral suspension at least 1 hour before or 2 hours after a meal.

Route	Onset	Peak	Duration
P.O.	Rapid	3 hr	24 hr

Adverse reactions
CNS: headache, lethargy, paresthesia, syncope, **seizures**
CV: hypotension, palpitations, chest pain, vasodilation
EENT: hearing loss
GI: nausea, vomiting, diarrhea, abdominal cramps, oral candidiasis, **pseudomembranous colitis**
GU: vaginal candidiasis, **nephrotoxicity**
Hematologic: lymphocytosis, eosinophilia, **bleeding tendency, hemolytic anemia, hypoprothrombinemia, neutropenia, thrombocytopenia, agranulocytosis, bone marrow depression**
Hepatic: hepatic failure, hepatomegaly
Musculoskeletal: arthralgia

Respiratory: dyspnea
Skin: urticaria, easy bruising, maculopapular or erythematous rash
Other: chills, fever, superinfection, **anaphylaxis, serum sickness**

Interactions
Drug-drug. *Aminoglycosides, loop diuretics:* increased risk of nephrotoxicity
Probenecid: decreased excretion and increased blood level of ceftibuten
Drug-diagnostic tests. *Alanine aminotransferase, alkaline phosphatase, aspartate aminotransferase, bilirubin, blood urea nitrogen, creatinine, eosinophils, gamma-glutamyltransferase, lactate dehydrogenase:* increased levels
Coombs' test, urinary 17-ketosteroids, nonenzyme-based urine glucose tests (such as Clinitest): false-positive results
Hemoglobin, platelets, white blood cells: decreased values
Drug-herbs. *Angelica, anise, arnica, asafetida, bogbean, boldo, celery, chamomile, clove, danshen, fenugreek, feverfew, garlic, ginger, ginkgo, ginseng, horse chestnut, horseradish, licorice, meadowsweet, onion, papain, passionflower, poplar, prickly ash, quassia, red clover, turmeric, wild carrot, wild lettuce, willow:* increased risk of bleeding

Patient monitoring
• Assess CBC and kidney and liver function test results.
• Monitor for signs and symptoms of superinfection and other serious adverse reactions.
• Be aware that cross-sensitivity to penicillins may occur.

Patient teaching
• Instruct patient to take oral suspension at least 1 hour before or 2 hours after a meal.

• Inform diabetic patient that oral suspension contains 1 g sucrose per teaspoon.

• Advise patient to continue to take full amount prescribed even when he feels better.

• Tell patient to report signs and symptoms of allergic response and other adverse reactions, such as rash, easy bruising, bleeding, severe GI problems, or difficulty breathing.

• As appropriate, review all other significant and life-threatening adverse reactions and interactions, especially those related to the drugs, tests, and herbs mentioned above.

ceftriaxone sodium
Rocephin

Pharmacologic class: Third-generation cephalosporin
Therapeutic class: Anti-infective
Pregnancy risk category B

Action
Interferes with bacterial cell-wall synthesis and division by binding to cell wall, causing cell to die. Active against gram-negative and gram-positive bacteria, with expanded activity against gram-negative bacteria. Exhibits minimal immunosuppressant activity.

Availability
Powder for injection: 250 mg, 500 mg, 1 g, 2 g
Premixed containers: 1 g/50 ml, 2 g/50 ml

⏀ Indications and dosages
➤ Infections of respiratory system, bones, joints, and skin; septicemia

Adults: 1 to 2 g/day I.M. or I.V. or in equally divided doses q 12 hours. Maximum daily dosage is 4 g.
➤ Uncomplicated gonorrhea
Adults: 250 mg I.M. as a single dose
➤ Surgical prophylaxis
Adults: 1 g I.V. as a single dose within 1 hour before start of surgical procedure
➤ Meningitis
Adults: 1 g to 2 g I.V. q 12 hours for 10 to 14 days
Children: Initially, 100 mg/kg/day I.M. or I.V. (not to exceed 4 g). Then 100 mg/kg/day I.M. or I.V. once daily or in equally divided doses q 12 hours (not to exceed 4 g) for 7 to 14 days.
➤ Otitis media
Children: 50 mg/kg I.M. as a single dose; maximum of 1 g/dose.
➤ Skin and skin-structure infections
Children: 50 to 75 mg/kg/day I.V. or I.M. once or twice daily. Maximum dosage is 2 g daily.
➤ Other serious infections
Children: 50 to 75 mg/kg/day I.V. or I.M. once or twice daily

Dosage adjustments
• Hepatic dysfunction with significant renal impairment

Off-label uses
• Disseminated gonorrhea
• Endocarditis
• Epididymitis
• Gonorrhea-associated meningitis
• Lyme disease
• *Neisseria meningitides* carriers
• Pelvic inflammatory disease

Contraindications
• Neonates (28 days or younger)

Precautions
Use cautiously in:
• hypersensitivity to cephalosporins or penicillins, allergies
• renal impairment, hepatic disease, gallbladder disease, phenylketonuria

- history of GI disease, diarrhea following antibiotic therapy
- pregnant or breastfeeding patients.

Administration

- Obtain specimens for culture and sensitivity testing as necessary before starting therapy.
- 🔊 Be aware that drug mustn't be given with or within 48 hours of calcium-containing I.V. solutions, including calcium-containing continuous infusions such as parenteral nutrition, because of risk of precipitation of ceftriaxone calcium salt (particularly in neonates).
- Know that drug for I.V. injection is compatible with sterile water, normal saline solution, dextrose 5% in water (D₅W), half-normal saline solution, and D₅W and normal saline solution.
- After reconstituting, dilute further to desired concentration for intermittent I.V. infusion. Infuse over 30 minutes.
- For I.M. use, reconstitute powder for injection with compatible solution by adding 0.9 ml of diluent to 250-mg vial, 1.8 ml to 500-mg vial, 3.6 ml to 1-g vial, or 7.2 ml to 2-g vial, to yield a concentration averaging 250 mg/ml.
- Divide high I.M. doses equally and administer in two separate sites. Inject deep into large muscle mass.

Route	Onset	Peak	Duration
I.V.	Rapid	End of infusion	12-24 hr
I.M.	Rapid	1-2 hr	12-24 hr

Adverse reactions

CNS: headache, confusion, hemiparesis, lethargy, paresthesia, syncope, **seizures**
CV: hypotension, palpitations, chest pain, vasodilation
EENT: hearing loss
GI: nausea, vomiting, diarrhea, abdominal cramps, oral candidiasis, **pseudomembranous colitis, pancreatitis, *Clostridium difficile*–associated diarrhea**
GU: vaginal candidiasis
Hematologic: lymphocytosis, eosinophilia, **bleeding tendency, hemolytic anemia, hypoprothrombinemia, neutropenia, thrombocytopenia, agranulocytosis, bone marrow depression**
Hepatic: jaundice, **hepatomegaly**
Musculoskeletal: arthralgia
Respiratory: dyspnea
Skin: urticaria, maculopapular or erythematous rash
Other: chills, fever, superinfection, pain at I.M. injection site, **anaphylaxis, serum sickness**

Interactions

Drug-drug. *Aminoglycosides, loop diuretics:* increased risk of nephrotoxicity
Calcium-containing solutions: possibly fatal reactions caused by ceftriaxone calcium precipitates
Probenecid: decreased excretion and increased blood level of ceftriaxone
Drug-diagnostic tests. *Alanine aminotransferase, alkaline phosphatase, aspartate aminotransferase, bilirubin, blood urea nitrogen, creatinine, eosinophils, gamma-glutamyltransferase, lactate dehydrogenase:* increased levels
Coombs' test, urinary 17-ketosteroids, nonenzyme-based urine glucose tests (such as Clinitest): false-positive results
Hemoglobin, platelets, white blood cells: decreased values
Drug-herbs. *Angelica, anise, arnica, asafetida, bogbean, boldo, celery, chamomile, clove, danshen, fenugreek, feverfew, garlic, ginger, ginkgo, ginseng, horse chestnut, horseradish, licorice, meadowsweet, onion, papain, passionflower, poplar, prickly ash, quassia, red clover, turmeric, wild carrot, wild lettuce, willow:* increased risk of bleeding.

Patient monitoring

◀€ Monitor for extreme confusion, tonic-clonic seizures, and mild hemiparesis when giving high doses.

• Monitor coagulation studies.

• Assess CBC and kidney and liver function test results.

• Monitor for signs and symptoms of superinfection and other serious adverse reactions.

• Be aware that cross-sensitivity to penicillins and cephalosporins may occur.

Patient teaching

• Instruct patient to report persistent diarrhea, bruising, or bleeding.

• Caution patient not to use herbs unless prescriber approves.

• As appropriate, review all other significant and life-threatening adverse reactions and interactions, especially those related to the drugs, tests, and herbs mentioned above.

---

cefuroxime axetil
Apo-Cefuroxime✦, Ceftin, Ratio-Cefuroxime✦, Zinnat⬢

cefuroxime sodium
Zinacef

Pharmacologic class: Second-generation cephalosporin
Therapeutic class: Anti-infective
Pregnancy risk category B

Action

Interferes with bacterial cell-wall synthesis and division by binding to cell wall, causing cell to die. Active against gram-negative and gram-positive bacteria, with expanded activity against gram-negative bacteria.

Exhibits minimal immunosuppressant activity.

Availability

Oral suspension: 125 mg/5 ml, 250 mg/5 ml
Powder for injection: 750 mg, 1.5 g, 7.5 g
Premixed containers: 750 mg/50 ml, 1.5 g/50 ml
Tablets: 125 mg, 250 mg, 500 mg

⬤ Indications and dosages

➤ Moderate to severe infections, including those of skin, bone, joints, urinary or respiratory tract, gynecologic infections

Adults and children ages 12 and older: 750 mg to 1.5 g I.M. or I.V. q 8 hours for 5 to 10 days or 250 to 500 mg P.O. q 12 hours

Children ages 3 months to 12 years: 50 to 100 mg/kg/day I.V. or I.M. in divided doses q 6 to 8 hours
➤ Gonorrhea

Adults: 750 mg to 1.5 g I.M. or I.V. as a single dose, or 1.5 g I.M. (750 mg in two separate sites), given with 1 g probenecid P.O.
➤ Bacterial meningitis

Adults and children ages 12 and older: Up to 3 g I.V. or I.M. q 8 hours

Children ages 3 months to 12 years: 200 to 240 mg/kg I.V. daily in divided doses q 6 to 8 hours
➤ Otitis media

Children ages 3 months to 12 years: 15 mg/kg P.O. q 12 hours (oral suspension) for 10 days, or 250 mg (tablets) P.O. q 12 hours for 10 days
➤ Pharyngitis; tonsillitis

Adults and children ages 13 and older: 250 mg P.O. b.i.d. for 10 days

Children ages 3 months to 12 years: 125 mg P.O. q 12 hours for 10 days, or 20 mg/kg/day P.O. in two divided doses for 10 days as oral suspension (maximum 500 mg/day)

Dosage adjustment
- Renal impairment (for injectable formulation)

Contraindications
- Hypersensitivity to cephalosporins or penicillins
- Carnitine deficiency

Precautions
Use cautiously in:
- renal or hepatic impairment
- pregnant or breastfeeding patients
- children.

Administration
- Reconstitute drug in vial with sterile water for injection.
- Give by direct I.V. injection over 3 to 5 minutes into large vein or flowing I.V. line.
- For intermittent I.V. infusion, reconstitute drug with 100 ml of dextrose 5% in water or normal saline solution; administer over 15 minutes to 1 hour. For continuous infusion, give in 500 to 1,000 ml of compatible solution; infuse over 6 to 24 hours.
- Inject I.M. doses deep into large muscle mass.
- Give oral form with food.
- Be aware that tablets and oral suspension are exchangeable on a milligram-for-milligram basis.

Route	Onset	Peak	Duration
P.O.	Unknown	2 hr	8-12 hr
I.V., I.M.	Rapid	End of infusion	6-12 hr

Adverse reactions
CNS: headache, hyperactivity, hypertonia, **seizures**
GI: nausea, vomiting, diarrhea, abdominal pain, dyspepsia, **pseudomembranous colitis**
GU: hematuria, vaginal candidiasis, **renal dysfunction, acute renal failure**
Hematologic: hemolytic anemia, aplastic anemia, hemorrhage

Hepatic: hepatic dysfunction
Metabolic: hyperglycemia
Skin: toxic epidermal necrolysis, **erythema multiforme, Stevens-Johnson syndrome**
Other: allergic reaction, drug fever, superinfection, **anaphylaxis**

Interactions
Drug-drug. *Antacids containing aluminum or magnesium, histamine$_2$-receptor antagonists:* increased cefuroxime absorption
Probenecid: decreased excretion and increased blood level of cefuroxime
Drug-diagnostic tests. *Blood glucose, Coombs' test, urine glucose tests using Benedict's solution:* false-positive results
Glucose, hematocrit: decreased levels
White blood cells in urine: increased level
Drug-food. *Moderate- or high-fat meal:* increased drug bioavailability

Patient monitoring
- Monitor patient for life-threatening adverse effects, including anaphylaxis, Stevens-Johnson syndrome, and pseudomembranous colitis.
- Monitor neurologic status, particularly for signs of impending seizures.
- Monitor kidney and liver function test results and intake and output.
- Monitor CBC with differential and prothrombin time; watch for signs and symptoms of blood dyscrasias.
- Monitor temperature; watch for signs and symptoms of superinfection.

Patient teaching
- Advise patient to immediately report rash or bleeding tendency.
- Instruct patient to take drug with food every 12 hours as prescribed.
- Teach patient how to recognize signs and symptoms of superinfection. Instruct him to report these right away.
- Advise patient to report CNS changes.

• As appropriate, review all other significant and life-threatening adverse reactions and interactions, especially those related to the drugs, tests, and foods mentioned above.

celecoxib
Celebrex

Pharmacologic class: Nonsteroidal cyclooxygenase-2 (COX-2) inhibitor, nonsteroidal anti-inflammatory drug (NSAID)

Therapeutic class: Antirheumatic

Pregnancy risk category C

FDA | BOXED WARNING

• Drug may increase risk of serious cardiovascular thrombotic events, myocardial infarction, and stroke (which can be fatal). Risk may increase with duration of use, and may be greater in patients who have cardiovascular disease or risk factors for it.
• Drug is contraindicated for perioperative pain in setting of coronary artery bypass graft surgery.
• Drug increases risk of serious GI adverse events, including bleeding, ulcers, and stomach or intestinal perforation, which can be fatal. These events can occur at any time during therapy and without warning. Elderly patients are at greater risk.

Action
Exhibits anti-inflammatory, analgesic, and antipyretic action due to inhibition of COX-2 enzyme

Availability
Capsules: 50 mg, 100 mg, 200 mg, 400 mg

Indications and dosages
➤ Ankylosing spondylitis, osteoarthritis
Adults: 200 mg/day P.O. as a single dose or 100 mg P.O. b.i.d.
➤ Rheumatoid arthritis
Adults: 100 to 200 mg P.O. b.i.d.
➤ Adjunctive treatment in familial adenomatous polyposis to decrease the number of adenomatous colorectal polyps
Adults: 400 mg P.O. b.i.d.
➤ Acute pain or primary dysmenorrhea
Adults: 400 mg P.O. once, plus one additional 200 mg-dose as needed on first day; then 200 mg b.i.d. as needed
➤ Juvenile rheumatoid arthritis
Children age 2 and older weighing 10 to 25 kg (22 to 55 lb): 50 mg P.O. b.i.d.
Children age 2 and older weighing 25 kg or more: 100 mg P.O. b.i.d.

Dosage adjustment
• Hepatic impairment
• Patients weighing less than 50 kg (110 lb)

Contraindications
• Hypersensitivity to drug, sulfonamides, or other NSAIDs
• Advanced renal disease
• Severe hepatic impairment
• Sensitivity precipitated by aspirin
• Third trimester of pregnancy
• Breastfeeding

Precautions
Use cautiously in:
• renal insufficiency, hypertension
• history of asthma, urticaria, renal disease, hepatic dysfunction, heart failure
• patients on long-term NSAID therapy
• elderly patients
• pregnant patients in first or second trimester
• children younger than age 18 (safety not established).

Reactions in **bold** are life-threatening.　　　◀╠ Clinical alert

Administration

• When administering doses higher than 200/mg daily, give with food or milk to improve drug absorption.

Route	Onset	Peak	Duration
P.O.	Unknown	3 hr	Unknown

Adverse reactions

CNS: dizziness, drowsiness, headache, insomnia, fatigue, **stroke**
CV: angina, tachycardia, peripheral edema, **myocardial infarction**
EENT: ophthalmic effects, tinnitus, epistaxis, pharyngitis, rhinitis, sinusitis
GI: nausea, diarrhea, constipation, abdominal pain, dyspepsia, flatulence, dry mouth, **GI bleeding**
GU: menorrhagia, **renal failure**
Hematologic: eosinophilia, ecchymosis, **neutropenia, leukopenia, pancytopenia, thrombocytopenia, agranulocytosis, granulocytopenia, aplastic anemia, bone marrow depression**
Hepatic: hepatotoxicity
Metabolic: hyperchloremia, hypophosphatemia
Musculoskeletal: back pain, leg cramps
Respiratory: upper respiratory tract infection
Skin: rash
Other: anaphylaxis

Interactions

Drug-drug. *Angiotensin-converting enzyme inhibitors, furosemide, thiazides:* reduced celecoxib efficacy
Antacids containing aluminum and magnesium: decreased celecoxib blood level
Aspirin (regular doses): increased risk of GI bleeding and GI ulcers
Fluconazole, lithium: increased blood levels of these drugs
Warfarin: increased risk of bleeding
Drug-diagnostic tests. *Alanine aminotransferase, aspartate aminotransferase, blood urea nitrogen:* increased levels
Hematocrit, hemoglobin: decreased values
Drug-herbs. *Dong quai, feverfew, garlic, ginger, horse chestnut, red clover:* increased risk of bleeding
White willow: increased risk of GI ulcers
Drug-behaviors. *Long-term alcohol use, smoking:* GI irritation and bleeding

Patient monitoring

• Monitor CBC, electrolyte levels, creatinine clearance, occult fecal blood test, and liver function test results every 6 to 12 months.

Patient teaching

🔊 Advise patient to immediately report bloody stools, vomiting of blood, or signs or symptoms of liver damage (nausea, fatigue, lethargy, pruritus, yellowing of eyes or skin, tenderness in upper right abdomen, or flulike symptoms).
• Instruct patient to take drug with food or milk.
• Tell patient to avoid aspirin and other NSAIDs (such as ibuprofen and naproxen) during therapy.
• As appropriate, review all other significant and life-threatening adverse reactions and interactions, especially those related to the drugs, tests, herbs, and behaviors mentioned above.

cephalexin

Apo-Cephalex✤, Biocef, Dom-Cephalexin✤, Keflex, Novo-Lexin✤, Nu-Cephalex✤, Panixine DisperDose, PMS-Cephalexin✤

Pharmacologic class: First-generation cephalosporin
Therapeutic class: Anti-infective
Pregnancy risk category B

✤ Canada   ⊕ UK   ☠ Hazardous drug   ⊗ High alert drug

Action
Interferes with bacterial cell-wall synthesis, causing cell to rupture and die. Active against many gram-positive bacteria; shows limited activity against gram-negative bacteria.

Availability
Capsules: 250 mg, 500 mg, 750 mg
Oral suspension: 125 mg/ 5 ml, 250 mg/5 ml
Tablets: 250 mg, 500 mg

⒤ Indications and dosages
➢ Respiratory tract infections caused by streptococci; skin and skin-structure infections caused by methicillin-sensitive staphylococci and streptococci; bone infections caused by methicillin-sensitive staphylococci or *Proteus mirabilis;* genitourinary infections caused by *Escherichia coli, P. mirabilis,* and *Klebsiella* species; *Haemophilus influenzae,* methicillin-sensitive staphylococcal, streptococcal, and *Moraxella catarrhalis* infections
Adults: 1 to 4 g P.O. daily in divided doses (usually 250 mg P.O. q 6 hours). For uncomplicated cystitis, skin and soft-tissue infections, and streptococcal pharyngitis, 500 mg P.O. q 12 hours.
Children: 25 to 50 mg/kg/day P.O. in divided doses
➢ Otitis media caused by *S. pneumoniae*
Children: 75 to 100 mg/kg/day P.O. in four divided doses

Dosage adjustment
• Renal impairment

Contraindications
• Hypersensitivity to cephalosporins or penicillin

Precautions
Use cautiously in:
• renal impairment, phenylketonuria
• history of GI disease
• debilitated or emaciated patients
• elderly patients
• pregnant or breastfeeding patients.

Administration
• Give with or without food.
• Refrigerate oral suspension.

Route	Onset	Peak	Duration
P.O.	Rapid	1 hr	6-12 hr

Adverse reactions
CNS: fever, headache, lethargy, paresthesia, syncope, **seizures**
CV: edema, hypotension, vasodilation, palpitations, chest pain
EENT: hearing loss
GI: nausea, vomiting, diarrhea, abdominal cramps, oral candidiasis, **pseudomembranous colitis**
GU: vaginal candidiasis, **nephrotoxicity**
Hematologic: lymphocytosis, eosinophilia, **bleeding tendency, hemolytic anemia, neutropenia, thrombocytopenia, agranulocytosis, bone marrow depression**
Musculoskeletal: joint pain
Respiratory: dyspnea
Skin: rash, maculopapular and erythematous urticaria
Other: superinfection, chills, pain, allergic reaction, hypersensitivity reactions including **anaphylaxis, serum sickness**

Interactions
Drug-drug. *Aminoglycosides, loop diuretics:* increased risk of nephrotoxicity
Chloramphenicol: antagonistic effect
Probenecid: increased cephalexin blood level
Drug-diagnostic tests. *Alanine aminotransferase, alkaline phosphatase, aspartate aminotransferase, bilirubin, blood urea nitrogen, creatinine, eosinophils, lactate dehydrogenase, lymphocytes:* increased values
Coombs' test: false-positive result (especially in neonates whose mothers received drug before delivery)
Granulocytes, neutrophils, white blood cells: decreased counts

---

Reactions in **bold** are life-threatening.   ◀€ Clinical alert

Patient monitoring
- Assess for signs and symptoms of serious adverse reactions, including hypersensitivity, severe diarrhea, and bleeding.
- During long-term therapy, monitor CBC and liver and kidney function test results.

Patient teaching
◀ Instruct patient to stop taking drug and contact prescriber immediately if he develops rash or difficulty breathing.
- Tell patient to take drug with full glass of water.
- Advise patient to report severe diarrhea.
- As appropriate, review all other significant and life-threatening adverse reactions and interactions, especially those related to the drugs and tests mentioned above.

cetirizine hydrochloride
All-Day Allergy, Aller-Relief♣, Allergy Relief♣, Benadryl Allergy Oral Solution⊕, Benadryl One a Day⊕, Piriteze⊕, Pollenshield Hayfever⊕, Reactine♣, Zirtec⊕, Zyrtec

Pharmacologic class: Histamine$_1$-receptor antagonist (peripherally selective)
Therapeutic class: Allergy, cold, and cough agent; antihistamine
Pregnancy risk category B

Action
Antagonizes histamine's effects at histamine$_1$-receptor sites, preventing allergic response. Also has mild bronchodilatory effects and blocks histamine-induced bronchoconstriction in asthma.

Availability
Syrup: 5 mg/5 ml
Tablets: 5 mg, 10 mg

⚡ Indications and dosages
➤ Allergic symptoms caused by histamine release
Adults and children older than age 6: 5 to 10 mg P.O. daily
Children ages 2 to 5: 2.5 to 5 mg P.O. daily

Dosage adjustment
- Renal impairment
- Hepatic impairment

Contraindications
- Hypersensitivity to drug or hydroxyzine
- Acute asthma attacks
- Angle-closure glaucoma
- Pyloroduodenal obstruction
- Breastfeeding

Precautions
Use cautiously in:
- renal impairment, significant hepatic dysfunction
- elderly patients
- pregnant patients
- children younger than age 2 (safety not established).

Administration
- Give with or without food.
- Administer at same time each day.

Route	Onset	Peak	Duration
P.O.	30 min	1-4 hr	24 hr

Adverse reactions
CNS: dizziness, drowsiness, fatigue
CV: palpitations, edema
EENT: pharyngitis
GI: nausea, vomiting, abdominal distress, dry mouth
Musculoskeletal: myalgia, joint pain
Respiratory: bronchospasm
Skin: photosensitivity, rash, **angioedema**
Other: fever

Interactions

Drug-drug. *CNS depressants:* additive CNS effects
Theophylline: decreased cetirizine clearance
Drug-diagnostic tests. *Allergy skin tests:* false-negative results
Drug-behaviors. *Alcohol use:* additive CNS effects
Sun exposure: photosensitivity

Patient monitoring

• Monitor creatinine levels in patients with renal dysfunction.
• Assess hepatic enzyme levels in patients with hepatic disease.

Patient teaching

• Tell patient to take with full glass of water.
• Inform patient that drug may impair alertness and that alcohol may exaggerate this effect.
• Caution patient to avoid driving and other hazardous activities until he knows how drug affects concentration and alertness.
• As appropriate, review all other significant and life-threatening adverse reactions and interactions, especially those related to the drugs, tests, and behaviors mentioned above.

certolizumab pegol

Cimzia

Pharmacologic class: Tumor necrosis factor (TNF) blocker
Therapeutic class: Immunomodulator
Pregnancy risk category B

FDA BOXED WARNING

Serious infections
• Patients treated with certolizumab are at increased risk for developing serious infections that may lead to hospitalization or death. Most patients who developed these infections were taking concomitant immunosuppressants, such as methotrexate or corticosteroids.
• Discontinue drug if patient develops serious infection or sepsis.
• Reported infections include active tuberculosis (TB), including reactivation of latent TB. Patients with TB have frequently presented with disseminated or extrapulmonary disease. Perform test for latent TB and if positive, start treatment for TB before starting drug. Monitor all patients for active TB during treatment, even if initial latent TB test is negative.
• Invasive fungal infections, including histoplasmosis, coccidioidomycosis, candidiasis, aspergillosis, blastomycosis, and pneumocystosis, have been reported. Patients with histoplasmosis or other invasive fungal infections may present with disseminated, rather than localized, disease. Antigen and antibody testing for histoplasmosis may be negative in some patients with active infection. Consider empiric antifungal therapy in patients at risk for invasive fungal infections who develop severe systemic illness.
• Bacterial, viral, and other infections due to opportunistic pathogens, including *Legionella* and *Listeria* species, have occurred.
• Carefully consider risks and benefits of treatment with certolizumab before initiating therapy in patients with chronic or recurrent infection.
• Closely monitor patients for signs and symptoms of infection during and after treatment with certolizumab.
• Lymphoma and other malignancies, some fatal, have been reported in children and adolescents treated with TNF blockers, of which certolizumab is a member.

• Drug isn't indicated for use in children.

Action
Binds to human TNF with a dissociation constant of 90 pM. TNF is a key proinflammatory cytokine with a central role in inflammatory processes. Selectively neutralizes TNF (IC90 of 4 ng/ml for inhibition of human TNF in the in vitro L929 murine fibrosarcoma cytotoxicity assay) but doesn't neutralize lymphotoxin.

Availability
Powder for reconstitution, lyophilized: 200 mg in single-use vials
Prefilled syringe: 200 mg/ml in 1-ml single-use prefilled syringes

⚡ Indications and dosages
➣ Moderate to severe Crohn's disease in patients with inadequate response to conventional therapy
Adults: Initially, 400 mg subcutaneously (given as two 200-mg injections), then at weeks 2 and 4. In patients with a clinical response, maintenance dosage is 400 mg q 4 weeks.
➣ Moderate to severe rheumatoid arthritis
Adults: Initially, 400 mg subcutaneously (given as two 200-mg injections), then at weeks 2 and 4 followed by 200 mg q other week. Consider 400 mg q 4 weeks for maintenance dosing.

Contraindications
None

Precautions
Use cautiously in:
• hypersensitivity reactions
• congestive heart failure (CHF)
• chronic or recurrent infection, serious infections
• chronic hepatitis B virus (HBV) carriers

• preexisting or recent-onset central or peripheral nervous system demyelinating disorders
• significant hematologic abnormalities
• development of positive antinuclear antibody (ANA) titers
• concurrent use of anakinra, abatacept, rituximab, natalizumab, other TNF blockers, or other biological disease-modifying antirheumatics (use not recommended)
• concurrent use of live or attenuated vaccines (don't use)
• immunosuppression and concurrent use of immunosuppressants, such as corticosteroids or methotrexate
• elderly patients (don't use)
• pregnant or breastfeeding patients
• children (safety and efficacy not established).

Administration
◀≣ Be aware that patients with active infections shouldn't start treatment with certolizumab. Also, consider risks and benefits of treatment before starting drug in patients with chronic or recurrent infection; in those who have been exposed to TB; in those with history of opportunistic infection; in those who have resided or traveled in areas of endemic TB or endemic mycoses, such as histoplasmosis, coccidioidomycosis, or blastomycosis; and in those with underlying conditions that may predispose to infection.
• Evaluate patients for TB risk factors and test for latent infection before starting drug.
◀≣ Evaluate patients at risk for HBV infection before initiating TNF-blocker therapy. Discontinue drug in patients who develop HBV reactivation and initiate effective antiviral therapy with appropriate supportive treatment. Know that safety of resuming TNF-blocker therapy after HBV reactivation has been controlled isn't known;

exercise caution when considering resumption of therapy.

◀€ Discontinue drug in patients who develop other serious infections or sepsis.

◀€ Discontinue drug in patients who develop signs and symptoms suggestive of a lupus-like syndrome following treatment.

• Consider discontinuing drug in patients with confirmed significant hematologic abnormalities.

◀€ Immediately discontinue drug if severe hypersensitivity reactions occur and initiate appropriate therapy.

Route	Onset	Peak	Duration
Subcutaneous	Unknown	54-171 hr	Unknown

Adverse reactions

CNS: headache, fatigue, anxiety, bipolar disorder, **suicide attempt, transient ischemic attack, stroke**

CV: hypertension, hypertensive heart disease, angina pectoris, **MI, myocardial ischemia, pericardial effusion, pericarditis, arrhythmias, atrial fibrillation, CHF**

EENT: optic neuritis, uveitis, retinal hemorrhage, nasopharyngitis, pharyngitis

GU: menstrual disorder, urinary tract infection, **nephrotic syndrome, renal failure**

Hematologic: anemia, leukopenia, pancytopenia, thrombophilia, bleeding, thrombophlebitis, vasculitis

Hepatic: elevated liver enzyme levels, **hepatitis**

Musculoskeletal: arthralgia, back pain

Respiratory: upper respiratory tract infection, acute bronchitis

Skin: rash, alopecia totalis, dermatitis, erythema nodosum, urticaria

Other: pyrexia, injection-site reactions, lymphadenopathy, **serious infections, malignancies, lupus-like syndrome, hypersensitivity**

Interactions

Drug-drug. *Abatacept, anakinra, natalizumab, rituximab, TNF blockers or other biological disease-modifying antirheumatics:* increased risk of serious infections

Live vaccines: increased risk of secondary transmission of disease and unknown response

Drug-diagnostic tests. ANA titers: increased risk of developing positive titers

APPT: elevated results

Patient monitoring

◀€ Continue to closely monitor patients for hypersensitivity reactions and treat appropriately.

• Closely monitor patients for infection during and after treatment. Know that patients who develop new infection during treatment should be closely monitored, undergo prompt and complete diagnostic workup appropriate for an immunocompromised patient, and be given appropriate antimicrobial therapy.

• Continue to evaluate patients for TB risk factors; test for latent infection periodically during therapy.

• For patients who reside or travel in regions where mycoses are endemic, suspect invasive fungal infection if serious systemic illness develops. Consider appropriate empiric antifungal therapy while a diagnostic workup is being performed. Antigen and antibody testing for histoplasmosis may be negative in some patients with active infection. When feasible, the decision to institute empiric antifungal therapy in these patients should be made in consultation with a physician with expertise in diagnosis and treatment of invasive fungal infections and should take into account both the risk of severe fungal infection and the risks of antifungal therapy.

• Observe for signs and symptoms of malignancies; be aware that

---

lymphomas, including Hodgkin's and non-Hodgkin's lymphoma, and leukemia have been reported.

◀﹦ Closely monitor patients with CHF during therapy.

• Closely monitor patients who are carriers of HBV and require treatment with certolizumab for clinical and laboratory signs of active HBV infection throughout therapy and for several months following termination of therapy.

◀﹦ Be aware that pancytopenia, including aplastic anemia, has been reported (rare) with TNF-blocker use. Watch for leukopenia, pancytopenia, or thrombocytopenia.

◀﹦ Watch for neurologic complications (rare), including new-onset or exacerbation of clinical symptoms or radiographic evidence of CNS demyelinating disease (including multiple sclerosis), peripheral demyelinating disease (including Guillain-Barré syndrome), seizure disorder, optic neuritis, and peripheral neuropathy.

Patient teaching

• Instruct patient who may self-inject on proper use of prefilled syringe, suitable injection sites (including thigh or abdomen), rotation of sites, and appropriate handling and disposal of syringe. Instruct patient to discard unused portions remaining in syringe.

◀﹦ Advise patient to seek immediate medical attention if signs or symptoms of severe allergic reactions occur.

• Advise patient to report new or worsening medical conditions, such as heart disease, neurologic disease, or autoimmune disorders, and to promptly report signs and symptoms suggestive of a cytopenia (such as bruising, bleeding, or persistent fever).

• Inform patient that drug may lower ability of immune system to fight infections. Instruct patient of importance of informing prescriber about

new or previous infections, including TB and reactivation of HBV infection.

• Counsel patient about possible risk of lymphoma and other malignancies while taking certolizumab.

• Tell patient to avoid taking live vaccines while using this drug.

• Advise breastfeeding patient that she should decide whether to discontinue breastfeeding or discontinue drug, taking into account importance of drug for her treatment.

• As appropriate, review all other significant and life-threatening adverse reactions and interactions, especially those related to the drugs and tests mentioned above.

cetuximab
Erbitux

Pharmacologic class: Epidermal growth factor receptor (EGFR) inhibitor

Therapeutic class: Antineoplastic

Pregnancy risk category C

FDA | BOXED WARNING

• Drug may cause severe infusion reactions. If severe reaction occurs, stop infusion immediately and discontinue therapy permanently.

• Cardiopulmonary arrest, sudden death, or both occurred in 2% of patients with squamous-cell carcinoma of head and neck who received drug plus radiation therapy and in 3% of patients with squamous-cell carcinoma of head and neck treated with European-approved cetuximab in combination with platinum-based therapy with 5-fluorouracil. Monitor serum electrolyte levels closely during and after therapy.

Action
Binds to EGFR, competitively inhibiting binding of epidermal growth factor and other ligands and blocking phosphorylation and activation of receptor-associated kinases. These actions lead to cell growth inhibition, apoptosis induction, and decreased matrix metalloproteinases and vascular endothelial growth factor.

Availability
Solution for injection: 50-ml single-use vial containing 100 mg (2 mg/ml), 100-ml single-use vial containing 200 mg (2 mg/ml)

Indications and dosages
➤ EGFR-expressing metastatic colorectal carcinoma, used alone in patients intolerant to irinotecan-based chemotherapy or in combination with irinotecan in patients refractory to irinotecan-based therapy
Adults: 400 mg/m^2 initial loading dose given as 120-minute I.V. infusion followed by maintenance dose of 250 mg/m^2 infused I.V. over 60 minutes
➤ Locally or regionally advanced squamous-cell carcinoma of head and neck, in combination with radiation therapy
Adults: 400 mg/m^2 as initial loading dose (first infusion) given as 120-minute I.V. infusion 1 week before initiation of radiation therapy. For recommended weekly maintenance dose (all other infusions), 250 mg/m^2 infused I.V. over 60 minutes weekly for duration of radiation therapy (6 to 7 weeks) given 1 hour before radiation therapy.
➤ Locally or regionally advanced squamous-cell carcinoma of head and neck in combination with platinum-based therapy plus 5-fluorouracil (5-FU)
Adults: Initially, 400 mg/m^2 on day of initiation of platinum-based therapy with 5-FU as a 120-minute I.V. infusion. Complete cetuximab administration 1 hour before platinum-based therapy with 5-FU. For recommended subsequent weekly doses (all other infusions), 250 mg/m^2 I.V. infusion over 60 minutes for duration of radiation therapy (6 to 7 weeks) or until disease progression or unacceptable toxicity occurs.
➤ Recurrent or metastatic squamous-cell carcinoma of head and neck (used alone) in patients for whom platinum-based therapy has failed
Adults: Initially, 400-mg/m^2 I.V. infusion followed by 250 mg/m^2 I.V. weekly until disease progresses or unacceptable toxicity occurs

Off-label uses
• Cancers that overexpress EGFR

Dosage adjustment
• Mild to moderate infusion (Grade 1 or 2) reaction
• Severe acneiform rash
• Acute onset or worsening of pulmonary symptoms

Contraindications
None

Precautions
Use cautiously in:
• hypersensitivity to murine proteins or drug components
• dermatologic or pulmonary toxicities
• patients receiving concurrent radiation therapy and cisplatin
• patients receiving concurrent radiation therapy who have history of coronary artery disease, arrhythmias, and congestive heart failure
• pregnant or breastfeeding patients
• children (safety and efficacy not established).

Administration
• As ordered, premedicate with histamine$_1$-antagonist (such as 50 mg diphenhydramine I.V.).

- Use low-protein-binding, 0.22 micrometer in-line filter placed as close to patient as possible.
◀€ Don't give by I.V. push or bolus.
◀€ Don't shake or dilute vial.
- Administer by I.V. infusion pump or syringe pump.
- Piggyback drug to patient's infusion line.
- Give initial dose over 2 hours at a rate of 10 mg/minute; give subsequent weekly doses over 1 hour. Maximum infusion rate shouldn't exceed 10 mg/minute.
- At end of infusion, flush I.V. lines with normal saline solution.
◀€ Be aware that 90% of infusion reactions occur with first infusion. Observe patient closely for 1 hour after infusion (or longer in patients who have experienced infusion reactions). Severe and life-threatening infusion reactions have occurred, including rapid-onset airway obstruction (bronchospasm, stridor, hoarseness), urticaria, and hypotension.
◀€ Permanently reduce infusion rate by 50% if patient experiences mild or moderate infusion reaction. Immediately and permanently discontinue drug in patient who experiences severe (Grade 3 or 4) infusion reaction.
- Make sure appropriate medical resources for treatment of severe infusion reactions are available during infusion.
- Expect patients with colorectal cancer to undergo immunohistochemical testing for EGFR expression using DakoCytomation EGFR pharmDx test kit.
- Interrupt therapy if patient develops acute onset or worsening of pulmonary symptoms. Discontinue therapy if pneumonitis or lung infiltrates are confirmed.
- For first occurrence of severe acneiform rash, delay infusion 1 to 2 weeks; if condition improves, continue therapy at 250 mg/m^2; if no improvement occurs, withdraw drug. For second occurrence, delay infusion

1 to 2 weeks; if condition improves, reduce dosage to 200 mg/m^2; if no improvement occurs, withdraw drug. For third occurrence, delay infusion for 1 to 2 weeks; if condition improves, reduce dosage to 150 mg/m^2; if no improvement occurs, withdraw drug. On fourth occurrence, withdraw drug.

Route	Onset	Peak	Duration
I.V.	Unknown	Unknown	Unknown

Adverse reactions
CNS: headache, insomnia, depression, malaise, asthenia
CV: cardiopulmonary arrest
EENT: conjunctivitis
GI: abdominal pain, diarrhea, nausea, vomiting, constipation, stomatitis, dyspepsia, anorexia
GU: renal failure
Hematologic: leukopenia, anemia
Metabolic: dehydration, electrolyte abnormalities
Musculoskeletal: back pain
Respiratory: dyspnea, increased cough, **interstitial lung disease, pulmonary embolus**
Skin: acneiform rash, alopecia, skin disorder, nail disorder, pruritus
Other: weight loss, fever, pain, infection, peripheral edema, **severe infusion reaction**

Interactions
Drug-diagnostic tests. *Calcium, magnesium:* decreased
Drug-behaviors. *Sun exposure:* exacerbated skin reactions

Patient monitoring
- Watch for signs and symptoms of infusion reaction.
- Monitor patient for hypomagnesemia and hypocalcemia during therapy and for 8 weeks afterward.
- Closely monitor serum electrolytes (including serum magnesium, potassium, and calcium) during therapy and after combination drug and radiation

therapy in patients with history of coronary artery disease, arrhythmias, and heart failure.

• Monitor patient with dermatologic toxicities for inflammatory or infectious sequelae.

• Watch for pulmonary toxicities in patient with history of interstitial pneumonitis or pulmonary fibrosis. Be prepared to interrupt or discontinue therapy and intervene appropriately.

• Monitor for potentially serious cardiotoxicity if patient is receiving drug in combination with radiation therapy and cisplatin.

• Stay alert for severe diarrhea and electrolyte depletion.

Patient teaching

◀ Urge patient to immediately report rash, which may indicate skin toxicity.

◀ Instruct patient to immediately report new or worsening respiratory or cardiovascular symptoms.

• Advise patient to use sunscreen and wear a hat when outdoors and to limit sun exposure, because sunlight can exacerbate skin reactions.

• Caution female with childbearing potential that drug may cause pregnancy loss or pose hazard to fetus.

• Advise female to discontinue breastfeeding during therapy and for 60 days after last dose.

• As appropriate, review all other significant and life-threatening adverse reactions and interactions, especially those related to the tests and behaviors mentioned above.

chlorambucil
Leukeran

Pharmacologic class: Alkylating agent, nitrogen mustard

Therapeutic class: Antineoplastic, immunosuppressant

Pregnancy risk category D

FDA BOXED WARNING

• Drug may suppress bone marrow function severely and is carcinogenic.

• Drug causes infertility and is probably mutagenic and teratogenic.

Action
Interacts with cellular DNA to produce cytotoxic cross-linkage, which disrupts cell function. Cell-cycle-phase nonspecific.

Availability
Tablets: 2 mg

Indications and dosages
➤ Chronic lymphocytic leukemia, malignant lymphoma, Hodgkin's disease

Adults: Initially, 0.1 to 0.2 mg/kg/day P.O. for 3 to 6 weeks as a single dose or in divided doses. Maintenance dosage is based on CBC but shouldn't exceed 0.1 mg/kg/day.

Off-label uses
• Idiopathic membranous nephropathy
• Meningoencephalitis associated with Behçet's disease
• Rheumatoid arthritis

Contraindications
• Hypersensitivity to drug or other alkylating agents
• Pregnancy or breastfeeding

Reactions in **bold** are life-threatening. ◀ Clinical alert

Precautions
Use cautiously in:
- hematopoietic depression, infection, other chronic debilitating diseases
- history of seizures or head trauma
- patients who have undergone radiation or other chemotherapy
- elderly patients
- females of childbearing age
- children (safety and efficacy not established).

Administration
- Before starting therapy, assess for history of seizures or head trauma.
- After full-course radiation or chemotherapy, wait 4 weeks before giving full doses (because of bone marrow vulnerability).
- To minimize GI effects, drug may be given at bedtime with antiemetic, especially if high dosage is prescribed.

Route	Onset	Peak	Duration
P.O.	Unknown	1 hr	Unknown

Adverse reactions
CNS: peripheral neuropathy, tremor, confusion, agitation, ataxia, flaccid paresis, **seizures**
EENT: keratitis
GI: nausea, vomiting, diarrhea
GU: sterile cystitis, amenorrhea, sterility, decreased sperm count
Hematologic: anemia, **leukopenia, thrombocytopenia, neutropenia, bone marrow depression**
Hepatic: jaundice, **hepatotoxicity**
Metabolic: hyperuricemia
Musculoskeletal: muscle twitching
Respiratory: interstitial pneumonitis, pulmonary fibrosis
Skin: rash, **erythema multiforme, epidermal necrolysis, Stevens-Johnson syndrome**
Other: drug fever, allergic reaction, **secondary malignancies**

Interactions
Drug-drug. *Anticoagulants, aspirin:* increased risk of bleeding
Immunosuppressants, myelosuppressants: additive bone marrow depression
Live-virus vaccines: decreased antibody response to vaccine, increased risk of adverse reactions
Drug-diagnostic tests. *Alanine aminotransferase, alkaline phosphatase, aspartate aminotransferase, uric acid:* increased levels (may reflect hepatotoxicity)
Granulocytes, hemoglobin, neutrophils, platelets, red blood cells, white blood cells (WBCs): decreased counts
Drug-herbs. *Astragalus, echinacea, melatonin:* interference with immunosuppressant action

Patient monitoring
🔊 Monitor CBC with white cell differential and platelet count weekly.
- Monitor WBC count every 3 to 4 days.
- Assess liver function test results.

Patient teaching
- Instruct patient to immediately report unusual bleeding or bruising, fever, nausea, vomiting, rash, chills, sore throat, cough, shortness of breath, seizures, amenorrhea, unusual lumps or masses, flank or stomach pain, joint pain, lip or mouth sores, or yellowing of skin or sclera.
- Tell patient to take drug with full glass of water.
- Inform patient that drug may increase his risk for infection. Advise him to wash hands frequently, wear a mask in public places, and avoid people with infections.
- Instruct patient to contact prescriber before receiving vaccines.
- Advise female patient to use reliable contraception.
- As appropriate, review all other significant and life-threatening adverse reactions and interactions, especially those related to the drugs, tests, and herbs mentioned above.

chlordiazepoxide hydrochloride
Apo-Chlordiazepoxide ✦

Pharmacologic class: Benzodiazepine
Therapeutic class: Anxiolytic, sedative-hypnotic
Controlled substance schedule IV
Pregnancy risk category D

Action
Unknown. May potentiate effects of gamma-aminobutyric acid (an inhibitory neurotransmitter) by increasing neuronal membrane permeability; may depress CNS at limbic and subcortical levels of brain. Anxiolytic effect occurs at doses well below those that cause sedation or ataxia.

Availability
Capsules: 5 mg, 10 mg, 25 mg
Injection: 100-mg ampules

🅸 Indications and dosages
➤ Mild to moderate anxiety
Adults: 5 to 10 mg P.O. three to four times daily
➤ Severe anxiety
Adults: Initially, 50 to 100 mg I.M. or I.V.; then 25 to 50 mg P.O. three to four times daily as needed
➤ Preoperative apprehension or anxiety
Adults: 5 to 10 mg P.O. three to four times daily for several days before surgery or 50 to 100 mg I.M. 1 hour before surgery
➤ Acute alcohol withdrawal
Adults: Initially, 50 to 100 mg I.V. or I.M. Repeat dose as needed up to 300 mg/day.

Dosage adjustment
• Hepatic impairment
• Age 65 or older

Contraindications
• Hypersensitivity to drug, other benzodiazepines, or tartrazine
• CNS depression
• Uncontrolled severe pain
• Porphyria
• Pregnancy or breastfeeding
• Children younger than age 6

Precautions
Use cautiously in:
• hepatic dysfunction, severe renal impairment
• debilitated or elderly patients.

Administration
• Dilute I.V. preparation with 5 ml of normal saline solution. Administer slowly over at least 1 minute.
• When giving I.M., use 2 ml of special I.M. diluent. Inject slowly and deeply into gluteus muscle.
• Don't use I.M. diluent for I.V. preparation.
• After I.V. or I.M. administration, observe patient closely and enforce bedrest for at least 3 hours.

Route	Onset	Peak	Duration
P.O.	Rapid	0.5-4 hr	Up to 24 hr
I.V.	1-5 min	Unknown	0.25-1 hr
I.M.	15-30 min	Unknown	Unknown

Adverse reactions
CNS: dizziness, drowsiness, hangover, headache, depression, paradoxical stimulation
EENT: blurred vision
GI: nausea, vomiting, constipation, diarrhea
Hematologic: agranulocytosis
Hepatic: jaundice
Skin: rash
Other: physical or psychological drug dependence, drug tolerance, pain at I.M. site

---

Interactions
Drug-drug. *Antidepressants, antihistamines, opioids:* additive CNS depression
Barbiturates, rifampin: decreased chlordiazepoxide efficacy
Cimetidine, disulfiram, fluoxetine, hormonal contraceptives, isoniazid, ketoconazole, metoprolol, propoxyphene, propranolol, valproic acid: enhanced chlordiazepoxide effect
Levodopa: decreased levodopa efficacy
Drug-diagnostic tests. *Alanine aminotransferase, aspartate aminotransferase, bilirubin:* increased levels
Granulocytes: decreased count
Metyrapone test: decreased response
Radioactive iodine uptake test (^{123}I or ^{131}I): decreased uptake
Urine 17-ketogenic steroids, urine 17-ketosteroids: altered test results
Drug-herbs. *Chamomile, hops, kava, skullcap, valerian:* increased CNS depression
Drug-behaviors. *Alcohol use:* increased CNS depression

Patient monitoring
• Monitor CBC and hepatic enzyme levels in prolonged therapy.
• Monitor renal and hepatic studies.
• Assess patient for apnea, bradycardia, and hypotension.

Patient teaching
• Caution patient to avoid driving and other hazardous activities until he knows how drug affects concentration and alertness.
• Advise patient to avoid alcohol during therapy.
• Tell patient not to stop taking drug abruptly. Instruct him to discuss dosage-tapering schedule with prescriber.
• Caution female patient not to take drug if she's pregnant or might become pregnant during therapy. Advise her to use reliable contraception.
• As appropriate, review all other significant and life-threatening adverse reactions and interactions, especially those related to the drugs, tests, herbs, and behaviors mentioned above.

chloroquine phosphate

Pharmacologic class: 4-aminoquinolone derivative
Therapeutic class: Antimalarial, amebicide
Pregnancy risk category C

FDA | BOXED WARNING

• Drug is indicated for treating malaria and extraintestinal amebiasis.
• Before prescribing, clinician should be familiar with complete package insert contents.

Action
Unknown. Antimalarial action may occur through inhibition of protein synthesis and alteration of DNA in susceptible parasites.

Availability
Tablets: 250 mg (150-mg base), 500 mg (300-mg base)

🖊 Indications and dosages
➤ Uncomplicated acute malarial attacks
Adults: Initially, 1 g (600-mg base) P.O., then an additional 500 mg (300-mg base) P.O. 6 hours later and a single dose of 500 mg (300-mg base) P.O. on second and third days. Or initially, 160- to 200-mg base I.M., repeated in 6 hours (800-mg base maximum dosage during first 24 hours); continue for 3 days until total dosage of 1.5-g base has been given. Switch to oral therapy as soon as possible.

Children: Initially, 10 mg (base)/kg P.O., then 5 mg (base)/kg 6 hours, 24 hours, and 36 hours later; don't exceed recommended adult dosage. Or initially, 5 mg (base)/kg I.M. repeated 6 hours later, 18 hours after second dose, and then 24 hours after third dose; don't exceed recommended adult dosage.

➤ Malaria prophylaxis

Adults: 500 mg (300-mg base) P.O. weekly 1 to 2 weeks before visiting endemic area and continued for 4 weeks after leaving area. If therapy starts after malaria exposure, initial dosage is 600-mg base P.O. in two divided doses given 6 hours apart.

Children: 5 mg (base)/kg P.O. weekly for 1 to 2 weeks before visiting endemic area and continued for 4 weeks after leaving area, to a maximum dosage of 300 mg weekly. If treatment starts after exposure, 10 mg (base)/kg P.O. in two divided doses 6 hours apart and continued for 8 weeks after leaving area.

➤ Extraintestinal amebiasis

Adults: Initially, 1 g (600-mg base) P.O. daily for 2 days, then 500 mg (300-mg base) daily for 2 to 3 weeks. When oral therapy isn't tolerated, give 160- to 200-mg base I.M. daily for 10 to 12 days; switch to oral therapy as soon as possible.

Children: 10 mg (base)/kg P.O. once daily for 2 to 3 weeks, to a maximum dosage of 300 mg (base) daily

Off-label uses
- Lupus erythematosus
- Rheumatoid arthritis

Contraindications
- Hypersensitivity to drug
- Retinal and visual field changes
- Porphyria

Precautions
Use cautiously in:
- severe GI, neurologic, or blood disorders; hepatic impairment; G6PD deficiency; neurologic disease; eczema; alcoholism
- pregnant patients
- children.

Administration
- For obese patient, determine weight-based dosages from lean body weight. (Drug is stored in body tissues and eliminated slowly.)

Route	Onset	Peak	Duration
P.O.	Unknown	1-3 hr	Unknown

Adverse reactions
CNS: mild and transient headache, personality changes, dizziness, vertigo neuropathy, **seizures**

CV: hypotension, ECG changes

EENT: blurred vision, difficulty focusing, reversible corneal changes, irreversible retinal damage leading to vision loss, scotomas, ototoxicity, tinnitus, nerve deafness

GI: nausea, vomiting, diarrhea, abdominal pain, stomatitis, anorexia

Hematologic: agranulocytosis, aplastic anemia, hemolytic anemia, thrombocytopenia

Skin: lichen planus eruptions, skin and mucosal pigmentation changes, pruritus, pleomorphic skin eruptions

Interactions
Drug-drug. *Aluminum and magnesium salts, kaolin:* decreased GI absorption of chloroquine

Ampicillin: reduced ampicillin bioavailability

Cimetidine: decreased hepatic metabolism of chloroquine

Cyclosporine: sudden increase in cyclosporine blood level

Drug-diagnostic tests. *Granulocytes, hemoglobin, platelets:* decreased values

Drug-behaviors. *Sun exposure:* exacerbation of drug-induced dermatoses

Patient monitoring
- Monitor hepatic enzyme levels in patients with hepatic disease.

Reactions in **bold** are life-threatening.

◀﹦ Clinical alert

- Assess creatinine levels in patients with renal insufficiency or failure.
- In long-term therapy (as for lupus or rheumatoid arthritis), be aware that desired effects may be delayed for up to 6 months.
- Be aware that drug is secreted in breast milk but not in sufficient amounts to prevent malaria in infant.

Patient teaching
- Tell patient to take drug with food at evenly spaced intervals.
- ◀€ Instruct patient to immediately report blurred vision or hearing changes.
- In areas where malaria is endemic, advise pregnant patient to consult prescriber about taking drug.
- Inform patient on long-term therapy that beneficial effects may take up to 6 months.
- As appropriate, review all other significant and life-threatening adverse reactions and interactions, especially those related to the drugs, tests, and behaviors mentioned above.

chlorpheniramine maleate
Ahist, Allercalm⊕, Allerief⊕, Calimol⊕, Chlorphen, Chlor-Trimeton, Chlor-Trimeton Allergy 4 Hour, Chlor-Trimeton Allergy 8 Hour, Chlor-Trimeton Allergy 12 Hour, Chlor-Tripolon♣, Diabetic Tussin Allergy Relief, Novo-Pheniram♣, Piriton⊕, Teldrin HBP

Pharmacologic class: Propylamine (nonselective)
Therapeutic class: Antihistamine; allergy, cold, and cough remedy
Pregnancy risk category B

Action
Antagonizes effects of histamine at histamine$_2$-receptor sites, preventing histamine-mediated responses

Availability
Capsules (sustained-release): 8 mg, 12 mg
Syrup: 1 mg/5 ml, 2 mg/5 ml, 2.5 mg/5 ml
Tablets: 4 mg, 8 mg, 12 mg
Tablets (chewable): 2 mg
Tablets (timed-release): 8 mg, 12 mg

⏺ Indications and dosages
➤ Allergy symptoms; management of anaphylaxis and transfusion reactions
Adults: 4 mg q 4 to 6 hours P.O. or 8 to 12 mg P.O. of sustained-release form q 8 to 12 hours. Maximum dosage is 24 mg/day.
Children ages 6 to 12: 2 mg P.O. q 4 to 6 hours daily. Maximum dosage is 12 mg/day.

Dosage adjustment
- Glaucoma
- Gastric ulcer
- Hyperthyroidism
- Heart disease

Contraindications
- Hypersensitivity to drug
- Acute asthma attacks
- Stenosing peptic ulcer
- Breastfeeding

Precautions
Use cautiously in:
- hepatic or renal disease, asthma, angle-closure glaucoma, prostatic hypertrophy
- elderly patients
- pregnant patients (safety not established).

Administration
- Don't crush or break timed-release tablets or sustained-release capsules.
- Discontinue drug 4 days before allergy skin tests. (Drug may cause false-negative reactions.)

Route	Onset	Peak	Duration
P.O.	15-30 min	1-2 hr	4-12 hr
P.O. (sustained)	Unknown	Unknown	Unknown

Adverse reactions

CNS: dizziness, drowsiness, excitation (in children), sedation, poor coordination, fatigue, confusion, restlessness, nervousness, tremor, headache, hysteria, tingling sensation, sensation of heaviness and weakness in hands
CV: palpitations, hypotension, bradycardia, tachycardia, extrasystoles, **arrhythmias**
EENT: blurred vision, diplopia, vertigo, tinnitus, acute labyrinthitis, nasal congestion, dry nose, dry throat, sore throat
GI: nausea, vomiting, diarrhea, constipation, epigastric distress, anorexia, dry mouth, **GI obstruction**
GU: urinary retention, urinary hesitancy, dysuria, early menses, decreased libido, erectile dysfunction
Hematologic: hemolytic anemia, hypoplastic anemia, thrombocytopenia, leukopenia, pancytopenia, agranulocytosis
Respiratory: thickened bronchial secretions, chest tightness, wheezing
Skin: urticaria, rash, photosensitivity, diaphoresis
Other: chills, increased appetite, weight gain, **anaphylactic shock**

Interactions

Drug-drug. *Anticholinergics, anticholinergic-like drugs (such as some antidepressants, atropine, haloperidol, phenothiazines, quinidine, disopyramide):* additive anticholinergic effects
CNS depressants (such as opioids, sedative-hypnotics): additive CNS depression
MAO inhibitors: intensified, prolonged anticholinergic effects
Drug-diagnostic tests. *Allergy skin tests:* false-negative reactions

Drug-behaviors. *Alcohol use:* additive CNS depression
Sun exposure: photosensitivity

Patient monitoring

• Assess for urinary retention and frequency.
• Monitor respiratory status throughout therapy.

Patient teaching

• Advise patient to take with full glass of water.
• Tell patient not to crush timed-release tablets or sustained-release capsules. Instruct him to swallow them whole.
• Caution patient to avoid driving and other hazardous activities until he knows how drug affects concentration and alertness.
• Advise parents to give dose to children in evening, because morning doses may cause inattention in school.
• As appropriate, review all other significant and life-threatening adverse reactions and interactions, especially those related to the drugs, tests, and behaviors mentioned above.

chlorpromazine hydrochloride
Apo-Chlorpromazine✦, Novo-Chlorpromazine✦

Pharmacologic class: Phenothiazine
Therapeutic class: Antipsychotic, anxiolytic, antiemetic
Pregnancy risk category C

Action

Unknown. May block postsynaptic dopamine receptors in brain and depress areas involved in wakefulness and emesis. Also possesses

---

anticholinergic, antihistaminic, and adrenergic-blocking properties.

Availability
Capsules (sustained-release): 30 mg, 75 mg, 150 mg, 200 mg, 300 mg
Injection: 25 mg/ml
Tablets: 10 mg, 25 mg, 50 mg, 100 mg, 200 mg

✿ Indications and dosages
➣ Acute schizophrenia or mania
Adults: *Hospitalized patients*—Initially, 25 mg I.M; if necessary, give an additional 25 to 50 mg in 1 hour. Increase dosage gradually, as needed, for several days (up to 400 mg q 4 to 6 hours in exceptionally severe cases) until symptoms are controlled; then give 500 mg P.O. daily. In less acutely disturbed patients, 25 mg P.O. t.i.d., increased gradually until effective dosage is reached (usually 400 mg P.O. daily). *Acutely disturbed outpatients*—Initially, 10 mg P.O. three or four times daily or 25 mg P.O. two or three times daily. In more severe cases, 25 mg P.O. t.i.d.; after 1 or 2 days, increase daily dosage by 20 to 50 mg at semiweekly intervals until effective dosage is reached.
Children ages 6 months to 12 years:
0.55 mg/kg P.O. (15 mg/m^2) q 4 to 6 hours as needed, or 0.55 mg/kg I.M. (15 mg/m^2) q 6 to 8 hours (not to exceed 40 mg/day in children ages 6 months to 5 years, or 75 mg/day in children ages 6 to 12)
➣ Nausea and vomiting
Adults: 10 to 25 mg P.O. q 4 to 6 hours, increased if necessary; or 25 mg I.M. If no hypertension occurs, give 25 to 50 mg I.M. q 3 to 4 hours as needed until vomiting stops; then switch to oral dosing
➣ Nausea and vomiting during surgery
Adults: 12.5 mg I.M., repeated in 30 minutes p.r.n. if no hypotension

occurs; or 2 mg I.V. at 2-minute intervals (not to exceed 25 mg)
Children ages 6 months to 12 years:
0.275 mg/kg I.M.; may repeat in 30 minutes as needed
➣ Preoperative sedation
Adults: 25 to 50 mg P.O. 2 to 3 hours before surgery, or 12.5 to 25 mg I.M. 1 to 2 hours before surgery
Children ages 6 months to 12 years:
0.55 mg/kg P.O. (15 mg/m^2) 2 to 3 hours before surgery, or 0.55 mg/kg I.M. 1 to 2 hours before surgery
➣ Intractable hiccups
Adults: 25 to 50 mg P.O. three to four times daily. If symptoms continue for 2 to 3 days, give 25 to 50 mg I.M.; if symptoms still persist, give 25 to 50 mg by slow I.V. infusion with patient positioned flat in bed.
➣ Acute intermittent porphyria
Adults: 25 to 50 mg P.O. three to four times daily. Drug is usually discontinued after several weeks, but some patients require maintenance doses. Or 25 mg I.M. t.i.d. until patient can tolerate oral doses.
➣ Tetanus
Adults: 25 to 50 mg P.O. three to four times daily (given with barbiturates, as prescribed). Total dosage and frequency determined by patient response.
Children ages 6 months to 12 years:
0.55 mg/kg I.M. or 0.55 mg/kg I.V. q 6 to 8 hours

Dosage adjustment
• Age over 60

Off-label uses
• Anxiety disorders
• Migraine
• Phencyclidine (PCP) psychosis

Contraindications
• Hypersensitivity to drug, other phenothiazines, sulfites (injection), benzyl alcohol (sustained-release capsules)
• Angle-closure glaucoma

- Bone marrow depression
- Severe hepatic or cardiovascular disease

Precautions
Use cautiously in:
- cardiac disease, diabetes mellitus, respiratory disease, prostatic hypertrophy, CNS tumors, epilepsy, intestinal obstruction
- elderly patients
- pregnant or breastfeeding patients
- children.

Administration
◄€ Know that I.V. infusion is recommended only for severe hiccups.
- When giving by I.V. infusion for intractable hiccups, dilute in 500 to 1,000 ml of normal saline solution and infuse slowly.
- For direct I.V. injection, dilute to 1 mg/ml using normal saline solution. Administer at a rate of at least 1 mg/minute for adults or 2 mg/minute for children.
- When giving I.M., use Z-track injection method to minimize tissue irritation.
- Don't inject subcutaneously.
- Know that in preoperative use, drug increases risk of neuromuscular excitation and hypotension when followed by barbiturate anesthetics.

Route	Onset	Peak	Duration
P.O.	30-60 min	Unknown	4-6 hr
P.O. (sustained)	30-60 min	Unknown	10-12 hr
I.V.	Rapid	Unknown	Unknown
I.M.	Unknown	Unknown	4-8 hr
P.R.	1-2 hr	Unknown	3-4 hr

Adverse reactions
CNS: sedation, drowsiness, extrapyramidal reactions, tardive dyskinesia, pseudoparkinsonism, **neuroleptic malignant syndrome, seizures**

CV: tachycardia, hypotension (especially with I.M. or I.V. use)
EENT: blurred vision, dry eyes, lens opacities, nasal congestion
GI: constipation, ileus, anorexia, dry mouth
GU: urinary retention, menstrual irregularities, galactorrhea, gynecomastia, inhibited ejaculation, priapism
Hematologic: eosinophilia, **agranulocytosis, leukopenia, hemolytic anemia, aplastic anemia, thrombocytopenia**
Hepatic: jaundice, **hepatitis**
Skin: rash, photosensitivity, pigmentation changes, sterile abscess
Other: allergic reactions, hyperthermia, pain at injection site

Interactions
Drug-drug. *Activated charcoal, adsorbent antidiarrheals, antacids:* decreased chlorpromazine absorption
Antidepressants, antihistamines, general anesthetics, MAO inhibitors, opioids, sedative-hypnotics: additive CNS depression
Antihistamines, disopyramide, quinidine, tricyclic antidepressants (TCAs): increased anticholinergic effects
Antihypertensives: additive hypotension
Barbiturates: increased metabolism and decreased efficacy of chlorpromazine
Bromocriptine: decreased bromocriptine efficacy
Epinephrine: antagonism of peripheral vasoconstriction, epinephrine reversal
Guanethidine: inhibition of antihypertensive effects
Lithium: disorientation, loss of consciousness, extrapyramidal symptoms
Meperidine: excessive sedation and hypotension
Norepinephrine: reduced pressor effect, elimination of bradycardia
Phenytoin: altered phenytoin blood level, lowered seizure threshold
Pimozide: increased risk of potentially serious CV reactions

Reactions in **bold** are life-threatening.   ◄€ Clinical alert

Propranolol: increased blood levels of both drugs

TCAs: increased TCA blood levels and effects

Valproic acid: decreased elimination and increased effects of valproic acid

Drug-diagnostic tests. *Alanine aminotransferase, alkaline phosphatase, aspartate aminotransferase, bilirubin:* increased levels

Granulocytes, hematocrit, hemoglobin, platelets, white blood cells: decreased values

Pregnancy tests: false-positive or false-negative result

Urine bilirubin: false-positive result

Drug-herbs. *Angel's trumpet, jimsonweed, scopolia:* increased anticholinergic effects

Chamomile, hops, kava, skullcap, valerian: increased CNS depression

St. John's wort: photosensitivity

Yohimbe: increased risk of toxicity

Drug-behaviors. *Alcohol use:* increased CNS depression

Sun exposure: increased risk of photosensitivity

Patient monitoring

• Monitor blood pressure closely during I.V. infusion.

🔊 Stay alert for signs and symptoms of neuroleptic malignant syndrome (hyperpyrexia, muscle rigidity, altered mental status, irregular pulse or blood pressure, tachycardia, diaphoresis, and arrhythmias). Stop drug immediately if these occur.

• Assess for extrapyramidal symptoms.

Patient teaching

• Tell patient to take capsules or tablets with a full glass of water, with or without food.

• Instruct patient not to crush sustained-release capsules.

• Tell patient to mix oral concentrate in juice, soda, applesauce, or pudding.

• Caution patient to avoid driving and other hazardous activities until he

knows how drug affects concentration and alertness.

• As appropriate, review all other significant and life-threatening adverse reactions and interactions, especially those related to the drugs, tests, herbs, and behaviors mentioned above.

chlorthalidone

Apo-Chlorthalidone✤, Hygroton⊕, Novo-Thalidone✤, Thalitone, Uridon✤

Pharmacologic class: Thiazide-like diuretic

Therapeutic class: Diuretic, antihypertensive

Pregnancy risk category B

Action

Unclear. Enhances excretion of sodium, chloride, and water by interfering with transport of sodium ions across renal tubular epithelium. Also may dilate arterioles.

Availability

Tablets: 15 mg, 25 mg, 50 mg, 100 mg

🖊 Indications and dosages

➢ Edema associated with heart failure, renal dysfunction, cirrhosis, corticosteroid therapy, and estrogen therapy

Adults: 50 to 100 mg/day (30 to 60 mg Thalitone) P.O. or 100 mg every other day (60 mg Thalitone) P.O., up to 200 mg/day (120 mg Thalitone) P.O.

➢ Management of mild to moderate hypertension

Adults: 25 mg/day (15 mg Thalitone) P.O. Based on patient response, may increase to 50 mg/day (30 to 50 mg Thalitone) P.O., then up to 100 mg/day (except Thalitone) P.O.

Contraindications
- Hypersensitivity to drug, other thiazides, sulfonamides, or tartrazine
- Renal decompensation

Precautions
Use cautiously in:
- renal or severe hepatic disease, abnormal glucose tolerance, gout, systemic lupus erythematosus, hyperparathyroidism, bipolar disorder
- elderly patients
- pregnant or breastfeeding patients.

Administration
- Know that dosages above 25 mg/day are likely to increase potassium excretion without further increasing sodium excretion or reducing blood pressure.

Route	Onset	Peak	Duration
P.O.	2 hr	4 hr	48-72 hr

Adverse reactions
CNS: dizziness, vertigo, drowsiness, lethargy, confusion, headache, insomnia, nervousness, paresthesia, asterixis, nystagmus, **encephalopathy**
CV: hypotension, ECG changes, chest pain, **arrhythmias, thrombophlebitis**
GI: nausea, vomiting, cramping, anorexia, pancreatitis
GU: polyuria, nocturia, erectile dysfunction, loss of libido
Hematologic: blood dyscrasias
Metabolic: gout attack, dehydration, hyperglycemia, hypokalemia, hypocalcemia, hypomagnesemia, hyponatremia, hypophosphatemia, hyperuricemia, hyperlipidemia, **hypochloremic alkalosis**
Musculoskeletal: muscle cramps, muscle spasms
Skin: flushing, photosensitivity, hives, rash, exfoliative dermatitis, **toxic epidermal necrolysis**
Other: fever, weight loss, hypersensitivity reactions

Interactions
Drug-drug. *Allopurinol:* increased risk of hypersensitivity reaction
Amphotericin B, corticosteroids, mezlocillin, piperacillin, ticarcillin: additive hypokalemia
Antihypertensives, barbiturates, nitrates, opiates: increased hypotension
Cholestyramine, colestipol: decreased chlorthalidone blood level
Digoxin: increased risk of hypokalemia
Lithium: increased risk of lithium toxicity
Nonsteroidal anti-inflammatory drugs: decreased diuretic effect
Drug-diagnostic tests. *Bilirubin, calcium, creatinine, uric acid:* increased levels
Glucose (in diabetic patients): increased blood and urine levels
Magnesium, potassium, protein-bound iodine, sodium, urine calcium: decreased levels
Drug-herbs. *Ginkgo:* decreased antihypertensive effects
Licorice, stimulant laxative herbs (aloe, cascara sagrada, senna): increased risk of potassium depletion
Drug-behaviors. *Acute alcohol ingestion:* additive hypotension
Sun exposure: increased risk of photosensitivity

Patient monitoring
- Closely monitor patient with renal insufficiency.
- Assess for signs and symptoms of hematologic disorders.
- Monitor CBC with white cell differential and serum uric acid and electrolyte levels.
- Assess for signs and symptoms of hypersensitivity reactions, especially dermatitis.
- Watch for fluid and electrolyte imbalances.

Patient teaching
- Instruct patient to consume a low-sodium diet containing plenty of

potassium-rich foods and beverages (such as bananas, green leafy vegetables, and citrus juice).
• Caution patient to avoid driving and other hazardous activities until he knows whether drug makes him dizzy or affects concentration and alertness.
• Tell patient with diabetes to check urine or blood glucose level frequently.
• As appropriate, review all other significant and life-threatening adverse reactions and interactions, especially those related to the drugs, tests, herbs, and behaviors mentioned above.

chlorzoxazone
Parafon Forte DSC, Strifon Forte✤

Pharmacologic class: Autonomic nervous system agent
Therapeutic class: Skeletal muscle relaxant (centrally acting)
Pregnancy risk category C

Action
Unclear. Thought to act on spinal cord and subcortical levels of brain, inhibiting multisynaptic reflex arcs responsible for skeletal muscle activity.

Availability
Caplets: 500 mg
Tablets: 250 mg, 500 mg

⚕ Indications and dosages
➤ Adjunct to rest and physical therapy in treatment of muscle spasms associated with acute, painful musculoskeletal conditions
Adults: 250 to 750 mg P.O. three to four times daily

Contraindications
• Hypersensitivity to drug
• Hepatic impairment

Precautions
Use cautiously in:
• underlying cardiovascular disease, renal impairment
• children (safety not established).

Administration
• If desired, crush tablets and mix contents with food or water.
• Don't withdraw drug abruptly.

Route	Onset	Peak	Duration
P.O.	30-60 min	1-2 hr	3-4 hr

Adverse reactions
CNS: dizziness, drowsiness, lightheadedness, malaise, headache, overstimulation, tremor
GI: nausea, vomiting, constipation, diarrhea, heartburn, abdominal distress, anorexia
GU: orange or purplish-red urine
Hepatic: hepatic dysfunction
Skin: allergic dermatitis, urticaria, erythema, pruritus, petechiae, ecchymosis, **angioedema**
Other: allergic reactions

Interactions
Drug-drug. *CNS depressants (including antihistamines, antidepressants, opioids, sedative-hypnotics):* increased risk of CNS depression
Drug-diagnostic tests. *Alanine aminotransferase, alkaline phosphatase, bilirubin:* increased levels
Drug-herbs. *Chamomile, hops, kava, skullcap, valerian:* increased CNS depression
Drug-behaviors. *Alcohol use:* increased sedation

Patient monitoring
◀€ Stay alert for signs and symptoms of hepatic dysfunction. Withhold drug and notify prescriber if these occur.
• Monitor hepatic enzyme and serum electrolyte levels.

Patient teaching

◀◈ Instruct patient to promptly report yellowing of eyes or skin.
• Caution patient not to consume alcohol during therapy.
• Instruct patient to avoid driving and other hazardous activities until he knows how drug affects concentration and alertness.
• Tell patient that drug may turn his urine orange or purplish-red.
• As appropriate, review all other significant and life-threatening adverse reactions and interactions, especially those related to the drugs, tests, herbs, and behaviors mentioned above.

cholestyramine

LoCHOLEST, LoCHOLEST Light, Novo-Cholamine✲, Novo-Cholamine Light✲, Prevalite, Questran, Questran Light

Pharmacologic class: Bile acid sequestrant
Therapeutic class: Lipid-lowering agent
Pregnancy risk category C

Action

Combines with bile acid in GI tract to form insoluble complex excreted in feces. Complex regulates and increases cholesterol synthesis, thereby decreasing serum cholesterol and low-density lipoprotein levels.

Availability

Powder for suspension; powder for suspension with aspartame: 4 g cholestyramine/packet or scoop

⦸ Indications and dosages

➤ Primary hypercholesterolemia and pruritus caused by biliary obstruction; primary hyperlipidemia

Adults: Initially, 4 g P.O. once or twice daily. May increase as needed and tolerated, up to 24 g/day in six divided doses.

Off-label uses

• Antibiotic-induced pseudomembranous colitis
• Adjunct in infantile diarrhea
• Digoxin toxicity

Contraindications

• Hypersensitivity to drug, its components, or other bile-acid sequestering resins
• Complete biliary obstruction
• Phenylketonuria (suspension containing aspartame)

Precautions

Use cautiously in:
• history of constipation or abnormal intestinal function
• pregnant patients
• children.

Administration

• Mix powder with soup, cereal, pulpy fruit, juice, milk, or water.
• Administer 1 hour before or 4 to 6 hours after other drugs.
• Be aware that fat-soluble vitamin supplements may be necessary with long-term drug use.

Route	Onset	Peak	Duration
P.O.	24-48 hr	1-3 wk	2-4 wk

Adverse reactions

CNS: headache, anxiety, vertigo, dizziness, insomnia, fatigue, syncope
EENT: tinnitus
GI: nausea, vomiting, constipation, abdominal discomfort, fecal impaction, flatulence, hemorrhoids, perianal irritation, steatorrhea
GU: hematuria, dysuria, diuresis, burnt odor to urine
Hematologic: anemia, ecchymosis
Hepatic: hepatic dysfunction

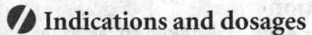

Reactions in **bold** are life-threatening. ◀◈ Clinical alert

Metabolic: vitamin A, D, E, and K deficiencies; **hyperchloremic acidosis**
Musculoskeletal: joint pain, arthritis, back pain, muscle pain
Respiratory: wheezing, asthma
Skin: hypersensitivity reaction (irritation, rash, urticaria)
Other: tongue irritation

Interactions

Drug-drug. *Acetaminophen, amiodarone, clindamycin, clofibrate, corticosteroids, digoxin, diuretics, fat-soluble vitamins (A, D, E, and K), gemfibrozil, glipizide, imipramine, methotrexate, methyldopa, mycophenolate, niacin, nonsteroidal anti-inflammatory drugs, penicillin, phenytoin, phosphates, propranolol, tetracyclines, tolbutamide, thyroid preparations, ursodiol, warfarin:* decreased absorption and effects of these drugs
Drug-diagnostic tests. *Alkaline phosphatase:* increased level
Hemoglobin: decreased value
Prothrombin time: increased

Patient monitoring

• Monitor CBC with white cell differential and liver function test results.
• If bleeding or bruising occurs, monitor prothrombin time. Drug may reduce vitamin K absorption.
• Watch for constipation, especially in patients with coronary artery disease. Take appropriate steps to prevent this problem.

Patient teaching

🔊 Instruct patient to immediately report yellowing of skin or eyes or easy bruising or bleeding.
• Tell patient to take drug 1 hour before or 4 to 6 hours after other drugs.
• Teach patient about role of diet in controlling cholesterol level and preventing constipation.

• Instruct patient to avoid inhaling or ingesting raw powder. Tell him to mix powder with food, juice, or milk before consuming.
• As appropriate, review all other significant and life-threatening adverse reactions and interactions, especially those related to the drugs and tests mentioned above.

cidofovir
Vistide

Pharmacologic class: Purine nucleotide cytosine analog
Therapeutic class: Antiviral
Pregnancy risk category C

FDA | BOXED WARNING

• Drug is indicated only for treatment of cytomegalovirus (CMV) retinitis in patients with AIDS.
• Renal impairment is major toxicity. As few as one or two doses have caused acute renal failure resulting in dialysis or contributing to death. To reduce possible nephrotoxicity, prehydrate with I.V. normal saline solution and give probenecid with each drug infusion. Monitor renal function within 48 hours before each dose, and modify dosage as indicated.
• Drug is contraindicated in patients receiving other nephrotoxic agents.
• Drug may cause neutropenia. Monitor neutrophil counts during therapy.
• In animal studies, drug was carcinogenic and teratogenic and caused hypospermia.

Action

Exerts antiviral effect by interfering with DNA synthesis of CMV, thereby inhibiting viral replication

---

Availability
Solution for injection: 75 mg/ml in 5-ml, single-use vials

⦿ Indications and dosages
➤ CMV retinitis in AIDS patients
Adults: 5 mg/kg I.V. infused over 1 hour q week for 2 continuous weeks; then 5 mg/kg I.V. once q 2 weeks as a maintenance dose

Dosage adjustment
• Renal impairment

Contraindications
• Hypersensitivity to drug, probenecid, or other sulfa-containing agents
• Creatinine level above 1.5 mg/dl, calculated creatinine clearance of 55 ml/minute or less, or urine protein level of 100 mg/dl or higher
• Concurrent use of nephrotoxic drugs

Precautions
Use cautiously in:
• renal impairment
• elderly patients
• pregnant or breastfeeding patients
• children younger than age 12 (safety and efficacy not established).

Administration
◀€ Be aware that drug carries a high risk of nephrotoxicity. Follow administration instructions carefully, including preinfusion and postinfusion hydration with I.V. normal saline solution.
• Premedicate with probenecid 2 g P.O., as prescribed, 3 hours before starting cidofovir infusion.
• Before starting infusion, give 1 L of normal saline solution over 1 to 2 hours.
• Mix I.V. dose in 100 ml of normal saline solution and infuse over 1 hour using infusion pump.
• Give 1 L of normal saline solution during or immediately after cidofovir infusion (unless contraindicated).

• Administer probenecid 1 g 2 hours and 8 hours after infusion ends, as prescribed.
◀€ If drug touches skin, flush thoroughly with water.

Route	Onset	Peak	Duration
I.V.	Rapid	End of infusion	Unknown

Adverse reactions
CNS: headache, **seizures, coma**
EENT: decreased intraocular pressure
GI: nausea, vomiting, diarrhea, anorexia, oral candidiasis
GU: proteinuria, **nephrotoxicity**
Hematologic: neutropenia
Hepatic: hepatomegaly
Metabolic: metabolic acidosis
Musculoskeletal: muscle contractions
Respiratory: dyspnea, increased cough
Skin: rash, alopecia
Other: pain, fever, chills, infection, pain at I.V. site

Interactions
Drug-drug. *Nephrotoxic drugs:* increased risk of nephrotoxicity
Drug-diagnostic tests. *Alanine aminotransferase, alkaline phosphatase, aspartate aminotransferase, blood urea nitrogen, creatinine, lactate dehydrogenase:* increased values
Bicarbonate, creatinine clearance, hemoglobin, neutrophils, platelets: decreased values

Patient monitoring
• Assess white blood cell count and creatinine and urine protein levels within 48 hours of each dose.
• Closely monitor intraocular pressure and visual acuity.
• Monitor hepatic enzyme levels in patients with hepatic disease.

Patient teaching
◀€ Tell patient to immediately report fever, vision changes, nausea, vomiting, rash, or urinary output changes.

Reactions in **bold** are life-threatening.　　　　◀€ Clinical alert

- Instruct patient to take probenecid, as prescribed, before each dose and to have regular eye examinations.
- Urge female patient of childbearing age to use effective contraception during and for 1 month after therapy.
- Instruct male patients to use barrier contraception during and for 3 months after therapy.
- As appropriate, review all other significant and life-threatening adverse reactions and interactions, especially those related to the drugs and tests mentioned above.

cilostazol
Pletal

Pharmacologic class: Quinolone derivative
Therapeutic class: Antiplatelet agent
Pregnancy risk category C

FDA | BOXED WARNING

- Drug and several of its metabolites inhibit phosphodiesterase III. Several drugs with this effect decreased survival in patients with class III-IV congestive heart failure (CHF). Drug is contraindicated in patients with CHF of any severity.

Action
Unclear. Thought to inhibit phosphodiesterase III by increasing cyclic adenosine monophosphate in platelets and blood vessels, causing vasodilation and enhancing cardiac contractility and coronary blood flow.

Availability
Tablets: 50 mg, 100 mg

Indications and dosages
➤ Intermittent claudication
Adults: 100 mg P.O. b.i.d. at least 30 minutes before or 2 hours after breakfast and dinner

Dosage adjustment
- Concurrent use of diltiazem, erythromycin, itraconazole, ketoconazole, or omeprazole

Contraindications
- Hypersensitivity to drug
- Heart failure

Precautions
Use cautiously in:
- cardiovascular disorders
- patients receiving other antiplatelet agents concurrently
- pregnant or breastfeeding patients
- children (safety and efficacy not established).

Administration
- Give with water 30 minutes before or 2 hours after patient consumes food or milk.
- Don't give with grapefruit juice.
- Be aware that although response may occur within 2 to 3 weeks, patient should continue therapy for up to 12 weeks or as prescribed.

Route	Onset	Peak	Duration
P.O.	Gradual	4-6 hr	Unknown

Adverse reactions
CNS: dizziness, headache, vertigo
CV: tachycardia
GI: abdominal pain, abnormal stools, dyspepsia, flatulence
EENT: rhinitis, pharyngitis
Musculoskeletal: back pain, myalgia
Respiratory: increased cough
Other: infection

Interactions
Drug-drug. *CYP3A4 and CYP2C19 inhibitors, diltiazem, erythromycin,*

macrolides, omeprazole: increased cilostazol blood level
Drug-food. *Grapefruit juice, high-fat meals:* increased cilostazol blood level
Drug-behaviors. *Smoking:* decreased exposure to cilostazol

Patient monitoring
• Monitor cardiovascular status.
• Closely monitor patient if he's receiving other antiplatelet drugs.

Patient teaching
• Instruct patient to take drug with full glass of water, 30 minutes before or 2 hours after food or milk.
• Advise patient to report nausea, vomiting, or abdominal pain.
• Instruct patient not to smoke, because smoking impedes drug effects.
• As appropriate, review all other significant adverse reactions and interactions, especially those related to the drugs, foods, and behaviors mentioned above.

cimetidine
Apo-Cimetidine✤, Dyspamet⊕, Galenmet⊕,Novo-Cimetine✤, Nu-Cimet✤, Tagamet HB

Pharmacologic class: Histamine₂-receptor antagonist
Therapeutic class: Antiulcer drug
Pregnancy risk category B

Action
Competitively inhibits histamine action at histamine₂-receptor sites of gastric parietal cells, thereby inhibiting gastric acid secretion

Availability
Oral liquid: 200 mg/5 ml, 300 mg/5 ml
Tablets: 200 mg, 300 mg, 400 mg, 600 mg, 800 mg

✓ Indications and dosages
➤ Active duodenal ulcer (short-term therapy)
Adults and children older than age 16: 800 mg P.O. at bedtime, or 300 mg P.O. q.i.d. with meals and at bedtime, or 400 mg P.O. b.i.d. Maintenance dosage is 400 mg P.O. at bedtime.
➤ Active benign gastric ulcer (short-term therapy)
Adults and children older than age 16: 800 mg P.O. at bedtime or 300 mg P.O. q.i.d. with meals and at bedtime
➤ Gastric hypersecretory conditions (such as Zollinger-Ellison syndrome); intractable ulcers
Adults and children older than age 16: 300 mg P.O. q.i.d. with meals and at bedtime
➤ Erosive gastroesophageal reflux disease
Adults and children older than age 16: 1,600 mg P.O. daily in divided doses (800 mg b.i.d. or 400 mg q.i.d.) for 12 weeks
➤ Heartburn; acid indigestion
Adults and children older than age 16: 200 mg (two tablets of over-the-counter product only) P.O. up to b.i.d. Give maximum dosage no longer than 2 weeks continuously, unless directed by prescriber.

Dosage adjustment
• Renal impairment

Off-label uses
• Acetaminophen overdose
• Adjunctive therapy in burns
• Barrett's esophagus
• Renal cancer
• Anaphylaxis

Contraindications
• Hypersensitivity to drug
• Alcohol intolerance

Precautions
Use cautiously in:
• renal impairment

Reactions in **bold** are life-threatening.   ◀€ Clinical alert

- elderly patients
- pregnant or breastfeeding patients.

Administration
- Give with meals.

Route	Onset	Peak	Duration
P.O.	30 min	45-90 min	4-5 hr

Adverse reactions
CNS: confusion, dizziness, drowsiness, hallucinations, agitation, psychosis, depression, anxiety, headache
GI: diarrhea
GU: reversible erectile dysfunction, gynecomastia

Interactions
Drug-drug. *Calcium channel blockers, carbamazepine, chloroquine, lidocaine, metformin, metronidazole, moricizine, pentoxifylline, phenytoin, propafenone, quinidine, quinine, some benzodiazepines, some beta-adrenergic blockers (chlordiazepoxide, diazepam, midazolam), sulfonylureas, tacrine, theophylline, triamterene, tricyclic antidepressants, valproic acid, warfarin:* decreased metabolism of these drugs, possible toxicity
Drug-diagnostic tests. *Creatinine, transaminases:* increased levels
Parathyroid hormone: decreased level
Skin tests using allergenic extracts: false-negative results (drug should be discontinued 24 hours before testing)
Drug-food. *Caffeine-containing foods and beverages (such as coffee, chocolate):* increased cimetidine blood level, increased risk of toxicity
Drug-herbs. *Pennyroyal:* change in formation rate of herb's toxic metabolite
Yerba maté: decreased yerba maté clearance, possible toxicity
Drug-behaviors. *Alcohol use:* increased blood alcohol level
Smoking: reversed cimetidine effects

Patient monitoring
- Monitor creatinine levels in patients with renal insufficiency or failure.

- Assess elderly or chronically ill patients for confusion (which usually resolves once drug therapy ends).

Patient teaching
- Inform patient with gastric ulcer that ulcer may take up to 2 months to heal. Advise him not to discontinue therapy, even if he feels better, without first consulting prescriber. Ulcer may recur if therapy ends too soon.
- Advise patient not to take over-the-counter cimetidine for more than 2 weeks continuously, except with prescriber's advice and supervision.
- As appropriate, review all other significant adverse reactions and interactions, especially those related to the drugs, tests, foods, herbs, and behaviors mentioned above.

cinacalcet hydrochloride
Mimpara ⊕, Sensipar

Pharmacologic class: Calcimimetic
Therapeutic class: Endocrine and metabolic agent
Pregnancy risk category C

Action
Directly lowers parathyroid hormone (PTH) levels by increasing sensitivity of calcium-sensing receptors to extracellular calcium

Availability
Tablets: 30 mg, 60 mg, 90 mg

⦸ Indications and dosages
➤ Secondary hyperparathyroidism in patients with chronic renal disease who are on dialysis
Adults: Dosage individualized; recommended starting dosage is 30 mg P.O. daily. Measure serum calcium and phosphorus levels within 1 week and

---

intact parathyroid hormone (iPTH) 1 to 4 weeks after initiation or dosage adjustment; titrate dosage no more often than every 2 to 4 weeks through sequential doses of 60 mg, 90 mg, 120 mg, and 180 mg P.O. once daily to recommended target iPTH for chronic renal disease patients on dialysis of 150 to 300 pg/ml.

➤ Hypercalcemia in patients with parathyroid carcinoma

Adults: Recommended starting dosage is 30 mg P.O. twice daily, titrated every 2 to 4 weeks through sequential doses of 60 mg and 90 mg twice daily, and 90 mg three or four times daily as needed to normalize serum calcium level.

Dosage adjustment

• Decreased calcium or iPTH level
• Concurrent use or discontinuation of strong CYP3A4 inhibitors (such as erythromycin, itraconazole, or ketoconazole)

Contraindications

• Hypersensitivity to drug or its components

Precautions

Use cautiously in:
• decreased serum calcium level, moderate or severe hepatic impairment
• pregnant or breastfeeding patients
• children (safety and efficacy not established).

Administration

• Don't initiate therapy if serum calcium level is less than lower limit of normal range (8.4 mg/dl).
• Administer tablets whole with food or shortly after a meal.
• If iPTH level decreases below recommended target range (150 to 300 pg/ml), reduce dosage of cinacalcet and vitamin D sterols or discontinue therapy.
• During titration, monitor serum calcium level frequently; if level drops below normal, take appropriate

measures to increase it, such as providing supplemental calcium, initiating or increasing dosage of calcium-based phosphate binder or vitamin D sterols, or withholding cinacalcet temporarily.
• Adjust dosage and closely monitor iPTH and calcium levels if patient is receiving or discontinuing a strong CYP3A4 inhibitor.

Route	Onset	Peak	Duration
P.O.	Unknown	2-6 hr	Unknown

Adverse reactions

CNS: dizziness, asthenia
CV: hypertension
GI: nausea, vomiting, diarrhea, anorexia
Musculoskeletal: myalgia
Other: chest pain (noncardiac)

Interactions

Drug-drug. *Amitriptyline:* increased amitriptyline and nortriptyline (active metabolite) exposure
Drugs metabolized by CYP4502D6 (such as flecainide, thioridazine, most tricyclic antidepressants, vinblastine): increased blood levels of either drug
Ketoconazole and other strong CYP3A4 inhibitors: increased cinacalcet exposure
Drug-diagnostic tests. *Calcium:* decreased

Patient monitoring

• Closely monitor iPTH and serum calcium levels throughout therapy in patients with moderate to severe hepatic impairment and in those who start or discontinue therapy with strong CYP3A4 inhibitor.
• Monitor iPTH level carefully to ensure that it doesn't fall below 100 pg/ml because adynamic bone disease may develop.
• Measure serum calcium and phosphorus levels within 1 week and iPTH level 1 to 4 weeks after initiation or dosage adjustment. Once maintenance dosage is established, measure serum

calcium and phosphorus levels approximately monthly and iPTH level every 1 to 3 months.

• Monitor serum calcium level closely in patient with history of seizure disorders.

Patient teaching
• Instruct patient to take tablets whole with food or shortly after a meal.
• As appropriate, review all other significant adverse reactions and interactions, especially those related to the drugs and tests mentioned above.

---

ciprofloxacin hydrochloride
Cetraxal, Ciloxan, Cipro, Cipro I.V., Ciproxin✛

Pharmacologic class: Fluoroquinolone
Therapeutic class: Anti-infective
Pregnancy risk category C

FDA | BOXED WARNING

• Fluoroquinolones for systemic use are associated with an increased risk of tendinitis and tendon rupture in all ages. This risk is further increased in patients usually over age 60, with concomitant use of corticosteroids, and in kidney, heart, and lung transplant recipients.

Action
Inhibits bacterial DNA synthesis by inhibiting DNA gyrase in susceptible gram-negative and gram-positive organisms

Availability
Injection: 200 mg/20 ml, 400 mg/40 ml, 200 mg/100 ml premixed in dextrose 5% in water (D_5W), 400 mg/200 ml premixed in D_5W, 1,200 mg/120-ml bulk package
Ophthalmic ointment: 3.5-g tube
Ophthalmic solution: 2.5-ml and 5-ml plastic dispensers
Otic solution: 0.2% (0.5 mg in 0.25 ml) in single-use container
Tablets: 250 mg, 500 mg, 750 mg

💊 Indications and dosages
➤ Acute sinusitis
Adults: 500 mg P.O. q 12 hours or 400 mg I.V. q 12 hours for 10 days
➤ Prostatitis
Adults: 500 mg P.O. q 12 hours or 400 mg I.V. q 12 hours for 28 days
➤ Intra-abdominal infections
Adults: 500 mg P.O. q 12 hours or 400 mg I.V. q 12 hours for 7 to 14 days
➤ Febrile neutropenic patients
Adults: 400 mg I.V. q 8 hours for 7 to 14 days
➤ Gonorrhea
Adults: 500 mg P.O. as a single dose
➤ Infectious diarrhea
Adults: 500 mg P.O. q 12 hours for 5 to 7 days
➤ Inhalation anthrax (postexposure)
Adults: 500 mg P.O. q 12 hours for 60 days or 400 mg I.V. q 12 hours for 60 days
Children: 15 mg/kg P.O. q 12 hours for 60 days (not to exceed 500 mg/dose), or 10 mg/kg I.V. q 12 hours for 60 days, not to exceed 400 mg/dose
➤ Infections of lower respiratory tract, skin and skin structures, bones, and joints
Adults: 500 to 750 mg P.O. q 12 hours or 400 mg I.V. q 8 hours for 7 to 14 days. Severe bone and joint infections may necessitate up to 6 weeks of therapy.
➤ Nosocomial pneumonia
Adults: 400 mg I.V. q 8 hours for 10 to 14 days
➤ Typhoid fever
Adults: 500 mg P.O. q 12 hours for 10 days

➤ Urinary tract infections

Adults: 250 to 500 mg P.O. q 12 hours or 200 to 400 mg I.V. q 12 hours for 3 days in acute uncomplicated infection or for 7 to 14 days in acute complicated infection

➤ Complicated urinary tract infections or pyelonephritis

Children ages 1 to 17: 6 to 10 mg/kg I.V. q 8 hours for 10 to 21 days (maximum, 400 mg/dose; not to be exceeded, even in patients weighing more than 51 kg [112 lb]). Or, 10 to 20 mg/kg P.O. q 12 hours for 10 to 21 days (maximum, 750 mg/dose; not to be exceeded, even in patients weighing more than 51 kg).

➤ Acute otitis externa

Adults: Instill contents of one single-use otic solution container (0.5 mg) into affected ear b.i.d. (approximately 12 hours apart) for 7 days

➤ Bacterial conjunctivitis caused by susceptible organisms

Adults: 0.5" ribbon of ophthalmic ointment applied to conjunctival sac t.i.d. on first 2 days, then 0.5" ribbon b.i.d. for 5 days. Or one to two drops of ophthalmic solution applied to conjunctival sac q 2 hours while awake for 2 days, then one or two drops q 4 hours while awake for 5 days.

➤ Corneal ulcers caused by susceptible organisms

Adults: Two drops of ophthalmic solution instilled into affected eye q 15 minutes for first 6 hours, then two drops into affected eye q 30 minutes for remainder of first day. On second day, two drops of ophthalmic solution hourly; on days 3 through 14, two drops q 4 hours.

Dosage adjustment
• Renal impairment or insufficiency

Off-label uses
• Chancroid
• Cystic fibrosis
• Pseudomembranous colitis caused by anti-infectives

Contraindications
• Hypersensitivity to drug or other fluoroquinolones
• Comcomitant administration of tizanidine

Precautions
Use cautiously in:
• cirrhosis, renal impairment, underlying CNS disease
• concurrent use of theophylline (risk of serious or fatal reactions, such as cardiac arrest, seizures, status epilepticus, and respiratory failure)
• elderly patients
• pregnant or breastfeeding patients
• children younger than age 18 (except for complicated urinary tract infection, pyelonephritis, and postexposure inhalation antrax only).

Administration
• Administer oral drug with or without food but not with dairy products or calcium-fortified juices alone; however, drug may be taken with a meal that contains these products.
• Infuse I.V. dose over at least 1 hour, using pump to ensure 1-hour duration.
◀€ Know that too-rapid I.V. infusion increases risk of anaphylaxis and other adverse reactions.
◀€ Know that treatment with ophthalmic solution may be continued after 14 days if corneal re-epithelialization hasn't occurred.

Route	Onset	Peak	Duration
P.O.	Rapid	1-2 hr	12 hr
I.V.	Rapid	End of infusion	12 hr
Ophthal.	Unknown	Unknown	Unknown
Otic	NA	NA	NA

Adverse reactions
CNS: agitation, headache, restlessness, confusion, delirium, peripheral neuropathy, **toxic psychosis**
CV: orthostatic hypotension, vasculitis

Reactions in **bold** are life-threatening.　　　　◀€ Clinical alert

EENT: nystagmus; with ophthalmic use—blurred vision; burning, stinging, irritation, itching, tearing, and redness of eyes; eyelid itching, swelling, or crusting; sensitivity to light

GI: nausea, vomiting, diarrhea, constipation, abdominal pain or discomfort, dyspepsia, dysphagia, flatulence, pancreatitis, **pseudomembranous colitis**

GU: albuminuria, candiduria, renal calculi

Hematologic: methemoglobinemia, agranulocytosis, hemolytic anemia

Hepatic: jaundice, **hepatic necrosis**

Metabolic: hyperglycemia, **hyperkalemia**

Musculoskeletal: myalgia, myoclonus, tendinitis, tendon rupture

Skin: rash, exfoliative dermatitis, toxic epidermal necrolysis, **erythema multiforme** photosensitivity

Other: injection-site reaction, altered taste, anosmia, exacerbation of myasthenia gravis, overgrowth of nonsusceptible organisms, hypersensitivity reactions including **anaphylaxis** and **Stevens-Johnson syndrome**

Interactions

Drug-drug. *Antacids, bismuth subsalicylate, iron salts, sucralfate, zinc salts:* decreased ciprofloxacin absorption

Cyclosporine: transient creatinine increase

Hormonal contraceptives: reduced contraceptive efficacy

Oral anticoagulants: increased anticoagulant effects

Phenytoin: increased or decreased phenytoin blood level

Probenecid: decreased renal elimination of ciprofloxacin, causing increased blood level

Theophylline: increased theophylline blood level, greater risk of toxicity

Tizanidine: significantly elevated tizanidine plasma level

Drug-diagnostic tests. *Alanine aminotransferase, alkaline phosphatase, aspartate aminotransferase, bilirubin, cholesterol, glucose, lactate dehydrogenase, potassium, triglycerides:* increased levels

Prothrombin time: prolonged

Drug-food. *Caffeine:* interference with caffeine clearance

Concurrent tube feedings, milk or yogurt (when consumed alone with ciprofloxacin): impaired drug absorption

Drug-herbs. *Fennel:* decreased drug absorption

Patient monitoring

• In patients with renal insufficiency, assess creatinine level before giving first dose and at least once a week during prolonged therapy. Monitor drug blood level closely.

🔊 Watch for signs and symptoms of serious adverse reactions, including GI problems, jaundice, tendon problems, and hypersensitivity reactions.

Patient teaching

• Tell patient to take drug with or without food at the same time each day.

• Advise patient not to take drug with dairy products or calcium-fortified juices alone or with caffeinated beverages.

• Advise patient to drink 8 oz of water every hour while awake to ensure adequate hydration.

🔊 Instruct patient to stop taking drug and notify prescriber at first sign of burning, numbness, or tingling in hands or feet; yellow eyes or skin; unusual tiredness; persistent diarrhea; rash; or tendon pain, swelling, or inflammation.

• Advise patient to avoid excessive exposure to sun or ultraviolet light and to discontinue drug and notify prescriber if phototoxicity (burning, erythema, exudation, vesicles, blistering, edema) occurs.

• Advise patient taking hormonal contraceptives to use supplemental birth control method, such as condoms,

because drug reduces contraceptive efficacy.
• Inform breastfeeding patient that drug is excreted in breast milk and can affect infant's bone growth. Advise her to consult prescriber before using drug.
• Teach patient how to use eye ointment or solution and tell patient not to touch eye dropper tip to any surface, to avoid contamination.
• Instruct patient how to use ear solution and to lie with affected ear upward for at least 1 minute after instilling solution.
• Caution patient with bacterial conjunctivitis not to wear contact lenses.
• As appropriate, review all other significant and life-threatening adverse reactions and interactions, especially those related to the drugs, tests, foods, and herbs mentioned above.

cisplatin
Platinex◆

Pharmacologic class: Alkylating agent, platinum coordination complex
Therapeutic class: Antineoplastic
Pregnancy risk category D

FDA | BOXED WARNING

• Give under supervision of physician experienced in cancer chemotherapy, in facility with adequate diagnostic and treatment resources.
• Drug may cause severe cumulative renal toxicity. Other major dose-related toxicities are myelosuppression, nausea, and vomiting.
• Drug may lead to significant ototoxicity (which may be more pronounced in children), high-frequency hearing loss, and deafness.

• Anaphylactic-like reactions may occur within minutes of administration.
• Use caution to prevent inadvertent overdose. Doses above 100 mg/m²/cycle once every 3 to 4 weeks are rarely used. Avoid inadvertent overdose stemming from confusion with Paraplatin (carboplatin) or failure to differentiate daily doses from total dose per cycle.

Action
Inhibits DNA synthesis by causing intrastrand and interstrand cross-linking of DNA

Availability
Injection: 1 mg/ml in 50-mg and 100-mg multidose vials

Indications and dosages
➤ Metastatic testicular tumors
Adults: 20 mg/m² I.V. daily for 5 days/cycle, repeated q 3 to 4 weeks
➤ Metastatic ovarian cancer
Adults: 75 to 100 mg/m² I.V., repeated q 4 weeks in combination with cyclophosphamide; or 100 mg/m² q 4 weeks as a single agent
➤ Advanced bladder cancer
Adults: 50 to 70 mg/m² I.V. q 3 to 4 weeks as a single agent; dosage depends on whether patient has undergone radiation or chemotherapy.

Off-label uses
• Cervical cancer
• Squamous cell carcinoma

Contraindications
• Hypersensitivity to drug or other platinum-containing compounds
• Severe impairment of renal function
• Severe myelosuppression
• Hearing impairment
• Pregnancy or breastfeeding

Reactions in **bold** are life-threatening.   ◀≋ Clinical alert

Precautions

Use cautiously in:

- mild to moderate renal impairment, active infection, myelosuppression, chronic debilitating illness, heart failure, electrolyte abnormalities
- females of childbearing age.

Administration

- Prepare drug with equipment that doesn't contain aluminum.
- Give 2 L of I.V. fluids, as prescribed, 8 to 12 hours before drug infusion to help prevent toxicity.
- Dilute each dose in 2 L of dextrose 5% in 1/4 or 1/2 saline solution or 0.9% normal saline solution. Do not use dextrose 5% in water.
- Infuse each liter over 3 to 4 hours to minimize toxicity. In well-hydrated patients with good renal function, infusions of 100 to 500 ml may be given over 30 minutes.
- Follow facility policy for handling and disposal of antineoplastics.
- ◀︎ If solution contacts skin, wash immediately and thoroughly with soap and water. If solution contacts mucosa, flush with water immediately.
- Protect drug from light.

Route	Onset	Peak	Duration
I.V.	Unknown	18-23 days	39 days

Adverse reactions

CNS: malaise, weakness, **seizures**
EENT: ototoxicity, tinnitus
GI: severe nausea, vomiting, diarrhea
GU: sterility, **nephrotoxicity**
Hematologic: anemia, **leukopenia, thrombocytopenia**
Hepatic: hepatotoxicity
Metabolic: hypocalcemia, hypokalemia, hypomagnesemia, hyperuricemia
Skin: alopecia
Other: phlebitis at I.V. site, **anaphylaxis**

Interactions

Drug-drug. *Amphotericin B, loop diuretics:* increased risk of hypokalemia and hypomagnesemia
Antineoplastics: additive bone marrow depression
Live-virus vaccines: decreased antibody response to vaccine, increased risk of adverse reactions
Nephrotoxic drugs (such as aminoglycosides): additive nephrotoxicity
Ototoxic drugs (such as loop diuretics): additive ototoxicity
Phenytoin: reduced phenytoin blood level
Drug-diagnostic tests. *Aspartate aminotransferase, bilirubin, blood urea nitrogen, creatinine, uric acid:* increased levels
Calcium, magnesium, phosphate, potassium, sodium: decreased levels
Coombs' test: positive result

Patient monitoring

- Before starting therapy and before each subsequent dose, assess renal function test results and CBC with white cell differential.
- Monitor neurologic status, hepatic enzyme and uric acid levels, and audiogram results.
- Monitor urine output closely.

Patient teaching

- Instruct patient to drink 8 oz of water every hour while awake.
- ◀︎ Advise patient to promptly report bleeding, bruising, hearing loss, yellowing of skin or eyes, decreased urine output, or suspected infection.
- Tell patient that drug may cause hair loss.
- Instruct female patient to use reliable contraception; drug can harm fetus.
- As appropriate, review all other significant and life-threatening adverse reactions and interactions, especially those related to the drugs and tests mentioned above.

---

citalopram hydrobromide
Celexa

Pharmacologic class: Selective serotonin reuptake inhibitor
Therapeutic class: Antidepressant
Pregnancy risk category C

FDA | BOXED WARNING

- Drug may increase risk of suicidal thinking and behavior in children and adolescents with major depressive disorder and other psychiatric disorders, especially during first few months of therapy. Risk must be balanced with clinical need, as depression itself increases suicide risk. With patient of any age, observe closely for clinical worsening, suicidality, and unusual behavior changes when therapy begins. Advise family to observe patient closely and communicate with prescriber as needed.
- Drug isn't approved for use in pediatric patients.

Action
Unclear. Thought to potentiate serotonergic activity in CNS by inhibiting neuronal uptake of serotonin.

Availability
Oral solution: 10 mg/5 ml
Tablets: 10 mg, 20 mg, 40 mg

Indications and dosages
➤ Depression
Adults: Initially, 20 mg P.O. daily; may increase to maximum recommended dosage of 40 mg/day at an interval of no less than 1 week.

Dosage adjustment
- Hepatic impairment
- CYP2C19 poor metabolizers or concurrent use of cimetidine or another CYP2C19 inhibitor
- Elderly patients

Off-label uses
- Alcoholism
- Panic disorder
- Premenstrual dysphoria
- Social phobia

Contraindications
- Hypersensitivity to drug or its components
- Concurrent use of MAO inhibitors or pimozide

Precautions
Use cautiously in:
- severe renal impairment, hepatic impairment
- bradycardia, hypokalemia, hypomagnesemia, hyponatremia, recent acute myocardial infarction, congenital long QT syndrome, or uncompensated heart failure (avoid use)
- concurrent use of drugs that prolong QTc interval (avoid use)
- concurrent use of serotonin precursors such as tryptophan (not recommended)
- concurrent use of aspirin, NSAIDs, warfarin, and other anticoagulants
- history of mania or seizure disorder
- elderly patients
- pregnant or breastfeeding patients
- children (safety not established).

Administration
- Administer drug in the morning or evening, with or without food.
- ◀ Don't give within 14 days of MAO inhibitor; life-threatening interactions may occur.
- ◀ Be aware that drug shouldn't be given at doses above 40 mg/day because of risk of QTc-interval prolongation.

🔊 Gradually reduce dosage rather than abruptly stopping drug.

Route	Onset	Peak	Duration
P.O.	1-4 wk	Unknown	Unknown

Adverse reactions

CNS: apathy, confusion, drowsiness, insomnia, migraine, weakness, agitation, amnesia, anxiety, dizziness, fatigue, poor concentration, tremor, paresthesia, deepening of depression, **suicide attempt, neuroleptic malignant syndrome-like reactions**

CV: orthostatic hypotension, tachycardia, ECG changes

Metabolic: hyponatremia

EENT: abnormal visual accommodation

GI: nausea, vomiting, diarrhea, abdominal pain, dyspepsia, flatulence, increased saliva, dry mouth, increased appetite, anorexia

GU: polyuria, amenorrhea, dysmenorrhea, ejaculatory delay, erectile dysfunction, decreased libido

Musculoskeletal: joint pain, myalgia

Respiratory: cough

Skin: rash, pruritus, diaphoresis, photosensitivity

Other: altered taste, fever, yawning, weight changes, **serotonin syndrome-like reactions**

Interactions

Drug-drug. *Aspirin, NSAIDs, warfarin, other anticoagulants:* increased risk of bleeding

Anti-infectives (such as gatifloxacin, moxifloxacin), antipsychotics (such as chlorpromazine, thioridazine), Class 1A antiarrhythmics (such as procainamide, quinidine), Class III antiarrhythmics (such as amiodarone, sotalol), CYP2C19 inhibitors (such as cimetidine), methadone, pentamidine: risk of prolonged QTc interval

Carbamazepine: decreased citalopram blood level

Centrally acting drugs (such as antihistamines, opioids, sedative-hypnotics): additive CNS effects

Erythromycin, itraconazole, ketoconazole, omeprazole: increased citalopram blood level

5-hydroxytryptamine₁ receptor agonists (such as sumatriptan, zolmitriptan): increased risk of adverse reactions

Lithium: potentiation of serotonergic effects

MAO inhibitors: life-threatening reactions

Tricyclic antidepressants (TCAs): altered TCA pharmacokinetics

Drug-diagnostic tests. *Serum sodium:* decreased level

Drug-herbs. *St. John's wort, S-adenosylmethionine (SAM-e):* increased risk of serotonergic reactions, including serotonin syndrome

Drug-behaviors. *Alcohol use:* additive CNS depression

Sun exposure: photosensitivity

Patient monitoring

• If patient is receiving lithium concurrently, watch closely for potentiation of serotonergic effects.

• Monitor patient for signs of mania or hypomania, bleeding, serotonin syndrome-like reactions (including mental status changes, such as agitation, hallucinations, coma), autonomic instability (such as tachycardia, labile blood pressure, hyperthermia), neuromuscular aberrations (such as hyperreflexia, incoordination), GI symptoms (such as nausea, vomiting, diarrhea) or neuroleptic malignant syndrome-like reactions (fever, muscle rigidity, mental status changes, irregular pulse or blood pressure, rapid heartbeats, excessive sweating).

• Monitor ECG and electrolyte levels in patients with cardiac conditions that may lead to QT-interval prolongation. Discontinue drug in patients with persistent QTc measurements of more than 500 ms.

• Be aware that drug should be discontinued in patients with symptomatic hyponatremia (headache, difficulty concentrating, memory impairment, confusion, weakness, unsteadiness). Signs and symptoms associated with more severe or acute cases have included hallucinations, syncope, seizures, coma, respiratory arrest, and death).

• When discontinuing drug, monitor patient for dysphoria, irritability, agitation, dizziness, sensory disturbances, anxiety, confusion, headache, lethargy, emotional lability, insomnia, and hypomania.

Patient teaching

• Instruct patient to take drug with full glass of water with or without food at same time every day.

◀€ Advise patient or caregiver (especially if drug is given to a child or adolescent) to immediately report suicidal thoughts or extreme depression.

• Instruct patient to move slowly when sitting up or standing, to avoid dizziness or light-headedness caused by sudden blood pressure decrease.

• Tell patient several weeks may pass before he starts to feel better.

• Instruct patient to immediately report irregular or rapid heartbeats, dizziness, fainting, palpitations, agitation, hallucinations, incoordination, nausea, vomiting, diarrhea, fever, muscle rigidity, altered mental status (including catatonic signs), excessive sweating, headache, difficulty concentrating, memory impairment, confusion, weakness, and unsteadiness.

• Tell patient about risk of bleeding associated with concomitant use of this drug and NSAIDs, aspirin, or other drugs that affect coagulation; tell patient to report bruising or other signs or symptoms of bleeding.

• Caution patient to avoid driving and other hazardous activities until drug's effects on concentration and alertness are known.

• Advise patient to avoid alcohol during therapy.

• Tell male patient he may experience inadequate filling of penile erectile tissue. Advise him to consult prescriber if he experiences adverse sexual effects.

• As appropriate, review all other significant and life-threatening adverse reactions and interactions, especially those related to the drugs, tests, herbs, and behaviors mentioned above.

clarithromycin

Biaxin Filmtab, Biaxin Granules, Biaxin XL Filmtab, Clarosip⊕, Klaricid⊕

Pharmacologic class: Macrolide

Therapeutic class: Anti-infective, antiulcer drug

Pregnancy risk category B

Action

Reversibly binds to 50S ribosomal subunit of susceptible bacterial organisms, blocking protein synthesis

Availability

Granules for oral suspension: 125 mg/5 ml, 250 mg/5 ml
Tablets: 250 mg, 500 mg
Tablets (extended-release): 500 mg

⍟ Indications and dosages

➤ Pharyngitis or tonsillitis caused by *Streptococcus pyogenes*
Adults: 250 mg P.O. q 12 hours for 10 days

➤ Acute maxillary sinusitis caused by *Haemophilus influenzae, Moraxella catarrhalis,* or *Streptococcus pneumoniae*
Adults: 500 mg P.O. q 12 hours for 14 days or two 500-mg extended-release tablets P.O. q 24 hours for 14 days

---

Children: 7.5 mg/kg P.O. q 12 hours for 10 days

➤ Acute exacerbation of chronic bronchitis caused by *H. influenzae, Haemophilus parainfluenzae, M. catarrhalis,* or *S. pneumoniae*
Adults: 500 mg P.O. q 12 hours for 7 to 14 days or two 500-mg extended-release tablets P.O. q 24 hours for 7 days

➤ Community-acquired pneumonia caused by *S. pneumoniae, Mycoplasma pneumoniae,* or *Chlamydia pneumoniae;* acute exacerbation of chronic bronchitis caused by *S. pneumoniae* or *M. catarrhalis*
Adults: 250 mg P.O. q 12 hours for 7 to 14 days or two 500-mg extended-release tablets P.O. q 24 hours for 7 days
Children: 7.5 mg/kg P.O. q 12 hours for 10 days

➤ Community-acquired pneumonia caused by *H. influenzae*
Adults: 250 mg P.O. q 12 hours for 7 days or two 500-mg extended-release tablets P.O. q 24 hours for 7 days

➤ Community-acquired pneumonia caused by *H. parainfluenzae* or *M. catarrhalis*
Adults: Two 500-mg extended-release tablets P.O. q 24 hours for 7 days

➤ Uncomplicated skin and skin-structure infections
Adults: 250 mg P.O. q 12 hours for 7 to 14 days

➤ Eradication of *Helicobacter pylori* as part of triple therapy with amoxicillin and omeprazole or lansoprazole
Adults: 500 mg P.O. q 12 hours for 10 to 14 days

➤ Eradication of *H. pylori* as part of dual therapy with omeprazole or ranitidine
Adults: 500 mg P.O. t.i.d. for 14 days

➤ Mycobacterial infections
Adults: 500 mg P.O. b.i.d.
Children: 7.5 mg/kg P.O. b.i.d., up to 500 mg b.i.d.

➤ Acute otitis media
Children: 7.5 mg/kg P.O. q 12 hours for 10 days

Dosage adjustment
• Renal or hepatic impairment

Off-label uses
• *Borrelia burgdorferi* infection

Contraindications
• Hypersensitivity to drug, erythromycin, or other macrolide anti-infectives
• Concurrent use of astemizole, cisapride, or pimozide
• Cardiac disease

Precautions
Use cautiously in:
• severe renal or hepatic impairment
• pregnant or breastfeeding patients.

Administration
• Obtain specimens for culture and sensitivity testing as appropriate before starting therapy.
• Give with or without food.
◀€ Don't give concurrently with astemizole (no longer available in United States), cisapride, or pimozide.
• Don't refrigerate oral suspension.

Route	Onset	Peak	Duration
P.O.	Unknown	2 hr	12 hr
P.O. (extended)	Unknown	4 hr	24 hr

Adverse reactions
CNS: headache
CV: ventricular arrhythmias
GI: nausea, diarrhea, abdominal pain or discomfort, dyspepsia
Other: abnormal taste

Interactions
Drug-drug. *Astemizole, cisapride, pimozide:* increased risk of arrhythmias and sudden death
Carbamazepine, digoxin, theophylline: increased blood levels of these drugs, greater risk of toxicity
Digoxin: increased digoxin blood level, causing digoxin toxicity
HMG-CoA reductase inhibitors (such as lovastatin, simvastatin): rhabdomyolysis

---

♣ Canada   ⊕ UK   ⚖ Hazardous drug   ⊗ High-alert drug

Zidovudine: increased or decreased peak zidovudine blood level

Drug-diagnostic tests. *Alkaline phosphatase, blood urea nitrogen:* increased values

Prothrombin time: increased

White blood cells: decreased count

Patient monitoring

• Monitor hepatic enzyme and creatinine levels during long-term therapy.

• Assess cardiovascular status.

Patient teaching

• Advise patient to take drug with full glass of water, either with food or on an empty stomach.

• Tell patient using oral suspension not to refrigerate it, and to discard it 14 days after mixing.

• Tell patient to swallow extended-release tablets whole.

• As appropriate, review all other significant and life-threatening adverse reactions and interactions, especially those related to the drugs and tests mentioned above.

clindamycin hydrochloride
Apo-Clindamycin✤, Cleocin, Dalacin C

clindamycin palmitate hydrochloride
Cleocin Pediatric, Dalacin C Flavored Granules✤

clindamycin phosphate
Cleocin Phosphate, Cleocin T, Clindagel, ClindaMax, Clindesse, Clindets, Dalacin C Phosphate✤, Dalacin T✤⊕, Evoclin, Zindaclin⊕

Pharmacologic class: Lincosamide
Therapeutic class: Anti-infective
Pregnancy risk category B

| **FDA** | **BOXED WARNING** |

• *Clostridium difficile*-associated diarrhea (CDAD) has been reported with use of nearly all antibacterial agents, including *Cleocin*, and may range in severity from mild diarrhea to fatal colitis. Treatment with antibacterial agents alters the normal flora of the colon, leading to overgrowth of *C. difficile.*

• Because *Cleocin* therapy has been associated with severe colitis that may be fatal, it should be reserved for serious infections for which less toxic *antimicrobials* are inappropriate. It shouldn't be used in patients with nonbacterial infections such as most upper respiratory tract infections.

• *C. difficile* produces toxins A and B, which contribute to the development of CDAD. Hypertoxin-producing strains of *C. difficile* cause increased morbidity and mortality because these infections can be refractory to antimicrobial therapy and may require *colectomy.* CDAD must be considered in all patients who present with diarrhea following antibiotic use. Careful medical history is necessary because CDAD has occurred more than 2 months after administration of antibacterial agents.

• If CDAD is suspected or confirmed, ongoing antibiotic use not directed against *C. difficile* may need to be discontinued. Appropriate fluid and electrolyte management, protein supplementation, antibiotic treatment of *C. difficile,* and surgical evaluation should be instituted as clinically indicated.

Action

Inhibits protein synthesis in susceptible bacteria at level of 50S ribosome, thereby inhibiting peptide bond formation and causing cell death

Availability

Aerosol foam: 1%
Capsules: 75 mg, 150 mg, 300 mg

Granules for oral suspension: 75 mg/5 ml
Injection: 150 mg base/ml
Topical: 1% gel, lotion, single-use
applicators, solution, and suspension
Vaginal cream: 2%
Vaginal suppositories (ovules): 100 mg

🚫 Indications and dosages
➤ Severe infections caused by sensitive organisms (such as *Bacteroides fragilis, Clostridium perfringens, Fusobacterium,* pneumococci, staphylococci, and streptococci)
Adults: 300 to 450 mg P.O. q 6 hours, or (for other than *C. perfringens*) 1.2 to 2.7 g/day I.M. or I.V. in two to four equally divided doses
Children: 16 to 20 mg/kg/day P.O. (hydrochloride) in three to four equally divided doses, or 13 to 25 mg/kg/day P.O. (palmitate hydrochloride) in three to four equally divided doses
Neonates younger than 1 month: 15 to 20 mg/kg/day I.M. or I.V. in three to four equally divided doses
➤ Acute pelvic inflammatory disease
Adults: 900 mg I.V. q 8 hours (given with gentamicin)
➤ Acne vulgaris
Adults and children older than age 12: Apply a thin film of topical gel, lotion, or solution locally to affected area b.i.d.

Off-label uses
• Bacterial vaginosis (phosphate)
• *Chlamydia trachomatis* infection in females
• CNS toxoplasmosis in AIDS patients (given with pyrimethamine)
• *Pneumocystis jiroveci* pneumonia (given with primaquine)
• Rosacea (lotion)

Contraindications
• Hypersensitivity to drug or lincomycin

Precautions
Use cautiously in:
• renal or hepatic impairment
• known alcohol intolerance
• pregnant patients
• neonates.

Administration
• Give oral doses with full glass of water, with or without food.
🔇 Don't give as I.V. bolus injection.
• Dilute I.V. solution to a concentration of 18 mg/ml using normal saline solution, dextrose 5% in water, or lactated Ringer's solution. Infuse no faster than 30 mg/minute.
• Don't administer I.M. dosages above 600 mg.
• Inject I.M. doses deep into large muscle mass to prevent induration and sterile abscess.

Route	Onset	Peak	Duration
P.O.	Rapid	45 min	6-8 hr
I.V.	Rapid	End of infusion	6-8 hr
I.M.	Rapid	1-3 hr	6-8 hr
Topical, vaginal	Unknown	Unknown	Unknown

Adverse reactions
GI: nausea, vomiting, diarrhea, abdominal pain, esophagitis, **pseudomembranous colitis**
Hematologic: neutropenia, leukopenia, agranulocytosis, thrombocytopenia purpura
Hepatic: jaundice, **hepatic dysfunction**
Skin: maculopapular rash, generalized morbilliform-like rash
Other: bitter taste (with I.V. use), phlebitis at I.V. site, induration and sterile abscess (with I.M. use), **anaphylaxis**

Interactions
Drug-drug. *Erythromycin:* antagonistic effect
Kaolin/pectin: decreased GI absorption of clindamycin
Hormonal contraceptives: decreased contraceptive efficacy

Neuromuscular blockers: enhanced neuromuscular blockade

Drug-diagnostic tests. *Alanine aminotransferase, alkaline phosphatase, aspartate aminotransferase, bilirubin, creatine kinase:* increased levels

Platelets, white blood cells: transient decrease in counts

Patient monitoring

• Monitor creatinine level closely in patients with renal insufficiency.

• Monitor hepatic enzyme levels in patients with hepatic disease.

• Assess for signs and symptoms of hypersensitivity reactions, including anaphylaxis.

• Assess for diarrhea and signs and symptoms of colitis.

Patient teaching

• Tell patient to take drug with food if it causes stomach upset.

◀€ Urge patient to contact prescriber immediately if he develops rash, unusual fatigue, or yellowing of skin or eyes or if diarrhea occurs during or after treatment.

• Tell patient that I.V. use may cause bitter taste. Reassure him that this effect will resolve on its own.

• Caution patient not to rely on condoms or diaphragm for contraception for 72 hours after using vaginal preparation; drug may weaken latex products and cause breakage.

• Instruct patient taking hormonal contraceptives to use supplemental birth control method, such as condoms (unless she's using a vaginal preparation); drug may reduce hormonal contraceptive efficacy.

• As appropriate, review all other significant and life-threatening adverse reactions and interactions, especially those related to the drugs and tests mentioned above.

clofarabine
Clolar, Evoltra ⊕

c

Pharmacologic class: Purine nucleoside antimetabolite

Therapeutic class: Antineoplastic

Pregnancy risk category D

Action

Inhibits DNA synthesis by decreasing cellular deoxynucleotide triphosphate pools through inhibitory action on ribonucleotide reductase, terminating DNA chain elongation, and inhibiting repair through incorporation into DNA chain by competitive inhibition of DNA polymerases. Drug is cytotoxic to rapidly proliferating and quiescent cancer cell types in vitro.

Availability

Solution for injection: 1 mg/ml (20 mg in 20-ml flint vials)

⊘ Indications and dosages

➤ Relapsed or refractory acute lymphoblastic leukemia after at least two previous regimens

Children and adults ages 1 to 21:
52 mg/m²/day by I.V. infusion over 2 hours daily for 5 consecutive days every 2 to 6 weeks, depending on toxicity and response

Dosage adjustment

• Hypotension
• Systemic inflammatory response syndrome (SIRS)
• Capillary leak syndrome (CLS)
• Substantial creatinine and bilirubin elevations

Contraindications

None

Precautions

Use cautiously in:
- renal or hepatic impairment, active infection, dehydration, hypotension
- adults older than age 21
- pregnant or breastfeeding patients.

Administration

- Filter through sterile 0.2-micron syringe filter, and dilute further with D_5W or normal saline solution for injection before I.V. infusion. Resulting admixture may be stored at room temperature but must be used within 24 hours of preparation.
- To prevent incompatibilities, don't give other drugs through same I.V. line.
- Administer continuous I.V. fluids throughout 5 days of treatment to reduce effects of tumor lysis and other adverse events. Give allopurinol, as ordered, if hyperuricemia is expected.
- Prophylactic steroids (such as 100 mg/m^2 hydrocortisone on days 1 through 3) may help prevent SIRS and CLS. If early signs or symptoms of these life-threatening syndromes occur, stop drug immediately and start appropriate supportive measures.
- Withdraw drug immediately if patient develops significant signs or symptoms of SIRS or CLS (such as hypotension); consider giving steroids, diuretics, and albumin. Drug may be reinstituted (generally at lower dosage) when patient is stable.
- Stop drug if hypotension occurs during 5 days of treatment. If hypotension is transient and resolves without pharmacologic intervention, reinstitute drug (generally at lower dosage).
- If creatinine or bilirubin level rises substantially, discontinue drug. Drug may be reinstituted (possibly at lower dosage) when patient is stable and organ function returns to baseline.
- Know that after recovery or return to baseline organ function, treatment cycles are repeated about every 2 to 6 weeks. Dosage is based on body surface area, calculated using actual height and weight before start of each cycle.
- Avoid concurrent administration of hepatotoxic or renotoxic drugs during 5 days of treatment.

Route	Onset	Peak	Duration
I.V.	Unknown	Unknown	Unknown

Adverse reactions

CNS: dizziness, headache, somnolence, tremor, anxiety, depression, lethargy, fatigue, irritability, rigors
CV: tachycardia, flushing, hypertension, hypotension
EENT: sore throat, epistaxis
GI: nausea, vomiting, diarrhea, constipation, abdominal pain, anorexia, gingival bleeding, oral candidiasis
GU: hematuria
Hematologic: febrile neutropenia, neutropenia, anemia, thrombocytopenia
Hepatic: hepatomegaly, jaundice
Musculoskeletal: arthralgia, back pain, myalgia, limb pain
Respiratory: pneumonia, cough, dyspnea, pleural effusion, respiratory distress
Skin: contusion, dermatitis, herpes simplex, dry skin, erythema, palmar-plantar erythrodysesthesia, petechiae, pruritus, cellulitis
Other: decreased appetite, weight loss, edema, injection site pain, mucosal inflammation, pain, fever, bacteremia, sepsis, staphylococcal infection, transfusion reaction

Interactions

Drug-drug. *Hepatotoxic or renotoxic drugs:* additive toxicity
Drug-diagnostic tests. *Alanine aminotransferase, aspartate aminotransferase, bilirubin:* increased
Drug-herbs. *Alpha-lipoic acid, coenzyme Q10:* decreased chemotherapeutic efficacy
Glutamine: possible increase in tumor growth

♦ Canada   ⊕ UK   ☣ Hazardous drug   ⊗ High-alert drug

Patient monitoring

• Assess hepatic and renal function before and during therapy.

• Closely monitor respiratory status and blood pressure during infusion.

• Monitor hematologic status carefully during therapy; drug may cause severe bone marrow depression, resulting in neutropenia, anemia, and thrombocytopenia.

• Monitor for signs and symptoms of tumor lysis syndrome or cytokine release (such as tachypnea, tachycardia, hypotension, and pulmonary edema), which could progress to SIRS, CLS, or organ dysfunction.

• Closely monitor patients receiving drugs that affect blood pressure or cardiac function.

Patient teaching

• Teach patient about appropriate measures to avoid dehydration caused by vomiting and diarrhea. Tell patient to seek medical advice if signs and symptoms of dehydration occur (such as dizziness, light-headedness, fainting spells, or decreased urine output).

• Advise female with childbearing potential to avoid pregnancy during therapy.

• Caution breastfeeding patient to discontinue breastfeeding during therapy.

• As appropriate, review all other significant and life-threatening adverse reactions and interactions, especially those related to the drugs, tests, and herbs mentioned above.

clomiphene citrate (clomifene⊕)

Clomid, Serophene

Pharmacologic class: Chlorotrianisene derivative

Therapeutic class: Fertility drug, ovulation stimulant

Pregnancy risk category X

Action

Binds with estrogen receptors in cytoplasm, increasing secretion of follicle-stimulating hormone, luteinizing hormone, and gonadotropin in hypothalamus and pituitary gland. These actions induce ovulation.

Availability

Tablets: 50 mg

⚡ Indications and dosages

➢ Ovarian failure

Adults: 50 mg/day P.O. for 5 days starting any time in patients with no recent uterine bleeding; or 50 mg/day P.O. starting on fifth day of menstrual cycle. If ovulation doesn't occur, increase to 100 mg/day P.O. for 5 days. Start next course of therapy as early as 30 days after previous course. If patient doesn't respond after three courses, no further doses are recommended.

Off-label uses

• Male sterility (controversial)

Contraindications

• Hepatic disease
• Organic intracranial lesions
• Uncontrolled thyroid or adrenal dysfunction
• Ovarian cyst
• Abnormal uterine bleeding or bleeding of undetermined origin
• Pregnancy

Reactions in **bold** are life-threatening.　　　　◀┋ Clinical alert

Precautions
None

Administration
• Obtain pregnancy test before therapy begins.
• Be aware that patient should undergo pelvic and eye examinations before starting therapy.

Route	Onset	Peak	Duration
P.O.	5-8 days	Unknown	6 wk

Adverse reactions
CNS: nervousness, insomnia, dizziness, light-headedness
CV: vasomotor flushing
EENT: visual disturbances
GI: nausea; vomiting; abdominal discomfort, distention, and bloating
GU: breast tenderness, ovarian enlargement, multiple pregnancies, birth defects in resulting pregnancies, **ovarian hyperstimulation syndrome, uterine bleeding**

Interactions
None significant

Patient monitoring
• Monitor patient for bleeding and other adverse reactions.

Patient teaching
◀€ Instruct patient to immediately report signs and symptoms of ovarian hyperstimulation syndrome, including nausea, vomiting, diarrhea, abdominal or pelvic pain, and swelling in hands or legs.
• Tell patient to report bleeding.
• Advise patient not to take drug if she is or may become pregnant.
• Inform patient that drug increases risk of multiple births, which heightens maternal risk.
• As appropriate, review all other significant and life-threatening adverse reactions.

clomipramine hydrochloride
Anafranil, Anafranil SR✚, Apo-Clomipramine✚, Co Clomipramine✚, Dom-Clomipramine, Gen-Clomipramine✚, Med-Clomipramine✚, Novo-Clopamine✚, PHL-Clomipramine✚, PMS-Clomipramine✚, Ratio Clomipramine✚

Pharmacologic class: Tricyclic antidepressant (TCA)
Therapeutic class: Antiobsessional agent, antidepressant
Pregnancy risk category C

FDA | BOXED WARNING
• Drug may increase risk of suicidal thinking and behavior in children and adolescents with major depressive disorder and other psychiatric disorders. Risk must be balanced with clinical need, as depression itself increases suicide risk. With patient of any age, observe closely for clinical worsening, suicidality, and unusual behavior changes when therapy begins. Advise family to observe patient closely and communicate with prescriber as needed.
• Drug isn't approved for use in pediatric patients, except those with obsessive-compulsive disorder.

Action
Unknown. Selectively inhibits norepinephrine and serotonin reuptake at presynaptic neurons in brain; also possesses moderate anticholinergic properties.

Availability
Aerosol foam: 1%
Capsules: 25 mg, 50 mg, 75 mg

⚠ Indications and dosages

➤ Obsessive-compulsive disorder
Adults: Initially, 25 mg/day P.O., increased over 2 weeks to 100 mg/day given in divided doses. May be increased further over several weeks, up to 250 mg/day given in divided doses.
Children ages 10 to 17: Initially, 25 mg/day P.O., increased over 2 weeks to 3 mg/kg/day or 100 mg/day (whichever is smaller) given in divided doses. May be increased further to 3 mg/kg/day or 200 mg/day (whichever is smaller) given in divided doses.

Dosage adjustment

• Elderly patients

Off-label uses

• Panic disorder

Contraindications

• Hypersensitivity to drug or other TCAs
• Recent myocardial infarction (MI)
• Concurrent MAO inhibitor or clonidine use

Precautions

Use cautiously in:
• glaucoma, hyperthyroidism, prostatic hypertrophy, preexisting cardiovascular disease
• elderly patients
• pregnant or breastfeeding patients
• children younger than age 10 (safety not established).

Administration

• Don't give with grapefruit juice.
• Once stabilizing dosage is reached, entire daily dose may be given at bedtime.

Route	Onset	Peak	Duration
P.O.	Unknown	2-6 hr	Unknown

Adverse reactions

CNS: lethargy, sedation, weakness, aggressive behavior, extrapyramidal reactions, poor concentration, feeling of unreality, delusions, anxiety, restlessness, panic, asthenia, syncope, insomnia, **seizures, suicidal ideation or behavior (especially in child or adolescent)**
CV: orthostatic hypotension, hypertension, ECG changes, tachycardia, palpitations, vasculitis, **arrhythmias, MI, precipitation of heart block**
EENT: blurred vision, dry eyes, vestibular disorder, nasal congestion, laryngitis
GI: nausea, vomiting, constipation, abdominal cramps, belching, epigastric distress, flatulence, dysphagia, increased salivation, stomatitis, parotid gland swelling, black tongue, dry mouth, **paralytic ileus**
GU: urinary retention, urinary hesitancy, urinary tract dilation, male sexual dysfunction, testicular swelling, gynecomastia, breast enlargement, menstrual irregularities, galactorrhea, libido changes
Hematologic: eosinophilia, purpura, anemia, **bone marrow depression, agranulocytosis, thrombocytopenia, leukopenia**
Metabolic: hyperthermia, hypothermia, **syndrome of inappropriate antidiuretic hormone secretion**
Musculoskeletal: muscle weakness
Skin: sweating, dry skin, photosensitivity, rash, pruritus, petechiae, flushing
Other: abnormal taste, chills, edema, increased appetite, weight gain

Interactions

Drug-drug. *Adrenergics, anticholinergics:* additive adrenergic or anticholinergic effects
Cimetidine, hormonal contraceptives, phenothiazines, selective serotonin reuptake inhibitors: increased clomipramine effects, greater risk of toxicity
Clonidine: hypertensive crisis

Reactions in **bold** are life-threatening.   ◀€ Clinical alert

CNS depressants (including antihistamines, opioid analgesics, sedative-hypnotics): additive CNS depression

Disulfiram: transient delirium

Guanethidine: interference with antihypertensive response

MAO inhibitors: severe or life-threatening adverse reactions

Levofloxacin, moxifloxacin: increased risk of adverse cardiovascular reactions

Drug-diagnostic tests. *Blood glucose, prolactin:* elevated levels

Drug-food. *Grapefruit juice:* increased clomipramine blood level and effects

Drug-herbs. *Chamomile, hops, kava, skullcap, valerian:* increased CNS depression

S-adenosylmethionine (SAM-e), St. John's wort: increased serotonergic effects, possibly causing serotonin syndrome

Drug-behaviors. *Alcohol use:* additive CNS depression

Nicotine use: increased metabolism and decreased efficacy of clomipramine

Sun exposure: photosensitivity

Patient monitoring

• Monitor patient for cardiovascular, CNS, and hematologic adverse reactions.

◀€ Assess for suicidal ideation. If necessary, institute suicide precautions.

Patient teaching

◀€ Advise patient (especially children or their parents) to immediately report suicidal thoughts or severe depression.

• Instruct patient not to drink grapefruit juice during therapy.

• Caution patient to avoid driving and other hazardous activities until he knows how drug affects concentration and alertness.

• Instruct patient to avoid alcohol, because it increases drowsiness.

• Tell patient to move slowly when sitting up or standing, to avoid dizziness

or light-headedness caused by sudden blood pressure drop.

• Caution patient not to stop taking drug abruptly, because this may cause nausea, headache, or malaise.

• As appropriate, review all other significant and life-threatening adverse reactions and interactions, especially those related to the drugs, tests, foods, herbs, and behaviors mentioned above.

clonazepam

Alti-Clonazepam♣, Apo-Clonazepam♣, Clonapam♣, Co Clonazepam♣, Dom-Clonazepam♣, Gen-Clonazepam♣, Klonopin, Novo-Clonazepam♣, PHL-Clonazepam♣, PMS-Clonazepam♣, Ratio Clonazepam♣, Rivotril♣⊕

Pharmacologic class: Benzodiazepine
Therapeutic class: Anticonvulsant
Controlled substance schedule IV
Pregnancy risk category D

Action

Unknown. May enhance activity of gamma-aminobutyric acid, an inhibitory neurotransmitter in CNS.

Availability

Tablets: 0.5 mg, 1 mg, 2 mg

✐ Indications and dosages

➢ Absence seizures (Lennox-Gastaut syndrome); akinetic and myoclonic seizures

Adults: Initially, 1.5 mg/day P.O. in three divided doses; may increase by 0.5 to 1 mg q 3 days until seizures are adequately controlled or drug intolerance occurs. Maximum dosage is 20 mg/day.

Infants and children ages 10 and younger or weighing 30 kg (66 lb) or

less: Initially, 0.01 to 0.03 mg/kg/day P.O. Give total dosage (not to exceed 0.05 mg/kg/day) in two to three equally divided doses. Increase by no more than 0.25 to 0.5 mg q 3 days until dosage of 0.1 to 0.2 mg/kg/day is reached, seizures are adequately controlled, or drug intolerance occurs.

Off-label uses

- Acute manic episodes of bipolar disorder
- Multifocal tic disorders
- Neuralgias
- Parkinsonian dysarthria
- Periodic leg movements occurring during sleep
- Adjunctive treatment of schizophrenia

Contraindications

- Hypersensitivity to drug or other benzodiazepines
- Severe hepatic disease
- Acute angle-closure glaucoma

Precautions

Use cautiously in:
- renal impairment, chronic respiratory disease, open-angle glaucoma
- history of porphyria
- pregnant or breastfeeding patients
- children.

Administration

◀ Be aware that overdose may cause fatal respiratory depression or cardiovascular collapse.

- Give tablets with water, and make sure patient swallows them whole.

Route	Onset	Peak	Duration
P.O.	20-60 min	1-2 hr	6-12 hr

Adverse reactions

CNS: ataxia, fatigue, drowsiness, behavioral changes, depression, dizziness, nervousness, reduced intellectual ability
CV: palpitations

EENT: abnormal eye movements, blurred vision, diplopia, nystagmus, sinusitis, rhinitis, pharyngitis
GI: constipation, diarrhea, hypersalivation
GU: dysuria, nocturia, urinary retention, dysmenorrhea, delayed ejaculation, erectile dysfunction
Hematologic: anemia, eosinophilia, **leukopenia, thrombocytopenia**
Hepatic: hepatitis
Musculoskeletal: myalgia
Respiratory: increased respiratory secretions, upper respiratory tract infection, cough, bronchitis, **respiratory depression**
Other: appetite changes, fever, physical or psychological drug dependence, drug tolerance, allergic reaction

Interactions

Drug-drug. *Antidepressants, antihistamines, opioids, other benzodiazepines:* additive CNS depression
Barbiturates, rifampin: increased metabolism and decreased efficacy of clonazepam
Cimetidine, disulfiram, fluoxetine, hormonal contraceptives, isoniazid, ketoconazole, metoprolol, propoxyphene, propranolol, valproic acid: decreased clonazepam metabolism
Phenytoin: decreased clonazepam blood level
Drug-diagnostic tests. *Eosinophils, liver function tests:* increased values
Platelets, white blood cells: decreased counts
Drug-herbs. *Chamomile, hops, kava, skullcap, valerian:* increased CNS depression
Drug-behaviors. *Alcohol use:* increased CNS depression

Patient monitoring

- Monitor patient for respiratory depression. Assess respiratory rate and quality, oxygen saturation (using pulse oximetry), and mental status.

C

Reactions in **bold** are life-threatening.　　　　◀ Clinical alert ·

• Monitor hematologic and liver function test results.

Patient teaching

🔊 Instruct patient to immediately report easy bleeding or bruising or yellowing of skin or eyes.

• Advise patient to avoid driving and other hazardous activities until he knows how drug affects concentration and alertness.

🔊 Caution patient not to stop taking drug abruptly. Advise him to consult prescriber for dosage-tapering schedule if he wishes to discontinue drug.

• Advise patient not to drink alcohol, which may increase drowsiness, dizziness, and risk of seizures.

• As appropriate, review all other significant and life-threatening adverse reactions and interactions, especially those related to the drugs, tests, herbs, and behaviors mentioned above.

---

clonidine
Catapres-TTS

clonidine hydrochloride
Apo-Clonidine✤, Catapres, Dixarit✤, Dom-Clonidine✤, Duraclon✜, Novo-Clonidine✤, Nu-Clonidine✤

Pharmacologic class: Centrally acting sympatholytic
Therapeutic class: Antihypertensive
Pregnancy risk category C

FDA | **BOXED WARNING**

• Before use, dilute clonidine hydrochloride 500-µg/mL strength product in appropriate solution.
• Epidural form (clonidine hydrochloride) isn't recommended for obstetric, postpartum, or perioperative pain management. In these cases, risk of hemodynamic instability may be unacceptable, except in rare patients for whom potential benefits may outweigh possible risks.

Action
Stimulates alpha-adrenergic receptors in CNS, decreasing sympathetic outflow, inhibiting vasoconstriction, and ultimately reducing blood pressure. Also prevents transmission of pain impulses by inhibiting pain pathway signals in brain.

Availability
Solution for epidural injection: 100 mcg/ml in 10-ml vials, 500 mcg/ml in 10-ml vials
Tablets: 100 mcg (0.1 mg), 200 mcg (0.2 mg), 300 mcg (0.3 mg)
Transdermal systems: 2.5 mg total released as 0.1 mg/24 hours (TTS 1), 5 mg total released as 0.2 mg/24 hours (TTS 2), 7.5 mg total released as 0.3 mg/24 hours (TTS 3)

💊 Indications and dosages
➤ Mild to moderate hypertension
Adults: 0.1 mg P.O. b.i.d. (morning and bedtime) alone or with other antihypertensives; increase in increments of 0.1 mg/day q week until desired response occurs. Or, one transdermal system applied once q 7 days to hairless area of intact skin on upper outer arm or chest.
➤ Severe pain in cancer patients unresponsive to opioids alone
Adults: Initially, 30 mcg/hour by continuous epidural infusion, titrated upward or downward depending on patient response

Dosage adjustment
• Renal impairment

Off-label uses
- Acute alcohol withdrawal
- Akathisia
- Diarrhea
- Prolonged surgical anesthesia

Contraindications
- Hypersensitivity to drug
- Hypersensitivity to components of adhesive layer (transdermal form)
- Infection at epidural injection site, bleeding problems (epidural use)
- Concurrent anticoagulant therapy

Precautions
Use cautiously in:
- renal insufficiency, serious cardiac or cerebrovascular disease
- elderly patients
- pregnant or breastfeeding patients.

Administration
- For epidural use, dilute drug solution in normal saline solution, as ordered.
- To minimize sedative effects, give largest portion of maintenance P.O. dose at bedtime.

Route	Onset	Peak	Duration
P.O.	30-60 min	2-4 hr	8-12 hr
Epidural	Rapid	19 min	Variable
Transdermal	Slow	2-3 days	7 days

Adverse reactions
CNS: drowsiness, depression, dizziness, nervousness, nightmares
CV: hypotension (especially with epidural use), palpitations, bradycardia
GI: nausea, vomiting, constipation, dry mouth
GU: urinary retention, nocturia, erectile dysfunction
Metabolic: sodium retention
Skin: rash, sweating, pruritus, dermatitis
Other: weight gain, withdrawal phenomenon

Interactions
Drug-drug. *Amphetamines, beta-adrenergic blockers, MAO inhibitors, prazosin, tricyclic antidepressants:* decreased antihypertensive effect
Beta-adrenergic blockers: increased withdrawal phenomenon
CNS depressants (including antihistamines, opioids, sedative-hypnotics): additive sedation
Epidurally administered local anesthetics: prolonged clonidine effects
Levodopa: decreased levodopa efficacy
Myocardial depressants (including beta-adrenergic blockers): additive bradycardia
Other antihypertensives, nitrates: additive hypotension
Verapamil: increased risk of adverse cardiovascular reactions
Drug-herbs. *Capsicum:* reduced antihypertensive effect
Drug-behaviors. *Alcohol use:* increased sedation

Patient monitoring
- Monitor patient for signs and symptoms of adverse cardiovascular reactions.
- Frequently assess vital signs, especially blood pressure and pulse.
- Monitor patient for drug tolerance and efficacy.

Patient teaching
- Instruct patient to move slowly when sitting up or standing, to avoid dizziness or light-headedness caused by sudden blood pressure decrease.
- 🔊 Caution patient not to stop taking drug abruptly.
- As appropriate, review all other significant adverse reactions and interactions, especially those related to the drugs, herbs, and behaviors mentioned above.

Reactions in **bold** are life-threatening.   🔊 Clinical alert

clopidogrel bisulfate
Plavix

Pharmacologic class: Platelet aggregation inhibitor
Therapeutic class: Antiplatelet drug
Pregnancy risk category B

FDA | BOXED WARNING

- Effectiveness of clopidogrel depends on activation to an active metabolite by the cytochrome P(CYP) 450 system, principally CYP2C19.
- Patients identified as CYP2C19 poor metabolizers treated with clopidogrel at recommended dosages exhibit higher cardiovascular event rates following acute coronary syndrome or percutaneous coronary intervention than patients with normal CYP2C19 function.
- Tests are available to identify a patient's CYP2C19 genotype and can be used as an aid in determining therapeutic strategy.
- Consider alternative treatment or treatment strategies in patients identified as CYP2C19 poor metabolizers.

Action
Inhibits platelet aggregation by blocking binding of adenosine diphosphate to platelets, thereby preventing thrombus formation

Availability
Tablets: 75 mg, 300 mg

Indications and dosages
➤ Recent myocardial infarction (MI) or stroke or established peripheral arterial disease
Adults: 75 mg/day P.O.
➤ Acute coronary syndrome (ACS)

Adults: 300 mg P.O. as a loading dose, then 75 mg/day P.O. in combination with aspirin (75 to 325 mg once daily) for patients with non-ST-segment elevation ACS (unstable angina, non-ST-elevation MI)
Adults: 75 mg P.O. once daily in combination with aspirin (75 to 325 mg once daily), with or without a loading dose and with or without thrombolytics for patients with ST-elevation MI

Contraindications
- Hypersensitivity to drug
- Active pathologic bleeding

Precautions
Use cautiously in:
- thrombotic thrombocytopenic purpura
- increased risk of bleeding
- concomitant use of drugs that inhibit CYP2C19 (such as esomeprazole, omeprazole)
- concomitant use of aspirin in patients with recent transient ischemic attack or cerebrovascular accident
- premature discontinuation of drug
- pregnant or breastfeeding patients
- children (safety and efficacy not established).

Administration
- Give with or without food.
- Know that drug may need to be discontinued 5 days before surgery.

Route	Onset	Peak	Duration
P.O.	Variable	60 min	3-4 hr

Adverse reactions
CNS: depression, dizziness, fatigue, headache
CV: chest pain, hypertension
EENT: epistaxis, rhinitis
GI: diarrhea, abdominal pain, dyspepsia, gastritis, **GI bleeding**
Hematologic: bleeding, neutropenia, thrombotic thrombocytopenic purpura

---

🍁 Canada   ⊕ UK   ⚕ Hazardous drug   ⊗ High-alert drug

Metabolic: hypercholesterolemia, gout
Musculoskeletal: joint pain, back pain
Respiratory: cough, dyspnea, bronchitis, upper respiratory tract infection, **bronchospasm**
Skin: pruritus, rash, angioedema
Other: hypersensitivity reactions, **anaphylactic reactions**

Interactions
Drug-drug. *Abciximab, aspirin, eptifibatide, heparin, heparinoids, nonsteroidal anti-inflammatory drugs (NSAIDs), thrombolytics, ticlopidine, tirofiban, warfarin:* increased risk of bleeding
CYP2C19 inhibitors (such as esomeprazole, omeprazole): significantly reduced clopidogrel antiplatelet activity
Fluvastatin, many NSAIDs, phenytoin, tamoxifen, tolbutamide, torsemide: interference with metabolism of these drugs
Drug-diagnostic tests. *Bilirubin, hepatic enzymes, nonprotein nitrogen, total cholesterol, uric acid:* increased levels
Platelets: decreased count
Drug-herbs. *Anise, arnica, chamomile, clove, fenugreek, feverfew, garlic, ginger, ginkgo, ginseng:* increased risk of bleeding

Patient monitoring
• Monitor hemoglobin and hematocrit periodically.
• Monitor patient for unusual bleeding or bruising; drug significantly increases risk of bleeding.
• Assess for occult GI blood loss if patient is receiving naproxen concurrently with clopidogrel.

Patient teaching
• Tell patient to take tablets with or without food.
◀≋ Advise patient to immediately report unusual or acute chest pain, respiratory difficulty, rash, purplish bruises on skin or in mouth, purple skin patches, unusual fatigue, fast heart rate, confusion, signs and symptoms of stroke (including weakness on one side, speech changes), low urine output, unresolved bleeding, diarrhea, GI distress, nosebleed, or acute headache.
◀≋ Instruct patient not to discontinue drug without consulting prescriber.
• Instruct patient to tell all health care providers that he's taking clopidogrel, especially if surgery is scheduled or new drugs are prescribed.
• Advise patient to contact prescriber before taking over-the-counter products, particularly nonsteroidal anti-inflammatory drugs.
• Tell patient drug may cause headache and dizziness. Caution him to avoid driving and other hazardous activities until he knows how drug affects concentration and alertness.
• Advise patient to minimize adverse GI effects by eating small, frequent meals or chewing gum.
• As appropriate, review all other significant and life-threatening adverse reactions and interactions, especially those related to the drugs, tests, and herbs mentioned above.

clorazepate dipotassium
Apo-Clorazepate❖, Novo-Clopate❖, Tranxene, Tranxene-SD, Tranxene-SD Half Strength, Tranxene-T

Pharmacologic class: Benzodiazepine
Therapeutic class: Anticonvulsant, anxiolytic
Controlled substance schedule IV
Pregnancy risk category D

Action
Unclear. Thought to potentiate effects of gamma-aminobutyric acid and other neurotransmitters, promoting inhibitory neurotransmission at excitatory synapses.

Reactions in **bold** are life-threatening.   ◀≋ Clinical alert

Availability

Tablets: 3.75 mg, 7.5 mg, 15 mg

⚠ Indications and dosages

➤ Anxiety
Adults: 7.5 to 15 mg P.O. two to four times daily
➤ Adjunctive therapy in partial seizure disorder
Adults and children older than age 12: Initially, 7.5 mg P.O. t.i.d.; increase by no more than 7.5 mg/week. Don't exceed 90 mg/day.
Children ages 9 to 12: Initially, 7.5 mg P.O. b.i.d.; increase by no more than 7.5 mg/week. Don't exceed 60 mg/day.
➤ Management of alcohol withdrawal
Adults: Initially, 30 mg P.O., followed by 15 mg P.O. two to four times daily on first day. On second day, give 45 to 90 mg P.O. in divided doses, then decrease gradually over subsequent days to 7.5 mg to 15 mg P.O. daily.

Dosage adjustment

• Elderly or debilitated patients

Contraindications

• Benzodiazepine hypersensitivity
• Acute angle-closure glaucoma
• Psychosis
• Concurrent ketoconazole or itraconazole therapy
• Children younger than age 9

Precautions

Use cautiously in:
• depression or suicidal ideation
• psychotic reaction
• elderly patients
• females of childbearing age
• pregnant or breastfeeding patients.

Administration

• If GI upset occurs, give with food.
• When discontinuing therapy after long-term use, taper dosage gradually over 4 to 8 weeks to avoid withdrawal symptoms.
• Take suicide precautions if patient is depressed or anxious.

Route	Onset	Peak	Duration
P.O.	Rapid	1-2 hr	Days

Adverse reactions

CNS: dizziness, drowsiness, lethargy, sedation, depression, fatigue, nervousness, confusion, irritability, headache, slurred speech, difficulty articulating words, stupor, rigidity, tremor, poor coordination
CV: hypertension, hypotension, palpitations
EENT: blurred or double vision
GI: dry mouth
Hematologic: neutropenia
Hepatic: jaundice
Skin: rash, diaphoresis
Other: weight gain or loss, drug dependence or tolerance

Interactions

Drug-drug. *Antacids:* altered clorazepate absorption rate
Antidepressants, antihistamines, opioids: additive CNS depression
Barbiturates, MAO inhibitors, other antidepressants, phenothiazines: potentiation of clorazepate effects
Cimetidine, disulfiram, fluoxetine, hormonal contraceptives, isoniazid, itraconazole, ketoconazole, metoprolol, propoxyphene, propranolol, valproic acid: decreased clorazepate metabolism, causing enhanced drug action or markedly increased CNS effects
Levodopa: decreased antiparkinsonian effect
Probenecid: rapid onset or prolonged action of clorazepate
Rifampin: increased metabolism and decreased efficacy of clorazepate
Theophylline: decreased sedative effect of clorazepate
Drug-diagnostic tests. *Alanine aminotransferase, alkaline phosphatase, aspartate aminotransferase:* increased levels
Drug-herbs. *Chamomile, hops, kava, skullcap, valerian:* increased CNS depression

Drug-behaviors. *Alcohol use:* increased CNS depression
Smoking: decreased drug absorption

Patient monitoring

• Assess for pregnancy before initiating therapy.
• Evaluate patient for depression, drug dependence, and drug tolerance.
• Monitor blood counts and liver function test results during long-term therapy; drug may cause neutropenia and jaundice.

Patient teaching

• Instruct patient to avoid driving and other hazardous activities until he knows how drug affects concentration and alertness.
• Tell patient to avoid smoking and use of alcohol or other CNS depressants.
◀€ Caution patient not to stop therapy abruptly, because withdrawal symptoms may occur.
• As appropriate, review all other significant and life-threatening adverse reactions and interactions, especially those related to the drugs, tests, herbs, and behaviors mentioned above.

clozapine

Apo-Clozapine❖, Clozaril, Denazapine⊕, Fazaclo ODT, Gen-Clozapine❖, PMS-Clozapine❖, Zaponex⊕

Pharmacologic class: Dibenzodiazepine derivative
Therapeutic class: Antipsychotic agent
Pregnancy risk category B

FDA | BOXED WARNING

• Because of significant agranulocytosis risk, use only to treat severely ill patients with schizophrenia who don't respond to standard antipsychotic drugs, or to reduce risk of recurrent suicidal behavior in patients with schizophrenia or schizoaffective disorder who risk reexperiencing suicidal behavior. Obtain baseline white blood cell (WBC) and absolute neutrophil counts before therapy, regularly during therapy, and for at least 4 weeks afterward.
• Drug is associated with seizures; likelihood increases at higher doses. Use caution when giving to patients with history of seizures or other predisposing factors. Instruct patient not to engage in activities in which sudden loss of consciousness could cause serious risk to self or others.
• Drug may increase risk of fatal myocarditis, especially during first month of therapy. Discontinue promptly if myocarditis is suspected.
• Orthostatic hypotension with or without syncope may occur. Rarely, collapse is profound and accompanied by respiratory or cardiac arrest, or both. Orthostatic hypotension is more likely during initial titration when dosage is raised rapidly. In patients who've had even brief interval off drug (2 or more days since last dose), start with 12.5 mg once or twice daily.
• During initial therapy, collapse and respiratory and cardiac arrest may occur. Use caution when initiating therapy.
• Drug increased risk of death in elderly patients with dementia-related psychosis; most deaths have been cardiovascular or infectious. Drug isn't approved for dementia-related psychosis.

Action

Unclear. Thought to interfere with dopamine binding in limbic system of CNS, with high affinity for dopamine$_4$ receptors. May antagonize adrenergic, cholinergic, histaminergic, and serotonergic receptors.

Availability

Tablets: 25 mg, 50 mg, 100 mg, 200 mg
Tablets (orally disintegrating): 12.5 mg, 25 mg, 100 mg

⑦ Indications and dosages

➤ Schizophrenia in patients unresponsive to other therapies
Adults: 12.5 mg P.O. daily or b.i.d.; increase daily in 25- to 50-mg increments, as tolerated, to target dosage of 300 to 450 mg/day by end of second week. Make subsequent dosage increases once or twice weekly in increments of 100 mg or less, to a maximum dosage of 900 mg/day P.O. in divided doses.

Dosage adjustment

- Renal impairment
- Elderly patients

Contraindications

- Hypersensitivity to drug
- Uncontrolled seizures
- Severe CNS depression or coma
- Paralytic ileus, myeloproliferative disorders, history of clozapine-induced agranulocytosis or severe granulocytopenia
- Concurrent use of drugs that cause agranulocytosis or bone marrow depression

Precautions

Use cautiously in:
- hypersensitivity to phenothiazines
- cardiac, hepatic, or renal impairment; CNS tumors; diabetes mellitus; history of seizures; prostatic hypertrophy; intestinal obstruction; angle-closure glaucoma, patients with a history of long QT syndrome or prolonged QT interval or other conditions that may increase risk of prolonged QT interval or sudden death
- elderly patients
- pregnant or breastfeeding patients
- children.

Administration

◀︎≣ Obtain WBC count before starting therapy. Don't give drug if WBC count is below 3,500/mm³.
- When discontinuing drug, taper dosage gradually over 1 to 2 weeks.
- Be aware that orally disintegrating tablets are meant to dissolve in mouth.

Route	Onset	Peak	Duration
P.O.	Unknown	2.5 hr	4-12 hr
P.O. (orally disint.)	Unknown	Unknown	Unknown

Adverse reactions

CNS: sedation, drowsiness, dizziness, vertigo, headache, tremor, insomnia, disturbed sleep, nightmares, agitation, lethargy, fatigue, weakness, confusion, anxiety, parkinsonism, slurred speech, depression, restlessness, extrapyramidal reactions, tardive dyskinesia, akathisia, syncope, **neuroleptic malignant syndrome, autonomic disturbances, seizures**
CV: hypotension, tachycardia, ECG changes, chest pain, **QT-interval prolongation, myocarditis**
EENT: blurred vision, dry eyes, nasal congestion, sinusitis
GI: nausea, vomiting, constipation, dyspepsia, salivation, dry mouth, anorexia
GU: urinary retention, urinary incontinence, urinary frequency and urgency, inhibited ejaculation
Musculoskeletal: muscle spasms, rigidity, back and muscle pain
Hematologic: agranulocytosis, leukopenia, hemolytic anemia, aplastic anemia, thrombocytopenia, neutropenia, eosinophilia
Respiratory: dyspnea, **respiratory arrest**
Skin: rash, sweating, **Stevens-Johnson syndrome**
Other: weight gain, fever

Interactions

Drug-drug. *Anticholinergics, antihypertensives, digoxin, warfarin:* increased effects of these drugs

Cimetidine, erythromycin: increased therapeutic and toxic effects of clozapine

Epinephrine: increased hypotension

Fluoxetine, fluvoxamine, paroxetine, sertraline: increased clozapine blood level

Phenytoin, rifampin: decreased clozapine blood level

Psychoactive drugs: additive psychoactive effect

Drug-diagnostic tests. *Granulocytes, hematocrit, hemoglobin, platelets, white blood cells:* decreased values

Liver function tests: abnormal values

Pregnancy test: false-positive result

Drug-food. *Caffeine:* increased clozapine blood level

Drug-herbs. *Angel's trumpet, Jimsonweed, scopolia:* increased anticholinergic effects

Nutmeg: decreased clozapine efficacy

St. John's wort: decreased clozapine blood level

Drug-behaviors. *Alcohol use:* increased CNS depression

Smoking: decreased clozapine blood level

Patient monitoring

◀€ Monitor WBC count weekly for first 6 months of therapy; if it's normal, WBC testing can be reduced to every other week. Notify prescriber immediately if WBC count decreases or agranulocytosis occurs.

• Monitor ECG and liver function test results.

• If drug must be withdrawn abruptly, monitor patient for psychosis and cholinergic rebound (headache, nausea, vomiting, diarrhea).

• Continue to monitor WBC count weekly for 4 weeks after therapy ends.

Patient teaching

• Tell patient to allow orally disintegrating tablet to dissolve in mouth.

• Teach patient about significant risk of agranulocytosis; tell him he'll need to undergo weekly blood testing to check for this blood disorder. Mention that clozapine tablets are available only through a special program that ensures required blood monitoring.

◀€ Advise patient to immediately report new onset of lethargy, weakness, fever, sore throat, malaise, mucous membrane ulcers, flulike symptoms, or other signs and symptoms of infection.

• As appropriate, review all other significant and life-threatening adverse reactions and interactions, especially those related to the drugs, tests, foods, herbs, and behaviors mentioned above.

coagulation factor VIIa (recombinant)
NovoSeven RT

Pharmacologic class: Coagulation factor VIIa

Therapeutic class: Antihemophilic agent

Pregnancy risk category C

FDA BOXED WARNING

• Arterial and venous thrombotic and thromboembolic events following administration of NovoSeven RT have been reported during postmarketing surveillance. Clinical studies have shown an increased risk of arterial thromboembolic adverse events with NovoSeven RT when administered outside the current approved indications. Fatal and nonfatal thrombotic events have been reported.

• Discuss the risks and explain the signs and symptoms of thrombotic and thromboembolic events to patients who will receive NovoSeven RT.

• Monitor patients for signs or symptoms of activation of the coagulation system and for thrombosis.

◀€ Clinical alert

• Safety and efficacy of NovoSeven RT haven't been established outside the approved indications.

Action
Promotes hemostasis by activating intrinsic pathway of coagulation cascade to form fibrin

Availability
Lyophilized powder for injection:
1 mg/vial, 2 mg/vial, 5 mg/vial

⊘ Indications and dosages
➤ Bleeding episodes in patients with hemophilia A or B who have inhibitors to factor VIII or IX and in patients with acquired hemophilia
Adults: For hemostatic dosing, 90 mcg/kg I.V. bolus q 2 hours until hemostasis occurs or therapy is deemed ineffective. For posthemostatic dosing, appropriate dosing duration hasn't been determined. For severe bleeds, continue dosing at 3- to 6-hour intervals after hemostasis is achieved, to maintain hemostatic plug.
➤ Prevention of bleeding in surgical interventions or invasive procedures in patients with hemophilia A or B who have inhibitors to factor VIII or IX and in patients with acquired hemophilia
Adults: Initially, 90 mcg/kg I.V. immediately before intervention and repeated at 2-hour intervals for duration of surgery. For minor surgery, administer postsurgical doses by I.V. bolus injection at 2-hour intervals for first 48 hours and then at 2- to 6-hour intervals until healing has occurred. For major surgery, administer postsurgical doses by I.V. injection at 2-hour intervals for 5 days, followed by 4-hour intervals until healing has occurred. Administer additional bolus doses, if required.
➤ Bleeding episodes or prevention of bleeding in surgical intervention or invasive procedures in patients with congenital factor VII deficiency
Adults: 15 to 30 mcg/kg I.V. q 4 to 6 hours until hemostasis is achieved. Effective treatment has been achieved with dosages as low as 10 mcg/kg.
➤ Bleeding episodes or surgery in patients with acquired hemophilia
Adults: 70 to 90 mcg/kg I.V., repeated q 2 to 3 hours until hemostasis is achieved

Contraindications
None

Precautions
Use cautiously in:
• hypersensitivity to drug, its components, or mouse, hamster, or bovine products
• prolonged use of drug
• concomitant use of activated or non-activated prothrombin complex concentrates (avoid use)
• patients with increased risk of thromboembolic complications (including advanced atherosclerotic disease, crush injury, septicemia, history of coronary heart disease, liver disease, disseminated intravascular coagulation, postoperative immobilization, elderly patients and neonates)
• pregnant or breastfeeding patients
• children.

Administration
• Monitor factor VII-deficient patients for prothrombin time and factor VII coagulant activity before administering drug.
◀€ Give by I.V. bolus only over 2 to 5 minutes, depending on dosage.
• Reconstitute only with specified volume of diluent supplied.
◀€ Don't mix with sterile water for injection or infusion solutions.
◀€ Don't inject diluent directly on the powder.
• Administer within 3 hours of reconstituting. If line needs to be flushed

before or after administering drug, use normal saline solution.

Route	Onset	Peak	Duration
I.V.	Unknown	Unknown	Unknown

Adverse reactions
CNS: headache, **cerebral artery occlusion, cerebrovascular accident**
CV: hypertension, hypotension, bradycardia, angina, superficial thrombophlebitis, **thrombophlebitis, deep vein thrombosis, coagulation disorder, disseminated intravascular coagulation (DIC), increased fibrinolysis, purpura**
GI: nausea, vomiting
GU: **renal dysfunction**
Hematologic: purpura, **hemorrhage, hemarthrosis, disseminated intravascular coagulation, coagulation disorders, decreased fibrinogen plasma, thrombosis**
Musculoskeletal: arthrosis, arthralgia
Respiratory: pneumonia, **pulmonary embolism**
Skin: pruritus, rash, urticaria
Other: fever, edema, pain, redness or reaction at injection site, **hypersensitivity reaction**

Interactions
Drug-drug. *Activated prothrombin complex concentrates, prothrombin complex concentrates:* risk of potential interaction (though not evaluated)

Patient monitoring
◀≋ Monitor for signs and symptoms of coagulation activation or thrombosis. If DIC or thrombosis is confirmed, reduce dosage or discontinue drug, depending on patient's symptoms.
• Monitor factor VII-deficient patients for prothrombin time and factor VII coagulant activity before and after administering drug. If factor VIIa activity fails to reach expected level, prothrombin time isn't corrected, or

bleeding isn't controlled after treatment with recommended dosages, antibody formation may be suspected and analysis for antibodies should be performed.
• Be aware that laboratory coagulation parameters may be used as adjunct to clinical evaluation of hemostasis to monitor drug efficacy and treatment schedule. However, these parameters lack direct correlation with achievement of hemostasis.
• Monitor renal function tests.

Patient teaching
◀≋ Instruct patient to immediately report signs and symptoms of hypersensitivity reactions (including hives, urticaria, chest tightness, or wheezing) and thrombosis (including new-onset swelling and pain in limbs or abdomen, new-onset chest pain, shortness of breath, loss of sensation, or altered consciousness or speech).
• Instruct patient to report swelling, pain, burning, or itching at infusion site.
• Tell patient to inform prescriber if she's pregnant or intends to become pregnant.
• As appropriate, review all other significant and life-threatening adverse reactions and interactions, especially those related to the drugs mentioned above.

codeine sulfate

Pharmacologic class: Opioid agonist
Therapeutic class: Opioid analgesic, antitussive
Controlled substance schedule II
Pregnancy risk category C

Action
Binds to opioid receptors in CNS, altering perception of painful stimuli. Causes generalized CNS depression, decreases cough reflex, and reduces GI motility.

Availability
Tablets: 15 mg, 30 mg, 60 mg

⏀ Indications and dosages
➤ Mild to moderately severe pain
Adults: 15 to 60 mg P.O. q 4 hours as needed. Doses above 60 mg may fail to give commensurate pain relief, and may be associated with an increased incidence of undesirable adverse effects.

Dosage adjustment
• Renal or hepatic impairment
• Elderly or debilitated patients

Contraindications
• Hypersensitivity to drug, its components, or other opioids
• Respiratory depression, severe bronchial asthma, hypercarbia
• Paralytic ileus or suspected paralytic ileus

Precautions
Use cautiously in:
• severe renal, hepatic, or pulmonary disease
• adrenal insufficiency, circulatory shock, hypotension, pancreatic or biliary tract disease, urethral stricture, seizures, head trauma, hypothyroidism, increased intracranial pressure, prostatic hypertrophy, undiagnosed abdominal pain, alcoholism
• concomitant use of alcohol, other opioids, illicit drugs
• elderly or debilitated patients
• pregnant or breastfeeding patients
• labor and delivery patients
• children younger than age 18 (safety and efficacy not established).

Administration
• If GI upset occurs, give with food.
• Titrate dosage for appropriate analgesic effect.
◀€ If overdose occurs, give naloxone I.V. as prescribed. Repeat administration as needed (up to manufacturer's recommended maximum dosage) to reverse toxic effects.

Route	Onset	Peak	Duration
P.O.	30-45 min	1-2 hr	4 hr

Adverse reactions
CNS: confusion, sedation, malaise, agitation, euphoria, floating feeling, headache, hallucinations, unusual dreams, apathy, mood changes
CV: hypotension, bradycardia, peripheral vasodilation, reduced peripheral resistance
EENT: blurred or double vision, miosis, reddened sclera
GI: nausea, vomiting, constipation, decreased gastric motility
GU: urinary retention, urinary tract spasms, urinary urgency
Respiratory: suppressed cough reflex, **respiratory depression**
Skin: flushing, sweating
Other: physical or psychological drug dependence, drug tolerance

Interactions
Drug-drug. *Antidepressants, antihistamines, sedative-hypnotics:* additive CNS depression
Nalbuphine, pentazocine: decreased analgesic effect
Opioid partial agonists (buprenorphine, butorphanol, nalbuphine, pentazocine): precipitation of opioid withdrawal in physically dependent patients
Drug-herbs. *Chamomile, hops, kava, skullcap, valerian:* increased CNS depression
Drug-behaviors. *Alcohol use:* increased CNS depression

♣ Canada   ⊕ UK   ☣ Hazardous drug   ⊗ High-alert drug

Patient monitoring
- Monitor vital signs and CNS status.
- Assess pain level and efficacy of pain relief.
- Evaluate patient for adverse reactions.
- ◀€ Stay alert for overdose signs and symptoms, such as CNS and respiratory depression, GI cramping, and constipation.
- Assess other drugs in patient's drug regimen for those that could cause additive or adverse interactions.
- Monitor patient for signs and symptoms of drug dependence or tolerance.

Patient teaching
- Teach patient to minimize adverse GI effects by taking doses with food or milk.
- ◀€ Tell patient to notify prescriber promptly if he experiences shortness of breath or difficulty breathing or if nausea, vomiting, or constipation become pronounced.
- Caution patient to avoid driving and other hazardous activities until he knows how drug affects concentration, alertness, vision, coordination, and physical dexterity.
- Instruct patient to move slowly when sitting up or standing, to avoid dizziness or light-headedness from sudden blood pressure decrease.
- As appropriate, review all other significant and life-threatening adverse reactions and interactions, especially those related to the drugs, herbs, and behaviors mentioned above.

colchicine
Colcrys

c

Pharmacologic class: Colchicum alkaloid
Therapeutic class: Antigout drug
Pregnancy risk category C

Action
Unclear. Antigout action may occur through white blood cell (WBC) migration and reduced lactic acid production by WBCs. This action in turn decreases uric acid deposition, kinetin formation, and phagocytosis, leading to reduction in inflammatory response.

Availability
Tablets: 0.6 mg

Ø Indications and dosages
➤ Prophylaxis of gout flares
Adults and adolescents age 16 and older: 0.6 mg P.O. daily or b.i.d. Maximum dosage, 1.2 mg/day.
➤ Treatment of gout flares
Adults and adolescents age 16 and older: 1.2 mg P.O. at first sign of a gout flare, followed by 0.6 mg 1 hour later. Wait 12 hours; then resume prophylactic dose.
➤ Familial Mediterranean fever
Adults and adolescents age 12 and older: 1.2 to 2.4 mg P.O. in one or two divided doses. Increase or decrease dosage as indicated and as tolerated in increments of 0.3 mg/day; not to exceed the maximum recommended daily dosage.
Children ages 6 to 12: 0.9 to 1.8 mg P.O. as a single dose or as divided doses b.i.d.
Children ages 4 to 6: 0.3 to 1.8 mg P.O. as a single dose or as divided doses b.i.d.

Dosage adjustment
• Mild hepatic or renal impairment

Off-label uses
• Hepatic cirrhosis
• Chronic progressive multiple sclerosis
• Pyoderma gangrenosum associated with Crohn's disease
• Psoriasis
• Dermatitis herpetiformis

Contraindications
• Hypersensitivity to drug
• Blood dyscrasias
• Serious GI, renal, hepatic, or cardiac disorders
• Concurrent use of P-glycoprotein or strong CYP3A4 inhibitors (including all protease inhibitors except fosamprenavir)

Precautions
Use cautiously in:
• renal impairment
• elderly or debilitated patients
• pregnant or breastfeeding patients
• children (safety not established).

Administration
• Give tablets without regard to meals.
• Know that GI reactions may be troublesome in patients with peptic ulcer or irritable bowel.

Route	Onset	Peak	Duration
P.O.	12 hr	24-72 hr	Unknown
I.V.	Rapid	Rapid	Rapid

Adverse reactions
CNS: peripheral neuritis, neuropathy
GI: nausea, vomiting, diarrhea, abdominal pain
GU: anuria, hematuria, reversible azoospermia, renal impairment
Hematologic: purpura, **agranulocytosis, aplastic anemia, thrombocytopenia**
Metabolic: vitamin B_{12} malabsorption
Musculoskeletal: myopathy
Skin: dermatosis, alopecia
Other: hypersensitivity reactions

Interactions
Drug-drug. *Cyclosporine:* colchicine-induced myopathy
Vitamin B_{12}: reversible vitamin malabsorption
Drug-diagnostic tests. *Alkaline phosphatase, aspartate aminotransferase:* increased levels
Hematocrit, hemoglobin, platelets: decreased values
Urine hemoglobin, urinary red blood cells: false-positive results
Drug-food. *Caffeine-containing foods and beverages:* decreased colchicine effect
Drug-herbs. *Herbal teas, St. John's wort:* decreased drug effect
Drug-behaviors. *Alcohol use:* increased uric acid level

Patient monitoring
◀≋ Monitor patient for signs and symptoms of toxicity (nausea, vomiting, abdominal pain, bloody diarrhea, burning sensation, muscle weakness, oliguria, hematuria, ascending paralysis, delirium, and seizures). Discontinue drug if these occur.
• Monitor CBC and renal function test results regularly.
• Be aware that patient may need opioids to control drug-induced diarrhea (especially if he's receiving maximum colchicine dosage).

Patient teaching
• Tell patient to take tablets with or without food.
• Instruct patient to report rash, sore throat, fever, tiredness, weakness, numbness, or tingling.
◀≋ Tell patient to immediately report muscle tremors, weakness, fatigue, bruising, bleeding, yellowing of eyes or skin, pale stools, dark urine, severe vomiting, watery or bloody diarrhea, or abdominal pain.
• Advise patient to increase fluid intake to prevent renal calculi (unless prescriber wants him to restrict fluids).

• Instruct patient to avoid alcohol, herbal teas, and caffeine during therapy.
• As appropriate, review all other significant and life-threatening adverse reactions and interactions, especially those related to the drugs, tests, foods, herbs, and behaviors mentioned above.

coleselevam hydrochloride
Cholestagel ⊕, Welchol

Pharmacologic class: Bile acid sequestrant
Therapeutic class: Antihyperlipidemic
Pregnancy risk category B

Action
Binds bile acids in GI tract and forms insoluble complex, impeding bile acid reabsorption and promoting its excretion. As a result, cholesterol and low-density lipoprotein (LDL) levels decrease.

Availability
Oral suspension: 3.75 g packet
Tablets: 625 mg

🖋 Indications and dosages
➤ Adjunct to diet and exercise to reduce LDL cholesterol in patients with primary hypercholesterolemia
Adults and children ages 10 to 17:
Three tablets (1,875 mg) P.O. b.i.d., or six tablets (3,750 mg) once daily; or, one 3.75-g packet P.O. once daily.
➤ Adjunct to diet and exercise to improve glycemic control in adults with type 2 diabetes mellitus
Adults: Three tablets (1,875 mg) P.O. b.i.d., or six tablets (3,750 mg) P.O. once daily; or, one 3.75-g packet P.O. once daily

Contraindications
• Hypersensitivity to drug
• Bowel obstruction
• Serum triglyceride level above 500 mg/dl or history of hypertriglyceridemia-induced pancreatitis

Precautions
Use cautiously in:
• susceptibility to vitamin K deficiency (such as patients on warfarin or those with malabsorption syndrome), concomitant use of fat-soluble vitamins
• patients with dysphagia or swallowing disorders, gastroparesis, other GI motility disorders; those who have had major GI tract surgery and who may be at risk for bowel obstruction
• children (safety and efficacy not established).

Administration
• Give with meals and fluids.
• Ensure that patient swallows tablets whole without crushing or chewing.
• Mix prescribed powder packet with 4 to 8 ounces of water, fruit juice, or diet soft drinks.
• Know that drug may be used alone or with HMG-CoA reductase inhibitor.

Route	Onset	Peak	Duration
P.O.	Unknown	2 wk	Unknown

Adverse reactions
CNS: headache, anxiety, vertigo, dizziness, insomnia, fatigue, syncope
EENT: tinnitus
GI: nausea, vomiting, diarrhea, constipation, abdominal discomfort, flatulence, fecal impaction, loose stools, fatty stools, rectal or hemorrhoidal bleeding, **other GI bleeding**
GU: increased libido
Hematologic: anemia, **bleeding tendency**
Metabolic: malabsorption of vitamins A, D, E, and K

Reactions in **bold** are life-threatening. ◀♬ Clinical alert

Musculoskeletal: back, muscle, or joint pain
Skin: bruising

Interactions

Drug-drug. *Fat-soluble vitamins (A, D, E, and K):* decreased vitamin absorption

Patient monitoring

• Monitor lipid levels before starting therapy and periodically thereafter.

Patient teaching

• Instruct patient to take drug with meals as directed.

• Instruct patient to mix powder packet for oral suspension with 4 to 8 ounces of water, fruit juice, or diet soft drinks; stir well, and drink. Tell patient not to take powder in its dry form.

• Instruct patient to take any vitamins at least 4 hours before taking this drug.

• Tell patient to report persistent GI upset, back or muscle pain or weakness, and respiratory problems.

• If drug causes constipation, instruct patient to increase exercise, drink plenty of fluids, consume more fruits and fiber, or take a stool softener.

• As appropriate, review all other significant and life-threatening adverse reactions and interactions, especially those related to the drugs mentioned above.

colestipol hydrochloride
Colestid

Pharmacologic class: Bile acid sequestrant
Therapeutic class: Antihyperlipidemic
Pregnancy risk category NR

Action

Binds bile acids in GI tract and forms insoluble complex, impeding bile acid reabsorption and promoting its excretion. As a result, cholesterol and low-density lipoprotein levels decrease.

Availability

Granules for suspension: 5 g/packet or scoop
Tablets: 1 g

🕖 Indications and dosages

➢ Primary hypercholesterolemia
Adults: *Granules*—5 g P.O. once or twice daily; may increase q 1 to 2 months up to 30 g/day P.O. given in one or two divided doses. *Tablets*—2 g P.O. once or twice daily; may increase q 1 to 2 months up to 16 g/day P.O. given in one or two divided doses.

Off-label uses

• Digoxin toxicity

Contraindications

• Hypersensitivity to drug

Precautions

Use cautiously in:
• history of constipation
• breastfeeding patients
• children (safety and efficacy not established).

Administration

• Mix granules with at least 90 ml of liquid, and stir until completely mixed.
• Give tablets with large amount of water.
• Administer other drugs 1 hour before or 4 hours after colestipol.

Route	Onset	Peak	Duration
P.O.	24-48 hr	1 mo	1 mo

Adverse reactions

CNS: dizziness, headache, vertigo, anxiety, syncope, fatigue
CV: chest pain
GI: nausea, vomiting, constipation, abdominal discomfort, fecal impaction, flatulence, fatty stools, hemorrhoids, perianal irritation, tongue irritation

Metabolic: deficiency of vitamins A, D, E, and K and folic acid, **hyperchloremic acidosis**
Musculoskeletal: osteoporosis, backache, muscle and joint pain, arthritis
Skin: irritation, rashes

Interactions
Drug-drug. *Amiodarone, corticosteroids, digoxin, diuretics, fat-soluble vitamins (A, D, E, K), folic acid, gemfibrozil, imipramine, methotrexate, mycophenolate, nonsteroidal anti-inflammatory drugs, penicillin G, phosphates, propranolol, tetracyclines, thyroid preparations, ursodiol:* decreased absorption of these drugs (when given orally)
Drug-diagnostic tests. *Alanine aminotransferase, alkaline phosphatase, aspartate aminotransferase, phosphorus:* increased levels
Prothrombin time: prolonged

Patient monitoring
• Monitor lipid levels frequently during first few months of therapy and periodically thereafter.
• Evaluate patient for signs and symptoms of abnormal bleeding.
• Be aware that prolonged use may increase bleeding tendency (from hypoprothrombinemia resulting from vitamin K deficiency). As prescribed and needed, give oral or parenteral vitamin K to reverse this effect.

Patient teaching
• Instruct patient to take granules with 3 to 4 oz of water, fruit juice, soup with high fluid content, cereal, or pulpy fruits (crushed).
• Tell patient to swallow tablets whole, one at a time, and not to crush, cut, or chew them.
• Inform patient that drug may interfere with absorption of many other drugs. Advise him to take other drugs 1 hour before or 4 hours after colestipol.
• As appropriate, review all other significant and life-threatening adverse reactions and interactions, especially those related to the drugs and tests mentioned above.

crizotinib
Xalkori

Pharmacologic class: Receptor tyrosine kinase inhibitor
Therapeutic class: Antineoplastic
Pregnancy risk category D

Action
Inhibits receptor tyrosine kinases, including ALK, hepatocyte growth factor receptor, and recepteur d'origine nantais. Translocations can affect the ALK gene, resulting in expression of oncogenic fusion proteins. Formation of ALK fusion proteins results in activation and dysregulation of the gene's expression and signaling, which can contribute to increased cell proliferation and survival in tumors expressing these proteins.

Availability
Capsules: 200 mg, 250 mg

ⓘ Indications and dosages
➤ Anaplastic lymphoma kinase-positive locally advanced or metastatic non-small-cell lung cancer (NSCLC)
Adults: 250 mg P.O. b.i.d. Dosing interruption or reduction to 200 mg P.O. b.i.d. may be required based on individual safety and tolerability; then 250 mg P.O. daily if further reduction is necessary.

Dosage adjustment
• Hepatotoxicity
• Hematologic toxicities
• Grade 3 QT interval prolongation

Contraindications
None

Precautions
Use cautiously in:
• hepatic impairment, severe renal impairment (creatinine clearance less than 30 ml/minute), end-stage renal disease
• congenital long QT syndrome (avoid use), congestive heart failure, brady-arrhythmias, electrolyte abnormalities, pulmonary disease
• concurrent use of drugs known to prolong QT interval (such as alfuzosin, amiodarone, ibutilide, or quetiapine)
• concurrent use of moderate CYP3A inhibitors
• concurrent use of strong CYP3A inducers or inhibitors (avoid use)
• concurrent use of CYP3A substrates with narrow therapeutic indices (avoid use)
• grapefruit, grapefruit juice, St. John's wort (avoid use)
• pregnant or breastfeeding patients
• children (safety and efficacy not established).

Administration
• Be aware that detection of ALK-positive NSCLC using an FDA-approved test is necessary before starting drug.
• Administer with or without food. Don't crush, dissolve, or open capsules.

Route	Onset	Peak	Duration
P.O.	Unknown	4-6 hr	Unknown

Adverse reactions
CNS: headache, fatigue, dizziness, neuropathy, insomnia
CV: bradycardia, **prolonged QT interval**
EENT: vision disorder
GI: nausea, vomiting, diarrhea, constipation, abdominal pain, esophageal disorder, stomatitis
GU: complex renal cysts
Hematologic: neutropenia, thrombocytopenia, lymphopenia
Hepatic: hepatotoxicity
Musculoskeletal: arthralgia, back pain
Respiratory: upper respiratory tract infection, dyspnea, cough, **pneumonia, pulmonary embolism**
Skin: rash
Other: edema, chest pain or discomfort, fever, decreased appetite, dysgeusia

Interactions
Drug-drug. *CYP3A substrates with narrow therapeutic indices (such as alfentanil, cyclosporine, dihydroergotamine, ergotamine, fentanyl, pimozide, quinidine, sirolimus, tacrolimus):* inhibited metabolism of these drugs, leading to potential for serious adverse reactions
Moderate CYP3A inhibitors (such as diltiazem): possible increased crizotinib plasma concentration
Strong CYP3A inducers (including but not limited to carbamazepine, phenobarbital, phenytoin, rifabutin, rifampin): decreased crizotinib plasma concentration
Strong CYP3A inhibitors (such as atazanavir, clarithromycin, indinavir, itraconazole, ketoconazole, nefazodone, nelfinavir, ritonavir, saquinavir, telithromycin, troleandomycin, voriconazole): increased crizotinib plasma concentration
Drug-diagnostic tests. *ALT, AST:* increased levels
Lymphocytes, neutrophils, platelets: decreased levels
Drug-food. *Grapefruit, grapefruit juice:* increased crizotinib plasma concentration
High-fat meal: decreased crizotinib area under the curve and C_{max}.
Drug-herbs. *St. John's wort:* decreased crizotinib plasma concentration

---

🍁 Canada   ⊕ UK   ☢ Hazardous drug   ⊗ High-alert drug

Patient monitoring

🔊 Monitor liver function tests (including ALT and total bilirubin) monthly and as clinically indicated, with more frequent testing in patients who develop transaminase elevations. Temporarily suspend drug, reduce dosage, or permanently discontinue drug as indicated.

• Monitor CBC with differential and renal function tests closely.

🔊 Monitor patient for pulmonary signs and symptoms indicative of pneumonitis; permanently discontinue drug in patients diagnosed with treatment-related pneumonitis.

🔊 Consider periodic ECGs and electrolyte monitoring in patients who have QT-interval prolongation or predisposition for QT-interval prolongation, or who are taking drugs known to prolong QT interval. Withhold drug in patients with Grade 3 QT-interval prolongation until recovery to Grade 1 or less; then resume at prescribed reduced dosage. Permanently discontinue drug if Grade 3 QT-interval prolongation recurs and in patients with Grade 4 QT-interval prolongation.

Patient teaching

• Tell patient to take drug with or without food, to avoid grapefruit and grapefruit juice, and not to crush, dissolve, or open capsules.

🔊 Instruct patient to immediately report signs and symptoms of liver disorder (such as weakness, fatigue, nausea, vomiting, right upper abdominal pain, jaundice, yellowing of skin or eyes, or dark urine).

🔊 Instruct patient to immediately report swelling of hands or feet, abnormal heartbeats, dizziness, or faintness.

• Inform patient that visual changes, such as perceived flashes of light, blurry vision, light sensitivity, and floaters, may occur and to report flashes or floaters to prescriber.

• Caution patient to use caution while driving and performing other hazardous activities, because of the risk of developing a vision disorder, dizziness, or fatigue while taking drug.

• Instruct patient to tell prescriber about all drugs he's taking, because some drugs have potential for serious drug interactions and shouldn't be taken with crizotinib.

• Advise patient not to use St. John's wort or other herbal supplements without consulting prescriber.

• Advise female patient of childbearing age to avoid becoming pregnant during treatment.

• Advise breastfeeding patient that she should decide whether to discontinue breastfeeding or discontinue drug, taking into account importance of drug for her treatment.

• As appropriate, review all other significant and life-threatening adverse reactions and interactions, especially those related to the drugs, tests, foods, and herbs mentioned above.

cromolyn sodium
Apo-Cromolyn✤, Gastrocrom, Nalcrom✤⊛, Nasalcrom, Nu-Cromolyn✤, Solu-Crom✤

Pharmacologic class: Chromone derivative
Therapeutic class: Mast cell stabilizer, antiasthmatic, ophthalmic decongestant
Pregnancy risk category B

Action

Inhibits release of histamine and reacting substances of anaphylaxis from mast cells, stabilizing the cell membrane and reducing the allergic response and inflammatory reaction

---

Availability
Nasal solution: 40 mg/ml (5.2 mg/spray) in 13-ml container (100 sprays) or 26-ml container (200 sprays)
Ophthalmic solution: 4%
Oral solution: 100 mg/5 ml
Solution for nebulization: 10 mg/ml

⃠ Indications and dosages
➤ Mastocytosis
Adults and children ages 13 and older: 200 mg P.O. q.i.d.
Children ages 2 to 12: 100 mg P.O. q.i.d.
➤ Vernal keratoconjunctivitis, vernal conjunctivitis, and vernal keratitis
Adults and children ages 4 and older: One to two drops of ophthalmic solution in each eye four to six times daily at regular intervals
➤ To prevent and relieve nasal symptoms of hay fever and other nasal allergies
Adults and children ages 2 and older: Spray once into each nostril. To prevent nasal allergy symptoms, use up to 1 week before contact with cause of allergy. To relieve nasal symptoms, repeat three to four times daily q 4 to 6 hours. If needed, may use up to six times per day. Use every day while in contact with allergen.
➤ Prevention of acute bronchospasm
Adults and children ages 2 and older: 20 mg q.i.d. via nebulization at regular intervals or no more than 1 hour before exposure to triggering event
➤ Management of bronchial asthma
Adults and children ages 2 and older: 20 mg via nebulization q.i.d. at regular intervals

Off-label uses
• Proctitis
• Ulcerative colitis
• Urticaria

Contraindications
• Hypersensitivity to drug
• Status asthmaticus

Precautions
Use cautiously in:
• renal or hepatic impairment, acute bronchospasm attacks
• pregnant or breastfeeding patients
• children younger than age 5.

Administration
• Administer oral form 30 minutes before meals and at bedtime.
• Before using nasal spray, have patient clear nasal passages by blowing nose.
• Don't expose solutions to direct sunlight.

Route	Onset	Peak	Duration
P.O., nasal, ophthalmic	<1 wk	2-4 wk	Unknown

Adverse reactions
CNS: headache, drowsiness, dizziness
EENT: nasal irritation, sneezing, epistaxis, postnasal drip (with nasal solution); stinging of eyes, lacrimation (with ophthalmic solution)
GI: nausea, diarrhea, stomachache, swollen parotid glands
GU: difficult or painful urination, urinary frequency
Musculoskeletal: myopathy
Respiratory: wheezing, cough, **bronchospasm**
Skin: erythema, rash, urticaria, angioedema
Other: altered taste, substernal burning, allergic reactions including **anaphylaxis, serum sickness**

Interactions
None significant

Patient monitoring
• Monitor pulmonary function periodically.

- Evaluate patient for signs and symptoms of overdose, including bronchospasm and difficult or painful urination.

Patient teaching
With nasal form—
- Teach patient how to instill nasal spray as directed.
- Tell patient that drug may cause unpleasant taste, but that rinsing mouth and performing frequent oral care may help. Also inform him that drug may cause headache.
- Advise patient to report increased sneezing; nasal burning, stinging, or irritation; sore throat; hoarseness; or nosebleed.
With oral form—
- Tell patient to take oral form 30 minutes before meals.
With ophthalmic form—
- Instruct patient to wash hands before using.
- Teach patient how to instill drops: Instruct him to tilt his head back and look up, place drops inside lower eyelid, close his eye, and roll eyeball in all directions. Tell him not to blink for about 30 seconds, and then to apply gentle pressure to inner corner of eye for 30 seconds.
- Caution patient not to let applicator tip touch eye or any other surface.
- Tell patient drug may cause temporary stinging of eye or blurred vision.
- Advise patient not to wear contact lenses during therapy.
With all forms—
- As appropriate, review all other significant adverse reactions.

cyclobenzaprine hydrochloride
Amrix, Apo-Cyclobenzaprine✚, Dom-Cyclobenzaprine✚, Fexmid, Flexeril, Novo-Cycloprine✚ PHL-Cyclobenzaprine✚, PMS-Cyclobenzaprine✚, Ratio-Cyclobenzaprine✚, Riva-Cyclobenzaprine✚

Pharmacologic class: Autonomic nervous system drug
Therapeutic class: Skeletal muscle relaxant (centrally acting)
Pregnancy risk category B

Action
Unclear. Thought to act primarily at brain stem (and to a lesser extent at spinal cord level) to relieve skeletal muscle spasms of local origin without altering muscle function.

Availability
Capsules (extended-release): 15 mg, 30 mg
Tablets: 5 mg, 7.5 mg, 10 mg

⬤ Indications and dosages
➤ Adjunct to rest and physical therapy to relieve muscle spasm associated with acute, painful musculoskeletal conditions
Adults: 5 mg P.O. t.i.d. (immediate-release tablet). May increase to 10 mg P.O. t.i.d. (immediate-release tablet) as needed. Or, 15 mg (extended-release capsule) P.O. daily; some patients may need up to 30 mg/day, given as one 30-mg (extended-release capsule) P.O. daily or two 15-mg (extended-release capsules) P.O. daily.

Contraindications
- Hypersensitivity to drug
- Acute recovery phase after myocardial infarction (MI)

Reactions in **bold** are life-threatening.   ◀€ Clinical alert

- Heart failure
- Arrhythmias
- Hyperthyroidism
- MAO inhibitor use within past 14 days

Precautions
Use cautiously in:
- cardiovascular disease, closed-angle glaucoma, hepatic impairment, increased intraocular pressure, urinary retention
- elderly patients
- pregnant or breastfeeding patients
- children younger than age 15.

Administration
🔊 Don't give within 14 days of MAO inhibitor. Drug interaction may cause hypertensive crisis and severe seizures.
- Give extended-release capsule at approximately the same time each day.
- Know that drug shouldn't be used for more than 3 weeks.
- Be aware that drug may not be first-line agent for elderly patients because of its anticholinergic effects.

Route	Onset	Peak	Duration
P.O. (capsules)	Unknown	7-8 hr	Unknown
P.O. (tablets)	1 hr	4-6 hr	12-24 hr

Adverse reactions
CNS: dizziness, drowsiness, syncope, confusion, fatigue, headache, nervousness, decreased mental acuity, irritability, weakness, insomnia, depression, disorientation, delusions, peripheral neuropathy, abnormal gait, Bell's palsy, EEG changes, extrapyramidal symptoms, **cerebrovascular accident**
CV: vasodilation, tachycardia, chest pain, hypotension, **MI, heart block**
EENT: blurred vision
GI: nausea, constipation, dyspepsia, swollen parotid glands, mouth inflammation, discolored tongue, dry mouth, **paralytic ileus**

GU: galactorrhea, urinary retention, urinary frequency, gynecomastia, testicular swelling, libido changes, erectile dysfunction
Hematologic: purpura, eosinophilia, **bone marrow depression, leukopenia, thrombocytopenia**
Metabolic: hyperglycemia, **hypoglycemia, syndrome of inappropriate diuretic hormone secretion**
Musculoskeletal: muscle ache
Respiratory: dyspnea
Skin: photosensitization, alopecia, angioedema
Other: unpleasant taste, weight gain or loss, edema

Interactions
Drug-drug. *Anticholinergics, anticholinergic-like drugs (including antidepressants, antihistamines, disopyramide, haloperidol, phenothiazines):* additive anticholinergic effects
Antihistamines, CNS depressants, opioids, sedative-hypnotics: additive CNS depression
Guanadrel, guanethidine: reduction in or blockage of these drugs' actions
MAO inhibitors: hyperpyretic crisis, seizures, death
Drug-herbs. *Chamomile, hops, kava, skullcap, valerian:* increased CNS depression
Drug-behaviors. *Alcohol use:* increased CNS depression

Patient monitoring
- Assess for adverse CNS effects, such as drowsiness, dizziness, and decreased mental acuity.
- Monitor patient for evidence of drug interactions, especially when giving drug with CNS depressants.

Patient teaching
- Tell patient to take extended-release capsule at approximately the same time each day.
- Tell patient that drug may cause dry mouth.

• Caution patient to avoid driving and other hazardous activities until he knows how drug affects concentration, alertness, and vision.
• Advise patient not to use alcohol, sedatives, pain medications, over-the-counter preparations, or herbs without consulting prescriber.
• As appropriate, review all other significant and life-threatening adverse reactions and interactions, especially those related to the drugs, herbs, and behaviors mentioned above.

cyclophosphamide
Endoxana⊕, Procytox✤

Pharmacologic class: Alkylating agent, nitrogen mustard
Therapeutic class: Antineoplastic
Pregnancy risk category D

Action
Unclear. Thought to prevent cell division by cross-linking DNA strands, thereby interfering with growth of susceptible cancer cells.

Availability
Powder for injection: 500 mg, 1 g, 2 g
Tablets: 25 mg, 50 mg

Indications and dosages
➤ Hodgkin's disease; malignant lymphoma; multiple myeloma; leukemia; advanced mycosis fungoides; neuroblastoma; ovarian cancer; breast cancer; and certain other tumors
Adults: Initially, 40 to 50 mg/kg I.V. in divided doses over 2 to 5 days, or 10 to 15 mg/kg I.V. q 10 days, or 3 to 5 mg/kg I.V. twice weekly.
Children: Initially, 2 to 8 mg/kg or 60 to 250 mg/m² P.O. or I.V. daily in divided doses for 6 or more days.

Maintenance dosage is 2 to 5 mg/kg or 50 to 150 mg/m² P.O. twice weekly.
➤ Biopsy-proven nephrotic syndrome in children
Children: 2.5 to 3 mg/kg/day P.O. for 60 to 90 days

Off-label uses
• Severe rheumatologic conditions
• Selected cases of severe progressive rheumatoid arthritis and systemic lupus erythematosus

Contraindications
• Hypersensitivity to drug
• Severe bone marrow depression

Precautions
Use cautiously in:
• renal or hepatic impairment, adrenalectomy, mild to moderate bone marrow depression, other chronic debilitating illnesses
• females of childbearing age
• pregnant patients
• breastfeeding patients (use not recommended).

Administration
• Verify that patient isn't pregnant before administering.
• Follow facility procedures for safe handling, administration, and disposal of chemotherapeutic drugs.
• Administer tablets on empty stomach. If drug causes severe GI upset, give with food.
• Don't cut or crush tablets.
• Know that dosage may need to be decreased if drug is given with other antineoplastics.
• Dilute each 100 mg of powder with 5 ml of sterile water for injection, to yield 20 mg/ml. Further dilute with compatible fluid, such as 5% dextrose injection, 5% dextrose and normal saline solution for injection, 5% dextrose and Ringer's injection, lactated Ringer's injection, or half-normal saline solution for injection.

• For I.V. injection, give each 100 mg over at least 1 minute. When giving dosages above 500 mg diluted in 100 to 250 ml of compatible solution, administer over 20 to 60 minutes.

• Use solution prepared with bacteriostatic water for injection within 24 hours if stored at room temperature or within 6 days if refrigerated.

• To minimize bladder toxicity, increase patient's fluid intake during therapy and for 1 to 2 days afterward. Most adults require fluid intake of at least 2 L/day.

Route	Onset	Peak	Duration
P.O., I.V.	7 days	7-15 days	21 days

Adverse reactions

CV: **cardiotoxicity**
GI: nausea, vomiting, diarrhea, abdominal pain or discomfort, stomatitis, oral mucosal ulcers, anorexia, **hemorrhagic colitis**
GU: urinary bladder fibrosis, hematuria, amenorrhea, decreased sperm count, sterility, **acute hemorrhagic cystitis, renal tubular necrosis, hemorrhagic ureteral inflammation**
Hematologic: anemia, **leukopenia, thrombocytopenia, bone marrow depression, neutropenia**
Hepatic: jaundice
Metabolic: hyperuricemia
Respiratory: **interstitial pulmonary fibrosis**
Skin: nail and pigmentation changes, alopecia
Other: poor wound healing, infections, allergic reactions including **anaphylaxis, secondary cancer**

Interactions

Drug-drug. *Allopurinol, thiazide diuretics:* increased risk of leukopenia
Digoxin: decreased digoxin blood level
Cardiotoxic drugs (such as cytarabine, daunorubicin, doxorubicin): additive cardiotoxicity

Chloramphenicol: prolonged cyclophosphamide half-life
Phenobarbital: increased risk of cyclophosphamide toxicity
Quinolones: decreased antimicrobial effect
Succinylcholine: prolonged neuromuscular blockade
Warfarin: increased anticoagulant effect
Drug-diagnostic tests. *Hemoglobin, platelets, pseudocholinesterase, red blood cells (RBCs), white blood cells:* decreased values
Uric acid: increased level

Patient monitoring

• Assess infusion site for signs of extravasation.

• Monitor hematologic profile to determine degree of hematopoietic suppression. Be aware that leukopenia is an expected drug effect and is used to help determine dosage.

• Monitor urine regularly for RBCs, which may precede hemorrhagic cystitis.

Patient teaching

• Tell patient to take tablets on empty stomach. However, if GI upset occurs, instruct him to take them with food.

🔊 Advise patient to promptly report unusual bleeding or bruising, fever, chills, sore throat, cough, shortness of breath, seizures, lack of menstrual flow, unusual lumps or masses, flank or stomach pain, joint pain, mouth or lip sores, or yellowing of skin or eyes.

• Instruct patient to drink 2 to 3 L of fluids daily (unless prescriber has told him to restrict fluids).

• Tell patient that drug may cause hair loss, but that hair usually grows back after treatment ends.

• Advise female patient to use barrier contraception during therapy and for 1 month afterward.

• Advise breastfeeding women not to breastfeed while taking this drug.

- As appropriate, review all other significant and life-threatening adverse reactions and interactions, especially those related to the drugs and tests mentioned above.

cyclosporine
Apo-Cyclosporine✳, Gengraf, Neoral, Sandimmune, Sandoz Cyclosporine

cyclosporine ophthalmic emulsion
Restasis, Sandimmun⊕

Pharmacologic class: Polypeptide antibiotic
Therapeutic class: Immunosuppressant
Pregnancy risk category C

FDA | BOXED WARNING

- Drug should be prescribed only by physicians experienced in managing systemic immunosuppressive therapy for indicated disease. At doses used for solid-organ transplantation, it should be prescribed only by physicians experienced in immunosuppressive therapy and management of organ transplant recipients. Patient should be managed in facility with adequate laboratory and medical resources. Physician responsible for maintenance therapy should have complete information needed for patient follow-up.
- Neoral may increase susceptibility to infection and neoplasia. In kidney, liver, and heart transplant patients, drug may be given with other immunosuppressants.
- Sandimmune should be given with adrenal corticosteroids but not other immunosuppressants. In transplant patients, increased susceptibility to infection and development of lymphoma and other neoplasms may result from increased immunosuppression.
- Sandimmune and Neoral aren't bioequivalent. Don't use interchangeably without physician supervision.
- In patients receiving Sandimmune soft-gelatin capsules and oral solution, monitor at repeated intervals (due to erratic absorption).

Action
Unclear. Thought to act by specific, reversible inhibition of immunocompetent lymphocytes in G_0-G_1 phase of cell cycle. Preferentially inhibits T lymphocytes; also inhibits lymphokine production. Ophthalmic action is unknown.

Availability
Capsules: 25 mg, 100 mg
Injection: 50 mg/ml
Oral solution: 100 mg/ml
Solution (ophthalmic): 0.05% (0.4 ml in 0.9 ml single-use vial)

⟐ Indications and dosages
➤ Psoriasis
Adults: *Neoral only*—1.25 mg/kg P.O. b.i.d. for 4 weeks. Based on patient response, may increase by 0.5 mg/kg/day once q 2 weeks, to a maximum dosage of 4 mg/kg/day.
➤ Severe active rheumatoid arthritis
Adults: *Neoral only*—1.25 mg/kg P.O. b.i.d. May adjust dosage by 0.5 to 0.75 mg/kg/day after 8 weeks and again after 12 weeks, to a maximum dosage of 4 mg/kg/day. If no response occurs after 16 weeks, discontinue therapy.
Gengraf only—2.5 mg/kg P.O. daily given in two divided doses; after 8 weeks, may increase to a maximum dosage of 4 mg/kg/day.

➤ To prevent organ rejection in kidney, liver, or heart transplantation
Adults and children: *Sandimmune only*—Initially, 15 mg/kg P.O. 4 to 12 hours before transplantation, then daily for 1 to 2 weeks postoperatively. Reduce dosage by 5% weekly to a maintenance level of 5 to 10 mg/kg/day. Or 5 to 6 mg/kg I.V. as a continuous infusion 4 to 12 hours before transplantation.

➤ To increase tear production in patients whose tear production is presumed to be suppressed due to ocular inflammation associated with keratoconjunctivitis sicca
Adults: 1 drop in each eye b.i.d. given 12 hours apart

Off-label uses
• Aplastic anemia
• Atopic dermatitis

Contraindications
• Hypersensitivity to drug and any ophthalmic components
• Rheumatoid arthritis, psoriasis in patients with abnormal renal function, uncontrolled hypertension, cancer (Gengraf, Neoral)
• Active ocular infections (ophthalmic use)

Precautions
Use cautiously in:
• hepatic impairment, renal dysfunction, active infection, hypertension
• herpes keratitis (ophthalmic use)
• pregnant or breastfeeding patients
• children younger than age 16 (safety and efficacy not established for ophthalmic use).

Administration
• For I.V. infusion, dilute as ordered with dextrose 5% in water or 0.9% normal saline solution. Administer over 2 to 6 hours.
• Mix Neoral solution with orange juice or apple juice to improve its taste.

• Dilute Sandimmune oral solution with milk, chocolate milk, or orange juice. Be aware that grapefruit and grapefruit juice affect drug metabolism.
• In postoperative patients, switch to P.O. dosage as tolerance allows.
• Be aware that Sandimmune and Neoral aren't bioequivalent. Don't use interchangeably.
• Before administering eyedrops, invert unit-dose vial a few times to obtain a uniform, white, opaque emulsion.
• Know that eyedrops can be used concomitantly with artificial tears, allowing a 15-minute interval between products.

Route	Onset	Peak	Duration
P.O.	Unknown	1.5-3.5 hr	Unknown
I.V.	Rapid	1-2 hr	Unknown
Ophthal. (undetectable blood levels)			

Adverse reactions
CNS: tremor, headache, confusion, paresthesia, insomnia, anxiety, depression, lethargy, weakness
CV: hypertension, chest pain, **myocardial infarction**
EENT: visual disturbances, hearing loss, tinnitus, rhinitis; (with ophthalmic use) ocular burning, conjunctival hyperemia, discharge, epiphora, eye pain, foreign body sensation, itching, stinging, blurring
GI: nausea, vomiting, diarrhea, constipation, abdominal discomfort, gastritis, peptic ulcer, mouth sores, difficulty swallowing, anorexia, **upper GI bleeding, pancreatitis**
GU: gynecomastia, hematuria, **nephrotoxicity, renal dysfunction, glomerular capillary thrombosis**
Hematologic: anemia, **leukopenia, thrombocytopenia**
Metabolic: hyperglycemia, hypomagnesemia, hyperuricemia, **hyperkalemia, metabolic acidosis**

🍁 Canada   ⊕ UK   ⚛ Hazardous drug   ⊗ High-alert drug

Musculoskeletal: muscle and joint pain
Respiratory: cough, dyspnea, ***Pneumocystis jiroveci* pneumonia**, **bronchospasm**
Skin: acne, hirsutism, brittle fingernails, hair breakage, night sweats
Other: gum hyperplasia, flulike symptoms, edema, fever, weight loss, hiccups, **anaphylaxis**

Interactions

The following interactions pertain to oral and I.V. routes only.
Drug-drug. *Acyclovir, aminoglycosides, amphotericin B, cimetidine, diclofenac, gentamicin, ketoconazole, melphalan, naproxen, ranitidine, sulindac, sulfamethoxazole, tacrolimus, tobramycin, trimethoprim, vancomycin:* increased risk of nephrotoxicity
Allopurinol, amiodarone, bromocriptine, clarithromycin, colchicine, danazol, diltiazem, erythromycin, fluconazole, imipenem and cilastatin, itraconazole, ketoconazole, methylprednisolone, nicardipine, prednisolone, quinupristin/dalfopristin, verapamil: increased cyclosporine blood level
Azathioprine, corticosteroids, cyclophosphamide: increased immunosuppression
Carbamazepine, isoniazid, nafcillin, octreotide, orlistat, phenobarbital, phenytoin, rifabutin, rifampin, ticlopidine: decreased cyclosporine blood level
Digoxin: decreased digoxin clearance
Live-virus vaccines: decreased antibody response to vaccine
Lovastatin: decreased lovastatin clearance, increased risk of myopathy and rhabdomyolysis
Potassium-sparing diuretics: increased risk of hyperkalemia
Drug-diagnostic tests. *Alanine aminotransferase, aspartate aminotransferase, bilirubin, blood urea nitrogen, creatinine, glucose, low-density lipoproteins:* increased levels

Hemoglobin, platelets, white blood cells: decreased values
Drug-food. *Grapefruit, grapefruit juice:* decreased cyclosporine metabolism, increased cyclosporine blood level
High-fat diet: decreased drug absorption (Neoral)
Drug-herbs. *Alfalfa sprouts, astragalus, echinacea, licorice:* interference with immunosuppressant action
St. John's wort: reduced cyclosporine blood level, possibly leading to organ rejection

Patient monitoring

• Observe patient for first 30 to 60 minutes of infusion. Monitor frequently thereafter.
• Monitor cyclosporine blood level, electrolyte levels, and liver and kidney function test results.
• Assess for signs and symptoms of hyperkalemia in patients receiving concurrent potassium-sparing diuretic.

Patient teaching

• Advise patient to dilute Neoral oral solution with orange or apple juice (preferably at room temperature) to improve its flavor.
• Instruct patient to use glass container when taking oral solution. Tell him not to let solution stand before drinking, to stir solution well and then drink all at once, and to rinse glass with same liquid and then drink again to ensure that he takes entire dose.
• Tell patient taking Neoral to avoid high-fat meals, grapefruit, and grapefruit juice.
• Advise patient to dilute Sandimmune oral solution with milk, chocolate milk, or orange juice to improve its flavor.
• Instruct patient to invert vial a few times to obtain a uniform, white, opaque emulsion before using

eyedrops and to discard vial immediately after use.

• Inform patient that eyedrops can be used with artificial tears but to allow 15-minute interval between products.

• Caution patient not to wear contact lenses because of decreased tear production; however, if contact lenses are used, advise patient to remove them before administering eyedrops and to reinsert 15 minutes after administration.

• Inform patient that he's at increased risk for infection. Caution him to avoid crowds and exposure to illness.

• Instruct patient not to take potassium supplements, herbal products, or dietary supplements without consulting prescriber.

• Tell patient he'll need to undergo repeated laboratory testing during therapy.

• As appropriate, review all other significant and life-threatening adverse reactions and interactions, especially those related to the drugs, tests, foods, and herbs mentioned above.

cyproheptadine hydrochloride

Periactin⊕, PMS-Cyproheptadine✿

Pharmacologic class: Piperidine (nonselective)
Therapeutic class: Antihistamine
Pregnancy risk category B

Action

Antagonizes effects of histamine at histamine$_1$-receptor sites, preventing histamine-mediated responses. Also blocks effects of serotonin, causing increased appetite.

Availability

Syrup: 2 mg/5 ml
Tablets: 4 mg

Indications and dosages

➢ Allergy symptoms caused by histamine release (including seasonal and perennial allergic rhinitis); chronic urticaria; angioedema; dermographism; cold urticaria; adjunctive therapy for anaphylactic reactions
Adults: Initially, 4 mg P.O. q 8 hours. Maintenance dosage is 4 to 20 mg/day in three divided doses, to a maximum dosage of 0.5 mg/kg/day.
Children ages 7 to 14: 2 to 4 mg P.O. q 12 hours. Don't exceed 16 mg/day.
Children ages 2 to 6: 2 mg P.O. q 12 hours. Don't exceed 12 mg/day.

Off-label uses

• Vascular cluster headaches
• Anorexia nervosa
• Cushing's syndrome

Contraindications

• Hypersensitivity to drug
• Alcohol intolerance (syrup only)
• Bladder neck obstruction
• Angle-closure glaucoma
• Ulcer disease
• Symptomatic prostatic hypertrophy
• MAO inhibitor use within past 14 days

Precautions

Use cautiously in:
• hepatic impairment
• elderly patients
• pregnant patients (safety not established)
• breastfeeding patients.

Administration

• Give with food or milk to decrease GI upset.

Route	Onset	Peak	Duration
P.O.	15-60 min	1-2 hr	8 hr

Adverse reactions
CNS: drowsiness, dizziness, excitation (especially in children), fatigue, sedation, hallucinations, disorientation, tremor
CV: palpitations, hypotension, **arrhythmias**
EENT: blurred vision, nasal dryness and congestion, dry throat
GI: constipation, dry mouth
GU: urinary retention, urinary frequency, ejaculatory inhibition, early menses
Respiratory: thickened bronchial secretions
Skin: rash, photosensitivity
Other: weight gain

Interactions
Drug-drug. *CNS depressants (including opioid analgesics, sedative-hypnotics):* increased CNS depression
MAO inhibitors: intensified, prolonged anticholinergic effects
Drug-diagnostic tests. *Allergy skin tests:* false-negative reactions
Drug-behaviors. *Alcohol use:* increased CNS depression

Patient monitoring
• Monitor patient for excessive anticholinergic effects.
• Assess for excessive CNS depression.
• Discontinue drug 4 days before diagnostic skin testing.

Patient teaching
• Advise patient to take drug with food to minimize GI upset.
• Caution patient not to use other CNS depressants, sleep aids, or alcohol during therapy.
• Instruct patient to avoid driving and other hazardous activities until he knows how drug affects concentration and alertness.
• As appropriate, review all other significant and life-threatening adverse reactions and interactions, especially those related to the drugs, tests, and behaviors mentioned above.

cytarabine
Cytosar✷, Cytosar-U,

cytarabine injection, lipid complex
DepoCyt, DepoCyte ⊕

Pharmacologic class: Antimetabolite, pyrimidine analog
Therapeutic class: Antineoplastic
Pregnancy risk category D

FDA | BOXED WARNING

• Drug should be given only by physicians experienced in cancer chemotherapy. For induction therapy, patients should be in facility with adequate resources to monitor drug tolerance and treat drug toxicity. Main toxic effect is bone marrow suppression with leukopenia, thrombocytopenia, and anemia. Less serious toxicities include nausea, vomiting, diarrhea, abdominal pain, oral ulcers, and hepatic dysfunction.
• Prescriber must weigh possible benefit against known toxic effects and should be familiar with complete package insert information.
• Give DepoCyt (liposomal injection) only under supervision of physician experienced with intrathecal cancer chemotherapy, in facility with adequate diagnostic and treatment resources. In all clinical studies, chemical arachnoiditis (manifested mainly by nausea, vomiting, headache, and fever) was common adverse event; unless treated, it may be fatal. Patients receiving DepoCyt should receive

---

dexamethasone concurrently to mitigate arachnoiditis symptoms.

Action
Unclear. Cytotoxic effect may stem from inhibition of DNA polymerase by drug's active metabolite.

Availability
Injection (conventional form): 20 mg
Liposomal injection for intrathecal use (sustained-release): 50 mg/5-ml vial
Powder for injection (conventional form): 100 mg, 500 mg, 1g, 2 g

⦸ Indications and dosages
➤ To induce remission of acute non-lymphocytic leukemia
Adults: Injection (conventional form)—100 mg/m²/day by continuous I.V. infusion on days 1 through 7, or 100 mg/m² I.V. q 12 hours on days 1 through 7, given with other antineoplastics
➤ Meningeal leukemia
Adults: Injection (conventional form)—5 to 75 mg/m²/day intrathecally for 4 days, or once q 4 days. Most common dosage is 30 mg/m² q 4 days until cerebrospinal fluid is normal.
➤ Lymphomatous meningitis
Adults: Liposomal injection—50 mg intrathecally q 14 days for two doses (at weeks 1 and 3); then q 14 days for three doses (at weeks 5, 7, and 9), with one additional dose at week 13; then q 28 days for four doses

Contraindications
• Hypersensitivity to drug
• Active meningeal infection (liposomal form)

Precautions
Use cautiously in:
• renal or hepatic disease, active infection, decreased bone marrow reserve, other chronic illnesses
• pregnant or breastfeeding patients.

Administration
• Follow facility procedures for safe handling, administration, and disposal of chemotherapeutic drugs.
• For I.V. injection, reconstitute each 100 mg with 5 ml of diluent (if necessary), and give each 100-mg dose over 1 to 3 minutes. For I.V. infusion, dilute further with 50 to 100 ml of dextrose 5% in water or normal saline solution, and infuse over 30 minutes to 24 hours (depending on dosage and concentration).
• Be aware that conventional and liposomal forms can be administered intrathecally.
◀€ Don't use intrathecal route for formulations containing benzyl alcohol.
• When giving conventional form intrathecally, reconstitute with autologous spinal fluid or preservative-free normal saline solution for injection. Use immediately.
• Patients receiving intrathecal cytarabine should be treated concurrently with dexamethasone to mitigate symptoms of chemical arachnoiditis.

Route	Onset	Peak	Duration
I.V.	Unknown	Unknown	Unknown
Intrathecal	Rapid	5 hr	14-28 hr

Adverse reactions
CNS: malaise, dizziness, headache, neuritis, **neurotoxicity, chemical arachnoiditis**
CV: chest pain, **thrombophlebitis**
EENT: conjunctivitis, **visual disturbances including permanent blindness (with liposomal form)**
GI: nausea, vomiting, diarrhea, abdominal pain, anal ulcers, esophagitis, esophageal ulcers, oral ulcers (in 5 to 10 days), anorexia, **bowel necrosis**
GU: urinary retention, **renal dysfunction**

✦ Canada   ⊕ UK   ☙ Hazardous drug   ⊗ High-alert drug

Hematologic: anemia, **megaloblastosis, reticulocytopenia, leukopenia, thrombocytopenia**
Hepatic: hepatic dysfunction
Metabolic: hyperuricemia
Musculoskeletal: muscle ache, bone pain
Respiratory: pneumonia, shortness of breath
Skin: rash, pruritus, freckling, skin ulcers, urticaria, alopecia
Other: flulike symptoms, edema, infection, fever, cellulitis at injection site, **anaphylaxis, infection (mild to fatal)**

Interactions

Drug-drug. *Digoxin:* decreased digoxin blood level
Fluorocytosine: decreased fluorocytosine blood level
Gentamicin: decreased gentamicin effects
Drug-diagnostic tests. *Hemoglobin, platelets, red blood cells, reticulocytes, white blood cells:* decreased values
Megaloblasts, uric acid: increased levels

Patient monitoring

• Observe for signs and symptoms of cytarabine syndrome (malaise, fever, muscle ache, bone pain, occasional chest pain, maculopapular rash, and conjunctivitis).
◀ When giving liposomal form, assess for signs and symptoms of chemical arachnoiditis, such as neck rigidity and pain, nausea, vomiting, headache, fever, and back pain.
• Monitor liver function test results, CBC with differential, platelet count, blood urea nitrogen, and serum creatinine and uric acid levels.
◀ Observe closely for signs and symptoms of infection, which could become severe and fatal.

Patient teaching

◀ Tell patient to contact prescriber immediately if he develops signs or symptoms of infection, cytarabine

syndrome (malaise, fever, muscle ache, bone pain, chest pain, rash, eye infection), or chemical arachnoiditis (neck rigidity or pain, nausea, vomiting, headache, fever, or back pain).
◀ Tell patient that drug makes him more susceptible to infection. Advise him to avoid crowds and exposure to illness.
• Advise patient to increase fluid intake, to promote uric acid excretion.
• As appropriate, review all other significant and life-threatening adverse reactions and interactions, especially those related to the drugs and tests mentioned above.

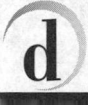

dacarbazine
DTIC✙, DTIC-Dome

Pharmacologic class: Alkylating drug, triazene
Therapeutic class: Antineoplastic
Pregnancy risk category C

FDA BOXED WARNING

• Give under supervision of physician experienced in cancer chemotherapy.
• Hematopoietic depression is most common toxicity; hepatic necrosis has also occurred.
• Drug is carcinogenic and teratogenic in animals.
• Prescriber must weigh potential benefit against toxicity risk.

Action
Unclear. Thought to inhibit DNA synthesis by acting as purine analog. Also causes alkylation and may interact with sulfhydryl groups.

Availability
Injection: 100-mg and 200-mg vials

⚡ Indications and dosages
➤ Hodgkin's disease
Adults: 150 mg/m² I.V. daily for 5 days in combination with other drugs, repeated q 4 weeks. Or 375 mg/m² I.V. on first day of combination therapy, repeated q 15 days.
➤ Metastatic malignant melanoma
Adults: 2 to 4.5 mg/kg I.V. daily for 10 days, repeated q 4 weeks. Or 250 mg/m² I.V. daily for 5 days, repeated q 3 weeks.

Off-label uses
• Malignant pheochromocytoma

Contraindications
• Hypersensitivity to drug

Precautions
Use cautiously in:
• hepatic dysfunction, impaired bone marrow function
• pregnant or breastfeeding patients
• children.

Administration
• Follow facility procedures for safe handling, administration, and disposal of chemotherapeutic drugs.
• Reconstitute with sterile water for injection according to manufacturer's directions.
• Further dilute reconstituted drug with 5% dextrose in water or normal saline solution.
◀€ Administer over 30 to 60 minutes by I.V. infusion only.
◀€ Take steps to prevent extravasation, which may cause tissue damage and severe pain.

Route	Onset	Peak	Duration
I.V.	Unknown	Unknown	Unknown

Adverse reactions
CNS: malaise, paresthesia
GI: nausea, vomiting, dyspepsia, anorexia

Hematologic: anemia, **leukopenia, thrombocytopenia, bone marrow depression**
Musculoskeletal: myalgia
Skin: dermatitis, erythematous or urticarial rash, alopecia, flushing, photosensitivity
Others: flulike symptoms, fever, **hypersensitivity reactions** including **anaphylaxis**

Interactions
Drug-diagnostic tests. *Platelets, red blood cells, white blood cells:* decreased counts
Drug-behaviors. *Sun exposure:* photosensitivity reaction

Patient monitoring
◀€ Frequently monitor CBC with white cell differential and platelet count. Know that hematopoietic depression is the most common toxicity and can be fatal.
• Assess infusion site closely for extravasation.

Patient teaching
◀€ Instruct patient to immediately report pain, burning, or swelling at infusion site; numbness in arms or legs; gait changes; respiratory distress; difficulty breathing; rash; or easy bruising or bleeding.
• Advise patient to minimize GI distress by eating small, frequent servings of healthy food and drinking plenty of fluids.
• Tell patient he'll undergo regular blood testing during therapy.
• As appropriate, review all other significant and life-threatening adverse reactions and interactions, especially those related to the tests and behaviors mentioned above.

dalfampridine
Ampyra

Pharmacologic class: Potassium channel blocker
Therapeutic class: Multiple sclerosis agent
Pregnancy risk category C

Action
Unknown. May increase conduction of action potentials in demyelinated axons through inhibition of potassium channels.

Availability
Tablets (extended release): 10 mg

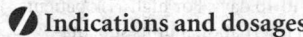 Indications and dosages
➤ To improve walking in patients with multiple sclerosis
Adults: 10 mg P.O. q 12 hours

Dosage adjustments
• Mild renal impairment

Contraindications
• History of seizures
• Moderate or severe renal impairment

Precautions
Use cautiously in:
• mild renal impairment
• pregnant or breastfeeding patients
• children younger than age 18 (safety and efficacy not established).

Administration
• Check creatinine clearance before starting drug.
• Administer with or without food.

Route	Onset	Peak	Duration
P.O.	Unknown	3-4 hr	Unknown

Adverse reactions
CNS: insomnia, dizziness, headache, asthenia, balance disorder, paresthesia, **seizures**
EENT: nasopharyngitis, pharyngolaryngeal pain
GI: nausea, constipation, dyspepsia
GU: urinary tract infection
Musculoskeletal: back pain
Other: multiple sclerosis relapse

Interactions
None

Patient monitoring
◀≣ Discontinue drug if seizure occurs.
• Monitor renal function tests regularly (especially creatinine clearance).

Patient teaching
• Instruct patient to take drug with or without food.
• Instruct patient to swallow tablet whole and not to break, crush, chew, or dissolve it.
◀≣ Advise patient to discontinue drug and immediately report to prescriber if seizures occur.
• Instruct patient to promptly report urinary tract problems.
• As appropriate, review all other significant and life-threatening adverse reactions.

dalteparin sodium
Fragmin

Pharmacologic class: Low-molecular-weight heparin
Therapeutic class: Anticoagulant
Pregnancy risk category B

FDA | BOXED WARNING

• Epidural or spinal hematomas may occur in patients who are anticoagulated with low-molecular-weight heparins or heparinoids and are receiving neuraxial anesthesia or undergoing spinal puncture. These hematomas may result in long-term or permanent paralysis. Consider these risks when scheduling patients for spinal procedures. Risk increases with use of indwelling epidural catheters, concomitant use of drugs affecting hemostasis (such as nonsteroidal anti-inflammatory drugs, platelet inhibitors, or other anticoagulants), traumatic or repeated epidural or spinal puncture, or history of spinal deformity or spinal surgery.

• Monitor patient frequently for signs and symptoms of neurologic impairment. If these occur, provide urgent treatment.

• Consider benefits and risks before neuraxial intervention in patients anticoagulated or to be anticoagulated for thromboprophylaxis.

Action
Inhibits thrombus and clot formation by blocking factor Xa and thrombin

Availability
Solution for injection (prefilled syringes): 12,500 units/0.5 ml, 15,000 units/0.6 ml, 18,000 units/0.72 ml, 5,000 units/0.2 ml, 7,500 units/0.3 ml, 10,000 units/0.4 ml
Solution for injection (multidose vials): 95,000 units/3.8 ml, 95,000 units/ 9.5 ml
Solution for injection (single-dose graduated syringe): 10,000 units/1 ml

⏀ Indications and dosages
➤ Extended treatment of symptomatic venous thromboembolism (VTE), including proximal deep vein thrombosis (DVT) and pulmonary embolism (PE) to reduce recurrence of VTE in patients with cancer
Adults: Recommended dosing: for first 30 days of treatment, give 200 international units/kg total body weight subcutaneously once daily. Give at dose of approximately 150 international units/kg subcutaneously once daily during months 2 through 6. Safety and efficacy beyond 6 months not established. Total daily dose shouldn't exceed 18,000 international units.

➤ To prevent DVT, which can lead to PE in patients undergoing hip and abdominal surgery who are at risk for thromboembolic complications
Adults: *Abdominal surgery*—2,500 international units subcutaneously 1 to 2 hours before surgery; then once daily for 5 to 10 days. For high-risk patients, 5,000 international units subcutaneously on evening before surgery; then once daily for 5 to 10 days. For cancer patients, 2,500 international units subcutaneously 1 to 2 hours before surgery; repeat dose 12 hours later, then give 5,000 international units subcutaneously every day for 5 to 10 days.

Hip replacement surgery—5,000 international units subcutaneously 10 to 14 hours before surgery; repeat dose 4 to 8 hours after surgery, then give 5,000 international units daily for 5 to 10 days. Or, 2,500 international units subcutaneously within 2 hours before surgery, followed by 2,500 international units subcutaneously 4 to 8 hours after surgery (allowing at least 6 hours between doses), followed by 5,000 international units subcutaneously daily for 5 to 10 days. Or, 2,500 international units subcutaneously 4 to 8 hours after surgery, followed by 5,000 international units subcutaneously daily for 5 to 10 days.

➤ Patients with severely restricted mobility during acute illness

Adults: 5,000 international units subcutaneously daily for 12 to 14 days

➤ Extended treatment of symptomatic venous thromboembolism in patients with cancer

Adults: For first 30 days of treatment, 200 international units/kg subcutaneously daily. Total daily dosage shouldn't exceed 18,000 international units. Give approximately 150 international units/kg subcutaneously daily during months 2 through 6. Total daily dosage shouldn't exceed 18,000 international units.

➤ To prevent ischemic complications in patients with unstable angina and non-Q-wave myocardial infarction

Adults: 120 international units/kg (not to exceed 10,000 international units) subcutaneously q 12 hours (concurrently with aspirin P.O.) for 5 to 8 days

Dosage adjustment
• Renal insufficiency
• Thrombocytopenia

Off-label uses
• Systemic anticoagulation

Contraindications
• Hypersensitivity to drug, heparin, pork products, sulfites, or benzyl alcohol
• Active major bleeding
• Thrombocytopenia
• Patients with unstable angina or non-Q-wave myocardial infarction who are undergoing regional anesthesia; cancer patients with symptomatic VTE who are undergoing regional anesthesia

Precautions
Use cautiously in:
• bacterial endocarditis, bleeding disorders, hemorrhagic stroke, severe uncontrolled hypertension, GI ulcer,

severe renal or hepatic insufficiency, hypertensive or diabetic retinopathy
• history of thrombocytopenia from heparin use
• history of congenital or acquired bleeding disorder
• recent CNS or ophthalmologic surgery
• recent GI disease
• spinal or epidural anesthesia
• pregnant or breastfeeding patients
• children (safety not established).

Administration
◀ɛ Know that dalteparin sodium is a high-alert drug.
◀ɛ Administer by subcutaneous route only. Don't give by I.M. or I.V. route.
• To minimize bruising at injection site, massage site with ice before giving injection.
• To give subcutaneous injection, have patient either sit up or lie down. Inject in U-shaped area around navel, upper outer side of thigh, or upper outer quadrangle of buttock. Rotate injection sites daily.
• Don't use interchangeably with heparin or other low-molecular-weight heparins.

Route	Onset	Peak	Duration
Subcut.	20-60 min	3-5 hr	12 hr

Adverse reactions
Hematologic: anemia, ecchymosis, **bleeding, thrombocytopenia, hemorrhage**
Skin: rash, urticaria
Other: pain, irritation, and hematoma at injection site; fever; edema

Interactions
Drug-drug. *Antiplatelet drugs (aspirin, clopidogrel, dipyridamole, ticlopidine), thrombolytics, warfarin:* increased risk of bleeding
Drug-diagnostic tests. *Alanine aminotransferase, aspartate aminotransferase:* increased levels

---

Reactions in **bold** are life-threatening.   ◀ɛ Clinical alert

Platelets: decreased count
Drug-herbs. *Anise, arnica, chamomile, clove, feverfew, garlic, ginger, ginkgo, ginseng:* increased risk of bleeding

Patient monitoring

🔊 Monitor patient for increased risk of bleeding if he's receiving concomitant drugs that affect platelet function.
• Monitor CBC and platelet count.
• Monitor stools for occult blood.

Patient teaching

• Teach patient proper injection technique if self-administering at home.
• Tell patient that drug may cause him to bleed easily. To avoid injury, advise him to brush teeth with soft toothbrush, use electric razor, and avoid scissors and sharp knives.
🔊 Advise patient to immediately report bleeding, bruising, dizziness, light-headedness, itching, rash, fever, swelling, or difficulty breathing.
• As appropriate, review all other significant and life-threatening adverse reactions and interactions, especially those related to the drugs, tests, and herbs mentioned above.

dantrolene sodium

Dantrium, Dantrium Intravenous

Pharmacologic class: Hydantoin derivative

Therapeutic class: Skeletal muscle relaxant (direct-acting), malignant hyperthermia agent

Pregnancy risk category C

FDA | BOXED WARNING

• Drug may be hepatotoxic and should be used only for recommended conditions. Daily doses of 400 mg are less likely to cause fatal and nonfatal hepatitis than daily doses above 800 mg. Overt hepatitis is most common during months 3 and 12, but may occur at any time; females, patients older than age 35, and those receiving concurrent therapy are at higher risk. Use only in conjunction with liver monitoring. Monitor liver function at baseline and regularly during therapy. Discontinue drug if values are abnormal.
• Use lowest possible effective dose. If no benefit occurs after 45 days, discontinue.

Action

Relaxes skeletal muscle by affecting excitation-contraction coupling response at site beyond myoneural junction, probably by interfering with calcium release from sarcoplasmic reticulum

Availability

Capsules: 25 mg, 50 mg, 100 mg
Powder for injection: 20 mg/vial

🕖 Indications and dosages

➤ Chronic spasticity resulting from upper motor neuron disorders, such as multiple sclerosis, cerebral palsy, or spinal cord injury
Adults: Initially, 25 mg P.O. daily, increased gradually in 25-mg increments, if needed, up to 100 mg two or three times daily, to a maximum dosage of 400 mg P.O. daily. Maintain dosage level for 4 to 7 days to gauge patient response.
Children: Initially, 0.5 mg/kg P.O. daily for 7 days, increased to 0.5 mg/kg P.O. t.i.d. for 7 days; then 1 mg/kg P.O. t.i.d. for 7 days; then 2 mg/kg t.i.d., as needed. Don't exceed 100 mg P.O. q.i.d.
➤ Malignant hyperthermic crisis
Adults and children: Initially, 1 mg/kg by I.V. push, repeated as needed up to a cumulative dosage of 10 mg/kg/day

---

➤ To prevent or minimize malignant hyperthermia in patients who require surgery

Adults and children: 4 to 8 mg/kg P.O. daily in three or four divided doses for 1 to 2 days before surgery; give last dose 3 to 4 hours before surgery. Or 2.5 mg/kg I.V. infused over 1 hour before anesthetics are given.

➤ To prevent recurrence of malignant hyperthermic crisis

Adults: 4 to 8 mg/kg daily P.O. in four divided doses for up to 3 days after initial hyperthermic crisis

Off-label uses
• Heat stroke
• Neuroleptic malignant syndrome

Contraindications
• Active hepatic disease (oral form)
• Patients who use spasticity to maintain posture or balance (oral form)
• Breastfeeding

Precautions
Use cautiously in:
• cardiac, hepatic, or respiratory dysfunction or impairment
• women (especially pregnant women)
• adults older than age 35
• children younger than age 5.

Administration
• For I.V. use, add 60 ml of sterile water for injection to each vial; shake until solution is clear. Protect from direct light and use within 6 hours.
• Give therapeutic or emergency dose by rapid I.V. push. Administer follow-up dose over 2 to 3 minutes.
• Prevent extravasation when giving I.V. Drug has high pH and causes tissue irritation.

Route	Onset	Peak	Duration
P.O.	Slow	Unknown	6-12 hr
I.V.	Rapid	Unknown	Unknown

Adverse reactions
CNS: dizziness, drowsiness, fatigue, malaise, weakness, confusion, depression, insomnia, nervousness, headache, light-headedness, speech disturbances, **seizures**

CV: tachycardia, blood pressure fluctuations, phlebitis, **heart failure**

EENT: double vision, excessive tearing

GI: nausea, vomiting, diarrhea, constipation, abdominal cramps, GI reflux and irritation, hematemesis, difficulty swallowing, anorexia, **GI bleeding**

GU: urinary frequency, dysuria, nocturia, urinary incontinence, hematuria, crystalluria, prostatitis

Hematologic: aplastic anemia, leukopenia, thrombocytopenia, lymphocytic lymphoma

Hepatic: hepatitis

Musculoskeletal: myalgia, backache

Respiratory: suffocating sensation, **respiratory depression, pleural effusion with pericarditis**

Skin: rash, urticaria, pruritus, eczema-like eruptions, sweating, photosensitivity, abnormal hair growth

Other: altered taste, chills, fever, edema

Interactions
Drug-drug. *CNS depressants:* increased CNS depression
Estrogen: increased risk of hepatotoxicity
Verapamil (I.V.): cardiovascular collapse (when given with I.V. dantrolene)
Drug-diagnostic tests. *Alanine aminotransferase, alkaline phosphatase, aspartate aminotransferase, bilirubin, blood urea nitrogen:* increased values
Drug-behaviors. *Alcohol use:* increased CNS depression
Sun exposure: phototoxicity

Patient monitoring
• Obtain baseline liver function test results; monitor periodically during therapy.
• Monitor ECG, serum electrolytes, and urine output regularly.

Reactions in **bold** are life-threatening. ◀€ Clinical alert

◀┊ With long-term oral therapy, monitor patient for signs and symptoms of hepatotoxicity. Be prepared to discontinue drug if these occur.

• Assess for muscle weakness, poor coordination, and reduced reflexes before and during therapy. Drug may weaken muscles and impair ambulation.

Patient teaching
◀┊ Instruct patient receiving prolonged oral therapy to immediately report weakness, malaise, fatigue, nausea, rash, itching, severe diarrhea, bloody or black tarry stools, or yellowing of skin or eyes.

• Inform patient that drug may cause drowsiness, dizziness, or light-headedness.

• Caution patient to avoid driving and other hazardous activities until he knows how drug affects concentration and alertness.

• As appropriate, review all other significant and life-threatening adverse reactions and interactions, especially those related to the drugs, tests, and behaviors mentioned above.

darbepoetin alfa
Aranesp

Pharmacologic class: Recombinant human erythropoietin
Therapeutic class: Hematopoietic
Pregnancy risk category C

FDA | BOXED WARNING

• In patients with chronic kidney disease, drug increases risk of death, serious cardiovascular events, and stroke when given to target hemoglobin level above 11 g/dl.

• No trial has identified a hemoglobin target level, darbepoetin alfa dosage, or dosing strategy that doesn't increase these risks.

• Use lowest dose sufficient to reduce need for red blood cell (RBC) transfusions.

• Drug may shorten overall survival or increase risk of tumor progression or recurrence in patients with breast, non-small-cell lung, head and neck, lymphoid, and cervical cancers.

• Prescribers and hospitals must enroll in and comply with the ESA APPRISE Oncology Program to prescribe or dispense this drug to patients with cancer.

• Use drug only for treatment of anemia due to myelosuppressive chemotherapy.

• Drug isn't indicated for patients receiving myelosuppressants when the anticipated outcome is cure.

• Discontinue drug following completion of a chemotherapy course.

Action
Stimulates erythropoiesis in bone marrow, increasing red blood cell production

Availability
Solution for injection: 25 mcg/ml, 40 mcg/ml, 60 mcg/ml, 100 mcg/ml, 200 mcg/ml, 300 mcg/ml, 500 mcg/ml, 150 mcg/0.75 ml in single-dose vials; 25 mcg/0.42ml, 40 mcg/0.4 ml, 60 mcg/0.3 ml, 100 mcg/0.5 ml, 150 mcg/0.3 ml, 200 mcg/0.4 ml, 300 mcg/0.6 ml, 500 mcg/1 ml in single-dose prefilled syringes

⍟ Indications and dosages
➣ Anemia caused by chronic kidney disease (CKD) in patients on dialysis
Adults: Initially, 0.45 mcg/kg I.V. or subcutaneously weekly, or 0.75 mcg/kg I.V. or subcutaneously q 2 weeks
➣ Anemia caused by CKD in patients not on dialysis

Adults: 0.45 mcg/kg I.V. or subcutaneously at 4-week intervals
➤ Chemotherapy-induced anemia in patients with nonmyeloid malignancies
Adults: 2.25 mcg/kg subcutaneously q week, or 500 mcg subcutaneously q 3 weeks.

Contraindications

- Serious allergic reactions to drug
- Uncontrolled hypertension
- Pure red cell aplasia that begins after treatment with darbepoetin alfa or other erythropoietin protein drugs

Precautions

Use cautiously in:
- latex allergy (needle cover of prefilled syringe contains dry natural rubber, a derivative of latex)
- anemia; thalassemia; porphyria; seizures; underlying hematologic disease, including hemolytic and sickle cell anemia
- lack or loss of response to drug
- pregnant or breastfeeding patients
- children.

Administration

- Give by subcutaneous or I.V. injection only. (I.V. route is recommended for patients on hemodialysis.)
- Evaluate iron status for all patients before and during treatment to ensure effective erythropoiesis.
- For patients with CKD on dialysis, start drug when hemoglobin level is less than 10 g/dl. If hemoglobin level approaches or exceeds 11 g/dl, reduce dosage or interrupt therapy.
- For patients with CKD not on dialysis, consider starting drug only when hemoglobin level is less than 10 g/dl and the following considerations apply: Rate of hemoglobin decline indicates likelihood of requiring an RBC transfusion and, reducing risk of alloimmunization or other RBC transfusion-related risks is a goal.

If hemoglobin level exceeds 10 g/dl, reduce dosage or interrupt therapy and use lowest dose sufficient to reduce need for RBC transfusions.
- Don't increase dosage more frequently than once q 4 weeks; dosage decreases can occur more frequently. Avoid frequent dosage adjustments.
- Don't dilute or give with other drug solutions.
- ◄€ Don't shake. Vigorous shaking may denature drug, making it biologically inactive.
- Give single I.V. dose over 1 minute.
- Discard unused portion. (Drug contains no preservative.)

Route	Onset	Peak	Duration
I.V., subcut.	2-6 wk	Unknown	Unknown

Adverse reactions

CNS: dizziness, headache, fatigue, weakness, **seizures, transient ischemic attack, cerebrovascular accident**
CV: hypertension, hypotension, chest pain, peripheral edema, **arrhythmias, heart failure, cardiac arrest, myocardial infarction, vascular access thrombosis**
GI: nausea, vomiting, diarrhea, constipation, abdominal pain
Metabolic: fluid overload
Musculoskeletal: myalgia; joint, back, and limb pain
Respiratory: cough, upper respiratory tract infection, dyspnea, bronchitis
Skin: pruritus
Other: fever, flulike symptoms, infection, pain at injection site

Interactions

None significant

Patient monitoring

- Assess hemoglobin concentration before starting therapy and then weekly during therapy.
- Observe closely for serious CNS and cardiovascular adverse reactions.

• Closely monitor blood pressure and renal function during therapy.
• Know that supplemental iron is recommended for patients with serum ferritin level below 100 mcg/ml or serum transferrin saturation below 20%.

Patient teaching
• Tell patient to report chest pain or other pain, muscle tremors, weakness, and cough or other respiratory symptoms.
• If patient will self-administer drug, tell him to follow exact directions for injection and needle disposal.
• Caution patient to avoid driving and other hazardous activities until he knows how drug affects concentration and alertness.
• Advise patient to minimize GI upset by eating small, frequent servings of healthy food and drinking plenty of fluids.
• Tell patient he'll undergo frequent blood testing during therapy to help determine correct dosage.
• As appropriate, review all other significant and life-threatening adverse reactions.

darifenacin hydrobromide
Emselex✛, Enablex

Pharmacologic class: Anticholinergic
Therapeutic class: Renal and genitourinary agent
Pregnancy risk category C

Action
Competitively antagonizes muscarinic receptors, reducing contractions of urinary bladder smooth muscle

Availability
Tablets (extended-release): 7.5 mg, 15 mg

⚡ Indications and dosages
➤ Overactive bladder with symptoms of urge urinary incontinence, urgency, and frequency
Adults: Initially, 7.5 mg P.O. daily; may increase to 15 mg P.O. daily as early as 2 weeks after therapy begins

Dosage adjustment
• Moderate hepatic impairment
• Concurrent use of potent CYP3A4 inhibitors (such as clarithromycin, itraconazole, ketoconazole, nefazodone, nelfinavir, and ritonavir)

Contraindications
• Hypersensitivity to drug or its components
• Urinary retention, gastric retention, uncontrolled angle-closure glaucoma, or increased risk for these conditions

Precautions
Use cautiously in:
• decreased GI motility (such as severe constipation, ulcerative colitis, or myasthenia gravis), controlled angle-closure glaucoma, hepatic impairment
• pregnant or breastfeeding patients
• children (safety and efficacy not established).

Administration
• Administer tablets whole with liquid (with or without food) once daily.
• Make sure patient doesn't chew, crush, or divide them.
• Know that drug isn't recommended for patients with severe hepatic impairment.

Route	Onset	Peak	Duration
P.O.	Unknown	5.2-7.6 hr	Unknown

Adverse reactions
CNS: dizziness, asthenia
CV: hypertension

EENT: dry eyes, abnormal vision, dry throat, bronchitis, pharyngitis, rhinitis, sinusitis

GI: nausea, vomiting, diarrhea, constipation, abdominal pain, dyspepsia, dry mouth

GU: urinary tract infection or disorder, vaginitis

Musculoskeletal: back pain, arthralgia

Skin: dry skin, rash, pruritus

Other: abnormal taste, weight gain, accidental injury, flulike syndrome, pain, peripheral edema, heat prostration

Interactions

Drug-drug. *Anticholinergics:* increased frequency or severity of adverse reactions

CYP4502D6 inhibitors: increased darifenacin exposure and blood level

Drugs metabolized by CYP2D6 (such as flecainide, thioridazine, and tricyclic antidepressants): increased blood levels of these drugs

Patient monitoring

• Monitor liver function tests frequently; withdraw drug if liver function tests show severe hepatic impairment.

• Monitor urinary function periodically.

Patient teaching

• Instruct patient to take tablets whole with liquid, with or without food. Tell him not to chew, divide, or crush them.

• Inform patient that some over-the-counter products such as antihistamines may increase risk of side effects.

• Caution patient that drug may cause heat prostration; describe signs and symptoms.

• As appropriate, review all other significant adverse reactions and interactions, especially those related to the drugs mentioned above.

darunavir ethanolate
Prezista

Pharmacologic class: Protease inhibitor

Therapeutic class: Antiretroviral

Pregnancy risk category B

Action
Inhibits human immunodeficiency virus-1 (HIV-1) protease, preventing formation of mature virus particles

Availability
Oral suspension: 100 mg/ml
Tablets: 75 mg, 150 mg, 400 mg, 600 mg

Indications and dosages

➤ HIV infection in treatment-naïve and treatment-experienced patients with no darunavir resistance-associated substitutions

Adults: 800 mg (two 400-mg tablets) or 8 ml (two 4-ml doses) oral suspension P.O. with ritonavir 100 mg P.O. daily

➤ HIV infection in treatment-experienced patients with at least one darunavir resistance-associated substitution

Adults: 600 mg (one 600-mg tablet) or 6 ml oral suspension P.O. b.i.d. with ritonavir 100 mg P.O. b.i.d.

➤ HIV infection (with ritonavir and other retrovirals)

Children age 3 to younger than 18 weighing 40 kg (88 lb) or more: 600 mg (tablets) or 6 ml (oral suspension) P.O. b.i.d. with ritonavir 100 mg (capsules or tablets) or 1.25 ml (oral solution) P.O. b.i.d.

Children age 3 to younger than 18 weighing 30 kg (66 lb) to less than 40 kg: 450 mg (tablets) or 4.6 ml (oral suspension) P.O. b.i.d. with ritonavir

60 mg (0.75 ml oral solution) P.O. b.i.d.

Children age 3 to younger than 18 weighing 15 kg (33 lb) to less than 30 kg: 375 mg (tablets) or 3.8 ml (oral suspension) P.O. b.i.d. with ritonavir 50 mg (0.6 ml oral solution) P.O. b.i.d.

Children age 3 to younger than 18 weighing 14 kg (31 lb) to less than 15 kg: 280 mg (2.8 ml oral suspension) P.O. b.i.d. with ritonavir 48 mg (0.6 ml oral solution) P.O. b.i.d.

Children age 3 to younger than 18 weighing 13 kg (29 lb) to less than 14 kg: 260 mg (2.6 ml oral suspension) P.O. b.i.d. with ritonavir 40 mg (0.5 ml oral solution) P.O. b.i.d.

Children age 3 to younger than 18 weighing 12 kg (26 lb) to less than 13 kg: 240 mg (2.4 ml oral suspension) P.O. b.i.d. with ritonavir 40 mg (0.5 ml oral solution) P.O. b.i.d.

Children age 3 to younger than 18 weighing 11 kg (24 lb) to less than 12 kg: 220 mg (2.2 ml oral suspension) P.O. b.i.d. with ritonavir 32 mg (0.4 ml oral solution) P.O. b.i.d.

Children age 3 to younger than 18 weighing 10 kg (22 lb) to less than 11 kg: 200 mg (2 ml oral suspension) P.O. b.i.d. with ritonavir 32 mg (0.4 ml oral solution) P.O. b.i.d.

Children's dosage shouldn't exceed treatment-experienced adult dosage.

Contraindications

• Concurrent administration with drugs (including alfuzosin, cisapride, dihydroergotamine, ergonovine, ergotamine, lovastatin, methylergonovine, midazolam, pimozide, rifampin, sildenafil, simvastatin, terfenadine, triazolam, and St. John's wort)

Precautions

Use cautiously in:
• hypersensitivity to drug or its components (including sulfa)
• severe hepatic impairment (use not recommended)

• diabetes mellitus, hemophilia, hepatic dysfunction or disease
• concurrent use of carbamazepine, phenobarbital, phenytoin (use not recommended)
• elderly patients
• pregnant or breastfeeding patients
• children younger than age 3 (safety and efficacy not established; don't use).

Administration

• Give with ritonavir and food.
• Before administering, assess children weighing 15 kg (33 lb) or more for the ability to swallow tablets. If a child is unable to reliably swallow a tablet, consider using oral suspension. Give 8-ml dose as two 4-ml administrations using the oral dosing syringe included.
🔊 Don't give concurrently with alfuzosin, cisapride, dihydroergotamine, ergonovine, ergotamine, methylergonovine, midazolam, pimozide, rifampin, sildenafil, simvastatin, terfenadine, terfenadine, or St. John's wort.
• Don't use once-daily dosing in children.

Route	Onset	Peak	Duration
P.O.	Unknown	2.5-4 hr	Unknown

Adverse reactions

CNS: asthenia, fatigue, headache, transient ischemic attack, confusion, disorientation, anxiety, irritability, altered mood, memory impairment, vertigo, rigors, peripheral neuropathy, paresthesia, hypoesthesia, somnolence, nightmares
CV: tachycardia, hypertension, **myocardial infarction**
EENT: nasopharyngitis
GI: nausea, vomiting, diarrhea, constipation, abdominal pain, dyspepsia, abdominal distention, flatulence, dry mouth, anorexia
GU: renal insufficiency, nephrolithiasis, polyuria, gynecomastia, **acute renal failure**

Metabolic: diabetes mellitus, polydipsia, obesity

Musculoskeletal: arthralgia, myalgia, extremity pain, osteopenia, osteoporosis

Respiratory: dyspnea, cough

Skin: allergic dermatitis, eczema, inflammation, toxic skin eruption, dermatitis medicamentosa, hyperhidrosis, folliculitis, maculopapular rash, alopecia, **erythema multiforme, Stevens-Johnson syndrome**

Other: body fat redistribution, lipoatrophy, decreased appetite, hiccups, pyrexia, night sweats, hyperthermia, peripheral edema, immune reconstitution syndrome (inflammatory response to indolent or residual opportunistic infections)

Interactions

Drug-drug. *Amiodarone, atorvastatin, bepridil, clarithromycin, cyclosporine, felodipine, fluticasone propionate (inhalation), lidocaine (systemic), nicardipine, nifedipine, pravastatin, quinidine, sildenafil, sirolimus, tacrolimus, tadalafil, trazodone, vardenafil:* increased blood levels of these drugs

Astemizole, cisapride, terfenadine: increased risk of serious or life-threatening reactions (such as arrhythmias)

Carbamazepine, dexamethasone (systemic), phenobarbital, phenytoin, rifampin: decreased darunavir blood level

Efavirenz: decreased blood levels of both drugs

Ergot derivatives (dihydroergotamine, ergonovine, ergotamine, methylergonovine): increased risk of acute ergot toxicity

Hormonal contraceptives: decreased ethinyl estradiol blood level; may decrease contraceptive efficacy

Itraconazole, ketoconazole: increased blood levels of these drugs and darunavir

Lopinavir/ritonavir, saquinavir: decreased effects of these drugs

Lovastatin, pimozide, simvastatin: increased risk of myopathy

Methadone, voriconazole, warfarin: decreased blood levels of these drugs

Midazolam, triazolam: increased risk of respiratory depression or increased sedation

Paroxetine, sertraline: decreased effects of these drugs

Rifabutin: increased rifabutin blood level, decreased darunavir blood level (when given with ritonavir)

Voriconazole: decreased voriconazole and increased darunavir blood levels

Drug-diagnostic tests. *Alanine aminotransferase, alkaline phosphatase, amylase, aspartate aminotransferase, gamma-glutamyltransferase, lipase, lipids, partial thromboplastin time, plasma prothrombin time, total cholesterol, triglycerides, uric acid:* increased levels

Bicarbonate, calcium, lymphocytes, platelets, total absolute neutrophils, white blood cells: decreased levels

Bilirubin, serum glucose, sodium: increased or decreased levels

Drug-food. *Any food:* increased drug absorption

Drug-herbs. *St. John's wort:* decreased darunavir blood level

Patient monitoring

• During initial treatment phase, stay alert for immune reconstitution syndrome.

• Monitor liver function studies frequently in patients with preexisting hepatic dysfunction or disease.

• Monitor blood glucose levels frequently in patients with diabetes mellitus.

• Carefully monitor patient receiving antiarrhythmics and HMG-CoA reductase inhibitors while taking this drug.

• Monitor International Normalized Ratio when giving drug with warfarin.

Patient teaching
• Instruct patient to take drug with ritonavir and food, as prescribed.
• Advise patient to inform prescriber of other drugs and supplements he's taking (including vitamins and herbs) before starting drug or taking new medication.
🔊 Urge patient to immediately report side effects (especially rash).
• Emphasize that drug doesn't cure HIV infection.
• Advise patient using hormonal contraceptives to use alternative contraceptive method while taking this drug.
• Advise patients who are pregnant or recently gave birth not to breastfeed because of risk of passing HIV infection to infant and potentially serious adverse drug reactions.
• As appropriate, review all other significant and life-threatening adverse reactions and interactions, especially those related to the drugs, tests, foods, and herbs mentioned above.

dasatinib
Sprycel

Pharmacologic class: Tyrosine kinase inhibitor
Therapeutic class: Antineoplastic
Pregnancy risk category D

Action
Inhibits growth of chronic myeloid leukemia (CML) and acute lymphoblastic leukemia (ALL) cell lines overexpressing BCR-ABL; this inhibition allows bone marrow to resume production of normal red cells, white cells, and platelets.

Availability
Tablets: 20 mg, 50 mg, 70 mg, 80 mg, 100 mg, 140 mg (film-coated)

Indications and dosages
➤ Newly diagnosed Philadelphia chromosome–positive (Ph+) chronic phase of CML
Adults: 100 mg P.O. daily in morning or evening; may increase dosage to 140 mg daily in patients who don't achieve a hematologic or cytogenetic response
➤ Chronic, accelerated or myeloid or lymphoid blast phase Ph+ CML in patients with resistance or intolerance to prior therapy, including imatinib; Philadelphia chromosome–positive acute lymphoblastic leukemia (Ph+ ALL) in patients with resistance or intolerance to prior therapy
Adults: 140 mg P.O. daily in two divided doses (70 mg b.i.d.) in morning and evening; may increase dosage to 180 mg daily in patients who don't achieve a hematologic or cytogenetic response

Dosage adjustment
• Myelosuppression
• Strong CYP3A4 inducers or inhibitors

Contraindications
None

Precautions
Use cautiously in:
• hepatic impairment
• myelosuppression
• comcomitant use of anticoagulants, aspirin, or NSAIDs
• patients with underlying cardiopulmonary disease
• concurrent use of strong CYP3A4 inducers or inhibitors (avoid use if possible)
• patients at risk for fluid retention or QT interval prolongation (including those with hypokalemia, hypomagnesemia, or congenital long-QT

syndrome; those taking antiarrhythmics or other drugs that lead to QT prolongation; and cumulative high-dose anthracycline therapy)
• concurrent use of histamine-2 (H_2) antagonists or proton pump inhibitors (not recommended)
• concurrent use of drugs that inhibit platelet function or anticoagulants
• pregnant or breastfeeding patients
• children younger than age 18 (safety and efficacy not established).

Administration

◀€ Evaluate patients for signs and symptoms of underlying cardiopulmonary disease before starting drug. If pulmonary arterial hypertension (PAH) is confirmed, permanently discontinue drug.
• Correct hypokalemia or hypomagnesemia before starting drug.
• Know that patients with CML or Ph+ ALL should have shown resistance to or intolerance of imatinib mesylate.
• Don't crush or cut tablets. Administer whole with or without food, but not with grapefruit juice.
• If tablets are inadvertently crushed or broken, wear disposable chemotherapy gloves. Pregnant personnel should avoid exposure to crushed or broken tablets.
• If patient needs antacid, give antacid at least 2 hours before or 2 hours after dasatinib.
• Know that hematopoietic growth factor may be used in patients with resistant myelosuppression.

Route	Onset	Peak	Duration
P.O.	Unknown	0.5-6 hr	Unknown

Adverse reactions

CNS: headache, fatigue, asthenia, neuropathy, peripheral neuropathy, dizziness, somnolence, insomnia, depression, malaise, **CNS bleeding**

CV: palpitations, flushing, hypertension, **prolonged QT interval, congestive heart failure, pericardial effusion, arrhythmia**
EENT: visual disorder, dry eye
GI: diarrhea, nausea, vomiting, mucositis, stomatitis, dyspepsia, abdominal distention, constipation, gastritis, oral soft-tissue disorder, colitis, enterocolitis, anorexia, appetite disturbances, dysphagia, abdominal pain, anal fissure, upper GI ulcer, esophagitis
Hematologic: myelosuppression (anemia, **neutropenia, thrombocytopenia, pancytopenia**), febrile neutropenia, **hemorrhage, GI bleeding**
Metabolic: fluid retention
Musculoskeletal: arthralgia, myalgia, inflammation, weakness
Respiratory: dyspnea, upper respiratory tract infection, pneumonia, pneumonitis, cough, lung infiltration, **pleural effusion, pulmonary edema, pulmonary hypertension**
Skin: rash, pruritus, acne, alopecia, dry skin, hyperhydrosis, urticaria, dermatitis
Other: fever, chills, infection, herpesvirus infection, ascites, generalized edema, pain, chest pain, dysgeusia, weight changes, temperature intolerance, contusion, **sepsis**

Interactions

Drug-drug. *Antacids:* reduced dasatinib plasma concentration
Anticoagulants, platelet inhibitors (such as aspirin, NSAIDs): increased risk of bleeding
CYP3A4 substrates with narrow therapeutic index (such as alfentanil, astemizole, cisapride, cyclosporine, ergot alkaloids, fentanyl, pimozide, quinidine, simvastatin, sirolimus, tacrolimus, terfenadine): potentially increased concentration of these drugs
H_2 antagonists or proton-pump inhibitors (such as famotidine, omeprazole), strong CYP3A4 inducers (such as carbamazepine, dexamethasone,

---

Reactions in **bold** are life-threatening.   ◀€ Clinical alert

phenobarbital, phenytoin, rifabutin, rifampin: reduced dasatinib blood level
Strong CYP3A4 inhibitors (such as atazanavir, clarithromycin, indinavir, itraconazole, ketoconazole, nefazodone, nelfinavir, ritonavir, saquinavir, telithromycin, voriconazole): increased dasatinib blood level

Drug-diagnostic tests. *Calcium, neutrophils, phosphorus, platelets:* decreased levels
ALT, AST, bilirubin, creatinine: increased levels

Drug-food. *Grapefruit juice:* increased dasatinib blood level

Drug-herbs. *St. John's wort:* unpredictable decrease in dasatinib blood level

Patient monitoring

🔊 Monitor patient for QT prolongation and hemorrhage.

• Be aware that severe thrombocytopenia, neutropenia, and anemia are more common in patients with advanced-phase CML or Ph+ ALL than in those with chronic-phase CML. Monitor complete blood count weekly for first 2 months and then monthly thereafter, or as indicated.

• Monitor hepatic function tests.

• Be prepared to manage transaminase or bilirubin elevations with dosage reduction or therapy interruption.

• Stay alert for fluid retention. Be prepared to manage with supportive care measures, such as diuretics or short courses of steroids.

• Monitor calcium levels. Some patients who develop Grade 3 or 4 hypocalcemia during therapy may recover with oral calcium supplementation.

🔊 Monitor patient for signs and symptoms of PAH (dyspnea, fatigue, hypoxia, fluid retention), which may occur anytime after initiation, including after more than 1 year of treatment.

Patient teaching

• Instruct patient to take tablet whole with or without food. Caution patient not to break, crush, or cut tablet.

• Advise patient to avoid grapefruit juice.

• Tell patient to take antacids (if needed) at least 2 hours before or 2 hours after dasatinib.

🔊 Instruct patient to immediately report fever or chills (and other signs or symptoms of infection), unusual bleeding or bruising, shortness of breath, fatigue, fluid retention, swelling, or weight gain.

• Instruct patient to report troublesome nausea, vomiting, diarrhea, headache, musculoskeletal pain, fatigue, or rash.

• Teach patient that drug may increase risk of infection. Advise patient to wash hands frequently, wear a mask in public places, and avoid people with infections.

• Inform lactose-intolerant patient that drug contains lactose.

• Advise patient to avoid St. John's wort, NSAIDs (such as ibuprofen), and over-the counter drugs that contain aspirin during therapy.

• Advise female patient that drug may harm fetus. Caution her to avoid becoming pregnant. If drug is used during pregnancy or patient becomes pregnant while taking it, inform her of potential hazard to fetus.

• Advise breastfeeding patient to discuss with prescriber whether to discontinue breastfeeding or drug, taking into account importance of drug to mother.

• Advise male taking drug to use condom, to avoid getting partner pregnant.

• As appropriate, review all other significant and life-threatening adverse reactions and interactions, especially those related to the drugs, tests, food, and herbs mentioned above.

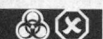

daunorubicin citrate liposome
DaunoXome

Pharmacologic class: Anthracycline glycoside
Therapeutic class: Antibiotic antineoplastic
Pregnancy risk category D

FDA   BOXED WARNING

- Monitor cardiac function regularly during therapy, because of potential cardiotoxicity and congestive heart failure. Also monitor cardiac function in patients who have cardiac disease or received previous anthracyclines.
- Severe myelosuppression may occur.
- Give under supervision of experienced physician.
- Reduce dosage in patients with hepatic impairment.
- Drug may cause triad of back pain, flushing, and chest tightness. Triad usually occurs within first 5 minutes of infusion, subsides with infusion interruption, and doesn't recur when infusion resumes at slower rate.

Action
Inhibits DNA synthesis and DNA-dependent RNA synthesis through intercalation. Formulation increases selectivity of daunorubicin for solid tumors; may increase permeability of tumor neovasculature to some particles in drug's size range.

Availability
Injection: 2 mg/ml

ⓘ Indications and dosages
➤ First-line cytotoxic therapy for advanced Kaposi's sarcoma associated with human immunodeficiency virus (HIV)
Adults: 40 mg/m^2 I.V. over 1 hour. Repeat q 2 weeks until evidence of disease progression or other complications occur.

Dosage adjustment
- Renal or hepatic impairment

Contraindications
- Hypersensitivity to drug

Precautions
Use cautiously in:
- renal or hepatic impairment, bone marrow depression, cardiac disease, gout, infections
- pregnant or breastfeeding patients.

Administration
- Follow facility policy for preparing and handling antineoplastics.
- Dilute 1:1 with 5% dextrose injection.
- Don't use in-line filter for I.V. infusion.
- If prescribed, premedicate with allopurinol to help prevent hyperuricemia.
- Take steps to prevent extravasation.
- Protect solution from light.

Route	Onset	Peak	Duration
I.V.	Unknown	Unknown	Unknown

Adverse reactions
CNS: headache, fatigue, malaise, confusion, depression, dizziness, drowsiness, emotional lability, anxiety, hallucinations, syncope, tremors, rigors, insomnia, neuropathy, amnesia, hyperactivity, abnormal thinking, **meningitis, seizures**
CV: hypertension, chest pain, palpitations, **myocardial infarction, cardiac arrest**
EENT: abnormal vision, conjunctivitis, eye pain, hearing loss, earache, tinnitus, rhinitis, sinusitis
GI: nausea, vomiting, diarrhea, constipation, abdominal pain, dyspepsia,

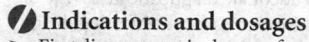

gastritis, enlarged spleen, fecal incontinence, hemorrhoids, tenesmus, melena, difficulty swallowing, dry mouth, mouth inflammation, **GI hemorrhage**
GU: dysuria, nocturia, polyuria
Hematologic: thrombocytopenia, neutropenia
Hepatic: hepatomegaly
Metabolic: hyperuricemia, dehydration
Musculoskeletal: joint pain, myalgia, muscle rigidity, back pain, abnormal gait
Respiratory: dyspnea, cough, hemoptysis, increased sputum, **pulmonary infiltrations, pulmonary hypertension**
Skin: pruritus, dry skin, seborrhea, folliculitis, alopecia, sweating
Other: bleeding gums, dental caries, altered taste, lymphadenopathy, opportunistic infections, fever, hot flashes, hiccups, thirst, infusion site inflammation, edema, allergic reactions

Interactions
Drug-diagnostic tests. *Granulocytes:* decreased count
Uric acid: increased level

Patient monitoring
• Assess cardiac, renal, and hepatic function before each course of treatment.
• Determine left ventricular ejection fraction before and during therapy.
• Evaluate CBC with white cell differential before each dose. Withhold dose if granulocyte count is below 750 cells/mm^3.
• Monitor serum uric acid level.

Patient teaching
◀ Instruct patient to immediately report swelling, pain, burning, or redness at infusion site, as well as persistent nausea, vomiting, diarrhea, chest pain, arm or leg swelling, difficulty breathing, palpitations, rapid heartbeat, yellowing of skin or eyes, abdominal pain, or bloody stools.

• Tell patient drug makes him more susceptible to infection. Advise him to avoid crowds and exposure to illness.
• Advise patient to minimize GI upset by eating small, frequent servings of healthy food, drinking plenty of fluids, and chewing gum.
• As appropriate, review all other significant and life-threatening adverse reactions and interactions, especially those related to the tests mentioned above.

daunorubicin hydrochloride
Cerubidine

Pharmacologic class: Anthracycline glycoside
Therapeutic class: Antibiotic antineoplastic
Pregnancy risk category D

FDA | **BOXED WARNING**

• Administer into rapidly flowing I.V. infusion; never give I.M. or subcutaneously. Severe local tissue necrosis results if extravasation occurs.
• Myocardial toxicity (manifested most severely as potentially fatal congestive heart failure) may occur during therapy or months to years afterward. Incidence increases with total cumulative dose exceeding 550 mg/m^2 in adults, 300 mg/m^2 in children older than age 2, or 10 mg/kg in children younger than age 2.
• Therapeutic doses cause severe myelosuppression. Drug should be given only by physician experienced in leukemia chemotherapy, in facility with adequate diagnostic and treatment resources for monitoring drug tolerance and treating toxicity. Physician and facility must be capable of

responding rapidly and completely to severe hemorrhagic conditions and overwhelming infection.
• Reduce dosage in patients with hepatic or renal impairment.

Action
Antimitotic and cytotoxic. Forms complexes with DNA by intercalation between base pairs. Inhibits topoisomerase II activity by stabilizing topoisomerase II complex; causes breaks in single- and double-stranded DNA. May also inhibit polymerase activity, influence regulation of gene expression, and cause free radical damage to DNA.

Availability
Injection: 5 mg/ml
Lyophilized powder for injection:
21.4 mg, 53.5 mg

⊘ Indications and dosages
➤ Acute nonlymphocytic leukemia
Adults older than age 60: 30 mg/m²/day I.V. on days 1, 2, and 3 of first course and on days 1 and 2 of subsequent courses; given with cytarabine I.V. infusion (7 days for first course, 5 days for subsequent courses)
Adults younger than age 60: 45 mg/m²/day I.V. on days 1, 2, and 3 of first course and on days 1 and 2 of subsequent courses; given with cytarabine I.V. infusion (7 days for first course, 5 days for subsequent courses)
➤ Acute lymphocytic leukemia
Adults: 45 mg/m²/day I.V. on days 1, 2, and 3; vincristine I.V. on days 1, 8, and 15; prednisone P.O. on days 1 through 22, then tapered between days 22 and 29; then asparaginase I.V. on days 22 to 32
Children ages 2 and older: 25 mg/m²/day I.V. on first day every week; may be given in combination with vincristine I.V. on first day every week and prednisone P.O. daily

Dosage adjustment
• Renal or hepatic impairment

Contraindications
• Hypersensitivity to drug

Precautions
Use cautiously in:
• renal or hepatic impairment, bone marrow depression, cardiac disease, gout, infections
• elderly patients
• pregnant or breastfeeding patients.

Administration
• Follow facility policy for preparing and handling antineoplastics.
• If prescribed, premedicate with allopurinol to help prevent hyperuricemia.
◀€ Give by I.V. route only.
• Reconstitute vial contents with 4 ml of sterile water for injection to yield 5 mg/ml solution.
• Don't mix with other drugs or heparin.
• Withdraw desired dosage into syringe containing 10 to 15 ml of normal saline solution; then inject into tubing or sidearm of compatible, rapidly flowing I.V. solution over 3 to 5 minutes. For intermittent infusion, mix with 100 ml of normal saline solution and infuse over 30 to 45 minutes.
◀€ Take care to prevent extravasation, because drug causes severe local tissue necrosis. If extravasation occurs, stop infusion immediately; according to facility policy, intervene to avoid severe tissue necrolysis, severe cellulitis, thrombophlebitis, and painful induration.

Route	Onset	Peak	Duration
I.V.	Unknown	Unknown	Unknown

Adverse reactions
CV: cardiotoxicity
GI: acute nausea, vomiting, GI mucosal inflammation
GU: urine discoloration

Reactions in **bold** are life-threatening.   ◀€ Clinical alert

Hematologic: bone marrow depression
Metabolic: hyperuricemia
Skin: rash, contact dermatitis, urticaria, reversible alopecia

Interactions
Drug-drug. *Other antineoplastic, hepatotoxic, or myelosuppressive drugs:* increased risk of toxicity
Drug diagnostic tests. *Granulocytes:* decreased count
Uric acid: increased level

Patient monitoring
◀€ Observe I.V. site closely for extravasation.
• Monitor cardiac, renal, and hepatic function before each course of treatment.
• Evaluate CBC with white cell differential before each dose. Withhold dose if granulocyte count is below 750 cells/mm³.
• Monitor serum uric acid level.

Patient teaching
◀€ Instruct patient to immediately report swelling, pain, burning, or redness at infusion site, as well as persistent nausea, vomiting, diarrhea, bloody stools, abdominal or chest pain, swollen arm or leg, difficulty breathing, palpitations, rapid heartbeat, or yellowing of skin or eyes.
• Inform patient that drug makes him more susceptible to infection. Caution him to avoid crowds and exposure to illness.
• Advise patient to minimize GI upset by eating small, frequent servings of healthy food, drinking plenty of fluids, and chewing gum.
• Tell patient that drug may redden his urine.
• As appropriate, review all other significant and life-threatening adverse reactions and interactions, especially those related to the drugs and tests mentioned above.

deferasirox
Exjade

Pharmacologic class: Iron-chelating agent
Therapeutic class: Antidote
Pregnancy risk category B

FDA BOXED WARNING

• Deferasirox may cause renal and hepatic impairment (including failure) and GI hemorrhage. In some reported cases, these reactions were fatal and were more frequently observed in patients with advanced age, high-risk myelodysplastic syndromes, underlying renal or hepatic impairment, or low platelet count (less than $50 \times 10^9/L$).
• Deferasirox therapy requires close patient monitoring, including measurement of serum creatinine and creatinine clearance before starting therapy and monthly thereafter.
• In patients with underlying renal impairment or risk factors for renal impairment, monitor serum creatinine and creatinine clearance weekly for the first month, then monthly thereafter.
• In patients with underlying hepatic impairment, monitor serum transaminase and bilirubin levels before starting therapy, every 2 weeks during first month, and monthly thereafter.

Action
Binds selectively to iron

Availability
Tablets for oral suspension: 125 mg, 250 mg, 500 mg

⚖️ Indications and dosages
➤ Chronic iron overload caused by blood transfusions

Adults and children ages 2 and older:
Initially, 20 mg/kg (calculated to nearest whole tablet) P.O. daily on empty stomach at least 30 minutes before a meal, preferably at same time each day. Don't exceed 30 mg/kg daily.

Dosage adjustment
• Serum creatinine elevation
• Severe, persistent liver enzyme elevations; moderate (Child-Pugh B) hepatic impairment
• Administration with potent UDP-glucuronosyltransferase (UGT) inducers or cholestyramine

Contraindications
• Hypersensitivity to drug or its components
• Creatinine clearance below 40 ml/minute or serum creatinine level above two times age-appropriate upper limit of normal
• Poor performance status and high-risk myelodysplastic syndromes or advanced malignancies
• Platelet count below 50×10^9/L

Precautions
Use cautiously in:
• serum creatinine elevation, liver enzyme elevation, severe rash
• severe hepatic impairment (Child-Pugh C) (avoid use)
• concurrent use of drugs with ulcerogenic or hemorrhagic potential, such as nonsteroidal anti-inflammatory drugs, corticosteroids, oral bisphosphonates, anticoagulants; or drugs metabolized by CYP3A4
• potent UGT inducers or cholestyramine (avoid use if possible)
• pregnant or breastfeeding patients.

Administration
◀᷉ Make sure patient doesn't swallow tablets whole.

• Disperse tablets completely in water, orange juice, or apple juice; have patient consume suspension immediately. If residue remains, resuspend it in small amount of liquid and have patient swallow it. Disperse doses lower than 1 g in 3.5 oz liquid; disperse doses higher than 1 g in 7 oz liquid.
• Adjust dosage every 3 to 6 months in increments of 5 to 10 mg/kg based on ferritin levels, treatment goals, and response.

Route	Onset	Peak	Duration
P.O.	Unknown	1.5-4 hr	Unknown

Adverse reactions
CNS: headache, fatigue, dizziness
EENT: cataract, retinal disorder, increased intraocular pressure, ear infection, hearing loss, rhinitis, nasopharyngitis, pharyngolaryngeal pain, pharyngitis, acute tonsillitis
GI: nausea, vomiting, diarrhea, abdominal pain, irritation, ulceration, **hemorrhage**
GU: renal dysfunction
Hematologic: cytopenias (agranulocytosis, neutropenia, thrombocytopenia)
Hepatic: liver dysfunction
Musculoskeletal: arthralgia, back pain
Respiratory: cough, respiratory tract infection, bronchitis
Skin: rash, urticaria, erythema multiforme
Other: fever, influenza **hypersensitivity reactions (including anaphylaxis, angioedema)**

Interactions
Drug-drug. *Aluminum-containing antacids:* possible binding with antacid
Cholestyramine, potent UGT inducers (such as phenobarbital, phenytoin, rifampin, ritonavir): decreased deferasirox systemic exposure (area under the curve)
Drugs metabolized by CYP3A4 (such as cyclosporine, hormonal contraceptives, simvastatin): possible decrease in CYP3A4 substrate concentration and

potential loss of effectiveness of these drugs

Drug-diagnostic tests. *Liver function tests, serum creatinine:* increased

Drug-food. *Any food:* increased deferasirox bioavailability

Patient monitoring

◀ Discontinue drug if hypersensitivity reactions are severe and institute appropriate medical intervention.

• Perform baseline auditory and ophthalmic testing; repeat every 12 months.

• Monitor serum ferritin levels monthly. If levels fall consistently below 500 mcg/L, consider temporarily interrupting therapy.

• Monitor serum creatinine level and creatinine clearance before starting drug and monthly thereafter. In patients with additional renal risk factors, monitor serum creatinine level and creatinine clearance weekly during first month after initiation or modification of therapy and monthly thereafter. Consider dosage reduction, therapy interruption, or drug discontinuation if levels increase.

• Monitor serum transaminase and bilirubin levels before starting drug, every 2 weeks during first month of therapy, and monthly thereafter. Consider dosage modifications or interruption of treatment for severe or persistent elevations.

• Monitor CBC regularly. Consider interrupting treatment in patients who develop unexplained cytopenia.

◀ Stay alert for signs and symptoms of GI ulceration and hemorrhage during therapy; promptly initiate additional evaluation and treatment if serious GI adverse event is suspected.

Patient teaching

• Instruct patient to take drug on empty stomach at least 30 minutes before food, preferably at same time each day.

• Instruct patient to place tablets in water, orange juice, or apple juice and stir until completely dissolved. Tell him not to chew or swallow them.

• Advise patient not to take aluminum-containing antacids during therapy.

• Tell patient drug may cause vision and hearing disturbances, necessitating routine ophthalmic and auditory testing.

• Caution patient to avoid driving and other hazardous activities until drug effects are known.

• As appropriate, review all other significant adverse reactions and interactions, especially those related to the drugs, tests, and foods mentioned above.

degarelix
Firmagon

Pharmacologic class: Gonadotropin-releasing hormone (GnRH) receptor antagonist

Therapeutic class: Antineoplastic

Pregnancy risk category X

Action

Binds reversibly to the pituitary GnRH receptors, thereby reducing the release of gonadotropins and consequently testosterone

Availability

Powder for injection: 80 mg/vial, 120 mg/vial

⚠ Indications and dosages

➤Advanced prostate cancer

Adults: Initially, 240 mg subcutaneously given as two injections of 120 mg each, followed by maintenance dose of 80 mg subcutaneously as a single injection every 28 days

Contraindications
- Hypersensitivity to drug or its components
- Females of childbearing potential

Precautions
Use cautiously in:
- moderate or severe renal impairment (creatinine clearance less than 50 ml/minute)
- severe hepatic dysfunction
- congenital long QT syndrome, electrolyte abnormalities, congestive heart failure, and in patients taking Class IA (such as quinidine, procainamide) or Class III (such as amiodarone, sotalol) antiarrhythmics
- children (safety and efficacy not established).

Administration
- Be aware that drug is intended for deep subcutaneous administration only and isn't to be administered I.V.
- Wear gloves during preparation and administration.
- Reconstitute powder with sterile water for injection. Don't use other solutions.
- Be aware that the treatment initiation pack contains two vials of Firmagon 120 mg that must be prepared for two subcutaneous injections; therefore, the instructions below need to be repeated a second time.
- For initial 120-mg dose, draw up 3 ml sterile water for injection using supplied reconstitution needle (21G, 2 inches) and slowly inject sterile water for injection into 120-mg vial to yield a concentration of 40 mg/ml.
- For 80-mg maintenance dose, draw up 4.2 ml sterile water for injection using supplied reconstitution needle (21G, 2 inches) and slowly inject sterile water for injection into 80-mg vial to yield a concentration of 20 mg/ml.
- Hold vial upright and swirl it very gently until liquid is clear and without undissolved powder or particles. If powder adheres to vial over the liquid surface, vial can be tilted slightly to dissolve powder. Don't shake vial, to prevent foam formation. A ring of small air bubbles on the surface of the liquid is acceptable. The reconstitution procedure may take up to 15 minutes.
- Tilt vial slightly and keep needle in lowest part of vial. Withdraw 3 ml of drug (120-mg dose) and 4 ml (80-mg dose) without turning vial upside down.
- Exchange reconstitution needle with administration needle for deep subcutaneous injection (27G, 1$^1/_4$ inches). Remove any air bubbles.
- Use reconstituted drug within 1 hour after addition of sterile water for injection.
- Give injection in abdomen in area that won't be exposed to pressure (such as not close to waistband or belt or close to ribs).

Route	Onset	Peak	Duration
Subcut.	Unknown	2 days	Unknown

Adverse reactions
CNS: fatigue, asthenia, dizziness, headache, insomnia
CV: hypertension, **prolonged QT interval**
GI: nausea, constipation
GU: urinary tract infection
Hepatic: abnormal hepatic function
Musculoskeletal: decreased bone density (with long-term therapy), back pain, arthralgia
Other: injection-site reactions, hot flashes, weight gain, fever, chills, night sweats, anti-degarelix antibody development

Interactions
Drug-diagnostic tests. *Gamma-glutamyltransferase, serum transaminases:* increased levels

Patient monitoring
- Monitor renal and hepatic function tests closely.

Reactions in **bold** are life-threatening. 🔊 Clinical alert

◀ Monitor patient on long-term androgen deprivation therapy for prolonged QT interval.

• Monitor testosterone concentration monthly until medical castration is achieved in patients with hepatic impairment; then consider every-other-month testosterone concentration measurement.

• Because this drug may suppress pituitary gonadal system, periodically monitor drug's therapeutic effect by measuring serum concentration of prostate-specific antigen (PSA). If PSA increases, measure serum testosterone concentration.

Patient teaching

• Advise patient to make sure injection site is free of pressure from belts, waistbands, or other types of clothing.

◀ Instruct patient to immediately report abnormal heartbeats, dizziness, or faintness.

• Tell patient that drug isn't indicated for use in women.

• Inform patient of possible adverse effects of androgen deprivation (hot flashes, skin flushing, increased weight, decreased sex drive, erectile dysfunction).

• As appropriate, review all other significant and life-threatening adverse reactions and interactions, especially those related to the tests mentioned above.

---

delavirdine mesylate
Rescriptor

Pharmacologic class: Nonnucleoside reverse transcriptase inhibitor
Therapeutic class: Antiretroviral
Pregnancy risk category C

Action
Binds to reverse transcriptase enzyme, blocking RNA-dependent and DNA-dependent DNA polymerase synthesis

Availability
Tablets: 100 mg, 200 mg

⚡ Indications and dosages
➤ Human immunodeficiency virus (HIV)-1 infection
Adults: 400 mg P.O. t.i.d.

Contraindications
• Hypersensitivity to drug
• Concurrent use of alprazolam, astemizole, ergot derivatives, midazolam, pimozide, terfenadine, or triazolam

Precautions
Use cautiously in:
• hepatic impairment
• pregnant or breastfeeding patients
• children younger than age 16 (safety and efficacy not established).

Administration
• Know that drug is usually given with at least two other antiretrovirals.
• If patient can't swallow tablets, dissolve 100-mg tablets in water by adding four tablets to at least 3 oz of water; let stand for a few minutes and then stir until completely dissolved. Have patient swallow entire mixture immediately. Then add small amount of water to glass and have him swallow this mixture to ensure that he consumes entire dose.
• Give 200-mg tablets intact; don't dissolve in water.
• If patient has achlorhydria, give drug with acidic beverage, such as orange juice.

◀ Don't give concurrently with alprazolam, astemizole or terfenadine (no longer available in United States), ergot derivatives, midazolam, pimozide, or triazolam.

Route	Onset	Peak	Duration
P.O.	Unknown	1 hr	Unknown

Adverse reactions

CNS: confusion, disorientation, dizziness, drowsiness, agitation, amnesia, changes in dreams, hallucinations, hyperesthesia, poor concentration, mania, nervousness, restlessness, paranoia, paresthesia, tremor, migraine, neuropathy, paralysis, **seizures**

CV: abnormal heart rate and rhythm, peripheral vascular disorder, peripheral edema, hypertension, orthostatic hypotension, cardiac insufficiency, **cardiomyopathy**

EENT: blurred or double vision, nystagmus, conjunctivitis, dry eyes, scleral yellowing, ear pain, otitis media, tinnitus, epistaxis, rhinitis

GI: nausea, diarrhea, constipation, abdominal pain or cramps, dyspepsia, abdominal distention, bloody stools, colitis, diverticulitis, enteritis, gastroenteritis, gastroesophageal reflux, mouth and tongue irritation and ulcers, increased saliva, difficulty swallowing, **GI bleeding, pancreatitis**

GU: hematuria, polyuria, chromaturia, proteinuria, nocturia, urinary tract infection, renal calculi, kidney pain, gynecomastia, erectile dysfunction, epididymitis, hemospermia, testicular pain, vaginal candidiasis, amenorrhea, irregular uterine bleeding

Hematologic: purpura, spleen disorders, eosinophilia, **granulocytosis, disseminated intravascular coagulation, leukopenia, neutropenia, pancytopenia, hemolytic anemia**

Hepatic: hepatotoxicity, hepatic failure, hepatomegaly

Metabolic: hypomagnesemia, hyperglycemia, hyperuricemia, hypocalcemia, hyponatremia, **hypoglycemia, hyperkalemia, metabolic acidosis**

Musculoskeletal: joint pain, arthritis, bone disorders, myalgia, muscle cramps, muscle weakness, bone pain, bone disorders, tendon disorders, tenosynovitis, neck pain and rigidity, limb pain, **tetany, rhabdomyolysis**

Respiratory: pulmonary congestion, dyspnea, pneumonia

Skin: pallor, bruising, yellowing of skin, dermal leukocytoblastic vasculitis, dermatitis, skin dryness and discoloration, erythema, folliculitis, herpes zoster or herpes simplex infection, petechiae, petechial or pruritic rash, seborrhea, alopecia, skin nodules, urticaria, sebaceous or epidermal cyst, angioedema, **erythema multiforme**

Other: tooth abscess, toothache, gingivitis, gum hemorrhage, weight gain or loss, fever, lymphadenopathy, adenopathy, increased thirst, hiccups, facial edema, pain, abscess, bacterial infection, *Mycobacterium tuberculosis* infection, body fat redistribution, hypersensitivity reaction, **sepsis, Stevens-Johnson syndrome**

Interactions

Drug-drug. *Alprazolam, astemizole, cisapride, ergot derivatives, midazolam, pimozide, terfenadine:* increased risk of serious or life-threatening adverse reactions

Antacids, histamine$_2$-receptor antagonists: reduced delavirdine absorption

Bepridil, clarithromycin, estrogen, hormonal contraceptives, indinavir, lopinavir-ritonavir, saquinavir, sildenafil, warfarin: increased blood levels of these drugs

Carbamazepine, phenobarbital, phenytoin, rifabutin, rifampin: loss of virologic response, resistance to delavirdine

Cholesterol-lowering HMG-CoA reductase inhibitors cleared by the CYP3A4 pathway: increased risk of myopathy and rhabdomyolysis

Dexamethasone: decreased delavirdine blood level

Didanosine: decreased blood levels of both drugs

Fluoxetine, ketoconazole: 50% increase in delavirdine blood level

Drug-diagnostic tests. *Alanine aminotransferase, alkaline phosphatase, aspartate aminotransferase, bilirubin, creatinine, lipase, gamma-glutamyl transpeptidase, triglycerides:* increased levels
Granulocytes, hemoglobin, neutrophils, platelets, red blood cells, white blood cells: decreased values
Partial thromboplastin time, prothrombin time: increased
Drug-herbs. *St. John's wort:* loss of virologic response or resistance to delavirdine

Patient monitoring
• Monitor liver function test results frequently when giving drug concurrently with saquinavir.
• Check electrolyte and uric acid levels regularly.
◀€ Monitor patient for serious hepatic, cardiovascular, and CNS problems and hypersensitivity reactions.

Patient teaching
• Tell patient he can take drug with or without food.
• If patient can't swallow tablets, teach him how to dissolve 100-mg tablets in water.
◀€ Tell patient to discontinue drug and consult prescriber immediately if he develops severe rash accompanied by fever, blistering, oral lesions, conjunctivitis, swelling, or muscle aches.
◀€ Tell patient to promptly report unusual fatigue, yellowing of skin or eyes, unusual bruising or bleeding, muscle weakness, or signs and symptoms of infection.
◀€ Advise patient that rash is a major adverse effect, usually occurring 1 to 3 weeks after therapy starts and resolving in 3 to 14 days. Instruct him to report rash promptly.
• Inform patient that drug doesn't cure HIV or reduce its transmission.
• As appropriate, review all other significant and life-threatening adverse reactions and interactions, especially those related to the drugs, tests, and herbs mentioned above.

denileukin diftitox
Ontak

Pharmacologic class: Biological response modifier
Therapeutic class: Antineoplastic
Pregnancy risk category C

FDA | BOXED WARNING

• Give only under supervision of physician experienced in cancer chemotherapy, in facility equipped and staffed for cardiopulmonary resuscitation where patient can be monitored closely.

Action
Recombinant DNA-derived cytotoxic protein. Interacts with interleukin-2 (IL-2) receptors on cell surface and inhibits cellular protein synthesis, causing cell death.

Availability
Frozen solution for injection: 150 mcg/ml

Indications and dosages
➢ Persistent or recurrent cutaneous T-cell lymphoma that expresses CD25 component of IL-2 receptor
Adults: 9 or 18 mcg/kg/day I.V. infused over 15 minutes for 5 consecutive days q 21 days

Contraindications
• Hypersensitivity to drug, its components, diphtheria toxin, or IL-2

Precautions
Use cautiously in:
• cardiovascular disease
• elderly patients

- pregnant or breastfeeding patients
- children (safety and efficacy not established).

Administration

- Follow facility procedures for safe handling, administration, and disposal of chemotherapeutic agents.
- 🔊 Administer by I.V. infusion only. Don't give by I.V. bolus.
- Dilute I.V. dose further with normal saline to concentration of at least 15 mcg/ml. Infuse over at least 15 minutes.
- Premedicate with acetaminophen, nonsteroidal anti-inflammatory drugs, and antihistamines, as ordered, to minimize infusion-related events.
- Gently swirl vial to mix, but avoid vigorous agitation.
- Don't mix with other drugs.
- Don't deliver through in-line filter.
- Infuse over at least 15 minutes.
- 🔊 During infusion, observe closely for signs and symptoms of hypersensitivity reaction.

Route	Onset	Peak	Duration
I.V.	Variable	Variable	Variable

Adverse reactions

CNS: dizziness, paresthesia, nervousness, confusion, insomnia, syncope, headache
CV: hypotension, hypertension, vasodilation, tachycardia, chest pain, **capillary leak syndrome** (with extravasation), **thrombosis, arrhythmias**
EENT: rhinitis, pharyngitis, **laryngospasm**
GI: nausea, vomiting, diarrhea, constipation, flatulence, dyspepsia, difficulty swallowing, anorexia
GU: hematuria, albuminuria, pyuria
Hematologic: anemia, **thrombocytopenia, leukopenia**
Musculoskeletal: myalgia, back or joint pain

Metabolic: hypoalbuminemia, hypocalcemia, hypokalemia, dehydration
Respiratory: dyspnea, cough, lung disorder
Skin: rash, pruritus, sweating
Other: weight loss, edema, flulike symptoms, injection site reaction, **hypersensitivity reactions** including **anaphylaxis**

Interactions

Drug-drug. *Live-virus vaccines:* decreased antibody reaction
Drug-diagnostic tests. *Albumin, calcium, potassium:* decreased levels
Urine creatinine: increased level

Patient monitoring

- Monitor patient closely during first infusion and for 24 hours afterward.
- Evaluate patient for vascular leak syndrome (marked by at least two of the following: edema, hypotension, hypoalbuminemia).
- Monitor CBC, blood chemistry panel, renal and hepatic function, and albumin level. Repeat all tests weekly during therapy.

Patient teaching

- 🔊 Instruct patient to immediately report chest pain, difficulty breathing, chills, burning at infusion site, or throat tightness, redness, swelling, or pain.
- Caution patient to avoid driving and other hazardous activities until he knows how drug affects concentration and alertness.
- Inform patient that drug makes him more susceptible to infection. Advise him to avoid crowds and exposure to illness.
- As appropriate, review all other significant and life-threatening adverse reactions and interactions, especially those related to the drugs and tests mentioned above.

Reactions in **bold** are life-threatening. 　　　　🔊 Clinical alert

desipramine hydrochloride
Apo-Desipramine✤, Dom-
Desipramine✤, Norpramin, Novo-
Desipramine✤, Nu-Desipramine✤,
PHL-Desipramine✤, PMS-
Desipramine✤, Ratio-Desipramine✤

Pharmacologic class: Tricyclic anti-
depressant
Therapeutic class: Antidepressant
Pregnancy risk category C

FDA | **BOXED WARNING**

- Drug may increase risk of suicidal
thinking and behavior in children and
adolescents with major depressive disorder and other psychiatric disorders.
Risk must be balanced with clinical
need, as depression itself increases suicide risk. With patient of any age,
observe closely for clinical worsening,
suicidality, and unusual behavior
changes when therapy begins. Advise
family to observe patient closely and
communicate with prescriber as needed.
- Drug isn't approved for use in pediatric patients.

Action
Inhibits norepinephrine or serotonin
reuptake at presynaptic neuron

Availability
Tablets: 10 mg, 25 mg, 50 mg, 75 mg,
100 mg, 150 mg

🖊 Indications and dosages
➢ Depression
Adults: Initially, 100 to 200 mg/day
P.O. Increase gradually if needed to a
maximum dosage of 300 mg/day.
Adolescents and elderly adults: 25 to
100 mg/day P.O. as a single dose or in
divided doses. Increase gradually if

needed to a maximum dosage of
150 mg/day.

Off-label uses
- Arthritis pain
- Cancer pain
- Diabetic or peripheral neuropathy
- Tic douloureux

Contraindications
- Hypersensitivity to drug
- Recovery phase of myocardial infarc-
tion (MI)
- MAO inhibitor use within past 14 days

Precautions
Use cautiously in:
- cardiovascular disorders, glaucoma,
thyroid disorders, history of seizure
disorders, mania, hypomania, adults
with major depressive disorder
- urinary retention
- adolescents and children.

Administration
- Before giving drug, measure patient's
sitting and supine blood pressure to
assess for orthostasis.
- Give full dose at bedtime to avoid
daytime drowsiness.
- Discontinue drug 2 days before
surgery.
🔊 Don't give within 14 days of MAO
inhibitor, because potentially fatal
reaction may occur.

Route	Onset	Peak	Duration
P.O.	Unknown	4-6 hr	Unknown

Adverse reactions
CNS: sedation, weakness, anxiety, restlessness, insomnia, delusions, confusion, agitation, hallucinations, disorientation, extrapyramidal reactions,
EEG changes, **neuroleptic malignant
syndrome, seizures, suicidal behavior
or ideation (especially in child or
adolescent)**

CV: hypotension, hypertension, tachycardia, palpitations, **arrhythmias, MI, heart block**
EENT: blurred vision, dry eyes, laryngitis
GI: nausea, vomiting, constipation, abdominal cramps, epigastric distress, difficulty swallowing, parotid gland swelling, mouth inflammation, dry mouth, black tongue
GU: urinary retention, delayed voiding, urinary tract dilation, testicular swelling, erectile or other male sexual dysfunction, gynecomastia, menstrual irregularities, galactorrhea, increased or decreased libido
Hematologic: purpura, eosinophilia, **bone marrow depression, agranulocytosis, thrombocytopenia**
Metabolic: syndrome of inappropriate antidiuretic hormone secretion
Musculoskeletal: muscle weakness
Skin: dry skin, photosensitivity, rash, pruritus, petechiae, sweating
Other: peculiar taste, weight gain, edema, hypothermia, flushing, withdrawal symptoms with abrupt drug cessation (dizziness, nausea, vomiting, headache, malaise, sleep disturbances, hyperthermia, irritability, worsening of depression), **sudden death (in children)**

Interactions

Drug-drug. *Adrenergics, anticholinergics:* additive adrenergic or anticholinergic effects
Cimetidine, phenothiazines, quinidine, selective serotonin reuptake inhibitors: increased desipramine effects, possible toxicity
Clonidine: hypertensive crisis
CNS depressants (antihistamines, opioid analgesics, sedative-hypnotics): additive CNS depression
MAO inhibitors: hyperpyretic crisis, severe seizures, death
Sparfloxacin: increased risk of adverse cardiovascular reactions

Drug-diagnostic tests. *Glucose:* increased or decreased level
Drug-food. *Grapefruit juice:* increased drug blood level and effects
Drug-herbs. *Chamomile, hops, kava, skullcap, valerian:* increased CNS depression
S-adenosylmethionine (SAM-e), St. John's wort: adverse serotonergic effects, including serotonin syndrome
Drug-behaviors. *Alcohol use:* increased response to alcohol
Smoking: increased metabolism and decreased efficacy of desipramine

Patient monitoring

◀€ Assess for suicidal tendencies before starting therapy.
• Monitor blood glucose level and CBC with white cell differential during therapy.
• Watch for severe CNS, cardiovascular, and hematologic adverse reactions.

Patient teaching

• Tell patient to take full dose at bedtime to avoid daytime drowsiness.
◀€ Urge patient to promptly report chest pain or easy bruising or bleeding.
• Inform patient that desired therapeutic effect may take 2 to 3 weeks.
◀€ Instruct patient or parent to immediately report increasing depression or suicidal ideation (especially in child or adolescent).
• Caution patient to avoid driving and other hazardous activities until he knows how drug affects alertness, vision, and coordination.
• As appropriate, review all other significant and life-threatening adverse reactions and interactions, especially those related to the drugs, tests, foods, herbs, and behaviors mentioned above.

---

desloratadine
Aerius✤, Clarinex, Clarinex Reditabs, Neoclarityn⊕

Pharmacologic class: Peripherally selective piperidine, selective histamine₁-receptor antagonist

Therapeutic class: Antihistamine (nonsedating, second generation)

Pregnancy risk category C

Action
Suppresses histamine release at peripheral histamine₁-receptor sites

Availability
Syrup: 2.5 mg/5 ml
Tablets: 5 mg
Tablets (orally disintegrating): 2.5 mg, 5 mg

⊘ Indications and dosages
➣ Seasonal and perennial allergic rhinitis; chronic idiopathic urticaria and allergies caused by indoor and outdoor allergens; pruritus; to reduce number and size of hives
Adults and children ages 12 and older: 5 mg/day P.O.
Children ages 6 to 11: 1 tsp (2.5 mg/ 5 ml syrup) P.O. once daily
Children ages 12 months to 5 years: ½ tsp (1.25 mg in 2.5 ml syrup) P.O. once daily
Children ages 6 to 11 months: 2 ml (1 mg syrup) P.O. once daily

Dosage adjustment
• Hepatic or renal impairment

Contraindications
• Hypersensitivity to drug, its components, or loratadine

Precautions
Use cautiously in:
• renal or hepatic impairment
• elderly patients
• pregnant or breastfeeding patients
• children younger than age 12 (safety and efficacy not established, except syrup).

Administration
• Give with or without food.

Route	Onset	Peak	Duration
P.O.	1 hr	3 hr	24 hr

Adverse reactions
CNS: dizziness, drowsiness, fatigue, headache
CV: tachycardia, palpitations
EENT: pharyngitis, dry throat
GI: nausea, dyspepsia, dry mouth
GU: dysmenorrhea
Musculoskeletal: myalgia
Other: flulike symptoms, hypersensitivity reaction

Interactions
Drug-diagnostic tests. *Bilirubin, hepatic enzymes:* increased values
Skin tests: interference with positive reaction to dermal reactivity indicators

Patient monitoring
• Monitor hepatic and renal function test results.

Patient teaching
• Tell patient he may take drug with or without food.
• Instruct patient to report rapid heartbeat, shortness of breath, rash, persistent flulike symptoms, or muscle ache.
• Caution patient to avoid driving and other hazardous activities until he knows how drug affects concentration and alertness.
• As appropriate, review all other significant adverse reactions and

---

✤ Canada   ⊕ UK   ☣ Hazardous drug   ⊗ High-alert drug

interactions, especially those related to the tests mentioned above.

desmopressin acetate (1-deamino-8-D-arginine vasopressin)

Apo-Desmopressin✸, DDAVP, DesmoMelt⊕, Desmospray⊕, Stimate

Pharmacologic class: Posterior pituitary hormone
Therapeutic class: Antidiuretic hormone
Pregnancy risk category B

Action

Enhances water reabsorption by increasing permeability of renal collecting ducts to adenosine monophosphate and water, thereby reducing urinary output and increasing urine osmolality. Also increases factor VIII (antihemophilic factor) activity.

Availability

Injection: 4 mcg/ml in single-dose 1-ml ampules and multidose 10-ml vials
Intranasal solution: 0.1 mg/ml, 1.5 mg/ ml
Intranasal spray (DDAVP): 0.1 mg/ml (10 mcg/spray) in 5-ml spray pump bottle
Tablets: 0.1 mg, 0.2 mg

💊 Indications and dosages

➤ Diabetes insipidus
Adults and children older than age 12:
0.05 mg P.O. b.i.d.; adjust dosage based on patient response. Or 0.1 to 0.4 ml (10 to 40 mcg) daily intranasally as a single dose or in two or three divided doses. Or 0.5 ml (2 mcg) to 1 ml (4 mcg) daily I.V. or subcutaneously, usually in two divided doses.

Children ages 3 months to 12 years:
0.05 to 0.3 ml/day intranasally in one or two divided doses
➤ Hemophilia A; von Willebrand's disease type I
Adults and children: 0.3 mcg/kg I.V.; may repeat dose if needed. Or 300 mcg of intranasal solution containing 1.5 mcg/ml; for patients weighing less than 50 kg (110 lb), total dosage of 150 mcg (one spray of solution containing 1.5 mg/ml into a single nostril) is usually sufficient. If needed to maintain hemostasis during surgery, give intranasal dose 2 hours before surgery or give I.V. dose 30 minutes before surgery.

Off-label uses

• Chronic autonomic failure (such as nocturnal polyuria, overnight weight loss, morning orthostatic hypotension)

Contraindications

• Hypersensitivity to drug
• Moderate to severe renal impairment
• Hemophilia A with factor VIII levels less than or equal to 5%
• Von Willebrand's disease type IIB
• Impaired level of consciousness (intranasal form)

Precautions

Use cautiously in:
• coronary artery disease, hypertensive cardiovascular disease, fluid and electrolyte imbalances
• breastfeeding patients.

Administration

• Adjust morning and evening dosages as appropriate to minimize frequent urination and risk of water intoxication.
• Give I.V. dose (diluted in normal saline solution) by infusion over 15 to 30 minutes.
• Monitor pulse and blood pressure throughout I.V. infusion
◀🎔 When giving to child with diabetes insipidus, carefully restrict fluid intake

---

◀🎔 Clinical alert

to prevent hyponatremia and water intoxication.

Route	Onset	Peak	Duration
P.O.	1 hr	1-5 hr	8-12 hr
I.V.	15-30 min	Unknown	4-12 hr
Intranasal	1 hr	1-1.5 hr	8-12 hr

Adverse reactions

CNS: headache, dizziness, insomnia
CV: slight blood pressure increase, chest pain, palpitations
EENT: rhinitis, epistaxis, sore throat
GI: nausea, abdominal pain
GU: vulvar pain
Respiratory: cough
Other: local erythema, flushing, swelling or burning after injection

Interactions

Drug-drug. *Carbamazepine, chlorpropamide, pressor drugs:* potentiation of desmopressin effects

Patient monitoring

• Monitor urine volume and specific gravity, plasma and urine osmolality, and electrolyte levels in patients with diabetes insipidus.
• Monitor factor VIII antigen levels, activated partial thromboplastin time, and bleeding time in patients with hemophilia.
🔊 When giving to child with diabetes insipidus, carefully monitor fluid intake and output.

Patient teaching

• Instruct patient to take drug exactly as prescribed and not to interchange strengths or delivery systems.
• Teach patient how to use prescribed delivery system if taking drug by other than oral route.
• Instruct patient with diabetes insipidus to avoid overhydration and to weigh himself daily. Tell him to report weight gain or swelling of arms or legs.

• If patient is using nasal spray, teach him to inspect nasal membranes regularly and to report increased nasal congestion or swelling.
• Caution elderly patient not to increase fluid intake beyond that sufficient to satisfy thirst.
• Instruct patient to report headache, respiratory difficulty, nausea, or abdominal pain to prescriber.
• As appropriate, review all significant adverse reactions and interactions, especially those related to the drugs mentioned above.

desvenlafaxine
Pristiq

Pharmacologic class: Selective serotonin reuptake inhibitor
Therapeutic class: Antidepressant
Pregnancy risk category C

FDA   BOXED WARNING

• Drug may increase risk of suicidal thinking and behavior in children and adolescents with major depressive disorder and other psychiatric disorders. Risk must be balanced with clinical need, as depression itself increases suicide risk. With patient of any age, observe closely for clinical worsening, suicidality, and unusual behavior changes when therapy begins. Advise family and caregivers to observe patient closely and communicate with prescriber as needed.
• Drug isn't approved for use in children.

Action

Potentiates serotonin and norepinephrine in CNS

Availability
Tablets (extended-release): 50 mg, 100 mg

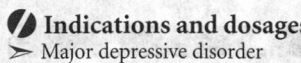 Indications and dosages
➤ Major depressive disorder
Adults: 50 mg P.O. daily

Dosage adjustment
• Severe renal impairment and end-stage renal disease
• Hepatic impairment (dosages above 100 mg daily not recommended)

Contraindications
• Hypersensitivity to drug, its components, or venlafaxine
• Within 14 days of an MAO inhibitor

Precautions
Use cautiously in:
• renal impairment, hypertension, cardiovascular or cerebrovascular disease, lipid metabolism disorders, abnormal bleeding, interstitial lung disease, eosinophilic pneumonia, seizure disorder, bipolar disorder or family history of mania or hypomania, increased intraocular pressure, increased risk of angle-closure glaucoma
• concurrent use of selective serotonin reuptake inhibitors (SSRIs) or serotonin norepinephrine reuptake inhibitors (SNRIs) (use not recommended)
• pregnant or breastfeeding patients
• children (safety and efficacy not established).

Administration
• Make sure hypertension is controlled before therapy starts.
• Give tablets whole with or without food at same time each day. Don't break, dissolve, or divide tablets.
• Reduce dosage gradually when discontinuing drug.

Route	Onset	Peak	Duration
P.O.	Unknown	7.5 hr	Unknown

Adverse reactions
CNS: dizziness, insomnia, somnolence, anxiety, fatigue, irritability, abnormal dreams, hypomania, mania, **seizures**
CV: hypertension
EENT: mydriasis, blurred vision, tinnitus
GI: nausea, vomiting, diarrhea, constipation, dry mouth
GU: male sexual function disorder
Hematologic: abnormal bleeding
Respiratory: interstitial lung disease, eosinophilic pneumonia
Skin: hyperhidrosis
Other: decreased appetite, weight loss

Interactions
Drug-drug. *Aspirin, NSAIDs, other drugs that affect coagulation:* increased risk of bleeding
Drugs metabolized by CYP2D6 (such as despiramine): increased blood levels of these drugs
Drugs metabolized by CYP3A4 (such as midazolam): decreased blood levels of these drugs
MAO inhibitors, serotonergics (lithium, SNRIs, SSRIs, tricyclic antidepressants, triptans), tramadol: potentially life-threatening serotonin syndrome
Potent CYP3A4 inhibitors: increased desvenlafaxine blood level
Drug-diagnostic tests. *Cholesterol, triglycerides:* increased levels
Sodium: decreased level
Urine protein: transient elevation
Drug-food. *Tryptophan supplements:* potentially life-threatening serotonin syndrome
Drug-herb. *St. John's wort:* potentially life-threatening serotonin syndrome

Patient monitoring
• Monitor patient's blood pressure regularly during therapy.
• Monitor cholesterol and triglyceride levels.
🔊 Monitor patient closely for clinical worsening, suicidality, and unusual behavior changes, especially during

d

---

first few months of therapy and after dosage changes.

◀◁ Monitor for progressive dyspnea, cough, or chest discomfort, which may signal serious lung disorders.

• Observe for signs and symptoms of hyponatremia (headache, poor concentration, memory impairment, confusion, weakness, and unsteadiness), especially in elderly patients.

◀◁ After discontinuing drug, monitor for dysphoric mood, irritability, agitation, dizziness, paresthesia, anxiety, confusion, headache, lethargy insomnia, tinnitus, and seizures.

Patient teaching
• Instruct patient to take tablets whole with or without food at same time each day. Caution patient not to chew, break, crush, dissolve, or divide tablets.
• Tell patient that full drug effects may take several weeks; advise patient not to stop taking drug.
• Caution patient not to discontinue drug abruptly.

◀◁ Advise patient's family or caregiver to monitor patient, especially for suicidality or new or worsening symptoms.

◀◁ Instruct patient to immediately report unusual bruising or bleeding.

• Advise patient not to take over-the-counter drugs containing aspirin or NSAIDs without consulting prescriber.
• Instruct patient to avoid herbs (especially St. John's wort) unless prescriber approves.
• Caution patient to avoid hazardous activities until drug's effects on concentration and alertness are known.
• Tell patient that inert matrix tablet may appear in stool, but active drug has already been absorbed.
• Advise female patient to notify prescriber if she is pregnant, intends to become pregnant, or is breastfeeding.
• As appropriate, review all other significant and life-threatening adverse reactions and interactions, especially those related to the drugs, tests, foods, and herbs mentioned above.

dexamethasone
Apo-Dexamethasone✢, Dexasone, Ozurdex

dexamethasone sodium phosphate

Pharmacologic class: Glucocorticoid
Therapeutic class: Anti-inflammatory
Pregnancy risk category C

Action
Unclear. Reduces inflammation by suppressing polymorphonuclear leukocyte migration, reversing increased capillary permeability, and stabilizing leukocyte lysosomal membranes. Also suppresses immune response (by reducing lymphatic activity), stimulates bone marrow, and promotes protein, fat, and carbohydrate metabolism.

Availability
Elixir: 0.5 mg/5 ml
Intravitreal implant: 0.7 mg
Oral solution: 0.5 mg/5 ml, 1 mg/ml
Solution for injection (sodium phosphate): 4 mg/ml, 10 mg/ml, 20 mg/ml, 24 mg/ml
Tablets: 0.25 mg, 0.5 mg, 0.75 mg, 1 mg, 1.5 mg, 2 mg, 4 mg, 6 mg

🕖 Indications and dosages
➢ Macular edema following branch retinal vein occlusion or central retinal vein occlusion; noninfectious uveitis affecting posterior segment of eye
Adults: 0.7 mg by intravitreal implant
➢ Allergic and inflammatory conditions
Adults: 0.75 to 9 mg/day (dexamethasone) P.O. as a single dose or in divided doses; in severe cases, much higher dosages may be needed. Dosage

requirements vary and must be individualized based on disease and patient response.

➤ Cerebral edema

Adults: Initially, 10 mg (sodium phosphate) I.V., followed by 4 mg I.M. q 6 hours. Then reduce dosage gradually over 5 to 7 days.

➤ Suppression test for Cushing's syndrome

Adults: 1 mg P.O. at 11 P.M. or 0.5 mg P.O. q 6 hours for 48 hours (with urine collection testing, as ordered)

Off-label uses

- Acute altitude sickness
- Bacterial meningitis
- Bronchopulmonary dysplasia in preterm infants
- Hirsutism
- Suppression test for detection, diagnosis, or management of depression

Contraindications

- Hypersensitivity to drug, benzyl alcohol, bisulfites, EDTA, creatinine, polysorbate 80, or methylparaben
- Systemic fungal infections
- Active or suspected ocular or periocular infections, advanced glaucoma (intravitreal implant)

Precautions

Use cautiously in:
- renal insufficiency, cirrhosis, diabetes mellitus, diverticulitis, GI disease, cardiovascular disease, hypoprothrombinemia, hypothyroidism, myasthenia gravis, glaucoma, osteoporosis, infections, underlying immunosuppression, psychotic tendencies
- pregnant or breastfeeding patients
- children.

Administration

- Give P.O. dose with food or milk.
- When giving I.M., inject deep into gluteal muscle; rotate sites as needed.
- For I.V. use, drug may be given undiluted as a single dose over 1 minute or

added to dextrose or I.V. saline solutions and given as an intermittent infusion at prescribed rate.

Route	Onset	Peak	Duration
P.O.	Unknown	1-2 hr	2.75 days
I.V.	1 hr	1 hr	Variable
I.M. (sodium phosphate)	1 hr	1 hr	6 days
Intravitreal implant	NA	NA	NA

Adverse reactions

CNS: headache, malaise, vertigo, psychiatric disturbances, **increased intracranial pressure, seizures**

CV: hypotension, **thrombophlebitis, myocardial rupture after recent myocardial infarction, thromboembolism**

EENT: cataracts; elevated intraocular pressure (IOP), conjunctival hemorrhage (with intravitreal implant)

GI: nausea, vomiting, abdominal distention, dry mouth, anorexia, **peptic ulcer, bowel perforation, pancreatitis, ulcerative esophagitis**

Metabolic: decreased carbohydrate tolerance, hyperglycemia, cushingoid appearance (moon face, buffalo hump), decreased growth (in children), latent diabetes mellitus, sodium and fluid retention, negative nitrogen balance, **adrenal suppression, hypokalemic alkalosis**

Musculoskeletal: muscle wasting, muscle pain, osteoporosis, aseptic joint necrosis, tendon rupture, long bone fractures

Skin: diaphoresis, angioedema, erythema, rash, pruritus, urticaria, contact dermatitis, acne, decreased wound healing, bruising, skin fragility, petechiae

Other: facial edema, weight gain or loss, increased susceptibility to infection, hypersensitivity reactions

---

Reactions in **bold** are life-threatening.　　　◀€ Clinical alert

Interactions

Drug-drug. *Barbiturates, phenytoin, rifampin:* decreased dexamethasone effects

Digoxin: increased risk of digoxin toxicity

Ephedrine: increased dexamethasone clearance

Estrogen, hormonal contraceptives: blocking of dexamethasone metabolism

Fluoroquinolones: increased risk of tendon rupture

Itraconazole, ketoconazole: increased dexamethasone blood level and effects

Live-virus vaccines: decreased antibody response to vaccine, increased risk of adverse reactions

Loop and thiazide diuretics: additive hypokalemia

Nonsteroidal anti-inflammatory drugs: increased risk of GI adverse effects

Somatrem, somatropin: decreased response to these drugs

Drug-diagnostic tests. *Calcium, potassium:* decreased levels

Cholesterol, glucose: increased levels

Nitroblue tetrazolium test: false-negative result

Drug-herbs. *Echinacea:* increased immune-stimulating effect

Ginseng: potentiation of immune-modulating response

Drug-behaviors. *Alcohol use:* increased risk of gastric irritation and GI ulcers

Patient monitoring

• Monitor blood glucose level closely in diabetic patients receiving drug orally.

• Monitor hemoglobin and potassium levels.

• Assess for occult blood loss.

◀€ In long-term therapy, never discontinue drug abruptly. Dosage must be tapered gradually.

• Monitor patient for increased IOP after intravitreal injection.

Patient teaching

◀€ Instruct patient to immediately report sudden weight gain, swelling of face or limbs, excessive nervousness or sleep disturbances, excessive body hair growth, vision changes, difficulty breathing, muscle weakness, persistent abdominal pain, or change in stool color.

• Tell patient to take oral drug with or after meals.

• Advise patient to report vision changes and if eye becomes red, sensitive to light, or painful after intravitreal implant, to promptly report this to ophthalmologist.

• Inform patient that drug makes him more susceptible to infection. Advise him to avoid crowds and exposure to illness.

◀€ Caution patient not to stop taking drug abruptly.

• As appropriate, review all other significant and life-threatening adverse reactions and interactions, especially those related to the drugs, tests, herbs, and behaviors mentioned above.

dexlansoprazole
Dexilant

Pharmacologic class: Proton pump inhibitor

Therapeutic class: GI agent

Pregnancy risk category B

Action

Suppresses gastric acid secretion by specific inhibition of (H+, K+)-ATPase in the gastric parietal cell.

Availability

Capsule: 30 mg, 60 mg

⚡ Indications and dosages

➤ Healing of all grades of erosive esophagitis (EE)

Adults: 60 mg P.O. daily for up to 8 weeks

➤ Maintaining healing of EE
Adults: 30 mg P.O. daily for up to 6 months

➤ Symptomatic nonerosive gastro-esophageal reflux disease (GERD)
Adults: 30 mg P.O. daily for up to 4 weeks

Dosage adjustment
• Moderate hepatic impairment

Contraindications
• Hypersensitivity to drug or its components

Precautions
Use cautiously in:
• moderate renal impairment
• pregnant or breastfeeding patients
• children younger than age 18 (safety and efficacy not established).

Administration
• Administer with or without food.

Route	Onset	Peak	Duration
P.O.	Unknown	1-2 hr and 4-5 hr (dual peaks)	Unknown

Adverse reactions
CNS: asthenia, dizziness, headache, migraine headache, memory impairment, paresthesia, psychomotor hyperactivity, tremor, trigeminal neuralgia, abnormal dreams, anxiety, depression, insomnia, **seizures**
CV: angina, bradycardia, chest pain, palpitations, tachycardia, hypertension, **deep vein thrombosis, arrhythmias, myocardial infarction**
EENT: eye irritation, eye swelling, ear pain, tinnitus, vertigo, nasopharyngitis, pharyngitis, sinusitis
GI: nausea; vomiting; diarrhea; abdominal pain, discomfort, tenderness; flatulence; abnormal feces; anal discomfort; Barrett's esophagus;

bezoar; abnormal bowel sounds; breath odor; microscopic colitis; colon and gastric polyps; constipation; dry mouth; duodenitis; dyspepsia; dysphagia; enteritis; eructation; esophagitis; gastritis; gastroenteritis; GI disorders; GI hypermotility disorders; GERD; ulcers and perforation; hematemesis; hematochezia; hemorrhoids; impaired gastric emptying; irritable bowel syndrome; mucus stools; oral mucosa blistering; painful defecation; proctitis; oral paresthesia; oral herpes; **rectal hemorrhage**
GU: vulvovaginal infection, libido changes, dysuria, micturition urgency, dysmenorrhea, dyspareunia, menorrhagia, menstrual disorder
Hematologic: anemia, lymphadenopathy
Hepatic: biliary colic, cholelithiasis, hepatomegaly
Metabolic: goiter
Musculoskeletal: arthralgia, arthritis, cramps, musculoskeletal pain, myalgia; hip, wrist, spine fracture (with long-term daily use)
Respiratory: upper respiratory tract infection, aspiration, asthma, bronchitis, cough, dyspnea, hyperventilation, respiratory tract congestion, sore throat
Skin: rash, sunburn, acne, dermatitis, erythema, pruritus, lesions, urticaria
Other: edema, chills, abnormal feeling, inflammation, mucosal inflammation, nodule, pain, pyrexia, candidal infection, viral infection, influenza, falls, overdose, procedural pain, weight gain, appetite changes, altered taste, hiccups, hot flushes, hypersensitivity

Interactions
Drug-drug. *Atazanavir:* decreased atazanavir level
Drugs with pH-dependent absorption (such as ampicillin esters, digoxin, iron salts, ketoconazole): interference with absorption of these drugs

---

Reactions in **bold** are life-threatening.　　　◀╟ Clinical alert

Tacrolimus: increased tacrolimus whole blood concentration
Warfarin: increased International Normalized Ratio and prothrombin time
Drug-diagnostic tests. *Alanine aminotransferase, alkaline phosphatase, aspartate aminotransferase, blood glucose, gastrin, potassium, serum creatinine, total protein:* increased levels
Bilirubin: increased or decreased level
Liver function tests: abnormal results
Platelets, serum calcium: decreased levels

Patient monitoring
• Monitor renal function tests closely.

Patient teaching
• Instruct patient to take drug with or without food.
• Tell patient to swallow capsule whole or open capsule and sprinkle contents on 1 tablespoon of applesauce and swallow immediately.
• Instruct patient to report allergic reactions (such as rash or itching) to prescriber.
• As appropriate, review all other significant and life-threatening adverse reactions and interactions, especially those related to the drugs and tests mentioned above.

dexmethylphenidate hydrochloride
Focalin, Focalin XR

Pharmacologic class: Methylphenidate derivative
Therapeutic class: CNS stimulant
Controlled substance schedule II
Pregnancy risk category C

FDA | **BOXED WARNING**

• Give cautiously to patient with history of drug dependence or alcoholism. Chronic abuse can cause marked tolerance and psychological dependence with abnormal behavior. Frank psychotic episodes may occur, especially with parenteral abuse. During withdrawal from abusive use, provide careful supervision, as severe depression may occur.
• Withdrawal after prolonged therapeutic use may unmask symptoms of underlying disorder that may require follow-up.

Action
Thought to block norepinephrine and dopamine reuptake, increasing the concentration of these neurotransmitters in extraneuronal space

Availability
Capsules (extended-release): 5 mg, 10 mg, 15 mg, 20 mg, 25 mg, 30 mg, 35 mg, 40 mg
Tablets: 2.5 mg, 5 mg, 10 mg

✪ Indications and dosages
➤ Attention deficit hyperactivity disorder
Adults and children older than age 6:
Tablets—In patients not receiving methylphenidate concurrently, 2.5 mg P.O. b.i.d. at least 4 hours apart; increase as needed in 2.5- to 5-mg increments to a maximum of 10 mg b.i.d. (Individualize dosage according to patient needs and response.) In patients receiving methylphenidate concurrently, start with half of methylphenidate dosage; maximum dosage is 10 mg P.O. b.i.d.
Capsules—In adults not receiving methylphenidate concurrently, 10 mg P.O. daily in morning; increase as needed in 10-mg increments

---

approximately weekly to maximum of 20 mg daily. In children not receiving methylphenidate concurrently, 5 mg daily in morning; increase as needed in 5-mg increments approximately weekly to maximum of 20 mg daily. In adults and children receiving methylphenidate concurrently, start with half of methylphenidate total daily dosage.

Contraindications
- Hypersensitivity to drug
- Glaucoma
- Anxiety, agitation, tension
- Family history or diagnosis of Tourette syndrome
- MAO inhibitor use within past 14 days

Precautions
Use cautiously in:
- hypertension, depression, seizures, cardiovascular disorders, psychosis, drug abuse
- pregnant or breastfeeding patients
- children under age 6 (safety and efficacy not established).

Administration
- Administer at same time each day without regard to meals.
- Give last dose at least 8 hours before bedtime to prevent insomnia.
- Know that regular-release tablets may be switched to same daily dosage as extended-release capsules.
- If necessary, open capsules, sprinkle contents over spoonful of applesauce, and administer immediately.
- Don't give within 14 days of MAO inhibitor use.

Route	Onset	Peak	Duration
P.O. (capsules)	Unknown	1.5-6.5 hr	Unknown
P.O. (tablets)	Variable	1-1.5 hr	Unknown

Adverse reactions
CNS: nervousness, insomnia, dizziness, drowsiness, headache, dyskinesia, chorea, Tourette syndrome, **toxic psychosis**
CV: increased or decreased heart rate and blood pressure, tachycardia, angina, palpitations, **arrhythmias**
EENT: blurred vision, visual accommodation problems
GI: nausea, abdominal pain
Hematologic: anemia, **leukopenia, thrombocytopenia**
Hepatic: hepatic dysfunction, hepatic coma
Skin: rash, alopecia
Other: fever, decreased appetite, weight loss, psychological drug dependence, drug tolerance, growth suppression in children (with long-term use)

Interactions
Drug-drug. *Anticoagulants, phenobarbital, phenytoin, primidone, selective serotonin reuptake inhibitors, tricyclic antidepressants:* inhibited metabolism and additive effects of these drugs
Antihypertensives, pressor agents (dopamine, epinephrine): decreased efficacy of these drugs
MAO inhibitors: severe hypertensive crisis

Patient monitoring
◀℈ Monitor blood pressure closely, especially in patients receiving antihypertensives concurrently.
- Evaluate cardiac status. Report palpitations and other signs and symptoms of arrhythmias.
- During prolonged therapy, regularly monitor CBC with white cell differential and platelet count.

Patient teaching
- Advise patient or parents that drug should be taken at same time each day.
- Instruct patient not to crush or chew capsule. If patient is unable to swallow capsules whole, advise him to open

capsules, sprinkle contents over spoonful of applesauce, and take immediately.

• Tell patient or parents that drug usually is discontinued if symptoms don't improve within 1 month.

• Instruct parents to monitor child's height and weight, because CNS stimulants have been associated with growth suppression.

• As appropriate, review all other significant and life-threatening adverse reactions and interactions, especially those related to the drugs mentioned above.

dextroamphetamine sulfate

Dexedrine Spansule, DextroStat

Pharmacologic class: Amphetamine

Therapeutic class: Sympathomimetic amine, CNS stimulant

Controlled substance schedule II

Pregnancy risk category C

FDA | BOXED WARNING

• Drug has high abuse potential. Prolonged use may lead to drug dependence. Stay alert for possibility of patient obtaining drug for nontherapeutic use or distribution. Drug should be prescribed sparingly.

• Misuse may cause sudden death and serious cardiovascular events.

Action

Produces CNS and respiratory stimulation by promoting release of norepinephrine from nerve terminals

Availability

Capsules (sustained-release): 5 mg, 10 mg, 15 mg

Oral solution: 5 mg/ml

Tablets: 5 mg, 10 mg

Indications and dosages

➤ Attention deficit hyperactivity disorder

Adults: 5 to 60 mg P.O. daily in divided doses until optimal response is obtained

Children ages 6 and older: 5 mg (capsules, oral solution, or tablets) P.O. once or twice daily, increased by 5 mg at weekly intervals until optimal response is obtained

Children ages 3 to 5: 2.5 mg (oral solution) P.O. daily, increased by 2.5 mg at weekly intervals until optimal response is obtained

➤ Narcolepsy

Adults: 5 to 60 mg P.O. daily as a single dose or in divided doses

Children ages 12 and older: 10 mg P.O. daily, increased by 10 mg at weekly intervals until desired response occurs or adult dosage is reached

Children ages 6 to 11: 5 mg P.O. daily, increased by 5 mg at weekly intervals until desired response occurs or adult dosage is reached

Contraindications

• Hypersensitivity to drug or tartrazine

• Glaucoma

• Psychotic disorders, agitated states

• Advanced arteriosclerosis, symptomatic cardiovascular disease, moderate to severe hypertension

• Hyperthyroidism

• MAO inhibitor use within past 14 days

• Pregnancy or breastfeeding

Precautions

Use cautiously in:

• cardiovascular disease, hypertension, diabetes mellitus

• history of substance abuse

• elderly patients.

Administration

• Make sure patient swallows sustained-release capsules whole without chewing or crushing.

• Before starting therapy, perform complete cardiac evaluation, including ECG and echocardiogram.
• Give last daily dose at least 6 hours before patient's bedtime.
◀€ Don't give within 14 days of MAO inhibitor, because potentially fatal reaction may occur.

Route	Onset	Peak	Duration
P.O.	1-2 hr	Unknown	2-10 hr
P.O. (sustained)	Unknown	Unknown	Up to 24 hr

Adverse reactions

CNS: hyperactivity, insomnia, restlessness, tremor, depression, dizziness, headache, irritability
CV: palpitations, tachycardia, hypertension, hypotension, **arrhythmias**
GI: nausea, vomiting, constipation, diarrhea, abdominal cramps, dry mouth
GU: erectile dysfunction, increased libido
Skin: urticaria
Other: metallic taste, decreased appetite, physical or psychological drug dependence

Interactions

Drug-drug. *Acetazolamide, sodium bicarbonate:* urine alkalization, leading to increased dextroamphetamine effects
Adrenergic blockers: additive effects
Ammonium chloride, ascorbic acid (large doses): urine acidification, leading to decreased dextroamphetamine effects
Beta-adrenergic blockers, tricyclic antidepressants: increased risk of adverse cardiovascular effects
Guanethidine: reversal of hypotensive effect
MAO inhibitors: hypertensive crisis
Phenothiazines: decreased dextroamphetamine effects
Selective serotonin reuptake inhibitors: increased risk of serotonin syndrome

Drug-diagnostic tests. *Plasma corticosteroids:* increased levels
Drug-food. *Caffeine:* increased stimulant effect
Drug-herbs. *Caffeine-containing herbs, ephedra (ma huang):* increased stimulant effect

Patient monitoring

• Interrupt therapy or reduce dosage periodically to assess drug efficacy in patients with behavior disorders.
• Monitor patient for new or worsening aggressive behavior.
• Monitor blood and urine glucose levels carefully in diabetic patient. Drug may alter regular insulin requirements.

Patient teaching

• Tell patient to swallow sustained-release capsules whole with liquid without chewing or crushing.
• Advise patient to take drug early in day to avoid insomnia.
◀€ Instruct patient to immediately notify prescriber if chest pain, irregular pulse, or worsening aggressive behavior occurs.
• Instruct patient to avoid driving and other hazardous activities until he knows how drug affects him.
• Caution patient not to stop therapy abruptly but to taper dosage gradually.
• As appropriate, review all other significant and life-threatening adverse reactions and interactions, especially those related to the drugs, tests, foods, and herbs mentioned above.

dextromethorphan hydrobromide

Adult Dry Cough⊕, Balminil DM✢, Broncho-Grippol-DM✢, Calmylin #1✢, Creo-Terpin, Creomulsion, Delsym, DexAlone, Hold DM, Koffex-DM✢, Neo-DM✢, Robitussin Children's Cough Long-Acting, Robitussin for Dry Coughs⊕, Robitussin Maximum Strength Cough Suppressant, Scot-Tussin Diabetes, Sedatuss✢, Triaminic Children's Long-Acting Cough, Trocal, Vicks DayQuil Cough, Vicks Vaposyrup for Dry Cough⊕, Vicks 44 Cough Relief

Pharmacologic class: Levorphanol derivative

Therapeutic class: Antitussive (nonnarcotic)

Pregnancy risk category C

Action

Depresses cough reflex through direct effect on cough center in medulla. Has no expectorant action and does not inhibit ciliary action. Although related to opioids structurally, lacks analgesic and addictive properties.

Availability

Gelcaps: 15 mg, 30 mg
Liquid: 3.5 mg/5 ml, 5 mg/5 ml, 7.5 mg/5 ml, 15 mg/5 ml
Lozenges: 5 mg, 7.5 mg
Oral suspension (extended-release): 30 mg/5 ml
Syrup: 7.5 mg/5 ml, 10 mg/15 ml

⚕ Indications and dosages

➤ Cough caused by minor viral upper respiratory tract infections or inhaled irritants

Adults and children over age 12: 10 to 20 mg P.O. q 4 hours, or 30 mg P.O. q 6 to 8 hours, or 60 mg of extended-release form P.O. b.i.d. (not to exceed 120 mg/day)

Children ages 6 to 12: 5 to 10 mg P.O. q 4 hours, or 15 mg P.O. q 6 to 8 hours, or 30 mg of extended-release form P.O. q 12 hours (not to exceed 60 mg/day)

Children ages 4 to 6: 2.5 to 7.5 mg (syrup) P.O. q 4 to 8 hours or 15 mg (extended-release form) P.O. b.i.d. Not to exceed 30 mg/day.

Dosage adjustment

• Elderly patients

Contraindications

• Hypersensitivity to drug
• Chronic productive cough
• MAO inhibitor use within past 14 days

Precautions

Use cautiously in:
• tartrazine sensitivity
• diabetes mellitus (with sucrose-containing drug products)
• pregnant or breastfeeding patients
• children younger than age 2 (safety not established).

Administration

• Don't administer lozenges to children younger than age 6.
🔊 Don't give within 14 days of MAO inhibitors.

Route	Onset	Peak	Duration
P.O.	15-30 min	Unknown	3-6 hr
P.O. (extended)	Unknown	Unknown	9-12 hr

Adverse reactions

CNS: dizziness and sedation
GI: nausea, vomiting, stomach pain

Interactions

Drug-drug. *Amiodarone, fluoxetine, quinidine:* increased dextromethorphan blood level, greater risk of adverse reactions

Antidepressants, antihistamines, opioids, sedative-hypnotics: additive CNS depression
MAO inhibitors, sibutramine: serotonin syndrome (nausea, confusion, blood pressure changes)
Drug-behaviors. *Alcohol use:* additive CNS depression

Patient monitoring
• Monitor cough frequency and type, and assess sputum characteristics.
• Assess hydration status. Increase patient's fluid input to help moisten secretions.

Patient teaching
• Advise patient to avoid irritants, such as smoking, dust, and fumes. Suggest use of humidifier to filter air pollutants.
• Inform patient that treatment aims to decrease coughing frequency and intensity without completely eliminating protective cough reflex.
• Instruct patient to contact health care provider if cough lasts more than 7 days.
• As appropriate, review all other significant adverse reactions and interactions, especially those related to the drugs and behaviors mentioned above.

dextrose (d-glucose)
BD Glucose, Glutose, Insta Glucose

Pharmacologic class: Monosaccharide
Therapeutic class: Carbohydrate caloric nutritional supplement
Pregnancy risk category C

Action
Prevents protein and nitrogen loss; promotes glycogen deposition and ketone accumulation (through osmotic diuretic action)

Availability
Injection: 2.5%, 5%, 10%, 20%, 25%, 30%, 40%, 50%, 60%, 70%
Oral gel: 40%
Tablets (chewable): 5 g

Indications and dosages
➤ Insulin-dependent hypoglycemia
Adults and children: Initially, 10 to 20 g P.O., repeated in 10 to 20 minutes if needed based on blood glucose level; or 20 to 50 ml by I.V. infusion or injection of 50% solution given at 3 ml/minute. Maintenance dosage is 10% to 15% solution by continuous I.V. infusion until blood glucose level reaches therapeutic range.
Infants and neonates: 2 ml/kg of 10% to 25% solution by slow I.V. infusion until blood glucose level reaches therapeutic range
➤ Calorie replacement
Adults and children: 2.5%, 5%, or 10% solution given through peripheral I.V. line, with dosage tailored to patient's need for fluid or calories; or 10% to 70% solution given through large central vein if needed (typically mixed with amino acids or other solution)

Off-label uses
• Varicose veins
• Insulin-secreting islet-cell adenoma

Contraindications
• Hypersensitivity to drug
• Hyperglycemia, diabetic coma
• Hemorrhage
• Heart failure

Precautions
Use cautiously in:
• renal, cardiac, or hepatic impairment; diabetes mellitus.

Administration
• Use aseptic technique when preparing solution. Bacteria thrive in high-glucose environments.
◄ Infuse concentrations above 10% through central vein.

Reactions in **bold** are life-threatening.　　　　　◄ Clinical alert

• Don't infuse concentrated solution rapidly, because doing so may cause hyperglycemia and fluid shifts.

◀€ Never stop infusion abruptly.

Route	Onset	Peak	Duration
P.O.	10-20 min	40 min	Unknown
I.V.	2-3 min	Unknown	Unknown

Adverse reactions

CNS: confusion, loss of consciousness
CV: hypertension, phlebitis, **venous thrombosis, heart failure**
GU: glycosuria, osmotic diuresis
Metabolic: hyperglycemia, hypervolemia, hypovolemia, electrolyte imbalances, **hyperosmolar coma**
Respiratory: pulmonary edema
Skin: flushing, urticaria
Other: chills, fever, dehydration, injection site reaction, infection

Interactions

Drug-drug. *Corticosteroids, corticotropin:* increased risk of fluid and electrolyte imbalances
Drug-diagnostic tests. *Glucose:* increased level

Patient monitoring

◀€ Monitor infusion site frequently to prevent irritation, tissue sloughing, necrosis, and phlebitis.
• Check blood glucose level at regular intervals.
• Monitor fluid intake and output.
• Weigh patient regularly.
• Assess patient for confusion.

Patient teaching

• Teach patient how to recognize signs and symptoms of hypoglycemia and hyperglycemia.
• Provide instructions on glucose self-monitoring.
• As appropriate, review all other significant and life-threatening adverse reactions and interactions, especially those related to the drugs and tests mentioned above.

diazepam

Apo-Diazepam✦, Bio-Diazepam✦, Dialar✛, Diastat, Diazemuls✦✛, Diazepam Intensol, Novo-Dipam✦, PMS-Diazepam✦, Stesolid✛, Tensium✛, Valclair✛, Valium, Vivol✦

Pharmacologic class: Benzodiazepine
Therapeutic class: Anxiolytic, anticonvulsant, sedative-hypnotic, skeletal muscle relaxant (centrally acting)
Controlled substance schedule IV
Pregnancy risk category D

Action

Produces anxiolytic effect and CNS depression by stimulating gamma-aminobutyric acid receptors. Relaxes skeletal muscles of spine by inhibiting polysynaptic afferent pathways. Controls seizures by enhancing presynaptic inhibition.

Availability

Injection: 5 mg/ml
Oral solution: 1 mg/ml, 5 mg/5 ml
Tablets: 2 mg, 5 mg, 10 mg

⏏ Indications and dosages

➤ Anxiety disorders
Adults: 2 to 10 mg P.O. two to four times daily, depending on symptom severity. Alternatively, for moderate anxiety, 2 to 5 mg I.V., repeated in 3 to 4 hours if needed. For severe anxiety, 5 to 10 mg I.V., repeated in 3 to 4 hours if needed.
Children age 6 months and older: 1 to 2.5 mg P.O. three to four times daily; may increase gradually as needed
➤ Before cardioversion
Adults: 5 to 15 mg I.V. 5 to 10 minutes before cardioversion
➤ Before endoscopy
Adults: Usually, 10 mg I.V. is sufficient; may be increased to 20 mg I.V.

Alternatively, 5 to 10 mg I.M. 30 minutes before endoscopy.

➤ Status epilepticus and severe recurrent convulsive seizures

Adults: 5 to 10 mg I.V. slowly, repeated as needed q 10 to 15 minutes, to a maximum of 30 mg; may repeat regimen if needed in 2 to 4 hours. May give I.M. if I.V. delivery is impossible.

Children ages 5 and older: 1 mg I.V. slowly q 2 to 5 minutes, to a maximum of 10 mg; repeat in 2 to 4 hours if needed. May give I.M. if I.V. delivery is impossible.

Children over 1 month to 5 years: 0.2 to 0.5 mg I.V. slowly q 2 to 5 minutes, to a maximum of 5 mg I.V. May give I.M. if I.V. delivery is impossible.

➤ Muscle spasm associated with local pathology, cerebral palsy, athetosis, "stiff-man" syndrome, or tetanus

Adults: 2 to 10 mg P.O. three to four times daily. Or initially, 5 to 10 mg I.V. or I.M., repeated in 3 to 4 hours if needed. Tetanus may necessitate higher dosages.

Elderly or debilitated patients: Initially, 2 to 2.5 mg P.O. once or twice daily, increased gradually as needed and tolerated

Children ages 5 and older: 5 to 10 mg I.M. or I.V., repeated q 3 to 4 hours as needed to control tetanus spasm

Children over 1 month to 5 years: 1 to 2 mg I.M. or I.V. slowly, repeated q 3 to 4 hours as needed to control tetanus spasm

➤ Acute alcohol withdrawal

Adults: Initially, 10 mg P.O. three to four times during first 24 hours, decreased to 5 mg P.O. three to four times daily p.r.n. Or initially, 10 mg I.M. or I.V.; then 5 to 10 mg I.M. or I.V. in 3 to 4 hours p.r.n.

Off-label uses
• Panic attacks
• Adjunct to general anesthesia

Contraindications
• Hypersensitivity to drug, other benzodiazepines, alcohol, or tartrazine
• Coma or CNS depression
• Narrow-angle glaucoma

Precautions
Use cautiously in:
• hepatic dysfunction, severe renal impairment
• elderly patients
• pregnant or breastfeeding patients (use not recommended)
• children.

Administration
• Give P.O. dose with or without food.
🔊 Administer I.V. infusion slowly into large vein, taking at least 1 minute for each 5 mg in adults or at least 3 minutes for each 0.25 mg/kg in children.
• Know that I.V. route is preferred over I.M. route because of slow or erratic I.M. absorption.
• Don't mix with other drugs or solutions in syringe or container.
• Enforce bed rest for at least 3 hours after I.V. injection.
• Give I.M. injection deeply and slowly into large muscle mass.
• If desired, mix oral solution with liquid or soft food.

Route	Onset	Peak	Duration
P.O.	30-60 min	1-2 hr	Up to 24 hr
I.V.	1-5 min	15-30 min	15-60 min
I.M.	Within 20 min	0.5-1.5 hr	Unknown

Adverse reactions
CNS: dizziness, drowsiness, lethargy, depression, light-headedness, disorientation, anger, manic or hypomanic episodes, restlessness, paresthesia, headache, slurred speech, dysarthria, stupor, tremor, dystonia, vivid dreams, extrapyramidal reactions, mild paradoxical excitation

---

CV: bradycardia, tachycardia, hypertension, hypotension, palpitations, **cardiovascular collapse**
EENT: blurred vision, diplopia, nystagmus, nasal congestion
GI: nausea, vomiting, diarrhea, constipation, gastric disorders, difficulty swallowing, increased salivation
GU: urinary retention or incontinence, menstrual irregularities, gynecomastia, libido changes
Hematologic: blood dyscrasias including eosinophilia, **leukopenia**, **agranulocytosis**, and **thrombocytopenia**
Hepatic: hepatic dysfunction
Musculoskeletal: muscle rigidity, muscular disturbances
Respiratory: respiratory depression
Skin: dermatitis, rash, pruritus, urticaria, diaphoresis
Other: weight gain or loss, decreased appetite, edema, hiccups, fever, physical or psychological drug dependence or tolerance

Interactions

Drug-drug. *Antidepressants, antihistamines, barbiturates, opioids:* additive CNS depression
Cimetidine, disulfiram, fluoxetine, hormonal contraceptives, isoniazid, ketoconazole, metoprolol, propoxyphene, propranolol, valproic acid: decreased metabolism and enhanced action of diazepam
Digoxin: increased digoxin blood level, possible toxicity
Levodopa: decreased levodopa efficacy
Rifampin: increased metabolism and decreased efficacy of diazepam
Theophylline: decreased sedative effect of diazepam
Drug-diagnostic tests. *Alanine aminotransferase, alkaline phosphatase, aspartate aminotransferase, lactate dehydrogenase:* increased levels
Neutrophils, platelets: decreased counts
Drug-herbs. *Chamomile, hops, kava, skullcap, valerian:* increased CNS depression

Drug-behaviors. *Alcohol use:* increased CNS depression

Patient monitoring

• Monitor vital signs and respiratory and neurologic status.
• Supervise ambulation, especially in elderly patients.
• Monitor CBC and kidney and liver function test results.
🔊 Avoid sudden drug withdrawal. Taper dosage gradually to termination of therapy.

Patient teaching

• Inform patient he may take drug with or without food; recommend taking it with food if it causes stomach upset.
• Caution patient to avoid driving and other hazardous activities until he knows how drug affects concentration and alertness.
🔊 Tell patient to notify prescriber immediately if easy bruising or bleeding occurs.
• Instruct patient to move slowly when sitting up or standing, to avoid dizziness from blood pressure decrease. Advise him to dangle legs briefly before getting out of bed.
🔊 Advise patient not to stop taking drug abruptly.
• Advise patient to avoid alcohol and other depressants such as sedatives while taking drug.
• Tell female patient not to take drug if she is pregnant or plans to breastfeed.
• As appropriate, review all other significant and life-threatening adverse reactions and interactions, especially those related to the drugs, tests, herbs, and behaviors mentioned above.

---

diclofenac epolamine
Flector Patch

diclofenac potassium
Cambia, Cataflam, Novo-Difenac-K✷, Novo-Difenac-SR✷, Zipsor

diclofenac sodium
Apo-Diclo✷, Dom-Diclofenac✷, Diclofex⬤, Fenactol⬤, Novo-Difenac✷, Nu-Diclo✷, Pennsaid, PMS-Diclofenac✷, Voltaren, Voltaren XR, Voltarol⬤

Pharmacologic class: Cyclooxygenase inhibitor, nonsteroidal anti-inflammatory drug (NSAID)

Therapeutic class: Nonopioid analgesic, antiarthritic

Pregnancy risk category C

FDA | BOXED WARNING

• Drug may increase risk of serious cardiovascular thrombotic events, myocardial infarction, and stroke. Risk may increase with duration of use. Patients with cardiovascular disease or risk factors for it may be at greater risk.
• Drug increases risk of serious GI adverse events, including bleeding, ulcers, and stomach or intestinal perforation. These events can occur at any time during use and without warning. Elderly patients are at greater risk.
• Drug is contraindicated for treatment of perioperative pain in setting of coronary artery bypass graft surgery.

Action
Unclear. Thought to block activity of cyclooxygenase, thereby inhibiting inflammatory responses of vasodilation and swelling and blocking transmission of painful stimuli.

Availability
diclofenac epolamine
Flector patch: 1.3%
diclofenac potassium
Capsules, liquid-filled: 25 mg
Powder for oral solution: 50 mg
Tablets: 50 mg
diclofenac sodium
Tablets (delayed-release): 25 mg, 50 mg, 75 mg
Tablets (extended-release): 100 mg
Topical gel: 1%
Topical solution: 1.5%

ⓥ Indications and dosages
➤ Acute migraine attacks
Adults: 50 mg P.O. (oral powder)
➤ Osteoarthritis pain of joints amenable to topical treatment
Adults: 2 g for each elbow, wrist, or hand; 4 g for each knee, ankle, or foot q.i.d. Maximum, 16 g daily to any single joint of lower extremities; maximum, 8 g daily to any single joint of upper extremities. Don't exceed 32 g/day over all affected joints.
➤ Osteoarthritis of knee
Adults: 40 drops on each painful knee q.i.d.
➤ Acute pain due to minor strains, sprains, and contusions (topical treatment)
Adults: One patch to most painful area b.i.d. Use lowest effective dosage for shortest duration consistent with individual patient's treatment goals.
➤ Analgesia; dysmenorrhea
Adults: Initially, 100 mg P.O., then 50 mg t.i.d. as needed
➤ Rheumatoid arthritis
Adults: Initially, 50 mg P.O. three to four times daily. After initial response, reduce to lowest dosage that controls symptoms. Usual maintenance dosage is 25 mg t.i.d.
➤ Osteoarthritis
Adults: Initially, 50 mg P.O. two to three times daily. After initial response, reduce to lowest dosage that controls symptoms.

Reactions in **bold** are life-threatening. ◀€ Clinical alert

➢ Ankylosing spondylitis
Adults: 25 mg P.O. four to five times daily. After initial response, reduce to lowest dosage that controls symptoms.

Dosage adjustment
• Renal impairment
• Elderly patients

Off-label uses
• Post-radial keratotomy symptoms
• Dental pain

Contraindications
• Hypersensitivity to drug or its components, other NSAIDs, or aspirin
• Active GI bleeding or ulcer disease
• Aspirin-sensitive asthma, urticaria
• Use as perioperative analgesia in coronary artery bypass graft surgery
• Use on nonintact or damaged skin (patch)

Precautions
Use cautiously in:
• severe cardiovascular (including patients taking diuretics or ACE inhibitors, patients with fluid retention, hypertension, or congestive heart failure), renal, or hepatic disease; bleeding tendency; dehydration
• advanced renal disease (not recommended)
• history of porphyria or preexisting asthma
• concurrent methotrexate or anticoagulant use; concurrent use of drugs known to be potentially hepatotoxic (such as acetaminophen, anti-infectives, or antiepileptics)
• concurrent use of aspirin (not recommended)
• concurrent use with oral NSAIDs (avoid use)
• elderly patients
• pregnant or breastfeeding patients
• children (safety and efficacy not established).

Administration
• Give on empty stomach 1 hour before or after a meal.

• If drug causes GI upset, give with milk or meals. Mix and give oral powder with 30 to 60 ml of water only.
• Make sure patient swallows extended-release and delayed-release forms whole without chewing or crushing.
• Know that oral powder isn't indicated for prophylactic migraine therapy or cluster headaches.
• Know that oral powder formulation isn't interchangeable with other oral forms.
• Don't apply patch to damaged or nonintact skin.
🔊 Avoid contact of patch with eyes and mucosa. If eye contact occurs, immediately wash eyes with water or saline solution

Route	Onset	Peak	Duration
P.O.	10 min	1 hr	8 hr
P.O. (delayed)	30 min	2-3 hr	8 hr
P.O. (extended)	Unknown	5-6 hr	Unknown
Patch	Unknown	10-20 hr	Unknown
Topical (gel, solution)	Unknown	10-14 hr	6 hr

Adverse reactions
CNS: dizziness, drowsiness, headache, paresthesia
CV: hypertension, **thrombosis**
EENT: tinnitus
GI: dyspepsia, diarrhea, abdominal pain, dyspepsia, heartburn, peptic ulcer, **GI bleeding, GI perforation**
GU: dysuria, frequent urination, hematuria, proteinuria, nephritis, **acute renal failure**
Hepatic: liver failure
Hematologic: prolonged bleeding time
Hepatic: hepatotoxicity
Skin: eczema, photosensitivity, rash, contact dermatitis, dry skin, exfoliation; application-site reactions, including pruritus, dermatitis, burning (with patch); **exfoliative dermatitis,**

Stevens-Johnson syndrome, toxic epidermal necrolysis
Other: dysgeusia, pain and redness allergic reactions (including edema), **anaphylaxis**

Interactions
Drug-drug. *Anticoagulants, antiplatelet agents, cephalosporins, plicamycin, thrombolytics:* increased risk of bleeding
Antihypertensives, diuretics: decreased efficacy of these drugs
Antineoplastics: increased risk of hematologic adverse reactions
Aspirin: increased adverse reactions
Colchicine, corticosteroids, other NSAIDs: additive adverse GI effects
Cyclosporine, probenecid: increased risk of diclofenac toxicity
Digoxin, lithium, methotrexate, phenytoin, theophylline: increased levels of these drugs, greater risk of toxicity
Diuretics (furosemide, thiazides): reduced natriuretic effect of these drugs
Potassium-sparing diuretics: increased risk of hyperkalemia
Voriconazole: increased diclofenac C_{max} and area under the curve
Drug-diagnostic tests. *Alanine aminotransferase, alkaline phosphatase, aspartate aminotransferase, blood urea nitrogen, creatinine, electrolytes, lactate dehydrogenase, urine uric acid:* increased values
Bleeding time: prolonged
Hematocrit, hemoglobin, platelets, serum uric acid, urine electrolytes, white blood cells: decreased values
Drug-herbs. *Anise, arnica, chamomile, clove, dong quai, fenugreek, feverfew, garlic, ginger, ginkgo, ginseng, and others:* increased risk of bleeding
Drug-behaviors. *Alcohol use:* increased risk of adverse GI effects

Patient monitoring
• Monitor hepatic and renal function.
• Observe for and report signs and symptoms of bleeding.
• Assess for hypertension.

• Monitor sodium and potassium levels in patients receiving potassium-sparing diuretics.
◀◢ Discontinue drug if rash or other signs of local skin reaction occur.
◀◢ Discontinue drug immediately if abnormal liver test values persist or worsen.
• Weigh patient to detect fluid retention. Report gain of more than 2 lb in 24 hours.

Patient teaching
• Instruct patient to take drug on empty stomach 1 hour before or after a meal.
• Advise patient not to lie down for 15 to 30 minutes after taking oral drug, to minimize esophageal irritation.
• Instruct patient to mix oral powder in 1 to 2 ounces of water only before taking.
• Tell patient to measure proper amount of gel using measuring dosing card supplied and to gently massage gel into skin of entire affected foot, knee, or ankle.
• Instruct patient to apply 10 drops of topical solution to clean, dry skin and to spread evenly around front, back, and sides of knee; then repeat this procedure until 40 drops have been applied and knee is completely covered with solution.
• Instruct patient not to apply gel, patch, or topical solution to open wounds and to avoid contact with eyes and mucous membranes.
• Advise patient to avoid exposing treated sites to bath water and sunlight, external heat, occlusive dressings or clothing, sunscreens, cosmetics, lotions, moisturizers, insect repellants, or other topical drugs.
• Instruct patient to wash hands thoroughly after applying topical solution, patch, or gel except when gel is applied to the hand. If gel is applied to a hand, advise patient to avoid washing treated hands for at least 1 hour after application.

• Tell patient to discard used patches out of the reach of children and pets.

◀€ Instruct patient to stop drug and immediately report wheezing and signs or symptoms of hypersensitivity reactions (rash, swelling of face or throat, shortness of breath) or liver impairment (unusual tiredness, weakness, nausea, yellowing of skin or eyes, tenderness on right upper side of abdomen, flulike symptoms).

◀€ Instruct patient to stop taking drug and contact prescriber promptly if he experiences ringing or buzzing in ears, dizziness, GI discomfort, or bleeding.

◀€ Inform patient that drug may cause serious CV side effects and to immediately report such signs and symptoms as unexplained weight gain, chest pain, shortness of breath, weakness, or slurred speech.

• Caution patient not to take over-the-counter analgesics during diclofenac therapy.

• Advise female patient to avoid pregnancy while taking this drug.

• Advise breastfeeding patient that she should decide whether to discontinue breastfeeding or discontinue drug, taking into account importance of drug for her treatment.

• As appropriate, review all other significant and life-threatening adverse reactions and interactions, especially those related to the drugs, tests, herbs, and behaviors mentioned above.

dicyclomine (dicycloverine✹)

Bentyl, Bentylol♣, Diclophen♣, Formulex♣, Lomine♣, Merbentyl✹, Protylol♣

Pharmacologic class: Anticholinergic
Therapeutic class: Antispasmodic
Pregnancy risk category B

Action
Thought to exert direct effect on GI smooth muscle by inhibiting acetylcholine at receptor sites, thereby reducing GI tract motility and tone

Availability
Capsules: 10 mg
Solution for injection: 10 mg/ml
Syrup: 10 mg/5 ml
Tablets: 20 mg

💊 Indications and dosages
➤ Irritable bowel syndrome in patients unresponsive to usual interventions
Adults: 20 mg P.O. or I.M. q.i.d.; may increase up to 160 mg/day

Contraindications
• Hypersensitivity to drug
• GI or genitourinary tract obstruction
• Severe ulcerative colitis
• Reflux esophagitis
• Unstable cardiovascular status
• Glaucoma
• Myasthenia gravis
• Breastfeeding
• Infants younger than 6 months

Precautions
Use cautiously in:
• hepatic or renal impairment, autonomic neuropathy, cardiovascular disease, prostatic hypertrophy
• elderly patients
• pregnant patients (safety not established).

Administration
• Give 30 to 60 minutes before meals; give bedtime dose at least 2 hours after evening meal.
◀€ Don't administer by I.V. route.
• Don't give by I.M. route for more than 2 days.

Route	Onset	Peak	Duration
P.O., I.M.	Unknown	Unknown	Unknown

♣ Canada   ✹ UK   🦶 Hazardous drug   ⊗ High-alert drug

Adverse reactions

CNS: confusion, drowsiness, light-headedness (with I.M. use), psychosis
CV: palpitations, tachycardia
EENT: blurred vision, increased intraocular pressure
GI: nausea, vomiting, constipation, heartburn, decreased salivation, dry mouth, **paralytic ileus**
GU: urinary hesitancy or retention, erectile dysfunction, decreased lactation
Skin: decreased sweating, rash, itching, urticaria
Other: pain and redness at I.M. site, allergic reactions including **anaphylaxis**

Interactions

Drug-drug. *Adsorbent antidiarrheals, antacids:* decreased dicyclomine absorption
Cyclopropane anesthetics: increased risk of cardiovascular adverse reactions
Oral drugs: altered absorption of these drugs
Potassium (oral): increased GI mucosal lesions
Other anticholinergics (including antihistamines, disopyramide, quinidine): additive anticholinergic effects
Drug-diagnostic tests. *Gastric acid secretion test:* antagonism of pentagastrin and histamine (testing agents)

Patient monitoring

◀€ Stay alert for anaphylaxis.
• Monitor vital signs and fluid intake and output. Ask patient about palpitations.
◀€ Assess for light-headedness, confusion, and rash after I.M. injection.
• Evaluate patient's vision, particularly for blurring and other signs and symptoms of increasing intraocular pressure.
• Assess bowel pattern, particularly for signs and symptoms of paralytic ileus.

Patient teaching

• Instruct patient to take drug 30 to 60 minutes before meals and to take bedtime dose at least 2 hours after evening meal.
• Advise patient not to take antacids or adsorbent antidiarrheals within 2 hours of dicyclomine.
◀€ Urge patient to promptly report rash, abdominal pain, decreased urinary output, or absence of bowel movements.
• Caution patient to avoid driving or other hazardous activities until he knows how drug affects concentration, vision, and alertness.
◀€ Instruct patient to avoid exposure to high temperatures and to immediately notify prescriber if fever and decreased sweating occur in high environmental temperature.
• Advise patient to minimize GI upset by eating small, frequent servings of healthy food and drinking plenty of fluids.
• As appropriate, review all other significant and life-threatening adverse reactions and interactions, especially those related to the drugs and tests mentioned above.

didanosine
(ddI, 2,3-dideoxyinosine)
Videx, Videx EC

Pharmacologic class: Nucleoside reverse transcriptase inhibitor
Therapeutic class: Antiretroviral, antiviral
Pregnancy risk category B

FDA BOXED WARNING

• Pancreatitis has occurred when drug was used alone or in combination regimens in treatment-naive or treatment-experienced patients. Suspend therapy in patients with suspected pancreatitis;

Reactions in **bold** are life-threatening. ◀€ Clinical alert

discontinue in patients with confirmed pancreatitis.

• Drug may cause lactic acidosis and severe hepatomegaly with steatosis when used alone or in combination with other antiretrovirals. Fatal lactic acidosis has occurred in pregnant women receiving didanosine-stavudine combination with other antiretrovirals. In pregnant patients, use this combination with caution and only if benefit clearly outweighs risk.

Action

Inhibits replication of human immunodeficiency virus (HIV) by disrupting synthesis of DNA polymerase, an enzyme crucial to DNA and RNA formation

Availability

Capsules (delayed-release): 125 mg, 200 mg, 250 mg, 400 mg
Powder for oral solution (pediatric): 2 g in 4-oz glass bottle, 4 g in 8-oz glass bottle

⚕ Indications and dosages

➤ HIV infection
Adults weighing 60 kg (132 lb) or more: 400 mg (capsules) P.O. once daily
Adults weighing less than 60 kg (132 lb): 250 mg (capsules) P.O. once daily
Children: 120 mg/m² (powder for oral solution, pediatric) P.O. q 12 hours

Dosage adjustment

• Renal impairment

Contraindications

• Hypersensitivity to drug
• Concurrent use of allopurinol or ribavirin

Precautions

Use cautiously in:
• renal or hepatic impairment, peripheral neuropathy, hyperuricemia
• elderly patients
• pregnant or breastfeeding patients
• children.

Administration

• Know that drug is usually given in conjunction with other antiretrovirals.
• Give on empty stomach 30 minutes before or 2 hours after a meal.
• Don't administer with fruit juice.
• Know that pharmacist must prepare pediatric powder for oral solution by diluting with water and antacid to a concentration of 10 mg/ml.
• Be aware that delayed-release capsules aren't intended for use in children.

Route	Onset	Peak	Duration
P.O.	Unknown	0.5-1 hr	Unknown

Adverse reactions

CNS: dizziness, anxiety, abnormal thinking, hypoesthesia, agitation, confusion, hypertonia, asthenia, peripheral neuropathy, **seizures, coma**
CV: peripheral coldness, palpitations, hypotension, bradycardia, weak pulse, pseudoaneurysm, incomplete atrioventricular (AV) block, **complete AV block, nodal arrhythmias, ventricular tachycardia, thrombophlebitis, embolism**
EENT: diplopia, abnormal vision, ocular hypotony, iritis, retinal detachment
GI: nausea, vomiting, diarrhea, abdominal enlargement, dyspepsia, ileus, GI reflux, hematemesis, dysphagia, dry mouth, **pancreatitis**
GU: urinary retention, frequency, or incontinence; dysuria; cystalgia; prostatitis; **renal dysfunction; nephrotoxicity**
Hematologic: anemia, **leukocytosis, thrombocytopenia, bleeding, neutropenia**
Hepatic: hepatomegaly with steatosis, noncirrhotic portal hypertension
Metabolic: diabetes mellitus, **hyperkalemia, lactic acidosis, noncirrhotic portal hypertension**
Musculoskeletal: muscle contractions

Respiratory: pneumonia, crackles, rhonchi, bronchitis, pleurisy, dyspnea, wheezing, **pleural effusion, pulmonary edema, pulmonary embolism, bronchospasm**
Skin: diaphoresis, pallor, rash, urticaria, pruritus, bullous eruption, petechiae, cellulitis, abscess
Other: edema, development of human antichimeric antibodies

Interactions
Drug-drug. *Allopurinol, ganciclovir (oral), ribavirin, tenofovir:* increased didanosine blood level
Amprenavir, delavirdine, indinavir, ritonavir, saquinavir: altered didanosine pharmacokinetics
Antacids, other drugs that increase gastric pH: increased risk of didanosine toxicity
Co-trimoxazole, pentamidine: increased risk of pancreatic toxicity
Dapsone, fluoroquinolones, ketoconazole: decreased blood levels of these drugs
Itraconazole: decreased itraconazole blood level
Methadone: 50% decrease in didanosine blood level
Drug-diagnostic tests. *Alanine aminotransferase, alkaline phosphatase, aspartate aminotransferase, bilirubin, uric acid:* increased levels
Granulocytes, hemoglobin, platelets, white blood cells: decreased values
Drug-food. *Any food:* decreased rate and extent of drug absorption

Patient monitoring
◀≋ Monitor patient for signs and symptoms of pancreatitis. Withhold drug in patients with signs or symptoms of pancreatitis and discontinue drug in patients with confirmed pancreatitis.
◀≋ Monitor patient for early signs and symptoms of portal hypertension (thrombocytopenia, splenomegaly). Discontinue drug in patients with evidence of noncirrhotic portal hypertension.

◀≋ Assess carefully for signs and symptoms of lactic acidosis, such as dizziness, light-headedness, and bradycardia.
• Monitor for signs and symptoms of peripheral neuropathy.
• In patients with renal impairment, watch for drug toxicity and hypermagnesemia (suggested by muscle weakness and confusion).

Patient teaching
• Tell patient to take drug on empty stomach.
• Advise patient using buffered powder to mix it with water, not juice, and to let powder dissolve for several minutes before taking.
◀≋ Instruct patient to immediately report abdominal pain, nausea, vomiting, tiredness, fast or irregular heartbeats, easy bruising, difficulty breathing, yellowing of skin or eyes, or dark urine.
• As appropriate, review all other significant and life-threatening adverse reactions and interactions, especially those related to the drugs, tests, and foods mentioned above.

digoxin
Apo-Digoxin❋, Digitek, Lanoxin, PMS Digoxin

Pharmacologic class: Cardiac glycoside
Therapeutic class: Inotropic, antiarrhythmic
Pregnancy risk category C

Action
Increases force and velocity of myocardial contraction and prolongs refractory period of atrioventricular (AV) node by increasing calcium entry into myocardial cells. Slows conduction

---

through sinoatrial and AV nodes and produces antiarrhythmic effect.

Availability

Oral solution (pediatric): 0.05 mg/ml
Injection: 0.05 mg/ml, 0.1 mg/ml, 0.25 mg/ml
Tablets: 0.125 mg, 0.25 mg, 0.5 mg

🖊 Indications and dosages

➤ Heart failure; tachyarrhythmias; atrial fibrillation and flutter; paroxysmal atrial tachycardia

Adults: For rapid digitalizing, 0.6 to 1 mg I.V. over 24 hours, with 50% of total dosage given initially and additional fractions given at 4- to 8-hour intervals; or digitalizing dose of 0.75 to 1.25 mg P.O. over 24 hours, with 50% of total dosage given initially and additional fractions given at 4- to 8-hour intervals. Maintenance dosage is 0.063 to 0.5 mg/day (tablets) or 0.35 to 0.5 mg/day (gelatin capsules), depending on lean body weight, renal function, and drug blood level.

Children older than age 10: For rapid digitalizing, 8 to 12 mcg/kg I.V. over 24 hours, with 50% of total dosage given initially and additional fractions given at 4- to 8-hour intervals; or digitalizing dose of 10 to 15 mcg/kg P.O. over 24 hours, with 50% of total dosage given initially and additional fractions given at 6- to 8-hour intervals. Maintenance dosage is 25% to 35% of loading dosage, given daily as a single dose (determined by renal function).

Children ages 5 to 10: For rapid digitalizing, 15 to 30 mcg/kg I.V. over 24 hours, with 50% of total dosage given initially and additional fractions given at 4- to 8-hour intervals; or digitalizing dose of 20 to 35 mcg/kg P.O. over 24 hours, with 50% of total dosage given initially and additional fractions given at 6- to 8-hour intervals. Maintenance dosage is 25% to 35% of loading

dosage, given daily in two divided doses (determined by renal function).

Children ages 2 to 5: For rapid digitalizing, 25 to 35 mcg/kg I.V. over 24 hours, with 50% of total dosage given initially and additional fractions given at 4- to 8-hour intervals; or digitalizing dose of 30 to 40 mcg/kg P.O. over 24 hours, with 50% of total dosage given initially and additional fractions given at 6- to 8-hour intervals. Maintenance dosage is 25% to 35% of loading dosage, given daily in two divided doses (determined by renal function).

Children ages 1 to 24 months: For rapid digitalizing, 30 to 50 mcg/kg I.V. over 24 hours, with 50% of total dosage given initially and additional fractions given at 4- to 8-hour intervals; or digitalizing dose of 35 to 60 mcg/kg P.O. over 24 hours, with 50% of total dosage given initially and additional fractions given at 6- to 8-hour intervals. Maintenance dosage is 25% to 35% of loading dosage, given daily in two divided doses (determined by renal function).

Infants (full-term): For rapid digitalizing, 20 to 30 mcg/kg I.V. over 24 hours, with 50% of total dosage given initially and additional fractions given at 4- to 8-hour intervals; or digitalizing dose of 25 to 35 mcg/kg P.O. over 24 hours, with 50% of total dosage given initially and additional fractions given at 6- to 8-hour intervals. Maintenance dosage is 25% to 35% of loading dosage, given daily in two divided doses (determined by renal function).

Infants (premature): For rapid digitalizing, 15 to 25 mcg/kg I.V. over 24 hours, with 50% of total dosage given initially and additional fractions given at 4- to 8-hour intervals; or digitalizing dose of 20 to 30 mcg/kg P.O. over 24 hours, with 50% of total dosage given initially and additional fractions given at 6- to 8-hour intervals. Maintenance dosage is 20% to 30% of loading dosage, given daily in two divided doses (determined by renal function).

Dosage adjustment
- Renal impairment
- Hyperthyroidism
- Elderly patients

Off-label uses
- Supraventricular tachyarrhythmias
- Intrauterine tachyarrhythmias

Contraindications
- Hypersensitivity to drug
- Uncontrolled ventricular arrhythmias
- AV block
- Idiopathic hypertrophic subaortic stenosis
- Constrictive pericarditis

Precautions
Use cautiously in:
- renal or hepatic impairment, electrolyte imbalances, myocardial infarction, thyroid disorders
- obesity
- elderly patients
- pregnant or breastfeeding patients.

Administration
- Administer I.V. drug undiluted, or dilute with sterile water for injection, normal saline solution, or dextrose 5% in water as directed.

◀€ Know that drug has narrow therapeutic index, so dosage must be monitored regularly and patient must be monitored for signs and symptoms of toxicity.
- Know that for rapid effect, initial digitalizing dose generally is given in several divided doses over 12 to 24 hours.
- Be aware that dosages used for atrial arrhythmias generally are higher than those used for inotropic effect.

Route	Onset	Peak	Duration
P.O.	0.5-2 hr	2-6 hr	2-4 days
I.V.	5-30 min	1-5 hr	2-4 days

Adverse reactions
CNS: fatigue, headache, asthenia
CV: bradycardia, ECG changes, **arrhythmias**
EENT: blurred or yellow vision
GI: nausea, vomiting, diarrhea
GU: gynecomastia
Hematologic: thrombocytopenia
Other: decreased appetite

Interactions
Drug-drug. *Amiodarone, cyclosporine, diclofenac, diltiazem, propafenone, quinidine, quinine, verapamil:* increased digoxin blood level, possibly leading to toxicity
Amphotericin B, corticosteroids, mezlocillin, piperacillin, thiazide and loop diuretics, ticarcillin: hypokalemia, increased risk of digoxin toxicity
Antacids, cholestyramine, colestipol, kaolin/pectin: decreased digoxin absorption
Beta-adrenergic blockers, other antiarrhythmics (including disopyramide, quinidine): additive bradycardia
Laxatives (excessive use): hypokalemia, increased risk of digoxin toxicity
Spironolactone: reduced digoxin clearance, increased risk of digoxin toxicity
Thyroid hormones: decreased digoxin efficacy
Drug-diagnostic tests. *Creatine kinase:* increased level
Drug-food. *High-fiber meal:* decreased digoxin absorption
Drug-herbs. *Coca seed, coffee seed, cola seed, guarana seed, horsetail, licorice, natural stimulants (such as aloe), yerba maté:* increased risk of digoxin toxicity and hypokalemia
Ephedra (ma huang): arrhythmias
Hawthorn: increased risk of adverse cardiovascular effects
Indian snakeroot: bradycardia
Psyllium: decreased digoxin absorption
St. John's wort: decreased blood level and effects of digoxin

d

Reactions in **bold** are life-threatening. ◀€ Clinical alert

Patient monitoring

• Assess apical pulse regularly for 1 full minute. If rate is less than 60 beats/minute, withhold dose and notify prescriber.

◀€ Monitor for signs and symptoms of drug toxicity (such as nausea, vomiting, visual disturbances, arrhythmias, and altered mental status). Be aware that therapeutic digoxin levels range from 0.5 to 2 ng/ml.

• Monitor ECG and blood levels of digoxin, potassium, magnesium, calcium, and creatinine.

• Stay alert for hypocalcemia. Know that this condition may predispose patient to digoxin toxicity and may decrease digoxin efficacy.

◀€ Watch closely for hypokalemia and hypomagnesemia. Know that digoxin toxicity may occur with these conditions despite digoxin blood levels below 2 ng/ml.

Patient teaching

• Tell patient to take drug at same time every day.

◀€ Instruct patient not to stop drug abruptly.

• Instruct patient not to take over-the-counter drugs without prescriber's approval.

◀€ Teach patient how to recognize and report signs and symptoms of digoxin toxicity.

• Stress importance of follow-up testing as directed by prescriber.

• As appropriate, review all other significant and life-threatening adverse reactions and interactions, especially those related to the drugs, tests, foods, and herbs mentioned above.

diltiazem hydrochloride

Adizem⊕, Angitil⊕, Apo-Diltiaz✦, Apo-Diltiazem✦, Calcicard⊕, Cardizem, Cardizem CD, Cardizem LA, Cartia XT, Dilacor-XR, Dilcardia⊕, Dilt-CD, Dilt-XR, Diltia XT, Diltzac, Dilzem⊕, Disogram⊕, Gen-Diltiazem✦, Med-Diltiazem✦, Novo-Diltiazem✦, Nu-Diltiaz✦, Optil⊕, Ratio-Diltiazem✦, Sandoz Diltiazem✦, Slozem⊕, Taztia XT, Tiazac, Tildiem⊕, Viazem⊕, Zemtard⊕

Pharmacologic class: Calcium channel blocker

Therapeutic class: Antianginal, antiarrhythmic (class IV), antihypertensive

Pregnancy risk category C

Action

Inhibits calcium from entering myocardial and vascular smooth-muscle cells, thereby depressing myocardial and smooth-muscle contraction and decreasing impulse formation and conduction velocity. As a result, systolic and diastolic pressures decrease.

Availability

Capsules (extended-release, sustained-release): 60 mg, 90 mg, 120 mg, 180 mg, 240 mg, 300 mg, 360 mg, 420 mg
Injection: 5 mg/ml in 10-ml vials, 100-mg Monovial
Tablets: 30 mg, 60 mg, 90 mg, 120 mg

⊘ Indications and dosages

➤ Angina pectoris and vasospastic (Prinzmetal's) angina; hypertension; supraventricular tachyarrhythmias; atrial flutter or fibrillation

Adults: 30 to 90 mg P.O. three to four times daily (tablets), or 60 to 120 mg P.O.

b.i.d. (sustained-release), or 180 to
240 mg P.O. once daily (extended-
release), adjusted after 14 days as
needed, up to a total daily dosage of
360 mg. Or 0.25 mg/kg by I.V. bolus
over 2 minutes; if response is inadequate after 15 minutes, may give 0.35
mg/kg over 2 minutes; may follow with
continuous I.V. infusion at 10 mg/hour
(at a range of 5 to 15 mg/hour) for up
to 24 hours.

Dosage adjustment
• Severe hepatic or renal impairment
• Elderly patients

Off-label uses
• Unstable angina, coronary artery
bypass graft surgery
• Tardive dyskinesia
• Migraine
• Hyperthyroidism
• Raynaud's phenomenon

Contraindications
• Hypersensitivity to drug
• Atrial flutter or fibrillation associated
with shortened refractory period
(Wolff-Parkinson-White syndrome,
with I.V. use)
• Recent myocardial infarction or pulmonary congestion
• Cardiogenic shock, concurrent I.V.
beta-blocker therapy, ventricular tachycardia, neonates (with I.V. use, because
of benzyl alcohol in syringe formulation)
• Sick sinus syndrome, second- or
third-degree atrioventricular block
(except in patients with ventricular
pacemakers)
• Hypotension (systolic pressure below
90 mm Hg)

Precautions
Use cautiously in:
• severe hepatic or renal impairment,
heart failure
• history of serious ventricular
arrhythmias
• concurrent use of I.V. diltiazem and
I.V. beta blockers
• elderly patients

• pregnant or breastfeeding patients
• children (safety not established).

Administration
• When giving I.V., dilute in dextrose
5% in water or normal saline solution.
• Give I.V. bolus dose over 2 minutes; a
second bolus may be given after
15 minutes.
• Administer continuous I.V. infusion
at a rate of 5 to 15 mg/hour.
🔊 When giving by continuous I.V.
infusion, make sure emergency equipment is available and that patient has
continuous ECG monitoring with frequent blood pressure monitoring.
• Don't crush tablets or sustained-
release capsules; they must be swallowed whole.
• Withhold dose if systolic blood pressure falls below 90 mm Hg, diastolic
pressure is below 60 mm Hg, or apical
pulse is slower than 60 beats/minute.

Route	Onset	Peak	Duration
P.O.	30 min	2-3 hr	6-8 hr
P.O. (sustained)	Unknown	Unknown	12 hr
P.O. (extended)	Unknown	14 hr	Up to 24 hr
I.V.	2-5 min	2-4 hr	Unknown

Adverse reactions
CNS: headache, abnormal dreams,
anxiety, confusion, dizziness, drowsiness, nervousness, psychiatric disturbances, asthenia, paresthesia, syncope,
tremor
CV: peripheral edema, bradycardia,
chest pain, hypotension, palpitations,
tachycardia, **arrhythmias, heart failure**
EENT: blurred vision, tinnitus, epistaxis
GI: nausea, vomiting, diarrhea, constipation, dyspepsia, dry mouth
GU: urinary frequency, dysuria, nocturia, polyuria, gynecomastia, sexual
dysfunction
Hematologic: anemia, **leukopenia,
thrombocytopenia**
Metabolic: hyperglycemia

Reactions in **bold** are life-threatening. 🔊 Clinical alert

Musculoskeletal: joint stiffness, muscle cramps
Respiratory: cough, dyspnea
Skin: rash, dermatitis, flushing, diaphoresis, photosensitivity, pruritus, urticaria, **erythema multiforme**
Other: unpleasant taste, gingival hyperplasia, weight gain, decreased appetite, **Stevens-Johnson syndrome**

Interactions
Drug-drug. *Beta-adrenergic blockers, digoxin, disopyramide, phenytoin:* bradycardia, conduction defects, heart failure
Carbamazepine, cyclosporine, quinidine: decreased diltiazem metabolism, increased risk of toxicity
Cimetidine, ranitidine: increased blood level and effects of diltiazem
Fentanyl, nitrates, other antihypertensives, quinidine: additive hypotension
HMG-CoA reductase inhibitors, imipramine, sirolimus, tacrolimus: increased blood levels of these drugs
Lithium: decreased lithium blood level, reduced antimanic control
Nonsteroidal anti-inflammatory drugs: decreased antihypertensive effect of diltiazem
Theophylline: increased theophylline effects
Drug-diagnostic tests. *Hepatic enzymes:* increased levels
Drug-food. *Grapefruit juice:* increased blood level and effects of diltiazem
Drug-behaviors. *Acute alcohol ingestion:* additive hypotension

Patient monitoring
• Check blood pressure and ECG before starting therapy, and monitor closely during dosage adjustment period. Withhold dose if systolic pressure is below 90 mm Hg.
🔊 Monitor for signs and symptoms of heart failure and worsening arrhythmias.
• Supervise patient during ambulation.

Patient teaching
• Instruct patient to swallow extended-release capsules whole and not to crush or chew them.
• Advise patient to change position slowly to minimize light-headedness and dizziness.
• Caution patient to avoid driving and other hazardous activities until he knows how drug affects concentration and alertness.
• As appropriate, review all other significant and life-threatening adverse reactions and interactions, especially those related to the drugs, tests, foods, and behaviors mentioned above.

dimenhydrinate
Apo-Dimenhydrinate✤, Arlevert✤, Dramamine, Dramanate✤, Gravol✤, PMS-Dimenhydrinate✤, Travamine✤, TripTone

Pharmacologic class: Anticholinergic
Therapeutic class: Antiemetic, antivertigo agent
Pregnancy risk category B

Action
Prevents nausea and vomiting by inhibiting vestibular stimulation of chemoreceptor trigger zone and inhibiting stimulation of vomiting center in brain

Availability
Injection: 50 mg/ml
Tablets: 50 mg
Tablets (chewable): 50 mg

🚫 Indications and dosages
➤ Prevention and treatment of nausea, vomiting, dizziness, and vertigo
Adults and children ages 12 and older: 50 to 100 mg P.O. q 4 hours (not to exceed 400 mg/day), or 50 mg I.M. or I.V. q 4 hours p.r.n.

Children ages 6 to 12: 25 to 50 mg P.O. q 6 to 8 hours (not to exceed 150 mg/day), or 1.25 mg/kg I.M. (37.5 mg/m²) q 6 hours p.r.n.

Children ages 2 to 6: 12.5 to 25 mg P.O. q 6 to 8 hours (not to exceed 75 mg/day)

Contraindications
• Hypersensitivity to drug or tartrazine
• Alcohol intolerance

Precautions
Use cautiously in:
• angle-closure glaucoma, seizure disorders, prostatic hypertrophy
• children younger than age 2.

Administration
• For I.V. use, dilute with dextrose 5% in water or normal saline solution.
• Give each 50-mg I.V. dose over 2 minutes.

◀€ Don't administer by I.V. route to premature or low-birth-weight infants. Solution contains benzyl alcohol, which can cause fatal "gasping" syndrome.

Route	Onset	Peak	Duration
P.O.	15-60 min	1-2 hr	3-6 hr
I.V.	Rapid	Unknown	3-6 hr
I.M.	20-30 min	1-2 hr	3-6 hr

Adverse reactions
CNS: drowsiness, dizziness, headache, paradoxical stimulation (in children)
CV: hypotension, palpitations
EENT: blurred vision, tinnitus
GI: diarrhea, constipation, dry mouth
GU: dysuria, urinary frequency
Skin: photosensitivity
Other: decreased appetite, pain at I.M. site

Interactions
Drug-drug. *Disopyramide, quinidine, tricyclic antidepressants:* increased anticholinergic effects
MAO inhibitors: intensified and prolonged anticholinergic effects

Other CNS depressants (such as antihistamines, opioids, sedative-hypnotics): additive CNS depression
Ototoxic drugs (such as aminoglycosides, ethacrynic acid): masking of signs or symptoms of ototoxicity
Drug-diagnostic tests. *Allergy skin tests:* false-negative results
Drug-behaviors. *Alcohol use:* increased CNS depression

Patient monitoring
• Assess for lethargy and drowsiness.
• Monitor for dizziness, nausea, and vomiting (possible indicators of drug toxicity).

Patient teaching
• To prevent motion sickness, advise patient to take drug 30 minutes before traveling and to repeat dose before meals and at bedtime.
• Instruct patient to avoid driving and other hazardous activities until he knows how drug affects concentration and alertness.
• Caution patient to avoid alcohol and sedative-hypnotics during therapy.
• As appropriate, review all other significant adverse reactions and interactions, especially those related to the drugs, tests, and behaviors mentioned above.

dinoprostone
(prostaglandin E₂, PGE₂)
Cervidil Vaginal Insert, Prepidil Endocervical Gel, Propress ⊕, Prostin E2 Vaginal Suppository

Pharmacologic class: Oxytocic, prostaglandin
Therapeutic class: Abortifacient, cervical ripening agent
Pregnancy risk category C

FDA | **BOXED WARNING**

- Dinoprostone vaginal suppository should be given only by trained personnel who adhere strictly to recommended dosages, in hospital that can provide immediate intensive care and acute surgical facilities.

Action

Initiates strong contractions of uterine smooth muscle by stimulating myometrium and promoting cervical softening, effacement, and dilation

Availability

Endocervical gel: 0.5 mg in 3-g gel vehicle in prefilled syringe with catheter
Vaginal insert: 10 mg
Vaginal suppositories: 20 mg

Ⓘ Indications and dosages

➤ Cervical ripening
Adults: 0.5 mg endocervical gel vaginally; if response is poor, may repeat in 6 hours (not to exceed 1.5 mg in 24 hours). Or one 10-mg vaginal insert.
➤ To induce abortion
Adults: One 20-mg vaginal suppository; repeat q 3 to 5 hours (not to exceed total dosage of 240 mg or duration of 48 hours).
➤ Nonmetastatic gestational trophoblastic disease (benign hydatidiform mole)
Adults: Insert one 20-mg suppository high into vagina; may repeat at 3- to 5-hour intervals for up to 2 days if necessary.

Contraindications

- Hypersensitivity to prostaglandins or additives in gel or suppository
- When vaginal delivery isn't indicated, such as with vasa previa or active genital herpes infection (Prepidil)
- Acute pelvic inflammatory disease
- Ruptured membranes, placenta previa, marked cephalopelvic disproportion, or unexplained vaginal bleeding during pregnancy
- When oxytocics are contraindicated or when prolonged contraction of uterus may be detrimental to fetal safety or uterine integrity, such as with previous cesarean section or major uterine surgery
- Concurrent use of I.V. oxytocics (Cervidil)
- Clinical suspicion or definite evidence of fetal distress when delivery isn't imminent (Cervidil, Prepidil)
- History of difficult labor or traumatic delivery, hyperactive or hypertonic uterine patterns (Prepidil)
- Obstetric emergencies in which benefit-to-risk ratio for either fetus or mother favors surgical intervention (Prepidil)
- Active cardiac, pulmonary, renal, or hepatic disease (Prostin E2 Vaginal Suppository)
- Multipara with six or more previous term pregnancies (Cervidil)
- Grand multipara with six or more previous term pregnancies with non-vertex presentation (Prepidil)

Precautions

Use cautiously in:
- history of pulmonary, cardiac, renal, or hepatic disease; asthma; jaundice; anemia; cervicitis; infected endocervical lesions; acute vaginitis; compromised (scarred) uterus; hypertension; hypotension; adrenal disorders; diabetes mellitus; epilepsy; glaucoma
- women age 30 or older, those with complications during pregnancy, and those with gestational age of more than 40 weeks are at increased risk of post-partum disseminated intravascular coagulation
- concurrent use of other oxytocics (not recommended).

Administration

- Keep patient supine for 15 to 30 minutes after gel administration and

for 10 minutes after administering suppository to prevent drug expulsion.
• Store suppositories in freezer; bring to room temperature before using.

Route	Onset	Peak	Duration
Vaginal (gel)	Rapid	30-45 min	Unknown
Vaginal (insert)	Rapid	Unknown	12 hr
Vaginal (suppository)	10 min	Unknown	2-3 hr

Adverse reactions

CNS: headache, drowsiness, syncope
CV: hypotension, hypertension
GI: nausea, vomiting, diarrhea
GU: urinary tract infection, vaginal or uterine pain, uterine contractile abnormalities, warm vaginal sensation, **uterine hypertonicity, uterine rupture**
Musculoskeletal. back pain
Respiratory: cough, dyspnea, wheezing
Other: allergic reactions including chills, fever, and **anaphylaxis**

Interactions

Drug-drug. *Other oxytocics:* increased oxytocic effects

Patient monitoring

◀€ Monitor uterine contractions and observe for excessive vaginal bleeding and cramping. Record sanitary pad count.
• Monitor vital signs and assess for drug-induced fever. Report significant blood pressure and pulse changes.
• Assess for wheezing, chest pain, and dyspnea.
• Evaluate for GI upset. To minimize, give antiemetic before dinoprostone therapy.

Patient teaching

• Advise patient to stay in supine position, as prescribed, after administration.
• Instruct patient to report fever, bleeding, or abdominal cramps.

• Tell patient to avoid douches, tampons, tub baths, and sexual intercourse for at least 2 weeks after receiving drug.
• As appropriate, review all other significant and life-threatening adverse reactions and interactions, especially those related to the drugs mentioned above.

d

diphenhydramine hydrochloride

Aler-Cap, Aler-Dryl, Allerdryl✤, AllerMax, Altaryl, Anti-Hist, Banophen, Benadryl, Benadryl Allergy, Benadryl Child Chesty Cough⊕, Benadryl Children's Allergy Fastmelt, Benadryl Dye-Free Allergy, Benadryl Itch Relief, Compoz Nighttime Sleep Aid, Dermamycin, Diphen, Diphenhist, Dytan, Genahist, Histapryn, Histergan⊕, Hydramine, Mandalyn Paedetriac⊕, Nightcalm, Nytol, PMS-Diphenhydramine✤, Siladryl, Simply Sleep, Sleepeaze⊕, Sleepettes D, Sleepinal, Sominex, Theraflu Thin Strips Multisymptom, Triaminic Thin Strips Children's Cough and Runny Nose, Twilite, Unisom Maximum Strength SleepGels

Pharmacologic class: Ethanolamine derivative, nonselective histamine₁-receptor antagonist

Therapeutic class: Antihistamine, antitussive, antiemetic, antivertigo agent, antidyskinetic

Pregnancy risk category B

Action

Interferes with histamine effects at histamine₁-receptor sites; prevents but doesn't reverse histamine-mediated response. Also possesses CNS depressant and anticholinergic properties.

Availability
Capsules: 25 mg, 50 mg
Elixir: 12.5 mg/5 ml
Injection: 10 mg/ml, 50 mg/ml
Strips (orally disintegrating): 12.5 mg, 25 mg
Syrup: 12.5 mg/5 ml
Tablets: 25 mg, 50 mg
Tablets (chewable): 12.5 mg, 25 mg
Tablets (orally disintegrating): 12.5 mg

⬤ Indications and dosages
➤ Allergy symptoms caused by histamine release (including anaphylaxis, seasonal and perennial allergic rhinitis, and allergic dermatoses); nausea; vertigo
Adults and children over age 12: 25 to 50 mg P.O. q 4 to 6 hours, or 10 to 50 mg I.V. or I.M. q 2 to 3 hours p.r.n. (Some patients may need up to 100 mg.) Don't exceed 400 mg/day.
Children ages 6 to 12: 12.5 to 25 mg P.O. q 4 to 6 hours, or 1.25 mg/kg (37.5 mg/m^2) I.M. or I.V. q.i.d. Don't exceed 150 mg/day.
Children ages 2 to 5: 6.25 mg P.O. q 4 to 6 hours. Don't exceed 37.5 mg/day.
➤ Cough
Adults: 25 mg P.O. q 4 hours p.r.n. Don't exceed 150 mg/day.
Children ages 6 to 12: 12.5 mg P.O. q 4 hours. Don't exceed 75 mg/day.
Children ages 2 to 5: 6.25 mg P.O. q 4 hours. Don't exceed 37.5 mg/24 hours.
➤ Dyskinesia; Parkinson's disease
Adults: Initially, 25 mg P.O. t.i.d.; may be increased to a maximum of 50 mg q.i.d.
➤ Mild nighttime sedation
Adults: 50 mg P.O. 20 to 30 minutes before bedtime

Dosage adjustment
• Elderly patients

Off-label uses
• Drug-induced extrapyramidal reactions

Contraindications
• Hypersensitivity to drug
• Alcohol intolerance
• Acute asthma attacks
• MAO inhibitor use within past 14 days
• Breastfeeding
• Neonates, premature infants

Precautions
Use cautiously in:
• severe hepatic disease, angle-closure glaucoma, seizure disorders, prostatic hypertrophy, cardiovascular disease, hyperthyroidism
• elderly patients
• pregnant patients (safety not established)
• children younger than age 2 (safety not established).

Administration
• For motion sickness, administer 30 minutes before activity.
• For I.V. use, check compatibility before mixing with other drugs.
• Inject I.M. dose deep into large muscle mass; rotate sites.
• Discontinue drug 4 days before allergy skin testing to avoid misleading results.
◀€ Don't give within 14 days of MAO inhibitors.

Route	Onset	Peak	Duration
P.O.	15-60 min	1-4 hr	4-8 hr
I.V.	Rapid	Unknown	4-8 hr
I.M.	20-30 min	1-4 hr	4-8 hr

Adverse reactions
CNS: drowsiness, dizziness, headache, paradoxical stimulation (especially in children)
CV: hypotension, palpitations, tachycardia
EENT: blurred vision, tinnitus
GI: diarrhea, constipation, dry mouth
GU: dysuria, urinary frequency or retention
Skin: photosensitivity

Other: decreased appetite, pain at I.M. injection site

Interactions
Drug-drug. *Antihistamines, opioids, sedative-hypnotics:* additive CNS depression
Disopyramide, quinidine, tricyclic antidepressants: increased anticholinergic effects
MAO inhibitors: intensified and prolonged anticholinergic effects
Drug-diagnostic tests. *Skin allergy tests:* false-negative results
Hemoglobin, platelets: decreased values
Drug-herbs. *Angel's trumpet, jimson weed, scopolia:* increased anticholinergic effects
Chamomile, hops, kava, skullcap, valerian: increased CNS depression
Drug-behaviors. *Alcohol use:* increased CNS depression

Patient monitoring
• Monitor cardiovascular status, especially in patients with cardiovascular disease.
• Supervise patient during ambulation. Use side rails as necessary.

Patient teaching
• Advise patient to avoid alcohol and other depressants such as sedatives while taking drug.
• Caution patient to avoid driving and other hazardous activities until he knows how drug affects concentration and alertness.
• As appropriate, review all other significant adverse reactions and interactions, especially those related to the drugs, tests, herbs, and behaviors mentioned above.

diphenoxylate hydrochloride and atropine sulfate (co-phenotrope⊕)
Lomotil, Lonox

d

Pharmacologic class: Anticholinergic, meperidine congener
Therapeutic class: Antidiarrheal
Controlled substance schedule V
Pregnancy risk category C

Action
Acts on smooth muscle of GI tract by decreasing peristalsis, which inhibits motility. (Small amount of atropine is added to reduce abuse potential.)

Availability
Liquid: 2.5 mg diphenoxylate and 0.025 mg atropine/5 ml
Tablets: 2.5 mg diphenoxylate and 0.025 mg atropine

⊘ Indications and dosages
➤ Diarrhea
Adults: Initially, 5 mg P.O. three to four times daily, then 5 mg/day as needed (not to exceed 20 mg/day). Decrease dosage when desired response occurs.
Children: Initially, 0.3 to 0.4 mg/kg P.O. (liquid only) daily in four divided doses. Decrease dosage when desired response occurs.

Dosage adjustment
• Elderly patients

Contraindications
• Hypersensitivity to drug
• Obstructive jaundice
• Diarrhea associated with pseudomembranous colitis or enterotoxin-producing bacteria
• Angle-closure glaucoma

Reactions in **bold** are life-threatening.   ◀€ Clinical alert

- Concurrent MAO inhibitor use
- Children younger than age 2

Precautions

Use cautiously in:
- inflammatory bowel disease; prostatic hypertrophy; severe hepatic disease (use with extreme caution)
- concurrent use of drugs that cause physical dependence; history of physical drug dependence
- elderly patients
- pregnant or breastfeeding patients
- children (safety not established in children younger than age 12).

Administration

🔊 Don't confuse brand name Lomotil with Lamictal (an anticonvulsant). Serious errors have been reported.
- Withhold drug if patient has severe fluid or electrolyte imbalance.
- Administer with food if GI upset occurs.

🔊 Don't give within 14 days of MAO inhibitors.

Route	Onset	Peak	Duration
P.O.	45-60 min	2 hr	3-4 hr

Adverse reactions

CNS: dizziness, confusion, drowsiness, headache, insomnia, nervousness
CV: tachycardia
EENT: blurred vision, dry eyes
GI: nausea, vomiting, constipation, epigastric distress, ileus, dry mouth
GU: urinary retention
Skin: flushing

Interactions

Drug-drug. *CNS depressants (including antihistamines, sedative-hypnotics, opioids):* increased CNS depression
Anticholinergic-like drugs (including tricyclic antidepressants, disopyramide): increased anticholinergic effects
MAO inhibitors: hypertensive crisis

Drug-diagnostic tests. *Amylase:* increased level
Drug-herbs. *Angel's trumpet, jimsonweed, scopolia:* increased anticholinergic effects
Drug-behaviors. *Alcohol use:* increased CNS depression

Patient monitoring

🔊 Assess for and report abdominal distention and signs or symptoms of decreased peristalsis.
- Watch for signs and symptoms of dehydration.
- Assess frequency and consistency of bowel movements.

Patient teaching

- Instruct patient to report persistent diarrhea.
- Caution patient to avoid driving and other hazardous activities until he knows how drug affects concentration and alertness.
- Tell patient that prolonged use may lead to dependence.
- As appropriate, review all other significant adverse reactions and interactions, especially those related to the drugs, tests, herbs, and behaviors mentioned above.

dipyridamole

Apo-Dipyridamole FC♣, Apo-Dipyridamole SC♣, Persantin✚, Persantine

Pharmacologic class: Platelet adhesion inhibitor

Therapeutic class: Antiplatelet agent, diagnostic agent (coronary vasodilator)

Pregnancy risk category B

Action
Unclear. May reduce platelet aggregation by inhibiting phosphodiesterase, adenosine uptake, or formation of thromboxane A_2.

Availability
Tablets: 25 mg, 50 mg, 75 mg

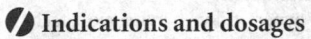 Indications and dosages
➤ To prevent thromboembolism in patients with prosthetic heart valves
Adults: 75 to 100 mg P.O. q.i.d.

Off-label uses
• Prevention of myocardial reinfarction (given with aspirin)
• Thrombotic thrombocytopenia purpura

Contraindications
• Hypersensitivity to drug

Precautions
Use cautiously in: .
• hypotension, hepatic insufficiency, severe coronary artery disease
• pregnant or breastfeeding patients
• children younger than age 12 (safety not established).

Administration
• Know that drug is usually given with warfarin when used to prevent thromboembolism.
• Give with a full glass of water at least 1 hour before or 2 hours after meals. If gastric distress occurs, give with food.

Route	Onset	Peak	Duration
P.O.	Unknown	Unknown	Unknown

Adverse reactions
CNS: dizziness, headache
CV: hypotension
GI: abdominal distress
Hepatic: hepatic failure
Skin: rash

Interactions
Drug-drug. *Adenosine:* increased adenosine plasma level and CV effects
Cholinesterase inhibitors: counteracts activity of cholinesterase inhibitors
Drug-diagnostic tests. *Hepatic enzymes:* increased levels
Drug-behaviors. *Alcohol use:* increased risk of hypotension

Patient monitoring
• Monitor for therapeutic efficacy, including improved exercise tolerance and decreased need for nitrates.
• Assess platelet and coagulation studies regularly.
• Monitor ECG and vital signs, especially blood pressure.
• Monitor hepatic function tests regularly.

Patient teaching
• Advise patient to take drug 1 hour before or 2 hours after meals for best absorption.
◀▌ Instruct patient to immediately report unusual tiredness, chest pain or other cardiac symptoms, upper right abdominal pain, yellowing of skin or eyes, or dark urine.
• As appropriate, review all other significant and life-threatening adverse reactions and interactions, especially those related to the drugs and tests mentioned above.

d

dobutamine hydrochloride

Pharmacologic class: Sympathomimetic, adrenergic
Therapeutic class: Inotropic
Pregnancy risk category B

Action
Stimulates $beta_1$-adrenergic receptors of heart, causing a positive inotropic

---

effect that increases myocardial contractility and stroke volume. Also reduces peripheral vascular resistance, decreases ventricular filling pressure, and promotes atrioventricular conduction.

Availability
Injection: 12.5 mg/ml in 20-ml vials

🚫 Indications and dosages
➣ Short-term treatment of cardiac decompensation caused by depressed contractility (such as during refractory heart failure); adjunct in cardiac surgery
Adults: 2.5 to 10 mcg/kg/minute I.V. as a continuous infusion, adjusted to hemodynamic response

Dosage adjustment
• Elderly patients

Off-label uses
• Adjunct in myocardial infarction (MI) and septic shock
• Diagnosis of coronary artery disease (echocardiography stress test, ventriculography, computed tomography)

Contraindications
• Hypersensitivity to drug
• Idiopathic hypertrophic subaortic stenosis

Precautions
Use cautiously in:
• hypertension, MI, atrial fibrillation, hypovolemia
• pregnant or breastfeeding patients
• children.

Administration
• As needed, correct hypovolemia before starting therapy by giving volume expanders, as prescribed.
• Use infusion pump or microdrip I.V. infusion set.
• Dilute with dextrose 5% in water or normal saline solution to at least 50 ml of solution. Know that drug is incompatible with alkaline solutions, such as sodium bicarbonate injection.

Route	Onset	Peak	Duration
I.V.	1-2 min	10 min	Brief

Adverse reactions
CNS: headache
CV: hypertension, hypotension, tachycardia, premature ventricular contractions, angina, palpitations, nonspecific chest pain, phlebitis
GI: nausea, vomiting
Metabolic: hypokalemia
Respiratory: dyspnea, **asthma attacks**
Skin: extravasation with tissue necrosis
Other: hypersensitivity reactions including **anaphylaxis**

Interactions
Drug-drug. *Beta-adrenergic blockers:* increased alpha-adrenergic effects
Bretylium: potentiation of vasopressor activity
Cyclopropane, halothane: serious arrhythmias
Guanethidine: decreased hypotensive effects
Thyroid hormone: increased cardiovascular effects
Tricyclic antidepressants: potentiation of cardiovascular and vasopressor effects
Drug-herbs. *Rue:* increased inotropic potential

Patient monitoring
• Monitor ECG and blood pressure continuously during administration.
• Monitor cardiac output, pulmonary capillary wedge pressure, and central venous pressure.
• Monitor fluid intake and output and watch for signs and symptoms of worsening heart failure.
🔊 Assess electrolyte levels. Stay especially alert for hypokalemia.

Patient teaching

- Instruct patient to report anginal pain, headache, leg cramps, and shortness of breath.
- Explain need for close observation and monitoring.
- As appropriate, review all other significant and life-threatening adverse reactions and interactions, especially those related to the drugs and herbs mentioned above.

docetaxel

Taxotere

Pharmacologic class: Mitosis inhibitor
Therapeutic class: Antineoplastic
Pregnancy risk category D

FDA BOXED WARNING

- Give under supervision of physician experienced in cancer chemotherapy, in facility with adequate diagnostic and treatment resources.
- Treatment-related death is more likely if patient has abnormal hepatic function, is receiving higher doses, or has non-small-cell lung cancer and history of platinum-based chemotherapy and is receiving drug as a single agent at dosage of 100 mg/m^2.
- Generally, drug shouldn't be given to patients with bilirubin level above upper limit of normal (ULN) or those with aspartate aminotransferase (AST) or alanine aminotransferase (ALT) above 1.5 × ULN concomitant with alkaline phosphatase (ALP) level above 2.5 × ULN. Bilirubin elevations or transaminase abnormalities concurrent with ALP abnormalities increases patient's risk for grade 4 neutropenia, febrile neutropenia, infections, severe thrombocytopenia, severe stomatitis, severe skin toxicity, and toxic death.

Patients with isolated transaminase elevations above 1.5 × ULN have higher rate of grade 4 febrile neutropenia, but without increased incidence of toxic death. Before each cycle, obtain bilirubin, ALT or AST, and ALP values and have physician review them.
- Don't give to patients with neutrophil count below 1,500 cells/mm^3. Obtain frequent blood cell counts to monitor for neutropenia (which may be severe and cause infection).
- Severe hypersensitivity reactions and fatal anaphylaxis (rare) have occurred in patients who received recommended 3-day dexamethasone premedication. If hypersensitivity reaction occurs, discontinue docetaxel immediately and give appropriate therapy. Don't give drug to patients with history of severe hypersensitivity reactions to it or other drugs containing polysorbate 80. Severe fluid retention may occur despite dexamethasone premedication regimen.

Action

Inhibits cellular mitosis by disrupting microtubular network

Availability

Injection concentrate: 20 mg, 80 mg

⏀ Indications and dosages

➤ Locally advanced or metastatic breast cancer unresponsive to previous regimens
Adults: 60 to 100 mg/m^2 I.V. over 1 hour q 3 weeks as single agent
➤ Adjuvant treatment of operable node-positive breast cancer
Adults: 75 mg/m^2 1 hour after doxorubicin 50 mg/m^2 and cyclophosphamide 500 mg/m^2 q 3 weeks for six courses
➤ Locally advanced or metastatic non-small-cell lung cancer (NSCLC) after platinum therapy failure
Adults: 75 mg/m^2 I.V. over 1 hour q 3 weeks as single agent

Reactions in **bold** are life-threatening.   ◀ Clinical alert

➤ Unresectable locally advanced or metastatic NSCLC in chemotherapy-naïve patients

Adults: 75 mg/m² I.V. over 1 hour q 3 weeks followed by cisplatin as ordered

➤ Androgen-independent (hormone refractory) metastatic prostate cancer

Adults: 75 mg/m² I.V. over 1 hour q 3 weeks with 5 mg prednisone P.O. b.i.d. continuously

➤ Gastric adenocarcinoma cancer

Adults: 75 mg/m² as a 1-hour infusion, followed by cisplatin as a 1- to 3-hour infusion (both on day 1 only), followed by fluorouracil given as a 24-hour continuous I.V. infusion for 5 days, starting at the end of the cisplatin infusion. Treatment is repeated q 3 weeks.

➤ Squamous cell carcinoma of head and neck

Adults: *Induction chemotherapy followed by radiotherapy*—75 mg/m² I.V. as 1-hour infusion followed by cisplatin 75 mg/m² I.V. over 1 hour (both on day 1 only), followed by fluorouracil 750 mg/m² given as 24-hour continuous I.V. infusion daily for 5 days, starting at end of cisplatin infusion. Treatment is repeated q 3 weeks for four cycles.

Adults: *Induction chemotherapy followed by chemoradiotherapy*—75 mg/m² I.V. as 1-hour infusion on day 1, followed by cisplatin 100 mg/m² I.V. as 30-minute to 3-hour infusion, followed by fluorouracil 1,000 mg/m²/day I.V. as continuous infusion from day 1 to day 4. Treatment is repeated q 3 weeks for three cycles.

Dosage adjustment

• Febrile neutropenia

Contraindications

• Hypersensitivity to drug or polysorbate 80
• Hepatic impairment
• Neutrophil count below 1,500 cells/mm³

Precautions

Use cautiously in:
• females of childbearing age
• pregnant or breastfeeding patients.

Administration

• Assess bilirubin, ALT, AST, and ALP levels before starting each cycle of drug therapy.
• Premedicate patient with oral corticosteroids before docetaxel administration to reduce fluid retention and severity of hypersensitivity reactions.
• Premedicate patient with antiemetics and hydrate with I.V. fluids, as prescribed, before cisplatin administration.
◀€ Don't let drug concentrate contact plasticized polyvinyl chloride equipment or devices.
• Know that when used for prostate cancer, drug must be given with prednisone, as prescribed.
• Dilute with accompanying diluent solution; rotate vial gently to mix. Once foam has largely dissipated, withdraw prescribed amount of drug and mix in glass or polypropylene bottle or in plastic bag with 250 ml of normal saline solution or dextrose 5% in water.
• Mix solution thoroughly and infuse over 1 hour, using polyethylene-lined infusion set.

Route	Onset	Peak	Duration
I.V.	Rapid	Unknown	7 days

Adverse reactions

CNS: fatigue, asthenia, neurosensory deficits, peripheral neuropathy
CV: peripheral edema, **cardiac tamponade, pericardial effusion**
GI: nausea, vomiting, diarrhea, stomatitis, ascites
Hematologic: anemia, **thrombocytopenia, leukopenia**
Musculoskeletal: myalgia, joint pain
Respiratory: bronchospasm, pulmonary edema

Skin: alopecia, rash, dermatitis, desquamation, erythema, nail disorders
Other: edema, hypersensitivity reactions including **anaphylaxis**

Interactions
Drug-drug. *Antineoplastics:* additive bone marrow depression
Cyclosporine, erythromycin, ketoconazole, troleandomycin: significant change in docetaxel effects
Live-virus vaccines: increased risk of infection

Patient monitoring
◀€ Watch for signs and symptoms of anaphylaxis or other hypersensitivity reactions, especially with first two doses.
• Monitor vital signs and fluid intake and output. Watch for signs and symptoms of fluid overload and bronchospasm.
• Monitor CBC, and assess for signs and symptoms of blood dyscrasias.
• Closely monitor neutrophil and platelet counts before and during therapy.
• Observe I.V. site frequently for extravasation.
• Assess neurologic status to detect neurosensory deficits and peripheral neuropathy.

Patient teaching
• Instruct patient to weigh himself daily and to immediately report sudden weight gain or difficulty breathing.
◀€ Tell patient to report signs and symptoms of blood dyscrasias. Inform him that he'll undergo frequent blood testing to monitor these effects.
◀€ Advise patient to immediately report rash or difficulty breathing.
• Inform patient that nail disorders and hair loss are common with docetaxel use, but that hair and nails will grow back after therapy ends.

• Advise female patient of childbearing age to use effective contraception during therapy and to notify prescriber if she suspects pregnancy.
• As appropriate, review all other significant and life-threatening adverse reactions and interactions, especially those related to the drugs mentioned above.

d

docusate calcium
Apo-Docusate Calcium✲, Calax✲, DC Softgels, Novo-Docusate Calcium✲, PMS-Docusate Calcium✲, Ratio-Docusate Calcium✲, Soflax C✲, Stool Softener DC, Surfak Liquigels

docusate sodium
Apo-Docusate Sodium✲, Colace, Correctol, Correctol Stool Softener✲, Diocto, Dioctyl⊕, Docusol⊕, Dom-Docusate Sodium✲, D.O.S. Softgels, Docu-Soft, DOK, D-S-S, DulcoEase⊕, Dulcolax Stool Softener, Enemeez, Genasoft Softgels, Norgalax⊕, Novo Docusate✲, PHL-Docusate Sodium✲, PMS-Docusate Sodium, Ratio-Docusate Sodium✲, Selax✲, Silace

Pharmacologic class: Emollient
Therapeutic class: Stool softener, surfactant
Pregnancy risk category C

Action
Increases absorption of liquid into stool, resulting in softening of fecal mass. Also promotes electrolyte and water secretion into colon.

Availability
docusate calcium
Capsules: 240 mg

Capsules (soft gels): 240 mg
Rectal solution: 283 mg/5 ml
docusate sodium
Capsules: 50 mg, 100 mg, 250 mg
Capsules (soft gels): 100 mg, 250 mg
Liquid: 150 mg/15 ml
Syrup: 50 mg/15 ml, 60 mg/15 ml,
20 mg/5 ml, 100 mg/30 ml, 150 mg/
15 ml
Tablets: 100 mg

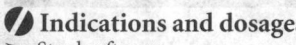 Indications and dosages

➤ Stool softener
Adults and children older than age 12:
240 mg (docusate calcium) or 50 to
200 mg (docusate sodium) P.O. daily
until bowel movements are normal
Children ages 6 to 12: 40 to 120 mg
(docusate sodium) P.O. daily
Children ages 3 to 6: 20 to 60 mg
(docusate sodium) P.O. daily

Contraindications

• Hypersensitivity to drug
• Abdominal pain, nausea, or vomiting
• Intestinal obstruction

Precautions

Use cautiously in:
• pregnant or breastfeeding patients.

Administration

• Give tablets and capsules with full
glass of water.
• Give liquid solution with milk or
fruit juice.
• Be aware that excessive or long-
term use may lead to laxative
dependence.

Route	Onset	Peak	Duration
P.O.	24-48 hr (up to 5 days)	Unknown	Unknown

Adverse reactions

EENT: throat irritation
GI: nausea, diarrhea, mild cramps
Skin: rash
Other: bitter taste, decreased appetite,
laxative dependence

Interactions

Drug-drug. *Mineral oil:* increased
mineral oil absorption, causing toxicity
Warfarin: decreased warfarin effects
(with high doses)

Patient monitoring

• If diarrhea occurs, withhold drug
and notify prescriber.
• Know that therapeutic efficacy usually becomes apparent 1 to 3 days after
first dose.

Patient teaching

• Instruct patient to drink sufficient
fluids with each dose and to increase
fluid intake during the day.
• Advise patient to prevent constipation
by increasing fluids and consuming more
dietary fiber (as in fruits and bran).
• Inform patient that excessive or
prolonged use may lead to laxative
dependence.
• As appropriate, review all other significant adverse reactions and interactions, especially those related to the
drugs mentioned above.

dolasetron mesylate
Anzemet

Pharmacologic class: Selective serotonin
subtype 3 (5-HT$_3$) receptor antagonist
Therapeutic class: Antiemetic
Pregnancy risk category B

Action

Blocks serotonin activation at receptor
sites in vagal nerve terminals and in
chemoreceptor trigger zone in CNS,
decreasing the vomiting reflex

Availability

Injection: 12.5 mg/0.625-ml ampules,
20 mg/ml in 5-ml vials
Tablets: 50 mg, 100 mg

⚠ Indications and dosages

➤ Chemotherapy-induced nausea and vomiting

Adults: 100 mg P.O. 1 hour before chemotherapy or 1.8 mg/kg I.V. 30 minutes before chemotherapy

Children ages 2 to 16: 1.8 mg/kg P.O. within 1 hour before chemotherapy or 1.8 mg/kg I.V. (not to exceed 100 mg) 30 minutes before chemotherapy

➤ Prevention or treatment of post-operative nausea and vomiting

Adults: 100 mg P.O. within 2 hours before surgery or 12.5 mg I.V. 15 minutes before cessation of anesthesia (for prevention) or as soon as nausea or vomiting begins (for treatment)

Children ages 2 to 16: 1.2 mg/kg P.O. (up to 100 mg/dose) within 2 hours before surgery or 0.35 mg/kg I.V. (up to 12.5 mg) 15 minutes before cessation of anesthesia (for prevention) or as soon as nausea or vomiting begins (for treatment)

Contraindications

• Hypersensitivity to drug
• Arrhythmias

Precautions

Use cautiously in:
• risk factors for prolonged cardiac conduction intervals
• pregnant or breastfeeding patients (safety not established).

Administration

• Give oral dose at least 1 hour before chemotherapy for best results.
• To prevent postoperative nausea, give oral dose within 2 hours before surgery.
• If patient has difficulty swallowing tablet, injection solution may be mixed with apple or apple-grape juice and given orally.
• For I.V. use, give 100 mg single dose undiluted over 30 seconds. For I.V. infusion, dilute in normal saline solution, dextrose 5% in water, or lactated Ringer's solution to 50 ml, and give

single dose over at least 15 minutes. Don't mix with other drugs.
• Flush I.V. line before and after infusion.

Route	Onset	Peak	Duration
P.O.	Unknown	1-2 hr	Up to 24 hr
I.V.	Unknown	15-30 min	Up to 24 hr

Adverse reactions

CNS: headache (increased in cancer patients), dizziness, fatigue, syncope
CV: bradycardia, tachycardia, ECG changes, hypertension, hypotension
GI: diarrhea, constipation, dyspepsia, abdominal pain
GU: urinary retention, **oliguria**
Skin: pruritus, rash
Other: chills, fever, decreased appetite

Interactions

Drug-drug. *Antiarrhythmics, anthracy-cline (high cumulative doses), diuretics,* drugs that prolong QTc interval: increased risk of conduction abnormalities
Drugs that affect hepatic microsomal enzymes: altered dolasetron blood level
Drug-diagnostic tests. *Alanine aminotransferase, aspartate aminotransferase:* increased levels

Patient monitoring

• Monitor closely for excessive diuresis.
◀ Watch for ECG changes, including prolonged PR interval and widened QRS complex, especially in patients receiving antiarrhythmics concurrently.

Patient teaching

• Instruct patient to take drug 1 to 2 hours before chemotherapy.
• Inform patient that drug commonly causes headache.
• As appropriate, review all other significant and life-threatening adverse reactions and interactions, especially those related to the drugs and tests mentioned above.

Reactions in **bold** are life-threatening. ◀ Clinical alert

donepezil hydrochloride
Aricept

Pharmacologic class: Acetylcholinesterase inhibitor
Therapeutic class: Anti-Alzheimer's agent
Pregnancy risk category C

Action
Reversibly inhibits acetylcholinesterase hydrolysis in CNS, leading to increased acetylcholine level and temporary cognitive improvement in patients with Alzheimer's disease

Availability
Tablets: 5 mg, 10 mg, 23 mg
Tablets (orally disintegrating): 5 mg, 10 mg

🖊 Indications and dosages
➤ Mild to moderate Alzheimer's disease
Adults: Initially, 5 mg P.O. daily. After 4 to 6 weeks, may increase dosage to 10 mg at bedtime.
➤ Moderate to severe Alzheimer's disease
Adults: Initially, 10 mg P.O. daily. After 3 months, may increase dosage to 23 mg.

Contraindications
• Hypersensitivity to drug or piperidine derivatives

Precautions
Use cautiously in:
• cardiovascular disease, chronic obstructive pulmonary disease (COPD), asthma, or sick sinus syndrome
• patients at risk for developing ulcers, such as those with history of ulcer disease or those concurrently receiving NSAIDs

• pregnant or breastfeeding patients
• children (safety and efficacy not established).

Administration
• Give with or without food.
• For best response, give at bedtime.

Route	Onset	Peak	Duration
P.O.	Unknown	3-4 hr	Unknown

Adverse reactions
CNS: headache, dizziness, vertigo, fatigue, depression, aggression, irritability, restlessness, nervousness, paresthesia, insomnia, abnormal dreams, tremor, aphasia, **seizures**
CV: chest pain, bradycardia, hypertension, hypotension, vasodilation, **atrial fibrillation, heart block**
EENT: cataracts, blurred vision, eye irritation, sore throat
GI: nausea, vomiting, diarrhea, anorexia, bloating, epigastric pain, fecal incontinence, **GI bleeding**
GU: urinary frequency, increased libido, bladder outflow obstruction
Metabolic: dehydration
Musculoskeletal: muscle cramps, arthritis, bone fracture
Respiratory: dyspnea, bronchitis
Skin: pruritus, urticaria, bruising, diaphoresis, rash, flushing
Other: toothache, decreased appetite, weight loss, hot flashes, influenza

Interactions
Drug-drug. *Anticholinergics:* reduced donepezil effects
Anticholinesterases, cholinomimetics: synergistic effects
Carbamazepine, dexamethasone, phenobarbital, phenytoin, rifampin: accelerated donepezil elimination
NSAIDs: increased risk of GI bleeding

Patient monitoring
◀ᶓ Watch closely for increased bronchoconstriction in patients with history of asthma or COPD.

• Assess cardiovascular status. Drug may cause bradycardia from increased vagal tone.
• Monitor closely for signs and symptoms of GI ulcers and bleeding, especially if patient takes NSAIDs concurrently.

Patient teaching

• Advise patient to take drug at bedtime with or without food.
• Instruct patient to allow orally disintegrating tablet to dissolve under tongue and then follow with a glass of water.
• Tell patient not to split, crush, or chew 23-mg tablet.
• Inform patient that drug may slow the heart rate, leading to fainting episodes.
◀€ Instruct patient to immediately report signs or symptoms of GI ulcers ("coffee-ground" vomitus, black tarry stools, and abdominal pain), or irregular heartbeat.
• As appropriate, review all other significant and life-threatening adverse reactions and interactions, especially those related to the drugs mentioned above.

dopamine hydrochloride
Intropin

Pharmacologic class: Catecholamine, adrenergic
Therapeutic class: Inotropic, vasopressor
Pregnancy risk category C

FDA | BOXED WARNING

• Dilute full-strength injection before administering.
• If extravasation occurs, infiltrate area promptly with 10 to 15 ml of saline solution containing 5 to 10 mg phentolamine to prevent sloughing and necrosis. Use syringe with fine hypodermic needle, and infiltrate solution liberally throughout area. Give phentolamine as soon as possible; its sympathetic blockade causes immediate local hyperemic changes if area is infiltrated within 12 hours.

Action

Causes norepinephrine release (mainly on dopaminergic receptors), leading to vasodilation of renal and mesenteric arteries. Also exerts inotropic effects on heart, which increases the heart rate, blood flow, myocardial contractility, and stroke volume.

Availability

Injection for dilution: 40 mg/ml, 80 mg/ml, 160 mg/ml
Premixed injection: 0.8 mg/ml, 1.6 mg/ml, 3.2 mg/ml in 250 ml and 500 ml of dextrose 5% in water

Indications and dosages

➤ Shock; hemodynamic imbalance; hypotension; heart failure
Adults and children: 2 to 5 mcg/kg/minute by I.V. infusion. Titrate dosage to desired response; may increase infusion by 1 to 4 mcg/kg/minute at 10- to 30-minute intervals. Maximum dosage is 50 mcg/kg/minute.

Contraindications

• Hypersensitivity to drug or bisulfites
• Tachyarrhythmias, ventricular fibrillation
• Pheochromocytoma

Precautions

Use cautiously in:
• hypovolemia, myocardial infarction, occlusive vascular disease, diabetic endarteritis, atrial embolism
• concurrent MAO inhibitor use
• pregnant or breastfeeding patients
• children.

Administration

- Give I.V. infusion using metered pump or other device that controls flow.
- Add 200 to 400 mg of dopamine to 250 to 500 ml of normal saline solution, 5% dextrose injection, 5% dextrose and half-normal saline solution, or 5% dextrose in lactated Ringer's solution.
- Infuse into large (preferably central) vein to minimize extravasation.

◀◤ Don't give concurrently with MAO inhibitors. Reduce dosage if patient has received MAO inhibitor recently.

Route	Onset	Peak	Duration
I.V.	1-2 min	Unknown	<10 min

Adverse reactions

CNS: headache
CV: palpitations, hypotension, angina, ECG changes, tachycardia, vasoconstriction, **arrhythmias**
EENT: mydriasis
GI: nausea, vomiting
Metabolic: azotemia, hyperglycemia
Respiratory: dyspnea, asthma attacks
Skin: piloerection
Other: irritation at injection site, **gangrene of extremities** (with high doses for prolonged periods or in occlusive vascular disease)

Interactions

Drug-drug. *Alpha- or beta-adrenergic blockers:* antagonism of dopamine effects
Ergot alkaloids: extreme blood pressure increase
Guanethidine: decreased cardiostimulatory effects
Inhalation anesthetics: increased risk of hypertension, arrhythmias
MAO inhibitors: hypertensive crisis
Oxytocics: severe, persistent hypotension
Phenytoin: seizures, severe hypotension, bradycardia

Tricyclic antidepressants: decreased pressor response
Drug-diagnostic tests. *Glucose, nitrogenous compounds, urine catecholamines:* increased levels

Patient monitoring

- Monitor blood pressure, pulse, urinary output, and pulmonary artery wedge pressure during infusion.

◀◤ Inspect I.V. site regularly for irritation. Avoid extravasation.

◀◤ Monitor color and temperature of extremities.

◀◤ Never stop infusion abruptly, because this may cause severe hypotension. Instead, taper gradually.

Patient teaching

- Explain the need for close observation during infusion.
- Instruct patient to report adverse reactions and I.V. site discomfort.
- As appropriate, review all other significant and life-threatening adverse reactions and interactions, especially those related to the drugs and tests mentioned above.

doripenem monohydrate
Doribax

Pharmacologic class: Carbapenem
Therapeutic class: Anti-infective
Pregnancy risk category B

Action

Acts against aerobic and anaerobic gram-positive and gram-negative bacteria

Availability

Powder for reconstitution for infusion: 500 mg single-use vials

---

Indications and dosages

➤ Complicated intra-abdominal infections caused by *Escherichia coli, Klebsiella pneumoniae, Pseudomonas aeruginosa, Bacteroides caccae, Bacteroides fragilis, Bacteroides thetaiotaomicron, Bacteroides uniformis, Bacteroides vulgatus, Streptococcus intermedius, Streptococcus constellatus,* and *Peptostreptococcus micros;* complicated urinary tract infections (UTIs), such as pyelonephritis caused by *E. coli* (including cases with concurrent bacteremia), *K. pneumoniae, Proteus mirabilis, P. aeruginosa,* and *Acinetobacter baumannii*

Adults ages 18 and older: 500 mg q 8 hours by I.V. infusion over 1 hour; continue for 5 to 14 days for complicated intra-abdominal infections and 10 days for complicated UTIs, with possible extension to 14 days for patients with concurrent bacteremia

Dosage adjustment

• Renal impairment

Contraindications

• Serious hypersensitivity to drug or other carbapenems
• History of anaphylactic reactions to beta-lactams

Precautions

Use cautiously in:
• renal impairment
• pregnant or breastfeeding patients
• children (safety and efficacy not established).

Administration

◀€ Don't use constituted suspension for direct injection; dilute further before giving by I.V. infusion.
• To prepare 500-mg dose, constitute vial with 10 ml sterile water for injection or normal saline solution for injection, and shake gently to form suspension; resulting concentration is 50 mg/ml. Withdraw suspension using syringe with 21G needle, and add it to infusion bag containing 100 ml normal saline solution or 5% dextrose; shake gently until clear. Final infusion solution concentration is 4.5 mg/ml.
• To prepare 250-mg dose, constitute vial with 10 ml sterile water for injection or normal saline solution for injection, and shake gently to form suspension. Resulting concentration is 50 mg/ml. Withdraw suspension using syringe with 21G needle, and add it to infusion bag containing 100 ml normal saline solution for injection or 5% dextrose; shake gently until clear. Remove 55 ml of this solution from bag and discard. Infuse remaining solution, which contains 250 mg (4.5 mg/ml).
• To prepare infusions in Baxter Minibag Plus infusion bags, see infusion bag manufacturer's instructions.
• Know that infusion solutions range from clear and colorless to clear and slightly yellow. Color variations within this range don't affect product potency.
• Don't mix with or physically add to solutions containing other drugs.
• Don't administer by inhalation.

Route	Onset	Peak	Duration
I.V.	Unknown	Unknown	Unknown

Adverse reactions

CNS: headache
CV: phlebitis
GI: nausea, diarrhea, oral candidiasis, ***Clostridium difficile*–associated diarrhea**
GU: vulvomycotic infection
Hematologic: anemia
Respiratory: pneumonitis (with inhalation use)
Skin: rash, allergic or bullous dermatitis, erythema, macular and papular eruptions, urticaria, erythema multiforme
Other: hypersensitivity reactions (including **anaphylaxis**)

Interactions

Drug-drug. *Probenecid:* reduced doripenem renal clearance

Valproic acid: decreased valproic acid level and loss of seizure control
Drug-diagnostic tests. *ALT, AST, liver enzymes, transaminases:* increased levels

Patient monitoring

• Closely monitor patient for diarrhea.

◀€ If allergic reaction occurs, discontinue drug and intervene for serious anaphylactic reactions by giving epinephrine and taking other emergency measures as ordered and needed, including oxygen, I.V. fluids and antihistamines, corticosteroids, pressor amines, and airway management.

• Monitor renal function in patients with moderate to severe renal impairment.

Patient teaching

◀€ Tell patient to immediately report rash, diarrhea, or difficulty breathing.

• As appropriate, review all other significant and life-threatening adverse reactions and interactions, especially those related to the drugs and tests mentioned above.

dornase alfa

Pulmozyme

Pharmacologic class: Recombinant human deoxyribonuclease I

Therapeutic class: Cystic fibrosis agent, mucolytic enzyme, respiratory inhalant

Pregnancy risk category B

Action

Selectively cleaves to DNA in sputum, decreasing viscosity of pulmonary secretions

Availability

Inhalation solution: 2.5-mg ampule (1 mg/ml)

⚠ Indications and dosages

➢ To reduce respiratory tract infections and improve pulmonary function in patients with cystic fibrosis

Adults and children: One ampule (2.5 mg) inhaled once daily; some patients may benefit from twice-daily dosing. Safety and efficacy of daily administration haven't been demonstrated for longer than 12 months.

Contraindications

• Hypersensitivity to drug, its components, or products derived from Chinese hamster ovary cells

Precautions

Use cautiously in:

• pregnant or breastfeeding patients.

Administration

• Don't shake, dilute, or mix with other drugs.

• Use only with approved nebulizer.

• Discard cloudy or discolored solution.

Route	Onset	Peak	Duration
Inhalation	Unknown	Unknown	Unknown

Adverse reactions

CV: chest pain

EENT: conjunctivitis, rhinitis, pharyngitis, hemoptysis, voice changes

Respiratory: dyspnea, increased sputum, wheezing

Skin: rash, urticaria, pruritus

Other: hypersensitivity reactions

Interactions

None known

Patient monitoring

• Assess patient periodically. Report improvement in dyspnea and sputum clearance.

• Monitor for signs and symptoms of hypersensitivity reaction.

Patient teaching
• Teach patient how to use nebulizer.
• Instruct patient to report rash, hives, and itching.
• As appropriate, review all other significant adverse reactions mentioned above.

doxapram hydrochloride
Dopram

Pharmacologic class: CNS and respiratory stimulant
Therapeutic class: Analeptic
Pregnancy risk category B

Action
Activates peripheral carotid, aortic, and other chemoreceptors to stimulate respiration. Increases tidal volume and respiratory rate by directly stimulating respiratory center in medulla oblongata.

Availability
Injection: 20 mg/ml

🚫 Indications and dosages
➤ Respiratory depression after anesthesia
Adults and adolescents: 5 mg/minute by I.V. infusion until desired response occurs; then reduce to 1 to 3 mg/minute, to a maximum cumulative dosage of 4 mg/kg (or 300 mg). Or 0.5 to 1 mg/kg I.V. injection, repeated q 5 minutes, if needed, to a maximum total dosage of 1.5 mg/kg.
➤ Chronic pulmonary disease related to acute hypercapnia
Adults: 1 to 2 mg/minute by I.V. infusion, using a concentration of 2 mg/ml, to a maximum of 3 mg/minute. Infusion shouldn't exceed 2 hours.
➤ Drug-induced CNS depression
Adults: Initially, 2 mg/kg I.V., repeated in 5 minutes and then q 1 to 2 hours until patient awakens, to a maximum daily dosage of 3 g. For infusion, priming dose of 2 mg/kg I.V.; if no response occurs, continue for 1 to 2 hours as needed; if some response occurs, give I.V. infusion of 250 mg in 250 ml of saline solution or dextrose 5% in water at 1 to 3 mg/minute until patient awakens. Don't infuse longer than 2 hours or give more than 3 g/day.

Off-label uses
• Laryngospasm secondary to postoperative tracheal extubation
• Apnea of prematurity
• Postoperative shivering

Contraindications
• Hypersensitivity to drug
• Cardiovascular disorders, severe hypertension
• Cerebrovascular accident
• Head injury, seizures
• Respiratory failure, restrictive respiratory disease
• Neonates

Precautions
Use cautiously in:
• bronchial asthma, arrhythmias, increased intracranial pressure, hyperthyroidism, pheochromocytoma, metabolic disorders
• concurrent use of mechanical ventilation
• pregnant or breastfeeding patients.

Administration
• Ensure adequate airway and oxygenation before administering.
• Give I.V. slowly to avoid hemolysis.
• Know that doxapram is compatible with 5% and 10% dextrose in water and with normal saline solution.
◀€ Don't mix with thiopental sodium, bicarbonate, or aminophylline, because precipitates or gas may form.

Route	Onset	Peak	Duration
I.V.	20-40 sec	1-2 min	5-12 min

Reactions in **bold** are life-threatening.   ◀€ Clinical alert

Adverse reactions
CNS: weakness, dizziness, drowsiness, headache, dysarthria, dysphonia, disorientation, hyperactivity, paresthesia, **loss of consciousness, seizures**
CV: hypotension, bradycardia, chest pain or tightness, heart rate changes, **thrombophlebitis, atrioventricular block, arrhythmias, cardiac arrest**
EENT: lacrimation, diplopia, miosis, conjunctival hyperemia, sneezing, **laryngospasm**
GI: nausea, vomiting, diarrhea, abdominal cramps, increased salivation, dysphagia
GU: urinary frequency or incontinence, albuminuria
Musculoskeletal: muscle cramps, fasciculations
Respiratory: dyspnea, increased secretions, cough, hyperventilation, tachypnea, rebound hypoventilation **bronchospasm**
Skin: rash, diaphoresis, flushing
Other: burning or hot sensation in genitalia and perineal areas, hiccups

Interactions
Drug-drug. *General anesthetics:* increased risk of self-limiting arrhythmias
MAO inhibitors, sympathomimetics: potentiation of adverse cardiovascular effects
Skeletal muscle relaxants: masking of residual effects of these drugs
Drug-diagnostic tests. *Blood urea nitrogen:* increased level
Erythrocytes, hematocrit, hemoglobin, red blood cells, white blood cells: decreased levels

Patient monitoring
• Assess blood pressure, pulse, deep tendon reflexes, airway, and arterial blood gas values before starting therapy and frequently during infusion.
• Monitor I.V. site frequently for irritation and thrombophlebitis.

◀€ Discontinue infusion immediately if hypotension or dyspnea suddenly develops.

Patient teaching
• Instruct patient to report adverse reactions promptly.
• As appropriate, review all other significant and life-threatening adverse reactions and interactions, especially those related to the drugs and tests mentioned above.

doxazosin mesylate
Cardozin XL✚, Cardura, Cardura XL, Doxadura✚

Pharmacologic class: Sympatholytic, peripherally acting antiadrenergic
Therapeutic class: Antihypertensive
Pregnancy risk category C

Action
Blocks alpha₁-adrenergic receptors, promoting vasodilation. Also reduces urethral resistance, relieving obstruction and improving urine flow and other symptoms of benign prostatic hypertrophy (BPH).

Availability
Tablets: 1 mg, 2 mg, 4 mg, 8 mg
Tablets (extended-release): 4 mg, 8 mg

❶ Indications and dosages
➤ Hypertension
Adults: 1 mg P.O. once daily. May increase dosage gradually q 2 weeks, up to 2 to 16 mg daily, as needed.
➤ BPH
Adults: 1 mg P.O. once daily. May increase dosage gradually, up to 8 mg daily, as needed. Or, initially 4 mg (extended-release) P.O. daily. May increase dosage to 8 mg daily, as needed, at 3- to 4-week intervals.

Off-label uses
• Pheochromocytoma
• Syndrome X

Contraindications
• Hypersensitivity to drug, its components, or quinazoline derivatives

Precautions
Use cautiously in:
• renal or mild or moderate hepatic impairment, coronary insufficiency, or preexisting severe GI narrowing
• severe hepatic impairment (extended-release form not recommended)
• intraoperative floppy iris syndrome
• concurrent use of strong CYP3A4 inhibitor (such as atazanavir, clarithromycin, indinavir, itraconazole, ketoconazole, nefazodone, nelfinavir, ritonavir, saquinavir, telithromycin, or voriconazole), phosphodiesterase-5 (PDE-5) inhibitors
• elderly patients
• pregnant or breastfeeding patients (extended-release form not recommended in breastfeeding patients)
• children (safety not established).

Administration
• Give initial immediate-release dose at bedtime to minimize orthostatic hypotension and syncope.
• Give initial extended-release dose at breakfast.
• Be aware that extended-release tablets aren't indicated for hypertension.
• Be aware that prostate carcinoma should be ruled out before giving drug for BPH.
• Know that incidence of orthostatic hypotension increases greatly when daily dosage exceeds 4 mg and that it usually occurs within 6 hours of administration.
◀≀ If new or worsening signs or symptoms of angina pectoris occur, discontinue drug.

Route	Onset	Peak	Duration
P.O.	1-2 hr	2-6 hr	24 hr
P.O. (extended)	Unknown	4.3-13.7 hr	Unknown

Adverse reactions
CNS: dizziness, vertigo, headache, depression, drowsiness, fatigue, nervousness, weakness, asthenia
CV: orthostatic hypotension, chest pain, palpitations, tachycardia, **arrhythmias**
EENT: abnormal or blurred vision, conjunctivitis, epistaxis, rhinitis, pharyngitis
GI: nausea, vomiting, diarrhea, constipation, abdominal discomfort, flatulence, dry mouth
GU: decreased libido, sexual dysfunction
Respiratory: dyspnea
Musculoskeletal: joint pain, arthritis, gout, myalgia
Skin: flushing, rash, pruritus
Other: edema

Interactions
Drug-drug. *Clonidine, nitrates, other antihypertensives:* decreased antihypertensive effect
Drugs that reduce GI motility leading to markedly prolonged GI retention times (such as anticholinergics): increased systemic exposure to doxazosin
PDE-5 inhibitors: increased risk of symptomatic hypotension
Drug-diagnostic tests. *Neutrophils, white blood cells:* decreased counts
Drug-food. *Any food:* increased drug plasma C_{max} (extended-release form)

Patient monitoring
• Monitor blood pressure with patient lying down and standing up every 2 to 6 hours after initial dose or after a dosage increase (when orthostatic hypotension is most likely to occur).

Reactions in **bold** are life-threatening.

◀≀ Clinical alert

Patient teaching

- Tell patient to swallow extended-release tablets whole and not to chew, divide, cut, or crush them.
- Caution patient not to drive or perform other activities requiring alertness for 12 to 24 hours after first dose.
- Tell patient to move slowly when sitting up or standing, to avoid dizziness or light-headedness from sudden blood pressure decrease.
- Advise patient to report episodes of dizziness or palpitations.
- As appropriate, review all other significant and life-threatening adverse reactions and interactions, especially those related to the drugs and tests mentioned above.

doxepin hydrochloride

Apo-Doxepin✢, Novo-Doxepin✢, Prudoxin, Silenor, Sinepin⊕, Xepin⊕, Zonalon

Pharmacologic class: Tricyclic antidepressant
Therapeutic class: Antidepressant, anxiolytic, antipruritic
Pregnancy risk category C

FDA | BOXED WARNING

- Drug may increase risk of suicidal thinking and behavior in children and adolescents with major depressive disorder and other psychiatric disorders. Risk must be balanced with clinical need, as depression itself increases suicide risk. With patient of any age, observe closely for clinical worsening, suicidality, and unusual behavior changes when therapy begins. Advise family and caregivers to observe patient closely and communicate with prescriber as needed.
- Drug isn't approved for use in pediatric patients.

Action

Unknown. May prevent reuptake of norepinephrine, serotonin, or both at presynaptic neurons, increasing levels of these neurotransmitters in CNS. Exact mechanism in pruritus also unknown, but drug is a potent histamine$_1$- and histamine$_2$-blocker.

Availability

Capsules: 10 mg, 25 mg, 50 mg, 75 mg, 100 mg, 150 mg
Cream (topical): 5% in 30-g tube
Oral concentrate: 10 mg/ml
Tablets: 3 mg, 6 mg

⦸ Indications and dosages

➤ Endogenous depression; anxiety
Adults: Initially, 25 mg P.O. t.i.d., increased as needed up to 150 mg daily in outpatients and 300 mg daily in hospitalized patients
Elderly adults: Initially, 25 to 50 mg P.O. daily; may be increased as needed
➤ Short-term relief of histamine-mediated pruritus of moderate severity accompanying such conditions as eczematous dermatitis
Adults: Apply a thin film of cream to skin q.i.d., with 3 to 4 hours between applications, for a maximum of 8 days.
➤ Insomnia
Adults: 6 mg P.O. daily 30 minutes before bedtime

Dosage adjustment

- Elderly patients

Contraindications

- Hypersensitivity to drug or other dibenzoxepins
- Glaucoma
- Predisposition to urinary retention
- MAO inhibitor use within past 14 days

Precautions
Use cautiously in:
- cardiovascular disease, prostatic enlargement, seizures
- severe sleep apnea (use not recommended)
- elderly patients
- pregnant or breastfeeding patients.

Administration
- If desired, mix contents of capsule with food.
- Dilute oral concentrate with 120 ml of water, milk, or juice. Be aware that drug is incompatible with carbonated beverages.
- Know that drug may be given at bedtime to prevent daytime sleepiness. If given for insomnia, avoid giving within 3 hours of a meal.

◀€ Don't give within 14 days of MAO inhibitor, because drug interaction may cause cardiovascular instability.

◀€ Avoid concurrent use of other CNS depressants, because inadvertent overdose may occur.
- With topical cream, don't apply to broken skin or use occlusive dressings, because doing so increases dermal absorption.
- Be aware that drug is usually given in conjunction with psychotherapy when used for depression.

Route	Onset	Peak	Duration
P.O.	Unknown	2 hr	Unknown
Topical	Unknown	Unknown	Unknown

Adverse reactions
CNS: fatigue, sedation, agitation, confusion, hallucinations, drowsiness, dizziness, extrapyramidal reactions, poor concentration, syncope, **seizures, cerebrovascular accident, increased risk of suicide or suicidal ideation** (especially in child or adolescent)
CV: hypotension, orthostatic hypotension, hypertension, vasculitis, ECG changes, tachycardia, palpitations, **arrhythmias, myocardial infarction, heart block**
EENT: blurred vision, increased intraocular pressure, lacrimation, tinnitus, nasal congestion
GI: nausea, constipation, dry mouth, **paralytic ileus**
GU: urinary retention, delayed voiding, urinary tract dilation, gynecomastia, galactorrhea, menstrual irregularities, testicular swelling, libido changes
Hematologic: purpura, **bone marrow depression, eosinophilia, agranulocytosis, thrombocytopenia, leukopenia**
Metabolic: hyperglycemia, **hypoglycemia**
Skin: photosensitivity, rash, urticaria, pruritus, diaphoresis, flushing, petechiae, alopecia, local burning, stinging, tingling, irritation, or rash (with topical use)
Other: increased appetite, weight gain or loss, hyperthermia, chills, edema, drug-induced fever, hypersensitivity reactions

Interactions
Drug-drug. *Barbiturates, CNS depressants (including antihistamines, clonidine, opioids, sedative-hypnotics):* additive CNS depression
Carbamazepine, class IC antiarrhythmics (flecainide, propafenone), other antidepressants, other CYP450-2D6 inhibitors (amiodarone, cimetidine, quinidine, ritonavir), phenothiazines: increased doxepin blood level and effects
Clonidine: hypertensive crisis
Guanethidine: antagonism of antihypertensive effects
Levodopa: delayed or decreased levodopa absorption, hypertension
MAO inhibitors: tachycardia, seizures, potentially fatal reactions
Rifamycin: decreased doxepin effects
Selective serotonin reuptake inhibitors: increased risk of toxicity

---

Reactions in **bold** are life-threatening. ◀€ Clinical alert

Drug-diagnostic tests. *Bilirubin, hepatic enzymes:* increased levels
Glucose: increased or decreased level
Liver function tests: altered results
Drug-herbs. *Angel's trumpet, jimson-weed, scopolia:* increased anticholinergic effects
Chamomile, hops, kava, skullcap, valerian: increased CNS depression
Evening primrose oil: additive or synergistic effects
S-adenosylmethionine (SAM-e), St. John's wort, yohimbe: serotonin syndrome
Drug-behaviors. *Alcohol use:* increased CNS depression
Smoking: increased drug metabolism and altered effects
Sun exposure: increased risk of photosensitivity reactions

Patient monitoring

◀≶ Record mood changes and watch for suicidal tendencies, especially in child or adolescent.
• Assess bowel elimination pattern. Increase fluids and administer stool softeners as ordered to ease constipation.
• Monitor fluid intake and output. Report changes in voiding pattern.
• Monitor liver function test results, CBC with white cell differential, and glucose level.

Patient teaching

• Tell patient to take drug 30 minutes before bedtime and not within 3 hours of a meal when taking for insomnia.
• Advise patient on long-term therapy not to stop taking drug abruptly because this may lead to nausea, headache, and malaise.
◀≶ Instruct patient and significant other, as appropriate, to monitor mental status carefully and to immediately report increased depression or suicidal thoughts or behavior (especially when used in child or adolescent).
◀≶ Tell patient to promptly report easy bruising or bleeding.

• Caution patient to avoid driving and other hazardous activities until he knows how drug affects concentration and alertness.
• Instruct patient to move slowly when sitting up or standing, to avoid dizziness or light-headedness from sudden blood pressure decrease.
• Explain that drowsiness and dizziness usually subside after several weeks.
• Tell patient that using topical cream on more than 10% of body surface area may cause drowsiness.
• Caution patient using topical cream not to apply it to broken skin and not to use occlusive dressings. Also tell him to avoid contact with eyes and to rinse eyes thoroughly with warm water if contact occurs.
• As appropriate, review all other significant and life-threatening adverse reactions and interactions, especially those related to the drugs, tests, herbs, and behaviors mentioned above.

doxorubicin hydrochloride
Adriamycin PFS, Adriamycin RDF, Rubex

Pharmacologic class: Anthracycline
Therapeutic class: Antibiotic antineoplastic
Pregnancy risk category D

FDA BOXED WARNING

• Administer I.V. only—never I.M. or subcutaneously. Extravasation causes severe local tissue necrosis.
• Myocardial toxicity may occur during therapy or months to years afterward. Risk factors (cardiovascular disease, previous or concurrent radiotherapy to mediastinal or pericardial area, previous therapy with

doxorubicin or other anthracyclines or anthracenediones, and concomitant use of other cardiotoxic drugs) may increase myocardial toxicity risk. Toxicity may occur at higher or lower cumulative doses even in patients without cardiac risk factors. Pediatric patients have increased risk of delayed cardiotoxicity.

• Secondary acute myelogenous leukemia (AML) may occur. Refractory secondary leukemia is more common when drug is given in combination with DNA-damaging antineoplastics, when patients have been heavily pretreated with cytotoxic drugs, and with dosage escalation. Pediatric patients also are at risk for secondary AML.

• Reduce dosage in hepatic impairment.

• Drug may cause severe myelosuppression.

• Give under supervision of physician experienced in cancer chemotherapy.

Action
Unclear. Thought to inhibit DNA and RNA synthesis by forming complex with DNA. Also exerts immunosuppressive activity. Cell-cycle–S-phase specific.

Availability
Injection (preservative-free): 2 mg/ml
Powder for injection: 10 mg, 20 mg, 50 mg

⊘ Indications and dosages
➤ Solid tumors, including bladder, breast, lung, stomach, and thyroid cancers; malignant lymphomas, including Hodgkin's disease; acute leukemia; chronic lymphocytic leukemia; multiple myeloma; Wilms' tumor; neuroblastoma
Adults: 60 to 75 mg/m² I.V. as a single dose at 21-day cycles, or 30 mg/m² I.V. as a single daily dose on first to third days of 4-week cycle, or 20 mg/m² I.V. once weekly. Maximum cumulative dosage is 550 mg/m².

Dosage adjustment
• Bone marrow depression
• Impaired cardiac or hepatic function

Off-label uses
• Endometrial carcinoma, islet cell carcinoma

Contraindications
• Hypersensitivity to drug
• Severe bone marrow depression
• Previous treatment with maximum cumulative doses of doxorubicin, other anthracyclines, or anthracenes

Precautions
Use cautiously in:
• cardiac disease, hepatic impairment, depressed bone marrow reserve, CNS metastases, brain tumor, malignant melanoma, renal carcinoma
• elderly patients
• females of childbearing age
• pregnant or breastfeeding patients
• children.

Administration
• Follow facility policy for handling and preparing antineoplastics.

◀﹦ Don't dilute solution with bacteriostatic diluent. Don't mix with other drugs.

• Dilute as directed with normal saline solution to a final concentration of 2 mg/ml.

• Administer slowly over 3 to 5 minutes into tubing of free-flowing I.V. infusion of normal saline solution or dextrose 5% in water.

• Deliver into large vein using butterfly needle. Avoid veins over joints or extremities with compromised venous or lymphatic drainage.

◀﹦ Avoid rapid infusion, because this may increase risk of acute infusion-related reactions (back pain, chest tightness, flushing).

◀﹦ If extravasation occurs, stop infusion immediately, apply ice, and notify prescriber.

d

Route	Onset	Peak	Duration
I.V.	Rapid	2 hr	24-36 days

Adverse reactions

CNS: drowsiness, dizziness, asthenia, fatigue, malaise, paresthesia, headache, depression, insomnia, anxiety, emotional lability

CV: chest pain, hypotension, tachycardia, peripheral edema, **cardiomyopathy, heart failure, arrhythmias, pericardial effusion**

GI: nausea, vomiting, diarrhea, constipation, enlarged abdomen, abdominal pain, dyspepsia, oral candidiasis, moniliasis, stomatitis, glossitis, esophagitis, dysphagia

GU: albuminuria, hyperuricosuria, red urine

Hematologic: anemia, **leukopenia, thrombocytopenia, neutropenia, bone marrow depression**

Metabolic: hyperglycemia, hypocalcemia

Musculoskeletal: myalgia, back pain

Respiratory: dyspnea, increased cough, pneumonia

Skin: rash, dry skin, pruritus, skin discoloration, alopecia, diaphoresis, exfoliative dermatitis, palmar-plantar erythrodysesthesia

Other: abnormal taste, infection, chills, fever, herpes zoster, injection site reactions, allergic reactions including **anaphylaxis, acute infusion-associated reactions**

Interactions

Drug-drug. *Antineoplastics:* additive bone marrow depression

Cyclophosphamide: increased risk of hemorrhagic cystitis, increased cardiotoxicity

Cyclosporine: profound and prolonged hematologic toxicity, increased risk of coma and seizures

Dactinomycin (in children): increased risk of pneumonitis

Live-virus vaccines: decreased antibody response to vaccine, increased risk of adverse reactions

Mercaptopurine: hepatitis

Paclitaxel (if given first): reduced doxorubicin clearance, increased incidence and severity of neutropenia and stomatitis

Phenobarbital: increased clearance and decreased effects of doxorubicin

Phenytoin: decreased phenytoin blood level

Progesterone: increased incidence and severity of neutropenia and thrombocytopenia

Streptozocin: increased doxorubicin half-life

Verapamil: increased doxorubicin blood level

Drug-diagnostic tests. *Alkaline phosphatase, bilirubin, glucose, prothrombin time, serum and urine uric acid:* increased levels

Calcium, hemoglobin, neutrophils, platelets, white blood cells (WBCs): decreased levels

Patient monitoring

◀€ Watch for acute life-threatening arrhythmias, which may occur during or within a few hours after administration.

◀€ Monitor for cardiomyopathy and subsequent heart failure with chronic overdose (more common in children).

• Stay alert for erythematous streaking along vein next to injection site, which may indicate too-rapid infusion.

• Watch for nausea and vomiting. Administer antiemetics as needed.

◀€ Check for superinfection or hemorrhage caused by persistent bone marrow depression (but expect WBC counts as low as 1,000/mm³ during therapy).

◀€ Watch closely for infusion-related reactions and anaphylaxis.

• Monitor CBC, hepatic profile, coagulation tests, ejection fraction, and glucose, uric acid, bilirubin, and calcium blood levels.

Patient teaching

◀€ Advise patient to promptly report irregular heartbeats, easy bruising or bleeding, or signs of hypersensitivity reaction, such as a rash.

• Caution patient to avoid people with colds, flu, or other contagious illnesses.

• Explain that drug may cause complete but reversible hair loss.

• Inform patient that drug may turn urine red for 1 or 2 days.

• As appropriate, review all other significant and life-threatening adverse reactions and interactions, especially those related to the drugs and tests mentioned above.

doxorubicin hydrochloride, liposomal
Caelyx✢⊕, Doxil, Myocet⊕

Pharmacologic class: Anthracycline
Therapeutic class: Antibiotic antineoplastic
Pregnancy risk category D

FDA | BOXED WARNING

• Drug may cause cardiotoxicity. Myocardial damage may lead to heart failure and may occur as total cumulative dose (which includes previous use of other anthracyclines or anthracenediones) approaches 550 mg/m². Toxicity may occur at lower cumulative doses in patients who have had previous mediastinal irradiation or are receiving concurrent cyclophosphamides.

• Acute infusion-related reactions occur in up to 10% of patients. They usually resolve over several hours to 1 day after infusion ends; in some patients, they resolve with slower infusion rate. Serious and sometimes life-threatening allergic or anaphylactoid-like infusion reactions may occur. Keep emergency equipment and drugs to treat reaction available for immediate use.

• Drug may cause severe myelosuppression.

• Reduce dosage in hepatic impairment.

• Accidental substitution of liposomal form for doxorubicin hydrochloride may cause severe adverse effects. Don't substitute on mg-per-mg basis.

Action
Unclear. Thought to inhibit DNA and RNA synthesis by forming complex with DNA. Also exerts immunosuppressive activity. Liposomal encapsulation increases uptake by tumors, prolongs drug action, and may decrease toxicity. Cell-cycle–S-phase specific.

Availability
Liposomal dispersion for injection: 2 mg/ml in 10-ml vial, 2 mg/ml in 25-ml vials

⫽ Indications and dosages
➤ AIDS-related Kaposi's sarcoma
Adults: 20 mg/m² I.V. once q 3 weeks
➤ Metastatic ovarian carcinoma
Adults: Initially, 50 mg/m² I.V. at a rate of 1 mg/minute q 4 weeks for at least four courses. If no adverse reactions occur, increase infusion rate to complete the infusion over 1 hour.

Dosage adjustment
• Hepatic impairment

Contraindications
• Hypersensitivity to drug
• Malignant melanoma
• CNS metastases
• Bone marrow depression
• Cardiac disease
• Breastfeeding

Precautions
Use cautiously in:
• hepatic impairment, brain tumor, renal carcinoma, myelosuppression
• elderly patients

- females of childbearing age
- pregnant patients
- children.

Administration

- Follow facility policy for handling and preparing antineoplastics.
- Dilute dose (up to 90 mg) in 250 ml of dextrose 5% in water. Don't use any other diluent.
- ◀◁ Don't dilute solution with bacteriostatic diluent. Don't mix with other drugs.
- Don't use in-line filter.
- Administer slowly by I.V. infusion at initial rate of 1 mg/minute. If no infusion reaction occurs, increase rate to complete infusion over 1 hour. Don't give as I.V. bolus.
- ◀◁ Avoid rapid infusion, which may increase the risk of infusion-related reactions (back pain, chest tightness, flushing).
- ◀◁ If extravasation occurs, stop infusion immediately, apply ice, and notify prescriber.
- Don't give I.M. or subcutaneously.
- Know that drug is a translucent red dispersion, not a clear solution.

Route	Onset	Peak	Duration
I.V.	10 days	14 days	21-24 days

Adverse reactions

CNS: drowsiness, dizziness, asthenia, fatigue, malaise, paresthesia, headache, depression, insomnia, anxiety, emotional lability
CV: chest pain, hypotension, tachycardia, peripheral edema, **cardiomyopathy, heart failure, arrhythmias, pericardial effusion**
GI: nausea, vomiting, diarrhea, constipation, abdominal pain, enlarged abdomen, dyspepsia, moniliasis, stomatitis, glossitis, oral candidiasis, esophagitis, dysphagia
GU: albuminuria, red urine

Hematologic: anemia, **leukopenia, thrombocytopenia, neutropenia, bone marrow depression**
Hepatic: jaundice
Metabolic: hypocalcemia, hyperglycemia
Musculoskeletal: myalgia, back pain, hand-foot syndrome
Respiratory: dyspnea, increased cough, pneumonia
Skin: rash, dry skin, pruritus, skin discoloration, alopecia, diaphoresis, exfoliative dermatitis, palmar-plantar erythrodysesthesia
Other: altered taste, fever, chills, infection, herpes zoster, injection site reactions, allergic reactions including **anaphylaxis, acute infusion reaction**

Interactions

Drug-drug. *Antineoplastics:* additive bone marrow depression
Cyclophosphamide: increased risk of hemorrhagic cystitis
Cyclosporine: profound and prolonged hematologic toxicity, increased risk of coma and seizures, increased cardiotoxicity
Dactinomycin (in children): increased risk of pneumonitis
Live-virus vaccines: decreased antibody response to vaccine, increased risk of adverse reactions
Mercaptopurine: hepatitis
Paclitaxel (if administered first): reduced doxorubicin clearance, increased incidence and severity of neutropenia and stomatitis
Phenobarbital: increased clearance and decreased effects of doxorubicin
Phenytoin: decreased phenytoin blood level
Progesterone: increased risk and severity of neutropenia and thrombocytopenia
Streptozocin: prolonged doxorubicin half-life
Verapamil: increased doxorubicin blood level
Drug-diagnostic tests. *Alkaline phosphatase, bilirubin, glucose, prothrombin*

---

time, serum and urine uric acid: increased levels
Calcium, hemoglobin, neutrophils, platelets, white blood cells: decreased levels

Patient monitoring

◀€ Observe patient closely for anaphylaxis and bleeding problems.

◀€ Stay alert for acute life-threatening arrhythmias, which may occur during or within a few hours after administration.

◀€ Assess for cardiomyopathy and subsequent heart failure with chronic overdose (more common in children).

◀€ Monitor closely for acute infusion reaction.

• Assess for and report liver engorgement and yellowing of skin or eyes.

• Check CBC, coagulation tests, hepatic profile, and bilirubin, glucose, calcium and uric acid levels.

• Watch for nausea and vomiting. Give antiemetics, as needed and prescribed.

• Assess for constipation and give fluids and stool softeners, as needed and prescribed.

Patient teaching

◀€ Instruct patient to immediately report shortness of breath; tingling or burning, redness, flaking, bothersome swelling, small blisters, or small sores on palms of hands or soles of feet; rash, chest pain, or palpitations.

• Advise patient to avoid people with colds, flu, or other contagious illnesses.

• As appropriate, review all other significant and life-threatening adverse reactions and interactions, especially those related to the drugs and tests mentioned above.

doxycycline
Adoxa, Oracea, Vibramycin

doxycycline calcium
Vibramycin Calcium

d

doxycycline hyclate
Alodox, Apo-Doxy✦, Doryx, Doxy 100, Doxytab, Novo-Doxylin✦, Oraxyl, Periostat, Vibramycin-D✦, Vibramycin Hyclate

doxycycline monohydrate
Monodox

Pharmacologic class: Tetracycline
Therapeutic class: Anti-infective
Pregnancy risk category D

Action
Unclear. Thought to inhibit bacterial protein synthesis at 30S and 50S ribosomal subunit and to alter cytoplasmic membrane of susceptible organisms.

Availability
Capsules: 50 mg, 100 mg, 150 mg
Capsules (coated pellets): 40 mg, 75 mg, 100 mg
Powder for injection: 100 mg, 200 mg
Powder for oral suspension: 25 mg/5 ml
Syrup: 50 mg
Tablets: 20 mg, 50 mg, 75 mg, 100 mg

⏀ Indications and dosages
➤ Rosacea
Adults: 40 mg P.O. daily in the morning
➤ Infections caused by various organisms, including *Mycoplasma, Chlamydia,* and *Rickettsia* organisms, and *Borrelia burgdorfer*
Adults and children weighing more than 45 kg (99 lb): 100 mg P.O. q 12 hours on first day, followed by 100 to

---

200 mg P.O. once daily; or 50 to 100 mg P.O. q 12 hours; or 200 mg I.V. once daily; or 100 mg I.V. q 12 hours on first day, followed by 100 to 200 mg I.V. once daily; or 50 to 100 mg I.V. q 12 hours
Children weighing 45 kg (99 lb) or less: 2.2 mg/kg P.O. q 12 hours on first day, followed by 2.2 to 4.4 mg/kg/day P.O. once daily; or 1.1 to 2.2 mg/kg P.O. q 12 hours; or 4.4 mg/kg I.V. once daily; or 2.2 mg/kg I.V. q 12 hours on first day, followed by 2.2 to 4.4 mg/kg I.V. once daily; or 1.1 to 2.2 mg/kg I.V. q 12 hours
➤ Gonorrhea in penicillin-allergic patients
Adults and children weighing more than 45 kg (99 lb): 100 mg P.O. q 12 hours for 7 days; or 300 mg P.O. initially, followed by another 300 mg P.O. 1 hour later
➤ Lyme disease
Adults and children weighing more than 45 kg (99 lb): 100 mg P.O. b.i.d. for 10 to 30 days
➤ Periodontitis
Adults and children weighing more than 45 kg (99 lb): 20 mg P.O. b.i.d. for up to 9 months
➤ Anthrax
Adults and children weighing more than 45 kg (99 lb): 100 mg P.O. b.i.d. for 60 days; or 100 mg I.V. q 12 hours for 60 days, changing to oral route when appropriate
Children weighing 45 kg (99 lb) or less: 2.2 mg/kg P.O. b.i.d. for 60 days; or 100 mg I.V. q 12 hours for 60 days, changing to oral route when appropriate
➤ Prevention of malaria caused by *Plasmodium falciparum* in short-term travelers (less than 4 months)
Adults: 100 mg/day P.O. starting 1 to 2 days before travel begins and continuing during and for 4 weeks after travel
Children: 2 mg/kg/day P.O., up to adult dosage of 100 mg/day, starting 1 to 2 days before travel begins and continuing during and for 4 weeks after travel

Off-label uses
• Traveler's diarrhea
• Pleural effusion

Contraindications
• Hypersensitivity to drug, other tetracyclines, or bisulfites (with some drug products)

Precautions
Use cautiously in:
• renal disease, hepatic impairment, nephrogenic diabetes insipidus, cachexia
• pregnant or breastfeeding patients
• children younger than age 8.

Administration
• Obtain specimens for culture and sensitivity testing, as ordered, before first dose.
◀≋ Don't give in conjunction with methoxyflurane anesthetic. Severe or fatal kidney damage may result.
• Reconstitute powder for injection with dextrose 5% in water, normal saline solution, lactated Ringer's solution, or dextrose 5% in lactated Ringer's solution.
• Don't infuse solutions with concentrations above 1 mg/ml.
• Infuse 100-mg dose over at least 1 hour.
• Complete infusion within 12 hours of dilution, unless diluted with lactated Ringer's solution or dextrose 5% in lactated Ringer's solution; in this case, complete infusion within 6 hours.
◀≋ Don't give during last half of pregnancy or to children under age 8 unless other drugs are likely to be ineffective or are contraindicated. Drug may retard bone growth and cause tooth discoloration and malformation.
• Be aware that capsules with coated pellets contain immediate- and delayed-release pellets.

Route	Onset	Peak	Duration
P.O.	1-2 hr	1.5-4 hr	12 hr
I.V.	Rapid	End of infusion	12 hr

Adverse reactions

CNS: paresthesia, **pseudotumor cerebri**

CV: phlebitis, **thrombophlebitis, pericarditis**

EENT: vestibular reactions, hoarseness, pharyngitis

GI: nausea, vomiting, diarrhea, esophagitis, epigastric distress, enterocolitis, anogenital lesions or inflammation, glossitis, oral candidiasis, black hairy tongue, **pancreatitis**

GU: dark yellow or brown urine, vaginal candidiasis

Hematologic: hemolytic anemia, neutropenia, thrombocytopenia

Hepatic: hepatotoxicity

Musculoskeletal: bone growth retardation (in children younger than age 8)

Skin: photosensitivity, maculopapular or erythematous rash, hyperpigmentation, urticaria

Other: tooth enamel defects, increased appetite, phlebitis at I.V. site, superinfection, hypersensitivity reactions including **anaphylaxis**

Interactions

Drug-drug. *Adsorbent antidiarrheals; antacids; calcium, iron, and magnesium preparations:* decreased doxycycline absorption

Barbiturates, carbamazepine, hormonal contraceptives containing estrogen, phenytoin, rifamycin: decreased doxycycline efficacy

Cholestyramine, colestipol: decreased oral absorption of doxycycline

Methoxyflurane: increased nephrotoxicity

Penicillin: decreased penicillin activity

Sucralfate: prevention of doxycycline absorption from GI tract

Warfarin: enhanced warfarin effects

Drug-diagnostic tests. *Alkaline phosphatase, alanine aminotransferase, amylase, aspartate aminotransferase, bilirubin, blood urea nitrogen (BUN), eosinophils:* increased levels

Hemoglobin, neutrophils, platelets, white blood cells: decreased levels

Urine catecholamines: false elevations

Drug-food. *Calcium-containing foods:* decreased drug absorption

Drug-behaviors. *Alcohol use:* decreased anti-infective effect of doxycycline

Sun exposure: increased risk of photosensitivity

Patient monitoring

• Evaluate I.V. site regularly. Apply cool compresses as needed.

◀€ Monitor for hypersensitivity reactions, including anaphylaxis.

• Monitor hepatic profile, CBC, BUN, and creatinine levels.

• Assess for hypercoagulability in patients taking warfarin concurrently.

• Monitor for digoxin toxicity in patients taking digoxin concurrently.

Patient teaching

• Advise patient to take with 8 oz of water to ensure passage into stomach.

• Tell patient to take on empty stomach at least 1 hour before meals or 2 hours afterwards.

• Instruct patient to take at least 1 hour before bedtime to prevent esophagitis.

◀€ Tell patient to immediately report painful swallowing, abdominal pain, easy bruising or bleeding, or signs of hypersensitivity (such as rash).

• Advise female patient to tell prescriber if she is pregnant.

• Instruct patient to avoid alcohol use and large amounts of calcium-containing foods (such as dairy products and some green leafy vegetables, such as spinach).

• Stress importance of good oral hygiene.

Reactions in **bold** are life-threatening.   ◀€ Clinical alert

• As appropriate, review all other significant and life-threatening adverse reactions and interactions, especially those related to the drugs, tests, foods, and behaviors mentioned above.

dronabinol
Marinol

Pharmacologic class: Cannabinoid
Therapeutic class: Antiemetic
Controlled substance III
Pregnancy risk category B

Action
Unknown. May exert antiemetic effect by inhibiting vomiting control mechanism in medulla oblongata.

Availability
Capsules: 2.5 mg, 5 mg, 10 mg

🕖 Indications and dosages
➤ Prevention of nausea and vomiting caused by chemotherapy
Adults and children: Initially, 5 mg/m² P.O. 1 to 3 hours before chemotherapy. Repeat dose q 2 to 4 hours after chemotherapy, up to four to six doses per day. If 5-mg/m² dose is ineffective and patient has no significant adverse reactions, dosage may be increased in increments of 2.5 mg/m² to a maximum dosage of 15 mg/m².
➤ Appetite stimulant
Adults and children: Initially, 2.5 mg P.O. b.i.d. May reduce dosage to 2.5 mg/day given as a single evening or bedtime dose. Maximum dosage is 10 mg P.O. b.i.d.

Contraindications
• Hypersensitivity to cannabinoids or sesame oil
• Breastfeeding

Precautions
Use cautiously in:
• hypertension, heart disease, bipolar disorder, schizophrenia, drug abuse, seizures
• pregnant patients.

Administration
• When used to stimulate appetite, give before lunch and dinner.

Route	Onset	Peak	Duration
P.O.	30-60 min	2-4 hr	4-6 hr

Adverse reactions
CNS: drowsiness, anxiety, impaired coordination, irritability, depression, headache, hallucinations, memory loss, paresthesia, ataxia, paranoia, disorientation, nightmares, speech difficulties, syncope, **suicidal ideation**
CV: tachycardia, hypotension, hypertension
EENT: visual disturbances, tinnitus
GI: dry mouth
Skin: facial flushing, diaphoresis

Interactions
Drug-drug. *Anticholinergics, antihistamines, tricyclic antidepressants:* increased tachycardia and hypertension
CNS depressants: increased CNS depression
Ritonavir: increased dronabinol blood level and risk of toxicity
Drug-behaviors. *Alcohol use:* increased CNS depression

Patient monitoring
• Monitor vital signs for hypotension and tachycardia.
◀€ Check for adverse CNS reactions. Report significant depression, paranoid reaction, or emotional lability.
• Monitor nutritional status and hydration.

Patient teaching
• Teach patient about drug's significant adverse CNS and cardiovascular

effects. Emphasize that he should take it only as prescribed and needed.

◀◗ Advise patient (and significant other) to immediately report depression, suicidal thoughts, paranoid reactions, seizures, and other serious CNS reactions.

• Caution patient to avoid driving and other hazardous activities until he knows how drug affects concentration and alertness.

• As appropriate, review all other significant and life-threatening adverse reactions and interactions, especially those related to the drugs and behaviors mentioned above.

dronedarone
Multaq

Pharmacologic class: Benzofuran derivative
Therapeutic class: Antiarrhythmic
Pregnancy risk category X

FDA BOXED WARNING

• In patients with symptomatic heart failure and recent decompensation requiring hospitalization or with New York Heart Association Class IV heart failure, dronedarone doubles risk of death and is contraindicated in these patients.

• In patients with permanent AF, dronedarone doubles risk of death, stroke, and hospitalization for heart failure. Dronedarone is contraindicated in patients with AF who won't or can't be cardioverted into normal sinus rhythm.

Action
Unknown.

Availability
Tablets: 400 mg

⚕ Indications and dosages
➤ To reduce risk of hospitalization for atrial fibrillation (AF) in patients in sinus rhythm with a history of paroxysmal or persistent AF
Adults: 400 mg P.O. b.i.d. with morning and evening meals

Contraindications
• Permanent AF (patients in whom normal sinus rhythm won't or can't be restored), symptomatic heart failure with recent decompensation requiring hospitalization or New York Heart Association Class IV symptoms, second- or third-degree atrioventricular (AV) block or sick sinus syndrome (except when used with a functioning pacemaker), bradycardia less than 50 beats/minute, QTc Bazett interval at or above 500 ms or PR interval above 280 ms

• Concomitant use of drugs or herbal products that prolong QT interval and may induce torsades de pointes (such as phenothiazine antipsychotics, tricyclic antidepressants, certain oral macrolide antibiotics, Class I and III antiarrhythmics)

• Concomitant use of a strong CYP3A inhibitor (such as clarithromycin, cyclosporine, itraconazole, ketoconazole, nefazodone, ritonavir, telithromycin, voriconazole)

• Hepatotoxicity related to the previous use of amiodarone and severe hepatic impairment

• Patients who are or may become pregnant

• Breastfeeding patients

Precautions
Use cautiously in:
• new or worsening heart failure during treatment, QT-interval prolongation
• hypokalemia, hypomagnesemia
• increased serum creatinine level
• children younger than age 18 (safety and efficacy not established).

Reactions in **bold** are life-threatening.   ◀◗ Clinical alert

Administration

🔊 Be aware that treatment with Class I or III antiarrhythmics or strong CYP3A inhibitors must be stopped before start of dronedarone.

• Note that hypokalemia or hypomagnesemia may occur with concomitant administration of potassium-depleting diuretics. Ensure that potassium levels are within normal range before starting drug.

• Administer with morning and evening meals but not with grapefruit juice.

Route	Onset	Peak	Duration
P.O.	Unknown	3-6 hr	Unknown

Adverse reactions

CNS: asthenia
CV: bradycardia, **QT-interval prolongation, new or worsening heart failure**
GI: diarrhea, nausea, vomiting, abdominal pain, dyspepsia
Hepatic: hepatocellular injury, acute liver injury
Metabolic: hypokalemia, hypomagnesemia, increased creatinine
Skin: rash (generalized, macular, maculopapular, erythematous), pruritus, eczema, dermatitis, allergic dermatitis

Interactions

Drug-drug. *Beta blockers, such as metoprolol, propranolol:* increased effects to these drugs, increased risk of bradycardia
Calcium channel blockers, with depressant effects on sinus and AV nodes, such as diltiazem, nifedipine, verapamil: increased dronedarone and calcium channel blocker effects; potentiated dronedarone effects on conduction
CYP3A inducers, such as carbamazepine, phenobarbital, phenytoin, rifampin: significantly decreased dronedarone effect
Digoxin: potentiated dronedarone electrophysiologic effects (such as decreased AV node conduction); increased digoxin level; increased GI disorders

Drugs that prolong QT interval: risk of torsades de pointes–type ventricular tachycardia
Other CYP2D6 substrates, such as other beta blockers, selective serotonin reuptake inhibitors, tricyclic antidepressants: increased effects of these drugs
Potent CYP3A inhibitors, such as clarithromycin, cyclosporine, itraconazole, ketoconazole, nefazodone, ritonavir, telithromycin, voriconazole: increased dronedarone effect and C_{max}
HMG-CoA reductase inhibitors, such as simvastatin: increased simvastatin effect
Sirolimus, tacrolimus, other CYP3A substrates with narrow therapeutic range: increased plasma concentrations of these drugs
Drug-diagnostic tests. *Serum creatinine:* increased level
Magnesium, potassium: decreased levels
Drug-food. *Any food:* increased drug bioavailability
Grapefruit juice: increased dronedarone effect and C_{max}
Drug-herbs. *St. John's wort:* significantly decreased dronedarone effect

Patient monitoring

🔊 Observe patient closely for worsening heart failure: If heart failure develops or worsens, consider suspending or discontinuing drug.
🔊 Discontinue drug if QT-interval prolongation occurs (QTc Bazett interval at or above 500 ms).
• Monitor patient for hypokalemia and hypomagnesemia, especially with concomitant administration of potassium-depleting diuretics. Maintain potassium and magnesium levels within normal range.
• Monitor renal function and watch for increase in serum creatinine level.

Patient teaching

• Instruct patient to take drug with morning and evening meals and to avoid grapefruit juice.

◀€ Advise patient to immediately notify prescriber if signs and symptoms of worsening heart failure develop, such as acute weight gain, edema in legs or feet, or increasing shortness of breath.

• Instruct patient to consult prescriber before taking other prescription or nonprescription drugs or herbal products, particularly St. John's wort.

• As appropriate, review all other significant and life-threatening adverse reactions and interactions, especially those related to the drugs, tests, foods, and herbs mentioned above.

droperidol
Inapsine

Pharmacologic class: Butyrophenone
Therapeutic class: General anesthetic, antiemetic
Pregnancy risk category C

FDA | BOXED WARNING

• QT prolongation and torsades de pointes may occur at or below recommended doses, even in patients with no known risk factors. (Risk factors for prolonged QT syndrome include heart failure, bradycardia, cardiac hypertrophy, hypokalemia, hypomagnesemia, age older than 65, alcohol abuse, and use of diuretics, drugs that prolong the QT interval, benzodiazepines, volatile anesthetics, or I.V. opioids.) Some cases have been fatal. Reserve drug for patients with refractory disease. Use with extreme caution in patients at risk for prolonged QT interval.

• Drug is contraindicated in patients with known or suspected QT prolongation.

Action
Produces marked sedation by directly blocking subcortical receptors. Produces antiemetic effect by blocking CNS receptors in chemoreceptor trigger zone.

Availability
Injection: 2.5 mg/ml in 1-ml, 2-ml, and 5-ml ampules and in 2-ml, 5-ml, and 10-ml vials

🖉 Indications and dosages
➤ Perioperative nausea and vomiting
Adults: Initially, 2.5 mg I.M. or I.V. Additional doses of 1.25 mg may be given. Dosages are highly individualized according to patient's age, weight, physical status, and underlying pathologic condition.
Children ages 2 to 12: Initially, 0.1 mg/kg I.M. or I.V. Additional doses up to a total of 2.5 mg may be given. Dosages are highly individualized according to patient's age, weight, physical status, and underlying clinical condition.

Dosage adjustment
• Elderly or debilitated patients
• High-risk patients (such as patients over age 65 and those with heart failure, alcohol abuse, or other factors that predispose to prolonged QT interval)
• Patients who have received other CNS depressants (such as analgesics or anesthetics)

Contraindications
• Hypersensitivity to drug
• Known or suspected QT-interval prolongation (more than 440 millisec in males or 450 millisec in females)

Precautions
Use cautiously in:
• severe cardiac or renal disease, diabetes mellitus, respiratory insufficiency, prostatic hypertrophy, angle-closure glaucoma, CNS depression, CNS tumors, intestinal obstruction, bone marrow depression

---

Reactions in **bold** are life-threatening. ◀€ Clinical alert

- elderly patients
- pregnant or breastfeeding patients
- children younger than age 2.

Administration
- Know that drug is indicated to ease perioperative nausea and vomiting only in patients who don't respond adequately to other treatment.
- Be aware that drug doesn't need to be diluted for I.V. or I.M. use.
- Give by slow I.V. injection, or inject I.M. into large muscle.

Route	Onset	Peak	Duration
I.V., I.M.	3-10 min	30 min	2-4 hr

Adverse reactions
CNS: weakness, dysarthria, dysphonia, dizziness, extrapyramidal reactions, headache, postoperative hallucinatory episodes with transient depression, tremor, irritability, paresthesia, aggression, vertigo, ataxia, **loss of consciousness, seizures, neuroleptic malignant syndrome**
CV: chest pain, hypertension, hypotension, vasodilation, **arrhythmias, atrial fibrillation**
EENT: cataracts, blurred vision, eye irritation, sore throat
GI: nausea, vomiting, diarrhea, abdominal cramps, bloating, epigastric pain, fecal incontinence, increased salivation, dysphagia
GU: urinary frequency, increased libido
Hepatic: cholestatic jaundice
Metabolic: dehydration
Musculoskeletal: muscle cramps, arthritis, bone fractures
Respiratory: bronchitis, dyspnea
Skin: bruising, rash, urticaria, facial sweating, diaphoresis, pruritus, flushing
Other: toothache, weight loss, hot flashes, influenza, chills

Interactions
Drug-drug. *Antihypertensives, nitrates:* additive hypertension
CNS depressants (including antidepressants, antihistamines, opioids): additive CNS depression
Drugs that induce hypokalemia or hypomagnesemia (such as diuretics and laxatives and supraphysiologic use of steroid hormones with mineralocorticoid activity): possible precipitation, QT interval prolongation
Drugs that prolong QTc interval (such as antidepressants, class I or III antiarrhythmics, antimalarials, calcium channel blockers, some antihistamines, some neuroleptics): increased risk of conduction abnormalities
Drug-herbs. *Chamomile, hops, kava, skullcap, valerian:* increased CNS depression
Drug-behaviors. *Alcohol use:* additive CNS depression

Patient monitoring
◀€ Monitor QT interval; report prolongation. Also watch for torsades de pointes.
◀€ Know that drug may cause sudden death at high doses (above 25 mg) in patients at risk for arrhythmias.
◀€ Monitor for signs and symptoms of neuroleptic malignant syndrome, such as hyperthermia, severe extrapyramidal symptoms, altered mental status, stupor, coma, hypertension, tachycardia, pallor, or diaphoresis. (However, this syndrome is rare.)
- Assess vital signs frequently. Stay alert for orthostatic hypotension and tachycardia. Keep I.V. fluids and vasopressors on hand to treat pronounced hypotension.
◀€ Don't place hypotensive patient in Trendelenburg position because this may deepen anesthesia, precipitating respiratory arrest.
- Avoid abrupt position changes.
- Observe for signs and symptoms of respiratory compromise if drug is used concurrently with narcotics.

Patient teaching
- Advise patient not to drink alcohol or take CNS depressants for 24 hours after receiving drug.

- Tell patient drug may cause extreme drowsiness for several days after administration.
- Caution patient not to drive or perform other activities requiring mental alertness.
- Instruct patient to change positions slowly.
- As appropriate, review all other significant and life-threatening adverse reactions and interactions, especially those related to the drugs, herbs, and behaviors mentioned above.

duloxetine hydrochloride
Cymbalta, Yentreve✦

Pharmacologic class: Selective serotonin and norepinephrine reuptake inhibitor

Therapeutic class: Antidepressant

Pregnancy risk category C

FDA | BOXED WARNING

- Drug may increase risk of suicidal thinking and behavior in children, adolescents, and young adults with major depressive disorder and other psychiatric disorders, especially during first few months of therapy. Risk must be balanced with clinical need, as depression itself increases suicide risk. With patient of any age, observe closely for clinical worsening, suicidality, and unusual behavior changes when therapy begins. Advise family and caregivers to observe patient closely and communicate with prescriber as needed.
- Drug isn't approved for use in children.

Action
Unknown. May potentiate serotonergic and noradrenergic activity in CNS.

Availability
Capsules (delayed-release): 20 mg, 30 mg, 60 mg

⚡ Indications and dosages
➤ Major depressive disorder
Adults: 40 mg/day (20 mg b.i.d.) P.O. to 60 mg/day (once daily or as 30 mg b.i.d.) P.O. If needed, start at 30 mg P.O. once daily for 1 week so patient can adjust to drug before increasing to 60 mg/day. If dosage is increased above 60 mg/day, use increments of 30 mg/day. Some patients may require maintenance dosage of 60 mg once daily for several months or longer.
➤ Generalized anxiety disorder
Adults: For most patients, recommended starting dose is 60 mg P.O. once daily. If needed, start at 30 mg P.O. once daily for 1 week so patient can adjust to drug before increasing to 60 mg/day. If dosage is increased above 60 mg/day, use increments of 30 mg/day.
➤ Diabetic peripheral neuropathic pain
Adults: 60 mg P.O. once daily. For patients with unknown tolerance, consider starting at lower dosage.
➤ Fibromyalgia, chronic musculoskeletal pain
Adults: Initially, 30 mg P.O. daily for 1 week so patient can adjust to drug before increasing to 60 mg P.O. once daily. Some patients may respond to starting dosage. Base continued therapy on patient response.

Dosage adjustment
- Renal impairment

Contraindications
- MAO inhibitor use within past 14 days
- Uncontrolled narrow-angle glaucoma

Precautions
Use cautiously in:
- hepatic insufficiency, severe renal impairment, or chronic hepatic disease (use not recommended)

Reactions in **bold** are life-threatening. ◀€ Clinical alert

- hyponatremia, seizure disorder, controlled narrow-angle glaucoma, conditions that slow gastric emptying, urinary hesitancy and frequency
- history of mania
- concurrent use of potent CYP1A2 inhibitors (such as fluoroquinolones, thioridazine, or serotonin precursors) (avoid use)
- concurrent use of 5-hydroxytryptamine receptor agonist (triptan) or other CNS-acting drugs
- heavy alcohol use
- pregnant patients
- breastfeeding patients (use not recommended)
- children, adolescents, and young adults.

Administration

- Assess blood pressure before starting therapy.
- Give without regard to meals.
- Make sure patient swallows capsule whole without chewing or crushing it. Don't sprinkle contents onto food or mix with liquids.

🔊 Don't give within 14 days of MAO inhibitors; don't give MAO inhibitors within 5 days of duloxetine withdrawal.

Route	Onset	Peak	Duration
P.O.	Unknown	6 hr	Unknown

Adverse reactions

CNS: fatigue, somnolence, dizziness, asthenia, headache, agitation, abnormal dreams, tremor, insomnia, anxiety, worsening of depression, increased risk of suicide or suicidal ideation (especially in child or adolescent)
CV: orthostatic hypotension, syncope
EENT: blurred vision, mydriasis, nasopharyngitis, laryngopharyngeal pain
GI: nausea, vomiting, diarrhea, constipation, dyspepsia, dysgeusia, dry mouth
GU: abnormal orgasm, erectile or ejaculatory dysfunction, delayed ejaculation, decreased libido, frequent daytime urination
Hematologic: abnormal bleeding (ecchymoses, hematomas, epistaxis, petechiae, **life-threatening hemorrhage**)
Hepatic: hepatotoxicity
Musculoskeletal: muscle cramp, pain, and spasms
Respiratory: cough, upper respiratory tract infection
Skin: increased sweating, hot flashes, rash, pruritus
Other: pyrexia, seasonal allergy, yawning, decreased appetite, weight loss, **serotonin syndrome**

Interactions

Drug-drug. *Aspirin, NSAIDs, other drugs that affect coagulation:* increased risk of bleeding
Drugs metabolized by CYP2D6 (such as phenothiazines, tricyclic antidepressants, type 1C antiarrhythmics): increased blood levels of these drugs
Highly protein-bound drugs: increased free concentrations of these drugs, potentially causing adverse reactions
MAO inhibitors: serious and potentially fatal interactions
Potent CYP1A2 inhibitors (such as cimetidine, fluvoxamine, quinolone antibiotics), potent CYP2D6 inhibitors (such as fluoxetine, paroxetine, quinidine): increased duloxetine blood level
Serotonergic drugs (such as linezolid, lithium, tramadol, triptans): increased risk of serotonin syndrome
Thioridazine: increased risk of serious ventricular arrhythmias and sudden death
Warfarin: altered anticoagulant effect, including increased bleeding
Drug-diagnostic tests. *ALP, ALT, AST, creatine kinase:* increased levels
Sodium: decreased level
Drug-herbs. *St. John's wort:* increased risk of serotonin syndrome
Drug-behaviors. *Alcohol use:* increased risk of hepatic damage

Smoking: decreased duloxetine bioavailability

Patient monitoring

🔊 Monitor patient's mental status carefully. Stay alert for mood changes and signs of suicidal ideation, especially in child or adolescent.

• Monitor liver function test results and creatinine level for evidence of hepatic impairment.

🔊 Watch for potentially life-threatening serotonin syndrome, especially with concomitant use of serotonergic drugs (including triptans) or drugs that impair serotonin metabolism (including MAO inhibitors). Signs and symptoms may include mental status changes (agitation, hallucinations, coma), autonomic instability (tachycardia, labile blood pressure, hyperthermia), neuromuscular aberrations (hyperreflexia, incoordination) and GI upset (nausea, vomiting, diarrhea).

• Monitor blood pressure periodically during therapy.

• Watch for signs and symptoms of hyponatremia, such as headache, poor concentration, memory impairment, confusion, weakness, and unsteadiness. If these occur, consider discontinuing drug and provide treatment as appropriate.

• Know that in diabetic patients, small increases in fasting blood glucose, glycosylated hemoglobin, and total cholesterol levels may occur.

• If concurrent triptan use is warranted, observe patient closely, especially at start of therapy and during dosage increases.

• Carefully monitor patient receiving warfarin when duloxetine is begun or discontinued.

🔊 Don't stop drug abruptly. Taper dosage gradually.

Patient teaching

• Advise patient to take drug without regard to meals.

• Instruct patient to swallow capsules whole without chewing or crushing. Tell patient not to sprinkle contents onto food or mix with liquids.

🔊 Advise patient (and parent or significant other as appropriate) to monitor mental status carefully and immediately report increased depression or suicidal thoughts or behavior (especially in child or adolescent).

🔊 Instruct patient to report signs and symptoms of liver damage (unexplained flulike symptoms, itching, right upper abdominal tenderness, dark urine, or yellow skin).

🔊 Tell patient not to stop taking drug abruptly and that dosage will be tapered gradually when drug is discontinued.

• Caution patient to avoid driving and other hazardous activities until drug's effects on concentration and alertness are known.

• Advise patient to rise slowly from a sitting or lying position to avoid sudden blood pressure drop.

• Instruct patient to avoid heavy alcohol use during therapy because of increased risk of liver damage.

• Caution patient to avoid NSAIDs, aspirin, and other drugs that affect coagulation unless prescriber approves.

• Instruct patient not to use herbs, especially St. John's wort, without consulting prescriber.

• Tell female patient to notify prescriber if she is pregnant or breastfeeding or plans to become pregnant or to breastfeed.

• As appropriate, review all other significant and life-threatening adverse reactions and interactions, especially those related to the drugs, tests, herbs, and behaviors mentioned above.

Reactions in **bold** are life-threatening.   🔊 Clinical alert

dutasteride
Avodart

Pharmacologic class: Synthetic 4-azasteroid compound
Therapeutic class: 5-alpha-reductase inhibitor, sex hormone
Pregnancy risk category X

Action
Inhibits 5-alpha-reductase, an intracellular enzyme present in liver, skin, and prostate that's required for conversion of testosterone to 5-alpha-dihydrotestosterone (DHT). DHT appears to be the principal androgen responsible for stimulating prostatic growth.

Availability
Capsules: 0.5 mg

Indications and dosages
➤ Symptomatic benign prostatic hypertrophy (alone or in combination with tamsulosin)
Adults: 0.5 mg P.O. daily

Contraindications
• Hypersensitivity to drug, its components, other 5-alpha-reductase inhibitors, xanthines (such as coffee, theobromine), or ethylenediamine
• Women
• Children

Precautions
Use cautiously in:
• hepatic impairment.

Administration
• Don't handle drug if you're pregnant or plan to become pregnant.
• Don't open or crush capsule.
• Give without regard to food.

Route	Onset	Peak	Duration
P.O.	Rapid	2-3 hr	Unknown

Adverse reactions
GI: dyspepsia
GU: decreased libido, decreased ejaculatory volume, erectile dysfunction, gynecomastia

Interactions
Drug-drug. *Cimetidine, ciprofloxacin, diltiazem, ketoconazole, other drugs metabolized by CYP450-3A4 pathway, ritonavir, verapamil:* increased dutasteride blood level
Drug-diagnostic tests. *Prostate-specific antigen (PSA):* decreased level
Thyroid-stimulating hormone: increased level

Patient monitoring
• Monitor fluid intake and output. Assess for ease of starting urine stream and for urinary urgency or frequency.
• Check baseline PSA level; reevaluate at 3 to 6 months.

Patient teaching
• Tell patient to take drug with full glass of water without crushing or opening capsule.
• Instruct patient not to take capsule if it's cracked or leaking.
• Inform patient that drug decreases testosterone production in prostate.
• Tell patient to report dysuria and urinary urgency.
🔊 Advise patient not to donate blood for at least 6 months after final dose.
• Inform patient that drug may decrease ejaculatory volume.
• Explain that sexual side effects eventually will subside.
• As appropriate, review all other significant adverse reactions and interactions, especially those related to the drugs and tests mentioned above.

efavirenz
Sustiva

Pharmacologic class: Nonnucleoside reverse transcriptase inhibitor
Therapeutic class: Antiretroviral
Pregnancy risk category D

Action
Inhibits human immunodeficiency virus (HIV) reverse transcriptase (required for transcription of HIV-1 RNA to DNA), leading to viral cell death

Availability
Capsules: 50 mg, 200 mg
Tablets: 600 mg

🖉 Indications and dosages
➤ HIV infection (given with one or more additional antiretrovirals)
Adults and children older than age 3 and weighing more than 40 kg (88 lb): 600 mg P.O. once daily
Children weighing 32.5 to 40 kg (71.5 to 88 lb): 400 mg P.O. once daily
Children weighing 25 to 32.5 kg (55 to 71.5 lb): 350 mg P.O. once daily
Children weighing 20 to 25 kg (44 to 55 lb): 300 mg P.O. once daily
Children weighing 15 to 20 kg (33 to 44 lb): 250 mg P.O. once daily
Children weighing 10 to 15 kg (22 to 33 lb): 200 mg P.O. once daily

Dosage adjustment
• Concurrent use of rifampin or voriconazole

Contraindications
• Hypersensitivity to drug
• Concurrent use of astemizole, cisapride, midazolam, triazolam, ergot derivatives, voriconazole, or bepridil

Precautions
Use cautiously in:
• hypercholesterolemia, hepatic impairment, concurrent use of hepatotoxic drugs, mental illness, or substance abuse
• concurrent use of St. John's wort (use not recommended)
• pregnant or breastfeeding patients
• children.

Administration
• Give on empty stomach.
• Know that drug is given with other antiretrovirals.

Route	Onset	Peak	Duration
P.O.	Rapid	3-5 hr	24 hr

Adverse reactions
CNS: dizziness, drowsiness, fatigue, insomnia, abnormal dreams, hypoesthesia, depression, headache, poor concentration, nervousness, anxiety, CNS depression, **suicidal ideation**
CV: arrhythmias
GI: nausea, diarrhea, flatulence, abdominal pain, dyspepsia
GU: hematuria, renal calculi
Hepatic: hepatotoxicity
Respiratory: respiratory depression
Skin: rash, diaphoresis, pruritus, **erythema multiforme, toxic epidermal necrolysis, Stevens-Johnson syndrome**
Other: increased appetite

Interactions
Drug-drug. *Azole antifungals (ketoconazole, voriconazole):* decreased antifungal plasma concentration, increased efavirenz plasma concentration
Calcium channel blockers: possible decreased calcium channel blocker concentration

Clarithromycin, indinavir: reduced blood levels of these drugs

CNS depressants (including antidepressants, antihistamines, opioids): increased CNS depression

CYP450 inducers (including phenobarbital, rifabutin, rifampin): increased clearance and decreased blood level of efavirenz

CYP450 inhibitors, ergot alkaloids, estrogen, midazolam, ritonavir, triazolam: increased blood levels of these drugs, greater risk of serious adverse reactions (including arrhythmias, CNS and respiratory depression, and hepatotoxicity)

HMG-CoA reductase inhibitors: decreased plasma concentration of atorvastatin, pravastatin, and simvastatin

Hormonal contraceptives: increased ethinyl estradiol blood level

Protease inhibitors: decreased plasma level and efficacy of these drugs

Saquinavir: decreased saquinavir blood level

Warfarin: increased or decreased warfarin effects

Drug-diagnostic tests. *Alanine aminotransferase, aspartate aminotransferase, gamma-glutamyltransferase, total cholesterol, triglycerides:* increased levels

Urine cannabinoid test: false-positive result

Drug-food. *High-fat meal:* increased drug absorption

Drug-herbs. *St. John's wort:* decreased efavirenz blood level and efficacy, drug resistance

Drug-behaviors. *Alcohol use:* increased CNS depression

Patient monitoring

• Monitor dietary intake and hepatic and lipid profile.

• Closely monitor patients with hepatic failure.

◀€ Record mood changes and stay alert for suicidal ideation or behavior.

• Be aware that drug may cause hypercholesterolemia.

• Know that amount of HIV in blood may increase if patient stops drug therapy even briefly.

Patient teaching

• Instruct patient to take with full glass of water, preferably at bedtime to improve tolerance of CNS effects. Also tell him to avoid taking drug with high-fat meals.

• Inform patient that drug must be taken in combination with other antiretrovirals.

• Tell patient that drug doesn't cure HIV or AIDS and that he can still transmit virus to others.

◀€ Advise patient to report suicidal thoughts and other psychiatric symptoms.

• Caution patient to avoid driving and other hazardous activities until he knows how drug affects concentration and alertness.

◀€ Tell female patient to immediately inform prescriber if she becomes pregnant.

• Advise female patient to use adequate contraceptive measures for 12 weeks after discontinuing drug.

• As appropriate, review all other significant and life-threatening adverse reactions and interactions, especially those related to the drugs, tests, foods, herbs, and behaviors mentioned above.

eletriptan hydrobromide
Relpax

Pharmacologic class: 5-hydroxytryptamine-1 (5-HT$_1$) receptor agonist

Therapeutic class: Antimigraine agent

Pregnancy risk category C

Action

Binds with serotonin 5-HT$_{1B}$ receptors on intracranial blood vessels and serotonin 5-HT$_{1D}$ receptors on sensory nerve endings, constricting cranial arteries and thereby relieving migraine

Availability
Tablets: 20 mg, 40 mg

ⓘ Indications and dosages
➤ Migraine with or without aura
Adults: Initially, 20 to 40 mg P.O.; may repeat in 2 hours if headache returns after initial improvement. Maximum recommended single dosage is 40 mg.

Contraindications
- Hypersensitivity to drug
- Basilar and hemiplegic migraine
- Severe hepatic disease
- Ischemic heart disease
- Peripheral vascular disease
- Cerebrovascular syndromes
- Uncontrolled hypertension
- Ischemic bowel disease
- Within 24 hours of another serotonin agonist or ergot-type drug

Precautions
Use cautiously in:
- hepatic or renal impairment, diabetes mellitus, hypercholesterolemia, cardiac disorders
- pregnant or breastfeeding patients
- children.

Administration
- Give first dose as soon as migraine symptoms arise.
- ◀ᯤ Be aware that first dose should be given under close supervision to patients with coronary artery disease.
- If headache improves but then recurs, give second dose at least 2 hours after first.
- Be aware that drug's safety in treating an average of more than three headaches within a 30-day period has not been established.

Route	Onset	Peak	Duration
P.O.	2 hr	2-3 hr	Unknown

Adverse reactions
CNS: dizziness, insomnia, drowsiness, headache, fatigue, anxiety, paresthesia, asthenia, **cerebrovascular ischemia**
CV: chest pain, palpitations, hypertension, **cardiovascular ischemia**
GI: nausea, vomiting, diarrhea, dry mouth
Musculoskeletal: muscle weakness
Respiratory: chest tightness or pressure
Skin: flushing
Other: hot or cold sensation

Interactions
Drug-drug. *Antihistamines, ergotamine, ergot derivatives:* increased vasospastic effects
CYP450-3A4 inhibitors (such as clarithromycin, ketoconazole, propranolol): increased eletriptan blood level
MAO inhibitors: increased eletriptan effects

Patient monitoring
- Monitor vital signs and assess for chest pain, tightness, or pressure.

Patient teaching
- Instruct patient to take first dose as soon as migraine symptoms occur. If headache improves but then recurs, advise him to take second dose at least 2 hours after first.
- Caution patient to avoid driving and other hazardous activities until drug no longer affects concentration and alertness.
- Tell patient to report chest pain, pressure, or tightness.
- Inform patient that drug won't prevent migraines and isn't effective against other headache types.
- As appropriate, review all other significant and life-threatening adverse

---

Reactions in **bold** are life-threatening.   ◀ᯤ Clinical alert reactions and interactions, especially those related to the drugs mentioned above.

emtricitabine
Emtriva

Pharmacologic class: Nucleoside reverse transcriptase inhibitor
Therapeutic class: Antiretroviral
Pregnancy risk category B

FDA | BOXED WARNING

- Drug has caused lactic acidosis and severe hepatomegaly with steatosis (including fatal cases) when used alone or in combination with other antiretrovirals.
- Drug isn't indicated for chronic hepatitis B virus (HBV) infection. Safety and efficacy haven't been established in patients co-infected with HBV and human immunodeficiency virus (HIV). Discontinuation has led to severe acute HBV exacerbations. Monitor hepatic function closely.

Action
Inhibits activity of HIV-1 reverse transcriptase by competing with natural substrate and by its incorporation into nascent viral DNA, thereby halting viral replication

Availability
Capsules: 200 mg
Oral solution: 10 mg/ml in 170-ml bottles

🕖 Indications and dosages
➣ HIV-1 infection, with other antiretrovirals

Adults ages 18 and older: 200-mg capsule P.O. daily or 240 mg (24 ml) oral solution P.O. once daily
Children ages 3 months to 17 years weighing more than 33 kg (73 lb): 200-mg capsule P.O. once daily
Children ages 3 months to 17 years weighing less than 33 kg (73 lb): 6 mg/kg oral solution P.O. daily to maximum of 240 mg (24 ml) once daily
Children ages 0 to 3 months: 3 mg/kg oral solution P.O. once daily

Dosage adjustment
- Renal impairment

Contraindications
- Hypersensitivity to drug or its components

Precautions
Use cautiously in:
- renal impairment
- increased risk for lactic acidosis or hepatic impairment
- obese patients
- elderly patients
- children (safety and efficacy not established).

Administration
- Give with or without food.
- Know that drug must be given with other antiretrovirals.
- Know that capsule can be given to child weighing more than 33 kg if child can swallow an intact capsule.

Route	Onset	Peak	Duration
P.O.	Rapid	1-2 hr	Unknown

Adverse reactions
CNS: dizziness, headache, insomnia, abnormal dreams, depression, peripheral neuritis or neuropathy, paresthesia
EENT: rhinitis
GI: nausea, vomiting, diarrhea, abdominal pain, dyspepsia
Hepatic: hepatotoxicity

Metabolic: cushingoid appearance (buffalo hump, moon face), **lactic acidosis**
Musculoskeletal: joint pain, myalgia
Respiratory: increased cough
Skin: rash, skin discoloration (hyperpigmentation on palms and soles)
Other: body fat redistribution

Interactions
Drug-drug. *Tenofovir disoproxil fumarate:* increased emtricitabine effect
Drug-diagnostic tests. *Alanine aminotransferase, amylase, aspartate aminotransferase, bilirubin, creatine kinase, lipase, triglycerides:* increased levels
Glucose: increased or decreased level
Neutrophils: decreased count

Patient monitoring
◀€ Monitor closely (especially in females and obese patients) for signs and symptoms of lactic acidosis and hepatotoxicity, even if patient doesn't have marked transaminase elevations.
• Assess neurologic status, checking especially for depression, peripheral neuropathy, and paresthesia.
• Monitor neutrophil count, lipid panel, liver function tests, and blood glucose level.
◀€ Monitor patient closely for several months after drug withdrawal. Severe, acute exacerbations of hepatitis B virus (HBV) have been reported after discontinuation in patients co-infected with HBV and HIV.
• Monitor nutritional and hydration status in light of GI adverse effects and underlying disease.
• Watch for cushingoid appearance and body fat redistribution.

Patient teaching
• Tell patient to take a missed dose as soon as he remembers. However, if it's almost time for next dose, tell him to

skip the missed dose and take next dose as scheduled.
◀€ Instruct patient not to change dosage or stop taking drug unless prescriber approves.
• Tell patient drug should be taken only in combination with other drugs that treat HIV.
◀€ Instruct patient not to take this drug if already taking Altripla (combination of efavirenz, emtricitabine, and tenofovir), Combivir (combination of lamivudine and zidovudine), Epivir (lamivudine), Epzicom (combination of abacavir and lamivudine), Trizivir (combination of abacavir, lamivudine, and zidovidine), or Truvada (combination of emtricitabine and tenofovir), because these drugs contain the same or similar ingredients.
◀€ Tell patient to immediately report signs or symptoms of lactic acidosis—unusual tiredness or muscle pain, difficulty breathing, stomach pain with nausea and vomiting, coldness, dizziness or light-headedness, or fast or irregular heartbeat.
◀€ Instruct patient to immediately report signs or symptoms of liver problems—unusual tiredness, yellowing of skin or eyes, dark urine, lightcolored feces, appetite loss, nausea, or pain in lower abdominal area.
• Advise patient to report adverse CNS reactions and to use good judgment about driving and other hazardous activities.
• Caution patient that drug may cause depression. Tell him to notify prescriber if he develops symptoms.
• Inform patient that drug may cause body fat redistribution, dark areas on palms and soles, and rash.
• Tell female patient to inform prescriber if she is pregnant or plans to become pregnant.
• Caution HIV-positive patient not to breastfeed.
• As appropriate, review all other significant and life-threatening adverse

e

reactions and interactions, especially those related to the drugs and tests mentioned above.

enalapril maleate
Apo-Enalapril✱, CO Enalapril✱, Gen-Enalapril✱, Innovace⊕, Novo-Enalapril✱, PMS-Enalapril✱, Ratio-Enalapril✱, Riva-Enalapril✱, Sandoz-Enalapril✱, Taro-Enalapril✱, Vasotec

enalaprilat
Vasotec IV

Pharmacologic class: Angiotensin-converting enzyme (ACE) inhibitor

Therapeutic class: Antihypertensive

Pregnancy risk category C (first trimester), *D* (second and third trimesters)

FDA | BOXED WARNING

- When used during second or third trimester of pregnancy, drug can cause fetal injury and even death. Discontinue as soon as pregnancy is detected.

Action
Inhibits conversion of angiotensin I to angiotensin II, a potent vasoconstrictor; inactivates bradykinin and prostaglandins. Also increases plasma renin and potassium levels and reduces aldosterone levels, resulting in systemic vasodilation.

Availability
Injection: 1.25 mg/ml
Tablets: 2.5 mg, 5 mg, 10 mg, 20 mg

🕖 Indications and dosages
➤ Hypertension
Adults: For patients not taking concomitant diuretics—initially, 5 mg P.O. once daily, increased after 1 to 2 weeks as needed to a maintenance dosage of 10 to 40 mg P.O. daily given as a single dose or in two divided doses; or 1.25 mg I.V. q 6 hours. For patients taking diuretics—initially, 2.5 mg P.O. or 0.625 mg I.V.

Children: 0.08 mg/kg P.O. once daily; may be increased based on blood pressure response up to 5 mg daily. Maximum dosage is 0.58 mg/kg/dose.
➤ Heart failure
Adults: Initially, 2.5 mg P.O. once or twice daily, increased after 1 to 2 weeks as needed to maintenance dosage of 5 to 40 mg P.O. daily given as a single dose or in two divided doses
➤ Asymptomatic left ventricular dysfunction
Adults: Initially, 2.5 mg P.O. once or twice daily, increased after 1 to 2 weeks as needed to a maximum of 20 mg/day in divided doses

Dosage adjustment
- Renal impairment

Off-label uses
- Diabetic nephropathy
- Hypertensive emergency

Contraindications
- Hypersensitivity to drug or other ACE inhibitors
- Angioedema
- Pregnancy

Precautions
Use cautiously in:
- renal or hepatic impairment, hypovolemia, hyponatremia, aortic stenosis, hypertrophic cardiomyopathy, cerebrovascular or cardiac insufficiency
- concurrent diuretic use
- elderly patients
- breastfeeding patients
- children.

� Canada   ⊕ UK   ✿ Hazardous drug   ⊗ High-alert drug

Administration

- Give oral doses with food or beverage.
- Discontinue diuretics for 2 to 3 days before starting drug, if possible.
- Know that I.V. administration is usually reserved for patients who cannot take P.O. form.
- Be aware that I.V. administration isn't recommended for pediatric patients.
- Administer I.V. dose either undiluted or diluted in 50 ml of dextrose 5% in water, normal saline solution, dextrose 5% in normal saline solution, or dextrose 5% in lactated Ringer's solution.
- Give single I.V. dose by push or piggyback over 5 minutes. If patient is at risk for hypotension, infusion may be given over 1 hour.
- Be aware that black patients have a higher risk of angioedema.

Route	Onset	Peak	Duration
P.O.	1 hr	4-6 hr	24 hr
I.V.	15 min	3-4 hr	6 hr

Adverse reactions

CNS: dizziness, fatigue, headache, insomnia, drowsiness, vertigo, asthenia, paresthesia, ataxia, confusion, depression, nervousness, **cerebrovascular accident**

CV: orthostatic hypotension, palpitations, angina pectoris, tachycardia, peripheral edema, **arrhythmias, cardiac arrest**

EENT: sinusitis

GI: nausea, vomiting, constipation, dyspepsia, abdominal pain, dry mouth, **pancreatitis**

GU: proteinuria, urinary tract infection, erectile dysfunction, decreased libido, **oliguria**

Hematologic: agranulocytosis, bone marrow depression

Hepatic: hepatitis

Metabolic: hyponatremia, **hyperkalemia**

Respiratory: cough, upper respiratory tract infection, asthma, bronchitis, dyspnea, **eosinophilic pneumonitis**

Skin: rash, alopecia, photosensitivity, diaphoresis, exfoliative dermatitis, angioedema, **erythema multiforme**

Other: altered taste, fever, increased appetite, anaphylactoid reactions

Interactions

Drug-drug. *Allopurinol:* increased risk of hypersensitivity reaction

Antacids: decreased enalapril absorption

Cyclosporine, indomethacin, potassium-sparing diuretics, potassium supplements: hyperkalemia

Digoxin, lithium: increased blood levels of these drugs, possible toxicity

Diuretics, nitrates, other antihypertensives, phenothiazines: additive hypotension

Nonsteroidal anti-inflammatory drugs: decreased antihypertensive response

Rifampin: decreased enalapril efficacy

Drug-diagnostic tests. *Alanine aminotransferase, alkaline phosphatase, aspartate aminotransferase, bilirubin, blood urea nitrogen (BUN), creatinine, potassium:* increased levels

Antinuclear antibodies: positive titer

Sodium: decreased level

Drug-food. *Salt substitutes containing potassium:* hyperkalemia

Drug-herbs. *Capsaicin:* increased incidence of cough

Drug-behaviors. *Acute alcohol ingestion:* additive hypotension

Sun exposure: photosensitivity reaction

Patient monitoring

◀€ Assess for rapid blood pressure drop leading to cardiovascular collapse, especially when giving with diuretics.

◀€ In patient with renal insufficiency or renal artery stenosis, monitor for worsening renal function.

- After initial dose, observe patient closely for at least 2 hours until blood pressure has stabilized. Then continue to observe for additional hour.

Reactions in **bold** are life-threatening.   ◀€ Clinical alert

- Monitor vital signs, fluid intake and output, and daily weight.
- Supervise patient during ambulation until effects of drug are known.
- Monitor liver function tests, BUN, and creatinine and electrolyte levels.

Patient teaching
- Inform patient that drug's full effect may not occur for several weeks.
- Advise patient to report persistent dry cough with nasal congestion.
- 📢 Tell patient to immediately report swelling of face, eye area, tongue, lips, hands, or feet; rash, hives, or severe itching; unexplained fever; unusual tiredness; yellowing of skin or eyes; abdominal pain; or easy bruising.
- Instruct patient to move slowly when sitting up or standing, to avoid dizziness or light-headedness from sudden blood pressure decrease.
- As appropriate, review all other significant and life-threatening adverse reactions and interactions, especially those related to the drugs, tests, foods, herbs, and behaviors mentioned above.

enfuvirtide
Fuzeon

Pharmacologic class: Human immunodeficiency-1 (HIV-1) fusion inhibitor
Therapeutic class: Antiretroviral
Pregnancy risk category B

Action
Interferes with entry of HIV-1 into cells by inhibiting fusion of viral and cellular membranes

Availability
Powder for injection: 90 mg/1-ml vial

⚡ Indications and dosages
➢ HIV-1 infection in adults in combination with other antiretrovirals
Adults: 90 mg subcutaneously b.i.d. in upper arm, anterior thigh, or abdomen
Children ages 6 to 16: 2 mg/kg subcutaneously b.i.d. in upper arm, anterior thigh, or abdomen. Maximum dosage is 90 mg b.i.d.

Contraindications
- Hypersensitivity to drug or its components

Precautions
Use cautiously in:
- increased risk of pneumonia
- injection site reaction
- concurrent use of anticoagulants
- hemophilia or other coagulant disorders
- elderly patients
- children younger than age 6 (safety and efficacy not established).

Administration
- Rotate injection sites.
- Be aware that preferred injection sites are upper arm, anterior thigh, and abdomen.
- Reconstitute with 1.1 ml of sterile water for injection, and gently tap vial for 10 seconds. Then gently roll vial between hands or allow vial to stand until product dissolves completely (could take up to 45 minutes).
- Know that drug is usually given with other antiretrovirals.
- Use reconstituted solution immediately.

Route	Onset	Peak	Duration
Subcut.	Unknown	4 hr	Unknown

Adverse reactions
CNS: fatigue, asthenia, insomnia, depression, anxiety, peripheral neuropathy
EENT: conjunctivitis, sinusitis
GI: nausea, diarrhea, upper abdominal pain, dry mouth, anorexia, pancreatitis
Hematologic: lymphadenopathy

Musculoskeletal: limb pain, myalgia
Respiratory: cough, pneumonia
Skin: folliculitis
Other: taste disturbance, decreased appetite, weight loss, herpes simplex infection, injection site reactions (erythema, induration, nodules, cysts, mild to moderate pain, infection), flulike illness, hypersensitivity reactions

Interactions

Drug-diagnostic tests. *Alanine aminotransferase, amylase, aspartate aminotransferase, creatine kinase, eosinophils, gamma-glutamyltransferase, lipase, triglycerides:* increased levels
Hemoglobin: decreased level

Patient monitoring

• Inspect injection sites frequently for adverse reactions.
• Monitor CBC with white cell differential, lipid panel, liver function test results, and gastric enzymes levels.
• Watch for hypersensitivity reactions.
• Monitor nutritional and hydration status in light of GI adverse effects and underlying disease.

Patient teaching

• Teach patient (or caregiver) how to reconstitute and self-administer drug, as appropriate.
◀€ Instruct patient not to change dosage or stop taking drug unless prescriber approves.
◀€ Tell patient to immediately report signs or symptoms of hypersensitivity reaction (such as rash, fever, nausea and vomiting, and chills).
• Teach patient how to recognize signs and symptoms of injection site reaction. Tell him to contact prescriber if these occur, especially if they last more than 7 days.
• Advise female patient to notify prescriber if she is pregnant or plans to become pregnant.
• Tell HIV-infected patient not to breastfeed.

• If patient misses a dose, instruct him to take it as soon as he remembers. However, if it's almost time for next dose, tell him to skip the missed dose and take next dose on schedule.
• As appropriate, review all other significant adverse reactions and interactions, especially those related to the tests mentioned above.

enoxaparin sodium
Clexane ⊕, Lovenox

Pharmacologic class: Low-molecular-weight heparin
Therapeutic class: Anticoagulant
Pregnancy risk category B

FDA BOXED WARNING

• During epidural or spinal anesthesia or puncture, patients receiving drug or scheduled to receive it for thromboprophylaxis are at risk for epidural or spinal hematoma, which can lead to long-term or permanent paralysis. Risk increases with use of indwelling epidural catheter for analgesia administration and with concurrent use of drugs affecting hemostasis (such as nonsteroidal anti-inflammatory drugs [NSAIDs], platelet inhibitors, and other anticoagulants). Risk also rises with traumatic or repeated epidural or spinal puncture or history of spinal deformity or spinal surgery. Before neuraxial intervention, physician should weigh drug's potential benefit against risk.
• Monitor patient frequently for signs and symptoms of neurologic impairment. If these occur, provide urgent treatment.

◀€ Clinical alert

Action

Inhibits thrombus and clot formation by blocking factor Xa and factor IIa. This inhibition accelerates formation of antithrombin III-thrombin complex (a coagulation inhibitor), thereby deactivating thrombin and preventing conversion of fibrinogen to fibrin.

Availability

Solution for injection: 30 mg/0.3 ml, 40 mg/0.4 ml, 60 mg/0.6 ml, 80 mg/0.8 ml, 120 mg/0.8 ml, 100 mg/1 ml, 150 mg/1 ml (all in prefilled syringes); 300 mg/3 ml (in multidose vials)

✱ Indications and dosages

➤ Patients at risk for thromboembolic complications due to severely restricted mobility during acute illness
Adults: 40 mg subcutaneously daily for up to 14 days
➤ Prevention of pulmonary embolism and deep-vein thrombosis (DVT) after abdominal surgery
Adults: 40 mg subcutaneously 2 hours before surgery, repeated 24 hours after initial dose (provided hemostasis has been established) and continued once daily for 7 to 10 days until risk of DVT has diminished
➤ Prevention of pulmonary embolism and DVT after hip or knee replacement surgery
Adults: 30 mg subcutaneously 12 to 24 hours after surgery (provided hemostasis has been established), repeated q 12 hours for 7 to 10 days until risk of DVT has diminished. Alternatively, hip-replacement patient may receive 40 mg subcutaneously 12 hours before surgery and then once daily for 3 weeks, for a total of 4 weeks of therapy.
➤ Prevention of ischemic complications of unstable angina or non-Q-wave myocardial infarction
Adults: 1 mg/kg subcutaneously q 12 hours, given with aspirin 100 to 325 mg P.O. once daily until patient is clinically stable
➤ Hospitalized patients with acute DVT with or without pulmonary embolism (PE) (given with warfarin sodium)
Adults: 1 mg/kg subcutaneously q 12 hours or 1.5 mg/kg subcutaneously once daily for 5 to 7 days until therapeutic effect is established. Warfarin therapy usually begins within 72 hours of enoxaparin injection.
➤ Outpatients with acute DVT without PE (given with warfarin sodium)
Adults: 1 mg/kg subcutaneously q 12 hours for 5 to 7 days until therapeutic effect is established. Warfarin therapy usually begins within 72 hours of enoxaparin injection.

Dosage adjustment

• Patients weighing less than 45 kg (99 lb)
• Creatinine clearance below 30 ml/minute

Off-label uses

• Prevention of clots associated with hemodialysis
• Prevention of thrombosis during pregnancy

Contraindications

• Hypersensitivity to drug, heparin, sulfites, benzyl alcohol, or pork products
• Thrombocytopenia
• Active major bleeding

Precautions

Use cautiously in:
• severe hepatic or renal disease, retinopathy (hypertensive or diabetic), uncontrolled hypertension, hemorrhagic stroke, bacterial endocarditis, GI bleeding or other bleeding disorders
• recent history of ulcer disease, history of congenital or acquired bleeding disorder, history of thrombocytopenia related to heparin use
• recent CNS surgery

- pregnant or breastfeeding patients
- children.

Administration

🔊 Be aware that enoxaparin is a high-alert drug.
- Use tuberculin syringe with multidose vial to ensure accurate dosage.
- Don't expel air bubble from syringe before administering.
- Inject drug deep subcutaneously with patient in supine position. Alternate left and right anterolateral and posterolateral abdominal wall sites.
- Don't rub injection site.

🔊 Don't give by I.M. or I.V. route.

Route	Onset	Peak	Duration
Subcut.	Unknown	3-5 hr	24 hr

Adverse reactions

CNS: dizziness, headache, insomnia, confusion, **cerebrovascular accident**
CV: edema, chest pain, **atrial fibrillation, heart failure**
GI: nausea, vomiting, constipation
GU: urinary retention
Hematologic: anemia, **bleeding tendency, thrombocytopenia, hemorrhage**
Metabolic: hyperkalemia
Skin: bruising, pruritus, rash, urticaria
Other: fever; pain, irritation, or erythema at injection site

Interactions

Drug-drug. *Warfarin, other drugs that affect platelet function (including abciximab, aspirin, clopidogrel, dextran, dipyridamole, eptifibatide, NSAIDs, some penicillins, ticlopidine, tirofiban):* increased risk of bleeding
Drug-diagnostic tests. *Hepatic enzymes:* reversible increases
Hemoglobin, platelets: decreased levels
Drug-herbs. *Anise, arnica, chamomile, clove, feverfew, garlic, ginger, ginkgo, ginseng:* increased risk of bleeding

Patient monitoring

- Monitor CBC and platelet counts. Watch for signs and symptoms of bleeding or bruising.
- Monitor fluid intake and output. Watch for fluid retention and edema.

Patient teaching

- If patient will self-administer drug, teach proper injection technique.

🔊 Instruct patient to promptly report irregular heart beat, unusual bleeding or bruising, rash, or hives.
- Teach patient safety measures to avoid bruising or bleeding.
- Advise patient to weigh himself regularly and to report gains.
- Instruct patient to inform dentists and other health care professionals about enoxaparin use.
- As appropriate, review all other significant and life-threatening adverse reactions and interactions, especially those related to the drugs, tests, and herbs mentioned above.

entacapone
Comtan, Comtess ⊕

Pharmacologic class: Catechol O-methyltransferase (COMT) inhibitor
Therapeutic class: Antidyskinetic
Pregnancy risk category C

Action

Inhibits COMT, the primary enzyme involved in metabolizing levodopa. This inhibition increases levodopa blood level and duration of action, easing symptoms of Parkinson's disease.

Availability

Tablets: 200 mg

Indications and dosages

➤ Adjunctive treatment of idiopathic Parkinson's disease in patients experiencing wearing off of carbidopa-levodopa effects

Adults: 200 mg P.O. with each carbidopa-levodopa dose, to a maximum of eight times daily (1,600 mg)

Contraindications

• Hypersensitivity to drug

Precautions

Use cautiously in:
• hepatic or renal dysfunction, hypertension, heart disease
• pregnant and breastfeeding patients.

Administration

• Give without regard to food.
• Administer at same time as carbidopa-levodopa. Make sure patient swallows tablet whole.

◀€ Don't withdraw drug abruptly.

Route	Onset	Peak	Duration
P.O.	Variable	1 hr	Unknown

Adverse reactions

CNS: dizziness, depression, drowsiness, disorientation, memory loss, agitation, delusions, hallucinations, paranoia, euphoria, dyskinesia, hyperkinesia, light-headedness, paresthesia, heaviness of limbs, numbness of fingers

CV: tachycardia, orthostatic hypotension, hypertension

GI: nausea, vomiting, epigastric pain, flatulence

GU: urine discoloration

Respiratory: upper respiratory tract infection, dyspnea, sinus congestion

Other: fever

Interactions

Drug-drug. *Ampicillin, chloramphenicol, cholestyramine, erythromycin, probenecid, rifampin:* decreased entacapone excretion

Bitolterol, dobutamine, dopamine, epinephrine, isoetherine, isoproterenol, methyldopa, norepinephrine: increased heart rate, increased risk of arrhythmias, excessive blood pressure changes

MAO inhibitors: increased risk of toxicity

Drug-behaviors. *Alcohol use:* increased risk of adverse reactions

Patient monitoring

• Monitor vital signs, watching especially for orthostatic hypotension.
• Evaluate neurologic status closely. Check for hallucinations and new onset or exacerbation of dyskinesia.
• Assess respiratory status, particularly for dyspnea and signs and symptoms of upper respiratory tract infection.
• Monitor nutritional and hydration status if patient experiences vomiting.

Patient teaching

• Instruct patient to swallow tablet whole and to take it at same time as carbidopa-levodopa.

◀€ Caution patient not to stop taking drug abruptly.

• Advise patient to move slowly when sitting up or standing, to avoid dizziness or light-headedness from sudden blood pressure decrease.
• Caution patient to avoid driving and other hazardous activities until drug no longer affects concentration and alertness.

◀€ Instruct patient (and caregiver) to institute safety measures at home to prevent injury related to disease or drug's adverse CNS effects.

• As appropriate, review all other significant adverse reactions and interactions, especially those related to the drugs and behaviors mentioned above.

♣ Canada   ⊕ UK   ❧ Hazardous drug   ⊗ High-alert drug

entecavir
Baraclude

Pharmacologic class: Guanosine nucleoside analogue
Therapeutic class: Antiviral
Pregnancy risk category C

FDA | BOXED WARNING

- Drug may cause lactic acidosis and severe hepatomegaly with steatosis (including fatal cases) when used alone or in combination with antiretrovirals.
- Severe acute hepatitis B exacerbations have occurred in patients who discontinued anti-hepatitis B therapy, including entecavir. Monitor hepatic function for at least several months after discontinuation. If appropriate, initiate anti-hepatitis B therapy.
- When used to treat chronic hepatitis B, drug may cause human immunodeficiency virus (HIV) resistance to HIV nucleoside reverse transcriptase inhibitors in patients with untreated HIV infection. Therapy isn't recommended for HIV/hepatitis B virus (HBV) co-infected patients except those also receiving highly active antiretroviral therapy.

Action
Competes with natural substrate deoxyguanosine triphosphate to inhibit HBV polymerase (reverse transcriptase)

Availability
Oral solution: 0.05 mg/ml
Tablets: 0.5 mg, 1 mg

⃠ Indications and dosages
➤ Chronic HBV infection with evidence of active viral replication and either persistent serum transaminase elevations or histologically active disease

Adolescents and adults ages 16 and older: In nucleoside-treatment-naïve patients with compensated liver disease, 0.5 mg P. O. once daily. In patients with a history of hepatitis B viremia while receiving lamivudine or known lamivudine or telbivudine resistance mutations rtM204I/V with or without rtL180M, rtL80I/V, or rtV173L, or patients with decompensated liver disease, 1 mg P.O. once daily.

Dosage adjustment
- Creatinine clearance below 50 ml/minute

Contraindications
- Hypersensitivity to drug or its components

Precautions
Use cautiously in:
- liver transplant recipients who are receiving or have received immunosuppressants that may affect renal function
- elderly patients
- pregnant or breastfeeding patients
- children younger than age 16.

Administration
- Administer at least 2 hours before or after a meal.

Route	Onset	Peak	Duration
P.O.	Unknown	0.5-1.5 hr	Unknown

Adverse reactions
CNS: headache, dizziness, fatigue
GI: nausea, diarrhea, dyspepsia, increased GI enzymes
Hematologic: hematuria
Hepatic: HBV exacerbation, **severe hepatomegaly**
Metabolic: glycosuria, **lactic acidosis**

Interactions
Drug-drug. *Drugs that reduce renal function or compete for active tubular secretion:* increased blood levels of either drug
Drug-diagnostic tests. *Alanine aminotransferase, amylase, aspartate*

Reactions in **bold** are life-threatening.   ◀ Clinical alert

aminotransferase, lipase, glucose, serum creatinine, total bilirubin: increased

Patient monitoring
• Monitor renal function before and during therapy, especially in liver transplant recipients who are receiving or have received immunosuppressants that may affect renal function.

◀£ Monitor liver function closely for evidence of HBV exacerbation for at least several months after drug discontinuation.

◀£ Monitor for lactic acidosis (associated with nucleoside analogues).

Patient teaching
• Instruct patient to take drug on empty stomach (at least 2 hours before or after a meal).

◀£ Teach patient about signs and symptoms of lactic acidosis and importance of contacting prescriber if these occur.

◀£ Instruct patient to immediately report worsening symptoms, such as increased yellowing of skin or eyes, dark urine, or fatigue.

• As appropriate, review all other significant and life-threatening adverse reactions and interactions, especially those related to the drugs and tests mentioned above.

⊗

epinephrine
Twinject

epinephrine hydrochloride
Adrenalin Chloride♣, Anapen⊕, Epi-E-Z Pen♣, EpiPen, EpiPen Jr.

Pharmacologic class: Sympathomimetic (direct acting)

Therapeutic class: Bronchodilator, mydriatic

Pregnancy risk category C

Action
Stimulates alpha- and beta-adrenergic receptors, causing relaxation of cardiac and bronchial smooth muscle and dilation of skeletal muscles. Also decreases aqueous humor production, increases aqueous outflow, and dilates pupils by contracting dilator muscle.

Availability
Auto-injector for I.M. injection: 1:2,000 (0.5 mg/ml)
Injection: 0.1 mg/ml, 0.5 mg/ml, 1 mg/ml
Ophthalmic drops: 0.5%, 1%, 2%
Solution for inhalation (as racepinephrine): 2.5% (equivalent to 1% epinephrine)

Indications and dosages
➤ Bronchodilation; anaphylaxis; hypersensitivity reaction
Adults: 0.1 to 0.5 ml of 1:1,000 solution subcutaneously or I.M., repeated q 10 to 15 minutes p.r.n. Or 0.1 to 0.25 ml of 1:10,000 solution I.V. slowly over 5 to 10 minutes; may repeat q 5 to 15 minutes p.r.n. or follow with a continuous infusion of 1 mcg/minute, increased to 4 mcg/minute p.r.n. For emergency treatment, EpiPen delivers 0.3 mg I.M. of 1:1,000 epinephrine.
Children: For emergency treatment, EpiPen Jr. delivers 0.15 mg I.M. of 1:2,000 epinephrine.
➤ Acute asthma attack
Adults and children ages 4 and older: One to three deep inhalations of inhalation solution with hand-held nebulizer, repeated q 3 hours p.r.n.
➤ To restore cardiac rhythm in cardiac arrest
Adults: 0.5 to 1 mg I.V., repeated q 3 to 5 minutes, if needed. If no response, may give 3 to 5 mg I.V. q 3 to 5 minutes.
➤ Chronic simple glaucoma
Adults: One drop in affected eye once or twice daily. Adjust dosage to meet patient's needs.

➤ To prolong local anesthetic effects
Adults and children: 1:200,000 concentration with local anesthetic

Contraindications
• Hypersensitivity to drug, its components, or sulfites
• Angle-closure glaucoma
• Cardiac dilatation, cardiac insufficiency
• Cerebral arteriosclerosis, organic brain syndrome
• Shock with use of general anesthetics and halogenated hydrocarbons or cyclosporine
• MAO inhibitor use within past 14 days
• Labor
• Breastfeeding

Precautions
Use cautiously in:
• hypertension, hyperthyroidism, diabetes, prostatic hypertrophy
• elderly patients
• pregnant patients
• children.

Administration
• In anaphylaxis, use I.M. route, not subcutaneous route, if possible.
◀𝄞 Inject EpiPen and EpiPen Jr. only into anterolateral aspect of thigh. Don't inject into buttocks or give I.V.
◀𝄞 Be aware that not all epinephrine solutions can be given I.V. Check manufacturer's label.
• For I.V. injection, give each 1-mg dose over at least 1 minute. For continuous infusion, use rate of 1 to 10 mcg/minute, adjusting to desired response.
• Use Epi-Pen Jr. for patients weighing less than 30 kg (66 lb).
◀𝄞 Don't give within 14 days of MAO inhibitors.

Route	Onset	Peak	Duration
I.V.	Immediate	5 min	Short
I.M.	Variable	Unknown	1-4 hr
Subcut.	5-15 min	0.5 hr	1-4 hr
Inhalation solution	Unknown	Unknown	Unknown

Adverse reactions
CNS: nervousness, anxiety, tremor, vertigo, headache, disorientation, agitation, drowsiness, fear, dizziness, asthenia, **cerebral hemorrhage, cerebrovascular accident (CVA)**
CV: palpitations, widened pulse pressure, hypertension, tachycardia, angina, ECG changes, **ventricular fibrillation, shock**
GI: nausea, vomiting
GU: decreased urinary output, urinary retention, dysuria
Respiratory: dyspnea, **pulmonary edema**
Skin: urticaria, pallor, diaphoresis, necrosis
Other: hemorrhage at injection site

Interactions
Drug-drug. *Alpha-adrenergic blockers:* hypotension from unopposed beta-adrenergic effects
Antihistamines, thyroid hormone, tricyclic antidepressants: severe sympathomimetic effects
Beta-adrenergic blockers (such as propranolol): vasodilation and reflex tachycardia
Cardiac glycosides, general anesthetics: increased risk of ventricular arrhythmias
Diuretics: decreased vascular response
Doxapram, mazindol, methylphenidate: enhanced CNS stimulation or pressor effects
Ergot alkaloids: decreased vasoconstriction
Guanadrel, guanethidine: enhanced pressor effects of epinephrine
Levodopa: increased risk of arrhythmias
Levothyroxine: potentiation of epinephrine effects
MAO inhibitors: increased risk of hypertensive crisis
Drug-diagnostic tests. *Glucose:* transient elevation
Lactic acid: elevated level (with prolonged use)

e

Reactions in **bold** are life-threatening.   ◀𝄞 Clinical alert

Patient monitoring

◀€ Monitor vital signs, ECG, and cardiovascular and respiratory status. Watch for ventricular fibrillation, tachycardia, arrhythmias, and signs and symptoms of shock. Ask patient about anginal pain.

• Assess drug's effect on underlying problem (such as anaphylaxis or asthma attack), and repeat dose as needed.

◀€ Monitor neurologic status, particularly for decreased level of consciousness and other signs and symptoms of cerebral hemorrhage or CVA.

• Monitor fluid intake and output, watching for urinary retention or decreased urinary output.

• Inspect injection site for hemorrhage or skin necrosis.

Patient teaching

• Teach patient who uses auto-injector how to use syringe correctly, when to inject drug, and when to repeat doses.

• Teach patient who uses hand-held nebulizer correct use of equipment and drug. Explain indications for both initial dose and repeat doses.

◀€ Inform patient that drug may cause serious adverse effects. Tell him which symptoms to report.

• If patient will self-administer drug outside of health care setting, explain need for prompt evaluation by a health care provider to ensure that underlying disorder has been corrected.

• As appropriate, review all other significant and life-threatening adverse reactions and interactions, especially those related to the drugs and tests mentioned above.

epirubicin hydrochloride
Ellence, Pharmorubicin PMS✤

Pharmacologic class: Anthracycline
Therapeutic class: Antibiotic antineoplastic
Pregnancy risk category D

FDA BOXED WARNING

• Extravasation during administration causes severe local tissue necrosis; don't give epirubicin hydrochloride by I.M. or subcutaneous route.

• Cardiac toxicity, including fatal congestive heart failure (CHF), may occur either during therapy or months to years after therapy ends. Probability of developing clinically evident CHF is estimated as approximately 0.9% at a cumulative dose of 550 mg/m², 1.6% at 700 mg/m², and 3.3% at 900 mg/m². In adjuvant treatment of breast cancer, maximum cumulative dose used in clinical trials was 720 mg/m². Risk of developing CHF increases rapidly with increasing total cumulative doses above 900 mg/m²; exceed this cumulative dose only with extreme caution. Active or dormant cardiovascular disease, previous or concurrent radiotherapy to mediastinal or pericardial area, previous anthracycline or anthracenedione therapy, or concurrent use of other cardiotoxic drugs may increase cardiac toxicity risk. Toxicity may occur at lower cumulative doses even if patient has no cardiac risk factors.

• Secondary acute myelogenous leukemia (AML) has been reported in breast cancer patients who have been treated with anthracyclines, including epirubicin. Refractory secondary leukemia is more common when such drugs are given in combination with

DNA-damaging antineoplastics, when patients have been heavily pretreated with cytotoxic drugs, or when epirubicin dosage has been escalated. Cumulative risk of developing treatment-related AML or myelodysplastic syndrome (MDS), in 7,110 patients with breast cancer who received adjuvant treatment with epirubicin-containing regimens, was estimated as 0.27% at 3 years, 0.46% at 5 years, and 0.55% at 8 years.

• Reduce dosage in patients with hepatic impairment.

• Drug may cause severe myelosuppression.

• Give under supervision of physician experienced in cancer chemotherapy.

Action

Unknown. Forms complex with DNA by intercalation with nucleotide base pairs, causing inhibition of DNA, RNA, and protein synthesis.

Availability

Injection: 2 mg/ml, in 5 ml-, 25 ml-, 75 ml-, and 100-ml vials

Powder for injection (lyophilized): 50-mg single-dose vial

⚕ Indications and dosages

➤ Adjunctive therapy in patients with axillary-node tumor involvement after resection of primary breast cancer

Adults: 100 to 120 mg/m^2 by I.V. infusion over 3 to 5 minutes on first day of each cycle or divided equally in two doses on days 1 and 8 of each cycle; repeat cycle q 3 to 4 weeks for six cycles in conjunction with cyclophosphamide and fluorouracil.

Dosage adjustment

• Hepatic and severe renal impairment

• Hematologic or Grade 3 or 4 non-hematologic toxicity and neutropenic fever

Off-label uses

• Cancer of bladder, lung, nasopharynx, endometrium, and ovaries

Contraindications

• Hypersensitivity to drug, other anthracyclines, or anthracenediones

• Severe myocardial insufficiency, recent myocardial infarction, severe arrhythmias

• Severe hepatic dysfunction

• Baseline neutrophil count below 1,500/mm^3

• Previous treatment with anthracyclines up to the maximum cumulative doses

Precautions

Use cautiously in:

• heart disease, hepatic, or renal disease

• previous or recent radiation therapy

• hyperuricemia

• concurrent use of cimetidine, other cardiotoxic drugs, or live or live-attenuated vaccines

• elderly patients (female patients age 70 and older)

• pregnant or breastfeeding patients

• children.

Administration

• Be aware that drug may be given with antibiotics.

• Know that previous anthracycline use must be considered when determining dosage because of increased risk of heart failure.

• Follow facility policy for administration and disposal of carcinogenic drugs.

• Assess blood counts, including absolute neutrophil count, serum creatinine, and liver function before and during each cycle of therapy.

• Consider prophylactic use of antiemetics before administration,

e

Reactions in **bold** are life-threatening.   ◀€ Clinical alert

particularly when given in conjunction with other emetogenic drugs.

◀€ Avoid extravasation. If patient complains of burning or stinging, switch infusion to a different vein.

• Administer premixed solution over 3 to 5 minutes into tubing of free-flowing I.V. line containing dextrose 5% in water or normal saline solution. Don't mix with other drugs in same syringe.

• Direct I.V. push is not recommended because of extravasation risk.

• If patient develops facial flushing or red streak in the vein being infused, slow infusion rate.

• Be aware that refrigerated storage of solution for injection can result in formation of a gelled product. Gelled product will return to a slightly viscous to mobile solution after 2- to a maximum of 4-hour equilibration at controlled room temperature (15° to 25° C [59° to 77° F]).

Route	Onset	Peak	Duration
I.V.	Unknown	Unknown	Unknown

Adverse reactions

CNS: lethargy
CV: cardiomyopathy, cardiotoxicity, heart failure
EENT: conjunctivitis, keratitis
GI: nausea, vomiting, diarrhea, mucositis
GU: reddish urine, amenorrhea
Hematologic: anemia, **leukopenia, neutropenia, thrombocytopenia secondary acute myelogenous leukemia, thrombophlebitis, thromboembolic phenomena**
Metabolic: hyperuricemia
Respiratory: pulmonary embolism
Skin: alopecia; rash; pruritus; darkening of soles, palms, or nails
Other: increased appetite, infection, fever, hot flashes, tissue necrosis, **injection-related reactions, tumor lysis syndrome**

Interactions

Drug-drug. *Cardioactive compounds that could cause heart failure (such as calcium channel blockers):* increased risk of heart failure
Cimetidine: increased epirubicin blood level
Live or live-attenuated vaccines: increased risk of serious or fatal infection
Trastuzumab, other cardiotoxic drugs: increased risk of cardiotoxicity
Drug-diagnostic tests. *Hemoglobin, neutrophils, platelets, white blood cells:* decreased values

Patient monitoring

◀€ Monitor vital signs, left ventricular ejection fraction, and cardiovascular status carefully. Watch for signs and symptoms of cardiomyopathy and heart failure.

• Assess nutritional status and hydration in light of GI adverse effects.

◀€ Monitor CBC with white cell differential and watch for signs and symptoms of blood dyscrasias.

• Check temperature. Stay alert for fever and other signs or symptoms of infection.

◀€ Consider the possibility of tumor lysis syndrome in potentially susceptible patients and monitor serum uric acid, potassium, calcium, phosphate, and creatinine levels immediately after initial chemotherapy. Be aware that hydration, urine alkalinization, and prophylaxis with allopurinol to prevent hyperuricemia may minimize potential complications of tumor lysis syndrome.

• Continue to monitor serum total bilirubin, AST, and serum creatinine levels during treatment.

Patient teaching

• Inform patient that drug may cause tissue damage at injection site. Tell him to report pain, burning, or swelling.

◀◤ Instruct patient to immediately report sudden weight gain, swelling, or shortness of breath.

◀◤ Tell patient to promptly report unusual bruising or bleeding, fever, or signs and symptoms of infection or tumor lysis syndrome.

• Advise patient to avoid receiving live vaccines while taking this drug.

• Explain that drug will cause hair loss but that hair should grow back within a few months after therapy.

• Advise female patient that drug may cause premature menopause or permanent cessation of menses.

• As appropriate, review all other significant and life-threatening adverse reactions and interactions, especially those related to the drugs and tests mentioned above.

eplerenone
Inspra

Pharmacologic class: Aldosterone receptor blocker
Therapeutic class: Antihypertensive
Pregnancy risk category B

Action
Binds to and blocks aldosterone receptors, disrupting normal sodium and water reabsorption and causing sodium and water excretion to increase. These actions reduce blood volume and blood pressure.

Availability
Tablets: 25 mg, 50 mg

⊘ Indications and dosages
➤ Hypertension
Adults: 50 mg/day P.O. as a single dose. After 4-week trial, may increase to 50 mg P.O. b.i.d. if necessary.

➤ Heart failure; post-myocardial infarction (MI)
Adults: Initially, 25 mg P.O. once daily. After 4 weeks, may increase to maximum dosage of 50 mg P.O. once daily.

Contraindications
• Hypersensitivity to drug
• Hyperkalemia
• Potassium supplements or potassium-sparing diuretics
• Type 2 diabetes mellitus with microalbuminuria
• Severe renal impairment

Precautions
Use cautiously in:
• hepatic impairment
• pregnant or breastfeeding patients
• children (safety and efficacy not established).

Administration
• Give with or without food.
• Know that drug may be given alone or with other antihypertensives.

Route	Onset	Peak	Duration
P.O.	Slow	1.5 hr	Unknown

Adverse reactions
CNS: headache, dizziness, fatigue
CV: angina, **MI**
GI: diarrhea, abdominal pain
GU: albuminuria, vaginal bleeding, changes in sexual function, gynecomastia and breast pain (in men)
Metabolic: hypercholesterolemia, **hyperkalemia**
Respiratory: cough
Other: flulike symptoms

Interactions
Drug-drug. *Angiotensin-converting enzyme inhibitors, potassium-sparing diuretics, potassium supplements:* increased risk of hyperkalemia
CYP450-3A4 inhibitors: serious toxic effects
Lithium: increased risk of toxicity

Nonsteroidal anti-inflammatory drugs: decreased hypertensive effect of eplerenone

Patient monitoring

• Monitor electrolyte levels, and watch for signs and symptoms of hyperkalemia.
• Check vital signs, and ask patient about chest pain.
• Monitor lipid panel.
• Assess for new onset of persistent dry cough or flulike symptoms.

Patient teaching

🔊 Advise patient to immediately report chest pain, flulike symptoms, or persistent dry cough.
• Caution patient to avoid driving and other hazardous activities until he knows how drug affects concentration and alertness.
• Inform patient that drug may affect sexual function. Encourage him to discuss this issue with prescriber.
• Advise female patient to discuss pregnancy or breastfeeding with prescriber before starting drug.
• As appropriate, review all other significant and life-threatening adverse reactions and interactions, especially those related to the drugs mentioned above.

epoetin alfa

Epogen, Eprex✤⊕, Procrit

Pharmacologic class: Recombinant human erythropoietin
Therapeutic class: Biological response modifier
Pregnancy risk category C

FDA | BOXED WARNING

• Erythropoiesis-stimulating agents (ESAs) increase risk of death, myocardial infarction, stroke, venous thromboembolism, thrombosis of vascular access, and tumor progression or recurrence.
• In controlled trials, patients with chronic kidney disease experienced greater risks of death, serious adverse cardiovascular reactions, and stroke when administered ESAs to target a hemoglobin level of greater than 11 g/dl.
• No trial has identified a hemoglobin target level, ESA dosage, or dosing strategy that doesn't increase these risks.
• Use lowest dosage sufficient to reduce need for red blood cell (RBC) transfusions.
• ESAs shortened overall survival or increased risk of tumor progression or recurrence in clinical studies of patients with breast, non-small-cell lung, head and neck, lymphoid, and cervical cancers.
• Because of these risks, prescribers and hospitals must enroll in and comply with the ESA APPRISE Oncology Program to prescribe or dispense epoetin to patients with cancer. To enroll in the ESA APPRISE Oncology Program, visit www.esa-apprise.com or call 1-866-284-8089 for further assistance.
• Because of increased risk of deep venous thrombosis (DVT), DVT prophylaxis is recommended.

Action

Binds to erythropoietin, stimulating mitotic activity of erythroid progenitor cells in bone marrow and causing release of reticulocytes from bone marrow into bloodstream, where they become mature RBCs

Availability

Injection: 2,000 units/ml, 3,000 units/ml, 4,000 units/ml, 10,000 units/ml; 10,000 units/ml and 20,000 units/ml in multidose vials

⦿ Indications and dosages

➤ Anemia associated with chronic kidney disease (CKD) in patients on dialysis or not on dialysis

Adults: Initially, 50 to 100 units/kg I.V. or subcutaneously three times weekly. Don't increase dosage more frequently than once q 4 weeks. May decrease dosage more frequently but avoid frequent dosage adjustments.

➤ Anemia in children with chronic CKD who are on dialysis

Children ages 1 month to 16 years: Initially, 50 units/kg I.V. or subcutaneously three times weekly. Don't increase dosage more frequently than once q 4 weeks. May decrease dosage more frequently but avoid frequent dosage adjustments.

➤ Anemia caused by zidovudine therapy in patients with human immunodeficiency virus infection

Adults: 100 units/kg I.V. or subcutaneously three times weekly for 8 weeks or until hematocrit level is adequate. If desired response isn't reached after 8 weeks, dosage may be increased by 50 to 100 units/kg I.V. or subcutaneously three times weekly; after 4 to 8 weeks, dosage may be further increased, as prescribed, to a maximum dosage of 300 units/kg I.V. or subcutaneously three times weekly.

➤ Anemia due to effects of concomitant myelosuppressive chemotherapy, and upon initiation, there is a minimum of two additional months of planned chemotherapy

Adults: 150 units/kg subcutaneously three times weekly until completion of a chemotherapy course, or 40,000 units subcutaneously weekly until completion of a chemotherapy course

Children ages 5 to 18: 600 units/kg I.V. weekly until completion of a chemotherapy course

➤ To reduce need for blood transfusion in surgical patients

Adults: 300 units/kg subcutaneously daily for 10 days before surgery, on day of surgery, and for 4 days after surgery; or 600 units/kg subcutaneously weekly starting 3 weeks before surgery, followed by additional dose on day of surgery

Contraindications

• Serious allergic reactions
• Uncontrolled hypertension
• Pure red cell aplasia that begins after treatment
• Use of multidose vials in neonates, infants, and pregnant and breastfeeding patients

Precautions

Use cautiously in:
• renal insufficiency, CV disease
• pregnant or breastfeeding patients
• children younger than age 1 month (safety and efficacy not established).

Administration

• Don't shake drug and don't use if it has been shaken or frozen.
• Don't dilute or mix with other drug solutions. However, preservative-free epoetin alfa from single-use vials may be admixed in a syringe with bacteriostatic 0.9% sodium chloride injection with benzyl alcohol 0.9% (bacteriostatic saline) in a 1:1 ratio using aseptic technique at time of administration; keep in mind that risks are associated with benzyl alcohol use in some patients.
• Don't reenter preservative-free vials.
• For patients with CKD on dialysis, start drug when hemoglobin level is less than 10 g/dl. If hemoglobin level approaches or exceeds 11 g/dl, reduce dosage or interrupt dosing.
• For patients with CKD not on dialysis, consider starting drug only when hemoglobin level is less than 10 g/dl and the following considerations

---

Reactions in **bold** are life-threatening.   ◀𝄚 Clinical alert apply: Rate of hemoglobin decline indicates the likelihood of requiring an RBC transfusion and reducing the risk of alloimmunization or other RBC transfusion-related risks is a goal. If hemoglobin level exceeds 10 g/dl, reduce dosage or interrupt dosing and use lowest dosage sufficient to reduce the need for RBC transfusions.

• Be aware that in patients undergoing surgery, deep venous thrombosis prophylaxis is strongly recommended during epoetin alfa therapy.

• For I.V. use, give single dose by direct I.V. injection over at least 1 minute, and follow with saline flush.

• If patient is on hemodialysis, administer drug into venous return line of dialysis tubing after patient completes dialysis session.

• Know that supplemental iron may be needed to support erythropoiesis and avoid iron depletion.

◀₣ Avoid using multidose vials in neonates, infants, and pregnant and breastfeeding patients because of benzyl alcohol content, which has been associated with serious adverse events and death, including "gasping syndrome."

Route	Onset	Peak	Duration
I.V.	Immediate	Immediate	Unknown
Subcut.	Unknown	5-24 hr	Unknown

Adverse reactions
CNS: headache, paresthesia, fatigue, dizziness, asthenia, **seizures**
CV: hypertension, increased clotting of arteriovenous grafts
GI: nausea, vomiting, diarrhea
Metabolic: hyperuricemia, hyperphosphatemia, **hyperkalemia**
Musculoskeletal: joint pain
Respiratory: cough, dyspnea
Skin: rash, urticaria
Other: fever, edema, injection site pain

Interactions
Drug-diagnostic tests. *Blood urea nitrogen, creatinine, phosphate, potassium, uric acid:* increased levels

Patient monitoring
• Monitor vital signs and cardiovascular status, especially for hypertension and edema.

• Assess arteriovenous graft for patency, because drug may increase clotting at graft.

• Monitor electrolyte and uric acid levels. Watch closely for hyperuricemia, hyperkalemia, and hyperphosphatemia.

• Check temperature for fever.

• Monitor neurologic status for signs and symptoms of impending seizure.

• Evaluate nutritional status and hydration in light of GI adverse effects.

Patient teaching
• Tell patient who will self-administer drug to follow exact directions for injection and needle disposal.

◀₣ Instruct patient to monitor weight and blood pressure regularly and to immediately report hypertension, sudden weight gain, or swelling.

• Caution patient to avoid driving and other hazardous activities until he knows how drug affects concentration, motor skills, and alertness.

• Tell patient to minimize GI upset by eating small, frequent servings of food and drinking plenty of fluids.

• Advise female patient to discuss pregnancy or breastfeeding with prescriber before starting drug.

• As appropriate, review all other significant and life-threatening adverse reactions and interactions, especially those related to the tests mentioned above.

eprosartan mesylate
Teveten

Pharmacologic class: Angiotensin II receptor antagonist
Therapeutic class: Antihypertensive
Pregnancy risk category C (first trimester), *D* (second and third trimesters)

FDA | BOXED WARNING

• Drugs that act directly on the renin-angiotensin system can cause injury and death to a developing fetus. When pregnancy is detected, discontinue drug as soon as possible.

Action
Blocks aldosterone-stimulating and vasoconstrictive effects of angiotensin II at receptor sites in vascular smooth muscles and adrenal glands, decreasing vascular resistance

Availability
Tablets: 400 mg, 600 mg

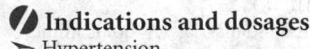 Indications and dosages
➤ Hypertension
Adults: 600 mg P.O. once daily or in divided doses b.i.d. Total daily dosage range is 400 to 800 mg.

Contraindications
• Hypersensitivity to drug or its components
• Pregnancy or breastfeeding

Precautions
Use cautiously in:
• hypotension, heart failure, renal or hepatic impairment, obstructive biliary disorders, volume or sodium depletion
• concurrent high-dose diuretic therapy

• females of childbearing age
• children younger than age 18 (safety not established).

Administration
• Give initial dose in supervised medical setting, and monitor blood pressure for 2 hours after administration.
• Know that drug may be given alone or with other antihypertensives.
• Be aware that black patients have a higher risk of angioedema.
• Be prepared to treat transient hypotension by placing patient in supine position and giving I.V. normal saline infusion as needed.

Route	Onset	Peak	Duration
P.O.	Unknown	6 hr	24 hr

Adverse reactions
CNS: dizziness, fatigue, headache, syncope
CV: hypotension, chest pain, peripheral edema
EENT: sinus disorders
GI: nausea, diarrhea, constipation, abdominal pain, dry mouth
GU: albuminuria, **renal failure**
Hepatic: hepatitis
Metabolic: gout, **hyperkalemia**
Musculoskeletal: joint pain, back pain, muscle weakness
Respiratory: upper respiratory tract infection, cough, bronchitis
Skin: angioedema
Other: dental pain, fever, facial edema

Interactions
Drug-drug. *Antihypertensives, diuretics:* increased risk of hypotension
Nonsteroidal anti-inflammatory drugs: decreased antihypertensive effect of eprosartan
Potassium-sparing diuretics, potassium supplements: increased risk of hyperkalemia

e

Reactions in **bold** are life-threatening.　　　◀€ Clinical alert

Drug-diagnostic tests. *Absolute neutrophil count, hemoglobin, platelets, white blood cells:* decreased
Albumin, creatinine, liver function tests, serum BUN: elevated levels
Drug-food. *Salt substitutes containing potassium:* increased risk of hyperkalemia
Drug-herbs. *Ephedra (ma huang):* antagonism of eprosartan action
Drug-behaviors. *Alcohol use:* increased CNS depression

Patient monitoring
• Monitor vital signs, particularly for hypotension after administration.
• Assess cardiovascular status, especially for chest pain, syncope, and edema.
• Monitor liver and kidney function test results, watching for drug-induced hepatitis or renal failure.
• Assess respiratory status. Stay alert for dry, persistent cough and signs and symptoms of respiratory infections.
• Monitor electrolyte levels, and watch for signs and symptoms of hyperkalemia.

Patient teaching
• Instruct patient to take drug at same time each day, with or without food.
◀≋ Inform patient that drug may cause angioedema. Instruct him to immediately report facial or lip swelling, fever, or sore throat.
◀≋ Advise patient to immediately report chest pain, fainting, decreased urine output, unusual tiredness, yellowing of skin or eyes, or swelling.
◀≋ Tell female patient to contact prescriber right away if she suspects she's pregnant.
• Caution female not to breastfeed while taking drug.
• As appropriate, review all other significant and life-threatening adverse reactions and interactions, especially those related to the drugs, tests, foods, herbs, and behaviors mentioned above.

eptifibatide
Integrilin

Pharmacologic class: Platelet aggregation inhibitor
Therapeutic class: Antiplatelet agent
Pregnancy risk category B

Action
Decreases platelet aggregation by binding to platelet-receptor glycoprotein, preventing binding of fibrinogen to platelets, which causes thrombus formation

Availability
Injection: 10-ml vial (2 mg/ml), 100-ml vial (0.75 mg/ml)

🕖 Indications and dosages
➤ Acute coronary syndrome (unstable angina or non-Q-wave myocardial infarction)
Adults: 180 mcg/kg I.V. bolus over 1 to 2 minutes, followed by a continuous infusion of 2 mcg/kg/minute for up to 72 hours
➤ Prevention of thrombosis related to percutaneous coronary intervention (PCI)
Adults: 180 mcg/kg I.V. bolus immediately before PCI, then a continuous infusion of 2 mcg/kg/minute, followed by a second 180-mcg/kg bolus 10 minutes after first bolus. Continue infusion until discharge or for up to 24 hours.

Dosage adjustment
• Renal impairment

Contraindications
• Hypersensitivity to drug or its components
• Severe hypertension
• Bleeding disorders or evidence of active abnormal bleeding within previous 30 days

- Renal dialysis
- Recent cerebrovascular accident
- Recent surgery
- Current or planned administration of another parenteral Gp IIb/IIIa inhibitor

Precautions
Use cautiously in:
- renal insufficiency
- creatinine level below 2 mg/dl
- platelet count below 100,000/mm³
- elderly patients
- pregnant or breastfeeding patients
- children (safety and efficacy not established).

Administration
- Withdraw single bolus dose from 10-ml vial into syringe, and give by I.V. push over 1 to 2 minutes. Follow single I.V. bolus dose with continuous I.V. infusion given undiluted from 100-ml vial spiked with infusion set connected to infusion control device.
- Don't administer through same I.V. line as furosemide.

Route	Onset	Peak	Duration
I.V.	Immediate	Immediate	4-6 hr

Adverse reactions
CNS: headache, dizziness, asthenia, syncope
CV: hypotension
GI: nausea, diarrhea, constipation
GU: hematuria
Hematologic: bleeding tendency, thrombocytopenia
Skin: flushing
Other: bleeding at femoral access site

Interactions
Drug-drug. *Clopidogrel, dipyridamole, nonsteroidal anti-inflammatory drugs, oral anticoagulants, thrombolytics, ticlopidine:* increased risk of bleeding
Other platelet aggregation inhibitors: serious bleeding

Drug-diagnostic tests. *Platelets:* decreased count
Drug-herbs. *Most commonly used herbs:* increased anticoagulant effect of eptifibatide

Patient monitoring
- Monitor vital signs and assess cardiovascular status, especially for syncope and hypotension.
- Monitor coagulation studies, CBC, and platelet count. Watch for signs and symptoms of abnormal bleeding or bruising and hematuria.
- Check carefully for bleeding at all sites of invasive procedures, particularly femoral access site.

Patient teaching
- Tell patient drug may cause serious adverse effects but can help prevent a heart attack. Reassure him that he'll be closely monitored during therapy.
- ◀€ Instruct patient to immediately report fainting or abnormal bruising or bleeding.
- Teach patient safety measures to avoid bruising or bleeding.
- As appropriate, review all other significant and life-threatening adverse reactions and interactions, especially those related to the drugs, tests, and herbs mentioned above.

eribulin
Halaven

Pharmacologic class: Non-taxane microtubule dynamics inhibitor
Therapeutic class: Antineoplastic
Pregnancy risk category D

Action
Inhibits growth phase of microtubules without affecting the shortening phase and sequesters tubulin into

---

nonproductive aggregates; exerts its effects via a tubulin-based antimitotic mechanism leading to G2/M cell-cycle block, disruption of mitotic spindles and, ultimately, apoptotic cell death after prolonged mitotic blockage

Availability
*Injection:*1 mg/2 ml (0.5 mg/ml) in single-use vials

⁄ Indications and dosages
➤ Metastatic breast cancer in patients who have previously received at least two chemotherapeutic regimens for metastatic disease
Adults: 1.4 mg/m² I.V. over 2 to 5 minutes on days 1 and 8 of 21-day cycle

Dosage adjustment
• Mild and moderate hepatic impairment, moderate renal impairment
• Hematologic toxicities
• Peripheral neuropathy

Contraindications
None

Precautions
Use cautiously in:
• hepatic or renal impairment
• neutropenia, neuropathy
• congenital long QT syndrome (avoid use)
• congestive heart failure, brady-arrhythmias, drugs known to prolong QT interval (including Class Ia and III antiarrhythmics), electrolyte abnormalities
• pregnant or breastfeeding patients
• children younger than age 18 (safety and efficacy not established).

Administration
• Don't dilute with dextrose-containing solutions or mix with other drugs.
• Obtain CBC before each dose; increase frequency in patients who develop Grade 3 or 4 cytopenias.

• Correct hypokalemia or hypomagnesemia before starting therapy.
◀€ Don't administer day-1 or day-8 dose if any of the following occurs: Absolute neutrophil count less than 1,000/mm³, platelet count less than 75,000/mm³, or Grade 3 or 4 non-hematologic toxicities. Delay day-8 dose for maximum of 1 week.
• If toxicities don't resolve or improve to Grade 2 severity by day 15, omit dose. If toxicities resolve or improve to Grade 2 severity by day 15, give drug at reduced dosage and initiate next cycle no sooner than 2 weeks later.
◀€ Delay drug administration and reduce subsequent doses in patients who experience febrile neutropenia or Grade 4 neutropenia lasting longer than 7 days.
• Withhold drug in patients who experience Grade 3 or 4 peripheral neuropathy until resolution to Grade 2 or less.
• Don't reescalate dosage after it has been reduced.

Route	Onset	Peak	Duration
I.V.	Unknown	Unknown	Unknown

Adverse reactions
CNS: headache, dizziness, asthenia, fatigue, peripheral neuropathy, insomnia, depression
CV: prolonged QT interval
EENT: increased lacrimation
GI: nausea, vomiting, diarrhea, constipation, anorexia, dyspepsia, abdominal pain, stomatitis, dry mouth
GU: urinary tract infection
Hematologic: anemia, neutropenia, **febrile neutropenia, thrombocytopenia**
Hepatic: liver function test abnormalities
Metabolic: hypokalemia
Musculoskeletal: arthralgia, myalgia, back pain, bone pain, extremity pain, muscle spasm, muscular weakness

Respiratory: cough, dyspnea, upper respiratory tract infection
Skin: alopecia, rash
Other: mucosal inflammation, pyrexia, weight loss, peripheral edema, dysgeusia

Interactions
Drug-diagnostic tests. *ALT:* increased level
Potassium: decreased level

Patient monitoring
• Monitor CBC with differential and renal and hepatic function tests closely.
• Monitor serum magnesium and potassium levels periodically during therapy.
• Monitor ECG in patients with congestive heart failure, bradyarrhythmias, or electrolyte abnormalities, or if patients are taking drugs known to prolong QT interval, including Class Ia and III antiarrhythmics.
• Monitor patients closely for signs and symptoms of peripheral motor and sensory neuropathy.

Patient teaching
◀ Instruct patient to immediately report abnormal heartbeats, dizziness, or faintness.
• Advise patient to promptly report fever, chills, burning or pain on urination, cough, or numbness, tingling, or burning of hands and feet.
• Advise female patient of childbearing age of potential hazard to fetus if drug is used during pregnancy and to inform prescriber if she becomes pregnant while taking drug.
• Advise breastfeeding patient that she should decide whether to discontinue breastfeeding or discontinue drug, taking into account importance of drug for her treatment.
• As appropriate, review all other significant and life-threatening adverse reactions and interactions, especially those related to the tests mentioned above.

erlotinib
Tarceva

Pharmacologic class: Epidermal growth factor receptor (EGFR) inhibitor
Therapeutic class: Antineoplastic
Pregnancy risk category D

e

Action
Unclear. Drug inhibits intracellular phosphorylation of tyrosine kinase associated with EGFR, which is expressed on cell surface of both normal cells and cancer cells.

Availability
Tablets: 25 mg, 100 mg, 150 mg

⚕ Indications and dosages
➤ Locally advanced or metastatic non-small-cell lung cancer after failure of at least one chemotherapy regimen; maintenance treatment in patients whose disease hasn't progressed after four cycles of platinum-based first-line chemotherapy
Adults: 150 mg P.O. at least 1 hour before or 2 hours after food ingestion, continued until disease progresses or unacceptable toxicity occurs
➤ First-line treatment of locally advanced, unresectable, or metastatic pancreatic cancer (given with gemcitabine)
Adults: 100 mg P.O. daily at least 1 hour before or 2 hours after food ingestion, continued until disease progresses or unacceptable toxicity occurs

Dosage adjustment
• Severe diarrhea
• Pretreatment with CYP3A4 inducers
• Concurrent use of potent CYP3A4 inhibitors (such as ketoconazole)
• Acute onset of new or progressing pulmonary symptoms

Reactions in **bold** are life-threatening.　　　◀ Clinical alert

Off-label uses
- Colorectal and renal cell cancer
- Malignant glioma

Contraindications
None

Precautions
Use cautiously in:
- hepatic impairment, diarrhea
- pulmonary symptoms, suspected interstitial lung disease (such as pneumonitis, interstitial pneumonia, obliterative bronchiolitis, pulmonary fibrosis, adult respiratory distress syndrome, or lung filtration)
- concomitant use of anti-angiogenic agents, corticosteroids, nonsteroidal anti-inflammatory drugs, or taxane-based chemotherapy; prior history of peptic ulceration or diverticular disease
- concurrent warfarin therapy
- pregnant or breastfeeding patients
- children (safety and efficacy not established).

Administration
- Give at least 1 hour before or 2 hours after food ingestion.
- ◀€ Interrupt therapy if patient develops acute onset of new or progressing pulmonary symptoms pending diagnostic evaluation. If interstitial lung disease develops, discontinue drug and administer appropriate interventions.
- ◀€ Be aware that some cases of hepatorenal syndrome, acute renal failure, and renal insufficiency may be secondary to baseline hepatic impairment while others may be associated with severe dehydration. Interrupt therapy and take appropriate measures to intensively rehydrate patient, as needed.
- ◀€ Discontinue drug if total bilirubin level is above three times upper limit of normal (ULN) or transaminase levels are above five times ULN versus pretreatment values; signs and symptoms

of GI perforation occur; severe bullous, blistering, or exfoliating conditions develop; or acute or worsening ocular disorders such as eye pain occur.

Route	Onset	Peak	Duration
P.O.	Unknown	4 hr	Unknown

Adverse reactions
CNS: fatigue
EENT: conjunctivitis, keratoconjunctivitis sicca **corneal perforation and ulceration**
GI: nausea, vomiting, diarrhea, abdominal pain, anorexia, stomatitis **GI perforation**
GU: renal insufficiency, acute renal failure
Hepatic: hepatorenal syndrome, hepatic failure
Respiratory: dyspnea, cough, **interstitial lung disease**
Skin: rash, pruritus, dry skin, **Stevens-Johnson syndrome, toxic epidermal necrolysis-like reactions**
Other: infection

Interactions
Drug-drug. *CYP3A4 inhibitors (such as clarithromycin, indinavir, itraconazole, ketoconazole, ritonavir, saquinavir, telithromycin):* increased erlotinib blood level
CYP3A4 inducers (such as carbamazepine, phenobarbital, phenytoin, rifampin): decreased erlotinib blood level
Warfarin, other coumarin anticoagulants: elevated INR, increased bleeding risk
Drug-diagnostic tests. *Alanine aminotransferase, aspartate aminotransferase, bilirubin:* increased
International Normalized Ratio: increased
Liver function tests: abnormal
Drug-food. *Any food:* increased erlotinib bioavailability
Drug-herb. *Coenzyme Q10:* decreased chemotherapy efficacy

St. John's wort: decreased erlotinib blood level

Drug-behaviors. *Smoking:* decreased erlotinib plasma concentration

Patient monitoring

◀€ Perform periodic serum electrolyte measurements and renal and liver function testing.

• Advise patient not to smoke while taking drug.

• Monitor INR and prothrombin time regularly in patients receiving warfarin, other coumarin anticoagulants, or nonsteroidal anti-inflammatory drugs.

◀€ Monitor for signs and symptoms of respiratory disorders and GI perforation.

Patient teaching

◀€ Advise patient to seek immediate medical attention for severe or persistent diarrhea, nausea, vomiting, anorexia, severe rash, eye pain, eye irritation, or onset or worsening of unexplained shortness of breath or cough.

• Advise patient not to smoke while taking drug.

• As appropriate, review all other significant and life-threatening adverse reactions and interactions, especially those related to the drugs, tests, foods, and herbs mentioned above.

ertapenem
Invanz

Pharmacologic class: Carbapenem
Therapeutic class: Anti-infective
Pregnancy risk category B

Action

Inhibits cell-wall synthesis in bacteria, causing cell death

Availability

Powder for infusion (lyophilized): 1 g/vial

🖉 Indications and dosages

➤ Community-acquired pneumonia; skin infections; complicated genitourinary (GU) infections; complicated intra-abdominal infections; acute pelvic infections

Adults and children older than age 13: 1 g I.M. or I.V. daily. Length of treatment varies with type of infection: community-acquired pneumonia, 10 to 14 days; skin and skin structures, 7 to 14 days; GU, 10 to 14 days; intra-abdominal, 5 to 14 days; acute pelvic, 3 to 10 days.

Children age 3 months to 12 years: 15 mg/kg twice daily (not to exceed 1 g/day). May be given by I.V. infusion for up to 14 days or I.M. injection for up to 7 days.

➤ Prophylaxis of surgical site infection in elective colorectal surgery

Adults: 1 g I.V. as single dose given 1 hour before surgical incision

Dosage adjustment

• Renal impairment

Contraindications

• Hypersensitivity to drug, its components, other carbapenems, or beta-lactams

• I.M. injection in patients allergic to lidocaine or other amide local anesthetics

Precautions

Use cautiously in:

• seizure disorder

• pregnant or breastfeeding patients

• children (not recommended in infants younger than age 3 months).

Administration

• Reconstitute for I.V. use by adding to vial 10 ml of sterile or bacteriostatic water or normal saline for injection. Don't use diluents containing dextrose.

Reactions in **bold** are life-threatening.   ◀€ Clinical alert

• Further dilute reconstituted drug in 50 ml of normal saline solution; infuse over 30 minutes. Don't mix or infuse with other drugs.
• Reconstitute for I.M. use by adding 3.2 ml of 1% lidocaine to vial and shaking well.
• Inject I.M. dose deep into large muscle mass, such as gluteus maximus or lateral thigh.

Route	Onset	Peak	Duration
I.V.	Rapid	30 min	Unknown
I.M.	10 min	2.3 hr	Unknown

Adverse reactions

CNS: headache, dizziness, asthenia, fatigue, insomnia, altered mental status, anxiety, **seizures**
CV: hypotension, hypertension, chest pain, phlebitis, **thrombophlebitis, arrhythmias, heart failure**
EENT: pharyngitis
GI: nausea, vomiting, diarrhea, constipation, abdominal pain, dyspepsia, gastroesophageal reflux disease, **pseudomembranous colitis**
GU: vaginitis
Hepatic: hepatotoxicity
Respiratory: crackles, cough, dyspnea, wheezing, **respiratory distress**
Skin: rash, **erythema multiforme, Stevens-Johnson syndrome, toxic epidermal necrolysis**
Other: fever, pain, induration, and inflammation at I.V. site; edema; hypersensitivity reactions including **anaphylaxis**

Interactions

Drug-drug. *Probenecid:* increased blood level and half-life of ertapenem

Patient monitoring

◀€ Monitor vital signs, ECG, and cardiovascular status closely. Stay alert for arrhythmias, edema, respiratory distress, and other signs and symptoms of heart failure.
◀€ Assess neurologic status, and watch for signs of impending seizure.

◀€ Monitor bowel pattern, and stay alert for signs and symptoms of pseudomembranous colitis.
• Inspect injection site for evidence of thrombophlebitis and induration.
◀€ Watch for indications of erythema multiforme (sore throat, rash, cough, iris lesions, mouth sores, fever). Report early signs before condition progresses to Stevens-Johnson syndrome, and stay alert for other hypersensitivity reactions (including anaphylaxis).

Patient teaching

• Tell patient to notify nurse right away if drug causes pain or swelling at injection site.
• Inform patient that drug can be toxic to many organ systems. Tell him to promptly report significant adverse reactions.
• Tell female patient to inform prescriber of pregnancy or breastfeeding before taking drug.
• As appropriate, review all other significant and life-threatening adverse reactions and interactions, especially those related to the drugs mentioned above.

---

erythromycin

Apo-Erythro❖, Apo-Erythro-EC, Diomycin❖, Erybid❖, Erymax⊕, Ery-Tab, Erythromid❖, PCE❖, Rommix⊕, Tiloryth⊕

erythromycin ethylsuccinate

Apo-Erythro-ES❖, E.E.S., EryPed

erythromycin lactobionate

Erythrocin

erythromycin stearate

Erythrocin Stearate

---

erythromycin (topical)
Akne-Mycin, A/T/S, E-Glades,
E-Solve 2, Erycette, Eryderm, Erygel,
Sans-Acne✜, Stiemycin⊕

Pharmacologic class: Macrolide
Therapeutic class: Anti-infective
Pregnancy risk category B

Action
Binds with 50S subunit of susceptible
bacterial ribosomes, suppressing
protein synthesis in bacterial cells and
causing cell death

Availability
erythromycin base
Capsules (delayed-release): 250 mg
Ointment (ophthalmic): 0.5%
Tablets: 250 mg, 500 mg
Tablets (delayed-release, enteric-coated):
250 mg, 333 mg, 500 mg
Tablets (particles in tablets): 333 mg,
500 mg
erythromycin ethylsuccinate
Oral suspension: 200 mg/5 ml, 400
mg/5 ml
Powder for suspension: 100 mg/2.5 ml,
200 mg/5 ml, 400 mg/5 ml
Tablets: 400 mg
erythromycin lactobionate
Powder for injection: 500 mg, 1 g
erythromycin stearate
Tablets (film-coated): 250 mg, 500 mg
erythromycin (topical)
Gel: 2%
Ointment: 2%
Solution: 2%
Swabs: 2%

⟪/⟫ Indications and dosages
➤ Pelvic inflammatory disease
Adults: 500 mg (base) I.V. q 6 hours
for 3 days, then 250 mg (base, estolate,
or stearate) or 400 mg (ethylsuccinate)
q 6 hours for 7 days
➤ Syphilis
Adults: 500 mg (base, estolate, or
stearate) P.O. q.i.d. for 14 days

➤ Most upper and lower respiratory
tract infections; otitis media; skin
infections; Legionnaires' disease
Adults: 250 mg P.O. q 6 hours, or 333
mg P.O. q 8 hours, or 500 mg P.O. q 12
hours (base, estolate, or stearate); or
400 mg P.O. q 6 hours or 800 mg P.O. q
12 hours (ethylsuccinate); or 250 to
500 mg I.V. (up to 1 g) q 6 hours (gluceptate or lactobionate)
Children: 30 to 50 mg/kg/day (base,
estolate, ethylsuccinate, or lactobionate) I.V. or P.O., in divided doses q 6
hours when giving I.V. and q 6 to 8
hours when giving P.O. Maximum
dosage is 2 g/day for base or estolate,
3.2 g/day for ethylsuccinate, and 4 g/
day for lactobionate.
➤ Intestinal amebiasis
Adults: 250 mg (base, estolate, or
stearate) or 400 mg (ethylsuccinate)
P.O. q 6 hours for 10 to 14 days
Children: 30 to 50 mg/kg/day (base,
estolate, ethylsuccinate, or stearate)
P.O. in divided doses over 10 to 14 days
➤ Prophylaxis of ophthalmia neona-
torum caused by *Neisseria gonorrhoeae*
or *Chlamydia trachomatis*
Neonates: 0.5- to 1-cm ribbon of ointment into each lower conjunctival sac
once
➤ Treatment of conjunctivitis of the
newborn caused by susceptible
organisms
Neonates: 50 mg/kg/day (ethylsuccinate) P.O. in four divided doses for at
least 14 days
➤ Pertussis
Children: 40 to 50 mg/kg/day (estolate
preferred) P.O. in four divided doses
for 14 days
➤ Pneumonia of infancy
Infants: 50 mg/kg/day (estolate or
ethylsuccinate) P.O. in four divided
doses for at least 3 weeks
➤ Acne
Adults and children older than age 12:
2% ointment, gel, or solution applied
topically b.i.d.

e

Reactions in **bold** are life-threatening.　　　◀€ Clinical alert

Dosage adjustment
• Hepatic impairment

Off-label uses
• Chancroid

Contraindications
• Hypersensitivity to drug or tartrazine
• Concurrent use of astemizole, cisapride, pimozide, or terfenadine
• Hepatic impairment (with estolate)
• Pregnancy (with estolate)

Precautions
Use cautiously in:
• myasthenia gravis
• hepatic disease.

Administration
◀◝ Be aware that ventricular arrhythmias and sudden death may occur if drug is given concurrently with potent CYP3A inhibitors (such as clarithromycin, diltiazem, nitroimidazole antifungal agents, protease inhibitors, verapamil, and troleandomycin).
• Give erythromycin ethylsuccinate and delayed-release products without regard to meals, but avoid giving with grapefruit juice.
• Give erythromycin base or stearate 1 hour before or 2 hours after meals for optimal absorption.
• Follow label directions to reconstitute drug for I.V. use. For intermittent infusion, infuse each 250 mg in at least 100 ml of normal saline solution over 20 to 60 minutes. Continuous infusion may be given over 6 to 24 hours as directed.

Route	Onset	Peak	Duration
P.O.	1 hr	1-4 hr	6-12 hr
I.V.	Rapid	End of infusion	6-12 hr

Adverse reactions
CV: torsades de pointes, arrhythmias
EENT: ototoxicity
GI: nausea, vomiting, diarrhea, abdominal pain or cramps
Hepatic: hepatic dysfunction, hepatitis
Skin: rash
Other: increased appetite, aggravation of weakness in myasthenia gravis, allergic reactions, superinfection, phlebitis at I.V. site

Interactions
Drug-drug. *Alfentanil, alprazolam, bromocriptine, buspirone, carbamazepine, clozapine, cyclosporine, diazepam, disopyramide, ergot alkaloids, felodipine, methylprednisolone, midazolam, tacrolimus, theophylline, triazolam, vinblastine, warfarin:* increased blood levels and risk of toxicity from these drugs
Clindamycin, lincomycin: antagonism of erythromycin's effects
CYP3A inhibitors: increased erythromycin blood level, with risk of ventricular arrhythmias and sudden death
Digoxin: increased digoxin blood level
HMG-CoA reductase inhibitors: increased risk of myopathy and rhabdomyolysis
Hormonal contraceptives: decreased contraceptive efficacy
Astemizole, cisapride, pimozide, sparfloxacin, terfenadine: increased risk of serious arrhythmias
Rifabutin, rifampin: decreased erythromycin effects, increased risk of adverse GI reactions
Theophylline: increased theophylline blood level, decreased erythromycin blood level
Drug-diagnostic tests. *Alanine aminotransferase, alkaline phosphatase, aspartate aminotransferase, bilirubin:* increased levels
Urine catecholamines: false elevations
Drug-food. *Grapefruit juice:* increased erythromycin blood level

Patient monitoring
• Check temperature, and watch for signs and symptoms of superinfection.

• Monitor liver function tests. Watch for signs and symptoms of hepatotoxicity.
• Assess patient's hearing for signs of ototoxicity.

Patient teaching
• Instruct patient to take with 8 oz of water 1 hour before or 2 hours after meals, and to avoid grapefruit juice.
• If drug causes GI upset, encourage patient to take it with food.
• Tell patient not to swallow chewable tablets whole and not to chew or crush enteric-coated tablets.
◀€ Advise patient to immediately report irregular heart beats, unusual tiredness, yellowing of skin or eyes, or signs and symptoms of new infection.
• Tell patient he'll undergo periodic blood tests to monitor liver function.
• As appropriate, review all other significant and life-threatening adverse reactions and interactions, especially those related to the drugs, tests, and foods mentioned above.

escitalopram oxalate
Cipralex ⊕, Lexapro

Pharmacologic class: Selective serotonin reuptake inhibitor
Therapeutic class: Antidepressant
Pregnancy risk category C

FDA **BOXED WARNING**

• Drug may increase risk of suicidal thinking and behavior in children and adolescents with major depressive disorder and other psychiatric disorders. Risk is greater during first few months of treatment, and must be balanced with clinical need, as depression itself increases suicide risk. With patient of any age, observe closely for clinical worsening, suicidality, and unusual behavior changes when therapy begins. Advise family to observe patient closely and communicate with prescriber as needed.
• Drug isn't approved for use in pediatric patients.

Action
Prevents serotonin reuptake by CNS neurons, making more serotonin available in brain and thereby relieving depression

Availability
Oral solution: 5 mg/5 ml
Tablets: 5 mg, 10 mg, 20 mg

🕖 Indications and dosages
➤ Major depression
Adults: Initially, 10 mg P.O. daily as a single dose. After at least 1 week, may increase to 20 mg P.O. daily, as needed.
Adolescents ages 12 to 17: Initially, 10 mg P.O. daily. After at least 3 weeks, may increase to 20 mg P.O. daily as needed.
Elderly adults and patients with hepatic impairment: Maximum dosage of 10 mg P.O. daily as a single dose
➤ Generalized anxiety disorder
Adults: Initially, 10 mg P.O. daily as a single dose. After at least 1 week, may increase to 20 mg P.O. daily as needed.

Dosage adjustment
• Hepatic impairment
• Elderly patients

Contraindications
• Hypersensitivity to drug
• Concurrent use of pimozide
• MAO inhibitor use within past 14 days

Precautions
Use cautiously in:
• renal or hepatic impairment, other conditions that cause altered

e

Reactions in **bold** are life-threatening.　　　　◀€ Clinical alert

metabolism or hemodynamic responses, history of mania or seizures, suicidal tendency
- concomitant use of nonsteroidal anti-inflammatory drugs (NSAIDs), aspirin, warfarin, or other drugs that affect coagulation
- elderly patients
- pregnant or breastfeeding patients
- children younger than age 12 with major depression and younger than age 18 with generalized anxiety disorder (safety and efficacy not established).

Administration
- Give with or without food in the morning or evening.
- 🔊 Don't give within 14 days of MAO inhibitor.

Route	Onset	Peak	Duration
P.O.	Slow	3.5-6.5 hr	Unknown

Adverse reactions
CNS: drowsiness, dizziness, insomnia, fatigue, **neuroleptic malignant syndrome-like reactions, increased risk of suicide or suicidal ideation** (especially in child or adolescent)
EENT: rhinitis, sinusitis
GI: nausea, vomiting, diarrhea, constipation, dyspepsia, abdominal pain, dry mouth
GU: ejaculatory disorders, erectile dysfunction, anorgasmia (in females), decreased libido
Metabolic: hyponatremia (in association with syndrome of inappropriate antidiuretic hormone secretion)
Other: increased appetite, flulike symptoms, **serotonin syndrome**

Interactions
Drug-drug. *Aspirin, NSAIDs, warfarin:* increased risk of bleeding
Carbamazepine, lithium: decreased effects of escitalopram

Citalopram: increased risk of serious toxic effects
MAO inhibitors: increased escitalopram blood level and risk of toxicity
Pimozide: prolonged QT interval
Triptans: weakness, hyperreflexia, incoordination
Drug-diagnostic tests. *Sodium:* decreased level
Drug-herbs. *Ginkgo, St. John's wort:* increased risk of adverse effects
Drug-behaviors. *Alcohol use:* increased motor impairment

Patient monitoring
🔊 Assess patient's mood closely. Watch for signs and symptoms of increased depression or suicidal ideation (especially in child or adolescent).
🔊 Monitor patient closely for serotonin syndrome or neuroleptic malignant syndrome-like reactions; immediately discontinue drug if these occur.
- Be aware that gradual dosage reduction rather than abrupt cessation is recommended. When drug is discontinued, monitor for dysphoric mood, irritability, agitation, dizziness, sensory disturbances, anxiety, confusion, headache, lethargy, emotional lability, and insomnia.

Patient teaching
- Advise patient to minimize GI upset by eating small, frequent servings of food and drinking plenty of fluids.
- Inform patient that full drug effect may take up to 4 weeks. Caution him not to overuse drug or stop drug abruptly.
🔊 Tell patient (and parent or significant other as appropriate) to contact prescriber immediately if depression worsens or suicidal thoughts develop (especially in child or adolescent).
🔊 Instruct patient to immediately discontinue drug and notify prescriber if the following symptoms occur: overheating, muscle rigidity, altered mental

status, irregular pulse or blood pressure, rapid or irregular heart beat, excessive sweating, involuntary muscle movements, fever, or seizures.

• Caution patient to avoid driving and other hazardous activities until he knows how drug affects concentration and alertness.

• As appropriate, review all other significant and life-threatening adverse reactions and interactions, especially those related to the drugs, tests, herbs, and behaviors mentioned above.

esmolol hydrochloride
Brevibloc

Pharmacologic class: Beta-adrenergic blocker (cardioselective)

Therapeutic class: Antiarrhythmic, antihypertensive

Pregnancy risk category C

Action
Blocks stimulation of beta-adrenergic receptors (primarily beta$_1$ receptors), thereby reducing atrioventricular conduction and cardiac output and decreasing blood pressure

Availability
Injection: 10 mg/ml

⚠ Indications and dosages
➤ Supraventricular tachycardia
Adults: Initially, a loading dose of 500 mcg/kg/minute by I.V. infusion over 1 minute, followed by a maintenance infusion of 50 mcg/kg/minute over 4 minutes. If desired response doesn't occur after 5 minutes, repeat loading dose and increase maintenance infusion to 100 mcg/kg/minute for 4 minutes. Repeat sequence as needed, with maintenance dosage increased in increments of 50 mcg/kg/minute, to a maximum maintenance infusion of 200 mcg/kg/minute for 48 hours.
➤ Sinus tachycardia or hypertension
Adults: Initially, 80 mg (1 mg/kg) by I.V. bolus over 30 seconds; then, if needed, 150 mcg/kg/minute by I.V. infusion, to a maximum of 300 mcg/kg/minute

Off-label uses
• Acute myocardial ischemia

Contraindications
• Hypersensitivity to drug
• Heart failure
• Heart block greater than third degree
• Sinus bradycardia
• Cardiogenic shock

Precautions
Use cautiously in:
• renal impairment, diabetes, bronchospasm, cardiac disease, cerebrovascular insufficiency, peripheral vascular disease, hyperthyroidism, myasthenic conditions
• pregnant or breastfeeding patients.

Administration
• Be aware that compatible solutions include 5% dextrose for injection, 5% dextrose in lactated Ringer's injection, 5% dextrose in Ringer's injection, 5% dextrose in 0.45% or 0.9% sodium chloride injection, and lactated Ringer's injection.
• Don't mix with 5% sodium bicarbonate injection.
• Large fluid volumes may be needed to infuse drug. Use caution when excessive fluids could be harmful.

Route	Onset	Peak	Duration
I.V.	Immediate	30 min	30 min after infusion

Adverse reactions
CNS: anxiety, depression, dizziness, drowsiness, headache, agitation, fatigue, confusion, speech disorders, asthenia

---

CV: peripheral ischemia, chest pain, bradycardia, hypotension
GI: nausea, vomiting, heartburn
GU: urinary retention
Respiratory: wheezing, dyspnea
Skin: flushing, pallor, erythema
Other: altered taste, fever, chills, edema, midscapular pain, inflammation or induration at infusion site

Interactions

Drug-drug. *Alpha$_1$-adrenergic blockers:* exaggerated antihypertensive effect
Catecholamines, reserpine: increased bradycardia and hypotension
Digoxin: increased digoxin blood level
Morphine: increased esmolol blood level
Succinylcholine: prolonged neuromuscular blockade
Drug-herbs. *Ephedra (ma huang), St. John's wort, yohimbe:* decreased antihypertensive effect

Patient monitoring

• Monitor vital signs and ECG, particularly for hypotension.
• Assess neurologic status, and institute safety measures as needed.
• Monitor fluid intake and output, watching for urinary retention.
• Check I.V. site regularly.

Patient teaching

• Explain to patient that drug is an emergency measure to control blood pressure, arrhythmias, or heart rate.
• Ensure patient he'll be closely monitored throughout drug therapy.
• Tell patient to report pain or redness at I.V. site.
• As appropriate, review all other significant adverse reactions and interactions, especially those related to the drugs and herbs mentioned above.

esomeprazole magnesium
Nexium

Pharmacologic class: Proton pump inhibitor
Therapeutic class: Antiulcer agent
Pregnancy risk category C

Action

Reduces gastric acid production by inhibiting enzyme activity in gastric parietal cells, preventing transport of hydrogen ions into gastric lumen

Availability

Capsules (delayed-release): 20 mg, 40 mg
Powder for delayed-release oral suspension: 2.5-mg, 5-mg, 10-mg, 20-mg, 40-mg packets

⚡ Indications and dosages

➤ Treatment of gastroesophageal reflux disease (GERD); healing of erosive esophagitis
Children ages 1 month to younger than 1 year weighing 3 kg (6.5 lb) to 5 kg: 2.5 mg P.O. daily for up to 6 weeks
Adults: 20 to 40 mg P.O. once daily for 4 to 8 weeks
Children ages 1 month to younger than 1 year weighing more than 7.5 kg to 12 kg (16.5 to 26 lb): 10 mg P.O. daily for up to 6 weeks
Children ages 1 month to younger than 1 year weighing more than 5 kg (11 lb) to 7.5 kg: 5 mg P.O. daily for up to 6 weeks
Children ages 1 to 11 weighing 20 kg (44 lb) or more: 10 or 20 mg P.O. daily for 8 weeks
Children ages 1 to 11 weighing less than 20 kg (44 lb): 10 mg P.O. daily for 8 weeks
➤ Treatment of GERD; maintenance of healing of erosive esophagitis

Adults: 20 mg P.O. once daily
➤ Symptomatic GERD
Adults: 20 mg P.O. once daily for
4 weeks
Children ages 12 to 17: 20 or 40 mg
P.O. daily for up to 8 weeks
Children ages 1 to 11: 10 mg P.O. daily
for up to 8 weeks
➤ *Helicobacter pylori* eradication to
decrease risk of duodenal ulcer
recurrence
Adults: 40 mg P.O. once daily for
10 days, given in combination with
amoxicillin 1,000 mg b.i.d. for 10 days
and with clarithromycin 500 mg b.i.d.
for 10 days
➤ Treatment of pathological hyper-
secretory conditions including
Zollinger-Ellison syndrome
Adults: 40 mg P.O. b.i.d.
➤ Risk reduction of NSAID-associated
gastric ulcer
Adults: 20 or 40 mg P.O. once daily for
up to 6 months

Contraindications
• Hypersensitivity to proton pump
inhibitors

Precautions
Use cautiously in:
• severe hepatic impairment
• increased risk of hip, wrist, and spine
fractures
• pregnant or breastfeeding patients
• children younger than age 18 (safety
not established).

Administration
• Give 1 hour before or 2 hours after a
meal.
• Know that contents of capsules may
be mixed with applesauce.
• Don't crush capsules or pellets.
• Be aware that hypomagnesemia has
been reported rarely in patients treated
with proton pump inhibitors for at
least 3 months. For patients expected
to be on prolonged treatment or who
take proton pump inhibitors with

drugs such as digoxin or drugs that
may cause hypomagnesemia (such as
diuretics), consider monitoring magnesium level before starting treatment.

Route	Onset	Peak	Duration
P.O.	Rapid	1.6 hr	24 hr

Adverse reactions
CNS: headache, dizziness, asthenia,
vertigo, apathy, anxiety, paresthesia,
insomnia, abnormal dreams
EENT: sinusitis, epistaxis
GI: nausea, vomiting, diarrhea, constipation, abdominal pain, flatulence, dry
mouth
Metabolic: hypomagnesemia
Musculoskeletal: hip, wrist, spine fractures (with long-term daily use)
Respiratory: upper respiratory tract
infection, cough
Skin: rash, inflammation, urticaria,
pruritus, alopecia, dry skin

Interactions
Drug-drug. *CYP2C19 or CYP3A4
inducers (such as rifampin):* reduced
esomeprazole level
Digoxin, iron salts, ketoconazole: altered
absorption and effects of these drugs
Methotrexate: increased serum
methotrexate level
Drug-diagnostic tests. *Alanine aminotransferase, alkaline phosphatase, aspartate aminotransferase, bilirubin, creatinine, uric acid:* increased levels
*Hemoglobin, platelets, potassium,
sodium, thyroxine, white blood cells:*
altered levels
Serum chromogranin A (CgA):
increased level (may cause false-
positive results in diagnostic investigations for neuroendocrine tumors)
Drug-herbs. *St. John's wort:* reduced
esomeprazole level

Patient monitoring
• Monitor neurologic status, especially
for dizziness, headache, paresthesia,
and asthenia.

- Watch for signs and symptoms of EENT and respiratory infections.
- Assess nutritional and hydration status in light of adverse GI effects.
- Check for rash and other signs of hypersensitivity.
- Monitor liver function test results if patient is on long-term therapy.
- Continue to monitor patients periodically who are expected to be on prolonged treatment or who take proton pump inhibitors with drugs such as digoxin or drugs that may cause hypomagnesemia.

Patient teaching
- Instruct patient to take drug 1 hour before or 2 hours after a meal.
- If patient has trouble swallowing capsule, tell him to open it, sprinkle pellets into soft food (such as applesauce), and take right away.
- Instruct patient to recognize and report signs or symptoms of hypomagnesemia.
- Caution patient to avoid driving and other hazardous activities until he knows how drug affects concentration and alertness.
- Advise female patient to tell prescriber if she's pregnant or breastfeeding.
- As appropriate, review all other significant adverse reactions and interactions, especially those related to the drugs and tests mentioned above.

estradiol
Bedol⊕, Elestrin, Elleste⊕, Elleste-Solo⊕, Estrace, Estring, Estrogel, Gynodiol, Innofem, Oestrogel⊕, Progynova⊕, Sandrena⊕, Vagifem, Zumenon⊕

estradiol acetate
Femring, Femtrace

estradiol cypionate
Depo-Estradiol

estradiol hemihydrate
Estrasorb

estradiol transdermal system
Alora, Climara, Estraderm, Estradot⊕, Evorel⊕, Fematrix⊕, Femseven⊕, Menostar, Vivelle

estradiol valerate
Climaval⊕, Delestrogen, Femogex♣

Pharmacologic class: Estrogen
Therapeutic class: Hormone
Pregnancy risk category X

FDA | BOXED WARNING
- Drug increases endometrial cancer risk in postmenopausal women.
- Drug may increase risk of cardiovascular disease, breast cancer, and dementia.
- Drug shouldn't be used during pregnancy.
- Warnings may vary somewhat among specific brands. See package insert for complete warning information.

Action
Binds to nuclear receptors in responsive tissues (such as female genital organs, breasts, and pituitary gland), enhancing DNA, RNA, and protein synthesis. In androgen-dependent prostate cancer, competes for androgen receptor sites, inhibiting androgen activity. Also decreases pituitary release of follicle-stimulating hormone and luteinizing hormone.

Availability
Injection (cypionate in oil): 5 mg/ml
Injection (valerate in oil): 10 mg/ml, 20 mg/ml, 40 mg/ml
Tablets: 0.5 mg, 1 mg, 1.5 mg, 2 mg

Tablets (film-coated): 25.8 mcg estradiol hemidrate (equivalent to 25 mcg estradiol)
Transdermal system: 25 mcg/24-hour release rate, 37.5 mcg/24-hour release rate, 50 mcg/24-hour release rate, 75 mcg/24-hour release rate, 100 mcg/24-hour release rate
Vaginal cream: 100 mcg/g
Vaginal ring: 2 mg released over 90 days
Vaginal tablets: 10 mcg

⊘ Indications and dosages

➤ Symptoms of menopause, atrophic vaginitis, female hypogonadism, ovarian failure, and osteoporosis
Adults: 0.5 to 2 mg (estradiol) P.O. daily continuously or cyclically. Or 1 to 5 mg (cypionate) or 10 to 20 mg (valerate) I.M. monthly. Or 50- or 100-mcg/24-hour transdermal patch applied twice weekly (Alora, Estraderm) or weekly (Climara). Or 25-mcg/24-hour patch applied q 7 days (FemPatch) or 37.5- to 100-mcg transdermal patch applied twice weekly (Vivelle). Or 2 to 4 g (0.2 to 0.4 mg) vaginal cream (estradiol) applied daily for 1 to 2 weeks, then decreased to 1 to 2 g/day for 1 to 2 weeks, then a maintenance dose of 1 g one to three times weekly for 3 weeks, then off for 1 week; repeat cycle once vaginal mucosa has been restored. Or 2-mg vaginal ring q 3 months or 10-mcg vaginal tablet once daily for 2 weeks, then twice weekly.
➤ Postmenopausal breast cancer
Adults: 10 mg P.O. t.i.d. (estradiol)
➤ Prostate cancer
Adults: 1 to 2 mg P.O. t.i.d. (estradiol) or 30 mg I.M. q 1 to 2 weeks (valerate)

Contraindications

• Hypersensitivity to drug or its components
• Thromboembolic disease (current or previous)
• Undiagnosed vaginal bleeding
• Breast or reproductive system cancer (except in metastatic disease)
• Estrogen-dependent neoplasms
• Pregnancy

Precautions

Use cautiously in:
• cardiovascular, hepatic, or renal disease
• breastfeeding patients.

Administration

• Inject I.M. dose deep into large muscle mass; rotate injection sites.
• If switching from oral to transdermal estrogen, apply patch 1 week after withdrawal of oral therapy.

Route	Onset	Peak	Duration
P.O.	Slow	Days	Unknown
I.M.	Unknown	Unknown	Unknown
Transdermal	Unknown	Unknown	3-4 days (Estraderm) 7 days (Climara)
Vaginal ring	Unknown	Unknown	90 days
Vaginal tablet	Unknown	Unknown	3-4 days

Adverse reactions

CNS: headache, dizziness, lethargy, depression
CV: hypertension, **myocardial infarction (MI), thromboembolism**
EENT: contact lens intolerance, worsening of myopia or astigmatism
GI: nausea, vomiting, **bowel obstruction with vaginal ring (rare)**
GU: amenorrhea, dysmenorrhea, breakthrough bleeding, cervical erosions, decreased libido, vaginal candidiasis, erectile dysfunction, testicular atrophy, gynecomastia, breast pain or tenderness
Hepatic: jaundice
Metabolic: sodium and fluid retention, hypercalcemia, hyperglycemia
Musculoskeletal: leg cramps
Skin: oily skin, acne, pigmentation changes, urticaria

Reactions in **bold** are life-threatening.   ◀€ Clinical alert

Other: weight loss or gain, edema, increased appetite, **toxic shock syndrome with vaginal ring (rare)**

Interactions

Drug-drug. *Insulin, oral hypoglycemics, warfarin:* altered requirements for these drugs

Drug-diagnostic tests. *Antithrombin III, folate, low-density lipoproteins, pyridoxine, total cholesterol, urine pregnanediol:* decreased levels

Cortisol; factors VII, VIII, IX, and X; glucose; high-density lipoproteins; phospholipids; prolactin; prothrombin; sodium; triglycerides: increased levels

Metyrapone test: false decrease

Thyroid function tests: false interpretation

Drug-behaviors. *Smoking:* increased risk of adverse CV reactions

Patient monitoring

◀€ Monitor vital signs and cardiovascular status, especially for hypertension, thromboembolism, and MI.

• Be aware that a few cases of ring adherence to the vaginal wall have occurred, which may require evaluation of wall ulceration and erosion.

• Assess vision.

• In diabetic patient, monitor blood glucose level and watch for signs and symptoms of hyperglycemia.

Patient teaching

• Instruct patient to place transdermal patch on clean, dry skin area.

• Teach proper technique for use of vaginal tablet, ring, or cream, as appropriate.

• Tell patient drug may cause loss of libido (in women) or erectile dysfunction (in men). Encourage patient to discuss these issues with prescriber.

◀€ Teach patient to recognize and immediately report signs and symptoms of thromboembolism.

◀€ Caution patient not to take drug if she is or plans to become pregnant.

• Advise patient that drug may worsen nearsightedness or astigmatism and make contact lenses uncomfortable.

• As appropriate, review all other significant and life-threatening adverse reactions and interactions, especially those related to the drugs, tests, and behaviors mentioned above.

estrogens, conjugated

C.E.S.♣, Congest♣, Premarin, Premarin Intravenous

Pharmacologic class: Estrogen

Therapeutic class: Replacement hormone, antineoplastic, antiosteoporotic

Pregnancy risk category X

FDA | BOXED WARNING

• Drug increases endometrial cancer risk in postmenopausal women who use unopposed estrogens. Adding a progestin to estrogen therapy has been shown to reduce risk of endometrial hyperplasia, which may be a precursor to endometrial cancer. Adequate diagnostic measures, including directed or random endometrial sampling when indicated, should be undertaken to rule out malignancy in postmenopausal women with undiagnosed persistent or recurring abnormal genital bleeding.

• Drug may increase risk of cardiovascular disease, breast cancer, and dementia. Estrogen-alone therapy shouldn't be used to prevent cardiovascular disease or dementia. The Women's Health Initiative (WHI) estrogen-alone substudy reported increased risks of stroke and deep vein thrombosis (DVT) in postmenopausal women (ages 50 to 79) during 6.8 years and 7.1 years, respectively, of treatment with daily oral conjugated estrogens 0.625 mg, relative to placebo. The estrogen plus progestin substudy of WHI reported increased risks of myocardial infarction, stroke, invasive breast cancer, pulmonary emboli, and DVT in postmenopausal women (ages 50 to 79) during 5.6 years of treatment with daily conjugated estrogen 0.625 mg combined with medroxyprogesterone acetate 2.5 mg, relative to placebo. The WHI Memory Study estrogen-alone ancillary study, a substudy of WHI, reported an increased risk of developing probable dementia in postmenopausal women age 65 or older. It's unknown if this finding applies to younger postmenopausal women.

• In the absence of comparable data, these risks should be assumed to be similar for other dosages of conjugated estrogens and other dosage forms of estrogens. Because of these risks, estrogens with or without progestins should be prescribed at lowest effective dosages and for shortest duration consistent with treatment goals and risks for the individual woman.

Action
Bind to nuclear receptors in responsive tissues (such as female genital organs, breasts, and pituitary gland), enhancing DNA, RNA, and protein synthesis. In androgen-dependent prostate cancer, compete for androgen receptor sites, inhibiting androgen activity. Also decrease pituitary release of follicle-stimulating and luteinizing hormones.

Availability
Powder for injection: 25 mg/5 ml
Tablets: 0.3 mg, 0.625 mg, 0.9 mg, 1.25 mg
Vaginal cream: 0.625 mg/g

✍ Indications and dosages
➤ Ovariectomy; primary ovarian failure
Adults: 1.25 mg P.O. daily continuously or in cycles of 3 weeks on and 1 week off
➤ Osteoporosis and menopausal symptoms
Adults: 0.3 to 1.25 mg P.O. daily continuously or in cycles of 3 weeks on and 1 week off
➤ Female hypogonadism
Adults: 0.3 to 0.625 mg P.O. daily, given in cycles of 3 weeks on and 1 week off
➤ Inoperable breast cancer in men and postmenopausal women
Adults: 10 mg P.O. t.i.d. for 3 months or more
➤ Inoperable prostate carcinoma
Adults: 1.25 to 2.5 mg P.O. t.i.d.
➤ Uterine bleeding caused by hormonal imbalance
Adults: 25 mg I.M. or I.V., repeated in 6 to 12 hours if necessary
➤ Atrophic vaginitis, kraurosis vulvae
Adults: 0.5 to 2 g (vaginal cream) intravaginally daily in cycles of 3 weeks on and 1 week off
➤ Moderate to severe dyspareunia
Adults: 0.5 g (vaginal cream) intravaginally daily in cycles of 3 weeks on and 1 week off

Contraindications
• Hypersensitivity to drug or its components
• Thromboembolic disease (current or previous)
• Undiagnosed vaginal bleeding
• Breast or reproductive system cancer (except metastatic disease)
• Estrogen-dependent neoplasms
• Pregnancy

Precautions
Use cautiously in:
• cardiovascular disease, severe hepatic or renal disease, asthma, bone disease, migraine, seizures, breast disease

---

- family history of breast or genital tract cancer
- breastfeeding patients.

Administration

- Know that drug is compatible with dextrose 5% in water and normal saline solution.

Route	Onset	Peak	Duration
P.O., I.M.	Unknown	Unknown	6-12 hr
I.V.	Rapid	Unknown	6-12 hr
Intravaginal	Unknown	Unknown	Unknown

Adverse reactions

CNS: headache, dizziness, lethargy, depression, asthenia, paresthesia, syncope, **cerebrovascular accident (CVA), seizures**

CV: hypertension, chest pain, **myocardial infarction (MI), thromboembolism**

EENT: contact lens intolerance, worsening of myopia or astigmatism, otitis media, sinusitis, rhinitis, pharyngitis

GI: nausea, vomiting, diarrhea, abdominal cramps, bloating, enlarged abdomen, dyspepsia, flatulence, gastritis, gastroenteritis, hemorrhoids, colitis, gallbladder disease, anorexia, **pancreatitis**

GU: urinary incontinence, dysuria, urinary tract infection, amenorrhea, dysmenorrhea, endometrial hyperplasia, vaginal candidiasis, leukorrhea, vaginal hemorrhage, genital eruptions, gynecomastia, breast tenderness, breast enlargement or secretion, reduced libido, erectile dysfunction, testicular atrophy, **increased risk of breast cancer, endometrial cancer, hemolytic uremic syndrome**

Hepatic: cholestatic jaundice, **hepatic adenoma**

Metabolic: hyperglycemia, hypercalcemia, sodium and fluid retention, reduced carbohydrate tolerance

Musculoskeletal: leg cramps, back pain, skeletal pain

Respiratory: upper respiratory tract infection, bronchitis, **pulmonary embolism**

Skin: acne, oily skin, pigmentation changes, urticaria, pruritus, erythema nodosum, hemorrhagic eruption, skin hypertrophy, hirsutism, alopecia, **erythema multiforme**

Other: edema, weight changes, increased appetite, hypersensitivity reaction, **angioedema**

Interactions

Drug-drug. *Corticosteroids:* enhanced corticosteroid effects

CYP450 inducers (such as barbiturates, rifampin): decreased estrogen efficacy

Hypoglycemics, warfarin: altered requirement for these drugs

Phenytoin: loss of seizure control

Tamoxifen: interference with tamoxifen effects

Tricyclic antidepressants: reduced antidepressant effects

Drug-diagnostic tests. *Antithrombin III, folate, low-density lipoproteins, pyridoxine, total cholesterol, urine pregnanediol:* decreased values

Cortisol; factors VII, VIII, IX, and X; glucose; high-density lipoproteins; phospholipids; prolactin; prothrombin; sodium; triglycerides: increased values

Metyrapone test: false decrease

Thyroid function tests: false interpretation

Drug-food. *Caffeine:* increased caffeine blood level

Drug-herbs. *Black cohosh:* increased risk of adverse reactions

Red clover: interference with estrogen effects

Saw palmetto: antiestrogenic effects

St. John's wort: decreased drug blood level and effects

Drug-behaviors. *Smoking:* increased risk of adverse cardiovascular reactions

---

Patient monitoring

• Monitor liver function test results and assess abdomen for enlarged liver.

• Evaluate patient for breast tenderness and swelling. As needed, give analgesics and apply cool compresses.

• Monitor fluid intake and output, and weigh patient daily.

◀℥ Know that drug increases risk of thromboembolism, CVA, and MI.

• Be aware that exogenous estrogens may induce or exacerbate symptoms of angioedema, particularly in women with hereditary angioedema.

• Check serum phosphatase level in patients with prostate cancer.

• Monitor calcium, glucose, and folic acid levels.

• Evaluate bone density annually.

Patient teaching

◀℥ Teach patient to recognize and report signs and symptoms of thromboembolism.

◀℥ Caution patient not to take drug if she is or plans to become pregnant.

• Tell patient to report breakthrough vaginal bleeding.

• Recommend that patient have routine breast examinations.

• As appropriate, review all other significant and life-threatening adverse reactions and interactions, especially those related to the drugs, tests, foods, herbs, and behaviors mentioned above.

estrogens, esterified
Menest

Pharmacologic class: Estrogen

Therapeutic class: Replacement hormone, antineoplastic, antiosteoporotic

Pregnancy risk category X

Action

Bind to nuclear receptors in responsive tissues (such as female genital organs, breasts, and pituitary gland), enhancing DNA, RNA, and protein synthesis. In androgen-dependent prostate cancer, compete for androgen receptor sites, inhibiting androgen activity. Also decrease pituitary release of follicle-stimulating hormone and luteinizing hormone.

Availability

Tablets: 0.3 mg, 0.625 mg, 1.25 mg, 2.5 mg

⍟ Indications and dosages

➤ Moderate to severe vasomotor symptoms or atrophic vaginitis

Adults: 0.3 to 1.25 mg P.O. daily, adjusted to lowest effective dosage; usually given in cycles of 3 weeks on, 1 week off

➤ Female hypogonadism

Adults: 2.5 to 7.5 mg P.O. daily in divided doses for 20 days, followed by 10-day rest period. If no bleeding occurs, repeat same dosing schedule. If bleeding occurs before end of rest period, start 20-day estrogen-progestin cycle, with progestin P.O. given during last 5 days of estrogen therapy.

➤ Inoperable prostate cancer

Adults: 1.25 to 2.5 mg P.O. t.i.d.

➤ Selected breast cancers (inoperable, progressing)

Adults: 10 mg P.O. t.i.d. for at least 3 months
➤ Prevention of osteoporosis
Adults: Initially, 0.3 mg P.O. daily, increased as needed to a maximum of 1.25 mg/day

Contraindications
• Hypersensitivity to drug or its components
• Thromboembolic disease (current or previous)
• Undiagnosed vaginal bleeding
• Breast and reproductive cancers (except metastatic disease)
• Estrogen-dependent neoplasms
• Pregnancy

Precautions
Use cautiously in:
• cardiovascular disease, severe hepatic or renal disease, asthma, bone disease, migraines, seizures, breast nodules, fibrocystic breasts
• family history of breast or genital tract cancer
• breastfeeding patients.

Administration
• Administer with food or fluids.
• Give cyclically as prescribed, except when used palliatively for cancer treatment.

Route	Onset	Peak	Duration
P.O.	Slow	Days	Unknown

Adverse reactions
CNS: headache, dizziness, lethargy, depression, asthenia, paresthesia, syncope, **increased risk of cerebrovascular accident (CVA), seizures**
CV: hypertension, chest pain, **myocardial infarction (MI), thromboembolism**
EENT: contact lens intolerance, worsening of myopia or astigmatism, otitis media, sinusitis, rhinitis, pharyngitis
GI: nausea, vomiting, diarrhea, dyspepsia, flatulence, gastritis, gastroenteritis, enlarged abdomen, hemorrhoids, colitis, gallbladder disease, anorexia, **pancreatitis**
GU: urinary incontinence, dysuria, amenorrhea, dysmenorrhea, endometrial hyperplasia, urinary tract infection, leukorrhea, vaginal discomfort or pain, vaginal hemorrhage, genital eruptions, gynecomastia, breast tenderness, breast enlargement or secretion, reduced libido, erectile dysfunction, testicular atrophy, **increased risk of breast cancer, endometrial cancer, hemolytic uremic syndrome**
Hepatic: cholestatic jaundice, **hepatic adenoma**
Metabolic: hyperglycemia, hypercalcemia, sodium and fluid retention, reduced carbohydrate tolerance
Musculoskeletal: leg cramps, back pain, skeletal pain
Respiratory: upper respiratory tract infection, bronchitis, **pulmonary embolism**
Skin: acne, increased pigmentation, urticaria, pruritus, erythema nodosum, hemorrhagic eruption, alopecia, hirsutism
Other: increased appetite, weight changes, edema, flulike symptoms, hypersensitivity reactions

Interactions
Drug-drug. *Corticosteroids:* enhanced corticosteroid effects
CYP450 inducers (such as barbiturates, rifampin): decreased estrogen efficacy
Hypoglycemics, warfarin: altered requirement for these drugs
Phenytoin: loss of seizure control
Tamoxifen: interference with tamoxifen efficacy
Tricyclic antidepressants: reduced antidepressant effect
Drug-diagnostic tests. *Antithrombin III, folate, low-density lipoproteins, pyridoxine, total cholesterol, urine pregnanediol:* decreased values
Cortisol; factors VII, VIII, IX, and X; glucose; high-density lipoproteins;

---

phospholipids; prolactin; prothrombin; sodium; triglycerides: increased values
Metyrapone test: false decrease
Thyroid function tests: false interpretation
Drug-food. *Caffeine:* increased caffeine blood level
Drug-herbs. *Black cohosh:* increased risk of adverse reactions
Red clover: interference with estrogen therapy
Saw palmetto: antiestrogenic effects
St. John's wort: decreased drug blood level and effects
Drug-behaviors. *Smoking:* increased risk of adverse cardiovascular reactions

Patient monitoring

• Monitor fluid intake and output, and weigh patient daily.
• Evaluate patient for breast tenderness and swelling. As needed, administer analgesics and apply cool compresses.
◀€ Know that drug increases risk of thromboembolism, CVA, and MI.
• Monitor liver function test results, and assess abdomen for enlarged liver.
• Check serum phosphatase level in patients with prostate cancer, and adjust dosage as appropriate.
• Monitor calcium, glucose, and folic acid levels.

Patient teaching

◀€ Teach patient to recognize and immediately report signs and symptoms of thromboembolism.
◀€ Caution patient not to take drug if she is or plans to become pregnant.
• Teach patient how to perform breast self-examination. Emphasize importance of monthly checks.
• Tell patient to report breakthrough vaginal bleeding.
• Mention that drug may cause contact lens intolerance. Advise patient to report vision changes.

• Inform male patient that drug may cause gynecomastia.
• As appropriate, review all other significant and life-threatening adverse reactions and interactions, especially those related to the drugs, tests, foods, herbs, and behaviors mentioned above.

eszopiclone
Lunesta

Pharmacologic class: Nonbenzodiazepine
Therapeutic class: Hypnotic
Controlled substance schedule IV
Pregnancy risk category C

Action

Unclear. Effect may result from interaction with GABA-receptor complexes at binding domains near or allosterically coupled with benzodiazepine receptors.

Availability

Tablets: 1 mg, 2 mg, 3 mg

Indications and dosages

➤ Insomnia

Nonelderly adults: 2 mg P.O. immediately before bedtime. Drug may be initiated at, or dosage may be increased to, 3 mg if indicated clinically. In patients also receiving potent CYP3A4 inhibitors, starting dosage shouldn't exceed 1 mg.

Elderly adults: 1 mg P.O. immediately before bedtime. Dosage may be increased to 2 mg if indicated clinically. If patient's chief complaint is difficulty staying asleep, recommended dosage is 2 mg P.O. immediately before bedtime.

Dosage adjustment

• Hepatic impairment
• Concomitant use of other CNS depressants

Reactions in **bold** are life-threatening.   ◀€ Clinical alert

Contraindications
None

Precautions
Use cautiously in:
- hepatic impairment, respiratory compromise, depression
- pregnant or breastfeeding patients
- children younger than age 18 (safety and efficacy not established).

Administration
- Don't give with or immediately after a heavy, high-fat meal because this may slow drug absorption and reduce efficacy.

Route	Onset	Peak	Duration
P.O.	Unknown	1 hr	6 hr

Adverse reactions
CNS: headache, anxiety, confusion, depression, dizziness, hallucinations, nervousness, abnormal dreams
CV: chest pain, peripheral edema
GI: nausea, vomiting, diarrhea, dyspepsia, cholelithiasis, dry mouth
GU: urinary tract infection, decreased libido, dysmenorrhea, gynecomastia (in males)
Respiratory: respiratory infection
Skin: rash, pruritus
Other: unpleasant taste, viral infection, neuralgia, facial edema, allergic reaction

Interactions
Drug-drug. *CYP3A4 inhibitors (such as itraconazole, ketoconazole, ritonavir, troleandomycin):* increased eszopiclone blood level
CYP3A4 inducers (such as rifampin): decreased eszopiclone blood level
Drug-food. *Heavy, high-fat meal:* slowed drug absorption and reduced efficacy
Drug-behaviors. *Alcohol use:* additive effects on psychomotor performance

Patient monitoring
- Before starting therapy, evaluate patient to help eliminate physical or psychiatric causes of insomnia.
- Know that after rapid dosage decrease or abrupt drug withdrawal, patient may experience signs and symptoms similar to those associated with withdrawal from other CNS depressants.

Patient teaching
- Instruct patient not to take drug with or immediately after a heavy, high-fat meal.
- Advise patient to take drug immediately before bedtime; otherwise, short-term memory impairment, hallucinations, incoordination, dizziness, and light-headedness may occur.
- Caution patient not to engage in hazardous activities after taking drug.
- Tell patient drug may have some effect the next day; advise him to use extreme care when driving or performing other hazardous activities until drug effects are known.
- Caution patient not to take drug with other psychotropics, anticonvulsants, antihistamines, or other drugs that cause CNS depression.
- Advise patient not to take drug with alcohol.
- As appropriate, review all other significant adverse reactions and interactions, especially those related to the drugs, foods, and behaviors mentioned above.

etanercept
Enbrel

Pharmacologic class: Immunomodulator
Therapeutic class: Antiarthritic
Pregnancy risk category B

• Patients treated with etanercept are at increased risk for developing serious infections that may lead to hospitalization or death. Most patients who developed these infections were taking concomitant immunosuppressants, such as methotrexate or corticosteroids. Etanercept should be discontinued if patient develops a serious infection or sepsis. Reported infections include:

Active tuberculosis (TB), including reactivation of latent TB. Patients have frequently presented with disseminated or extrapulmonary disease. Patients should be tested for latent TB before etanercept use and during therapy. Treatment for latent infection should be initiated before etanercept use.

Invasive fungal infections, including histoplasmosis, coccidioidomycosis, candidiasis, aspergillosis, blastomycosis, and pneumocystosis. Patients with histoplasmosis or other invasive fungal infections may present with disseminated, rather than localized, disease. Antigen and antibody testing for histoplasmosis may be negative in some patients with active infection. Empiric antifungal therapy should be considered in patients at risk for invasive fungal infections who develop severe systemic illness.

Bacterial, viral, and other infections due to opportunistic pathogens, including *Legionella* and *Listeria* species.

• Risks and benefits of treatment with etanercept should be carefully considered before starting therapy in patients with chronic or recurrent infection.

• Closely monitor patients for signs and symptoms of infection during and after treatment with etanercept, including the possible development of TB in patients who tested negative for latent TB before starting therapy.

• Lymphoma and other malignancies, some fatal, have been reported in children and adolescents treated with tumor necrosis factor blockers, including etanercept.

Action
Reacts with and deactivates free-floating tumor necrosis factor, responsible for inflammation

Availability
Powder for injection: 25 mg in multiple-use vial
Prefilled syringe (single-use): 50 mg/ml

⊘ Indications and dosages
➤ Moderately to severely active rheumatoid arthritis; ankylosing spondylitis; psoriatric arthritis
Adults: 50 mg subcutaneously q week given as a single injection. Dosages above 50 mg/week are not recommended.
➤ Chronic moderate to severe plaque psoriasis
Adults ages 18 and older: 50 mg subcutaneously twice weekly (given 3 or 4 days apart) for 3 months, followed by reduction to a maintenance dosage of 50 mg weekly
➤ Polyarticular-course juvenile rheumatoid arthritis
Children ages 4 to 17: 0.8 mg/kg subcutaneously q week, to a maximum of 50 mg weekly

Contraindications
• Hypersensitivity to drug or its components
• Sepsis

Precautions
Use cautiously in:
• immunosuppression, chronic infection, heart failure

- latex allergy (needle cover of diluent syringe contains latex)
- elderly patients
- pregnant or breastfeeding patients
- children younger than age 4.

Administration

- Inject subcutaneously into thigh, abdomen, or upper arm.
- For adult, use single-use, 50 mg/ml prefilled syringe.
- For child weighing 63 kg (138 lb) or more, use single-use, 50 mg/ml pre-filled syringe for weekly dose; for child weighing 31 to 62 kg (68 to 137 lb), administer total weekly dose from multiple-use vial as two injections on same day or 3 or 4 days apart; for child weighing less than 31 kg (68 lb), give as a single weekly injection using multiple-use vial.
- Rotate injection sites.

Route	Onset	Peak	Duration
Subcut.	Slow	72 hr	Unknown

Adverse reactions

CNS: asthenia, headache, depression, dizziness, paresthesia, fatigue, demyelinating disorders (such as multiple sclerosis and myelitis), **cerebral hemorrhage, seizures, cerebrovascular accident (CVA)**

CV: hypotension, hypertension, chest pain, **deep-vein thrombosis, thrombophlebitis, myocardial ischemia, myocardial infarction (MI), heart failure**

EENT: ocular inflammation, pharyngitis, rhinitis, sinusitis

GI: nausea, vomiting, diarrhea, abdominal pain, dyspepsia, anorexia, cholecystitis, **abdominal abscess, GI hemorrhage, intestinal perforation, pancreatitis**

GU: pyelonephritis, membranous glomerulonephropathy

Hematologic: anemia, **aplastic anemia, leukopenia, pancytopenia, thrombocytopenia**

Metabolic: hypomagnesemia

Musculoskeletal: bursitis, polymyositis, joint pain

Respiratory: cough, congestion, dyspnea, bronchitis, pneumonia, **pulmonary embolism, interstitial lung disease**

Skin: flushing, cellulitis, pruritus, rash, cutaneous vasculitis, urticaria, alopecia, angioedema

Other: altered taste, weight gain, adenopathy, fever, irritation at injection site, peripheral edema, flulike symptoms, autoantibody formation, **lupus-like syndrome, serious infections, malignancies**

Interactions

None significant

Patient monitoring

◀€ Watch for signs and symptoms of malignancies, pancytopenia and infection.

◀€ Monitor for evidence of GI bleeding, lupus-like syndrome, and serious hypersensitivity reactions. Stop therapy immediately if these occur.

- Monitor CBC and coagulation studies.

◀€ Check for signs and symptoms of cardiac compromise and cerebrovascular events.

- Monitor pulmonary function test results periodically to assess lung status.
- Assess patient's ability to self-administer drug.
- Check for irritation at injection site. As needed, apply cool compresses.
- Examine eyes for conjunctival dryness. As needed, apply artificial tears.

Patient teaching

◀€ Tell patient to withhold dose and contact prescriber if he develops signs or symptoms of infection or is exposed to anyone with chickenpox.

◀◤ Tell patient to immediately report hypersensitivity reaction, neurologic or respiratory problems, sudden weight gain, chest pain, or easy bruising or bleeding.
• Teach patient or caregiver how to administer drug and handle and dispose of equipment.
• Caution patient not to get live-virus vaccines.
• Tell female to inform prescriber if she is pregnant or breastfeeding.
• Advise patient to expect redness, swelling, and pain at injection site. Assure him that these problems will diminish over time.
• As appropriate, review all other significant and life-threatening adverse reactions mentioned above.

ethambutol hydrochloride
Etibi✸, Myambutol

Pharmacologic class: Synthetic anti-tubercular
Therapeutic class: Antitubercular, antileprotic
Pregnancy risk category B

Action
Unknown. Thought to interfere with RNA synthesis of bacterial metabolites, decreasing mycobacterial replication.

Availability
Tablets: 100 mg, 400 mg

🕭 Indications and dosages
➢ Adjunct in tuberculosis and atypical mycobacterial infection caused by *Mycobacterium tuberculosis*
Adults and adolescents: In patients who haven't received previous antitubercular therapy, 15 mg/kg P.O. daily. In patients who have received previous antitubercular therapy, 25 mg/kg P.O. daily, decreased after 60 days to 15 mg/kg daily.

Dosage adjustment
• Renal impairment

Contraindications
• Hypersensitivity to drug

Precautions
Use cautiously in:
• impaired renal or hepatic function, cataracts, optic neuritis, recurrent eye inflammation, diabetic retinopathy, gout
• pregnant patients
• children younger than age 13.

Administration
• Obtain specimens for culture and sensitivity testing, as necessary, before starting therapy and periodically throughout therapy.
• Give with food.

Route	Onset	Peak	Duration
P.O.	Rapid	2-4 hr	24 hr

Adverse reactions
CNS: confusion, disorientation, malaise, dizziness, hallucinations, headache, peripheral neuritis
EENT: optic neuritis, blurred vision, decreased visual acuity, red-green color blindness, eye pain
GI: nausea, vomiting, abdominal pain, GI upset, anorexia
Hematologic: eosinophilia, **thrombocytopenia**
Hepatic: transient hepatic impairment
Metabolic: hyperuricemia, **hypoglycemia**
Musculoskeletal: joint pain, gouty arthritis
Respiratory: bloody sputum, **pulmonary infiltrates**
Skin: rash, pruritus, toxic epidermal necrolysis
Other: fever, **anaphylactoid reactions**

e

Reactions in **bold** are life-threatening.   ◀◤ Clinical alert

Interactions
Drug-drug. *Aluminum salts:* delayed and reduced ethambutol absorption
Other neurotoxic drugs: increased risk of neurotoxicity
Drug-diagnostic tests. *Alanine aminotransferase, aspartate aminotransferase, bilirubin, uric acid:* increased levels
Glucose: decreased level

Patient monitoring
◀℥ Watch for serious adverse reactions, such as thrombocytopenia, respiratory problems, and anaphylactoid reactions.
• Monitor liver function tests, CBC, and blood urea nitrogen, creatinine glucose, and serum uric acid levels.
• Give analgesics for drug-induced pain, as prescribed.
• Observe for signs and symptoms of gout.

Patient teaching
• Instruct patient to take with 8 oz of water. If stomach upset occurs, advise him to take with food.
• If patient must take antacids, advise him to take only aluminum-free antacids.
◀℥ Tell patient to immediately report easy bruising or bleeding, respiratory problems, or signs and symptoms of hypersensitivity reactions.
• Advise patient to report vision changes and to have annual eye exams. Reassure him that visual disturbances will subside within several weeks to months after drug is discontinued.
• As appropriate, review all other significant and life-threatening adverse reactions and interactions, especially those related to the drugs and tests mentioned above.

etidronate disodium
Didronel, Didronel PMO ✙

Pharmacologic class: Bisphosphonate
Therapeutic class: Bone resorption inhibitor, hypocalcemic agent
Pregnancy risk category B

Action
Blocks calcium absorption, slowing bone metabolism and reducing bone resorption and formation

Availability
Tablets: 200 mg, 400 mg

🔥 Indications and dosages
➤ Paget's disease
Adults: 5 to 10 mg/kg P.O. daily as a single dose for up to 6 months, or 11 to 20 mg/kg P.O. daily for up to 3 months
➤ Heterotopic ossification after hip replacement
Adults: 20 mg/kg P.O. daily for 1 month before and 3 months after surgery
➤ Heterotopic ossification in spinal cord injury
Adults: Initially, 20 mg/kg P.O. daily for 2 weeks, decreased to 10 mg/kg P.O. daily for 10 weeks

Dosage adjustment
• Decreased glomerular filtration rate

Contraindications
• Hypersensitivity to drug or its components
• Abnormalities of esophagus, such as stricture or achalasia, that delay esophageal emptying
• Osteomalacia

Precautions
Use cautiously in:
• renal impairment, long bone fractures, active upper GI condition (such as Barrett's esophagus, dysphagia,

other esophageal diseases, gastritis, duodenitis, or ulcers)
• pregnant or breastfeeding patients
• children (safety not established).

Administration

• Give with 6 to 8 oz of water 2 hours before first meal.
• Make sure patient doesn't eat for 2 hours after receiving dose.
• Know that therapy longer than 3 months is not recommended.

Route	Onset	Peak	Duration
P.O. (Paget's)	1 mo	Unknown	1 yr
P.O. (ossif.)	Unknown	Unknown	Several mo

Adverse reactions

GI: nausea, constipation, stomatitis, diarrhea, esophageal irritation
Metabolic: hyperphosphatemia
Musculoskeletal: bone pain and tenderness, fractures, osteonecrosis of the jaw
Skin: rash

Interactions

Drug-drug. *Warfarin:* increased prothrombin time
Drug-diagnostic tests. *Serum phosphorus:* increased level

Patient monitoring

• Monitor fluid intake and output.
• Monitor patient for GI discomfort. Divide doses as needed to ease symptoms.
• Assess bowel pattern. If constipation occurs, increase fluids and administer stool softeners, as prescribed.
• Closely monitor renal function tests and serum phosphorus level.

Patient teaching

• Instruct patient to take drug first thing in morning on an empty stomach, with 6 to 8 oz of water only and to stay upright for at least 30 minutes afterward.
• Instruct patient not to take drug with food because of decreased drug absorption.
• Tell patient not to consume high-calcium products, such as milk or antacids, or vitamins and mineral supplements high in calcium, iron, magnesium, or aluminum, within 2 hours of taking dose.
◀≶ Tell patient to immediately discontinue drug and notify prescriber if severe chest pain, difficulty or painful swallowing, or new or worsening heartburn occurs.
• Advise patient to report bone pain or decreased range of motion.
• As appropriate, review all other significant adverse reactions and interactions, especially those related to the drugs and tests mentioned above.

etodolac

Apo-Etodolac✦, Eccoxolac⊕, Gen-Etodolac✦, Taro-Ultradol, Ultradol✦

Pharmacologic class: Pyranocarboxylic acid, nonsteroidal anti-inflammatory drug (NSAID)

Therapeutic class: Nonopioid analgesic

Pregnancy risk category C (first and second trimesters), *D* (third trimester)

FDA BOXED WARNING

• Drug may increase risk of serious cardiovascular thrombotic events, myocardial infarction, and stroke, which can be fatal. Risk may increase with duration of use. Patients with cardiovascular disease or risk factors for it may be at greater risk.

- Drug is contraindicated for perioperative pain in setting of coronary artery bypass graft surgery.
- Drug increases risk of serious adverse GI events, including bleeding, ulcers, and perforation of stomach or intestines, which can be fatal. Elderly patients are at greater risk.

Action
Blocks activity of cyclooxygenase (which is needed for prostaglandin synthesis), easing pain and reducing inflammation

Availability
Capsules: 200 mg, 300 mg
Tablets: 400 mg, 500 mg
Tablets (extended-release): 400 mg, 500 mg, 600 mg

⦸ Indications and dosages
➤ Osteoarthritis; rheumatoid arthritis
Adults: 300 mg P.O. two or three times daily; or 400 mg, 500 mg, or 600 mg P.O. b.i.d.; or 400 to 1,000 mg P.O. (extended-release tablets) once daily
➤ Mild to moderate pain
Adults: 200 to 400 mg P.O. q 6 to 8 hours, not to exceed 1,200 mg/day

Contraindications
- Hypersensitivity to drug or its components
- Concurrent use of other NSAIDs
- Active GI bleeding or ulcer disease

Precautions
Use cautiously in:
- severe cardiovascular, renal, or hepatic disease
- elderly patients
- breastfeeding patients
- children (safety not established).

Administration
- Give with food or antacids to reduce GI upset.

- Make sure patient swallows extended-release tablets whole without crushing or chewing.
- Withhold drug several days before invasive surgery, as ordered.

Route	Onset	Peak	Duration
P.O.	30 min	1-2 hr	4-12 hr
P.O. (extended)	Unknown	3-12 hr	6-12 hr

Adverse reactions
CNS: dizziness, malaise, weakness, depression, nervousness
CV: hypertension
EENT: blurred vision, tinnitus
GI: nausea, vomiting, constipation, diarrhea, flatulence, dyspepsia, peptic ulcer, duodenitis, intestinal ulceration, gastritis, melena
GU: dysuria, urinary frequency, polyuria, **renal failure**
Hematologic: thrombocytopenia
Hepatic: cholestatic jaundice, **cholestatic hepatitis, hepatic necrosis**
Skin: rash, skin peeling, cutaneous vasculitis with purpura, hyperpigmentation
Other: fluid retention, chills, fever, allergic reaction

Interactions
Drug-drug. *Aminoglycosides:* elevated aminoglycoside blood level (in premature infants)
Anticoagulants: prolonged prothrombin time
Beta-adrenergic blockers: reduced antihypertensive effect
Bisphosphonates: increased risk of gastric ulcers
Cholestyramine: decreased etodolac absorption
Cyclosporine: increased risk of nephrotoxicity
Diuretics: decreased diuretic effect
Lithium: increased lithium blood level, greater risk of toxicity
Methotrexate: increased risk of methotrexate toxicity

Phenylbutazone: increased etodolac effects

Phenytoin: increased phenytoin blood level

Salicylates: decreased etodolac blood level

Drug-diagnostic tests. *Bleeding time:* prolonged

Blood urea nitrogen (BUN), creatinine, hepatic enzymes: increased levels

Urine bilirubin, urine ketones: false-positive results

Drug-herbs. *Arnica, chamomile, clove, dong quai, feverfew, garlic, ginkgo, ginseng:* increased risk of bleeding

White willow: increased etodolac effects

Drug-behaviors. *Alcohol use:* increased risk of adverse effects

Sun exposure: phototoxicity

Patient monitoring

• Monitor CBC, liver function tests, BUN, creatinine level, and coagulation studies.

• Assess for GI bleeding and gastric upset. Administer antacids as needed and prescribed.

• Know that drug may cause false-positive urine bilirubin and urine ketone test results.

◀€ Monitor patient for signs and symptoms of thrombocytopenia and increased bleeding time.

• Assess for fluid retention and weigh patient daily.

• Watch for decreased blood pressure control in hypertensive patients.

Patient teaching

• Instruct patient to take with meals if possible.

• Tell patient to swallow extended-release tablets whole without crushing or chewing.

◀€ Instruct patient to immediately report unusual bleeding or bruising, change in urination pattern, unusual tiredness, or yellowing of skin or eyes.

• Advise patient to avoid activities that can cause injury.

• As appropriate, review all other significant and life-threatening adverse reactions and interactions, especially those related to the drugs, tests, herbs, and behaviors mentioned above.

etonogestrel and ethinyl estradiol vaginal ring
NuvaRing

Pharmacologic class: Sex hormone

Therapeutic class: Contraceptive

Pregnancy risk category X

FDA BOXED WARNING

• Cigarette smoking increases risk of serious cardiovascular adverse effects from combination oral contraceptive use. This risk increases with age and with heavy smoking (15 or more cigarettes daily) and is quite marked in women older than age 35. Women who use combination hormonal contraceptives, including NuvaRing, should be strongly advised not to smoke.

Action

Inhibits ovulation by altering cervical mucosa and endometrium of uterus. This inhibition prevents sperm from entering the uterus, thereby preventing implantation.

Availability

Vaginal ring: 0.12 mg etonogestrel and 0.015 mg ethinyl estradiol delivered daily over 3 weeks

⍟ Indications and dosages

➤ To prevent pregnancy

Adults: Place one ring into vagina and leave in place for 3 weeks, then remove

---

Reactions in **bold** are life-threatening.   ◀€ Clinical alert

for 1 week. Insert next ring on same day of week as in previous cycle.

Contraindications
- Hypersensitivity to drug or its components
- Breast and uterine cancers or other known or suspected estrogen-dependent neoplasms
- Valvular heart disease with complications
- Thromboembolic disease (current or previous)
- Severe hypertension
- Diabetes with vascular involvement
- Headache with focal neurologic symptoms
- Hepatic tumors, cholestatic jaundice
- Major surgery with prolonged immobilization
- Undiagnosed vaginal bleeding
- Patients older than age 35 who smoke more than 15 cigarettes daily
- Pregnancy or breastfeeding

Precautions
Use cautiously in:
- underlying cardiovascular disease, severe hepatic or renal disease, asthma, bone disease, migraines, breast disease, seizures, sexually transmitted diseases
- family history of breast or genital tract cancers.

Administration
- Be aware that the best way to insert ring is with patient lying down, squatting, or standing and one leg raised.

Route	Onset	Peak	Duration
Vaginal	Rapid	Unknown	Unknown

Adverse reactions
CNS: headache, migraines, dizziness, lethargy, depression, **increased risk of cerebrovascular accident, seizures**
CV: hypertension, **myocardial infarction, thromboembolism**
EENT: worsening of myopia or astigmatism

GI: nausea, vomiting, abdominal cramps, bloating, **pancreatitis**
GU: amenorrhea, dysmenorrhea, cervical erosion, breakthrough bleeding, loss of libido, vaginal candidiasis, erectile dysfunction, testicular atrophy, breast tenderness, breast enlargement or secretion, **increased risk of endometrial and breast cancer**
Hepatic: cholestatic jaundice, **hepatic adenoma**
Metabolic: sodium and fluid retention
Respiratory: pulmonary embolism
Other: increased appetite, weight changes, edema

Interactions
Drug-drug. *Acetaminophen:* decreased acetaminophen blood level
Anti-infectives, barbiturates, carbamazepine, fosphenytoin, rifampin: decreased contraceptive efficacy
Corticosteroids: increased corticosteroid effects
Cyclosporine: increased risk of cyclosporine toxicity
CYP3A4 inhibitors (such as itraconazole, ketoconazole): increased hormone levels
Dantrolene, other hepatotoxic drugs: increased risk of hepatotoxicity
Hypoglycemics, warfarin: altered requirements for these drugs
Miconazole (vaginal capsules): increased hormone levels
Phenytoin: loss of seizure control
Protease inhibitors: increased contraceptive metabolism
Tamoxifen: interference with tamoxifen efficacy
Tricyclic antidepressants: reduced antidepressant effects
Drug-diagnostic tests. *Antithrombin III, folate, low-density lipoproteins, pyridoxine, total cholesterol:* decreased levels
Cortisol; factors VII, VIII, IX, and X; glucose; high-density lipoproteins; phospholipids; prolactin; prothrombin; sodium; triglycerides: increased levels
Drug-food. *Caffeine:* increased caffeine blood level

♣ Canada   ⊕ UK   ⚕ Hazardous drug   ⊗ High-alert drug

Drug-herbs. *Black cohosh:* increased risk of adverse reactions
Red clover: interference with contraceptive action
Saw palmetto: antiestrogenic effects
St. John's wort: decreased contraceptive blood level and effects
Drug-behaviors. *Smoking:* increased risk of adverse cardiovascular reactions

Patient monitoring

◀≶ Monitor CNS status. Report adverse CNS reactions immediately.

◀≶ Assess blood pressure frequently. If significant elevation of blood pressure occurs, discontinue NuvaRing.

• Monitor patient for depression.

◀≶ Watch for jaundice and liver engorgement; be aware that combination hormonal contraceptives may worsen existing gallbladder disease and may accelerate development of this disease in previously asymptomatic women. Discontinue drug if jaundice develops.

◀≶ Be aware that retinal thrombosis has been associated with the use of hormonal contraceptives. Discontinue NuvaRing if unexplained partial or complete loss of vision, onset of proptosis or diplopia, papilledema, or retinal vascular lesions occur. Take appropriate diagnostic and therapeutic measures immediately.

• Monitor glucose, calcium, and electrolyte levels and lipid profile.

Patient teaching

• Explain that for continued contraception, a new implant must be inserted exactly 1 week after old one is removed, even if patient is menstruating.

• Tell patient to insert and remove ring on same day of week and at same time of day.

• Tell patient that if ring slips out, she should replace it within 3 hours to ensure adequate contraceptive protection.

• Inform patient that smoking during therapy may increase risk of blood clots, phlebitis, and stroke.

◀≶ Tell patient to immediately report signs and symptoms of depression, sudden chest pain, difficulty breathing, or yellowing of skin or eyes.

◀≶ Tell patient to stop drug and immediately report unexplained partial or complete loss of vision, onset of proptosis or diplopia, papilledema, or retinal vascular lesions.

• Teach patient how to perform breast self-examinations. Emphasize importance of monthly checks.

• Tell patient that this product doesn't protect against HIV infection (AIDS) and other sexually transmitted diseases.

• As appropriate, review all other significant and life-threatening adverse reactions and interactions, especially those related to the drugs, tests, foods, herbs, and behaviors mentioned above.

etoposide (VP-16-213)
Eposin ⊕, Toposar, VePesid

etoposide phosphate
Etopophos

Pharmacologic class: Podophyllotoxin derivative

Therapeutic class: Antineoplastic

Pregnancy risk category D

FDA BOXED WARNING

• Give under supervision of physician experienced in cancer chemotherapy. Severe myelosuppression may occur, resulting in infection or bleeding.

Action

Damages DNA before mitosis by inhibiting topoisomerase II enzyme. This action impairs DNA synthesis and inhibits selected cancer cell growth. Cell-cycle-phase specific.

Availability

Capsules: 50 mg
Injection: 20 mg/ml
Powder for injection (phosphate): 100 mg in single-dose vials

𝟘 Indications and dosages

➢ Testicular cancer
Adults: 50 to 100 mg/m² I.V. daily for 5 days. Or 100 mg/m² I.V. on days 1, 3, and 5, with course repeated q 3 to 4 weeks.
➢ Small-cell carcinoma of lung
Adults: 70 mg/m² (rounded up or down to nearest 50 mg) P.O. daily for 4 days, then a maximum of 100 mg/m² (rounded up or down to nearest 50 mg) P.O. daily for 5 days every 3 to 4 weeks. Alternatively, 35 mg/m² I.V. daily for 4 days, then a maximum of 50 mg/m² I.V. daily for 5 days q 3 to 4 weeks.

Dosage adjustment

• Renal impairment

Off-label uses

• AIDS-related Kaposi's sarcoma
• Wilms' tumor
• Neuroblastoma
• Malignant lymphoma
• Hodgkin's disease
• Ovarian neoplasms

Contraindications

• Hypersensitivity to drug or its components

Precautions

Use cautiously in:
• active infections, decreased bone marrow reserve, renal or hepatic impairment
• pregnant patients and patients with childbearing potential
• breastfeeding patients
• children (safety and efficacy not established).

Administration

• For I.V. concentrations above 0.4 mg/ml, mix each 100 mg with 250 to 500 ml of dextrose 5% in water or normal saline solution, to help prevent crystallization.
• Give I.V. infusion over 30 to 60 minutes. Don't use in-line filter.
🔊 Avoid rapid infusion, which may cause severe hypotension and bronchospasm.
• Administer with antiemetics, as prescribed.
• Wear disposable gloves when handling. If drug comes into contact with skin, wash thoroughly with soap and water.
• Be aware that drug is given with other chemotherapeutic agents.

Route	Onset	Peak	Duration
P.O., I.V.	7-14 days	9-16 days	20 days

Adverse reactions

CNS: drowsiness, fatigue, headache, vertigo, peripheral neuropathy
CV: hypotension (with I.V. use), **heart failure, myocardial infarction**
GI: nausea, vomiting, stomatitis
GU: sterility
Hematologic: anemia, **leukopenia, thrombocytopenia, bone marrow depression**
Hepatic: hepatotoxicity
Metabolic: hyperuricemia
Musculoskeletal: muscle cramps
Respiratory: pulmonary edema, bronchospasm
Other: alopecia, fever, phlebitis at I.V. site, allergic reactions including **anaphylaxis**

Interactions

Drug-drug. *Live-virus vaccines:* increased risk of adverse reactions
Other antineoplastics: additive bone marrow depression

Drug-diagnostic tests. *Hemoglobin, neutrophils, platelets, red blood cells, white blood cells:* decreased values
Uric acid: increased level

Patient monitoring

◀╠ Monitor blood pressure during and after infusion. Stop infusion if severe hypotension occurs.

• With I.V. use, monitor infusion rate closely to prevent infusion reactions.

• Throughout infusion, check I.V. site for extravasation, which may cause thrombophlebitis.

◀╠ Keep diphenhydramine, hydrocortisone, epinephrine, and artificial airway at hand in case anaphylaxis occurs.

• Assess for CNS adverse effects. Assist patient during ambulation as needed.

◀╠ Monitor for signs and symptoms of bone marrow depression.

• Monitor CBC, liver function tests, and blood urea nitrogen and creatinine levels. Report platelet count below 50,000/mm³ or neutrophil count below 500/mm³.

Patient teaching

• Instruct patient to inspect mouth daily for ulcers and bleeding gums.

◀╠ Tell patient to immediately report difficulty breathing or signs and symptoms of allergic reaction.

◀╠ Caution female of childbearing age to avoid pregnancy and breastfeeding during drug therapy.

• Instruct patient to move slowly when sitting up or standing, to avoid light-headedness or dizziness from sudden blood pressure decrease.

• Tell patient drug may cause hair loss.

• As appropriate, review all other significant and life-threatening adverse reactions and interactions, especially those related to the drugs and tests mentioned above.

etravirine
Intelence

Pharmacologic class: Nonnucleoside reverse transcriptase inhibitor (NNRTI)
Therapeutic class: Antiretroviral
Pregnancy risk category B

Action
Blocks human immunodeficiency virus (HIV) reverse transcriptase, an enzyme necessary for HIV replication. Blockade leads to reduced viral load and increased CD4+ cell count, which in turn help prevent other infections when drug is given with other antiretrovirals.

Availability
Tablets: 25 mg, 100 mg, 200 mg

⁄ Indications and dosages
➤ HIV-1 infection in antiretroviral treatment-experienced patients age 6 and older who have evidence of viral replication and HIV-1 strains resistant to an NNRTI and other antiretrovirals, given in combination with other antiretrovirals
Adults and children ages 6 to younger than 18 weighing 30 kg (66 lb) or more: 200 mg P.O. b.i.d.
Children ages 6 to younger than 18 weighing 25 kg (55 lb) to less than 30 kg: 150 mg P.O. b.i.d.
Children ages 6 to younger than 18 weighing 20 kg (44 lb) to less than 25 kg: 125 mg P.O. b.i.d.
Children ages 6 to younger than 18 weighing 16 kg (35 lb) to less than 20 kg: 100 mg P.O. b.i.d.
Children's dosages shouldn't exceed the recommended adult dosage.

Contraindications
None

Precautions

Use cautiously in:
- elderly patients
- pregnant or breastfeeding patients
- children younger than age 6 (safety and efficacy not established).

Administration

- Administer after a meal.
- 🔇 Don't give with tipranavir/ritonavir, fosamprenavir/ritonavir, atazanavir/ritonavir, protease inhibitors administered without ritonavir, other NNRTIs, or St. John's wort.

Route	Onset	Peak	Duration
P.O.	Unknown	2.5-4 hr	Unknown

Adverse reactions

CNS: paresthesia, somnolence, seizure, hypoesthesia, amnesia, hypersomnia, tremor, disorientation, insomnia, anxiety, sleep disorder, abnormal dreams, confusional state, nervousness, nightmares, fatigue, peripheral neuropathy, headache, **hemorrhagic stroke**

CV: syncope, angina pectoris, hypertension, **myocardial infarction, atrial fibrillation**

EENT: blurred vision, vertigo

GI: nausea, vomiting, diarrhea, constipation, abdominal pain, gastroesophageal reflux disease, flatulence, gastritis, abdominal distention, retching, hematemesis, stomatitis, pancreatitis, anorexia, dry mouth

GU: gynecomastia, **renal failure**

Hematologic: anemia, **hemolytic anemia**

Hepatic: cytolytic hepatitis, hepatic steatosis, hepatitis, hepatomegaly

Metabolic: diabetes mellitus, dyslipidemia, body fat redistribution or accumulation

Respiratory: exertional dyspnea, bronchospasm

Skin: rash, hyperhidrosis, prurigo, dry skin, lipohypertrophy, lipodystrophy, **Stevens-Johnson syndrome, erythema multiforme**

Other: sluggishness, night sweats, facial edema, immune reconstitution syndrome, hypersensitivity reaction, **angioneurotic edema**

Interactions

Drug-drug. *Amiodarone, bepridil, disopyramide, flecainide, lidocaine (systemic), lovastatin, mexiletine, propafenone, quinidine, simvastatin:* decreased blood levels of these drugs

Atazanavir/ritonavir: significant decrease in atazanavir blood level with loss of atazanavir therapeutic effect

Atorvastatin: possible increase in effects of both drugs

Carbamazepine, dexamethasone (systemic), efavirenz, nevirapine, phenobarbital, phenytoin, rifabutin, rifampin, rifapentine, ritonavir, tipranavir/ritonavir: significant decrease in etravirine blood level and loss of therapeutic effect

Clarithromycin: decreased clarithromycin blood level

Diazepam, fluvastatin, voriconazole, warfarin: increased blood levels of these drugs

Fluconazole, lopinavir/ritonavir, posaconazole: increased etravirine blood level

Immunosuppressants (cyclosporine, sirolimus, tacrolimus): possible change in blood levels of these drugs

Itraconazole, ketoconazole: decreased blood levels of these drugs, increased etravirine blood level

Methadone: possible change in methadone effects

Protease inhibitors (amprenavir, atazanavir, indinavir, nelfinavir) given without low-dose ritonavir: significant change in blood levels of these drugs

Saquinavir/ritonavir: reduced etravirine blood level

Sildenafil: possible decrease in sildenafil effect

Drug-diagnostic tests. *ALP, amylase, AST, cholesterol, creatinine, glucose, lipase, low-density lipoproteins, triglycerides:* increased levels
Hemoglobin, neutrophils, platelets: decreased levels
Drug-food. *Any food:* increased etravirine levels
Drug-herbs. *St. John's wort:* significant decrease in etravirine blood level and loss of therapeutic effect

Patient monitoring

◀ Monitor patient closely for rash; discontinue therapy if severe rash develops.

• Be aware that immune reconstitution syndrome may occur in patients receiving combination antiretroviral therapy. During initial phase of therapy, patient whose immune system responds may develop inflammatory response to indolent or residual opportunistic infections (such as *Mycobacterium avium* complex, cytomegalovirus, *Pneumocystis jiroveci* pneumonia, and tuberculosis), which may necessitate further evaluation and treatment.

• Monitor International Normalized Ratio when giving drug concomitantly with warfarin.

• Watch for new-onset diabetes mellitus, exacerbation of preexisting diabetes, and hyperglycemia.

Patient teaching

• Tell patient to take drug after a meal exactly as prescribed.

• Instruct patient unable to swallow tablets whole to disperse tablets in glass of water, stir dispersion well, drink it immediately, then rinse glass with water several times and completely swallow each rinse to ensure that entire dose is consumed.

• Inform patient that drug doesn't cure HIV infection or reduce risk of passing HIV to others through sexual contact, needle sharing, or blood exposure.

• Advise patient that drug may interact with many other drugs and herbs (especially St. John's wort). Tell patient to discuss use of other drugs and herbs with prescriber.

◀ Advise patient to immediately report rash or new infections.

• Inform patient that drug may lead to body fat redistribution or accumulation and that the cause and long-term effects of these conditions are unknown.

• Advise female patient to notify prescriber if she is pregnant or intends to become pregnant.

• Because of potential HIV transmission and adverse reactions in breastfeeding infants, instruct women receiving this drug not to breastfeed.

• As appropriate, review all other significant and life-threatening adverse reactions and interactions, especially those related to the drugs, tests, foods, and herbs mentioned above.

everolimus
Afinitor, Zortress

Pharmacologic class: mTOR inhibitor
Therapeutic class: Antineoplastic, macrolide immunosuppressant
Pregnancy risk category D (Afinitor), C (Zortress)

FDA BOXED WARNING

• Only physicians experienced in immunosuppressive therapy and management of transplant patients should prescribe Zortress. Manage patient receiving this drug in a facility equipped and staffed with adequate laboratory and supportive medical

---

resources. Physician responsible for maintenance therapy should have complete information requisite for patient follow-up.

• Increased susceptibility to infection and possible development of malignancies may result from Zortress-induced immunosuppression.

• Increased nephrotoxicity can occur with use of standard doses of cyclosporine in combination with Zortress. Therefore, reduced doses of cyclosporine should be used to reduce nephrotoxicity. Closely monitor cyclosporine and Zortress whole blood trough concentrations.

• An increased risk of kidney arterial and venous thrombosis, resulting in graft loss, was reported in patients taking Zortress, mostly within first 30 days after transplantation.

• Increased mortality, often associated with serious infections, within first 3 months after transplantation was observed in a clinical trial of de novo heart transplant patients receiving immunosuppressive regimens with or without induction therapy. Use in heart transplantation isn't recommended.

Action
Binds to intracellular proteins, resulting in an inhibitory (Afinitor) or immunosuppressive (Zortress) complex resulting in inhibition of mTOR kinase

Availability
Tablets (Afinitor): 2.5 mg, 5 mg, 7.5 mg, 10 mg
Tablets (Zortress): 0.25 mg, 0.5 mg, 0.75 mg

⊘ Indications and dosages
➤ Metastatic, locally advanced, or unresectable progressive neuroendocrine tumors of pancreatic origin; advanced renal cell carcinoma after failure of treatment with sunitinib or sorafenib; renal angiomyolipoma and tuberous sclerosis complex

Adults: 10 mg (Afinitor) P.O. daily continued as long as clinical benefit is observed or until unacceptable toxicity occurs

➤Subependymal giant cell astrocytoma (SEGA) requiring intervention in patients who aren't candidates for surgical intervention

Adults and children age 3 and older with body surface area (BSA) of 2.2 m² or more: 7.5 mg (Afinitor) P.O. daily

Adults and children age 3 and older with BSA of 1.3 to 2.1 m²: 5 mg (Afinitor) P.O. daily

Adults and children age 3 and older with BSA of 0.5 to 1.2 m²: 2.5 mg (Afinitor) P.O. daily

➤Prophylaxis of organ rejection in kidney transplant patients at low-to-moderate immunologic risk

Adults: Initially, 0.75 mg (Zortress) P.O. b.i.d. in combination with basiliximab induction and concurrently with reduced doses of cyclosporine and corticosteroids. Adjust maintenance dosage to achieve Zortress trough concentration within 3- to 8-ng/ml target range at 4- to 5-day intervals. Start doses as soon as possible after transplant.

Dosage adjustment
• Moderate hepatic impairment (Zortress)
• Mild, moderate, or severe hepatic impairment; change in hepatic status during therapy (Afinitor)
• Patients with SEGA who have severe hepatic impairment (Afinitor not recommended)
• Concurrent use of CYP3A4 inducers or inhibitors (Afinitor, Zortress)
• Concurrent use of moderate inhibitors of CYP3A4 or p-glycoprotein (PgP) (Afinitor)
• Strong CYP3A4 inducers (Afinitor)

- When switching cyclosporine formulations or when cyclosporine dosage is reduced according to recommended target concentrations (Zortress)
- Possible dosage adjustment based on everolimus blood concentrations achieved, tolerability, individual response, and change in concomitant medications (Afinitor, Zortress)

Contraindications

- Hypersensitivity to drug, other rapamycin derivatives, or any of its components

Precautions

Afinitor
Use cautiously in:
- moderate hepatic impairment, renal failure
- severe hepatic impairment (use not recommended)
- noninfectious pneumonitis, infection, oral ulceration
- concurrent use of strong CYP3A4 inhibitors or inducers (avoid use)
- concurrent use of moderate CYP3A4 or PgP inhibitors
- concurrent use of live vaccines, close contact with those who have received live vaccines (avoid use)
- grapefruit, grapefruit juice, other foods known to inhibit CYP450 and PgP activity, St. John's wort
- pregnant or breastfeeding patients
- children with SEGA younger than age 3 or with BSA less than 0.58 m^2 (safety and efficacy not established).

Zortress
Use cautiously in:
- moderate hepatic impairment, renal dysfunction
- noninfectious pneumonitis, infection, oral ulceration
- lymphoma, other malignancies
- rare hereditary problems of galactose intolerance, Lapp lactase deficiency, glucose-galactose malabsorption (avoid use)

- wound healing, fluid accumulation, hyperlipidemia, proteinuria, polyoma virus infections, noninfectious pneumonitis, **thrombotic microangiopathy, thrombotic thrombocytopenic purpura, hemolytic uremic syndrome,** new-onset diabetes, male infertility
- prolonged exposure to ultraviolet light and sunlight (avoid use)
- concurrent use of CYP3A4 and CYP2D6 substrates with narrow therapeutic index
- concurrent use of strong CYP3A4 inducer rifampin (not recommended)
- concurrent use of ACE inhibitors
- concurrent use of standard doses of cyclosporine (avoid use)
- concurrent use of HMG-CoA reductase inhibitors (such as simvastatin, lovastatin) in transplant patients receiving cyclosporine
- concurrent use of live vaccines, close contact with those who have received live vaccines (avoid use)
- pregnant or breastfeeding patients
- children younger than age 18 (safety and efficacy not established).

Administration

- Administer tablets whole with a glass of water and food (not grapefruit juice or grapefruit products) or give consistently without food.
- Administer Zortress consistently approximately 12 hours apart to minimize variability in absorption and at same time as cyclosporine.
- For patient unable to swallow Afinitor tablets: Immediately before administering, disperse tablets completely in a glass of water (containing approximately 30 ml) by gently stirring. Rinse glass with same volume of water and have patient completely swallow rinse to ensure entire dose is administered.
- Before starting Afinitor, obtain CBC, renal function tests (including BUN, serum creatinine, or urinary protein), and fasting serum glucose and lipid

profile (when possible ensure optimal glucose and lipid control).

◀€ Discontinue Afinitor therapy in patients with signs and symptoms of severe noninfectious pneumonitis.

◀€ Before starting Afinitor, complete treatment of preexisting invasive fungal infections. During treatment, be vigilant for signs and symptoms of infection. If diagnosis of infection is made, institute appropriate treatment promptly and consider interrupting or discontinuing therapy. If diagnosis of invasive systemic fungal infection is made, discontinue drug and treat with appropriate antifungal therapy.

• Be aware that Afinitor isn't recommended for use in patients with SEGA who have severe hepatic impairment.

• Be aware that patients with galactose intolerance, Lapp lactase deficiency, or glucose-galactose malabsorption shouldn't take Zortress as this may result in diarrhea and malabsorption of drug.

Route	Onset	Peak	Duration
P.O.	Unknown	1-2 hr	Unknown

Adverse reactions
Afinitor
CNS: headache, migraine headache, fatigue, malaise, asthenia, dizziness, insomnia, paresthesia, personality change, somnolence, anxiety, **seizures**
CV: hypertension, tachycardia, **deep vein thrombosis, cardiac arrest, congestive heart failure**
EENT: eyelid edema, conjunctivitis, ocular hyperemia, otitis media, otitis externa, nasopharyngitis, rhinitis, allergic rhinitis, epistaxis, sinusitis, oropharyngeal pain, pharyngolaryngeal pain, rhinorrhea, pharyngitis, pharyngeal inflammation, nasal congestion
GI: nausea, vomiting, diarrhea, abdominal pain, stomatitis, oral ulcers, constipation, dry mouth, anorexia, hemorrhoids, dysphagia, gastroenteritis, gastric infection, gastritis

GU: urinary tract infection, proteinuria, **nephrotoxicity, acute renal failure**
Hematologic: anemia, decreased hemoglobin, leukopenia, lymphopenia, neutropenia, pancytopenia, **thrombocytopenia, hemorrhage**
Hepatic: hepatic failure
Metabolic: hyperglycemia, increased ALP, hypercholesterolemia, decreased bicarbonate, hypophosphatemia, increased AST and ALT, hypertriglyceridemia, hypocalcemia, hypokalemia, hyperkalemia, hyponatremia, increased serum creatinine, decreased albumin, increased bilirubin, new-onset exacerbation of preexisting diabetes mellitus
Musculoskeletal: arthralgia, back pain, extremity pain, muscle spasms, jaw pain
Respiratory: cough, upper respiratory tract infection, dyspnea, exertional dyspnea, **pneumonia, noninfectious pneumonitis, acute respiratory distress, pulmonary embolus, respiratory failure, pleural effusion**
Skin: rash, nail disorders, pruritus, dry skin, impaired wound healing, erythema, skin lesion, acneiform dermatitis, cellulitis, tinea, skin infection, contact dermatitis, acne, excoriation, pityriasis rosea
Other: mucosal inflammation, edema, peripheral edema, fluid accumulation, dehydration, fever, infections, weight loss, decreased appetite, dysgeusia, chest pain, chills, abnormal chest X-ray, palmar-plantar erythrodysesthesia syndrome, **sepsis, death (cause unknown), hypersensitivity reactions (including, but not limited to, anaphylaxis, dyspnea, flushing, chest pain, angioedema)**

Zortress
CNS: fatigue, headache, tremor, insomnia
CV: hypertension
GI: nausea, vomiting, constipation, diarrhea, abdominal pain, dyspepsia

---

GU: urinary tract infection, proteinuria, male infertility, hematuria, dysuria
Hematologic: anemia, leukopenia, **graft thrombosis, thrombotic microangiopathy, TTP, hemolytic uremic syndrome**
Hepatic: increased hepatic enzymes and bilirubin
Metabolic: hyperlipidemia, increased serum creatinine, new-onset diabetes mellitus, exacerbation of preexisting diabetes mellitus, hyperkalemia, hypokalemia, hypercholesterolemia, dyslipidemia, hypomagnesemia, hypophosphatemia, hyperglycemia
Musculoskeletal: back pain, extremity pain
Respiratory: cough, upper respiratory tract infection, **noninfectious pneumonitis**
Skin: impaired wound healing
Other: peripheral edema, incision and procedural pain, fluid accumulation, fever, **serious infections, polyoma virus infections, lymphomas and other malignancies, angioedema, hypersensitivity**

Interactions
Afinitor
Drug-drug. *Depot octreotide:* increased octreotide C_{min}
Moderate CYP3A4 and PgP inhibitors (such as amprenavir, aprepitant, diltiazem, erythromycin, fluconazole, fosamprenavir, verapamil): significantly increased everolimus exposure
Strong CYP3A4 inducers (such as carbamazepine, phenobarbital, phenytoin, rifabutin, rifampin, rifapentine): decreased everolimus exposure
Strong CYP3A4 inhibitors (such as atazanavir, clarithromycin, indinavir, itraconazole, ketoconazole, nefazodone, nelfinavir, ritonavir, saquinavir, telithromycin, voriconazole): significantly increased everolimus exposure
Drug-diagnostic tests. *ALP, ALT, AST, blood glucose, cholesterol, serum*

bilirubin, serum creatinine, lipids, triglycerides, urine proteins: increased levels
Bicarbonates, calcium, hemoglobin, platelets, serum albumin, serum phosphorus, sodium, WBCs: decreased levels
Potassium: decreased or increased level
Drug-food. *Grapefruit, grapefruit juice, other foods known to inhibit CYP450 and PgP:* increased everolimus exposure
Drug-herbs. *St. John's wort:* decreased everolimus exposure
Zortress
Drug-drug. *CYP3A substrates (such as cyclosporine) and CYP2D6 substrates with narrow therapeutic indices:* potentially increased concentrations of these drugs
CYP3A4 and PgP substrates (verapamil): significantly increased everolimus C_{max} and area under the curve
Moderate CYP3A4 and PgP inhibitors (such as amprenavir, diltiazem, fluconazole, indinavir, macrolide antibiotics, nicardipine): increased everolimus blood concentration
PgP inhibitors (such as cyclosporine, digoxin): increased everolimus blood concentration
Strong CYP3A4 inducers (such as carbamazepine, efavirenz, nevirapine, phenobarbital, phenytoin, rifampin): decreased everolimus exposure
Strong CYP3A4 inhibitors (such as clarithromycin, itraconazole, ketoconazole, ritonavir, telithromycin, voriconazole): significantly increased everolimus exposure
Drug-diagnostic tests. *Blood glucose, cholesterol, lipids, magnesium, hepatic enzymes, serum bilirubin, serum creatinine, serum phosphorus:* increased levels
Hemoglobin, platelets: decreased levels
Potassium: decreased or increased level
Drug-food. *Grapefruit, grapefruit juice:* increased everolimus exposure
Drug-herbs. *St. John's wort:* decreased everolimus exposure

Patient monitoring

- Closely monitor CBC with differential.

◀€ Monitor renal function, including BUN, urinary protein, and serum creatinine, closely.

- Closely monitor drug blood concentration in patients with hepatic impairment; during concomitant administration of CYP3A4 inducers/inhibitors, or PgP substrates; when switching cyclosporine formulations; and when cyclosporine dosage is reduced according to recommended target concentrations.

- Watch for increases in serum cholesterol, triglyceride, and blood glucose levels.

◀€ Closely monitor patients for hypersensitivity reactions, serious infections, respiratory or cardiac signs and symptoms, signs or symptoms of bleeding or thrombosis, seizures, and palmar-plantar erythrodysesthesia.

- Be aware that patients are at increased risk for delayed wound healing and fluid accumulation; particularly monitor incision sites to minimize complications.

Patient teaching

- Tell patient to take drug at same time each day with a whole glass of water, either consistently with food or without food.

- For patient taking Afinitor: Instruct patient to swallow tablets whole and not to chew or crush them. Tell patient unable to swallow tablets to disperse drug completely (by gently stirring) in a glass of water (containing approximately 1 ounce) immediately before drinking, then rinse with same volume of water and completely swallow rinse to ensure entire dose is taken.

- Tell patient to avoid grapefruit juice and grapefruit products during therapy.

- Inform patient of the need to monitor blood chemistry and hematologic values before starting therapy and periodically thereafter.

◀€ Instruct patient to immediately seek medical attention for difficulty breathing or new or worsening respiratory signs or symptoms, flushing, chest pain, swelling of airway or tongue, fever or other signs or symptoms of infection, urinary problems, or bleeding.

- For patient taking Afinitor: Instruct patient to report signs and symptoms of palmar-plantar erythrodysesthesia (such as redness, swelling, tenderness, or tingling of palms of hands or soles of feet).

◀€ For patient taking Zortress: Inform patient of increased risk of developing lymphomas and other malignancies, particularly of the skin. Tell patient to avoid prolonged exposure to ultraviolet light and sunlight during therapy.

◀€ For patient taking Zortress: Inform patient of risk of a clot in the blood vessels of the transplanted kidney and to immediately seek medical attention if pain in the groin, lower back, side, or abdomen; change in urination; blood in urine or dark-colored urine; fever; nausea; or vomiting occurs.

- Advise patient to manage oral ulcerations with mouthwashes (without alcohol or peroxide) and topical treatments, as prescribed.

- Instruct patient to tell prescriber about all drugs he's taking, because some drugs have potential for serious drug interactions and shouldn't be taken with everolimus.

- Tell patient to avoid live vaccines and close contact with those who have received live vaccines during therapy.

- Advise patient to avoid use of St. John's wort during therapy.

- For patient taking Zortress: Advise female patient of childbearing age that drug may cause fetal harm and to use an effective method of contraception during therapy and for 8 weeks after treatment ends.

• For patient taking Afinitor: Advise breastfeeding patient that she should decide whether to discontinue breastfeeding or discontinue drug, taking into account importance of the drug for her treatment.

• For patient taking Zortress: Advise female patient of childbearing age to avoid breastfeeding during therapy.

• For patient taking Zortress: Inform male patient of potential risk of infertility with therapy.

• As appropriate, review all other significant and life-threatening adverse reactions and interactions, especially those related to the drugs, tests, foods, and herbs mentioned above.

exemestane
Aromasin

Pharmacologic class: Aromatase inhibitor
Therapeutic class: Hormonal antineoplastic
Pregnancy risk category D

Action
Inhibits conversion of androgens to estrogen, which reduces estrogen concentrations and limits cancer cell growth in estrogen-dependent breast tumors

Availability
Tablets: 25 mg

Ⓘ Indications and dosages
➣ Advanced breast cancer
Adults: 25 mg P.O. once daily after a meal

Contraindications
• Hypersensitivity to drug or its components

• Premenopausal women, including pregnant women

Precautions
Use cautiously in:
• moderate to severe hepatic insufficiency or renal impairment
• concurrent use of estrogen-containing drugs
• breastfeeding patients
• children (safety and efficacy not established).

Administration
• Administer after meals with a full glass of water.
• Know that drug shouldn't be taken by premenopausal women or by patients receiving drugs that contain estrogen.

Route	Onset	Peak	Duration
P.O.	Unknown	1-2 hr	24 hr

Adverse reactions
CNS: headache, dizziness, confusion, asthenia, fatigue, weakness, hypoesthesia, paresthesia, pain, anxiety, insomnia, depression
CV: hypertension, chest pain
EENT: sinusitis
GI: nausea, vomiting, diarrhea, constipation, abdominal pain, dyspepsia, anorexia
GU: urinary tract infection
Musculoskeletal: pathologic fractures, arthritis, back pain, skeletal pain
Respiratory: dyspnea, cough, bronchitis, upper respiratory tract infection
Skin: rash, itching, alopecia, diaphoresis
Other: increased appetite, fever, hot flashes, infection, flulike symptoms, edema, lymphedema

Interactions
Drug-drug. *CYP3A4 inducers:* decreased exemestane blood level

---

Patient monitoring
- Monitor vital signs, especially blood pressure.
- Check for adverse GI reactions. Give antiemetics, as prescribed, for nausea and vomiting.
- Assess bowel elimination pattern. Increase fluids and administer stool softeners, as needed, to ease constipation.
- Monitor pain level. Administer analgesics, as prescribed, to relieve pain.
- Monitor liver function tests, CBC, and blood urea nitrogen, creatinine, and electrolyte levels.

Patient teaching
- Advise patient to take with full glass of water after a meal.
- Tell patient to report depression, insomnia, or excessive anxiety.
- Instruct patient to wear cotton clothing to let skin breathe if drug causes increased sweating or hot flashes.
- As appropriate, review all other significant adverse reactions and interactions, especially those related to the drugs mentioned above.

exenatide acetate
Byetta, Bydureon

Pharmacologic class: Incretin mimetic
Therapeutic class: Hypoglycemic
Pregnancy risk category C

FDA | **BOXED WARNING**

- It isn't known whether exenatide extended-release (Bydureon) causes thyroid C-cell tumors, including medullary thyroid carcinoma (MTC), in humans, because human relevance couldn't be determined by clinical or nonclinical studies
- Bydureon is contraindicated in patients with personal or family history of MTC and in patients with multiple endocrine neoplasia syndrome type 2.
- Routine serum calcitonin or thyroid ultrasound monitoring is of uncertain value in patients treated with Bydureon.
- Counsel patient regarding risk and signs and symptoms of thyroid tumors.

Action
Enhances glucose-dependent insulin secretion by the pancreatic beta cells, suppresses inappropriately elevated glucagon secretion, and slows gastric emptying

Availability
Solution for injection: 250 mcg/ml as 60 doses in 5-mcg-per-dose/1.2-ml prefilled pen, 250 mcg/ml as 60 doses in 10-mcg-per-dose/2.4-ml prefilled pen
Suspension for injection (extended-release): 2 mg/vial

Indications and dosages
➤ Adjunct to diet and exercise to improve glycemic control in patients with type 2 diabetes mellitus
Adults: 5 mcg (Byetta) injected subcutaneously in thigh, abdomen, or upper arm twice daily within 60 minutes before morning and evening meals. Dosage can be increased to 10 mcg after 1 month of therapy, based on clinical response. Or, 2 mg (Bydureon) injected subcutaneously once q 7 days (weekly) at any time of day, with or without meals.

Dosage adjustment
- Concurrent sulfonylurea use (Byetta)

Contraindications
- Hypersensitivity to drug or its components
- Personal or family history of medullary thyroid carcinoma; multiple

endocrine neoplasia syndrome type 2 (Bydureon)

Precautions

Use cautiously in:
• severe renal impairment or end-stage renal disease, history of pancreatitis
• severe GI disease (use not recommended)
• type 1 diabetes or diabetic ketoacidosis (avoid use)
• drugs that have narrow therapeutic index or require rapid GI absorption
• concurrent use of insulin (Bydureon use not recommended); concurrent use of prandial insulin (Byetta use not recommended); or concurrent use of other glucose-independent insulin secretagogues (Byetta)
• elderly patients
• pregnant or breastfeeding patients
• children (safety and efficacy not established).

Administration

• Administer oral drugs 1 hour before exenatide. For oral drugs that must be taken with food, administer these with a light meal or snack when exenatide isn't given.
• Discard pen 30 days after first use, even if some drug remains. Don't freeze, and don't use drug if it has been frozen.
• Be aware that Bydureon is intended for patient self-administration and must be administered immediately after powder is suspended.
• Don't coadminister Bydureon and Byetta

Route	Onset	Peak	Duration
Subcut. (immediate)	Unknown	2.1 hr	Unknown
Subcut. (extended)	Unknown	2-7 wk	Unknown

Adverse reactions

CNS: dizziness, headache, asthenia, jitteriness
GI: nausea, vomiting, diarrhea, dyspepsia, gastroesophageal reflux disease, **acute pancreatitis**
Metabolic: hypoglycemia (especially with concurrent sulfonylurea)
Skin: excessive sweating
Other: decreased appetite, general injection site reaction, hypersensitivity reaction

Interactions

Drug-drug. *Anti-infectives, hormonal contraceptives:* possible slowing of GI transit time
Drug-behaviors. *Alcohol use:* reduced blood glucose level

Patient monitoring

• Monitor serum glucose level frequently, especially in patients also receiving sulfonylureas.
• Monitor renal function tests periodically.
◀◗ Be aware that Bydureon hasn't been studied with warfarin; however, postmarketing reports indicate increased INR, sometimes associated with bleeding, occurs with concomitant use of warfarin and Byetta. Monitor prothrombin time more frequently in patients taking warfarin after starting or altering therapy. Once a stable prothrombin time has been documented, prothrombin times can be monitored at intervals usually recommended for patients on warfarin.
◀◗ Be aware that exenatide has been associated with acute pancreatitis, including fatal and nonfatal hemorrhagic or necrotizing pancreatitis. If pancreatitis is suspected, promptly discontinue drug and initiate appropriate management. If pancreatitis is confirmed, don't restart drug.

Reactions in **bold** are life-threatening.   ◀◗ Clinical alert

Patient teaching
• Instruct patient to take Byetta within 1 hour before morning and evening meals meals (or before the two main meals of the day, approximately 6 hours or more apart).

• Teach patient how to self-administer Byetta with prefilled pen. Tell patient to do a new pen set-up one time only, when starting a new prefilled pen. Advise patient to discard pen 30 days after first use, even if some drug remains.

◀፡ Instruct patient to inject Bydureon subcutaneously once every 7 days at any time of day, with or without a meal.

◀፡ Tell patient that Bydureon is provided in a single-dose tray containing one 2-mg vial of drug, one vial connector, one prefilled diluent syringe, and two needles (one provided as a spare). Instruct patient not to substitute needles or any other components in tray. Tell patient to follow manufacturer's directions precisely for preparing the drug for injection and that the drug must be injected immediately after the powder is suspended in the diluent and transferred to the syringe.

• Caution patient not to freeze drug and not to use it if it has been frozen.

◀፡ Teach patient to recognize and immediately report signs and symptoms of hypoglycemia and diabetic ketoacidosis.

◀፡ Teach patient how to recognize and to promptly report signs and symptoms of pancreatitis.

• Advise patient to avoid alcohol during therapy.

• Instruct breastfeeding patient to either discontinue breastfeeding or stop taking drug.

• As appropriate, review all other significant and life-threatening adverse reactions and interactions, especially those related to the drugs and behaviors mentioned above.

ezetimibe
Ezetrol⊕, Zetia

Pharmacologic class: Cholesterol absorption inhibitor
Therapeutic class: Antihyperlipidemic
Pregnancy risk category C

Action
Inhibits cholesterol absorption in the intestine, decreasing intestinal delivery of cholesterol to the liver and increasing systemic cholesterol clearance. Net effect is decreased serum cholesterol level.

Availability
Tablets: 10 mg

ⓓ Indications and dosages
➤ Adjunct to diet to reduce elevated total cholesterol (total-C), low-density lipoprotein cholesterol (LDL-C), non-high-density lipoprotein cholesterol (non-HDL-C), and apolipoprotein B (Apo B) in patients with primary hyperlipidemia, alone or in combination with HMG-CoA reductase inhibitor; to reduce elevated total-C, LDL-C, Apo B, and non-HDL-C in patients with mixed hyperlipidemia, in combination with fenofibrate; to reduce elevated total-C and LDL-C in patients with homozygous familial hypercholesterolemia, in combination with atorvastatin or simvastatin; to reduce elevated sitosterol and campesterol in patients with homozygous sitosterolemia
Adults: 10 mg/day P.O.

Contraindications
• Hypersensitivity to drug or its components

• Active hepatic disease or unexplained, persistent transaminase elevations (when given with a statin)
• Women who are pregnant or may become pregnant (when given with a statin)
• Breastfeeding patients (when given with a statin)

Precautions
Use cautiously in:
• moderate or severe hepatic impairment (use not recommended)
• skeletal muscle toxicity
• concurrent use of cyclosporine or fibrates other than fenofibrate (use not recommended)
• elderly patients
• pregnant or breastfeeding patients not receiving HMG-CoA reductase inhibitors
• children younger than age 10.

Administration
• Give with or without food.
• Be aware that drug may be given concurrently with HMG-CoA reductase inhibitor (such as atorvastatin or simvastatin).
• Give at least 2 hours before or 4 hours after bile acid sequestrant (if prescribed).

Route	Onset	Peak	Duration
P.O.	Moderate	4-12 hr	Unknown

Adverse reactions
CNS: headache, dizziness, fatigue
EENT: nasopharyngitis, sinusitis
GI: diarrhea
Musculoskeletal: back pain, myalgia, joint pain, extremity pain, **rhabdomyolysis**
Respiratory: upper respiratory tract infection

Interactions
Drug-drug. *Cholestyramine:* decreased ezetimibe blood level
Cyclosporine, fenofibrate, gemfibrozil: increased ezetimibe blood level
Fibrates: increased risk of cholesterol excretion into gallbladder leading to cholelithiasis
Drug-diagnostic tests. *Liver function tests:* increased values

Patient monitoring
• Monitor hepatic and lipid profiles.
• Monitor cyclosporine concentration in patients receiving drug concurrently with cyclosporine.
• Monitor International Normalized Ratio if patient also receiving warfarin.
• Assess for and report unexplained muscle pain.
• If cholelithiasis is suspected in patient also receiving fenofibrate, obtain gallbladder studies and consider alternative lipid-lowering therapy.

Patient teaching
• Teach patient about the role of diet, exercise, and weight loss in lowering cholesterol levels.
◀€ Instruct patient to immediately report unexplained muscle pain, tenderness, or weakness while taking this drug.
• Advise breastfeeding patient not to take this drug while taking a statin.
• Advise female patient of childbearing age to use effective contraception while taking this drug concurrently with a statin and if she becomes pregnant to stop taking ezetimibe and statin and call her prescriber.
• As appropriate, review all other significant and life-threatening adverse reactions and interactions, especially those related to the drugs and tests mentioned above.

factor IX (human)
AlphaNine SD, Immune VH✤, Mononine

factor IX (recombinant)
BeneFix

factor IX complex
Bebulin VH, Defix⊕, Hipfix⊕,
Octaplex✤, Profilnine SD, Proplex T
(heat-treated), Replenine⊕

Pharmacologic class: Blood modifier
Therapeutic class: Antihemophilic
Pregnancy risk category C

Action
Converts fibrinogen to fibrin, increasing levels of clotting factors

Availability
Powder for injection: Various strengths; units specified on label

⚕ Indications and dosages
➤ Factor IX deficiency (hemophilia B or Christmas disease); anticoagulant overdose
Adults and children: Dosage individualized; drug administered I.V. Use following equations to calculate approximate units needed:
Human product—1 unit/kg times body weight (in kg) times desired increase in factor IX level, expressed as percentage of normal
Recombinant product—1.2 units/kg times body weight (in kg) times desired increase in factor IX level, expressed as percentage of normal
Proplex T—0.5 unit/kg times body weight (in kg) times desired increase in factor IX level, expressed as percentage of normal

Off-label uses
• Hepatic dysfunction
• Esophagitis
• Unspecified GI hemorrhage (human product)

Contraindications
• Hypersensitivity to mouse or hamster protein (with BeneFix)
• Fibrinolysis

Precautions
Use cautiously in:
• recent surgery
• pregnant patients
• children younger than age 6 (safety and efficacy not established).

Administration
◀€ Give by slow I.V. infusion. Average infusion rate is 100 units (2 to 3 ml)/minute; don't exceed 10 ml/minute.
• If prescribed, administer hepatitis B vaccine before giving factor IX.
• Know that dosage is highly individualized according to degree of factor IX deficiency, patient's weight, and bleeding severity.
• Don't use glass syringe. Don't shake reconstituted solution or mix with other I.V. solutions.

Route	Onset	Peak	Duration
I.V.	Immediate	10-30 min	Unknown

Adverse reactions
CNS: light-headedness, paresthesia, headache
CV: blood pressure changes, **thromboembolic reactions, myocardial infarction (MI)**
EENT: allergic rhinitis
GI: nausea, vomiting
Hematologic: disseminated intravascular coagulation (DIC)
Respiratory: pulmonary embolism

Skin: rash, flushing, diaphoresis, pruritus, urticaria

Other: altered taste, fever, chills, burning sensation in jaw and skull, pain at I.V. injection site, hypersensitivity reactions including **anaphylaxis**

Interactions

Drug-drug. *Aminocaproic acid:* increased risk of thrombosis

Patient monitoring

• Be aware that factor IX complex may transmit hepatitis.

• Closely monitor vital signs during infusion.

◀€ Observe for hemolytic reaction. If it occurs, stop infusion, flush line with saline solution, and notify prescriber immediately.

• Monitor I.V. injection site closely.

◀€ Monitor coagulation studies closely. Know that drug may cause thromboembolic disorders, including MI and DIC.

Patient teaching

• Inform patient that drug may transmit diseases.

◀€ Tell patient to immediately report signs and symptoms of hypersensitivity reaction, including rash, hives, tightness in chest, wheezing, shortness of breath, and swelling of throat or lips.

◀€ Advise patient to immediately report unusual bleeding or bruising.

• Caution patient to avoid activities that can cause injury.

• Tell patient to wear medical identification stating that he has a blood-clotting disorder.

• Instruct patient to notify surgeon or dentist of his blood-clotting disorder before surgery or invasive dental procedures.

• As appropriate, review all other significant and life-threatening adverse reactions and interactions, especially those related to the drugs mentioned above.

famciclovir

Apo-Famciclovir✤, Famvir, PMS-Famciclovir✤, Sandoz Famciclovir✤

Pharmacologic class: Synthetic nucleoside
Therapeutic class: Antiviral
Pregnancy risk category B

Action

Converts to penciclovir and selectively inhibits DNA polymerase and viral DNA synthesis

Availability

Tablets: 125 mg, 250 mg, 500 mg

Indications and dosages

➤ Acute herpes zoster infection (shingles)
Adults: 500 mg P.O. q 8 hours for 7 days
➤ Recurrent genital herpes in immunocompetent patients
Adults: 1,000 mg P.O. b.i.d. for 1 day, starting as soon as symptoms appear
➤ Suppression of recurrent genital herpes
Adults: 250 mg P.O. b.i.d. for up to 1 year
➤ Recurrent herpes simplex infection in patients with human immunodeficiency virus
Adults: 500 mg P.O. b.i.d. for 7 days
➤ Herpes labialis (oral herpes simplex) in immunocompetent patients
Adults: 1,500 mg P.O. as a one-time dose given as soon as symptoms appear

Dosage adjustment

• Renal impairment

Contraindications
• Hypersensitivity to drug or its components

Precautions
Use cautiously in:
• renal or hepatic impairment
• elderly patients
• pregnant or breastfeeding patients
• children younger than age 18.

Administration
• Know that for best response, therapy should begin within 6 hours of onset of genital herpes symptoms or lesions.
• Give with or without food.

Route	Onset	Peak	Duration
P.O.	Unknown	1 hr	Unknown

Adverse reactions
CNS: headache, fatigue, dizziness, drowsiness, paresthesia, insomnia
EENT: pharyngitis, sinusitis
GI: nausea, vomiting, diarrhea, constipation, abdominal pain, anorexia
Musculoskeletal: back pain, joint pain
Skin: pruritus, rash
Other: fever

Interactions
Drug-drug. *Digoxin:* increased digoxin blood level, increased risk of toxicity
Probenecid: increased blood level of penciclovir (active antiviral compound of famciclovir)

Patient monitoring
• When giving concurrently with digoxin, monitor digoxin blood level and evaluate for digoxin toxicity.
• Monitor CBC, blood urea nitrogen, creatinine, and electrolyte levels.
• Be aware that drug may take several weeks to reach therapeutic level.
• Know that renal failure may raise blood drug level, increasing the risk of adverse reactions.

• Avoid direct contact with infected areas. Wash hands frequently and wear gloves during patient contact.

Patient teaching
• Instruct patient to take with food or milk to avoid upset stomach.
• Inform patient that drug doesn't cure herpes but only decreases pain and itching by allowing sores to heal and preventing new ones from forming.
• Advise patient to wear loose-fitting clothing to avoid irritating lesions.
• Tell patient to report rash or itching.
• Instruct female patient to tell prescriber if she is pregnant or breastfeeding.
• As appropriate, review all other significant adverse reactions and interactions, especially those related to the drugs mentioned above.

famotidine
Apo-Famotidine✚, Gen-Famotidine✚, Maalox H2 Acid Controller, Mylanta AR, Novo-Famotidine✚, Nu-Famotidine✚, Pepcid, Pepcid AC, Ulcidine✚, Ultra Heartburn Relief⊕

Pharmacologic class: Histamine₂-receptor antagonist
Therapeutic class: Antiulcer drug
Pregnancy risk category B

Action
Blocks action of histamine at histamine₂-receptor sites in gastric parietal cells, inhibiting gastric acid secretion and stabilizing pepsin

Availability
Gelcaps: 10 mg
Oral suspension: 40 mg/5 ml

Solution for injection: 10 mg/ml,
20 mg/50 ml of normal saline solution
Tablets: 10 mg, 20 mg, 40 mg
Tablets (chewable): 10 mg
Tablets (orally disintegrating): 20 mg,
40 mg

ⓘ Indications and dosages

➤ Active duodenal ulcers and benign
gastric ulcers
Adults: 40 mg P.O. once daily at bedtime or 20 mg P.O. b.i.d. for up to
8 weeks
➤ Prophylaxis of duodenal ulcers
Adults: 20 mg P.O. once daily at bedtime
➤ Gastroesophageal reflux disease
Adults: 20 mg P.O. b.i.d. for up to 6
weeks. Maximum dosage is 40 mg
b.i.d. for up to 12 weeks.
Children ages 1 to 16: 1 mg/kg P.O.
daily in two divided doses, to a maximum of 40 mg b.i.d.
Infants ages 3 months to 1 year: 0.5
mg/kg P.O. b.i.d. for up to 8 weeks
Infants younger than age 3 months:
0.5 mg/kg P.O. once daily for up to 8
weeks
➤ Gastric hypersecretory conditions
(such as Zollinger-Ellison syndrome)
Adults: Initially, 20 mg P.O. q 6 hours,
increased as needed to 160 mg q 6
hours
➤ Hospitalized patients with pathologic hypersecretory conditions or
ulcers; patients who can't take oral
drugs
Adults: 20 mg I.V. q 12 hours
➤ Prevention or treatment of heartburn, acid indigestion, and sour stomach (Pepcid AC only)
Adults: For prevention, 10 mg P.O. 1
hour before eating, or 10-mg chewable
tablet 15 minutes before eating, to a
maximum of 20 mg/24 hours for up to
2 weeks. For symptomatic treatment,
10 mg P.O. once or twice daily.

Dosage adjustment

• Renal impairment

Contraindications

• Hypersensitivity to drug or other his-
tamine$_2$-receptor antagonists

Precautions

Use cautiously in:
• renal impairment with prolonged
QT interval and seizures (very rare)
• elderly patients
• pregnant or breastfeeding patients.

Administration

• Be aware that drug usually is given in
one daily dose to patients with renal
insufficiency.
• Give P.O. form with foods or liquids.
• Dilute I.V. form with 10 ml dextrose
5% in water or normal saline solution
(100 ml) for I.V. piggyback
administration.
• Deliver by I.V. push over 2 minutes or
intermittent infusion over 30 minutes.
• Know that drug may cause transient
irritation at I.V. site.

Route	Onset	Peak	Duration
P.O.	Within 1 hr	1-4 hr	6-12 hr
I.V.	Rapid	0.5-3 hr	8-15 hr

Adverse reactions

CNS: dizziness, headache, paresthesia,
asthenia, fatigue, insomnia, somnolence, psychic disturbances
CV: palpitations, **arrhythmias, AV
block**
GI: nausea, vomiting, diarrhea, constipation, dry mouth, anorexia, cholestatic jaundice, abdominal pain
GU: decreased libido
**Hematologic: agranulocytosis, pancy-
topenia, leukopenia, thrombocytopenia (rare)**
Hepatic: liver enzyme abnormalities,
hepatitis
EENT: orbital edema, conjunctival
redness, tinnitus
Musculoskeletal: musculoskeletal
pain, muscle cramps, arthralgia
**Respiratory: bronchospasm, intersti-
tial pneumonia**

Reactions in **bold** are life-threatening. 🔊 Clinical alert

Skin: flushing, acne, dry skin, rash, urticaria, alopecia, pruritus; **epidermal necrolysis and Stevens-Johnson syndrome (very rare)**
Other: altered taste, fever, pain at injection site, **hypersensitivity reactions including anaphylaxis and angioedema**

Interactions
Drug-diagnostic tests. *Liver enzymes:* altered levels

Patient monitoring
• Assess patient for GI signs and symptoms.
• Monitor blood urea nitrogen and creatinine levels in patients with renal impairment.
◀≋ Monitor patient for prolonged QT interval and seizures, which have been reported very rarely in patients with impaired renal function whose famotidine dosage or dosing interval may not have been adjusted appropriately. Also monitor patient for arrhythmia and AV block.
◀≋ Monitor patient for signs and symptoms of epidermal necrolysis, Stevens-Johnson syndrome, and hematologic or respiratory changes.

Patient teaching
• Tell patient that drug is most effective when taken at bedtime.
• Inform patient that pain relief may not begin until several days after therapy starts.
◀≋ Instruct patient to take drug exactly as prescribed and to immediately report cardiovascular signs and symptoms, seizures, and hematologic or respiratory changes.
• Tell female patient to inform prescriber if she is pregnant or breastfeeding.
• As appropriate, review all other significant and life-threatening adverse reactions and interactions, especially those related to the tests mentioned above.

febuxostat
Uloric

Pharmacologic class: Xanthine oxidase inhibitor
Therapeutic class: Antigout agent
Pregnancy risk category C

Action
Decreases serum uric acid level

Availability
Tablets: 40 mg, 80 mg

⃠ Indications and dosages
➤ Long-term management of hyperuricemia in patients with gout
Adults: Initially, 40 mg P.O. daily; for patients who don't achieve serum uric acid level of less than 6 mg/dl after 2 weeks with 40 mg, give 80 mg P.O. daily

Contraindications
• Concomitant use of azathioprine, mercaptopurine

Precautions
Use cautiously in:
• severe hepatic or renal impairment
• patients with greatly increased rate of urate formation, such as in malignant disease and its treatment and Lesch-Nyhan syndrome (use not recommended)
• concurrent use of theophylline
• pregnant or breastfeeding patients
• children younger than age 18 (safety and efficacy not established).

Administration
• Administer with or without food.

Route	Onset	Peak	Duration
P.O.	Unknown	Unknown	Unknown

🍁 Canada   ⊕ UK   ☣ Hazardous drug   ⊗ High-alert drug

Adverse reactions

CNS: dizziness, **nonfatal cerebrovascular accident (CVA)**
CV: cardiovascular thromboembolic events (nonfatal myocardial infarction [MI], deaths)
GI: nausea
Hepatic: liver function abnormalities
Musculoskeletal: arthralgia
Skin: rash

Interactions

Drug-drug. *Drugs metabolized by xanthine oxidase (such as azathioprine, mercaptopurine):* may increase plasma concentrations of these drugs, leading to severe toxicity
Theophylline: altered theophylline metabolism
Drug-diagnostic tests. *Alanine aminotransferase, aspartate aminotransferase:* increased levels

Patient monitoring

◀€ Monitor patient for signs and symptoms of MI or CVA.
• Be aware that gout flares (caused by reduction in serum uric acid levels resulting in mobilization of urate from tissue deposits) may occur. To prevent such flares, provide concurrent prophylactic treatment with a nonsteroidal anti-inflammatory drug or colchicine, as prescribed.
• Monitor liver function tests 2 months and 4 months after starting therapy and periodically thereafter.

Patient teaching

• Instruct patient to take drug with or without food.
◀€ Instruct patient to immediately report cardiovascular symptoms (such as shortness of breath or chest pain) or strokelike symptoms (such as headache or dizziness) to prescriber.
• Tell patient to inform prescriber of increased gout symptoms or rash.
• As appropriate, review all other significant and life-threatening adverse reactions and interactions, especially those related to the drugs and tests mentioned above.

felodipine
Cardioplen ⊕, Felotens ⊕, Keloc ⊕, Neofel ⊕, Plendil, Renedil ✿, Vascalpha ⊕

f

Pharmacologic class: Calcium channel blocker
Therapeutic class: Antihypertensive, antianginal
Pregnancy risk category C

Action

Impedes extracellular calcium ion movement across membranes of myocardial muscle cells, depressing myocardial contractility and impulse formation; slows impulse conduction velocity and dilates coronary arteries and peripheral arterioles. Net effect is reduced cardiac workload and lower blood pressure.

Availability

Tablets (extended-release): 2.5 mg, 5 mg, 10 mg

🕊 Indications and dosages

➤ Hypertension
Adults: Initially, 5 mg P.O. daily. Depending on response, may decrease to 2.5 mg or increase to a maximum of 10 mg P.O. daily at 2-week intervals.

Dosage adjustment

• Hepatic impairment
• Elderly patients

Off-label uses

• Heart failure
• Angina pectoris or vasospastic (Prinzmetal's) angina

Reactions in **bold** are life-threatening.   ◀€ Clinical alert

Contraindications
- Hypersensitivity to drug

Precautions
Use cautiously in:
- cardiac disease, arrhythmias, severe hepatic or renal impairment
- elderly patients
- pregnant or breastfeeding patients
- children (safety not established).

Administration
- Give without regard to meals.
- Make sure patient swallows tablet whole without crushing or chewing.

Route	Onset	Peak	Duration
P.O.	1 hr	2-4 hr	Up to 24 hr

Adverse reactions
CNS: headache, drowsiness, dizziness, syncope, nervousness, anxiety, psychiatric disturbances, paresthesia, insomnia, asthenia, confusion, irritability

CV: chest pain, peripheral edema, hypotension, palpitations, tachycardia, angina, **arrhythmias, myocardial infarction, atrioventricular block**

EENT: rhinorrhea, sneezing, pharyngitis

GI: nausea, vomiting, diarrhea, constipation, abdominal discomfort, dyspepsia, abdominal cramps, flatulence, dry mouth

Hematologic: anemia

Musculoskeletal: back pain

Respiratory: bronchitis

Skin: dermatitis, rash, pruritus, urticaria, erythema

Other: dysgeusia, gingival hyperplasia, facial edema, thirst, warm sensation

Interactions
Drug-drug. *Antifungals, cimetidine, erythromycin, propranolol, ranitidine:* increased felodipine blood level, increased risk of toxicity

Barbiturates, hydantoins: decreased felodipine blood level

Beta-adrenergic blockers, digoxin, disopyramide, phenytoin: bradycardia, conduction defects, heart failure

Fentanyl, nitrates, other antihypertensives, quinidine: additive hypotension

Nonsteroidal anti-inflammatory drugs: decreased antihypertensive effects

Drug-food. *Grapefruit juice:* increased felodipine blood level and effects

Drug-behaviors. *Acute alcohol ingestion:* additive hypotension

Patient monitoring
🔊 Don't give to patient with heart block unless he has a pacemaker.

🔊 Use extreme caution when administering to patients with pulmonary hypertension, renal insufficiency, heart failure, or compromised ventricular function (especially those receiving beta-adrenergic blockers concurrently).

- Monitor fluid intake and output, and weigh patient daily.
- Monitor ECG and vital signs. Assess for signs and symptoms of heart block.
- Assess for reflex tachycardia, angina, and sustained hypotension.
- Check hepatic profile and alkaline phosphatase level in patients with hepatic impairment.

Patient teaching
- Tell patient drug controls but doesn't cure high blood pressure, so he should keep taking it even if he feels well.
- Instruct patient to move slowly when rising, to avoid light-headedness or dizziness from sudden blood pressure decrease.
- Explain that exercise and hot weather may increase drug's hypotensive effects.
- Tell patient to report peripheral edema, persistent headache, or flushing.
- Advise patient to use hard candy or gum if dry mouth or thirst occurs.
- Tell female patient to inform prescriber if she is pregnant or breastfeeding.

- As appropriate, review all other significant and life-threatening adverse reactions and interactions, especially those related to the drugs, foods, and behaviors mentioned above.

fenofibrate

Antara, Apo-Fenofibrate✙, Fenogal⊕, Lipantil⊕, Lipofen, Lofibra, Nu-Fenofibrate✙, Tricor, Triglide, Supralip⊕

Pharmacologic class: Fibric acid derivative
Therapeutic class: Antihyperlipidemic
Pregnancy risk category C

Action
Inhibits triglyceride synthesis in liver, reducing levels of low- and very-low-density lipoproteins. Also increases uric acid secretion.

Availability
Capsules: 50 mg, 150 mg
Capsules (micronized): 43 mg, 67 mg, 130 mg, 134 mg, 200 mg
Tablets: 48 mg, 50 mg, 54 mg, 145 mg, 160 mg

⏀ Indications and dosages
➤ Adjunct to dietary therapy to reduce elevated low-density lipoproteins (LDL)-C, total cholesterol, triglycerides, and apolipoprotein B; to increase high-density lipoprotein-C level in adult patients with primary hypercholesterolemia or mixed dyslipidemia (Fredrickson Types IIa and IIb)
Adults: 1 tablet (145 or 160 mg), 1 capsule (150 mg), or 1 micronized capsule (130 or 200 mg) P.O. daily
➤ Hypertriglyceridemia
Adults: Initially, 50 to 150 mg P.O. daily (capsule); 43 to 200 mg P.O. daily

(micronized capsule); 48 to 160 mg P.O. daily (tablet)

Dosage adjustment
- Renal impairment
- Elderly patients

Off-label uses
- Polymetabolic syndrome X

Contraindications
- Hypersensitivity to drug
- Hepatic disease or unexplained, persistent liver function test abnormalities
- Severe renal impairment
- Gallbladder disease
- Breastfeeding

Precautions
Use cautiously in:
- pancreatitis, cholelithiasis
- patients receiving warfarin concurrently
- pregnant patients
- children.

Administration
◀€ Before giving, be aware of potentially serious interactions, such as with nephrotic drugs.
- Administer with meals.
- Give bile acid sequestrants at least 1 hour before or 4 to 6 hours after fenofibrate.

Route	Onset	Peak	Duration
P.O.	Variable	6-8 hr	Unknown

Adverse reactions
CNS: drowsiness, dizziness, fatigue, headache, migraine, insomnia, depression, vertigo, nervousness, anxiety, paresthesia, hypotonia, neuralgia
CV: tachycardia, varicose veins, phlebitis, angina, hypertension, hypotension, peripheral vascular disease, vasodilation, ECG abnormalities, coronary artery disease, **arrhythmias,**

Reactions in **bold** are life-threatening.   ◀€ Clinical alert

ventricular extrasystoles, myocardial infarction, atrial fibrillation

EENT: conjunctivitis, abnormal vision, cataracts, refraction disorder, otitis media, rhinitis, sinusitis, pharyngitis, laryngitis

GI: nausea, vomiting, diarrhea, constipation, abdominal pain, flatulence, dyspepsia, gastritis, gastroenteritis, esophagitis, duodenal or peptic ulcer, colitis, cholelithiasis, cholecystitis, rectal disorder, **rectal hemorrhage**

GU: urinary frequency, dysuria, cystitis, urolithiasis, prostatic disorder, gynecomastia, vaginal candidiasis, decreased libido, **renal dysfunction**

Hematologic: eosinophilia, anemia, lymphadenopathy, **thrombocytopenia, leukopenia**

Hepatic: fatty liver deposits

Metabolic: hyperuricemia, gout, **hypoglycemia**

Musculoskeletal: back, muscle, or joint pain; myositis; arthritis; tenosynovitis; arthrosis; bursitis

Respiratory: respiratory disorders, bronchitis, increased cough, dyspnea, pneumonia, **asthma**

Skin: rash, pruritus, urticaria, bruising, acne, eczema, diaphoresis, dermatitis, herpes simplex, herpes zoster, alopecia, nail disorder

Other: weight loss or gain, edema, fever, flulike symptoms, hypersensitivity reactions

Interactions

Drug-drug. *Bile acid sequestrants (resins):* decreased absorption and efficacy of fenofibrate

Immunosuppressants, other nephrotoxic drugs: increased risk of renal toxicity

Oral anticoagulants: increased risk of bleeding

Statins (such as simvastatin): rhabdomyolysis, acute renal failure

Drug-diagnostic tests. *Alanine aminotransferase, alkaline phosphatase, aspartate aminotransferase, blood urea nitrogen, creatinine, gamma-glutamyltransferase, uric acid:* increased values

Granulocytes, hemoglobin, neutrophils, platelets, white blood cells (WBCs): decreased values

Liver function tests: abnormal results

Drug-food. *Any food:* increased drug absorption

Drug-behaviors. *Alcohol use:* elevated triglyceride level

Patient monitoring

• Assess creatine kinase and lipid levels and liver function test results.

• Monitor CBC and WBC count. Expect these to decrease at start of therapy, then stabilize.

Patient teaching

• Instruct patient to take with meals for best effect.

• Remind patient that he still needs to follow a triglyceride-lowering diet.

• Caution patient to avoid driving and other hazardous activities until he knows how drug affects concentration and alertness.

• Advise patient to minimize GI upset by eating frequent, small servings of food and drinking plenty of fluids.

• Tell patient that drug may take up to 2 months to alter lipid values.

• Inform breastfeeding patient that she must choose between taking fenofibrate and breastfeeding.

• Tell female patient to inform prescriber if she is pregnant.

• Inform patient that he'll undergo regular blood testing.

• As appropriate, review all other significant and life-threatening adverse reactions and interactions, especially those related to the drugs, tests, foods, and behaviors mentioned above.

---

fenofibric acid
Trilipix

Pharmacologic class: Fibric acid derivative
Therapeutic class: Antihyperlipidemic
Pregnancy risk category C

Action
Increases lipolysis and elimination of triglyceride-rich particles from plasma by activating lipoprotein lipase and reducing production of Apo CII (an inhibitor of lipoprotein lipase activity)

Availability
Capsules (delayed-release): 45 mg, 135 mg

Indications and dosages
➤ Adjunct to diet in combination with a statin in patients with mixed dyslipidemia and coronary heart disease (CHD) or a risk equivalent; adjunct to diet in patients with primary hyperlipidemia or mixed dyslipidemia
Adults: 135 mg P.O. daily
➤ Adjunct to diet in patients with severe hypertriglyceridemia
Adults: 45 to 135 mg P.O. daily

Dosage adjustment
• Mild to moderate renal impairment

Contraindications
• Hypersensitivity to drug, choline fenofibrate, or fenofibrate
• Severe renal impairment, including patients receiving dialysis
• Active liver disease, gallbladder disease
• Breastfeeding

Precautions
Use cautiously in:
• myositis, myopathy
• administration with maximum dosage of a statin (avoid use unless benefit outweighs risk)
• administration with oral anticoagulants
• pregnant patients
• children (safety and efficacy not established).

Administration
• Administer with or without food (but not with large amounts of grapefruit juice) and have patient swallow capsule whole.
• Be aware that drug isn't indicated for patients with elevated chylomicron and plasma triglyceride levels but with normal very-low-density lipoprotein level.

Route	Onset	Peak	Duration
P.O.	Unknown	4-5 hr	Unknown

Adverse reactions
CNS: fatigue, dizziness, headache, insomnia
CV: hypertension
EENT: nasopharyngitis, sinusitis, pharyngolaryngeal pain, rhinitis
GI: nausea, constipation, diarrhea, dyspepsia, abdominal pain, **pancreatitis**
GU: urinary tract infection
Musculoskeletal: back pain, muscle spasms, extremity pain, arthralgia, myalgia, musculoskeletal pain, myositis, myopathy, **rhabdomyolysis**
Respiratory: upper respiratory tract infection, bronchitis, cough, respiratory disorder
Skin: rash, **Stevens-Johnson syndrome, toxic epidermal necrolysis (rare)**
Other: pain, influenza, **acute hypersensitivity**

f

Reactions in **bold** are life-threatening.   ◀€ Clinical alert

Interactions

Drug-drug. *Bile acid resins:* decreased fenofibric acid absorption

Immunosuppressants (such as cyclosporine): increased risk of nephrotoxicity

Oral anticoagulants: prolonged prothrombin time or International Normalized Ratio

Drug-diagnostic tests. *Alanine aminotransferase (ALT), aspartate aminotransferase, creatine kinase (CK), hepatic enzymes, serum creatinine:* elevated levels

Hematocrit, hemoglobin, WBC: decreased levels

Drug-food. *Grapefruit juice (more than 1 qt daily):* increased risk of myopathy when fenofibric acid is taken with statins

Drug-behaviors. *Alcohol use (excessive):* exacerbation of hypertriglyceridemia

Patient monitoring

◀€ Monitor CK level; discontinue drug if markedly elevated CK level occurs or myopathy or myositis is diagnosed.

◀€ Regularly monitor liver function tests, including serum ALT; discontinue drug if levels persist above three times upper limit of normal.

◀€ Be aware that drug may increase cholesterol excretion into bile, potentially leading to cholelithiasis. Discontinue drug if gallstones develop.

• Monitor serum lipid levels periodically.

• Monitor renal function tests closely in patients at risk for renal insufficiency, such as elderly patients and those with diabetes mellitus.

Patient teaching

• Instruct patient to take drug with or without food (but not with large amounts of grapefruit juice) and to swallow capsule whole.

• Instruct patient that if drug is prescribed with another cholesterol-lowering drug called a statin, these drugs should be taken together.

◀€ Instruct patient to promptly inform prescriber if unexplained muscle pain, tenderness, or weakness occurs, particularly if accompanied by malaise or fever.

◀€ Instruct patient to promptly inform prescriber if skin blistering, peeling, or loosening; red lesions; severe rash; fever; or chills occur because these signs and symptoms may signal a serious skin disorder.

• Advise patient not to take other prescription or nonprescription drugs or herbal or vitamin supplements without first discussing with prescriber.

• As appropriate, review all other significant and life-threatening adverse reactions and interactions, especially those related to the drugs, tests, foods, and behaviors mentioned above.

fentanyl
Subsys

fentanyl citrate
Abstral, Actiq, Duragesic, Durogesic ⊕, Fentanyl Oralet, Fentora, Lazanda, Matrifen✤, Onsolis, Ran-Fentanyl✤, Ratio-Fentanyl✤, Sublimaze

Pharmacologic class: Opioid agonist

Therapeutic class: Opioid analgesic, anesthesia adjunct

Controlled substance schedule II

Pregnancy risk category C

FDA BOXED WARNING

• Abstral, Actiq, Fentora, Lazanda, Onsolis, and Subsys are contraindicated for managing acute or postoperative pain (including headache or migraine), because life-threatening hypoventilation can arise at any dosage in patients not taking long-term opioids. Don't administer to opioid-nontolerant patients, including those with only as-needed prior exposure.

• Because of differences in pharmacokinetic profiles, substitution of one transmucosal fentanyl product for another may result in fatal overdose and substitution on a mcg-per-mcg basis isn't recommended.

• Inform patients and caregivers that Actiq, Fentora, Lazanda, and Onsolis can be fatal to a child. Instruct them to keep all units out of children's reach and to discard opened units properly.

• Abstral, Fentora, Duragesic, Lazanda, Onsolis, and Subsys are for use only in opioid-tolerant patients. They contain a high concentration of potent Schedule II opioid agonist, with highest potential for abuse and risk of fatal overdose due to respiratory depression. These drugs are subject to criminal diversion. High fentanyl content in patches may be a particular target for abuse and diversion. When prescribing or dispensing these drugs, consider the increased risk of misuse, abuse, or diversion.

• Serious adverse events (including deaths) in patients treated with Abstral, Fentora, Lazanda, Onsolis, and Subsys have been reported. Deaths occurred as a result of improper patient selection (such as use in opioid nontolerant patients) or improper dosing.

• Fentanyl levels for Duragesic generally peak between 20 and 72 hours of treatment; serious or life-threatening hypoventilation may arise during initial Duragesic application period.

• Concomitant use of Abstral, Duragesic, Fentora, Lazanda, Onsolis, or Subsys with potent CYP450 3A4 inhibitors may raise fentanyl blood level, possibly increasing or prolonging adverse effects and causing potentially fatal respiratory depression. Closely monitor patients receiving this combination for an extended time; adjust dosage if needed.

• Duragesic safety hasn't been established in children younger than age 2. Administer only to opioid-tolerant children age 2 or older.

• Overestimating Duragesic dosage when converting patients from another opioid can lead to fatal overdose with first dose. Patients who have had serious adverse events (including overdose) must be monitored and treated for at least 24 hours.

• Use of damaged or cut Duragesic patch can lead to rapid release of contents and absorption of potentially fatal dose.

• Because of the risk of misuse, abuse, addiction, and overdose, Abstral, Actiq, Fentora, Lazanda, Onsolis, Subsys, and approved generic equivalents are available only through a restricted program required by the Food and Drug Administration called Transmucosal Immediate Release Fentanyl (TIRF) Risk Evaluation and Mitigation Strategy (REMS).

Action

Binds to specific opioid receptors in CNS, inhibiting pain pathways, altering pain perception, and increasing pain threshold

Availability

Buccal soluble film: 200 mcg, 400 mcg, 600 mcg, 800 mcg, 1,200 mcg
Buccal tablets: 100 mcg, 200 mcg, 400 mcg, 600 mcg, 800 mcg
Injection: 0.05 mg/ml
Nasal spray: 100 mcg, 400 mcg in 5-ml bottle

Sublingual spray: 100 mcg, 200 mcg, 400 mcg, 600 mcg, 800 mcg
Tablets (buccal): 100 mcg, 200 mcg, 300 mcg, 400 mcg, 600 mcg, 800 mcg
Tablets (sublingual): 100 mcg, 200 mcg, 300 mcg, 400 mcg, 600 mcg, 800 mcg
Transdermal system: 12 mcg/hour, 25 mcg/hour, 50 mcg/hour, 75 mcg/hour, 100 mcg/hour
Transmucosal lozenges: 200 mcg, 400 mcg, 600 mcg, 800 mcg, 1,200 mcg, 1,600 mcg

⚕ Indications and dosages

➣ **Breakthrough pain in opioid-tolerant patients with cancer**
Adults: One 200-mcg lozenge (Actiq) dissolved in mouth over 15 minutes; additional unit may be given 15 minutes later. If patient needs more than 1 unit per episode (evaluated over several episodes), dosage may be increased; for optimal use or titration, don't exceed 4 units daily. For patient not being converted from Actiq, give 100 mcg (Fentora). For patient being converted from Actiq, follow dosing recommendations below for Fentora.

Current Actiq (lozenges) dosage (mcg)	Initial Fentora (tablets) dosage (mcg)
200	100
400	100
600	200
800	200
1,200	2 × 200
1,600	2 × 200

If breakthrough pain doesn't ease after 30 minutes, give another dose once, using same strength previously given. Administer maximum of two doses for any breakthrough episode. Wait at least 4 hours before giving Fentora for another breakthrough episode.

For patients receiving sublingual tablets (Abstral), initially 100 mcg.
Individually titrate to a tolerable dose that provides adequate analgesia. Give no more than two doses per breakthrough pain episode. Wait at least 2 hours before treating another episode of breakthrough pain with Abstral. Limit consumption to treat four or fewer breakthrough pain episodes per day once a successful dose is found.

For patients receiving buccal soluble film (Onsolis), 200 mcg as initial starting dose; titrate using 200-mcg increments (up to a maximum of four 200-mcg films or a single 1,200-mcg film) to provide adequate analgesia without undue adverse effects. Maximum is one dose per episode, no more than four doses per day; separate by at least 2 hours.

For patients receiving sublingual spray (Subsys), initially 100 mcg. Individually titrate to a tolerable dose that provides adequate analgesia using a single dose per breakthrough pain episode. For each breakthrough pain episode treated, if pain isn't relieved after 30 minutes, patients may take only one additional dose of the same strength for that episode; patients should take a maximum of two doses of Subsys for any breakthrough pain episode. Patients must wait at least 4 hours before treating another episode of breakthrough pain. If necessary, increase dose to next highest strength (200 mcg). Subsequent titration steps are 400 mcg, 600 mcg, 800 mcg, 1,200 mcg, and 1,600 mcg. For maintenance, once dosage has been titrated to a level that provides adequate pain relief and tolerable adverse effects, patients should generally use only one dose of the appropriate strength per breakthrough pain episode.

For patients receiving nasal spray, initially 100 mcg (a single spray into one nostril or a single spray into each nostril). Individually titrate to an effective dose, from 100 mcg to 200 mcg to 400 mcg, up to a maximum of 800 mcg, that provides adequate analgesia with tolerable adverse effects. Maximum dose is a single spray into one nostril or single spray into each nostril per episode; no more than four doses per 24 hours. Wait at least 2 hours before treating another episode of breakthrough pain with Lazanda. During any episode, if adequate pain relief isn't achieved within 30 minutes, patients may use a rescue drug as directed by prescriber.

Patients must require and use around-the-clock opioids when taking Abstral, Actiq, Fentora, Lazanda, Onsolis, or Subsys.

➤ Management of chronic pain in patients requiring opioid analgesics
Adults: Initially, 25 mcg/hour (transdermal system); no more than 25 mcg/hour in patients who haven't been receiving opioids. To calculate dosage for patients already receiving opioids, assess 24-hour requirement for current opioid. Using equianalgesic table in prescribing information, convert to equivalent amount of morphine per 24 hours; then convert morphine dosage to appropriate dosage of transdermal fentanyl. During initial application, keep short-acting opioids on hand to treat breakthrough pain; morphine 10 mg I.M. or 60 mg P.O. q 4 hours (60 mg/24 hours I.M. or 360 mg/24 hours P.O.) is roughly equivalent to transdermal fentanyl 100 mcg/hour. For most patients, transdermal patch lasts 72 hours, but some require new patch q 48 hours.

➤ Short-term analgesia during anesthesia and immediate preoperative and postoperative periods
Adults: Individualized; 0.05 to 0.1 mg (Sublimaze) I.M. 30 to 60 minutes before surgery and as adjunct to general anesthesia; total dosage is 0.002 mg/kg. Maintenance dosage during surgery is 0.025 to 0.1 mg I.V. or I.M. Postoperatively, 0.05 to 0.1 mg I.M. to control pain, tachypnea, or emergence delirium; repeat in 1 to 2 hours if needed.

Children ages 2 to 12: Individualized; 2 to 3 mcg/kg (Sublimaze) I.V. depending on vital signs, or 5 to 15 mcg/kg (Fentanyl Oralet) transmucosally
➤ General anesthesia (with oxygen only)
Adults: Individualized; 0.05 to 0.1 mg/kg (Sublimaze) I.V. for high-dose therapy. Up to 0.12 mg/kg may be necessary.
➤ Adjunct to regional anesthesia
Adults: Individualized; 0.05 to 0.1 mg (Sublimaze) I.M. or slow I.V. over 1 to 2 minutes

Dosage adjustment
• Elderly patients

Contraindications
• Hypersensitivity to drug or transdermal adhesive (with fentanyl transdermal)
• Opioid-nontolerant patient
• Intermittent pain (on as-needed basis)
• Management of acute or mild pain
• Management of postoperative pain (except for injection form)
• Acute or severe bronchial asthma (Duragesic), significant respiratory depression, especially in unmonitored settings without resuscitation equipment
• Known or suspected paralytic ileus

Precautions
Use cautiously in:
• diabetes mellitus, severe or chronic pulmonary or hepatic disease, cardiovascular disease, CNS tumors, adrenal insufficiency, hypothyroidism, renal impairment, head injury or increased intracranial pressure (use with extreme caution)
• concurrent use of CNS depressants
• alcoholism or drug abuse
• MAO inhibitor use within 14 days (not recommended)
• elderly patients

f

Reactions in **bold** are life-threatening.　　　◀€ Clinical alert

- pregnant patients
- labor and delivery
- breastfeeding patients (not recommended)
- children younger than age 2 (Duragesic, Sublimaze), younger than age 16 (Actiq), or younger than age 18 (Abstral, Fentora, Lazanda, Onsolis, Subsys) (safety not established).

Administration

- Before applying transdermal patch, clip hair at site; don't use razor. Wash area with clean water only; dry well.
- Apply transdermal patch to nonirritated, nonirradiated flat surface. Press firmly in place for 30 seconds.
- In elderly patients, don't initiate fentanyl patch at dosages above 25 mcg/hour unless patient is already receiving more than 135 mg/day of oral morphine or equivalent.
- Don't open buccal tablet blister pack until ready to administer; don't push tablet through blister backing.
- Open buccal soluble film and spray packages immediately before use.
- Be aware that in some patients, dosages of both Fentora and maintenance (around-the-clock) opioid analgesic may need to be adjusted to provide ongoing relief of breakthrough pain. Generally, Fentora dosage should be increased if patient needs more than one dose per breakthrough pain episode for several consecutive episodes.
- Inject I.V. dose slowly over 3 to 5 minutes.
- 🔊 Keep opioid antagonist (naloxone) and emergency equipment available when giving drug I.V.
- Administer sublingual tablets on floor of mouth directly under tongue and allow to completely dissolve.
- Prime nasal spray device before use as directed by manufacturer.
- For patients no longer requiring opioid therapy, consider discontinuing sublingual tablets or nasal spray along with gradual downward titration of

other opioids to minimize possible withdrawal effects. For patients who continue to take long-term opioid therapy for persistent pain but no longer require treatment for breakthrough pain, sublingual tablets or nasal spray can usually be discontinued immediately.

- Be aware that drug isn't recommended for control of mild or intermittent pain.
- Be aware that fentanyl products are generally not interchangeable or substitutable on a mcg-per-mcg basis with other fentanyl products.

Route	Onset	Peak	Duration
I.V.	1-2 min	3-5 min	0.5-1 hr
I.M.	7-8 min	20-30 min	1-2 hr
Buccal film	Unknown	1 hr	Unknown
Nasal spray	Unknown	15-21 min	Unknown
Sub-lingual spray	Unknown	1.5 hr	Unknown
Trans-dermal	6 hr	12-24 hr	72 hr
Trans-mucosal	Rapid	15-30 min	Several hr

Adverse reactions

CNS: headache, dizziness, vertigo, floating feeling, lethargy, confusion, light-headedness, nervousness, hallucinations, delirium, insomnia, anxiety, fear, mood changes, tremor, sedation, coma, seizures

CV: palpitations, hypotension, hypertension, tachycardia, bradycardia, **arrhythmias, circulatory depression, cardiac arrest, shock**

EENT: blurred vision, diplopia, pharyngolaryngeal pain, **laryngospasm**

GI: nausea, vomiting, constipation, biliary tract spasm, dry mouth, anorexia

GU: urinary retention or hesitancy, ureteral or vesical sphincter spasm, decreased libido, erectile dysfunction

Musculoskeletal: skeletal and thoracic muscle rigidity

Respiratory: epistaxis, cough, nasal discomfort, rhinorrhea, nasal congestion, postnasal drip (Lazanda), dyspnea, slow and shallow respirations, suppressed cough reflex, **apnea, bronchospasm**

Skin: local skin irritation (with transdermal system), rash, urticaria, pruritus, diaphoresis, flushing, erythema, cold sensitivity

Other: oral mucosal reactions (at application site with buccal tablets), physical or psychological drug dependence, drug tolerance, pain or phlebitis at injection site, hypersensitivity, **anaphylaxis** (with oral transmucosal forms)

Interactions

Drug-drug. *Barbiturate anesthetics:* decreased effects of both drugs

Buprenorphine, dezocine, nalbuphine: decreased analgesic effect

CNS depressants (antidepressants, general anesthetics, other opioid analgesics, sedating antihistamines, sedative-hypnotics, skeletal muscle relaxants), CYP4503A4 inhibitors: profound sedation, hypoventilation, and hypotension

CYP4503A4 inducers (such as phenytoin, rifabutin, rifapentin): possible decrease in fentanyl blood level

CYP4503A4 inhibitors (such as amiodarone, amprenavir, aprepitant, clarithromycin, diltiazem, erythromycin, fluconazole, fosamprenavir, itraconazole, ketoconazole, nefazodone, nelfinavir, ritonavir, troleandomycin, verapamil): increased fentanyl blood level with increased adverse reactions, leading to greater risk of toxicity (including fatal respiratory depression)

MAO inhibitors: severe, unpredictable reactions

Opioid antagonists, partial-antagonist opioid analgesics: withdrawal in physically dependent patients

Drug-diagnostic tests. *Amylase, lipase:* increased levels

Granulocytes, hemoglobin, neutrophils, platelets, white blood cells: decreased levels

Drug-food. *Grapefruit, grapefruit juice:* increased fentanyl blood level, increased risk of toxicity

Drug-herbs. *Chamomile, hops, kava, skullcap, valerian:* increased CNS depression

Drug-behaviors. *Alcohol use:* profound sedation, hypoventilation, and hypotension

Patient monitoring

◀≋ Assess for muscle rigidity in patients receiving high doses; discuss need for neuromuscular blockers with prescriber. Patient receiving blocker will need ventilator.

• Monitor respiratory and cardiovascular function and urine output.

• With transdermal system, monitor patient's pain level often to determine if patch is effective for 72 hours or needs to be replaced after 48 hours. Know that drug level rises gradually for first 24 hours after patch is applied; supplemental analgesics may be needed then.

• If patient develops fever, assess for signs and symptoms of opioid toxicity, as more drug is absorbed at higher body temperatures.

• If adverse reactions to transdermal system occur, monitor patient for at least 12 hours after patch removal.

• Carefully monitor hematologic studies and hepatic enzyme levels.

Patient teaching

◀≋ Caution patient to keep transmucosal (lozenge) form out of children's reach even though it is supplied in individually sealed, child-resistant

---

pouch. One lozenge can be fatal to a child.

• Instruct patient to place lozenge between cheek and gum and suck on it for 15 minutes without chewing or swallowing.

• Teach patient proper technique for applying and disposing of transdermal patch.

• Tell patient that transdermal form is absorbed more rapidly if skin is warm from fever or hot environment. Instruct patient to avoid electric blankets, heating pads, heat lamps, hot tubs, and heated water beds and to promptly report fever or a move to a hot climate.

• Instruct patient not to open buccal tablet blister pack until ready to use. Teach patient to peel back blister backing to expose buccal tablet and not to push tablet through blister.

• Caution patient not to break, suck, chew, or swallow buccal tablet.

• Instruct patient to place buccal tablet between upper cheek and gum near rear molar until it dissolves, and to swallow remnants with a glass of water after 30 minutes.

• Instruct patient to use alternate sides of mouth when taking subsequent doses of buccal tablets.

• Instruct patient to open buccal soluble film or spray packages immediately before use.

• Instruct patient to rinse mouth with water to wet area for placement of buccal soluble film. Tell patient to place entire buccal soluble film near tip of a dry finger with pink side facing up and to place pink side of film against inside of cheek; then to press and hold film in place for 5 seconds, after which film should stay in place on its own. Tell patient that liquids may be consumed after 5 minutes. Instruct patient that film will dissolve in 15 to 30 minutes and not to chew, swallow, or manipulate film with tongue or fingers or eat food until film has dissolved. Advise

patient or caregiver to properly dispose of Onsolis film because drug can be fatal to children.

• Tell patient to place sublingual tablets on floor of mouth directly under tongue immediately after removal from blister unit. Tell patient not to chew, suck, or swallow tablets and allow tablets to completely dissolve in the sublingual cavity. Instruct patient not to eat or drink anything until tablets have completely dissolved. Advise patient who has a dry mouth that water may be used to moisten buccal mucosa before taking tablets.

• Instruct patient to carefully spray contents of sublingual spray unit into mouth underneath tongue. Tell patient or caregiver to dispose of used unit-dose systems immediately after use. Also tell patient to dispose of any unneeded unit-dose systems remaining from a prescription as soon as they are no longer needed. Consumed units represent a special risk because they are no longer protected by the child-resistant blister package, yet may contain enough drug to be fatal to children.

• Instruct patient on proper use of nasal spray and to press down firmly on finger grips until a "click" is heard and number in counting window advances by one. Tell patient that the fine mist spray isn't always felt on nasal mucosal membrane and to rely on the audible click and advancement of dose counter to confirm that a spray has been administered. Advise patient or caregiver that nasal spray contains an amount of drug that could be fatal to children, to individuals for whom it isn't prescribed, and to those who aren't opioid-tolerant.

• Tell patient to avoid grapefruit and grapefruit juice while taking drug.

• Advise patient not to breastfeed while taking drug.

• Caution patient to avoid driving and other hazardous activities until drug's

effects on concentration and alertness are known.
• As appropriate, review all other significant and life-threatening adverse reactions and interactions, especially those related to the drugs, tests, foods, herbs, and behaviors mentioned above.

fesoterodine fumarate
Toviaz

Pharmacologic class: Competitive muscarinic receptor antagonist
Therapeutic class: Urinary tract agent
Pregnancy risk category C

Action
Inhibits muscarinic receptors, thereby inhibiting contraction of bladder smooth muscle

Availability
Tablets (extended-release): 4 mg, 8 mg

⬥ Indications and dosages
➤ Treatment of overactive bladder with symptoms of urge urinary incontinency, urgency, and frequency
Adults: 4 mg P.O. daily; may increase to 8 mg daily based on response and tolerability

Dosage adjustment
• Severe renal impairment (creatinine clearance of less than 30 ml/minute)
• Coadministration of potent CP3A4 inhibitors (such as clarithromycin, itraconazole, and ketoconazole; dosages above 4 mg not recommended)

Contraindications
• Hypersensitivity to drug or its components
• Urinary or gastric retention
• Uncontrolled narrow-angle glaucoma

Precautions
Use cautiously in:
• severe hepatic impairment (use not recommended)
• severe renal impairment, clinically significant bladder outlet obstruction
• decreased GI motility, such as with severe constipation
• concurrent treatment of narrow-angle glaucoma
• myasthenia gravis
• concurrent use of CYP3A4 inhibitors
• pregnant or breastfeeding patients
• children (safety and efficacy not established).

Administration
• Administer with fluids and have patient swallow tablet whole.

Route	Onset	Peak	Duration
P.O.	Unknown	Approx. 5 hr	Unknown

Adverse reactions
CNS: insomnia
EENT: blurred vision, dry eyes, dry throat
GI: dry mouth, constipation, dyspepsia, nausea, upper abdominal pain
GU: urinary retention, urinary tract infection, dysuria
Musculoskeletal: back pain
Respiratory: cough, upper respiratory tract infection
Skin: decreased sweating, rash
Other: heat prostration, peripheral edema, **angioedema**

Interactions
Drug-drug. *CP3A4 inhibitors (such as clarithromycin, itraconazole, ketoconazole):* increased fesoterodine C_{max} and area under the curve (AUC)
Rifampin: decreased active metabolite of fesoterodine C_{max} and AUC
Other antimuscarinics: increased frequency or severity of adverse effects

(such as dry mouth, constipation, urinary retention)
Drug-diagnostic tests. *Alanine aminotransferase, gamma-glutamyltransferase:* increased levels
Drug-behaviors. *Alcohol use:* increased drowsiness

Patient monitoring
• Monitor kidney and liver function tests closely.
◀︎⑀ Be aware that life-threatening angioedema of the face, lips, tongue, and larynx has been reported with fesoterodine. In some cases, angioedema occurred after first dose. If involvement of the tongue, hypopharynx, or larynx occurs, promptly discontinue drug and initiate appropriate therapy and measures to ensure patent airway.

Patient teaching
• Instruct patient to take drug with fluids and to swallow tablet whole.
◀︎⑀ Instruct patient to immediately stop drug and seek medical attention if difficulty breathing or swelling of the face, lips, or tongue occurs.
• Inform patient that drug may cause constipation and urinary retention.
• Caution patient to avoid driving and other hazardous activities until drug's effects on concentration and alertness are known.
• Advise patient to avoid excessive exercise in hot weather.
• Advise patient to avoid alcohol use while taking drug.
• As appropriate, review all other significant adverse reactions and interactions, especially those related to the drugs, tests, and behaviors mentioned above.

fexofenadine hydrochloride
Allegra, Allegra ODT, Telfast⊕

Pharmacologic class: Peripherally selective piperidine, selective histamine₁-receptor antagonist
Therapeutic class: Antihistamine (nonsedating type), second-generation
Pregnancy risk category C

Action
Blocks effects of histamine at peripheral histamine₁-receptor sites, decreasing allergy signs and symptoms

Availability
Capsules: 60 mg
Oral suspension: 30 mg/5 ml (6 mg/ml)
Tablets: 30 mg, 60 mg, 180 mg
Tablets (orally disintegrating): 30 mg

🕖 Indications and dosages
➤ Seasonal allergic rhinitis; chronic idiopathic urticaria
Adults and children age 12 and older: 60 mg P.O. b.i.d. or 180 mg once daily (conventional tablets)
Children ages 6 to 11: 30 mg P.O. b.i.d. (conventional tablets or ODT tablets)
➤ Seasonal allergic rhinitis
Children ages 2 to 11: 30 mg P.O. b.i.d. (oral suspension and ODT)
➤ Chronic idiopathic urticaria
Children ages 6 months to less than 2 years: 15 mg P.O. b.i.d.(oral suspension and ODT)

Dosage adjustment
• Renal impairment

Contraindications
• Hypersensitivity to drug, terfenadine, or their components

Precautions

Use cautiously in:
- renal impairment
- concurrent ketoconazole or erythromycin therapy
- elderly patients
- pregnant or breastfeeding patients.

Administration

- Give capsules and conventional tablets with water; don't give with apple, orange, or grapefruit juice.
- Don't remove orally disintegrating tablets from original blister package until time of administration.
- Administer orally disintegrating tablets on an empty stomach; allow tablets to disintegrate on the tongue and then have patient swallow tablets with or without water.
- Don't break or use partial orally disintegrating tablets
- Know that orally disintegrating tablets contain phenylalanine.
- Don't give antacids within 2 hours of fexofenadine.

Route	Onset	Peak	Duration
P.O.	Within 1 hr	2-3 hr	12-24 hr

Adverse reactions

CNS: drowsiness, fatigue, headache
EENT: otitis media
GI: nausea, dyspepsia
Metabolic: dysmenorrhea
Respiratory: upper respiratory tract infection
Other: viral infection

Interactions

Drug-drug. *Antacids containing aluminum and magnesium:* decreased absorption and efficacy of fexofenadine
Drug-diagnostic tests. *Skin allergy tests:* false-negative results
Drug-food. *Apple, orange, and grapefruit juice:* decreased absorption and efficacy of fexofenadine

Patient monitoring

- Monitor renal function.
- Watch for signs and symptoms of viral infection.

Patient teaching

- Instruct patient to take conventional tablets with water, and not with apple, orange, or grapefruit juice.
- Instruct patient not to remove orally disintegrating tablets from original blister package until time of administration.
- Instruct patient to take orally disintegrating tablets on an empty stomach at least 1 hour before or 2 hours after a meal, to allow tablet to disintegrate on the tongue, and then to swallow with or without water. Advise patient not to chew tablets.
- Tell patient not to break or use partial orally disintegrating tablets.
- Tell patient to stop taking drug 4 days before diagnostic skin tests, to avoid interference with test results.
- Advise patient to report signs or symptoms of viral infection, especially upper respiratory tract infection.
- Caution patient to avoid driving and other hazardous activities until he knows how drug affects concentration and alertness.
- Advise female patient to inform prescriber if she is pregnant or breastfeeding.
- As appropriate, review all other significant adverse reactions and interactions, especially those related to the drugs, tests, and foods mentioned above.

fidaxomicin

Dificid

Pharmacologic class: Macrolide
Therapeutic class: Anti-infective
Pregnancy risk category B

f

Reactions in **bold** are life-threatening.   ◀€ Clinical alert

Action

Bactericidal against *Clostridium difficile* in vitro, inhibiting RNA synthesis by RNA polymerases

Availability

Tablets: 200 mg

🚫 Indications and dosages

➤ *C. difficile*–associated diarrhea

Adults: 200-mg tablet P.O. b.i.d. for 10 days

Contraindications

None

Precautions

Use cautiously in:
- systemic infections or absence of proven or strongly suspected *C. difficile* infection
- pregnant or breastfeeding patients
- children younger than age 18 (safety and efficacy not established).

Administration

- Administer with or without food.
- Be aware that using drug in absence of proven or strongly suspected *C. difficile* infection is unlikely to provide benefit to patient and increases risk of development of drug-resistant bacteria.
- Be aware that drug has minimal systemic absorption and isn't effective in treatment of systemic infections.

Route	Onset	Peak	Duration
P.O.	Unknown	2 hr	Unknown

Adverse reactions

GI: nausea, vomiting, abdominal pain, **GI hemorrhage**

Hematologic: anemia, neutropenia

Interactions

Drug-drug. *Cyclosporine:* increased plasma concentrations of fidaxomicin and its metabolite

Patient monitoring

- Monitor CBC periodically.
- Observe patient for signs and symptoms of GI hemorrhage.

Patient teaching

- Tell patient to take drug with or without food.
- Inform patient that drug only treats *C. difficile*–associated diarrhea and shouldn't be used to treat other infections.
- Inform patient that although it's common to feel better early in the course of therapy, the drug should be taken exactly as directed. Skipping doses or not completing full course of therapy may decrease effectiveness of immediate treatment and increase likelihood that bacteria will develop resistance and won't be treatable by this drug or other antibacterials in the future.

🔊 Instruct patient to promptly report signs and symptoms of GI bleeding.

- As appropriate, review all other significant and life-threatening adverse reactions and interactions, especially those related to the drugs mentioned above.

filgrastim
Neupogen

Pharmacologic class: Granulocyte colony–stimulating factor

Therapeutic class: Hematopoietic stimulator, antineutropenic

Pregnancy risk category C

Action

Induces formation of neutrophil progenitor cells by binding directly to receptor on surface granulocyte, stimulating cell proliferation and differentiation. Also potentiates effects of mature neutrophils and reduces fever and risk of infection associated with severe neutropenia.

Availability
SingleJect prefilled syringes: 300 mcg, 480 mcg
Vial for injection: 300 mcg/ml, 480 mcg/1.6 ml

✪ Indications and dosages
➤ To prevent infection after myelo-suppressive chemotherapy
Adults: 5 mcg/kg/day by subcutaneous injection or I.V. infusion over 15 to 30 minutes, or continuous subcutaneous or continuous I.V. infusion, increased by 5 mcg/kg with each chemotherapy cycle if needed
➤ Neutropenia after bone marrow transplantation
Adults: 10 mcg/kg/day I.V. over 4 or 24 hours or as a continuous subcutaneous infusion over 24 hours
➤ To enhance peripheral blood progenitor cell collection in autologous hematopoietic stem cell transplantation
Adults: 10 mcg/kg/day by subcutaneous injection or as continuous subcutaneous infusion, starting 4 days before first leukapheresis procedure and continuing until last day of leukapheresis
➤ Neutropenia in congenital neutropenia
Adults: 6 mcg/kg subcutaneously b.i.d.
➤ Neutropenia in idiopathic or cyclic neutropenia
Adults: 5 mcg/kg/day subcutaneously

Off-label uses
• AIDS
• Aplastic anemia
• Hairy cell leukemia
• Myelodysplasia

Contraindications
• Hypersensitivity to drug, its components, or *Escherichia coli*–derived proteins

Precautions
Use cautiously in:
• patients receiving lithium or other drugs that can potentiate neutrophil release
• breastfeeding patients.

Administration
• Know that drug may be injected into venous return line of dialysis tubing after dialysis is completed.
◀€ To dilute for I.V. administration, use dextrose 5% in water. Never use saline solution, because it may cause drug to precipitate.
• Administer single dose intermittently over 15 to 30 minutes or by continuous infusion over 4 to 24 hours.
• Don't mix with other drugs, and don't shake.
• Don't give within 24 hours of chemotherapy, bone marrow transplantation, or radiation therapy.

Route	Onset	Peak	Duration
I.V.	5-60 min	24 hr	1-7 days
Subcut.	5-60 min	2-8 hr	1-7 days

Adverse reactions
CNS: headache, weakness
CV: chest pain, hypotension, transient supraventricular tachycardia, **myocardial infarction, arrhythmias**
EENT: sore throat
GI: nausea, vomiting, diarrhea, constipation, abdominal pain, splenomegaly, stomatitis
GU: bleeding
Hematologic: leukocytosis, sickle cell crisis, thrombocytopenia, splenic rupture
Metabolic: hyperuricemia
Musculoskeletal: bone, joint, muscle, arm, or leg pain
Respiratory: dyspnea, cough
Skin: pruritus, rash, erythema, alopecia, **cutaneous necrotic vasculitis**
Other: fever, mucositis, pain at injection site, edema, hypersensitivity reactions

---

Reactions in **bold** are life-threatening.   ◀€ Clinical alert

Interactions

Drug-drug. *Lithium:* increased neutrophil production
Topotecan: prolonged neutropenia
Vincristine: increased risk of severe atypical peripheral neuropathy
Drug-diagnostic tests. *Alkaline phosphatase, creatinine, lactate dehydrogenase, uric acid:* increased levels
Platelets: decreased count

Patient monitoring

• Obtain CBC with platelet count before starting therapy; monitor these counts often thereafter.
• Monitor cardiovascular status carefully.
• Assess for signs and symptoms of sickle cell crisis and splenic rupture.

Patient teaching

• Teach patient how to recognize and promptly report signs and symptoms of allergic response.
• Caution patient to avoid driving and other hazardous activities until he knows how drug affects concentration and alertness.
• Advise patient to discuss possible need for iron supplements, vitamin B_{12}, and folic acid with prescriber.
• Teach patient how to monitor blood pressure at home.
• Advise patient to minimize GI upset by eating small, frequent servings of food and drinking adequate fluids.
• Tell female patient to inform prescriber if she is breastfeeding.
• Inform patient that he'll undergo regular blood testing during therapy.
• As appropriate, review all other significant and life-threatening adverse reactions and interactions, especially those related to the drugs and tests mentioned above.

finasteride
Propecia, Proscar

Pharmacologic class: Androgen inhibitor
Therapeutic class: Sex hormone, hair regrowth stimulant
Pregnancy risk category X

Action
Suppresses dihydrotestosterone levels by inhibiting the hepatic enzyme 5-alpha reductase, which converts testosterone to dihydrotestosterone in prostate, liver, and skin

Availability
Tablets: 1 mg (Propecia), 5 mg (Proscar)

💊 Indications and dosages
➤ Symptomatic benign prostatic hypertrophy (BPH)
Adults: 5 mg P.O. daily
➤ To reduce risk of progression of BPH symptoms
Adults: 5 mg P.O. daily (Proscar) given with doxazosin
➤ Male-pattern baldness
Adults: 1 mg P.O. daily

Off-label uses
• Acne in women
• Hirsutism

Contraindications
• Hypersensitivity to drug or its components
• Pregnant patients, women who may potentially be pregnant

Precautions
Use cautiously in:
• hepatic impairment, obstructive uropathy, increased risk of high-grade prostate cancer, decrease in serum prostate-specific antigen (PSA) level

---

- women (not indicated)
- children (not indicated).

Administration

- Give with or without food.
- Know that female patients who are or may be pregnant shouldn't handle crushed or broken tablets. (Tablets are coated, so handling of intact tablets doesn't pose a problem.)

Route	Onset	Peak	Duration
P.O. (BPH)	Unknown	8 hr	24 hr
P.O. (baldness)	3 mo	Unknown	Unknown

Adverse reactions

CNS: dizziness, headache, asthenia
EENT: lip swelling
GU: erectile dysfunction, decreased ejaculate volume, decreased libido, testicular pain, gynecomastia
Musculoskeletal: back pain
Skin: rash

Interactions

Drug-drug. *Theophylline:* increased theophylline clearance
Drug-diagnostic tests. *PSA:* 50% decrease

Patient monitoring

- Carefully evaluate sustained PSA increases during therapy.
- Monitor fluid intake and output closely.

Patient teaching

- Tell patient he may take drug with or without food.
- Caution patient to avoid driving and other hazardous activities until he knows how drug affects concentration and alertness.
- Inform patient that he may experience erectile dysfunction and decreased ejaculate. Advise him to discuss these issues with prescriber.

- Caution female caregiver or companion who is or may be pregnant not to handle crushed or broken tablets.
- Tell patient he may need at least 6 months of therapy for BPH treatment and at least 3 months to see improvement in male-pattern baldness.
- Inform patient with BPH that he'll undergo periodic digital rectal exams.
- Instruct patient not to donate blood for at least 1 month after last dose.
- As appropriate, review all other significant adverse reactions and interactions, especially those related to the drugs and tests mentioned above.

fingolimod
Gilenya

Pharmacologic class: Sphingosine 1-phosphate receptor modulator
Therapeutic class: Immunologic agent
Pregnancy risk category C

Action

Blocks capacity of lymphocytes to egress from lymph nodes, reducing number of lymphocytes in peripheral blood. Mechanism by which fingolimod exerts therapeutic effects in multiple sclerosis (MS) is unknown, but may involve reduction of lymphocyte migration into CNS.

Availability

Capsules: 0.5 mg

Indications and dosages

➢ Relapsing forms of MS
Adults: 0.5 mg P.O. daily

Contraindications

- Recent (within last 6 months) occurrence of myocardial infarction, unstable angina, stroke, transient ischemic attack, decompensated heart failure requiring hospitalization, Class III/IV heart failure

• History or presence of Mobitz Type II second- or third-degree AV block or sick sinus syndrome, unless patient has pacemaker

• Baseline QTc interval 500 ms or greater

• Treatment with Class Ia or Class III antiarrhythmics

Precautions

Use cautiously in:

• hepatic or severe renal impairment

• compromised respiratory function, AV conduction abnormalities, bradycardia, hypertension

• infections, macular edema

• patients without history of chickenpox or without vaccination against varicella zoster virus (VZV)

• concurrent use of drugs that slow heart rate or AV conduction

• concurrent use of vaccines (avoid use during treatment and for 2 months after treatment)

• concurrent use of antineoplastics, immunosuppressants, or immunomodulators

• elderly patients

• pregnant or breastfeeding patients

• children younger than age 18 (safety and efficacy not established).

Administration

• Administer with or without food.

• Be aware that patients with active acute or chronic infections shouldn't start treatment until infection is resolved.

• Before starting treatment, make sure recent CBC (within 6 months) is available.

• Before starting treatment, obtain liver enzyme values, particularly transaminase and bilirubin levels (within 6 months).

• Before starting treatment, test patient without history of chickenpox or without vaccination against VZV for

antibodies to VZV. Consider VZV vaccination of antibody-negative patients before beginning treatment, after which initiation of fingolimod treatment should be postponed for 1 month to allow for full effect of vaccination.

• Be aware that decrease in heart rate and AV conduction may occur after first dose. To identify underlying risk factors for bradycardia and AV block before starting therapy: If a recent ECG (within 6 months) isn't available, obtain an ECG in patients using antiarrhythmics (including beta blockers and calcium channel blockers), in those with cardiac risk factors, and in those who on examination have a slow or irregular heartbeat.

• Obtain baseline ophthalmologic evaluation.

Route	Onset	Peak	Duration
P.O.	Unknown	12-16 hr	Unknown

Adverse reactions

CNS: headache, dizziness, paresthesia, migraine, asthenia, depression, **vascular events (including posterior reversible encephalopathy syndrome)**

CV: hypertension, bradycardia, AV conduction abnormalities, **vascular events (including ischemic and hemorrhagic strokes, peripheral arterial occlusive disease)**

EENT: macular edema, blurred vision, eye pain, sinusitis

GI: gastroenteritis, diarrhea

Hematologic: lymphopenia, leukopenia, **lymphomas**

Hepatic: increased liver enzyme levels

Metabolic: increased triglyceride levels

Musculoskeletal: back pain

Respiratory: dyspnea, bronchitis, cough

Skin: alopecia, eczema, pruritus

Other: influenza-type viral infections, herpes viral infections, tinea infections

Interactions

Drug-drug. *Antineoplastics, immunomodulators, immunosuppressants:* increased risk of immunosuppression

Beta blockers (atenolol), Class Ia (such as procainamide, quinidine) or Class III (such as amiodarone, sotalol) antiarrhythmics: decreased heart rate

Ketoconazole: increased fingolimod and fingolimod-phosphate blood levels

Vaccines: reduced vaccine effectiveness

Live attenuated vaccines: increased risk of infection

Drug-diagnostic tests. *Lymphocytes:* reduced levels

Serum transaminases: elevated levels

Patient monitoring

• Continue to closely monitor CBC with differential; be aware that because drug reduces blood lymphocyte counts via redistribution in secondary lymphoid organs, peripheral blood lymphocyte counts can't be utilized to evaluate lymphocyte status during therapy.

◀€ Be aware that patient with preexisting liver disease may be at increased risk for developing elevated liver enzyme levels. Closely monitor liver enzyme levels if hepatic injury is suspected. Discontinue drug if significant hepatic injury is confirmed.

• Monitor renal function tests in patients with renal impairment.

◀€ At start of therapy, carefully watch for reduced heart rate in patients receiving concurrent beta blockers or heart rate-lowering calcium channel blockers, such as diltiazem, verapamil, or digoxin.

◀€ Observe patient for 6 hours after first dose for bradycardia. Should postdose bradyarrhythmia-related signs and symptoms occur, initiate appropriate management and continue observation until signs and symptoms have resolved.

◀€ Closely monitor patients receiving Class Ia or Class III antiarrhythmics for bradycardia for development of torsades de pointes.

• Monitor patient for conduction abnormalities, which are usually transient and asymptomatic. Such abnormalities may resolve within first 24 hours of treatment, but occasionally may require treatment.

• Monitor blood pressure during treatment.

◀€ Monitor patient for infection during treatment and for 2 months after discontinuation of drug. Consider suspending treatment if patient develops serious infection; reassess benefits and risks before restarting therapy.

• Be aware that patients who develop unexplained dyspnea during therapy should have spirometric evaluation of respiratory function and evaluation of diffusion lung capacity for carbon monoxide if clinically indicated.

• Monitor visual acuity 3 to 4 months after treatment initiation; be aware that patients with diabetes mellitus or history of uveitis are at increased risk and should have regular ophthalmologic evaluations.

• Closely monitor patients taking fingolimod and systemic ketoconazole concomitantly, because risk of adverse reactions is greater.

Patient teaching

• Tell patient to take drug with or without food.

• Inform patient that he will need to be observed for 6 hours after first dose.

• Advise patient who hasn't had chickenpox or VZV vaccination to consider vaccination before treatment begins.

• Advise patient to avoid live attenuated vaccines during treatment and for 2 months post treatment because of risk of infection.

• Tell patient not to discontinue drug without first discussing with prescriber.

◀€ Advise patient to promptly report unexplained nausea, vomiting, abdominal pain, dizziness, fatigue, anorexia, dark urine, yellowing of skin or eyes, fever, infection, slow or irregular heartbeat, or unexplained shortness of breath.

◀€ Advise patient to have eye examinations 3 to 4 months after beginning therapy and to contact prescriber if vision changes occur. Instruct patient to immediately report blurriness or shadows in center of vision, blind spot in center of vision, sensitivity to light, or unusually colored (tinted) vision.

• Instruct patient to tell prescriber about all drugs he's taking because some drugs have potential for serious drug interactions and shouldn't be taken with fingolimod.

• Advise female patient of childbearing age to use effective contraception to avoid pregnancy during therapy and for 2 months after treatment ends.

• Advise breastfeeding patient that she should decide whether to discontinue breastfeeding or discontinue drug, taking into account importance of the drug for her treatment.

• As appropriate, review all other significant and life-threatening adverse reactions and interactions, especially those related to the drugs and tests mentioned above.

flecainide acetate
Apo-Flecainide✤, Tambocor, Tambocor XL⊕

Pharmacologic class: Cardiac benzamide local anesthetic

Therapeutic class: Antiarrhythmic (class IC)

Pregnancy risk category C

Action
Inhibits fast sodium channels of myocardial cell membrane. Also slows conduction, shortens action potential, stops paroxysmal reentrant supraventricular tachycardia, and decreases conduction in accessory pathways in Wolff-Parkinson-White syndrome.

Availability
Tablets: 50 mg, 100 mg, 150 mg

⚡ Indications and dosages
➤ Supraventricular tachyarrhythmias (including paroxysmal supraventricular tachycardia and paroxysmal atrial fibrillation or flutter)
Adults: Initially, 50 mg P.O. q 12 hours, increased by 50 mg b.i.d. q 4 days until desired response occurs or maximum daily dosage of 300 mg is reached
➤ Sustained, life-threatening ventricular tachycardia
Adults: Initially, 100 mg P.O. q 12 hours, increased by 50 mg b.i.d. q 4 days until desired response occurs or maximum daily dosage of 400 mg is reached

Dosage adjustment
• Heart failure
• Renal impairment

Off-label uses
- Ventricular arrhythmias
- Wolff-Parkinson-White syndrome

Contraindications
- Hypersensitivity to drug
- Preexisting atrioventricular block or right bundle-branch block
- Recent MI
- Cardiogenic shock

Precautions
Use cautiously in:
- heart failure, renal impairment
- patients taking concurrent amiodarone, beta-adrenergic blockers, disopyramide, or verapamil
- pregnant or breastfeeding patients
- children (safety not established).

Administration
- Initiate therapy only in hospital setting with trained personnel and continuous ECG monitoring.
- Before giving, correct hypokalemia or hyperkalemia.
- Be aware that dosage may be reduced once arrhythmias have been adequately controlled.

Route	Onset	Peak	Duration
P.O.	Unknown	2-3 hr	12 hr

Adverse reactions
CNS: dizziness, anxiety, fatigue, headache, depression, malaise, tremor, weakness, hypoesthesia, paresthesia
CV: chest pain, palpitations, **second- or third-degree heart block, heart failure, new or worsening arrhythmias**
EENT: blurred vision, visual disturbances, corneal deposits
GI: nausea, vomiting, constipation, abdominal pain, dyspepsia, anorexia
Hepatic: hepatitis
Respiratory: dyspnea
Skin: rash, diaphoresis
Other: edema, fever

Interactions
Drug-drug. *Acidifying drugs:* increased renal elimination, decreased efficacy of flecainide (with urine pH below 5)
Alkalizing drugs: increased flecainide blood level, possible toxicity
Amiodarone: doubling of flecainide blood level
Beta-adrenergic blockers: increased blood levels of both drugs
Beta-adrenergic blockers, disopyramide, verapamil: additive myocardial depressant effect
Digoxin: 15% to 25% increase in digoxin blood level
Other antiarrhythmics (including calcium channel blockers): increased risk of arrhythmias
Drug-diagnostic tests. *Alkaline phosphatase:* increased level (with prolonged therapy)
Drug-food. *Foods that decrease urine pH below 5 (such as acidic juices):* increased renal elimination and possibly decreased efficacy of drug
Foods that increase urine pH above 7 (as in strict vegetarian diets): increased drug blood level
Drug-behaviors. *Smoking:* increased plasma clearance and decreased efficacy of drug

Patient monitoring
◀€ Monitor ECG for worsening arrhythmias.
- Measure pacing threshold 1 week before therapy starts and again after 1 week of therapy.
- Monitor potassium and flecainide blood levels.
- Assess respiratory status regularly.
- Monitor hepatic function tests.

Patient teaching
◀€ Instruct patient to immediately report cardiac or respiratory symptoms, unusual tiredness, or yellowing of skin or eyes.

Reactions in **bold** are life-threatening.   ◀€ Clinical alert

- Tell patient drug may cause numbness. Advise him to avoid injury to areas with sensory impairment.
- Caution patient to avoid driving and other hazardous activities until he knows how drug affects concentration, alertness, and vision.
- Advise patient to minimize GI upset by eating small, frequent servings of food and drinking adequate fluids.
- Tell female patient to inform prescriber if she is pregnant or breastfeeding.
- Inform patient that he'll undergo regular blood testing during therapy.
- As appropriate, review all other significant and life-threatening adverse reactions and interactions, especially those related to the drugs, tests, foods, and behaviors mentioned above.

fluconazole

Apo-Fluconazole✤, Canesten Oral⊕, Co Fluconazole✤, Diflucan, Dom-Fluconazole✤, Gen-Fluconazole✤, Novo-Fluconazole✤, PHL-Fluconazole✤, PMS-Fluconazole✤, Riva-Fluconazole✤

Pharmacologic class: Synthetic azole
Therapeutic class: Systemic antifungal
Pregnancy risk category C

Action
Alters cellular membrane, increasing permeability and leakage of essential elements needed for fungal growth. At higher concentrations, may be fungicidal.

Availability
Injection: 2 mg/ml in 100- or 200-ml bottles or containers

Powder for oral suspension: 50 mg/ 5 ml in 35-ml bottle, 200 mg/5 ml in 35-ml bottle
Tablets: 50 mg, 100 mg, 150 mg, 200 mg

Indications and dosages
➤ Oropharyngeal candidiasis
Adults: 200 mg P.O. or I.V. on first day, followed by 100 mg/day for at least 2 weeks
Children: 6 mg/kg P.O. or I.V. on first day, followed by 3 mg/kg/day for at least 2 weeks
➤ Esophageal candidiasis
Adults: 200 mg P.O. or I.V. on first day, followed by 100 mg/day for 3 weeks and then for 2 weeks after symptom resolution. Up to 400 mg/day may be used in severe cases.
Children: 6 mg/kg P.O. or I.V. on first day, followed by 3 mg/kg/day for 3 weeks and for at least 2 weeks after symptom resolution
➤ Candidal urinary tract infection; peritonitis
Adults: 50 to 200 mg P.O. or I.V. daily
➤ Systemic candidiasis
Adults: 400 mg P.O. or I.V. on first day, followed by 200 mg/day for 4 weeks and for at least 2 weeks after symptom resolution
Children: 6 to 12 mg/kg/day P.O. or I.V.
➤ Vaginal candidiasis
Adults: 150 mg P.O. as a single dose
➤ Cryptococcal meningitis
Adults: 400 mg P.O. or I.V. on first day, followed by 200 or 400 mg/day for 10 to 12 weeks after cerebrospinal fluid (CSF) is negative
Children: 12 mg/kg P.O. or I.V. on first day, followed by 6 mg/kg/day for 10 to 12 weeks after CSF is negative
➤ Suppression of cryptococcal meningitis in patients with AIDS
Adults: 200 mg/day P.O. or I.V.
➤ To prevent candidiasis after bone marrow transplantation

✤ Canada   ⊕ UK   ⚱ Hazardous drug   ⊗ High-alert drug

Adults: 400 mg/day P.O. or I.V. for several days before and 7 days after neutrophil count rises above 1,000 cells/mm^3

Dosage adjustment
• Renal impairment
• Elderly patients

Contraindications
• Hypersensitivity to drug or its components
• Concurrent use of terfenadine (not available in U.S.) in patients receiving fluconazole at multiple doses of 400 mg or higher and other drugs known to prolong QT interval and that are metabolized via CYP3A4, such as cisapride, astemizole (not available in U.S.), pimozide, and quinidine

Precautions
Use cautiously in:
• hypersensitivity to other azole antifungals
• renal impairment or hepatic disease
• potentially proarrhythmic conditions
• concurrent use of erythromycin because of potential for increased risk of prolonged QT interval, torsades de pointes, and consequently sudden death (avoid use)
• pregnant or breastfeeding patients
• children younger than 6 months.

Administration
🔊 Limit single I.V. infusion to 200 mg/hour or less, using infusion pump.
• Don't piggyback with other I.V. infusions.
• Keep overwrap on I.V. bag until just before use.
• Know that plastic container may be opaque (from moisture absorbed during sterilization). This doesn't affect drug and will decrease over time.
• Be aware that powder for oral suspension contains sucrose and shouldn't be used in patients with hereditary fructose intolerance, glucose-galactose malabsorption, and sucrase-isomaltase deficiency.

Route	Onset	Peak	Duration
P.O.	Slow	1-2 hr	2-4 days
I.V.	Rapid	1 hr	2-4 days

Adverse reactions
CNS: headache, dizziness
CV: QT interval prolongation, torsades de pointes
GI: nausea, vomiting, diarrhea, dyspepsia, abdominal discomfort
Hematologic: leukopenia, thrombocytopenia
Hepatic: hepatotoxicity
Skin: rash, pruritus, exfoliative skin disorders (including **Stevens-Johnson syndrome**)
Other: altered taste, **anaphylaxis**

Interactions
Drug-drug. *Alfentanil, cyclosporine, phenytoin, rifabutin, tacrolimus, theophylline, zidovudine:* increased blood levels of these drugs, greater risk of toxicity
Benzodiazepines, buspirone, losartan, nisoldipine, tricyclic antidepressants, zolpidem: increased blood levels and effects of these drugs
CYP3A4 inducers: inhibited CYP3A4 enzyme system, altered actions of CYP3A4 inducers (with fluconazole dosages above 200 mg/day)
Glipizide, glyburide, tolbutamide: increased hypoglycemic effect of these drugs
Rifampin: increased rifampin blood level, decreased fluconazole blood level
Thiazide diuretics: increased fluconazole blood level
Warfarin: increased warfarin activity
Drug-diagnostic tests. *Alanine aminotransferase, alkaline phosphatase, bilirubin, gamma-glutamyltransferase, hepatic enzymes:* increased levels
Platelets, white blood cells: decreased counts

f

Patient monitoring

◀€ Stay alert for signs and symptoms of anaphylaxis. Stop drug immediately if these occur.

◀€ Monitor liver function test results and hematologic studies; discontinue drug if clinical signs and symptoms consistent with liver disease develop that may be attributable to fluconazole.

◀€ Assess for rash; if lesions develop, monitor patient. Stop drug and notify prescriber if lesions progress (may signal Stevens-Johnson syndrome).

• Be aware that patients with human immunodeficiency virus have greater risk of adverse reactions.

Patient teaching

◀€ Teach patient how to recognize and immediately report signs and symptoms of allergic response.

• Urge patient to contact prescriber if rash occurs, to determine whether Stevens-Johnson syndrome is developing.

• Caution patient to avoid driving and other hazardous activities until he knows how drug affects concentration and alertness.

• Advise patient to minimize GI upset by eating frequent, small servings of food and drinking adequate fluids.

• Tell female patient to inform prescriber if she is pregnant or breastfeeding.

• As appropriate, review all other significant and life-threatening adverse reactions and interactions, especially those related to the drugs and tests mentioned above.

flucytosine
Ancobon, Ancotil ⊕

Pharmacologic class: Fluorinated pyrimidine analog
Therapeutic class: Antifungal
Pregnancy risk category C

FDA | BOXED WARNING

• Use with extreme caution in renal impairment. Closely monitor hematologic, renal, and hepatic status of all patients. Review instructions thoroughly before administration.

Action

Unclear. Thought to interfere with protein synthesis in cells of susceptible fungi after conversion to fluorouracil.

Availability

Capsules: 250 mg, 500 mg

ⓘ Indications and dosages

➤ Severe fungal infections caused by susceptible strains of *Candida* species (including septicemia, endocarditis, urinary tract infections [UTIs]), and pulmonary infections) and *Cryptococcus* species (including meningitis, pulmonary infections, and UTIs)
Adults: 50 to 150 mg/kg P.O. daily in four equally divided doses q 6 hours

Dosage adjustment

• Renal impairment (glomerular filtration rate below 50 ml/minute)

Off-label uses

• Chromomycosis

Contraindications

• Hypersensitivity to drug or other antifungals

Precautions

Use cautiously in:
• renal impairment, underlying hepatic disease, bone marrow depression
• pregnant or breastfeeding patients
• children (safety not established).

Administration

• Give capsules a few at a time over 15 minutes to minimize nausea and vomiting.

♣ Canada   ⊕ UK   ⚕ Hazardous drug   ⊗ High-alert drug

• Know that drug is rarely used alone. Expect to give another antifungal or amphotericin B concurrently.

Route	Onset	Peak	Duration
P.O.	Variable	2 hr	10-12 hr

Adverse reactions

CNS: headache, dizziness, confusion, hallucinations, vertigo, psychosis, ataxia, paresthesia, parkinsonism, peripheral neuropathy
CV: chest pain, **cardiac arrest**
EENT: hearing loss
GI: nausea, vomiting, diarrhea, dyspepsia, ulcerative colitis, abdominal discomfort, anorexia, duodenal ulcer, **hemorrhage**
GU: azotemia, crystalluria, **renal failure**
Hematologic: eosinophilia, anemia, **leukopenia, aplastic anemia, thrombocytopenia, bone marrow depression, agranulocytosis**
Hepatic: jaundice
Metabolic: hypokalemia, **hypoglycemia**
Respiratory: dyspnea, **respiratory arrest**
Skin: rash, pruritus, urticaria, photosensitivity

Interactions

Drug-drug. *Amphotericin B:* synergistic effects, increased risk of toxicity
Drug-diagnostic tests. *Alanine aminotransferase, alkaline phosphatase, aspartate aminotransferase, bilirubin, gammaglutamyltransferase:* increased levels
Glucose, granulocytes, hemoglobin, platelets, potassium, white blood cells: decreased levels

Patient monitoring

• Monitor kidney and liver function test results.
• Carefully monitor blood glucose level and hematologic test results.
◀€ Assess for serious cardiovascular, renal, respiratory, and hematologic adverse reactions.
• Evaluate electrolyte levels, particularly potassium.

• Assess for signs and symptoms of bleeding.

Patient teaching

• Advise patient to take capsules over 15-minute period to reduce GI upset.
◀€ Instruct patient to immediately report unusual bleeding or bruising.
• Caution patient to avoid driving and other hazardous activities until he knows how drug affects concentration and alertness.
• Instruct patient to minimize GI upset by eating frequent, small servings of food and drinking adequate fluids.
• Advise female patient to inform prescriber if she is pregnant or breastfeeding.
• Tell patient he'll undergo regular blood testing during therapy.
• As appropriate, review all other significant and life-threatening adverse reactions and interactions, especially those related to the drugs and tests mentioned above.

flunisolide

APO-Flunisolide✢, Nasarel, PMS-Flunisolide✢, Ratio-Flunisolide✢, Rhinalar Nasal Mist✢

Pharmacologic class: Intranasal steroid
Therapeutic class: Respiratory inhalant
Pregnancy risk category C

Action

Unknown. Thought to diminish capillary permeability and suppress migration of polymorphonuclear leukocytes, decreasing inflammation.

Availability

Spray solution: 25 ml (each actuation delivers approximately 25 mcg)

⚕ Indications and dosages

➤ Relief of seasonal or perennial rhinitis

Adults: Two sprays in each nostril b.i.d.; may increase to two sprays in each nostril t.i.d. Maximum daily dose is eight sprays in each nostril. For maintenance, after desired clinical effect occurs, reduce dosage to smallest amount needed to control symptoms.

Children ages 6 to 14: One spray in each nostril t.i.d. or two sprays in each nostril b.i.d.; maximum daily dose is four sprays in each nostril. For maintenance, after desired clinical effect occurs, reduce dosage to smallest amount needed to control symptoms.

Contraindications

• Hypersensitivity to drug or its components
• Untreated local infections of nasal mucosa

Precautions

Use cautiously in:
• localized *Candida albicans* infection; tuberculosis; untreated fungal, bacterial, or systemic viral infections; ocular herpes simplex
• patients receiving immunosuppressive therapy.

Administration

• Don't increase dosage or discontinue drug abruptly.

Route	Onset	Peak	Duration
Inhalation (nasal)	Unknown	10-30 min	Unknown

Adverse reactions

CNS: headache, light-headedness, nervousness, dizziness
EENT: cataracts; glaucoma; blurred vision; conjunctivitis; increased intraocular pressure; lacrimation; dry, irritated eyes; tinnitus; otitis; otitis media; rhinorrhea; rhinitis; nasal irritation, burning, and dryness; nasal stuffiness and pain; sneezing; nasal ulcer; epistaxis; localized *Candida albicans* nasal infections; nasal mucosa ulcerations; nasal septum perforation; throat discomfort, soreness, and dryness; mild nasopharyngeal irritation; pharyngitis; dry mucous membranes; nasal and sinus congestion; sinusitis; hoarseness, voice changes
GI: nausea, vomiting, diarrhea, abdominal pain, dyspepsia, dry mouth
Metabolic: hyperadrenocorticism
Musculoskeletal: myalgia, arthralgia, aseptic necrosis of femoral head
Respiratory: wheezing, dyspnea, increased cough, bronchitis, **bronchospasm, asthma symptoms**
Skin: rash, pruritus, urticaria, contact dermatitis, alopecia, herpes simplex infection
Other: altered taste and smell, facial edema, fever, flulike symptoms, aches and pains, infections, **angioedema, anaphylaxis**

Interactions

Drug-diagnostic tests. *Aspartate aminotransferase:* increased level

Patient monitoring

◀€ Monitor patient closely for serious adverse reactions, including anaphylaxis, angioedema, hyperadrenocorticism, and serious infections.

Patient teaching

◀€ Teach patient to recognize and immediately report serious adverse reactions.
• Teach patient proper use of drug. Caution him not to use more than prescribed amount; doing so may cause serious side effects.
• Tell patient maximum drug effects may not occur for several weeks.
• Tell patient to avoid people with measles, chickenpox, and other transmissible infections.

• Caution patient to withhold dose and contact prescriber if infection occurs.

• Instruct female patient to tell prescriber if she becomes pregnant.

• Tell female patient not to breastfeed without consulting prescriber.

• As appropriate, review all other significant and life-threatening adverse reactions and interactions, especially those related to the tests mentioned above.

fluorouracil
(5-fluorouracil, 5-FU)
Adrucil, Efudex, Fluoroplex

Pharmacologic class: Antimetabolite
Therapeutic class: Antineoplastic
Pregnancy risk category D

FDA | **BOXED WARNING**

• Patient should be hospitalized during first course of treatment, as drug may cause severe toxic reactions.

Action
Inhibits DNA and RNA synthesis, leading to death of rapid-growing neoplastic cells. Cell-cycle–S-phase specific.

Availability
Cream: 1%, 5%
Injection: 50 mg/ml in 10-ml ampules and 10-, 20-, and 100-ml vials
Solution: 1%, 2%, 5%

Indications and dosages
➤ Advanced colorectal cancer
Adults: 370 mg/m² I.V. for 5 days, preceded by leucovorin 200 mg/m² daily for 5 days; may be repeated q 4 to 5 weeks. No single daily dose should exceed 800 mg.

➤ Colon, rectal, breast, gastric, and pancreatic cancer
Adults: Initially, 12 mg/kg/day I.V. for 4 days; then 6 mg/kg I.V. on days 6, 8, 10, and 12. Maximum dosage is 800 mg/day. For maintenance, start 30 days after last dose. If no toxicity, use dosage from first course. If toxicity occurs, give 10 to 15 mg/kg/week as single dose after toxicity subsides. Don't exceed 1 g/week.
➤ Actinic (solar) keratoses
Adults: 1% solution or cream applied once or twice daily to lesions on head, neck, or chest; 2% to 5% solution or cream may be needed for other areas.
➤ Superficial basal cell carcinoma
Adults: 5% solution or cream applied b.i.d. for 3 to 6 weeks (up to 12 weeks)

Contraindications
• Hypersensitivity to drug or its components
• Bone marrow depression
• Dihydropyrimidine dehydrogenase enzyme deficiency (with topical route)
• Poor nutritional status
• Serious infection
• Pregnancy or breastfeeding

Precautions
Use cautiously in:
• renal or hepatic impairment, infections, edema, ascites
• obese patients.

Administration
◀≣ Consult facility's cancer protocols to ensure correct dosage, administration technique, and cycle length.
• Give antiemetic before fluorouracil, as ordered, to reduce GI upset.
• Know that drug may be given without dilution by direct I.V. injection over 1 to 3 minutes.
• For I.V. infusion, dilute with dextrose 5% in water, sterile water, or normal saline solution in plastic bag (not glass

---

Reactions in **bold** are life-threatening.   ◀≣ Clinical alert

bottle). Infusion may be given over a period of 24 hours or more.

◀€ Be aware of the importance of leucovorin rescue with fluorouracil therapy, if prescribed.

• Check infusion site frequently to detect extravasation.

• Use nonmetal applicator or appropriate gloves to apply topical form.

• Avoid applying topical form to mucous membranes or irritated skin.

• Don't use occlusive dressings over topical form.

• Know that pyridoxine may be given with fluorouracil to reduce risk of palmar-plantar erythrodysesthesia (hand-foot syndrome).

Route	Onset	Peak	Duration
I.V.	1-9 days	9-21 days	30 days
Topical	Unknown	Unknown	Unknown

Adverse reactions

CNS: confusion, disorientation, euphoria, ataxia, headache, weakness, malaise, **acute cerebellar syndrome or dysfunction**

CV: angina, **myocardial ischemia, thrombophlebitis**

EENT: vision changes, photophobia, lacrimation, lacrimal duct stenosis, nystagmus, epistaxis

GI: nausea, vomiting, diarrhea, stomatitis, anorexia, GI ulcer, **GI bleeding**

Hematologic: anemia, **leukopenia, thrombocytopenia**

Skin: alopecia, maculopapular rash, melanosis of nails, nail loss, palmar-plantar erythrodysesthesia, photosensitivity, local inflammation reaction (with cream), dermatitis

Other: fever, **anaphylaxis**

Interactions

Drug-drug. *Bone marrow depressants (including other antineoplastics):* additive bone marrow depression
Irinotecan: dehydration, neutropenia, sepsis

Leucovorin calcium: increased risk of fluorouracil toxicity
Live-virus vaccines: decreased antibody response to vaccine, increased risk of adverse reactions

Drug-diagnostic tests. *Alanine aminotransferase, alkaline phosphatase, aspartate aminotransferase, bilirubin, lactate dehydrogenase, urinary 5-hydroxyindoleacetic acid:* increased levels
Albumin, granulocytes, platelets, red blood cells, white blood cells (WBCs): decreased levels

Drug-behaviors. *Sun exposure:* increased risk of phototoxicity

Patient monitoring

◀€ Watch for signs and symptoms of toxicity, especially stomatitis and diarrhea. If these occur, stop drug and notify prescriber. Note that toxicity may take 1 to 3 weeks to develop.

• Monitor CBC, WBC and platelet counts, and kidney and liver function test results.

• Assess fluid intake and output.

• With long-term use, watch for serious rash on hands and feet. If it occurs, consult prescriber regarding need for pyridoxine.

• Assess for bleeding tendency.

• Monitor blood glucose level in patients at risk for hyperglycemia.

Patient teaching

◀€ Emphasize importance of taking leucovorin as prescribed with high-dose therapy.

◀€ Instruct patient to report signs and symptoms of toxicity, particularly stomatitis and diarrhea. Tell him that these may not occur for 1 to 3 weeks.

• Caution patient to avoid driving and other hazardous activities until he knows how drug affects concentration and alertness.

• Tell patient to avoid activities that can cause injury. Instruct him to use

---

soft toothbrush and electric razor to avoid gum and skin injury.

• Advise patient to minimize GI upset by eating frequent, small servings of food and drinking adequate fluids.

• Tell patient that drug may cause reversible hair loss.

• Inform patient that he'll undergo regular blood testing during therapy.

◀╠ Advise female to inform prescriber immediately if she is pregnant. Caution her not to breastfeed.

• As appropriate, review all other significant and life-threatening adverse reactions and interactions, especially those related to the drugs, tests, and behaviors mentioned above.

fluoxetine hydrochloride

Prozac, Prozac Weekly, Prozit✚, Sarafem

Pharmacologic class: Selective serotonin reuptake inhibitor
Therapeutic class: Antidepressant
Pregnancy risk category B

FDA | BOXED WARNING

• Drug may increase risk of suicidal thinking and behavior in children and adolescents with major depressive disorder (MDD) and other psychiatric disorders, especially during first few months of therapy. Risk must be balanced with clinical need, as depression itself increases suicide risk. With patient of any age, observe closely for clinical worsening, suicidality, and unusual behavior changes when therapy begins. Advise family and caregivers to observe patient closely and communicate with prescriber as needed.

• Prozac is approved for use in pediatric patients with MDD and obsessive-compulsive disorder.

Action

Selectively inhibits serotonin reuptake in CNS; has little to no effect on norepinephrine and dopamine reuptake

Availability

Capsules: 10 mg, 15 mg, 20 mg, 40 mg
Capsules (delayed-release): 90 mg
Oral solution: 20 mg/5 ml
Tablets: 10 mg, 15 mg, 20 mg

💊 Indications and dosages

➤ Major depressive disorder (MDD)
Adults: 20 mg/day P.O. in morning. After several weeks, may increase by 20 mg/day at weekly intervals. Give dosages above 20 mg/day in two divided doses (morning and noon); don't exceed 80 mg/day. Patients stabilized on 20 mg/day may be switched to 90-mg/week delayed-release capsules (Prozac Weekly) 7 days after last 20-mg dose.

Children ages 8 to 18: Initially, 10 to 20 mg/day P.O. After 1 week at 10 mg daily, dosage should be increased to 20 mg/day. However, because of higher plasma levels in lower-weight children, starting and target dose in this group may be 10 mg/day. Dosage increase to 20 mg/day may be considered after several weeks if insufficient clinical improvement occurs.

➤ Obsessive-compulsive disorder (OCD)
Adults: Initially, 20 mg/day P.O. in morning. After several weeks, may increase dosage. Give doses above 20 mg/day once daily (morning) or in two divided doses b.i.d. (morning and noon). Dosage range of 20 to 60 mg/day is recommended; however, dosages of up to 80 mg/day have been well tolerated. Don't exceed 80 mg/day.

Children ages 7 to 17: Initially, 10 mg/day P.O. in morning in adolescents and higher-weight children; after 2 weeks, may increase dosage to 20 mg/day. Additional dosage increases may be considered after several more weeks if insufficient clinical improvement occurs. Dosage range of 20 to 60 mg/day is recommended. Initially, 10 mg/day P.O. in lower-weight children; may increase dosage after several more weeks if insufficient clinical improvement occurs. Dosage range of 20 to 30 mg/day is recommended. Experience with daily doses greater than 20 mg is very minimal; there is no experience with doses greater than 60 mg.

➤ Acute treatment of depressive episodes associated with bipolar I disorder

Adults: Initially, 20 mg fluoxetine P.O. with 5 mg olanzapine P.O. daily; dosage range of fluoxetine is 20 to 50 mg; olanzapine, 5 to 12.5 mg. Safety of fluoxetine doses above 75 mg and olanzapine doses above 18 mg haven't been established

➤ Bulimia nervosa

Adults: 60 mg/day P.O.; may be titrated upward over several days

➤ Panic disorder

Adults: 10 mg/day P.O. for 1 week; then, if needed, increase to 20 mg/day. Dosage increases of up to 60 mg/day may be considered after several weeks if patient doesn't respond to lower dosage.

➤ Premenstrual dysphoric disorder

Adults: 20 mg/day (Sarafem) P.O., not to exceed 80 mg/day

Dosage adjustment
• Hepatic impairment
• Concurrent disease or multiple concomitant medications
• Pregnant women during third trimester
• Elderly patients

Off-label uses
• Diabetic peripheral neuropathy
• Alcoholism
• Bipolar II disorder
• Borderline personality disorder
• Narcolepsy
• Posttraumatic stress disorder
• Schizophrenia
• Social phobia

Contraindications
• Hypersensitivity to drug
• MAO inhibitor use within past 14 days
• Concurrent use of thioridazine or within 5 weeks of discontinuing fluoxetine
• Concurrent use of pimozide

Precautions
Use cautiously in:
• hepatic or renal impairment, diabetes mellitus, cardiovascular disease, concomitant illness, acute narrow-angle glaucoma
• history of seizures, serotonin syndrome or neuroleptic malignant syndrome, clinical worsening and suicidal thinking and behavior, activation of mania or hypomania
• hyponatremia in association with syndrome of inappropriate antidiuretic hormone secretion
• concurrent use of NSAIDs, aspirin, warfarin, or other drugs that affect coagulation
• concurrent use of tryptophan (use not recommended)
• pregnant patients (third trimester)
• breastfeeding patients (use not recommended)
• children younger than age 7 (in OCD use), younger than age 8 (in MDD use), younger than age 18 for all other uses (safety and efficacy not established).

Administration
◀€ Be aware that drug should be discontinued 5 weeks before MAO

inhibitor or thioridazine therapy begins.

• Give before 2 P.M. to prevent night-time insomnia.

• Be aware that drug should be gradually reduced rather than abruptly stopped whenever possible.

Route	Onset	Peak	Duration
P.O.	Unknown	6-8 hr	Unknown

Adverse reactions

CNS: anxiety, drowsiness, headache, insomnia, abnormal dreams, dizziness, fatigue, nervousness, hypomania, mania, weakness, tremor, **seizures, suicidal ideation**

CV: chest pain, palpitations, **prolonged QTc interval**

EENT: visual disturbances, stuffy nose, sinusitis, pharyngitis

GI: nausea, vomiting, diarrhea, constipation, abdominal pain, dyspepsia, dry mouth, anorexia

GU: urinary frequency, sexual dysfunction, dysmenorrhea

Metabolic: hypouricemia, hypocalcemia, hyponatremia, hyperglycemia, **hypoglycemia**

Musculoskeletal: joint, back, or muscle pain

Respiratory: cough, upper respiratory tract infection, dyspnea, **respiratory distress**

Skin: diaphoresis, pruritus, erythema nodosum, flushing, rash

Other: abnormal taste, weight loss, fever, flulike symptoms, hot flashes, **serotonin syndrome, neuroleptic malignant syndrome (NMS),** allergic reactions, hypersensitivity reactions

Interactions

Drug-drug. *Adrenergics:* increased sensitivity to adrenergics, increased risk of serotonin syndrome

Alprazolam: decreased metabolism and increased effects of alprazolam

Antihistamines, opioids, other antidepressants, sedative-hypnotics: additive CNS depression

Aspirin, NSAIDs, warfarin, other drugs that affect coagulation: increased risk of GI or other bleeding

Buspirone: potentiation of fluoxetine effects, increased risk of seizures

Carbamazepine, clozapine, digoxin, haloperidol, lithium, phenytoin, warfarin: increased blood levels of these drugs, greater risk of adverse reactions

CYP450-2D6 inducers: increased effects of these drugs

Cyproheptadine: decrease in or reversal of fluoxetine effects

Digoxin, warfarin, other highly protein-bound drugs: increased risk of adverse reactions to either drug

Efavirenz, ritonavir, saquinavir, other CYP450 inhibitors: serotonergics, triptans: increased risk of serotonin syndrome

MAO inhibitors: confusion, agitation, seizures, hypertension, and hyperpyrexia (serotonin syndrome)

Pimozide: increased risk of drug interaction or QTc-interval prolongation

Thioridazine: increased risk of QTc-interval prolongation or potential for elevated thioridazine plasma level

Other antidepressants, phenothiazines, risperidone, tryptophan: increased risk of adverse reactions

Ritonavir: increased ritonavir blood level

Drug-diagnostic tests. *Alanine aminotransferase, alkaline phosphatase, blood urea nitrogen, creatine kinase, electrolytes, glucose:* increased levels

Sodium: decreased level

Drug-herbs. *St. John's wort:* increased risk of serotonin syndrome

Drug-behaviors. *Alcohol use:* additive CNS depression

Patient monitoring

◀€ Monitor patient for signs and symptoms of depression. Assess for suicidal ideation.

Reactions in **bold** are life-threatening.　　　　◀€ Clinical alert

◀╠ Evaluate neurologic status, watching especially for seizures.

◀╠ Monitor cardiovascular status, particularly for prolonged QTc interval.

• Assess weight regularly. Watch for signs of eating disorders.

◀╠ Monitor patient for signs and symptoms of allergic reactions, serotonin syndrome, or NMS-like reactions. Discontinue drug immediately and initiate supportive treatment if these reactions occur.

Patient teaching

• Encourage patient to establish effective bedtime routine to minimize sleep disorders.

• Tell patient drug may take 4 weeks or longer to be fully effective.

◀╠ Instruct patient to contact prescriber if he develops worsening depression or has suicidal thoughts.

◀╠ Instruct patient to immediately stop drug and report signs and symptoms of allergic reactions (rash), serotonin syndrome, or neuroleptic malignant syndrome–like reactions.

• Caution patient to avoid driving and other hazardous activities until he knows how drug affects concentration and alertness.

• Tell female patient to inform prescriber if she is pregnant or breastfeeding.

• As appropriate, review all other significant and life-threatening adverse reactions and interactions, especially those related to the drugs, tests, herbs, and behaviors mentioned above.

fluphenazine decanoate
Fluphenazine Omega❦, Modecate, Modecate❦⊕

fluphenazine hydrochloride
Apo-Fluphenazine❦, Moditen⊕, PMS-Fluphenazine❦

Pharmacologic class: Phenothiazine, dopaminergic blocker

Therapeutic class: Anxiolytic, antipsychotic

Pregnancy risk category C

Action
Unclear. May alter postsynaptic mesolimbic dopamine receptors in brain and reduce release of hypothalamic and hypophyseal hormones thought to depress reticular activating system, thereby preventing psychotic symptoms.

Availability
fluphenazine decanoate
Depot injection: 25 mg/ml
fluphenazine hydrochloride
Elixir: 2.5 mg/5 ml
Injection: 2.5 mg/ml
Oral concentrate: 5 mg/ml
Tablets: 1 mg, 2.5 mg, 5 mg, 10 mg

🖉 Indications and dosages
➤ Psychotic disorders
Adults: 2.5 to 10 mg/day (hydrochloride) P.O. in divided doses q 6 to 8 hours or as a single dose at bedtime; typical daily dosage is 1 to 5 mg; give oral doses above 20 mg/day with caution. Or initially, 1.25 mg I.M., divided and given q 6 to 8 hours. Parenteral hydrochloride dosage is one-third to one-half of oral dosage. Or 12.5 to 25 mg I.M. or subcutaneously (decanoate); base subsequent dosage and dosing intervals of 1 to 4 weeks on patient response; don't exceed 100 mg.

Dosage adjustment
• Elderly patients

Contraindications
- Hypersensitivity to drug, sulfites (with injectable form), or benzyl alcohol
- Angle-closure glaucoma
- Bone marrow depression
- Severe hepatic or cardiovascular disease

Precautions
Use cautiously in:
- diabetes, respiratory disease, prostatic hypertrophy, CNS tumors
- elderly patients
- pregnant or breastfeeding patients (safety not established)
- children with acute illnesses, infections, gastroenteritis, or dehydration.

Administration
◀€ Be aware that parenteral form is for I.M. and subcutaneous use only. Don't give I.V.
- Don't give parenteral form to comatose or severely depressed patient.
- Use gloves when handling. To prevent contact dermatitis, keep drug away from clothing and skin.
- Dilute concentrated oral forms in juice, milk, or semisolid food just before administering.
- Give long-acting, oil-based preparations with dry needle of at least 21G.
- Be aware that antacids and adsorbent antidiarrheals may decrease adsorption of fluphenazine. Give 1 hour before or 2 hours after fluphenazine.

Route	Onset	Peak	Duration
P.O.	<1 hr	0.5 hr	6-8 hr
I.M. (HCl)	1 hr	1.5-2 hr	6-8 hr
I.M.	24-72 hr	Unknown	1-6 wk
Subcut.	Unknown	Unknown	Unknown

Adverse reactions
CNS: drowsiness, sedation, extrapyramidal reactions, tardive dyskinesia, pseudoparkinsonism, **neuroleptic malignant syndrome, seizures**
CV: hypotension, tachycardia

EENT: blurred vision, dry eyes, lens opacities, nasal congestion
GI: constipation, dry mouth, anorexia, **paralytic ileus**
GU: urinary retention, menstrual irregularities, inhibited ejaculation, priapism, gynecomastia, lactation
Hematologic: eosinophilia, **hemolytic anemia, aplastic anemia, agranulocytosis, leukopenia, thrombocytopenia**
Hepatic: jaundice, **hepatitis**
Metabolic: galactorrhea, hyperthermia
Skin: photosensitivity, rash
Other: allergic reactions, pain at injection site, sterile abscess

Interactions
Drug-drug. *Activated charcoal, adsorbent antidiarrheals, antacids:* decreased fluphenazine adsorption
Anticholinergics: decreased fluphenazine effects
Antidepressants, antihistamines, general anesthetics, MAO inhibitors, opioid analgesics, sedative-hypnotics: additive CNS depression
Antihistamines, disopyramide, quinidine, tricyclic antidepressants (TCAs): increased risk of anticholinergic effects
Antihypertensives: additive hypotension
Barbiturates: increased fluphenazine metabolism and decreased efficacy
Bromocriptine: decreased bromocriptine efficacy
Guanethidine: inhibition of antihypertensive effects
Lithium: disorientation, unconsciousness, extrapyramidal symptoms
Meperidine: excessive sedation and hypotension
Ofloxacin: increased QTc interval
Phenytoin: increased or decreased phenytoin blood level
Pimozide: increased risk of potentially serious cardiovascular reactions
Propranolol: increased blood levels of both drugs
TCAs: increased blood levels and effects of TCAs

Reactions in **bold** are life-threatening. ◀€ Clinical alert

Drug-diagnostic tests. *Alanine aminotransferase, alkaline phosphatase, aspartate aminotransferase, bilirubin:* increased levels

Granulocytes, hematocrit, hemoglobin, leukocytes, platelets: decreased values

Pregnancy tests: false-positive or false-negative result

Urine bilirubin: false-positive result

Drug-herbs. *Angel's trumpet, jimsonweed, scopolia:* increased anticholinergic effects

Chamomile, hops, kava, skullcap: increased CNS depression

St. John's wort: photosensitivity

Yohimbe: fluphenazine toxicity

Drug-behaviors. *Alcohol use:* increased CNS depression

Sun exposure: increased risk of photosensitivity

Patient monitoring

◀≀ Monitor patient for signs and symptoms of neuroleptic malignant syndrome (extrapyramidal symptoms, hyperthermia, autonomic symptoms).

◀≀ Stop giving drug and notify prescriber immediately if patient shows signs or symptoms of blood dyscrasias (fever, infection, sore throat, cellulitis, or weakness).

• Observe for tardive dyskinesia.

• Watch for bleeding tendency.

• Monitor CBC, bilirubin level, and liver function test results.

• Assess kidney function and ophthalmic test results in patients on long-term therapy.

Patient teaching

◀≀ Tell patient not to stop taking drug suddenly, because serious adverse effects may occur.

• Advise patient to report urinary retention or constipation.

◀≀ Instruct patient to immediately report unusual bleeding or bruising.

• Caution patient to avoid driving and other hazardous activities until he

knows how drug affects concentration, alertness, and vision.

• Tell patient to avoid activities that can cause injury. Advise him to use soft toothbrush and electric razor to avoid gum and skin injury.

• Inform patient that he'll undergo regular blood testing during therapy.

• Tell female patient to inform prescriber if she is pregnant or breastfeeding.

• As appropriate, review all other significant and life-threatening adverse reactions and interactions, especially those related to the drugs, tests, herbs, and behaviors mentioned above.

flurazepam hydrochloride

Apo-Flurazepam✤, Bio-Flurazepam, Dalmane, Novo-Flupam✤, PMS-Flurazepam✤, Somnol✤, Som Pam✤

Pharmacologic class: Benzodiazepine
Therapeutic class: Sedative-hypnotic
Controlled substance IV
Pregnancy risk category X

Action

Depresses CNS at limbic, thalamic, and hypothalamic levels by enhancing inhibitory neurotransmitter effect of gamma-aminobutyric acid on neuronal excitability

Availability

Capsules: 15 mg, 30 mg

⊘ Indications and dosages

➤ Short-term management of insomnia (less than 4 weeks)
Adults: 15 to 30 mg P.O. at bedtime

Dosage adjustment

• Elderly or debilitated patients

Contraindications
• Hypersensitivity to drug or other benzodiazepines
• Preexisting CNS depression
• Angle-closure glaucoma
• Pregnancy or breastfeeding

Precautions
Use cautiously in:
• hepatic dysfunction
• history of suicide attempt or drug dependence
• elderly patients
• children younger than age 15 (safety not established).

Administration
• Before starting therapy, evaluate patient's mental status and check kidney and liver function tests and CBC.

Route	Onset	Peak	Duration
P.O.	15-45 min	0.5-1 hr	7-8 hr

Adverse reactions
CNS: dizziness, daytime drowsiness, headache, lethargy, confusion, poor concentration, depression, paradoxical excitation, ataxia
EENT: blurred vision
GI: nausea, vomiting, diarrhea, constipation, dyspepsia, abdominal pain
Respiratory: sleep apnea
Skin: rash
Other: abnormal taste, hangover, physical or psychological drug dependence, drug tolerance

Interactions
Drug-drug. *Antidepressants, antihistamines, opioids:* additive CNS depression
Barbiturates, rifampin: increased flurazepam metabolism, decreased efficacy
Cimetidine, disulfiram, fluoxetine, hormonal contraceptives, isoniazid, ketoconazole, metoprolol, propoxyphene, propranolol, valproic acid: decreased flurazepam metabolism, enhanced efficacy

Levodopa: decreased levodopa efficacy
Theophylline: decreased sedative effects of flurazepam
Drug-diagnostic tests. *Alanine aminotransferase, alkaline phosphatase, aspartate aminotransferase, total and direct bilirubin:* increased levels
Drug-herbs. *Chamomile, hops, kava, skullcap, valerian:* additive CNS depression
Drug-behaviors. *Alcohol use:* additive CNS depression
Smoking: increased drug metabolism and clearance

Patient monitoring
• With long-term use, watch for signs and symptoms of physical or psychological dependence.
• Monitor patient's mental status, especially for depression and suicidal ideation.
• Watch for signs of drug hoarding or overuse.
• Monitor CBC and liver and kidney function tests.

Patient teaching
◀€ Urge patient (and significant other as appropriate) to report signs and symptoms of depression or suicidal thoughts or actions.
◀€ Advise female patient to immediately tell prescriber if she is pregnant. Caution her not to breastfeed.
• Inform patient that drug may cause physical or psychological dependence.
• Advise patient to minimize GI upset by eating frequent, small servings of food and drinking adequate fluids.
• As appropriate, review all other significant and life-threatening adverse reactions and interactions, especially those related to the drugs, tests, herbs, and behaviors mentioned above.

Reactions in **bold** are life-threatening.   ◀€ Clinical alert

flutamide
APO-Flutamide♣, Drogenil⊕,
Euflex♣, Novo-Flutamide♣,
PMS-Flutamide♣

Pharmacologic class: Antiandrogen
Therapeutic class: Antineoplastic
Pregnancy risk category D

FDA | BOXED WARNING

- Postmarketing hospitalizations and deaths from hepatic failure have occurred. Evidence of hepatic injury includes elevated serum transaminase levels, jaundice, hepatic encephalopathy, and death related to acute hepatic failure. In some patients, hepatic injury reversed after drug withdrawal. Approximately half of reported cases occurred within first 3 months of therapy.
- Measure serum transaminase levels before therapy begins. Drug isn't recommended if alanine aminotransferase (ALT) values exceed twice the upper limit of normal (ULN). Once therapy begins, measure transaminase levels monthly for first 4 months and periodically thereafter. Obtain liver function tests at first sign of hepatic dysfunction. If patient has jaundice or ALT level exceeding 2 x ULN, discontinue drug immediately and follow liver function tests closely until they resolve.

Action
Exerts potent antiandrogenic activity at cellular level by inhibiting androgen uptake or nuclear binding of androgen

Availability
Capsules: 125 mg

⚕ Indications and dosages
➢ Metastatic prostate cancer

Adults: 250 mg P.O. t.i.d. q 8 hours, given with luteinizing hormone-releasing hormone (LHRH) analog. Total daily dosage is 750 mg.

Off-label uses
- Benign prostatic hypertrophy

Contraindications
- Hypersensitivity to drug
- Severe hepatic impairment
- Sleep apnea
- Women

Precautions
None

Administration
- Be aware that leuprolide acetate is the most common LHRH analog given with flutamide.

Route	Onset	Peak	Duration
P.O.	Variable	2 hr	72 hr

Adverse reactions
CNS: drowsiness, confusion, depression, anxiety, nervousness, paresthesia
CV: peripheral edema, hypertension
GI: nausea, vomiting, diarrhea, constipation, abdominal pain, dyspepsia, anorexia, dry mouth
GU: erectile dysfunction, loss of libido, gynecomastia, hot flashes
Hematologic: anemia, **leukopenia, thrombocytopenia**
Hepatic: hepatitis
Skin: rash, photosensitivity

Interactions
Drug-drug. *Warfarin:* increased prothrombin time
Drug-diagnostic tests. *Alkaline phosphatase, alanine aminotransferase, aspartate aminotransferase, blood urea nitrogen, creatine kinase:* increased levels
Hemoglobin, platelets, white blood cells: decreased levels
Drug-herbs. *Chaparral, comfrey, eucalyptus, germander, pennyroyal, skullcap, valerian:* increased risk of hepatotoxicity
Drug-behaviors. *Sun exposure:* increased risk of photosensitivity

---

Patient monitoring

• Monitor CBC and liver function tests.

◀€ Watch for bleeding tendency and signs and symptoms of hepatic damage (jaundice, vomiting, dark yellow or brown urine).

• Monitor blood pressure.

Patient teaching

◀€ Instruct patient to immediately report unusual bleeding or bruising.

• Tell patient to avoid activities that can cause injury. Advise him to use soft toothbrush and electric razor to avoid gum and skin injury.

• Caution patient to avoid driving and other hazardous activities until he knows how drug affects concentration and alertness.

• Instruct patient to minimize GI upset by eating frequent, small servings of healthy food.

• Tell patient he'll undergo regular blood testing during therapy.

• As appropriate, review all other significant and life-threatening adverse reactions and interactions, especially those related to the drugs, tests, herbs, and behaviors mentioned above.

fluticasone propionate

Cutivate, Flixonase⊕, Flixotide⊕, Flonase, Flovent Diskus, Flovent HFA

fluticasone furoate

Avamys✲, Veramyst

Pharmacologic class: Corticosteroid

Therapeutic class: Respiratory inhalant (Flovent, Flonase), anti-inflammatory drug (Cutivate)

Pregnancy risk category C

Action

Unknown. Has potent vasoconstrictive and anti-inflammatory properties.

Availability

fluticasone propionate

Inhalation aerosol, metered (Flovent HFA): 44 mcg, 110 mcg, 220 mcg

Inhalation powder, metered (Flovent Diskus): 50 mcg, 100 mcg, 250 mcg

Nasal spray (Flonase): 50 mcg

Topical cream (Cutivate): 0.005%

Topical ointment (Cutivate): 0.005%

fluticasone furoate

Nasal spray (Veramyst): 27.5 mcg fluticasone furoate in each 50-microliter spray in 10-g bottle containing 120 sprays

⦿ Indications and dosages

➤ Prophylaxis of asthma and treatment of asthma for patients requiring oral corticosteroid therapy (Flovent HFA and Flovent Diskus)

Adults and children age 4 and older: Recommended starting dosage and highest recommended dosage, based on prior asthma therapy, are listed in charts below.

Recommended Flovent FHA dosages

Previous Therapy	Starting dosage	Highest dosage
For Adults and adolescents age 12 and older		
Bronchodilators alone	88 mcg b.i.d.	440 mcg b.i.d.
Inhaled corticosteroids	88-220 mcg b.i.d.[1]	440 mcg b.i.d.
Oral corticosteroids[2]	440 mcg b.i.d.	880 mcg b.i.d.
Children ages 4 to 11[3]	88 mcg b.i.d.	88 mcg b.i.d.

1. Consider starting dosages above 88 mcg b.i.d. for patients with poorer asthma control or those who have previously required doses of inhaled corticosteroids in the higher range for the specific agent.
2. For patients currently receiving long-term oral corticosteroid therapy, reduce prednisone dosage no faster than 2.5 to 5 mg/day on a weekly basis beginning after at least 1 week of therapy with Flovent HFA. Once prednisone reduction is complete, reduce dosage to lowest effective dosage.
3. Recommended pediatric dosage is 88 mcg b.i.d. regardless of prior therapy.

Reactions in **bold** are life-threatening.

◀€ Clinical alert

Recommended Flovent Diskus dosages

Previous Therapy	Starting dosage	Highest dosage
Adults and adolescents age 12 and older		
Bronchodilators alone	100 mcg b.i.d.	500 mcg b.i.d.
Inhaled corticosteroids	100-250 mcg b.i.d.[1]	500 mcg b.i.d.
Oral corticosteroids[2]	500-1,000 mcg b.i.d.[3]	1,000 mcg b.i.d.
Children ages 4 to 11[4]	50 mcg b.i.d.	100 mcg b.i.d.

1. Consider starting dosages above 100 mcg b.i.d. (adults and adolescents) and 50 mcg b.i.d. (children ages 4 to 11) for patients with poorer asthma control or who have previously required doses of inhaled corticosteroids in the higher range for the specific agent.
2. For patients currently receiving long-term oral corticosteroid therapy, reduce prednisone dosage no faster than 2.5 to 5 mg/day on a weekly basis beginning after at least 1 week of therapy with Flovent Diskus. Once prednisone reduction is complete, reduce dosage to lowest effective dosage.
3. Choose starting dosage based on individual patient assessment. Inability to decrease oral corticosteroid dosage further during corticosteroid reduction may indicate the need to increase fluticasone propionate dosage to maximum of 1,000 mcg b.i.d.
4. Because individual responses may vary, children previously maintained on other inhaled corticosteroids may require dosage adjustments upon transfer to Flovent Diskus.

➤ Seasonal and perennial allergic and nonallergic rhinitis (Flonase)
Adults: Two sprays in each nostril daily or one spray in each nostril b.i.d. After first few days, may reduce dosage to one spray in each nostril daily; some patients may find p.r.n. use of two sprays in each nostril daily effective for symptom control. Maximum dosage is 200 mcg daily (two sprays in each nostril).

Adolescents and children ages 4 and older: Initially, one spray in each nostril daily. If patient doesn't respond, may increase to two sprays in each nostril. Once adequate control is achieved, reduce dosage to one spray in each nostril daily.

➤ Symptoms of seasonal and perennial allergic rhinitis (Veramyst)
Adults and adolescents age 12 and older: 110 mcg (2 sprays per nostril) once daily
Children ages 2 to 11: 55 mcg (1 spray per nostril) once daily
➤ Inflammatory and pruritic manifestations of corticosteroid-responsive atopic dermatoses
Adults and children ages 3 months and older: Apply thin film of Cutivate cream to affected skin area once or twice daily.
➤ Other corticosteroid-responsive dermatoses
Adults and children ages 3 months and older: Apply thin film of Cutivate cream to affected skin area b.i.d.

Contraindications

• Hypersensitivity to drug or its components
• Primary treatment of status asthmaticus or other acute asthma episodes necessitating intensive measures (Flovent FHA, Flovent Diskus)
• Severe allergy to milk proteins (Flovent Diskus)

Precautions

Use cautiously in:
• recurrent epistaxis, recent nasal septal ulcer, nasal surgery, or trauma
• severe hepatic disease (Veramyst)
• glaucoma and cataracts
• tuberculosis; respiratory tract infection; fungal, bacterial, viral, or parasitic infections; ocular herpes simplex
• hypercorticism and adrenal suppression (when used at higher than recommended dosages or in susceptible persons)
• concurrent use of other CYP3A inhibitors (such as ketoconazole; use not recommended with ritonavir)
• *Candida albicans* infection (Flovent, Veramyst)
• elderly patients (Flonase, Veramyst)

- pregnant or breastfeeding patients (Flovent, Flonase, Veramyst)
- children younger age than 4 (Flonase, Flovent)
- children younger than age 2 (Veramyst).

Administration

- Know that Flonase may cause immediate hypersensitivity reaction (contact dermatitis).
- Be aware that topical ointment should be used in adults only.
- Prime Veramyst nasal spray before first use, when not used for more than 30 days, or if cap has been left off bottle for 5 days or more.
- Administer inhalation powder by oral inhalation only.

Route	Onset	Peak	Duration
Oral or nasal inhalation, topical	Unknown	Unknown	Unknown

Adverse reactions

CNS: *Cutivate ointment*—lightheadedness; *Flonase*—headache, dizziness; *Flovent*—headache, dizziness, giddiness; *Veramyst*—headache
EENT: *Flonase*—cataract, glaucoma, increased intraocular pressure, epistaxis, nasal burning or irritation, bloody nasal mucus, runny nose, pharyngitis; *Flovent*—cataract, glaucoma, nasal congestion, nasal septum perforation, nasal discharge, nasal sinus pain, sinusitis, rhinitis, allergic rhinitis, pharyngitis, dysphonia; *Veramyst*—cataract, glaucoma, increased intraocular pressure, epistaxis, pharyngolaryngeal pain, nasal ulceration
GI: *Flonase*—nausea, vomiting, diarrhea, abdominal pain; *Flovent*—nausea, vomiting, diarrhea, dyspepsia, stomach disorder, oral candidiasis
GU: *Flovent*—dysmenorrhea
Metabolic: *Flovent, Veramyst*—hypercorticism and adrenal suppression

Musculoskeletal: *Flonase*—aches and pains; *Flovent*—joint pain, limb pain, sprain, strain, aches and pains, reduced bone mineral density; *Veramyst*—back pain
Respiratory: *Flonase*—asthma symptoms, cough, bronchitis, wheezing (rare); *Flovent*—upper respiratory tract infection, influenza, bronchitis, chest congestion, **bronchospasm;** *Veramyst*—cough
Skin: *Cutivate cream*—pruritus, skin dryness, skin burning, erythematous rash, dusky erythema, eczema exacerbation, skin irritation, urticaria; *Cutivate ointment*—skin burning or irritation, hypertrichosis, increased erythema, hives; *Flovent*—urticaria, rash, skin eruption
Other: *Cutivate cream or ointment*—numbness of fingers, facial or nonfacial telangiectasia; *Flonase*—fever, flulike symptoms, hypersensitivity reaction; *Flovent*—dental problems, fever, *C. albicans* infection, immunosuppression, immediate or delayed hypersensitivity reactions, **angioedema;** anaphylaxis; *Veramyst*—pyrexia

Interactions

Drug-drug. *Ketoconazole, other strong CYP3A inhibitors:* increased fluticasone exposure (with Flonase, Flovent, Veramyst)
Ritonavir: increased systemic corticosteroid effects (with Flonase, Flovent, Veramyst)
Drug-diagnostic tests. *Adrenocorticotropic hormone stimulation test, plasma cortisol test, urinary free cortisol test:* interference with test results

Patient monitoring

- Monitor patient for withdrawal symptoms after Flovent is discontinued.
- Stay alert for systemic corticosteroid effects when administering Flovent, Flonase, or Veramyst.

- Observe for reduced growth rate in child or adolescent using Flovent, Flonase, or Veramyst.
- When giving Flovent, watch for eosinophilic conditions, such as Churg-Strauss syndrome.

◀€ When giving Flonase, assess for epistaxis, wheezing, nasal septum perforation, cataracts, glaucoma, and increased intraocular pressure (rare reaction).

◀€ When giving Veramyst, assess for epistaxis, nasal septum perforation, cataracts, glaucoma, and increased intraocular pressure (rare reaction).

Patient teaching

- Tell patient to take drug exactly as prescribed.
- Teach patient proper use of prescribed form.

◀€ Advise patient to immediately report signs of allergic reaction.

- Caution patient to avoid exposure to people with chickenpox or measles.
- Advise female patient taking Flonase, Flovent, or Veramyst to inform prescriber if she is pregnant or breastfeeding.
- As appropriate, review all other significant and life-threatening adverse reactions and interactions, especially those related to the drugs and tests mentioned above.

fluvastatin sodium
Lescol, Lescol XL

Pharmacologic class: HMG-CoA reductase inhibitor
Therapeutic class: Antihyperlipidemic
Pregnancy risk category X

Action

Competitively inhibits HMG-CoA reductase, an enzyme needed to synthesize cholesterol. This inhibition reduces cholesterol concentration in hepatic cells, which in turn increases synthesis of low-density lipoprotein (LDL) receptors, enhances LDL uptake, and ultimately reduces plasma cholesterol concentration.

Availability
Capsules: 20 mg, 40 mg
Tablets (extended-release): 80 mg

🕖 Indications and dosages

➤ Adjunctive therapy to diet to reduce elevated total cholesterol (TC), LDL-C, apolipoprotein B (Apo B), and triglyceride levels; to increase HDL-C in patients with primary hypercholesterolemia and mixed dyslipidemia; to reduce risk of undergoing revascularization procedures in patients with clinically evident coronary heart disease (CHD); to slow progression of atherosclerosis in patients with CHD
Adults: Initially, 40 mg (capsule) P.O. in evening or b.i.d. Don't give two 40-mg capsules at one time. Or, 80 mg (extended-release tablet) P.O. as a single dose at any time of day.

➤ Adjunctive therapy to diet to reduce elevated TC, LDL-C, and Apo B levels in boys and postmenarchal girls with heterozygous familial hypercholesterolemia after failing adequate trial of diet therapy
Children ages 10 to 16: Initially, 20 mg (capsule) P.O. May increase dosage to maximum daily dose: 40 mg (capsule) P.O. b.i.d. or one 80-mg extended-release tablet once daily at 6-week intervals. Individualize dosages according to goal of therapy.

Dosage adjustment
- Concurrent use of cyclosporine, fluconazole, or lipid-modifying doses (1 g/day or greater) of niacin

Contraindications

- Hypersensitivity to drug or its components
- Active hepatic disease or unexplained, persistent serum transaminase elevations
- Patients who are pregnant or may become pregnant
- Breastfeeding patients

Precautions

Use cautiously in:

- severe renal impairment, history of liver disease or heavy alcohol use, uncontrolled hypothyroidism
- concurrent use of gemfibrozil (avoid use)
- concurrent use of cyclosporine, other fibrates, drugs that may decrease levels of endogenous steroid hormones (such as ketoconazole, spironolactone, cimetidine)
- elderly patients (advanced age a predisposing factor for myopathy)
- children younger than age 9 (safety not established).

Administration

- Know that before starting drug, patient should be on standard cholesterol-lowering diet and weight-control and physical exercise programs, if appropriate.
- Check liver enzyme test values before starting drug.
- Give with or without food.
- If patient is also receiving bile-acid resin, give fluvastatin at bedtime at least 4 hours after resin.

Route	Onset	Peak	Duration
P.O.	Unknown	1 hr	Unknown
P.O. (extended)	Unknown	2.5-3 hr	Unknown

Adverse reactions

CNS: headache, dizziness, insomnia, fatigue

CV: syncope, hypertension, intermittent claudication, **atrial fibrillation**
EENT: sinusitis, nasopharyngitis
GI: nausea, vomiting, diarrhea, constipation, dyspepsia, flatulence, abdominal pain, gastric disorder
GU: urinary tract infection, **myoglobinuria, acute renal failure**
Hepatic: abnormal liver function tests **hepatitis** (rare), **hepatic failure**
Metabolic: hyperglycemia
Musculoskeletal: joint pain, arthritis, extremity pain, myalgia, myopathy, **rhabdomyolysis**
Respiratory: exertional dyspnea, bronchitis
Other: flulike symptoms, tooth disorder, accidental trauma, peripheral edema, allergic reaction

Interactions

Drug-drug. *Cholestyramine:* decreased fluvastatin blood level
Antifungals, erythromycin, colchicine, gemfibrozil and other fibrates, lipid-modifying doses of niacin, other HMG-CoA inhibitors: increased risk of myopathy
Cimetidine, diclofenac, omeprazole, ranitidine: increased fluvastatin blood level
Cyclosporine, fluconazole: increased fluvastatin exposure
Glyburide, phenytoin: increased blood levels of both drugs
Rifampin: increased fluvastatin metabolism, decreased blood level
Drug-diagnostic tests. *Alanine aminotransferase, aspartate aminotransferase, creatine kinase, fasting serum glucose, HbA1c:* increased levels
Drug-behaviors. *Alcohol use:* increased risk of hepatotoxicity

Patient monitoring

- Watch for allergic reaction to drug.
- ◀€ Assess for myositis. If patient has muscle pain, monitor CK level. Discontinue drug if myopathy is diagnosed or suspected.

Reactions in **bold** are life-threatening.   ◀€ Clinical alert

- Monitor lipid levels and liver function test results, particularly in patients with history of liver disease or heavy alcohol use.
- Be aware that bleeding or increased prothrombin times have occurred in patients taking coumarin anticoagulants concurrently with other HMG-CoA reductase inhibitors. Monitor prothrombin times closely in patients receiving warfarin-type anticoagulants when fluvastatin is initiated or dosage is changed. Watch for bleeding tendencies.
- In patients receiving phenytoin, or glyburide, closely monitor drug's effects on phenytoin or glyburide levels when fluvastatin is initiated or fluvastatin dosage is changed.

Patient teaching

- Instruct patient to take once-daily dosages in evening for best effect.
- Tell patient to take drug with or without food.
- Tell patient not to open capsules and not to break, crush, or chew extended-release tablets.
- Advise patient to maintain standard cholesterol-lowering diet and weight-control and physical exercise programs, as appropriate.
- ◀€ Instruct patient to immediately report irregular heart beat, muscle aches or pains, yellowing of eyes or skin, or unusual tiredness.
- ◀€ Teach patient how to recognize and report signs and symptoms of allergic response, renal dysfunction, or myopathy.
- Advise patient to notify prescriber if he drinks more than two glasses of alcohol daily.
- Advise women of childbearing age to use effective contraception and to stop drug immediately and notify prescriber if pregnancy occurs.
- Tell patient that full effect of drug may take up to 4 weeks.

- As appropriate, review all other significant and life-threatening adverse reactions and interactions, especially those related to the drugs, tests, and behaviors mentioned above.

fluvoxamine maleate

Apo-Fluvoxamine✲, Co Fluvoxamine✲, Dom-Fluvoxamine✲, Faverin⊕, Luvox CR, Novo-Fluvoxamine✲, Nu-Fluvoxamine✲, PHL-Fluvoxamine✲, PMS-Fluvoxamine✲, Ratio-Fluvoxamine✲, Riva-Fluvoxamine✲, Sandoz Fluvoxamine✲

Pharmacologic class: Selective serotonin reuptake inhibitor (SSRI)
Therapeutic class: Antidepressant, antiobsessive agent
Pregnancy risk category C

FDA BOXED WARNING

- Drug may increase risk of suicidal thinking and behavior in children and adolescents with major depressive disorder and other psychiatric disorders, especially during first few months of therapy. Risk must be balanced with clinical need, as depression itself increases suicide risk. With patient of any age, observe closely for clinical worsening, suicidality, and unusual behavior changes when therapy begins. Advise family and caregivers to observe patient closely and communicate with prescriber as needed.
- Drug isn't approved for use in pediatric patients except those with obsessive-compulsive disorder.

Action
Selectively inhibits serotonin reuptake in neurons. This inhibition is thought to relieve depression and reduce behaviors related to obsessive-compulsive disorder (OCD).

Availability
Capsules (extended-release): 100 mg, 150 mg
Tablets: 25 mg, 50 mg, 100 mg

⏀ Indications and dosages
➤ OCD
Adults: Initially, 50 mg P.O. daily at bedtime; may increase by 50 mg q 4 to 7 days until desired effect occurs (not to exceed 300 mg/day). If daily dosage exceeds 100 mg, give in two equally divided doses; if doses aren't equal, give larger dose at bedtime. As needed, adjust dosage periodically to maintain lowest effective dosage that controls symptoms (immediate-release formulation)
Children ages 8 to 17: Initially, 25 mg at bedtime; may increase by 25 mg/day q 4 to 7 days until desired effect occurs (up to 200 mg/day for patients up to age 11 or up to 300 mg for adolescents). If daily dosage exceeds 50 mg, give in divided doses, with larger dose at bedtime (immediate-release formulation).
➤ OCD; social anxiety disorder
Adults: 100 mg P.O. once daily at bedtime; titrate in 50-mg increments weekly, to a maximum of 300 mg/day (extended-release formulation).

Dosage adjustment
• Hepatic impairment
• Elderly patients

Off-label uses
• Autism
• Anxiety disorders

Contraindications
• Hypersensitivity to drug or other SSRIs
• MAO inhibitor use within past 14 days

Precautions
Use cautiously in:
• cardiovascular disease, hepatic or renal impairment, mania, seizures, suicidal tendency
• elderly patients
• labor and delivery
• pregnant or breastfeeding patients.

Administration
• Give with or without food.
• Discontinue 5 weeks before MAO inhibitor therapy is set to begin.

Route	Onset	Peak	Duration
P.O.	Rapid	2-8 hr	Unknown

Adverse reactions
CNS: dizziness, drowsiness, headache, insomnia, nervousness, anxiety, apathy, manic or psychotic reactions, depression, hypokinesia or hyperkinesia, tremor, **suicide or suicidal ideation** (especially in child or adolescent)
CV: hypertension, orthostatic hypotension, palpitations, tachycardia
EENT: sinusitis
GI: nausea, vomiting, diarrhea, constipation, dyspepsia, flatulence, dry mouth, dysphagia, anorexia
GU: decreased libido, sexual dysfunction, anorgasmia
Musculoskeletal: hypertonia, myoclonus, twitching
Respiratory: cough, dyspnea
Skin: diaphoresis
Other: abnormal taste, tooth disorder, dental caries, edema, weight gain or loss, chills, fever, flulike symptoms, yawning, hot flashes, allergic reactions, hypersensitivity reaction

Interactions
Drug-drug. *Beta-adrenergic blockers (such as propranolol), carbamazepine, lithium, L-tryptophan, methadone, some benzodiazepines, theophylline, tolbutamide, warfarin:* decreased fluvoxamine metabolism, increased effects

---

Reactions in **bold** are life-threatening.   ◀€ Clinical alert

Clozapine: increased clozapine blood level and risk of toxicity
MAO inhibitors: serotonin syndrome
Tricyclic antidepressants: increased fluvoxamine blood level
Drug-tests. *Hepatic enzyme levels:* increased
Drug-behaviors. *Smoking:* decreased fluvoxamine efficacy

Patient monitoring

◀€ Watch closely for signs and symptoms of depression and suicidal ideation (especially in child or adolescent).

• Assess patient's appetite. Report weight gain or loss.

• Monitor liver function test results.

• Monitor cardiovascular status, particularly blood pressure.

Patient teaching

• Instruct patient to swallow extended-release capsules whole and not to break, crush, or chew them.

◀€ Instruct patient or caregiver (especially with child or adolescent patient) to recognize and immediately report signs of suicidal intent or expressions of suicidal ideation.

• Inform patient that drug may take several weeks to be fully effective.

• Recommend establishing effective bedtime routine to minimize insomnia.

• Instruct female patient to notify prescriber if she becomes or intends to become pregnant. Caution her not to breastfeed.

• Caution patient to avoid driving and other hazardous activities until he knows how drug affects concentration and alertness.

• As appropriate, review all other significant and life-threatening adverse reactions and interactions, especially those related to the drugs, tests, and behaviors mentioned above.

fondaparinux sodium
Arixtra

Pharmacologic class: Selective factor Xa inhibitor

Therapeutic class: Anticoagulant, antithrombotic

Pregnancy risk category B

FDA | BOXED WARNING

• During epidural or spinal anesthesia or puncture, patients receiving drug or scheduled to receive it for thromboprophylaxis are at risk for epidural or spinal hematoma, which can lead to long-term or permanent paralysis. Risk increases with use of indwelling epidural catheter for analgesia administration and with concurrent use of drugs affecting hemostasis (such as nonsteroidal anitinflammatory drugs, platelet inhibitors, and other anticoagulants). Risk also rises with traumatic or repeated epidural or spinal puncture or history of spinal deformity or spinal surgery. Before neuraxial intervention, physician should weigh drug's potential benefit against risk.

• Monitor patient frequently for signs and symptoms of neurologic impairment. If these occur, provide urgent treatment.

Action

Selectively inhibits factor Xa, disrupting blood coagulation and inhibiting thrombin formation and thrombus development

Availability

Injection: 2.5 mg/0.5 ml in single-dose syringe

---

❶ Indications and dosages

➤ Prevention of deep-vein thrombosis after hip fracture surgery or hip or knee replacement surgery

Adults: 2.5 mg subcutaneously 6 to 8 hours after surgery, once hemostasis occurs; usual duration is 5 to 9 days (up to 11 days) given daily. After hip fracture surgery, extended prophylactic course of up to 24 additional days is recommended; some patients have tolerated a total course of 32 days.

➤ Deep-vein thrombosis and pulmonary emboli

Adults: 5 mg subcutaneously once daily for patients weighing less than 50 kg (110 lb), 7.5 mg subcutaneously for patients weighing 50 to 100 kg (110 to 220 lb) or 10 mg subcutaneously for patients weighing more than 100 kg (220 lb) for 5 days and until therapeutic oral anticoagulant effect occurs (as shown by International Normalized Ratio of 2 to 3). Usual duration of therapy is 5 to 9 days, but may continue for up to 26 days.

Dosage adjustment

• Renal impairment

Contraindications

• Hypersensitivity to drug
• Bacterial endocarditis
• Severe renal disease
• Active major bleeding
• Patients weighing less than 50 kg (110 lb) who have undergone hip fracture, hip replacement, or knee replacement surgery

Precautions

Use cautiously in:
• diabetic retinopathy, hepatic disease, blood dyscrasias, heparin-induced thrombocytopenia, severe hypertension, alcoholism
• patients older than age 75
• pregnant or breastfeeding patients
• children (safety and efficacy not established).

Administration

◀≋ Withhold for at least 6 to 8 hours after surgery, to minimize risk of major bleeding.

◀≋ Give by subcutaneous injection only. Don't give I.M.

• Rotate injection sites among fatty tissue areas on left and right anterolateral and posterolateral abdominal walls.

• Don't expel air bubble from syringe; doing so may reduce amount of drug delivered.

• Listen for slight click when plunger is fully released. After drug has been injected, needle retracts and white safety indicator is visible.

• Don't mix with other injections or infusions.

• Know that when drug is used to treat deep-vein thrombosis and pulmonary emboli, concomitant warfarin treatment should begin as soon as possible (usually within 72 hours).

Route	Onset	Peak	Duration
Subcut.	Rapid	3 hr	72 hr

Adverse reactions

CNS: depression, dizziness, asthenia, headache, abnormal thinking, confusion, insomnia, neuropathy
CV: hypotension
GI: nausea, vomiting, diarrhea, constipation, abdominal pain, dyspepsia, dry mouth, anorexia
GU: urinary retention, urinary tract infection
Hematologic: anemia, hematoma, purpura, minor bleeding, **major bleeding, thrombocytopenia, retroperitoneal hemorrhage, postoperative hemorrhage**
Metabolic: hypokalemia
Skin: bullous eruption
Other: increased wound drainage, injection site bleeding, pain, edema, fever

Interactions

Drug-drug. *Anticoagulants:* increased risk of bleeding

Drug-herbs. *Anise, astragalus, bilberry, black currant, bladder wrack, bogbean, boldo, borage, buchu, capsaicin, cat's claw, celery, chaparral, cinchona, clove oil, dandelion, dong quai, fenugreek, feverfew, garlic, ginger, ginkgo, papaya, red clover, rhubarb, safflower oil, skullcap, tan-shen:* additive anticoagulant effect

St. John's wort: reduced anticoagulant effect

Patient monitoring

• Monitor CBC, platelet count, creatinine level, and renal function tests. Assess stools for occult blood.

• Monitor vital signs, temperature, and fluid intake and output.

◀ Stay alert for bleeding tendency, especially postoperative hemorrhage.

• Check for increased wound drainage after surgery.

◀ In patient undergoing concomitant neuraxial anesthesia or spinal puncture, watch for neurologic impairment (indicating possible spinal or epidural hematoma).

◀ Discontinue drug if severe renal impairment occurs.

Patient teaching

◀ Instruct patient to immediately report bleeding.

• Caution patient to avoid activities that can cause injury. Tell him to use soft toothbrush and electric razor to avoid gum and skin injury.

• Tell patient that he'll undergo regular blood testing during therapy.

• As appropriate, review all other significant and life-threatening adverse reactions and interactions, especially those related to the drugs and herbs mentioned above.

formoterol fumarate

Atimos Modulite⊕, Foradil⊕, Foradil Aerolizer, Oxeze♣, Oxis⊕, Perforomist

Pharmacologic class: Sympathomimetic; long-acting, selective beta$_2$-adrenergic receptor agonist

Therapeutic class: Bronchodilator

Pregnancy risk category C

FDA | BOXED WARNING

• Drug may increase risk of asthma-related death. Give only as additional therapy for patients not adequately controlled on other asthma-controller medications or whose disease severity clearly warrants treatment with two maintenance therapies.

• In large placebo-controlled study, increase in asthma-related deaths occurred in patients receiving salmeterol; this finding may apply to formoterol.

Action

Stimulates intracellular adenylate cyclase, relaxing bronchial smooth muscle and inhibiting release of mediators of immediate hypersensitivity

Availability

Capsules for oral inhalation (used with Aerolizer inhaler): 12 mcg

ⓘ Indications and dosages

➤ Long-term maintenance of asthma; prevention or long-term maintenance of bronchospasm in patients with chronic obstructive pulmonary disease

Adults and children ages 5 and older: Contents of 1 capsule inhaled orally via Aerolizer q 12 hours

➤ Acute prevention of exercise-induced bronchospasm (on occasional, as-needed basis)

Adults and children ages 5 and older: Contents of 1 capsule inhaled orally via Aerolizer at least 15 minutes before start of exercise. Wait 12 hours after initial dose before giving repeat dose.

Contraindications

• Hypersensitivity to drug or its components
• Tachyarrhythmias

Precautions

Use cautiously in:
• acute asthma symptoms, deteriorating asthma, cardiovascular disorders, seizure disorders, thyrotoxicosis, diabetes, possible hypokalemia
• patients older than age 75
• labor
• pregnant or breastfeeding patients
• children younger than age 5.

Administration

• Be aware that drug is not intended for acute asthma attacks.
• Use capsules only with Aerolizer inhaler supplied.
• Keep capsules in blister until immediately before use.
◀ᕯ Make sure patient doesn't swallow capsules.

Route	Onset	Peak	Duration
Inhalation	Rapid	5 min	12 hr

Adverse reactions

CNS: tremor, dizziness, insomnia, anxiety
CV: chest pain
EENT: sinusitis, pharyngitis, tonsillitis
GI: dry mouth
Metabolic: hypokalemia, hyperglycemia
Musculoskeletal: muscle cramps, back pain, leg cramps

Respiratory: bronchitis, chest infection, dyspnea, upper respiratory tract infection, increased sputum
Skin: pruritus, rash
Other: dysphonia, viral infection, fever

Interactions

Drug-drug. *Adrenergics:* potentiation of formoterol's sympathomimetic effects
Beta-adrenergic blockers: partial or total inhibition of formoterol's effects
Cardiac glycosides, methylxanthines, potassium-wasting diuretics, steroids: potentiation of formoterol's hypokalemic effects, increased risk of arrhythmias
Disopyramide, MAO inhibitors, quinidine, phenothiazines, procainamide, tricyclic antidepressants: prolonged QTc interval, increased risk of ventricular arrhythmias
Halogenated hydrocarbon anesthetics: increased risk of arrhythmias
Levodopa, levothyroxine, oxytocin: impaired cardiac tolerance of formoterol
Drug-diagnostic tests. *Blood glucose:* increased level
Potassium: decreased level
Drug-behaviors. *Alcohol use:* impaired cardiac tolerance of formoterol

Patient monitoring

• Monitor pulmonary function test results.
• Monitor potassium and glucose levels.

Patient teaching

• Teach patient how to use capsules and Aerolizer inhaler provided.
• Instruct patient to keep capsules in blisters until immediately before use.
• Caution patient not to swallow capsules.
• Tell patient not to use drug for acute asthma attacks.
◀ᕯ Instruct patient to contact prescriber immediately if difficulty in

---

breathing persists after using drug or if condition worsens.

• Caution patient to take drug exactly as prescribed and not to stop therapy even if he feels better.

• Tell patient to consult prescriber if he has been taking inhaled, short-acting drugs on a regular basis.

• Advise female patient to tell prescriber if she is pregnant or breastfeeding or if she plans to become pregnant.

• Caution patient to avoid alcohol during therapy.

• As appropriate, review all other significant adverse reactions and interactions, especially those related to the drugs, tests, and behaviors mentioned above.

fosamprenavir calcium
Lexiva, Telzir✚⊕

Pharmacologic class: Human immunodeficiency virus (HIV) protease inhibitor

Therapeutic class: Antiretroviral

Pregnancy risk category C

Action
Blocks HIV reverse transcriptase, an enzyme necessary for HIV replication. Blockade leads to reduced viral load and increased CD4+ cell count, helping to ward off other infections when drug is given with other antiretrovirals.

Availability
Oral suspension: 50 mg/ml
Tablets: 700 mg

🚺 Indications and dosages
➤ HIV-1 infection, given in combination with other antiretrovirals

Adults (therapy-naive): 1,400 mg P.O. b.i.d. or 1,400 mg P.O. daily given with

rotonavir 200 mg daily; or 1,400 mg P.O. daily with ritonavir 100 mg daily; or 700 mg b.i.d. with ritonavir 100 mg b.i.d.

Adults (protease inhibitor– experienced): 700 mg P.O. b.i.d. with ritonavir 100 mg b.i.d.

Children ages 2 and older: Calculate dosage based on weight, but don't exceed adult dosage. When given in combination with ritonavir, fosamprenavir tablets may be used for children weighing at least 39 kg (86 lb); ritonavir capsules may be used for those weighing at least 33 kg (73 lb). See table below for more information.

Pediatrice dosages	
Therapy-naive children ages 2 to 5	30 mg/kg (oral suspension) P.O. b.i.d., not to exceed adult dosage of 1,400 mg b.i.d.
Therapy-naive children ages 6 and older	30 mg/kg P.O. b.i.d. or 18 mg/kg plus ritonavir 3 mg/kg b.i.d., not to exceed adult dosage of fosamprenavir 700 mg plus ritonavir 100 mg b.i.d.*
Therapy-experienced children ages 6 and older	18 mg/kg (oral suspension) P.O. plus ritonavir 3 mg/kg b.i.d., not to exceed adult dosage of fosamprenavir 700 mg b.i.d. plus ritonavir 100 mg b.i.d. Or 1,400 mg (tablets) P.O. b.i.d. for children weighing at least 47 kg when given without ritonavir.*

*Patients weighing at least 39 kg (86 lb) who are also taking ritonavir may receive oral suspension or tablets; those weighing at least 47 kg (104 lb) who aren't taking ritonavir may receive oral suspension or tablets.

Dosage adjustment
• Mild, moderate and severe hepatic impairment

Contraindications
• Hypersensitivity to drug or amprenavir

• Concomitant use of drugs that depend highly on CYP3A4 for clearance and for which elevated blood levels may lead to serious or

---

life-threatening events (such as some antiarrhythmics, antimycobacterials, ergot derivatives, GI motility agents, HMG co-reductase inhibitors, neuroleptics, nonnucleoside reverse transcriptase inhibitors, and sedative-hypnotics)
• Coadministration with ritonavir in patients receiving flecainide or propafenone
• Concomitant use of St. John's wort

Precautions

Use cautiously in:
• sulfa allergy
• hepatic impairment
• diabetes mellitus
• elderly patients
• pregnant or breastfeeding patients
• children younger than age 2 (safety and efficacy not established).

Administration

• Assess cholesterol and triglyceride levels and hepatic function tests before starting therapy.
• Give oral suspension to adults without food and to children with food.
• Administer tablets with or without food.

Route	Onset	Peak	Duration
P.O.	Unknown	1.5-4 hr	Unknown

Adverse reactions

CNS: headache
GI: nausea, vomiting, diarrhea, abdominal pain
GU: nephrolithiasis
Hematologic: spontaneous bleeding (in hemophiliacs), acute hemolytic anemia
Metabolic: diabetes mellitus, body fat redistribution or accumulation
Skin: pruritus, maculopapular rash, **severe or life-threatening skin reactions**
Other: immune reconstitution syndrome

Interactions

Drug-drug. *Alfuzosin:* increased alfuzosin level, resulting in hypotension
Antimycobacterials (rifampin): decreased fosamprenavir blood level, possible loss of virologic response and possible resistance to fosamprenavir or to its protease inhibitor class (concomitant rifampin use contraindicated)
Amitriptyline, amlodipine, atorvastatin, benzodiazepines (alprazolam, clorazepate, diazepam, flurazepam), bepridil, cyclosporine, diltiazem, esomeprazole, felodipine, fluticasone, imipramine, isradipine, itraconazole, ketoconazole, lidocaine (systemic), nicardipine, nifedipine, nimodipine, nisoldipine, quinidine, rapamycin, rosuvastatin, tacrolimus, trazodone, verapamil: increased blood levels of these drugs
Carbamazepine, cimetidine, dexamethasone, efavirenz, famotidine, nizatidine, phenobarbital, phenytoin, ranitidine, saquinavir: decreased fosamprenavir blood levels
Cisapride, pimozide: possible serious or life-threatening reactions, such as arrhythmias (concomitant use with fosamprenavir contraindicated)
CYP3A4 inducers: significant decrease in fosamprenavir blood level and reduced therapeutic effect
CYP3A4 inhibitors: increased fosamprenavir blood level and increased incidence of adverse effects
Delavirdine: possible loss of virologic response and possible resistance to delavirdine
Ergot derivatives (dihydroergotamine, ergonovine, ergotamine, methylergonovine): serious or life-threatening reactions such as acute ergot toxicity (concomitant use with fosamprenavir contraindicated)
Flecainide, propafenone: increased risk of serious, life-threatening cardiac arrhythmias (concomitant use contraindicated)

f

Reactions in **bold** are life-threatening. ◀€ Clinical alert

HIV protease inhibitors (lopinavir/ritonavir): decreased blood levels of both drugs

Hormonal contraceptives: possible changes in hormone levels and liver enzyme elevations (if used in combination with fosamprenavir and ritonavir)

Indinavir, nelfinavir: increased fosamprenavir blood level

Lovastatin, simvastatin: increased risk of serious reactions such as myopathy, including rhabdomyolysis (concomitant use with fosamprenavir contraindicated)

Methadone: decreased methadone blood level

Midazolam, triazolam: serious or life-threatening reactions, such as prolonged or increased sedation or respiratory depression (concomitant use with fosamprenavir contraindicated)

Nevirapine: decreased fosamprenavir and increased nevirapine blood levels

Paroxetine (in combination with fosamprenavir and ritonavir): decreased paroxetine blood level

PDE5 inhibitors (such as sildenafil): increased risk of adverse reactions (such as hypotension, visual changes, priapism)

Phenytoin (in combination with fosamprenavir and ritonavir): increased fosamprenavir, decreased phenytoin blood level

Rifabutin: increased rifabutin and metabolite blood levels

Warfarin: altered blood levels

Drug-diagnostic tests. *ALT, AST, glucose, lipase, triglycerides:* increased levels

Drug-food. *High-fat meal:* reduced fosamprenavir effect

Drug-herbs. *St. John's wort:* significant decrease in fosamprenavir blood level with loss of therapeutic effect and possible resistance to fosamprenavir or its protease inhibitor class (concomitant use contraindicated)

Patient monitoring

◀€ Monitor patient closely for rash; discontinue drug if severe rash or moderate rash plus systemic symptoms develops.

• Be aware that immune reconstitution syndrome has occurred in patients treated with combination antiretroviral therapy. During initial phase of such therapy, patients whose immune system responds may develop inflammatory response to indolent or residual opportunistic infections (such as *Mycobacterium avium* complex, cytomegalovirus, *Pneumocystis jiroveci* pneumonia, and tuberculosis), which may necessitate further evaluation and treatment.

• Closely monitor International Normalized Ratio if patient is receiving warfarin concomitantly.

• Closely monitor hepatic function tests during therapy.

• Periodically monitor cholesterol and triglyceride levels.

• Watch for new-onset diabetes mellitus, exacerbation of preexisting diabetes, and hyperglycemia.

Patient teaching

• Advise adult patient to take oral suspension without food.

• Tell caregivers to give oral suspension with food to child.

• Instruct patient to shake oral suspension bottle vigorously before each use; mention that refrigeration may improve taste.

• Instruct patient to take tablets with or without food.

◀€ Advise patient to immediately report new infections or rash, which may become severe and potentially life-threatening.

• Inform patient that drug doesn't cure HIV infection or reduce risk of passing HIV to others through sexual contact, needle sharing, or blood exposure.

• Tell patient that drug may cause body fat redistribution or accumulation and that the cause and long-term health effects of this condition aren't known.

• Advise patient that drug may interact with many drugs and herbs (especially St. John's wort). Caution patient to discuss use of herbs and other drugs with prescriber.

• Advise male receiving PDE5 inhibitors (such as sildenafil, tadalafil, vardenafil) that he may be at increased risk for adverse events, including hypotension, visual changes, and priapism. Instruct him to promptly report symptoms.

• Advise patient taking hormonal contraceptives to use alternative contraception during therapy because hormone levels may be altered and liver enzyme levels may increase.

• Advise female to notify prescriber if she is pregnant or intends to become pregnant.

• Instruct women not to breastfeed while taking drug.

• As appropriate, review all other significant and life-threatening adverse reactions and interactions, especially those related to the drugs, tests, food, and herbs mentioned above.

fosinopril sodium

APO-Fosinopril✸, Gen-Fosinopril✸, Lin-Fosinopril✸, Monopril, Novo-Fosinopril✸, PMS-Fosinopril✸, Ran-Fosinopril✸, Ratio-Fosinopril✸, Riva-Fosinopril✸, Staril⊕

Pharmacologic class: Angiotensin-converting enzyme (ACE) inhibitor
Therapeutic class: Antihypertensive
Pregnancy risk category C (first trimester), **D** (second and third trimesters)

FDA BOXED WARNING

• When used during second or third trimester of pregnancy, drug may cause fetal injury or even death. Discontinue as soon as pregnancy is detected.

Action

Prevents conversion of angiotensin I to the vasoconstrictor angiotensin II, thereby reducing sodium and water retention and enhancing blood flow in circulatory system

Availability

Tablets: 10 mg, 20 mg, 40 mg

ⓕ Indications and dosages

➤ Hypertension
Adults: 10 mg P.O. daily. May increase as required up to 80 mg/day; typical range is 20 to 40 mg P.O. daily.
➤ Heart failure
Adults: 10 mg P.O. daily. May increase over several weeks up to 40 mg/day; typical range is 20 to 40 mg/day.

Dosage adjustment

• Renal impairment

Off-label uses

• Adjunct in myocardial infarction
• Nephropathy

Contraindications

• Hypersensitivity to drug or other ACE inhibitors
• Angioedema (hereditary or idiopathic)
• Pregnancy

Precautions

Use cautiously in:
• aortic stenosis, cardiomyopathy, cerebrovascular or cardiac insufficiency, renal or hepatic impairment, hyponatremia, hypovolemia

---

- black patients with hypertension
- patients receiving diuretics concurrently
- elderly patients
- breastfeeding patients (safety not established)
- children (safety not established).

Administration

- Don't administer within 2 hours of antacids.
- Give with or without food, but avoid giving with high-potassium foods or potassium supplements.

Route	Onset	Peak	Duration
P.O.	Within 1 hr	2-6 hr	24 hr

Adverse reactions

CNS: dizziness, drowsiness, fatigue, headache, insomnia, weakness, vertigo
CV: hypotension, angina pectoris, tachycardia
EENT: sinusitis
GI: nausea, vomiting, diarrhea, anorexia
GU: proteinuria, erectile dysfunction, decreased libido, **renal failure**
Hematologic: agranulocytosis, bone marrow depression
Metabolic: hyperkalemia
Respiratory: cough, bronchitis, dyspnea, **asthma, eosinophilic pneumonitis**
Skin: rash, **angioedema**
Other: altered taste, fever, hypersensitivity reactions including **anaphylaxis**

Interactions

Drug-drug. *Allopurinol:* increased risk of hypersensitivity reaction
Antacids: decreased fosinopril absorption
Antihypertensives, diuretics, general anesthetics, nitrates, phenothiazines: additive hypotension
Cyclosporine, indomethacin, potassium-sparing diuretics, potassium supplements: hyperkalemia
Digoxin, lithium: increased blood levels of these drugs, greater risk of toxicity

Indomethacin: decreased hypotensive effects
Drug-diagnostic tests. *Alanine aminotransferase, alkaline phosphatase, aspartate aminotransferase, bilirubin, blood urea nitrogen, creatinine, potassium:* increased levels
Antinuclear antibody titer: false-positive result
Sodium: decreased level
Drug-food. *Salt substitutes containing potassium:* hyperkalemia
Drug-herbs. *Capsaicin:* increased incidence of cough
Drug-behaviors. *Acute alcohol ingestion:* additive hypotension

Patient monitoring

- Monitor cardiovascular, respiratory, and neurologic status.
- Monitor CBC and liver and kidney function tests.
- Measure blood pressure to assess drug efficacy and detect hypotension.
- Assess patient's potassium intake; monitor serum potassium level.
- ◀€ Monitor for signs and symptoms of angioedema and anaphylaxis. If these occur, withdraw drug and contact prescriber immediately.

Patient teaching

- ◀€ Instruct patient to immediately report rash or difficulty breathing.
- Tell patient to report dizziness, fainting, bleeding tendency, change in urination pattern, swelling, or persistent cough.
- Encourage patient to drink enough fluids to stay well hydrated.
- Caution patient to avoid driving and other hazardous activities until he knows how drug affects concentration and alertness.
- Instruct female patient to notify prescriber if she suspects she is pregnant.
- Tell patient that he will undergo regular blood testing during therapy.
- As appropriate, review all other significant and life-threatening adverse

reactions and interactions, especially those related to the drugs, tests, foods, herbs, and behaviors mentioned above.

fosphenytoin sodium
Cerebyx, Pro-Epanutin ✤

Pharmacologic class: Hydantoin
Therapeutic class: Anticonvulsant
Pregnancy risk category D

Action
Thought to regulate neuronal membrane by promoting sodium excretion from neurons. This action prevents hyperexcitability and excessive stimulation, which inhibits spread of seizure activity. Lacks general CNS depressant effect.

Availability
Injection: 150 mg in 2-ml vials (100 mg phenytoin sodium), 750 mg in 10-ml vials (500 mg phenytoin sodium)

🕖 Indications and dosages
➤ Status epilepticus
Adults: 15 to 20 mg phenytoin sodium equivalent (PE)/kg I.V. at 100 to 150 mg PE/minute as a loading dose, then 4 to 6 mg (PE)/kg I.V. daily for maintenance
➤ To prevent seizures during neurosurgery
Adults: 10 to 20 mg PE/kg I.M. or I.V. as a loading dose, then 4 to 6 mg PE/kg I.M. or I.V. daily for maintenance

Dosage adjustment
• Hepatic disease
• Renal impairment
• Elderly patients

Contraindications
• Hypersensitivity to drug
• Adams-Stokes syndrome
• Arrhythmias

Precautions
Use cautiously in:
• hepatic or renal impairment, severe cardiac or respiratory disease
• elderly patients
• pregnant or breastfeeding patients (safety not established).

Administration
• Know that drug is a phenytoin prodrug and is given in PE units to avoid the need to perform molecular weight-based adjustments when converting between fosphenytoin and phenytoin sodium doses.
• For I.V. use, dilute in dextrose 5% in water or normal saline solution.
• Don't give faster than 150 mg PE/minute. Too-rapid infusion causes hypotension.
◀🔊 Check ECG, vital signs, and overall patient status continuously during infusion and for 10 to 20 minutes afterward.
• When giving I.M., rotate injection sites.

Route	Onset	Peak	Duration
I.V.	Rapid	Unknown	Up to 24 hr
I.M.	Unknown	30 min	Up to 24 hr

Adverse reactions
CNS: ataxia, agitation, dizziness, drowsiness, dysarthria, dyskinesia, speech disorder, extrapyramidal syndrome, headache, nervousness, weakness, confusion, hyperesthesia, paresthesia, **cerebral edema, coma, intracranial hypertension**
CV: hypotension, tachycardia
EENT: diplopia, nystagmus, tinnitus
GI: nausea, vomiting, constipation, dry mouth, anorexia
GU: pink, red, or reddish-brown urine
Hematologic: lymphadenopathy, **aplastic anemia, agranulocytosis, leukopenia, megaloblastic anemia, thrombocytopenia**
Hepatic: hepatitis

Reactions in **bold** are life-threatening.   ◀🔊 Clinical alert

Metabolic: hypocalcemia, hypokalemia, hyperglycemia, increased glucose tolerance

Musculoskeletal: back or pelvic pain, osteomalacia

Skin: hypertrichosis, rash, pruritus, exfoliative dermatitis, **Stevens-Johnson syndrome**

Other: gingival hyperplasia, altered taste, fever, facial edema, weight loss, injection site pain, allergic reactions

Interactions

Drug-drug. *Amiodarone, benzodiazepines, chloramphenicol, cimetidine, disulfiram, estrogens, felbamate, fluconazole, fluoxetine, halothane, influenza vaccine, isoniazid, itraconazole, ketoconazole, methylphenidate, miconazole, omeprazole, phenothiazines, phenylbutazone, salicylates, sulfonamides, tolbutamide, trazodone:* increased fosphenytoin blood level

Antidepressants, antihistamines, opioids, sedative-hypnotics: additive CNS depression

Barbiturates, carbamazepine, reserpine: decreased fosphenytoin blood level

Corticosteroids, cyclosporine, doxycycline, estrogens, felbamate, methadone, quinidine, rifampin: altered effects of these drugs

Dopamine: additive hypotension

Lidocaine, propranolol: additive cardiac depression

Streptozocin, theophylline: decreased efficacy of these drugs

Warfarin: initial increase in warfarin effects in patients stabilized on warfarin therapy, followed by decreased response to warfarin

Drug-diagnostic tests. *Alkaline phosphatase, glucose, hepatic enzymes:* increased levels

Dexamethasone, metyrapone: test interference

Glucose tolerance test: decreased tolerance

Potassium, thyroxine: decreased levels

Thyroid function tests: decreased values

Drug-behaviors. *Acute alcohol ingestion:* increased drug blood level, additive CNS depression

Chronic alcohol ingestion: decreased drug blood level

Patient monitoring

• Be prepared to slow administration or stop therapy if significant cardiovascular reactions occur.

• Monitor neurologic status carefully, especially for evidence of increasing intracranial pressure.

◀€ Assess for rash. Withhold drug and notify prescriber if it occurs.

• Monitor phenytoin blood level after drug has metabolized to phenytoin (about 2 hours after I.V. dose or 4 hours after I.M. dose).

• Monitor electrolyte levels.

• Evaluate blood glucose level. Watch for hyperglycemia in patients with diabetes.

Patient teaching

• Inform patient that he may experience sensory disturbances during I.V. administration.

◀€ Advise patient to immediately report adverse effects, particularly rash.

• Tell patient that drug may turn his urine pink, red, or reddish brown.

• As appropriate, review all other significant and life-threatening adverse reactions and interactions, especially those related to the drugs, tests, and behaviors mentioned above.

frovatriptan succinate
Frova, Migard✠

Pharmacologic class: Serotonin 5-hydroxytryptamine (5-HT)$_1$-receptor agonist

Therapeutic class: Antimigraine agent

Pregnancy risk category C

Action
Binds selectively to serotonin receptors on cranial arteries, causing vasoconstriction and decreased blood flow

Availability
Tablets: 2.5 mg

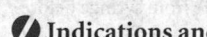 Indications and dosages
➤ Acute migraine
Adults: 2.5 mg P.O. as a single dose at first symptom of migraine. If migraine returns, may repeat after 2 hours. Maximum of three doses in 24 hours (7.5 mg/day).

Contraindications
• Hypersensitivity to drug or its components
• Cerebrovascular disorders
• Ischemic heart disease or history of myocardial infarction
• Uncontrolled hypertension
• Peripheral vascular disease
• Hemiplegic or basilar migraine
• Within 24 hours of another 5-HT$_1$-receptor agonist or ergotamine-containing or ergot-type drug

Precautions
Use cautiously in:
• patients receiving selective serotonin reuptake inhibitors (SSRIs) or serotonin norepinephrine reuptake inhibitors (SNRIs)
• pregnant or breastfeeding patients
• children (safety and efficacy not established).

Administration
• Give one tablet with plenty of fluids at first symptom of migraine.
• If headache returns, administer another tablet after 2 hours.
• Don't exceed three tablets in 24-hour period.
• Give first dose under close supervision if patient has coronary artery disease or other risk factors.

• Don't give within 24 hours of another 5-HT$_1$-receptor agonist or ergotamine-containing or ergot-type drug.

Route	Onset	Peak	Duration
P.O.	Variable	2-4 hr	Unknown

Adverse reactions
CNS: dizziness, headache, anxiety, malaise, fatigue, weakness, drowsiness, paresthesia, sensation loss
CV: palpitations, tightness in chest, **myocardial infarction (MI)**
EENT: abnormal vision, tinnitus, rhinitis
GI: nausea, diarrhea, dyspepsia, abdominal pain
Musculoskeletal: skeletal or muscle pain
Skin: flushing, diaphoresis, photosensitivity
Other: altered taste, hot or cold sensations

Interactions
Drug-drug. *Ergot alkaloids, other serotonin 5-HT$_1$-receptor agonists:* prolonged vasoactive reactions
Hormonal contraceptives, propranolol: increased frovatriptan bioavailability
SSRIs, SNRIs: serotonin syndrome (including mental status changes, hyperreflexia, nausea, vomiting)
Drug-behaviors. *Sun exposure:* increased risk of photosensitivity

Patient monitoring
• Assess for cardiovascular reactions, especially signs and symptoms of MI.
• Monitor neurologic status, particularly for indications of cerebrovascular accident.
• Check for rash and itching.

Patient teaching
• Instruct patient to take one tablet with plenty of fluids at first symptom of migraine.

f

Reactions in **bold** are life-threatening.   ◀€ Clinical alert

• Tell patient he may take second tablet 2 hours after first if migraine returns.
◀€ Advise patient to immediately report chest pain.

• Caution patient to avoid driving and other hazardous activities until he knows how drug affects concentration and alertness.

• As appropriate, review all other significant and life-threatening adverse reactions and interactions, especially those related to the drugs and behaviors mentioned above.

fulvestrant
Faslodex

Pharmacologic class: Estrogen receptor antagonist
Therapeutic class: Antineoplastic
Pregnancy risk category D

Action
Inhibits cell division by binding with and downgrading estrogen receptor protein in breast cancer cells

Availability
Prefilled syringes: 125 mg/2.5 ml, 250 mg/5 ml

Indications and dosages
➤ Hormone receptor–positive advanced metastatic breast cancer in postmenopausal women with disease progression who have received anti-estrogen therapy
Adults: 250 mg I.M. q month as a single 5-ml injection or two concomitant 2.5-ml injections

Contraindications
• Hypersensitivity to drug
• Pregnancy

Precautions
Use cautiously in:
• bleeding disorders, hepatic dysfunction, thrombocytopenia
• breastfeeding patients.

Administration
• Expel air bubble from syringe before giving injection.
• Administer I.M. injection slowly.

Route	Onset	Peak	Duration
I.M.	Slow	2-3 days	Unknown

Adverse reactions
CNS: depression, light-headedness, dizziness, headache, hallucinations, vertigo, insomnia, paresthesia, anxiety, weakness
CV: chest pain, vasodilation, peripheral edema
EENT: pharyngitis
GI: nausea, vomiting, diarrhea, constipation, abdominal pain, anorexia
GU: urinary tract infection, pelvic pain
Hematologic: anemia
Musculoskeletal: back pain, bone pain, arthritis
Respiratory: dyspnea, increased cough
Skin: flushing, rash, diaphoresis
Other: food distaste, fever, hot flashes, injection site reactions, pain, flulike symptoms

Interactions
Drug-drug. *Anticoagulants:* increased bleeding risk

Patient monitoring
• Monitor CBC.
• Assess liver function test results.

Patient teaching
• Advise patient to report signs and symptoms of infection, especially urinary tract infection.
• Caution patient to avoid driving and other hazardous activities until she knows how drug affects concentration and alertness.

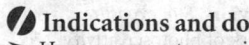

🔊 Tell patient to notify prescriber immediately if she thinks she is pregnant.
• Teach patient comfort measures to minimize hot flashes and rash.
• Instruct patient to minimize GI upset and sore throat by eating frequent, small servings of healthy food and drinking adequate fluids.
• Tell patient that drug may cause headache, muscle aches, or bone pain. Encourage her to discuss activity recommendations and pain management with prescriber.
• Advise patient to establish effective bedtime routine to minimize sleep disorders.
• As appropriate, review all other significant adverse reactions and interactions, especially those related to the drugs mentioned above.

furosemide

Apo-Furosemide✤, Bio-Furosemide✤, Dom-Furosemide✤, Frusol❋, Lasix, Lasix Special✤, Novosemide✤, Nu-Furosemide✤, PMS-Furosemide✤

Pharmacologic class: Sulfonamide loop diuretic
Therapeutic class: Diuretic, antihypertensive
Pregnancy risk category C

Action

Unclear. Thought to inhibit sodium and chloride reabsorption from ascending loop of Henle and distal renal tubules. Increases potassium excretion and plasma volume, promoting renal excretion of water, sodium, chloride, magnesium, hydrogen, and calcium.

Availability

Injection: 10 mg/ml
Oral solution: 10 mg/ml, 40 mg/5 ml
Tablets: 20 mg, 40 mg, 80 mg

Indications and dosages

➢ Acute pulmonary edema
Adults: 40 mg I.V. given over 1 to 2 minutes. If adequate response doesn't occur within 1 hour, give 80 mg I.V. over 1 to 2 minutes.
➢ Edema caused by heart failure, hepatic cirrhosis, or renal disease
Adults: Initially, 20 to 80 mg/day P.O. as a single dose; may increase in 20- to 40-mg increments P.O. q 6 to 8 hours until desired response occurs. Thereafter, may give once or twice daily. For maintenance, dosage may be reduced in some patients or carefully titrated upward to 600 mg P.O. daily in severe edema. Usual I.M. or I.V. dosage is 20 to 40 mg as a single injection; if response inadequate, second and each succeeding dose may be increased in 20-mg increments and given no more often than q 2 hours until desired response occurs. Single dose may then be given once or twice daily.
Infants and children: 2 mg/kg P.O. (oral solution) as a single dose. As necessary, increase in increments of 1 or 2 mg/kg q 6 to 8 hours to a maximum of 6 mg/kg/dose. For maintenance, give minimum effective dosage.
➢ Hypertension
Adults: 40 mg P.O. b.i.d. If satisfactory response doesn't occur, other antihypertensives may be added before furosemide dosage is increased. However, dosage may be titrated upward as needed and tolerated to a maximum of 240 mg P.O. daily in two or three divided doses.

Off-label uses

• Hypercalcemia associated with cancer

Contraindications

- Hypersensitivity to drug or other sulfonamides
- Anuria

Precautions

Use cautiously in:
- diabetes mellitus, severe hepatic disease
- elderly patients
- pregnant or breastfeeding patients
- neonates.

Administration

- Know that I.V. or I.M. injection is given when patient requires rapid onset of diuresis or can't receive oral doses.
- Be aware that I.V. dose may be given by direct injection over 1 to 2 minutes.
- For I.V. infusion, dilute in dextrose 5% in water, normal saline solution, or lactated Ringer's solution.
- 🔊 Don't infuse more than 4 mg/minute.
- Give oral doses in morning with food. If second dose is prescribed, give in afternoon.

Route	Onset	Peak	Duration
P.O.	30-60 min	1-2 hr	6-8 hr
I.V.	5 min	20-60 min	2 hr
I.M.	10-30 min	30 min	4-8 hr

Adverse reactions

CNS: dizziness, headache, vertigo, weakness, lethargy, paresthesia, drowsiness, restlessness, light-headedness
CV: hypotension, orthostatic hypotension, tachycardia, volume depletion, **necrotizing angiitis, thrombophlebitis, arrhythmias**
EENT: blurred vision, xanthopsia, hearing loss, tinnitus
GI: nausea, vomiting, diarrhea, constipation, dyspepsia, oral and gastric irritation, cramping, anorexia, dry mouth, **acute pancreatitis**

GU: excessive and frequent urination, nocturia, glycosuria, bladder spasm, **oliguria, interstitial nephritis**
Hematologic: anemia, purpura, **leukopenia, thrombocytopenia, hemolytic anemia**
Hepatic: jaundice
Metabolic: hyperglycemia, hyperuricemia, dehydration, hypokalemia, hypomagnesemia, hypocalcemia, **hypochloremic alkalosis**
Musculoskeletal: muscle pain, muscle cramps
Skin: photosensitivity, rash, diaphoresis, urticaria, pruritus, exfoliative dermatitis, **erythema multiforme**
Other: fever, transient pain at I.M. injection site

Interactions

Drug-drug. *Aminoglycosides, ethacrynic acid, other ototoxic drugs:* increased risk of ototoxicity
Amphotericin B, corticosteroids, corticotropin, potassium-wasting diuretics, stimulant laxatives: additive hypokalemia
Antihypertensives, diuretics, nitrates: additive hypotension
Cardiac glycosides: increased risk of glycoside toxicity and fatal arrhythmias
Clofibrate: exaggerated diuretic response, muscle pain and stiffness
Hydantoins, nonsteroidal anti-inflammatory drugs, probenecid: diuresis inhibition
Insulin, oral hypoglycemics: decreased hypoglycemic effect
Lithium: decreased lithium excretion, possible toxicity
Norepinephrine: decreased arterial response to norepinephrine
Propranolol: increased propranolol blood level
Salicylates: increased risk of salicylate toxicity at lower dosages than usual
Succinylcholine: potentiation of succinylcholine effect
Sucralfate: decreased naturietic and antihypertensive effects of furosemide

---

Sulfonylureas: decreased glucose tolerance, resulting in hyperglycemia
Theophyllines: altered, enhanced, or inhibited theophylline effects
Tubocurarine: antagonism of tubocurarine effects
Drug-diagnostic tests. *Blood urea nitrogen (BUN):* transient increase
Calcium, magnesium, platelets, potassium, sodium: decreased levels
Cholesterol, creatinine, glucose, nitrogenous compounds: increased levels
Drug-herbs. *Dandelion:* interference with drug's diuretic effect
Ephedra (ma huang), ginseng: decreased furosemide efficacy
Licorice: rapid potassium loss
Drug-behaviors. *Acute alcohol ingestion:* additive hypotension
Sun exposure: increased risk of photosensitivity

Patient monitoring

• Watch for signs and symptoms of ototoxicity.
◀€ Assess for other evidence of drug toxicity (arrhythmias, renal dysfunction, abdominal pain, sore throat, fever).
• Monitor CBC, BUN, and electrolyte, uric acid, and CO_2 levels.
• Monitor blood pressure, pulse, fluid intake and output, and weight.
• Assess blood glucose levels in patients with diabetes mellitus.
• Monitor dietary potassium intake. Watch for signs and symptoms of hypokalemia.

Patient teaching

• Instruct patient to take in morning with food (and second dose, if prescribed, in afternoon), to prevent nocturia.
• Tell patient that drug may cause serious interactions with many common drugs. Instruct him to tell all prescribers he's taking it.
• Instruct patient to report signs and symptoms of ototoxicity (hearing loss,

ringing in ears, vertigo) and other drug toxicities.
• Caution patient to avoid driving and other hazardous activities until he knows how drug affects concentration and alertness.
• Instruct patient to move slowly when rising, to avoid dizziness from sudden blood pressure decrease.
• Encourage patient to discuss need for potassium and magnesium supplements with prescriber.
• Caution patient to avoid alcohol and herbs while taking this drug.
• Inform patient that he'll undergo regular blood testing during therapy.
• As appropriate, review all other significant and life-threatening adverse reactions and interactions, especially those related to the drugs, tests, herbs, and behaviors mentioned above.

gabapentin

Apo-Gabapentin✦, Co Gabapentin✦, Dom-Gabapentin✦, Gen-Gabapentin✦, Gralise, Neurontin, Novo-Gabapentin✦, PHL-Gabapentin✦, PMS-Gabapentin✦, Ratio-Gabapentin✦, Riva-Gabapentin✦

gabapentin enacarbil

Horizant

Pharmacologic class: 1-amino-methyl cyclohexoneacetic acid
Therapeutic class: Anticonvulsant
Pregnancy risk category C

Action

Unknown. Possesses properties resembling those of other anticonvulsants, which appear to stabilize cell membranes by altering cation (sodium, calcium, and potassium) transport, thereby decreasing excitability and suppressing seizure discharge or focus.

Availability

Capsules: 100 mg, 300 mg, 400 mg
Oral solution: 250 mg/5 ml
Tablets: 300 mg, 600 mg, 800 mg
Tablets (extended-release): 300 mg, 600 mg

ⓘ Indications and dosages

➤ Adjunctive treatment of partial seizures

Adults and children older than age 12: Initially, 300 mg P.O. t.i.d. Usual range is 900 to 1,800 mg/day in three divided doses.

Children ages 5 to 12: Initially, 10 to 15 mg/kg/day P.O. in three divided doses, titrated upward over 3 days to 25 to 35 mg/kg/day in three divided doses

Children ages 3 to 4: Initially, 10 to 15 mg/kg/day P.O. in three divided doses, titrated upward over 3 days to 40 mg/kg/day in three divided doses

➤ Postherpetic neuralgia

Adults: Initially, 300 mg P.O. as a single dose on day 1; then 600 mg in two divided doses on day 2 and 900 mg in three divided doses on day 3. Then titrate upward as needed to 1,800 mg/day given in three divided doses. Or, titrate to a maximum of 1,800 mg (Gralise) P.O. daily as 300 mg on day 1, 600 mg on day 2, 900 mg on days 3 to 6, 1,200 mg on days 7 to 10, 1,500 mg on days 11 to 14, and 1,800 mg on day 15. Or initially, 600 mg (Horizant) P.O. in morning for 3 days; then increase to 600 mg b.i.d. beginning on day 4.

➤ Moderate to severe primary restless legs syndrome

Adult: 600 mg (Horizant) P.O. daily with food in evening

Dosage adjustment

• Renal impairment

Off-label uses

• Bipolar disorder
• Migraine prophylaxis
• Tremor associated with multiple sclerosis

Contraindications

• Hypersensitivity to drug or its components (other than Horizant)

Precautions

Use cautiously in:
• renal insufficiency
• creatinine clearance less than 15 ml/minute (Horizant) or less than 30 ml/minute (Gralise), patients on hemodialysis (avoid use)
• patients with suicidal thoughts or behavior
• elderly patients
• pregnant or breastfeeding patients
• children younger than age 3 (safety not established for partial seizures)
• children (safety not established for Horizant)
• children younger than age 18 (safety not established for Gralise).

Administration

• Give with or without food (other than Horizant and Gralise).
• Give Gralise and Horizant whole with evening meal.
• Administer first dose at bedtime to reduce adverse effects (other than Gralise and Horizant).
• Don't give within 2 hours of antacids.
• Give daily doses no more than 12 hours apart (other than Gralise and Horizant).
• Be aware that seizures may increase in patients with seizure disorders if drug is rapidly discontinued. Withdraw drug gradually over a minimum of 1 week.

• Be aware that Gralise and Horizant aren't interchangeable with other forms of gabapentin and safety and effectiveness of Gralise in patients with seizures hasn't been established.

Route	Onset	Peak	Duration
P.O.	Rapid	2-4 hr	8 hr
P.O. (Gralise)	Unknown	8 hr	Unknown
P.O. (extended)	Unknown	Unknown	Unknown

Adverse reactions

CNS: somnolence, headache, drowsiness, anxiety, dizziness, malaise, vertigo, weakness, ataxia, altered reflexes, hyperkinesia, paresthesia, tremor, amnesia, abnormal thinking, difficulty concentrating, hostility, emotional lability, **suicidal thoughts or behavior**
CV: hypertension, peripheral edema
EENT: abnormal vision, nystagmus, diplopia, amblyopia, rhinitis, pharyngitis, dry throat
GI: nausea, vomiting, constipation, flatulence, dyspepsia, anorexia, dry mouth
GU: erectile dysfunction
Hematologic: leukopenia
Musculoskeletal: joint, back, or muscle pain; fractures
Respiratory: cough
Skin: pruritus, abrasion
Other: dental abnormalities, gingivitis, facial edema, increased appetite, weight gain, **multiorgan hypersensitivity**

Interactions

Note: Apply to all forms other than Horizant
Drug-drug. *Antacids:* decreased gabapentin absorption
Antihistamines, CNS depressants, sedative-hypnotics: increased risk of CNS depression
Hydrocodone: decreased hydrocodone C_{max} and area under the curve (AUC), increased gabapentin AUC

Morphine: increased gabapentin concentration
Drug-diagnostic tests. *Urinary protein dipstick test:* false-positive result
White blood cells (WBCs): decreased count
Drug-behaviors. *Alcohol use:* increased risk of CNS depression

Patient monitoring

◀┋ Evaluate neurologic status (including observing for emergence or worsening of depression, suicidal thoughts or behavior, or unusual changes in mood or behavior) and motor function.
• Assess WBC count.
• Monitor blood pressure.
◀┋ Monitor patients for early signs and symptoms of hypersensitivity, such as fever or lymphadenopathy (although rash may not present). Discontinue drug if an alternative etiology for the signs or symptoms can' be established.

Patient teaching

• Tell patient he may take with or without food and to take first dose at bedtime to reduce adverse effects (other than Gralise and Horizant).
• Tell patient taking Gralise or Horizant to take drug with evening meal, to swallow tablet whole, and not to crush, split, or chew tablets.
◀┋ Caution patient not to stop taking drug suddenly. Dosage must be tapered to minimize seizure risk.
• Instruct patient to avoid driving and other hazardous activities until he knows how drug affects concentration, alertness, motor function, and vision.
• Tell patient that drug may cause joint pain, muscle aches, or bone pain. Encourage him to discuss activity recommendations and pain management with prescriber.
◀┋ Advise patient or caregiver to immediately report emergence or worsening of depression, suicidal

g

thoughts or behavior, or unusual changes in mood or behavior.

◀€ Instruct patient or caregiver to immediately report early signs and symptoms of hypersensitivity, such as fever or enlarged lymph nodes.

• Advise patient not to drink alcohol while taking gabapentin.

• As appropriate, review all other significant and life-threatening adverse reactions and interactions, especially those related to the drugs, tests, and behaviors mentioned above.

galantamine hydrobromide
Razadyne, Razadyne ER, Reminyl✚, Reminyl XL✚✚

Pharmacologic class: Cholinesterase inhibitor

Therapeutic class: Anti-Alzheimer's agent

Pregnancy risk category B

Action
Unclear. May reversibly inhibit acetylcholinesterase, increasing concentration of acetylcholine (necessary for nerve impulse transmission) in brain synapses.

Availability
Capsules (extended-release): 8 mg, 16 mg, 24 mg
Oral solution: 4 mg/ml
Tablets: 4 mg, 8 mg, 12 mg

⚕ Indications and dosages
➤ Mild to moderate dementia of Alzheimer's disease
Adults: Initially, 4 mg P.O. b.i.d. If patient tolerates dosage well after at least 4 weeks of therapy, increase to 8 mg P.O. b.i.d. May increase to 12 mg P.O. b.i.d. after at least 4 weeks at previous dosage. Recommended range is 16 to 24 mg daily in two divided doses. Or initially, 8 mg P.O. daily (Razadyne ER). If patient tolerates dosage after at least 4 weeks, increase to 16 mg P.O. daily. Further increase to 24 mg P.O. daily should be attempted after minimum of 4 weeks at 16 mg/day.

Dosage adjustment
• Moderate hepatic or renal impairment

Off-label uses
• Vascular dementia

Contraindications
• Hypersensitivity to drug
• Severe hepatic or renal impairment
• Pregnancy or breastfeeding
• Children

Precautions
Use cautiously in:
• asthma, chronic obstructive pulmonary disease, GI bleeding, moderate hepatic or renal impairment, Parkinson's disease, seizures.

Administration
• Before giving, make sure patient is well hydrated, to minimize GI upset.
• Give with morning and evening meals.
• Give with antiemetics as needed.
• Use pipette to add oral solution to beverage; have patient drink it right away.

Route	Onset	Peak	Duration
P.O.	Unknown	1 hr	Unknown

Adverse reactions
CNS: depression, dizziness, headache, tremor, insomnia, drowsiness, fatigue, syncope
CV: bradycardia
EENT: rhinitis
GI: nausea, vomiting, diarrhea, abdominal pain, dyspepsia, anorexia

GU: urinary tract infection, hematuria
Hematologic: anemia
Other: weight loss

Interactions
Drug-drug *Anticholinergics:* antagonism of anticholinergic activity
Cholinergics: synergistic effects
Cimetidine, erythromycin, ketoconazole, paroxetine: increased galantamine bioavailability

Patient monitoring
• Assess fluid intake and output to ensure adequate hydration, which helps reduce GI upset.
• Monitor cognitive status.
• Evaluate patient for cardiac conduction abnormalities. Assess pulse regularly for bradycardia.
• Observe for bleeding tendencies.
◀§ Assess for depression and suicidal ideation.

Patient teaching
• Instruct caregiver in proper technique for using oral pipette.
• Teach caregiver how to measure patient's pulse. Tell him to report slow pulse right away.
• Recommend frequent, small servings of healthy food and adequate fluids to minimize GI upset.
◀§ Tell patient or caregiver to watch for and report signs and symptoms of depression.
• Advise patient or caregiver to establish effective bedtime routine.
• Caution caregiver to prevent patient from performing hazardous activities until adverse reactions are known.
• As appropriate, review all other significant adverse reactions and interactions, especially those related to the drugs mentioned above.

ganciclovir (DHPG)
Cymevene⊕, Cytovene, Valcyte✴, Vitrasert

Pharmacologic class: Acyclic purine nucleoside analog of 2′-deoxyguanosine
Therapeutic class: Antiviral
Pregnancy risk category C

FDA | BOXED WARNING

• Drug may lead to granulocytopenia, anemia, and thrombocytopenia. In animal studies, it was carcinogenic and teratogenic and caused aspermatogenesis.
• Drug is indicated only to treat cytomegalovirus (CMV) retinitis in immunocompromised patients and to prevent CMV disease in at-risk transplant patients.

Action
Inhibits binding of deoxyguanosine triphosphate to DNA polymerase by terminating DNA synthesis, thereby inhibiting viral replication

Availability
Capsules: 250 mg, 500 mg
Injection: 500 mg/vial
Intravitreal implant: 4.5 mg

🖉 Indications and dosages
➤ Prevention of CMV in advanced human immunodeficiency virus (HIV) infection
Adults: 1,000 mg P.O. t.i.d.
➤ Prevention of CMV in transplant recipients
Adults: 5 mg/kg I.V. q 12 hours for 7 to 14 days; then 5 mg/kg/day 7 days per week or 6 mg/kg/day 5 days per week
➤ CMV retinitis in immunocompromised patients

Adults and children ages 9 and older: Intravitreal implant (4.5 mg) placed during intraocular surgery

Adults and children older than 3 months: Initially, 5 mg/kg I.V. q 12 hours for 14 to 21 days, followed by a maintenance dosage of 5 mg/kg/day 7 days per week or 6 mg/kg 5 days per week. For P.O. maintenance, 1,000 mg P.O. t.i.d. or 500 mg P.O. q 3 hours while patient is awake.

Dosage adjustment
- Renal impairment
- Elderly patients

Off-label uses
- CMV gastroenteritis, CMV pneumonia

Contraindications
- Hypersensitivity to drug or acyclovir
- Neutropenia or thrombocytopenia
- Contraindications for intraocular surgery, such as external infections or thrombocytopenia (with intravitreal implant)
- Breastfeeding

Precautions
Use cautiously in:
- renal impairment
- history of cytopenic reactions
- pregnant patients
- children younger than age 9 (with intravitreal implant).

Administration
◀€ Follow facility policy for handling and disposing of antineoplastic drugs. (Drug shares some properties with antitumor agents.)
- Be aware that safety and efficacy of I.V. use haven't been established for congenital or neonatal CMV disease, treatment of established CMV disease other than retinitis, or use in nonimmunocompromised individuals.
◀€ Don't let powder in capsules or I.V. solution contact skin, eyes, or mucous membranes. If contact occurs, wash skin thoroughly with soap and water, or flush eyes with water.
- Reconstitute 500-mg vial with 10 ml of sterile water; shake vial to dissolve drug. Then dilute drug again in 50 to 250 ml of compatible I.V. solution.
- If patient is on fluid restriction, dilute to a concentration of 10 mg/ml or less.
◀€ Administer a single dose by I.V. infusion slowly (over at least 1 hour), using infusion pump or microdrip (60 gtt/ml).
- Give I.V. solution within 24 hours of dilution to reduce risk of bacterial contamination.
◀€ Don't give by I.V. bolus or by I.M. or subcutaneous route.
- Administer oral doses with food.
- Be aware that intravitreal implant is designed to release drug over 5 to 8 months. Once drug is depleted (as shown by retinitis progression), implant may be removed and replaced.
◀€ Handle intravitreal implant carefully by suture tab only, to avoid damage to polymer coating. (Damage could increase rate of drug release.)

Route	Onset	Peak	Duration
P.O.	Slow	2-4 hr	Unknown
I.V., intravit.	Unknown	Unknown	Unknown

Adverse reactions
CNS: ataxia, confusion, dizziness, headache, drowsiness, tremor, abnormal thinking, agitation, amnesia, neuropathy, paresthesia, **seizures, coma**
CV: hypertension, hypotension, phlebitis, **arrhythmias**
EENT: vision loss for 2 to 4 weeks, vitreous loss, vitreous hemorrhage, cataract, retinal detachment, uveitis, endophthalmitis (all with intravitreal implant)

GI: nausea, vomiting, diarrhea, abdominal pain, dyspepsia, flatulence, anorexia, dry mouth
Hematologic: anemia, **agranulocytosis, thrombocytopenia, leukopenia**
Respiratory: pneumonia
Skin: rash, diaphoresis, pruritus
Other: fever; infection; chills; inflammation, pain, and phlebitis at injection site; **sepsis**

Interactions

Drug-drug. *Amphotericin B, cyclosporine, other nephrotoxic drugs:* increased risk of renal impairment and ganciclovir toxicity
Cilastatin, imipenem: increased seizure activity
Cytotoxic drugs: increased toxic effects
Immunosuppressants: increased immunologic and bone marrow depression
Probenecid: increased ganciclovir blood level
Zidovudine: increased risk of agranulocytosis
Drug-diagnostic tests. *Alanine aminotransferase, alkaline phosphatase, aspartate aminotransferase, creatinine, gamma-glutamyltransferase:* increased values
Granulocytes, hemoglobin, neutrophils, platelets, white blood cells: decreased values
Liver function tests: abnormal results

Patient monitoring

• Monitor liver function test results.
• Monitor neutrophil and platelet counts.
• Assess fluid intake and output to ensure adequate hydration.
• Make sure patient has regular ophthalmic examinations during both induction and maintenance therapy.
◀ Monitor neurologic status closely; watch for seizures and coma.
◀ Check for signs and symptoms of infection, particularly sepsis.

Patient teaching

◀ Advise patient to immediately report signs and symptoms of infection, including those at infusion site.
◀ Instruct patient to immediately report easy bruising or bleeding.
• Instruct patient to avoid driving and other hazardous activities until he knows how drug affects concentration and alertness.
• Caution female patient not to breastfeed.
• Inform patient that drug may cause birth defects. Tell females to use effective birth control during therapy; advise males to use barrier contraception during and for 90 days after therapy.
◀ Caution patient not to open or crush capsule. If powder from capsule contacts skin or eyes, tell him to wash skin thoroughly with soap and water or flush eyes with water.
• Instruct patient to minimize GI upset by eating frequent, small servings of healthy food.
• Tell patient he'll undergo regular blood testing during therapy.
• Explain that drug doesn't cure CMV retinitis and that patient should have eye exams every 4 to 6 weeks during therapy.
• As appropriate, review all other significant and life-threatening adverse reactions and interactions, especially those related to the drugs and tests mentioned above.

ganirelix acetate
Orgalutran✽⊕

Pharmacologic class: Gonadotropin-releasing hormone (GnRH) antagonist
Therapeutic class: Sex hormone
Pregnancy risk category X

Action
Competitively blocks GnRH receptors on pituitary gonadotroph, suppressing secretion of gonadotropin and luteinizing hormone (LH) and thereby preventing ovulation

Availability
Prefilled syringe: 250 mcg/0.5 ml

ⓘ Indications and dosages
➤ To inhibit premature LH surges during controlled ovarian hyperstimulation
Adult women: 250 mcg subcutaneously daily during early to mid-follicular phase

Contraindications
• Hypersensitivity to drug, its components, GnRH, or GnRH analogs
• Known or suspected pregnancy

Precautions
Use cautiously in:
• GnRH sensitivity
• latex sensitivity (packaging contains natural rubber latex)
• breastfeeding patients.

Administration
◄𝄞 Know that pregnancy must be excluded before therapy begins.
• Inject into abdomen (around navel) or upper thigh.
• Be aware that drug is given with follicle-stimulating hormone (FSH). After starting FSH on day 2 or 3 of menstrual cycle, patient receives ganirelix on morning of day 7 or 8 and continues this drug until adequate follicular response occurs. Then human chorionic gonadotropin is given and FSH and ganirelix are discontinued.

Route	Onset	Peak	Duration
Subcut.	Unknown	Unknown	Unknown

Adverse reactions
CNS: headache
GI: nausea, abdominal pain of GI tract origin
GU: abdominal pain of gynecologic origin, vaginal bleeding, **ovarian hyperstimulation syndrome**
Other: injection site reaction, **fetal death**

Interactions
Drug-diagnostic tests. *Hematocrit, total bilirubin:* decreased values
Neutrophils: altered count (8.3/mm³ or greater)

Patient monitoring
◄𝄞 Monitor patient for adverse effects, especially ovarian hyperstimulation.
• Monitor total bilirubin level and CBC with white cell differential.

Patient teaching
• Inform patient about possible adverse reactions.
• Teach patient about duration of treatment and required monitoring procedures.
◄𝄞 Urge patient to tell prescriber if she is pregnant before starting drug.
• As appropriate, review all other significant and life-threatening adverse reactions and interactions, especially those related to the tests mentioned above.

gemcitabine hydrochloride
Gemzar

Pharmacologic class: Antimetabolite (pyrimidine analog)
Therapeutic class: Antineoplastic
Pregnancy risk category D

Action
Kills malignant cells undergoing DNA synthesis; arrests progression of cells at G1/S border

Availability
Powder for injection: 200 mg in 10-ml vial, 1 g in 50-ml vial

⏀ Indications and dosages
➤ Pancreatic cancer
Adults: 1,000 mg/m² I.V. q week for 7 weeks, followed by 1 week of rest. May continue with cycles of once-weekly administration for 3 weeks, followed by 1 week of rest.
➤ Non-small-cell lung cancer (given with cisplatin)
Adults: 1,000 mg/m² I.V. on days 1, 8, and 15 of 28-day cycle; or 1,250 mg/m² on days 1 and 8 of 21-day cycle. Cisplatin also given on day 1.
➤ Breast cancer (combined with pac-litaxel after failure of anthracycline-containing adjuvant chemotherapy, unless anthracyclines were contraindicated)
Adults: 1,250 mg/m² I.V. over 30 minutes on days 1 and 8 of 21-day cycle, with paclitaxel given on day 1 before gemcitabine
➤ Advanced ovarian cancer after 6-month failure on platinum-based therapy (combined with carboplatin)
Adults: 1,000 mg/m² I.V. over 30 minutes on days 1 and 8 of each 21-day cycle, with carboplatin given on day 1 after gemcitabine administration.

Dosage adjustment
• Bone marrow depression

Off-label uses
• Bladder cancer

Contraindications
• Hypersensitivity to drug

Precautions
Use cautiously in:
• hepatic or renal impairment
• females of childbearing age
• pregnant or breastfeeding patients.

Administration
• Follow facility policy for preparing, handling, and administering carcino-genic, mutagenic, and teratogenic drugs.
• Add 5 ml of preservative-free normal saline solution to 200-mg vial, or add 25 ml of this solution to 1-g vial. Shake vial to dissolve drug.
• Reconstitute drug to a concentration of 40 mg/ml. If necessary, dilute fur-ther to a concentration of 1 mg/ml.
◀€ Infuse each dose over 30 minutes. (Infusions lasting longer than 1 hour increase toxicity risk.)

Route	Onset	Peak	Duration
I.V.	Unknown	Unknown	Unknown

Adverse reactions
CNS: paresthesia
GI: nausea, vomiting, diarrhea, stom-atitis
GU: hematuria, proteinuria, **hemolytic uremic syndrome, renal failure**
Hematologic: anemia, **leukopenia, thrombocytopenia**
Respiratory: dyspnea, **bronchospasm**
Skin: alopecia, rash, cellulitis
Other: flulike symptoms, fever, edema, injection site reactions, **anaphylactoid reactions**

Interactions
Drug-drug. *Live-virus vaccines:* decreased antibody response to vac-cine, increased risk of adverse reactions
Other antineoplastics: additive bone marrow depression
Drug-diagnostic tests. *Alanine amino-transferase, alkaline phosphatase, aspar-tate aminotransferase, bilirubin:* tran-sient increases
Blood urea nitrogen, serum creatinine: increased levels

Reactions in **bold** are life-threatening. ◀€ Clinical alert

Patient monitoring

◀€ Stop infusion and notify prescriber immediately if patient has signs or symptoms of allergic reaction.

• Monitor liver and kidney function test results.

◀€ Monitor CBC with white cell differential (particularly neutrophil and platelet counts) before each dose.

• Assess degree of bone marrow depression. Expect dosage changes based on blood counts.

◀€ Watch for signs and symptoms of infection and bleeding tendencies, even after drug therapy ends.

• Evaluate respiratory status regularly.

• Monitor temperature, especially during first 12 hours of therapy.

Patient teaching

◀€ Instruct patient to stop taking drug and immediately report signs or symptoms of allergic reaction.

◀€ Advise patient to immediately report signs or symptoms of infection (especially flulike symptoms).

◀€ Instruct patient to report unusual bleeding or bruising, change in urination pattern, or difficulty breathing.

• Caution patient to avoid driving and other hazardous activities until he knows how drug affects concentration and alertness.

• Advise patient to avoid activities that can cause injury. Tell him to use soft toothbrush and electric razor to avoid gum and skin injury.

• Tell patient to minimize GI upset by eating frequent, small servings of healthy food.

• Inform patient that he'll undergo blood testing periodically throughout therapy.

• As appropriate, review all other significant and life-threatening adverse reactions and interactions, especially those related to the drugs and tests mentioned above.

gemfibrozil

Apo-Gemfibrozil✦, Dom-Gemfibrozil✦, Gen-Gemfibrozil✦, Lopid, Novo-Gemfibrozil✦, Nu-Gemfibrozil✦, PMS-Gemfibrozil✦, Riva-Gemfibrozil✦

Pharmacologic class: Fibric acid derivative
Therapeutic class: Antihyperlipidemic
Pregnancy risk category C

Action

Inhibits peripheral lipolysis, resulting in decreased triglyceride levels. Also inhibits synthesis and increases clearance of very-low-density lipoproteins.

Availability

Tablets: 600 mg

🕖 Indications and dosages

➤ Type IIb hyperlipidemia in patients without coronary artery disease who don't respond to other treatments; adjunctive therapy for types IV and V hyperlipidemia

Adults: 1,200 mg P.O. daily in two divided doses

Contraindications

• Hypersensitivity to drug
• Gallbladder disease
• Severe renal dysfunction
• Hepatic dysfunction

Precautions

Use cautiously in:

• renal impairment, cholelithiasis, diabetes, hypothyroidism
• pregnant or breastfeeding patients
• children (safety not established).

Administration

• Give 30 minutes before a meal.

- Know that before starting drug and throughout therapy, patient should use dietary measures and exercise, as appropriate, to control hyperlipidemia.

Route	Onset	Peak	Duration
P.O.	2-5 days	4 wk	Unknown

Adverse reactions

CNS: fatigue, hypoesthesia, paresthesia, drowsiness, syncope, vertigo, dizziness, headache, **seizures**
CV: vasculitis
EENT: cataracts, blurred vision, retinal edema, hoarseness
GI: nausea, vomiting, diarrhea, abdominal or epigastric pain, heartburn, flatulence, gallstones, dry mouth
GU: dysuria, erectile dysfunction, decreased male fertility
Hematologic: eosinophilia, anemia, **bone marrow hypoplasia, leukopenia, thrombocytopenia**
Hepatic: hepatotoxicity
Metabolic: hypoglycemia
Musculoskeletal: joint, back, or muscle pain; myasthenia; myopathy; synovitis; myositis; **rhabdomyolysis**
Respiratory: cough
Skin: alopecia, rash, urticaria, eczema, pruritus, angioedema
Other: abnormal taste, chills, weight loss, increased risk of bacterial and viral infection, lupuslike syndrome, **anaphylaxis**

Interactions

Drug-drug. *Chenodiol, ursodiol:* decreased gemfibrozil efficacy
Cyclosporine: decreased cyclosporine effects
HMG-CoA reductase inhibitors: increased risk of rhabdomyolysis
Sulfonylureas: increased hypoglycemic effects
Warfarin: increased bleeding risk
Drug-diagnostic tests. *Alanine aminotransferase, alkaline phosphatase, aspartate aminotransferase, bilirubin,*

creatine kinase (CK), glucose, lactate dehydrogenase: increased values
Hematocrit, hemoglobin, potassium, white blood cells: decreased values

Patient monitoring

- Monitor kidney and liver function test results and serum lipid levels.
🔊 Watch for signs and symptoms of adverse reactions, especially bleeding tendency and hypersensitivity reaction.
- Monitor periodic blood counts during first year of therapy.
- Check CK level if myopathy occurs.

Patient teaching

- Tell patient to take drug 30 minutes before breakfast and dinner.
🔊 Advise patient to immediately report signs or symptoms of anaphylaxis (such as difficulty breathing or rash) or other allergic reactions.
🔊 Instruct patient to immediately report unusual bleeding or bruising or muscle pain.
- Caution patient to avoid driving and other hazardous activities until he knows how drug affects concentration and alertness.
- Stress importance of diet and exercise in lowering lipid levels.
- Inform patient that he'll undergo regular blood testing during therapy.
- As appropriate, review all other significant and life-threatening adverse reactions and interactions, especially those related to the drugs and tests mentioned above.

gemifloxacin mesylate
Factive

Pharmacologic class: Quinolone
Therapeutic class: Broad-spectrum anti-infective
Pregnancy risk category C

Reactions in **bold** are life-threatening.   🔊 Clinical alert

• Fluoroquinolones for systemic use are associated with an increased risk of tendinitis and tendon rupture in all ages. This risk is further increased in patients usually over age 60, with concomitant use of corticosteroids, and in kidney, heart, and lung transplant recipients.

Action
Inhibits DNA synthesis by inhibiting DNA gyrase and topoisomerase IV, enzymes needed for bacterial growth

Availability
Tablets: 320 mg

🖊 Indications and dosages
➤ Acute exacerbation of chronic bronchitis caused by susceptible organisms
Adults: 320 mg P.O. daily for 5 days
➤ Mild to moderate community-acquired pneumonia caused by susceptible organisms
Adults: 320 mg P.O. daily for 5 days

Dosage adjustment
• Renal impairment

Contraindications
• Hypersensitivity to drug
• History of prolonged QTc interval

Precautions
Use cautiously in:
• epilepsy or history of seizures
• pregnant or breastfeeding patients
• children younger than age 18 (safety not established).

Administration
• Give at same time every day with plenty of fluids, with or without food.
• Make sure patient swallows tablet whole without chewing.
• Don't give iron, multivitamins, didanosine, sucralfate, or antacids containing magnesium or aluminum within 3 hours of gemifloxacin.

Route	Onset	Peak	Duration
P.O.	Unknown	0.5-2 hr	Unknown

Adverse reactions
CNS: fatigue, headache, insomnia, drowsiness, nervousness, dizziness, tremor, vertigo, **seizures, loss of consciousness**
CV: hypotension, **prolonged QTc interval, cardiovascular collapse, shock**
EENT: vision abnormality, pharyngitis
GI: nausea, vomiting, diarrhea, constipation, abdominal pain, dyspepsia, gastritis, gastroenteritis, flatulence, anorexia, dry mouth, **pseudomembranous colitis**
GU: genital candidiasis, vaginitis, **acute renal insufficiency or failure, interstitial nephritis**
Hematologic: eosinophilia, anemia, **leukopenia, granulocytopenia, thrombocytopenia**
Hepatic: jaundice, **hepatitis, acute hepatic necrosis, hepatic failure**
Metabolic: hyperglycemia
Musculoskeletal: joint, back, or muscle pain; leg cramps; tendinitis; rupture of shoulder, hand, or Achilles tendon
Respiratory: dyspnea, pneumonia
Skin: rash, urticaria, pruritus, eczema, flushing, photosensitivity, angioedema
Other: altered taste, hot flashes, fungal infection, hypersensitivity reaction

Interactions
Drug-drug. *Antacids containing aluminum or magnesium, didanosine, iron, multivitamins, sucralfate:* reduced gemifloxacin absorption
Antiarrhythmics (class IA, such as quinidine and procainamide, and class III, such as amiodarone and sotalol), antipsychotics, erythromycin, tricyclic antidepressants: increased risk of prolonged QTc interval

---

Sucralfate: decreased gemifloxacin bioavailability

Drug-diagnostic tests. *Alanine aminotransferase, aspartate aminotransferase, bilirubin:* increased levels

Drug-behaviors. *Sun exposure:* increased risk of photosensitivity

Patient monitoring

• Stay alert for signs and symptoms of hypersensitivity reaction and other serious adverse reactions.

• Monitor ECG in patients at risk for prolonged QTc interval.

◀ Watch for signs and symptoms of tendinitis or tendon rupture.

Patient teaching

• Instruct patient to take drug at same time each day, with or without food.

• Teach patient how to recognize and report signs and symptoms of allergic response.

• Advise patient to take iron, vitamins, antacids, didanosine, or sucralfate 3 hours before or 2 hours after gemifloxacin.

◀ Instruct patient to stop taking drug and immediately report signs or symptoms of hypersensitivity reaction, severe diarrhea, change in urination pattern, easy bruising or bleeding, unusual tiredness, or yellowing of eyes or skin.

◀ Advise patient to stop taking drug and immediately report sudden severe pain in shoulder, hand, or Achilles tendon.

• Caution patient to avoid driving and other hazardous activities until he knows how drug affects concentration and alertness.

• As appropriate, review all other significant and life-threatening adverse reactions and interactions, especially those related to the drugs, tests, and behaviors mentioned above.

gentamicin sulfate
Alcomicin✦, Cidomycin✦⊕, Diogent✦, Garamycin✦, Gentacidin, Gentak, Genticin⊕, PMS-Gentamicin✦, Ratio-Gentamicin✦

Pharmacologic class: Aminoglycoside
Therapeutic class: Anti-infective
Pregnancy risk category D (parenteral), *C* (topical)

FDA | BOXED WARNING

• Observe patient closely for potential ototoxicity and nephrotoxicity. Safety isn't established in therapy exceeding 14 days.

• Neuromuscular blockade and respiratory paralysis have occurred after administration.

• Monitor renal function and eighth-nerve function closely, especially in patients with known or suspected renal impairment at onset of therapy, as well as those with initially normal renal function who develop signs of renal dysfunction during therapy.

• Avoid concurrent use with potent diuretics (such as furosemide and ethacrynic acid), because diuretics may cause ototoxicity. Also, I.V. diuretics may increase gentamicin toxicity by altering antibiotic serum and tissue levels.

• Avoid concurrent and sequential systemic, oral, or topical use of other neurotoxic or nephrotoxic products and other aminoglycosides. Advanced age and dehydration also may increase toxicity risk.

• Drug may harm fetus when given to pregnant women.

Action
Destroys gram-negative bacteria by irreversibly binding to 30S subunit of

bacterial ribosomes and blocking protein synthesis, resulting in misreading of genetic code and separation of ribosomes from messenger RNA

Availability
Cream: 0.1%
Injection: 10 mg/ml (pediatric), 40 mg/ml (adult)
I.V. infusion (premixed in normal saline solution): 40 mg, 60 mg, 70 mg, 80 mg, 90 mg, 100 mg, 120 mg
Ointment: 0.1%
Ointment (ophthalmic): 0.3% (base)
Solution (ophthalmic): 0.3% (base)

⒤ Indications and dosages
➤ Serious infections caused by *Pseudomonas aeruginosa, Escherichia coli,* and *Proteus, Klebsiella, Serratia, Enterobacter, Citrobacter,* or *Staphylococcus* species
Adults: 3 mg/kg/day in three divided doses I.M. or I.V. infusion q 8 hours. For life-threatening infections, up to 5 mg/kg/day in three to four divided doses; reduce to 3 mg/kg/day as indicated.
Children: 2 to 2.5 mg/kg q 8 hours I.M. or I.V. infusion
Infants older than 1 week: 2.5 mg/kg q 8 hours I.M. or I.V. infusion
Neonates younger than 1 week, preterm infants: 2.5 mg/kg q 12 hours I.M. or I.V. infusion. In preterm infants of less than 32 weeks' gestational age, 2.5 mg/kg q 18 hours or 3 mg/kg q 24 hours also may produce satisfactory peak and trough blood levels.
➤ Endocarditis prophylaxis before surgery
Adults: 1.5 mg/kg I.M. or I.V. 30 minutes before surgery, to a maximum of 80 mg. As prescribed, give with ampicillin or vancomycin.
Children: 2 mg/kg I.M. or I.V. 30 minutes before surgery, to a maximum of 80 mg
➤ External ocular infections caused by susceptible organisms

Adults and children: One to two drops of ophthalmic solution in eye q 4 hours. For serious infections, up to two drops q hour, or ophthalmic ointment applied to lower conjunctival sac two to three times daily.
➤ Treatment and prevention of superficial burns caused by susceptible bacteria
Adults and children older than age 1: Gently rub small a amount of drug topically on affected area three or four times daily.

Dosage adjustment
• Renal impairment
• Cystic fibrosis

Contraindications
• Hypersensitivity to drug or other aminoglycosides

Precautions
Use cautiously in:
• neuromuscular disease, renal impairment, hearing impairment
• sulfite sensitivity (with parenteral use)
• obese patients
• elderly patients
• pregnant or breastfeeding patients
• infants, neonates, and premature infants.

Administration
• Before starting therapy, obtain specimens as needed for culture and sensitivity testing.
• For I.V. infusion, dilute with 50 to 200 ml of dextrose 5% in water (D_5W) or normal saline solution, and administer over 30 minutes to 2 hours.
• After infusion, flush line with normal saline solution or D_5W.
• Obtain peak drug blood level 30 minutes after 30-minute infusion; obtain trough level within 30 minutes of next scheduled dose.
• Give cephalosporin or parenteral penicillin 1 hour before or after gentamicin, as prescribed.

- Know that for topical treatment of burns, gauze dressings may be applied.

Route	Onset	Peak	Duration
I.V.	Immediate	30-90 min	Unknown
I.M.	Unknown	30-90 min	Unknown
Topical, ophthalmic	Unknown	Unknown	Unknown

Adverse reactions

CNS: dizziness, vertigo, tremors, numbness, depression, confusion, lethargy, headache, paresthesia, **neuromuscular blockade, seizures, neurotoxicity**
EENT: visual disturbances, dry eyes, nystagmus, photophobia, ototoxicity, hearing loss, tinnitus
GI: nausea, vomiting, stomatitis, increased salivation, splenomegaly, anorexia
GU: increased urinary casts, polyuria, dysuria, erectile dysfunction, azotemia, **nephrotoxicity**
Hematologic: eosinophilia, **leukemoid reaction, hemolytic anemia, aplastic anemia, neutropenia, agranulocytosis, leukopenia, thrombocytopenia, pancytopenia**
Hepatic: hepatomegaly, hepatotoxicity, hepatic necrosis
Musculoskeletal: joint pain, muscle twitching
Respiratory: apnea
Skin: exfoliative dermatitis, rash, pruritus, urticaria, purpura, alopecia
Other: weight loss, superinfection, pain and irritation at I.M. injection site

Interactions

Drug-drug. *Acyclovir, amphotericin B, carboplatin, cephalosporins, cisplatin, loop diuretics, vancomycin, other ototoxic or nephrotoxic drugs:* increased risk of ototoxicity and nephrotoxicity
Dimenhydrinate, other antiemetics: masking of ototoxicity symptoms
General anesthetics, neuromuscular blockers: increased activity of these drugs
Indomethacin: increased gentamicin peak and trough levels

Penicillins (such as ampicillin, ticarcillin): synergistic effect
Tacrolimus: nephrotoxicity
Drug-diagnostic tests. *Alanine aminotransferase, aspartate aminotransferase, bilirubin, blood urea nitrogen (BUN), creatinine, lactate dehydrogenase:* increased values
Granulocytes, hemoglobin, platelets, white blood cells: decreased values
Reticulocytes: increased or decreased count

Patient monitoring

- Watch for signs and symptoms of hypersensitivity reactions.
- ◄€ Know that drug blood level monitoring is especially important in therapy lasting more than 5 days, acute or chronic renal impairment, extracellular fluid volume changes, obesity, infants younger than 3 months, concomitant use of nephrotoxic drugs, patients requiring higher doses or dosage interval adjustments (such as those with cystic fibrosis, endocarditis, or critical illness), and patients with signs or symptoms of nephrotoxicity or ototoxicity.
- Assess fluid intake and output, urine specific gravity, and urinalysis for signs of nephrotoxicity.
- Monitor CBC, BUN, creatinine level, and creatinine clearance.
- Weigh patient regularly.
- Assess for signs and symptoms of ototoxicity (hearing loss, tinnitus, ataxia, and vertigo).

Patient teaching

- ◄€ Teach patient to recognize and immediately report signs and symptoms of hypersensitivity reaction, infection, unusual tiredness, yellowing of skin or eyes, and muscle twitching.
- Advise patient to report signs and symptoms of ototoxicity (hearing loss, ringing in ears, vertigo).
- Instruct patient to drink plenty of fluids to ensure adequate urine output.

Reactions in **bold** are life-threatening.   ◄€ Clinical alert

- Tell patient to monitor urine output and report significant changes.
- Caution patient to avoid driving and other hazardous activities until he knows how drug affects concentration and alertness.
- As appropriate, review all other significant and life-threatening adverse reactions and interactions, especially those related to the drugs and tests mentioned above.

glatiramer acetate
Copaxone

Pharmacologic class: Immunomodulator

Therapeutic class: Multiple sclerosis agent

Pregnancy risk category B

Action
Unknown. Thought to alter immune processes believed to be responsible for pathogenesis of multiple sclerosis.

Availability
Injection: 20 mg lyophilized glatiramer acetate and 40 mg mannitol in single-use 2-ml vial (1-ml vial of sterile water for injection included for reconstitution)

🚺 Indications and dosages
➤ To reduce frequency of relapses in relapsing-remitting multiple sclerosis
Adults: 20 mg/day subcutaneously

Contraindications
- Hypersensitivity to drug

Precautions
Use cautiously in:
- pregnant or breastfeeding patients
- children (safety and efficacy not established).

Administration
- Give only by subcutaneous injection into arms, abdomen, hips, or thighs.
- Administer immediately after preparing. Discard unused portion.

Route	Onset	Peak	Duration
Subcut.	Slow	Unknown	Unknown

Adverse reactions
CNS: abnormal dreams, agitation, anxiety, confusion, emotional lability, migraine, nervousness, speech disorder, stupor, tremor, weakness, vertigo
CV: chest pain, hypertension, palpitations, tachycardia, peripheral edema
EENT: eye disorder, nystagmus, ear pain, rhinitis
GI: nausea, vomiting, diarrhea, anorexia, gastroenteritis, other GI disorder, oral candidiasis, salivary gland enlargement, ulcerative stomatitis
GU: urinary urgency, hematuria, erectile dysfunction, amenorrhea, dysmenorrhea, menorrhagia, abnormal Papanicolaou smear, vaginal candidiasis, **vaginal hemorrhage**
Hematologic: ecchymosis, lymphadenopathy
Musculoskeletal: joint, back, or neck pain; foot drop; hypertonia
Respiratory: bronchitis, dyspnea, hyperventilation
Skin: eczema, erythema, diaphoresis, pruritus, rash, skin atrophy, skin nodules, urticaria, warts
Other: dental caries, facial edema, weight gain, herpes simplex, herpes zoster, cysts, chills, flulike symptoms, pain at injection site

Interactions
None reported

Patient monitoring
◀🗲 Assess for immediate postinjection reaction, including flushing, chest pain, anxiety, breathing problems, and hives.

♣ Canada   ✠ UK   ⚕ Hazardous drug   ⊗ High-alert drug

- Watch for transient chest pain, but be aware that this problem doesn't seem to be clinically significant.
- Check for vaginal bleeding.
- Watch for signs and symptoms of infection.

Patient teaching

- Teach patient how to prepare and self-administer drug. Supervise him the first time he does so.
- ◀€ Teach patient to recognize and immediately report signs and symptoms of postinjection reaction. Tell him this reaction may occur right away or up to several months after first dose.
- Caution patient to avoid driving and other hazardous activities until he knows how drug affects concentration and alertness.
- ◀€ Instruct patient to report signs or symptoms of infection or vaginal hemorrhage.
- Provide dietary counseling. Refer patient to dietitian if adverse GI effects significantly affect food intake.
- As appropriate, review all other significant and life-threatening adverse reactions.

---

glimepiride

Amaryl, Apo-Glimepiride✣, CO Glimepiride✣, Novo-Glimepiride✣, PMS-Glimepiride✣, Ratio-Glimepiride✣, Sandoz Glimepiride✣

Pharmacologic class: Sulfonylurea
Therapeutic class: Hypoglycemic
Pregnancy risk category C

Action

Lowers blood glucose level by stimulating insulin release from pancreas, increasing insulin sensitivity at receptor sites, and decreasing hepatic

glucose production. Also increases peripheral tissue sensitivity to insulin and causes mild diuresis.

Availability

Tablets: 1 mg, 2 mg, 4 mg

Indications and dosages

➤ Adjunct to diet and exercise to lower blood glucose level in type 2 (non-insulin-dependent) diabetes mellitus

Adults: Initially, 1 to 2 mg P.O. daily given with first main meal; usual maintenance dosage is 1 to 4 mg P.O. daily. When patient reaches 2 mg/day, increase no more than 2 mg q 1 to 2 weeks, depending on glycemic control. Maximum dosage is 8 mg/day.

Dosage adjustment

- Renal or hepatic impairment
- Adrenal or pituitary insufficiency

Contraindications

- Hypersensitivity to drug
- Diabetic coma or ketoacidosis
- Severe renal, hepatic, or endocrine disease
- Pregnancy or breastfeeding

Precautions

Use cautiously in:
- mild to moderate hepatic or renal disease; cardiovascular disease; impaired thyroid, pituitary, or adrenal function
- elderly patients.

Administration

- Check baseline creatinine level for normal renal function before giving first dose.
- Give with first meal of day.

Route	Onset	Peak	Duration
P.O.	1 hr	2-3 hr	>24 hr

Adverse reactions

CNS: dizziness, drowsiness, headache, weakness

CV: increased CV mortality risk

EENT: blurred vision

GI: nausea, vomiting, diarrhea, constipation, cramps, heartburn, epigastric distress, anorexia

Hematologic: aplastic anemia, leukopenia, pancytopenia, thrombocytopenia, agranulocytosis

Hepatic: cholestatic jaundice, **hepatitis**

Metabolic: hyponatremia, **hypoglycemia**

Skin: rash, erythema, maculopapular eruptions, urticaria, eczema, angioedema, photosensitivity

Other: increased appetite

Interactions

Drug-drug. *Androgens (such as testosterone), chloramphenicol, clofibrate, guanethidine, MAO inhibitors, nonsteroidal anti-inflammatory drugs (except diclofenac), salicylates, sulfonamides, tricyclic antidepressants:* increased risk of hypoglycemia

Beta-adrenergic blockers: altered response to glimepiride, necessitating dosage change; prolonged hypoglycemia (with nonselective agents)

Calcium channel blockers, corticosteroids, estrogens, hydantoins, hormonal contraceptives, isoniazid, nicotinic acid, phenothiazines, phenytoin, rifampin, sympathomimetics, thiazide diuretics, thyroid preparations: decreased hypoglycemic effect of glimepiride

Warfarin: initially increased, then decreased, effects of both drugs

Drug-diagnostic tests. *Alanine aminotransferase, alkaline phosphatase, aspartate aminotransferase, bilirubin, blood urea nitrogen, cholesterol, liver function tests:* increased values

Glucose, granulocytes, hemoglobin, platelets, white blood cells: decreased values

Drug-herbs. *Agoral marshmallow, aloe (oral), bitter melon, burdock, chromium, coenzyme Q10, dandelion, eucalyptus, fenugreek:* additive hypoglycemic effects

Glucosamine: impaired glycemic control

Drug-behaviors. *Alcohol use:* disulfiram-like reaction

Sun exposure: increased risk of photosensitivity

Patient monitoring

• Monitor CBC with white cell differential, electrolyte levels, and blood chemistry results.

• Monitor blood glucose level regularly. Assess glycosylated hemoglobin level every 3 to 6 months.

• Evaluate kidney and liver function test results frequently, especially in patients with impairments.

• Assess neurologic status. Report cognitive or sensory impairment.

Patient teaching

• Instruct patient to self-monitor his blood glucose level as prescribed.

• Teach patient how to recognize signs and symptoms of hypoglycemia and hyperglycemia.

• Stress importance of diet and exercise to help control diabetes.

• Instruct patient to wear or carry medical identification describing his condition.

• Advise patient to keep sugar source readily available at all times in case of hypoglycemia.

• Caution patient to avoid driving and other hazardous activities until he knows how drug affects concentration and alertness.

• Tell patient he will undergo regular blood testing during therapy.

• As appropriate, review all other significant and life-threatening adverse reactions and interactions, especially those related to the drugs, tests, herbs, and behaviors mentioned above.

golimumab
Simponi

Pharmacologic class: Tumor necrosis factor (TNF) blocker
Therapeutic class: Immunomodulator
Pregnancy risk category B

FDA | BOXED WARNING

- Serious infections leading to hospitalization or death, including tuberculosis (TB), bacterial sepsis, invasive fungal (such as histoplasmosis), and other opportunistic infections have occurred in patients receiving golimumab.
- Discontinue drug if patient develops a serious infection or sepsis.
- Perform test for latent TB and, if positive, start treatment for TB before starting golimumab.
- Monitor all patients for active TB during treatment, even if initial latent TB test is negative.
- Lymphoma and other malignancies, some fatal, have been reported in children and adolescents treated with TNF blockers, of which this drug is a member.

Action
A human monoclonal antibody that binds to both the soluble and transmembrane bioactive forms of human TNF. This interaction prevents binding of TNF to its receptors, thereby inhibiting biological activity of TNFα (a cytokine protein). Elevated TNF levels in blood, synovium, and joints have been implicated in the pathophysiology of several chronic inflammatory diseases, such as rheumatoid arthritis, psoriatic arthritis, and ankylosing spondylitis. TNF is an important mediator of articular inflammation characteristic of these diseases.

Availability
Injection: 50 mg/0.5 ml in single-dose prefilled SmartJect® Autoinjector; 50 mg/0.5 ml in single-dose prefilled syringe

Indications and dosages
➤ Moderate to severe rheumatoid arthritis (with methotrexate); psoriatic arthritis, ankylosing spondylitis (with or without methotrexate or other nonbiological disease-modifying antirheumatics)
Adults: 50 mg subcutaneously monthly

Contraindications
None

Precautions
Use cautiously in:
- hypersensitivity reactions
- congestive heart failure (CHF)
- patients at risk for infection
- chronic hepatitis B virus (HBV) carriers
- central or peripheral nervous system demyelinating disorders
- cytopenia, including pancytopenia, leukopenia, neutropenia, aplastic anemia, and thrombocytopenia
- concurrent use of abatacept or anakinra (use not recommended)
- concurrent use of immunosuppressants, such as corticosteroids or methotrexate
- concurrent use of live vaccines (don't use)
- patients switching from other disease-modifying antirheumatics
- elderly patients
- pregnant or breastfeeding patients
- children younger than age 18 (safety and efficacy not established).

Administration
◀€ Be aware that patients with active infections shouldn't start treatment with golimumab. Also, consider risks and benefits of starting golimumab in

g

patients with chronic or recurrent infection, in those who have been exposed to TB, in those with a history of opportunistic infection, in those who have resided or traveled in areas of endemic TB or endemic mycoses (such as histoplasmosis, coccidioidomycosis, or blastomycosis), and in patients with underlying conditions that may predispose to infection. Be aware that when switching from one biological agent to another, overlapping biological activity may further increase risk of infection. Discontinue drug if patients develop other serious infections or sepsis.

◀€ Test for HBV infection before initiating TNF-blocker therapy. Discontinue drug in patients who develop HBV reactivation and initiate effective antiviral therapy with appropriate supportive treatment. Know that safety of resuming TNF-blocker therapy after HBV reactivation has been controlled isn't known; therefore, exercise caution when considering resumption of therapy.

• Before starting treatment, evaluate patient for TB risk factors and test for latent infection. Consider induration of 5 mm or greater with tuberculin skin testing a positive test when assessing if treatment for latent TB is needed, even for patient who has previously received bacille Calmette-Guérin vaccine. Treatment of latent TB infection before therapy with TNF blockers has been shown to reduce risk of TB reactivation during therapy.

• Consider anti-TB therapy before starting golimumab in patients with history of latent or active TB in whom adequate course of treatment can't be confirmed and in patients with negative test for latent TB but with risk factors for TB infection.

◀€ Consider discontinuing drug if central or peripheral nervous system demyelinating disorders develop.

◀€ Immediately discontinue drug if severe hypersensitivity reactions occur and initiate appropriate therapy.

Route	Onset	Peak	Duration
Sub-cutaneous	Unknown	2-6 days	Unknown

Adverse reactions

CNS: dizziness, paresthesia, **central or peripheral nervous system demyelinating disorders**
CV: hypertension, **CHF**
EENT: nasopharyngitis, pharyngitis, laryngitis, rhinitis, sinusitis
GI: constipation
Hematologic: pancytopenia, leukopenia, neutropenia, aplastic anemia, thrombocytopenia
Hepatic: hepatic dysfunction, **acute hepatic failure**
Respiratory: upper respiratory tract infection, bronchitis
Skin: urticaria, bruising, pruritus, irritation, induration
Other: injection-site reactions, viral infections, superficial fungal infections, pain, **serious infections, malignancies,** hypersensitivity reactions including **anaphylaxis**

Interactions

Drug-drug. *Abatacept, anakinra:* increased risk of serious infection
Anakinra: increased risk of neutropenia and serious infection
CYP450 substrates: possible altered golimumab level due to antagonized TNFα activity
Live vaccines: increased risk of infection
Drug-diagnostic tests. *ALT, AST:* increased levels

Patient monitoring

• Monitor CBC with differential and hepatic function tests closely.
• Continue to watch for signs and symptoms of TB and test for latent TB periodically during therapy. Strongly

consider TB in patients who develop new infection during treatment, especially in those who have previously or recently traveled to countries with high prevalence of TB or who have had close contact with a person with active TB.

• Closely observe for signs and symptoms of infection during and after treatment. Know that patients who develop new infection during treatment should be closely monitored, undergo prompt and complete diagnostic workup appropriate for immunocompromised patients, and be given appropriate antimicrobial therapy.

• Observe for signs and symptoms of malignancies. Be aware that lymphomas, including Hodgkin's and non-Hodgkin's lymphoma, and leukemia have been reported.

◀╞ Closely monitor patients with CHF during therapy. Discontinue drug if new or worsening CHF signs and symptoms develop.

• Closely monitor patients who are carriers of HBV and require treatment with golimumab for clinical and laboratory signs of active HBV infection throughout therapy and for several months after treatment ends.

• Continue to monitor patients for hypersensitivity reactions.

◀╞ Observe for signs and symptoms (although rare) of new-onset or exacerbation of CNS demyelinating diseases, including multiple sclerosis, and of peripheral demyelinating diseases, including Guillain-Barré syndrome.

Patient teaching

• Instruct patient who may self-inject on proper use of prefilled syringe, suitable sites for injection (including thigh and abdomen), rotation of sites, appropriate handling and disposal of syringe, and discarding unused portions of drug remaining in syringe.

• Advise latex-sensitive patient that needle cover on prefilled syringe and prefilled syringe in prefilled SmartJect Autoinjector contain dry natural rubber (a latex derivative).

◀╞ Advise patient to seek immediate medical attention if signs and symptoms of severe allergic reactions occur.

◀╞ Advise patient to promptly report new or worsening medical conditions (such as heart disease, neurological disease, or autoimmune disorders) and to promptly report signs and symptoms suggestive of cytopenia (such as bruising, bleeding, or persistent fever).

• Inform patient that drug may lower ability of immune system to fight infection and of importance of informing prescriber about new or previous infections, including TB and reactivation of HBV infection.

• Counsel patient about possible risk of lymphoma and other malignancies during therapy.

• Tell patient to avoid live vaccines during golimumab therapy.

• Advise breastfeeding patient that she should decide whether to discontinue breastfeeding or discontinue drug, taking into account importance of drug for her treatment.

• As appropriate, review all other significant and life-threatening adverse reactions and interactions, especially those related to the drugs and tests mentioned above.

glipizide
Glibenese ⊕, Glucotrol, Glucotrol XL, Minodiab ⊕

Pharmacologic class: Sulfonylurea
Therapeutic class: Hypoglycemic
Pregnancy risk category C

Action
Lowers blood glucose level by stimulating insulin release from pancreas, increasing insulin sensitivity at receptor sites, and decreasing hepatic glucose production. Also increases peripheral tissue sensitivity to insulin and causes mild diuresis.

Availability
Tablets: 5 mg, 10 mg
Tablets (extended-release): 5 mg, 10 mg

⦸ Indications and dosages
➢ To control blood glucose in type 2 (non-insulin-dependent) diabetes mellitus in patients who have some pancreatic function and don't respond to diet therapy
Adults: 5 mg/day P.O. initially, increased as needed after several days (range is 2.5 to 40 mg/day). Give extended-release tablet once daily; maximum dosage is 20 mg/day. Give daily dosage above 15 mg in two divided doses.
➢ Conversion from insulin therapy
Adults: With insulin dosage above 20 units/day, start with usual glipizide dosage and reduce insulin dosage by 50%. With insulin dosage of 20 units/day or less, insulin may be discontinued when glipizide therapy starts.

Dosage adjustment
• Hepatic or renal impairment
• Elderly patients

Contraindications
• Hypersensitivity to drug
• Severe renal, hepatic, thyroid, or other endocrine disease
• Uncontrolled infection, serious burns, or trauma
• Diabetic ketoacidosis
• Pregnancy or breastfeeding

Precautions
Use cautiously in:
• mild to moderate hepatic, renal, or cardiovascular disease; impaired thyroid, pituitary, or adrenal function
• elderly patients.

Administration
• Check baseline creatinine level for normal renal function before giving first dose.
• Give daily dose (extended-release) at breakfast.
• Administer immediate-release tablets 30 minutes before a meal (preferably breakfast). If patient takes two daily doses, give second dose before dinner.

Route	Onset	Peak	Duration
P.O.	15-30 min	1-2 hr	Up to 24 hr

Adverse reactions
CNS: dizziness, drowsiness, headache, weakness
CV: increased CV mortality risk
EENT: blurred vision
GI: nausea, vomiting, diarrhea, constipation, cramps, heartburn, epigastric distress, anorexia
Hematologic: aplastic anemia, agranulocytosis, leukopenia, pancytopenia, thrombocytopenia
Hepatic: cholestatic jaundice, **hepatitis**
Metabolic: hyponatremia, **hypoglycemia**
Skin: rash, pruritus, erythema, urticaria, eczema, angioedema, photosensitivity
Other: increased appetite

Interactions
Drug-drug. *Androgens (such as testosterone), chloramphenicol, clofibrate, guanethidine, MAO inhibitors, nonsteroidal anti-inflammatory drugs (except diclofenac), salicylates, sulfonamides, tricyclic antidepressants:* increased risk of hypoglycemia
Beta-adrenergic blockers: altered response to glipizide, requiring dosage change; prolonged hypoglycemia (with nonselective beta blockers)

Calcium channel blockers, corticosteroids, estrogens, hydantoins, hormonal contraceptives, isoniazid, nicotinic acid, phenothiazines, phenytoin, rifampin, sympathomimetics, thiazide diuretics, thyroid preparations: decreased hypoglycemic effect

Warfarin: initially increased, then decreased, effects of both drugs

Drug-diagnostic tests. *Alanine aminotransferase, alkaline phosphatase, aspartate aminotransferase, bilirubin, blood urea nitrogen, cholesterol:* increased values

Glucose, granulocytes, hemoglobin, platelets, white blood cells: decreased values

Drug-herbs. *Aloe (oral), bitter melon, burdock, chromium, coenzyme Q10, dandelion, eucalyptus, fenugreek:* additive hypoglycemic effects

Glucosamine: impaired glycemic control

Drug-behaviors. *Alcohol use:* disulfiram-like reaction

Patient monitoring

• Monitor blood glucose level, especially during periods of increased stress.
• Evaluate CBC and renal function tests.
• If patient is ill or has abnormal laboratory values, monitor electrolyte, ketone, glucose, pH, lactate dehydrogenase, and pyruvate levels.
• Monitor cardiovascular status.

Patient teaching

• Advise patient to take daily dose of extended-release tablets with breakfast or immediate-release tablet 30 minutes before breakfast (and second dose, if prescribed, before dinner).
• Advise patient to monitor blood glucose level as instructed by prescriber.
• Tell patient he may need supplemental insulin during times of stress or when he can't maintain adequate oral intake.

• Teach patient how to recognize signs and symptoms of hypoglycemia and hyperglycemia.
• Stress importance of diet and exercise to help control diabetes.
• Instruct patient to wear or carry medical identification describing his condition.
• Advise patient to keep sugar source at hand at all times in case of hypoglycemia.
• Caution patient to avoid driving and other hazardous activities until he knows how drug affects concentration and alertness.
• Tell patient he'll undergo regular blood testing during therapy.
• As appropriate, review all other significant and life-threatening adverse reactions and interactions, especially those related to the drugs, tests, herbs, and behaviors mentioned above.

glucagon
GlucaGen

Pharmacologic class: Antihypoglycemic
Therapeutic class: Insulin antagonist
Pregnancy risk category B

Action

Increases blood glucose concentration by converting glycogen in liver to glucose. Also relaxes GI smooth muscle.

Availability

Powder for injection: 1-mg vials

⚠ Indications and dosages

➤ Severe hypoglycemia

Adults and children weighing more than 20 kg (44 lb): 1 mg subcutaneously, I.M., or I.V.

Children weighing 20 kg (44 lb) or less: 20 to 30 mcg/kg or 0.5-mg dose subcutaneously, I.M., or I.V.

➤ Diagnostic aid for radiologic examination

Adults: 0.25 to 2 mg I.V. or 1 to 2 mg I.M. before radiologic procedure

Contraindications

• Hypersensitivity to drug
• Pheochromocytoma

Precautions

Use cautiously in:
• cardiac disease, adrenal insufficiency, chronic hypoglycemia
• history suggesting insulinoma or pheochromocytoma
• elderly patients
• pregnant or breastfeeding patients.

Administration

◀᛫ Use only in hypoglycemic emergencies for patients with diabetes mellitus.
• Mix drug in 1-mg vial with 1 ml of diluent supplied by manufacturer.
• For I.V. injection, give 1 mg over 1 minute.
• Use drug immediately after preparing; discard unused portion.
◀᛫ Patient should respond within 15 minutes. Because of potential serious adverse reactions linked to prolonged cerebral hypoglycemia, give I.V. glucose if patient fails to respond to glucagon.
• Give patient carbohydrate-rich foods as soon as he's alert.
• Dilute diagnostic aid doses above 2 mg with sterile water for injection.

Route	Onset	Peak	Duration
I.V.	Immediate	30 min	60-90 min
I.M., subcut.	4-10 min	Unknown	12-32 min

Adverse reactions

CV: hypotension
GI: nausea, vomiting
Metabolic: hypokalemia (with overdose)

Respiratory: bronchospasm, respiratory distress
Skin: urticaria, rash

Interactions

Drug-drug. *Anticoagulants:* enhanced anticoagulant effect
Drug-diagnostic tests. *Potassium:* decreased level

Patient monitoring

• Monitor blood glucose level.
• Monitor patient for aspiration.
• Assess blood pressure, electrolyte levels, and respiratory status.

Patient teaching

• Teach patient and family members the proper technique and timing for using this emergency drug.
◀᛫ Emphasize importance of contacting prescriber right away if hypoglycemic emergency occurs.
◀᛫ Tell caregiver or family member to arouse patient immediately and give additional carbohydrate by mouth as soon as patient can tolerate it.
• As appropriate, review all other significant and life-threatening adverse reactions and interactions, especially those related to the drugs and tests mentioned above.

glyburide (glibenclamide⊕)

Apo-Glyburide♣, Daonil⊕, DiaBeta, Dom-Glyburide*, Euglucon♣, Gen-Glybe♣, Glynase PresTab, Micronase, Novo-Glyburide♣, Nu-Glyburide♣, PMS-Glyburide♣, Ratio-Glyburide♣, Riva-Glyburide♣, Sandoz Glyburide♣, Semi-Daonil⊕

Pharmacologic class: Sulfonylurea
Therapeutic class: Hypoglycemic
Pregnancy risk category B

Action
Increases insulin binding and sensitivity at receptor sites, stimulating insulin release from beta cells in pancreas and reducing blood glucose level. Also decreases production of basal glucose in liver, enhances sensitivity of peripheral tissue to insulin, inhibits platelet aggregation, and causes mild diuresis.

Availability
Tablets: 1.25 mg, 2.5 mg, 5 mg
Tablets (micronized): 1.5 mg, 3 mg, 6 mg

⚕ Indications and dosages
➤ To control blood glucose in type 2 (non-insulin-dependent) diabetes mellitus in patients who have some pancreatic function and don't respond to diet therapy
Adults: Initially, 2.5 to 5 mg (regular tablets) P.O. daily; range is 1.25 to 20 mg/day as a single dose or in divided doses. Or initially, 1.5 to 3 mg (micronized tablets) P.O. daily, with range of 0.75 to 12 mg/day; give dosages above 6 mg in two divided doses.
➤ Conversion from insulin therapy
Adults: If patient takes less than 20 units of insulin daily, give 2.5 to 5 mg glyburide daily; with insulin dosage of 20 to 40 units/day, give 5 mg glyburide; with insulin dosage above 40 units/day, give 5 mg glyburide daily or 3 mg (micronized tablets) P.O. daily and reduce insulin dosage by 50%.

Dosage adjustment
• Hepatic or renal failure
• Elderly patients

Contraindications
• Hypersensitivity to drug
• Type 1 (insulin-dependent) diabetes
• Severe renal, hepatic, thyroid or other endocrine disease
• Pregnancy or breastfeeding

Precautions
Use cautiously in:
• mild to moderate hepatic, renal, or cardiovascular disease; impaired thyroid, pituitary, or adrenal function
• infection, stress, or dietary changes
• elderly patients.

Administration
◀€ Know that micronized glyburide is not bioequivalent to regular glyburide.
• Check baseline creatinine level for normal renal function before giving first dose.
• Give daily dose at breakfast; for patient receiving drug b.i.d., give second dose at dinner.
• Adjust dosage slowly if patient is taking metformin.

Route	Onset	Peak	Duration
P.O.	45-60 min	1.5-3 hr	24 hr

Adverse reactions
CNS: dizziness, drowsiness, headache, weakness
CV: increased CV mortality risk
EENT: visual accommodation changes, blurred vision
GI: nausea, vomiting, diarrhea, constipation, cramps, heartburn, epigastric distress, anorexia
Hematologic: aplastic anemia, leukopenia, thrombocytopenia, agranulocytosis, pancytopenia
Hepatic: cholestatic jaundice, **hepatitis**
Metabolic: hyponatremia, **hypoglycemia**
Skin: rash, pruritus, urticaria, eczema, erythema, photosensitivity, angioedema
Other: increased appetite

Interactions
Drug-drug. *Androgens (such as testosterone), chloramphenicol, clofibrate, guanethidine, MAO inhibitors, nonsteroidal anti-inflammatory drugs (except diclofenac), salicylates,*

---

sulfonamides, tricyclic antidepressants: increased risk of hypoglycemia

Beta-adrenergic blockers: altered response to glyburide, requiring increased or decreased dosage; prolonged hypoglycemia (with nonselective agents)

Calcium channel blockers, corticosteroids, estrogens, hydantoins, hormonal contraceptives, isoniazid, nicotinic acid, phenothiazines, phenytoin, rifampin, sympathomimetics, thiazide diuretics, thyroid preparations: decreased hypoglycemic effect of glyburide

Warfarin: initially increased, then decreased, effects of both drugs

Drug-diagnostic tests. *Alanine aminotransferase, alkaline phosphatase, aspartate aminotransferase, bilirubin, blood urea nitrogen, cholesterol:* increased values

Glucose, granulocytes, hemoglobin, platelets, white blood cells: decreased values

Drug-herbs. *Agoral marshmallow, aloe (oral), bitter melon, burdock, chromium, coenzyme Q10, dandelion, eucalyptus, fenugreek:* increased hypoglycemic effect

Glucosamine: impaired glycemic control

Drug-behaviors. *Alcohol use:* disulfiram-like reaction

Patient monitoring

• Monitor blood glucose level, especially during periods of increased stress.

• Monitor CBC and renal function test results.

• If patient is ill or has abnormal laboratory findings, monitor electrolyte, ketone, glucose, pH, lactate dehydrogenase, and pyruvate levels.

• Evaluate cardiovascular status.

Patient teaching

• Advise patient to take daily dose with breakfast (and second dose, if prescribed, with dinner).

• Teach patient how to self-monitor his glucose level as prescribed; tell him to report significant changes.

• Inform patient that he may need supplemental insulin during times of stress or when he can't maintain adequate oral intake.

• Teach patient how to recognize signs and symptoms of hypoglycemia and hyperglycemia.

• Instruct patient to keep sugar source available at all times.

• Encourage patient to drink plenty of fluids.

• Stress importance of diet and exercise in helping to control diabetes.

• Advise patient to wear or carry medical identification stating he has diabetes.

• Caution patient to avoid driving and other hazardous activities until he knows how drug affects concentration and alertness.

• Tell patient he'll undergo regular blood testing during therapy.

• As appropriate, review all other significant and life-threatening adverse reactions and interactions, especially those related to the drugs, tests, herbs, and behaviors mentioned above.

glycopyrrolate (glycopyrronium⊕)
Robinul, Robinul Forte

Pharmacologic class: Anticholinergic

Therapeutic class: Antispasmodic, antimuscarinic, parasympatholytic

Pregnancy risk category B

Action

Inhibits action of acetylcholine on muscarinic receptors that mediate effects of parasympathetic postganglionic impulses. This inhibition relaxes cardiac smooth muscle, inhibits vagal reflexes, and decreases tracheal and bronchial secretions.

Availability
Injection: 0.2 mg/ml
Tablets: 1 mg, 2 mg

Indications and dosages
➤ Adjunct in peptic ulcer disorders
Adults: 1 mg P.O. t.i.d. or 2 mg (Forte) two to three times daily, to a maximum of 8 mg/day; or 0.1 to 0.2 mg I.M. or I.V. three or four times daily
➤ To diminish secretions and block cardiac vagal reflexes before surgery
Adults and children ages 2 and older: 0.0044 mg/kg I.M. 30 to 60 minutes before anesthesia
Children ages 1 month to 2 years: 0.0088 mg/kg I.M. 30 to 60 minutes before anesthesia
➤ To diminish secretions and block cardiac vagal reflexes during surgery
Adults: 0.1 mg I.V. May repeat as needed at 2- to 3-minute intervals.
Children: 0.004 mg/kg I.V., not to exceed 0.1 mg as a single dose. May repeat at 2- to 3-minute intervals.
➤ To diminish or block cholinergic effects caused by anticholinesterase
Adults and children: 0.2 mg I.V. for each 1 mg neostigmine or 5 mg pyridostigmine. May give I.V. undiluted or with dextrose injection by infusion.

Off-label uses
• Sweating

Contraindications
• Hypersensitivity to drug
• Arrhythmias
• Chronic obstructive pulmonary disease
• GI disease, infection, atony or ileus
• Myasthenia gravis
• Glaucoma
• Obstructive uropathy
• Severe prostatic hypertrophy

Precautions
Use cautiously in:
• cardiovascular disease, heart failure, hypertension, renal or hepatic disease, Down syndrome, hyperthyroidism, hiatal hernia, ulcerative colitis, mild to moderate prostatic hypertrophy, autonomic neuropathy, spasticity, suspected brain damage
• pregnant or breastfeeding patients.

Administration
• Give oral dose 30 to 60 minutes before meals.
• For I.V. injection, give either undiluted or diluted with dextrose 5% or 10% in water or saline solution. Give each 0.2 mg over 1 to 2 minutes.
◀ Keep resuscitation equipment on hand to treat curare-like effects of overdose.

Route	Onset	Peak	Duration
P.O.	Unknown	Unknown	8-12 hr
I.V.	1 min	Unknown	3-7 hr
I.M., subcut.	15-30 min	30-45 min	3-7 hr

Adverse reactions
CNS: weakness, nervousness, insomnia, drowsiness, dizziness, headache, confusion, excitement
CV: palpitations, tachycardia
EENT: blurred vision, photophobia, mydriasis, increased intraocular pressure, cycloplegia
GI: nausea, vomiting, constipation, abdominal distention, epigastric distress, heartburn, gastroesophageal reflux, dry mouth, **paralytic ileus**
GU: urinary hesitancy or retention, lactation suppression, erectile dysfunction
Skin: urticaria, decreased sweating or anhidrosis
Other: loss of taste, fever, allergic reaction, irritation at I.M. injection site, **anaphylaxis, malignant hyperthermia**

Reactions in **bold** are life-threatening.   ◀ Clinical alert

Interactions
Drug-drug. *Amantadine, antihistamines, antiparkinsonian drugs, disopyramide, glutethimide, meperidine, phenothiazines, procainamide, quinidine, tricyclic antidepressants:* additive anticholinergic effects

Patient monitoring
◀€ Check for signs and symptoms of anaphylaxis and malignant hyperthermia.
• Monitor neurologic and cardiovascular status.
◀€ Assess for curare-like effects (neuromuscular blockade leading to muscle weakness and possible paralysis), which indicate overdose.
• Assess fluid intake and output. Have patient void before each dose to avoid urinary retention.

Patient teaching
• Advise patient to take oral dose 30 to 60 minutes before meals.
◀€ Tell patient to immediately report signs and symptoms of serious adverse effects, especially anaphylaxis.
• Caution patient to avoid driving and other hazardous activities until he knows how drug affects concentration, vision, and alertness.
• Tell patient to minimize GI upset by eating frequent, small servings of food and drinking adequate fluids.
• Advise patient to report urinary hesitancy or retention.
• As appropriate, review all other significant and life-threatening adverse reactions and interactions, especially those related to the drugs mentioned above.

goserelin acetate
Zoladex, Zoladex LA✤❋, Zoladex 3-Month

Pharmacologic class: Gonadotropin-releasing hormone (GnRH) analog
Therapeutic class: Antineoplastic, hormone
Pregnancy risk category D (breast cancer), *X* (endometriosis)

Action
Synthetic form of luteinizing hormone-releasing hormone (LHRH); inhibits gonadotropin production by acting directly on pituitary gland. Enhances release of luteinizing hormone (LH), follicle-stimulating hormone (FSH), and testosterone, lowering testosterone and estradiol levels.

Availability
Implant: 3.6 mg, 10.8 mg (in preloaded syringes)

⏀ Indications and dosages
➤ Palliative treatment of advanced prostate cancer
Adults: 3.6 mg subcutaneously q 4 weeks or 10.8 mg subcutaneously q 12 weeks into upper abdominal wall
➤ Adjunct to radiation therapy and flutamide in stage B2-C prostate cancer
Adults: 3.6 mg subcutaneously q 4 weeks starting on day 1 of radiation or during last week of radiation. Alternatively, 3.6 mg subcutaneously 8 weeks before radiation, then 10.8 mg on day 28 or 3.6 mg at 4-week intervals starting 8 weeks before radiation, for a total of four doses (two depots before and two during radiation therapy).
➤ Palliative treatment of advanced breast cancer in pre- and perimenopausal women

---

Adults: 3.6 mg subcutaneously q 4 weeks. If serum estradiol doesn't fall to postmenopausal levels, may increase to 7.2 mg q 4 weeks.

➤ Endometriosis

Adults ages 18 and older: 3.6 mg subcutaneously q 4 weeks, continued for 6 months

➤ Endometrial thinning before ablation for dysfunctional uterine bleeding

Adults: 3.6 mg subcutaneously 4 weeks before surgery. Alternatively, initial 3.6-mg dose may be followed 4 weeks later by a second 3.6-mg dose, with surgery 2 to 4 weeks after second dose.

Contraindications

• Hypersensitivity to drug or its components or to GnRH, GnRH agonist analogs
• Pregnant patients

Precautions

Use cautiously in:
• risk factors for osteoporosis
• chronic alcohol or tobacco use
• patients receiving drugs that affect bone density
• hyperglycemia, cardiovascular risk factors
• breastfeeding patients
• children younger than age 18 (safety not established).

Administration

• Administer pretreatment pregnancy test to female of childbearing age.
• Know that drug should be given only by a clinician experienced in its use.
• Implant is placed subcutaneously into upper abdominal wall using aseptic technique. Give local anesthetic and stretch skin with one hand. Insert needle into subcutaneous fat, then change needle angle until it parallels abdominal wall. Push needle in until hub touches patient's skin, and withdraw about 1 ml before depressing plunger all the way.

• Don't aspirate after inserting needle. Blood will be visible in syringe if needle enters blood vessel.
◀€ Don't give by I.V. route.
• Be aware that 10.8-mg implant should not be used in women.
• Be aware that if implant must be removed, it can be located by ultrasound.

Route	Onset	Peak	Duration
Subcut.	Unknown	2-4 wk	End of therapy

Adverse reactions

CNS: headache, anxiety, depression, dizziness, fatigue, insomnia, lethargy, pain, emotional lability, weakness, **cerebrovascular accident, spinal cord compression**

CV: vasodilation, chest pain, hypertension, palpitations, peripheral edema, **myocardial infarction, arrhythmias, sudden cardiac death**

EENT: blurred vision

GI: nausea, vomiting, diarrhea, constipation, ulcer, anorexia

GU: urinary obstruction, lower urinary tract symptoms, breast swelling or tenderness, vaginitis, amenorrhea, infertility, decreased libido, erectile dysfunction, other sexual dysfunction, decreased testicular size, **renal insufficiency**

Hematologic: anemia

Musculoskeletal: increased bone pain, joint pain, decreased bone density

Metabolic: gout, hyperglycemia, hypercalcemia

Respiratory: dyspnea, chronic obstructive pulmonary disease, upper respiratory tract infection

Skin: rash, acne, diaphoresis, seborrhea

Other: hirsutism, chills, fever, hot flashes, infection, weight gain, **tumor flare phenomenon, hypersensitivity, antibody formation, acute anaphylactic reactions**

Interactions
Drug-diagnostic tests. *Calcium, glucose, high- and low-density lipoproteins, triglycerides:* increased levels
FSH, LH: initially increased, then decreased, levels

Patient monitoring
• Assess menstrual symptoms and watch for breakthrough bleeding.
◀᷍ Monitor neurologic status. Watch closely for signs and symptoms of cerebrovascular accident.
◀᷍ Closely monitor cardiovascular and respiratory status.
• Monitor blood glucose and glycosylated hemoglobin periodically.

Patient teaching
• Advise female patient to avoid pregnancy and to use a nonhormonal contraceptive method.
• Instruct patient to call prescriber if menstrual bleeding persists or breakthrough bleeding occurs.
• Inform patient that menstruation may be delayed after therapy ends.
◀᷍ Instruct patient to recognize and immediately report signs and symptoms of hyperglycemia, and cardiovascular or neurological adverse reactions.
• As appropriate, review all other significant and life-threatening adverse reactions and interactions, especially those related to the tests mentioned above.

granisetron hydrochloride
Granisol, Kytril, Sancuso

Pharmacologic class: 5-hydroxy-tryptamine₃ antagonist
Therapeutic class: Antiemetic
Pregnancy risk category B

Action
Binds to serotonin receptors in chemoreceptor trigger zone and vagal nerve terminals, blocking serotonin release and controlling nausea and vomiting

Availability
Injection: 1 mg/ml
Oral solution: 2 mg/10 ml in 30-ml bottles
Tablets: 1 mg
Transdermal system (patch): 52-cm² patch (containing 34.3 mg granisetron delivering 3.1 mg/24 hours)

⚡ Indications and dosages
➤ To prevent nausea and vomiting caused by chemotherapy
Adults and children ages 2 to 16: For I.V. use, 10 mcg/kg I.V. within 30 minutes before chemotherapy. For P.O. use (adults only), 1 mg P.O. b.i.d., with first dose given at least 1 hour before chemotherapy and second dose given 12 hours later on days when chemotherapy is administered; or 2 mg P.O. daily at least 1 hour before chemotherapy. For transdermal use (adults only), apply patch for up to 7 days.
➤ To prevent nausea and vomiting caused by radiation therapy
Adults: 2 mg P.O. daily within 1 hour of radiation therapy
➤ Acute postoperative nausea and vomiting
Adults: 1 mg I.V. undiluted, administered over 30 seconds

Contraindications
• Hypersensitivity to drug

Precautions
Use cautiously in:
• pregnant or breastfeeding patients
• children younger than age 18 (safety of P.O. and transdermal use not established)

• children younger than age 2 (safety of I.V. use not established).

Administration

• For I.V. infusion, dilute with 20 to 50 ml of normal saline solution or dextrose 5% in water.
• Infuse I.V. over 5 minutes, starting 30 minutes before chemotherapy.
• For direct I.V. injection, give undiluted over 30 seconds.
• Don't mix I.V. form with other drugs.
• For P.O. use, give first dose 1 hour before chemotherapy and second dose 12 hours after first.
• Apply a single transdermal patch to upper outer arm for 24 to 48 hours before chemotherapy.
• Remove patch a minimum of 24 hours after chemotherapy completion. Patch may be worn up to 7 days depending on duration of chemotherapy.

Route	Onset	Peak	Duration
P.O.	Rapid	1 hr	24 hr
I.V.	Rapid	30 min	Up to 24 hr
Transdermal	Unknown	48 hr	Unknown

Adverse reactions

CNS: headache, anxiety, stimulation, weakness, drowsiness, dizziness
CV: hypertension
GI: nausea, vomiting, diarrhea, constipation, abdominal pain
Hematologic: anemia, **leukopenia, thrombocytopenia**
Skin: alopecia, application site reactions (patch)
Other: altered taste, decreased appetite, fever, chills, shivering

Interactions

Drug-diagnostic tests. *Alanine aminotransferase, aspartate aminotransferase:* increased levels
Electrolytes: altered levels
Hemoglobin, platelets, white blood cells: decreased levels

Drug-herbs. *Horehound:* enhanced serotonergic effects

Patient monitoring

• Monitor hepatic enzyme levels and CBC with white cell differential.
• Monitor temperature and blood pressure. Have patient use caution when ambulating, to avoid orthostatic hypotension.
• Know that patch may be degraded by direct exposure to natural or artificial sunlight.

Patient teaching

• Instruct patient to apply a single transdermal patch to upper outer arm 24 to 48 hours before chemotherapy.
• Instruct patient to remove patch by gently peeling it off in a minimum of 24 hours after chemotherapy completion.
• Instruct patient to remove patch if a severe or generalized skin reaction (such as rash or itching) occurs.
• Advise patient to avoid direct exposure of application site to natural or artificial sunlight by covering site with clothing while wearing patch and for 10 days after patch removal.
• Caution patient to avoid driving and other hazardous activities until he knows how drug affects concentration and alertness.
• Advise patient to minimize GI upset by eating frequent, small servings of healthy food.
• Tell patient he'll undergo regular blood testing during therapy.
• As appropriate, review all other significant and life-threatening adverse reactions and interactions, especially those related to the tests and herbs mentioned above.

g

guaifenesin (glyceryl guaiacolate)

Balminil Expectorant✱, Benilyn Childrens Chesty Coughs✚, Benylin-E✱, Calmylin Expectorant✱, Diabetic Tussin EX, Genatuss, Koffex Expectorant✱, Mucinex, Organidin NR, Phanacin XPECT, Pneumomist, Resyl✱, Robitussin, Robitussin Chesty Cough✚, Scot-tussin Expectorant, Siltussin SA, Tixylix Chesty Cough✚, Venos for Kids✚, Vicks Vaposyrup for Chesty Coughs✚

Pharmacologic class: Propanediol derivative
Therapeutic class: Expectorant
Pregnancy risk category C

Action

Exerts vasoconstrictive action that leads to decreased edema and congestion. Also increases respiratory secretions and reduces mucus viscosity.

Availability

Capsules: 200 mg
Oral solution: 100 mg/5 ml, 200 mg/5 ml
Syrup: 100 mg/5 ml
Tablets: 100 mg, 200 mg, 400 mg
Tablets (extended-release): 600 mg

⊘ Indications and dosages

➤ Cough due to upper respiratory tract infection

Adults: 200 to 400 mg P.O. q 4 hours (not to exceed 2,400 mg/day), or 600 to 1,200 mg P.O. (extended-release tablets) q 12 hours (not to exceed 2,400 mg/day)

Children ages 6 to 12: 100 to 200 mg P.O. q 4 hours (not to exceed 1,200 mg/day), or 600 mg P.O. (extended-release) q 12 hours (not to exceed 1,200 mg/day)

Children ages 2 to 6: 50 to 100 mg P.O. q 4 hours (not to exceed 600 mg/day)

Contraindications

- Hypersensitivity to drug
- Alcohol intolerance (with some products)

Precautions

Use cautiously in:
- diabetes mellitus, cough lasting more than 1 week or accompanied by fever, rash, or headache
- patients receiving disulfiram concurrently
- pregnant patients.

Administration

- Give with full glass of water.

Route	Onset	Peak	Duration
P.O.	30 min	Unknown	4-6 hr
P.O. (extended)	Unknown	Unknown	12 hr

Adverse reactions

CNS: headache, dizziness
GI: nausea, vomiting, diarrhea, stomach pain
Skin: rash, urticaria

Interactions

Drug-diagnostic tests. *Urinary 5-hydroxyindoleacetic acid, vanillylmandelic acid:* inaccurate results

Patient monitoring

- Assess cough quality and productivity. Reevaluate treatment if cough persists and is accompanied by fever or headache.

Patient teaching

- Tell patient to take with 8 oz of water and to drink plenty of fluids.
- Instruct patient to contact prescriber if cough lasts more than 1 week.

✱ Canada   ✚ UK   ⚚ Hazardous drug   ⊗ High-alert drug

- Caution patient to avoid driving and other hazardous activities until he knows how drug affects concentration and alertness.
- As appropriate, review all other significant adverse reactions and interactions, especially those related to the tests mentioned above.

guanfacine
Intuniv

Pharmacologic class: Centrally acting antiadrenergic
Therapeutic class: Antiadrenergic-sympatholytic, antihypertensive
Pregnancy risk category B

Action
Stimulates central alpha$_2$-adrenergic receptors, reducing sympathetic nerve impulses from vasomotor center to heart and blood vessels

Availability
Tablets: 1 mg, 2 mg
Tablets (extended-release): 1 mg, 2 mg, 3 mg, 4 mg

💊 Indications and dosages
➤ Management of hypertension (used alone or in combination with other agents, especially thiazide diuretics)
Adults: 1 mg (immediate-release) P.O. at bedtime. If response unsatisfactory after 3 to 4 weeks, increase to 2 mg (immediate-release) P.O. at bedtime.
➤ Attention deficit hyperactivity disorder (ADHD) as monotherapy and as adjunctive therapy to stimulants
Adults and children age 6 and older: 1 mg (extended-release) P.O. daily; adjust in increments of no more than 1 mg/week. Maintain dosage within 1 to 4 mg/day, depending on clinical response and tolerability. Consider

dosing on a mg/kg basis. Improvements have been observed starting at dosages of 0.05 to 0.08 mg/kg once daily. Dosages up to 0.12 mg/kg once daily may provide additional benefit. Dosages above 4 mg/day haven't been studied. If switching from immediate-release guanfacine, discontinue immediate-release treatment and titrate with extended-release, as directed.

Dosage adjustment
- Hepatic or renal impairment (immediate-release form)
- Concurrent use of CYP3A4 inducers such as rifampin (immediate-release form)

Off-label uses
- Attention deficit hyperactivity disorder (immediate-release form)
- Treatment of heroin withdrawal
- Hypertension in pregnancy

Contraindications
- Hypersensitivity to drug, its components, or other products containing guanfacine

Precautions
Use cautiously in:
- hepatic or renal impairment
- severe coronary insufficiency, cardiovascular or cerebovascular disease
- history of syncope, patients at risk for hypotension, bradycardia, heart block, or syncope, such as those taking antihypertensives (immediate-release form)
- concurrent use of CNS depressants
- concurrent use of antihypertensives, other products containing guanfacine, or CYP3A4/5 inhibitors such as ketoconazole (immediate-release form)
- elderly patients
- sedated patients (especially when given with centrally acting depressants)
- pregnant or breastfeeding patients
- children younger than age 6 (extended-release form) or 12 (immediate-release form).

Reactions in **bold** are life-threatening.   🔊 Clinical alert

Administration

- Measure heart rate and blood pressure before starting drug and after dosage increases.
- Give at bedtime to reduce daytime sleepiness (immediate-release form).
- Don't administer with high-fat meals (extended-release form).
- Know that therapy shouldn't be stopped abruptly, because this may cause rebound plasma and urinary catecholamines, anxiety, hypertension, and increase in blood pressure. When discontinuing, taper dosage in decrements of no more than 1 mg every 3 to 7 days.
- Be aware that drug may be used alone or with other agents, especially thiazide diuretics (immediate-release form).
- Be aware that for adolescents and children age 6 and older, efficacy beyond 9 weeks and safety beyond 2 years of treatment haven't been established.
- Don't substitute extended-release tablet for immediate-release tablet on a milligram-per-milligram basis, because of differing pharmacokinetic profiles.

Route	Onset	Peak	Duration
P.O.	Unknown	2.6 hr	Unknown
P.O. (extended)	Unknown	4-8 hr	Unknown

Adverse reactions

CNS: somnolence, insomnia, dizziness, postural dizziness, lethargy, irritability, agitation, anxiety, nightmares, headache, fatigue, amnesia, confusion, depression, hypokinesia, asthenia, malaise, paresthesia, paresis, **seizures**
CV: hypertension, hypotension, syncope, bradycardia, palpitations, substernal pain, **AV block, sinus arrhythmia**
EENT: conjunctivitis, iritis, vision disturbance, tinnitus, rhinitis
GI: nausea, vomiting, diarrhea, constipation, abdominal pain, dyspepsia, dysphagia, dry mouth
GU: erectile dysfunction, decreased libido, increased urinary frequency, enuresis
Musculoskeletal: leg cramps
Respiratory: dyspnea, asthma
Skin: dermatitis, pruritus, purpura, sweating, pallor, rash
Other: taste perversion, decreased appetite, weight gain, chest pain, hypersensitivity

Interactions

Drug-drug. *Antihypertensives:* increased risk of additive pharmacodynamic effects, such as hypotension and syncope
CNS depressants: (such as antipsychotics, barbiturates, benzodiazepines, sedative-hypnotics): additive sedation
CYP3A4 inducers (such as rifampin): decreased guanfacine plasma concentration
CYP3A4/5 inhibitors (such as ketoconazole), valproic acid: increased guanfacine plasma concentration
Phenobarbital, phenytoin: decreased elimination half-life and blood level of guanfacine
Valproic acid: increased serum valproic acid concentration
Drug-diagnostic tests. *Alanine aminotransferase:* increased level
Drug-food. *High-fat meal:* increased guanfacine C_{max} and area under the curve
Drug-behaviors. *Alcohol use:* additive sedation

Patient monitoring

- Monitor patient for evidence of drug efficacy.
- Monitor patient closely during drug withdrawal.
- ◀ Continue to monitor heart rate and blood pressure periodically during therapy. Watch for hypotension, bradycardia, syncope, and heart block, especially in patients taking antihypertensives.

◀ŧ Be aware that rash with exfoliation has occurred in a few patients. Should rash occur, discontinue drug and monitor patient appropriately.

Patient teaching
• Tell patient to take immediate-release tablets at bedtime to reduce daytime sleepiness.
• Tell patient to take extended-release tablets whole with water, milk, or other liquid but not to take with high-fat meals.
• Tell patient not to crush, chew, or break extended-release tablets before swallowing.
• Caution patient not to stop taking drug abruptly.
◀ŧ Instruct patient how to recognize and immediately report signs and symptoms of serious cardiovascular disorders.
◀ŧ Instruct patient to immediately report development of a rash.
• Advise patient to avoid driving and other hazardous activities until he knows how drug affects concentration and alertness.
• Tell patient to avoid alcohol during therapy.
• Advise patient to avoid dehydration or overheating.
• As appropriate, review all other significant adverse reactions and interactions, especially those related to the drugs, tests, foods, and behaviors mentioned above.

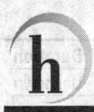

haloperidol
Apo-Haloperidol✹, Dozic⬡, Novo-Peridol✹, Peridol✹, PMS Haloperidol✹, Serenace⬡

haloperidol decanoate
Haldol Decanoate 50, Haloperidol LA Omega✹

haloperidol lactate
Haldol

Pharmacologic class: Butyrophenone
Therapeutic class: Antipsychotic
Pregnancy risk category C

FDA | BOXED WARNING

• Drug increased mortality in elderly patients with dementia-related psychosis. Although causes of death were varied, most appeared to be cardiovascular or infectious. Drug isn't approved for treatment of dementia-related psychosis.

Action
Unknown. Thought to block postsynaptic dopamine receptors in brain and increase dopamine turnover rate, inhibiting signs and symptoms of psychosis.

Availability
Injection (decanoate): 50 mg/ml, 100 mg/ml
Injection (lactate): 5 mg/ml
Oral concentrate (lactate): 2 mg/ml
Tablets: 0.5 mg, 1 mg, 2 mg, 5 mg, 10 mg, 20 mg

⊘ Indications and dosages
➤ Symptomatic treatment of psychotic disorders or Tourette syndrome
Adults: For moderate symptoms, 0.5 to 2 mg P.O. two to three times daily. For severe symptoms or chronic or resistant disorder, 3 to 5 mg P.O. two to three times daily, to a maximum of 100 mg daily if needed. Adjust subsequent dosages carefully based on response and tolerance. Alternatively, 2 to 5 mg I.M. (lactate) may be given for

prompt control of acutely agitated patient with moderate to severe symptoms; based on response, subsequent doses may be given q hour.

➤ Schizophrenia in patients who need prolonged parenteral antipsychotic therapy

Adults: For patient previously stabilized on oral haloperidol, initial I.M. dose (decanoate) is 10 to 20 times the previous daily P.O. haloperidol equivalent, depending on patient's stability on low or high P.O. dosage. Initially, I.M. dosage shouldn't exceed 100 mg. If conversion requires dosage above 100 mg, give balance in 3 to 7 days. Maintenance dosage is 10 to 15 times the previous daily P.O. dosage, depending on response.

➤ Psychotic disorders

Children ages 3 to 12 or weighing 15 to 40 kg (33 to 88 lb): 0.05 to 0.15 mg/kg/day P.O. in two or three divided doses. May be increased by 0.5 mg daily given in two or three divided doses at 5- to 7-day intervals, depending on response and tolerance.

➤ Nonpsychotic behavior disorder; Tourette syndrome; hyperactivity

Children ages 3 to 12 or weighing 15 to 40 kg (33 to 88 lb): 0.05 to 0.075 mg/kg/day P.O. in two or three divided doses

Dosage adjustment
• Elderly or debilitated patients

Off-label uses
• Nausea and vomiting
• Infantile autism
• Intractable hiccups

Contraindications
• Hypersensitivity to drug, tartrazine, sesame oil, or benzyl alcohol (with some products)
• Severe CNS depression or comatose states
• Parkinson's disease

Precautions
Use cautiously in:
• torsades de pointes, QT interval prolongation
• patients with allergies
• hepatic disease, bone marrow depression, cardiac disease, respiratory insufficiency, CNS tumors
• history of seizures, patients receiving anticonvulsants, EEG abnormalities
• concurrent anticoagulant use
• elderly patients
• pregnant or breastfeeding patients
• children (parenteral form not recommended).

Administration
• Be aware that torsades de pointes and QT interval prolongation have occurred in patients receiving haloperidol, especially when drug is given I.V. or in doses higher than recommended. Haloperidol isn't approved for I.V. use.
◄€ Don't give decanoate form I.V.
• Administer decanoate form by deep I.M. injection using 21G needle. Two injections may be necessary; maximum volume shouldn't exceed 3 ml.
• Know that recommended interval between I.M. injections is 4 weeks.
• Dilute oral concentrate in water, soda, or juice (orange, apple, tomato) immediately before administering.
• Be aware that patient should be switched from parenteral form to oral form as soon as possible.
• Know that parenteral form is not recommended in children.

Route	Onset	Peak	Duration
P.O.	Unknown	3-6 hr	Unknown
I.V. (lactate)	Unknown	Unknown	Unknown
I.M. (decanoate)	20-30 min	30-45 min	4-8 hr

Adverse reactions
CNS: confusion, drowsiness, restlessness, extrapyramidal reactions,

sedation, lethargy, insomnia, vertigo, tardive dyskinesia, **seizures, neuroleptic malignant syndrome**

CV: hypotension, hypertension, tachycardia, ECG changes, **torsades de pointes** (with I.V. use)

EENT: blurred vision, dry eyes

GI: constipation, ileus, dry mouth, anorexia

GU: urinary retention, menstrual irregularities, gynecomastia, priapism

Hematologic: anemia, **leukocytosis, leukopenia**

Hepatic: jaundice, **drug-induced hepatitis**

Metabolic: galactorrhea

Respiratory: dyspnea, **respiratory depression, bronchospasm, laryngospasm**

Skin: diaphoresis, photosensitivity, rash

Other: hyperpyrexia, hypersensitivity reactions

Interactions

Drug-drug. *Antidepressants, antihistamines, atropine, disopyramide, phenothiazines, quinidine, other anticholinergics:* additive anticholinergic effects

Antihypertensives, nitrates: additive hypotension

CNS depressants (including antihistamines, opioid analgesics, sedative-hypnotics): additive CNS depression

Epinephrine: severe hypotension and tachycardia

Levodopa, pergolide: decreased therapeutic effects of haloperidol

Lithium: acute encephalopathic syndrome

Methyldopa: dementia

Rifampin: decreased haloperidol plasma level

Drug-diagnostic tests. *Alanine aminotransferase, aspartate aminotransferase, thyroid function tests:* increased values

Arterial blood gases, bicarbonate: altered values

White blood cells: increased or decreased count

Drug-herbs. *Angel's trumpet, jimsonweed, scopolia:* antagonism of cholinergic effects

Chamomile, hops, kava, skullcap, valerian: increased CNS depression

Nutmeg: reduced haloperidol efficacy

Drug-behaviors. *Acute alcohol ingestion:* additive hypotension

Patient monitoring

◀€ Monitor CNS status closely, especially for seizures and neuroleptic malignant syndrome (shown by extrapyramidal symptoms, hyperthermia, and autonomic disturbances).

◀€ Monitor cardiovascular status, particularly for ECG changes, blood pressure changes, torsades de pointes, and atypical rapid ventricular tachycardia, which may progress to ventricular fibrillation (with I.V. use).

• Assess respiratory status.

• Monitor liver function test results and CBC with white cell differential.

• With prolonged use, assess for tardive dyskinesia (which may occur months or even years after starting drug).

Patient teaching

• Tell patient to dilute oral concentrate with water, cola, or juice immediately before taking.

◀€ Instruct patient to immediately report signs or symptoms of serious adverse reactions, such as unusual weakness, yellowing of skin or eyes, difficulty breathing, or symptoms of neuroleptic malignant syndrome (such as fever, muscle pain or rigidity, rapid or irregular pulse, increased sweating, change in urination pattern, or decreased mental acuity).

• Advise patient to minimize GI upset by eating frequent, small servings of food and drinking adequate fluids.

• As appropriate, review all other significant and life-threatening adverse reactions and interactions, especially those related to the drugs, tests, herbs, and behaviors mentioned above.

h

---

heparin sodium
Calciparine⊕, Canusal⊕, Hepalean♥,
Heparin Leo♥, Hep-Lock♥, Hep-
Lock U/P, Hepsal⊕, Monoparin⊕,
Multiparin⊕

Pharmacologic class: Antithrombotic
Therapeutic class: Anticoagulant
Pregnancy risk category C

Action
Inhibits thrombus by preventing conversion of prothrombin to thrombin
and fibrinogen to fibrin, preventing
clot formation. Doesn't lyse existing
clot, but prevents clot enlargement and
extension.

Availability
Solution for flushes: 1-unit/ml,
2-units/ml, 10-units/ml, 100-units/ml
syringes; 100-units/ml vials
Solution for injection: 1,000 units/ml,
10,000 units/ml, 20,000 units/ml,
40,000 units/ml in single-dose vials;
1,000 units/ml, 2,000 units/ml, 5,000
units/ml, 10,000 units/ml, 20,000
units/ml in multidose vials; 1,000
units/ml, 2,500 units/ml, 5,000
units/ml, 10,000 units/ml in unit-dose
syringes

ⓘ Indications and dosages
➢ Therapeutic anticoagulation
Adults: 10,000 units I.V. by intermittent bolus, then 5,000 to 10,000 units
I.V. q 4 to 6 hours. Or 5,000 units by
I.V. injection, then 20,000 to 40,000
units I.V. over 24 hours (about 1,000
units/hour or 15 to 18 units/kg/hour).
Or 5,000 units I.V., followed by initial
deep subcutaneous dose of 10,000 to
20,000 units, then 8,000 to 10,000 units
q 8 hours or 15,000 to 20,000 units q
12 hours.

Children: Initially, 50 units/kg by I.V.
drip, then 100 units/kg by I.V. drip q 4
hours. Or 20,000 units/m²/24 hours by
continuous I.V. infusion.
➢ To prevent thromboembolism
Adults: 5,000 units subcutaneously q 8
to 12 hours (may begin 2 hours before
surgery) given for 7 days or until
patient is fully ambulatory
➢ To prevent blood clotting during
cardiovascular surgery
Adults: At least 150 units/kg I.V. (300
units/kg if procedure less than
60 minutes; 400 units/kg if more than
60 minutes)
➢ I.V. flush
Adults and children: 10 to 100 units/
ml I.V. heparin sodium solution to fill
heparin lock set

Off-label uses
• Prophylaxis of left ventricular thrombi
• Prophylaxis of cerebrovascular acci-
dent after myocardial infarction

Contraindications
• Hypersensitivity to drug
• Bleeding disorders
• Severe thrombocytopenia
• Patients who can't undergo regular
blood coagulation tests

Precautions
Use cautiously in:
• severe hepatic or renal disease, bacterial endocarditis, hypertension, brain
injury, retinopathy, ulcer disease
• recent CNS or ophthalmic surgery
• immediate postpartum period
• women older than age 60
• pregnant patients.

Administration
◀≶ Know that I.V. heparin sodium is a
high-alert drug.
• Draw baseline blood sample for clot-
ting studies before starting drug.
◀≶ Use infusion pump to administer
I.V. dose. Check regularly to ensure
that infusion rate is correct.

• For I.V. use, give each 1,000-unit dose or single-dose injection over at least 1 minute. Give continuous infusion over 4 to 24 hours, depending on dose and volume of infusion solution.

• Draw blood for partial thromboplastin time (PTT) from opposite arm 4 hours after continuous I.V. infusion begins.

• Put note at patient's bedside to remind personnel to apply pressure dressings after withdrawing blood.

• With intermittent I.V. drug infusion, withdraw blood 30 minutes before dose, using arm without I.V. infusion.

• For subcutaneous dose, inject slowly between iliac crests in lower abdomen, deep into subcutaneous fat layer. Leave needle in place for 10 seconds before withdrawing. Don't massage area after injection. Alternate subcutaneous sites every 12 hours.

• Have protamine available as heparin agonist.

◀ℰ Don't give I.M.

◀ℰ Don't give heparin products containing benzyl alcohol to premature infants.

Route	Onset	Peak	Duration
I.V.	Immediate	5-10 min	2-6 hr
Subcut.	20-60 min	2-4 hr	8-12 hr

Adverse reactions

EENT: rhinitis

Hematologic: anemia, **thrombocytopenia, bleeding, severely prolonged clotting time**

Hepatic: hepatitis

Metabolic: hyperkalemia

Musculoskeletal: osteoporosis (with long-term use)

Skin: irritation, rash, urticaria, hematoma, ulceration, cutaneous or subcutaneous necrosis, pruritus, alopecia (with long-term use)

Other: fever, pain at injection site, hypersensitivity reactions, **white clot syndrome, anaphylactoid reactions**

Interactions

Drug-drug. *Antihistamines, digoxin, nicotine, tetracyclines:* decreased anticoagulant effect of heparin

Cefamandole, cefmetazole, cefoperazone, cefotetan, plicamycin, quinidine, valproic acid, other drugs that cause hypoprothrombinemia; drugs that affect platelet function (including abciximab, aspirin, clopidogrel, dextran, dipyridamole, eptifibitide, nonsteroidal anti-inflammatory drugs, some penicillins, thrombolytics, ticlopidine, tirofiban): increased bleeding risk

Drug-diagnostic tests. *Alanine aminotransferase, aspartate aminotransferase, free fatty acids, thyroxine, triiodothyronine resin:* increased levels

Cholesterol, triglycerides: decreased levels

^{125}I *fibrinogen uptake:* false-negative result

Prothrombin time: prolonged

Drug-herbs. *Anise, arnica, chamomile, clove, dong quai, feverfew, garlic, ginger, ginseng:* increased bleeding risk

Drug-behaviors. *Smoking:* increased bleeding risk

Patient monitoring

• Monitor infusion rate closely, even when using infusion pump.

• Evaluate patient's vital signs.

◀ℰ Watch for signs and symptoms of anaphylactoid reaction.

◀ℰ Assess for white clot syndrome (new thrombus formation in association with thrombocytopenia caused by irreversible platelet aggregation).

◀ℰ Stay alert for signs and symptoms of bleeding tendency.

• Check hematocrit, PTT, and platelet count frequently.

• Monitor liver function test results.

• In long-term therapy, periodically assess stool for occult blood.

• Monitor potassium level in patients with diabetes or renal disease. (Drug may cause hyperkalemia.)

h

Reactions in **bold** are life-threatening.　　　◀ℰ Clinical alert

Patient teaching

- If patient will self-administer drug, teach proper technique and emphasize need to rotate injection sites.
- 🔊 Advise patient that nosebleed, blood in urine, or black stools may be first sign of overdose and should be reported immediately.
- 🔊 Tell patient to immediately report other unusual bleeding or bruising.
- Urge patient to avoid activities that can cause injury. Advise him to use soft toothbrush and electric razor to avoid gum and skin injury.
- Tell patient he will undergo regular blood testing during therapy.
- As appropriate, review all other significant and life-threatening adverse reactions and interactions, especially those related to the drugs, tests, herbs, and behaviors mentioned above.

hydralazine hydrochloride

Apo-Hydralazine♣, Apresoline, Novo-Hylazin♣, Nu-Hydral♣

Pharmacologic class: Peripheral vaso-dilator
Therapeutic class: Antihypertensive
Pregnancy risk category C

Action

Relaxes vascular smooth muscles of arteries and arterioles, causing peripheral vasodilation and decreasing peripheral vascular resistance. These actions decrease blood pressure and increase heart rate, stroke volume, and cardiac output.

Availability

Injection: 20 mg/ml
Tablets: 10 mg, 25 mg, 50 mg, 100 mg

💊 Indications and dosages

➤ Hypertension

Adults: Initially, 10 mg P.O. q.i.d. After 2 to 4 days, may increase to 25 mg P.O. q.i.d. for remainder of first week; may then increase further to 50 mg P.O. q.i.d., up to 300 mg/day. Once maintenance dosage is established, may give in two daily doses.

Children: Initially, 0.75 mg/kg/day P.O. in four divided doses; may increase gradually over 3 to 4 weeks to 7.5 mg/kg or 200 mg/day

Neonates: 0.5 mg/kg P.O., I.M., or I.V. q 4 to 6 hours

Contraindications

- Hypersensitivity to drug or tartrazine
- Coronary artery disease
- Mitral valvular rheumatic heart disease

Precautions

Use cautiously in:
- suspected CV or cerebrovascular disease, severe renal or hepatic disease
- pregnant or breastfeeding patients
- children.

Administration

- Administer oral form with food.
- 🔊 Inject I.V. form slowly over 1 minute. Monitor blood pressure response continuously.
- Draw up and use parenteral drug immediately; solution changes color after contact with metal needle.

Route	Onset	Peak	Duration
P.O.	45 min	2 hr	3-8 hr
I.V.	10-20 min	15-30 min	3-8 hr
I.M.	10-30 min	1 hr	3-8 hr

Adverse reactions

CNS: dizziness, drowsiness, headache, peripheral neuritis
CV: tachycardia, angina, orthostatic hypotension, **arrhythmias**
EENT: lacrimation, nasal congestion
GI: nausea, vomiting, diarrhea, constipation, anorexia
Metabolic: sodium retention

Musculoskeletal: joint pain, arthritis
Skin: rash, blisters, flushing, pruritus, urticaria
Other: chills, fever, lymphadenopathy, edema, lupuslike syndrome

Interactions

Drug-drug. *Antihypertensives, nitrates:* additive hypotension
Epinephrine: reduced pressor response to epinephrine
Metoprolol, propranolol: increased blood levels of both drugs
MAO inhibitors: increased hypotension
Drug-diagnostic tests. *Coombs' test:* positive result
Granulocytes, hemoglobin, neutrophils, platelets, red blood cells, white blood cells: decreased levels
Drug-behaviors. *Alcohol use:* additive hypotensive response

Patient monitoring

• Monitor CBC, lupus erythematosus cell studies, and antinuclear antibody titers before and periodically during therapy.
• Monitor blood pressure, pulse rate and regularity, and daily weight.
• To avoid rapid blood pressure drop, taper dosage gradually before discontinuing.
◄€ Assess for lupuslike signs and symptoms, including joint pain, fever, myalgia, pharyngitis, and splenomegaly.
• Watch for peripheral neuritis. If it occurs, expect to give pyridoxine.

Patient teaching

• Tell patient to take tablets with food.
• Instruct patient to move slowly when rising (especially in morning on awakening), to avoid dizziness from sudden blood pressure decrease.
◄€ Instruct patient to immediately report fever, muscle and joint aches, or sore throat.
• Tell patient to report chest pain or numbness or tingling of hands or feet.

• To minimize GI upset, advise patient to eat small, frequent meals.
• Caution patient not to discontinue drug abruptly, because severe hypertension may result.
• As appropriate, review other significant and life-threatening adverse reactions and interactions, especially those related to the drugs, tests, and behaviors mentioned above.

hydrochlorothiazide

Apo-Hydro✲, Diuchlor H✲, Hydro-Par, Microzide, Neo-Codema✲, Novo-Hydrazide✲, PMS-Hydrochlorothiazide✲, Urozide✲

h

Pharmacologic class: Thiazide diuretic
Therapeutic class: Diuretic, antihypertensive
Pregnancy risk category B

Action

Increases sodium and water excretion by inhibiting sodium reabsorption in distal tubules; promotes excretion of chloride, potassium, magnesium, and bicarbonate. Also may produce arteriolar dilation, reducing blood pressure.

Availability

Capsules: 12.5 mg
Oral solution: 10 mg/ml, 100 mg/ml
Tablets: 12.5 mg, 25 mg, 50 mg, 100 mg

⊘ Indications and dosages

➤ Edema caused by heart failure, renal dysfunction, cirrhosis, corticosteroid therapy, or estrogen therapy
Adults: 25 to 100 mg P.O. daily as a single dose or in divided doses. Maximum dosage is 200 mg/day.
➤ Mild to moderate hypertension
Adults: Initially, 12.5 mg daily P.O.; then, based on blood pressure response, may give 12.5 to 50 mg/day

P.O. Higher dosages may be given in refractory cases.

Children ages 2 to 12: 1 to 2 mg/kg/day P.O. in single dose or two divided doses, not to exceed 100 mg/day

Children younger than age 2: 1 to 2 mg/kg P.O. as single dose or divided doses, not to exceed 37.5 mg/day; infants less than age 6 months may require dosage of 3 mg/kg/day in two divided doses.

Off-label uses

- Hypercalcemia
- Ménière's disease

Contraindications

- Hypersensitivity to drug, other thiazides, sulfonamides, or tartrazine
- Renal decompensation or anuria

Precautions

Use cautiously in:

- renal or severe hepatic impairment, fluid or electrolyte imbalances, gout, systemic lupus erythematosus, hyperparathyroidism, glucose tolerance abnormalities, bipolar disorder
- elderly patients
- pregnant or breastfeeding patients.

Administration

- Give with food or milk if GI upset occurs.
- Administer early in day so diuretic effect doesn't disturb sleep.

Route	Onset	Peak	Duration
P.O.	2 hr	3-6 hr	6-12 hr

Adverse reactions

CNS: dizziness, drowsiness, lethargy, headache, insomnia, nervousness, vertigo, asthenia, asterixis, paresthesias, confusion, fatigue, **encephalopathy**

CV: chest pain, orthostatic hypotension, ECG changes, **thrombophlebitis, arrhythmias**

EENT: nystagmus

GI: nausea, vomiting, epigastric distress, anorexia, **pancreatitis**

GU: polyuria, nocturia, erectile dysfunction, loss of libido, **renal failure**

Hematologic: anemia, **hemolytic anemia, agranulocytosis, leukopenia, thrombocytopenia**

Hepatic: jaundice, **hepatitis**

Metabolic: dehydration, gout, hyperglycemia, hypokalemia, hypocalcemia, hypovolemia, hypomagnesemia, hyponatremia, hypophosphatemia, hyperuricemia, **hypochloremic alkalosis**

Musculoskeletal: muscle cramps

Skin: photosensitivity, urticaria, rash, dermatitis, purpura, alopecia, flushing

Other: fever, weight loss, **anaphylaxis**

Interactions

Drug-drug. *Adrenocorticotropic hormone, corticosteroids:* increased risk of intensified electrolyte depletion, particularly hypokalemia

Allopurinol: increased risk of hypersensitivity reaction

Amphotericin B, corticosteroids, digoxin, mezlocillin, piperacillin, ticarcillin: increased risk of hypokalemia

Antihypertensives, barbiturates, nitrates, opioids: increased hypotension

Cholestyramine, colestipol: decreased hydrochlorothiazide absorption

Digoxin: increased risk of hypokalemia

Insulin, oral hypoglycemics: possible decreased hypoglycemic effect

Lithium: decreased excretion and increased blood level of lithium

Nondepolarizing skeletal muscle relaxants (such as tubocurarine): increased skeletal muscle relaxant effect

Nonsteroidal anti-inflammatory drugs: decreased hydrochlorothiazide efficacy

Vasopressors: decreased pressor effect

Drug-diagnostic tests. *Bilirubin, blood and urine glucose (in diabetic patients), calcium, creatinine, uric acid:* increased levels

Cholesterol, low-density lipoproteins, magnesium, potassium, protein-bound

---

iodine, sodium, triglycerides, urinary calcium: decreased levels

Drug-herbs. *Dandelion:* interference with diuretic activity

Ginkgo: decreased antihypertensive effect

Licorice, stimulant laxative herbs (aloe, cascara sagrada, senna): increased risk of hypokalemia

Drug-behaviors. *Alcohol use:* increased hypotension

Sun exposure: increased risk of photosensitivity

Patient monitoring

• Monitor blood pressure, fluid intake and output, and daily weight.

• Assess electrolyte levels, especially potassium. Monitor for signs and symptoms of hypokalemia.

• Monitor blood urea nitrogen and creatinine levels.

• Check blood glucose level in diabetic patients.

• Assess for signs and symptoms of gout attacks in patients with gouty arthritis.

Patient teaching

• Advise patient to take with food or milk if GI upset occurs.

• Tell patient to take early in day to avoid nighttime urination.

• Instruct patient to track intermittent doses on calendar.

• Tell patient to weigh himself daily, at same time on same scale and wearing same clothes.

◀€ Instruct patient to report decreased urination, swelling, unusual bleeding or bruising, dizziness, fatigue, numbness, and muscle weakness or cramping.

• Instruct patient to move slowly when sitting up or standing, to avoid dizziness from sudden blood pressure decrease.

• Caution patient to avoid driving and other hazardous activities until he knows how drug affects concentration and alertness.

• As appropriate, review all other significant and life-threatening adverse reactions and interactions, especially those related to the drugs, tests, herbs, and behaviors mentioned above.

hydrocodone bitartrate and acetaminophen

Anexsia, Ceta-Plus, Co-Gesic, Hydrocet, Lortab, Norco, Stagesic, Vicodin, Vicodin ES, Vicodin HP, Xodol, Zydone

hydrocodone bitartrate and aspirin

hydrocodone bitartrate and ibuprofen

Vicoprofen

hydrocodone bitartrate and homatropine methylbromide

Hycodan

Pharmacologic class: Opioid agonist/nonopioid analgesic combination

Therapeutic class: Opioid analgesic; allergy, cold, and cough remedy (antitussive)

Controlled substance schedule III

Pregnancy risk category C

Action

Blocks release of inhibitory neurotransmitters, altering perception of and emotional response to pain. Hydrocodone/ibuprofen combination raises pain threshold by nonselectively inhibiting cyclooxygenase; prostaglandin synthesis then decreases and anti-inflammatory and analgesic effects occur.

Availability
hydrocodone bitartrate and acetaminophen
Capsules: 5 mg hydrocodone (hyd.)/ 500 mg acetaminophen (acet.)
Elixir/oral solution: 2.5 mg hyd./167 mg acet./5 ml
Tablets: 2.5 mg hyd./500 mg acet.; 5 mg hyd./325 mg acet.; 5 mg hyd./400 mg acet.; 5 mg hyd./500 mg acet.; 7.5 mg hyd./325 mg acet.; 7.5 mg hyd./400 mg acet.; 7.5 mg hyd./500 mg acet.; 7.5 mg hyd./650 mg acet.; 7.5 mg hyd./750 mg acet.; 10 mg hyd./325 mg acet.; 10 mg hyd./400 mg acet.; 10 mg hyd./500 mg acet.; 10 mg hyd./650 mg acet.; 10 mg hyd./660 mg acet.; 10 mg hyd./750 mg acet.
hydrocodone bitartrate and aspirin
Tablets: 5 mg hyd./500 mg aspirin
hydrocodone bitartrate and ibuprofen
Tablets: 7.5 mg hyd./200 mg ibuprofen
hydrocodone bitartrate and homatropine methylbromide
Syrup: 1.5 mg/5 ml, 5 mg/5 ml
Tablets: 1.5 mg, 5 mg

❷ Indications and dosages
➤ Moderate to severe pain
Adults: 2.5 to 10 mg P.O. q 4 to 6 hours p.r.n. When giving hydrocodone/acetaminophen, don't exceed 60 mg/day; when giving hydrocodone/ibuprofen, don't exceed 37.5 mg/day.
Children: 0.15 to 0.2 mg/kg P.O. q 6 hours
➤ Cough
Adults: One tablet or 5 ml (syrup) q 4 to 6 hours as needed; don't exceed 6 tablets or 30 ml syrup in 24 hours.
Children ages 6 to 12: One-half tablet or 2.5 ml (syrup) q 4 to 6 hours as needed; don't exceed 3 tablets or 15 ml syrup in 24 hours.

Contraindications
• Hypersensitivity to hydrocodone, acetaminophen, aspirin, ibuprofen, or homatropine methylbromide (for corresponding combination products) or to alcohol, aspartame, saccharine, sugar, or tartrazine (with some products)

Precautions
Use cautiously in:
• severe renal, hepatic, or pulmonary disease; increased intracranial pressure; hypothyroidism; adrenal insufficiency; prostatic hypertrophy; thrombocytopenia; alcoholism
• elderly patients
• pregnant or breastfeeding patients.

Administration
◀€ In patients receiving concurrent MAO inhibitors, know that hydrocodone may produce severe, unpredictable reactions. Initial dosage may need to be 25% lower than usual dosage.

Route	Onset	Peak	Duration
P.O.	10-30 min	30-60 min	4-6 hr

Adverse reactions
CNS: confusion, drowsiness, sedation, dysphoria, euphoria, floating feeling, hallucinations, headache, anxiety, depression, fatigue, insomnia, lethargy, nervousness, slurred speech, tremor, asthenia, unusual dreams
CV: orthostatic hypotension, bradycardia, peripheral edema, palpitations, **arrhythmias**
EENT: blurred vision, vision changes, diplopia, miosis, tinnitus, pharyngitis, rhinitis, sinusitis
GI: nausea, vomiting, constipation, dysphagia, esophagitis, dyspepsia, flatulence, gastritis, gastroenteritis, mouth ulcers, dry mouth, anorexia
GU: urinary retention or frequency, erectile dysfunction
Respiratory: respiratory depression, bronchitis, dyspnea
Skin: pruritus, urticaria, diaphoresis, flushing
Other: physical or psychological drug dependence, drug tolerance

Interactions

Drug-drug. *Angiotensin-converting enzyme inhibitors:* decreased therapeutic effects of these drugs

Antihistamines, sedative-hypnotics: additive CNS depression

Buprenorphine, butorphanol, nalbuphine, pentazocine: precipitation of opioid withdrawal in physically dependent patients

Buprenorphine, pentazocine: decreased analgesia

Lithium: increased lithium blood level (with hydrocodone/ibuprofen only)

MAO inhibitors: severe, unpredictable reactions

Methotrexate: increased methotrexate blood level

Naloxone: withdrawal symptoms

Oral anticoagulants: increased risk of GI bleeding (with hydrocodone/ibuprofen only)

Drug-diagnostic tests. *Amylase, lipase:* increased levels

Drug-herbs. *Chamomile, hops, kava, skullcaps, valerian:* increased CNS depression

Drug-behaviors. *Alcohol use:* increased CNS depression

Patient monitoring

• In prolonged use, monitor for psychological and physical dependence.

• Watch closely for withdrawal symptoms when drug is discontinued.

• Assess elderly patients carefully for adverse reactions.

◀≋ Monitor for signs and symptoms of drug overdose, including nausea, vomiting, blurred vision, cool and clammy skin, dizziness, confusion, dyspnea, respiratory depression, bradycardia, hearing loss, tinnitus, headache, and mood or behavior changes.

Patient teaching

• Tell patient drug may cause drowsiness. Caution him to avoid driving and other hazardous activities until CNS effects are known.

• Inform patient that prolonged use may lead to physical or psychological dependence.

• Caution patient to avoid alcohol during therapy.

• Instruct patient to move slowly when sitting up or standing, to avoid dizziness from sudden blood pressure decrease.

• As appropriate, review all other significant and life-threatening adverse reactions and interactions, especially those related to the drugs, tests, herbs, and behaviors mentioned above.

h

hydrocortisone
Ala-Cort, Ala-Scalp, Cetacort, Colocort, Cortef, Cortenema, Hi-Cor, Hycort✲, Hytone, Stie-Cort, Synacort, Texacort

hydrocortisone acetate
Cortifoam, Hydrocortistab✇

hydrocortisone butyrate
Locoid

hydrocortisone sodium succinate
A-hydroCort, Solu-Cortef

hydrocortisone valerate
Westcort

Pharmacologic class: Short-acting corticosteroid

Therapeutic class: Anti-inflammatory (steroidal)

Pregnancy risk category C

Action

Suppresses inflammatory and immune responses, mainly by inhibiting migration of leukocytes and

---

Reactions in **bold** are life-threatening.   ◀≋ Clinical alert

phagocytes and decreasing inflammatory mediators

Availability

Cream, gel, lotion, ointment, solution: various strengths
Injection: 25 mg/ml, 50 mg/ml; 100 mg/vial, 250 mg/vial, 500 mg/vial, 1,000 mg/vial
Intrarectal aerosol foam: 90 mg
Oral suspension: 10 mg/5 ml
Retention enema: 100 mg/60 ml
Spray (topical): 1%
Tablets: 5 mg, 10 mg, 20 mg

⦸ Indications and dosages

➤ Replacement therapy in adrenocortical insufficiency; hypercalcemia due to cancer; arthritis; collagen diseases; dermatologic diseases; autoimmune and hematologic disorders; trichinosis; ulcerative colitis; multiple sclerosis; proctitis; nephrotic syndrome; aspiration pneumonia
hydrocortisone, hydrocortisone cypionate—
Adults and children: 20 to 240 mg/day P.O.
hydrocortisone acetate (suspension)—
Adults and children: 5 to 75 mg by intra-articular injection (depending on joint size) q 2 to 3 weeks
hydrocortisone acetate (intrarectal foam)—
Adults and children: One applicatorful of intrarectal foam daily or b.i.d. for 2 to 3 weeks; then one applicatorful every other day
hydrocortisone sodium phosphate—
Adults and children: 15 to 240 mg/day subcutaneously, I.M., or I.V., adjusted according to response
hydrocortisone sodium succinate—
Adults and children: 100 to 500 mg I.M. or I.V.; may repeat at 2-, 4-, or 6-hour intervals, depending on response and condition
hydrocortisone retention enema—
Adults and children: 100 mg P.R. at bedtime for 21 nights or until desired response; patient should retain enema for at least 1 hour.
➤ Itching and inflammation caused by skin conditions
Adults and children: Thin film of topical preparation applied to affected area one to four times daily, depending on drug form and severity of condition

Off-label uses

- Phlebitis
- Stomatitis

Contraindications

- Hypersensitivity to drug, alcohol, bisulfites, or tartrazine (with some products)
- Systemic fungal infections
- Concurrent use of other immunosuppressant corticosteroids
- Concurrent administration of live-virus vaccines

Precautions

Use cautiously in:
- hypertension, osteoporosis, glaucoma, renal or GI disease, hypothyroidism, cirrhosis, thromboembolic disorders, myasthenia gravis, heart failure
- pregnant or breastfeeding patients
- children ages 6 and younger (safety not established).

Administration

- Give oral form with food or milk to avoid GI upset.
- Give I.V. injection of sodium succinate form over 30 seconds to a few minutes.
- Know that drug may be given as intermittent or continuous I.V. infusion. Dilute in normal saline solution, dextrose 5% in water, or dextrose 5% in normal saline solution.
- Inject I.M. deep into gluteal muscle. Rotate injection sites to prevent muscle atrophy.

- Be aware that subcutaneous administration may cause muscle atrophy or sterile abscess.
◀℈ Never abruptly discontinue high-dose or long-term systemic therapy.
- Know that systemic forms typically are used for adrenal replacement rather than inflammation.
- Be aware that occlusive dressings, heat, hydration, inflammation, denuding, and thinning of skin increase topical drug absorption.

Route	Onset	Peak	Duration
P.O.	1-2 hr	1-2 hr	1-1.5 days
I.V.	Immediate	Unknown	1-1.5 days
I.M.	Rapid	4-8 hr	1-1.5 days
P.R.	Slow	3-5 days	4-6 days
Spray (topical), subcut.	Unknown	Unknown	Unknown

Adverse reactions

CNS: headache, nervousness, depression, euphoria, personality changes, psychoses, vertigo, paresthesia, insomnia, restlessness, conus medullaris syndrome, **meningitis, increased intracranial pressure, seizures**
CV: hypotension, hypertension, **thrombophlebitis, heart failure, shock, fat embolism, thromboembolism, arrhythmias**
EENT: cataracts, glaucoma, increased intraocular pressure, epistaxis, nasal congestion, perforated nasal septum, dysphonia, hoarseness, nasopharyngeal or oropharyngeal fungal infections
GI: nausea, vomiting, esophageal candidiasis or ulcer, abdominal distention, dry mouth, **rectal bleeding, peptic ulceration, pancreatitis**
Hematologic: purpura
Metabolic: sodium and fluid retention, hypokalemia, hypocalcemia, hyperglycemia, hypercholesterolemia, amenorrhea, growth retardation, diabetes mellitus, cushingoid appearance, **hypothalamic-pituitary-adrenal suppression with secondary adrenal insufficiency** (with abrupt withdrawal or high-dose, prolonged use)
Musculoskeletal: osteoporosis, aseptic joint necrosis, muscle pain or weakness, steroid myopathy, loss of muscle mass, tendon rupture, spontaneous fractures
Respiratory: cough, wheezing, rebound congestion, **bronchospasm**
Skin: rash, pruritus, urticaria, contact dermatitis, acne, bruising, hirsutism, petechiae, striae, acneiform lesions, skin fragility and thinness, angioedema
Other: altered taste; anosmia; appetite changes; weight gain; facial edema; increased susceptibility to infection; masking or aggravation of infection; adhesive arachnoiditis; injection site pain, burning, or atrophy; immunosuppression; hypersensitivity reactions including **anaphylaxis**

Interactions

Drug-drug. *Amphotericin B, loop and thiazide diuretics, mezlocillin, piperacillin, ticarcillin:* additive hypokalemia
Fluoroquinolones: increased risk of tendon rupture
Hormonal contraceptives: prolonged half-life and increased effects of hydrocortisone
Insulin, oral hypoglycemics: increased requirements for these drugs
Live-virus vaccines: decreased antibody response to vaccine, increased risk of adverse reactions
Nonsteroidal anti-inflammatory drugs: increased risk of adverse GI reactions
Phenobarbital, phenytoin, rifampin: decreased hydrocortisone efficacy
Somatrem: inhibition of growth-promoting effect
Drug-diagnostic tests. *Calcium, potassium, thyroxine, triiodothyronine:* decreased levels
Cholesterol, glucose: increased levels
Digoxin assays: false elevation (with some test methods)
Nitroblue tetrazolium test: false-negative result

h

Drug-herbs. *Echinacea:* increased immunostimulation
Ginseng: potentiation of immunomodulation
Drug-behaviors. *Alcohol use:* increased risk of gastric irritation and GI ulcers

Patient monitoring

◀≋ In high-dose therapy (which should not exceed 48 hours), watch closely for signs and symptoms of depression or psychotic episodes.
• Monitor blood pressure, weight, and electrolyte levels regularly.
• Assess blood glucose levels in diabetic patients. Expect to increase insulin or oral hypoglycemic dosage.
◀≋ Monitor patient's response during weaning from drug. Watch for adrenal crisis, which may occur if drug is discontinued too quickly.

Patient teaching

• Instruct patient to take daily P.O. dose with food by 8 A.M.
◀≋ Urge patient to immediately report unusual weight gain, face or leg swelling, epigastric burning, vomiting of blood, black tarry stools, irregular menstrual cycles, fever, prolonged sore throat, cold or other infection, or worsening of symptoms.
• Tell patient using topical form not to apply occlusive dressing unless instructed by prescriber.
• Advise patient to discontinue topical drug and notify prescriber if local irritation occurs.
• Instruct patient to eat small, frequent meals and to take antacids as needed to minimize GI upset.
• Tell patient that response to drug will be monitored regularly.
◀≋ Caution patient not to stop taking drug abruptly.
• In long-term use, instruct patient to have regular eye exams.
• Instruct patient to wear medical identification stating that he's taking this drug.

• As appropriate, review all other significant and life-threatening adverse reactions and interactions, especially those related to the drugs, tests, herbs, and behaviors mentioned above.

hydromorphone hydrochloride

Dilaudid, Dilaudid-5, Dilaudid-HP, Hydromorph Contin✤, Hydromorph-IR✤, Palladone⊕, Palladone SR⊕, PHL-Hydromorphone✤, PMS-Hydromorphone✤

Pharmacologic class: Opioid agonist
Therapeutic class: Opioid analgesic, antitussive
Controlled substance schedule II
Pregnancy risk category C (with long-term use or at term with high doses: *D*)

FDA | BOXED WARNING

• Drug is a potent Schedule II opioid agonist with highest abuse potential and risk of causing respiratory depression. Alcohol, other opioids, and CNS depressants potentiate respiratory depressant effects, increasing risk of potentially fatal respiratory depression.

Action

Binds to opiate receptors in spinal cord and CNS, altering perception of and response to painful stimuli while producing generalized CNS depression. Also subdues cough reflex and decreases GI motility.

Availability

Injection: 1 mg/ml, 2 mg/ml, 4 mg/ml, 10 mg/ml

Powder for injection (lyophilized):
250-mg vials (high-potency)
Oral solution: 5 mg/5 ml
Rectal suppositories: 3 mg
Tablets: 2 mg, 3 mg, 4 mg, 8 mg

ⓘ Indications and dosages
➤ Moderate to severe pain
**Adults weighing more than 50 kg
(110 lb):** 2 mg P.O. (tablets) q 4 to 6
hours p.r.n. For more severe pain, 4 mg
P.O. (tablets) may be given q 4 to
6 hours. If pain increases in severity,
analgesia isn't adequate, or tolerance
develops, a gradual increase in dosage
may be required. Or 2.5 to 10 mg P.O.
(oral solution) q 4 to 6 hours p.r.n. as
directed by clinical situation. Or 1 to 2
mg subcutaneously, I.M., or I.V. q 4 to
6 hours p.r.n.; or 3 mg P.R. q 6 to 8
hours p.r.n. Adjust dosage based on
pain severity, underlying disease, and
patient's age and size.

Contraindications
• Hypersensitivity to narcotics or
bisulfites
• Acute or severe bronchial asthma or
upper respiratory tract obstruction

Precautions
Use cautiously in:
• increased intracranial pressure; severe
renal, hepatic, or pulmonary disease;
hypothyroidism; adrenal insufficiency;
prostatic hypertrophy; alcoholism
• concurrent use of MAO inhibitors
• elderly patients
• pregnant or breastfeeding patients.

Administration
◀₣ Be aware that high-potency hydromorphone (Dilaudid-HP) is a highly
concentrated solution and shouldn't be
confused with standard parenteral formulations of hydromorphone or other
opioids. Overdose and death may result.
• Know that high-potency formulation
is recommended for opioid-tolerant
patients who require larger than usual

doses of opioids to gain adequate pain
relief.
• For maximal analgesic effect, give
before pain becomes severe.
• For I.V. infusion, mix with dextrose
5% in water, normal saline solution, or
lactated Ringer's solution.
• Give single-dose I.V. injection slowly,
over 2 to 5 minutes for each 2-mg dose.
• Rotate I.M. and subcutaneous sites to
prevent muscle atrophy.
• Give oral form with food to avoid GI
upset.

Route	Onset	Peak	Duration
P.O.	30 min	90-120 min	4 hr
I.V.	10-15 min	15-30 min	2-3 hr
I.M., subcut.	15 min	30-60 min	4-5 hr
P.R.	15-30 min	30-90 min	4-5 hr

Adverse reactions
CNS: confusion, sedation, dysphoria,
euphoria, floating feeling, hallucinations, headache, unusual dreams, anxiety, dizziness, drowsiness
CV: hypotension, hypertension, palpitations, bradycardia, tachycardia
EENT: blurred vision, diplopia, miosis,
nystagmus, tinnitus, laryngeal edema,
laryngospasm
GI: nausea, vomiting, constipation,
abdominal cramps, biliary tract spasm,
anorexia
GU: urinary retention, dysuria
Hepatic: hepatotoxicity
Respiratory: dyspnea, wheezing, **bronchospasm, respiratory depression**
Skin: flushing, diaphoresis
Other: physical or psychological drug
dependence; drug tolerance; injection
site pain, redness, or swelling

Interactions
Drug-drug. *Antidepressants, antihistamines, MAO inhibitors, sedative-
hypnotics:* additive CNS depression
*Antihypertensives, diuretics, guanadrel,
guanethidine, mecamylamine:* increased
risk of hypotension

h

Reactions in **bold** are life-threatening.   ◀₣ Clinical alert

Atropine, belladonna alkaloids, difenoxin, diphenoxylate, kaolin and pectin, loperamide, paregoric: increased risk of CNS depression, severe constipation

Barbiturates: increased sedation

Buprenorphine, butorphanol, nalbuphine, pentazocine: precipitation of opioid withdrawal in physically dependent patients

Nalbuphine, pentazocine: decreased analgesia

Drug-diagnostic tests. *Amylase, lipase:* increased levels

Drug-herbs. *Chamomile, hops, kava, skullcap, valerian:* increased CNS depression

Drug-behaviors. *Alcohol use:* increased CNS depression

Patient monitoring

◀€ With I.V. use, monitor for respiratory depression. Keep resuscitation equipment and naloxone nearby.

• Assess for signs and symptoms of physical or psychological drug dependence.

• Monitor for constipation.

Patient teaching

◀€ Instruct patient to take drug exactly as prescribed before pain becomes severe, but caution him that drug may be habit-forming.

• Tell patient to take oral form with food to avoid GI upset.

• Advise patient to report difficulty breathing, nausea, vomiting, or dizziness.

• Caution patient to avoid driving and other hazardous activities until he knows how drug affects concentration and alertness.

• Tell patient to avoid alcohol while taking drug.

• As appropriate, review all other significant and life-threatening adverse reactions and interactions, especially those related to the drugs, tests, herbs, and behaviors mentioned above.

hydroxychloroquine sulfate

Apo-Hydroxychloroquine✤,
Gen-Hydroxychloroquine✤, Plaquenil

Pharmacologic class: 4-aminoquinolone

Therapeutic class: Antimalarial, antirheumatic, anti-inflammatory (disease-modifying)

Pregnancy risk category C

FDA | BOXED WARNING

• Familiarize yourself completely with contents of the manufacturer's package insert before administering or prescribing this drug.

Action

Unknown. Thought to interfere with inhibition of protein synthesis and DNA replication, leading to parasitic death.

Availability

Tablets: 200 mg (155 mg base); 200 mg hydroxychloroquine sulfate is equivalent to 155 mg of hydroxychloroquine base

⏀ Indications and dosages

➤ Malaria prophylaxis (dosages expressed as mg of base)

Adults: 310 mg P.O. q week, starting 1 to 2 weeks before entering endemic area and continuing for 4 weeks after leaving area

Children: 5 mg/kg P.O. q week, starting 1 to 2 weeks before entering endemic area and continuing for 4 weeks after leaving area

➤ Acute malarial attack (dosages expressed as mg of base)

Adults: Initially, 620 mg P.O., then 310 mg 6 hours, 24 hours, and 48 hours later

---

Children: Initially, 10 mg/kg P.O., then 5 mg/kg 6 hours, 24 hours, and 48 hours later

➤ Rheumatoid arthritis

Adults: 400 to 600 mg/day P.O. for 4 to 12 weeks, then reduced by 50%

➤ Systemic lupus erythematosus

Adults: 400 mg P.O. once or twice daily for several months, then reduced to 200 to 400 mg daily, depending on response

Contraindications

• Hypersensitivity to drug or chloroquine
• Retinal or visual field changes
• Long-term therapy in children

Precautions

Use cautiously in:
• hepatic or renal impairment, G6PD deficiency, psoriasis, bone marrow depression, alcoholism
• obese patients
• pregnant or breastfeeding patients
• children.

Administration

• Give with food or milk.
• For malaria prophylaxis, schedule doses on same day each week.

Route	Onset	Peak	Duration
P.O.	Unknown	2-4.5 hr	Unknown

Adverse reactions

CNS: anxiety, apathy, confusion, fatigue, headache, psychoses, mood swings, irritability, neuromyopathy, peripheral neuritis, **seizures**
CV: ECG changes, hypotension
EENT: visual disturbances, retinopathy, keratopathy, ototoxicity, tinnitus
GI: nausea, vomiting, diarrhea, abdominal cramps, anorexia
Hematologic: leukopenia, **agranulocytosis, aplastic anemia, thrombocytopenia**
Hepatic: jaundice, **hepatotoxicity**

Musculoskeletal: muscle weakness
Skin: dermatoses, rash, pruritus, pigmentation changes, pleomorphic skin eruption, worsened psoriasis, alopecia, bleaching of hair
Other: weight loss

Interactions

Drug-diagnostic tests. *Granulocytes, hemoglobin, platelets:* decreased values
Drug-behaviors. *Sun exposure:* exacerbation of drug-induced dermatoses

Patient monitoring

◀€ Monitor for signs and symptoms of overdose, such as nausea, vomiting, drowsiness, visual disturbances, cardiovascular collapse, and seizures.
• Watch for adverse reactions.

Patient teaching

• Advise patient to take with food or milk.
◀€ Instruct patient to immediately report such adverse reactions as vision changes, nausea, vomiting, drowsiness, mental changes, mood swings, headache, ringing in ears, muscle weakness, rash, bleeding, bruising, and yellowing of skin and eyes.
• In long-term therapy, advise patient to have regular eye exams.
• As appropriate, review all other significant and life-threatening adverse reactions and interactions, especially those related to the drugs, tests, and behaviors mentioned above.

hydroxyurea
Droxia, Hydrea

Pharmacologic class: Antimetabolite
Therapeutic class: Antineoplastic
Pregnancy risk category D

◀€ Clinical alert

FDA **BOXED WARNING**

- Drug may cause severe and even life-threatening adverse effects. Administer under supervision of physician experienced in using drug to treat sickle cell anemia.
- Drug damages genes, chromosomes, and DNA and may be carcinogenic. Secondary leukemias have occurred in patients receiving it as long-term therapy for myeloproliferative disorders. Prescriber and patient must carefully weigh potential benefits against undefined risk of secondary cancers.

Action

Unknown. May inhibit enzyme necessary for DNA synthesis without disrupting RNA or protein synthesis.

Availability

Capsules: 200 mg, 300 mg, 400 mg, 500 mg

🖉 Indications and dosages

➤ Head and neck cancer; ovarian cancer; malignant melanoma
Adults: 60 to 80 mg/kg (2 to 3 g/m^2) P.O. as a single daily dose q 3 days, or 20 to 30 mg/kg/day P.O. as a single dose. Begin therapy 7 days before radiation.
➤ Resistant chronic myelogenous leukemia
Adults: 20 to 30 mg/kg/day P.O. in one or two divided doses
➤ Sickle cell anemia
Adults and children: 15 mg/kg/day P.O. as a single dose. May increase by 5 mg/kg/day P.O. q 12 weeks, up to 35 mg/kg/day.

Off-label uses

- Thrombocythemia
- Human immunodeficiency virus

Contraindications

- Hypersensitivity to drug or tartrazine

- Bone marrow depression
- Severe anemia or thrombocytopenia

Precautions

Use cautiously in:
- renal or hepatic impairment
- obese patients
- females of childbearing age
- elderly patients.

Administration

- Provide frequent mouth care.

Route	Onset	Peak	Duration
P.O.	Unknown	2 hr	24 hr

Adverse reactions

CNS: drowsiness, malaise, confusion, dizziness, headache
GI: nausea, vomiting, diarrhea, constipation, stomatitis, anorexia
GU: dysuria, hyperuricemia, infertility, **renal tubular dysfunction**
Hematologic: anemia, **megaloblastosis, leukopenia, thrombocytopenia, bone marrow depression**
Hepatic: hepatitis
Metabolic: hyperuricemia
Skin: alopecia, erythema, pruritus, rash, urticaria, exacerbation of post-radiation erythema
Other: chills, fever

Interactions

Drug-drug. *Live-virus vaccines:* decreased antibody response to vaccine, increased risk of adverse reactions
Myelosuppressants: additive bone marrow depression
Drug-diagnostic tests. *Blood urea nitrogen, creatinine, uric acid:* increased values
Hemoglobin, platelets, red blood cells, white blood cells: decreased values
Mean corpuscular volume: transient increase

Patient monitoring

- Assess CBC weekly.

- Closely monitor patient with renal or hepatic impairment. Check kidney and liver function tests often.
- Assess fluid status. Make sure patient drinks 10 to 12 glasses of water daily.

Patient teaching

- Advise patient to mark dates for drug doses, diagnostic tests, and treatments on calendar.
- ◀︎ Instruct patient to immediately report easy bruising, bleeding, unusual tiredness, or yellowing of skin or eyes.
- Tell patient to report such adverse effects as appetite loss, nausea, vomiting, oral lesions, constipation, diarrhea, confusion, dizziness, headache, and rash.
- Instruct female patient to use barrier contraception.
- Tell patient he will undergo regular blood testing to monitor drug effects.
- As appropriate, review all other significant and life-threatening adverse reactions and interactions, especially those related to the drugs and tests mentioned above.

hydroxyzine hydrochloride

Apo-Hydroxyzine✤, Atarax✤⊕,
Novo-Hydroxyzin✤,
Nu-Hydroxyzine✤, PMS-
Hydroxyzine✤, Riva-Hydroxyzine✤,
Ucerax⊕

hydroxyzine pamoate
Vistaril

Pharmacologic class: Piperazine derivative
Therapeutic class: Anxiolytic, antihistamine, sedative-hypnotic
Pregnancy risk category NR

Action
Unknown. Anxiolytic and sedative effects may stem from suppression of activity in subcortical levels of CNS. Antihistamine effects may result from histamine suppression at cellular receptor sites.

Availability
Capsules: 25 mg, 50 mg, 100 mg (pamoate)
Injection: 25 mg/ml, 50 mg/ml
Oral suspension: 25 mg/5 ml (pamoate)
Syrup: 10 mg/5 ml
Tablets: 10 mg, 25 mg, 50 mg

🖊 Indications and dosages
➤ Psychiatric emergencies; acute or chronic alcoholism
Adults: 50 to 100 mg I.M. immediately, then q 4 to 6 hours p.r.n.
➤ Nausea and vomiting; adjunct in pre- and postoperative sedation
Adults: 25 to 100 mg I.M. q 4 to 6 hours
Children: 1.1 mg/kg I.M. q 4 to 6 hours
➤ Anxiety
Adults and children ages 6 and older: 50 to 100 mg P.O. q.i.d.
Children younger than age 6: 50 mg P.O. daily in divided doses
➤ Pruritus
Adults: 25 mg P.O. three or four times daily
Children ages 6 and older: 50 to 100 mg P.O. daily in divided doses
Children younger than age 6: 50 mg P.O. daily in divided doses

Off-label uses
- Seasonal allergic rhinitis

Contraindications
- Hypersensitivity to drug or cetirizine
- Early pregnancy

Precautions
Use cautiously in:
- severe hepatic dysfunction
- elderly patients.

Reactions in **bold** are life-threatening.　　　　◀︎ Clinical alert

Administration

🔊 Don't administer I.V. or subcutaneously (may cause tissue necrosis).
• Use Z-track method for I.M. injection. Inject deep into large muscle (preferably, upper outer quadrant of buttock).

Route	Onset	Peak	Duration
P.O., I.M.	15-30 min	2-4 hr	4-6 hr

Adverse reactions

CNS: drowsiness, agitation, dizziness, headache, asthenia, ataxia
GI: nausea, constipation, dry mouth
GU: urinary retention
Respiratory: wheezing
Skin: flushing
Other: bitter taste, hypersensitivity reaction, pain or abscess at I.M. injection site

Interactions

Drug-drug. *Anticholinergics, antidepressants, antihistamines, phenothiazines, quinidine:* additive effects of these drugs
Antidepressants, antihistamines, opioids, sedative-hypnotics, other CNS depressants: additive CNS depression
Drug-diagnostic tests. *Skin tests using allergen extracts:* false-negative results
Drug-herbs. *Angel's trumpet, jimsonweed, scopolia:* increased anticholinergic effects
Chamomile, hops, kava, skullcap, valerian: increased CNS depression
Drug-behaviors. *Alcohol use:* increased CNS depression

Patient monitoring

• Monitor closely for CNS depression and oversedation, especially if patient is receiving other CNS depressants.
• Assess for adverse effects, especially in elderly patients.
• Monitor liver function test results in patients with hepatic impairment.

Patient teaching

• Tell patient to contact prescriber if he experiences wheezing, muscle spasms, or incoordination.
• Caution patient to avoid driving and other hazardous activities until he knows how drug affects concentration and alertness.
• Instruct patient to avoid alcohol while taking drug.
• As appropriate, review all other significant adverse reactions and interactions, especially those related to the drugs, tests, herbs, and behaviors mentioned above.

hyoscyamine
Cystospaz

hyoscyamine sulfate
Anaspaz, Hyospaz, Levsin, Levsin/SL, Symax, Symax-SL, Symax-SR

Pharmacologic class: Anticholinergic
Therapeutic class: Antispasmodic
Pregnancy risk category C

Action

Competitively inhibits acetylcholine action at autonomic nerve sites, relaxing smooth muscle and decreasing glandular secretions

Availability

hyoscyamine
Tablets: 0.15 mg
hyoscyamine sulfate
Capsules (timed-release): 0.375 mg
Elixir: 0.125 mg/5 ml
Injection: 0.5 mg/ml
Oral solution: 0.125 mg/ml
Tablets: 0.125 mg
Tablets (extended-release): 0.375 mg
Tablets (orally disintegrating): 0.125 mg
Tablets (sublingual): 0.125 mg

⊘ Indications and dosages

➤ Adjunct in GI tract disorders; pain and hypersecretion in pancreatitis; cystitis; renal colic; infant colic; acute rhinitis; rigidity, tremors, and hyperhidrosis in Parkinson's disease; partial heart block due to vagal activity

Adults and children ages 12 and older: 0.125 to 0.25 mg (sulfate) P.O. or S.L. two to four times daily, or 0.375 to 0.75 mg (extended-release sulfate) P.O. q 12 hours, or 0.25 to 0.5 mg (sulfate) subcutaneously, I.M., or I.V. two to four times daily p.r.n.

Children ages 2 to 12: In children weighing approximately 50 kg (110 lb), 0.125 mg (sulfate) P.O. q 4 hours p.r.n.; in children weighing approximately 20 kg (40 lb), 0.0625 mg P.O. (sulfate); in children weighing approximately 10 kg (22 lb), 0.031 to 0.033 mg (sulfate) P.O. Don't exceed 0.75 mg/day.

Children ages 2 and younger: In children weighing approximately 7 kg (15 lb), 0.025 (sulfate) P.O. q 4 hours p.r.n.; in children weighing approximately 5 kg (11 lb), 0.0208 mg (sulfate) P.O. q 4 hours p.r.n.; in children weighing approximately 3.4 kg (7.5 lb), 0.0167 mg (sulfate) P.O. q 4 hours p.r.n.; in children weighing approximately 2.3 kg (5 lb), 0.0125 mg (sulfate) P.O. q 4 hours p.r.n.

➤ Before endoscopy or hypotonic duodenography

Adults: 0.25 to 0.5 mg (sulfate) subcutaneously, I.M., or I.V. 5 to 10 minutes before procedure

➤ Preoperatively to inhibit salivation and excessive respiratory secretions

Adults and children older than age 2: 5 mcg/kg (sulfate) I.M., I.V., or subcutaneously 30 to 60 minutes before anesthesia induction

➤ Muscarinic toxicity

Adults: 1 to 2 mg (sulfate) I.V. Additional 1-mg doses may be given I.M. or I.V. q 3 to 10 minutes until muscarinic signs and symptoms subside; doses may be repeated if needed. Patient may need up to 25 mg during first 24 hours. For maintenance, 0.5 to 1 mg P.O. at intervals of several hours until signs and symptoms disappear.

Contraindications

• Hypersensitivity to anticholinergics, alcohol, sulfites, or tartrazine
• Angle-closure glaucoma, synechia
• GU or GI obstructive disease, severe ulcerative colitis
• Renal or hepatic disease
• Neonates or premature infants

Precautions

Use cautiously in:
• cardiovascular disease, prostatic hypertrophy, reflux esophagitis, brain damage, autonomic neuropathy, hyperthyroidism, glaucoma, Down syndrome, spastic paralysis
• elderly patients
• pregnant (safety not established) or breastfeeding patients
• infants and small children.

Administration

• Administer 30 to 60 minutes before meals and at bedtime.
• Give bedtime dose at least 2 hours after last evening meal or snack.
• Be aware that hyoscyamine is given P.O. only, whereas hyoscyamine sulfate may be given P.O., I.M., I.V., sublingually, or subcutaneously.
• Know that a cholinerase reactivator (pralidoxime) is given concomitantly to treat muscarinic toxicity.

Route	Onset	Peak	Duration
P.O.	20-30 min	0.5-1 hr	4-12 hr
P.O. (extended)	20-30 min	40-90 min	12 hr
I.V.	2 min	15-30 min	4 hr
I.M., subcut.	Unknown	15-30 min	4-12 hr
S.L.	5-20 min	0.5-1 hr	4 hr

Adverse reactions

CNS: confusion, excitement, nervousness, dizziness, light-headedness, headache, insomnia
CV: palpitations, tachycardia
EENT: blurred vision, cycloplegia, increased intraocular pressure, mydriasis, photophobia
GI: nausea, vomiting, constipation, bloating, dry mouth, **paralytic ileus**
GU: urinary hesitancy or retention, erectile dysfunction, lactation suppression
Skin: flushing, decreased sweating, urticaria, local irritation (with I.M., I.V., or subcutaneous use)
Other: altered taste, allergic reactions (including fever), heat intolerance, **anaphylaxis**

Interactions

Drug-drug. *Amantadine, antihistamines, antiparkinsonian drugs, disopyramide, glutethimide, meperidine, procainamide, quinidine, tricyclic antidepressants:* increased anticholinergic effects
Antacids: decreased hyoscyamine absorption
Atenolol: increased atenolol effects
Ketoconazole: interference with absorption of both drugs
Methotrimeprazine: increased risk of extrapyramidal effects
Phenothiazines: decreased phenothiazine effects, increased anticholinergic effects
Drug-herbs. *Jimsonweed:* adverse cardiovascular effects

Patient monitoring

• Watch for adverse reactions.
• Check for mental status changes, such as confusion.
• Evaluate fluid intake and output.
• Assess patient's response to temperature changes (especially hot weather). Drug may cause heat intolerance, predisposing patient to heat stroke.

Patient teaching

• Tell patient to take on empty stomach 30 to 60 minutes before meals and at least 2 hours after last evening meal or snack.
• Instruct patient with urinary hesitancy to empty bladder before taking.
• Caution patient to avoid driving and other hazardous activities until he knows how drug affects concentration and alertness.
• As appropriate, review all other significant and life-threatening adverse reactions and interactions, especially those related to the drugs and herbs mentioned above.

ibandronate sodium
Boniva, Boniva Injection, Bonviva ⊕

ibandronic acid ⊕

Pharmacologic class: Bisphosphonate
Therapeutic class: Calcium regulator
Pregnancy risk category C

Action

Inhibits osteoclast activity and reduces bone resorption and turnover; in postmenopausal women, reduces elevated bone turnover rate, leading to (on average) net gain in bone mass

Availability

Solution for injection: 3 mg/3 ml in single-use prefilled glass syringes
Tablets (film-coated): 2.5 mg, 150 mg

⚡ Indications and dosages

➤ Osteoporosis treatment and prevention in postmenopausal women
Adults: 2.5-mg tablet P.O. daily, or 150-mg tablet P.O. once monthly on same date each month
➤ Osteoporosis treatment in postmenopausal women

🍁 Canada   ⊕ UK   ☣ Hazardous drug   ⊗ High-alert drug

Adults: 3 mg I.V. injection every 3 months

Contraindications
• Hypersensitivity to drug or its components
• Uncorrected hypocalcemia
• Inability to stand or sit upright for at least 60 minutes (after oral administration)
• Abnormalities of esophagus, such as stricture or achalasia, that delay esophageal emptying (tablets)

Precautions
Use cautiously in:
• severe renal impairment (not recommended)
• active upper GI disease (such as Barrett's esophagus, dysphagia, other esophageal diseases, gastritis, duodenitis, or ulcers)
• patients who develop jaw osteonecrosis during therapy
• concurrent use of aspirin, nonsteroidal anti-inflammatory drugs (NSAIDs), or other bisphosphonates
• pregnant or breastfeeding patients
• children younger than age 18 (safety and efficacy not established).

Administration
• With patient standing or sitting upright, give oral dose with 6 to 8 oz water at least 60 minutes before first food or drink (other than water) of day or before administering other oral drugs or supplements (including calcium, antacids, and vitamins).
• Give with plain water only; some mineral waters may have higher calcium concentration and shouldn't be used.
• Don't let patient chew or suck tablet because this may cause oropharyngeal ulcers.
• Keep patient upright for at least 60 minutes after oral dose to avoid serious esophageal irritation.

• Give parenteral formulation only by I.V. injection over 15 to 30 seconds.
• Don't mix parenteral formulation with calcium-containing solutions or other I.V. drugs.
• If patient misses I.V. dose, give it as soon as possible; thereafter, give dose every 3 months from date of last injection. Don't administer more often than every 3 months.

Route	Onset	Peak	Duration
P.O.	0.5-2 hr	Unknown	Unknown
I.V.	Rapid	Unknown	Unknown

Adverse reactions
CNS: insomnia, asthenia, headache, fatigue, dizziness, vertigo, nerve root lesion
CV: hypertension
EENT: pharyngitis
GI: constipation, diarrhea, vomiting, abdominal pain, dysphagia, esophagitis, esophageal irritation (tablets), gastric ulcer, dyspepsia, gastritis, **esophageal ulcer**
GU: urinary tract infection
Metabolic: hypercholesterolemia, hypocalcemia
Musculoskeletal: osteonecrosis (mainly in jaw), localized osteoarthritis and muscle cramp, joint disorder, joint pain, muscle pain, back pain, extremity pain, arthritis
Respiratory: upper respiratory tract infection, bronchitis, pneumonia
Skin: rash
Other: tooth disorder, influenza, infection, injection site reaction, allergic reaction

Interactions
Drug-drug. *Aspirin, NSAIDs:* additive GI irritation
Drugs containing calcium and other multivalent cations (such as aluminum, iron, magnesium), including antacids, supplements, and vitamins: interference with ibandronate absorption

i

Reactions in **bold** are life-threatening.　　　◀€ Clinical alert

Drug-diagnostic tests. *Alkaline phosphatase, calcium:* decreased
Bone-imaging agents: interference with test results
Drug-food. *Milk, mineral water, other foods and beverages:* interference with ibandronate absorption, reducing drug's bioavailability and effect on bone mineral density (when patient consumes food or beverage less than 60 minutes after ibandronate dose)

Patient monitoring

• Monitor creatinine clearance in patients with mild or moderate renal impairment.

◀€ Monitor for signs and symptoms of GI irritation (including ulcers) after oral administration; discontinue drug if new or worsening symptoms occur.

• Evaluate serum calcium and phosphate levels.

• Monitor for hypocalcemia and other disturbances of bone and mineral metabolism; administer effective treatment before therapy starts.

• Monitor patient for adequate intake of supplemental calcium and vitamin D during therapy, as appropriate.

Patient teaching

• Advise patient to read patient information leaflet carefully before starting drug.

• Instruct patient to take drug first thing in morning on empty stomach with 6 to 8 oz of plain water only.

◀€ Caution patient not to chew or suck tablet because this may cause throat ulcers.

• Instruct patient not to eat, drink, or take other oral medications for 60 minutes after taking tablet.

◀€ Caution patient not to lie down for at least 60 minutes after taking drug.

• Advise patient to take once-monthly tablet (150 mg) on same date each month.

• If patient misses once-monthly dose and next scheduled dose is more than

7 days away, instruct her to take one 150-mg tablet in morning after the day she remembers it and then resume taking one 150-mg tablet every month in morning of chosen day, per original schedule. However, if next scheduled dose is only 1 to 7 days away, tell her to wait until next scheduled dose.

◀€ Instruct patient to stop drug and immediately report heartburn, serious vomiting, severe chest or abdominal pain, difficulty swallowing, severe bone, joint, or muscle pain.

• If drug is prescribed for injection, tell patient she will receive it every 3 months.

• Advise patient to take supplemental calcium and vitamin D as prescribed, if dietary intake is inadequate.

• Teach patient to take only those pain relievers recommended by prescriber. Point out that some over-the-counter pain preparations (such as aspirin and NSAIDs) may worsen adverse effects.

• As appropriate, review all other significant and life-threatening adverse reactions and interactions, especially those related to the drugs, tests, and foods mentioned above.

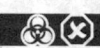

ibritumomab tiuxetan
Zevalin

Pharmacologic class: Monoclonal antibody
Therapeutic class: Antineoplastic
Pregnancy risk category D

FDA | BOXED WARNING

• Deaths have occurred within 24 hours of rituximab infusion, an essential component of Zevalin therapeutic regimen. These fatalities were associated with hypoxia, pulmonary infiltrates, acute respiratory distress syndrome, myocardial infarction, ventricular fibrillation, or cardiogenic shock. Most fatalities (80%) occurred with first rituximab infusion. Discontinue rituximab and Y-90 Zevalin infusions in patients who develop severe infusion reactions.

• Y-90 Zevalin administration causes severe and prolonged cytopenias in most patients. Don't administer Y-90 Zevalin to patients with 25% or greater lymphoma marrow involvement or impaired bone marrow reserve.

• Severe cutaneous and mucocutaneous reactions, some fatal, can occur with the Zevalin therapeutic regimen. Discontinue rituximab and Y-90 Zevalin infusions in patients experiencing severe cutaneous or mucocutaneous reactions.

• Dosage of Y-90 Zevalin shouldn't exceed 32.0 mCi (1,184 MBq).

Action
Binds indium-111 (In-111) or yttrium-90 (Y-90) with free amino groups of lysines and arginines within antibody; binds specifically to CD20 antigen, found on surface of normal and malignant B lymphocytes. Radioactive component of Y-90 causes cellular damage via free radicals in target cells.

Availability
Injection: 3.2 mg/2 ml (two Zevalin kits containing four vials each)

🟡 Indications and dosages
➤ Relapsed or refractory, low-grade or follicular B-cell non-Hodgkin's lymphoma (NHL); previously untreated follicular NHL in patients who achieve partial or complete response to first-line chemotherapy
Adults: Two-step regimen that includes pre-dose of rituximab
Step 1: Single I.V. infusion of 250 mg/m^2 rituximab at 50 mg/hour; in absence of infusion reactions, increase rate in 50-mg/hour increments q 30 minutes, to a maximum of 400 mg/hour. Immediately stop rituximab infusion for serious infusion reactions and discontinue Zevalin therapeutic regimen. Temporarily slow or interrupt rituximab infusion for less severe infusion reactions. If symptoms improve, continue infusion at one-half the previous rate.
Step 2: On day 7, 8, or 9, rituximab 250 mg/m^2 I.V. at initial rate of 100 mg/hour. Increase rate by 100-mg/hour increments at 30-minute intervals, to a maximum of 400 mg/hour as tolerated. If infusion reactions occurred during rituximab infusion on day 1 of treatment, administer rituximab at initial rate of 50 mg/hour and escalate infusion rate in 50-mg/hour increments every 30 minutes to a maximum of 400 mg/hour. Administer Y-90 Zevalin injection through free-flowing I.V. line within 4 hours after completion of rituximab infusion. Use a 0.22-micron, low-protein-binding in-line filter between syringe and infusion port. After injection, flush line with at least 10 ml of normal saline.

If platelet count is 150,000/mm^3 or greater, administer Y-90 Zevalin over 10 minutes as an I.V. injection at a dose of Y-90 0.4 mCi/kg (14.8 MBq/kg) actual body weight. If platelet count is 100,000/mm^3 to 149,000/mm^3 in relapsed or refractory patients, administer Y-90 Zevalin over 10 minutes as an I.V. injection at a dose of Y-90 0.3 mCi/kg (11.1 MBq/kg) actual body weight. Don't administer more than 32 mCi (1,184 MBq) Y-90 Zevalin dose regardless of patient's body weight.

Contraindications
None

Precautions
Use cautiously in:
• cardiac conditions
• elderly patients
• pregnant or breastfeeding patients.

Reactions in **bold** are life-threatening.　　◀€ Clinical alert

Administration

🔊 Don't administer to patients with lymphoma marrow involvement at or above 25% or impaired bone marrow reserve.

🔊 Assess for human antimurine antibody before treatment. If result is positive, patient may experience hypersensitivity reaction.

• Premedicate patient with acetaminophen and diphenhydramine, as ordered, before each rituximab infusion.

• Know that ibritumomab should be used only as part of a regimen that combines ibritumomab and rituximab.

🔊 Give ibritumomab by slow I.V. infusion over 10 minutes; monitor closely.

🔊 Don't give by I.V. push.

🔊 Take steps to prevent extravasation of Y-90 Zevalin. If extravasation occurs, immediately stop infusion and restart in another vein.

• Don't give Y-90 Zevalin if platelet count is less than 100,000/mm³.

🔊 Immediately and permanently discontinue drug if severe infusion reaction occurs (urticaria, hypotension, angioedema, hypoxia, bronchospasm, pulmonary infiltrates, acute respiratory distress syndrome, MI, ventricular fibrillation, cardiogenic shock). Temporarily slow or interrupt rituximab infusion for less severe infusion reactions.

🔊 Discontinue drug if severe cutaneous or mucocutaneous reactions develop.

• Follow facility policy on radiation precautions to protect patients, visitors, and medical personnel from radiation exposure.

Route	Onset	Peak	Duration
I.V.	Unknown	Unknown	Unknown

Adverse reactions

CNS: dizziness, anxiety, headache, insomnia, asthenia

CV: hypotension, peripheral edema

EENT: rhinitis, epistaxis, throat irritation

GI: nausea, vomiting, diarrhea, constipation, anorexia, dyspepsia, abdominal pain or enlargement, melena

Hematologic: anemia, **thrombocytopenia, neutropenia, pancytopenia, hemorrhage, myelodysplastic syndrome, acute myelogenous leukemia**

Musculoskeletal: joint pain, myalgia, back pain

Respiratory: increased cough, dyspnea, **apnea, bronchospasm**

Skin: flushing, bruising, diaphoresis, petechiae, pruritus, rash, urticaria, angioedema, **erythema multiforme, Stevens-Johnson syndrome, toxic epidermal necrolysis, bullous dermatitis, exfoliative dermatitis**

Other: bacterial infection, I.V. site irritation, fever, chills, generalized pain, tumor pain, hypersensitivity reactions including **anaphylaxis, myeloid malignancies, dysplasias, serious infusion reactions**

Interactions

None significant

Patient monitoring

🔊 Institute infection control protocols. Protect patient from potential sources of infection.

🔊 Assess CBC and platelet count before starting therapy. Monitor regularly during and after therapy.

🔊 Monitor patient for hypersensitivity reactions, which can be fatal and usually occur within 30 minutes to 2 hours of administration.

• Be alert for unusual bleeding or bruising.

Patient teaching

🔊 Instruct patient to promptly report difficulty breathing, rash, fever, chills, severe GI distress, black tarry stools, illness or injury, or unusual bleeding or bruising.

• Tell patient that drug increases his risk of infection. Instruct him to avoid crowds and potential or known sources of infection.
• Advise patient to eat small, frequent meals and take antiemetic drugs to control nausea and vomiting, as needed and prescribed.
• Advise patient that he'll undergo blood testing during therapy to monitor drug effects.
• Advise patient not to receive live viral vaccines during or immediately after taking this drug.
• As appropriate, review all other significant and life-threatening adverse reactions mentioned above.

ibuprofen

Actiprofen Caplets✷, Advil, Advil Extra Strength✷, Advil Migraine, Advil Pediatric Drops, Anadin Ibuprofen⊕, Anadin Ultra⊕, Apo-Ibuprofen✷, Arthrofen⊕, Brufen⊕, Caldolor, Calprofen⊕, Children's Advil, Children's Motrin, Cuprofen⊕, Extra Strength Motrin IB✷, Hedex Ibuprofen⊕, Ibugel⊕, Ibuleve⊕, Ibumousse⊕, Ibuspray⊕, Junior Strength Advil, Junior Strength Motrin, Motrin, Motrin IB, Motrin Infant, NeoProfen, Novo-Profen, Nu-Ibuprofen✷, Nurofen⊕, PMS-Ibuprofen✷

Pharmacologic class: Nonsteroidal anti-inflammatory drug (NSAID)
Therapeutic class: Analgesic, antipyretic, anti-inflammatory
Pregnancy risk category B (third trimester: *D*)

• Drug may increase risk of serious cardiovascular thrombotic events, myocardial infarction, and stroke. Risk may increase with duration of use, and may be greater in patients who have cardiovascular disease or risk factors for it.
• Drug is contraindicated for perioperative pain in setting of coronary artery bypass graft surgery.
• Drug increases risk of serious GI adverse events, including bleeding, ulcers, and stomach or intestinal perforation, which can be fatal. These events can occur at any time during therapy and without warning. Elderly patients are at greater risk.

Action
Unknown. Thought to inhibit cyclooxygenase, an enzyme needed for prostaglandin synthesis.

Availability
Capsules (liquigels): 200 mg
Injection: 400 mg/4-ml, 800 mg/8-ml vials
Oral suspension: 100 mg/5 ml
Pediatric drops: 50 mg/1.25 ml
Tablets: 100 mg, 200 mg, 400 mg, 600 mg, 800 mg
Tablets (chewable): 50 mg, 100 mg

💊 Indications and dosages
➤ Rheumatoid arthritis; osteoarthritis
Adults: 1.2 to 3.2 g/day P.O. in three to four divided doses
➤ Mild to moderate pain
Adults: 400 mg P.O. q 4 to 6 hours p.r.n. or 400 to 800 mg I.V. over 30 minutes q 6 hours, as necessary
➤ Moderate to severe pain as adjunct to opioid analgesics
Adults: 400 to 800 mg I.V. over 30 minutes q 6 hours, as necessary

---

Reactions in **bold** are life-threatening.   ◀€ Clinical alert

➢Fever reduction
Adults: 400 mg I.V. over 30 minutes, followed by 400 mg P.O. q 4 to 6 hours or 100 to 200 mg P.O. q 4 hours as necessary
➢ Primary dysmenorrhea
Adults: 400 mg P.O. q 4 hours p.r.n.
➢ Juvenile arthritis
Children: 30 to 40 mg/kg/day P.O. in three or four divided doses. Daily dosages above 50 mg/kg aren't recommended.
➢ Fever reduction; pain relief
Children ages 6 to 12: 5 mg/kg P.O. if temperature is below 102.5 °F (39.2 °C) or 10 mg/kg if temperature is above 102.5 °F. Maximum daily dosage is 40 mg/kg.

Off-label uses
• Migraine and tension headaches

Contraindications
• Hypersensitivity to drug or other NSAIDs
• Perioperative use in coronary artery bypass graft surgery

Precautions
Use cautiously in:
• severe cardiovascular, renal, or hepatic disease; GI disease; asthma; chronic alcohol use
• elderly patients
• pregnant (avoid use after 30 weeks' gestation) or breastfeeding patients
• children younger than age 17 (safety and efficacy not established).

Administration
• Ideally, give oral form 1 hour before or 2 hours after meal. If GI upset occurs, give with meals.
• Be aware that patients must be well hydrated before I.V. form is administered.
• Dilute injection form before administering.

Route	Onset	Peak	Duration
P.O. (analgesic)	30 min	1-2 hr	4-6 hr
P.O. (anti-inflam.)	7 days	1-2 wk	Unknown

Adverse reactions
CNS: headache, dizziness, drowsiness, nervousness, **aseptic meningitis**
CV: hypertension, **arrhythmias**
EENT: amblyopia, blurred vision, tinnitus
GI: nausea, vomiting, constipation, dyspepsia, abdominal discomfort, **GI bleeding**
GU: cystitis, hematuria, azotemia, **renal failure**
Hematologic: anemia, **prolonged bleeding time, aplastic anemia, neutropenia, pancytopenia, thrombocytopenia, leukopenia, agranulocytosis**
Hepatic: hepatitis
Metabolic: hyperglycemia, **hypoglycemia**
Respiratory: bronchospasm
Skin: rash, pruritus, urticaria, **Stevens-Johnson syndrome**
Other: edema, allergic reactions including **anaphylaxis**

Interactions
Drug-drug. *Antihypertensives, diuretics:* decreased efficacy of these drugs
Aspirin and other NSAIDs, corticosteroids: additive adverse GI effects
Cefamandole, cefoperazone, cefotetan, drugs affecting platelet function (including abciximab, clopidogrel, eptifibatide, ticlopidine, tirofiban), plicamycin, thrombolytics, valproic acid, warfarin: increased risk of bleeding
Cyclosporine: increased risk of nephrotoxicity
Digoxin: slightly increased digoxin blood level
Lithium: increased lithium blood level, greater risk of lithium toxicity
Methotrexate: increased risk of methotrexate toxicity

Probenecid: increased risk of ibuprofen toxicity

Drug-diagnostic tests. *Alanine aminotransferase, alkaline phosphatase, aspartate aminotransferase, blood urea nitrogen, creatinine, lactate dehydrogenase, potassium:* increased values
Bleeding time: prolonged
Creatinine clearance, glucose, hematocrit, hemoglobin, platelets, white blood cells: decreased values
Drug-herbs. *Anise, arnica, chamomile, clove, dong quai, fenugreek, feverfew, garlic, ginger, ginkgo, ginseng, licorice:* increased risk of bleeding
White willow: additive adverse GI effects
Drug-behaviors. *Alcohol use:* additive adverse GI effects
Sun exposure: phototoxicity

Patient monitoring
• Monitor for desired effect.
• Watch for GI upset, adverse CNS effects (such as headache and drowsiness), and hypersensitivity reaction.
• Stay alert for GI bleeding and ulcers, especially in long-term therapy.
• In long-term therapy, assess renal and hepatic function regularly.
• Monitor blood pressure closely during treatment.

Patient teaching
• Tell patient to take oral drug with full glass of water, with food, or after meals to minimize GI upset.
• To help prevent esophageal irritation, instruct patient to avoid lying down for 30 to 60 minutes after taking dose.
◀ Instruct patient to immediately report irregular heartbeats, black tarry stools, vision changes, unusual tiredness, yellowing of skin or eyes, change in urination pattern, difficulty breathing, finger or ankle swelling, weight gain, itching, rash, fever, or sore throat.
• Caution patient to avoid driving and other hazardous activities until he knows how drug affects concentration, alertness, and balance.
• As appropriate, review all other significant and life-threatening adverse reactions and interactions, especially those related to the drugs, tests, herbs, and behaviors mentioned above.

ibutilide fumarate
Corvert

Pharmacologic class: Ibutilide derivative
Therapeutic class: Antiarrhythmic (class III)
Pregnancy risk category C

FDA BOXED WARNING

• Drug can cause potentially fatal arrhythmias—particularly sustained polymorphic ventricular tachycardia, usually in association with QT prolongation (torsades de pointes). In studies, these arrhythmias arose within several hours of administration. They can be reversed if treated promptly. Drug must be given in setting of continuous ECG monitoring and by personnel trained in identifying and treating acute ventricular arrhythmias. Patients with atrial fibrillation of more than 2 to 3 days' duration must be adequately anticoagulated, generally for at least 2 weeks.
• Patients with chronic atrial fibrillation tend to revert after conversion to sinus rhythm, and treatments to maintain sinus rhythm carry risks. Therefore, patients to be treated with drug should be selected carefully, with expected benefits of maintaining sinus rhythm outweighing drug's immediate risks and risks of maintenance therapy, and with drug offering benefits over alternative management.

Reactions in **bold** are life-threatening.   ◀ Clinical alert

Action
Prolongs myocardial action potential by slowing repolarization and atrioventricular (AV) conduction

Availability
Solution: 0.1 mg/ml in 10-ml vials

🚫 Indications and dosages
➤ To convert atrial fibrillation or flutter to sinus rhythm
Adults weighing more than 60 kg (132 lb): 1 vial (1 mg) by I.V. infusion over 10 minutes. May repeat after 10 minutes if arrhythmia persists.
Adults weighing less than 60 kg (132 lb): 0.1 mg/kg (0.01 mg/kg) by I.V. infusion over 10 minutes. May repeat after 10 minutes if arrhythmia persists.

Contraindications
• Hypersensitivity to drug or its components

Precautions
Use cautiously in:
• ventricular and AV arrhythmias
• pregnant or breastfeeding patients.

Administration
◀€ Monitor ECG continuously during and after infusion. Stop infusion immediately if ventricular tachycardia occurs.
• As appropriate, administer diluted or undiluted. To dilute, add 10-ml vial to 50 ml of normal saline solution or dextrose 5% in water, to yield a concentration of 0.017 mg/ml.
• Infuse over 10 minutes.
◀€ Don't give with amiodarone, disopyramide, quinidine, procainamide, or sotalol, because of increased risk of dangerous arrhythmias.

Route	Onset	Peak	Duration
I.V.	Immediate	10 min	Unknown

Adverse reactions
CNS: headache, light-headedness, dizziness, numbness or tingling in arms

CV: hypotension, hypertension, bradycardia, **bundle-branch block, ventricular extrasystoles, ventricular arrhythmias, ventricular tachycardia, AV heart block, heart failure**
GI: nausea
GU: renal failure

Interactions
Drug-drug. *Amiodarone, disopyramide, quinidine, procainamide, sotalol:* increased risk of dangerous arrhythmias
Antihistamines, phenothiazines, tricyclic antidepressants: increased proarrhythmic effect (prolonged QT interval)

Patient monitoring
• Before giving, assess electrolyte levels and correct abnormalities (especially involving potassium and magnesium), because hypokalemia and hypomagnesemia can lead to arrhythmias.
◀€ Watch for premature ventricular contractions, sinus tachycardia, sinus bradycardia, and heart block.
• Monitor ECG during and for at least 4 hours after infusion.
◀€ Keep emergency equipment (defibrillator, emergency cart and drug box, oxygen, suction, and intubation equipment) at hand during and for at least 4 hours after infusion.
• Monitor prothrombin time, International Normalized Ratio, and activated partial thromboplastin time if patient is receiving anticoagulant therapy.

Patient teaching
◀€ Instruct patient to immediately report chest pain, dizziness, numbness, palpitations, headache, or difficulty breathing.
• Tell patient he'll be monitored closely for at least 4 hours after drug administration.

---

idarubicin hydrochloride
Idamycin PFS, Zavedos ⊕

Pharmacologic class: Anthracycline antibiotic
Therapeutic class: Antineoplastic
Pregnancy risk category D

FDA BOXED WARNING

• Administer slowly I.V.—never I.M. or subcutaneously. Extravasation may cause severe local tissue necrosis.
• Drug may cause myocardial toxicity leading to heart failure, especially in patients who have received prior anthracyclines or have preexisting cardiac disease.
• Severe bone marrow depression can occur when drug is used at effective therapeutic doses.
• Reduce dosage in hepatic or renal impairment.
• Give under supervision of physician experienced in using leukemia chemotherapeutic drugs, in facility with adequate diagnostic and treatment resources.

Action
Inhibits nucleic acid synthesis by disrupting DNA and RNA polymerase, causing cell death

Availability
Injection: 1 mg/ml

⧸ Indications and dosages
➤ Acute myeloid leukemia
Adults: 12 mg/m²/day by slow I.V. injection over 10 to 15 minutes for 3 days. As prescribed, give with cytarabine by continuous I.V. infusion for 7 days, or give cytarabine as I.V. bolus followed by 5 days of cytarabine by continuous I.V. infusion. Second course may be given, depending on response.

Dosage adjustment
• Renal or hepatic impairment
• Severe mucositis

Off-label uses
• Acute nonlymphocytic and chronic myelogenous leukemias
• Non-Hodgkin's lymphoma
• Breast cancer

Contraindications
• Hypersensitivity to drug
• Pregnancy or breastfeeding

Precautions
Use cautiously in:
• renal or hepatic impairment
• bone marrow depression
• previous treatment with anthracyclines or cardiotoxic drugs
• cardiac disease.

Administration
◀€ When preparing, wear goggles and gloves, because exposure may cause severe skin reaction. If exposure occurs, wash affected area immediately with soap and water. For eye exposure, follow standard eye irrigation procedure.
• Reconstitute 5-, 10-, or 20-mg vial with 5, 10, or 20 ml of normal saline solution, respectively, to yield a concentration of 1 mg/ml.
• Give slowly over 10 to 15 minutes into I.V. tubing that is infusing normal saline solution or dextrose 5% in water.
◀€ Don't administer subcutaneously or I.M. (may cause tissue necrosis).
• If severe mucositis occurs, delay second course (if prescribed) until full recovery; then reduce dosage by 25%.

Route	Onset	Peak	Duration
I.V.	Immediate	Several min	Unknown

Reactions in **bold** are life-threatening.   ◀€ Clinical alert

Adverse reactions

CNS: headache, mental status changes, peripheral neuropathy, **seizures**
CV: chest pain, **heart failure, atrial fibrillation, myocardial infarction, arrhythmias**
GI: nausea, vomiting, diarrhea, cramps, mucositis, **GI hemorrhage**
GU: red urine, **renal failure**
Hematologic: bone marrow depression
Hepatic: hepatic function changes
Metabolic: hyperuricemia
Skin: alopecia, urticaria, bullous erythematous rash on palms and soles, erythema at previously irradiated site, tissue necrosis or urticaria at injection site
Other: fever, infection, hypersensitivity reaction

Interactions

Drug-drug. *Alkaline solutions, heparin:* incompatibility

Patient monitoring

◀€ Evaluate injection site for burning, stinging, and extravasation. If extravasation occurs, stop infusion and restart in another vein. Then rinse area with normal saline solution and apply cold compress. (Local infiltration with corticosteroids may be indicated.)
• Monitor patient's response to therapy regularly.
• Assess serum uric acid level and CBC.
• Monitor hemodynamic status and cardiac output. Assess for S_3 heart sound (which signals heart failure).
• Assess fluid intake and output. Make sure patient is adequately hydrated, to prevent hyperuricemia.

Patient teaching

◀€ Instruct patient to immediately report unusual bleeding or bruising, difficulty breathing, or sudden weight gain.
• Tell patient to eat small, frequent meals.
• Advise patient to keep follow-up appointments for assessment, regular blood testing, and monitoring of drug effects.
• As appropriate, review all other significant and life-threatening adverse reactions and interactions, especially those related to the drugs mentioned above.

ifosfamide
Ifex, Mitoxana ⊕

Pharmacologic class: Alkylating agent, nitrogen mustard
Therapeutic class: Antineoplastic
Pregnancy risk category D

FDA | BOXED WARNING

• Give under supervision of physician experienced in using cancer chemotherapy, in facility with adequate diagnostic and treatment resources. Adverse urotoxic effects (especially hemorrhagic cystitis) and CNS toxicities (such as confusion and coma) have occurred; these effects may warrant drug discontinuation.
• Severe myelosuppression may occur.

Action
Alkylates DNA, interfering with replication and synthesis of susceptible cells and ultimately causing cell death

Availability
Injection: 1 g or 3 g in single-dose vials

⊘ Indications and dosages
➤ Germ-cell testicular cancer
Adults: 1.2 g/m²/day by I.V. infusion over 30 minutes for 5 days. May repeat q 3 weeks or after recovery from hematologic toxicity.

Off-label uses
• Acute leukemia
• Breast, lung, ovarian, and pancreatic cancer

- Malignant lymphomas
- Sarcomas

Contraindications
- Hypersensitivity to drug
- Severe bone marrow depression
- Pregnancy or breastfeeding

Precautions
Use cautiously in:
- impaired renal or hepatic function, mild to moderate bone marrow depression.

Administration
- Follow facility policy for handling antineoplastic agents.
- Know that drug is usually given with other antineoplastics and hemorrhagic cystitis agent.
- To reconstitute, add sterile water or bacteriostatic water to vial, and shake gently.
- Mix 20 ml of diluent with 1-g vial or 60 ml of diluent with 3-g vial, to yield a concentration of 50 mg/ml. For smaller concentrations, dilute solution further with normal saline solution, dextrose 5% in water, lactated Ringer's solution, or sterile water.
- Administer I.V. slowly over at least 30 minutes.

Route	Onset	Peak	Duration
I.V.	Immediate	Unknown	Unknown

Adverse reactions
CNS: drowsiness, confusion, ataxia, hallucinations, depressive psychosis, dizziness, disorientation, cranial nerve dysfunction, **coma, seizures**
CV: phlebitis
GI: nausea, vomiting, diarrhea, anorexia, stomatitis
GU: hematuria, bladder fibrosis, gonadal suppression, **nephrotoxicity, hemorrhagic cystitis**
Hematologic: anemia, **leukopenia, thrombocytopenia, bone marrow depression**

Metabolic: metabolic acidosis
Skin: alopecia
Other: infection, **secondary neoplasms**

Interactions
Drug-diagnostic tests. *Hepatic enzymes, uric acid:* increased levels
Platelets, white blood cells: decreased counts

Patient monitoring
- Monitor hematopoietic function tests (such as CBC with white cell differential) before therapy and weekly during therapy.
- Assess fluid intake and output. Ensure fluid intake of at least 2 L daily to prevent bladder toxicity.
- ◀€ Monitor urine output for hematuria and hemorrhagic cystitis. Administer mesna (protective drug), as indicated and prescribed.

Patient teaching
- ◀€ Tell patient to immediately report jaundice, unusual bleeding or bruising, bloody urine, pain on urination, fever, chills, sore throat, cough, difficulty breathing, unusual lumps or masses, mouth sores, or pain in flank, stomach, or joints.
- Instruct patient to maintain adequate hydration and nutrition. Advise him to drink 10 to 12 glasses of fluid each day.
- Inform patient that drug may cause hair loss.
- Advise both male and female patients to use reliable contraception during and immediately after therapy, because drug may cause severe birth defects.
- Urge patient to keep regular follow-up appointments for blood tests and monitoring of drug effects.
- As appropriate, review other significant and life-threatening adverse reactions and interactions, especially those related to the drugs and tests mentioned above.

Reactions in **bold** are life-threatening.　　　　◀€ Clinical alert

iloperidone
Fanapt

Pharmacologic class: Piperidinyl-benzisoxazole derivative
Therapeutic class: Antipsychotic
Pregnancy risk category C

FDA | BOXED WARNING

• Elderly patients with dementia-related psychosis treated with antipsychotics are at increased risk for death. Analyses of 17 placebo-controlled trials (modal duration of 10 weeks), largely in patients taking atypical antipsychotics, revealed a risk of death in the drug-treated patients of between 1.6 and 1.7 times the risk of death in placebo-treated patients. Over the course of a typical 10-week controlled trial, the rate of death in drug-treated patients was about 4.5%, compared to a rate of about 2.6% in the placebo group. Although causes of death were varied, most of the deaths appeared to be either cardiovascular (for example, heart failure, sudden death) or infectious (for example, pneumonia) in nature.

• Observational studies suggest that, similar to atypical antipsychotics, treatment with conventional antipsychotics may increase mortality. The extent to which findings of increased mortality in observational studies may be attributed to the antipsychotic as opposed to some characteristic(s) of the patients isn't clear.

• Iloperidone isn't approved for treatment of patients with dementia-related psychosis.

Action
Unknown

Availability
Tablets: 1 mg, 2 mg, 4 mg, 6 mg, 8 mg, 10 mg, 12 mg

🛈 Indications and dosages
➤ Acute treatment of schizophrenia
Adults: Initially, 1 mg P.O. daily; may increase by daily adjustments to 2 mg b.i.d., 4 mg b.i.d., 6 mg b.i.d., 8 mg b.i.d., 10 mg b.i.d., and 12 mg b.i.d. on days 2, 3, 4, 5, 6, and 7, respectively, to reach target dosage range of 6 to 12 mg P.O. b.i.d.

Dosage adjustment
• Concomitant use of strong CYP2D6 inhibitors (such as fluoxetine, paroxetine) and strong CYP3A inhibitors (such as clarithromycin, ketoconazole)

Contraindications
• Hypersensitivity to drug or its components

Precautions
Use cautiously in:
• hepatic impairment (use not recommended)
• congenital long QTc syndrome, history of cardiac arrhythmias (avoid use)
• known cardiovascular disease, cerebrovascular disease, or conditions that predispose patient to hypotension
• seizures or conditions that lower seizure threshold (such as Alzheimer's dementia)
• history of neuroleptic malignant syndrome
• preexisting low WBC count, history of drug-induced leukopenia or neutropenia
• possibility of conditions contributing to an elevated core body temperature (strenuous exercise, exposure to extreme heat, concomitant medication with anticholinergic activity, dehydration)
• concomitant use of drugs known to prolong QTc interval, including Class 1A antiarrhythmics (such as

---

♦ Canada   ⊕ UK   ☣ Hazardous drug   ⊗ High-alert drug

procainamide quinidine), Class III antiarrhythmics (such as amiodarone, sotalol), antipsychotics (such as chlorpromazine, thioridazine), antibiotics (such as gatifloxacin, moxifloxacin), or other drug classes known to prolong QTc interval (avoid use)

• conditions that may increase risk of torsades de pointes or sudden death in association with use of drugs that prolong QTc interval, including bradycardia, hypokalemia, hypomagnesemia, recent acute myocardial infarction, uncompensated heart failure, and cardiac arrhythmia (avoid use)

• concomitant use of drugs that inhibit iloperidone metabolism, patients with reduced CYP2D6 activity

• concomitant use of other centrally acting drugs

• patients at risk for suicide or aspiration pneumonia

• pregnant or breastfeeding patients

• children and adolescents (safety and efficacy not established).

Administration

• Determine baseline serum potassium and magnesium levels in patients at risk for significant electrolyte imbalance before starting drug.

• Perform fasting glucose testing in patients at risk for diabetes mellitus before starting drug.

• Administer without regard to meals.

• Be aware that drug must be titrated slowly to avoid orthostatic hypotension.

• Follow initiation schedule if an interval between dosing of more than 3 days occurs.

Route	Onset	Peak	Duration
P.O.	Unknown	2-4 hr	Unknown

Adverse reactions

CNS: fatigue, tardive dyskinesia, dizziness, somnolence, tremor, lethargy, extrapyramidal disorder, **seizures, neuroleptic malignant syndrome**

CV: hypotension, orthostatic hypotension, tachycardia, **prolonged QTc interval**

EENT: blurred vision, nasopharyngitis, nasal congestion

GI: nausea, diarrhea, dry mouth, abdominal discomfort, dysphagia

GU: ejaculation failure

Hematologic: leukopenia, neutropenia, **agranulocytosis**

Metabolic: hyperprolactinemia, **hyperglycemia (with associated ketoacidosis, hyperosmolar coma, or death)**

Musculoskeletal: arthralgia, stiffness

Respiratory: upper respiratory tract infection, dyspnea

Skin: rash

Other: weight gain, altered body temperature regulation, hypersensitivity (including pruritus, urticaria)

Interactions

Drug-drug. *Drugs known to prolong QTc interval:* increased risk of life-threatening arrhythmia

Strong CYP2D6 inhibitors (such as fluoxetine, paroxetine), strong CYP3A inhibitors (such as clarithromycin, ketoconazole): inhibited iloperidone elimination resulting in increased blood levels

Drug-diagnostic tests. *Blood glucose:* increased level

Prolactin: increased level

White blood cells (WBCs): decreased levels

Drug-behaviors. *Alcohol use:* increased CNS effects

Patient monitoring

◀€ Discontinue drug in patient with persistent QTc measurements above 500 ms.

◀€ Initiate further evaluation, including cardiac monitoring, if patient develops signs and symptoms of cardiac arrhythmias (such as dizziness, palpitations, or syncope).

◀€ Monitor patient for signs and symptoms of neuroleptic malignant syndrome, such as hyperpyrexia, muscle rigidity, altered mental status (including catatonic signs), and evidence of autonomic instability (irregular pulse or blood pressure, tachycardia, diaphoresis, cardiac arrhythmia, elevated creatine kinase level, myoglobinuria from rhabdomyolysis, and renal failure). If such signs and symptoms occur, immediately discontinue drug and treat appropriately.

◀€ Frequently monitor CBC with differential, especially during first few months of therapy in patient with preexisting low WBC count or history of drug-induced leukopenia or neutropenia. Discontinue drug at first sign of decline in WBC count in absence of other causative factors.

◀€ Discontinue drug if patient develops severe neutropenia (absolute neutrophil count below $1,000/mm^3$) and continue to monitor WBC count until recovery.

• Periodically perform fasting glucose testing in patient at risk for diabetes mellitus; watch closely for worsening of glucose control in patient with diabetes mellitus.

• Periodically monitor serum potassium and magnesium levels; hypokalemia and hypomagnesemia may increase risk of QTc interval prolongation.

• Consider discontinuing drug if signs and symptoms of tardive dyskinesia occur (such as repetitive, involuntary, purposeless movements; grimacing; tongue protrusion; or lip smacking).

• Carefully evaluate patient for history of drug abuse; if history exists, observe patient for signs and symptoms of misuse or abuse (such as drug-seeking behavior and increases in dosage). Also evaluate patient for risk of suicide.

Patient teaching

• Instruct patient to take drug with or without food.

◀€ Instruct patient to immediately report signs and symptoms of cardiac arrhythmias (such as dizziness, palpitations, or syncope).

◀€ Instruct patient to immediately report signs and symptoms of neurologic malignant syndrome, such as fever, muscle rigidity, altered mental status (including catatonic signs), irregular pulse or blood pressure, rapid heartbeat, and excessive sweating.

• Tell patient to promptly report fever or other signs and symptoms of infection.

• Tell patient to promptly report signs and symptoms of tardive dyskinesia (such as repetitive, involuntary, purposeless movements; grimacing; tongue protrusion; or lip smacking).

• Tell patient to report signs and symptoms of high blood glucose level (such as weakness, or excessive thirst, hunger, or urination).

• Advise patient to move slowly on rising to avoid sudden drop in blood pressure.

• Advise patient to avoid excessive exercise, exposure to extreme heat, and dehydration.

• Caution patient to avoid driving and other hazardous activities until drug's effects on concentration and alertness are known.

• Advise patient to avoid alcohol use while taking drug.

• Advise patient to consult prescriber before taking other prescription or nonprescription drugs.

• As appropriate, review all other significant and life-threatening adverse reactions and interactions, especially those related to the drugs, tests, and behaviors mentioned above.

imatinib mesylate
Gleevec, Glivec⊕

Pharmacologic class: Protein-tyrosine kinase inhibitor
Therapeutic class: Antineoplastic
Pregnancy risk category D

Action
Inhibits proliferation of Bcr-Abl tyrosine kinase, an abnormal chromosome protein found in most patients with chronic myeloid leukemia (CML). This inhibition suppresses tumor growth.

Availability
Tablets: 100 mg, 400 mg

⃠ Indications and dosages
➤ Philadelphia chromosome–positive (Ph+) CML
Adults: During chronic phase, 400 mg P.O. daily as a single dose; during accelerated phase or blast crisis, 600 mg P.O. daily as a single dose. May increase to 600 mg P.O. daily during chronic phase or to 800 mg P.O. daily (400 mg b.i.d.) during accelerated phase or blast crisis in absence of severe adverse drug reaction and severe non-leukemia-related neutropenia or thrombocytopenia in following circumstances: disease progression at any time, failure to achieve satisfactory hematologic response after at least 3 months of treatment, failure to achieve cytogenetic response after 6 to 12 months of treatment, or loss of previously achieved hematologic or cytogenetic response.
➤ Newly diagnosed Ph+ CML
Children: 340 mg/m²/day P.O. as once-daily dose; or, daily dose may be split into two (once in morning and once in evening). Daily dose not to exceed 600 mg.

➤ Ph+ chronic-phase CML recurrent after stem cell transplant or resistant to interferon-alpha therapy
Children: 260 mg/m²/day P.O. as once-daily dose; or, daily dose may be split into two (once in morning and once in evening).
➤ Relapsed/refractory Ph+ acute lymphoblastic leukemia
Adults: 600 mg P.O. daily as single dose
➤ Myelodysplastic/myeloproliferative diseases
Adults: 400 mg P.O. daily as single dose
➤ Aggressive systemic mastocytosis (ASM)
Adults: Recommended dosage is 400 mg P.O. daily as single dose for patients without D816V c-Kit mutation. If c-Kit mutational status is unknown or unavailable, 400 mg daily may be considered for patients with ASM not responding satisfactorily to other therapies. For patients with ASM associated with eosinophilia, a starting dose of 100 mg P.O. daily is recommended. Dosage increase from 100 to 400 mg for these patients may be considered in absence of adverse drug reactions if assessments show insufficient response to therapy.
➤ Hypereosinophilic syndrome/ chronic eosinophilic leukemia
Adults: Recommended dosage is 400 mg P.O. daily as single dose
➤ Dermatofibrosarcoma protuberans
Adults: Recommended dosage is 800 mg P.O. daily (given as 400 mg twice daily)
➤ Kit (CD117)-positive unresectable or metastatic malignant GI stromal tumors
Adults: 400 to 600 mg P.O. daily

Dosage adjustment
• Hepatic or hematologic impairment
• Concurrent use of potent CYP3A4 inducers, such as rifampin or phenytoin

Contraindications
• Hypersensitivity to drug or its components

Precautions
Use cautiously in:
• renal or hepatic impairment
• pregnant or breastfeeding patients
• children younger than age 2 (safety and efficacy not established).

Administration
• Give with meal and large glass of water.
• Disperse tablets in glass of water or apple juice for patients unable to swallow tablets. Place required number of tablets in appropriate volume of beverage (approximately 50 ml for 100-mg tablet, and 200 ml for 400-mg tablet) and stir with spoon. Administer suspension immediately after complete disintegration of tablets.

Route	Onset	Peak	Duration
P.O.	Unknown	2-4 hr	Unknown

Adverse reactions
CNS: headache, fatigue, asthenia, malaise, insomnia, headache, **cerebral hemorrhage**
CV: heart failure, ventricular dysfunction
GI: nausea, vomiting, diarrhea, constipation, anorexia, abdominal pain or cramps, dyspepsia, **GI hemorrhage**
Hematologic: anemia, **hemorrhage, neutropenia, thrombocytopenia, gastrointestinal perforation**
Hepatic: hepatotoxicity
Metabolic: hypokalemia, fluid retention
Musculoskeletal: myalgia, muscle cramps, musculoskeletal or joint pain
Respiratory: cough, dyspnea, pneumonia
Skin: rash, pruritus, night sweats, petechiae **bullous dermatitis, reactions (erythema multiforme, Stevens-Johnson syndrome)**
Other: weight gain, edema, fever

Interactions
Drug-drug. *Cyclosporine, dihydropyridine calcium channel blockers, pimozide, some HMG-CoA reductase inhibitors, triazolobenzodiazepines:* increased blood levels of these drugs
CYP450-3A4 inducers (such as carbamazepine, dexamethasone, phenobarbital, phenytoin): increased metabolism and decreased blood level of imatinib
CYP450-3A4 inhibitors (such as clarithromycin, erythromycin, itraconazole, ketoconazole): decreased metabolism and increased blood level of imatinib
Warfarin: altered warfarin metabolism
Drug-diagnostic tests. *Alanine aminotransferase, alkaline phosphatase, aspartate aminotransferase, bilirubin, creatinine, hepatic enzymes:* increased values
Hemoglobin, neutrophils, platelets, potassium: decreased values
Drug-herbs. *St. John's wort:* decreased imatinib effects

Patient monitoring
• Monitor for GI distress. Provide small, frequent meals; consult dietitian if nausea and vomiting persist.
◀£ Monitor CBC before therapy starts and regularly during therapy. Expect to adjust dosage if bone marrow depression occurs.
◀£ Evaluate for signs and symptoms of bleeding, edema, and fluid retention.
• Measure daily weight and fluid intake and output.
• Monitor liver function tests.

Patient teaching
• Advise patient to take with a meal and a large glass of water.
• Instruct patient to avoid potential sources of infection, such as crowds and people with known infections.
• Tell patient drug may cause sudden weight gain and fluid retention. Instruct him to weigh himself daily.
◀£ Advise patient to immediately report sudden weight gain, swelling,

difficulty breathing, signs or symptoms of infection, unusual bleeding or bruising, or jaundice.
• Tell patient he'll undergo frequent blood testing to monitor drug effects.
• As appropriate, review all other significant and life-threatening adverse reactions and interactions, especially those related to the drugs, tests, and herbs mentioned above.

imipenem and cilastatin sodium
Primaxin

Pharmacologic class: Carbapenem
Therapeutic class: Anti-infective
Pregnancy risk category C

Action
Acts against many gram-positive and gram-negative organisms by binding to bacterial cell wall, causing cell death. Addition of cilastatin prevents renal inactivation of imipenem, resulting in increased urinary concentration. Imipenem resists actions of many enzymes that degrade most other penicillins and penicillin-like drugs.

Availability
Powder for I.M. injection: 500 mg imipenem/500 mg cilastatin, 750 mg imipenem/750 mg cilastatin
Powder for I.V. injection: 250 mg imipenem/250 mg cilastatin, 500 mg imipenem/500 mg cilastatin

⚠ Indications and dosages
➤ Lower respiratory tract infections, urinary tract infections, abdominal infections, gynecologic infections, skin infections, bone and joint infections, endocarditis, and polymicrobial infections

Adults: For mild infections, 250 to 500 mg I.V. q 6 hours; for moderate infections, 500 mg I.V. q 6 to 8 hours or 1 g I.V. q 8 hours; for serious infections, 500 mg I.V. q 6 hours to 1 g q 6 to 8 hours or 500 to 750 mg I.M. q 12 hours
Children: 15 to 25 mg/kg I.V. q 6 hours or 10 to 15 mg/kg I.M. q 6 hours
Infants ages 4 weeks to 3 months: 25 mg/kg I.V. q 6 hours
Infants ages 1 to 4 weeks: 25 mg/kg I.V. q 8 hours
Infants age 1 week and younger: 25 mg/kg I.V. q 12 hours

Dosage adjustment
• Renal impairment

Contraindications
• Hypersensitivity to drug, penicillins, or cephalosporins

Precautions
Use cautiously in:
• seizure disorders, renal impairment
• history of multiple hypersensitivity reactions
• elderly patients
• pregnant or breastfeeding patients.

Administration
• For I.V. use, reconstitute each 250- or 500-mg vial with 10 ml of diluent; shake well.
• For piggyback infusion, add 250- or 500-mg I.V. dose to 100 ml of diluent; shake solution until clear and drug has dissolved completely.
• Infuse doses of 500 mg or less over 20 to 30 minutes; infuse doses of 750 to 1,000 mg over 40 to 60 minutes.
• Slow infusion rate if patient experiences nausea, vomiting, dizziness or sweating.
• For I.M. use, inject into large muscle.

Route	Onset	Peak	Duration
I.V.	Rapid	End of infusion	6-8 hr
I.M.	Rapid	1-2 hr	12 hr

Reactions in **bold** are life-threatening.   ◀€ Clinical alert

Adverse reactions

CNS: dizziness, drowsiness, **seizures**
CV: hypotension
GI: nausea, vomiting, diarrhea, **pseudomembranous colitis**
Hematologic: eosinophilia
Skin: rash, pruritus, diaphoresis, urticaria
Other: phlebitis at I.V. site, fever, superinfection, allergic reactions including **anaphylaxis**

Interactions

Drug-drug. *Cyclosporine, ganciclovir:* increased risk of seizures
Probenecid: decreased renal excretion of imipenem
Drug-diagnostic tests. *Alanine aminotransferase, alkaline phosphatase, aspartate aminotransferase, bilirubin, blood urea nitrogen, creatinine, lactate dehydrogenase:* increased values
Direct Coombs' test: positive result
Hematocrit, hemoglobin: decreased

Patient monitoring

◀℥ Stay alert for seizures in patients with brain lesions, head trauma, or other CNS disorders and in those receiving more than 2 g daily.
◀℥ Monitor closely for severe diarrhea and hypersensitivity reaction.
• Assess tissue or fluid culture results obtained before and during therapy.
• Monitor for signs and symptoms of infection, such as fever and elevated white blood cell count. Also evaluate for bacterial and fungal superinfection.
• Monitor electrolyte levels, especially sodium.

Patient teaching

• Caution patient to report discomfort at I.V. site.
◀℥ Instruct patient to report rash, hives, difficulty breathing, and signs or symptoms of superinfection (such as diarrhea, mouth sores, and vaginal itching or discharge).

• As appropriate, review all other significant and life-threatening adverse reactions and interactions, especially those related to the drugs and tests mentioned above.

imipramine hydrochloride

Apo-Imipramine✿, Impril✿, Novopramine✿, PMS-Imipramine✿, Tofranil

imipramine pamoate

Tofranil-PM

Pharmacologic class: Dibenzazepine derivative
Therapeutic class: Tricyclic antidepressant
Pregnancy risk category C

FDA   BOXED WARNING

• Drug may increase risk of suicidal thinking and behavior in children and adolescents with major depressive disorder and other psychiatric disorders, especially during first few months of therapy. Risk must be balanced with clinical need, as depression itself increases suicide risk. With patient of any age, observe closely for clinical worsening, suicidality, and unusual behavior changes when therapy begins. Advise family and caregivers to observe patient closely and communicate with prescriber as needed.
• Drug isn't approved for use in pediatric patients.

Action

Unknown. May block reuptake of norepinephrine and serotonin at neuronal membrane, potentiating their effects.

Availability
Capsules: 75 mg, 100 mg, 125 mg, 150 mg (pamoate)
Tablets: 10 mg, 25 mg, 50 mg (hydrochloride)

🕧 Indications and dosages
➤ Endogenous depression
Adults: 75 to 100 mg P.O. daily in divided doses. Don't exceed 200 mg/day for outpatients or 300 mg/day for inpatients.
Elderly patients, adolescents: 30 to 40 mg P.O. daily in divided doses, up to 100 mg/day
➤ Functional enuresis
Children: 25 mg P.O. daily 1 hour before bedtime. If necessary, increase by 25 mg/day at weekly intervals, up to 75 mg P.O. daily in children ages 12 and older or up to 50 mg P.O. daily in children younger than age 12.
➤ Attention deficit hyperactivity disorder
Children ages 6 and older: 2 to 5 mg/kg P.O. daily in two or three divided doses

Off-label uses
• Diabetic neuropathy

Contraindications
• Hypersensitivity to drug or bisulfites
• Untreated angle-closure glaucoma
• MAO inhibitor use within past 14 days

Precautions
Use cautiously in:
• cardiovascular disease, prostatic enlargement, seizures, urinary retention
• elderly patients
• pregnant or breastfeeding patients.

Administration
◀€ Don't give concurrently with MAO inhibitors. Interaction may lead to hypotension, tachycardia, and potentially fatal reactions.
• Give with food or milk if GI upset occurs.

Route	Onset	Peak	Duration
P.O.	Unknown	30 min-2 hr	2-6 wk

Adverse reactions
CNS: fatigue, sedation, agitation, confusion, hallucinations, drowsiness, dizziness, syncope, extrapyramidal effects, poor concentration, **cerebrovascular accident, seizures, suicidal behavior or ideation** (especially in child or adolescent)
CV: hypotension, ECG changes, hypertension, vasculitis, palpitations, tachycardia, **arrhythmias, myocardial infarction, heart block**
EENT: blurred vision, increased intraocular pressure (IOP), lacrimation, tinnitus, nasal congestion
GI: diarrhea, dry mouth, **paralytic ileus**
GU: urinary retention, urinary tract dilation, gynecomastia, menstrual irregularities, galactorrhea, testicular swelling, libido changes, erectile dysfunction
Hematologic: eosinophilia, purpura, **bone marrow suppression, agranulocytosis, thrombocytopenia, leukopenia**
Hepatic: hepatitis
Metabolic: hyperthermia, hyperglycemia, **hypoglycemia**
Skin: flushing, diaphoresis, photosensitivity, rash, urticaria, pruritus, petechiae, alopecia
Other: increased appetite, weight gain or loss, edema, drug fever, chills, hypersensitivity reactions

Interactions
Drug-drug. *Adrenergics:* increased hypertensive effect
Carbamazepine, class IC antiarrhythmics, other antidepressants, phenothiazines: additive effects of imipramine
CNS depressants: additive CNS depression
Clonidine: decreased clonidine effects

Reactions in **bold** are life-threatening.   ◀€ Clinical alert

CYP450-2D6 inhibitors (such as amio-darone, cimetidine, quinidine, riton-avir): increased imipramine effects
Guanethidine: prevention of therapeutic response to imipramine
Levodopa: delayed or decreased levodopa absorption, hypertension
MAO inhibitors: hypotension, tachycardia, potentially fatal reactions
Selective serotonin reuptake inhibitors: increased imipramine blood level
Sparfloxacin: increased risk of cardiovascular reactions
Drug-diagnostic tests. Alkaline phosphatase, bilirubin: elevated levels
Glucose: increased or decreased level
Liver function tests: altered values
Drug-herbs. Angel's trumpet, jimson-weed, scopolia: increased anticholinergic effects
Chamomile, hops, kava, skullcap, valerian: increased CNS depression
Evening primrose oil: additive or synergistic effects
S-adenosylmethionine (SAM-e), St. John's wort: serotonin syndrome
Drug-behaviors. Alcohol use: increased CNS depression
Smoking: increased metabolism and altered effects of imipramine
Sun exposure: increased risk of photosensitivity

Patient monitoring

◀€ Closely monitor patient's mood and assess his risk for self-harm. Limit drug access if he may be suicidal.

• Assess for urinary retention and increased IOP in patients with history of urinary retention or angle-closure glaucoma.

◀€ Monitor blood pressure before and during therapy and before dosage increases.

• Watch for arrhythmias in patients with history of cardiac disease.

• During withdrawal, monitor for adverse effects, such as headache, malaise, nausea, vomiting, and sleep disturbances.

• Assess for signs and symptoms of infection. Monitor CBC with white cell differential.

Patient teaching

◀€ Teach patient or caregiver to recognize and immediately report signs of suicidal intent or expressions of suicidal ideation (especially in child or adolescent).

• Instruct patient to eat small, frequent meals to minimize GI upset.

• Inform patient that drug may cause changes in sexual function, such as erectile dysfunction and decreased libido.

◀€ Tell patient to immediately report seizure, chest pain, abdominal pain or bloating, easy bruising or bleeding, unusual tiredness, or yellowing of skin or eyes.

• Advise patient to report fever, chills, sore throat, dry mouth, excessive sedation, difficulty urinating, or palpitations.

• Caution patient to avoid driving and other hazardous activities until he knows how drug affects concentration and alertness.

• As appropriate, review all other significant and life-threatening adverse reactions and interactions, especially those related to the drugs, tests, herbs, and behaviors mentioned above.

immune globulin for I.M. use (IGIM)
GammaSTAN S/D

immune globulin for I.V. use, human (IGIV)
Carimune NF, Flebogamma, Gammagard S/D, Gammar-P IV, Gamunex, Octagam, Polygam S/D, Privigen, Sandoglobulin, Vivaglobulin

immune globulin for I.V. and subcutaneous use, human
Gamunex-C

immune globulin for subcutaneous use, human
Hizentra

Pharmacologic class: Immune serum
Therapeutic class: Antibody-production stimulator
Pregnancy risk category C

FDA BOXED WARNING

• IGIV (human) products have been linked to renal dysfunction, acute renal failure (ARF), osmotic nephrosis, and death. Patients predisposed to ARF include those with preexisting renal insufficiency, diabetes mellitus, age older than 65, volume depletion, sepsis, or paraproteinemia and those receiving known nephrotoxic drugs. In these patients, give drug at minimum rate of infusion feasible. IGIV products containing sucrose accounted for disproportionate share of renal dysfunction and acute renal failure reports.

Action
Improves immunity by binding to and neutralizing pathogens, thereby increasing antibodies against bacterial, viral, parasitic, and mycoplasmic antigens. Acts through antimicrobial and antitoxin neutralization.

Availability
Injection: 2- and 10-ml vials (IGIM)
Powder for injection: 1-, 2.5-, 3-, 5-, 6-, 10-, and 12-g vials (IGIV)
Solution (5%): 10-, 50-, 100-, 200-, and 250-ml vials (IGIV)
Solution (10%): 10-, 25-, 50-, 100-, and 200-ml vials (IGIV)

⚕ Indications and dosages
➤ To prevent hepatitis A
Adults traveling to areas where hepatitis A is common: 0.02 ml/kg I.M. if staying less than 3 months; 0.06 ml/kg repeated q 4 to 6 months if staying 3 months or longer
Adults with household or institutional contacts: 0.02 ml/kg I.M.
➤ To prevent or reduce severity of measles in susceptible persons
Adults and children: 0.2 ml/kg to 0.25 ml/kg I.M. within 6 days of exposure to measles
➤ Exposure to measles in immunocompromised children
Children: 0.5 ml/kg I.M. as soon as possible after exposure
➤ Varicella in immunocompromised patients
Adults: 0.6 to 1.2 ml/kg I.M. as soon as possible if varicella-zoster immune globulin is unavailable
➤ To reduce risk of infection and fetal damage in females exposed to rubella during early pregnancy
Adults: 0.55 ml/kg I.M.
➤ Immunoglobulin deficiency
Adults: Initially, 1.3 ml/kg I.M., followed in 3 to 4 weeks by 0.66 ml/kg, up to 100 mg/kg q 3 to 4 weeks
➤ Immunodeficiency
Gamimune N—
Adults and children: 100 to 200 mg/kg I.V. or 2 to 4 ml/kg (10%) I.V. monthly
Gammagard S/D—
Adults and children: 200 to 400 mg/kg I.V., then monthly in doses based on response
Gammar-P IV—
Adults: 200 to 400 mg/kg I.V. q 3 to 4 weeks
Children and adolescents: 200 mg/kg I.V. q 3 to 4 weeks
Iveegam EN—

i

Adults and children: 200 mg/kg I.V. monthly; may increase up to 800 mg/kg/month based on response
Panglobulin—
Adults and children: 200 mg/kg I.V. monthly, increased to 300 mg/kg/month. In some patients, infusion frequency may be increased.
Panglobulin NF/Carimune NF—
Adults and children: 0.2 g/kg I.V. monthly. If response inadequate, dosage may be increased to 0.3 g/kg or infusion frequency may be increased.
Polygam S/D—
Adults and children: 100 to 400 mg/kg I.V. monthly
Sandoglobulin—
Adults and children: 100 to 400 mg/kg I.V. monthly. In patients with previously untreated agammaglobulinemia or hypogammaglobulinemia, first infusion may be increased to 300 mg/kg or infusion frequency may be increased.
Venoglobulin—
Adults and children: 200 mg/kg I.V. monthly, increased up to 400 mg/kg/month. In some patients, infusion frequency may be increased.
➤ Idiopathic thrombocytopenic purpura
Gamimune N—
Adults and children: 400 mg/kg I.V. for 5 consecutive days, or 1,000 mg/kg/day for 1 day or for 2 consecutive days
Gammagard S/D—
Adults and children: 1,000 mg/kg I.V. Up to three doses may be given on alternating days, dependent on platelet count.
Panglobulin—
Adults and children: Initially, 0.4 g/kg I.V. for 2 to 5 consecutive days
Polygam S/D—
Adults and children: 1 g/kg I.V. Depending on response, additional doses may be given.
Venoglobulin-S—
Adults and children: 2,000 mg/kg I.V. over 5 days or less for induction

therapy; then 1,000 mg/kg p.r.n. to maintain platelet count of 30,000/mm^3 in children or 20,000/mm^3 in adults or to prevent bleeding episodes between infusions
➤ Kawasaki disease
Gammagard S/D—
Adults and adolescents: 1 g/kg I.V. as a single dose; alternatively, 400 mg/kg/day for 4 consecutive days with aspirin
Iveegam EN—
Adults and children: 400 mg/kg/day I.V. with aspirin
Polygam S/D—
Adults and children: 1 g/kg I.V. as a single dose, or 400 mg/kg I.V. for 4 consecutive days starting within 7 days of fever onset. Give with aspirin, as prescribed.
Sandoglobulin—
Adults and children: 400 mg/kg I.V. for 2 to 5 consecutive days. If platelet count falls below 30,000/mm^3 or significant bleeding occurs, may give 0.4 g/kg as a single infusion, increased to 0.8 or 1 g/kg as a single infusion, depending on response.
Venoglobulin S—
Adults and children: 2 g/kg I.V. infused over 10 to 12 hours with aspirin
➤ To prevent bacterial infection in patients with hypogammaglobulinemia or recurrent bacterial infection associated with B-cell chronic lymphocytic leukemia
Adults and adolescents: 400 mg/kg I.V. (Gammagard S/D or Polygam S/D) q 3 to 4 weeks
➤ To reduce risk of graft-versus-host disease, interstitial pneumonia, septicemia, and other infections during first 100 days after bone marrow transplantation
Adults ages 20 and older: 500 mg/kg I.V. (Gamimune N) 7 days before and 2 days before transplantation, then weekly through 90th day after transplantation

➤ To prevent bacterial infection in children with human immunodeficiency virus
Children: 400 mg/kg I.V. (Gamimune N) q 28 days

Off-label uses

• Chronic inflammatory demyelinating polyneuropathy
• Guillain-Barré syndrome

Contraindications

• Hypersensitivity to drug or its components
• Selective immunoglobulin A deficiency

Precautions

Use cautiously in:
• bleeding disorders, renal impairment
• pregnant patients.

Administration

◀ᚷ Before giving, determine if patient has risk factors for acute renal failure (such as use of nephrotoxic drugs; history of diabetes mellitus, renal insufficiency, sepsis, volume depletion, or paraproteinemia; age 65 or older).
• For I.V. use, decrease infusion rate by 50% to 25% for patients at risk for renal dysfunction.
◀ᚷ Give IGIM by I.M. route only; give IGIV by I.V. route only.
• If sterile laminar airflow conditions aren't available for drug reconstitution, administer immediately; discard unused portion.
• Don't shake vigorously, because foaming may occur. Know that cold drug or diluent may take up to 20 minutes to dissolve.

Route	Onset	Peak	Duration
I.V.	Unknown	Unknown	21-28 days
I.M.	Unknown	2 days	Unknown

Adverse reactions

CNS: headache, malaise
CV: chest pain, tachycardia, **thromboembolism**
GI: nausea, vomiting, abdominal pain
Musculoskeletal: joint pain, back pain, myalgia
Respiratory: dyspnea
Skin: pruritus
Other: chills, lymphadenopathy, pain at injection site, **anaphylaxis**

Interactions

Drug-drug. *Live-virus vaccines:* decreased antibody response to vaccine

Patient monitoring

◀ᚷ Watch for acute inflammatory reaction in patients receiving drug for first time (usually appears within 30 to 60 minutes after infusion begins), in those whose last treatment was more than 8 weeks earlier, and when initial infusion rate exceeds 1 ml/minute.
• Monitor vital signs continuously during I.V. infusion. Stay alert for hypotension.
• Assess fluid volume status and blood urea nitrogen and creatinine levels.
• After infusion ends, monitor patient closely for nausea, vomiting, drowsiness, and severe headache.

Patient teaching

• Instruct patient to report symptoms occurring during or after therapy.
• Advise patient to avoid live-virus vaccines for 3 months after therapy; drug may delay or inhibit body's response to vaccine.
• As appropriate, review all significant and life-threatening adverse reactions and interactions, especially those related to the drugs mentioned above.

i

Reactions in **bold** are life-threatening.   ◀ᚷ Clinical alert

indapamide
Apo-Indapamide✦, Dom-
Indapamide✦, Gen-Indapamide✦,
Lozide✦, Lozol, Natrilix✚, Nindaxa✚,
Novo-Indapamide✦, Nu-
Indapamide✦, PHL-Indapamide✦,
PMS-Indapamide✦, Riva-
Indapamide✦

Pharmacologic class: Thiazide-like
diuretic
Therapeutic class: Diuretic, antihypertensive
Pregnancy risk category B

Action
Increases sodium and water excretion
by inhibiting sodium reabsorption in
distal tubule; enhances excretion of
sodium, chloride, potassium, and
water. May cause arteriolar
vasodilation.

Availability
Tablets: 1.25 mg, 2.5 mg

🚺 Indications and dosages
➤ Edema caused by heart failure
Adults: 2.5 mg P.O. daily in morning.
After 1 week, may increase to 5 mg/day.
➤ Mild to moderate hypertension
Adults: 1.25 mg P.O. daily in morning.
May increase q 4 weeks, up to 5 mg/day.

Contraindications
• Hypersensitivity to drug, other
thiazide-like drugs, or tartrazine
• Anuria

Precautions
Use cautiously in:
• renal or severe hepatic impairment,
ascites, fluid or electrolyte imbalances,
gout, systemic lupus erythematosus,
impaired glucose tolerance, hyperparathyroidism, bipolar disorder
• pregnant or breastfeeding patients.

Administration
• Administer with food or milk to
reduce GI upset.
• Give early in day to avoid nocturia.

Route	Onset	Peak	Duration
P.O. (single dose)	1-2 hr	2 hr	36 hr

Adverse reactions
CNS: dizziness, light-headedness,
headache, restlessness, insomnia,
lethargy, fatigue, drowsiness, asthenia,
depression, anxiety, nervousness,
paresthesia, irritability, agitation
CV: orthostatic hypotension, palpitations, premature ventricular contractions, **arrhythmias**
EENT: blurred vision, rhinorrhea
GI: nausea, vomiting, diarrhea, constipation, bloating, epigastric distress,
gastric irritation, abdominal pain or
cramps, dry mouth, anorexia
GU: nocturia, polyuria, glycosuria,
erectile dysfunction
Metabolic: dehydration, gout, hyperglycemia, hypokalemia, hypocalcemia,
hypomagnesemia, hyponatremia,
hypovolemia, hypophosphatemia,
hyperuricemia, **hypochloremic
alkalosis**
Musculoskeletal: muscle cramps and
spasms
Skin: flushing, rash, urticaria, pruritus,
photosensitivity, cutaneous vasculitis,
necrotizing vasculitis
Other: weight loss

Interactions
Drug-drug. *Amphotericin B, corticosteroids:* additive hypokalemia
Antihypertensives, nitrates: additive
hypotension
Cholestyramine, colestipol: decreased
indapamide absorption

Lithium: decreased lithium excretion, increased risk of lithium toxicity
Sulfonylureas: decreased hypoglycemic efficacy
Drug-diagnostic tests. *Bilirubin, blood and urine glucose (in diabetic patients), blood urea nitrogen (BUN), calcium, creatinine, uric acid:* increased values
Cholesterol, low-density lipoproteins, magnesium, potassium, protein-bound iodine, sodium, triglycerides, urinary calcium: decreased values
Drug-herbs. *Ginkgo:* decreased antihypertensive effect
Licorice, stimulant laxative herbs (aloe, cascara sagrada, senna): increased risk of hypokalemia
Drug-behaviors. *Acute alcohol ingestion:* additive hypotension
Sun exposure: increased risk of photosensitivity

Patient monitoring

◀€ Assess for signs and symptoms of hypokalemia, including ventricular arrhythmias, muscle weakness, and cramping.
• Monitor BUN, creatinine, and electrolyte levels.
• Assess daily weight and fluid intake and output.
• Monitor blood pressure response to drug.
• Watch for signs and symptoms of orthostatic hypotension.

Patient teaching

• Advise patient to consume potassium-rich foods, such as oranges, bananas, potatoes, and spinach.
• Instruct patient to move slowly when sitting up or standing, to avoid dizziness from sudden blood pressure decrease.
• Tell patient to weigh himself daily on same scale at same time of day while wearing similar clothing. Instruct him to report gain of more than 2 lb (0.9 kg) in 1 day or 5 lb (2.2 kg) in 1 week.
• Caution patient to avoid driving and other hazardous activities until he

knows how drug affects concentration and alertness.
• As appropriate, review all other significant and life-threatening adverse reactions and interactions, especially those related to the drugs, tests, herbs, and behaviors mentioned above.

indinavir sulfate
Crixivan

Pharmacologic class: Protease inhibitor
Therapeutic class: Antiretroviral
Pregnancy risk category C

Action
Inhibits replication, function, and maturation of human immunodeficiency virus (HIV) protease, an enzyme essential to formation of infectious virus. As a result, further spread of virus is prevented.

Availability
Capsules: 100 mg, 200 mg, 333 mg, 400 mg

Indications and dosages
➤ HIV infection
Adults: 800 mg P.O. q 8 hours

Dosage adjustment
• Mild to moderate hepatic insufficiency secondary to cirrhosis

Contraindications
• Hypersensitivity to drug or its components
• Concurrent use of amiodarone, ergot derivatives, cisapride, pimozide, or oral midazolam, triazolam, alprazolam, alfuzosin, sildenafil

---

Precautions

Use cautiously in:
- renal or severe hepatic impairment, history of renal calculi
- pregnant or breastfeeding patients
- children.

Administration

- Know that drug is usually given with other antiretrovirals.
- Give with full glass of water on empty stomach 1 hour before or 2 hours after meals.
- If GI upset occurs, give with a light meal.

◀ Don't give concurrently with alfuzosin, amiodarone, sildenafil, cisapride (not available in U.S.), ergot derivatives, midazolam, pimozide, or triazolam.

Route	Onset	Peak	Duration
P.O.	Rapid	0.8 hr	8 hr

Adverse reactions

CNS: depression, dizziness, headache, drowsiness, malaise, asthenia
CV: angina, **myocardial infarction**
EENT: oral paresthesia
GI: nausea, vomiting, diarrhea, abdominal pain or distention, dyspepsia, acid regurgitation, **pancreatitis**
GU: dysuria, crystalluria, nephrolithiasis or urolithiasis leading to **renal insufficiency or failure, interstitial nephritis**
Hematologic: anemia, **acute hemolytic anemia, increased spontaneous bleeding** (in hemophiliacs)
Hepatic: jaundice, **hepatic dysfunction, hepatic failure**
Metabolic: new onset or exacerbation of diabetes mellitus, hyperglycemia
Musculoskeletal: joint or back pain
Respiratory: cough, dyspnea
Skin: urticaria, rash, pruritus
Other: abnormal taste, increased or decreased appetite, body fat redistribution or accumulation, fever, **anaphylactoid reactions**

Interactions

Drug-drug. *Azole antifungals, delavirdine, interleukins:* elevated indinavir blood level, greater risk of toxicity
Cisapride, ergot derivatives, midazolam, pimozide, triazolam: CYP3A4 inhibition by indinavir, leading to increased blood levels of these drugs and dangerous reactions
Didanosine, efavirenz, rifamycins: decreased indinavir effects
Drug-diagnostic tests. *Alanine aminotransferase, amylase, aspartate aminotransferase, bilirubin, cholesterol, glucose, triglycerides:* increased values
Hemoglobin, neutrophils, platelets: decreased values
Drug-food. *Any food:* decreased indinavir absorption
Drug-herbs. *St. John's wort:* decreased indinavir blood level

Patient monitoring

- Assess fluid intake and output to ensure adequate hydration and help prevent nephrolithiasis or urolithiasis.
- Monitor for adverse GI and CNS effects.
- Evaluate liver function test results. Assess for hyperbilirubinemia.
- Monitor cholesterol, glucose, and CBC with white cell differential.

Patient teaching

- Tell patient to take 1 hour before or 2 hours after meals with a full glass of water.
- If GI upset occurs, advise patient to take with a light meal.

◀ Instruct patient to report severe nausea or diarrhea, fever, chills, flank pain, urine or stool color changes, yellowing of skin or eyes, or personality changes.

- Tell patient that drug doesn't cure HIV infection and that its long-term effects are largely unknown.

• As appropriate, review all other significant and life-threatening adverse reactions and interactions, especially those related to the drugs, tests, foods, and herbs mentioned above.

indomethacin
(indometacin⊕)

Apo-Indomethacin✻, Flexin, Indameth✻, Indocid-R⊕, Indomax SR⊕, Indocid✻, Indocid PDA⊕, Indocin SR, Indolar SR⊕, Indotec✻, Novo-Methacin✻, Nu-Indo✻, Pardelprin⊕, Pro-Indo✻, Ratio-Indomethacin✻, Rheumacin⊕, Rhodacine✻, Rimacid⊕, Sandoz Indomethacin✻, Slo-Indo⊕

Pharmacologic class: Nonsteroidal anti-inflammatory drug (NSAID)

Therapeutic class: Anti-inflammatory, analgesic, antipyretic

Pregnancy risk category B (third trimester: *D*)

FDA | **BOXED WARNING**

• Drug may increase risk of serious cardiovascular thrombotic events, myocardial infarction, and stroke (which can be fatal). Risk may increase with duration of use, and may be greater in patients who have cardiovascular disease or risk factors for it.
• Drug is contraindicated for perioperative pain in setting of coronary artery bypass graft surgery.
• Drug increases risk of serious GI adverse events, including bleeding, ulcers, and stomach or intestinal perforation, which can be fatal. These events can occur at any time during therapy and without warning. Elderly patients are at greater risk.

Action
Unknown. Thought to inhibit cyclooxygenase, an enzyme needed for prostaglandin synthesis.

Availability
Capsules: 25 mg, 50 mg
Capsules (sustained-release): 75 mg
Oral suspension: 25 mg/5 ml

⚔ Indications and dosages
➤ Rheumatoid arthritis; osteoarthritis; ankylosing spondylitis
Adults: 25 to 50 mg P.O. two or three times daily, not to exceed 200 mg daily; or one 75-mg sustained-release capsule P.O. once or twice daily
➤ Acute gouty arthritis
Adults: 50 mg P.O. t.i.d. until pain is tolerable; then reduce dosage rapidly and, finally, discontinue drug. Don't give sustained-release form.
➤ Acute bursitis or tendinitis of shoulder
Adults: 75 to 150 mg P.O. daily in three or four divided doses. Discontinue once inflammation is controlled.

Off-label uses
• Bartter's syndrome
• Pericarditis

Contraindications
• Hypersensitivity to drug, its components, or other NSAIDs
• Active GI bleeding
• Concurrent diflunisal use

Precautions
Use cautiously in:
• severe cardiovascular, renal, or hepatic disease
• history of ulcer disease
• elderly patients
• pregnant or breastfeeding patients
• children ages 14 and younger (efficacy not established).

Reactions in **bold** are life-threatening. ◀≦ Clinical alert

Administration
- Give with food, full glass of water, or antacids to reduce GI upset.
- Don't open or crush capsules.
- For arthritis, give up to 100 mg of daily dose at bedtime as needed to reduce nighttime pain and morning stiffness.
- Don't give sustained-release form to patients with gouty arthritis.

Route	Onset	Peak	Duration
P.O. (analgesic)	30 min	0.5-2 hr	4-6 hr
P.O. (sustained, analgesic)	30 min	Unknown	4-6 hr
P.O. (regular or sustained, anti-inflam.)	Up to 7 days	1-2 wk	Unknown

Adverse reactions
CNS: headache, dizziness, drowsiness, fatigue, vertigo, depression, **seizures**
EENT: tinnitus
GI: nausea, vomiting, diarrhea, constipation, abdominal pain or cramps, dyspepsia, ulcers, **GI bleeding**
Other: allergic reactions including **anaphylaxis**

Interactions
Drug-drug. *Antihypertensives, diuretics:* decreased efficacy of these drugs
Corticosteroids, other NSAIDs: additive adverse GI reactions
Cyclosporine: increased risk of nephrotoxicity
Diflunisal: potentially fatal GI hemorrhage
Lithium, methotrexate, zidovudine: increased risk of toxicity from these drugs
Probenecid: increased risk of indomethacin toxicity
Drug-diagnostic tests. *Dexamethasone suppression test:* false-negative result
Drug-herbs. *Anise, arnica, chamomile, clove, dong quai, feverfew, garlic, ginger, ginkgo, ginseng:* increased bleeding risk

Patient monitoring
- Assess for dizziness, drowsiness, headache, fatigue, and exacerbation of depression, epilepsy, or parkinsonism.
- Monitor for drug efficacy, indicated by improved joint mobility, pain relief, and decreased inflammation.
- Monitor urine output for marked reduction.
- Watch for signs and symptoms of GI bleeding and ulcers.

Patient teaching
- Tell patient to take with food, full glass of water, or antacid to reduce GI upset.
- Advise patient not to open or crush capsules.
- Inform breastfeeding patient that indomethacin enters breast milk and may cause seizures in infant. Advise her to use a different infant feeding method during therapy.
- Caution patient to avoid driving and other hazardous activities until he knows how drug affects concentration, balance, and alertness.
- As appropriate, review all other significant and life-threatening adverse reactions and interactions, especially those related to the drugs, tests, and herbs mentioned above.

infliximab
Remicade

Pharmacologic class: Monoclonal antibody
Therapeutic class: Antirheumatic, GI anti-inflammatory
Pregnancy risk category B

FDA | **BOXED WARNING**

- Patients treated with infliximab are at increased risk for developing serious infections, including tuberculosis (TB),

---

♦ Canada   ⊕ UK   ⚗ Hazardous drug   ⊗ High-alert drug

bacterial sepsis, invasive fungal infections (such as histoplasmosis, coccidioidomycosis, candidiasis, aspergillosis, blastomycosis, and pneumocystosis), and infections due to other opportunistic pathogens (including *Legionella* and *Listeria* species), that may lead to hospitalization or death. Most patients who developed these infections were taking concomitant immunosuppressants (such as methotrexate or corticosteroids).

• Carefully consider risks and benefits of treatment with infliximab before starting therapy in patients with chronic or recurrent infection.

• TB includes active TB and reactivation of latent TB. Patients with TB have frequently presented with disseminated or extrapulmonary disease. Patients should be tested for latent TB before starting infliximab and during therapy. Treatment for latent infection should be started before initiating infliximab.

• Patients with histoplasmosis or other invasive fungal infections may present with disseminated, rather than localized, disease. Antigen and antibody testing for histoplasmosis may be negative in some patients with active infection. Consider empiric antifungal therapy in patients at risk for invasive fungal infections who develop severe systemic illness.

• Closely monitor patients for signs and symptoms of infection during and after treatment with infliximab, including possible development of TB in patients who tested negative for latent TB before starting infliximab.

• Discontinue drug if patient develops a serious infection or sepsis.

• Lymphoma and other malignancies, some fatal, have been reported in children and adolescents treated with tumor necrosis factor (TNF) blockers, including infliximab. Postmarketing cases of hepatosplenic T-cell lymphoma, a rare type of T-cell lymphoma, have been reported in patients treated with TNF blockers, including infliximab. All cases occurred in patients with Crohn's disease and ulcerative colitis, the majority of whom were adolescent or young adult males. This rare, aggressive T-cell lymphoma is fatal. All of these patients had received treatment with azathioprine or 6-mercaptopurine concomitantly with infliximab at or before diagnosis.

Action
Neutralizes and prevents activity of tumor necrosis factor-alpha (TNF-alpha) by binding to soluble and transmembrane forms of TNF and inhibiting its receptors, resulting in antiinflammatory and antiproliferative activity. Reduces rate of joint destruction in rheumatoid arthritis and eases symptoms of Crohn's disease.

Availability
Powder for injection: 100 mg/vial

Indications and dosages
➤ Rheumatoid arthritis (given with methotrexate)

Adults: Initially, 3 mg/kg I.V., followed by 3 mg/kg 2 and 6 weeks after initial dose, then q 8 weeks. In partial responders, dosage may be adjusted up to 10 mg/kg or treatment may be repeated as often as q 4 weeks.

➤ Crohn's disease

Adults and children age 6 and older: 5 mg/kg I.V. as a single infusion, starting as induction regimen at 0, 2, and 6 weeks, then a maintenance regimen of 5 mg/kg q 8 weeks. For some adults patients who respond initially but then stop responding, dosage of 10 mg/kg may be warranted.

➤ Ulcerative colitis

Adults and children age 6 and older: 5 mg/kg I.V. infusion given as induction therapy at 0, 2, and 6 weeks, followed by maintenance regimen of 5 mg/kg I.V. q 8 weeks thereafter

➤Ankylosing spondylitis

Adults: 5 mg/kg I.V. infusion at 0, 2, and 6 weeks, followed by maintenance regimen of 5 mg/kg q 6 weeks thereafter

➤Psoriatic arthritis

Adults: 5 mg/kg I.V. infusion (with or without methotrexate) given as induction therapy at 0, 2, and 6 weeks, followed by maintenance regimen of 5 mg/kg q 8 weeks thereafter

➤Plaque psoriasis

Adults: 5 mg/kg I.V. infusion given as induction therapy at 0, 2, and 6 weeks, followed by maintenance regimen of 5 mg/kg q 8 weeks thereafter

Off-label uses
• Sarcoidosis

Contraindications
• Hypersensitivity to drug, murine proteins, or other drug components
• Dosages above 5 mg/kg for patients with moderate to severe heart failure

Precautions
Use cautiously in:
• history of tuberculosis (TB), active infection, or exposure to TB; patients who have resided in or traveled in areas of endemic TB or endemic mycoses, such as histoplasmosis, coccidioidomycosis, or blastomycosis
• chronic or recurrent infection or underlying conditions that may predispose to infection; history of opportunistic infection; hepatitis B virus (HBV) carriers
• jaundice or marked liver enzyme elevations, cytopenias
• neurologic disorders (including CNS manifestation of systemic vasculitis, seizures), new-onset or exacerbation of demyelinating disorders (including multiple sclerosis and optic neuritis) and peripheral demyelinating disorders (including Guillain-Barré syndrome)
• male patients with Crohn's disease or ulcerative colitis who are receiving azathioprine or 6-mercaptopurine treatment
• concurrent use of live vaccines, tocilizumab (avoid use)
• concurrent use of anakinra or abatacept (use not recommended)
• when switching between biological disease-modifying antirheumatics (overlapping biological activity may further increase risk of infection)
• elderly patients
• pregnant or breastfeeding patients
• children younger than age 6 (safety not established).

Administration
• Know that latent TB should be treated before infliximab therapy begins.
• To reconstitute, use 21G or smaller needle to add 10 ml of sterile water to each vial. To mix, swirl (don't shake). Solution may foam and appear clear or light yellow.
• Withdraw volume equal to amount of reconstituted drug from 250-ml polypropylene or polyolefin infusion bag or glass bottle of normal saline solution. Slowly add reconstituted drug to infusion bag or bottle, and gently mix. Use within 3 hours.
• Know that concentration of infusion should be 0.4 mg/ml to 4 mg/ml.
• Give I.V. infusion over at least 2 hours. Use polyethylene-lined infusion set equipped with in-line filter, with pore size of 1.2 microns or less.
• Premedicate with antihistamines, acetaminophen, and corticosteroids, as prescribed.

◀€ Watch for infusion reactions, especially after first infusion. Be aware that mild to moderate infusion reactions may improve after slowing or suspension of infusion. Upon resolution of reaction, restart infusion at lower infusion rate or administer antihistamines, acetaminophen, or corticosteroids. Discontinue drug in patients who don't tolerate infusion following these interventions; permanently discontinue drug in patients who have severe infusion-related hypersensitivity reactions.

• Discard unused portions of infusion solution.

• Don't give to patient with active infection.

• Be aware that patient who doesn't respond by week 14 isn't likely to respond, and therapy should cease.

Route	Onset	Peak	Duration
I.V.	1-2 wk	Unknown	12-48 wk

Adverse reactions

CNS: fatigue, headache, anxiety, depression, dizziness, insomnia, CNS manifestation of systemic vasculitis, seizures, new-onset or exacerbation of demyelinating disorders (including multiple sclerosis, optic neuritis, Guillain-Barré syndrome)

CV: chest pain, hypertension, hypotension, tachycardia, peripheral edema, **worsening of heart failure**

EENT: conjunctivitis, rhinitis, sinusitis, laryngitis, pharyngitis

GI: nausea, vomiting, diarrhea, constipation, abdominal pain, dyspepsia, flatulence, ulcerative stomatitis, **intestinal obstruction**

GU: dysuria, urinary frequency, urinary tract infection

Hematologic: hematoma, anemia, **hemolytic anemia, pancytopenia**

Hepatic: HBV reactivation, **hepatotoxicity**

Musculoskeletal: arthritis, joint pain, back pain, myalgia, involuntary muscle contractions

Respiratory: upper respiratory tract infection, bronchitis, cough, dyspnea

Skin: acne, diaphoresis, dry skin, bruising, eczema, erythema, flushing, pruritus, urticaria, rash, alopecia

Other: oral pain, tooth pain, moniliasis, chills, hot flashes, flulike symptoms, herpes simplex, herpes zoster, **autoimmunity**, lupuslike syndrome, serious infections, **malignancies, infusion reactions,** hypersensitivity reaction including **anaphylaxis or serum sickness-like reactions**

Interactions

Drug-drug. *Abatacept, anakinra:* increased risk of infections

Tocilizumab: increased immunosuppression and increased risk of infection

Vaccines: decreased antibody response to vaccine

Drug-diagnostic tests. *Antinuclear antibodies:* positive titer

Hepatic enzymes: increased values

Hemoglobin: decreased value

Patient monitoring

◀﹦ Stay alert for signs and symptoms of hypersensitivity and infusion reactions, including fever, chills, itching, rash, chest pain, dyspnea, facial flushing, and headache.

◀﹦ Watch for evidence of infection, especially in patients who have chronic infections or are receiving immunosuppressants. Drug increases risk of life-threatening opportunistic infections and TB.

• Monitor platelets and CBC with white cell differential.

◀﹦ Assess for heart failure in patients with history of cardiac disease.

◀﹦ Be aware that CNS disorders (such as seizures, new-onset or exacerbation of demyelinating disorders), malignancies including lymphoma, HBV reactivation, hepatotoxicity, and cytopenias may occur.

Patient teaching

◀﹦ Instruct patient to report signs or symptoms of hypersensitivity reaction, such as fever, chills, itching, rash, chest pain, dyspnea, and facial flushing (may occur up to 12 days after therapy).

Reactions in **bold** are life-threatening.　　　　◀﹦ Clinical alert

◀€ Tell patient to report infection symptoms, such as fever, burning on urination, cough, or sore throat.
• Advise patient to avoid potential infection sources, such as crowds and people with known infections.
• Advise patient not to receive live vaccines while receiving infliximab.
◀€ Instruct patient how to recognize and immediately report signs and symptoms of blood dyscrasias, hepatotoxicity, or other new or worsening symptoms.
• As appropriate, review all other significant and life-threatening adverse reactions and interactions, especially those related to the drugs and tests mentioned above.

insulin, regular (insulin injection)

Humulin R, Humulin-R Regular U-500 (concentrate), Insulin-Toronto✤

insulin (lispro)

Humalog, Humalog Pen

insulin glulisine, recombinant

Apidra, Apidra SoloSTAR

insulin lispro protamine, human

Humalog Mix 50/50, Humalog Mix 75/25

isophane insulin suspension (NPH insulin)

Humulin N, Novolin N

isophane insulin suspension (NPH) and insulin injection (regular)

Humulin 70/30 (70% isophane insulin and 30% insulin injection), Humulin 70/30 PenFill, Novolin 70/30, Novolin 70/30 PenFill

Pharmacologic class: Pancreatic hormone
Therapeutic class: Hypoglycemic
Pregnancy risk category B

Action

Promotes glucose transport, which stimulates carbohydrate metabolism in skeletal and cardiac muscle and adipose tissue. Also promotes phosphorylation of glucose in liver, where it is converted to glycogen. Directly affects fat and protein metabolism, stimulates protein synthesis, inhibits release of free fatty acids, and indirectly decreases phosphate and potassium.

Availability

Glulisine, recombinant: 100 units/ml in 10-ml vials, 100 units/ml in 3-ml cartridge system, 100 units/ml in 3-ml prefilled pen
Isophane suspension, injection (regular): 70 units NPH and 30 units regular insulin/ml (100 units/ml total), 50 units NPH and 50 units regular insulin/ml (100 units/ml total)
Isophane suspension (NPH insulin): 100 units/ml
Lispro: 100 units/ml in 10-ml vials and 1.5-ml cartridges
Regular insulin injection: 100 units/ml
Regular U-500 (concentrated), insulin human injection: 500 units/ml
Zinc suspension, extended (ultralente): 100 units/ml
Zinc suspension (lente insulin): 100 units/ml

✋ Indications and dosages

➤ Type 1 (insulin-dependent) diabetes mellitus; type 2 (non-insulin-dependent) diabetes mellitus unresponsive to diet and oral hypoglycemics

Adults and children: In newly diagnosed diabetes, total of 0.5 to 1 unit/kg/day subcutaneously as part of multidose regimen of short- and long-acting insulin. Dosage individualized based on patient's glucose level, adjusted to premeal and bedtime glucose levels. Reserve concentrated insulin (500 units/ml) for patients requiring more than 200 units/day.

➤ Diabetic ketoacidosis

Adults and children: Loading dose of 0.15 units/kg (nonconcentrated regular insulin) I.V. bolus, followed by continuous infusion of 0.1 unit/kg/hour until glucose level drops. Then administer subcutaneously, adjusting dosage according to glucose level.

Contraindications

- Hypersensitivity to drug or its components
- Hypoglycemia

Precautions

Use cautiously in:

- hepatic or renal impairment, hypothyroidism, hyperthyroidism
- elderly patients
- pregnant or breastfeeding patients
- children.

Administration

◀﹦ Be aware that insulin is a high-alert drug whether given subcutaneously or I.V.

◀﹦ Don't give insulin I.V. (except nonconcentrated regular insulin), because anaphylactic reaction may occur.

- When mixing two types of insulin, draw up regular insulin into syringe first.

- For I.V. infusion, mix regular insulin only with normal or half-normal saline solution, as prescribed, to yield a concentration of 1 unit/ml. Give every 50 units I.V. over at least 1 minute.
- Rotate subcutaneous injection sites to prevent lipodystrophy.
- Administer mixtures of regular and NPH or regular and lente insulins within 5 to 15 minutes of mixing.

Route	Onset	Peak	Duration
I.V. (regular)	10-30 min	15-30 min	Unknown
Subcut. (glulisine)	Rapid	Unknown	Short
Subcut. (lente)	1-2.5 hr	7-15 hr	24 hr
Subcut. (lispro)	15 min	30-90 min	6-8 hr
Subcut. (lispro/ protamine mix; regular U-500 conc.)	Unknown	Unknown	Unknown
Subcut. (NPH)	1-1.5 hr	4-12 hr	24 hr
Subcut. (regular)	30-60 min	2-4 hr	Unknown
Subcut. (ultralente)	8 hr	10-30 hr	>36 hr

Adverse reactions

Metabolic: hypokalemia, sodium retention, **hypoglycemia, rebound hyperglycemia (Somogyi effect)**

Skin: urticaria, rash, pruritus

Other: edema; lipodystrophy; lipohypertrophy; erythema, stinging, or warmth at injection site; allergic reactions including **anaphylaxis**

Interactions

Drug-drug. *Acetazolamide, albuterol, antiretrovirals, asparaginase, calcitonin, corticosteroids, cyclophosphamide, danazol, dextrothyroxine, diazoxide, diltiazem, diuretics, dobutamine, epinephrine, estrogens, hormonal contraceptives, isoniazid, morphine, niacin,*

Reactions in **bold** are life-threatening. ◀﹦ Clinical alert

phenothiazines, phenytoin, somatropin, terbutaline, thyroid hormones: decreased hypoglycemic effect

Anabolic steroids, angiotensin-converting enzyme inhibitors, calcium, chloroquine, clofibrate, clonidine, disopyramide, fluoxetine, guanethidine, mebendazole, MAO inhibitors, octreotide, oral hypoglycemics, phenylbutazone, propoxyphene, pyridoxine, salicylates, sulfinpyrazone, sulfonamides, tetracyclines: increased hypoglycemic effect

Beta-adrenergic blockers (nonselective): masking of some hypoglycemia symptoms, delayed recovery from hypoglycemia

Lithium carbonate: decreased or increased hypoglycemic effect

Pentamidine: increased hypoglycemic effect, possibly followed by hyperglycemia

Drug-diagnostic tests. *Glucose, inorganic phosphate, magnesium, potassium:* decreased levels

Liver and thyroid function tests: interference with test results

Urine vanillylmandelic acid: increased level

Drug-herbs. *Basil, burdock, glucosamine, sage:* altered glycemic control

Chromium, coenzyme Q10, dandelion, eucalyptus, fenugreek, marshmallow: increased hypoglycemic effect

Garlic, ginseng: decreased blood glucose level

Drug-behaviors. *Alcohol use:* increased hypoglycemic effect

Marijuana use: increased blood glucose level

Smoking: increased blood glucose level, decreased response to insulin

Patient monitoring

• Monitor glucose level frequently to assess drug efficacy and appropriateness of dosage.

• Watch blood glucose level closely if patient is converting from one insulin type to another or is under unusual stress (as from surgery or trauma).

◀€ Monitor for signs and symptoms of hypoglycemia. Keep glucose source at hand in case hypoglycemia occurs.

◀€ Assess for signs and symptoms of hyperglycemia, such as polydipsia, polyphagia, polyuria, and diabetic ketoacidosis (as shown by blood and urinary ketones, metabolic acidosis, extremely elevated blood glucose level).

• Monitor for glycosuria.

• Closely evaluate kidney and liver function test results in patients with renal or hepatic impairment.

Patient teaching

• Teach patient how to administer insulin subcutaneously as appropriate.

• Advise patient to draw up regular insulin into syringe first when mixing two types of insulin. Caution him not to change order of mixing insulins.

• Instruct patient to rotate subcutaneous injection sites and keep a record of sites used, to prevent fatty tissue breakdown.

◀€ Teach patient how to recognize and report signs and symptoms of hypoglycemia and hyperglycemia. Advise him to carry a glucose source at all times.

• Instruct patient to store insulin in refrigerator (not freezer).

• Teach patient how to monitor and record blood glucose level and, if indicated, urine glucose and ketone levels.

• Tell patient that dietary changes, activity, and stress can alter blood glucose level and insulin requirements.

• Instruct patient to wear medical identification stating that he is diabetic and takes insulin.

• Advise patient to have regular medical, vision, and dental exams.

• As appropriate, review all other significant and life-threatening adverse reactions and interactions, especially those related to the drugs, tests, herbs, and behaviors mentioned above.

insulin aspart
(rDNA origin)
NovoLog

insulin aspart and insulin aspart protamine
NovoLog Mix 70/30

Pharmacologic class: Pancreatic hormone
Therapeutic class: Hypoglycemic
Pregnancy risk category C

Action
Short-acting insulin form. Promotes glucose transport, which stimulates carbohydrate metabolism in skeletal and cardiac muscle and adipose tissue. Also promotes phosphorylation of glucose in liver, where it's converted to glycogen. Directly affects fat and protein metabolism, stimulates protein synthesis, inhibits release of free fatty acids, and indirectly decreases phosphate and potassium.

Availability
Injection (NovoLog): 100 units/ml in 10-ml vials and 3-ml PenFill cartridges
Injection (NovoLog Mix 70/30): 100 units/ml in 10-ml vials, 3-ml PenFill cartridges, and 3-ml FlexPen prefilled syringes

💊 Indications and dosages
➤ Type 1 (insulin-dependent) diabetes mellitus; type 2 (non-insulin-dependent) diabetes mellitus
Adults and children ages 6 and older:
Insulin aspart—Dosage tailored to patient's needs, given subcutaneously in divided doses 5 to 10 minutes before meals. Insulin aspart provides 50% to 70% of dose; intermediate or long-acting insulin provides remainder.

Dosage range is 0.5 to 1 unit/kg/day in divided doses based on meals. *Insulin aspart and insulin aspart protamine*—Give subcutaneously b.i.d., 15 minutes before morning and evening meals. For monotherapy, initial dosage is 0.4 to 0.6 unit/kg/day in two divided doses. Titrate in increments of 2 to 4 units q 3 to 4 days to achieve target fasting plasma glucose level. When given with oral hypoglycemics, initial dosage is 0.2 to 0.3 unit/kg/day.

Contraindications
• Hypersensitivity to drug or its components
• Hypoglycemia

Precautions
Use cautiously in:
• hepatic or renal impairment, hypothyroidism, hyperthyroidism
• elderly patients
• pregnant or breastfeeding patients
• children.

Administration
◀€ Be aware that insulin is a high-alert drug.
• Know that drug is bioavailable as regular human insulin but has a faster onset and shorter duration.
• Give by subcutaneous route only, 5 to 10 minutes (15 minutes for Novolog Mix 70/30) before a meal.
• When mixing insulin aspart with intermediate or long-acting insulin, draw up insulin aspart into syringe first.
◀€ Don't mix insulin aspart protamine with any other insulin.
• When giving insulin aspart by pump, don't mix with other insulins.
• Rotate injection sites to prevent lipodystrophy.

Route	Onset	Peak	Duration
Subcut.	15 min	1-3 hr	3-5 hr

i

Adverse reactions

Metabolic: hypokalemia, sodium retention, **hypoglycemia, rebound hyperglycemia (Somogyi effect)**
Musculoskeletal: myalgia
Skin: urticaria, rash, pruritus
Other: edema; lipodystrophy; lipohypertrophy; redness, warmth, or stinging at injection site; allergic reactions including **anaphylaxis**

Interactions

Drug-drug. *Acetazolamide, albuterol, antiretrovirals, asparaginase, calcitonin, corticosteroids, cyclophosphamide, danazol, dextrothyroxine, diazoxide, diltiazem, diuretics, dobutamine, epinephrine, estrogens, hormonal contraceptives, isoniazid, morphine, niacin, phenothiazines, phenytoin, somatropin, terbutaline, thyroid hormones:* decreased hypoglycemic effect
Anabolic steroids, angiotensin-converting enzyme inhibitors, calcium, chloroquine, clofibrate, clonidine, disopyramide, fluoxetine, guanethidine, mebendazole, MAO inhibitors, octreotide, oral hypoglycemics, phenylbutazone, propoxyphene, pyridoxine, salicylates, sulfinpyrazone, sulfonamides, tetracyclines: increased hypoglycemic effect
Beta-adrenergic blockers (nonselective): masking of some hypoglycemia signs and symptoms, delayed recovery from hypoglycemia
Lithium carbonate: decreased or increased hypoglycemic effect
Pentamidine: increased hypoglycemic effect, possibly followed by hyperglycemia
Drug-diagnostic tests. *Glucose, inorganic phosphate, magnesium, potassium:* decreased levels
Liver and thyroid function studies: test interference
Urine vanillylmandelic acid: increased level
Drug-herbs. *Basil, bee pollen, burdock, glucosamine, sage:* altered glycemic control

Chromium, coenzyme Q10, dandelion, eucalyptus, fenugreek, marshmallow: increased hypoglycemic effect
Garlic, ginseng: decreased blood glucose level
Drug-behaviors. *Alcohol use:* increased hypoglycemic effect
Marijuana use: increased blood glucose level
Smoking: increased blood glucose level, decreased response to insulin

Patient monitoring

• Monitor blood glucose level frequently to gauge drug efficacy and appropriateness of dosage.
• Watch blood glucose level closely if patient is converting from one insulin type to another or is under unusual stress (as from surgery or trauma).
◀ Stay alert for signs and symptoms of hypoglycemia. Keep glucose source at hand.
◀ Assess for evidence of hyperglycemia, such as polydipsia, polyphagia, polyuria, and diabetic ketoacidosis (as shown by urine and blood ketones, metabolic acidosis, extremely elevated blood glucose level, and hypovolemia).
• Monitor for glycosuria.
• Closely monitor kidney and liver function test results in patients with renal or hepatic impairment.

Patient teaching

• Teach patient how to administer insulin subcutaneously or by injection pen.
• If patient must mix insulin aspart with intermediate or long-acting insulin, instruct him to draw up insulin aspart into syringe first.
◀ Tell patient not to mix any other insulin with mixture of insulin aspart and insulin aspart protamine.
• Advise patient to rotate subcutaneous injection sites and keep a record of sites used, to help prevent fatty tissue breakdown.

◀≣ Teach patient how to recognize and report signs and symptoms of hypoglycemia and hyperglycemia. Advise him to always carry a glucose source.

• Inform patient that changes in diet, activity, and stress level affect blood glucose levels and insulin requirements.

• Teach patient how to monitor and record blood glucose level and, if indicated, urine glucose and ketone levels.

• Tell patient to wear medical identification stating that he is diabetic and takes insulin.

• Instruct patient to have regular medical, vision, and dental exams.

• Tell female patient to contact prescriber if she is pregnant or plans to become pregnant.

• Advise patient to store insulin in refrigerator, not freezer.

• As appropriate, review all other significant and life-threatening adverse reactions and interactions, especially those related to the drugs, tests, herbs, and behaviors mentioned above.

ⓧ

insulin glargine (rDNA origin)
Lantus

Pharmacologic class: Pancreatic hormone
Therapeutic class: Hypoglycemic
Pregnancy risk category C

Action
Long-acting insulin form. Promotes glucose transport, which stimulates carbohydrate metabolism in skeletal and cardiac muscle and adipose tissue. Also promotes phosphorylation of glucose in liver, where it's converted to glycogen. Directly affects fat and protein metabolism, stimulates protein synthesis, inhibits release of free fatty acids, and indirectly decreases phosphate and potassium.

Availability
Injection: 100 units/ml in 10-ml vials and 3-ml cartridges

Indications and dosages
➤ Type 1 (insulin-dependent) diabetes mellitus and type 2 (non-insulin-dependent) diabetes mellitus in patients who need long-acting insulin
Adults and children ages 6 and older: Subcutaneous injection daily at same time each day, with dosage based on blood glucose level
➤ Conversion from another insulin type in patients with type 1 diabetes mellitus who need long-acting insulin
Adults and children ages 6 and older: For patients switching from once-daily NPH or ultralente human insulin, start glargine at same dosage as current insulin dosage. For patients taking twice-daily NPH or ultralente human insulin, reduce initial glargine dosage by approximately 20% of current insulin dosage during week 1; then adjust based on blood glucose level.
➤ Type 2 diabetes mellitus in patients receiving oral hypoglycemics
Adults: Dosage highly individualized based on glucose levels and response

Contraindications
• Hypersensitivity to drug or its components
• Hypoglycemia

Precautions
Use cautiously in:
• pregnant or breastfeeding patients
• children.

Administration
◀≣ Be aware that insulin is a high-alert drug.
• Give by subcutaneous route only, at same time each day.

i

Reactions in **bold** are life-threatening.   Clinical alert

◀€ Don't mix in solution with other drugs, including other insulins.

• Before drawing up insulin into syringe, roll vial between hands to ensure uniform dispersion; don't shake.

• Rotate injection sites to prevent lipodystrophy.

Route	Onset	Peak	Duration
Subcut.	1.1 hr	5 hr	24 hr

Adverse reactions

Metabolic: rebound hyperglycemia (Somogyi effect), hypoglycemia
Skin: urticaria, rash, pruritus, redness, stinging, or warmth at injection site
Other: edema, lipodystrophy, lipohypertrophy, allergic reactions including **anaphylaxis**

Interactions

Drug-drug. *Acetazolamide, albuterol, antiretrovirals, asparaginase, calcitonin, corticosteroids, cyclophosphamide, danazol, dextrothyroxine, diazoxide, diltiazem, diuretics, dobutamine, epinephrine, estrogens, hormonal contraceptives, isoniazid, morphine, niacin, phenothiazines, phenytoin, somatropin, terbutaline, thyroid hormones:* decreased hypoglycemic effect
Anabolic steroids, angiotensin-converting enzyme inhibitors, calcium, chloroquine, clofibrate, clonidine, disopyramide, fluoxetine, guanethidine, mebendazole, MAO inhibitors, octreotide, oral hypoglycemics, phenylbutazone, propoxyphene, pyridoxine, salicylates, sulfinpyrazone, sulfonamides, tetracyclines: increased hypoglycemic effect
Beta-adrenergic blockers (nonselective): masking of some hypoglycemia signs and symptoms, delayed recovery from hypoglycemia
Lithium carbonate: altered hypoglycemic effect

Pentamidine: increased hypoglycemic effect, possibly followed by hyperglycemia
Drug-diagnostic tests. *Glucose, inorganic phosphate, magnesium, potassium:* decreased levels
Liver and thyroid function studies: test interference
Urine vanillylmandelic acid: increased level
Drug-herbs. *Basil, bee pollen, burdock, glucosamine, sage:* altered glycemic control
Chromium, coenzyme Q10, dandelion, eucalyptus, fenugreek, marshmallow: increased hypoglycemic effect
Garlic, ginseng: decreased blood glucose level
Drug-behaviors. *Alcohol use:* increased hypoglycemic effect
Marijuana use: increased blood glucose level
Smoking: increased blood glucose level, decreased response to insulin

Patient monitoring

• Monitor blood glucose level frequently to assess drug efficacy and appropriateness of dosage.

• Watch blood glucose level closely if patient is converting from one insulin type to another or is under unusual stress (as from surgery or trauma).

◀€ Check for signs and symptoms of hypoglycemia (such as CNS changes). Keep glucose source at hand.

◀€ Monitor for signs and symptoms of hyperglycemia, such as polydipsia, polyphagia, polyuria, and diabetic ketoacidosis (blood and urine ketones, metabolic acidosis, extremely elevated glucose level, hypovolemia).

• Monitor for glycosuria.

• Closely monitor kidney and liver function test results in patients with renal or hepatic impairment.

Patient teaching

• Instruct patient how to administer insulin subcutaneously.

◀◝ Teach patient how to recognize and report signs and symptoms of hypoglycemia and hyperglycemia. Advise him to always carry glucose source.

• Advise patient to rotate subcutaneous injection sites and keep a record of sites used.

• Teach patient how to monitor and record blood glucose level and, if indicated, urine glucose and ketone levels.

• Inform patient that changes in diet, activity, and stress level can affect blood glucose level and insulin requirements.

• Advise patient to wear medical identification stating that he is diabetic and takes insulin.

• As appropriate, review all other significant and life-threatening adverse reactions and interactions, especially those related to the drugs, tests, herbs, and behaviors mentioned above.

interferon alfa-2b, recombinant
Intron A, Viraferon⊕

Pharmacologic class: Biological response modifier
Therapeutic class: Antineoplastic, antiviral
Pregnancy risk category C

FDA BOXED WARNING

• Drug may cause or worsen fatal or life-threatening neuropsychiatric, autoimmune, ischemic, and infectious disorders. Monitor patient closely with periodic clinical and laboratory evaluations. Discontinue drug in patients with persistently severe or worsening signs or symptoms of these conditions. In many cases, these disorders resolve after withdrawal.

Action
Unknown. Antitumor and antiviral activity may stem from direct antiproliferative action against tumor or viral cells, inhibition of viral replication, and modulation of host immune response.

Availability
Injection: 3 million international units/0.5-ml vial, 5 million international units/0.5-ml vial, 10 million international units/1-ml vial; 18 million international units/3.2-ml vial, 25 million international units/ 3.2-ml vial
Powder for injection (vial with diluent): 3 million, 5 million, 10 million, 18 million, 25 million, and 50 million international units

💊 Indications and dosages
➤ Chronic hepatitis C
Adults: 3 million international units subcutaneously or I.M. three times weekly. If patient tolerates therapy and alanine aminotransferase (ALT) level is normal after 16 weeks, continue for 18 to 24 weeks. If ALT doesn't normalize, drug may be withdrawn.
➤ Chronic hepatitis B
Adults: 30 to 35 million international units subcutaneously or I.M. weekly for 16 weeks, given as 5 million international units daily or 10 million international units three times weekly
➤ Hairy cell leukemia
Adults: 2 million international units/ m² I.M. or subcutaneously three times weekly for 6 months or longer
➤ AIDS-related Kaposi's sarcoma
Adults: 30 million international units/ m² subcutaneously or I.M. three times weekly. Continue dosage unless intolerance occurs or disease advances rapidly.
➤ Malignant melanoma (as adjunct to surgery)
Adults: 20 million international units/m² I.V. for 5 consecutive days per

week for 4 weeks; then a maintenance dosage of 10 million international units/m² subcutaneously three times weekly for 48 weeks. Withhold drug if adverse reactions occur; when reactions ease, resume at half of previous dosage. Withdraw if reactions persist.
➤ Condyloma acuminatum (genital or venereal warts)
Adults: 1 million international units/lesion given intralesionally three times weekly for 3 weeks
➤ Aggressive follicular non-Hodgkin's lymphoma
Adults: 5 million international units subcutaneously three times weekly for up to 18 months (given with chemotherapy regimen containing anthracycline)

Off-label uses
• Adjuvant treatment of malignant melanoma
• Hepatitis D

Contraindications
• Hypersensitivity to drug or its components
• Autoimmune disorders
• Female partners of males receiving drug

Precautions
Use cautiously in:
• cardiac or pulmonary disease; bone marrow, autoimmune, seizure, or psychiatric disorders
• diabetic patients prone to ketoacidosis
• pregnant or breastfeeding patients
• children.

Administration
• Administer by subcutaneous, I.M., I.V., or intralesional route. For I.V. use, reconstitute with diluent provided by manufacturer (bacteriostatic water for injection), according to chart provided. Mix gently, draw drug up into sterile syringe, and inject into 100 ml of normal saline solution. Infuse slowly over 20 minutes.
• Give antiemetics, as needed and prescribed, for nausea and vomiting.

Route	Onset	Peak	Duration
I.V.	Unknown	15-60 min	4 hr
I.M.	Unknown	2-12 hr	Unknown
Subcut.	Unknown	3-12 hr	Unknown
Intrales.	Unknown	Unknown	Unknown

Adverse reactions
CNS: dizziness, confusion, paresthesia, rigors, lethargy, depression, difficulty thinking or concentrating, insomnia, anxiety, fatigue, asthenia, amnesia, malaise, nervousness, drowsiness, **suicidal ideation**
CV: chest pain, hypertension, palpitations, **arrhythmias**
EENT: visual disturbances, stye, hearing disorders, nasal congestion, sinusitis, rhinitis, pharyngitis
GI: nausea, vomiting, diarrhea, constipation, abdominal pain, dyspepsia, flatulence, eructation, stomatitis, dry mouth, **intestinal obstruction**
GU: gynecomastia, impaired fertility in women, transient erectile dysfunction
Hematologic: anemia, **leukopenia, thrombocytopenia, neutropenia**
Metabolic: hyperglycemia, hypocalcemia
Musculoskeletal: joint pain, back pain, myalgia
Respiratory: cough, dyspnea
Skin: flushing, rash, dry skin, pruritus, alopecia, dermatitis, diaphoresis
Other: gingivitis, flulike symptoms, candidiasis, edema, weight loss

Interactions
Drug-drug. *Aminophylline, theophylline:* reduced clearance of these drugs
CNS depressants: additive CNS effects
Live-virus vaccines: decreased antibody response to vaccine, increased risk of adverse reactions
Zidovudine: synergistic effects

Drug-diagnostic tests. *Alkaline phosphatase, ALT, aspartate aminotransferase, bilirubin, blood urea nitrogen, calcium, creatinine, fasting glucose, lactate dehydrogenase, neutralizing antibodies, phosphate, uric acid:* increased levels
Hemoglobin, platelets, white blood cells: decreased values
International Normalized Ratio, partial thromboplastin time, prothrombin time: increased values

Patient monitoring

◀€ Before therapy and monthly during therapy, assess CBC with white cell differential, bone marrow hairy cells, glucose and electrolyte levels, and liver and kidney function tests.

• Discontinue therapy if neutrophil count drops below 500 cells/mm^2.

• Monitor fluid intake and output. Keep patient well hydrated.

• Assess for GI upset. Provide small, frequent meals and antiemetics to ease severe nausea and vomiting.

◀€ Monitor for mental status changes, depression, and suicidal ideation.

• Assess for bleeding and bruising.

• Institute infection-control measures. Monitor for signs and symptoms of infection.

Patient teaching

• Teach patient or caregiver how to prepare and give drug subcutaneously or I.M., rotate injection sites, and track dosing schedule and injection sites on calendar.

• Caution patient to avoid driving and other hazardous activities until he knows how drug affects concentration, alertness, and vision.

• Inform female patient that drug is linked to fetal abnormalities. Advise her not to get pregnant during therapy, and to use barrier contraception.

• Tell female patient not to breastfeed.

• Advise patient to avoid potential infection sources, such as crowds and people with known infections.

• Tell patient to eat small, frequent meals to combat nausea, vomiting, and loss of appetite.

• Inform male patient that drug may cause transient erectile dysfunction.

◀€ Instruct patient to immediately report depression, suicidal thoughts, mental status changes, signs or symptoms of infection (such as fever, chills, sore throat), unusual bleeding or bruising, dizziness, palpitations, or chest pain.

• Tell patient he'll need regular follow-up examinations and blood tests to gauge drug effects.

• As appropriate, review all other significant and life-threatening adverse reactions and interactions, especially those related to the drugs and tests mentioned above.

interferon alfacon-1
Infergen

Pharmacologic class: Biological response modifier
Therapeutic class: Antiviral
Pregnancy risk category C (monotherapy), X (with ribavirin)

FDA   BOXED WARNING

• Drug may cause or worsen fatal or life-threatening neuropsychiatric, autoimmune, ischemic, and infectious disorders. Monitor patient closely with periodic clinical and laboratory evaluations. Discontinue drug in patients with persistently severe or worsening signs or symptoms of these conditions. In many cases, these disorders resolve after withdrawal.

• If drug is used with ribavirin, birth defects or death of the fetus may occur. Female patients and female partners of male patients must take extreme care to avoid pregnancy. Ribavirin also causes hemolytic anemia, which may result in a worsening of cardiac disease. Ribavirin is genotoxic and mutagenic and should be considered a potential carcinogen.

Action
Binds to membrane receptors on viral cells, inducing protein synthesis, inhibiting viral replication, and suppressing cell proliferation. Increases phagocytosis, enhances expression of human leukocyte antigen, and augments lymphocyte cytotoxicity.

Availability
Injection: 9-mcg/0.3-ml vials, 15-mcg/0.5-ml vials

❶ Indications and dosages
➤ Chronic hepatitis C
Adults: Initially as monotherapy, 9 mcg subcutaneously as a single dose three times weekly for 24 weeks; for patients who tolerated previous interferon therapy and didn't respond or relapsed following its discontinuation, 15 mcg subcutaneously as a single injection three times weekly for up to 48 weeks. For combination therapy, 15 mcg subcutaneously daily as a single injection with weight-based ribavirin at 1,000 to 1,200 mg (less than 75 kg to 75 kg or more, respectively) P.O. daily in two divided doses for up to 48 weeks.

Dosage adjustment
• Hematologic toxicities
• Patients with depression
• Serious adverse reactions

Off-label uses
• Hairy cell leukemia

Contraindications
• Hypersensitivity to drug, its components, or ribavirin
• Hepatic decompensation (Child-Pugh score above 6), autoimmune hepatitis
• Patients with creatinine clearance below 50 ml/minute (combination therapy with ribavirin)
• Hemoglobinopathies, such as thalassemia major and sickle cell anemia (combination therapy with ribavirin)
• Pregnant patients and men whose female partners are pregnant (combination therapy with ribavirin)

Precautions
Use cautiously in:
• cardiac disease, severe psychiatric disorders, ischemic and hemorrhagic cerebrovascular events, pulmonary disorders, chronic hepatitis C infection with cirrhosis, renal insufficiency, colitis, pancreatitis, ophthalmologic disorders, endocrine disorders, any abnormal test values
• history of significant or unstable cardiac disease (avoid use)
• other autoimmune disorders
• abnormally low peripheral blood cell counts or concurrent use of agents known to cause myelosuppression
• combination therapy with ribavirin in patients with low baseline neutrophil count (less than 1,500/mm^3)
• transplant patients or other chronically immunosuppressed patients
• combination of interferon alfacon-1 and ribavirin in treatment-naïve patients or in patients co-infected with hepatitis B virus or HIV-1 (safety and efficacy not established)
• breastfeeding patients
• children age 18 and younger.

Administration
• Give by subcutaneous route only.
• Give antiemetics for nausea and vomiting, as needed and prescribed.

Route	Onset	Peak	Duration
Subcut.	Unknown	24-36 hr	Unknown

• Be aware that female patients must have a negative pregnancy test before starting combination therapy with ribavirin.

• Be aware that patients who have pre-existing cardiac abnormalities should have an ECG before starting treatment with interferon alfacon-1 and ribavirin combination.

• Be aware that laboratory tests are recommended for all patients before starting therapy. Entrance criteria that may be considered as a guideline to acceptable baseline values for initiation of treatment are shown below:

Test	Baseline value
Absolute neutrophil count	$\geq 1{,}500 \times 10^6/L$
Bilirubin	≤ 1.4 mg/dl (except patients with Gilbert's syndrome)
Hemoglobin concentration	≥ 10 g/dl
Platelet count	$\geq 75 \times 10^9/L$
Serum albumin concentration	≥ 25 g/L
Serum creatinine concentration	< 180 µmol/L (< 2 mg/dl) or creatinine clearance > 0.83 ml/second (> 50 ml/minute)
Thyroid-stimulating hormone, T_4	Within normal limits

Adverse reactions

CNS: dizziness, confusion, rigors, headache, emotional lability, hypoesthesia, paresthesia, lethargy, depression, difficulty thinking or concentrating, insomnia, anxiety, fatigue, amnesia, nervousness, drowsiness, asthenia, malaise, **suicidal ideation, stroke**
CV: chest pain, hypertension, palpitations, hypotension, tachycardia, angina pectoris, **cardiomyopathy, myocardial infarction, arrhythmias**
EENT: visual disturbances, stye, retinopathy including macular edema, retinal artery or vein thrombosis, retinal hemorrhages and cotton wool spots, optic neuritis, papilledema, retinal detachment, hearing disorders, nasal congestion, rhinitis, sinusitis, pharyngitis
GI: nausea, vomiting, diarrhea, constipation, abdominal pain, flatulence, eructation, stomatitis, dry mouth, anorexia, **intestinal obstruction, hemorrhagic and ischemic colitis, pancreatitis**
GU: impaired fertility in women, gynecomastia, erectile dysfunction, **renal failure**
Hematologic: anemia, **leukopenia, thrombocytopenia, neutropenia, severe cytopenias, hemolytic anemia**
Hepatic: hepatic decompensation
Metabolic: hyperglycemia, diabetes mellitus, hypothyroidism, hyperthyroidism
Musculoskeletal: joint pain, back pain, limb pain, neck pain, myalgia
Respiratory: cough, dyspnea, **pulmonary infiltrates, pneumonia, bronchiolitis obliterans, interstitial pneumonitis, pulmonary hypertension, sarcoidosis**
Skin: rash, dryness, pruritus, flushing, alopecia, candidiasis, dermatitis, diaphoresis
Other: gingivitis, flulike symptoms, edema, weight loss, fever, body pain, injection-site erythema, infections, hypersensitivity including urticaria, **autoimmune disorders, angioedema, bronchoconstriction, anaphylaxis**

Interactions

Drug-diagnostic tests. *Alkaline phosphatase, aspartate aminotransferase, bilirubin, creatinine, lactate dehydrogenase, neutralizing antibodies,*

serum creatinine, thyroid-stimulating hormone, triglycerides, uric acid: increased values
Granulocytes, hematocrit, hemoglobin, platelets, serum albumin, thyroxine white blood cells: decreased values

Patient monitoring

◀≋ Before and regularly during therapy, assess CBC with white cell differential and hepatitis C virus antibodies.

• Assess fluid intake and output. Keep patient well hydrated.

◀≋ Stay alert for depression, mental status changes, psychosis, and suicidal ideation (especially in patients with history of mental illness).

• Assess for bleeding and bruising.

• Institute infection-control measures. Monitor for signs and symptoms of infection.

• Watch for flulike symptoms.

◀≋ Monitor patient for hypersensitivity reactions; discontinue drug immediately and institute appropriate treatment if severe signs and symptoms (such as urticaria, angioedema, bronchoconstriction, or anaphylaxis) occur.

◀≋ Monitor patient for signs and symptoms of pancreatitis. Suspend treatment if signs and symptoms occur; discontinue treatment in patients diagnosed with pancreatitis.

◀≋ Closely watch for and discontinue treatment if patient develops persistent or unexplained pulmonary infiltrates or pulmonary function impairment. Be aware that respiratory failure has been observed with interferon rechallenge.

◀≋ Be aware that patients with chronic hepatitis C with cirrhosis may be at risk for hepatic decompensation when treated with this drug. Closely monitor hepatic function during treatment. Treatment should be immediately discontinued if signs and symptoms of hepatic decompensation, such as jaundice, ascites, coagulopathy, or decreased serum albumin, are observed.

• Monitor renal function (particularly increases in serum creatinine level) during therapy.

◀≋ Be aware that hemorrhagic and ischemic colitis, sometimes fatal, has been observed within 12 weeks of initiation of therapy. Discontinue drug immediately in patients who develop signs and symptoms of colitis.

◀≋ Be aware that development or exacerbation of autoimmune disorders (such as autoimmune thrombocytopenia, idiopathic thrombocytopenic purpura, psoriasis, rheumatoid arthritis, thyroiditis, interstitial nephritis, and systemic lupus erythematosus have occurred in patients receiving interferon alpha therapies.

• Monitor patients for vision impairment; be aware that patient who develop ocular signs and symptoms should receive a prompt and complete eye examination. Discontinue therapy in patients who develop new or worsening ophthalmologic disorders.

• For patients receiving combination therapy, discontinue ribavirin in patients who temporarily or permanently discontinue interferon alfacon-1.

Patient teaching

• Teach patient or caregiver how to administer drug subcutaneously, rotate injection sites, and track dosing schedule and injection sites on calendar.

• Advise patient to avoid sources of potential infection, such as crowds and people with known infections.

• Caution patient to avoid driving and other hazardous activities until he knows how drug affects concentration, alertness, and vision.

• Tell female patient that drug is linked to fetal abnormalities. Advise her not to get pregnant during therapy, and to use barrier contraception.

■€ Instruct patient to immediately report signs and symptoms of infection, unusual bleeding or bruising, mental status changes, dizziness, palpitations, vision impairment, diarrhea, abdominal pain, respiratory signs and symptoms, rash, hives, or new or worsening symptoms.

• Tell patient he'll need regular follow-up examinations and blood tests to gauge drug effects.

• As appropriate, review all other significant and life-threatening adverse reactions and interactions, especially those related to the drugs and tests mentioned above.

interferon beta-1a
Avonex, Rebif

interferon beta-1b
Betaferon⊕, Betaseron, Extavia

Pharmacologic class: Biological response modifier
Therapeutic class: Antiviral, immunoregulator
Pregnancy risk category C

Action
Binds and competes with specific receptors on cell surface, inducing various interferon-induced gene products. Also inhibits proliferation of T cells.

Availability
Lyophilized powder for injection (beta-1a): 22 mcg (6 million international units; Rebif), 33 mcg (6.6 million international units; Avonex), 44 mcg (12 million international units; Rebif)
Lyophilized powder for injection (beta-1b): 0.3 mg in glass, single-use, 3-ml vial

Powder for injection (beta-1b): 0.3 mg (9.6 million international units; Betaseron)
Prefilled syringes (beta-1a): 30 mcg/ 0.5 ml (Avonex)

⚕ Indications and dosages
➤ To reduce frequency of exacerbations in relapsing-remitting multiple sclerosis
Adults ages 18 and older: 8.8 mcg Rebif subcutaneously three times weekly, increased over a 4-week period to 44 mcg three times weekly. Or 30 mcg Avonex I.M. once a week. Or 8 million international units (0.25 mg) Betaseron subcutaneously every other day. Or initially, 0.0625 mg (0.25 ml) (Extavia) subcutaneously every other day, increased over 6 weeks to 0.25 mg (1 ml) every other day.

Contraindications
• Hypersensitivity to drug, its components, or albumin

Precautions
Use cautiously in:
• cardiac disease, seizure disorders, mental disorders, depression, suicidal tendencies
• women of childbearing age
• pregnant or breastfeeding patients
• children ages 18 and younger.

Administration
• Reconstitute Avonex (I.M. injection) and Rebif (subcutaneous injection) using diluent provided, according to instructions provided.
• Reconstitute Betaseron (subcutaneous injection) using 1.2 ml of diluent supplied by manufacturer, to yield a concentration of 0.25 mg/ml. Swirl gently to mix; don't shake. Use reconstituted drug within 3 hours; discard unused portion.
• Reconstitute Extavia (subcutaneous injection) by attaching prefilled, single-use syringe containing 1.2 ml of diluent supplied by manufacturer to vial

using vial adapter. Slowly inject 1.2 ml of diluent into vial to yield a concentration of 0.25 mg/ml. Swirl gently to mix; don't shake. Use reconstituted drug within 3 hours; discard unused portion.

Route	Onset	Peak	Duration
I.M.	Unknown	Unknown	Unknown
Subcut.	Unknown	1-8 hr	Unknown

Adverse reactions

CNS: dizziness, confusion, rigors, paresthesia, lethargy, depression, difficulty thinking or concentrating, insomnia, anxiety, fatigue, amnesia, nervousness, drowsiness, asthenia, malaise, **suicidal ideation**

CV: chest pain, hypertension, palpitations, **arrhythmias**

EENT: visual disturbances, stye, hearing disorders, nasal congestion, sinusitis, rhinitis, pharyngitis

GI: nausea, vomiting, diarrhea, constipation, abdominal pain, dyspepsia, flatulence, eructation, stomatitis, dry mouth, **intestinal obstruction**

GU: gynecomastia, breast pain, early or delayed menses, menstrual bleeding or spotting, shortened duration of menstrual flow, menorrhagia

Hematologic: anemia, **neutropenia, leukopenia, thrombocytopenia**

Metabolic: hypocalcemia

Musculoskeletal: joint pain, back pain, myalgia, myasthenia

Respiratory: cough, dyspnea

Skin: rash, dry skin, pruritus, flushing, alopecia, dermatitis, diaphoresis

Other: gingivitis, flulike symptoms, weight loss, edema, candidiasis, lymphadenopathy, inflammation, pain

Interactions

Drug-diagnostic tests. *Alanine aminotransferase, alkaline phosphatase, aspartate aminotransferase, bilirubin, blood urea nitrogen, creatinine, glucose, lactate dehydrogenase, neutralizing antibodies, phosphorus, uric acid:* increased values *Hemoglobin, neutrophils, white blood cells:* decreased values

Patient monitoring

◀€ Before therapy and monthly during therapy, assess CBC with white cell differential, glucose and electrolyte levels, and liver and kidney function tests.

• Assess fluid intake and output. Keep patient well hydrated.

• Watch for GI upset. Provide small, frequent meals to minimize nausea and vomiting.

◀€ Monitor for mental status changes, depression, and suicidal ideation.

• Evaluate for bleeding and bruising.

• Institute infection-control measures. Monitor for infection symptoms.

Patient teaching

• Teach patient or caregiver how to administer drug subcutaneously or I.M., rotate injection sites, and track dosing schedule and injection sites on calendar.

• Advise patient to avoid sources of potential infection, such as crowds and people with known infections.

• Tell patient to eat small, frequent meals to combat nausea, vomiting, and appetite loss.

• Caution patient to avoid driving and other hazardous activities until he knows how drug affects concentration, alertness, and vision.

◀€ Tell patient to contact prescriber immediately if depression or suicidal ideation occurs.

• Inform female patient that drug is linked to fetal abnormalities. Advise her not to get pregnant during therapy, and to use barrier contraception. Tell her to consult prescriber before breastfeeding.

◀€ Instruct patient to immediately report signs or symptoms of infection (such as fever, chills, sore throat, achiness), unusual bleeding or bruising,

mental status changes, dizziness, palpitations, or chest pain.
• Tell patient he'll need regular follow-up examinations and blood tests to monitor drug effects.
• As appropriate, review all other significant and life-threatening adverse reactions and interactions, especially those related to the tests mentioned above.

interferon gamma-1b
Actimmune, Immukin🍁

Pharmacologic class: Biological response modifier
Therapeutic class: Antineoplastic
Pregnancy risk category C

Action
Enhances cellular toxicity and killer cell activity and promotes generation of oxygen metabolites in phagocytes, resulting in destruction of microorganisms.

Availability
Injection: 100 mcg (2 million international units)/0.5-ml vial

🕖 Indications and dosages
➤ Chronic granulomatous disease; severe malignant osteoperosis
Adults with body surface area (BSA) above 0.5 m²: 50 mcg/m² (1 million international units/m²) subcutaneously three times weekly
Adults with BSA of 0.5 m² or less: 1.5 mcg/kg subcutaneously three times weekly in deltoid or anterior thigh

Contraindications
• Hypersensitivity to drug, its components, or *Escherichia coli*–derived products

Precautions
Use cautiously in:
• thyroid disorders, bone marrow depression, hepatic or cardiac disease, seizure disorders, compromised CNS function
• pregnant or breastfeeding patients
• children ages 18 and younger.

Administration
• Administer into deltoid muscle by subcutaneous route only.
• Give at bedtime if flulike symptoms occur.
• Provide antiemetics to ease nausea and vomiting, as prescribed.

Route	Onset	Peak	Duration
Subcut.	Unknown	7 hr	Unknown

Adverse reactions
CNS: dizziness, confusion, paresthesia, lethargy, depression, difficulty thinking or concentrating, insomnia, anxiety, fatigue, amnesia, nervousness, drowsiness, asthenia, malaise
CV: chest pain, hypertension, palpitations, **arrhythmias**
GI: nausea, vomiting, diarrhea, constipation, abdominal pain, **pancreatitis**
GU: proteinuria
Hematologic: anemia, **leukopenia, thrombocytopenia, neutropenia**
Musculoskeletal: joint pain, back pain, myalgia
Skin: flushing, rash, dry skin, erythema
Other: flulike symptoms, weight loss, edema, hypersensitivity reaction

Interactions
Drug-drug. *Bone marrow depressants:* increased bone marrow depression
Zidovudine: increased zidovudine blood level
Drug-diagnostic tests. *Hepatic enzymes:* increased levels
Neutrophils, platelets: decreased counts

Patient monitoring

◀≋ Before and monthly during therapy, assess CBC with white cell differential, glucose and electrolyte levels, and liver and kidney function tests.

• Assess fluid intake and output. Keep patient well hydrated.

• Monitor for GI upset. Provide small, frequent meals or antiemetics to ease severe nausea and vomiting.

◀≋ Monitor patient for mental status changes and depression.

• Assess for flulike symptoms. If these occur, give drug at bedtime and provide supportive care, such as rest and acetaminophen for headache and fever.

Patient teaching

• Teach patient or caregiver how to administer drug subcutaneously, rotate injection sites, and track dosing schedule and injection sites on calendar.

◀≋ Tell patient to contact prescriber immediately if depression occurs.

• Advise patient to eat small, frequent meals to combat nausea, vomiting, and appetite loss.

• Caution patient to avoid driving and other hazardous activities until he knows how drug affects concentration and alertness.

• Inform female patient that drug is linked to fetal abnormalities. Advise her not to get pregnant during therapy, and to use barrier contraception.

• Tell female patient to consult prescriber before breastfeeding.

• Tell patient he'll need regular follow-up examinations and blood tests to monitor drug effects.

• As appropriate, review all other significant and life-threatening adverse reactions and interactions, especially those related to the drugs and tests mentioned above.

irbesartan

Aprovel✙, Avapro

Pharmacologic class: Angiotensin II receptor antagonist

Therapeutic class: Antihypertensive

Pregnancy risk category D

FDA | BOXED WARNING

• When used during second or third trimester of pregnancy, drug may cause fetal injury and even death. Discontinue as soon as pregnancy is detected.

Action

Blocks aldosterone-secreting and potent vasoconstrictive effects of angiotensin II at tissue receptor sites, which reduces vasoconstriction and lowers blood pressure

Availability

Tablets: 75 mg, 150 mg, 300 mg

⚡ Indications and dosages

➤ Hypertension

Adults: 150 mg/day P.O.; may increase to 300 mg/day

➤ Nephropathy in patients with type 2 diabetes and hypertension

Adults: 300 mg P.O. once daily

Dosage adjustment

• Volume-depleted or hemodialysis patients receiving diuretics

Contraindications

• Hypersensitivity to drug or its components

Precautions

Use cautiously in:

• heart failure, volume or sodium depletion, renal disease, hepatic impairment

- black patients
- females of childbearing age
- pregnant or breastfeeding patients
- children ages 18 and younger (safety not established).

Administration

- Administer with or without food.
- Know that drug may be given with other antihypertensive drugs.

Route	Onset	Peak	Duration
P.O.	Unknown	Within 2 hr	24 hr

Adverse reactions

CNS: dizziness, fatigue, headache, syncope
CV: orthostatic hypotension, chest pain, peripheral edema
EENT: conjunctivitis, vision disturbance, ear pain, sinus disorders
GI: nausea, diarrhea, constipation, abdominal pain, dry mouth
GU: albuminuria, **renal failure**
Metabolic: gout, **hyperkalemia**
Musculoskeletal: joint pain, back pain, muscle weakness
Respiratory: upper respiratory tract infection, cough, bronchitis
Other: dental pain

Interactions

Drug-drug. *Diuretics, other antihypertensives:* increased risk of hypotension
Lithium: increased lithium blood level
Nonsteroidal anti-inflammatory drugs: decreased antihypertensive effects
Potassium-sparing diuretics, potassium supplements: increased risk of hyperkalemia
Drug-diagnostic tests. *Albumin:* increased level
Drug-food. *Salt substitutes containing potassium:* increased risk of hyperkalemia

Patient monitoring

- Monitor vital signs, especially blood pressure.
- Watch for signs and symptoms of orthostatic hypotension.

- Watch blood pressure closely when volume depletion may cause hypotension (as in diaphoresis, nausea, vomiting, diarrhea, and postoperative period).
- Assess fluid intake and output. Keep patient well hydrated, especially if he's receiving diuretics concurrently.
- Monitor blood urea nitrogen and creatinine levels.

Patient teaching

- Tell patient he may take with or without food.
- Instruct patient to change position slowly and to stay well hydrated, to minimize blood pressure decrease when rising.
- Caution patient to avoid driving and other hazardous activities until he knows how drug affects concentration and alertness.
- Tell female patient that drug has been linked to fetal injury and deaths. Caution her not to get pregnant during therapy. Advise her to use barrier contraception.
- Instruct female patient to report pregnancy.
- Instruct patient to report fever, chills, dizziness, severe vomiting, diarrhea, and dehydration.
- As appropriate, review all other significant and life-threatening adverse reactions and interactions, especially those related to the drugs, tests, and foods mentioned above.

irinotecan hydrochloride
Campto ✦, Camptosar

Pharmacologic class: Topoisomerase inhibitor
Therapeutic class: Hormonal antineoplastic
Pregnancy risk category D

FDA | BOXED WARNING

- Give under supervision of physician experienced in using cancer chemotherapy, in facility with adequate diagnostic and treatment resources.
- Drug can cause both early and late forms of diarrhea that may be severe. Early diarrhea (arising during or shortly after drug infusion) may be accompanied by cholinergic symptoms of rhinitis, increased salivation, miosis, lacrimation, diaphoresis, flushing, and intestinal hyperperistalsis that can cause abdominal cramping. Atropine may prevent or relieve such symptoms. Late diarrhea (generally arising more than 24 hours after administration) can be life-threatening and prolonged, and may lead to dehydration, electrolyte imbalance, or sepsis. For late diarrhea, give loperamide promptly. Carefully monitor patients with diarrhea and provide fluid and electrolyte replacement if they become dehydrated or antibiotic therapy if they develop ileus, fever, or severe neutropenia. Interrupt administration of irinotecan and reduce subsequent doses if severe diarrhea occurs.
- Drug may cause severe myelosuppression.

Action

Inhibits topoisomerase 1 (an enzyme that allows DNA replication) by binding to it. This action prevents religation of DNA strand, which results in breakage of double-stranded DNA and cell death.

Availability

Injection: 20 mg/ml in 2-ml and 5-ml vials

⦸ Indications and dosages

➢ Metastatic colorectal cancer or recurrence or progression of metastatic colorectal cancer after fluorouracil (5-FU) therapy

Adults: 125 mg/m² I.V. infused over 90 minutes on days 1, 8, 15, and 22, followed by a 2-week rest; given with leucovorin and 5-FU. Or, 180 mg/m² I.V. infused over 90 minutes on days 1, 15, and 29 with leucovorin, 5-FU bolus, and 5-FU infusion followed by a 2-week rest. Or as monotherapy, 125 mg/m² I.V. infused over 90 minutes weekly for 4 weeks, followed by a 2-week rest period; or, 350 mg/m² I.V. infused over 90 minutes q 3 weeks as long as tolerable. Adjust dosage in increments based on tolerance and age.

Off-label uses

- Most cancers

Contraindications

- Hypersensitivity to drug
- Concurrent atazanavir use
- Pregnancy or breastfeeding

Precautions

Use cautiously in:
- bone marrow depression, severe diarrhea
- patients undergoing radiation therapy
- elderly patients
- children.

Administration

◀€ Follow facility policy for handling antineoplastics. If skin contact occurs, wash with soap and water immediately and thoroughly. If mucous membrane contact occurs, flush with water.
- Dilute in dextrose 5% in water or normal saline solution, to a concentration of 0.12 to 1.1 mg/ml.
- Infuse within 6 hours if drug is stored at room temperature or within 24 hours if refrigerated.
- Give single dose by I.V. infusion over 90 minutes.
- Administer antiemetic to ease nausea and vomiting, as needed and prescribed.

Route	Onset	Peak	Duration
I.V.	Immediate	1-2 hr	Unknown

Adverse reactions

CNS: insomnia, dizziness, asthenia, headache, akathisia

CV: vasodilation, orthostatic hypotension

EENT: rhinitis

GI: nausea, vomiting, constipation, diarrhea, flatulence, dyspepsia, abdominal pain or enlargement, stomatitis, anorexia

Hematologic: anemia, **neutropenia, leukopenia, thrombocytopenia**

Hepatic: hepatotoxicity

Metabolic: dehydration

Musculoskeletal: back pain

Respiratory: dyspnea, increased cough

Skin: alopecia, diaphoresis, rash

Other: weight loss, edema, fever, pain, chills, minor infections

Interactions

Drug-drug. *Dexamethasone:* increased risk of lymphocytopenia

Diuretics: increased risk of dehydration

Laxatives: increased risk of diarrhea

Other antineoplastics: additive adverse effects

Drug-diagnostic tests. *Alkaline phosphatase:* increased level

Hemoglobin, neutrophils, white blood cells: decreased values

Patient monitoring

◀≷ Assess CBC before each infusion. Withhold dose if neutrophil count is below 1,500 cells/mm³.

• Monitor infusion site for extravasation; if it occurs, flush with sterile water and apply ice.

• Assess fluid intake and output. Keep patient well hydrated.

• Monitor oral intake. Evaluate for nausea and vomiting.

• Assess for diarrhea. In severe diarrhea, expect to decrease dosage or withhold dose.

• Institute infection-control protocols to help prevent infection.

• Monitor liver function test results.

Patient teaching

• Inform patient that blood tests will be done before each dose.

• Instruct patient to report pain at infusion site; severe nausea or vomiting; severe, increased, or bloody diarrhea; infection; or injury.

◀≷ Instruct patient to immediately report unusual tiredness or yellowing of skin or eyes.

• Tell patient that drug increases his risk of infection. Advise him to avoid crowds and other potential infection sources.

• Caution female patient not to breastfeed or become pregnant during therapy. Recommend barrier contraception.

• As appropriate, review all other significant and life-threatening adverse reactions and interactions, especially those related to the drugs and tests mentioned above.

iron dextran
Cosmofer⊕, DexFerrum, InFeD

Pharmacologic class: Trace element
Therapeutic class: Iron supplement
Pregnancy risk category C

FDA │ BOXED WARNING

• Parenteral use has caused anaphylactic-type reactions, some resulting in death. Use only in patients with clearly established indications when laboratory tests confirm iron deficiency not amenable to oral iron therapy. Give drug only where resuscitation techniques and treatment of anaphylactic and anaphylactoid shock are readily available.

Reactions in **bold** are life-threatening.   ◀≷ Clinical alert

Action
Replenishes depleted stores of iron (a component of hemoglobin) in bone marrow

Availability
Injection: 50 mg/ml

🔷 Indications and dosages
➤ Iron-deficiency anemia in patients who can't tolerate oral iron
Adults and children weighing more than 15 kg (33 lb): Dosage individualized based on patient's weight and hemoglobin (Hgb) value, using the following formula: Dosage (ml) = 0.0442 (desired Hgb minus patient's Hgb) times lean body weight (LBW) plus the product of 0.26 times LBW

Give test dose before starting I.V. or I.M. therapy: For I.V. use, administer test dose of 0.5 ml (25 mg) I.V. over 30 seconds to 5 minutes; if no reactions occur within 1 hour, give remainder of therapeutic dose I.V.; repeat this dose daily. For I.M. use, give test dose of 0.5 ml (25 mg) by Z-track method; if no reactions occur, give daily doses not exceeding 100 mg I.M. in adults, 50 mg I.M. in children weighing more than 10 kg (22 lb), or 25 mg in infants weighing less than 5 kg (11 lb).
➤ Iron replacement caused by blood loss
Adults: Dosage individualized based on the following formula: Replacement iron (in mg) = blood loss (in ml) times hematocrit

Contraindications
• Hypersensitivity to drug, alcohol, tartrazine, or sulfites
• Acute phase of infectious renal disease or hemolytic anemia

Precautions
Use cautiously in:
• autoimmune disorders, arthritis, severe hepatic impairment
• elderly patients
• breastfeeding patients
• children.

Administration
• For I.M. administration, inject by Z-track method into upper outer quadrant of gluteal muscle.
• For intermittent I.V. infusion, administer undiluted at a rate no faster than 1 ml/minute.
• Don't give with oral iron preparations.

Route	Onset	Peak	Duration
I.V., I.M.	4 days	1-2 wk	Wks-mos

Adverse reactions
CNS: dizziness, headache, syncope, **seizures**
CV: chest pain, tachycardia, hypotension
GI: nausea, vomiting
Hematologic: hemochromatosis, hemolysis, **hemosiderosis**
Musculoskeletal: joint pain, myalgia
Respiratory: dyspnea
Other: abnormal or metallic taste, tooth discoloration, fever, lymphadenopathy, hypersensitivity reactions including **anaphylaxis**

Interactions
None significant

Patient monitoring
🔊 Monitor for hypersensitivity reaction. Keep epinephrine and other emergency supplies on hand in case reaction occurs.
• Assess serum ferritin levels regularly, because these levels correlate with iron stores.
• In patients with rheumatoid arthritis, monitor for acute exacerbation of joint pain and swelling. Provide appropriate comfort measures.
• Watch for signs and symptoms of iron overload, including decreased activity, sedation, and GI or respiratory tract bleeding.

Patient teaching
• Caution patient not to take oral iron preparations or vitamins containing iron during therapy.
• Instruct patient to report difficulty breathing, itching, or rash.
• Tell patient he'll undergo periodic blood testing to monitor his response to therapy.
• As appropriate, review all other significant and life-threatening adverse reactions mentioned above.

iron sucrose
Venofer

Pharmacologic class: Trace element
Therapeutic class: Iron supplement
Pregnancy risk category B

Action
Replenishes depleted stores of iron (a component of hemoglobin) in bone marrow

Availability
Aqueous complex for injection: 20 mg elemental iron/ml in 5-ml single-use vials (100 mg of elemental iron)

⊘ Indications and dosages
➤ Iron-deficiency anemia in hemodialysis patients concurrently receiving erythropoietin
Adults: 100 mg of elemental iron (5 ml) I.V. directly into dialysis line or by slow injection or infusion during dialysis session (up to three times weekly) for 10 doses (total of 1,000 mg)

Off-label uses
• Autologous blood donation
• Bloodless surgery

Contraindications
• Hypersensitivity to drug, alcohol, tartrazine, or sulfites
• Hemolytic anemias and other anemias not caused by iron deficiency
• Primary hemochromatosis

Precautions
Use cautiously in:
• autoimmune disorders, arthritis, severe hepatic impairment
• elderly patients
• breastfeeding patients
• children.

Administration
• Give test dose only if ordered: 50 mg (2.5 ml) I.V. over 3 to 10 minutes.
• Dilute 100 mg of elemental iron in no more than 100 ml of normal saline solution; infuse slowly I.V. over at least 15 minutes.
• Administer I.V. directly into dialysis line or by infusion at 20 mg/minute, not to exceed 100 mg/injection.
• Don't give with oral iron preparations.

Route	Onset	Peak	Duration
I.V.	4 days	1-2 wk	Wks-mos

Adverse reactions
CNS: dizziness, headache, syncope, **seizures**
CV: chest pain, tachycardia, hypotension
GI: nausea, vomiting
Hematologic: hemochromatosis, hemolysis, **hemosiderosis**
Musculoskeletal: muscle cramps, aches, or weakness; joint pain
Respiratory: dyspnea
Other: abnormal or metallic taste, tooth discoloration, fever, lymphadenopathy, allergic reactions including **anaphylaxis**

Interactions
None significant

◀€ Clinical alert

Patient monitoring

◀€ Monitor for hypersensitivity reaction. Keep epinephrine and other emergency supplies available in case reaction occurs.

• Assess hemoglobin, hematocrit, serum ferritin, and transferrin saturation levels before, during, and after therapy.

◀€ Monitor blood pressure. Stay alert for hypotension.

• Watch for signs and symptoms of iron overload, such as decreased activity, sedation, and GI or respiratory tract bleeding.

Patient teaching

• Caution patient not to take oral iron preparations or vitamin supplements containing iron during therapy.

• Instruct patient to report dyspnea, itching, or rash.

• Tell patient he'll undergo periodic blood testing to monitor his response to therapy.

• As appropriate, review all other significant and life-threatening adverse reactions mentioned above.

isoniazid (INH)

Dom-Isoniazid♣, Isotamine♣, PMS Isoniazid♣, Rifater⊕, Rifinah⊕, Rimactazid⊕

Pharmacologic class: Isonicotinic acid hydrazide

Therapeutic class: Antitubercular

Pregnancy risk category C

FDA | BOXED WARNING

• Severe and sometimes fatal hepatitis has occurred, even after many months of treatment. Risk increases with age until 64, then decreases after age 65.

Risk also rises with daily alcohol consumption. Monitor patients carefully and interview them monthly. For persons aged 35 and older, also measure liver enzymes before therapy starts and periodically throughout. Isoniazid-associated hepatitis usually arises during first 3 months of therapy. Hepatitis risk also increases with daily alcohol use, chronic hepatic disease, and injection drug use. Recent report suggests increased risk of fatal hepatitis among women; risk also may increase during postpartum period. If adverse effects or signs and symptoms of hepatic damage occur, discontinue drug promptly.

• Tuberculosis patients with isoniazid-associated hepatitis should receive appropriate treatment with alternative drugs. If isoniazid must be restarted, do so only after symptoms and laboratory abnormalities resolve. Restart in small and gradually increasing doses, and withdraw drug immediately at any indication of recurrent liver involvement. Defer preventive treatment in patients with acute hepatic disease.

Action

Inhibits cell-wall biosynthesis by interfering with lipid and nucleic acid DNA synthesis in tubercle bacilli cells

Availability

Injection: 100 mg/ml
Syrup: 50 mg/5 ml
Tablets: 100 mg, 300 mg

🖊️ Indications and dosages

➤ Active tuberculosis (TB)

Adults: 5 mg/kg P.O. or I.M. (maximum of 300 mg/day) daily as a single dose, or 15 mg/kg (maximum of 900 mg/day) two to three times weekly; given with other agents

Children: 10 to 15 mg/kg P.O. or I.M. (maximum of 300 mg/day) daily as a single dose, or 20 to 40 mg/kg (maximum of 900 mg/day) two to three times weekly

➣ To prevent TB in patients exposed to active disease

Adults: 300 mg P.O. daily as a single dose for 6 to 12 months

Children and infants: 10 mg/kg P.O. daily as a single dose for up to 12 months

Off-label uses

• *Mycobacterium kansasii* infection

Contraindications

• Hypersensitivity to drug
• Acute hepatic disease or previous hepatitis caused by isoniazid therapy

Precautions

Use cautiously in:
• severe renal impairment, diabetes, diabetic retinopathy, ocular defects, chronic alcoholism, hepatic damage
• Black or Hispanic women
• pregnant or breastfeeding patients
• children ages 13 and younger.

Administration

• Give on empty stomach 1 hour before or 2 hours after meals. If GI upset occurs, administer with food.
• Administer parenterally only if patient can't receive oral form.
• Use cautiously in diabetic or alcoholic patients and those at risk for neuropathy.

Route	Onset	Peak	Duration
P.O., I.M.	Rapid	1-2 hr	Up to 24 hr

Adverse reactions

CNS: peripheral neuropathy, dizziness, memory impairment, slurred speech, psychosis, **toxic encephalopathy, seizures**

EENT: visual disturbances

GI: nausea, vomiting

GU: gynecomastia

Hematologic: eosinophilia, **methemoglobinemia, hemolytic anemia,** **aplastic anemia, agranulocytosis, thrombocytopenia**

Hepatic: hepatitis

Metabolic: pyridoxine deficiency, hyperglycemia, **metabolic acidosis**

Respiratory: dyspnea

Other: fever, pellagra, lupuslike syndrome, injection site irritation, hypersensitivity reaction

Interactions

Drug-drug. *Aluminum-containing antacids:* decreased isoniazid absorption

Bacille Calmette-Guérin vaccine: ineffective vaccination

Carbamazepine: increased carbamazepine blood level

Disulfiram: psychotic reactions, incoordination

Hepatotoxic drugs: increased risk of hepatotoxicity

Ketoconazole: decreased ketoconazole blood level and efficacy

Other antituberculars: additive CNS toxicity

Phenytoin: inhibition of phenytoin metabolism

Drug-diagnostic tests. *Albumin:* increased level

Drug-food. *Foods containing tyramine:* hypertensive crisis, other severe reactions

Drug-behaviors. *Alcohol use:* increased risk of hepatitis

Patient monitoring

• Assess hepatic enzyme levels.
• Watch for adverse reactions, such as peripheral neuropathy.

Patient teaching

• Advise patient to take once daily on empty stomach, 1 hour before or 2 hours after meals. If GI upset occurs, tell him to take with small amount of food.
• Caution patient to avoid foods containing tyramine (such as cheese, fish, salami, red wine, and yeast extracts), because drug-food interaction may cause chills, diaphoresis, and palpitations.

i

• Teach patient with peripheral neuropathy to take care to prevent burns and other injuries.
• Instruct patient to report anorexia, nausea, vomiting, jaundice, dark urine, and numbness or tingling of hands or feet.
• Tell patient he'll need periodic medical and eye examinations and blood tests to gauge drug effects.
• As appropriate, review all other significant and life-threatening adverse reactions and interactions, especially those related to the drugs, tests, foods, and behaviors mentioned above.

---

isoproterenol hydrochloride
Isuprel

Pharmacologic class: Sympathomimetic, beta$_1$-adrenergic and beta$_2$-adrenergic agonist
Therapeutic class: Vasopressor, bronchodilator, antiasthmatic
Pregnancy risk category C

Action
Acts on beta$_2$-adrenergic receptors, causing relaxation of bronchial smooth muscle; acts on beta$_1$-adrenergic receptors in heart, causing positive inotropic and chronotropic effects and increasing cardiac output. Also lowers peripheral vascular resistance in skeletal muscle and inhibits antigen-induced histamine release.

Availability
Injection: 20 mcg/ml, 200 mcg/ml

⚠ Indications and dosages
➤ Shock
Adults and children: 0.5 to 5 mcg/minute by continuous I.V. infusion

➤ Heart block; ventricular arrhythmias
Adults: Initially, 0.02 to 0.06 mg I.V., then 0.01 to 0.2 mg I.V. or 5 mcg/minute I.V. Or initially, 0.2 mg I.M., then 0.02 to 1 mg I.M., depending on response. Or initially, 0.2 mg subcutaneously, then 0.15 to 0.2 mg subcutaneously, depending on response.
➤ Bronchospasm during anesthesia
Adults: 0.01 to 0.02 mg I.V., repeated when necessary

Contraindications
• Angina pectoris
• Angle-closure glaucoma
• Tachyarrhythmias
• Tachycardia or heart block caused by digitalis intoxication
• Ventricular arrhythmias that warrant inotropic therapy
• Labor, delivery, breastfeeding

Precautions
Use cautiously in:
• renal impairment, unstable vasomotor disorders, hypertension, coronary insufficiency, chronic obstructive pulmonary disease, diabetes mellitus, hyperthyroidism
• history of cerebrovascular accident or seizures
• elderly patients.

Administration
• Give each 0.02-mg I.V. dose by direct injection over 1 minute, or by I.V. infusion, as ordered. Always use continuous infusion pump to deliver infusion.

Route	Onset	Peak	Duration
I.V.	Immediate	Unknown	<1 hr
I.M.	Unknown	Unknown	Unknown
Subcut.	Immediate	Unknown	2 hr

Adverse reactions
CNS: tremors, anxiety, insomnia, headache, dizziness, asthenia, nervousness

---

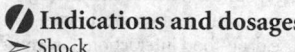

CV: palpitations, tachycardia, angina, rapid blood pressure changes, **arrhythmias, cardiac arrest, Stokes-Adams attacks**
EENT: pharyngitis, visual blurring
GI: nausea, vomiting, heartburn
Metabolic: hyperglycemia
Respiratory: bronchitis, dyspnea, increased sputum, **pulmonary edema, bronchospasm**
Skin: diaphoresis
Other: parotid gland swelling (with prolonged use), pallor

Interactions
Drug-drug. *Cyclopropane, epinephrine, halogenated general anesthetics:* increased risk of arrhythmias
Propranolol, other beta-adrenergic blockers: antagonism of bronchodilating effects
Drug-diagnostic tests. *Glucose:* increased level

Patient monitoring
• During I.V. administration, monitor ECG and vital signs carefully.
• Assess patient's response to drug and adjust I.V. infusion rate accordingly.
• Closely monitor arterial blood gas values, urine output, and central venous pressure.
◀€ Stay alert for rebound bronchospasm.

Patient teaching
• Assure patient that he'll be monitored closely.

isosorbide dinitrate
Angitak ⊕, Apo-ISDN ✤, Cedocard ⊕, Cedocard-SR ✤, Dilatrate-SR, Isochron, Isoket ⊕, Isordil Titradose, Novo-Sorbide ✤, PMS-Isosorbide ✤, Soni-Slo SR, Sorbid

isosorbide mononitrate
Angeze ⊕, Chemydur ⊕, Cibral ⊕, Cibral XL ⊕, Dynamin ⊕, Dynamin XL ⊕, Elantan ⊕, Elantan LA ⊕, Imazin XL ⊕, Imdur ⊕, Imo LA ⊕, Isib ⊕, ISMO, Isodur ⊕, Ketanodur ⊕, Modisal ⊕, Monigen ⊕, Monigen XL ⊕, Monit ⊕, Monit LS ⊕, Monoket, Monomax ⊕, Monomax SR ⊕, Monomax XL ⊕, Monomil ⊕, Monosorb ⊕, Trangina ⊕, Trangina XL ⊕, Xismox ⊕, Zemon ⊕, Zemon XL ⊕

Pharmacologic class: Nitrate
Therapeutic class: Antianginal
Pregnancy risk category C

Action
Promotes peripheral vasodilation and reduces preload and afterload, decreasing myocardial oxygen consumption and increasing cardiac output. Also dilates coronary arteries, increasing blood flow and improving collateral circulation.

Availability
isosorbide dinitrate
Capsules: 40 mg
Capsules (extended-release): 40 mg
Tablets: 2.5 mg, 5 mg, 10 mg, 20 mg, 30 mg, 40 mg
Tablets (chewable): 5 mg, 10 mg
Tablets (extended-release): 20 mg, 40 mg
Tablets (sublingual): 2.5 mg, 5 mg, 10 mg
isosorbide mononitrate
Tablets: 10 mg, 20 mg
Tablets (extended-release): 30 mg, 60 mg, 120 mg

⒤ Indications and dosages
➤ Treatment and prophylaxis in situations likely to provoke acute angina pectoris
Adults: 2.5 to 5 mg S.L. May repeat dose q 5 to 10 minutes for a total of three doses in 15 to 30 minutes.

Reactions in **bold** are life-threatening.   ◀€ Clinical alert

➤ Prophylaxis of angina pectoris
Adults: 5 to 40 mg P.O. (dinitrate conventional tablets) two to three times daily. Or 5 to 20 mg (mononitrate conventional tablets) b.i.d. Or 30 to 60 mg (mononitrate extended-release tablets) once daily. After several days, dosage may be increased to 120 mg (given as single 120-mg tablet or two 60-mg tablets) once daily. Rarely, 240 mg/day (mononitrate extended-release tablets) may be needed.

Off-label uses
- Heart failure

Contraindications
- Hypersensitivity to drug
- Severe anemia
- Acute myocardial infarction
- Angle-closure glaucoma
- Concurrent sildenafil therapy

Precautions
Use cautiously in:
- head trauma, volume depletion
- elderly patients
- pregnant or breastfeeding patients
- children.

Administration
- Give oral form 30 minutes before or 1 to 2 hours after a meal. Make sure patient swallows tablets or capsules whole.
- Have patient wet S.L. tablet with saliva before placing it under tongue. To avoid tingling sensation, have him place tablet in buccal pouch.

Route	Onset	Peak	Duration
P.O. (dinitrate)	15-40 min	Unknown	4 hr
P.O. (dinitrate, extended)	30 min	Unknown	≤12 hr
P.O. (mononitrate)	30-60 min	Unknown	7 hr
P.O. (mononitrate, extended)	Unknown	Unknown	12 hr
S.L. (dinitrate)	2-5 min	Unknown	1-2 hr

Adverse reactions
CNS: dizziness, headache, apprehension, asthenia, syncope
CV: orthostatic hypotension, tachycardia, paradoxical bradycardia, rebound hypertension
EENT: sublingual burning (with S.L. route)
GI: nausea, vomiting, dry mouth, abdominal pain
Skin: flushing

Interactions
Drug-drug. *Aspirin:* increased isosorbide blood level and effects
Beta-adrenergic blockers, calcium channel blockers, phenothiazines: additive hypotension
Dihydroergotamine: antagonism of dihydroergotamine effects
Sildenafil: severe and potentially fatal hypotension
Drug-diagnostic tests. *Cholesterol:* decreased level
Methemoglobin, urine vanillylmandelic acid: increased levels

Patient monitoring
- Monitor ECG and vital signs closely, especially blood pressure.
- 🔊 In suspected overdose, assess for signs and symptoms of increased intracranial pressure.
- Monitor arterial blood gas values and methemoglobin levels.

Patient teaching
- Teach patient to take oral drug 30 minutes before or 1 to 2 hours after a meal.
- Inform patient that drug may cause headache. Advise him to treat headache as usual and not to alter drug schedule. If headache persists, tell him to contact prescriber.
- Instruct patient to move slowly when sitting up or standing, to avoid dizziness or light-headedness from sudden blood pressure decrease.

• As appropriate, review all other significant adverse reactions and interactions, especially those related to the drugs and tests mentioned above.

isradipine
DynaCirc CR, Prescal ⊕

Pharmacologic class: Calcium channel blocker
Therapeutic class: Antihypertensive
Pregnancy risk category C

Action
Inhibits calcium ion movement across cell membranes of cardiac and arterial muscles, relaxing coronary and peripheral vascular smooth muscle. This action reduces diastolic blood pressure, enhances left ventricular function, and improves ejection rates; it also reduces mean vascular and systemic vascular resistance, increasing cardiac output and improving stroke volume.

Availability
Capsules: 2.5 mg, 5 mg
Tablets (controlled-release): 5 mg, 10 mg

⏀ Indications and dosages
➤ Hypertension
Adults: Initially, 2.5 mg P.O. b.i.d. as monotherapy or combined with a thiazide diuretic (regular-release capsules); may increase in increments of 5 mg/day at 2- to 4-week intervals, to a maximum of 20 mg/day. Or, 5 to 10 mg P.O. (controlled-release) daily as monotherapy or combined with a thiazide diuretic.

Contraindications
• Hypersensitivity to drug or other calcium channel blockers

Precautions
Use cautiously in:
• heart disease, hypotension, hepatic or renal disease, GI hypermotility or obstruction (controlled-release form)
• concurrent use of beta-adrenergic blockers
• elderly patients
• pregnant or breastfeeding patients
• children.

Administration
• Give with or without food.
• Don't give with grapefruit juice.
• Don't crush or break controlled-release tablets. Make sure patient swallows them whole.

Route	Onset	Peak	Duration
P.O.	2 hr	Unknown	Unknown
P.O. (controlled)	Unknown	Unknown	Unknown

Adverse reactions
CNS: dizziness, headache, fatigue, syncope, sleep disturbances
CV: peripheral edema, tachycardia, hypotension, chest pain, **arrhythmias**
GI: nausea, vomiting, constipation, abdominal pain or distention, dry mouth
GU: nocturia, urinary frequency
Hematologic: leukopenia
Hepatic: hepatitis
Skin: rash, pruritus, urticaria
Other: flushing

Interactions
Drug-drug. *Atracurium, gallamine, pancuronium, tubocurarine, vecuronium:* increased respiratory depression
Beta-adrenergic blockers: increased cardiac depression
Carbamazepine, digoxin, prazosin, quinidine: increased blood levels of these drugs
Drug-food. *Grapefruit juice:* increased drug absorption

Patient monitoring

- Monitor vital signs closely, especially blood pressure.
- Assess liver function test results.
- Monitor for arrhythmias and peripheral edema.

Patient teaching

- Tell patient he may take with or without food, but not with grapefruit juice.
- Instruct patient to move slowly when sitting up or standing, to avoid dizziness or light-headedness from sudden blood pressure decrease.
- Caution patient to avoid driving and other hazardous activities until he knows how drug affects concentration and alertness.
- Teach patient with heart, kidney, or liver disease to watch for and promptly report adverse reactions.
- As appropriate, review all other significant and life-threatening adverse reactions and interactions, especially those related to the drugs and foods mentioned above.

itraconazole

Sporanox

Pharmacologic class: Synthetic triazole
Therapeutic class: Antifungal
Pregnancy risk category C

FDA   BOXED WARNING

- Don't administer capsules to treat onychomycosis in patients with evidence of ventricular dysfunction, such as current or previous heart failure. If heart failure signs or symptoms occur during therapy, discontinue drug.
- Concurrent use of cisapride, dofetilide, levacetylmethadol (levomethadyl), pimozide, or quinidine with itraconazole capsules or oral solution is contraindicated. Itraconazole is a potent CYP3A4 inhibitor and may raise blood levels of drugs metabolized by this pathway. Serious cardiovascular events (including QT prolongation, torsades de pointes, ventricular tachycardia, cardiac arrest, and sudden death) have occurred in patients taking these drugs concurrently with itraconazole.

Action

Prevents ergosterol synthesis in fungal cell membranes, altering membrane permeability

Availability

Capsules: 100 mg
Oral solution: 10 mg/ml

Indications and dosages

➤ Aspergillosis; blastomycosis; histoplasmosis
Adults: 200 to 400 mg P.O. daily for at least 3 months until patient is cured. In life-threatening infections, loading dose of 200 mg P.O. t.i.d. for 3 days, then 200 to 400 mg P.O. daily until cured.
➤ Esophageal candidiasis
Adults: 100 to 200 mg of oral solution daily, swished in mouth for several seconds and swallowed, for at least 3 weeks; continue for 2 weeks after symptoms resolve.
➤ Oropharyngeal candidiasis
Adults: 200 mg of oral solution daily, swished in mouth for several seconds and swallowed, for 1 to 2 weeks
➤ Onychomycosis; tinea unguium
Adults: For toenails, 200 mg P.O. daily for 12 weeks. For fingernails, 200 mg b.i.d. for 1 week; wait 3 weeks, then repeat dosage for 1 week.

Contraindications

- Hypersensitivity to drug or its components
- Ventricular dysfunction, congestive heart failure (CHF) or history of CHF (in onychomycosis use)

• Concomitant use of astemizole, cisapride, dofetilide, ergot alkaloids (such as dihydroergotamine, ergonovine, ergotamine, and methylergonovine), lovastatin, midazolam, pimozide, quinidine, simvastatin, or triazolam
• Pregnancy or anticipated pregnancy (in onychomycosis use)

Precautions

Use cautiously in:
• hypersensitivity to other azole derivatives
• renal impairment (with I.V. use), hepatic disorders, achlorhydria, hypochlorhydria
• breastfeeding patients
• children (safety and efficacy not established).

Administration

• Obtain specimens for fungal cultures, as needed, before starting therapy.
• Administer capsule with a full meal.
• Give oral solution without food when possible.
• Be aware that liquid and tablets aren't interchangeable.

Route	Onset	Peak	Duration
P.O.	Slow	4-6 hr	4-6 days

Adverse reactions

CNS: dizziness, headache, fatigue, malaise
CV: peripheral edema, tachycardia, **heart failure**
EENT: rhinitis, transient or permanent hearing loss
GI: nausea, vomiting, constipation, abdominal pain, flatulence, anorexia, dyspepsia, **GI bleeding, pancreatitis**
GU: albuminuria, erectile dysfunction
Hepatic: jaundice, **hepatotoxicity** (including **hepatic failure and death**)
Metabolic: hypokalemia
Musculoskeletal: myalgia, bursitis, **rhabdomyolysis**

Respiratory: pulmonary edema
Skin: flushing, rash, pruritus, urticaria, increased sweating, herpes zoster infection
Other: fever, pain

Interactions

Drug-drug. *Alfentanil, antihistamines (minimally sedating agents, such as fexofenadine, loratadine), antineoplastics (busulfan, docetaxel, vinca alkaloids), anxiolytics, benzodiazepines, cyclosporine, delavirdine, digoxin, immunosuppressants, methylprednisolone, protease inhibitors, tacrolimus, tolterodine, tretinoin:* increased blood levels of these drugs
Amiodarone, anabolic steroids, androgens, antithyroid drugs, carmustine, chloroquine, dantrolene, daunorubicin, disulfiram, estrogens, gold salts, hormonal contraceptives, hydroxychloroquine, mercaptopurine, methotrexate, methyldopa, naltrexone (with long-term use), valproic acid: increased risk of hepatic damage
Amphotericin B: reduced or inhibited amphotericin B effects
Antacids, anticonvulsants, antimycobacterials, cyclobenzaprine, histamine$_2$-receptor blockers, isoniazid, proton pump inhibitors (such as lansoprazole, omeprazole), reverse transcriptase inhibitors, sucralfate: reduced itraconazole blood level
Antipsychotics, antiarrhythmics (such as quinidine, dofetilide), anxiolytics, astemizole, cisapride: increased risk of serious cardiovascular effects
Calcium channel blockers: increased risk of edema, possible increase in itraconazole's effect
Carbamazepine, carbidopa, levodopa: altered blood levels of these drugs
Didanosine, vinblastine, vincristine, xanthine bronchodilators: decreased efficacy of these drugs
Digoxin: increased digoxin blood level, possible digoxin toxicity

---

HMG-CoA reductase inhibitors, miconazole: inhibited metabolism of these drugs, increased risk of skeletal muscle toxicity (including rhabdomyolysis)
Macrolide antibiotics: increased itraconazole blood level
Oral hypoglycemics: severe blood glucose decrease
Quetiapine, sildenafil: increased efficacy of these drugs
Warfarin: enhanced anticoagulant effect
Drug-diagnostic tests. *Alanine aminotransferase, alkaline phosphatase, aspartate aminotransferase, blood urea nitrogen, gamma-glutamyltransferase, serum creatinine:* increased levels
Potassium, magnesium: decreased levels
Drug-food. *Any food, cola:* increased itraconazole blood level
Grapefruit juice: decreased blood level and reduced therapeutic effects of itraconazole
Drug-herbs. *Chaparral, comfrey, germander, jin bu huan, kava*: increased risk of hepatic damage
Drug-behaviors. *Alcohol consumption:* toxic reaction, hepatic damage

Patient monitoring

• In patient with hepatic dysfunction, monitor hepatic enzyme levels.

◀€ Monitor for signs and symptoms of hearing loss, pancreatitis, hepatic dysfunction (jaundice, fatigue, nausea, vomiting, dark urine, pale stools), heart failure, muscle disorder, and pulmonary or peripheral edema.

• Monitor potassium level. Stay alert for hypokalemia.

Patient teaching

• Tell patient he may take capsule with a full meal. If he's using oral solution, advise him to take it without food.

• Inform patient that drug interacts with many other drugs. Advise him to tell all prescribers he's taking it.

◀€ Teach patient to recognize and immediately report signs and symptoms of hearing loss, pancreatitis,

hepatic dysfunction, persistent muscle pain, and heart failure.

• Caution patient to avoid driving and other hazardous activities until he knows how drug affects concentration and alertness.

• Advise female patient of childbearing potential to use effective contraception during and for 1 month after therapy. Caution her not to breastfeed.

• As appropriate, review all other significant and life-threatening adverse reactions and interactions, especially those related to the drugs, tests, foods, herbs, and behaviors mentioned above.

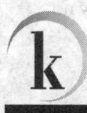

ketoconazole

Apo-Ketoconazole✣, Dactarin Gold⊕, Dandrazol⊕, Extina, Kryoxolr, Nizoral, Nizoral A-D, Novo-Ketoconazole✣, Nu-Ketocon✣, Nu-Ketoconazole✣, Ratio-Ketoconazole✣, Xolegel

Pharmacologic class: Imidazole
Therapeutic class: Antifungal
Pregnancy risk category C

FDA | **BOXED WARNING**

• Oral form has been linked to hepatic toxicity, including some deaths. Inform patient of this risk, and monitor closely.
• Concurrent use of astemizole, cisapride, or terfenadine with ketoconazole tablets is contraindicated, because serious cardiovascular adverse events (including death, ventricular tachycardia, and torsades de pointes) have occurred.

Action
Alters fungal cell membranes, resulting in increased permeability, growth inhibition, and ultimately, cell death

Availability
Cream: 2%
Shampoo: 1%, 2%
Tablets: 200 mg

🕛 Indications and dosages
➤ Blastomycosis; chronic mucocutaneous candidiasis; oral thrush; candiduria; coccidioidomycosis; histoplasmosis; chromomycosis; paracoccidioidomycosis; mucocutaneous or vaginal candidiasis
Adults: 200 to 400 mg P.O. daily
Children ages 2 and older: 3.3 to 6.6 mg/kg P.O. as a single daily dose. Duration depends on infection: for candidiasis, 1 to 2 weeks; other systemic mycoses, 6 months; recalcitrant dermatophyte infections involving glabrous skin, 4 weeks. Chronic mucocutaneous candidiasis requires maintenance therapy.
➤ Scaling caused by dandruff or seborrheic dermatitis
Adults: 2% shampoo applied topically twice weekly for 4 weeks, then as needed to control symptoms, with at least 3 days between applications; or 1% shampoo applied topically q 3 to 4 days for up to 8 weeks, then as needed to control dandruff
➤ Tinea corporis; tinea cruris; tinea versicolor; tinea pedis, cutaneous candidiasis
Adults: 2% cream applied topically to affected areas daily for 2 weeks (except for tinea pedis, which may require 6 weeks of therapy)

Contraindications
• Hypersensitivity to drug or its components
• Concurrent oral astemizole, cisapride, triazolam, or terfenadine therapy

Precautions
Use cautiously in:
• renal or hepatic disease, achlorhydria
• pregnant or breastfeeding patients
• children younger than age 2.

Administration
• Apply cream to damp skin of affected area and wide surrounding area.
• To use shampoo, wet hair, then apply shampoo and massage into scalp for 1 minute. Leave on for 5 minutes before rinsing. Rinse and repeat, this time leaving shampoo on scalp for 3 minutes before rinsing.
• Don't apply shampoo to broken or inflamed skin.
• In achlorhydria, dissolve 200-mg tablet in 4 ml of 0.2N hydrochloric acid solution.
• Withhold antacids for at least 2 hours after giving oral ketoconazole.
🔊 Don't give concurrently with cisapride, available in U.S. for compassionate use only. (Astemizole and terfenadine are not available in U.S.)

Route	Onset	Peak	Duration
P.O.	Unknown	1-2 hr	Unknown
Topical	Unknown	Unknown	Unknown

Adverse reactions
CNS: headache, nervousness, dizziness, drowsiness, severe depression, **suicidal ideation**
EENT: photophobia
GI: nausea, vomiting, diarrhea, abdominal pain, anorexia
GU: erectile dysfunction, gynecomastia
Hematologic: purpura, **hemolytic anemia, thrombocytopenia, leukopenia**
Hepatic: hepatotoxicity
Metabolic: hyperlipidemia
Skin: pruritus, rash, dermatitis, urticaria, severe irritation, stinging,

k

---

alopecia, abnormal hair texture, scalp pustules, oily skin, dry hair and scalp
Other: fever, chills, allergic reaction

Interactions
Drug-drug. *Antacids, anticholinergics, histamine$_2$-receptor antagonists:* decreased ketoconazole absorption
Cyclosporine: increased cyclosporine blood level
Isoniazid, rifampin: increased ketoconazole metabolism
Theophylline: decreased theophylline blood level
Topical corticosteroids: increased corticosteroid absorption
Triazolam (oral): increased triazolam effects
Drug-diagnostic tests. *Alanine aminotransferase, alkaline phosphatase, aspartate aminotransferase:* increased levels
Hemoglobin, platelets, white blood cells: decreased levels
Drug-herbs. *Yew:* inhibited ketoconazole metabolism

Patient monitoring
◀ᴇ Assess for suicidal ideation and signs and symptoms of depression.
◀ᴇ Monitor for evidence of hepatotoxicity, such as nausea, fatigue, jaundice, dark urine, and pale stools.
• With long-term therapy, stay alert for adrenal crisis.

Patient teaching
◀ᴇ Advise patient to watch for signs and symptoms of depression and to immediately report suicidal thoughts.
◀ᴇ Teach patient to recognize and immediately report signs and symptoms of hepatotoxicity, such as unusual tiredness or yellowing of skin or eyes.
• Advise patient not to take antacids for at least 2 hours after oral ketoconazole.

• Instruct patient to apply cream to damp skin of affected area and wide surrounding area.
• Tell patient to wet hair before applying shampoo and to massage into scalp for 1 minute; then leave on for 5 minutes before rinsing off. Tell him to shampoo again, leaving it on for 3 minutes this time before rinsing.
• Caution patient not to apply shampoo to broken or inflamed skin.
• As appropriate, review all other significant and life-threatening adverse reactions and interactions, especially those related to the drugs, tests, and herbs mentioned above.

ketorolac tromethamine
Acular, Acular LS, Apo-Ketorolac✦

Pharmacologic class: Nonsteroidal anti-inflammatory drug (NSAID)
Therapeutic class: Analgesic, antipyretic, anti-inflammatory
Pregnancy risk category C (first and second trimesters), *D* (third trimester)

FDA **BOXED WARNING**

• Drug is indicated for short-term management (up to 5 days in adults) of moderately severe acute pain that requires opioid-level analgesia. It's not indicated for minor or chronic painful conditions. Drug carries many risks; NSAID-related adverse events can be serious in certain patients, especially when used inappropriately. Raising dosage beyond recommendations increases risk of serious adverse events and won't provide better efficacy.
• Drug can cause peptic ulcers, GI bleeding, and perforation and is

contraindicated in patients with active peptic ulcer disease, recent GI bleeding or perforation, or history of peptic ulcer disease or GI bleeding.

• Drug is contraindicated in advanced renal impairment and patients at risk for renal failure.

• Drug inhibits platelet function and is contraindicated in patients with suspected or confirmed cerebrovascular bleeding, hemorrhagic diathesis, incomplete hemostasis, or high risk of bleeding.

• Drug is contraindicated as prophylactic analgesic before major surgery, and intraoperatively when hemostasis is critical.

• Hypersensitivity reactions ranging from bronchospasm to anaphylactic shock have occurred. Ensure that appropriate counteractive measures are available when giving first dose of injection form. Drug is contraindicated in known hypersensitivity to ketorolac or allergic reaction to aspirin or other NSAID.

• Drug is contraindicated for intrathecal or epidural administration (due to alcohol content), during labor and delivery (may impede fetal circulation and inhibit uterine contractions), in breastfeeding women (due to potential adverse effects of prostaglandin-inhibiting drugs on neonates), and in patients currently receiving aspirin or NSAIDs (due to cumulative risk of serious NSAID-related adverse effects).

• Tablet form is indicated only as continuation therapy to injection form, and combined duration of use of both forms mustn't exceed 5 days.

• For tablets, recommended total daily dose (maximum 40 mg) is significantly lower than for injection (maximum 120 mg).

• Adjust dosage in patients age 65 and older, those weighing less than 50 kg (110 lb), and those with moderately elevated serum creatinine level. With injection form, don't exceed 60 mg (total daily dose) in these patients.

Injection form is indicated as single-dose therapy in pediatric patients, not to exceed 30 mg for I.M. use or 15 mg for I.V. use.

Action
Interferes with prostaglandin biosynthesis by inhibiting cyclooxygenase pathway of arachidonic acid metabolism; also acts as potent inhibitor of platelet aggregation

Availability
Injection: 15 mg/ml in 1-ml preloaded syringes, 30 mg/ml in 1- and 2-ml preloaded syringes
Ophthalmic solution: 0.4%, 0.5%
Tablets: 10 mg

⚕ Indications and dosages
➤ Moderately severe acute pain
Adults younger than age 65: Initially, 30 mg I.V. or 60 mg I.M. as a single dose, or 30 mg I.M. or I.V. q 6 hours, not to exceed 120 mg/day. To switch to P.O. therapy, give 20 mg P.O. initially for patients who received single 30-mg I.V. or 60-mg I.M. dose, followed by 10 mg P.O. q 4 to 6 hours as needed (not to exceed 40 mg/day or 5 days).
Children ages 2 to 16: 1 mg/kg I.M. as a single dose, to a maximum of 30 mg; or one dose of 0.5 mg/kg I.V., to a maximum of 15 mg
➤ Ocular itching caused by seasonal allergic conjunctivitis
Adults and children ages 3 and older: One drop of 0.5% ophthalmic solution (Acular) instilled into affected eye q.i.d.
➤ Postoperative ocular inflammation related to cataract extraction
Adults and children ages 3 and older: One drop of 0.5% ophthalmic solution (Acular) instilled into operative eye q.i.d., starting 24 hours after surgery and continuing for 2 weeks
➤ To reduce ocular pain, burning, or stinging after corneal refractive surgery

k

Adults and children ages 3 and older:
One drop of 0.4% ophthalmic solution
(Acular LS) instilled into operative eye
q.i.d. for up to 4 days

Dosage adjustment
- Mild to moderate renal impairment
- Elderly patients
- Patients weighing less than 50 kg

Contraindications
- Hypersensitivity to drug, its components, aspirin, or other NSAIDs
- Concurrent use of aspirin, other NSAIDs, or probenecid
- Peptic ulcer disease
- GI bleeding or perforation
- Advanced renal impairment, risk of renal failure
- Increased risk of bleeding, suspected or confirmed cerebrovascular bleeding, hemorrhagic diathesis, incomplete hemostasis
- Prophylactic use before major surgery, intraoperative use when hemostasis is critical
- Labor and delivery
- Breastfeeding

Precautions
Use cautiously in:
- mild to moderate renal impairment, cardiovascular disease
- elderly patients
- pregnant patients
- children.

Administration
- Be aware that oral therapy is indicated only as continuation of parenteral therapy.
- 🔊 Know that parenteral therapy shouldn't exceed 20 doses in 5 days.
- For I.V. use, dilute with normal saline solution, dextrose 5% in water, dextrose 5% and normal saline solution, Ringer's solution, or lactated Ringer's solution.
- Administer single I.V. bolus over 1 to 2 minutes.
- Inject I.M. dose slowly and deeply.

- Don't give by epidural or intrathecal injection.

Route	Onset	Peak	Duration
P.O.	Unknown	2-3 hr	≥4-6 hr
I.V., I.M.	10 min	1-2 hr	≥6 hr
Ophthalmic	Unknown	Unknown	Unknown

Adverse reactions
CNS: drowsiness, headache, dizziness
CV: hypertension
EENT: tinnitus
GI: nausea, vomiting, diarrhea, constipation, flatulence, dyspepsia, epigastric pain, stomatitis
Hematologic: thrombocytopenia
Skin: rash, pruritus, diaphoresis
Other: excessive thirst, edema, injection site pain

Interactions
Drug-drug. *Angiotensin-converting enzyme inhibitors, beta-adrenergic blockers:* decreased antihypertensive effect
Anticoagulants: prolonged prothrombin time
Aspirin: altered ketorolac distribution, metabolism, and excretion; increased risk of serious adverse reactions
Cholestyramine: decreased ketorolac absorption
Corticosteroids, other NSAIDs: additive adverse GI effects
Diuretics: decreased diuretic effect
Hydantoins, lithium: increased blood levels and greater risk of toxicity of these drugs
Methotrexate: increased risk of methotrexate toxicity
Probenecid: increased risk of ketorolac toxicity
Drug-diagnostic tests. *Bleeding time:* prolonged for 24 to 48 hours after therapy ends
Drug-herbs. *Anise, arnica, chamomile, clove, dong quai, feverfew, garlic, ginger, ginkgo, ginseng:* increased risk of bleeding

---

🍁 Canada   ⊕ UK   ☙ Hazardous drug   ⊗ High-alert drug

Patient monitoring
• Monitor for adverse reactions, especially prolonged bleeding time and CNS reactions.
• Check I.M. injection site for hematoma and bleeding.
• Monitor fluid intake and output.

Patient teaching
• Inform patient that drug is meant only for short-term pain management.
◀€ Tell patient to immediately report bleeding and adverse CNS reactions.
• Advise patient to minimize GI upset by eating small, frequent servings of healthy foods.
• Instruct patient to avoid aspirin products and herbs during therapy.
• Teach patient how to use eye drops, if prescribed.
• Caution female patient not to take drug if she is breastfeeding.
• Advise patient to avoid driving and other hazardous activities until he knows how drug affects concentration and alertness.
• As appropriate, review all other significant and life-threatening adverse reactions and interactions, especially those related to the drugs, tests, and herbs mentioned above.

labetalol hydrochloride
Trandate

Pharmacologic class: Beta-adrenergic blocker (nonselective), alpha-adrenergic blocker (selective)
Therapeutic class: Antihypertensive
Pregnancy risk category C

Action
Blocks stimulation of beta$_1$- and beta$_2$-adrenergic receptor sites and alpha$_1$-adrenergic receptors, decreasing myocardial contractile force and enhancing coronary artery blood flow and myocardial perfusion. Net effect is decreased heart rate and blood pressure.

Availability
Injection: 5 mg/ml
Tablets: 100 mg, 200 mg, 300 mg

Indications and dosages
➤ Hypertension
Adults: Initially, 100 mg P.O. b.i.d., alone or combined with a diuretic; may increase by 100 mg b.i.d. q 2 to 3 days as needed. Usual range is 400 to 800 mg/day in two divided doses; up to 2.4 g/day have been given.
➤ Hypertensive crisis
Adults: Initially, 20 mg I.V. bolus over 2 minutes, then I.V. injection of 40 to 80 mg q 10 minutes until blood pressure falls to desired level; maximum dosage is 300 mg. Alternatively, 50 to 200 mg by continuous I.V. infusion at 2 mg/minute; continue infusion until desired blood pressure is reached. Follow I.V. dosing with P.O. dosing.
➤ Conversion from I.V. to P.O. dosing
Hospitalized adults: Discontinue I.V. therapy when desired blood pressure is reached; start P.O. dosing when supine diastolic pressure begins to rise. Initial P.O. dosage is 200 mg, followed 6 to 12 hours later with additional dose of 200 to 400 mg P.O., depending on blood pressure response. Then titrate at 1-day intervals to dosage ranging from 400 to 2,400 mg/day P.O. in two or three divided doses.

Dosage adjustment
• Chronic hepatic disease
• Elderly patients

Off-label uses

- Hypertension secondary to pheochromocytoma or clonidine withdrawal

Contraindications

- Hypersensitivity to drug
- Bronchospastic disease
- Overt heart failure, cardiogenic shock
- Second- or third-degree atrioventricular block
- Severe bradycardia
- Conditions associated with severe and prolonged hypotension

Precautions

Use cautiously in:
- hepatic impairment, pulmonary disease, diabetes mellitus, hyperthyroidism, thyrotoxicosis
- elderly patients
- pregnant or breastfeeding patients
- children.

Administration

- Know that drug may be given as I.V. bolus or continuous infusion.
- Be aware that drug may be given undiluted for I.V. bolus injection. For continuous infusion, dilute in dextrose 5% in water or normal saline solution, and deliver with infusion control pump.
- Don't mix with 5% sodium bicarbonate injection.
- Give direct I.V. injection over 2 minutes at 10-minute intervals.

Route	Onset	Peak	Duration
P.O.	20 min-2 hr	1-4 hr	8-12 hr
I.V.	2-5 min	5 min	16-18 hr

Adverse reactions

CNS: fatigue, asthenia, anxiety, depression, dizziness, paresthesia, drowsiness, insomnia, memory loss, nightmares, mental status changes
CV: orthostatic hypotension, peripheral vasoconstriction, bradycardia, **arrhythmias, heart failure**

EENT: blurred vision, dry eyes, nasal congestion
GI: nausea, diarrhea, constipation
GU: erectile dysfunction, decreased libido
Hematologic: purpura, **agranulocytosis, thrombocytopenia**
Metabolic: hyperglycemia, **hypoglycemia**
Musculoskeletal: joint pain, back pain, muscle cramps
Respiratory: wheezing, **bronchospasm, pulmonary edema**
Skin: rash, pruritus

Interactions

Drug-drug. *Adrenergic bronchodilators, theophylline:* decreased efficacy of these drugs
Antihypertensives, nitrates: additive hypotension
Cimetidine, propranolol: increased labetalol effects
Digoxin: additive bradycardia
Dobutamine, dopamine: reduced beneficial cardiovascular effects of these drugs
General anesthetics, verapamil: additive myocardial depression
Insulin, oral hypoglycemics: altered hypoglycemic efficacy
MAO inhibitors: hypertension
Nonsteroidal anti-inflammatory drugs: decreased antihypertensive action
Drug-diagnostic tests. *Alanine aminotransferase, alkaline phosphatase, antinuclear antibodies, aspartate aminotransferase, blood urea nitrogen, glucose, liver function tests, low-density lipoproteins, potassium, triglycerides, uric acid:* increased values

Patient monitoring

- Monitor ECG and vital signs, especially blood pressure.
- Assess cardiovascular, respiratory, and neurologic status closely to detect adverse reactions.
- Monitor CBC, blood glucose level, and liver function tests.

Patient teaching

◀€ Instruct patient to immediately report adverse reactions, such as easy bruising or bleeding or respiratory problems.

• Tell patient he may feel dizzy when starting therapy, especially if he's also taking a diuretic.

• Advise patient to move slowly when sitting up or standing, to avoid dizziness or light-headedness from sudden blood pressure decrease.

• Caution patient to avoid driving and other hazardous activities until he knows how drug affects concentration, vision, and alertness.

• Emphasize need for follow-up care and regular blood pressure monitoring.

◀€ Caution patient not to stop taking drug abruptly, because this may cause myocardial infarction or worsen angina.

• As appropriate, review all other significant and life-threatening adverse reactions and interactions, especially those related to the drugs and tests mentioned above.

lactulose

Apo-Lactulose✿, Consulose, Duphalac⊕, Enulose, Euro-Lac✿, Generlac, Gen-Lac✿, GPI-Lactulose✿, Kristalose, Lactugal⊕, Lactulax✿, Lemlax⊕, PMS-Lactulose✿, Ratio-Lactulose✿, Regulose⊕

Pharmacologic class: Osmotic
Therapeutic class: Laxative
Pregnancy risk category B

Action

Produces osmotic effect, which increases water content in colon and enhances peristalsis. Breakdown products in colon lead to acidification of colonic contents, softening of feces, and decreased ammonia absorption from colon to systemic circulation. These effects reduce blood ammonia level in portal-system encephalopathy.

Availability

Powder (single-use packets): 10 g, 20 g
Syrup: 10 g/15 ml

⚕ Indications and dosages

➤ Constipation
Adults: 10 to 20 g (15 to 30 ml) P.O. daily; may increase to 60 ml daily p.r.n.
➤ Portal-system encephalopathy
Adults: 20 to 30 g (30 to 45 ml) P.O. three or four times daily until two or three soft stools are produced daily. Therapy may continue over long term. Or, 300 ml P.O. with 700 ml of water or normal saline solution. Or, as retention enema by rectal balloon catheter, repeated q 4 to 6 hours.

Contraindications

• Patients requiring low-galactose diet

Precautions

Use cautiously in:
• diabetes mellitus
• elderly patients
• pregnant or breastfeeding patients
• children.

Administration

• Don't give concurrently with other laxatives.
• Dissolve contents of single-use packet in 4 oz of water or juice.
• Dilute syrup with water or fruit juice to mask taste.

Route	Onset	Peak	Duration
P.O.	24-48 hr	Unknown	Unknown

Adverse reactions

GI: nausea, vomiting, diarrhea, intestinal cramps, abdominal distention, flatulence

Metabolic: hyperglycemia (in diabetic patients), hypokalemia, hypernatremia

Interactions

Drug-drug. *Anti-infectives:* decreased lactulose efficacy
Other laxatives: interference with response to lactulose (in patients with hepatic encephalopathy)
Drug-diagnostic tests. *Blood ammonia:* 25% to 50% decrease
Glucose: increased level (in diabetic patients)
Potassium: decreased level
Sodium: increased level

Patient monitoring

• Watch for adverse GI reactions.
• Check stool consistency and frequency.
• Monitor electrolyte levels, especially in elderly patients.
• Check blood glucose level in diabetic patients.

Patient teaching

• Instruct patient to dissolve contents of single-use packet in 4 oz of water or juice.
• Suggest that patient dilute syrup with water or juice to mask taste.
• Tell patient drug may cause flatulence and intestinal cramps at first, but these symptoms usually subside.
• Inform patient that excessive use may cause diarrhea and excessive fluid loss.
• Encourage patient to drink adequate fluids and to report signs and symptoms of dehydration.
• As appropriate, review all other significant adverse reactions and interactions, especially those related to the drugs and tests mentioned above.

lamivudine

Epivir, Epivir-HBV, 3TC✦, Heptovir✦, Zeffix⊕

Pharmacologic class: Nucleoside reverse transcriptase inhibitor
Therapeutic class: Antiretroviral
Pregnancy risk category C

FDA   BOXED WARNING

• Lactic acidosis and severe hepatomegaly with steatosis (including fatal cases) have occurred when drug was used alone or in combination with other nucleoside analogues.
• Epivir tablets and oral solution (used to treat human immunodeficiency virus [HIV] infection) contain higher dose of active ingredient (lamivudine) than Epivir-HBV tablets and oral solution (used to treat chronic hepatitis B). Patients with HIV should receive only dosing forms appropriate for HIV treatment.
• After Epivir discontinuation, severe acute hepatitis B exacerbations have occurred in patients co-infected with hepatitis B virus (HBV) and HIV. Monitor hepatic function closely for at least several months in these patients. If appropriate, begin anti–hepatitis B therapy.

Action

Inhibits HIV reverse transcription by viral DNA chain termination. Impedes RNA- and DNA-dependent DNA polymerase activities.

Availability

Oral solution: 5 mg/ml and 10 mg/ml in 240-ml bottles
Tablets: 100 mg, 150 mg, 300 mg

⟐ Indications and dosages

➤ HIV infection (given with other antiretrovirals)

Adults and children older than age 16: 150 mg P.O. b.i.d. or 300 mg P.O. daily

Children ages 3 months to 16 years: 4 mg/kg P.O. b.i.d. to a maximum of 150 mg P.O. b.i.d.

➤ Chronic HBV

Adults: 100 mg (Epivir-HBV) P.O. once daily

Children ages 2 to 17: 3 mg/kg (Epivir-HBV) P.O. once daily, to a maximum of 100 mg P.O. daily

Dosage adjustment

• Renal impairment

Contraindications

• Hypersensitivity to drug or its components

Precautions

Use cautiously in:
• impaired renal function, history of hepatic disease, obesity, granulocyte count below 1,000/mm³
• long-term therapy
• elderly patients
• women (especially if pregnant)
• children.

Administration

• Give with or without food.

◀≋ Be aware that Epivir contains 150 mg lamivudine and Epivir-HBV contains 100 mg lamivudine. Strengths are not interchangeable.

◀≋ Know that when given to patients with unrecognized or untreated HIV, Epivir-HBV is likely to cause rapid emergence of HIV resistance.

Route	Onset	Peak	Duration
P.O.	Unknown	0.9 hr	12 hr

Adverse reactions

CNS: fatigue, headache, insomnia, malaise, asthenia, depression, dizziness, paresthesia, peripheral neuropathy, **seizures**

GI: nausea, vomiting, diarrhea, anorexia, abdominal discomfort, dyspepsia, splenomegaly, **pancreatitis**

Hematologic: anemia, **neutropenia**

Hepatic: hepatomegaly with steatosis

Metabolic: hyperglycemia, **lactic acidosis**

Musculoskeletal: muscle, joint, or bone pain; muscle weakness; myalgia; **rhabdomyolysis**

Respiratory: cough, abnormal breath sounds, wheezing

Skin: alopecia, rash, urticaria, **erythema multiforme, Stevens-Johnson syndrome**

Other: lymphadenopathy, body fat redistribution, hypersensitivity reactions including **anaphylaxis; immune reconstitution syndrome**

Interactions

Drug-drug. *Co-trimoxazole:* increased lamivudine blood level

Zalcitabine: interference with effects of both drugs

Drug-diagnostic tests. *Alanine aminotransferase, alkaline phosphatase, aspartate aminotransferase, bilirubin, creatine kinase, liver function tests:* increased levels

Hemoglobin, hematocrit, neutrophils: decreased levels

Patient monitoring

• Check vital signs regularly.
• Monitor CBC and platelet count frequently. Watch for evidence of bone marrow toxicity.
• Monitor blood glucose level and kidney and liver function test results.
• Assess neurologic and mental status. Report signs or symptoms of depression.
• Closely monitor obese patients, women, and patients with a history of hepatic disease; they're at increased risk for lactic acidosis and severe hepatomegaly with steatosis.

Reactions in **bold** are life-threatening. ◀≋ Clinical alert

- Monitor HIV patients for co-infection with HBV (which may recur when drug is withdrawn).
🔊 Monitor patients for signs and symptoms of immune reconstitution syndrome.

Patient teaching
- Tell patient he may take with or without food.
- Advise patient to minimize GI upset by eating small, frequent servings of healthy food and drinking plenty of fluids.
- Tell HIV patient that drug doesn't cure virus or prevent its transmission and that opportunistic infections may occur. Advise him to take appropriate precautions during sex.
- Teach patient how to recognize and immediately report signs and symptoms of immune reconstitution syndrome.
- Caution patient to avoid driving and other hazardous activities until he knows how drug affects concentration and alertness.
- Caution HIV patient not to breast-feed, because of risk of passing infection to infant.
- As appropriate, review all other significant and life-threatening adverse reactions and interactions, especially those related to the drugs and tests mentioned above.

lamotrigine
Apo-Lamotrigine✤, Gen-Lamotrigine✤, Lamictal, Lamictal Chewable Dispersible, Lamictal ODT, Lamictal XR, Novo-Lamotrigine✤, PMS-Lamotrigine✤, Ratio-Lamotrigine✤

Pharmacologic class: Phenyltriazine
Therapeutic class: Anticonvulsant
Pregnancy risk category C

FDA BOXED WARNING

- Lamotrigine has caused life-threatening serious rashes, including Stevens-Johnson syndrome, toxic epidermal necrolysis, and rash-related death. Rate of serious rash is greater in children than in adults. Additional factors that may increase risk of rash include concurrent use with valproate, exceeding lamotrigine recommended initial dose, or exceeding lamotrigine recommended dosage escalation.
- Drug also causes benign rashes; however, it's impossible to predict which rashes will prove to be serious or life-threatening. Discontinue drug at first sign of rash, unless rash is clearly not drug-related.

Action
Unknown. Thought to block sodium channel membranes, which in turn inhibits release of the neurotransmitters glutamate and aspartate in brain.

Availability
Tablets: 25 mg, 100 mg, 150 mg, 200 mg
Tablets (chewable): 2 mg, 5 mg, 25 mg
Tablets (extended-release): 25 mg, 50 mg, 100 mg, 200 mg, 250 mg, 300 mg
Tablets (orally disintegrating): 25 mg, 50 mg, 100 mg, 200 mg

💊 Indications and dosages
➤ Partial seizures, generalized seizures of Lennox-Gastaut syndrome, and primary generalized tonic-clonic seizures in patients receiving valproate
Adults and children ages 12 and older: 25 mg immediate-release P.O. every other day during weeks 1 and 2; then 25 mg daily during weeks 3 and 4. Then week 5 onwards to maintenance, increase dosage by 25 to 50 mg/day every 1 to 2 weeks. Usual maintenance dosage is 100 to 400 mg/ day in one or two divided doses. For those taking

valproate alone, maximum dosage is 200 mg/day.

Children ages 2 to 12: 0.15 mg/kg/day immediate-release P.O. (rounded down to nearest whole tablet) in one or two divided doses during weeks 1 and 2; then 0.3 mg/kg/day P.O. (rounded down to nearest whole tablet) in one or two divided doses during weeks 3 and 4. Then week 5 onwards to maintenance, increase every 1 to 2 weeks as 0.3 mg/kg/day (rounded down to nearest whole tablet) added to previously administered daily dose. Usual maintenance dosage is 1 to 5 mg/kg/day. Maximum dosage is 200 mg/day in one or two divided doses. For patients taking valproate alone, maintenance dosage is 1 to 3 mg/kg/day. May need to increase maintenance dose by as much as 50% in patients weighing less than 30 kg (66 lb), based on clinical response.

➤ Partial seizures, generalized seizures of Lennox-Gastaut syndrome, and primary generalized tonic-clonic seizures in patients receiving antiepileptic drugs (AEDs) other than carbamazepine, phenytoin, phenobarbital, primidone, or valproate

Adults and children ages 12 and older: 25 mg immediate-release P.O. every day during weeks 1 and 2; then 50 mg daily during weeks 3 and 4. Increase by 50 mg/day every 1 to 2 weeks. Usual maintenance dosage is 225 to 375 mg/day in two divided doses.

Children ages 2 to 12: 0.3 mg/kg/day immediate-release P.O. in one or two divided doses (rounded down to nearest whole tablet) during weeks 1 and 2; then 0.6 mg/kg/day P.O. in two divided doses (rounded down to nearest whole tablet) during weeks 3 and 4. Then week 5 onwards to maintenance, increase every 1 to 2 weeks as 0.6 mg/kg/day (rounded down to nearest whole tablet) added to previously administered daily dose. Usual maintenance dosage is 4.5 to 7.5 mg/kg/day (maximum, 300 mg/day) in two

divided doses. May need to increase maintenance dose by as much as 50% in patients weighing less than 30 kg, based on clinical response.

➤ Partial seizures, generalized seizures of Lennox-Gastaut syndrome, and primary generalized tonic-clonic seizures in patients receiving carbamazepine, phenytoin, phenobarbital, or primidone, but not receiving valproate

Adults and children ages 12 and older: 50 mg/day immediate-release P.O. during weeks 1 and 2; then 100 mg/day in two divided doses during weeks 3 and 4. Then week 5 onwards to maintenance, increase by 100 mg/day every 1 to 2 weeks. Usual maintenance dosage is 300 to 500 mg/day in two divided doses.

Children ages 2 to 12: 0.6 mg/kg/day immediate-release P.O. in two divided doses (rounded down to nearest whole tablet) during weeks 1 and 2; then 1.2 mg/kg/day in two divided doses (rounded down to nearest whole tablet) during weeks 3 and 4. Then week 5 onwards to maintenance, increase every 1 to 2 weeks as 1.2 mg/kg/day (rounded down to nearest whole tablet) added to previously administered daily dose. Usual maintenance dosage is 5 to 15 mg/kg/day (maximum, 400 mg/day) in two divided doses. May need to increase maintenance dose by as much as 50% in patients weighing less than 30 kg, based on clinical response.

➤ Adjunctive therapy for primary generalized tonic-clonic seizures and partial-onset seizures with or without secondary generalization in patients receiving valproate

Adults and children ages 13 and older: 25 mg P.O. (Lamictal XR) every other day during weeks 1 and 2; 25 mg daily during weeks 3 and 4; 50 mg daily week 5; 100 mg daily week 6; then 150 mg daily week 7. Usual

---

maintenance dose starting week 8 and onward is 200 to 250 mg every day.

➤ Adjunctive therapy for primary generalized tonic-clonic seizures and partial-onset seizures with or without secondary generalization in patients not receiving carbamazepine, phenytoin, phenobarbital, primidone, or valproate

Adults and children ages 13 and older: 25 mg P.O. (Lamictal XR) daily during weeks 1 and 2; 50 mg daily during weeks 3 and 4; 100 mg daily week 5; 150 mg daily week 6; then 200 mg daily week 7. Usual maintenance dose starting week 8 and onward is 300 to 400 mg every day.

➤ Adjunctive therapy for primary generalized tonic-clonic seizures and partial-onset seizures with or without secondary generalization in patients receiving carbamazepine, phenytoin, phenobarbital, or primidone, but *not* receiving valproate

Adults and children ages 13 and older: 50 mg P.O. (Lamictal XR) daily during weeks 1 and 2; 100 mg daily during weeks 3 and 4; 200 mg daily week 5; 300 mg daily week 6; then 400 mg daily week 7. Usual maintenance dose starting week 8 and onward is 400 to 600 mg every day.

➤ Conversion to monotherapy for partial-onset seizures in patients receiving valproate

Adults and children ages 13 and older: 25 mg P.O. (Lamictal XR) every other day during weeks 1 and 2; 25 mg daily during weeks 3 and 4; 50 mg daily week 5; 100 mg daily week 6; then 150 mg daily week 7 while maintaining established valproate dose. Then maintain Lamictal XR at 150 mg daily while decreasing valproate dosage by decrements no greater than 500 mg/day/week and then maintain valproate for 1 week. Increase Lamictal XR to 200 mg/day and simultaneously decrease valproate to 250 mg/day and maintain for 1 week. Increase Lamictal

XR to 250 or 300 mg/day and discontinue valproate.

➤ Conversion from adjunctive therapy of carbamazepine, phenytoin, phenobarbital, or primidone to monotherapy with Lamictal XR in patients with primary generalized tonic-clonic seizures and partial-onset seizures with or without secondary generalization

Adults and children ages 13 and older: After achieving a dosage of 500 mg/day P.O. of Lamictal XR, the concomitant enzyme-inducing antiepileptic drug (AED) should be withdrawn by 20% decrements each week over 4-week period. Two weeks after completion of withdrawal of the enzyme-inducing AED, the dosage of Lamictal XR may be decreased no faster than 100 mg/day each week to achieve the monotherapy maintenance dosage range of 250 to 300 mg/day.

➤ Conversion from adjunctive therapy with AEDs other than carbamazepine, phenytoin, phenobarbital, primidone, or valproate to monotherapy with Lamictal XR

Adults and children ages 13 and older: After achieving a dosage of 250 to 300 mg/day P.O. of Lamictal XR, the concomitant AED should be withdrawn by 20% decrements each week over 4-week period.

➤ Conversion to monotherapy for seizures in patients receiving carbamazepine, phenytoin, phenobarbital, primidone, or valproate as a single agent

Adults and children ages 16 and older: Usual maintenance dosage is 500 mg/day immediate-release P.O. in two divided doses.

➤ Conversion from carbamazepine, phenytoin, phenobarbital, or primidone to monotherapy with lamotrigine for seizures

Adults and children ages 16 and older: 50 mg/day immediate-release P.O. during weeks 1 and 2; then 100 mg/day in two divided doses during weeks 3 and 4.

Then week 5 onwards to maintenance, increase by 100 mg/day every 1 to 2 weeks. Usual maintenance dosage is 300 to 500 mg/day in two divided doses. After achieving lamotrigine maintenance dosage of 500 mg/day P.O., withdraw concomitant AED by 20% decrements each week over 4-week period.

➤ Conversion from adjunctive therapy with valproate to monotherapy with lamotrigine for seizures

Adults and children ages 16 and older: Achieve lamotrigine dosage of 200 mg/day immediate-release P.O. and maintain previous stable valproate dosage. Maintain lamotrigine dosage of 200 mg/day and decrease valproate dosage to 500 mg/day by decrements no greater than 500 mg/day; maintain regimen for 1 week. Then increase lamotrigine dosage to 300 mg/day while simultaneously decreasing valproate to 250 mg/day; maintain regimen for 1 week. Then discontinue valproate completely and increase lamotrigine dosage by 100 mg/day every week to 500 mg/day.

➤ Maintenance treatment of bipolar I disorder to delay time to occurrence of mood episodes in patients treated with standard therapy for acute mood episodes

Adults: Target dosage is 200 mg immediate-release P.O. daily titrated over 7 weeks (or 100 mg daily in patients taking valproate, or 400 mg daily in patients not taking valproate who are receiving carbamazepine, rifampin, phenytoin, phenobarbital, or primidone). If other psychotropic drugs are withdrawn following stabilization, adjust lamotrigine dosage as indicated.

Dosage adjustment
• Moderate to severe hepatic dysfunction
• Renal impairment
• Heart disease

• Starting or stopping estrogen-containing oral hormonal contraceptives
• Concurrent use of valproate

Off-label uses
• Drug-resistant seizures
• Mood stabilization in rapid-cycling bipolar II disorder

Contraindications
• Hypersensitivity to drug or its components

Precautions
Use cautiously in:
• renal or hepatic impairment or other diseases or conditions that affect metabolism or elimination
• concurrent use of other anticonvulsants or estrogen-containing oral contraceptives
• history of allergy to or rash from other AEDs
• clinical worsening, emergence of new symptoms, and suicidal ideation or behaviors
• aseptic meningitis, multiorgan hypersensitivity reactions, blood dyscrasias, ophthalmologic effects
• pregnant or breastfeeding patients
• children younger than age 2; children younger than age 13 (extended-release form); children younger than age 18 with mood disorders (safety and efficacy not established).

Administration
• Give with or without food.
• Don't crush or break regular tablets; make sure patient swallows them whole.
• Crush chewable tablets or mix in diluted fruit juice if patient can't chew them.
• Know that patients may be converted directly from immediate-release form to extended-release form, with the initial extended-release dose matching the total daily immediate-release dose.

- Be aware that effectiveness of drug in treating acute mood episodes hasn't been established.

◀℥ Be aware that abrupt drug withdrawal may induce seizures. If drug must be discontinued, decrease dosage by 50% per week over at least 2 weeks.

◀℥ Don't confuse Lamictal with other drugs having sound-alike names (such as Lamisil, Lomotil, and Ludiomil).

Route	Onset	Peak	Duration
P.O.	Unknown	1.4-4.8 hr	Unknown

Adverse reactions

CNS: dizziness, vertigo, headache, drowsiness, ataxia, incoordination, insomnia, sleep disorders, tremor, depression, anxiety, irritability, impaired memory, poor concentration, emotional lability, racing thoughts, dysarthria, malaise, asthenia, somnolence, amnesia, hypoesthesia, decreased or increased reflexes, fatigue, migraine, dream abnormality, **suicidal ideation, seizures, aseptic meningitis**

CV: palpitations, **hemorrhage**

EENT: diplopia, nystagmus, blurred vision, possible long-term ophthalmologic effects, ear disorder, rhinitis, epistaxis, sinusitis, pharyngitis

GI: nausea, vomiting, diarrhea, constipation, abdominal pain, dyspepsia, dry mouth, anorexia, peptic ulcer, flatulence, **rectal hemorrhage**

GU: dysmenorrhea, amenorrhea, vaginitis, increased libido, urinary tract infection, urinary frequency, penis disorder

Hematologic: blood dyscrasias (such as neutropenia, thrombocytopenia, pancytopenia)

Musculoskeletal: muscle spasm, neck pain, back pain, arthralgia, myalgia

Respiratory: cough, dyspnea, bronchitis, bronchospasm

Skin: pruritus, contact dermatitis, dry skin, sweating, photosensitivity, eczema, alopecia, rash, urticaria, **erythema multiforme, toxic epidermal necrolysis, Stevens-Johnson syndrome**

Other: infection, pain, weight changes, chest pain, accidental injury, lymphadenopathy, flulike syndrome, fever, tooth disorder, edema, peripheral edema, facial edema, hypersensitivity reactions (rare) including **anaphylaxis; multiorgan hypersensitivity reactions**

Interactions

Drug-drug. *Carbamazepine, phenobarbital, phenytoin, primidone:* decreased lamotrigine steady-state level

Estrogen-containing oral contraceptives, rifampin: increased lamotrigine clearance

Folate inhibitors (such as methotrexate, co-trimoxazole): additive effects of lamotrigine

Topiramate: increased topiramate concentrations

Valproate: decreased lamotrigine clearance, increased steady-state level

Drug-diagnostic tests. *All blood cells:* decreased levels

Liver function tests: abnormal

Drug-behaviors. *Sun exposure:* photosensitivity

Patient monitoring

- Monitor renal and hepatic function.

◀℥ Watch for signs and symptoms of hypersensitivity reaction (Stevens-Johnson syndrome or anaphylaxis) and potentially fatal or life-threatening multiorgan hypersensitivity reactions (early signs may include rash, fever, and lymphadenopathy); discontinue drug if alternative etiology for this reaction isn't found.

◀℥ Monitor patient with bipolar disorder closely for clinical worsening and suicidality.

- Monitor vital signs regularly.
- Monitor CNS status carefully, noting adverse reactions and changes in seizure pattern.

- Monitor patient for signs and symptoms of anemia, unexpected infection, or bleeding.
- Be aware that because drug binds to melanin, it could accumulate over time in the eye and other melanin-containing tissues.
- Monitor lamotrigine blood levels, especially during dosage adjustments.

Patient teaching
- Tell patient or caregiver that drug may be taken with or without food.
- Instruct patient or caregiver that immediate- and extended-release tablets must be swallowed whole without crushing or breaking.
- Instruct patient or caregiver that orally disintegrating tablets should be placed on the tongue and moved around in the mouth; the tablets will disintegrate rapidly. Then they can be swallowed with or without water, and can be taken with or without food.
- Instruct patient or caregiver to crush chewable tablets or mix them in diluted fruit juice if patient can't chew them. Tell patient to add dispersed tablets to approximately 1 teaspoon of liquid in glass or spoon, mix solution when tablets are completely dispersed, and then take entire amount immediately.
- Inform patient or caregiver not to stop drug abruptly and that dosage is adjusted slowly, as indicated.
- ◀€ Advise patient or caregiver to stop drug and notify prescriber immediately at first sign of rash or enlarged lymph nodes.
- Instruct patient or caregiver to immediately report unexpected infection, unusual fatigue, bleeding, headache, fever, nausea, vomiting, or nuchal rigidity.
- Tell patient or caregiver to report vision changes.
- Caution patient to avoid driving and other hazardous activities until he knows how drug affects concentration and alertness.

- As appropriate, review all other significant and life-threatening adverse reactions and interactions, especially those related to the drugs, tests, and behaviors mentioned above.

lansoprazole
Prevacid, Prevacid SoluTab, Prevacid 24HR, Zoton ✠

Pharmacologic class: Gastric acid pump inhibitor
Therapeutic class: Antiulcer drug
Pregnancy risk category B

Action
Inhibits activity of proton pump in gastric parietal cells, decreasing gastric acid production

Availability
Capsules (delayed-release): 15 mg, 30 mg
Granules for oral suspension (delayed-release, enteric-coated): 15 mg, 30 mg
Prevpac (combination product for Helicobacter pylori *infection):* daily pack containing two 30-mg lansoprazole capsules, four 500-mg amoxicillin capsules, and two 500-mg clarithromycin tablets
Prevacid NapraPAC 375 (combination product for reducing risk of ulcers from nonsteroidal anti-inflammatory drugs [NSAIDs]): weekly pack containing seven 15-mg Prevacid capsules and fourteen 375-mg Naprosyn tablets
Prevacid NapraPAC 500 (combination product for reducing risk of ulcers from NSAIDs): weekly pack containing seven 15-mg Prevacid capsules and fourteen 500-mg Naprosyn tablets
Prevacid SoluTab (delayed-release, orally disintegrating tablet): 15 mg, 30 mg

❶ Indications and dosages

➤ Active duodenal ulcer

Adults: 15 mg P.O. daily for 4 weeks

➤ Maintenance of healed duodenal ulcer

Adults: 15 mg P.O. daily

➤ *H. pylori* eradication, to reduce risk of duodenal ulcer recurrence

Adults: In triple therapy, 30 mg lansoprazole P.O., 1 g amoxicillin P.O., and 500 mg clarithromycin P.O. q 12 hours for 10 or 14 days. In dual therapy, 30 mg lansoprazole P.O. and 1 g amoxicillin P.O. q 8 hours for 14 days.

➤ Benign gastric ulcer

Adults: 30 mg P.O. daily for up to 8 weeks

➤ Gastric ulcer associated with NSAIDs

Adults: 30 mg P.O. once daily for up to 8 weeks

➤ To reduce risk of NSAID-associated gastric ulcer

Adults: 15 mg P.O. daily for up to 12 weeks

➤ Gastroesophageal reflux disease

Adults and children ages 12 to 17: 15 mg P.O. daily for up to 8 weeks

Children ages 1 to 11 weighing more than 30 kg (66 lb): 30 mg P.O. daily for up to 12 weeks

Children ages 1 to 11 weighing 30 kg (66 lb) or less: 15 mg P.O. daily for up to 12 weeks

➤ Erosive esophagitis

Adults and children ages 12 to 17: 30 mg P.O. daily for up to 8 weeks. Some patients may require 8 additional weeks.

Children ages 1 to 11 weighing more than 30 kg (66 lb): 30 mg P.O. daily for up to 12 weeks

Children ages 1 to 11 weighing 30 kg (66 lb) or less: 15 mg P.O. daily for up to 12 weeks

➤ To maintain healing of erosive esophagitis

Adults: 15 mg P.O. daily

➤ Pathologic hypersecretory conditions (including Zollinger-Ellison syndrome)

Adults: Initially, 60 mg P.O. daily, to a maximum of 90 mg P.O. b.i.d. Divide daily dosages over 120 mg.

➤ Frequent heartburn (two or more times a week)

Adults: 15 mg P.O. (delayed-release capsule) daily up to 14 days

Dosage adjustment

• Significant hepatic insufficiency

Contraindications

• Hypersensitivity to drug or its components

Precautions

Use cautiously in:

• phenylketonuria (orally disintegrating tablets), severe hepatic impairment

• elderly patients

• pregnant or breastfeeding patients

• children younger than age 18.

Administration

• Give oral form before meals.

• If patient has difficulty swallowing delayed-release capsule, open it and sprinkle contents onto small amount of soft food, such as applesauce or pudding. Don't crush or let patient chew drug.

• When giving orally disintegrating tablet, place tablet on patient's tongue and let it disintegrate until particles can be swallowed.

• Know that orally disintegrating tablet contains phenylalanine.

• When giving oral suspension, empty packet contents into container with 2 tbsp water. Stir contents well, and have patient drink immediately. Don't give oral suspension through nasogastric (NG) tube.

• When injecting contents of delayed-release capsule through NG tube, open capsule and mix granules with 40 ml

---

apple juice. Then rinse tube with additional apple juice to clear.

Route	Onset	Peak	Duration
P.O.	Rapid	Unknown	>24 hr

Adverse reactions

CNS: headache, confusion, anxiety, malaise, paresthesia, abnormal thinking, depression, dizziness, syncope, **cerebrovascular accident**
CV: chest pain, hypertension, hypotension, **myocardial infarction, shock**
EENT: visual field deficits, otitis media, tinnitus, epistaxis
GI: nausea, diarrhea, abdominal pain, cholelithiasis, ulcerative colitis, esophageal ulcer, hematemesis, stomatitis, dysphagia, **GI hemorrhage**
GU: renal calculi, erectile dysfunction, abnormal menses, breast tenderness, gynecomastia
Hematologic: anemia
Musculoskeletal: hip, wrist, spine fractures (with long-term daily use)
Respiratory: cough, bronchitis, **asthma**
Skin: urticaria, alopecia, acne, pruritus, photosensitivity

Interactions

Drug-drug. *Drugs requiring acidic pH (such as ampicillin esters, digoxin, iron salts, itraconazole, ketoconazole):* decreased absorption of these drugs
Sucralfate: decreased lansoprazole absorption
Theophylline: increased theophylline clearance
Drug-food. *Any food:* decreased rate and extent of GI drug absorption
Drug-herbs. *Male fern:* inactivation of herb
St. John's wort: increased risk of photosensitivity

Patient monitoring

• Monitor for GI adverse reactions.
• Assess nutritional status and fluid balance to identify significant problems.

Patient teaching

• Instruct patient to take before meals.
• If patient has difficulty swallowing, tell him to open delayed-release capsule and sprinkle contents onto small amount of soft food (such as applesauce or pudding). Emphasize that he must not crush or chew drug.
• Tell patient to take orally disintegrating tablet by placing it on tongue and letting it disintegrate.
• Instruct patient to take oral suspension by emptying packet contents into container with 2 tbsp water. Tell him to stir contents well and drink immediately.
• Advise patient to minimize GI upset by eating small, frequent servings of food and drinking plenty of fluids.
• As appropriate, review all other significant and life-threatening adverse reactions and interactions, especially those related to the drugs, foods, and herbs mentioned above.

lanthanum carbonate
Fosrenol

Pharmacologic class: Phosphate binder
Therapeutic class: Renal and genitourinary agent
Pregnancy risk category C

Action

Dissociates in acidic environment of upper GI tract to release lanthanum ions, which bind dietary phosphate released from food during digestion and inhibit phosphate absorption by forming highly insoluble lanthanum phosphate complexes

Availability

Tablets (chewable): 500 mg, 750 mg, 1,000 mg

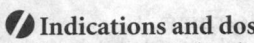 Indications and dosages

➤ To reduce serum phosphate level in patients with end-stage renal disease
Adults: Initially, 1,500 mg P.O. (chewed) daily in divided doses with meals; titrate every 2 to 3 weeks until serum phosphate falls to acceptable level.

Contraindications

• Bowel obstruction, ileus, or fecal impaction

Precautions

Use cautiously in:
• acute peptic ulcer, Crohn's disease, ulcerative colitis
• pregnant or breastfeeding patients
• children (safety and efficacy not established).

Administration

• Give before meals; ensure that patient chews tablets completely before swallowing to reduce risk of serious adverse GI events.

Route	Onset	Peak	Duration
P.O.	Unknown	Unknown	Unknown

Adverse reactions

CNS: headache
CV: hypotension
GI: nausea, vomiting, diarrhea, constipation, abdominal pain
Metabolic: hypercalcemia
Respiratory: bronchitis, rhinitis
Other: dialysis graft complication or occlusion

Interactions

Drug-diagnostic tests. *Serum calcium:* increased

Patient monitoring

• Monitor serum calcium and phosphorus levels periodically.

Patient teaching

• Instruct patient to take drug with or immediately after meals and to chew tablets completely before swallowing.
• Advise patient to discuss any planned dietary changes with prescriber.
• Inform female patient with childbearing potential that drug isn't recommended during pregnancy.
• Instruct female patient to tell prescriber if she's breastfeeding.
• As appropriate, review all other significant adverse reactions and interactions, especially those related to the tests mentioned above.

lapatinib
Tykerb

Pharmacologic class: 4-Anilinoquinazoline kinase inhibitor
Therapeutic class: Antineoplastic
Pregnancy risk category D

Action

Lapatinib is a 4-anilinoquinazoline kinase inhibitor of the intracellular tyrosine kinase domains of both Epidermal Growth Factor Receptor (EGFR [ErbB1]) and of Human Epidermal Receptor Type 2 (HER2 [ErbB2]) receptors (estimated K_i^{app} values of 3nM and 13nM, respectively) with a dissociation half-life of ≥300 minutes. Lapatinib inhibits ErbB-driven tumor cell growth in vitro and in various animal models.

Availability

Tablets: 250 mg

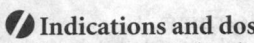 Indications and dosages

➤ Advanced or metastatic breast cancer in patients whose tumors overexpress HER2 and who have received

prior therapy, including an anthracycline, a taxane, and trastuzumab
Adults: 1,250 mg P.O. daily on days 1
to 21 continuously in combination
with capecitabine on days 1 to 14 in
repeating 21-day cycle
➤ Postmenopausal women with hormone receptor-positive metastatic
breast cancer that overexpresses HER2
receptor, for whom hormonal therapy
is indicated
Adults: 1,500 mg P.O. daily continuously in combination with letrozole

Dosage adjustment
• Severe hepatic impairment
• Cardiac toxicity
• Grade 2 or greater NCI CTCAE
toxicity
• Concurrent use of strong CYP3A4
inducers/inhibitors

Contraindications
• Hypersensitivity to drug or its
components

Precautions
Use cautiously in:
• severe hepatic impairment (Child-
Pugh Class C)
• decreased left ventricular ejection
fraction (LVEF), patients who have or
may develop prolongation of QT interval (including patients with
hypokalemia, hypomagnesemia, congenital long QT syndrome; patients
taking antiarrhythmics or other products leading to QT-interval prolongation; and cumulative high-dose
anthracycline therapy)
• Grade 2 or greater NCI CTCAE
toxicity
• interstitial lung disease and pneumonitis, diarrhea
• strong CYP3A4 inducers including
St. John's wort, strong CYP3A4
inhibitors (avoid use)
• concurrent use of CYP3A4, CYP2C8,
and P-glycoprotein (PgP) substrates
• grapefruit, grapefruit products
(avoid use)

• pregnant or breastfeeding patients
• children (safety and efficacy not
established).

Administration
• Administer at least 1 hour before or
1 hour after a meal, but give
capecitabine with food or within 30
minutes after food. Don't give with
grapefruit or grapefruit juice. Don't
divide daily doses.
• Correct hypokalemia or hypomagnesemia before lapatinib administration.
• Assess serum digoxin concentration
before starting drug. If digoxin serum
concentration is greater than 1.2 ng/ml,
reduce digoxin dosage as prescribed.
• Evaluate LVEF before starting lapatinib treatment to ensure patient has
baseline LVEF within institution's normal limits. Be aware that drug should
be discontinued in patients with
decreased LVEF that is Grade 2 or
greater NCI CTCAE toxicity and in
patients with LVEF that drops below
institution's lower limit of normal.
Lapatinib in combination with
capecitabine may be restarted at
reduced dosage of 1,000 mg/day and in
combination with letrozole may be
restarted at reduced dosage of 1,250
mg/day after minimum of 2 weeks if
LVEF recovers to normal and patient is
asymptomatic.
◀€ Obtain liver function test results
(transaminases, bilirubin, and ALP)
before starting treatment. Consider
reducing dosage in patients with severe
hepatic impairment from 1,250
mg/day to 750 mg/day (HER2-positive
metastatic breast cancer indication) or
from 1,500 mg/day to 1,000 mg/day
(hormone receptor-positive, HER2-
positive breast cancer indication) to
adjust area under the curve (AUC) to
normal range. In patients who develop
severe hepatotoxicity during therapy,
discontinue drug and don't restart.
◀€ Discontinue drug in patients who
experience pulmonary signs and

Reactions in **bold** are life-threatening.   ◀€ Clinical alert

symptoms indicative of interstitial lung disease/pneumonitis that are Grade 3 or greater (NCI CTCAE).

• If patient must receive a strong CYP3A4 inhibitor concurrently, consider reducing lapatinib dosage to 500 mg/day. This dosage is predicted to adjust lapatinib AUC to the range observed without inhibitors. If the strong inhibitor is discontinued, a washout period of approximately 1 week should be allowed before lapatinib dosage is adjusted upward to indicated dosage.

• If patient must receive a strong CYP3A4 inducer concurrently, consider titrating lapatanib dosage gradually from 1,250 mg/day up to 4,500 mg/day (HER2-positive metastatic breast cancer indication) or from 1,500 mg/day up to 5,500 mg/day (hormone receptor–positive, HER2-positive breast cancer indication) based on tolerability. This dosage is predicted to adjust lapatinib AUC to the range observed without inducers. If the strong inducer is discontinued, lapatinib dosage should be reduced to indicated dosage.

• Be aware that severe diarrhea may require administration of oral or I.V. electrolytes and fluids and interruption or discontinuation of therapy.

Route	Onset	Peak	Duration
P.O.	Unknown	4 hr	Unknown

Adverse reactions

CNS: headache, fatigue, insomnia, asthenia
CV: prolonged QT interval
EENT: epistaxis
GI: nausea, vomiting, diarrhea, anorexia, dyspepsia, stomatitis
Hepatic: hepatotoxicity
Musculoskeletal: extremity pain, back pain
Respiratory: dyspnea, **interstitial lung disease, pneumonitis**

Skin: rash, dry skin, alopecia, pruritus, nail disorder, palmar-plantar erythrodysesthesia
Other: mucosal inflammation

Interactions

Drug-drug. *CYP3A4 substrates (midazolam), CYP2C8 and PgP substrates (paclitaxel), PgP substrates (digoxin):* increased exposure of these drugs
Strong CYP3A4 inducers (such as carbamazepine, dexamethasone, phenobarbital, phenytoin, rifabutin, rifampin, rifapentin): decreased lapatinib systemic exposure
Strong CYP3A4 inhibitors (such as atazanavir, clarithromycin, indinavir, itraconazole, ketoconazole, nefazodone, nelfinavir, ritonavir, saquinavir, telithromycin, voriconazole): increased lapatinib systemic exposure and half-life
Drug-diagnostic tests. *ALT, AST, total bilirubin:* increased levels
Hemoglobin, neutrophils, platelets: decreased levels
Drug-food. *Any food:* increased lapatinib systemic exposure
Grapefruit: increased lapatinib plasma concentration
High-fat meal: increased AUC value
Drug-herbs. *St. John's Wort:* decreased lapatinib systemic exposure

Patient monitoring

• Monitor CBC with differential and hepatic function tests closely.
• Monitor serum digoxin concentration throughout coadministration with lapatinib.
🔊 Continue to monitor patient for prolonged QT interval, interstitial lung disease, and pneumonitis.

Patient teaching

• Tell patient to take lapatinib at least 1 hour before or 1 hour after a meal but if capecitabine is also prescribed to take capecitabine with food or within 30 minutes after food. Advise patient not to take lapatinib with grapefruit or grapefruit juice or divide daily doses.

 Instruct patient to immediately report tiredness, dizziness, shortness of breath, pounding or racing heartbeats, itching, yellowing of skin or eyes, dark urine, right upper abdominal pain or discomfort, or red, painful hands and feet.

• Teach patient how to prevent and manage diarrhea, which may be severe; instruct patient to inform prescriber of changes in bowel pattern or severe diarrhea.

• Instruct patient to tell prescriber about all drugs he's taking, because some drugs have potential for serious drug interactions and shouldn't be taken with lapatinib.

• Advise patient not to use St. John's wort or other herbal supplements without consulting prescriber.

• Advise female patient of childbearing age to avoid becoming pregnant during therapy.

• Advise breastfeeding patient that she should decide whether to discontinue breastfeeding or discontinue drug, taking into account importance of drug for her treatment.

• As appropriate, review all other significant and life-threatening adverse reactions and interactions, especially those related to the drugs, tests, foods, and herbs mentioned above.

leflunomide

Apo-Leflunomide✖, Arava, Novo-Leflunomide✖, PMS-Leflunomide✖, Sandoz Leflunomide✖

Pharmacologic class: Immune modulator
Therapeutic class: Antirheumatic
Pregnancy risk category X

FDA BOXED WARNING

• Rule out pregnancy before starting therapy. Drug is contraindicated in pregnant women and in women of childbearing age who don't use reliable contraception. Caution patient to avoid pregnancy during therapy or before completing drug elimination procedure after treatment.

• Be aware that severe liver injury, including fatal liver failure, has been reported in some patients treated with leflunomide. Know that patients with preexisting acute or chronic liver disease, or those with serum alanine aminotransferase (ALT) level of more than two times the upper limit of normal (ULN) before initiating treatment, shouldn't be treated with leflunomide. Use caution when giving drug with other potentially hepatotoxic drugs. Monitor ALT level at least monthly for first 6 months of therapy, and every 6 to 8 weeks thereafter. If ALT elevation is more than three times ULN, interrupt therapy while investigating the probable cause of the ALT elevation by close observation and additional tests. If ALT elevation is likely leflunomide-induced, start cholestyramine washout and monitor liver tests weekly until normalized. If leflunomide-induced liver injury is unlikely (because another probable cause has been found), resumption of therapy may be considered.

Action

Inhibits T-cell pyrimidine biosynthesis, tyrosine kinases, and dihydroorotate dehydrogenase, blocking structural damage caused by inflammatory response to autoimmune process. Also shows analgesic, antipyretic, and histamine-blocking activity.

Availability

Tablets: 10 mg, 20 mg, 100 mg

⚕ Indications and dosages

➤ Active rheumatoid arthritis

Adults: 100 mg P.O. daily for 3 days, then a maintenance dosage of 20 mg daily. If intolerance occurs, decrease to 10 mg daily.

Route	Onset	Peak	Duration
P.O.	1 mo	3-6 mo	Unknown

Dosage adjustment

- Hepatic enzyme elevations

Contraindications

- Hypersensitivity to drug or its components
- Women who are or may become pregnant

Precautions

Use cautiously in:
- renal insufficiency
- patients with severe immunodeficiency, bone marrow dysplasia, or severe, uncontrolled infections (not recommended)
- new-onset or worsening pulmonary symptoms
- concurrent use of potentially hepatotoxic drugs
- concurrent use of live-virus vaccines (not recommended)
- men attempting to father a child
- breastfeeding patients
- children younger than age 18.

Administration

- Before starting drug, screen patients for latent tuberculosis (TB) infection with a tuberculin skin test. Treat patients who test positive for TB with standard medical practice before starting leflunomide.
- Obtain baseline platelet and white blood cell (WBC) counts, and hemoglobin or hematocrit.
- Check patient's blood pressure before starting leflunomide
- Give with or without food.
- Be aware that drug has a long half-life. To eliminate from bloodstream, give 8 g cholestyramine P.O. t.i.d. for 11 days.

Adverse reactions

CNS: headache, dizziness, asthenia
CV: chest pain, hypertension
EENT: rhinitis, sinusitis, pharyngitis
GI: nausea, vomiting, diarrhea, abdominal pain, dyspepsia, gastroenteritis, mouth ulcers, anorexia
GU: urinary tract infection
Hematologic: pancytopenia, agranulocytosis, thrombocytopenia (rare)
Hepatic: hepatotoxicity
Metabolic: hypokalemia
Musculoskeletal: joint pain or disorders, back pain, leg cramps, synovitis, tenosynovitis
Respiratory: bronchitis, increased cough, pneumonia, respiratory infection, **fatal interstitial lung disease**
Skin: alopecia, rash, dry skin, eczema, pruritus, **Stevens-Johnson syndrome, toxic epidermal necrolysis**
Other: weight loss, pain, infection, allergic reactions, flulike symptoms

Interactions

Drug-drug. *Activated charcoal, cholestyramine:* rapid, steep drop in blood level of leflunomide's active metabolite
Methotrexate, other hepatotoxic drugs: increased risk of hepatotoxicity
Rifampin: increased blood level of leflunomide's active metabolite
Drug-diagnostic tests. *Alanine aminotransferase (ALT); aspartate aminotransferase:* increased levels
Hematocrit, hemoglobin, platelets, WBCs: decreased levels

Patient monitoring

- Check vital signs closely.
- Monitor platelet and WBC counts and hemoglobin or hematocrit monthly for 6 months after initiation of therapy and every 6 to 8 weeks thereafter. If evidence of bone marrow suppression occurs, discontinue drug

and treat as indicated to reduce plasma concentration of leflunomide's active metabolite.

◀€ Watch for signs and symptoms of hepatotoxicity.

◀€ Be aware that rare cases of Stevens-Johnson syndrome and toxic epidermal necrolysis have been reported in patients receiving leflunomide. If patient develops either condition, discontinue drug by using the recommended drug elimination procedure.

• Periodically assess cardiovascular status, including blood pressure, carefully to detect adverse reactions.

• Be aware that interstitial lung disease has been reported during leflunomide therapy and has been associated with fatal outcomes. New-onset or worsening pulmonary symptoms, such as cough and dyspnea with or without associated fever, may be cause for discontinuing drug and for further investigation as appropriate. If stopping drug is necessary, consider initiation of wash-out procedures.

• Monitor electrolyte levels.

• Monitor ALT level at least monthly for 6 months after starting drug, and every 6 to 8 weeks thereafter. If ALT level is more than three times the upper limit of normal, interrupt therapy while investigating the probable cause of the ALT elevation by close observation and additional tests. If leflunomide therapy is likely cause, start cholestyramine washout and monitor liver tests weekly until normalized. If leflunomide-induced liver injury is unlikely because another probable cause has been found, consider resuming drug therapy.

• Stay alert for signs and symptoms of infection. If a serious infection occurs, it may be necessary to interrupt therapy and administer cholestyramine or charcoal, as indicated.

• Observe patient closely after dosage reduction. Metabolite levels may take several weeks to fall.

Patient teaching

• Tell patient he may take with or without food.

◀€ Advise patient to immediately report unusual tiredness or yellowing of skin or eyes.

◀€ Instruct patient to recognize and report signs or symptoms of infection, respiratory problems, Stevens-Johnson syndrome, and toxic epidermal necrolysis.

• Advise patient to avoid vaccination with live-virus vaccines.

• Caution patient to avoid driving and other hazardous activities until he knows how drug affects concentration and alertness.

◀€ Inform female of childbearing age that drug may harm fetus. Tell her to contact prescriber immediately if she suspects pregnancy.

• Caution female not to breastfeed without consulting prescriber.

• Advise male planning to father a child to consult prescriber, because drug may harm fetus.

• Tell patient he'll undergo regular blood testing to check liver function.

• As appropriate, review all other significant and life-threatening adverse reactions and interactions, especially those related to the drugs and tests mentioned above.

lenalidomide
Revlimid

Pharmacologic class: Thalidomide analogue

Therapeutic class: Antineoplastic, immunomodulator

Pregnancy risk category X

• If taken during pregnancy, drug may cause fetal death or severe, life-threatening birth defects. Advise females to avoid pregnancy. Drug is available only under RevAssist distribution program, in which only registered prescribers and pharmacists can prescribe and dispense it to registered patients who meet certain conditions. For information, visit www.REVLIMID.com or call 1-888-423-5436.

• Drug has been linked to hematologic toxicity (including significant neutropenia and thrombocytopenia); 80% of patients with myelodysplastic syndrome (MDS) associated with deletion 5q cytogenic abnormality have required dose delays or dosage reductions. For patients with these syndromes, monitor complete blood count (CBC) weekly for first 8 weeks of therapy and at least monthly thereafter. Patients may require dose delay, dosage reduction, or both and require blood product support, growth factors, or both.

• Drug may increase risk of deep vein thrombosis and pulmonary embolism in patients with multiple myeloma who receive it in combination with dexamethasone. Stay alert for signs and symptoms, such as shortness of breath, chest pain, and arm or leg swelling. Prescriber must consider patient's risk factors when deciding whether to use prophylaxis.

Action
Inhibits secretion of proinflammatory cytokines and increases secretion of anti-inflammatory cytokines from peripheral mononuclear cells

Availability
Capsules: 5 mg, 10 mg, 15 mg, 25 mg

⚕ Indications and dosages
➤ Transfusion-dependent anemia caused by low- or intermediate-1-risk MDS associated with deletion 5q cytogenic abnormality (with or without additional cytogenic abnormalities)
Adults: 10 mg P.O. daily
➤ Multiple myeloma, in patients who have received at least one prior therapy given with dexamethasone
Adults: 25 mg P.O. daily with water given as single 25-mg capsule on days 1 to 21 of repeated 28-day cycles. Recommended dexamethasone dosage is 40 mg/day on days 1 to 4, 9 to 12, and 17 to 20 of each 28-day cycle for first four cycles of therapy, then 40 mg P.O. daily on days 1 to 4 every 28 days.

Dosage adjustment
• Thrombocytopenia
• Neutropenia
• Moderate to severe renal impairment and patients on dialysis

Contraindications
• Hypersensitivity to drug or its components
• Pregnancy

Precautions
Use cautiously in:
• renal impairment
• history of Grade 4 rash associated with thalidomide treatment (use not recommended)
• elderly patients
• patients with childbearing potential
• breastfeeding patients
• children (safety and efficacy not established).

Administration
• Be aware that patient must be able to reliably follow instructions and must understand conditions of RevAssist program to be eligible for drug.
• Administer drug with water.
• Know that before drug is prescribed, female patient should have two

negative pregnancy tests (with sensitivity of at least 50 mIU/ml).

◀€ Be aware that patients with history of Grade 4 rash associated with thalidomide treatment shouldn't receive drug.

Route	Onset	Peak	Duration
P.O.	Unknown	40 min -1.5 hr	Unknown

Adverse reactions

CNS: dizziness, headache, hypoesthesia, peripheral neuropathy, insomnia, depression, rigors, fatigue
CV: hypertension, palpitations, **deep vein thrombosis**
EENT: epistaxis, rhinitis, pharyngitis, nasopharyngitis, sinusitis
GI: diarrhea, loose stools, constipation, nausea, vomiting, abdominal pain, anorexia, dry mouth, dysgeusia
GU: urinary tract infection, dysuria
Hematologic: anemia, **thrombocytopenia, neutropenia, leukopenia, febrile neutropenia, granulocytopenia, pancytopenia**
Metabolic: hypokalemia, hypomagnesemia, hypothyroidism
Musculoskeletal: arthralgia, back pain, muscle cramps, limb pain, myalgia
Respiratory: cough, dyspnea, exertional dyspnea, bronchitis, upper respiratory tract infection, pneumonia, **respiratory distress, pulmonary embolism**
Skin: pruritus, rash, dry skin, contusion, ecchymosis, erythema, **angioedema, Stevens-Johnson syndrome, toxic epidermal necrolysis**
Other: fever, peripheral edema, pain, chest pain, cellulitis, night sweats, increased sweating, sepsis, **tumor lysis syndrome**

Interactions

Drug-drug. *Digoxin:* increased digoxin level
Drug-diagnostic tests. *Magnesium, potassium, thyroid function:* decrease in levels or function

Patient monitoring

• Monitor CBC weekly for first 3 months, then at least monthly.
• Watch carefully for electrolyte disorders and abnormal thyroid function tests.

◀€ Monitor patient closely for signs and symptoms of serious dermatologic reactions; interrupt therapy for Grade 2 to 3 rash. Discontinue drug for angioedema, Grade 4 rash, or exfoliative or bullous rash, or if Stevens-Johnson syndrome or toxic epidermal necrolysis is suspected; don't resume drug in these patients.

◀€ Monitor patient closely for signs and symptoms of tumor lysis syndrome (irregular heartbeat, shortness of breath, high potassium or uric acid levels, impairment of mental ability, renal failure) and take appropriate measures.

Patient teaching

• Instruct patient to swallow capsules whole with water and not to open, chew, or crush them.
• Advise patient to report unusual symptoms or persistence or worsening of known symptoms.
• Urge female patient to use two effective contraceptive methods simultaneously for at least 4 weeks before starting therapy, during therapy, during dosage interruptions, and for 4 weeks after therapy ends. Emphasize that she must use contraception even if she has a history of infertility (unless she has had a hysterectomy).
• Instruct female patient to stop taking drug if she misses a period, has unusual menstrual bleeding, stops using contraception, or suspects pregnancy.
• Advise patient to immediately report unprotected sexual contact or suspected pregnancy.
• Instruct male patient to use latex condom during sexual contact with female of childbearing potential.

Reactions in **bold** are life-threatening. ◀€ Clinical alert

• Inform patients they can't donate blood during therapy.

• Tell male patients they can't donate sperm or semen during therapy.

• As appropriate, review all other significant or life-threatening adverse reactions and interactions, especially those related to the drugs and tests mentioned above.

letrozole
Femara

Pharmacologic class: Aromatase inhibitor
Therapeutic class: Antineoplastic
Pregnancy risk category D

Action
Inhibits aromatase, an enzyme that promotes conversion of estrogen precursors to estrogen. This inhibition reduces circulating estrogen levels and stops progression of breast cancer.

Availability
Tablets: 2.5 mg

Indications and dosages
➢ Metastatic or advanced breast cancer in postmenopausal women; early breast cancer in postmenopausal women who have received 5 years of antiestrogen therapy
Adults: 2.5 mg P.O. daily

Contraindications
• Hypersensitivity to drug or its components

Precautions
Use cautiously in:
• severe hepatic impairment
• pregnant or breastfeeding patients
• children (safety not established).

Administration
• Give with or without meals.

Route	Onset	Peak	Duration
P.O.	Unknown	2-3 days	Unknown

Adverse reactions
CNS: anxiety, depression, dizziness, drowsiness, fatigue, headache, vertigo, asthenia
CV: chest pain, hypertension
EENT: blurred vision
GI: nausea, vomiting, diarrhea, constipation, abdominal pain, dyspepsia, anorexia
Metabolic: hypercalcemia
Musculoskeletal: musculoskeletal or joint pain, fractures
Respiratory: cough, dyspnea, **pleural effusion**
Skin: alopecia, pruritus, rash, diaphoresis
Other: hot flashes, edema, weight gain, **angioedema, anaphylactic reactions**

Interactions
Drug-diagnostic tests. *Cholesterol, gamma-glutamyltransferase:* increased levels

Patient monitoring
• Check vital signs and assess cardiovascular and respiratory status.
• Monitor renal and hepatic function, electrolyte levels, and lipid panels.
• Assess for adverse CNS effects, including depression. Institute safety measures as needed to prevent injury.

Patient teaching
• Tell patient she can take with or without food.
• Instruct patient to weigh herself regularly and report significant changes.
• Advise patient and family to watch for signs and symptoms of depression.
• Tell patient to minimize GI upset by eating small, frequent servings of healthy food and drinking plenty of fluids.
• Caution patient to avoid driving and other hazardous activities until she

knows how drug affects concentration and alertness.
• Inform patient that treatment is long term. Urge her to keep follow-up appointments with prescriber.
• Tell patient to inform prescriber if she is pregnant or breastfeeding.
• As appropriate, review all other significant and life-threatening adverse reactions and interactions, especially those related to the tests mentioned above.

leucovorin calcium (citrovorum factor, folinic acid)
Calcium Folinate✛, Lederfolin✛, Refolinon✛

Pharmacologic class: Water-soluble vitamin

Therapeutic class: Vitamin, antidote to folic acid antagonist, antianemic, antineoplastic adjunct

Pregnancy risk category C

Action
Counteracts therapeutic and toxic effects of folic acid antagonists; may enhance therapeutic and toxic effects of fluoropyrimidines used in cancer therapy. Also supplements folic acid in folic acid deficiency.

Availability
Injection (expressed as base): 10 mg/vial, 50 mg/vial, 100 mg/vial, 200 mg/vial, 350 mg/vial, 500 mg/vial
Injection, preservative-free (expressed as base): 10 mg/vial, 50 mg/vial, 200 mg/vial, 350 mg/vial, 500 mg/vial
Tablets: 5 mg, 15 mg, 25 mg

🕖 Indications and dosages
➤ Leucovorin rescue after high-dose methotrexate therapy

Adults: 15 mg (approximately 10 mg/m²) P.O., I.M., or I.V. q 6 hours, starting 24 hours after methotrexate infusion begins and continuing until serum methotrexate level drops below 10^{-8} M. If 24-hour serum creatinine level rises 50% over baseline or if 24-hour methotrexate level exceeds 5×10^{-6} M or 48-hour level exceeds 9×10^{-7} M, increase leucovorin dosage to 100 mg/m² I.V. q 3 hours and continue hydration and urinary alkalization until methotrexate level drops below 10^{-8} M.
➤ To reduce toxicity and counteract effects of impaired methotrexate elimination or inadvertent overdose of folic acid antagonist
Adults: 15 mg (roughly 10 mg/m²) I.M., I.V., or P.O. q 6 hours until serum methotrexate level drops below 10^{-8} M. If 24-hour serum creatinine level rises 50% over baseline or if 24-hour methotrexate level exceeds 5×10^{-6} M or 48-hour level exceeds 9×10^{-7} M, increase leucovorin dosage to 100 mg/m² I.V. q 3 hours and continue hydration and urinary alkalization until methotrexate level drops below 10^{-8} M.
➤ Advanced colorectal cancer
Adults: Usually given in one of the following regimens: 200 mg/m² slow I.V. injection over at least 3 minutes, followed by I.V. injection of 5-fluorouracil (5-FU); or 20 mg/m² I.V. injection, followed by I.V. injection of 5-FU. Treatment is repeated daily for 5 days, and may then be repeated at 28-day intervals for two courses and then at 4- to 5-week intervals, as prescribed.
➤ Megaloblastic anemia secondary to folic acid deficiency
Adults: Up to 1 mg I.M. daily

Dosage adjustment
• In leucovorin rescue after high-dose methotrexate therapy: delayed early or late methotrexate elimination (serum methotrexate level still above 0.2 µM

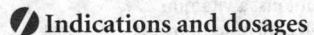

at 72 hours and above 0.05 μM [5 × 10^{-8}] at 96 hours after administration)
• Evidence of acute renal injury

Contraindications
• Treatment of pernicious anemia and other megaloblastic anemias caused by vitamin B_{12} deficiency

Precautions
Use cautiously in:
• anemia (when vitamin B_{12} deficiency has been ruled out)
• patients receiving 5-FU concomitantly
• pregnant or breastfeeding patients
• children.

Administration
◀ℰ Recheck leucovorin dosage in current published protocols before giving as methotrexate rescue.
• Give parenterally in patients with GI toxicity, nausea, or vomiting.
• Reconstitute leucovorin injection with sterile or bacteriostatic water for injection containing benzyl alcohol. (When giving with 5-FU for colorectal cancer in dosages above 10 mg/m², reconstitute only with sterile water for injection.)
◀ℰ Don't mix leucovorin injection with 5-FU, because precipitation will occur.
◀ℰ Give I.V. leucovorin slowly (no faster than 160 mg/minute) because of calcium content. Large doses may be infused over 1 to 6 hours as directed.
◀ℰ Don't give intrathecally; drug may be harmful or fatal by this route.
• Be aware that P.O. dosages above 25 mg are not recommended.

Route	Onset	Peak	Duration
P.O.	20-30 min	6-90 min	3-6 hr
I.V.	<5 min	Unknown	3-6 hr
I.M.	10-20 min	35-60 min	3-6 hr

Adverse reactions
Skin: urticaria
Other: allergic sensitization reactions, **anaphylactoid reactions**

Interactions
Drug-drug. *5-FU:* enhanced fluorouracil toxicity
Methotrexate, other folic acid antagonists: negated therapeutic and toxic effects of these drugs
Phenobarbital, phenytoin, primidone: negated anticonvulsant effect, increased frequency of seizures in susceptible children

Patient monitoring
◀ℰ Monitor serum creatinine and methotrexate levels every 24 hours.
◀ℰ Monitor closely for adverse reactions. Continue leucovorin therapy, hydration, and urinary alkalization until serum methotrexate level drops below 10^{-8} M.
◀ℰ Monitor CBC with white cell differential and platelet count before leucovorin/5-FU therapy starts. Repeat weekly during first two courses and then once each cycle at anticipated white blood cell nadir.
• Check electrolyte levels and liver function tests before each treatment for first three cycles. Thereafter, check before every other cycle.
• Assess for adequate hydration when giving with 5-FU or high-dose methotrexate.
• Watch for hypersensitivity reactions, especially anaphylactoid reactions.

Patient teaching
• Teach patient about drug and protocol.
◀ℰ Stress importance of taking leucovorin as prescribed with high-dose methotrexate therapy. Emphasize that it's not just a vitamin.
• Tell patient to immediately report signs or symptoms of allergic reaction, such as hives.

- As appropriate, review all other significant and life-threatening adverse reactions and interactions, especially those related to the drugs mentioned above.

leuprolide acetate (leuprorelin⊕)

Eligard, Lupron, Lupron Depot, Lupron Depot-Ped, Lupron Depot-3 Month, Lupron Depot-4 Month, Lupron-3 Month SR Depot, Prostap⊕

Pharmacologic class: Gonadotropin-releasing hormone (GnRH) analog
Therapeutic class: Antineoplastic
Pregnancy risk category X

Action
Inhibits and desensitizes GnRH receptors, thus inhibiting gonadotropin secretion when given continuously. This inhibition causes initial increase and then profound decrease in luteinizing hormone and follicle-stimulating hormone levels and, ultimately, reduces testosterone and estrogen sex hormones.

Availability
Eligard Depot: 7.5 mg, 22.5 mg, 30 mg, 45 mg
Injection: 1 mg/0.2 ml
Lupron Depot injection: 3.75 mg/ml, 7.5 mg/ml
Lupron Depot-3 month injection: 11.25 mg, 22.5 mg
Lupron Depot-4 month injection: 30 mg
Lupron Depot-Ped injection: 7.5 mg, 11.25 mg, 15 mg

💋 Indications and dosages
➤ Advanced prostate cancer
Adults: 1 mg subcutaneously daily (1 mg/0.2-ml formulation). For Lupron Depot formulation, 7.5 mg I.M. monthly, 22.5 mg I.M. q 3 months, or 30 mg I.M. q 4 months. For Eligard formulation, 7.5 mg subcutaneously monthly, 22.5 mg subcutaneously q 3 months, 30 mg subcutaneously q 4 months, or 45 mg subcutaneously q 6 months.
➤ Endometriosis
Adults: 3.75 mg I.M. (depot injection) as a single injection once monthly, or 11.25 mg I.M. q 3 months. Duration is up to 6 months.
➤ Adjunct to iron therapy in anemia caused by uterine leiomyomas
Adults: 3.75 mg I.M. monthly or 11.25 mg I.M. q 3 months as a single dose. Recommended duration is 6 months or less.
➤ Central precocious puberty
Children: 50 mcg/kg/day subcutaneously as a single injection, increased in increments of 10 mcg/kg/day as needed
Children weighing more than 37.5 kg (82.5 lb): Initially, 15 mg of Depot-Ped I.M. q 4 weeks, increased in increments of 3.75 mg q 4 weeks as needed
Children weighing 25 to 37.5 kg (55 to 82.5 lb): Initially, 11.25 mg of Depot-Ped I.M. q 4 weeks, increased in increments of 3.75 mg q 4 weeks as needed
Children weighing less than 25 kg (55 lb): Initially, 7.5 mg of Depot-Ped I.M. q 4 weeks, increased in increments of 3.75 mg q 4 weeks as needed

Contraindications
- Hypersensitivity to drug, its components, GnRH, or other GnRH analogs
- Undiagnosed abnormal vaginal bleeding
- Pregnancy or breastfeeding

Precautions
Use cautiously in:
- renal, hepatic, or cardiac impairment.

Administration
- Give Eligard within 30 minutes of mixing. After this time, discard.
- Administer Lupron injection immediately after mixing. Otherwise, discard.
- Administer Lupron Depot-Ped only under prescriber's supervision.

Route	Onset	Peak	Duration
I.M. depot	4 hr	Variable	1, 3, 4 mo
Subcut. (prec. puberty)	1 wk	Unknown	4-12 wk after therapy
Subcut. (endo-metriosis, cancer)	2-4 wk	After 1-2 mo	2-3 mo after therapy

Adverse reactions
CNS: anxiety, depression, dizziness, drowsiness, asthenia, fatigue, headache, vertigo, syncope, mood changes
CV: palpitations, angina, **arrhythmias, myocardial infarction**
EENT: blurred vision
GI: nausea, vomiting, diarrhea, constipation, abdominal pain, dyspepsia, anorexia
GU: urinary frequency, hematuria, decreased testes size, erectile dysfunction, decreased libido, gynecomastia
Hematologic: anemia, **thrombocytopenia**
Respiratory: dyspnea, pleural rub, **worsening of pulmonary fibrosis, pulmonary embolism**
Skin: alopecia, pruritus, rash, diaphoresis
Other: sour taste, edema, hot flashes, **anaphylaxis**

Interactions
Drug-diagnostic tests. *Blood urea nitrogen, creatinine:* increased levels
Pituitary-gonadal system tests: misleading results during and for up to 3 months after therapy

Patient monitoring
- Observe injection site for local reactions.
- ◀€ Monitor cardiovascular and respiratory status carefully to detect serious adverse reactions.
- Evaluate neurologic status. Institute safety measures as needed to prevent injury.
- Periodically monitor serum testosterone and prostate-specific antigen levels.

Patient teaching
- Inform patient that localized reaction may occur at injection site. Tell him to contact prescriber if symptoms don't resolve.
- Advise patient and family to watch for and report signs or symptoms of depression.
- Tell patient drug may cause libido changes or erectile dysfunction. Encourage him to discuss these problems with prescriber.
- Teach patient to minimize GI upset by eating small, frequent servings of food and drinking plenty of fluids.
- ◀€ Instruct female of childbearing age to use reliable contraception during therapy. Tell her to stop drug immediately and contact prescriber if she suspects pregnancy.
- ◀€ Tell female patient not to breastfeed.
- Caution patient to avoid driving and other hazardous activities until he knows how drug affects concentration and alertness.
- As appropriate, review all other significant and life-threatening adverse reactions and interactions, especially those related to the tests mentioned above.

levalbuterol hydrochloride
Xopenex HFA

Pharmacologic class: Adrenergic beta$_2$ agonist
Therapeutic class: Bronchodilator
Pregnancy risk category C

Action
Binds to beta$_2$-adrenergic receptors on bronchial cell membrane, stimulating the intracellular enzyme adenylate cyclase to convert adenosine triphosphate to cyclic-3′,5′-adenosine monophosphate. This action relaxes smooth muscles, dilates bronchioles, and increases diuresis.

Availability
Solution for inhalation: 0.31 mg/3 ml, 0.63 mg/3 ml, 1.25 mg/3 ml

🚫 Indications and dosages
➣ Prevention and treatment of bronchospasm
Adults and children ages 12 and older: 0.63 to 1.25 mg by oral inhalation via nebulizer q 6 to 8 hours
Children ages 6 to 11: 0.31 to 0.63 mg by oral inhalation via nebulizer t.i.d.

Contraindications
• Hypersensitivity to drug or racemic albuterol

Precautions
Use cautiously in:
• renal, hepatic, or cardiac impairment; hyperthyroidism; diabetes mellitus; hypertension; prostatic hypertrophy; angle-closure glaucoma; seizures
• pregnant patients.

Administration
• Use only with nebulizer system designed for this drug.

• Keep unopened vials in foil pouch. Once pouch is opened, use within 2 weeks.
• If vial is removed from pouch, protect from light and use within 1 week.

Route	Onset	Peak	Duration
Inhalation	10-17 min	1.5 hr	5-6 hr

Adverse reactions
CNS: anxiety, dizziness, hypertonia, insomnia, migraine, headache, nervousness, paresthesia, syncope, tremor
CV: chest pain, hypertension, hypotension, tachycardia
EENT: rhinitis, sinusitis, dry throat
GI: nausea, vomiting, diarrhea, constipation, abdominal pain, dyspepsia, anorexia, dry mouth
Metabolic: hypokalemia
Musculoskeletal: muscle cramps, myalgia
Respiratory: cough, dyspnea, **asthma exacerbation, paradoxical bronchospasm**
Other: sour taste, flulike symptoms, lymphadenopathy, chills

Interactions
Drug-drug. *Aerosol bronchodilators:* increased action of both drugs
Antidepressants: increased risk of adverse cardiovascular effects
Beta-adrenergic blockers: inhibition of levalbuterol effect
Digoxin: decreased digoxin blood level
Loop and thiazide diuretics: increased risk of hypokalemia
Drug-food. *Caffeine-containing foods and beverages:* increased stimulation
Drug-herbs. *Cola nut, ephedra (ma huang), guarana, yerba maté:* increased stimulation

Patient monitoring
• Monitor vital signs and ECG closely.
• Assess cardiovascular and neurologic status. Institute safety measures as needed to prevent injury.

Reactions in **bold** are life-threatening.   🔊 Clinical alert

◀€ Monitor for paradoxical broncho-spasm. If it occurs, stop drug therapy and notify prescriber immediately.
• Check electrolyte levels for hypo-kalemia.
• Assess patient's response to drug. Contact prescriber if patient needs more frequent doses for same effect.

Patient teaching
• Teach patient how to prepare drug, administer it with nebulizer, and main-tain and clean nebulizer.
• Advise patient to continue treat-ment for about 5 to 15 minutes or until mist no longer forms in nebu-lizer reservoir.
◀€ Tell patient to immediately report increased difficulty breathing or tight-ness in chest.
• Caution patient to avoid driving and other hazardous activities until he knows how drug affects concentration and alertness.
• As appropriate, review all other sig-nificant and life-threatening adverse reactions and interactions, especially those related to the drugs, foods, and herbs mentioned above.

levetiracetam

Apo-Levetiracetam✷, Co Levetiracetam✷, Dom-Levetiracetam✷, Keppra, Keppra XR, PHL-Levetiracetam, PMS-Levetiracetam✷

Pharmacologic class: Pyrrolidine derivative
Therapeutic class: Anticonvulsant
Pregnancy risk category C

Action
Unknown. Thought to prevent seizures by inhibiting nerve impulses in hippocampus of brain. Chemically unrelated to other anticonvulsants.

Availability
Oral solution: 100 mg/ml
Solution for injection: 500 mg/5 ml in single-use 5-ml vial
Tablets: 250 mg, 500 mg, 750 mg, 1,000 mg
Tablets (extended-release): 500 mg

✪ Indications and dosages
➤ Adjunctive treatment of partial-onset seizures in patients with epilepsy
Adults and children ages 16 and older: Initially, 500 mg P.O. (immediate-release preparations) b.i.d. May increase by 1,000 mg/day q 2 weeks to a maximum daily dosage of 3,000 mg, as needed. Or, initially 1,000 mg P.O. (extended-release tablets) once daily. Adjust in increments of 1,000 mg q 2 weeks to a maximum daily dosage of 3,000 mg, as appropriate. Or, when oral administration is temporarily not feasible, give initial daily I.V. dosage equivalent to total daily dosage and frequency of oral drug.
Children ages 4 to 15: Initially, 20 mg/kg/day P.O. (immediate-release preparations) in two divided doses (10 mg/kg b.i.d.). Increase daily dosage every 2 weeks by increments of 20 mg/kg to recommended daily dosage of 60 mg/kg (30 mg/kg b.i.d.). If patient can't tolerate daily dosage of 60 mg/kg, reduce daily dosage.
➤ Myoclonic seizures in patients with juvenile myoclonic epilepsy
Children ages 16 and older: Initially, 500 mg I.V. b.i.d. Increase dosage by 1,000 mg/day every 2 weeks to recom-mended total daily dosage of 3,000 mg.
Children ages 12 and older: Initially, 500 mg P.O. (immediate-release tablets or oral solution) b.i.d. Increase dosage by 1,000 mg/day every 2 weeks to the recommended total daily dose of 3,000 mg.

➤ Primary generalized tonic-clonic seizures

Adults and children ages 16 and older: Initially, 1,000 mg P.O. b.i.d. Increase dosage by 1,000 mg/day every 2 weeks to the recommended total daily dose of 3,000 mg.

Children ages 6 to 15: Initially, 10 mg/kg P.O. b.i.d. Increase daily dosage every 2 weeks by increments of 20 mg/kg to recommended total daily dosage of 60 mg/kg (30 mg/kg b.i.d.).

Dosage adjustment
• Renal impairment (especially in dialysis patients)

Contraindications
• Hypersensitivity to drug or its components

Precautions
Use cautiously in:
• renal, hepatic, or cardiac impairment
• psychosis
• pregnant or breastfeeding patients
• children younger than age 16 (safety and efficacy not established).

Administration
• Give oral form with or without food.
• Know that patients weighing 44 lb (20 kg) or less should be given oral solution.
• Be aware that injection form is intended for temporary use when oral route isn't feasible.
◀℥ Be aware that injection form is for I.V. use only and must be diluted before administering.
• Dilute 500 mg/ml in 100 ml 0.9% normal saline injection, lactated Ringer's injection, or dextrose 5% injection. Withdraw 5 ml, 10 ml, or 15 ml for 500-mg, 1,000-mg, or 1,500-mg dose, respectively.
• Administer as a 15-minute I.V. infusion.
◀℥ Don't discontinue suddenly. Instead, taper dosage gradually.

Route	Onset	Peak	Duration
P.O.	Rapid	1 hr	Unknown
P.O. (ext-rel.)	Unknown	4 hr	Unknown
I.V.	Rapid	Unknown	Unknown

Adverse reactions
CNS: aggression, anger, irritability, mental or mood changes, asthenia, ataxia, dizziness, drowsiness, somnolence, fatigue, nervousness, depression, anxiety, amnesia, hostility, coordination difficulties, headache, paresthesia, vertigo
EENT: diplopia, pharyngitis, rhinitis, sinusitis
GI: nausea, vomiting, anorexia
Hematologic: neutropenia, leukopenia
Respiratory: cough
Other: infection, pain

Interactions
Drug-herbs. *Evening primrose oil:* lowered seizure threshold

Patient monitoring
• Measure temperature and watch for signs and symptoms of infection.
◀℥ Monitor neurologic status. Report signs that patient is dangerous to himself or others.
• Evaluate nutritional status. Report signs of anorexia.

Patient teaching
• Tell patient to take with or without food.
• Instruct patient to swallow extended-release tablets whole and not to chew, break, or crush them.
◀℥ Advise family to contact prescriber if patient poses a danger to himself or others.
◀℥ Caution patient not to stop taking drug abruptly, because doing so may increase seizure activity.
• Teach patient and family about adverse CNS reactions, and tell them to report these promptly. Urge them

---

Reactions in **bold** are life-threatening.   ◀℥ Clinical alert

to take safety measures to prevent injury.
- Instruct patient to avoid activities that require mental alertness until CNS reactions are known.
- Inform patient that he'll undergo periodic blood testing during therapy.
- As appropriate, review all other significant and life-threatening adverse reactions and interactions, especially those related to the herbs mentioned above.

levocetirizine

levocetirizine dihydrochloride
Xyzal

Pharmacologic class:
Histamine$_1$(H$_1$)–receptor antagonist
Therapeutic class: Antihistamine
Pregnancy risk category B

Action
Exerts principal antihistaminic effects via selective inhibition of H$_1$ receptors

Availability
Oral solution: 2.5 mg/5 ml (0.5 mg/ml)
Tablets: 5 mg

🖊 Indications and dosages
➤ Symptoms of allergic rhinitis (seasonal and perennial); uncomplicated skin manifestations of chronic idiopathic urticaria
Adults and children ages 12 and older: 5 mg P.O. daily in evening
Children ages 6 to 11: 2.5 mg P.O. daily in evening; don't exceed recommended dosage.

Dosage adjustment
- Renal impairment.
- Hepatic impairment

Contraindications
- Hypersensitivity to drug, its components, or cetirizine
- End-stage renal disease
- Hemodialysis
- Renal impairment (children ages 6 to 11)

Precautions
Use cautiously in:
- renal impairment
- pregnant patients
- elderly patients
- breastfeeding patients (use not recommended)
- children younger than age 6 (safety and efficacy not established).

Administration
- Give with or without food.

Route	Onset	Peak	Duration
P.O.	Unknown	0.5 hr	Unknown

Adverse reactions
CNS: somnolence; fatigue, asthenia
EENT: epistaxis (children), nasopharyngitis, pharyngitis
GI: dry mouth
Respiratory: cough (children)
Other: pyrexia (children)

Interactions
Drug-drug. *Ritonavir:* increased levocetirizine blood level and half-life, decreased clearance
Drug-behaviors. *Alcohol use:* increased risk of impaired CNS function

Patient monitoring
- Stay alert for excessive CNS depression.
- Closely monitor renal function tests in patients with renal impairment.

Patient teaching
- Tell patient drug can be taken with or without food.

- Instruct patient to avoid alcohol and other depressants, such as sleeping pills, unless prescriber approves.
- Caution patient to avoid hazardous activities until drug's effects on concentration and alertness are known.
- Advise female patient to notify prescriber if she is pregnant or intends to become pregnant.
- Tell breastfeeding patient to discontinue breastfeeding during therapy.
- As appropriate, review all other significant adverse reactions and interactions, especially those related to the drugs and behaviors mentioned above.

levofloxacin
Iquix, Levaquin, Novo-
Levofloxacin✿, Oftaquix✤, Quixin,
Tavanic✤

Pharmacologic class: Fluoroquinolone
Therapeutic class: Anti-infective
Pregnancy risk category C

FDA BOXED WARNING

Fluoroquinolones for systemic use are associated with an increased risk of tendinitis and tendon rupture in all ages. This risk is further increased in patients usually over age 60, with concomitant use of corticosteroids, and in kidney, heart, and lung transplant recipients.

Action
Inhibits the enzyme DNA gyrase in susceptible gram-negative and gram-positive aerobic and anaerobic bacteria, interfering with bacterial DNA synthesis

Availability
Ophthalmic solution: Quixin—0.5%
(5 mg/ml), Iquix—1.5%
Premixed solution for injection: 250 mg/
50 ml, 500 mg/100 ml, 750 mg/150 ml
Solution for injection (concentrated):
500 mg/20 ml
Tablets: 250 mg, 500 mg, 750 mg

🕗 Indications and dosages
➤ Acute bacterial exacerbation of chronic bronchitis
Adults: 500 mg I.V. or P.O. q 24 hours for 7 days
➤ Community-acquired pneumonia
Adults: 500 mg I.V. or P.O. q 24 hours for 7 to 14 days, or 750 mg I.V. or P.O. q 24 hours for 5 days
➤ Nosocomial pneumonia caused by methicillin-susceptible strains of *Staphylococcus aureus, Pseudomonas aeruginosa, Serratia marcescens, Escherichia coli, Klebsiella pneumoniae, Haemophilus influenzae,* or *Streptococcus pneumoniae;* complicated skin and skin-structure infections
Adults: 750 mg I.V. or P.O. q 24 hours for 7 to 14 days
➤ Acute bacterial sinusitis caused by *S. pneumoniae, H. influenzae,* or *Moraxella catarrhalis*
Adults: 500 mg I.V. or P.O. q 24 hours for 10 to 14 days or 750 mg P.O. or I.V. q 24 hours for 5 days
➤ Uncomplicated skin and skin-structure infections
Adults: 500 mg I.V. or P.O. q 24 hours for 7 to 10 days
➤ Complicated urinary tract infections; acute pyelonephritis caused by *E. coli*
Adults: 250 mg I.V. or P.O. q 24 hours for 10 days or 750 mg P.O. or I.V. q 24 hours for 5 days
➤ Uncomplicated urinary tract infections
Adults: 250 mg I.V. or P.O. q 24 hours for 3 days

Reactions in **bold** are life-threatening. 🔊 Clinical alert

➤ Chronic bacterial prostatitis
Adults: 500 mg I.V. or P.O. q 24 hours for 28 days.
➤ Conjunctivitis
Adults and children ages 1 and older: One or two drops of 0.5% ophthalmic solution into affected eye q 2 hours while awake on days 1 and 2 (up to eight times daily); then one or two drops q 4 hours while awake on days 3 through 7 (up to four times daily)
➤ Corneal ulcers
Adults and children ages 6 and older: On days 1 to 3, one or two drops of 1.5% ophthalmic solution instilled into affected eye(s) q 30 minutes to 1 hour while awake and q 4 to 6 hours after retiring; thereafter, one or two drops q 1 to 4 hours while awake until treatment completion
➤ Inhalational anthrax (postexposure)
Adults and children ages 6 months and older weighing more than 50 kg (110 lb): 500 mg P.O. or I.V. q 24 hours for 60 days
Children ages 6 months and older weighing less than 50 kg (110 lb): 8 mg/kg P.O. or I.V., not to exceed 250 mg/dose q 12 hours for 60 days

Dosage adjustment
• Renal impairment

Contraindications
• Hypersensitivity to drug, its components, or other quinolones

Precautions
Use cautiously in:
• bradycardia, acute myocardial ischemia, prolonged QTc interval, cirrhosis, renal impairment, underlying CNS disease, uncorrected hypocalcemia
• elderly patients
• pregnant or breastfeeding patients
• children younger than age 18 (except in ophthalmic use).

Administration
• Be aware that oral and I.V. dosages are identical.
• Give parenteral form by I.V. route only. Drug isn't for I.M., subcutaneous, intrathecal, or intraperitoneal use.
• To prepare I.V. infusion, use compatible solution, such as 0.9% sodium chloride injection, dextrose 5% and 0.9% sodium chloride injection, dextrose 5% in water, or dextrose 5% in lactated Ringer's solution.
• Infuse over 60 to 90 minutes, depending on dosage. Don't infuse with other drugs.
◀€ Avoid rapid or bolus I.V. administration, because this may cause severe hypotension
• Flush I.V. line before and after infusion.
• Give oral doses 2 hours before or after sucralfate, iron, antacids containing magnesium or aluminum, or multivitamins with zinc.
• Give oral form without regard to food, but don't give with milk or yogurt alone.
• Be aware that the two ophthalmic preparations have different indications.

Route	Onset	Peak	Duration
P.O.	Rapid	1-2 hr	24 hr
I.V.	Rapid	End of infusion	24 hr
Ophth.	Unknown	Unknown	Unknown

Adverse reactions
CNS: dizziness, headache, insomnia, **seizures**
CV: chest pain, palpitations, hypotension
EENT: photophobia, sinusitis, pharyngitis
GI: nausea, vomiting, diarrhea, constipation, abdominal pain, dyspepsia, flatulence, **pseudomembranous colitis**
GU: vaginitis
Hematologic: lymphocytopenia
Metabolic: hyperglycemia, **hypoglycemia**

Musculoskeletal: back pain, tendon rupture, tendinitis

Skin: photosensitivity

Other: altered taste, reaction and pain at I.V. site, hypersensitivity reactions including **Stevens-Johnson syndrome**

Interactions

Drug-drug. *Antacids containing aluminum or magnesium, didanosine (tablets), iron salts, sucralfate, zinc salts:* decreased levofloxacin absorption

Cimetidine: interference with levofloxacin elimination

Nonsteroidal anti-inflammatory drugs: increased risk of CNS stimulation and seizures

Drug-diagnostic tests. *Glucose:* increased or decreased level

Lymphocytes: decreased count

EEG: abnormal findings

Drug-food. *Concurrent tube feedings, milk, yogurt:* impaired levofloxacin absorption

Drug-herbs. *Dong quai, St. John's wort:* phototoxicity

Fennel: decreased levofloxacin absorption

Drug-behaviors. *Sun exposure:* phototoxicity

Patient monitoring

• Check vital signs, especially blood pressure. Too-rapid infusion can cause hypotension.

• Closely monitor patients with renal insufficiency.

• Monitor blood glucose level closely in diabetic patients.

◀€ Assess for severe diarrhea, which may indicate pseudomembranous colitis.

◀€ Watch for hypersensitivity reaction. Discontinue drug immediately if rash or other signs or symptoms occur.

◀€ Watch for signs and symptoms of tendinitis or tendon rupture.

Patient teaching

◀€ Tell patient to stop taking drug and contact prescriber if he experiences signs or symptoms of hypersensitivity reaction (rash, hives, or other skin reactions) or severe diarrhea (which may indicate pseudomembranous colitis).

◀€ Instruct patient to stop taking drug and notify prescriber immediately if tendon pain, swelling, or inflammation occurs.

• Instruct patient not to take with milk, yogurt, multivitamins containing zinc or iron, or antacids containing aluminum or magnesium.

• Teach patient proper use of eye drops. Tell him to avoid touching applicator tip to eye, finger, or any other object.

• Caution patient to avoid driving and other activities that require mental alertness until CNS effects of drug are known.

• As appropriate, review all other significant and life-threatening adverse reactions and interactions, especially those related to the drugs, tests, foods, herbs, and behaviors mentioned above.

levonorgestrel

Levonelle⊕, Mirena, Plan B One-Step

Pharmacologic class: Contraceptive, intrauterine device (Mirena); oral contraceptive, progestin-only pill (Plan B)

Therapeutic class: Contraceptive

Pregnancy risk category X (Mirena), *NR* (Plan B)

Action

Unclear. Mirena may enhance local contraceptive efficacy by thickening the cervical mucus (which prevents passage of sperm into uterus), inhibiting sperm capacitation or survival, and altering the endometrium. Plan B is thought to prevent ovulation or fertilization.

Availability
Intrauterine system (Mirena): 52 mg levonorgestrel
Tablets (Plan B): 1.5 mg

⃠ Indications and dosages
➤ Intrauterine contraception for up to 5 years; heavy menstrual bleeding for women who choose to use intrauterine contraception
Adults: One intrauterine system (Mirena) inserted into uterus for up to 5 years
➤ Emergency contraception to prevent pregnancy
Adults: 1.5 mg (Plan B) P.O. as soon as possible within 72 hours after unprotected intercourse

Contraindications
Mirena—
• Hypersensitivity to drug or its components
• Known or suspected pregnancy
• Congenital or acquired uterine anomaly
• Acute pelvic inflammatory disease (PID) or history of PID (unless patient had subsequent intrauterine pregnancy)
• Postpartum endometritis or infected abortion within past 3 months
• Known or suspected uterine or cervical neoplasia or unresolved abnormal Papanicolaou (Pap) test
• Untreated acute cervicitis or vaginitis
• Acute hepatic disease or hepatic tumor (benign or malignant)
• Genital bleeding of unknown cause
• Conditions associated with increased risk of infection
• Genital actinomycosis
• Previously inserted intrauterine device that has not been removed
• Known or suspected breast cancer

• History of ectopic pregnancy or conditions that predispose to it
Plan B —
• Hypersensitivity to drug or its components
• Known or suspected pregnancy
• Undiagnosed abnormal genital bleeding

Precautions
Use Mirena cautiously in:
• diabetes mellitus
• breastfeeding patients.
Use Plan B cautiously in:
• coagulopathy
• diabetes mellitus
• patients receiving anticoagulants concurrently.

Administration
• Know that Mirena should be inserted under aseptic conditions by health care professional familiar with procedure.
• Verify that patient isn't pregnant before Mirena insertion.
• Know that Plan B should be given as soon as possible within 72 hours of unprotected sexual intercourse. Drug isn't suitable as long-term contraceptive.

Route	Onset	Peak	Duration
P.O.	Unknown	1.6 ± 0.7 hr	Unknown
Intra-uterine	No peaks or troughs		

Adverse reactions
CNS: headache (Mirena, Plan B), fatigue, dizziness (Plan B), severe headache, migraine, nervousness, depression (Mirena)
CV: hypertension (Mirena)
EENT: sinusitis (Mirena)
GI: nausea, vomiting, abdominal pain (Mirena, Plan B), diarrhea (Plan B), **intestinal perforation or obstruction** (Mirena)
GU: breast tenderness (Mirena, Plan B); lighter or heavier menstrual bleeding (Plan B); breast pain; increased

progesterone levels; ovarian cysts; dysmenorrhea; amenorrhea; spotting; erratic or prolonged menstrual bleeding; pelvic infection; vaginitis; cervicitis; dyspareunia; leukorrhea; decreased libido; abnormal Pap smear; expulsion, embedment in myometrium, adhesions, **cervical or ureteral perforation** (Mirena)

Hematologic: anemia (Mirena)
Hepatic: jaundice (Mirena)
Musculoskeletal: back pain (Mirena)
Respiratory: upper respiratory tract infection (Mirena)
Skin: skin disorder, acne, eczema, hair loss (Mirena)
Other: water retention, weight gain, **sepsis** (Mirena)

Interactions

Drug-drug. *Hepatic enzyme-inducing drugs (such as barbiturates, carbamazepine, phenytoin, rifampin):* decreased Plan B efficacy
Drug-diagnostic tests. *Glucose:* altered level (Mirena)

Patient monitoring

• Monitor blood pressure.
• Watch for adverse reactions, especially changes in menstrual bleeding.
• Monitor blood glucose level in diabetic patients.
• Check liver function tests frequently.

Patient teaching

• Tell patient taking either product that drug does not prevent HIV or other sexually transmitted diseases.
• Teach patient using Mirena how to check (after menstrual period) to make sure thread still protrudes from cervix. Caution her not to pull on thread, because this could cause displacement.
◀ Instruct patient using Mirena to immediately report fever, chills, unusual vaginal discharge, or abdominal or pelvic pain or tenderness.

• Explain that for maximum efficacy, patient should take Plan B as soon as possible after unprotected sex.
• Inform patient that Plan B isn't intended for routine contraception and doesn't terminate existing pregnancy.
• Tell patient to report adverse reactions.
• As appropriate, review all other significant and life-threatening adverse reactions and interactions, especially those related to the drugs and tests mentioned above.

levorphanol tartrate

Pharmacologic class: Synthetic opioid agonist
Therapeutic class: Opioid analgesic
Controlled substance schedule II
Pregnancy risk category C

Action

Inhibits adenylate cyclase, which regulates release of pain neurotransmitters (acetylcholine, dopamine, substance P, and gamma-aminobutyric acid). Also stimulates mu and kappa opioid receptors, altering perception of and emotional response to pain.

Availability

Tablets: 2 mg

Indications and dosages

➤ Moderate to severe pain
Adults: 2 mg P.O. q 6 to 8 hours p.r.n., provided patient is assessed for hypoventilation and excessive sedation. If necessary, may increase dosage to up to 3 mg q 6 to 8 hours, after adequate evaluation of patient response. Higher doses may be appropriate in opioid-tolerant patients. Adjust dosage

---

Reactions in **bold** are life-threatening.　　　　◀ Clinical alert

according to patient's severity of pain, age, weight, physical status, underlying diseases, and use of concomitant medications. Total oral daily doses of more than 6 to 12 mg in 24 hours are generally not recommended as starting doses in nonopioid-tolerant patients.

Dosage adjustment
- Hepatic or renal insufficiency
- Elderly patients

Contraindications
- Hypersensitivity to drug or other opioid agonists
- Bronchial asthma
- Increased intracranial pressure
- Respiratory depression
- Acute alcoholism

Precautions
Use cautiously in:
- renal or hepatic dysfunction, chronic obstructive pulmonary disease, acute abdominal conditions, cardiovascular disease, seizure disorders, cerebral arteriosclerosis, Addison's disease, prostatic hypertrophy, toxic psychosis
- pregnant or breastfeeding patients
- children.

Administration
◄€ Make sure resuscitation equipment is available before starting therapy.

Route	Onset	Peak	Duration
P.O.	10-60 min	90-120 min	4-5 hr

Adverse reactions
CNS: personality disorders, nervousness, insomnia, hypokinesia, dyskinesia, drowsiness, light-headedness, dizziness, depression, delusions, confusion, amnesia, sedation, euphoria, delirium, mood changes, **coma, seizures**
CV: palpitations, hypotension, tachycardia, bradycardia, **shock, peripheral circulatory collapse, cardiac arrest**
EENT: diplopia, abnormal vision

GI: nausea, vomiting, constipation, abdominal pain, dyspepsia, increased colonic motility (in patients with chronic ulcerative colitis), dry mouth
GU: dysuria, urinary retention or hesitancy, ureteral or vesicle sphincter spasms, decreased libido, **oliguria**
Hepatic: biliary tract spasms, **hepatic failure**
Respiratory: suppressed cough reflex, hyperventilation, **periodic apnea**
Skin: urticaria, rash, pruritus, cyanosis, facial flushing
Other: physical or psychological drug dependence

Interactions
Drug-drug. *Alfentanil, fentanyl, sufentanil, other CNS depressants:* increased CNS and respiratory depression, increased risk of hypotension
Anticholinergics: increased risk of severe constipation
Antidiarrheals (such as atropine, difenoxin, kaolin, loperamide), antihypertensives: increased risk of hypotension
Buprenorphine, naloxone, naltrexone: decreased levorphanol efficacy
Metoclopramide: antagonism of metoclopramide effects
Neuromuscular blockers: increased risk of prolonged CNS and respiratory depression
Drug-diagnostic tests. *Amylase, lipase:* increased levels
Drug-behaviors. *Alcohol use:* increased CNS depression

Patient monitoring
- Check vital signs and respiratory status, and monitor ECG carefully.
- Evaluate fluid intake and output.
- Assess neurologic status. Institute safety precautions as needed to prevent injury.
- Watch for signs and symptoms of depression.
- Monitor liver and kidney function tests.

Patient teaching

🔊 Instruct patient or caregiver to report adverse reactions immediately.

• Tell patient or caregiver to use safety measures as needed to prevent injury and to report significant problems.

• Advise patient to avoid alcohol while taking this drug.

• Caution patient to avoid driving and other hazardous activities until he knows how drug affects concentration and alertness.

• As appropriate, review all other significant and life-threatening adverse reactions and interactions, especially those related to the drugs, tests, and behaviors mentioned above.

levothyroxine sodium (L-thyroxine, T₄)

Eltroxin✣⊕, Euthyrox✣, Evotrox⊕, Levo-T, Levolet, Levothroid, Levoxyl, Nu-Thyro✣, Soloxine, Synthroid, Unithroid

Pharmacologic class: Synthetic thyroxine hormone
Therapeutic class: Thyroid hormone replacement
Pregnancy risk category A

FDA | BOXED WARNING

• Drug shouldn't be used alone or with other agents to treat obesity or weight loss. In euthyroid patients, doses within range of daily hormonal requirements are ineffective for weight loss. Larger doses may cause serious or life-threatening toxicity, particularly when given with sympathomimetic amines (such as those used for anorectic effects).

Action

Synthetic form of thyroxine that replaces endogenous thyroxine, increasing thyroid hormone levels. Thyroid hormones help regulate cell growth and differentiation and increase metabolism of lipids, protein, and carbohydrates.

Availability

Powder for injection: 200 mcg/vial in 6- and 10-ml vials, 500 mcg/vial in 6- and 10-ml vials
Tablets: 25 mcg, 50 mcg, 75 mcg, 88 mcg, 100 mcg, 112 mcg, 125 mcg, 137 mcg, 150 mcg, 175 mcg, 200 mcg, 300 mcg

⦿ Indications and dosages

➤ Hypothyroidism; treatment or prevention of euthyroid goiter
Adults: For healthy adults younger than age 50 and those over age 50 who have recently been treated or undergone short-term therapy, start at full replacement dosage of 1.7 mcg/kg P.O. daily, given 30 minutes to 1 hour before breakfast. For patients older than age 50 or younger than age 50 with heart disease, 25 to 50 mcg P.O. daily, increased q 4 to 6 weeks. In severe hypothyroidism, initial dosage is 12.5 to 25 mcg P.O. daily, adjusted by 25 mcg daily q 2 to 4 weeks. For patients who can't tolerate oral doses, adjust I.M. or I.V. dosage to roughly half of oral dosage.
➤ Congenital hypothyroidism
Children older than age 12 who have completed puberty and growth: 1.7 mcg/kg P.O. daily
Children older than age 12 who have not completed puberty and growth: Up to 150 mcg or 2 to 3 mcg/kg P.O. daily
Children ages 6 to 12: 4 to 5 mcg/kg P.O. daily
Children ages 1 to 5: 5 to 6 mcg/kg P.O. daily
Infants ages 6 to 12 months: 6 to 8 mcg/kg P.O. daily

Infants ages 3 to 6 months: 8 to 10 mcg/kg P.O. daily
Infants up to 3 months old: 10 to 15 mcg/kg P.O. daily
➤ Myxedema coma or stupor
Adults: 200 to 500 mcg I.V. as a solution containing 100 mcg/ml. Additional 100 to 300 mcg may be given on day 2 if significant improvement has not occurred. Convert to P.O. therapy when patient is clinically stable.
➤ Thyroid-stimulating hormone suppression in well-differentiated thyroid cancers and thyroid nodules
Adults: Dosage individualized based on disease and patient

Dosage adjustment
• Cardiovascular disease
• Psychosis or agitation
• Elderly patients

Contraindications
• Hypersensitivity to drug, its components, or tartrazine
• Acute myocardial infarction
• Thyrotoxicosis
• Adrenal insufficiency

Precautions
Use cautiously in:
• cardiovascular disease, severe renal insufficiency, diabetes mellitus
• elderly patients
• pregnant or breastfeeding patients.

Administration
• Be aware that all dosages are highly individualized.
• Give tablets on an empty stomach 30 minutes to 1 hour before first meal of day.
• If patient can't swallow tablets, crush them and sprinkle onto small amount of food, such as applesauce. For infants and children, dissolve tablets in small amount of water, nonsoybean formula, or breast milk and administer immediately.

• Don't give oral form within 4 hours of bile acid sequestrants or antacids.
• Reconstitute Synthroid powder for injection with 5 ml of 0.9% sodium chloride injection. Shake until clear and use immediately.
• For I.V. administration, give each 100 mcg over at least 1 minute.
• Be aware that the various levothyroxine preparations aren't bioequivalent. Patient should consistently use same brand or generic product, with dosing based on weight, age, physical condition, and symptom duration.
• When drug is given for thyroid-stimulating hormone (TSH) suppression test, TSH suppression level is not well established and radioactive iodine (^{131}I) is given before and after treatment course.

Route	Onset	Peak	Duration
P.O.	Unknown	Unknown	Unknown
I.V.	6-8 hr	24 hr	Unknown
I.M.	Unknown	Unknown	Unknown

Adverse reactions
CNS: insomnia, irritability, nervousness, headache
CV: tachycardia, angina pectoris, hypotension, hypertension, increased cardiac output, **arrhythmias, cardiovascular collapse**
GI: vomiting, diarrhea, abdominal cramps
GU: menstrual irregularities
Metabolic: hyperthyroidism
Musculoskeletal: accelerated bone maturation (in children), decreased bone density (in women on long-term therapy)
Skin: alopecia (in children), diaphoresis
Other: heat intolerance, weight loss

Interactions
Drug-drug. *Aminoglutethimide, amiodarone, anabolic steroids, antithyroid drugs, asparaginase, barbiturates, carbamazepine, chloral hydrate, cholestyramine, clofibrate, colestipol, corticosteroids,*

danazol, diazepam, estrogens, ethionamide, fluorouracil, heparin (with I.V. use), insulin, lithium, methadone, mitotane, nitroprusside, oxyphenbutazone, perphenazine, phenylbutazone, phenytoin, propranolol, salicylates (large doses), sulfonylureas, thiazides: altered thyroid function test results

Antacids, bile acid sequestrants: interference with levothyroxine absorption

Anticoagulants: increased anticoagulant action

Beta-adrenergic blockers (selected): decreased beta blocker action

Cardiac glycosides: decreased cardiac glycoside blood level

Cholestyramine, colestipol: levothyroxine inefficacy

Theophyllines: decreased theophylline clearance

Drug-diagnostic tests. *Thyroid function tests:* decreased values

Drug-food. *Foods high in iron or fiber, soybeans:* decreased drug absorption

Patient monitoring
• Check vital signs and ECG routinely.
• Monitor thyroid and liver function tests.

◀◶ Evaluate for signs and symptoms of overdose, including those of hyperthyroidism (weight loss, cardiac symptoms, abdominal cramps).
• Monitor closely for drug efficacy.
• Check patients with Addison's disease or diabetes mellitus for worsening of these conditions.

◀◶ Watch for signs and symptoms of bleeding tendency, especially in patients receiving anticoagulants concurrently.

Patient teaching
• Explain that patient may require lifelong therapy and must undergo regular blood testing.
• Tell patient or parent to report adverse effects, including signs or symptoms of hyperthyroidism or hypothyroidism.

• Caution patient to avoid driving and other hazardous activities until he knows how drug affects concentration and alertness.
• Advise patient to avoid getting overheated, as in hot environments or during vigorous exercise.
• Tell parents that child being treated may lose hair during first few months of therapy. Reassure them that this effect usually is transient.
• As appropriate, review all other significant and life-threatening adverse reactions and interactions, especially those related to the drugs, tests, and foods mentioned above.

lidocaine hydrochloride
Anesticaine, Anesticon, Laryng-O-Jet✛, Lidodan❖, Lidoderm, Lidomax❖, LidoPen Auto-Injector, LTA Pediatric, Lurocaine❖, Xylocaine, Xylocaine-MPF, Xylocard❖

Pharmacologic class: Amide
Therapeutic class: Antiarrhythmic (class IB), local anesthetic
Pregnancy risk category B

Action
Suppresses automaticity of ventricular cells, decreasing diastolic depolarization and increasing ventricular fibrillation threshold. Produces local anesthesia by reducing sodium permeability of sensory nerves, which blocks impulse generation and conduction.

Availability
Injection for I.M. use: 300 mg/3 ml (automatic injection device)
Injection for direct I.V. use: 1% and 2% in syringes and vials

---

Reactions in **bold** are life-threatening. ◀◶ Clinical alert

Injection for I.V. infusion: 2 mg/ml, 4 mg/ml, 8 mg/ml
Injection for I.V injection admixtures: 40 mg/ml, 100 mg/ml, 200 mg/ml
Patch: 5%
Topical cream: 0.5%, 4%
Topical gel: 0.5%, 2.5%
Topical jelly: 2%
Topical liquid, ointment: 2.5%, 5%
Topical solution: 4%
Topical solution (viscous): 2%
Topical spray: 0.5%

⃠ Indications and dosages

➤ Ventricular arrhythmias
Adults: Initially, 50 to 100 mg I.V. bolus given at rate of 25 to 50 mg/minute. If desired response doesn't occur after 5 minutes, give repeat dose at 25 to 50 mg/minute; maximum dosage is 300 mg given over 1 hour. Maintenance dosage is 1 to 4 mg/minute by continuous I.V. infusion for no more than 24 hours.
Children: Initially, 1 mg/kg I.V. bolus, then repeated based on patient response; don't exceed 5 mg/kg. Maintenance dosage is 30 mcg/kg/minute by continuous I.V. infusion.
➤ Caudal anesthesia (without epinephrine)
Adults: For obstetric analgesia, 200 to 300 mg caudally as 1% solution. For surgical anesthesia, 225 to 300 mg as 1.5% solution. For continuous caudal anesthesia, don't repeat maximum dosage at intervals of less than 90 minutes.
➤ Epidural anesthesia (without epinephrine)
Adults: For lumbar analgesia, 250 to 300 mg epidurally as 1% solution, 225 to 300 mg as 1.5% solution, or 200 to 300 mg as 2% solution. For thoracic anesthesia, 200 to 300 mg as 1% solution. For continuous epidural anesthesia, don't repeat maximum dosage at intervals of less than 90 minutes.
➤ I.V. regional infiltration (without epinephrine)

Adults: 50 to 300 mg I.V. as 0.5% solution. For I.V. regional anesthesia, maximum dosage is 4 mg/kg.
➤ I.V. local infiltration (without epinephrine)
Children: Up to 4.5 mg/kg I.V. as 0.25% to 1% solution
➤ Spinal anesthesia (without epinephrine)
Adults: For obstetric low-spinal or saddle-block anesthesia (normal vaginal delivery), 50 mg of 5% Xylocaine-MPF with glucose 7.5%, or 9 to 15 mg of 1.5% Xylocaine-MPF with dextrose 7.5%. For cesarean section, 75 mg of 5% Xylocaine-MPF with glucose 7.5%. For surgical anesthesia, 75 to 100 mg of 5% Xylocaine-MPF with glucose 7.5%.
➤ Paracervical anesthesia (without epinephrine)
Adults: For obstetric analgesia, 100 mg paracervically as 1% solution (each side). For paracervical block, maximum dosage is 200 mg over each 90-minute period (half administered on each side).
➤ Peripheral nerve block
Adults: For brachial nerve block, 225 to 300 mg as 1.5% solution. For dental nerve block, 20 to 100 mg as 2% solution with epinephrine 1:100,000 or 1:50,000. For intercostal nerve block, 30 mg as 1% solution. For pudendal nerve block, 100 mg as 1% solution. For paravertebral nerve block, 30 mg to 50 mg as 1% solution.
➤ Sympathetic nerve block (without epinephrine)
Adults: For cervical nerve block, 50 mg as 1% solution. For lumbar nerve block, 50 to 100 mg as 1% solution.
➤ Dental anesthesia
Adults: 1 to 5 ml of lidocaine 2% with epinephrine 1:50,000 or 1:100,000. Maximum dosage is less than 500 mg (7 mg/kg).
Children: 20 to 30 mg as 2% solution with epinephrine 1:100,000

➤ Topical anesthesia for skin or mucous membranes

Adults: Apply thin layer of gel, jelly, or ointment to skin or mucous membranes as needed before procedure; or apply 5% patch to most painful areas and intact skin (up to three patches at a time for up to 12 hours within a 24-hour period). For new denture fittings, use 5-g ointment (250 mg) per single dose or 20 g/day. For oropharyngeal use, apply to desired area or to instrument before insertion.

Children: Apply thin layer of ointment to skin or mucous membranes p.r.n. before procedure. Maximum dosage is 2.5 g ointment per 6 hours or 4.5 mg/kg.

➤ Prevention or treatment of pain during procedures involving male or female urethra

Adults: For female urethral examination, apply 3 to 5 ml of 2% jelly topically several minutes before exam. For male sounding or cystoscopy, apply 5 to 10 ml of 2% jelly topically before procedure, or apply 30 ml to fill or dilate urethra in divided doses using penile clamp for several minutes between doses. For male catheterization, apply 5 to 10 ml of 2% jelly to anterior urethra before procedure. Don't use more than 600 mg/12 hours.

➤ Oral cavity disorders; pharyngeal disorders

Adults: For oral cavity disorders, 300 mg (15 ml) of viscous oral topical solution swished and then expelled, or applied with cotton swab q 3 hours p.r.n. For pharyngeal disorders, use same dosage, but solution may be swallowed.

Children older than age 3: Dosage individualized based on age, weight, and physical condition. Maximum dosage is 4.5 mg/kg q 3 hours.

Children up to age 3: 1.25 ml applied with swab q 3 hours

➤ Local anesthesia (oral or nasal mucosa)

Adults: 0.6 to 3 mg/kg or 40 to 200 mg of 4% topical solution, not to exceed 4.5 mg/kg or 300 mg (7.5 ml)

Children: Dosage individualized

Off-label uses

• Pediatric patients with cardiac arrest who develop frequent premature ventricular contractions
• Status epilepticus

Contraindications

• Hypersensitivity to drug, its components, or other amide local anesthetics
• Heart failure, cardiogenic shock, second- or third-degree heart block, intraventricular block in absence of a pacemaker
• Wolff-Parkinson-White or Adams-Stokes syndrome
• Severe hemorrhage, shock, or heart block (lidocaine with dextrose)
• Local infection at puncture site (lidocaine with dextrose)
• Septicemia (lidocaine with dextrose)

Precautions

Use cautiously in:
• renal or hepatic disorders, inflammation or sepsis in injection area
• labor or delivery
• breastfeeding patients.

Administration

◀᪥ Know that I.V. lidocaine is a high-alert drug.

◀᪥ Make sure resuscitation equipment and oxygen are available before giving I.V. lidocaine.

• Dilute injection in additive syringe and single-use vial according to manufacturer's instructions before administering as I.V. infusion.

• Add 1 g lidocaine to 1 L dextrose 5% in water to yield a solution of 1 mg/ml.

• For I.V. bolus injection, give doses of 25 to 50 mg over at least 1 minute. Deliver continuous infusion by infusion pump no faster than 4 mg/minute.

Reactions in **bold** are life-threatening.   ◀᪥ Clinical alert

◀€ Know that too-rapid infusion may cause seizures.
• Be aware that drug can be given I.M. using 10% parenteral solution only.

Route	Onset	Peak	Duration
I.V.	45-90 sec	Immediate	10-20 min
I.M.	5-15 min	Unknown	60-90 min
Topical	2-5 min	Unknown	30-60 min

Adverse reactions

CNS: anxiety; confusion; difficulty speaking; dizziness; hallucinations; lethargy; paresthesia; light-headedness; fatigue; drowsiness; headache; persistent sensory, motor, or **autonomic deficit of lower spinal segment; septic meningitis; seizures**
CV: bradycardia, hypotension, new or worsening **arrhythmias, cardiac arrest**
EENT: diplopia, abnormal vision
GI: nausea, vomiting, dry mouth
GU: urinary retention
Metabolic: methemoglobinemia
Respiratory: suppressed cough reflex, **respiratory depression, respiratory arrest**
Skin: rash; urticaria; pruritus; erythema; contact dermatitis; cutaneous lesions; tissue irritation, sloughing, and necrosis
Other: fever; edema; infection, burning, stinging, tenderness, and swelling at injection site; **anaphylaxis**

Interactions

Drug-drug. *Beta-adrenergic blockers, cimetidine:* increased lidocaine blood level
MAO inhibitors, tricyclic antidepressants: prolonged hypertension
Mexiletine, tocainide: additive cardiac effects
Phenytoin, procainamide: increased cardiac depression
Drug-diagnostic tests. *Creatine kinase:* increased level (with I.M. use)

Patient monitoring

◀€ Monitor vital signs and ECG continuously. Watch for cardiac depression.
◀€ Evaluate level of consciousness closely.
◀€ Watch for adverse reactions, particularly anaphylaxis.
◀€ Stay alert for seizures.
◀€ Monitor neurologic status for lower spinal segment deficits.
• Give supportive oxygen therapy, as indicated and prescribed.
• Monitor electrolyte, blood urea nitrogen, and creatinine levels.
• Assess topical site for adverse reactions.

Patient teaching

• Discuss reason for drug therapy with patient and family, when appropriate.
• Explain that patient will be monitored continuously during therapy.
◀€ Instruct patient to promptly report discomfort at I.V. site as well as adverse effects, especially cardiovascular, respiratory, or neurologic problems or allergic reactions.
• As appropriate, review all other significant and life-threatening adverse reactions and interactions, especially those related to the drugs and tests mentioned above.

lindane
Hexit Lotion✤, Hexit Shampoo 1✤, PMS-Lindane LOT 1✤, PMS-Lindane SHP 1✤

Pharmacologic class: Chlorinated hydrocarbon
Therapeutic class: Scabicide, pediculocide
Pregnancy risk category C

FDA | BOXED WARNING

- Use only in patients who can't tolerate or have failed first-line treatment with safer drugs.
- Seizures and deaths have occurred with repeat or prolonged application, and in rare cases after a single application used as directed. Use cautiously in infants, children, elderly patients, persons with other skin conditions, and in those weighing less than 110 lb (50 kg).
- Drug is contraindicated in premature infants and patients with uncontrolled seizure disorders.
- Instruct patient about proper drug use, amount to apply, how long to leave it on, and importance of avoiding retreatment.

Action
Absorbed through parasitic ova and arthropods, which stimulates parasitic nervous system and results in seizures and death of parasite

Availability
Lotion: 1%
Shampoo: 1%

⚕ Indications and dosages
➣ Secondary treatment of scabies
Adults and children: Apply enough lotion on dry skin to cover entire surface from neck down. Rub in well, and leave in place 12 hours. Then wash skin thoroughly.
➣ Secondary treatment of *Pediculosis capitis* (head lice) or *Pediculosis pubis* (pubic lice)
Adults and children: Apply enough shampoo to dry hair (1 oz or less for short hair, 1½ oz for medium length hair, up to 2 oz for long hair) to thoroughly wet hair and skin or scalp of affected and surrounding hairy areas. Leave in place 12 hours. Then wash hair thoroughly.

Contraindications
- Hypersensitivity to drug or its components
- Seizure disorder
- Crusted (Norwegian) scabies and other conditions that may increase systemic drug absorption
- Premature neonates

Precautions
Use cautiously in:
- conditions that increase seizure risk (such as history of seizures, head injury, AIDS)
- skin conditions
- concurrent use of skin creams, oils, or ointments
- patients weighing less than 50 kg (110 lb)
- elderly patients
- breastfeeding patients
- infants or children.

Administration
- To apply, wear gloves made of nitrile, latex with neoprene, or sheer vinyl.
- Before applying lindane shampoo, use regular shampoo without conditioner; rinse and dry hair completely. Wait 1 hour before using lindane shampoo.
- Don't use lindane lotion or shampoo with other lotions, creams, or oils.
- Thoroughly wash skin after lotion has been in place for 12 hours.

Route	Onset	Peak	Duration
Topical	Unknown	6 hr	Unknown

Adverse reactions
CNS: dizziness, seizures, headache, anxiety, paresthesia
EENT: irritation of eyes, nose, and throat (from vapor inhalation)
GI: nausea and vomiting (from vapor inhalation)
Hematologic: aplastic anemia (with prolonged use)
Skin: dermatitis, urticaria, pruritus, alopecia
Other: pain

Reactions in **bold** are life-threatening.   ◄€ Clinical alert

Interactions
Drug-drug. *Drugs that lower seizure threshold, antidepressants:* increased seizure activity

Patient monitoring
• Monitor drug efficacy.

Patient teaching
◀€ Emphasize that drug is for external use only, and that ingesting even small amounts can be fatal.
• If drug will be applied by another person, tell patient that this person must wear gloves made of nitrile, latex with neoprene, or sheer vinyl.
• Instruct patient using lindane lotion to wash, rinse, and dry skin well before applying lindane if skin has cream, lotion, ointment, or oil on it. If he takes a warm bath or shower before applying lindane, instruct him to let skin dry and cool down. Then tell him to apply lindane to dry skin, rub in well, leave on skin for 8 to 12 hours, and then remove it by washing thoroughly.
• Instruct patient using lindane shampoo to apply enough shampoo to dry hair to thoroughly wet the hair and skin or scalp of affected and surrounding hairy areas, and then rub shampoo thoroughly into hair and skin or scalp and let it sit for 4 minutes. Then tell him to add just enough water to work up a good lather, then rinse thoroughly and dry hair with clean towel. When hair is completely dry, instruct him to comb it with a fine-toothed comb to remove any remaining nits or nit shells. Tell him not to use shampoo in combination with oils, lotions, or creams.
• To avoid reinfestation, instruct patient to launder all recently worn or used clothing, bed linens, and towels in hot water.
• Caution patient to avoid contact with eyes when applying lotion or shampoo.
• Tell patient with scabies that sexual contacts and other close personal contacts should be examined and, if necessary, treated.
• Advise female patient to inform prescriber if she plans to breastfeed.
• As appropriate, review all other significant and life-threatening adverse reactions and interactions, especially those related to the drugs mentioned above.

linezolid
Zyvox, Zyvoxam✤

Pharmacologic class: Oxazolidinone
Therapeutic class: Anti-infective
Pregnancy risk category C

Action
Selectively binds to bacterial 23S ribosomal RNA of 50S subunit, preventing formation of essential component of bacterial protein synthesis. Bacteriostatic or bactericidal against gram-positive and some gram-negative bacteria.

Availability
Injection: 2-mg/ml
Powder for oral suspension: 100 mg/5 ml
Tablets: 400 mg, 600 mg

⍟ Indications and dosages
➤ Vancomycin-resistant *Enterococcus faecium* infections
Adults and children ages 12 and older: 600 mg P.O. or I.V. infusion q 12 hours for 14 to 28 days
Children from birth to age 11: 10 mg/kg I.V. q 8 hours for 14 to 28 days
➤ Nosocomial pneumonia; community-acquired pneumonia; complicated skin and skin-structure infections
Adults and children ages 12 and older: 600 mg P.O. or I.V. infusion q 12 hours for 10 to 14 days

Children from birth to age 11: 10 mg/kg P.O. or I.V. q 8 hours for 10 to 14 days

➤ Uncomplicated skin and soft-tissue infections

Adults: 400 mg P.O. q 12 hours for 10 to 14 days

Adolescents: 600 mg P.O. or I.V. q 12 hours for 10 to 14 days

Children ages 5 to 11: 10 mg/kg P.O. or I.V. q 12 hours for 10 to 14 days

Children younger than age 5: 10 mg/kg P.O. or I.V. q 8 hours for 10 to 14 days

Contraindications

• Hypersensitivity to drug or its components

Precautions

Use cautiously in:

• hepatic dysfunction, hypertension, hyperthyroidism, pheochromocytoma, bone marrow depression, pseudomembranous colitis

• phenylketonuria (oral suspension only)

• pregnant or breastfeeding patients.

Administration

• Give oral drug with or without food.

• For I.V. injection, use single-use, ready-to-use infusion bag. Check for particulate matter before giving. Infuse over 30 minutes to 2 hours.

• For I.V. infusion, mix with dextrose 5% in water, normal saline solution, or lactated Ringer's injection.

• Flush I.V. line before and after administering, to avoid incompatibilities.

Route	Onset	Peak	Duration
P.O.	Rapid	1-2 hr	Unknown
I.V.	Unknown	Unknown	Unknown

Adverse reactions

CNS: anxiety, confusion, difficulty speaking, dizziness, hallucinations, lethargy, paresthesia, light-headedness, fatigue, drowsiness, headache, **seizures**

GI: nausea, vomiting, diarrhea, gastritis, anorexia, dry mouth, **pseudomembranous colitis**

Hematologic: thrombocytopenia

Skin: rash, photosensitivity, diaphoresis

Other: fever, fungal infections

Interactions

Drug-drug. *Antiplatelet drugs (such as aspirin, dipyridamole, nonsteroidal anti-inflammatory drugs):* increased bleeding risk

MAO inhibitors, pseudoephedrine: increased risk of hypertension and associated adverse effects

Serotonergics: serotonin syndrome

Drug-diagnostic tests. *Prothrombin time:* altered

Drug-food. *Tyramine-containing foods and beverages (such as beer; Chianti and certain other red wines; aged cheese; bananas; aged, cured, or spoiled meats; salted herring and other dried fish; avocado; bean curd; red plums; soy sauce; spinach; tofu, tomatoes; yeast):* hypertension

Patient monitoring

• Monitor neurologic status. Institute safety measures as needed to prevent injury.

• Check I.V. site for infiltration.

◀❬ Watch for bleeding and signs and symptoms of other adverse reactions (especially pseudomembranous colitis).

• Monitor CBC, coagulation studies, and culture and sensitivity tests.

Patient teaching

• Tell patient he may take with or without food, but should avoid foods containing tyramine.

◀❬ Tell patient to promptly report bleeding or severe diarrhea.

• Instruct patient to minimize adverse GI effects by eating small, frequent servings of healthy food.

Reactions in **bold** are life-threatening.   Clinical alert

- Caution patient to avoid driving and other hazardous activities until he knows how drug affects concentration and alertness.
- As appropriate, review all other significant and life-threatening adverse reactions and interactions, especially those related to the drugs, tests, and foods mentioned above.

liothyronine sodium (T₃)
Cytomel, Tertroxin✚, Triostat

Pharmacologic class: Synthetic thyroxine hormone

Therapeutic class: Thyroid hormone replacement

Pregnancy risk category A

FDA | BOXED WARNING

- Drug has been used (alone or with other agents) to treat obesity. In euthyroid patients, doses within range of daily hormonal requirements are ineffective for weight loss. Larger doses may cause serious or life-threatening toxicity, particularly when given with sympathomimetic amines (such as those used for anorectic effects).

Action
Synthetic form of triiodothyronine (T_3). Regulates cell growth and differentiation; increases metabolism of lipids, proteins, and carbohydrates; and enhances aerobic mitochondrial function. Also reduces tissue lactic acidosis.

Availability
Injection: 10 mcg/ml in 1-ml vials
Tablets: 5 mcg, 25 mcg, 50 mcg

Indications and dosages
➤ Thyroid hormone replacement in mild hypothyroidism
Adults: All dosages individualized. Initially, 25 mcg P.O. daily; may increase in increments of 12.5 to 25 mcg/day q 1 to 2 weeks. Usual maintenance dosage is 25 to 75 mcg P.O. daily.
➤ Myxedema
Adults: All dosages individualized. Initially, 5 mcg P.O. daily; increase in increments of 5 to 10 mcg/day q 1 to 2 weeks, up to 25 mcg/day. If response still isn't adequate, increase by 5 mcg to 25 mcg P.O. daily q 1 to 2 weeks until desired response occurs. Usual maintenance dosage is 50 to 100 mcg/day P.O.
➤ Myxedema coma
Adults: Initially, 25 to 50 mcg I.V.; after 4 hours, reassess patient's need for subsequent doses (up to 65 mcg in 24 hours). In cardiovascular disease, initial dosage is 10 to 20 mcg I.V.
➤ Simple goiter
Adults: All dosages individualized. Initially, 5 mcg P.O. daily. Increase by 5 to 10 mcg/day q 1 to 2 weeks, up to 25 mcg/day; then increase by 12.5 to 25 mcg P.O. daily q week until desired effect occurs. Usual maintenance dosage is 75 mcg P.O. daily.
Children or elderly adults: Initially, 5 mcg P.O once daily. Increase by 5 mcg q 1 to 2 weeks until desired effect occurs.
➤ T_3 suppression test to distinguish hyperthyroidism from thyroid gland autonomy
Adults: 75 to 100 mcg P.O. daily for 7 days in conjunction with radioactive iodine

Dosage adjustment
- Severe, long-standing hypothyroidism
- Cardiovascular disease
- Psychosis or agitation
- Elderly patients

Contraindications
• Hypersensitivity to drug or its components
• Acute myocardial infarction
• Untreated thyrotoxicosis
• Uncorrected adrenal insufficiency and coexisting hypothyroidism
• Artificial rewarming (I.V. form only)

Precautions
Use cautiously in:
• cardiovascular disease, severe renal insufficiency, uncorrected adrenocortical disorders, diabetes mellitus
• elderly patients
• pregnant or breastfeeding patients.

Administration
• Know that all dosages are highly individualized.
• Administer single oral dose in morning with or without food.
• Injectable form is for I.V. use only. Don't give I.M.
• Infuse each 10-mcg dose over 1 minute.
• Give repeat I.V. doses more than 4 hours but less than 12 hours apart.
• Be aware that in T_3 suppression test, radioactive iodine (^{131}I) is given before and after 7-day liothyronine course.

Route	Onset	Peak	Duration
P.O.	Unknown	24-72 hr	72 hr
I.V.	Unknown	Unknown	Unknown

Adverse reactions
CNS: insomnia, irritability, nervousness, headache
CV: tachycardia, angina pectoris, hypotension, hypertension, increased cardiac output, **arrhythmias, cardiovascular collapse**
GI: vomiting, diarrhea, cramps
GU: menstrual irregularities
Metabolic: hyperthyroidism, hyperglycemia
Musculoskeletal: accelerated bone maturation (in children), decreased bone density (with long-term use in women)
Skin: alopecia (in children), diaphoresis
Other: weight loss, heat intolerance

Interactions
Drug-drug. *Anabolic steroids, antithyroid drugs, asparaginase, barbiturates, carbamazepine, chloral hydrate, clofibrate, corticosteroids, danazol, estrogens, fluorouracil, heparin (with I.V. use), lithium, methadone, mitotane, oxyphenbutazone, perphenazine, phenylbutazone, phenytoin, propranolol, salicylates (large doses), sulfonylureas:* altered thyroid function test results
Anticoagulants: increased anticoagulant action
Beta-adrenergic blockers (selected): impaired beta blocker action
Cardiac glycosides: decreased cardiac glycoside blood level
Cholestyramine, colestipol: liothyronine inefficacy
Theophyllines: decreased theophylline clearance
Drug-diagnostic tests. *Thyroid function tests:* altered values
Drug-food. *Foods high in iron or fiber, soybeans:* decreased drug absorption

Patient monitoring
◀€ Monitor for evidence of overdose, including signs and symptoms of hyperthyroidism (weight loss, cardiac symptoms, and abdominal cramps).
• In patients with Addison's disease or diabetes mellitus, assess for evidence that these conditions are worsening. In diabetic patients, also monitor blood glucose level.
• Monitor vital signs and ECG routinely.
• Check thyroid and liver function tests.

Patient teaching
• Teach patient to take in morning with or without food.

- Explain that patient may require life-long therapy and will need to undergo regular blood testing.
- Caution patient to avoid driving and other hazardous activities until he knows how drug affects concentration and alertness.
- Inform parents that hair loss may occur in children during first few months but that this effect is usually transient.
- As appropriate, review all other significant and life-threatening adverse reactions and interactions, especially those related to the drugs, tests, and foods mentioned above.

liotrix
Thyrolar

Pharmacologic class: Synthetic thyroid hormone

Therapeutic class: Thyroid hormone replacement

Pregnancy risk category A

FDA | BOXED WARNING

- Drug has been used (alone or with other agents) to treat obesity. In euthyroid patients, doses within range of daily hormonal requirements are ineffective for weight loss. Larger doses may produce serious or even life-threatening toxicity, particularly when given with sympathomimetic amines (such as those used for anorectic effects).

Action
Increases basal metabolic rate, helps regulate cell growth and differentiation, and enhances metabolism of lipids, proteins, and carbohydrates

Availability
Tablets: 12.5 mcg levothyroxine sodium and 3.1 mcg liothyronine sodium (Thyrolar-¼); 25 mcg levothyroxine sodium and 6.25 mcg liothyronine sodium (Thyrolar-½); 50 mcg levothyroxine sodium and 12.5 mcg liothyronine sodium (Thyrolar-1); 100 mcg levothyroxine sodium and 25 mcg liothyronine sodium (Thyrolar-2); 150 mcg levothyroxine sodium and 37.5 mcg liothyronine sodium (Thyrolar-3)

⚕ Indications and dosages
➤ Hypothyroidism
Adults: All dosages individualized. Initially, one tablet Thyrolar-½ P.O., increased by one tablet Thyrolar-¼ P.O. daily until desired effect occurs. Usual maintenance dosage is one tablet Thyrolar-1 or Thyrolar-2 P.O. daily, adjusted within first 4 weeks based on laboratory results.
➤ Congenital hypothyroidism
Children older than age 12: 18.75/75 mcg P.O. daily
Children ages 6 to 11: 12.5/50 to 18.75/75 mcg P.O. daily
Children ages 1 to 5: 9.35/37.5 to 12.5/50 mcg P.O. daily
Children ages 6 to 12 months: 6.25/25 to 9.35/37.5 mcg P.O. daily
Children up to 6 months: 3.1/12.5 to 6.25/25 mcg (Thyrolar-¼) P.O. daily

Dosage adjustment
- Severe, long-standing hypothyroidism
- Cardiovascular disease
- Psychosis or agitation
- Elderly patients

Contraindications
- Hypersensitivity to drug or its components
- Acute myocardial infarction
- Uncorrected thyrotoxicosis
- Uncorrected adrenal insufficiency and coexisting hypothyroidism

---

Precautions

Use cautiously in:
- cardiovascular disease, severe renal insufficiency, diabetes mellitus, uncorrected adrenocortical disorders
- elderly patients
- pregnant or breastfeeding patients.

Administration

- Know that all dosages are highly individualized.
- Administer single daily dose in morning with or without food.

Route	Onset	Peak	Duration
P.O. (levothyroxine)	Unknown	Unknown	Unknown
P.O. (liothyronine)	Unknown	24-72 hr	72 hr

Adverse reactions

CNS: insomnia, irritability, nervousness, headache
CV: angina pectoris, hypotension, hypertension, increased cardiac output, tachycardia, **arrhythmias, cardiovascular collapse**
GI: vomiting, diarrhea, cramps
GU: menstrual irregularities
Metabolic: hyperthyroidism
Musculoskeletal: accelerated bone maturation (in children), decreased bone density (with long-term use in women)
Skin: alopecia (in children), diaphoresis
Other: weight loss, heat intolerance

Interactions

Drug-drug. *Aminoglutethimide, amiodarone, anabolic steroids, antithyroid drugs, asparaginase, barbiturates, carbamazepine, chloral hydrate, cholestyramine, clofibrate, colestipol, corticosteroids, danazol, diazepam, estrogens, ethionamide, fluorouracil, heparin (with I.V. use), insulin, lithium, methadone, mitotane, nitroprusside, oxyphenbutazone, P-aminosalicyclic acid, perphenazine, phenylbutazone, phenytoin, propranolol, salicylates (large doses), sulfonylureas, thiazides:* altered thyroid function test results
Anticoagulants: increased anticoagulant action
Beta-adrenergic blockers (selected): decreased beta blocker action
Cardiac glycosides: decreased cardiac glycoside blood level
Cholestyramine, colestipol: liotrix inefficacy
Theophyllines: decreased theophylline clearance
Drug-diagnostic tests. *Thyroid function tests:* decreased values
Drug-food. *Foods high in iron or fiber, soybeans:* decreased drug absorption

Patient monitoring

- Monitor for evidence of overdose, such as signs and symptoms of hyperthyroidism (weight loss, cardiac symptoms, abdominal cramps).
- Watch closely for signs and symptoms of undertreatment.
- In patients with Addison's disease or diabetes mellitus, assess for signs that these conditions are worsening. In diabetic patients, monitor blood glucose level.
- Check vital signs and ECG routinely.
- Monitor thyroid and liver function tests.
- Assess for signs and symptoms of bleeding tendency, especially if patient's taking anticoagulants.

Patient teaching

- Inform patient or parents that drug should be taken in morning with or without food.
- Explain that patient may require lifelong therapy and will need to undergo regular blood testing.
- Advise diabetic patient (or his parents) to monitor patient's blood glucose level closely.

Reactions in **bold** are life-threatening.   ◀€ Clinical alert

- Caution patient to avoid driving and other hazardous activities until he knows how drug affects concentration and alertness.
- Inform parents that hair loss may occur in children during first few months of therapy but that this effect is usually transient.
- As appropriate, review all other significant and life-threatening adverse reactions and interactions, especially those related to the drugs, tests, and foods mentioned above.

liraglutide
Victoza

Pharmacologic class: Glucagon-like peptide-1 (GLP-1) receptor agonist
Therapeutic class: Hypoglycemic
Pregnancy risk category C

FDA BOXED WARNING

- Liraglutide causes dose-dependent and treatment-duration-dependent thyroid C-cell tumors at clinically relevant exposures in both genders of rats and mice. It's unknown whether drug causes thyroid C-cell tumors, including medullary thyroid carcinoma (MTC), in humans, as human relevance couldn't be ruled out by clinical or nonclinical studies.
- Drug is contraindicated in patients with personal or family history of MTC and in patients with multiple endocrine neoplasia syndrome type 2 (MEN 2).

Action
Activates GLP-1 receptor, a membrane-bound cell-surface receptor coupled to adenylyl cyclase by the stimulatory G-protein, Gs, in pancreatic beta cells and increases intracellular cyclic AMP, leading to insulin release in the presence of elevated glucose levels; also decreases glucagon secretion in a glucose-dependent manner. Mechanism of blood-glucose lowering also involves a delay in gastric emptying.

Availability
Injection: 0.6 mg, 1.2 mg, 1.8 mg (6 mg/ml, 3 ml) in prefilled, multidose pens

Indications and dosages
➤ Adjunct to diet and exercise to improve glycemic control in adults with type 2 diabetes mellitus
Adults: Initially, 0.6 mg subcutaneously daily for 1 week. After 1 week, increase dosage to 1.2 mg daily. If 1.2-mg dose doesn't result in acceptable glycemic control, dosage can be increased to 1.8 mg daily.

Contraindications
- Personal or family history of medullary thyroid carcinoma
- MEN 2

Precautions
Use cautiously in:
- hepatic or renal impairment
- history of pancreatitis
- concomitant use of oral hypoglycemics
- breastfeeding patients
- children (safety and efficacy not established).

Administration
- Administer without regard to meals.
- Be aware that initial dose is intended to reduce GI symptoms and isn't effective for glycemic control.
- When initiating drug, consider reducing dosage of concomitantly administered oral hypoglycemics to reduce risk of hypoglycemia.

Route	Onset	Peak	Duration
Subcut.	Unknown	Unknown	Unknown

Adverse reactions
CNS: dizziness, headache
CV: hypertension
EENT: sinusitis, nasopharyngitis
GI: nausea, vomiting, diarrhea, constipation, **pancreatitis**
GU: urinary tract infection
Metabolic: hypoglycemia, **hyperosmolar coma, death**
Musculoskeletal: back pain
Respiratory: upper respiratory tract infection
Other: influenza

Interactions
Drug-drug. *Insulin secretagogues (such as sulfonylureas):* increased risk of hypoglycemia
Oral drugs: decreased absorption of these drugs
Drug-diagnostic tests. *Blood glucose:* decreased level

Patient monitoring
◀≋ If pancreatitis is suspected, discontinue drug promptly, perform confirmatory tests, and treat appropriately. If pancreatitis is confirmed, don't restart drug.

◀≋ Monitor patient for signs and symptoms of thyroid tumor.

Patient teaching
• Instruct patient to take drug without regard to meals.

◀≋ Instruct patient to discontinue drug and immediately notify prescriber if persistent severe abdominal pain occurs that may radiate to the back and may or may not be accompanied by vomiting.

◀≋ Instruct patient to immediately notify prescriber if signs and symptoms of thyroid tumor occur (such as persistent hoarseness, mass in the neck, difficulty swallowing, or difficulty breathing).

• As appropriate, review all other significant and life-threatening adverse reactions and interactions, especially those related to the drugs and tests mentioned above.

lisdexamfetamine dimesylate
Vyvanse

Pharmacologic class: Amphetamine prodrug
Therapeutic class: CNS stimulant
Controlled substance schedule II
Pregnancy risk category C

FDA | BOXED WARNING

• Drug has high abuse potential. Prolonged use may lead to drug dependence. Stay alert for possibility of persons obtaining it for nontherapeutic use or distribution. Drug should be prescribed or dispensed sparingly.
• Drug misuse may cause sudden death and serious cardiovascular adverse events.

Action
Rapidly absorbed and converted to dextroamphetamine, which is responsible for CNS activity. Therapeutic action in attention deficit hyperactivity disorder (ADHD) is unknown.

Availability
Capsules: 20 mg, 30 mg, 40 mg, 50 mg, 60 mg, 70 mg

ⓘ Indications and dosages
➤ ADHD
Adults and Children ages 6 to 12: Individualize dosage based on therapeutic needs and response. For child starting treatment for first time or switching from another drug,

recommended dosage is 30 mg P.O. once daily in morning. If daily dosage will be increased above 30 mg, adjust in increments of 10 to 20 mg/day at approximately weekly intervals. Maximum recommended dosage is 70 mg/day.

Contraindications
• Hypersensitivity or idiosyncratic reaction to sympathomimetic amines
• Advanced arteriosclerosis, symptomatic cardiovascular disease, moderate to severe hypertension, hyperthyroidism, glaucoma, agitated state
• History of drug abuse
• During or within 14 days of MAO inhibitor therapy

Precautions
Use cautiously in:
• concurrent use of other sympathomimetics
• tics, Tourette syndrome, hypertension or other cardiovascular conditions, preexisting psychosis (such as bipolar disorder)
• electroencephalogram (EEG) abnormalities or seizures
• pregnant and breastfeeding patients
• adults
• children younger than age 6 or older than age 12 (safety and efficacy not established).

Administration
• Administer with or without food.
• Give in morning to avoid insomnia.
• Give capsules whole, or open and dissolve entire contents in glass of water. When using solution method, don't divide single-capsule dose; make sure patient consumes solution immediately.
• ◀€ Don't give within 14 days of MAO inhibitors.

Route	Onset	Peak	Duration
P.O.	Unknown	1 hr	Unknown

Adverse reactions
CNS: dizziness, headache, somnolence, insomnia, irritability, labile affect, manic symptoms, dysphoria, euphoria, aggression, restlessness, tics, dyskinesia, psychomotor hyperactivity, psychotic episodes, depression, tremor, **seizure, stroke**
CV: palpitations, tachycardia, hypertension, **ventricular hypertrophy, myocardial infarction, cardiomyopathy, sudden death**
EENT: visual disturbances
GI: abdominal pain, nausea, vomiting, diarrhea, constipation, dry mouth, unpleasant taste
GU: libido changes, erectile dysfunction
Skin: rash, toxic epidermal necrolysis, urticaria, **Stevens-Johnson syndrome**
Other: decreased appetite, weight loss, growth suppression, fever, amphetamine tolerance and dependency, hypersensitivity reactions including **angioedema** and **anaphylaxis**

Interactions
Drug-drug. *Adrenergic blockers:* inhibited adrenergic blocker action
Antihistamines: decreased sedative effect of antihistamine
Antihypertensives: antagonism of antihypertensive effect
Chlorpromazine: inhibited stimulant effect
Desipramine, protriptyline (and possibly other tricyclic antidepressants): enhanced antidepressant activity, causing sustained rise in d-amphetamine concentration in brain
Ethosuximide: delayed intestinal absorption of this drug
Haloperidol: inhibited central stimulant effects
Lithium carbonate: inhibited anorectic and stimulatory effects of lisdexamfetamine

MAO inhibitors: slowed lisdexamfetamine metabolism, possibly leading to hypertensive crises

Meperidine: potentiated analgesic effect of meperidine

Methenamine therapy: increased amphetamine urinary excretion, causing reduced lisdexamfetamine blood level and efficacy

Norepinephrine: enhanced norepinephrine adrenergic effect

Phenobarbital, phenytoin: possible delayed intestinal absorption of these drugs, possible synergistic anticonvulsant action

Propoxyphene: increased risk of potentiated CNS stimulation (leading to life-threatening seizures in propoxyphene overdosage)

Drug-diagnostic tests. *Plasma corticosteroids:* increased levels

Urinary steroids: interference with results

Drug-herbs. Veratrum *alkaloids, such as* Veratrum album *(white hellebore),* V. eschsholtzii *(American hellebore), and* V. luteum *(false unicorn):* inhibited hypotensive effect of these herbs

Patient monitoring

• Before initiating therapy, evaluate patient and family for history of cardiovascular abnormalities, tics or Tourette syndrome (or exacerbation of these), EEG abnormalities, and seizures. Drug may lower seizure threshold.

• During early treatment phase, stay alert for worsening of aggressive behavior or hostility.

• Monitor blood pressure and pulse.

• Know that when possible, drug therapy should be interrupted occasionally to determine if behavioral symptoms recur to extent that necessitates continued therapy.

• Monitor patient for appropriate growth and weight gain.

• Watch for signs and symptoms of drug tolerance, dependence, and abuse.

Patient teaching

• Inform patient or caregiver that drug can be taken with or without food. Advise them that it should be taken in morning to help avoid insomnia.

• Instruct patient to take capsule whole, or to open it and dissolve entire contents in glass of water, and consume solution immediately.

• Advise patient or caregiver to watch for and report seizures, worsening of aggressive behavior, tics, or inappropriate growth or weight gain.

• Instruct patient to avoid using herbs unless prescriber approves.

• Caution patient to avoid hazardous activities until drug's effects on concentration, coordination, and vision are known.

• As appropriate, review all other significant and life-threatening adverse reactions and interactions, especially those related to the drugs, tests, and herbs mentioned above.

lisinopril

Apo-Lisinopril✱, Carace⊕, Co-Lisinopril✱, Dom-Lisinopril✱, Gen-Lisinopril✱, Novo-Lisinopril✱, PHL-Lisinopril✱, Prinivil, Ratio-Lisinopril✱, Riva-Lisinopril✱, Zestril

Pharmacologic class: Angiotensin-converting enzyme (ACE) inhibitor

Therapeutic class: Antihypertensive

Pregnancy risk category C (first trimester), *D* (second and third trimesters)

- When used during second or third trimester of pregnancy, drug may cause fetal harm or death. Discontinue as soon as pregnancy is detected.

Action

Inhibits conversion of angiotensin I to angiotensin II (a potent vasoconstrictor), decreasing systemic vascular resistance, blood pressure, preload, and afterload. Also inactivates bradykinin and other vasodilatory prostaglandins, increases plasma renin levels, and reduces aldosterone levels.

Availability

Tablets: 2.5 mg, 5 mg, 10 mg, 20 mg, 30 mg, 40 mg

ⓘ Indications and dosages

➤ Hypertension

Adults: Initially, 10 mg P.O. daily, increased to a maintenance dosage of 20 to 40 mg/day. Maximum daily dosage is 80 mg. In patients on diuretics, start with 5 mg/day P.O.

➤ Heart failure

Adults: 5 mg/day P.O. (Prinivil), increased in increments, as ordered, to a maximum of 20 mg/day as a single dose. Or 5 to 40 mg P.O. (Zestril) as a single daily dose given with digitalis and diuretics, increased in increments of no more than 10 mg at intervals of at least 2 weeks, to highest dosage tolerated; maximum dosage is 40 mg/day P.O.

➤ Adjunctive therapy after acute myocardial infarction

Adults: Initially, 5 mg P.O., followed by 5 mg after 24 hours, 10 mg after 48 hours, and then 10 mg daily for 6 weeks (given with standard thrombolytic, aspirin, or beta-adrenergic blocker therapy). If systolic pressure is 120 mm Hg or lower, initial dosage is 2.5 mg for 2 days, then 2.5 to 5 mg/day.

Dosage adjustment

- Impaired renal function
- Heart failure with hyponatremia

Contraindications

- Hypersensitivity to drug or other ACE inhibitors
- Angioedema (hereditary, idiopathic, or ACE-inhibitor induced)
- Pregnancy (second and third trimesters)

Precautions

Use cautiously in:

- renal impairment, hypertension, cerebrovascular or cardiac insufficiency
- family history of angioedema
- concurrent diuretic therapy
- black patients (in whom drug may be less effective in treating hypertension)
- elderly patients
- pregnant patients in first trimester
- breastfeeding patients
- children (safety not established).

Administration

- Give once a day in morning, with or without food.

🔊 Measure blood pressure before administering. Withhold drug, if appropriate, according to prescriber's blood pressure parameters. Adjust dosage according to blood pressure response.

- Expect prescriber to add low-dose diuretic if lisinopril alone doesn't control blood pressure.

Route	Onset	Peak	Duration
P.O.	1 hr	6 hr	24 hr

Adverse reactions

CNS: dizziness, fatigue, headache, asthenia
CV: hypotension, orthostatic hypotension, syncope, chest pain, angina pectoris
GI: nausea, diarrhea, abdominal pain, anorexia
GU: erectile dysfunction, decreased libido, **renal dysfunction**
Metabolic: hyponatremia, **hyperkalemia**
Musculoskeletal: myalgia

Respiratory: cough, upper respiratory tract infection, bronchitis, dyspnea, **asthma**
Skin: rash, pruritus, angioedema
Other: altered taste, fever, **anaphylaxis**

Interactions

Drug-drug. *Cyclosporine, potassium-sparing diuretics, potassium supplements:* hyperkalemia
Diuretics, other antihypertensives: excessive hypotension
Indomethacin: reduced antihypertensive effect
Lithium: increased lithium blood level, greater risk of lithium toxicity
Nonsteroidal anti-inflammatory drugs: further deterioration in patients with renal compromise, decreased antihypertensive effects
Thiazides: hypokalemia
Drug-diagnostic tests. *Blood urea nitrogen, creatinine, hematocrit, hemoglobin:* slightly increased levels
Liver function tests, potassium: increased levels
Sodium: decreased level
Drug-food. *Salt substitutes containing potassium:* hyperkalemia
Drug-herbs. *Capsaicin:* cough
Ephedra (ma huang), licorice, yohimbine: antagonistic effects
Drug-behaviors. *Acute alcohol ingestion:* excessive hypotension

Patient monitoring

• Before and periodically during therapy, monitor CBC with white cell differential and kidney and liver function tests.
◀€ Monitor for signs and symptoms of angioedema or anaphylaxis. If these occur, discontinue drug and contact prescriber immediately.
• Check blood pressure frequently to assess drug efficacy. Monitor closely for hypotension, especially in patients also taking diuretics.
• Check vital signs and ECG regularly. Assess cardiovascular status carefully.

• Monitor respiratory and neurologic status.
• Assess potassium intake and blood potassium level.

Patient teaching

• Advise patient to take once a day in morning, with or without food.
◀€ Tell patient to immediately report fainting, continuing cough, rash, itching, swelling (especially of face, lips, tongue, or throat), severe dizziness, difficulty breathing, extreme tiredness, or continuing nausea.
◀€ Instruct female patient to notify prescriber if she becomes pregnant.
• Tell patient that drug may cause temporary blood pressure decrease if he stands up suddenly. Advise him to rise slowly and carefully.
• Explain that drug may cause muscle aches or headache. Encourage patient to discuss activity recommendations and pain relief with prescriber.
• Caution patient to avoid driving and other hazardous activities until he knows how drug affects concentration and alertness.
• Instruct patient to avoid potassium-based salt substitutes or potassium supplements.
• Tell patient he'll undergo regular blood testing during therapy.
• As appropriate, review all other significant and life-threatening adverse reactions and interactions, especially those related to the drugs, tests, foods, herbs, and behaviors mentioned above.

lithium carbonate

Apo-Lithium Camcolit✚, Apo-Lithium Carbonate✱, Carbolith✱, Duralith✱, Euro-Lithium✱, Liskonum✚, Lithane, Lithobid, Lithonate✚, PHL-Lithium Carbonate✱, PMS-Lithium Carbonate✱, Priadel✚

---

lithium citrate
PMS-Lithium Citrate✶

Pharmacologic class: Miscellaneous CNS drug
Therapeutic class: Antimanic drug
Pregnancy risk category D

FDA | BOXED WARNING

• Lithium toxicity is closely related to lithium blood level and can occur at doses close to therapeutic levels. Before starting therapy, ensure that resources for prompt, accurate blood lithium testing are available.

Action
Unknown. Thought to disrupt sodium exchange and transport in nerves and muscles and control reuptake of neurotransmitters.

Availability
Capsules: 150 mg, 300 mg, 600 mg
Syrup (citrate): 300 mg (8 mEq lithium)/5 ml
Tablets: 300 mg
Tablets (extended-release): 300 mg, 450 mg
Tablets (slow-release): 300 mg

💊 Indications and dosages
➢ Manic episodes of bipolar disorder
Adults and children ages 12 and older: 900 to 1,800 mg P.O. daily in divided doses (for example, 300 to 600 mg t.i.d. or 450 to 900 mg b.i.d. of controlled- or slow-release form) to achieve blood level of 1 to 1.5 mEq/L; measure blood level twice weekly until patient stabilizes. Maintenance dosage is 900 to 1,200 mg/day in divided doses (for example, 300 to 400 mg t.i.d. or 450 to 600 mg b.i.d. of controlled- or slow-release form) to maintain blood level of 0.6 to 1.2 mEq/L. Monitor blood level at least q 2 months.

Dosage adjustment
• Impaired renal function
• Elderly patients

Off-label uses
• Acute manic episodes in children
• Corticosteroid-induced psychosis
• Neutropenia secondary to antineoplastic therapy
• Tardive dyskinesia
• Alcoholism
• Bulimia

Contraindications
None

Precautions
Use cautiously in:
• hepatic or thyroid disease, severe cardiovascular or renal disease, diabetes mellitus, seizure disorders, systemic infections, brain trauma, organic brain syndrome, urinary retention, severe sodium depletion
• elderly patients
• pregnant or breastfeeding patients
• children (safety not established).

Administration
🔊 Be aware that dosages are individualized according to lithium blood level and response.
• Give with food or milk to minimize GI upset.
• Make sure patient swallows slow-release tablet whole without chewing or crushing.
• When switching patient from immediate-release to controlled- or slow-release form, give same total daily dosage.

Route	Onset	Peak	Duration
P.O.	Unknown	0.5-3 hr	Unknown
P.O. (controlled, slow-release)	Unknown	3-12 hr	Unknown

Adverse reactions
CNS: dizziness, drowsiness, headache, tremor, tics, EEG changes, ataxia, choreoathetotic movements, abnormal

tongue movements, extrapyramidal reactions, cogwheel rigidity, blackout spells, psychomotor retardation, slow mental functioning, slurred speech, startled response, restlessness, agitation, confusion, hallucinations, poor memory, worsening of organic brain syndrome, stupor, **coma, epileptiform seizures**

CV: bradycardia, ECG changes, hypotension, **sinus node dysfunction with severe bradycardia and syncope, arrhythmias, peripheral circulatory collapse**

EENT: blurred vision, nystagmus, tinnitus

GI: nausea, vomiting, diarrhea, abdominal pain, fecal incontinence, gastritis, flatulence, dyspepsia, anorexia, increased salivation, salivary gland swelling, dry mouth

GU: urinary incontinence, glycosuria, albuminuria, erectile or other sexual dysfunction, polyuria or other signs of nephrogenic diabetes insipidus, **oliguria**

Hematologic: leukocytosis

Metabolic: hypothyroidism or hyperthyroidism, goiter, hyperglycemia, hypercalcemia, hyponatremia, hyperparathyroidism

Musculoskeletal: swollen or painful joints, muscle weakness, muscle fasciculations and twitching, clonic arm or leg movements, hypertonicity, hyperactive deep tendon reflexes, polyarthralgia

Skin: dry thin hair, alopecia, diminished or absent skin sensations, chronic folliculitis, eczema with dry skin, new onset or exacerbation of psoriasis, pruritus (with or without rash), cutaneous ulcers, angioedema

Other: altered, metallic, or salty taste; dental caries; weight gain; excessive thirst; polydipsia; fever; edema of lips, ankles, and wrists

Interactions

Drug-drug. *Acetazolamide, alkalinizing agents (such as sodium bicarbonate), urea, verapamil, xanthines:* decreased lithium blood level

Calcium channel blockers, carbamazepine, haloperidol, methyldopa: increased risk of neurotoxicity

Diuretics: increased sodium loss, increased risk of lithium toxicity

Fluoxetine, loop diuretics, metronidazole, nonsteroidal anti-inflammatory drugs: increased risk of lithium toxicity

Iodide salts: synergistic effects, increased risk of hypothyroidism

Neuromuscular blockers: prolonged neuromuscular blockade, severe respiratory depression

Phenothiazines: decreased phenothiazine blood level or increased lithium blood level, greater risk of neurotoxicity

Selective serotonin reuptake inhibitors: increased risk of tremor, confusion, dizziness, agitation, and diarrhea

Sympathomimetics: decreased pressor sensitivity

Tricyclic antidepressants: increased antidepressant effects

Drug-diagnostic tests. *Albumin, creatinine, sodium, thyroxine, triiodothyronine:* decreased levels

Calcium, glucose, ^{131}I uptake, white blood cells (WBCs): increased levels

Drug-food. *Caffeine-containing foods and beverages:* decreased lithium blood level and efficacy

Drug-herbs. *Caffeine-containing herbs (cola nut, guarana, yerba maté):* decreased lithium blood level and efficacy

Patient monitoring

• Obtain baseline ECG and electrolyte levels before and periodically during therapy.

• Assess neurologic and psychiatric status. Institute safety measures as needed to prevent injury.

• Monitor lithium blood level, WBC count, and thyroid and kidney function tests.

• Assess cardiovascular status regularly.

• Monitor fluid intake and output. Watch for edema and weight gain.

Patient teaching
• Advise patient to take with food or milk to minimize GI upset.
• Instruct patient to swallow slow-release tablet whole without chewing or crushing.
• Tell patient that beneficial effects may take 1 to 3 weeks to appear.
• Advise patient to limit foods and beverages containing caffeine, because they may interfere with drug action.
• Tell patient to maintain adequate fluid intake.
• Explain that drug may cause adverse CNS effects. Advise patient to avoid activities requiring mental alertness until effects are known.
◀€ Emphasize importance of having regular blood tests, to help detect and prevent serious adverse reactions.
• Instruct patient to carry appropriate medical identification at all times.
• As appropriate, review all other significant and life-threatening adverse reactions and interactions, especially those related to the drugs, tests, foods, and herbs mentioned above.

lomustine
CeeNU

Pharmacologic class: Alkylating drug (nitrosourea)
Therapeutic class: Antineoplastic
Pregnancy risk category D

FDA BOXED WARNING

• Give under supervision of physician experienced in cancer chemotherapy, in facility with adequate diagnostic and treatment resources. Most common and severe toxic effect is bone marrow suppression, which may contribute to bleeding and overwhelming infections in already compromised patients. Delayed bone marrow suppression is major toxicity, so monitor blood counts weekly for at least 6 weeks after dose. At recommended dosage, don't give courses more often than every 6 weeks. Bone marrow toxicity is cumulative; consider adjusting dosage based on nadir blood counts from previous dose.

Action
Inactivates neoplastic cells by alkylating DNA, causing DNA structural modification and fragmentation. Thought to act in late G1 or early S phase of cell cycle.

Availability
Capsules: 10 mg, 40 mg, 100 mg
Dose pack: two 10-mg capsules, two 40-mg capsules, and 100-mg capsules

Indications and dosages
➤ Adjunctive therapy in primary and metastatic brain tumors; secondary therapy in Hodgkin's disease
Adults and children: As monotherapy, 130 mg/m² P.O. as a single dose q 6 weeks in previously untreated patients. In bone marrow suppression, initial dosage is 100 mg/m² P.O. q 6 weeks; don't repeat dose until platelet count exceeds 100,000/mm³ and white blood cell (WBC) count exceeds 4,000/mm³. When given with other myelosuppressive drugs, adjust dosage accordingly.

Dosage adjustment
• Bone marrow depression (based on WBC and platelet counts)

Contraindications
• Hypersensitivity to drug

Precautions

Use cautiously in:
- renal or hepatic dysfunction, bone marrow depression
- pregnant or breastfeeding patients.

Administration

- Obtain CBC with white cell differential before starting therapy.
- Administer antiemetic before giving drug, as prescribed, to minimize nausea.
- Give 2 to 4 hours after meals to enhance absorption.
- If vomiting occurs shortly after administration, notify prescriber.

Route	Onset	Peak	Duration
P.O.	10 min	3 hr	48 hr

Adverse reactions

CNS: anxiety, confusion, dizziness, hallucinations, lethargy, headache, paresthesia, light-headedness, drowsiness, fatigue, **seizures**

GI: nausea; vomiting; anorexia; sore mouth, lips, and throat; **GI bleeding**

GU: amenorrhea, azoospermia, progressive azotemia, **nephrotoxicity, renal failure**

Hematologic: anemia, **leukopenia, thrombocytopenia, bone marrow depression**

Hepatic: hepatotoxicity

Skin: alopecia

Other: secondary cancers

Interactions

Drug-drug. *Anticoagulants, nonsteroidal anti-inflammatory drugs:* increased bleeding risk

Myelosuppressants: increased bone marrow depression

Drug-diagnostic tests. *Hemoglobin, platelets, red blood cells, WBCs:* decreased values

Liver function tests, nitrogenous compounds: increased values

Patient monitoring

◀€ Watch for evidence of overdose, including bone marrow depression, nausea, and vomiting.

◀€ Monitor CBC and platelet counts closely. Watch for signs and symptoms of bleeding and bruising.

- Avoid I.M. injections if platelet count is below 100,000/mm^3.
- Check kidney, liver, and pulmonary function tests frequently.
- Assess neurologic status carefully. Institute safety measures as needed to prevent injury.

◀€ Watch for signs and symptoms of secondary cancers.

Patient teaching

- Instruct patient to contact prescriber if he vomits shortly after taking drug.

◀€ Tell patient to immediately report easy bruising or bleeding, which may signal low platelet count.

- Advise patient to report changes in urination pattern.
- Instruct patient to avoid exposure to people with infections, because drug may make him more susceptible to infection.

◀€ Caution female of childbearing age to use reliable contraception and to immediately report suspected or confirmed pregnancy.

- Advise female patient to inform prescriber if she is breastfeeding.
- Caution patient to avoid driving and other hazardous activities until he knows how drug affects concentration and alertness.
- Advise patient to minimize GI side effects by eating small, frequent servings of healthy food.
- Inform patient that drug may cause hair loss.
- Tell patient he'll undergo frequent blood testing during therapy.
- As appropriate, review all other significant and life-threatening adverse reactions and interactions, especially those related to the drugs and tests mentioned above.

Reactions in **bold** are life-threatening.   ◀€ Clinical alert

loperamide hydrochloride

Apo-Loperamide❖, Arret⊕,
Diah-Limit⊕, Diamode, Diaquitte⊕,
Diareze⊕, Diarr-Eze❖, Diarrhea
Relief❖, Diocalm Ultra⊕, Diocaps⊕,
Dom-Loperamide❖, Entocalm⊕,
Imodium, Imodium A-D, K-Pek II,
Loperacap❖, Norimode⊕,
Normaloe⊕, Novo-Loperamide❖,
PHL-Loperamide❖, PMS-
Loperamine❖, Riva-Loperamine❖,
Sandoz Loperamide

Pharmacologic class: Piperidine derivative

Therapeutic class: Antidiarrheal
Pregnancy risk category B

Action
Inhibits peristalsis of intestinal wall musculature and intestinal contents. Also reduces fecal volume, increases fecal bulk, and minimizes fluid and electrolyte loss.

Availability
Capsules: 2 mg
Solution: 1 mg/5 ml
Tablets: 2 mg
Tablets (chewable): 2 mg

⦸ Indications and dosages
➤ Acute diarrhea
Adults: Initially, 4 mg P.O., then 2 mg after each loose stool. Usual maintenance dosage is 4 to 8 mg P.O. daily in divided doses, not to exceed 16 mg daily.
Children ages 8 to 12 or weighing more than 30 kg (66 lb): Initially, 2 mg P.O. t.i.d., then 1 mg/10 kg after each loose stool, not to exceed 6 mg daily
Children ages 6 to 8 or weighing 20 to 30 kg (44 to 66 lb): Initially, 2 mg P.O.

b.i.d., then 1 mg/10 kg after each loose stool, not to exceed 4 mg daily
Children ages 2 to 5 or weighing 13 to 20 kg (29 to 44 lb): Initially, 1 mg P.O. t.i.d., then 1 mg/10 kg after each loose stool, not to exceed 3 mg daily
➤ Acute diarrhea (treated with over-the-counter loperamide)
Adults and children ages 12 and older: Two caplets with 4 to 8 oz water after first loose stool, then one caplet (with 4 to 8 oz water) after each subsequent loose stool. Don't exceed four caplets in 24 hours. Or give equivalent dosage in liquid form.
Children ages 9 to 11 who weigh 27 to 43 kg (60 to 95 lbs): One caplet with 4 to 8 oz water after first loose stool, then ½ caplet (with 4 to 8 oz water) after each subsequent loose stool. Don't exceed three caplets in 24 hours. Or give equivalent dosage in liquid form.
Children ages 6 to 8 who weigh 22 to 27 kg (48 to 59 lbs): One caplet with 4 to 8 oz water after first loose stool, then ½ caplet with 4 to 8 oz water after each subsequent loose stool. Don't exceed two caplets in 24 hours. Or give equivalent dosage in liquid form.
Children younger than age 6: Consult physician.
➤ Chronic diarrhea
Adults: Initially, 4 mg P.O., then 2 mg after each loose stool; reduce dosage as tolerated. Don't exceed 16 mg daily for more than 10 days.

Contraindications
• Hypersensitivity to drug
• Abdominal pain of unknown cause (especially with fever)
• Acute diarrhea caused by enteroinvasive *Escherichia coli*, *Salmonella*, or *Shigella*
• Acute ulcerative colitis
• Bloody diarrhea with temperature above 38.3 °C (101 °F) (with OTC product)

❖ Canada   ⊕ UK   ⚕ Hazardous drug   ⊗ High-alert drug

- Pseudomembranous colitis associated with broad-spectrum anti-infectives
- Children younger than age 6

Precautions
Use cautiously in:
- hepatic disease
- elderly patients
- pregnant or breastfeeding patients
- children.

Administration
- Use patient's weight to determine appropriate dosage (especially in children).

Route	Onset	Peak	Duration
P.O.	1 hr	2.5-5 hr	10 hr

Adverse reactions
CNS: drowsiness, dizziness
GI: nausea; vomiting; constipation; abdominal pain, distention, or discomfort; dry mouth; **toxic megacolon** (in patients with acute ulcerative colitis)
Other: allergic reactions

Interactions
Drug-drug. *Antidepressants, antihistamines, other anticholinergics:* additive anticholinergic effects
CNS depressants (including antihistamines, opioid analgesics, sedative-hypnotics): additive CNS depression
Drug-herbs. *Chamomile, hops, kava, skullcap, valerian:* increased CNS depression
Drug-behaviors. *Alcohol use:* increased CNS depression

Patient monitoring
◀≶ Watch for signs and symptoms of abdominal distention, which may signal toxic megacolon in patient with ulcerative colitis.
- Assess bowel movements to evaluate drug efficacy and determine need for repeat doses.

- Monitor stool cultures as indicated.
- Check stool for occult blood as indicated.
- Evaluate fluid intake and output.
- Stay alert for CNS effects, especially in children.

Patient teaching
- Stress importance of maintaining high fluid intake to prevent dehydration.
◀≶ Instruct patient or parents to report fever, mucus in stool, or history of hepatic disease before using drug.
◀≶ Caution patient or parents to discontinue drug if symptoms worsen or diarrhea lasts longer than 2 days.
- As appropriate, review all other significant and life-threatening adverse reactions and interactions, especially those related to the drugs, herbs, and behaviors mentioned above.

loratadine
Aerius✤, Alavert, Allertin, Claritin, Claritin RediTabs, Clarityn⊕

Pharmacologic class: Histamine₁-receptor antagonist (second-generation)
Therapeutic class: Antihistamine (nonsedating)
Pregnancy risk category B

Action
Selective histamine₁-receptor antagonist. Blocks peripheral effects of histamine release during allergic reactions, decreasing or preventing allergy symptoms.

Availability
Syrup: 1 mg/ml
Tablets: 10 mg
Tablets (rapidly disintegrating): 10 mg

Reactions in **bold** are life-threatening. ◀≶ Clinical alert

Indications and dosages

➤ Seasonal allergies; chronic idiopathic urticaria

Adults and children ages 6 and older: 10 mg P.O. daily

Children ages 2 to 5: 5 mg P.O. daily

Dosage adjustment

• Renal or hepatic impairment

Contraindications

• Hypersensitivity to drug

Precautions

Use cautiously in:
• renal or hepatic impairment
• elderly patients
• pregnant patients
• children younger than age 2 (safety not established).

Administration

• Give once a day on empty stomach.
• Place rapidly disintegrating tablet on tongue; give with or without water.
• Use rapidly disintegrating tablets within 6 months of opening foil pouch and immediately after opening individual tablet blister.

Route	Onset	Peak	Duration
P.O.	1-3 hr	8-12 hr	>24 hr

Adverse reactions

CNS: headache, nervousness, insomnia
EENT: conjunctivitis, earache, epistaxis, pharyngitis
GI: abdominal pain; dry mouth; diarrhea, stomatitis (in children)
Skin: rash, photosensitivity, angioedema
Other: tooth disorder (in children), fever, flulike symptoms, viral infections

Interactions

Drug-food. *Any food:* increased drug absorption

Patient monitoring

• Watch for adverse reactions, especially in children.
• Assess patient's response to drug.
• Watch for new symptoms or exacerbation of existing symptoms.

Patient teaching

• Advise patient to take exactly as prescribed, once a day on empty stomach.
• Tell patient to report persistent or worsening symptoms.
• Instruct patient to report adverse reactions, such as headache or nervousness.
• Caution patient to avoid driving and other hazardous activities until he knows how drug affects concentration and alertness.
• As appropriate, review all other significant adverse reactions and interactions, especially those related to the foods mentioned above.

---

lorazepam

Apo-Lorazepam✤, Ativan, Dom-Lorazepam✤, Novo-Lorazem✤, Nu-Loraz✤, PHL-Lorazepam✤, PMS-Lorazepam✤, Pro-Lorazepam✤

Pharmacologic class: Benzodiazepine
Therapeutic class: Anxiolytic
Controlled substance schedule IV
Pregnancy risk category D

Action

Unknown. Thought to depress CNS at limbic system and disrupt neurotransmission in reticular activating system.

Availability

Injection: 2 mg/ml, 4 mg/ml
Solution (concentrated): 2 mg/ml
Tablets: 0.5 mg, 1 mg, 2 mg

Indications and dosages

➤ Anxiety

Adults: 2 to 3 mg P.O. daily in two or three divided doses. Maximum dosage is 10 mg daily.

➤ Insomnia

Adults: 2 to 4 mg P.O. at bedtime

➤ Premedication before surgery (as antianxiety agent, sedative-hypnotic, or amnestic)

Adults: 0.05 mg/kg (not to exceed 4 mg) deep I.M. injection at least 2 hours before surgery, or 0.044 mg/kg (not to exceed 2 mg) I.V. 15 to 20 minutes before surgery. For greater amnestic effect, give up to 0.05 mg/kg (not to exceed 4 mg) I.V. 15 to 20 minutes before surgery.

➤ Status epilepticus

Adults: 4 mg I.V. given slowly (no faster than 2 mg/minute). If seizures continue or recur after 10 to 15 minutes, repeat dose. If seizure control isn't established after second dose, other measures should be used. Don't exceed 8 mg in 12 hours.

Dosage adjustment

• Elderly or debilitated patients

Off-label uses

• Acute alcohol withdrawal syndrome

Contraindications

• Hypersensitivity to drug, other benzodiazepines, polyethylene or propylene glycol, or benzyl alcohol
• Acute angle-closure glaucoma
• Coma or CNS depression
• Hepatic or renal failure

Precautions

Use cautiously in:
• hepatic or renal impairment
• history of suicide attempt, drug abuse, depressive disorder, or psychosis
• elderly patients
• pregnant or breastfeeding patients.

Administration

• For I.V. use, dilute with equal volume of compatible diluent, such as normal saline solution or dextrose 5% in water. Keep resuscitation equipment and oxygen at hand.

◀€ Give each 2 mg of I.V. dose slowly, over 2 to 5 minutes. Don't exceed rate of 2 mg/minute.

• Don't give parenteral form to children younger than age 18.

Route	Onset	Peak	Duration
P.O.	15-45 min	1-6 hr	Up to 48 hr
I.V.	Rapid	15-20 min	Up to 48 hr
I.M.	15-30 min	1-2 hr	Up to 48 hr

Adverse reactions

CNS: amnesia, agitation, ataxia, depression, disorientation, dizziness, drowsiness, headache, incoordination, asthenia

CV (with too rapid I.V. administration): hypotension, bradycardia, tachycardia, apnea, **cardiac arrest, cardiovascular collapse**

EENT: blurred vision, diplopia, nystagmus

GI: nausea, abdominal discomfort

Other: increased or decreased appetite

Interactions

Drug-drug. *CNS depressants (including antidepressants, antihistamines, benzodiazepines, sedative-hypnotics):* additive CNS depression

Hormonal contraceptives: increased lorazepam clearance

Drug-herbs. *Chamomile, hops, kava, skullcap, valerian:* increased CNS depression

Drug-behaviors. *Alcohol use:* increased CNS depression

Smoking: increased metabolism and decreased efficacy of lorazepam

Patient monitoring

◀€ During I.V. administration, monitor ECG and cardiovascular and respiratory status.

Reactions in **bold** are life-threatening.   ◀€ Clinical alert

- Monitor vital signs closely.
- Evaluate for amnesia.
- Watch closely for CNS depression. Institute safety precautions as needed to prevent injury.
- 🔊 Monitor for signs and symptoms of overdose (such as confusion, hypotension, coma, and labored breathing).
- Assess liver function tests and CBC.

Patient teaching
- Tell patient and family about drug's possible CNS effects. Recommend appropriate safety precautions.
- Explain that with long-term use, drug must be discontinued slowly (typically over 8 to 12 weeks).
- Instruct patient to avoid alcohol, because it increases drowsiness and other CNS effects.
- Caution patient to avoid smoking, because it speeds drug breakdown in body.
- Advise female patient to inform prescriber if she is pregnant or breast-feeding.
- As appropriate, review all other significant and life-threatening adverse reactions and interactions, especially those related to the drugs, herbs, and behaviors mentioned above.

losartan potassium
Cozaar

Pharmacologic class: Angiotensin II receptor antagonist

Therapeutic class: Antihypertensive

Pregnancy risk category C (first trimester), *D* (second and third trimesters)

| FDA | BOXED WARNING |

- When used during second or third trimester of pregnancy, drug may cause fetal harm or death. Discontinue as soon as pregnancy is detected.

Action
Blocks vasoconstricting and aldosterone-secreting effects of angiotensin II at various receptor sites, including vascular smooth muscle and adrenal glands. Also increases urinary flow and enhances excretion of chloride, magnesium, calcium, and phosphate.

Availability
Tablets: 25 mg, 50 mg, 100 mg

🜚 Indications and dosages
➤ Hypertension
Adults: Initially, 50 mg/day P.O.; range is 25 to 100 mg/day as a single dose or in two divided doses. May be used alone or with other drugs.
Children ages 6 and older: 0.7 mg/kg P.O. daily, up to total of 50 mg
➤ To prevent cerebrovascular accident (stroke) in hypertensive patients with left ventricular hypertrophy (LVH)
Adults: Initially, 50 mg P.O. daily, increased to 100 mg P.O. daily. May be given concurrently with hydrochlorothiazide.
➤ Nephropathy in patients with type 2 diabetes
Adults: 50 mg/day P.O.; increase to 100 mg/day based on blood pressure response.

Dosage adjustment
- Hepatic impairment
- Concurrent diuretic therapy

Contraindications
- Hypersensitivity to drug or its components
- Pregnancy (second and third trimesters)

Precautions

Use cautiously in:
- heart failure, renal or hepatic impairment, obstructive biliary disorders
- high-dose diuretic therapy
- black patients
- pregnant patients (first trimester) or breastfeeding patients
- children younger than age 6 (safety not established).

Administration

- Administer with or without food.
- Know that if drug efficacy (measured at trough) is inadequate with once-daily dosing, prescriber may switch to twice-daily regimen using same or higher daily dosage.
- Be aware that drug may take 3 to 6 weeks to reach maximal efficacy.

Route	Onset	Peak	Duration
P.O.	Unknown	1 hr	Unknown

Adverse reactions

CNS: dizziness, insomnia, headache, asthenia, fatigue
CV: hypotension
EENT: sinus disorders
GI: nausea, vomiting, diarrhea, dyspepsia, abdominal pain
Metabolic: hyperkalemia
Musculoskeletal: joint pain, back pain, muscle cramps
Respiratory: symptoms of upper respiratory infection, dry cough
Other: hypersensitivity reactions including **angioedema**

Interactions

Drug-drug. *Diuretics, other antihypertensives:* increased risk of hypotension
Fluconazole: inhibited losartan metabolism, increased antihypertensive effects
Indomethacin: decreased losartan effects
Lithium: decreased lithium metabolism
Nonsteroidal anti-inflammatory drugs: decreased renal function
Potassium-sparing diuretics, potassium supplements: hyperkalemia

Rifamycins: enhanced losartan metabolism, decreased antihypertensive effects
Drug-diagnostic tests. *Albumin:* increased level
Drug-food. *Salt substitutes containing potassium:* hyperkalemia

Patient monitoring

🔊 Watch for angioedema and other hypersensitivity reactions.
- Monitor blood pressure to evaluate drug efficacy.
- Assess liver and kidney function tests and electrolyte levels.
- Stay alert for oliguria, progressive azotemia, and renal failure in patients with severe heart failure whose renal function depends on the renin-angiotensin-aldosterone system.
- Know that in black patients, losartan and other ACE inhibitors may be ineffective when used alone. Drug isn't indicated for stroke prevention in black hypertensive patients with LVH.
- Be aware that drug may cause fetal injury or death when used during second or third trimester of pregnancy.

Patient teaching

- Instruct patient to avoid potassium supplements and salt substitutes containing potassium, unless directed by prescriber.
🔊 Caution female patient not to take drug during second or third trimester of pregnancy. Advise her to contact prescriber immediately if she suspects pregnancy.
- Tell female patient to discuss breastfeeding with prescriber before taking.
🔊 Instruct patient to immediately report hypersensitivity reactions, especially lip or eyelid swelling, throat tightness, and difficulty breathing.
- As appropriate, review all other significant and life-threatening adverse reactions and interactions, especially those related to the drugs, tests, and foods mentioned above.

Reactions in **bold** are life-threatening.　　🔊 Clinical alert

lovastatin

Altoprev, Apo-Lovastatin✤, Co
Lovastatin✤, Dom-Lovastatin✤,
Gen-Lovastatin✤, Mevacor, Novo-
Lovastatin✤, Nu-Lovastatin✤, PHL-
Lovastatin✤, PMS-Lovastatin✤,
Ran-Lovastatin✤, Ratio-Lovastatin✤,
Sandoz Lovastatin✤

Pharmacologic class: HMG-CoA
reductase inhibitor
Therapeutic class: Antihyperlipidemic
Pregnancy risk category X

Action
Inhibits HMG-CoA reductase, an
enzyme crucial to cholesterol synthesis.
Decreases total cholesterol and low-
density lipoprotein (LDL) levels and
increases high-density lipoprotein
level.

Availability
Tablets: 10 mg, 20 mg, 40 mg
Tablets (extended-release): 10 mg,
20 mg, 40 mg, 60 mg

ⓘ Indications and dosages
➤ To reduce LDL, total cholesterol,
triglyceride, and apolipoprotein B
levels
Adults: Initially, 20 mg P.O. daily. May
be increased, as needed, at 4-week intervals to a maximum of 80 mg/day as a
single dose or in divided doses. Or 20 mg
P.O. (extended-release) daily. May be
increased, as needed, at 4-week intervals
to a maximum daily dosage of 60 mg.
➤ Heterozygous familial hypercholesterolemia in boys and postmenarchal
girls ages 10 and older who have high
LDL and cholesterol levels despite adequate trial of diet therapy
Adolescents ages 10 to 17: 10 to 40 mg
P.O. daily, with adjustments made at
4-week intervals

Dosage adjustment
• Severe renal insufficiency

Off-label uses
• High-risk patients with diabetic dyslipidemia, familial dysbetalipoproteinemia, familial combined hyperlipidemia, or nephrotic hyperlipidemia

Contraindications
• Hypersensitivity to drug, its components, or angiotensin-converting
enzyme inhibitors
• Active hepatic disease or unexplained persistent hepatic enzyme
elevation
• Concurrent gemfibrozil or azole
antifungal therapy
• Pregnancy or breastfeeding

Precautions
Use cautiously in:
• cerebral arteriosclerosis, heart disease, renal impairment, severe acute
infection, severe hypotension or
hypertension, uncontrolled seizures,
myopathy, visual disturbances, major
surgery, trauma, alcoholism
• severe metabolic, endocrine, or electrolyte problems
• women of childbearing age
• children.

Administration
• Give daily dose with evening meal.
• Increase dosage at intervals of
4 weeks or longer, as ordered.
• Don't give with grapefruit juice (may
increase drug blood level).
◀⅋ Discontinue if alanine aminotransferase (ALT) or aspartate aminotransferase (AST) level exceeds three times
the upper limit of normal.

Route	Onset	Peak	Duration
P.O.	Unknown	2 hr	Unknown
P.O. (extended)	Unknown	Unknown	Unknown

Adverse reactions

CNS: headache, dizziness, asthenia
EENT: blurred vision, eye irritation
GI: nausea, vomiting, constipation, diarrhea, abdominal pain or cramps, dyspepsia, flatulence
Hepatic: hepatotoxicity
Musculoskeletal: myalgia, cramps, **rhabdomyolysis**
Skin: pruritus, rash, photosensitivity
Other: hypersensitivity reaction

Interactions

Drug-drug. *Azole antifungals, cyclosporine, erythromycin, folic acid derivatives, gemfibrozil, niacin:* increased risk of myopathy and rhabdomyolysis
Bile acid sequestrants: decreased lovastatin blood level
Isradipine: increased lovastatin clearance
Warfarin: increased prothrombin time, bleeding
Drug-diagnostic tests. *ALT, AST:* increased levels
Drug-food. *Grapefruit juice:* increased lovastatin blood level
Drug-herbs. *Red yeast rice:* increased risk of adverse reactions
Chaparral, comfrey, germander, jin bu huan, kava, pennyroyal, St. John's wort: increased risk of hepatotoxicity

Patient monitoring

• Obtain liver function tests before starting therapy, 6 and 12 weeks after therapy begins or dosage is increased, and periodically thereafter.

Patient teaching

• Tell patient to take immediate-release tablets with evening meal or extended-release tablets at bedtime.
• Instruct patient not to break, crush, or chew extended-release tablets.
• Emphasize importance of cholesterol-lowering diet and other therapies, such as exercise and weight control.
◀≷ Instruct patient to report unexplained muscle pain, tenderness, or weakness, as well as signs or symptoms of hepatotoxicity (fever, malaise, abdominal pain, yellowing of skin or eyes, clay-colored stools, or tea-colored urine).
◀≷ Advise patient to contact prescriber immediately if she is breastfeeding or suspects pregnancy.
• Tell patient not to use herbs without consulting prescriber.
• Inform patient that drug may cause photosensitivity. Caution him to avoid excessive sun or heat lamp light.
• As appropriate, review all other significant and life-threatening adverse reactions and interactions, especially those related to the drugs, tests, foods, and herbs mentioned above.

loxapine succinate

Apo-Loxapine✤, Dom-Loxapine✤, Loxapac✤, Nu-Loxapine✤, PHL-Loxapine✤, PMS-Loxapine✤

Pharmacologic class: Tricyclic dibenzoxazepine derivative
Therapeutic class: Antipsychotic
Pregnancy risk category C

Action

Unknown. Thought to block neurotransmission of postsynaptic dopamine receptors in brain, alleviating psychotic symptoms.

Availability

Capsules: 5 mg, 10 mg, 25 mg, 50 mg

🖊 Indications and dosages

➤ Schizophrenia
Adults: 10 mg P.O. b.i.d. Dosage may be increased over first 7 to 10 days, up to 100 mg/day P.O. in two to four divided doses. Maximum dosage is 250 mg/day.

Dosage adjustment
- Elderly patients

Contraindications
- Hypersensitivity to drug or other dibenzoxazepines
- Coma or severe drug-induced CNS depression

Precautions
Use cautiously in:
- seizures, cerebral arteriosclerosis, severe hypotension, hypertension, glaucoma, breast cancer, hepatic disease, bone marrow depression, Parkinson's disease, blood dyscrasias, urinary retention, concurrent use of other CNS active drugs or anticholinergics
- pregnant or breastfeeding patients
- children younger than age 16.

Administration
- Give with or without food.

Route	Onset	Peak	Duration
P.O.	30 min	1.5-3 hr	12 hr

Adverse reactions
CNS: drowsiness, insomnia, vertigo, headache, dizziness, weakness, akinesia, staggering or shuffling gait, slurred speech, agitation, extrapyramidal reactions, sedation, syncope, tardive dyskinesia, numbness, confusion, pseudoparkinsonism, EEG changes, **seizures, neuroleptic malignant syndrome**
CV: orthostatic hypotension, hypertension, ECG changes
EENT: blurred vision, ptosis, nasal congestion
GI: nausea, vomiting, constipation, dry mouth, **paralytic ileus**
GU: urinary retention
Hematologic: leukopenia, agranulocytosis, thrombocytopenia
Hepatic: hepatocellular injury with hepatic enzyme elevations
Metabolic: polydipsia
Musculoskeletal: muscle twitching

Skin: rash, pruritus, seborrhea, photosensitivity, alopecia
Other: weight gain or loss, hyperpyrexia, facial edema, hypersensitivity reactions

Interactions
Drug-drug. *Anticholinergics, CNS depressants:* additive effects
Epinephrine: severe hypotension, tachycardia, decreased epinephrine effects
Drug-diagnostic tests. *Granulocytes, platelets, white blood cells:* decreased counts
Liver function tests: increased values
Drug-behaviors. *Alcohol use:* increased CNS depression

Patient monitoring
- Measure blood pressure before and periodically during therapy.
- Monitor hematologic studies and liver function tests.
- 🔊 Stay alert for evidence of neuroleptic malignant syndrome (extrapyramidal symptoms, hyperpyrexia, muscle rigidity, altered mental status, irregular pulse or blood pressure, tachycardia, arrhythmias, diaphoresis).
- Assess for tardive dyskinesia (involuntary jerky movements of face, tongue, jaws, trunk, arms, and legs), especially in elderly women.

Patient teaching
- Tell patient to take with or without food.
- Inform patient that drug may cause tardive dyskinesia. Describe symptoms.
- Caution patient to avoid activities requiring mental concentration until drug's effects are known.
- 🔊 Teach patient to immediately report sore throat, fever, rash, impaired vision, tremors, involuntary muscle twitching, muscle stiffness, or yellowing of eyes or skin.

🍁 Canada   ⊕ UK   ⚗ Hazardous drug   ⊗ High-alert drug

• Instruct patient to move slowly when sitting up or standing, to avoid dizziness from sudden blood pressure decrease.
• Caution patient to avoid alcohol use.
• As appropriate, review all other significant and life-threatening adverse reactions and interactions, especially those related to the drugs, tests, and behaviors mentioned above.

lubiprostone
Amitiza

Pharmacologic class: Chloride channel activator
Therapeutic class: GI motility enhancer
Pregnancy risk category C

Action
Enhances chloride-rich intestinal fluid secretion without altering sodium and potassium serum concentrations; increases intestinal fluid secretion and intestinal motility, which promotes stool passage and relieves symptoms of chronic idiopathic constipation

Availability
Soft gelatin capsules: 8 mcg, 24 mcg

Indications and dosages
➤ Chronic idiopathic constipation
Adults: 24 mcg P.O. twice daily
➤ Treatment of irritable bowel syndrome with constipation in women
Adults ages 18 and older: 8 mcg P.O. b.i.d.

Dosage adjustment
• Moderate to severe hepatic impairment

Contraindications
• Hypersensitivity to drug or its components
• History of mechanical GI obstruction

Precautions
Use cautiously in:
• severe diarrhea, hepatic or renal dysfunction
• pregnant or breastfeeding patients.

Administration
• Administer with food and water.

Route	Onset	Peak	Duration
P.O.	Unknown	1.14 hr	Unknown

Adverse reactions
CNS: headache, dizziness, hypoesthesia, fatigue, depression, anxiety, insomnia
CV: chest discomfort or pain, hypertension
EENT: sinusitis, nasopharyngitis, pharyngolaryngeal pain
GI: nausea, vomiting, diarrhea, constipation, abdominal distention, abdominal pain or discomfort, flatulence, dyspepsia, gastroesophageal reflux disease, gastroenteritis, dry mouth
GU: urinary tract infection
Musculoskeletal: arthralgia, back pain, extremity pain, muscle cramp
Respiratory: upper respiratory tract infection, influenza, bronchitis, dyspnea, cough
Other: weight gain, peripheral edema, fever, viral infection

Interactions
None

Patient monitoring
• Evaluate patient for signs and symptoms of mechanical obstruction before therapy begins.
• Assess patient periodically for continuing need for therapy.

Patient teaching
• Instruct patient not to break or chew capsule.
• Instruct patient not to take drug during episodes of severe diarrhea.

Reactions in **bold** are life-threatening. Clinical alert

• Advise patient to report side effects, such as severe nausea, diarrhea, and dyspnea, to prescriber.
• Caution female patient with child-bearing potential that drug may pose hazard to fetus.
• Advise breastfeeding patient that she should decide whether to discontinue breastfeeding or stop taking drug.
• As appropriate, review all other significant adverse reactions.

lymphocyte immune globulin (antithymocyte globulin equine, ATG, ATG equine, LIG)
Atgam

Pharmacologic class: Immunoglobulin
Therapeutic class: Immunosuppressant
Pregnancy risk category C

FDA | BOXED WARNING

• Give drug under supervision of physician experienced in immunosuppressive therapy for treatment of renal transplant or asplastic anemia patients, in facility with adequate laboratory and supportive resources

Action
Unknown. Thought to inhibit cell-mediated immune response by altering function of or eliminating T lymphocytes in circulation.

Availability
Injection: 50 mg/ml in 5-ml ampules

🚫 Indications and dosages
➤ To prevent acute renal allograft rejection

Adults and children: 15 mg/kg/day I.V. for 14 days, then switch to alternate-day dosing for 14 days (for a total of 21 doses in 28 days). Give first dose within 24 hours of transplantation.
➤ Acute renal allograft rejection
Adults and children: 10 to 15 mg/kg/day I.V. for 14 days, then may switch to alternate-day dosing for 14 days (for a total of 21 doses in 28 days). Start therapy at first sign of rejection.
➤ Aplastic anemia in patients ineligible for bone marrow transplantation
Adults and children: 10 to 20 mg/kg/day I.V. for 8 to 14 days; then may give additional alternate-day doses for a total of up to 21 doses in 28 days

Off-label uses
• Bone marrow, liver, and heart transplantation
• Multiple sclerosis
• Myasthenia gravis
• Scleroderma

Contraindications
• History of severe systemic reaction to lymphocyte immune globulin or other equine preparation

Precautions
Use cautiously in:
• severe renal or hepatic disease
• pregnant or breastfeeding patients
• children.

Administration
🔊 Know that drug should be given only by health care professionals experienced in immunosuppressive therapy for treating aplastic anemia or renal transplant patients, in facilities equipped and staffed with adequate laboratory and supportive resources.
🔊 Because of high risk of anaphylaxis, perform intradermal skin test before first dose. Inject 0.1-ml dose of 1:1,000 dilution of LIG intradermally; a control test using 0.9% sodium chloride injection is injected

contralaterally. Observe site every 15 to 20 minutes during first hour after injection, and monitor patient for systemic manifestations. Local reaction of 10 mm or greater with wheal, erythema, or both (with or without pseudopod formation and itching or marked local swelling) indicates positive test (which warrants consideration of alternate therapy). Systemic reaction (such as tachycardia, dyspnea, hypotension, or anaphylaxis) precludes LIG therapy.

• Premedicate with antipyretic, antihistamine, or corticosteroid, as prescribed, to minimize reactions.

• For I.V. infusion, dilute prescribed dose in 250 to 1,000 ml of 0.45% or 0.9% sodium chloride injection. (Don't dilute in dextrose solutions or highly acidic solutions.) Final concentration shouldn't exceed 4 mg/ml. Infuse total daily dose over at least 4 hours.

• When adding drug to infusion container, invert container so air doesn't enter. Gently swirl or rotate container to mix solution.

• Using in-line filter with pore size of 0.2 to 1 micron, infuse into central vein, shunt, or arteriovenous fistula over at least 4 hours.

• Be aware that drug is usually given concurrently with azathioprine and corticosteroids when used for allograft rejection.

Route	Onset	Peak	Duration
I.V.	Unknown	Unknown	Unknown

Adverse reactions

CNS: malaise, agitation, headache, dizziness, weakness, syncope, **encephalitis, seizures**

CV: hypotension, hypertension, chest pain, bradycardia, tachycardia, cardiac irregularities, phlebitis, **myocarditis, thrombophlebitis, heart failure**

EENT: periorbital edema

GI: nausea, vomiting, diarrhea, stomatitis

Hematologic: leukopenia, agranulocytosis, thrombocytopenia, aplastic anemia

Hepatic: hepatosplenomegaly

Metabolic: hyperglycemia

Musculoskeletal: joint pain or stiffness, myalgia, back pain

Respiratory: dyspnea, **pleural effusion**

Skin: rash, pruritus, urticaria, diaphoresis, night sweats

Other: burning soles and palms, fever, chills, pain at infusion site, edema, lymphadenopathy, hypersensitivity reactions including **serum sickness** and **anaphylaxis**

Interactions

Drug-diagnostic tests. *Creatinine, glucose, hepatic enzymes:* increased values
Hemoglobin, platelets, white blood cells: decreased values
Kidney and liver function tests: abnormal results

Patient monitoring

◀≋ During infusion, watch for signs and symptoms of hypersensitivity reaction, such as rash, respiratory distress, or chest, flank, or back pain. Be aware that this reaction may occur even with a negative skin test.

◀≋ Discontinue drug if renal transplant patient develops signs or symptoms of anaphylaxis or severe thrombocytopenia or leukopenia.

• Be aware that product derives from equine and human blood components and may transmit infections.

• Monitor for signs and symptoms of infection, such as fever, malaise, and sore throat (caused by immunosuppression).

Patient teaching

◀≋ Tell patient to immediately report adverse reactions during infusion (such as pain at infusion site) as well as

---

Reactions in **bold** are life-threatening.   ◀≋ Clinical alert

systemic complaints (such as easy bruising or bleeding or signs of hypersensitivity reaction).

• Instruct patient to avoid sources of infection, such as people with known infections. Tell him to promptly report signs or symptoms of infection.

◀≣ Advise patient to immediately report evidence of serum sickness, including fever, joint pain, nausea, vomiting, lymphadenopathy, and rash.

◀≣ Caution female patient not to take drug if she is pregnant.

• Tell female patient to inform prescriber if she is breastfeeding.

• As appropriate, review all other significant and life-threatening adverse reactions and interactions, especially those related to the tests mentioned above.

magnesium chloride

magnesium citrate
Citramag ⊕ , Citro-Mag ✤ , Citroma

magnesium gluconate
Mag G, Magonate

magnesium hydroxide
Dulcolax Milk of Magnesia, Phillips Milk of Magnesia, Phillips Milk of Magnesia Concentrate

magnesium oxide
Mag-ox, Uro-Mag

magnesium sulfate
Epsom Salts

Pharmacologic class: Mineral

Therapeutic class: Electrolyte replacement, laxative, antacid, anticonvulsant

Pregnancy risk category A (magnesium sulfate), *NR* (magnesium citrate, hydroxide, oxide), *unknown* (magnesium chloride, gluconate)

Action
Increases osmotic gradient in small intestine, which draws water into intestines and causes distention. These effects stimulate peristalsis and bowel evacuation. In antacid action, reacts with hydrochloric acid in stomach to form water and increase gastric pH. In anticonvulsant action, depresses CNS and blocks transmission of peripheral neuromuscular impulses.

Availability
magnesium chloride
Injection: 20%
magnesium citrate
Oral solution: 240-ml, 296-ml, and 300-ml bottles
magnesium gluconate
Liquid: 1,000 mg/5 ml
Tablets: 500 mg
magnesium hydroxide
Liquid: 400 mg/5 ml
Liquid concentrate: 800 mg/5 ml
Tablets (chewable): 300 mg
magnesium oxide
Capsules: 140 mg
Tablets: 250 mg, 400 mg, 420 mg, 500 mg
magnesium sulfate
Granules (for oral use): 120 g, 4 lb
Injection: 10%, 12.5%, 25%, 50%

🕖 Indications and dosages
➤ Mild magnesium deficiency
Adults: 1 g (2 ml of 50% sulfate solution) I.M. q 6 hours for four doses

➤ Severe hypomagnesemia

Adults: 250 mg (2 mEq)/kg (sulfate) I.M. within 4-hour period, or 5 g (approximately 40 mEq) in 1 liter 5% dextrose injection or 0.9% sodium chloride solution by I.V. infusion over 3 hours

➤ Hypomagnesemia treatment

Adults and children: Dosage individualized based on severity of deficiency; may give citrate, gluconate, hydroxide, oxide, or sulfate.

➤ Hypomagnesemia prophylaxis

Adults and children: Dosage based on normal recommended daily magnesium intake; may give citrate, gluconate, hydroxide, oxide, or sulfate.

➤ Supplemental magnesium in total parenteral nutrition (TPN)

Adults: 8 to 24 mEq/day (sulfate) by I.V. infusion, added to TPN solution

➤ Constipation

Adults and children ages 12 and older: 15 g (sulfate granules) in 240 ml water; or 30 to 60 ml/day P.O. (hydroxide) given with water; or a single dose of 10 to 30 ml P.O. (hydroxide concentrate); or one bottle of oral solution (citrate), as directed

Children ages 6 to 11: 5 to 10 g (sulfate granules) in 120 ml water; or a single dose of 2.5 to 5 ml P.O. (sulfate) in a half-glass of water; or 15 to 30 ml P.O. daily (hydroxide) given with water; or a single dose of 7.5 to 15 ml P.O. (hydroxide concentrate); or three to four tablets (hydroxide); or 50 to 100 ml, as directed, of oral solution (citrate)

Children ages 2 to 5: Single dose of 5 to 15 ml P.O. (hydroxide); or 2.5 to 7.5 ml P.O. daily (hydroxide concentrate); or one to two tablets (hydroxide); or 4 to 12 ml oral solution (citrate), as directed

➤ Indigestion

Adults and children ages 12 and older: 5 to 15 ml P.O. (hydroxide liquid) up to q.i.d. with water; or 2.5 to 7.5 ml P.O. (hydroxide liquid concentrate) up to q.i.d. with water; or 622 to 1,244 mg P.O. (hydroxide tablets) up to q.i.d.; or 400 to 800 mg P.O. (oxide tablets) daily

➤ To prevent and control seizures in preeclampsia or eclampsia

Adults: 4 to 5 g 50% sulfate solution I.M. q 4 hours, as necessary; or 4 g 10% to 20% sulfate solution I.V., not to exceed 1.5 ml/minute of 10% solution; or 4 to 5 g I.V. infusion in 250 ml of 5% dextrose or sodium chloride solution, not to exceed 3 ml/minute

➤ Acute nephritis to control hypertension, encephalopathy, and seizures in children

Children: 100 mg/kg 50% sulfate solution I.M. q 4 to 6 hours as needed; or 20 to 40 mg/kg 20% solution I.M., repeated as necessary

Off-label uses

• Bronchodilation in some asthmatic patients
• Post–myocardial infarction hypomagnesemia

Contraindications

• Hypermagnesemia
• Heart block
• Myocardial damage
• Active labor or within 2 hours of delivery

Precautions

Use cautiously in:
• renal insufficiency, abdominal pain, nausea and vomiting, rectal bleeding, anuria, hypocalcemia
• pregnant patients.

Administration

◀❬ Be aware that magnesium sulfate injection is a high-alert drug.
• Know that I.V. use is reserved for life-threatening seizures.
• When giving magnesium sulfate I.V., don't exceed concentration of 20% or infusion rate of 150 mg/minute, except in seizures caused by severe eclampsia. Too-rapid I.V. infusion may cause hypotension and asystole.

m

• When giving magnesium sulfate I.M. to adults, use concentration of 25% to 50%; when giving to infants and children, don't exceed 20%.

Route	Onset	Peak	Duration
P.O.	3-6 hr	4 hr	Unknown
I.V.	Immediate	Unknown	30 min
I.M.	60 min	Unknown	3-4 hr

Adverse reactions

CNS (with I.V. use): confusion, decreased reflexes, dizziness, syncope, sedation, hypothermia, **paralysis**
CV (with I.V. use): hypotension, **arrhythmias, circulatory collapse**
GI: nausea, vomiting, cramps, flatulence, anorexia
Metabolic: hypermagnesemia, hypocalcemia
Musculoskeletal (with I.V. use): muscle weakness, flaccidity
Respiratory: respiratory paralysis
Skin: diaphoresis
Other: allergic reaction, injection site reaction, laxative dependence (with repeated or prolonged use)

Interactions

Drug-drug. *Aminoquinolones, nitrofurantoin, penicillamine, tetracyclines:* decreased absorption of these drugs (with oral magnesium)
CNS depressants: additive effects
Digoxin: heart block, conduction changes (with I.V. use)
Enteric-coated drugs: faster dissolution of these drugs
Neuromuscular blockers: increased effects of these drugs (with I.V. use)
Drug-diagnostic tests. *Calcium, magnesium:* increased levels (with I.V. use)

Patient monitoring

◀€ When giving prolonged or repeated I.V. infusions, assess patellar reflex and monitor for respiratory rate of 16 breaths/minute or more.
◀€ With I.V. use, monitor blood magnesium level (desired level is 3 to 6 mg/dl or 2.5 to 5 mEq/L). Check for signs

and symptoms of magnesium toxicity (hypotension, nausea, vomiting, ECG changes, muscle weakness, mental or respiratory depression, coma). Keep injectable calcium on hand to counteract magnesium toxicity.
• Monitor urine output, which should measure 100 ml or more every 4 hours.
◀€ If I.V. magnesium was given before delivery, assess neonate for signs and symptoms of magnesium toxicity, such as neuromuscular or respiratory depression.
• Monitor electrolyte levels and liver function tests.

Patient teaching

◀€ Teach patient about adverse reactions. Instruct him to report symptoms that occur during I.V. administration.
• Advise patient to consult prescriber before using magnesium if he's taking other drugs. Magnesium may delay or enhance absorption of other drugs.
• Inform patient that repeated or prolonged use of magnesium citrate, hydroxide, or sulfate may cause laxative dependence. Inform him that healthy diet and exercise can reduce need for laxatives.
• Tell pregnant female to make sure prescriber knows she is pregnant before taking drug.
• As appropriate, review all other significant and life-threatening adverse reactions and interactions, especially those related to the drugs and tests mentioned above.

mannitol
Osmitrol, Polyfusor ⊕, Resectisol

Pharmacologic class: Osmotic diuretic
Therapeutic class: Diuretic
Pregnancy risk category C

Action
Increases osmotic pressure of plasma in glomerular filtrate, inhibiting tubular reabsorption of water and electrolytes (including sodium and potassium). These actions enhance water flow from various tissues and ultimately decrease intracranial and intraocular pressures; serum sodium level rises while potassium and blood urea levels fall. Also protects kidneys by preventing toxins from forming and blocking tubules.

Availability
Injection: 5%, 10%, 15%, 20%, 25%
Solution: 5 g/100 ml

🕖 Indications and dosages
➤ Test dose for marked oliguria or suspected inadequate renal function
Adults: 0.2 g/kg I.V. infusion (approximately 50 ml of 25% solution, 75 ml of 20% solution, or 100 ml of 15% solution) over 3 to 5 minutes. If urine flow doesn't increase, second dose may be given; if response is inadequate after second dose, reevaluate patient.
➤ To prevent oliguria during cardiovascular and other surgeries
Adults: 50 to 100 g I.V. infusion as 5% to 15% solution
➤ Acute oliguria
Adults: Up to 100 g I.V. infusion as 15% to 25% solution
Children: 0.25 to 2 g/kg I.V. or 60 mg/m^2 as 15% to 20% solution over 2 to 6 hours
➤ To reduce intracranial pressure and brain mass
Adults: 0.5 to 2 g/kg I.V. infusion as 15% to 25% solution given over 30 to 60 minutes
Children: 1 to 2 g/kg I.V. or 30 to 60 g/m^2 over 30 to 60 minutes. Small or debilitated patients may require smaller dose of 500 mg/kg.
➤ To reduce intraocular pressure
Adults: 0.5 to 2 g/kg I.V. infusion as 15% to 25% solution given over 30 to 60 minutes. For preoperative use, give 60 to 90 minutes before surgery.

Children: 1 to 2 g/kg I.V. or 30 to 60 g/m^2 over 30 to 60 minutes. Small or debilitated patients may require smaller dose of 500 mg/kg.
➤ To promote diuresis in drug toxicity
Adults: 5% to 25% solution by I.V. infusion given continuously to maintain high urine output
Children: 2 g/kg I.V. of 5% to 10% solution given continuously to maintain high urine output
➤ Irrigation during transurethral resection of prostate
Adults: 2.5% to 5% solution instilled into bladder via indwelling urethral catheter, as needed

Contraindications
• Active intracranial bleeding (except during craniotomy)
• Anuria secondary to severe renal disease
• Progressive heart failure, pulmonary congestion, renal damage, or renal dysfunction after mannitol therapy begins
• Severe pulmonary congestion or pulmonary edema
• Severe dehydration

Precautions
Use cautiously in:
• severe renal disease, heart failure, mild to moderate dehydration
• pregnant or breastfeeding patients.

Administration
◀€ Withhold drug until adequate renal function and urinary output are established.
• When administering for drug toxicity, give fluids and electrolytes to match fluid loss.
• Be aware that at low temperatures, solution may crystallize (especially concentrations above 15%). If crystals form, warm bottle in hot-water bath or dry-heat oven or autoclave, then cool to body temperature or lower before giving.
• Don't give electrolyte-free mannitol solutions with blood; when giving blood with mannitol, add 20 mEq or

m

Reactions in **bold** are life-threatening.   ◀€ Clinical alert

more of sodium chloride solution to each liter of mannitol solution to avoid pseudoagglutination.

• Know that drug may be given as continuous or intermittent I.V. infusion. Infuse at prescribed rate using infusion device and in-line filter. Give single I.V. dose over 30 to 90 minutes in adults.

◀€ Avoid extravasation, because it may cause local edema and tissue necrosis.

Route	Onset	Peak	Duration
I.V. (diuresis)	1-3 hr	Unknown	Up to 8 hr
I.V. (intraocular press.)	Unknown	Unknown	4-8 hr
I.V. (intracranial press.)	30 min	Unknown	3-8 hr

Adverse reactions

CNS: dizziness, headache, **seizures**
CV: chest pain, hypotension, hypertension, tachycardia, **thrombophlebitis, heart failure, vascular overload**
EENT: blurred vision, rhinitis
GI: nausea, vomiting, diarrhea, dry mouth
GU: polyuria, urinary retention, **osmotic nephrosis**
Metabolic: dehydration, water intoxication, hypernatremia, hyponatremia, hypovolemia, hypokalemia, **hyperkalemia, metabolic acidosis**
Respiratory: pulmonary congestion
Skin: rash, urticaria
Other: chills, fever, thirst, edema, extravasation with edema and tissue necrosis

Interactions

Drug-drug. *Digoxin:* increased risk of digoxin toxicity
Diuretics: increased therapeutic effects of mannitol
Lithium: increased urinary excretion of lithium
Drug-diagnostic tests. *Electrolytes:* increased or decreased levels

Patient monitoring

◀€ Monitor I.V. site carefully to avoid extravasation and tissue necrosis.
• In comatose patient, insert indwelling urinary catheter as ordered to monitor urine output.
• Monitor renal function tests, urinary output, fluid balance, central venous pressure, and electrolyte levels (especially sodium and potassium).
◀€ Watch for excessive fluid loss and signs and symptoms of hypovolemia and dehydration.
◀€ Assess for evidence of circulatory overload, including pulmonary edema, water intoxication, and heart failure.

Patient teaching

• Teach patient about importance of monitoring exact urinary output.
◀€ Advise patient to report pain at infusion site as well as adverse reactions, such as increased shortness of breath or pain in back, legs, or chest.
• Tell patient drug may cause thirst or dry mouth. Emphasize that fluid restrictions are necessary, but that frequent mouth care should ease these symptoms.
• As appropriate, review all other significant and life-threatening adverse reactions and interactions, especially those related to the drugs and tests mentioned above.

meclizine hydrochloride (meclozine ⊕)

Antivert, Bonamine✤, Bonine, Dramamine Less Drowsy Formula, Sea-Legs⊕, Traveleeze⊕

Pharmacologic class: Anticholinergic
Therapeutic class: Antiemetic, anti-vertigo drug
Pregnancy risk category B

✤ Canada   ⊕ UK   ✺ Hazardous drug   ⊗ High-alert drug

Action
Decreases excitability of middle-ear labyrinth and depresses conduction in vestibular-cerebellar pathways

Availability
Tablets: 12.5 mg, 25 mg, 50 mg
Tablets (chewable): 25 mg

Indications and dosages
➤ Motion sickness
Adults: 25 to 50 mg P.O. 1 hour before travel. May repeat q 24 hours for duration of travel.
➤ Vertigo associated with diseases affecting the vestibular system
Adults: 25 to 100 mg P.O. daily in divided doses

Contraindications
• Hypersensitivity to drug

Precautions
Use cautiously in:
• prostatic hypertrophy, stenosing peptic ulcer, bladder neck obstruction, pyloroduodenal obstruction, arrhythmias, angle-closure glaucoma, bronchial asthma
• pregnant or breastfeeding patients
• children (younger than age 12).

Administration
• Know that tablets may be chewed or swallowed whole.

Route	Onset	Peak	Duration
P.O.	1 hr	Unknown	8-24 hr

Adverse reactions
CNS: drowsiness, fatigue, confusion, excitement, euphoria, nervousness, restlessness, insomnia, vertigo, visual and auditory hallucinations, **seizures**
CV: hypotension, palpitations, tachycardia
EENT: blurred vision, diplopia, tinnitus, dry nose, dry throat
GI: nausea, vomiting, diarrhea, constipation, dry mouth, anorexia
GU: difficulty urinating, urinary retention, urinary frequency
Skin: rash, urticaria

Interactions
Drug-drug. *Anticholinergics (including some antihistamines, antidepressants, atropine, haloperidol, phenothiazines):* additive anticholinergic effects
Antihistamines, CNS depressants (such as opioids, sedative-hypnotics): additive CNS depression
Drug-diagnostic tests. *Skin tests using allergen extracts:* false-negative results
Drug-behaviors. *Alcohol use:* additive CNS depression

Patient monitoring
• Discontinue drug, as ordered, at least 4 days before skin testing.
• Know that drug has anticholinergic effects.

Patient teaching
• Tell patient to take as prescribed to minimize adverse effects.
• Caution patient to avoid driving and other hazardous activities until he knows how drug affects concentration and alertness.
• Advise patient to relieve dry mouth with hard candy or frequent sips of fluids.
• As appropriate, review all other significant and life-threatening adverse reactions and interactions, especially those related to the drugs, tests, and behaviors mentioned above.

m

medroxyprogesterone acetate

Apo-Medroxy✤, Climanor⊕, Depo-Provera, Depo-SUBQ-Provera 104, Dom-Medroxyprogesterone✤, Gen-Medroxy✤, Novo-Medrone✤, PMS-Medroxyprogesterone✤, Provera, Ratio-MPA

Pharmacologic class: Hormone
Therapeutic class: Progestin
Pregnancy risk category X

FDA | BOXED WARNING

• Injection form may cause significant bone density loss. Loss increases with duration of use and may not be completely reversible. It is unknown if use during adolescence or early adulthood reduces peak bone mass and increases risk for osteoporotic fracture later in life.
• Injection form should be used as long-term contraceptive (more than 2 years) only if other contraceptive methods are inadequate.

Action

Inhibits pituitary gonadotropin secretion, preventing follicular maturation, ovulation, and pregnancy

Availability

Suspension for depot injection: 150 mg/ml, 400 mg/ml
Suspension for depot subcutaneous injection: 104 mg/0.65 ml in prefilled single-use syringes
Tablets: 2.5 mg, 5 mg, 10 mg

⊘ Indications and dosages

➤ Secondary amenorrhea

Adults: 5 to 10 mg/day P.O. for 5 to 10 days, starting at any time during menstrual cycle
➤ Dysfunctional uterine bleeding; menses induction
Adults: 5 to 10 mg/day P.O. for 5 to 10 days, starting on day 16 or 21 of menstrual cycle
➤ To prevent estrogen-related endometrial changes in postmenopausal women
Adults: 2.5 to 5 mg/day P.O. given with 0.625 mg conjugated estrogens P.O. (monophasic regimen); or 5 mg/day P.O. on days 15 to 28 of cycle, given with 0.625 mg conjugated estrogens P.O. daily throughout cycle (biphasic regimen)
➤ Management of endometriosis-associated pain
Adults: 104 mg (Depot-subcutaneous-Provera) in anterior thigh or abdomen q 12 to 14 weeks
➤ To prevent pregnancy
Adults: 150 mg (Depo-Provera) deep I.M. injection q 13 weeks or 104 mg (Depot-subcutaneous-Provera) in anterior thigh or abdomen q 12 to 14 weeks. Give first injection during first 5 days of normal menstrual period or first 5 postpartal days if patient isn't breastfeeding, or during sixth postpartal week if patient is breastfeeding exclusively.
➤ Renal or endometrial cancer
Adults: 400 to 1,000 mg I.M.; may repeat weekly. If improvement occurs, decrease to 400 mg q month.

Off-label uses

• Advanced breast cancer

Contraindications

• Hypersensitivity to drug or its components
• Cerebrovascular or thromboembolic disease
• Hepatic dysfunction or disease
• Breast or genital cancer
• Undiagnosed vaginal bleeding
• Known or suspected pregnancy

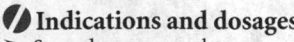

Precautions

Use cautiously in:

- seizure disorder, renal or cardiovascular disease, asthma, diabetes mellitus, depression, migraine
- history of hepatic disease.

Administration

- Before starting therapy, obtain thorough history and physical examination, with emphasis on breast and pelvic organs. Also obtain Pap smear, and repeat annually during therapy.
- With contraceptive use, rule out pregnancy before first dose and when more than 14 weeks have passed since previous dose.
- For I.M. injection, inject deep into gluteal, deltoid, or anterior thigh muscle. Rotate injection sites.
- Be aware that when drug is used to prevent estrogen-related endometrial changes in postmenopausal women, lowest dosage should be used for shortest time, because treatment exceeding 1 year correlates with cancer. (Some combination products have 0.3 mg estrogen/1.5 mg progesterone or 0.45 mg estrogen/1.5 mg progesterone.)

Route	Onset	Peak	Duration
P.O.	Unknown	Unknown	Unknown
I.M.	Wks-1 mo	1 mo	Unknown
Subcut.	Unknown	Unknown	Unknown

Adverse reactions

CNS: insomnia, migraine, nervousness, drowsiness, dizziness, fatigue, depression, mood changes
CV: thrombophlebitis, thromboembolism
EENT: diplopia, proptosis, retinal vascular lesions, **papilledema**
GI: abdominal pain, bloating
GU: amenorrhea, leukorrhea, spotting, cervical secretions, galactorrhea, breast tenderness and secretion, cervical erosions, pelvic pain, infertility
Hepatic: jaundice

Metabolic: fluid retention, hyperglycemia
Musculoskeletal: leg cramps, back pain
Respiratory: pulmonary embolism
Skin: pruritus, urticaria, rash, acne, alopecia, hirsutism, chloasma, melasma, sterile abscesses, induration at I.M. site
Other: weight and appetite changes, edema, angioedema, allergic reactions including **anaphylaxis**

Interactions

Drug-drug. *Bromocriptine:* decreased bromocriptine efficacy
Carbamazepine, phenobarbital, phenytoin, rifampin: decreased contraceptive efficacy
Drug-diagnostic tests. *Alkaline phosphatase, low-density lipoproteins:* increased levels
High-density lipoproteins, pregnanediol excretion: decreased levels
Thyroid hormone assays: altered results
Drug-behaviors. *Alcohol use:* additive CNS depression

Patient monitoring

- Monitor patient for fluid retention and for signs and symptoms of thrombophlebitis, including pain, swelling, and redness of lower legs.
- 🔊 Assess for visual disturbances and headache. If ocular exam shows papilledema or retinal vascular lesions, drug should be discontinued.
- Evaluate liver function tests.
- 🔊 Watch for abdominal pain, fever, malaise, jaundice, darkened urine, and clay-colored stools.

Patient teaching

- Advise patient that drug may cause nausea, vomiting, headache, abdominal pain, painful breast swelling, and abnormal bleeding pattern. Instruct her to report these effects if pronounced.
- 🔊 Tell patient to promptly report bloating, swelling, appetite loss, rash,

---

Reactions in **bold** are life-threatening.　　　　🔊 Clinical alert

yellowed skin, mood changes or depression, nervousness, dizziness, chest pain, shortness of breath, visual disturbances, or severe headache.
• Teach patient how to perform breast self-exams.
• Tell patient she must undergo yearly physical examinations with Pap smear.
• As appropriate, review all other significant and life-threatening adverse reactions and interactions, especially those related to the drugs, tests, and behaviors mentioned above.

mefloquine hydrochloride
Apo-Mefloquine ✤, Lariam

Pharmacologic class: 4-quinoline-methanol derivative, quinine analog
Therapeutic class: Antimalarial
Pregnancy risk category C

Action
Unknown. Thought to increase intravesicular pH in parasite acid vesicles and form complexes with hemin, inhibiting parasite development.

Availability
Tablets: 250 mg

🕖 Indications and dosages
➤ Acute malarial infection
Adults: 1,250 mg P.O. as a single dose
Children: 20 to 25 mg/kg P.O. in two divided doses given 6 to 8 hours apart
➤ Malaria prophylaxis
Adults and children weighing more than 45 kg (99 lb): 250 mg P.O. once weekly on same day each week, starting 1 week before entering endemic area and continuing for 4 weeks after leaving area
Children weighing 30 to 45 kg (66 to 99 lb): 187.5 mg P.O. q week
Children weighing 20 to 30 kg (44 to 66 lb): 125 mg P.O. q week

Children weighing 10 to 20 kg (22 to 44 lb): 62.5 mg P.O. q week
Children weighing 5 to 10 kg (11 to 22 lb): 31.25 mg P.O. q week

Contraindications
• Hypersensitivity to drug, related agents (quinine, quinidine), or excipients
• Prophylactic use in patients with active depression, recent history of depression, generalized anxiety disorder, psychosis, schizophrenia, other psychiatric disorders, or history of seizures

Precautions
Use cautiously in:
• cardiac disorders, seizure disorders
• pregnant or breastfeeding patients
• children.

Administration
• Don't give on empty stomach. Administer with at least 240 ml of water.
• Know that after completing mefloquine therapy for acute malarial infection, patient should receive primaquine (or other 8-aminoquinolone) to prevent relapse.

Route	Onset	Peak	Duration
P.O.	Unknown	7-24 hr	Unknown

Adverse reactions
CNS: dizziness, syncope, headache, psychotic changes, depression, hallucinations, confusion, anxiety, fatigue, vertigo, **seizures**
EENT: blurred vision, tinnitus
GI: nausea, vomiting, diarrhea, loose stools, abdominal discomfort, anorexia
Hematologic: leukopenia, **thrombocytopenia**
Musculoskeletal: myalgia
Skin: rash
Other: fever, chills

✤ Canada   ✦ UK   ⚗ Hazardous drug   ⊗ High-alert drug

Interactions
Drug-drug. *Beta-adrenergic blockers, quinidine, quinine:* ECG abnormalities, cardiac arrest
Chloroquine, quinine: increased risk of seizures
Valproic acid: decreased valproic acid blood level, loss of seizure control
Drug-diagnostic tests. *Hematocrit, platelets, white blood cells:* decreased values
Transaminases: transient increases

Patient monitoring
◀፝ Monitor patient with acute *Plasmodium vivax* malaria who is at high risk for relapse. Because drug doesn't eliminate exoerythrocytic (hepatic-phase) parasites, patient should receive primaquine after mefloquine therapy.
◀፝ Watch for psychiatric symptoms, such as acute anxiety, depression, restlessness, or confusion. These may precede more serious psychiatric events.
• Evaluate hepatic function during prolonged prophylactic therapy.
◀፝ In patients receiving related drugs (such as quinine, quinidine, or chloroquine) concurrently, be alert for ECG abnormalities and seizures. Separate administration times by at least 12 hours.
◀፝ Closely monitor patients with serious or life-threatening *Plasmodium falciparum* infection. Be aware that they should receive I.V. antimalarial drugs and that mefloquine may be used to complete course of therapy.

Patient teaching
• Tell patient to take with full glass of water and not on empty stomach.
• In prophylactic use, instruct patient to take first dose 1 week before departure and to continue therapy as prescribed upon return. Tell him to take drug on same day each week.
• Advise patient to report fever after returning from malarious area.

• Inform patient that malaria prophylaxis should include protective clothing, insect repellent, and bed netting.
◀፝ Tell patient to immediately report psychiatric symptoms (such as acute anxiety, depression, restlessness, or confusion) and to stop taking drug.
• Caution patient to avoid driving and other hazardous activities because drug may cause dizziness.
• Instruct patient to have periodic ophthalmic exams, because drug may cause eye damage.
• Tell female patient to inform prescriber if she is pregnant.
• Advise female patient not to breast-feed while taking drug.
• As appropriate, review all other significant and life-threatening adverse reactions and interactions, especially those related to the drugs and tests mentioned above.

megestrol acetate
Apo-Megestrol✦, Megace, Megace ES, Megace-OS✦, Nu-Megestrol

Pharmacologic class: Hormone
Therapeutic class: Progestin, antineoplastic, appetite stimulant
Pregnancy risk category D (tablets), *X* (suspension)

Action
Unknown. Thought to suppress growth of progestin-sensitive breast and endometrial tumors by inhibiting pituitary and adrenal function.

Availability
Oral suspension: 40 mg/ml
Oral suspension (concentrate): 625 mg/ 5 ml
Tablets: 20 mg, 40 mg

ⓘ Indications and dosages

➤ Breast cancer
Adults: 160 mg/day P.O. given as 40 mg P.O. q.i.d.
➤ Endometrial cancer
Adults: 40 to 320 mg/day P.O. in divided doses
➤ Anorexia, cachexia, or unexplained significant weight loss in AIDS patients
Adults: 800 mg (oral suspension only) P.O. daily, or 625 mg (oral suspension concentrate) P.O. daily

Off-label uses

• Endometriosis, endometrial hyperplasia
• Prostatic hypertrophy
• Contraception

Contraindications

• Hypersensitivity to drug or its components
• Known or suspected pregnancy (suspension only)

Precautions

Use cautiously in:
• diabetes mellitus, severe hepatic disease, renal disease, cardiovascular disease, seizure disorders, cerebral hemorrhage, migraine, asthma, undiagnosed vaginal bleeding, depression
• history of thrombophlebitis
• breastfeeding.

Administration

• Give with meals if GI upset occurs.

Route	Onset	Peak	Duration
P.O.	Unknown	3-5 hr	Unknown

Adverse reactions

CNS: headache, insomnia, drowsiness, asthenia, confusion, neuropathy, hyperesthesia, abnormal thinking, paresthesias, depression, **seizures**
CV: hypertension, chest pain, **thrombophlebitis, deep vein thrombosis**

EENT: amblyopia, retinal thrombosis, pharyngitis
GI: nausea, vomiting, constipation, abdominal pain, flatulence, dyspepsia, dry mouth, increased salivation, oral candidiasis
GU: breast tenderness, breakthrough bleeding, decreased libido
Hematologic: anemia, **leukopenia**
Hepatic: hepatomegaly
Metabolic: hyperglycemia
Musculoskeletal: carpal tunnel syndrome, back pain
Respiratory: dyspnea, cough, pneumonia, **pulmonary embolism**
Skin: alopecia, rash, pruritus, sweating
Other: edema, fever, weight gain, herpes infection

Interactions

Drug-diagnostic tests. *Lactate dehydrogenase:* increased level

Patient monitoring

◀€ Watch for signs and symptoms of thromboembolic disorders.
◀€ Stay alert for visual disturbances, headache, abdominal pain, and hepatomegaly.
• Monitor glucose level in diabetic patients.

Patient teaching

• Inform patient that drug may cause back or abdominal pain, headache, nausea, vomiting, or breast tenderness.
◀€ Tell patient to immediately report pain, swelling or redness of lower legs, chest or back pain, or shortness of breath.
• Advise patient to contact prescriber if adverse effects become pronounced or if other troublesome signs or symptoms occur.
• Urge patient to use reliable contraception.
◀€ Instruct patient to immediately report suspected pregnancy.
• Caution female patient to avoid breastfeeding.

- Advise diabetic patient to monitor blood glucose level.
- As appropriate, review all other significant and life-threatening adverse reactions and interactions, especially those related to the tests mentioned above.

meloxicam

Apo-Meloxicam✤, Co Meloxicam✤, Dom-Meloxicam✤, Gen-Meloxicam✤, Mobic, Mobicox✤, Novo-Meloxicam✤, PHL-Meloxicam✤, Ratio-Meloxicam✤

Pharmacologic class: Nonopioid analgesic, nonsteroidal anti-inflammatory drug (NSAID)

Therapeutic class: Analgesic, anti-inflammatory drug

Pregnancy risk category C

FDA | BOXED WARNING

- Drug may increase risk of serious cardiovascular thrombotic events, myocardial infarction (MI), and stroke. Risk may increase with duration of use. Patients with cardiovascular disease or risk factors for it may be at greater risk.
- Drug increases risk of serious GI adverse events, including bleeding, ulcers, and stomach or intestinal perforation. These events can occur at any time during use and without warning. Elderly patients are at greater risk.
- Drug is contraindicated for treatment of perioperative pain in setting of coronary artery bypass graft surgery.

Action

Unknown. Thought to reduce inflammation and pain by inhibiting prostaglandin synthesis of the enzyme cyclooxygenase.

Availability

Oral suspension: 7.5 mg/5 ml
Tablets: 7.5 mg, 15 mg

⚕ Indications and dosages

➤ Osteoarthritis; rheumatoid arthritis
Adults: 7.5 mg P.O. once daily; may increase to 15 mg/day
➤ Juvenile arthritis
Children ages 2 and older: 0.125 mg/kg P.O. once daily, up to a maximum of 7.5 mg

Contraindications

- Hypersensitivity to drug, its components, or other NSAIDs

Precautions

Use cautiously in:
- bleeding disorders, GI or cardiac disorders, severe renal impairment, severe hepatic disease, asthma, peptic ulcer disease
- concurrent aspirin, oral anticoagulant, or corticosteroid therapy
- elderly or debilitated patients
- pregnant or breastfeeding patients.

Administration

- Before starting therapy, ask patient about aspirin sensitivity and allergies to other NSAIDs. If patient is dehydrated, provide adequate fluids.

Route	Onset	Peak	Duration
P.O.	Unknown	5-6 hr	24 hr

Adverse reactions

CNS: headache, dizziness, syncope, malaise, fatigue, asthenia, depression, confusion, nervousness, drowsiness, insomnia, vertigo, tremor, paresthesia, anxiety, **seizures**
CV: hypertension, hypotension, palpitations, angina, vasculitis, **heart failure, arrhythmias**, MI
EENT: abnormal vision, conjunctivitis, hearing loss, tinnitus, pharyngitis
GI: nausea, vomiting, diarrhea, constipation, colitis, GI ulcers with

m

Reactions in **bold** are life-threatening.

◀€ Clinical alert

perforation, abdominal pain, dyspepsia, gastroesophageal reflux, esophagitis, flatulence, ulcerative stomatitis, dry mouth, **pancreatitis, GI hemorrhage**
GU: urinary frequency, urinary tract infection, albuminuria, hematuria, **renal failure**
Hematologic: anemia, purpura, **leukopenia, thrombocytopenia**
Hepatic: hepatitis
Musculoskeletal: joint pain, back pain
Metabolic: dehydration
Respiratory: upper respiratory infection, dyspnea, coughing, asthma, **bronchospasm**
Skin: rash, urticaria, pruritus, bullous eruption, sweating, alopecia, photosensitivity, angioedema
Other: altered taste, increased appetite, weight gain or loss, hot flashes, fluid retention and edema, masking of infection symptoms, hypersensitivity reactions including **anaphylaxis**

Interactions
Drug-drug. *Angiotensin-converting enzyme inhibitors:* decreased antihypertensive effect
Anticoagulants: increased risk of bleeding
Aspirin: increased meloxicam blood level, increased risk of toxicity
Cholestyramine: decreased meloxicam blood level
Furosemide, thiazides: decreased diuretic effect
Lithium: increased lithium blood level
Drug-diagnostic tests. *Alanine aminotransferase, aspartate aminotransferase, bilirubin, blood urea nitrogen, creatinine, gamma-glutamyl transferase:* increased levels
Hemoglobin, platelets, white blood cells: decreased values
Drug-behaviors. *Alcohol use, smoking:* increased risk of GI irritation and bleeding

Patient monitoring
◀€ Closely monitor patient with aspirin-sensitivity asthma, because of risk of severe bronchospasm.
• In prolonged therapy, monitor CBC and kidney and liver function tests.
◀€ Assess for cardiovascular disorders and hepatotoxicity.
• Monitor patient for fluid retention and weight gain.

Patient teaching
◀€ Instruct patient to immediately report signs and symptoms of hepatotoxicity, including right upper quadrant pain, nausea, fatigue, lethargy, pruritus, and jaundice.
• Tell patient to report abdominal pain, blood in stool or emesis, or black tarry stools.
• Instruct patient to avoid alcohol and smoking.
• Caution pregnant patient to avoid drug, especially during third trimester.
• Tell patient to consult prescriber before taking over-the-counter preparations.
• As appropriate, review all other significant and life-threatening adverse reactions and interactions, especially those related to the drugs, tests, and behaviors mentioned above.

melphalan (L-PAM, L-phenylalanine mustard, L-sarcolysin)
Alkeran

melphalan hydrochloride
Alkeran

Pharmacologic class: Alkylator
Therapeutic class: Antineoplastic
Pregnancy risk category D

BOXED WARNING

• Give under supervision of physician experienced in cancer chemotherapy, in facility with adequate diagnostic and treatment resources.

• Drug may cause severe bone marrow suppression leading to infection or bleeding. I.V. use causes greater myelosuppression than oral use, and also may lead to hypersensitivity reactions (including anaphylaxis).

• Drug may cause leukemia and is potentially mutagenic.

Action

Forms cross-links between strands of cellular DNA, disrupting DNA and RNA transcription and causing cell death

Availability

Powder for injection (melphalan hydrochloride): 50 mg
Tablets: 2 mg

🖊 Indications and dosages

➤ Multiple myeloma

Adults: Initially, 6 mg P.O. daily for 2 to 3 weeks, then discontinue drug for up to 4 weeks or until white blood cell (WBC) and platelet counts increase; then give maintenance dosage of 2 or 10 mg/day for 7 to 10 days, then withhold until WBC recovery followed by 2 mg/day maintenance or 0.15 mg/kg/day P.O. for 7 days or 0.25 mg/kg for 4 days, repeated q 4 to 6 weeks. For those who can't tolerate oral therapy, 16 mg/m^2 by I.V. infusion over 15 to 20 minutes at 2-week intervals for four doses (usually with prednisone); I.V. dose can be repeated q 4 weeks after recovery from toxicity.

➤ Nonresectable advanced ovarian cancer

Adults: 0.2 mg/kg/day P.O. for 5 days q 4 to 5 weeks

Dosage adjustment

• Renal impairment

Contraindications

• Hypersensitivity to drug
• Patients whose disease has shown previous drug resistance

Precautions

Use cautiously in:
• bone marrow depression, infection, renal disease
• previous radiation therapy
• patients with childbearing potential
• pregnant or breastfeeding patients
• children (safety and efficacy not established).

Administration

• Before starting therapy, obtain CBC with white cell differential and platelet count. Repeat periodically before each course.

• For I.V. use, reconstitute by rapidly injecting 10 ml of supplied diluent into vial with lyophilized powder. Shake until solution is clear (yields a concentration of 5 mg/ml).

• Dilute desired dosage in 0.9% sodium chloride injection to a concentration no greater than 0.45 mg/ml. Administer over 15 minutes, being sure to give entire dose within 60 minutes of reconstitution.

🔊 Minimize time between reconstitution, dilution, and administration, because solution is unstable.

Route	Onset	Peak	Duration
P.O.	5 days	2-3 wk	5-6 wk
I.V.	Unknown	Unknown	Unknown

Adverse reactions

CV: hypotension, tachycardia, vasculitis
GI: nausea, vomiting, diarrhea, oral ulcers, stomatitis
GU: hyperuricemia, amenorrhea, gonadal suppression, infertility

Hematologic: anemia, purpura, **bone marrow depression, leukopenia, thrombocytopenia**
Hepatic: hepatotoxicity
Metabolic: hyperuricemia
Respiratory: dyspnea, **interstitial pneumonitis, bronchospasm, fibrosis**
Skin: rash, urticaria, pruritus, alopecia, sweating
Other: edema, extravasation at I.V. site, allergic reactions including **anaphylaxis**

Interactions

Drug-drug. *Carmustine:* increased pulmonary toxicity
Cimetidine: decreased GI absorption of melphalan
Cisplatin: increased risk of renal dysfunction, decreased melphalan clearance
Cyclosporine: increased risk of nephrotoxicity, severe renal failure
Interferon alfa: decreased melphalan blood level
Live-virus vaccines: decreased antibody response to vaccine
Myelosuppressants: additive toxicity
Nalidixic acid: increased risk of severe hemorrhagic necrotic enterocolitis (in children)
Drug-diagnostic tests. *Hemoglobin, platelets, red blood cells, WBCs:* decreased values
Nitrogenous compounds: increased levels
Drug-food. *Any food:* decreased absorption of oral melphalan

Patient monitoring

◀€ Monitor patient for thrombocytopenia and leukopenia. If platelet count exceeds 100,000/mm³ or WBC count is below 3,000/mm³, discontinue drug until peripheral blood counts recover.
◀€ Watch closely for indications of bone marrow depression, including infection, anemia, and bleeding.
◀€ After multiple courses, watch for acute hypersensitivity reaction. If it

occurs, discontinue drug and administer volume expanders, corticosteroids, or antihistamines, as prescribed.
• Watch for signs and symptoms of GI or pulmonary toxicity.
• Evaluate renal and hepatic function.

Patient teaching

• Tell patient to take oral tablets without food, because food may decrease drug absorption.
• Instruct patient to take entire daily oral dose at one time on empty stomach.
◀€ Advise patient to immediately report unusual bleeding or bruising, fever, chills, sore throat, shortness of breath, yellowing of skin or eyes, persistent cough, flank or stomach pain, joint pain, black tarry stools, rash, or unusual lumps or masses.
• Tell patient to consult prescriber before using over-the-counter medications.
• Advise patient to use reliable contraception.
• Caution patient to avoid breastfeeding.
• As appropriate, review all other significant and life-threatening adverse reactions and interactions, especially those related to the drugs, tests, and foods mentioned above.

memantine
Ebixa✲⊕, Namenda

Pharmacologic class: N-methyl-D-aspartate receptor antagonist (NMDA)
Therapeutic class: Anti-Alzheimer's agent
Pregnancy risk category B

Action

Unclear. Thought to act as a low- to moderate-affinity NMDA receptor antagonist, binding to NMDA receptor-operated channels. (Activation of these channels is thought to contribute to Alzheimer's symptoms.)

Availability
Oral solution: 2 mg/ml
Tablets: 5 mg, 10 mg
Tablets (titration pack): 28 tablets of 5 mg and 21 tablets of 10 mg

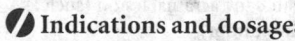 Indications and dosages
➣ **Moderate to severe Alzheimer's-type dementia**
Adults: Initially, 5 mg P.O. daily. Then titrate at intervals of at least 1 week in 5-mg increments, to a maximum of 10 mg P.O. b.i.d.

Dosage adjustment
• Moderate renal impairment

Contraindications
• Hypersensitivity to drug or its components

Precautions
Use cautiously in:
• neurologic conditions, moderate to severe renal impairment, genitourinary conditions that increase pH
• pregnant or breastfeeding patients.

Administration
• Give with or without food.

Route	Onset	Peak	Duration
P.O.	Unknown	3-7 hr	Unknown

Adverse reactions
CNS: dizziness, headache, syncope, aggressive reaction, confusion, somnolence, hallucinations, agitation, insomnia, vertigo, ataxia, abnormal gait, hypokinesia, anxiety, **transient ischemic attack, cerebrovascular accident (CVA)**
CV: hypertension, **cardiac failure**
EENT: cataract, conjunctivitis
GI: nausea, vomiting, diarrhea, constipation, anorexia
GU: frequent voiding, urinary incontinence, urinary tract infection
Hematologic: anemia
Musculoskeletal: back pain, arthralgia
Respiratory: cough, dyspnea, bronchitis, pneumonia
Skin: rash
Other: weight loss, fatigue, pain, falls, flulike symptoms, peripheral edema

Interactions
Drug-drug. *Cimetidine, hydrochlorothiazide, nicotine, quinidine, ranitidine, triamterene:* altered blood levels of both drugs
Urine-alkalizing drugs (carbonic anhydrase inhibitors, sodium bicarbonate): decreased memantine elimination
Drug-diagnostic tests. *Alkaline phosphatase:* increased level

Patient monitoring
◀€ Check for heart failure and signs and symptoms of CVA.
• Monitor kidney function tests.

Patient teaching
• Tell patient to take with or without food.
• Instruct patient or caregiver not to mix solution with other liquids and to take or give oral solution only with included dosing device.
• Make sure patient or caregiver understands dose escalation.
• As appropriate, review all other significant and life-threatening adverse reactions and interactions, especially those related to the drugs and tests mentioned above.

menotropins
Menopur, Repronex

Pharmacologic class: Hormone
Therapeutic class: Exogenous gonadotropin
Pregnancy risk category X

Action
Simulates action of follicle-stimulating hormone (FSH) by promoting follicular growth and maturation

Availability
Injection (powder or pellet for reconstitution): 75 international units luteinizing hormone (LH); 150 international units LH and 150 international units FSH activity/vial

🖉 Indications and dosages
➤ Controlled ovarian stimulation in patients with oligoanovulation
Women: Dosage individualized. Recommended dosage is 150 international units I.M. or subcutaneously daily during first 5 days of treatment, with subsequent dosages adjusted based on response. Adjust dosage no more often than every 2 days, and don't exceed 75 to 150 international units per adjustment. Maximum daily dosage is 450 international units. Dosing beyond 12 days is not recommended. If response is appropriate, human chorionic gonadotropin (hCG) should be given I.M. 1 day after last menotropins dose.
➤ Assisted reproductive technologies
Women: In patients who've received gonadotropin-releasing hormone agonists or antagonist pituitary suppression, recommended initial dosage is 225 international units I.M. or subcutaneously, with subsequent dosage adjustments based on response. Adjust dosage no more often than every 2 days, and don't exceed 75 to 150 international units per adjustment. Maximum daily dosage is 450 international units. Dosing beyond 12 days isn't recommended. Once adequate follicular development appears, hCG is given to induce follicular maturation in preparation for oocyte retrieval.

Contraindications
• Hypersensitivity to drug
• High FSH levels (indicating primary ovarian failure)
• Abnormal bleeding of undetermined origin
• Uncontrolled thyroid or adrenal dysfunction
• Organic intracranial lesion (such as pituitary tumor)
• Causes of infertility other than anovulation (unless patient is candidate for in vitro fertilization)
• Ovarian cysts or enlargement not caused by polycystic ovarian syndrome
• Pregnancy

Precautions
Use cautiously in:
• renal or hepatic insufficiency (safety and efficacy not established)
• breastfeeding patients.

Administration
• Know that drug may be given either I.M. or subcutaneously.
• To reconstitute powder or pellet for injection, add accompanying 2 ml of 0.9% sodium chloride injection to vial.
• Inject immediately after reconstitution. Discard unused portion.
• Rotate injection sites.
• Use lower abdomen for subcutaneous injection.
• Withhold hCG if serum estradiol level exceeds 2,000 pg/ml or abdominal pain occurs.

Route	Onset	Peak	Duration
I.M.	Unknown	Unknown	Unknown
Subcut.	Unknown	Unknown	Unknown

Adverse reactions
CNS: headache, malaise, dizziness, **cerebrovascular accident**
CV: tachycardia, **venous thrombophlebitis, arterial occlusion, arterial thromboembolism**

GI: nausea, vomiting, diarrhea, abdominal cramps and distention, **hemoperitoneum**

GU: ovarian enlargement with pain, gynecomastia, ovarian cysts, multiple births, **ovarian hyperstimulation syndrome (OHSS), ectopic pregnancy**

Metabolic: electrolyte imbalances

Musculoskeletal: muscle aches, joint pain

Respiratory: dyspnea, tachypnea, **atelectasis, adult respiratory distress syndrome, pulmonary embolism, pulmonary infarction**

Skin: rash

Other: fever, hypersensitivity reaction, **anaphylaxis**

Interactions
None significant

Patient monitoring
• Know that before starting menotropins/hCG therapy to induce ovulation and pregnancy, patient should undergo gynecologic and endocrine evaluation with hysterosalpingogram to rule out pregnancy and neoplastic lesions.

• Assess patient to confirm anovulation. Obtain urinary gonadotropin levels as ordered to rule out primary ovarian failure. (Male partner's fertility should be evaluated, also).

• In older females (who have greater risk of anovulatory disorders and endometrial cancer), assess cervical dilation and curettage results.

• Evaluate patient for expected ovarian stimulation without hyperstimulation.

◀᠁ Monitor for early indications of OHSS—severe pelvic pain, nausea, vomiting, and weight gain. OHSS usually occurs 2 weeks after treatment ends, peaks 7 to 10 days after ovulation, and resolves with menses onset.

◀᠁ If OHSS occurs, drug is withdrawn and patient is hospitalized for bed rest, fluid and electrolyte management, and analgesics. Monitor daily fluid intake and output, weight, abdominal girth, hematocrit, serum and urinary electrolytes, urine specific gravity, blood urea nitrogen, and creatinine. Watch for hemoconcentration caused by fluid loss into peritoneal, pleural, and pericardial cavities.

◀᠁ Stay alert for pulmonary and thromboembolic complications.

• Assess male patient for pituitary insufficiency as possible cause of infertility.

Patient teaching
• Before therapy, teach patient about duration of treatment and necessary monitoring.

• Inform patient about risk of multiple births with menotropins and hCG use.

• For infertile females, encourage daily intercourse starting on day before hCG administration.

• As appropriate, review all other significant and life-threatening adverse reactions.

meperidine hydrochloride (pethidine hydrochloride)
Demerol, Meperitab

Pharmacologic class: Opioid agonist

Therapeutic class: Analgesic, adjunct to anesthesia

Controlled substance schedule II

Pregnancy risk category C

Action
Binds to and depresses opiate receptors in spinal cord and CNS, altering perception of and response to pain

Availability
Injection: 10 mg/ml, 25 mg/ml, 50 mg/ml, 75 mg/ml, 100 mg/ml
Oral solution: 500 mg/5 ml
Syrup: 50 mg/5 ml
Tablets: 50 mg, 100 mg

⏀ Indications and dosages

➤ Moderate to severe pain

Adults: 50 to 150 mg P.O., I.M., or subcutaneously q 3 to 4 hours as needed

Children: 1.1 to 1.8 mg/kg P.O., I.M., or subcutaneously q 3 to 4 hours, not to exceed 100 mg/dose

➤ Preoperative sedation

Adults: 50 to 100 mg I.M. or subcutaneously 30 to 90 minutes before anesthesia

Children: 1 to 2.2 mg/kg I.M. or subcutaneously 30 to 90 minutes before anesthesia. Don't exceed adult dosage.

➤ Support of anesthesia

Adults: Fractional doses (such as 10 mg/ml) by repeated slow I.V. injections or continuous I.V. infusion of a more dilute solution (such as 1 mg/ml). Dosages should be individualized.

➤ Analgesia during labor

Adults: 50 to 100 mg I.M. or subcutaneously when contractions are regular. May repeat q 1 to 3 hours.

Contraindications

• Hypersensitivity to drug or bisulfites (with some injectable products)
• MAO inhibitor use within past 14 days

Precautions

Use cautiously in:
• head trauma; increased intracranial pressure (ICP); severe renal, hepatic, or pulmonary disease; hypothyroidism; adrenal insufficiency; extensive burns; alcoholism; supraventricular tachycardia; seizure disorders
• undiagnosed abdominal pain or prostatic hyperplasia
• elderly or debilitated patients
• pregnant patients (not recommended before labor)
• labor (drug may cause respiratory depression in neonate)
• breastfeeding patients
• children.

Administration

• Give I.M. injection slowly into large muscle. Preferably, use diluted solution.
• Give oral solution or syrup in a halfglass of water to avoid topical anesthetic effect on mucous membranes.
• Be aware that drug is compatible with 5% dextrose and lactated Ringer's solution, dextrose-saline solution combinations, and 2.5%, 5%, or 10% dextrose in water.
◀﹦ Know that drug is not compatible with soluble barbiturates, aminophylline, heparin, morphine sulfate, methicillin, phenytoin, sodium bicarbonate, iodide, sulfadiazine, or sulfisoxazole.
• Don't give for chronic pain control, because of potential toxicity and dependence.

Route	Onset	Peak	Duration
P.O.	15 min	60 min	2-4 hr
I.V.	Immediate	5-7 min	2-4 hr
I.M.	10-15 min	30-50 min	2-4 hr
Subcut.	10-15 min	40-60 min	2-4 hr

Adverse reactions

CNS: confusion, sedation, dysphoria, euphoria, floating feeling, hallucinations, headache, unusual dreams, **seizures**

CV: hypotension, **bradycardia, cardiac arrest, shock**

EENT: blurred vision, diplopia, miosis

GI: nausea, vomiting, constipation, ileus, biliary tract spasms

GU: urinary retention

Respiratory: respiratory depression, respiratory arrest

Skin: flushing, sweating, induration

Other: pain at injection site, local irritation, physical or psychological drug dependence, drug tolerance

Interactions

Drug-drug. *Antihistamines, sedativehypnotics:* additive CNS depression

---

Barbiturates, cimetidine, protease inhibitor antiretrovirals: increased respiratory and CNS depression

Chlorpromazine, thioridazine: increased risk of meperidine toxicity

MAO inhibitors, procarbazine: potentially fatal reaction

Opioid agonist-antagonists: precipitation of opioid withdrawal in physically dependent patients

Phenytoin: increased meperidine metabolism and decreased effects

Drug-diagnostic tests. *Amylase, lipase:* increased levels

Drug-herbs. *Chamomile, hops, kava, skullcap, valerian:* increased CNS depression

Drug-behaviors. *Alcohol use:* increased CNS depression

Patient monitoring

◀︎≋ Monitor vital signs. Don't give drug if patient has significant respiratory or CNS depression.

• Reassess patient's pain level after administration.

◀︎≋ Watch for seizures, agitation, irritability, nervousness, tremors, twitches, and myoclonus in patients at risk for normeperidine accumulation (such as those with renal or hepatic impairment).

◀︎≋ Use with extreme caution in patients with head injury. Drug may increase ICP and cause adverse reactions that obscure clinical course.

• Closely monitor patients with acute abdominal pain. Drug may obscure diagnosis and clinical course of GI condition.

• Evaluate bowel and bladder function.

• With long-term or repeated use, watch for psychological and physical drug dependence and tolerance.

◀︎≋ With pediatric patients, stay alert for increased risk of seizures.

Patient teaching

• Tell patient using oral solution or syrup to take drug with a half-glass of water to minimize local anesthetic effect.

• Caution patient to avoid driving and other hazardous activities, because drug may cause dizziness or drowsiness.

• Advise patient to avoid alcohol.

• Instruct ambulatory patient to change position slowly to avoid orthostatic hypotension.

• Tell female patient to inform prescriber if she is pregnant or breastfeeding.

• As appropriate, review all other significant and life-threatening adverse reactions and interactions, especially those related to the drugs, tests, herbs, and behaviors mentioned above.

mercaptopurine (6-mercaptopurine, 6-MP)
Purinethol, Puri-Nethol ✚

m

Pharmacologic class: Antimetabolite
Therapeutic class: Antineoplastic
Pregnancy risk category D

FDA | **BOXED WARNING**

• Don't give drug unless diagnosis of acute lymphatic leukemia is confirmed and responsible physician knows how to assess response to chemotherapy.

Action
Inhibits DNA and RNA synthesis, suppressing growth of certain cancer cells

Availability
Tablets: 50 mg

🖊 Indications and dosages
➤ Maintenance therapy for acute lymphatic (lymphocytic, lymphoblastic) leukemia

Adults and children: On complete hematologic remission, 1.5 to 2.5 mg/kg/day P.O. as a single dose (combined with other agents as prescribed).

Contraindications

• Hypersensitivity to drug or its components
• Prior resistance to drug or thioguanine
• Breastfeeding

Precautions

Use cautiously in:
• renal or hepatic impairment
• decreased platelet or neutrophil counts after chemotherapy or radiation
• inherited thiopurine methyltransferase deficiency
• pregnant patients.

Administration

• Follow facility protocols regarding proper handling and disposal of drug.
◀€ Don't handle drug if you are pregnant.
• Be aware that total daily dosage is calculated to nearest multiple of 25 mg and given once daily.
◀€ Be aware that when mercaptopurine is given with allopurinol, mercaptopurine dosage must be reduced to one-third to one-fourth of usual dosage to avoid severe toxicity.
◀€ Withdraw drug immediately if white blood cell (WBC) or platelet count falls rapidly or steeply.

Route	Onset	Peak	Duration
P.O.	Unknown	2 hr	Unknown

Adverse reactions

GI: nausea, vomiting, anorexia, diarrhea, GI ulcers, painful oral ulcers, **pancreatitis**
Hematologic: anemia, **leukopenia, thrombocytopenia**
Hepatic: jaundice, **hepatotoxicity**

Metabolic: hyperuricemia
Skin: rash, hyperpigmentation

Interactions

Drug-drug. *Allopurinol (more than 300 mg), aminosalicylate derivatives (mesalazine, olsalazine, sulfasalazine):* increased bone marrow depression
Warfarin: decreased anticoagulant effect
Drug-diagnostic tests. *Hemoglobin, platelets, red blood cells, uric acid, WBCs:* increased values

Patient monitoring

◀€ Watch for signs and symptoms of hepatotoxicity.
• Monitor weekly CBC with white cell differential and platelet count.
• Assess bone marrow aspiration and biopsy results, as necessary, to aid assessment of disease progression, resistance to therapy, and drug-induced marrow hypoplasia.
• Monitor serum uric acid level.
• Evaluate fluid intake and output.
• Monitor liver function tests and bilirubin level weekly at start of therapy, then monthly.

Patient teaching

◀€ Instruct patient to immediately report fever, sore throat, increased bleeding or bruising, or signs or symptoms of liver problems (right-sided abdominal pain, yellowing of skin or eyes, nausea, vomiting, clay-colored stools, or dark urine).
• Advise both male and female patients to use reliable contraception.
• Encourage patient to maintain adequate fluid intake.
• Caution patient not to get vaccinations without consulting prescriber.
• As appropriate, review all other significant and life-threatening adverse reactions and interactions, especially those related to the drugs and tests mentioned above.

meropenem
Meronem ⊕, Merrem I.V.

Pharmacologic class: Carbapenem
Therapeutic class: Anti-infective
Pregnancy risk category B

Action
Inhibits bacterial cell-wall synthesis and penetrates gram-negative and gram-positive bacteria

Availability
Powder for injection: 500-mg and 1-g vials

💋 Indications and dosages
➤ Intra-abdominal infections
Adults: 1 g I.V. q 8 hours over 15 to 30 minutes by infusion or over 3 to 5 minutes as a bolus injection
Children weighing 50 kg (110 lb) or more: 1 g I.V. q 8 hours over 15 to 30 minutes by infusion or over 3 to 5 minutes as a bolus injection
Children ages 3 months and older weighing less than 50 kg (110 lb): 20 mg/kg q 8 hours over 15 to 30 minutes by infusion or over 3 to 5 minutes as a bolus injection
➤ Bacterial meningitis
Children weighing 50 kg (110 lb) or more: 2 g I.V. q 8 hours over 15 to 30 minutes by infusion or over 3 to 5 minutes as a bolus injection
Children ages 3 month and older weighing less than 50 kg (110 lb): 40 mg/kg q 8 hours over 15 to 30 minutes by infusion or over 3 to 5 minutes as a bolus injection, to a maximum of 2 g q 8 hours
➤ Complicated skin and skin-structure infections
Adults: 500 mg I.V. q 8 hours

Dosage adjustment
• Renal impairment

Off-label uses
• Acute pulmonary exacerbation caused by respiratory tract infection with susceptible organisms in cystic fibrosis patients

Contraindications
• Hypersensitivity to drug, its components, or other beta-lactams

Precautions
Use cautiously in:
• sulfite sensitivity, renal disease, seizure disorder
• pregnant or breastfeeding patients
• children.

Administration
• For I.V. bolus, add 10 or 20 ml of sterile water to 500-mg or 1-g vial, respectively, to yield a concentration of 50 mg/ml. Shake until clear. Administer single dose over 3 to 5 minutes.
• For intermittent I.V. infusion, piggyback vials can be reconstituted with compatible I.V. solution (0.9% sodium chloride or 5% dextrose) to yield a concentration of 2.5 to 50 mg/ml. Or vials can be reconstituted as for direct I.V. injection and added to compatible I.V. solution for further dilution. To reconstitute and administer ADD-Vantage systems, follow manufacturer's instructions. Infuse drug over 15 to 30 minutes.
• Use diluted solution immediately, if possible.

Route	Onset	Peak	Duration
I.V.	Unknown	1 hr	Unknown

Adverse reactions
CNS: headache, insomnia, dizziness, drowsiness, weakness, **seizures**
CV: hypotension, phlebitis, palpitations, **heart failure, cardiac arrest, myocardial infarction**
GI: nausea, vomiting, diarrhea, constipation, tongue discoloration, oral candidiasis, glossitis, **pseudomembranous colitis**

m

Reactions in **bold** are life-threatening. ◀€ Clinical alert

GU: vaginal candidiasis
Hematologic: anemia, eosinophilia, **leukopenia, bone marrow depression, thrombocytopenia, neutropenia**
Musculoskeletal: myoclonus
Respiratory: chest discomfort, dyspnea, hyperventilation
Skin: rash, urticaria, pruritus, erythema at injection site
Other: altered taste, fever, pain, fungal infection, **anaphylaxis**

Interactions
Drug-drug. *Probenecid:* increased meropenem blood level
Drug-diagnostic tests. *Alanine aminotransferase, alkaline phosphatase, amylase, aspartate aminotransferase, bilirubin, blood urea nitrogen, eosinophils, gamma-glutamyl transpeptidase, lactate dehydrogenase, lipase:* increased values
Hematocrit, hemoglobin, platelets, neutrophils, white blood cells: decreased values
International Normalized Ratio, partial thromboplastin time, prothrombin time: increased or decreased values

Patient monitoring
• Collect specimens for culture and sensitivity testing as needed. However, be aware that drug therapy may start pending results.
◀≷ Monitor patient for hypersensitivity reaction or anaphylaxis. If either occurs, stop infusion immediately and initiate emergency treatment.
• Monitor for CNS irritability and seizures.
• In prolonged therapy, evaluate hematopoietic, renal, and hepatic function and watch for overgrowth of nonsusceptible organisms.
• If diarrhea occurs, check for pseudomembranous colitis and obtain stool cultures.
• Obtain hearing tests in child being treated for bacterial meningitis.

Patient teaching
• Advise patient to report such adverse reactions as CNS irritability, diarrhea, rash, shortness of breath, or pain at infusion site.
• As appropriate, review all other significant and life-threatening adverse reactions and interactions, especially those related to the drugs and tests mentioned above.

mesalamine (5-aminosalicylic acid, 5-ASA, mesalazine, mesalazine⊕)
Apriso, Asacol, Asacol HD, Canasa, Ipocol⊕, Lialda, Mesasal♣, Mesren⊕, Mezavant♣, Novo-5-ASA-Ect♣, Pentasa, Rowasa, Salofalk♣⊕

Pharmacologic class: 5-amino-2-hydroxybenzoic acid
Therapeutic class: GI anti-inflammatory drug
Pregnancy risk category B

Action
Unknown. Thought to act in colon, where it blocks cyclooxygenase and inhibits prostaglandin synthesis.

Availability
Capsules (extended-release): 250 mg, 500 mg, 0.375 g (Apriso)
Rectal suspension: 4 g/60 ml
Suppositories: 1,000 mg
Tablets (delayed-release): 400 mg (Pentasa), 800 mg (Asacol HD), 1.2 g (Lialda)

🕖 Indications and dosages
➤ Active ulcerative colitis
Adults: 800 mg P.O. (Asacol delayed-release tablets) t.i.d. for 6 weeks

➤ To induce remission in mildly to moderately active ulcerative colitis
Adults: 1 g P.O. (Pentasa extended-release capsules) q.i.d. for a total dosage of 4 g daily for up to 8 weeks. Or, two to four 1.2 g (Lialda) extended-release tablets P.O. once daily for total daily dose of 2.4 or 4.8 g for up to 8 weeks.

➤ Active distal ulcerative colitis, proctosigmoiditis, or proctitis
Adults: 4-g enema (Rowasa 60 ml) P.R. daily at bedtime, retained for 8 hours. Continue for 3 to 6 weeks.

➤ Active ulcerative proctitis
Adults: 500 mg (Canasa suppository) P.R. b.i.d., increased to t.i.d. if response inadequate after 2 weeks. Or 1,000 mg (suppository) P.R. at bedtime, continued for 3 to 6 weeks.

➤ To maintain remission of ulcerative colitis
Adults: 1.6 g (Asacol) P.O. daily in divided doses. Or, 1.5 g (Apriso) P.O. daily in the morning.

Contraindications
• Hypersensitivity to drug, its components, or salicylates

Precautions
Use cautiously in:
• severe hepatic or renal impairment
• allergy to sulfasalazine
• pyloric stenosis (delayed-release tablets)
• conditions predisposing to development of myocarditis or pericarditis
• pregnant or breastfeeding patients
• children younger than age 18 (safety and efficacy not established).

Administration
• Give Apriso capsules with or without food. Don't give concurrently with antacids.
• Give Lialda tablets with meal.
• Make sure patient swallows tablets whole without crushing or chewing.

• For best effect, have patient retain suppository for 1 to 3 hours.

Route	Onset	Peak	Duration
P.O.	Unknown	Unknown	6-8 hr
P.R.	Unknown	Unknown	24 hr

Adverse reactions
CNS: headache, dizziness, malaise, weakness
CV: chest pain, **mesalamine-induced cardiac hypersensitivity reactions (myocarditis and pericarditis)**
EENT: rhinitis, pharyngitis
GI: nausea, vomiting, diarrhea, eructation, flatulence, anal irritation (with rectal use), **pancreatitis**
GU: interstitial nephritis, renal failure
Musculoskeletal: back pain
Skin: alopecia, rash
Other: fever, acute intolerance syndrome, **anaphylaxis, acute intolerance syndrome**

Interactions
Drug-drug. *Antacids:* increased risk of dissolution of coating of Apriso granules
Azathioprine, 6-mercaptopurine: increased potential for blood disorders
Nephrotoxic drugs (including nonsteroidal anti-inflammatory agents): increased risk of renal adverse reactions

Patient monitoring
◄€ Monitor carefully for mesalamine-induced cardiac hypersensitivity reactions (myocarditis and pericarditis).
◄€ Closely monitor patients with history of allergic reactions to sulfasalazine or sulfite sensitivity (if using enema).
• Assess kidney and liver function before and periodically during therapy.
• Monitor for suppository efficacy, which should appear in 3 to 21 days. However, know that treatment usually continues for 3 to 6 weeks.
◄€ Watch for signs and symptoms of intolerance syndrome, such as

m

Reactions in **bold** are life-threatening.　　　　◄€ Clinical alert

cramping, acute abdominal pain, bloody diarrhea, fever, headache, and rash. If these occur, discontinue drug and notify prescriber.

🔊 Watch for signs and symptoms of intolerance syndrome, such as cramping, acute abdominal pain, bloody diarrhea, fever, headache, and rash. If these occur, discontinue drug. Drug may be restarted later only if clearly needed, under close medical supervision and at reduced dosage.

Patient teaching
• Instruct patient to swallow tablets or capsules whole.
• Tell patient to contact prescriber if partially intact tablets repeatedly appear in stools.
• Advise patient using suppository to avoid excessive handling and to retain suppository for 1 to 3 hours or longer for maximum benefit.
• Teach patient about proper enema administration. Tell him to stay in position for at least 30 minutes and, if possible, retain medication overnight.

🔊 Advise patient to immediately report breathing difficulties, allergic symptoms, cramping, acute abdominal pain, bloody diarrhea, fever, headache, or rash.
• As appropriate, review all other significant and life-threatening adverse reactions, especially those related to the drugs mentioned above.

mesna
Mesnex, Uromitexan♣⊕

Pharmacologic class: Detoxifying agent
Therapeutic class: Hemorrhagic cystitis inhibitor
Pregnancy risk category B

Action
Reacts in kidney with urotoxic ifosfamide metabolites (acrolein and 4-hydroxy-ifosfamide), resulting in their detoxification. Also binds to double bonds of acrolein and to other urotoxic metabolites.

Availability
Injection: 100 mg/ml in 10-ml vials
Tablets (coated): 400 mg

🖊 Indications and dosages
➢ To prevent hemorrhagic cystitis in patients receiving ifosfamide
Adults: *Combination I.V. and P.O. regimen*—Single I.V. bolus dose of mesna at 20% of ifosfamide dosage, given at same time as ifosfamide, followed by two doses of mesna tablets P.O. at 40% of ifosfamide dosage given 2 and 6 hours after ifosfamide dose. *I.V. regimen*—I.V. bolus of mesna at 20% of ifosfamide dosage given at same time as ifosfamide, repeated 4 and 8 hours after each ifosfamide dose.

Dosage adjustment
• Children

Contraindications
• Hypersensitivity to drug or other thiol compounds

Precautions
Use cautiously in:
• autoimmune disorders
• pregnant or breastfeeding patients.

Administration
• Dilute with dextrose 5% in water, dextrose 5% in normal saline solution, dextrose 5% in 0.2% sodium chloride solution, dextrose 5% in 0.33% sodium chloride solution, dextrose 5% in 0.45% sodium chloride solution, normal saline solution, or lactated Ringer's solution for injection.

• Give I.V. bolus over at least 1 minute with ifosfamide dose and at prescribed intervals after ifosfamide doses.

◀€ Don't use multidose vial (contains benzyl alcohol) in neonates or infants. In older children, use with caution.

• If patient vomits within 2 hours of oral mesna dose, repeat oral dose or switch to I.V. route.

Route	Onset	Peak	Duration
P.O.	Unknown	4-8 hr	24 hr
I.V.	Unknown	1 hr	24 hr

Adverse reactions

CNS: fatigue, malaise, irritability, headache, dizziness, drowsiness, hyperesthesia, rigors

CV: hypertension, hypotension, ST-segment elevation, tachycardia

EENT: conjunctivitis, pharyngitis, rhinitis

GI: nausea, vomiting, diarrhea, constipation, anorexia, flatulence

Hematologic: hematuria

Musculoskeletal: back pain, joint pain, myalgia

Respiratory: coughing, tachypnea, **bronchospasm**

Skin: flushing, rash

Other: arm or leg pain, injection site reactions, fever, flulike symptoms, allergic reactions

Interactions

Drug-diagnostic tests. *Hepatic enzymes:* increased levels

Urinary erythrocytes: false-positive or false-negative results

Urine tests using Ames Multistix: false-positive for ketonuria

Patient monitoring

• Monitor nutritional and hydration status.

• Monitor vital signs and ECG. Watch closely for blood pressure changes and tachycardia.

• Assess body temperature. Stay alert for fever, flulike symptoms, and EENT infections.

• Monitor respiratory status carefully. Watch closely for cough, bronchospasm, and tachypnea.

Patient teaching

• Inform patient that drug may cause significant adverse effects. Reassure him that he will be monitored closely.

• Encourage patient to request analgesics or other pain-relief measures for headache, back or joint pain, hyperesthesia, or muscle ache.

◀€ Advise patient to immediately report breathing difficulties and allergic symptoms.

• Inform patient about drug's adverse CNS effects. Explain safety measures used to prevent injury.

• As appropriate, review all other significant and life-threatening adverse reactions and interactions, especially those related to the tests mentioned above.

m

⊗

metformin hydrochloride

Apo-Metformin✶, Co Metformin✶, Dom-Metformin✶, Fortamet, Gen-Metformin✶, Glucophage, Glucophage XR, Glumetza, Glycon✶, Med Metformin✶, Metsol⊕, Novo-Metformin✶, Nu-Metformin✶, PHL-Metformin✶, PMS-Metformin✶, Ran-Metformin✶, Ratio-Metformin✶, Rhoxal-Metformin✶, Riomet, Riva-Metformin✶, Sandoz Metformin✶

Pharmacologic class: Biguanide
Therapeutic class: Hypoglycemic
Pregnancy risk category B

Reactions in **bold** are life-threatening.   ◀€ Clinical alert

- Lactic acidosis is rare but serious (50% mortality) metabolic complication that can result from drug accumulation. Lactic acidosis is also linked to such conditions as diabetes mellitus and significant tissue hypoperfusion and hypoxemia. Lactic acidosis incidence in patients receiving drug is low; cases have occurred mainly in diabetics with significant renal insufficiency. Patients with unstable or acute heart failure at risk of hypoperfusion and hypoxemia are at increased lactic acidosis risk.
- Lactic acidosis risk rises with age and degree of renal dysfunction, and may decrease significantly through regular renal monitoring and by using lowest effective dosage. Perform careful renal monitoring, especially in elderly patients. Withhold drug promptly if patient develops condition linked to hypoxemia, dehydration, or sepsis. Avoid giving drug to patients with hepatic disease, as hepatic impairment may significantly limit lactate clearance. Caution patient against excessive alcohol use during therapy, as alcohol potentiates drug effects on lactate metabolism. Temporarily withdraw drug before intravascular radiocontrast study or surgical procedure.
- Lactic acidosis onset commonly is subtle and accompanied only by nonspecific symptoms. Instruct patient to notify physician immediately if symptoms occur; withdraw drug until situation is clarified.
- Suspect lactic acidosis in diabetic patient with metabolic acidosis who lacks evidence of ketoacidosis.
- Lactic acidosis requires emergency treatment. Discontinue metformin immediately and begin general supportive measures promptly. Prompt hemodialysis is recommended to correct acidosis and remove accumulated drug, and can lead to prompt symptom reversal and recovery.

Action
Increases insulin sensitivity by decreasing glucose production and absorption in liver and intestines and enhancing glucose uptake and utilization

Availability
Oral solution: 100 mg/ml, 500 mg/5 ml
Tablets: 500 mg, 850 mg, 1,000 mg
Tablets (extended-release): 500 mg, 750 mg

⏀ Indications and dosages
➢ Adjunct to diet and exercise to improve glycemic control in type 2 (non-insulin-dependent) diabetes mellitus
Adults and children ages 17 and older: Initially, 500 mg P.O. b.i.d.; may increase by 500 mg/week, up to 2,000 mg/day. If patient needs more than 2,000 mg/day, give in three divided doses (not to exceed 2,500 mg/day). Alternatively, 850 mg P.O. daily, increased by 850 mg q 2 weeks, up to 2,550 mg/day in divided doses (850 mg t.i.d.). *Extended-release tablets*—500 mg/day P.O. with evening meal; may increase by 500 mg weekly, up to 2,000 mg/day. If 2,000 mg once daily is inadequate, 1,000 mg may be given b.i.d.
Children ages 10 to 16: 500 mg P.O. b.i.d. Increase in increments of 500 mg weekly to a maximum of 2,000 mg daily in divided doses.
➢ Concurrent use with sulfonylurea or insulin in type 2 diabetes mellitus
Adults and children ages 17 and older: If patient hasn't responded to maximum metformin dosage of 2,000 mg/day in 4 weeks, sulfonylurea may be added while metformin therapy continues at highest dosage (even if patient experienced primary or secondary failure on sulfonylurea). Adjust dosages of both drugs until glycemic control adequate. If response inadequate within 1 to 3 months of concurrent therapy, consider alternatives.
➢ Concurrent use with insulin in type 2 diabetes mellitus

🍁 Canada   ⊕ UK   ☣ Hazardous drug   ⊗ High-alert drug

Adults ages 17 and older: Continue current insulin dosage while starting metformin at 500 mg P.O. once daily. If response inadequate, increase metformin dosage by 500 mg after approximately 1 week and then by 500 mg weekly until glycemic control is achieved. Maximum metformin dosage is 2,500 mg. Optimally, decrease insulin dosage 10% to 25% when fasting plasma glucose level is below 120 mg/dl. Individualize dosage adjustments based on glycemic response.

Dosage adjustment
• Elderly or debilitated patients

Contraindications
• Hypersensitivity to drug
• Acute or chronic metabolic acidosis (including diabetic ketoacidosis) with or without coma
• Underlying renal dysfunction
• Heart failure requiring drug therapy

Precautions
Use cautiously in:
• renal impairment, myocardial infarction, cerebrovascular accident, hypoxia, sepsis, pituitary deficiency or hyperthyroidism, dehydration, hypoxemia, chronic alcohol use
• elderly or debilitated patients
• pregnant or breastfeeding patients
• children (safety not established).

Administration
• Administer with a meal.
• Make sure patient swallows extended-release tablets whole without crushing or chewing.
• Don't administer extended-release tablets to children.
• Know that drug is given with diet therapy, sulfonylureas, or both.

Route	Onset	Peak	Duration
P.O.	Unknown	2-4 hr	12 hr
P.O. (extended)	Unknown	4-8 hr	24 hr

Adverse reactions
GI: diarrhea, nausea, vomiting, abdominal bloating
Metabolic: lactic acidosis
Other: unpleasant metallic taste, decreased vitamin B_{12} level

Interactions
Drug-drug. *Amiloride, calcium channel blockers, digoxin, morphine, procainamide, quinidine, ranitidine, triamterene, trimethoprim, vancomycin:* altered response to metformin
Cimetidine, furosemide, nifedipine: increased metformin effects
Iodinated contrast media: increased risk of lactic acidosis
Drug-diagnostic tests. *Urine ketones:* false-positive results
Drug-herbs. *Glucosamine:* decreased glycemic control
Chromium, coenzyme Q10, fenugreek: additive hypoglycemic effects
Drug-behaviors. *Alcohol use:* increased metformin effects

Patient monitoring
• When switching from chlorpropamide, stay alert for hypoglycemia during first 2 weeks of metformin therapy; chlorpropamide may stay in body for prolonged time. Conversion from other standard oral hypoglycemics requires no transition period.
• Monitor blood glucose level closely. If it isn't controlled after 4 weeks at maximum dosage, oral sulfonylurea may be added.
• Monitor kidney and liver function tests, particularly in elderly patients.
• Assess hematologic parameters and vitamin B_{12} levels at start of therapy and periodically thereafter.
◀€ Watch for signs and symptoms of lactic acidosis. Stop drug if acidosis occurs. To aid differential diagnosis, check electrolyte, ketone, glucose, blood pH, lactate, and metformin blood levels.

m

• Periodically monitor glucose and glycosylated hemoglobin levels to evaluate drug efficacy.

Patient teaching

• Teach patient about diabetes and importance of proper diet, exercise, weight control, and blood glucose monitoring.

• Inform patient that drug may cause diarrhea, nausea, and upset stomach. Advise him to take it with meals to reduce these effects, and tell him that adverse effects often subside over time.

◀፡ Teach patient to recognize and immediately report signs and symptoms of acidosis, such as weakness, fatigue, muscle pain, dyspnea, abdominal pain, dizziness, light-headedness, and slow or irregular heartbeat.

• Advise patient to report changes in health status (such as infection, persistent vomiting and diarrhea, or need for surgery). These may warrant dosage decrease or drug withdrawal.

• As appropriate, review all other significant and life-threatening adverse reactions and interactions, especially those related to the drugs, tests, herbs, and behaviors mentioned above.

methadone hydrochloride eptadone⊕

Dolophine, Metadol, Methadone HCl Intensol, Methadose, Physeptone⊕, Synastone⊕

Pharmacologic class: Opioid agonist
Therapeutic class: Analgesic, opioid detoxification adjunct
Controlled substance schedule II
Pregnancy risk category C

FDA BOXED WARNING

• Deaths have occurred during drug initiation for opioid dependence. In some cases, deaths apparently resulted from respiratory or cardiac effects of methadone and too-rapid titration without considering drug accumulation. Make sure you understand drug's pharmacokinetics, and be vigilant during treatment initiation and dosage titration. Caution patients against self-medicating with CNS depressants at start of therapy.

• Prolonged QT intervals and serious arrhythmia (torsades de pointes) have occurred. Most cases involved patients being treated for pain with large, multiple daily doses.

• Federal law requires that when drug is used to treat opioid addiction in detoxification or maintenance programs, it can be dispensed only by treatment programs certified by the Substance Abuse and Mental Health Services Administration and approved by designated state authority. Certified treatment programs must dispense and use drug in oral form only and according to treatment requirements stipulated in Federal Opioid Treatment Standards. Failure to abide by regulations may lead to criminal prosecution, drug seizure, revocation of program approval, and injunction precluding program operation.

Action

Binds to and depresses opiate receptors in spinal cord and CNS, altering perception of and response to pain

Availability

Injection: 10 mg/ml
Oral solution: 5 mg/5 ml, 10 mg/5 ml, 10 mg/ml (concentrate)
Tablets: 5 mg, 10 mg
Tablets (dispersible diskettes): 40 mg

⚡ Indications and dosages

➤ Opioid detoxification

Adults: Initially, 15 to 20 mg/day P.O. to suppress withdrawal. Additional doses may be necessary if symptoms aren't suppressed or if they reappear. Most patients are adequately stabilized on total daily dosage of 40 mg given in single or divided doses; however, some may need higher dosages. When patient is stable for 2 to 3 days, decrease dosage gradually at 2-day intervals. If patient can't tolerate oral doses, give I.M. or subcutaneously (usually at about 25% of total daily P.O. dosage) in two injections.

➤ To maintain opioid abstinence

Adults: Oral dosage highly individualized based on control of abstinence symptoms without respiratory depression or marked sedation. If patient can't tolerate oral doses, give I.M. or subcutaneously (usually at about 25% of total daily P.O. dosage) in two injections.

➤ Chronic and severe pain

Adults: For chronic pain, 2.5 to 10 mg P.O., I.M., or subcutaneously q 3 to 4 hours as needed; adjust dosage and dosing interval as needed. For severe chronic pain (as in terminal illness), 5 to 20 mg P.O. q 6 to 8 hours.

Children: Dosage individualized.

Contraindications

• Hypersensitivity to drug or other opioid agonists

Precautions

Use cautiously in:

• head trauma; severe renal, hepatic, or pulmonary disease; hypothyroidism; adrenal insufficiency; undiagnosed abdominal pain; prostatic hypertrophy; urethral stricture; toxic psychosis; Addison's disease; cor pulmonale; increased intracranial pressure; severe inflammatory bowel disease; severe CNS depression; hypercapnia; seizures; fever; alcoholism

• recent renal or hepatic surgery
• elderly or debilitated patients
• pregnant patients, patients in labor, or breastfeeding patients.

Administration

• Mix dispersible tablets with 120 ml of water or orange juice, citrus Tang, or other acidic fruit beverage.

• Dilute 10 mg/ml of oral solution with water or other liquid to at least 30 ml. In detoxification and maintenance of opioid withdrawal, dilute solution in at least 90 ml of fluid.

• When used parenterally, I.M. route is preferred. Rotate injection sites.

• For detoxification and maintenance, give oral solution only, to reduce potential for parenteral abuse, hoarding, and accidental ingestion.

• Know that patients who can't take oral drugs because of nausea or vomiting during detoxification or maintenance should be hospitalized and given methadone parenterally.

Route	Onset	Peak	Duration
P.O.	30-60 min	1.5-2 hr	4-6 hr
I.M., subcut.	10-20 min	1-2 hr	4-5 hr

Adverse reactions

CNS: amnesia, anxiety, confusion, poor concentration, delirium, delusions, depression, dizziness, drowsiness, euphoria, fever, hallucinations, headache, insomnia, lethargy, lightheadedness, malaise, psychosis, restlessness, sedation, clouded sensorium, syncope, tremor, **seizures, coma**

CV: hypotension, palpitations, edema, bradycardia, **shock, cardiac arrest**

EENT: visual disturbances

GI: nausea, vomiting, constipation, ileus, biliary tract spasm, gastroesophageal reflux, indigestion, dysphagia, dry mouth, anorexia

GU: urinary hesitancy, urinary retention, prolonged labor, difficult ejaculation, erectile dysfunction

---

Reactions in **bold** are life-threatening.   ◀€ Clinical alert

Hematologic: anemia, **leukopenia, thrombocytopenia**
Musculoskeletal: joint pain
Respiratory: depressed cough reflex, hypoventilation, wheezing, **asthma exacerbation, atelectasis, pulmonary edema, bronchospasm, respiratory depression or arrest, apnea**
Skin: urticaria, pruritus, flushing, pallor, diaphoresis
Other: allergic reaction, hiccups, facial or injection site edema, pain, physical or psychological drug dependence, withdrawal symptoms

Interactions

Drug-drug. *Amitriptyline, antihistamines, chloral hydrate, clomipramine, glutethimide, methocarbamol, MAO inhibitors, nortriptyline:* increased CNS and respiratory depression
Anticholinergics: increased risk of severe constipation leading to ileus
Antiemetics, general anesthetics, phenothiazines, sedative-hypnotics, tranquilizers: coma, hypotension, respiratory depression, severe sedation
Ascorbic acid, phenytoin, phosphate, potassium, rifampin: decreased methadone blood level
Cimetidine, fluvoxamine, protease inhibitors: increased analgesia, CNS and respiratory depression
Diuretics: increased diuresis
Hydroxyzine: increased analgesia, CNS depression, and hypotension
Paregoric, loperamide: increased CNS depression, severe constipation
Naloxone: antagonism of methadone's analgesic, CNS, and respiratory effects
Naltrexone: induction or worsening of withdrawal symptoms (when given within 7 days of methadone)
Neuromuscular blockers: increased or prolonged respiratory depression
Drug-diagnostic tests. *Amylase, liver function tests:* increased levels
Drug-behaviors. *Alcohol use:* increased CNS and respiratory depression

Patient monitoring

• Assess patient for relief of severe, chronic pain requiring around-the-clock dosing. Tailor dosage to patient's pain level and drug tolerance.
• Monitor CNS, respiratory, and cardiovascular status.
• Watch for deepening sedation, which may increase with successive doses.
• Evaluate bowel and bladder function. Give laxatives if appropriate.
• Monitor detoxification treatment closely. Short-term detoxification shouldn't exceed 30 days; long-term detoxification, 180 days.
• Assess patient on maintenance therapy for successful rehabilitation. Know that maintenance therapy should be part of comprehensive treatment plan that includes medical, vocational rehabilitative, employment, educational, and counseling services.

Patient teaching

◀€ Instruct patient to promptly report severe adverse reactions.
• Tell patient he may take drug with food if GI upset occurs.
• Tell ambulatory patient to change positions slowly to avoid orthostatic hypotension.
◀€ Caution patient not to discontinue drug abruptly.
• Advise patient to avoid driving and other hazardous activities, because drug may cause drowsiness or dizziness.
• Tell female patient to inform prescriber if she's pregnant or breastfeeding.
• As appropriate, review all other significant and life-threatening adverse reactions and interactions, especially those related to the drugs, tests, and behaviors mentioned above.

methimazole
Apo-Methimazole✤, Tapazole

Pharmacologic class: Thiomidazole derivative
Therapeutic class: Antithyroid drug
Pregnancy risk category D

Action
Directly interferes with thyroid synthesis by preventing iodine from combining with thyroglobulin, leading to decreased thyroid hormone levels

Availability
Tablets: 5 mg, 10 mg

💊 Indications and dosages
➤ Mild hyperthyroidism
Adults and adolescents: Initially, 15 mg P.O. daily in three equally divided doses at approximately 8-hour intervals. For maintenance, 5 to 15 mg/day in equally divided doses at approximately 8-hour intervals.
Children: Initially, 0.4 mg/kg/day in three divided doses at 8-hour intervals. For maintenance, approximately 0.2 mg/kg/day in three divided doses at 8-hour intervals.
➤ Moderate hyperthyroidism
Adults and adolescents: Initially, 30 to 40 mg P.O. daily in three equally divided doses at approximately 8-hour intervals. For maintenance, 5 to 15 mg/day in three equally divided doses at approximately 8-hour intervals.
Children: 0.4 mg/kg/day P.O. as a single dose or in divided doses at 8-hour intervals. For maintenance, approximately 0.2 mg/kg/day as a single dose or in three divided doses at 8-hour intervals.
➤ Severe hyperthyroidism
Adults and adolescents: Initially, 60 mg/day P.O. in three equally divided doses at approximately 8-hour intervals. For maintenance, 5 to 15 mg/day in three equally divided doses at approximately 8-hour intervals.
Children: Initially, 0.4 mg/kg/day P.O. as a single dose or in three divided doses at 8-hour intervals. For maintenance, approximately 0.2 mg/kg/day as a single dose or in three divided doses at 8-hour intervals.

Contraindications
- Hypersensitivity to drug
- Breastfeeding

Precautions
Use cautiously in:
- bone marrow depression
- patients older than age 40
- pregnant patients.

Administration
- Give with meals as needed to reduce GI upset.

Route	Onset	Peak	Duration
P.O.	30-40 min	60 min	2-4 hr

Adverse reactions
CNS: headache, vertigo, paresthesia, neuritis, depression, neuropathy, CNS stimulation
GI: nausea, vomiting, constipation, epigastric distress, ileus, salivary gland enlargement, dry mouth, anorexia
GU: nephritis
Hematologic: thrombocytopenia, agranulocytosis, leukopenia, aplastic anemia
Hepatic: jaundice, **hepatic dysfunction, hepatitis**
Metabolic: hypothyroidism
Musculoskeletal: joint pain, myalgia
Skin: rash, urticaria, skin discoloration, pruritus, erythema nodosum, exfoliative dermatitis, abnormal hair loss
Other: fever, lymphadenopathy, lupus-like syndrome

m

Reactions in **bold** are life-threatening. 🔊 Clinical alert

Interactions

Drug-drug. *Aminophylline, oxtriphylline, theophylline:* decreased clearance of both drugs

Amiodarone, iodine, potassium iodide: decreased response to methimazole

Anticoagulants: altered requirements for both drugs

Beta-adrenergic blockers: altered beta blocker clearance

Digoxin: increased digoxin blood level

Drug-diagnostic tests. *Granulocytes, hemoglobin, platelets, white blood cells:* decreased values

Patient monitoring

• Check for agranulocytosis in patients older than age 40 and in those receiving more than 40 mg/day.

• Assess hematologic studies. Agranulocytosis usually occurs within first 2 months of therapy and is rare after 4 months.

• Monitor thyroid function tests periodically. Once hyperthyroidism is controlled, elevated thyroid-stimulating factor indicates need for dosage decrease.

• Assess liver function tests and check for signs and symptoms of hepatic dysfunction.

• Monitor patient for fever, sore throat, and other evidence of infection as well as for unusual bleeding or bruising.

• Assess patient for signs and symptoms of hypothyroidism, such as hard edema of subcutaneous tissue, drowsiness, slow mentation, dryness or loss of hair, decreased temperature, hoarseness, and muscle weakness.

Patient teaching

• Tell patient to take with meals if GI upset occurs.

• Advise patient to take exactly as prescribed to maintain constant blood level.

• Tell patient to report rash, fever, sore throat, unusual bleeding or bruising, headache, rash, yellowing of skin or eyes, abdominal pain, vomiting, or flu-like symptoms.

• Caution female patient not to breast-feed while taking drug.

• As appropriate, review all other significant and life-threatening adverse reactions and interactions, especially those related to the drugs and tests mentioned above.

methocarbamol

PMS-Methocarbamol♣, Robaxin

Pharmacologic class: Autonomic nervous system agent

Therapeutic class: Skeletal muscle relaxant (centrally acting)

Pregnancy risk category C

Action

Unknown. Thought to depress central perception of pain without directly relaxing skeletal muscles or directly affecting motor endplate or motor nerves.

Availability

Injection: 100 mg/ml in 10-ml ampules, 100 mg/ml in 10-ml vials

Tablets: 500 mg, 750 mg

Indications and dosages

➤ Adjunct in muscle spasms caused by acute, painful musculoskeletal conditions

Adults: Initially, 1.5 g P.O. q.i.d. (up to 8 g/day) for 2 to 3 days, then 4 to 4.5 g/day P.O. in three to six divided doses; or 750 mg P.O. q 4 hours or 1 g P.O. q.i.d. or 1.5 g P.O. t.i.d. If oral dosing isn't feasible or if condition is severe, give 1 to 3 g/day I.M. or I.V. for maximum of 3 days.

Off-label uses

• Tetanus

Contraindications
• Hypersensitivity to drug, its components, or polyethylene glycol (with parenteral form)
• Renal impairment (with parenteral form)

Precautions
Use cautiously in:
• seizure disorders (with parenteral use)
• pregnant or breastfeeding patients
• children (safety not established).

Administration
• For direct I.V. injection, administer slowly. Keep patient supine for 10 to 15 minutes afterward.
• For I.V. infusion, dilute 1 g with up to 250 ml 5% dextrose or 0.9% sodium chloride injection.
• Avoid extravasation; drug is hypertonic.
• Don't give subcutaneously.
• For I.M. use, inject no more than 500 mg (5 ml of 10% injection) into each gluteal area.
• Don't use parenteral form in patients with renal impairment. Polyethylene glycol vehicle may irritate kidneys.
• When giving for tetanus, crush and suspend tablets in water or saline solution, and give via nasogastric tube, if necessary.
• Be aware that drug is usually given as part of regimen that includes rest and physical therapy.

Route	Onset	Peak	Duration
P.O.	30 min	2 hr	Unknown
I.V.	Immediate	End of infusion	Unknown
I.M.	Unknown	Unknown	Unknown

Adverse reactions
CNS: dizziness, light-headedness, drowsiness, syncope, **seizures** (with I.V. use)
CV: bradycardia or hypotension (with I.V. use)

EENT: blurred vision, conjunctivitis, nasal congestion
GI: nausea, GI upset, anorexia
GU: brown, black, or green urine
Musculoskeletal: mild muscle incoordination (with I.V. or I.M. use)
Skin: flushing (with I.V. use), pruritus, rash, urticaria
Other: fever, pain at I.M. injection site, phlebitis at I.V. site, allergic reactions including **anaphylaxis** (with I.M. or I.V. use)

Interactions
Drug-drug. *Antihistamines, CNS depressants (such as opioids, sedative-hypnotics):* additive CNS depression
Drug-diagnostic tests. *Urinary 5-hydroxyindoleacetic acid, urine vanillylmandelic acid:* false elevations
Drug-herbs. *Chamomile, hops, kava, skullcap, valerian:* increased CNS depression
Drug-behaviors. *Alcohol use:* increased CNS depression

Patient monitoring
• Assess for orthostatic hypotension, especially with parenteral use. Keep patient supine for 10 to 15 minutes after I.V. administration.
◀€ Watch for anaphylaxis after I.M. or I.V. administration.
◀€ Stay alert for bradycardia and syncope after I.V. or I.M. dose. As needed and prescribed, give epinephrine, corticosteroids, or antihistamines.
• Monitor I.V. site frequently to prevent sloughing and thrombophlebitis.

Patient teaching
• Tell patient that drug may turn urine brown, black, or green.
• Caution patient to avoid driving and other hazardous activities, because drug may cause drowsiness or dizziness.
• Instruct patient to move slowly when changing position, to avoid dizziness from sudden blood pressure decrease.

Reactions in **bold** are life-threatening.   ◀€ Clinical alert

• As appropriate, review all other significant and life-threatening adverse reactions and interactions, especially those related to the drugs, tests, herbs, and behaviors mentioned above.

methotrexate (amethopterin, MTX)
Apo-Methotrexate✤, Maxtrex⊕, Trexall

methotrexate sodium
Metoject✤⊕, Ratio-Methotrexate Sodium

Pharmacologic class: Antimetabolite, folic acid antagonist
Therapeutic class: Antineoplastic
Pregnancy risk category X

FDA BOXED WARNING

• Give drug under supervision of physician experienced in antimetabolite use.
• Use drug only in life-threatening neoplastic diseases or in patients with severe, recalcitrant, disabling psoriasis that responds inadequately to other therapies.
• Deaths have occurred when drug was used to treat cancer and psoriasis.
• Monitor patient closely for bone marrow, liver, lung, and kidney toxicities. Explain risks involved, and stress importance of adequate follow-up.
• Use caution when giving high-dose regimen for osteosarcoma. (High-dose regimens for other cancers are investigational.)
• Don't use preserved forms and diluents containing preservatives for intrathecal or high-dose therapy.
• Don't give to pregnant women or women with childbearing potential unless medical evidence suggests benefits may outweigh risks. Drug has caused fetal death and congenital anomalies.
• Drug elimination is reduced in patients with renal impairment, ascites, or pleural effusions. Monitor them carefully for toxicity; dosage may need to be reduced or drug may need to be stopped.
• Unexpectedly severe (sometimes fatal) bone marrow suppression and GI toxicity have occurred in patients receiving drug (usually in high doses) concurrently with nonsteroidal anti-inflammatory drugs (NSAIDs).
• Drug causes hepatotoxicity, fibrosis, and cirrhosis, but generally only after prolonged use. Acute liver enzyme elevations are common but usually transient and asymptomatic. Perform periodic liver biopsies in psoriasis patients receiving long-term therapy.
• Potentially dangerous lung disease may arise acutely at any time during therapy. Not always fully reversible, it has occurred at dosages as low as 7.5 mg/week.
• Interrupt therapy for diarrhea and ulcerative stomatitis; otherwise, hemorrhagic enteritis and death from intestinal perforation may occur.
• Malignant lymphomas may occur at low dosages and may not require cytotoxic treatment. Discontinue drug first; if lymphoma doesn't regress, begin appropriate treatment.
• Drug may induce tumor lysis syndrome in patients with rapidly growing tumors.
• Severe and occasionally fatal skin reactions have occurred within days of single or multiple P.O., I.M., I.V., or intrathecal doses. Drug withdrawal has led to recovery.
• Potentially fatal opportunistic infections may occur.
• When given concomitantly with radiation therapy, drug may increase risk of soft-tissue necrosis and osteonecrosis.

Action
Binds to dihydrofolate reductase, interfering with folic acid metabolism and inhibiting DNA synthesis and cellular replication

Availability
Injection: 20-mg, 25-mg, 50-mg, 100-mg, 250-mg, and 1,000-mg vials *(lyophilized powder, preservative-free)*
Tablets: 2.5 mg, 5 mg, 7.5 mg, 10 mg, 15 mg

🄸 Indications and dosages
➣ Acute lymphoblastic leukemia
Adults and children: 3.3 mg/m² P.O. or I.M. daily for 4 to 6 weeks, then 20 to 30 mg/m² P.O. or I.M. weekly in two divided doses; given with corticosteroid. Alternatively, 2.5 mg/kg I.V. q 14 days.
➣ Meningeal leukemia
Adult and children: 12 mg/m² (maximum of 15 mg) intrathecally at intervals of 2 to 5 days, repeated until cerebrospinal fluid cell count is normal
➣ Burkitt's lymphoma
Adults: In stages I and II, 10 to 25 mg P.O. daily for 4 to 8 days; in stage III, combined with other neoplastic drugs. Patients in all stages usually require several courses of therapy, with 7- to 10-day rest periods between courses.
➣ Mycosis fungoides
Adults: 2.5 to 10 mg/day P.O. or 50 mg I.M. q week or 25 mg I.M. twice weekly
➣ Osteosarcoma
Adults: As part of adjunctive regimen with other antineoplastics, initially 12 g/m² I.V. as 4-hour infusion, then 12 to 15 g/m² I.V. in subsequent 4-hour infusions given at weeks 4, 5, 6, 7, 11, 12, 15, 16, 29, 30, 44, and 45 until peak blood level reaches 1,000 micromoles. Leucovorin rescue must start 24 hours after methotrexate infusion begins; if patient can't tolerate oral leucovorin, dose must be given I.M. or I.V. on same schedule.

➣ Trophoblastic tumors (choriocarcinoma, hydatidiform mole)
Adults: 15 to 30 mg P.O. or I.M. daily for 5 days. Repeat course three to five times as required, with rest periods of at least 1 week between courses, until toxic symptoms subside.
➣ Lymphosarcoma (stage III)
Adults: 0.625 to 2.5 mg/kg/day P.O., I.M., or I.V.
➣ Psoriasis
Adults: After test dose, 2.5 mg P.O. at 12-hour intervals for three doses weekly, to a maximum of 30 mg weekly. Alternatively, 10 to 25 mg P.O., I.M., or I.V. as a single weekly dose, to a maximum of 30 mg weekly; decrease dosage when adequate response occurs.
➣ Rheumatoid arthritis
Adults: 7.5 mg P.O. weekly as a single dose or divided as 2.5 mg q 12 hours for three doses weekly. May gradually increase, if needed, up to 20 mg/week; decrease when adequate response occurs.

Dosage adjustment
• Renal or hepatic impairment
• Elderly patients

Off-label uses
• Relapsing-remitting multiple sclerosis
• Refractory Crohn's disease

Contraindications
• Hypersensitivity to drug
• Psoriasis or rheumatoid arthritis in pregnant patients
• Breastfeeding

Precautions
Use cautiously in:
• severe myocardial, hepatic, or renal disease; decreased bone marrow reserve; active infection; hypotension; coma
• elderly patients
• patients with childbearing potential
• young children.

m

Administration

🔊 Be aware that methotrexate is a high-alert drug when used orally for nonchemotherapeutic use.

🔊 Know that patient must be adequately hydrated before therapy and urine must be alkalized using sodium bicarbonate.

• Follow facility policy for handling, preparing, and administering carcinogenic, mutagenic, and teratogenic drugs.

• Be aware that oral administration is preferred. Give oral dose 1 hour before or 2 hours after meals. (Food decreases absorption of tablets and reduces peak blood level.)

• Reconstitute powder for injection with preservative-free solution, such as 5% dextrose solution or 0.9% sodium chloride injection. Reconstitute 20-mg and 50-mg vials to yield a concentration no greater than 25 mg/ml. Reconstitute 1-g vial with 19.4 ml to yield a concentration of 50 mg/ml.

• For high-dose I.V. infusion, dilute in 5% dextrose solution. Administer each 10 mg over 1 minute or by infusion over 30 minutes to 4 hours as directed.

• For intrathecal use, reconstitute immediately before administration, using preservative-free solution (such as 0.9% sodium chloride for injection), to a concentration of 1 mg/ml.

🔊 For intrathecal or high-dose therapy, use preservative-free injection form.

• Avoid I.M. injections if platelet count is below 50,000/mm^3.

🔊 For osteosarcoma, make sure leucovorin rescue is used appropriately in patients receiving high methotrexate doses. Rescue usually starts 24 hours after methotrexate infusion begins.

Route	Onset	Peak	Duration
P.O.	Unknown	1-2 hr	Unknown
I.V.	Immediate	Immediate	Unknown
I.M.	Unknown	0.5-1 hr	Unknown
Intrathecal	Unknown	Unknown	Unknown

Adverse reactions

CNS: malaise, fatigue, drowsiness, dizziness, headache, aphasia, hemiparesis, demyelination, **seizures, leukoencephalopathy, chemical arachnoiditis** (with intrathecal use)

EENT: blurred vision, pharyngitis

GI: nausea, vomiting, stomatitis, hematemesis, melena, GI ulcers, enteritis, gingivitis, pharyngitis, anorexia, **GI bleeding**

GU: hematuria, cystitis, infertility, menstrual dysfunction, defective spermatogenesis, abortion, **tubular necrosis, severe nephropathy, renal failure**

Hematologic: anemia, **leukopenia, thrombocytopenia, severe bone marrow depression**

Hepatic: hepatotoxicity

Metabolic: hyperuricemia, diabetes mellitus

Musculoskeletal: joint pain, myalgia, osteonecrosis, osteoporosis (with long-term use in children)

Respiratory: dry nonproductive cough, **pneumonitis, pulmonary fibrosis, pulmonary interstitial infiltrates**

Skin: pruritus, rash, urticaria, alopecia, painful plaque erosions, photosensitivity

Other: chills, fever, increased susceptibility to infection, **septicemia, anaphylaxis, sudden death**

Interactions

Drug-drug. *Activated charcoal:* decreased blood level of oral or I.V. methotrexate

Folic acid derivatives: antagonism of methotrexate effects

Fosphenytoin, phenytoin: decreased blood levels of these drugs

Hepatotoxic drugs: increased risk of hepatotoxicity

NSAIDs, phenylbutazone, probenecid, salicylates, sulfonamides: increased methotrexate toxicity

---

Oral antibiotics: decreased methotrexate absorption
Penicillin, sulfonamide: increased methotrexate blood level
Procarbazine: increased nephrotoxicity
Theophylline: increased theophylline level
Vaccines: vaccine inefficacy
Drug-diagnostic tests. *Hemoglobin, platelets, red blood cells, white blood cells:* decreased values
Pregnancy tests: false-positive result
Protein-bound iodine, transaminases, uric acid: increased levels
Drug-food. *Any food:* delayed methotrexate absorption and decreased peak blood level
Drug-herbs. *Astragalus, echinacea, melatonin:* interference with methotrexate-induced immunosuppression
Drug-behaviors. *Alcohol use:* increased hepatotoxicity
Sun exposure: photosensitivity

Patient monitoring

• Watch for vomiting, diarrhea, or stomatitis, which may cause dehydration.

◀͟ Know that high-dose therapy may cause nephrotoxicity. Monitor renal function, hydration status, urine alkalization (for pH above 6.5), and methotrexate blood level.

◀͟ Assess for fever, sore throat, bleeding, increased bruising, and other signs and symptoms of hematologic compromise or infection.

• With high-dose or intrathecal therapy, watch for CNS toxicity.

◀͟ Monitor creatinine and methotrexate blood levels 24 hours after therapy starts and then daily. Adjust leucovorin dosage as prescribed.

• Check hematologic studies at least monthly; blood or platelet transfusions may be necessary.

• Monitor liver and kidney function studies every 1 to 3 months. Evaluate uric acid levels.

◀͟ Watch for signs and symptoms of pulmonary toxicity, such as fever, dry nonproductive cough, dyspnea, hypoxemia, and infiltrates on chest X-ray.

• Know that methotrexate exits slowly from third-space compartments (ascites, pleural effusions). Before therapy starts, fluid should be evacuated; during therapy, monitor drug blood level.

Patient teaching

◀͟ Review dosing instructions carefully with patient to avoid toxicity. Tell patient with rheumatoid arthritis or psoriasis to take doses weekly.

• Advise patient to take oral doses 1 hour before or 2 hours after meals.

• Instruct patient to report diarrhea, abdominal pain, clay-colored or black tarry stools, fever, chills, sore throat, unusual bleeding or bruising, sores in or around mouth, cough or shortness of breath, yellowing of skin or eyes, dark or bloody urine, swelling of feet or legs, or joint pain.

• Tell patient to take temperature daily and to report fever or other signs or symptoms of infection.

• Instruct patient to drink 2 to 3 L of fluid each day.

• Advise male patients to use reliable contraception during and for at least 3 months after therapy. Advise female patients to use reliable contraception during and for one ovulatory cycle after therapy; also caution them not to breastfeed.

• Advise patient to avoid sun exposure and to use sunscreen and protective clothing (especially if he has psoriasis).

• Instruct patient to avoid alcohol.

• Tell patient he'll need to undergo blood tests during therapy.

• As appropriate, review all other significant and life-threatening adverse

m

reactions and interactions, especially those related to the drugs, tests, foods, herbs, and behaviors mentioned above.

Route	Onset	Peak	Duration
P.O.	12-24 hr	<3 days	Unknown

Adverse reactions
GI: nausea; vomiting; diarrhea; severe constipation; abdominal distention; cramps; esophageal, gastric, small-intestine, or colonic strictures (with dry form); **GI obstruction**
Other: laxative dependence (with long-term use)

Interactions
Drug-drug. *Antibiotics, digitalis, nitrofurantoin, oral anticoagulants, salicylates, tetracyclines:* decreased absorption and action of these drugs

Patient monitoring
• Assess patient's dietary habits. Consider factors that promote constipation, such as certain diseases and medications.
• Monitor patient for signs and symptoms of esophageal obstruction.
• Evaluate fluid and electrolyte balance in patients using laxatives excessively.

Patient teaching
• Instruct patient to take with a full glass (8 oz) of water.
• Advise patient to prevent or minimize constipation through adequate fluid intake (four to six glasses of water daily), proper diet, increased fiber intake, daily exercise, and prompt response to urge to defecate.
◀€ Instruct patient to report chest pain or pressure, vomiting, and difficulty breathing (possible symptoms of GI obstruction).
• Caution patient not to use drug for more than 1 week without prescriber's approval.
• Inform patient that chronic laxative use may lead to dependence.
• Tell patient to contact prescriber if constipation persists or if rectal bleeding or symptoms of electrolyte

methylcellulose
Celevac⊕, Citrucel, Entrocel✿

Pharmacologic class: Semisynthetic cellulose derivative
Therapeutic class: Bulk laxative
Pregnancy risk category NR

Action
Stimulates peristalsis by promoting water absorption into fecal matter and increasing bulk, resulting in bowel evacuation

Availability
Powder: 105 mg/g, 196 mg/g

🖊 Indications and dosages
➤ Chronic constipation
Adults and children ages 12 and older: Up to 6 g P.O. daily in divided doses of 0.45 to 3 g
Children ages 6 to 11: Up to 3 g P.O. daily in divided doses of 0.45 to 1.5 g

Contraindications
• Signs or symptoms of appendicitis or undiagnosed abdominal pain
• Partial bowel obstruction
• Dysphagia

Precautions
Use cautiously in:
• hepatitis
• intestinal ulcers
• laxative-dependent patients.

Administration
• Give with 8 oz of fluid.
• If patient is receiving maximum daily dosage, give in divided doses to reduce risk of esophageal obstruction.

---

imbalance (muscle cramps, weakness, dizziness) occur.

• As appropriate, review all other significant and life-threatening adverse reactions and interactions, especially those related to the drugs mentioned above.

methyldopa

Aldomet ⊕, Apo-Methyldopa♣, Novomedopa♣, Nu-Medopa♣

methyldopate hydrochloride

Pharmacologic class: Centrally acting antiadrenergic
Therapeutic class: Antihypertensive
Pregnancy risk category B

Action

Stimulates CNS alpha-adrenergic receptors, decreasing sympathetic stimulation to heart and blood vessels. Also reduces arterial pressure and plasma renin.

Availability

Injection: 50 mg/ml in 5- and 10-ml vials
Oral suspension (contains bisulfites): 250 mg/5 ml
Tablets: 125 mg, 250 mg, 500 mg

💊 Indications and dosages

➤ Hypertension
Adults: 250 mg P.O. two to three times daily for 2 days (not to exceed 500 mg/day in divided doses if used with other agents); may increase q 2 days as needed. Usual maintenance dosage is 500 mg to 2 g/day (not to exceed 3 g/day) P.O. in two to four divided doses or 250 to 500 mg I.V. q 6 hours (up to 1 g q 6 hours).

Children: 10 mg/kg/day (300 mg/m²/day) P.O. in two to four divided doses. May increase q 2 days up to 65 mg/kg/day (2 g/m²/day), or 3 g/day in divided doses (whichever is lower) or 5 to 10 mg/kg I.V. q 6 hours; up to 65 mg/kg/day (2 g/m²/day), or 3 g/day in divided doses (whichever is lower).

Contraindications

• Hypersensitivity to drug or its components
• Pheochromocytoma
• Active hepatic disease or history of methyldopa-associated hepatic disorders
• MAO inhibitor use within past 14 days

Precautions

Use cautiously in:
• heart failure, edema, hemolytic anemia, hypotension, severe bilateral cerebrovascular disease
• dialysis patients
• elderly patients
• pregnant or breastfeeding patients.

Administration

◀𝄞 Don't give within 14 days of MAO inhibitors.
• To prepare I.V. infusion, add prescribed dosage to 100 ml 5% dextrose injection. Or administer in 5% dextrose injection in a concentration of 100 mg/10 ml. Give each dose over 30 to 60 minutes.
• Dilute and administer ADD-Vantage vials containing 50 mg/ml according to manufacturer's instructions.
◀𝄞 Don't stop drug therapy abruptly.

Route	Onset	Peak	Duration
P.O.	Unknown	4-6 hr	24-48 hr
I.V.	Unknown	4-6 hr	10-16 hr

Adverse reactions

CNS: headache, asthenia, weakness, dizziness, sedation, decreased mental acuity, depression, paresthesia,

---

parkinsonism, Bell's palsy, involuntary choreoathetotic movements
CV: bradycardia, edema, orthostatic hypotension, **myocarditis**
EENT: nasal congestion
GI: nausea, vomiting, diarrhea, constipation, abdominal distention, colitis, dry mouth, sialadenitis, sore or black tongue, **pancreatitis**
GU: breast enlargement, gynecomastia, failure to ejaculate, erectile dysfunction
Hematologic: eosinophilia, **hemolytic anemia**
Hepatic: hepatitis
Other: fever

Interactions

Drug-drug. *Adrenergics, MAO inhibitors:* excessive sympathetic stimulation
Amphetamines, barbiturates, nonsteroidal anti-inflammatory drugs, phenothiazines, tricyclic antidepressants: decreased antihypertensive effect
Anesthestics, antihypertensives, nitrates: additive hypotension
Ferrous gluconate, ferrous sulfate: decreased methyldopa blood level
Haloperidol: increased haloperidol effects, increased risk of psychoses
Levodopa: additive hypotension and CNS toxicity
Lithium: increased risk of lithium toxicity
Nonselective beta-adrenergic blockers: paradoxical hypertension
Tolbutamide: increased tolbutamide effects
Drug-diagnostic tests. *Alanine aminotransferase, alkaline phosphatase, aspartate aminotransferase, bilirubin, blood urea nitrogen, creatinine, potassium, prolactin, sodium, uric acid:* increased levels
Direct Coombs' test: positive result
Liver function tests: abnormal results
Prothrombin time: prolonged
Drug-herbs. *Capsicum:* reduced antihypertensive effects

Drug-behaviors. *Alcohol use:* increased hypotension

Patient monitoring

• Obtain direct Coombs' test before therapy starts and 6 and 12 months later.
• Monitor periodic blood counts to detect adverse hematologic reactions.
• Monitor liver function tests and check for signs and symptoms of hepatic dysfunction (particularly during first 6 to 12 weeks of therapy).
• Check for edema or weight gain to help determine if diuretic should be added to regimen.
• Monitor blood pressure. Drug tolerance may occur during second and third months of therapy.

Patient teaching

• Tell patient that sedation usually occurs when therapy starts and during dosage titration. To lessen this effect, advise him to begin dosage titration in evening.
◀€ Tell patient not to stop taking drug abruptly.
◀€ Instruct patient to report fever, yellowing of skin or eyes, fatigue, abdominal pain, flulike symptoms, swelling, or significant weight gain.
• Inform patient that urine may darken after exposure to air.
• Advise patient to move slowly when changing position, to avoid dizziness from sudden blood pressure decrease.
• Caution patient to avoid driving and other hazardous activities until effects of drug are known or dosage titration is completed.
• As appropriate, review all other significant and life-threatening adverse reactions and interactions, especially those related to the drugs, tests, herbs, and behaviors mentioned above.

methylergonovine maleate
Methergine

Pharmacologic class: Ergot alkaloid
Therapeutic class: Oxytocic
Pregnancy risk category C

Action
Directly stimulates vascular smooth-muscle contractions in uterus and cervix and decreases bleeding after delivery

Availability
Injection: 0.2 mg/ml
Tablets: 0.2 mg

𝟂 Indications and dosages
➤ Prevention and treatment of post-partum hemorrhage
Adults: 0.2 mg I.M.; repeat q 2 to 4 hours as needed to a total of five doses. In emergencies, 0.2 mg I.V. over 1 minute. After initial I.M. or I.V. dose, 0.2 mg P.O. q 6 to 8 hours for 2 to 7 days; decrease dosage if cramping occurs.

Contraindications
• Hypersensitivity to drug
• Hypertension
• Toxemia
• Pregnancy (except during third stage of labor)

Precautions
Use cautiously in:
• severe hepatic or renal disease, vascular disease, jaundice, sepsis
• patients in second stage of labor.

Administration
• Be aware that drug isn't routinely given I.V. because of risk of severe hypertension and cerebrovascular accident (CVA). Monitor blood pressure and uterine contractions during administration.

• If I.V. use is necessary, give dose over 1 minute. Dose may be diluted in 5 ml of 0.9% sodium chloride injection.
• Be aware that prolonged therapy should be avoided because of ergotism risk.

Route	Onset	Peak	Duration
P.O.	5-10 min	30 min	3 hr
I.V.	Immediate	Unknown	45 min
I.M.	2-5 min	Unknown	3 hr

Adverse reactions
CNS: dizziness, headache, hallucination, **seizures, CVA** (with I.V. use)
CV: hypertension, hypotension, transient chest pain, palpitations, **thrombophlebitis**
EENT: tinnitus, nasal congestion
GI: nausea, vomiting, diarrhea
GU: hematuria
Musculoskeletal: leg cramps
Respiratory: dyspnea
Skin: diaphoresis, rash, allergic reactions
Other: foul taste

Interactions
Drug-drug. *Dopamine, ergot alkaloids, oxytocin, regional anesthetics, vasoconstrictors:* excessive vasoconstriction
Drug-diagnostic tests. *Prolactin:* increased level

Patient monitoring
◀€ Know that if used during third stage of labor, drug increases risk of hemorrhage and infection.
• When giving I.V., closely monitor blood pressure, pulse, uterine contractions, and bleeding.
• Monitor patient for adverse effects.

Patient teaching
• Inform patient and family of reason for using drug, and provide reassurance.
• Tell patient drug may cause nausea, vomiting, dizziness, increased blood pressure, headache, ringing in ears,

---

Reactions in **bold** are life-threatening.   ◀€ Clinical alert

chest pain, or shortness of breath. Advise her to report severe or troublesome symptoms.

• As appropriate, review all other significant and life-threatening adverse reactions and interactions, especially those related to the drugs and tests mentioned above.

methylnaltrexone bromide
Relistor

Pharmacologic class: Mu-opioid receptor antagonist (peripherally acting)
Therapeutic class: Opioid
Pregnancy risk category B

Action
Selectively antagonizes opioid binding at mu-opioid receptors (such as those in GI tract) while having restricted ability to cross blood-brain barrier, thereby decreasing constipating effects of opioids without altering analgesic effects on CNS

Availability
Solution for injection: 12 mg/0.6 ml in single-use vials

🕖 Indications and dosages
➤ Opioid-induced constipation in patients with advanced illness who are receiving palliative care and haven't responded adequately to laxatives

Adults weighing 62 to less than 114 kg (136 to less than 251 lb): 12 mg subcutaneously every other day as needed, but no more frequently than one dose in 24 hours

Adults weighing 38 to less than 62 kg (84 to less than 136 lb): 8 mg subcutaneously every other day as needed, but no more frequently than one dose in 24 hours

Adults weighing outside above ranges: 0.15 mg/kg subcutaneously every other day as needed, but no more frequently than one dose in 24 hours

Dosage adjustment
• Severe renal impairment (creatinine clearance less than 30 ml/minute)

Contraindications
• Known or suspected mechanical GI obstruction

Precautions
Use cautiously in:
• renal impairment
• severe or persistent diarrhea, known or suspected GI tract lesions
• pregnant or breastfeeding patients
• children (safety and efficacy not established).

Administration
• Once drawn into syringe, if drug won't be given immediately, store at ambient room temperature and administer within 24 hours.

Route	Onset	Peak	Duration
P.O.	Rapid	0.5 hr	Unknown

Adverse reactions
CNS: dizziness, malaise
GI: nausea, abdominal pain, diarrhea, flatulence abdominal cramping, **GI perforation**
Other: flushing, pain, diaphoresis

Interactions
None

Patient monitoring
◀≋ Monitor patient for severe or persistent diarrhea and signs and symptoms of GI perforation. Discontinue drug if either occurs.

Patient teaching
• Teach patient who will take drug at home how to prepare and administer it and discard supplies properly.

- Tell patient that if drug won't be administered immediately after it's drawn into syringe, it should be stored at ambient room temperature and administered within 24 hours.
- Inform patient that solution should be clear and colorless to pale yellow.
- Advise patient to stay near toilet facilities after receiving drug.
◀ᚸ Instruct patient to stop taking drug if severe or persistent diarrhea or severe, persistent, or worsening abdominal signs or symptoms occur.
- Tell patient that common side effects include transient abdominal pain, nausea, and vomiting. Advise patient to contact prescriber if these symptoms persist or worsen.
- Instruct patient to stop taking drug if opioid pain medication is discontinued.
- As appropriate, review all other significant adverse reactions mentioned above.

methylphenidate hydrochloride

Apo-Methylphenidate✦, Biphentin✦, Concerta, Concerta XL⊕, Daytrana, Equasym⊕, Equasym XL⊕, Medikinet⊕, Medikinet XL⊕, Metadate CD, Metadate ER, PHL-Methylphenidate✦, PMS-Methylphenidate✦, Ratio-Methylphenidate✦, Ritalin, Ritalin LA, Ritalin-SR

Pharmacologic class: Piperidine derivative
Therapeutic class: CNS stimulant
Controlled substance schedule II
Pregnancy risk category C

FDA | BOXED WARNING

- Give cautiously to patients with history of drug dependence or alcoholism. Chronic abuse can cause marked tolerance and psychological dependence with abnormal behavior. Frank psychotic episodes may occur, especially with parenteral abuse. Supervise carefully during withdrawal from abusive use, as severe depression may occur. Withdrawal after prolonged therapeutic use may unmask symptoms of underlying disorder, possibly requiring follow-up.

Action

Increases release of norepinephrine, which stimulates impulse transmission in respiratory system and CNS. Net effect is increased mental alertness.

Availability

Capsules (extended-release): 10 mg, 20 mg, 30 mg, 40 mg, 50 mg, 60 mg
Solution (oral): 5 mg/5 ml, 10 mg/10 ml
Tablets (chewable): 2.5 mg, 5 mg, 10 mg
Tablets (extended-release): 10 mg, 18 mg, 20 mg, 27 mg, 36 mg, 54 mg
Tablets (prompt-release): 5 mg, 10 mg, 20 mg
Tablets (sustained-release): 20 mg
Transdermal patch: 10 mg/9 hours, 15 mg/9 hours, 20 mg/9 hours, 30 mg/9 hours

🕔 Indications and dosages

➤ Adjunctive treatment of attention deficit hyperactivity disorder (ADHD)
Adults: 5 to 20 mg P.O. (prompt-release tablets) two to three times daily. Or, 20 to 30 mg (oral solution) P.O. daily. Once maintenance dosage is determined, may switch to extended-release.
Children older than age 6: Initially, 5 mg P.O. (prompt-release tablets or oral solution) before breakfast and

m

◀ᚸ Clinical alert

lunch; increase by 5 to 10 mg at weekly intervals, not to exceed 60 mg/day. Once maintenance dosage is determined, may switch to extended-release.

If previous methylphenidate dosage was 10 mg b.i.d. or 20 mg sustained-release, give Ritalin LA 20 mg P.O. once daily. If previous dosage was 15 mg b.i.d., give Ritalin LA 30 mg P.O. once daily. If previous dosage was 20 mg b.i.d. or 40 mg sustained-release, give Ritalin LA 40 mg P.O. once daily. If previous dosage was 30 mg b.i.d. or 60 mg sustained-release, give Ritalin LA 60 mg P.O. once daily.

In all patients, Ritalin-SR or Metadate ER may be prescribed instead of prompt-release tablets when 8-hour dosage of those forms corresponds to titrated 8-hour dosage of prompt-release tablets.

Concerta—
Adults: If new to methylphenidate, initially 18 or 36 mg/day. Increase dosage by 18 mg/day at weekly intervals, not to exceed 72 mg/day. For patients currently using methylphenidate, dosing is based on current dosage regimen and clinical judgment.

Children ages 6 and older who haven't used methylphenidate previously: Initially, 18 mg P.O. once daily in morning; may be titrated weekly up to 54 mg/day

Children ages 6 and older using other methylphenidate forms: 18 mg P.O. once daily in morning if previous dosage was 5 mg two to three times daily, or 20 mg P.O. daily (sustained-release); 36 mg once daily in morning if previous dosage was 10 mg two to three times daily or 40 mg daily (sustained-release); or 54 mg once daily in morning if previous dosage was 15 mg two to three times daily or 60 mg once daily (sustained-release)

Metadate CD—
Children ages 6 and older: Initially, 20 mg once daily; may adjust in weekly increments of 10 to 20 mg, to a maximum of 60 mg/day taken in morning

➤ Adjunctive treatment of attention deficit hyperactivity disorder (ADHD)
Daytrana—
Children ages 6 and older: Apply patch to hip area 2 hours before effect is needed; remove 9 hours after application; titrate dosages as needed.

➤ Narcolepsy
Adults: 10 mg P.O. (Ritalin, Ritalin SR, or Metadate ER) two to three times daily, 30 to 45 minutes before a meal. Some patients may require up to 60 mg daily.

Off-label uses

• Depression in ill, elderly patients (such as those with cerebrovascular accident)
• To enhance analgesia and sedation in patients receiving opioids

Contraindications

• Hypersensitivity to drug or its components, including sucrose (Metadate CD)
• Glaucoma
• Motor tics, Tourette syndrome (or family history of syndrome)
• Marked anxiety, tension, agitation
• Severe hypertension, angina, arrhythmias, heart failure, recent myocardial infarction, hyperthyroidism, thyrotoxicosis
• Concurrent use of halogenated anesthetics
• MAO inhibitor use within past 14 days

Precautions

Use cautiously in:
• hypertension, seizure disorders
• psychosis
• suicidal or homicidal tendencies
• slow growth (children)
• elderly or debilitated patients
• pregnant or breastfeeding patients
• children younger than age 6.

Administration

🔊 Be aware that Metadate CD contains sucrose. Don't give to patients with rare hereditary problems of fructose intolerance, glucose-galactose malabsorption, or sucrase-isomaltase insufficiency.

• Don't give Metadate CD on day of surgery.

• Don't crush extended-release tablets or extended-release trilayer core tablets (Concerta).

• Have patient swallow extended-release capsules (Metadate CD, Ritalin LA) intact; or, if desired, sprinkle entire contents onto small amount (1 tbsp) of applesauce immediately before administration. (However, don't sprinkle Ritalin LA onto warm applesauce because its release properties may be affected.) Give water after patient swallows dose.

• Don't give extended-release tablets to initiate therapy or for daily use until dosage has been titrated using conventional tablets.

• Apply patch immediately after opening pouch to a clean, dry hip area and alternate hips daily.

🔊 Don't give within 14 days of MAO inhibitor use.

• To help prevent insomnia, give last daily dose of conventional tablets several hours before bedtime.

• Discontinue drug periodically in children who have responded to therapy, to assess patient's condition. After withdrawal, improvement may be temporary or permanent.

• Be aware that therapy shouldn't continue indefinitely.

Route	Onset	Peak	Duration
P.O.	Unknown	1-3 hr	4-6 hr
P.O. (extended)	Unknown	Unknown	Up to 8 hr
Transdermal	Unknown	Unknown	Unknown

Adverse reactions

CNS: restlessness, tremor, dizziness, headache, irritability, hyperactivity, insomnia, akathisia, dyskinesia, reversible ischemic neurologic deficit, **toxic psychosis**

CV: hypertension, hypotension, palpitations, tachycardia, Raynaud's phenomenon, **sudden death** (patients with structural cardiac abnormalities or other serious heart problems)

EENT: blurred vision

GI: nausea, vomiting, diarrhea, constipation, cramps, dry mouth, anorexia

Skin: rash, contact sensitization

Other: metallic taste, fever, suppression of weight gain (in children), hypersensitivity reactions, physical or psychological drug dependence, drug tolerance, peripheral coldness

Interactions

Drug-drug. *Anticonvulsants, phenylbutazone, selective serotonin reuptake inhibitors, tricyclic antidepressants, warfarin:* inhibited metabolism and increased effects of these drugs

Guanethidine: antagonism of hypotensive effect

Halogenated anesthetics: sudden blood pressure increase

MAO inhibitors, vasopressors: hypertensive crisis

Drug-food. *Caffeine-containing foods and beverages (such as coffee, cola, chocolate):* increased CNS stimulation

Drug-herbs. *Ephedra (ma huang), caffeine-containing herbs (such as cola nut, guarana, maté):* increased CNS stimulation

Drug-behaviors. *Alcohol use:* additive hypotension

Patient monitoring

• Monitor patient periodically for drug tolerance and psychological dependence.

• Watch for adverse effects. Know that these usually can be controlled by adjusting schedule or dosage.

- Monitor for contact sensitization (erythema accompanied by edema, papules, vesicles) that does not significantly improve within 48 hours or spreads beyond the patch site. Discontinue drug if this occurs.
- Stay alert for tachycardia, abdominal pain, insomnia, anorexia, and weight loss (more common in children).
- Consider periodic hematologic and liver function tests, especially during prolonged therapy.
- Monitor blood pressure, especially in patients with history of hypertension.
- Evaluate child's weight and growth patterns.
- Assess child for tics, which may develop in 15% to 30% of children using drug.

Patient teaching

- Inform patient or parent that last daily dose should be taken several hours before bedtime to avoid insomnia.
- Make sure patient or parent understands how drug should be taken.
- Tell patient taking Concerta not to be concerned if tablet-like substance appears in stool.
- Teach caregiver how to use patch and to make sure that skin is clean, dry, and free of cuts or irritation.
- Tell caregiver not to allow child to use heat sources, such as heating pads or electric blankets, while wearing the patch.
- Instruct caregiver to report redness accompanied by swelling or solid bumps or blisters on the skin that do not significantly improve within 48 hours or spread beyond the patch site.
- Tell caregiver to replace the patch if it falls off, but total wear time for the day should remain 9 hours.
- Advise patient or parent to report insomnia, palpitations, vomiting, fever, or rash.
- Caution patient or parent that continual use may lead to psychological or physical dependence.

- Instruct patient to avoid driving and other hazardous tasks until drug effects are known.
- As appropriate, review all other significant and life-threatening adverse reactions and interactions, especially those related to the drugs, foods, herbs, and behaviors mentioned above.

methylprednisolone
Medrol, Medrone⊕

methylprednisolone acetate
Depo-Medrol, Depo-Medrone⊕, Unimed✤

methylprednisolone sodium succinate
A-Methapred, Solu-Medrol, Solu-Medrone⊕

Pharmacologic class: Glucocorticoid

Therapeutic class: Antiasthmatic, anti-inflammatory (steroidal), immunosuppressant

Pregnancy risk category C

Action

Unclear. Reduces inflammation and prevents edema by stabilizing membranes and reducing permeability of leukocytic cells. Suppresses immune system by interfering with antigen-antibody interactions of macrophages and T cells.

Availability

Solution for injection: 40 mg, 125 mg, 500 mg, 1 g, 2 g
Suspension for injection: 20 mg/ml, 40 mg/ml, 80 mg/ml
Tablets: 2 mg, 4 mg, 8 mg, 16 mg, 24 mg, 32 mg

⬤ Indications and dosages

➤ **Diseases and disorders of endocrine system, collagen, skin, eye, GI tract, respiratory system, or hematologic system; neoplastic diseases; allergies; edema; multiple sclerosis; tuberculous meningitis; trichinosis; rheumatic disorders; osteoarthritis; bursitis; localized inflammatory lesions**

Adults: *Methylprednisolone*—4 to 160 mg P.O. daily in four divided doses, depending on disease or disorder.

Acetate—40 to 120 mg I.M., or 4 to 80 mg by intra-articular or soft-tissue injection, or 20 to 60 mg by intralesional injection (depending on type, size, and location of inflammation); may be repeated at 1 to 5 weeks.

Sodium succinate high-dose therapy—30 mg/kg I.V. over at least 30 minutes. May be repeated q 4 to 6 hours for 48 hours.

Off-label uses

• Lupus nephritis
• *Pneumocystis jiroveci* pneumonia in AIDS patients

Contraindications

• Hypersensitivity to drug or its component
• Systemic fungal infections
• Use in premature infants (with sodium succinate form, which contains benzyl alcohol)

Precautions

Use cautiously in:
• cardiovascular, hepatic, renal, or GI disease; active untreated infections; thromboembolitic tendency; idiopathic thrombocytopenic purpura; osteoporosis; myasthenia gravis; hypothyroidism; glaucoma; ocular herpes simplex; vaccinia or varicella; seizure disorders; metastatic cancer
• pregnant or breastfeeding patients
• children.

Administration

• As needed and prescribed, give prophylactic antacids to prevent peptic ulcers in patients receiving high doses.
• When methylprednisolone acetate is substituted for oral form, know that I.M. dosage should equal oral dosage and should be given once daily.
• Know that methylprednisolone acetate is not for I.V. use. It may be given I.M. or by intra-articular, intralesional, or soft-tissue injection.
• Be aware that methylprednisolone sodium succinate may be given I.M. or I.V. Reconstitute with bacteriostatic water for injection containing 0.9% benzyl alcohol, per manufacturer's instructions.
• In long-term methylprednisolone therapy, alternate-day therapy should be considered.
• For direct I.V. injection, inject each 500-mg dose over 2 to 3 minutes or more. For I.V. infusion, further dilute in compatible I.V. solution (such as 5% dextrose, 0.9% sodium chloride, or 5% dextrose in 0.9% sodium chloride injection) and give over 10 to 20 minutes.
• Maintain patient on lowest effective dosage, to minimize adverse effects.

Route	Onset	Peak	Duration
P.O.	Rapid	2-3 hr	30-36 hr
I.M., I.V. (succinate)	Rapid	Unknown	Unknown
I.M. (acetate)	6-48 hr	4-8 days	1-4 wk

Adverse reactions

CNS: headache, restlessness, nervousness, depression, euphoria, personality changes, psychoses, vertigo, paresthesias, insomnia, adhesive arachnoiditis, conus medullaris syndrome, **increased intracranial pressure, seizures, meningitis**

CV: hypotension, hypertension, **arrhythmias, heart failure, shock,**

---

fat embolism, thrombophlebitis, thromboembolism

EENT: cataracts, glaucoma, increased intraocular pressure, nasal irritation, nasal septum perforation, sneezing, epistaxis, nasopharyngeal or oropharyngeal fungal infection, dysphonia, hoarseness, throat irritation

GI: nausea, vomiting, abdominal distention, rectal bleeding, dry mouth, anorexia, esophageal candidiasis, **esophageal ulcer, peptic ulcer, pancreatitis**

GU: amenorrhea, irregular menses

Respiratory: cough, wheezing, **bronchospasm**

Metabolic: decreased growth (in children), reduced carbohydrate tolerance, diabetes mellitus, hyperglycemia, sodium and fluid retention, hypokalemia, hypocalcemia, cushingoid state (with long-term use), **hypothalamic-pituitary-adrenal suppression** (with systemic use beyond 5 days), **adrenal suppression** (with long-term, high-dose use), **acute adrenal insufficiency** (with abrupt withdrawal)

Musculoskeletal: muscle wasting, osteoporosis, osteonecrosis, tendon rupture, aseptic joint necrosis, muscle pain and weakness, steroid myopathy, spontaneous fractures (with long-term use)

Skin: facial edema, rash, pruritus, urticaria, contact dermatitis, acne, decreased wound healing, bruising, hirsutism, thin and fragile skin, petechiae, purpura, striae, subcutaneous fat atrophy, skin atrophy, acneiform lesions, angioedema

Other: anosmia, bad taste, increased appetite, weight gain (with long-term use), Churg-Strauss syndrome, increased susceptibility to infection, aggravation or masking of infections, impaired wound healing, atrophy at injection site, local pain and burning, irritation, hypersensitivity reaction

Interactions

Drug-drug. *Amphotericin B, mezlocillin, piperacillin, thiazide and loop diuretics, ticarcillin:* additive hypokalemia

Fluoroquinolones: increased risk of tendon rupture

Isoniazid, phenobarbital, phenytoin, rifampin: decreased methylprednisolone efficacy

Ketoconazole: decreased methylprednisolone clearance

Live-virus vaccines: decreased antibody response to vaccine, increased risk of adverse reactions

Nonsteroidal anti-inflammatory drugs: increased risk of adverse GI effects

Oral anticoagulants: altered anticoagulant requirement

Drug-diagnostic tests. *Calcium, potassium, thyroxine, triiodothyronine:* decreased levels

Cholesterol, glucose: increased levels

Nitroblue tetrazolium test for bacterial infection: false-negative result

Drug-herbs. *Echinacea:* increased immune stimulation

Ginseng: immunomodulation

Drug-behaviors. *Alcohol use:* increased risk of gastric irritation and ulcers

Patient monitoring

• Monitor fluid and electrolyte balance, weight, and blood pressure.

• With long-term or high-dose use, assess for cushingoid effects, such as moon face, central obesity, acne, abdominal striae, hypertension, osteoporosis, myopathy, hyperglycemia, fluid and electrolyte imbalances, and increased susceptibility to infection.

🔊 Check for signs and symptoms of steroid-induced psychosis (delirium, euphoria, insomnia, mood swings, personality changes, and depression).

• Monitor growth and development in children on prolonged therapy.

• Know that therapy beyond 6 months increases risk of osteoporosis. Obtain

---

baseline bone density mass, and provide teaching about lifestyle factors (such as weight-bearing exercise, proper diet, moderation of alcohol intake, and smoking cessation) and possible need for calcium, vitamin D, or bisphosphonate therapy.

• With long-term use, withdraw drug gradually.

◀≶ After dosage reduction or drug withdrawal, monitor patient for signs and symptoms of adrenal insufficiency.

Patient teaching

• Tell patient to take with food to minimize GI upset.

• Advise patient on chronic therapy to have periodic eye exams and to carry medical identification that states he's taking drug.

• Inform patient that drug increases risk for infection. Urge him to avoid exposure to people with infections such as measles and chickenpox. Tell him to contact prescriber if exposure occurs.

• Advise patient to report unusual weight gain, swelling, muscle weakness, black tarry stools, vomiting of blood, menstrual irregularities, sore throat, fever, or infection.

◀≶ Tell patient to immediately report signs or symptoms of adrenal insufficiency (including fatigue, appetite loss, nausea, vomiting, diarrhea, weight loss, weakness, and dizziness) after dosage reduction or drug withdrawal.

• Advise diabetic patient to monitor blood glucose level carefully.

• As appropriate, review all other significant and life-threatening adverse reactions and interactions, especially those related to the drugs, tests, herbs, and behaviors mentioned above.

metoclopramide hydrochloride

Apo-Metoclop✣, Gastrobid⊕, Gastromax⊕, Maxeran✣, Maxolon⊕, Maxolon SR⊕, Metozolv ODT, Nu-Metoclopramide✣, Paramax⊕, PMS-Metoclopramide, Reglan

Pharmacologic class: Dopamine antagonist

Therapeutic class: Antiemetic, GI stimulant

Pregnancy risk category B

FDA | BOXED WARNING

• Drug can cause tardive dyskinesia, a serious movement disorder that's often irreversible. Risk of developing tardive dyskinesia increases with duration of treatment and total cumulative dose.

• Discontinue drug in patients who develop signs or symptoms of tardive dyskinesia, which has no known treatment. In some patients, signs and symptoms may lessen or resolve after drug is stopped.

• Avoid using metoclopramide for longer than 12 weeks except in rare cases in which potential benefit outweighs risk of developing tardive dyskinesia.

Action

Blocks dopamine receptors by disrupting CNS chemoreceptor trigger zone, increasing peristalsis and promoting gastric emptying

Availability

Injection: 5 mg/ml
Solution: 5 mg/5 ml
Solution (concentrated): 10 mg/ml
Tablets: 5 mg, 10 mg

m

Tablets (orally disintegrating): 5 mg, 10 mg

✒ Indications and dosages

➤ To prevent chemotherapy-induced vomiting

Adults: 1 to 2 mg/kg I.V. 30 minutes before chemotherapy, then q 2 hours for two doses, then q 3 hours for three additional doses

➤ To facilitate small-bowel intubation; radiologic examination when delayed gastric emptying interferes

Adults and children older than age 14: 10 mg I.V. as a single dose

Children ages 6 to 14: 2.5 to 5 mg I.V. as a single dose

Children younger than age 6: 0.1 mg/kg I.V. as a single dose

➤ Diabetic gastroparesis

Adults: 10 mg P.O. 30 minutes before meals and at bedtime for 2 to 8 weeks. If patient can't tolerate P.O. doses, give same dosage I.V. or I.M.

➤ Gastroesophageal reflux

Adults: 10 to 15 mg P.O. 30 minutes before meals and at bedtime for up to 12 weeks. For prevention, single dose of 20 mg (some patients may respond to doses as small as 5 mg).

➤ Prevention of postoperative nausea and vomiting

Adults: 10 to 20 mg I.M. near end of surgical procedure. Repeat dose q 4 to 6 hours, as needed.

Dosage adjustment
• Renal impairment

Off-label uses
• Hiccups

Contraindications
• Hypersensitivity to drug
• Pheochromocytoma
• Parkinson's disease
• Suspected GI obstruction, perforation, or hemorrhage
• History of seizure disorders

Precautions
Use cautiously in:
• diabetes mellitus, renal dysfunction
• history of depression
• elderly patients
• pregnant or breastfeeding patients
• children.

Administration
• Mix oral solution with water, juice, carbonated beverage, or semisolid food (such as applesauce or pudding) just before administration.
• Remove orally disintegrating tablets with dry hands immediately before administering. After removing, place tablet on patient's tongue, where it will dissolve in approximately 1 minute. Tell patient to swallow saliva.
• Give I.M. or direct I.V. without further dilution.
• Administer low doses (10 mg or less) by direct I.V. injection slowly over 2 minutes. (Rapid injection may cause intense anxiety and restlessness followed by drowsiness.)
• For I.V. infusion, dilute with 50 ml of 5% dextrose in 0.9% sodium chloride solution, 5% dextrose in 0.45% sodium chloride solution, or lactated Ringer's solution. Infuse over at least 15 minutes.

Route	Onset	Peak	Duration
P.O.	30-60 min	Unknown	1-2 hr
I.V.	1-3 min	Immediate	1-2 hr
I.M.	10-15 min	Unknown	1-2 hr

Adverse reactions
CNS: drowsiness, restlessness, anxiety, depression, irritability, fatigue, lassitude, insomnia, tardive dyskinesia, parkinsonian-like reactions, extrapyramidal reactions, akathisia, dystonia
CV: hypertension, hypotension, **arrhythmias, neuroleptic malignant syndrome**
GI: nausea, constipation, diarrhea, dry mouth
GU: gynecomastia

Interactions

Drug-drug. *Anticholinergics, opioids:* antagonism of metoclopramide's GI motility effect

Antidepressants, antihistamines, other CNS depressants (such as opioids, sedative-hypnotics): additive CNS depression

Cimetidine, digoxin: decreased blood levels of these drugs

General anesthetics: exaggerated hypotension

Haloperidol, phenothiazines: increased risk of extrapyramidal reactions

Levodopa: decreased metoclopramide efficacy

MAO inhibitors: increased catecholamine release

Drug-diagnostic tests. *Aldosterone, prolactin:* increased levels

Drug-behaviors. *Alcohol use:* increased blood alcohol level, increased CNS depression

Patient monitoring

• Monitor blood pressure during I.V. administration.

• Stay alert for depression and other adverse CNS effects.

◀€ Watch for extrapyramidal reactions, which usually occur within first 24 to 48 hours of therapy. To reverse these symptoms, give diphenhydramine 50 mg I.M. or benztropine 1 to 2 mg I.M., as prescribed.

• Check for development of parkinsonian-like symptoms, which may occur within first 6 months of therapy and usually subside within 2 to 3 months after withdrawal.

◀€ With long-term use, assess patient for tardive dyskinesia and discontinue drug if signs or symptoms of tardive dyskinesia develop. Avoid treatment for longer than 12 weeks in all but rare cases in which therapeutic benefit outweighs risk of developing tardive dyskinesia.

◀€ Monitor patient closely for signs and symptoms of neuroleptic malignant syndrome (hyperthermia, muscle rigidity, altered consciousness, and evidence of autonomic instability [irregular pulse or blood pressure, tachycardia, diaphoresis, and cardiac arrhythmias]); immediately discontinue drug if these symptoms occur.

• In diabetic patient, stay alert for gastric stasis. Insulin dosage may need to be adjusted.

Patient teaching

• Tell patient to take 30 minutes before meals.

• Tell patient taking orally disintegrating tablets to remove tablet with dry hands immediately before use. Instruct patient to place tablet on tongue, where it will dissolve in approximately 1 minute, and then swallow saliva.

◀€ Instruct patient to report involuntary movements of face, eyes, or limbs; muscle rigidity; altered consciousness; irregular pulse or blood pressure; rapid or irregular heartbeats; or excessive sweating.

• Caution patient to avoid driving and other hazardous activities until drug's effects are known.

• As appropriate, review all other significant and life-threatening adverse reactions and interactions, especially those related to the drugs, tests, and behaviors mentioned above.

metolazone
Metenix⊕, Zaroxolyn

Pharmacologic class: Thiazide-like diuretic

Therapeutic class: Diuretic, antihypertensive

Pregnancy risk category B

Action

Inhibits electrolyte reabsorption from ascending loop of Henle and decreases reabsorption of sodium and potassium in distal renal tubules, increasing plasma osmotic pressure and promoting diuresis

Availability
Tablets: 2.5 mg, 5 mg, 10 mg

Indications and dosages
➤ Hypertension
Adult: 2.5 to 5 mg P.O. daily.
➤ Edema caused by heart failure or renal disease
Adults: 5 to 20 mg P.O. daily

Contraindications
• Hypersensitivity to drug
• Hepatic coma or precoma
• Anuria

Precautions
Use cautiously in:
• severe hepatic or renal impairment, gout, hyperparathyroidism, glucose tolerance abnormalities, fluid or electrolyte imbalances, bipolar disorders
• elderly patients
• pregnant or breastfeeding patients
• children (safety not established).

Administration
• Give in morning to avoid frequent nighttime urination.
• Discontinue drug before parathyroid function tests are performed.
• Be aware that metolazone is the only thiazide-like diuretic that may cause diuresis in patients with glomerular filtration rates below 20 ml/minute.

Route	Onset	Peak	Duration
P.O.	1 hr	2 hr	12-24 hr

Adverse reactions
CNS: drowsiness, lethargy, vertigo, paresthesia, weakness, headache, fatigue
CV: chest pain, hypotension, palpitations, **venous thrombosis, arrhythmias**
GI: nausea, vomiting, bloating, cramping, anorexia, **pancreatitis**
GU: polyuria, nocturia, erectile dysfunction, decreased libido
Hematologic: aplastic anemia, leukopenia, agranulocytosis
Hepatic: hepatitis
Metabolic: dehydration, hypercalcemia, hypomagnesemia, hyponatremia, hypophosphatemia, hypovolemia, hyperglycemia, hyperuricemia, **hypokalemia, hypochloremic alkalosis**
Musculoskeletal: muscle cramps
Skin: photosensitivity, rashes
Other: chills

Interactions
Drug-drug. *Amphotericin B, corticosteroids, mezlocillin, piperacillin, ticarcillin:* additive hypokalemia
Antigout drugs: increased uric acid level
Antihypertensives, nitrates: additive hypotension
Digoxin: increased risk of digoxin toxicity
Lithium: decreased lithium excretion, increased risk of lithium toxicity
Drug-diagnostic tests. *Bilirubin, calcium, cholesterol, creatinine, low-density lipoproteins, triglycerides, uric acid:* increased levels
Blood glucose, urine glucose: increased levels in diabetic patients
Magnesium, potassium, protein-bound iodine, sodium, urinary calcium: decreased levels
Drug-food. *Any food:* increased metolazone absorption
Drug-herbs. *Aloe, cascara sagrada, senna:* increased risk of hypokalemia
Drug-behaviors. *Sun exposure:* increased risk of photosensitivity

Patient monitoring
• Monitor baseline and periodic electrolyte, blood urea nitrogen, glucose, and uric acid levels.
• Evaluate blood pressure regularly.
◀€ Watch for signs and symptoms of hypokalemia, which may necessitate potassium supplements, potassium-rich diet, or potassium-sparing diuretic. Hypokalemia is particularly

dangerous to patients who are on digitalis or have had ventricular arrhythmias.

• Assess patient for fluid and electrolyte imbalances.

Patient teaching

• Advise patient to take in morning to avoid frequent nighttime urination.

• Tell patient he may take with food or milk to prevent GI upset.

◀€ Instruct patient to report muscle pain, weakness, or cramps; nausea; vomiting; diarrhea; dizziness; restlessness; excessive thirst; fatigue; drowsiness; increased pulse; or irregular heart beats.

• Inform patient that drug may cause gout attacks. Advise him to report sudden joint pain.

• Instruct patient to use sunscreen and protective clothing to avoid photosensitivity.

• As appropriate, review all other significant and life-threatening adverse reactions and interactions, especially those related to the drugs, tests, foods, herbs, and behaviors mentioned above.

---

metoprolol succinate
Toprol-XL

metoprolol tartrate
Apo-Metoprolol✦, Betaloc✦⊕, Betaloc Durules✦, Dom-Metoprolol✦, Gen-Metoprolol✦, Lopresor⊕, Lopresor SR✦, Lopressor, Novo-Metoprol✦, Nu-Metop✦, PHL-Metoprolol, PMS-Metoprolol-L✦, Sandoz Metoprolol✦

Pharmacologic class: Beta-adrenergic blocker (selective)

Therapeutic class: Antihypertensive, antianginal

Pregnancy risk category C

• Exacerbations of angina pectoris and myocardial infarction (MI) may follow abrupt withdrawal of some beta blockers. When discontinuing long-term therapy, particularly in patients with ischemic heart disease, reduce dosage gradually over 1 to 2 weeks and monitor patient carefully. If angina worsens markedly or acute coronary insufficiency develops, reinstate drug promptly (at least temporarily) and take other appropriate measures to manage unstable angina. Caution patient not to interrupt or discontinue therapy without prescriber's advice. Because coronary artery disease is common and may be unrecognized, it may be prudent not to discontinue drug abruptly even in patients treated only for hypertension.

Action
Blocks stimulation of beta₁ (myocardial) adrenergic receptors, usually without affecting beta₂ (pulmonary, vascular, uterine) adrenergic receptor sites

Availability
Injection (tartrate): 1 mg/ml
Tablets: 50 mg, 100 mg
Tablets (extended-release, succinate): 25 mg, 50 mg, 100 mg, 200 mg

Indications and dosages
➤ Hypertension

Adults: 50 to 100 mg P.O. daily as a single dose or in two divided doses (conventional tablets) or once daily (extended-release tablets). May be increased q 7 days as needed, up to 450 mg/day (tartrate) or 400 mg (succinate extended-release).

➤ Angina pectoris

Adults: 100 mg P.O. daily as a single dose or in two divided doses (conventional tablets) or once daily

---

(extended-release tablets). May be increased q 7 days as needed, up to 400 mg.

➤ MI

Adults: Three bolus injections of 5 mg I.V. given at 2-minute intervals. If patient tolerates I.V. dose, give 50 mg P.O. 15 minutes after last I.V. dose, and continue P.O. doses q 6 hours for 48 hours. For maintenance, 100 mg P.O. b.i.d. If patient doesn't tolerate full I.V. dose, give 25 to 50 mg P.O. (depending on degree of intolerance), starting 15 minutes after last I.V. dose or when clinical condition allows; discontinue drug if patient shows severe intolerance. As late treatment, 100 mg P.O. b.i.d. when clinical condition allows, continued for at least 3 months.

➤ Symptomatic heart failure

Adults: 25 mg P.O. daily (extended-release tablets) in patients with NYHA Class II heart failure. Dosage may be doubled q 2 weeks, up to 200 mg/day or until highest tolerated dosage is reached. For more severe heart failure, start with 12.5 mg P.O. daily.

Off-label uses
• Ventricular arrhythmias, tachycardia
• Tremors
• Anxiety

Contraindications
• Sinus bradycardia, heart block greater than first degree, cardiogenic shock, overt cardiac failure (with Lopressor used for hypertension or angina)
• Heart rate below 45 beats/minute, second- or third-degree heart block, significant first-degree heart block; systolic pressure below 100 mm Hg; or moderate-to-severe cardiac failure (when Lopressor is used for MI)
• Hypersensitivity to drug or its components, severe bradycardia, heart block greater than first degree, cardiogenic shock, decompensated cardiac failure, sick sinus syndrome (unless permanent pacemaker is in place) (with Toprol-XL)

Precautions
Use cautiously in:
• renal or hepatic impairment, pulmonary disease, diabetes mellitus, thyrotoxicosis
• MAO inhibitor use within past 14 days
• pregnant or breastfeeding patients
• children (safety not established).

Administration
• Give metoprolol tartrate with or immediately after meals, because food enhances its absorption.
• Know that succinate extended-release tablets are scored and can be divided. However, tablet or half-tablet should be swallowed whole and not crushed or chewed.
• For I.V. administration, give each dose undiluted by direct injection over at least 1 minute.

Route	Onset	Peak	Duration
P.O.	15 min	1 hr	6-12 hr
P.O. (extended)	15 min	6-12 hr	24 hr
I.V.	Immediate	20 min	5-8 hr

Adverse reactions
CNS: fatigue, weakness, anxiety, depression, dizziness, drowsiness, insomnia, memory loss, mental status changes, nervousness, nightmares
CV: orthostatic hypotension, peripheral vasoconstriction, bradycardia, **heart failure, pulmonary edema**
EENT: blurred vision, stuffy nose
GI: nausea, vomiting, constipation, diarrhea, flatulence, gastric pain, heartburn, dry mouth
GU: urinary frequency, erectile dysfunction, decreased libido
Hepatic: hepatitis
Metabolic: hyperglycemia, **hypoglycemia**
Respiratory: wheezing, **bronchospasm**
Musculoskeletal: back pain, joint pain
Skin: rash
Other: drug-induced lupus syndrome

Interactions

Drug-drug. *Amphetamines, ephedrine, epinephrine, norepinephrine, phenylephrine, pseudoephedrine:* unopposed alpha-adrenergic stimulation (excessive hypertension, bradycardia)
Antihypertensives, nitrates: additive hypotension
Digoxin: additive bradycardia
Dobutamine, dopamine: reduced cardiovascular benefits of these drugs
General anesthetics, phenytoin (I.V.), verapamil: additive myocardial depression
Insulin, oral hypoglycemics: altered efficacy of these drugs
MAO inhibitors: hypertension
Drug-diagnostic tests. *Alanine aminotransferase, alkaline phosphatase, aspartate aminotransferase, blood urea nitrogen, glucose, lactate dehydrogenase, lipoproteins, potassium, triglycerides, uric acid:* increased levels
Drug-food. *Any food:* enhanced drug absorption
Drug-behaviors. *Acute alcohol ingestion:* additive hypotension
Cocaine use: unopposed alpha-adrenergic stimulation (excessive hypertension, bradycardia)

Patient monitoring

• Measure blood pressure closely when starting therapy and titrating dosage. Once patient stabilizes, measure blood pressure every 3 to 6 months.
• Monitor blood pressure and pulse before I.V. administration. If patient is hypotensive or has bradycardia, consult prescriber before giving dose.
• Watch for orthostatic hypotension in at-risk patients, particularly the elderly.
• Assess glucose levels in diabetic patient. Be aware that drug may mask signs and symptoms of hypoglycemia.
• Monitor for signs and symptoms of hyperthyroidism. Know that drug may mask these. Reduce dosage gradually in hyperthyroid patients.

🔊 When discontinuing drug, reduce dosage gradually over 1 to 2 weeks.

Patient teaching

• Advise patient to take with or immediately after meals.
• Tell patient that extended-release tablets are scored and can be divided, but that he should swallow tablets or half-tablets whole and not crush or chew them.
🔊 Advise patient with heart failure to report signs or symptoms of worsening condition, including weight gain and increasing shortness of breath.
• Caution patient to avoid driving and other hazardous activities until drug effects are known.
• Instruct patient to notify health care providers (including dentists) that he is taking drug before having surgery.
• As appropriate, review all other significant and life-threatening adverse reactions and interactions, especially those related to the drugs, tests, foods, and behaviors mentioned above.

metronidazole

Acea , Anabact ✦, Apo-Metronidazole ✦, Elyzol ✦, Flagyl, Flagyl ER, Flagystatin ✦, Florazole ER, MetroCream, MetroGel, MetroGel-Vaginal, MetroLotion, Metrolyl ✦, Metrosa ✦, Metrotop ✦, Metrozol ✦, Neutratop ✦, Nidagel ✦, Noritate, Novo-Nidazol ✦, PMS-Metronidazole ✦, Rosasol ✦, Rozex, Zidoval ✦, Zyomet ✦

---

metronidazole hydrochloride
Flagyl IV

Pharmacologic class: Nitroimidazole derivative
Therapeutic class: Anti-infective, antiprotozoal
Pregnancy risk category B

Action
Disturbs DNA synthesis in susceptible bacterial organisms

Availability
Capsules: 375 mg
Powder for injection: 5 mg/ml, 500-mg vials
Premixed injection: 500 mg/100 ml
Tablets: 250 mg, 500 mg
Tablets (extended-release): 750 mg
Topical cream, topical gel: 0.75% in 28.4-g tubes
Topical lotion: 0.75% in 59-ml bottle
Vaginal gel: 0.75% (37.5 mg/5-g applicator) in 70-g tubes

ⓘ Indications and dosages
➤ Trichomoniasis
Adults: 2 g P.O. as a single dose or in two 1-g doses given on same day. Alternatively, 500 mg P.O. b.i.d. for 7 days.
➤ Bacterial infections
Adults: Initially, 15 mg/kg I.V., followed by 7.5 mg/kg I.V. q 6 hours, not to exceed 4 g/day for 7 to 10 days
➤ Amebiasis
Adults: 750 mg P.O. q 8 hours for 5 to 10 days
➤ Amebic liver abscess

Adults: 500 to 750 mg P.O. t.i.d. for 5 to 10 days. If drug can't be given orally, administer 500 mg I.V. q 6 hours for 10 days.
Children: 35 to 50 mg/kg/day P.O. in three divided doses for 10 days, to a maximum of 750 mg/dose
➤ Bacterial vaginosis
Adults: In nonpregnant patients, 750 mg/day P.O. (extended-release) for 7 days or 5 g of 0.75% vaginal gel b.i.d. for 5 days. In pregnant patients, 250 mg P.O. t.i.d. for 7 days.
➤ Perioperative prophylaxis in colorectal surgery
Adults: Initially, 15 mg/kg I.V. infusion over 30 to 60 minutes, completed 1 hour before surgery; if necessary, 7.5 mg/kg I.V. infusion over 30 to 60 minutes at 6 and 12 hours after initial dose
➤ Rosacea
Adults: Rub a thin layer of topical lotion, gel, or cream onto entire affected area morning and evening. Improvement should occur within 3 weeks.

Contraindications
• Hypersensitivity to drug, other nitroimidazole derivatives, or parabens (topical form only)
• First-trimester pregnancy in patients with trichomoniasis

Precautions
Use cautiously in:
• severe hepatic impairment
• history of blood dyscrasias, seizures, or other neurologic problems
• breastfeeding patients
• children.

Administration
• Reconstitute powder for injection by adding 4.4 ml of sterile or bacteriostatic water for injection, 0.9% sodium chloride injection, or bacteriostatic sodium chloride injection to 500-mg vial. Further dilute resulting

concentration (100 mg/ml) in 0.9% sodium chloride injection, 5% dextrose injection, or lactated Ringer's injection solution to a concentration of 8 mg/ml or less. Infuse each I.V. dose over 1 hour.

• Be aware that for I.V. injection, drug need not be diluted or neutralized.

• Don't use equipment containing aluminum to reconstitute or transfer reconstituted solution to diluent; solution may turn reddish-brown.

• Don't interchange vaginal gel with topical gel, cream, or lotion.

Route	Onset	Peak	Duration
P.O.	Rapid	1-3 hr	8 hr
P.O. (extended)	Rapid	Unknown	Up to 24 hr
I.V.	Rapid	End of infusion	6-8 hr
Topical	Unknown	6-12 hr	Unknown
Vaginal	Unknown	6-12 hr	12 hr

Adverse reactions

CNS: dizziness, headache, ataxia, vertigo, incoordination, insomnia, fatigue
EENT: rhinitis, sinusitis, pharyngitis
GI: nausea, vomiting, diarrhea, abdominal pain, furry tongue, glossitis, dry mouth, anorexia
GU: dysuria, dark urine, incontinence
Hematologic: leukopenia
Skin: rash, urticaria, burning, mild skin dryness, skin irritation, transient redness (with topical forms)
Other: unpleasant or metallic taste, superinfection, phlebitis at I.V. site

Interactions

Drug-drug. *Azathioprine, fluorouracil:* increased risk of leukopenia
Cimetidine: decreased metronidazole metabolism, increased risk of toxicity
Disulfiram: acute psychosis and confusion
Lithium: increased lithium blood level
Phenobarbital: increased metronidazole metabolism, decreased efficacy

Warfarin: increased warfarin effects
Drug-diagnostic tests. *Alanine aminotransferase, aspartate aminotransferase, lactate dehydrogenase:* altered levels
Drug-behaviors. *Alcohol use:* disulfiram-like reaction

Patient monitoring

• Monitor I.V. site. Avoid prolonged use of indwelling catheter.

• Evaluate hematologic studies, especially in patients with history of blood dyscrasias.

Patient teaching

• Advise patient to take drug with food if it causes GI upset. However, instruct him to take extended-release tablets 1 hour before or 2 hours after meals.

• Tell patient with trichomoniasis to refrain from sexual intercourse or to have male partner wear a condom to prevent reinfection. Explain that asymptomatic sex partners should be treated simultaneously.

• Advise patient to report fever, sore throat, bleeding, or bruising.

• Inform patient that drug may cause metallic taste and may discolor urine deep brownish-red.

• Tell patient using topical form to clean area thoroughly with mild cleanser before use and then wait 15 to 20 minutes before applying drug. Tell her she may apply cosmetics to skin after applying drug; with topical lotion, instruct her to let skin dry at least 5 minutes before applying cosmetics.

• Tell female patient to consult prescriber if she is pregnant or plans to become pregnant.

• As appropriate, review all other significant and life-threatening adverse reactions and interactions, especially those related to the drugs, tests, and behaviors mentioned above.

m

---

micafungin sodium
Mycamine

Pharmacologic class: Semisynthetic lipopeptide (echinocandin)
Therapeutic class: Antifungal
Pregnancy risk category C

Action
Inhibits synthesis of 1,3-β-D-glucan, an essential component of fungal cell walls

Availability
Powder for reconstitution for infusion (lyophilized): 50-mg and 100-mg single-use vials

ⓘ Indications and dosages
➤ Candidemia, acute disseminated candidiasis, *Candida* peritonitis and abscesses
Adults: 100 mg daily by I.V. infusion over 1 hour for 15 days (range, 10 to 47 days)
➤ Esophageal candidiasis
Adults: 150 mg daily by I.V. infusion over 1 hour for 15 days (range, 10 to 30 days)
➤ Prophylaxis of *Candida* infections in patients undergoing hematopoietic stem-cell transplantation
Adults: 50 mg daily by I.V. infusion over 1 hour for 19 days (range, 6 to 51 days)

Contraindications
• Hypersensitivity to drug, its components, or other echinocandins

Precautions
Use cautiously in:
• renal or hepatic disease
• pregnant or breastfeeding patients
• children (safety and efficacy not established).

Administration
• Administer by I.V. infusion only.
• Reconstitute with 5 ml normal saline solution injection (without bacteriostatic agent) or dextrose 5% injection added to 50-mg or 100-mg vial to yield approximately 10 mg/ml or 20 mg/ml, respectively.
• To minimize excessive foaming, gently dissolve powder by swirling vial. Don't shake vigorously.
• Protect diluted solution from light.
• Add reconstituted solution to 100 ml normal saline solution or 100 ml dextrose 5% before infusing.
• Flush existing I.V. line with normal saline solution before infusing drug.
• Infuse over 1 hour. Be aware that more rapid infusion increases risk of histamine-mediated reactions (rash, pruritus, facial swelling, vasodilation).
🔊 If serious hypersensitivity (anaphylaxis or anaphylactoid) reaction occurs, immediately discontinue infusion and provide appropriate interventions.

Route	Onset	Peak	Duration
P.O.	Unknown	Unknown	Unknown

Adverse reactions
CNS: headache, insomnia, fatigue, rigors, dizziness, anxiety
CV: vasodilation, hypotension, hypertension, bradycardia, tachycardia, phlebitis, flushing, **atrial fibrillation**
EENT: epistaxis
GI: nausea, vomiting, diarrhea, constipation, abdominal pain, dyspepsia, anorexia, decreased appetite
Hematologic: anemia, **thrombocytopenia, aggravated anemia, neutropenia, febrile neutropenia**
Metabolic: fluid retention, **fluid overload**
Musculoskeletal: back pain
Respiratory: pneumonia, cough, dyspnea
Skin: rash, pruritus, decubitus ulcers, erythema

🍁 Canada   ⊕ UK   ☣ Hazardous drug   ⊗ High-alert drug

Other: facial swelling, injection-site reaction, infection, bacteremia, fever, mucosal inflammation, peripheral edema, **sepsis, septic shock, hypersensitivity reaction** (including **anaphylaxis, anaphylactoid reactions,** and **shock**)

Interactions
Drug-drug. *Itraconazole, nifedipine, sirolimus:* increased risk of toxicity
Drug-diagnostic tests. *ALP, ALT, AST, sodium:* increased levels
Calcium, glucose, magnesium, potassium: decreased levels
Liver function tests: abnormal

Patient monitoring
• If patient develops clinical or laboratory evidence of hematologic abnormalities, abnormal liver function tests, or electrolyte disorders, monitor closely for signs or symptoms that these conditions are getting worse. Risks against benefits of continuing therapy should be considered.

Patient teaching
• Instruct patient to contact prescriber if unusual symptoms develop or if pre-existing symptoms persist or get worse.
• As appropriate, review all other significant and life-threatening adverse reactions and interactions, especially those related to the drugs and tests mentioned above.

midazolam hydrochloride
Apo-Midazolam ✦, Hypnovel ⊕

Pharmacologic class: Benzodiazepine
Therapeutic class: Anxiolytic, sedative-hypnotic, adjunct for general anesthesia induction
Controlled substance schedule IV
Pregnancy risk category D

• I.V. form is linked to respiratory depression and respiratory arrest, especially when used for sedation in non-critical care settings. In some cases, where this wasn't recognized promptly and treated effectively, death or hypoxic encephalopathy resulted. Use I.V. form only in hospital or ambulatory care setting that provides continuous monitoring of respiratory and cardiac function. Ensure immediate availability of resuscitative drugs and equipment as well as personnel trained in their use and skilled in airway management. For deeply sedated pediatric patient, dedicated individual should monitor patient throughout procedure.
• Patients who are debilitated, older than age 60, or receiving concurrent opioids or other CNS depressants require lower dosages. Slowly titrate initial dose and all subsequent doses; give over at least 2 minutes and allow 2 or more additional minutes to fully evaluate sedative effect. In pediatric patients, calculate dosage on mg/kg basis, and titrate slowly.
• Don't give by rapid injection to neonates. Severe hypotension and seizures may result.

Action
Unknown. Thought to suppress CNS stimulation at limbic and subcortical levels by enhancing the effects of gamma-aminobutyric acid, an inhibitory neurotransmitter.

Availability
Injection: 1 mg/ml, 5 mg/ml
Syrup: 2 mg/ml

⚕ Indications and dosages
➢ To induce general anesthesia
Adults younger than age 55: 0.3 to 0.35 mg/kg I.V. over 20 to 30 seconds if patient hasn't received premedication, or 0.15 to 0.35 mg/kg (usual dosage of

m

0.25 mg/kg) I.V. over 20 to 30 seconds if patient has received premedication. Wait 2 minutes to evaluate effect. Additional increments of 25% of initial dosage may be needed to complete induction.

➤ Continuous infusion to initiate sedation

Adults: When rapid sedation is required, give loading dose of 0.01 to 0.05 mg/kg I.V. slowly; repeat dose q 10 to 15 minutes until adequate sedation occurs. To maintain sedation, infuse at initial rate of 0.02 to 0.10 mg/kg/hour (1 to 7 mg/hour). Adjust infusion rate as needed.

➤ Preoperative sedation, anxiolysis, and amnesia

Adults: 0.07 to 0.08 mg/kg I.M. 30 minutes to 1 hour before surgery. For I.V. administration in healthy adults younger than age 60, give initial dose of 1 mg and titrate slowly to effect. Some patients may respond adequately to 1-mg dose. Don't give more than 2.5 mg over a 2-minute period. Total dosage above 5 mg is rarely necessary. Wait at least 2 minutes after additional doses to assess effect.

➤ Anxiolysis and amnesia before diagnostic, therapeutic, and endoscopic procedures or anesthesia induction

Children: 0.25 to 0.5 mg/kg P.O. as a single dose. Maximum dosage is 20 mg.

Dosage adjustment
• Elderly patients
• Children or neonates

Contraindications
• Hypersensitivity to drug, its components, or other benzodiazepines
• Acute closed-angle glaucoma
• Allergy to cherries (syrup preparation)

Precautions
Use cautiously in:
• pulmonary disease, heart failure, renal impairment, severe hepatic impairment
• obese pediatric patients
• elderly or debilitated patients
• pregnant or breastfeeding patients
• children and neonates.

Administration
🔊 Keep oxygen and resuscitation equipment at hand in case severe respiratory depression occurs.
• Inject I.M. deep into large muscle mass.
• Know that drug may be mixed in same syringe as meperidine, atropine, scopolamine, or morphine.
• Dilute concentrate for I.V. infusion to 0.5 mg/ml using dextrose 5% in water or normal saline solution. Infuse over at least 2 minutes; then wait at least 2 minutes before giving second dose. Be aware that excessive dosage or rapid I.V. delivery may cause severe respiratory depression.
• Give oral form with liquid, but never with grapefruit juice.

Route	Onset	Peak	Duration
P.O.	10-20 min	45-60 min	2-6 hr
I.V.	1.5-5 min	Rapid	2-6 hr
I.M.	15 min	15-60 min	2-6 hr

Adverse reactions
CNS: headache, oversedation, drowsiness, agitation and excitement (in children)
CV: hypotension, irregular pulse, bradycardia, **arrhythmias, cardiac arrest**
GI: nausea, vomiting
Respiratory: decreased respiratory rate, hiccups, **apnea, respiratory arrest**
Other: pain and tenderness at injection site

Interactions
Drug-drug. *CNS depressants (such as some antidepressants, antihistamines, barbiturates, opioids, tranquilizers), respiratory depressants:* potentiation of CNS effects of these drugs
Diltiazem, verapamil: increased midazolam blood level
Erythromycin: decreased midazolam clearance

Hormonal contraceptives: prolonged midazolam half-life
Rifampin: decreased midazolam blood level
Theophylline: increased sedative effect of midazolam
Drug-food. *Grapefruit juice:* increased bioavailability of oral midazolam
Drug-herbs. *Chamomile, kava, skullcap, valerian:* increased CNS depression
Drug-behaviors. *Alcohol use:* potentiation of midazolam effects

Patient monitoring
• Monitor vital signs, ECG, respiratory status, and oxygen saturation.
• Assess neurologic status closely, especially in pediatric patient.
• Watch for nausea and vomiting.

Patient teaching
• Advise patient that drug causes perioperative amnesia.
• If patient will use oral drug at home, instruct him to take it with liquid but never grapefruit juice.
• Caution patient to avoid driving and other hazardous activities until he knows how drug affects concentration and alertness.
• Tell female patient to inform prescriber is she is pregnant or breastfeeding.
• As appropriate, review all other significant and life-threatening adverse reactions and interactions, especially those related to the drugs, foods, herbs, and behaviors mentioned above.

midodrine hydrochloride
Amatine✱, Apo-Midodrine✱, Orvaten, ProAmatine

Pharmacologic class: Alpha$_1$-adrenergic agonist
Therapeutic class: Antihypotensive, vasopressor
Pregnancy risk category C

FDA BOXED WARNING

• Drug can markedly increase supine blood pressure, and should be used in patients whose lives are considerably impaired despite standard clinical care. Indication for its use in treating symptomatic orthostatic hypotension rests mainly on an increase in systolic pressure measured 1 minute after standing. Currently, drug's clinical benefits (mainly improved ability to perform activities of daily living) haven't been verified.

Action
Forms active metabolite, desglymidodrine, an alpha$_1$-adrenergic agonist that activates alpha-adrenergic receptors in arteriolar and venous vasculature. This effect increases vascular resistance and ultimately raises blood pressure.

Availability
Tablets: 2.5 mg, 5 mg

⟋ Indications and dosages
➢ Symptomatic orthostatic hypotension
Adults: 10 mg P.O. t.i.d. during daytime hours with patient in upright position. Give first dose when patient arises in morning, second dose at midday, and third dose in late afternoon.

Dosage adjustment
• Renal impairment

Contraindications
• Severe coronary artery disease or organic heart disease
• Acute renal disease, urinary retention
• Pheochromocytoma
• Thyrotoxicosis
• Persistent, excessive supine hypertension

Precautions
Use cautiously in:
• renal or hepatic impairment, diabetes mellitus, vision problems
• pregnant or breastfeeding patients.

Reactions in **bold** are life-threatening. ◀€ Clinical alert

Administration

• Don't give within 4 hours of bedtime.

Route	Onset	Peak	Duration
P.O.	Rapid	1-2 hr	Unknown

Adverse reactions

CNS: paresthesia
CV: vasodilation, bradycardia, **supine hypertension**
GI: abdominal pain, dry mouth
GU: urinary retention, frequency, or urgency
Skin: rash, pruritus, piloerection
Other: chills, increased pain

Interactions

Drug-drug. *Alpha- and beta-adrenergic blockers, cardiac glycosides, steroids:* increased risk of bradycardia, atrioventricular block
Alpha-adrenergic blockers, fludrocortisone: increased risk of supine hypertension

Patient monitoring

• Monitor supine and sitting blood pressures closely. Report marked rise in supine blood pressure.
• Stay alert for paresthesias.
• Monitor kidney function studies and fluid intake and output. Watch for urinary frequency, urgency, or retention.

Patient teaching

◀€ Instruct patient to take while in upright position.
• Tell patient to take first dose as soon as he arises for the day, second dose at midday, and third dose in late afternoon (before 6 P.M.). Stress that doses must be taken at least 3 hours apart. Advise patient not to take drug after dinner or within 4 hours of bedtime.
◀€ Instruct patient to promptly report symptoms of supine hypertension (pounding in ears, blurred vision, headache).
• Caution patient to avoid driving and other hazardous activities until he knows how drug affects concentration, vision, and alertness.
• As appropriate, review all other significant and life-threatening adverse reactions and interactions, especially those related to the drugs mentioned above.

mifepristone (RU-486)

Korlym, Mifegyne✚,
Mifeprex

Pharmacologic class: Synthetic steroid
Therapeutic class: Antiprogestational agent, abortifacient
Pregnancy risk category NR

FDA | BOXED WARNING

• Rare cases of serious and sometimes fatal infections and bleeding have followed spontaneous, surgical, and medical abortions, including after mifepristone use. Before starting drug, inform patient of risk of these serious events and discuss medication guide and patient agreement. Ensure that patient knows whom to call and what to do, including going to emergency department (ED) if none of provided contacts are reachable; if she experiences sustained fever, severe abdominal pain, prolonged heavy bleeding, or syncope; or if she has abdominal pain or discomfort or general malaise (including weakness, nausea, vomiting, or diarrhea) more than 24 hours after taking drug.
• Patients with serious bacterial infections and sepsis may present without fever, bacteremia, or significant pelvic examination findings after abortion.

Rare deaths have occurred in patients without fever, with or without abdominal pain, but with leukocytosis with marked left shift, tachycardia, hemoconcentration, and general malaise. Maintain high index of suspicion to rule out serious infection and sepsis.

• Advise patient to take medication guide with her if she visits ED or another health care provider who didn't prescribe drug, so provider will be aware that patient is undergoing medical abortion.

• Be aware that pregnancy must be excluded before initiation of treatment with Korlym. Patients must avoid pregnancy during treatment and for 1 month after therapy ends by using a nonhormonal, medically acceptable method of contraception; if patient has had a surgical sterilization, no additional contraception is needed. Pregnancy must also be excluded if treatment is interrupted for more than 14 days in females of childbearing potential.

Action
Antagonizes progesterone receptor sites, inhibiting activity of endogenous and exogenous progesterone and stimulating uterine contractions, which causes fetus to separate from placental wall

Availability
Tablets: 200 mg, 300 mg

🕖 Indications and dosages
➤ Termination of intrauterine pregnancy through day 49 of pregnancy
Adults: On day 1, mifepristone 600 mg P.O. as a single dose. On day 3, misoprostol 400 mcg P.O. (unless abortion has been confirmed).
➤ Hyperglycemia secondary to hypercortisolism in adults with endogenous Cushing's syndrome who have type 2 diabetes or glucose

intolerance and have failed surgery or aren't candidates for surgery
Adults: Initially, 300 mg P.O. daily; increase based on clinical response and tolerability in 300-mg increments to a maximum of 1,200 mg daily. Don't exceed 20 mg/kg/day.

Dosage Adjustment
• Renal impairment (Korlym)
• Mild to moderate hepatic impairment (Korlym)
• Concurrent use of strong P450 CYP3A inhibitors (Korlym)

Contraindications
• Hypersensitivity to drug, misoprostol, or other prostaglandins
• Confirmed or suspected ectopic pregnancy or adnexal mass
• Chronic adrenal failure
• Bleeding disorders
• Concurrent anticoagulant therapy or long-term corticosteroid therapy
• Presence of intrauterine device (IUD)
• Inherited porphyrias
• Concomitant treatment with systemic corticosteroids for serious medical conditions or illnesses (Korlym)
• Concurrent use of simvastatin or lovastatin and CYP3A substrates with narrow therapeutic range (Korlym)
• History of unexplained vaginal bleeding or endometrial hyperplasia with atypia or endometrial carcinoma (Korlym)
• Pregnancy (Korlym)

Precautions
Use cautiously in:
• cardiovascular, respiratory, renal, or hepatic disorders; hypertension; type 1 diabetes mellitus; anemia; jaundice; seizure disorder; cervicitis; infected endocervical lesions; acute vaginitis; uterine scarring
• hypokalemia, underlying heart conditions including heart failure and coronary vascular disease (Korlym)

m

- hemorrhagic disorders or concurrent use of anticoagulants (Korlym)
- concurrent use of QT interval-prolonging drugs, patients with potassium channel variants resulting in long QT interval (avoid Korlym use)
- concurrent use of drugs metabolized by CYP2B6 and moderate CYP3A inhibitors (Korlym)
- concurrent use of CYP3A inducers (such as rifampin, rifabutin, rifapentin, phenobarbital, phenytoin, carbamazepine, and St. John's wort) or hormonal contraceptives (avoid use)
- concurrent use of strong CYP3A inhibitors (use Korlym with extreme caution and only when necessary; limit dosage to 300 mg)
- concurrent use of drugs metabolized by CYP2C8/2C9 (use lowest dose of CYP2C8/2C9 substrates when used with Korlym)
- breastfeeding patients (Korlym)
- children (Korlym; safety and efficacy not established).

Administration

- Before giving dose for termination of pregnancy, make sure patient doesn't have an IUD in place.
- Correct hypokalemia before starting Korlym.
- Give for termination of pregnancy only in health care facility under supervision of health care provider qualified to assess pregnancy stage and rule out ectopic pregnancy.
- Administer with fluids, but not with grapefruit juice.
- When giving for termination of pregnancy, confirm pregnancy termination 14 days after initial dose.

Route	Onset	Peak	Duration
P.O.	Rapid	90 min	11 days

Adverse reactions

CNS: dizziness, fainting, headache, weakness, fatigue, insomnia, asthenia, anxiety, syncope, rigors

CV: hypertension, **QT-interval prolongation** (Korlym)
EENT: sinusitis
GI: nausea, vomiting, diarrhea, abdominal cramping, dyspepsia
GU: vaginitis, leukorrhea, uterine cramping, pelvic pain; endometrial hypertrophy, cystic dilatation of endometrial glands, vaginal bleeding (Korlym); **uterine hemorrhage**
Hematologic: anemia
Metabolic: hypokalemia, adrenal insufficiency (Korlym)
Musculoskeletal: leg pain, back pain, arthralgia
Skin: rash (Korlym)
Other: viral infections; fever, decreased appetite, peripheral edema, opportunistic infections (Korlym)

Interactions

Drug-drug. *CYP2C8/2C9 substrates:* increased plasma concentrations of these drugs
CYP3A inducers (such as carbamazepine, phenobarbital, phenytoin, rifabutin, rifampin, rifapentin): decreased mifepristone concentrations
CYP3A substrates with narrow therapeutic range (such as cyclosporine, dihydroergotamine, ergotamine, fentanyl, pimozide, quinidine, sirolimus, tacrolimus): increased exposure of these drugs and effects
Drugs metabolized by CYP2B6 (bupropion, efavirenz): significantly increased exposure of these drugs
Drugs metabolized by CYP3A (lovastatin, simvastatin): increased risk of myopathy and rhabdomyolysis
Glucocorticoids: antagonized glucocorticoid effect
Moderate CYP3A inhibitors (such as amprenavir, aprepitant, atazanavir, ciprofloxacin, darunavir/ritonavir, diltiazem, erythromycin, fluconazole, imatinib, verapamil), strong CYP3A inhibitors (such as amprenavir, boceprevir, clarithromycin, conivaptan, fosamprenavir, indinavir, itraconazole,

---

lopinavir, mibefradil, nefazodone, nelfinavir, posaconazole, ritonavir, saquinavir, telaprevir, telithromycin, voriconazole): increased plasma mifepristone concentration

Oral contraceptives: decreased oral contraceptive effectiveness

Drug-diagnostic tests. *Hematocrit, hemoglobin:* decreased values

Potassium: decreased level

Red blood cells: decreased count

Drug-food. *Grapefruit juice:* increased mifepristone blood level and effects

Drug-herbs. *St. John's wort:* decreased mifepristone blood level and effects

Patient monitoring

• Assess vital signs, breath sounds, and bowel sounds.

• Monitor uterine contractions and type and amount of vaginal bleeding.

• Evaluate CBC.

• Monitor serum potassium level 1 to 2 weeks after starting or increasing Korlym dosage and periodically thereafter.

🔊 Closely monitor patient taking Korlym for signs and symptoms of adrenal insufficiency, including weakness, nausea, increased fatigue, hypotension, and hypoglycemia. If adrenal insufficiency is suspected, discontinue drug immediately and administer glucocorticoids without delay. May resume Korlym at a lower dosage after resolution of adrenal insufficiency.

• Be aware that patients with endogenous Cushing's syndrome are at risk for opportunistic infections such as *Pneumocystis jiroveci* pneumonia while taking Korlym. Monitor patient for respiratory distress shortly after Korlym initiation. Initiate appropriate diagnostic tests and treat *P. jiroveci* as indicated.

Patient teaching

When used for termination of pregnancy:

• After administration, tell patient she will need to return in 48 hours for a prostaglandin drug or to verify pregnancy termination.

• Tell patient she will have contractions for 3 or more hours after receiving drug and that vaginal bleeding may last 9 to 16 days.

🔊 Instruct patient to contact prescriber if she has persistent or extremely heavy vaginal bleeding, extreme fatigue, or orthostatic hypotension.

Caution patient that vaginal bleeding does not prove that complete abortion has occurred. Tell her she will need follow-up appointment 2 weeks later to verify pregnancy termination.

• Inform patient that she is at risk for pregnancy right after abortion is complete. Encourage appropriate contraceptive decision.

When used for hyperglycemia secondary to hypercortisolism in patients with endogenous Cushing's syndrome:

🔊 Instruct patient to recognize and report signs and symptoms of hypokalemia, respiratory infections, and adrenal insufficiency.

• Advise patient not to take drug with grapefruit juice and not to use herbal products without consulting prescriber.

When used for either indication:

• As appropriate, review all other significant and life-threatening adverse reactions and interactions, especially those related to the drugs, tests, foods, and herbs mentioned above.

miglitol
Glyset

Pharmacologic class: Alphaglucosidase inhibitor

Therapeutic class: Hypoglycemic

Pregnancy risk category B

Action

Inhibits alpha-glucosidases, which convert oligosaccharides and disaccharides to glucose. This inhibition causes blood glucose reduction (especially in postprandial hyperglycemia).

Availability

Tablets: 25 mg, 50 mg, 100 mg

⬤ Indications and dosages

➤ Adjunct to diet in non-insulin-dependent (type 2) diabetes mellitus or combined with a sulfonylurea when diet plus either miglitol or a sulfonylurea alone doesn't control hyperglycemia

Adults: 25 mg P.O. t.i.d. with first bite of each main meal. After 4 to 8 weeks, may increase to 50 mg P.O. t.i.d. After 3 months, adjust dosage further based on glycosylated hemoglobin (HbA1c) level, to a maximum of 100 mg P.O. t.i.d.

Contraindications

• Hypersensitivity to drug or its components

• Insulin-dependent (type 1) diabetes mellitus, diabetic ketoacidosis

• Chronic intestinal disorder associated with marked digestive or absorptive disorders or conditions that may deteriorate due to increased gas formation

• Inflammatory bowel disease, colonic ulceration, partial intestinal obstruction, or predisposition to intestinal obstruction

Precautions

Use cautiously in:

• significant renal impairment (safety not established)

• fever, infection, trauma, stress

• pregnant or breastfeeding patients

• children (safety not established).

Administration

• Give with first bite of three main meals.

Route	Onset	Peak	Duration
P.O.	Unknown	2-3 hr	Unknown

Adverse reactions

GI: abdominal pain, diarrhea, flatulence
Skin: rash

Interactions

Drug-drug. *Digestive enzyme preparations (such as amylase), intestinal absorbents (such as charcoal):* reduced miglitol efficacy
Digoxin, propranolol, ranitidine: decreased bioavailability of these drugs
Drug-diagnostic tests. *Serum iron:* below-normal level
Drug-food. *Carbohydrates:* increased diarrhea

Patient monitoring

• Monitor CBC, blood glucose, and HBA1c levels.

• Watch for hyperglycemia or hypoglycemia, especially if patient also takes insulin or oral sulfonylureas.

Patient teaching

• Instruct patient to take drug three times daily with first bite of three main meals.

• Advise patient to take drug as prescribed. If appropriate, tell him he may need insulin during periods of increased stress, infection, or surgery.

• Teach patient about diabetes. Stress importance of proper diet, exercise, weight control, and blood glucose monitoring.

• Inform patient that sucrose (as in table sugar) and fruit juice don't effectively treat miglitol-induced hypoglycemia. Advise him to use dextrose or glucagon instead to raise blood glucose level quickly.

• Tell patient drug may cause abdominal pain, diarrhea, and gas. Reassure him that these effects usually subside after several weeks.

• As appropriate, review all other significant adverse reactions and interactions, especially those related to the drugs, tests, and foods mentioned above.

milnacipran hydrochloride
Savella

Pharmacologic class: Selective serotonin and norepinephrine reuptake inhibitor
Therapeutic class: Antidepressant
Pregnancy risk category C

FDA | BOXED WARNING

- Drug causes increased risk of suicidal ideation, thinking, and behavior in children, adolescents, and young adults taking antidepressants for major depressive disorder and other psychiatric disorders.
- Drug isn't approved for use in children.

Action
Unknown

Availability
Tablets: 12.5 mg, 25 mg, 50 mg, 100 mg

ⓘ Indications and dosages
➤ Management of fibromyalgia
Adults: Initially, 12.5 mg P.O. on day 1; increase to 100 mg daily over 1 week by giving 12.5 mg b.i.d. on days 2 and 3; then 25 mg b.i.d. on days 4 to 7; after day 7, give 50 mg b.i.d.; may increase to 100 mg b.i.d. based on patient response

Dosage adjustment
- Severe renal impairment

Contraindications
- Monoamine oxidase (MAO) inhibitor use within past 14 days
- Uncontrolled narrow-angle glaucoma

Precautions
Use cautiously in:
- severe hepatic or moderate renal impairment
- seizures, significant hypertension, cardiac disease
- history of mania, patients with depressive symptoms, those at risk for suicide
- controlled narrow-angle glaucoma
- concomitant use of serotonin precursors (such as tryptophan) and selective serotonin reuptake inhibitors and selective norepinephrine reuptake inhibitors (use not recommended)
- concomitant use of drugs that increase blood pressure or heart rate
- concomitant use of I.V. digoxin
- concomitant use of nonsteroidal anti-inflammatory drugs (NSAIDs), aspirin, or other drugs that affect coagulation
- significant alcohol use or chronic hepatic disease (avoid use)
- obstructive uropathies (in males)
- elderly patients
- pregnant or breastfeeding patients
- children (safety and efficacy not established).

Administration
- Check blood pressure and pulse rate before starting drug.
- Administer with or without food.
- ◀ Don't give concurrently or within 14 days of MAO inhibitor therapy; allow 5 days after stopping drug before starting MAO inhibitor.

Route	Onset	Peak	Duration
P.O.	Unknown	Unknown	Unknown

Adverse reactions
CNS: headache, tension headache, migraine, dizziness, insomnia, paresthesia, hypoesthesia, tremor, anxiety, fatigue, irritability, somnolence,

m

depression, stress, **seizures, neuroleptic malignant syndrome, suicidal behavior or ideation** (especially in child or adolescent)

CV: increased heart rate, hypertension, tachycardia, palpitations, peripheral edema

EENT: blurred vision

GI: nausea, vomiting, constipation, dry mouth, abdominal pain, decreased appetite, diarrhea, dyspepsia, gastroesophageal reflux disease, flatulence, abdominal distention

GU: dysuria; ejaculation disorder; ejaculation failure; erectile dysfunction; decreased libido; prostatitis; scrotal, testicular, and urethral pain; testicular swelling; urinary hesitation and retention; decreased urine flow (males); urinary tract infection, cystitis

Hematologic: bleeding

Hepatic: fulminant hepatitis (rare)

Metabolic: hyponatremia, hypercholesterolemia

Respiratory: upper respiratory tract infection, dyspnea

Skin: rash, pruritus

Other: hot flushes, flushing, hyperhidrosis, chest pain or discomfort, chills, weight loss or gain, pyrexia, injury, poisoning, procedural complications, abnormal taste, night sweats, **serotonin syndrome**

Interactions

Drug-drug. *Catecholamines (such as epinephrine, norepinephrine):* increased risk of paroxysmal hypertension, cardiac arrhythmias

Clonidine: inhibited clonidine antihypertensive effects

Digoxin (I.V.): increased risk of adverse hemodynamic effects (such as orthostatic hypotension, tachycardia)

Drugs that affect coagulation (such as *aspirin, NSAIDS):* increased risk of bleeding

Drugs that affect serotonergic neurotransmitter system (such as antipsychotics, dopamine antagonists, lithium, triptans, tryptophan, and inhibitors of serotonin uptake [such as citalopram, escitalopram, fluoxetine, fluvoxamine, paroxetine, sertraline]): increased risk of serotonin syndrome or neuroleptic malignant syndrome–like reactions, increased risk of hypertension, coronary artery vasoconstriction

MAO inhibitors (such as isocarboxazid, phenelzine, tranylcypromine): increased risk of potentially fatal reactions (hyperthermia, myoclonus, autonomic instability)

Other centrally acting drugs: increased risk of CNS effects

Drug-diagnostic tests. *Alanine aminotransferase, aspartate aminotransferase, cholesterol:* increased levels

Sodium: decreased level

Drug-behaviors. *Substantial alcohol use:* aggravation of preexisting hepatic disease

Patient monitoring

◀€ Monitor patient's mental status carefully. Stay alert for mood changes and indications of suicidal ideation, especially in child or adolescent.

◀€ Discontinue drug and provide appropriate treatment if signs and symptoms of serotonin syndrome or neuroleptic malignant syndrome occur.

◀€ Discontinue drug if signs and symptoms of hepatic dysfunction occur; don't restart drug unless another cause can be determined.

• Consider discontinuing drug if symptomatic hyponatremia occurs.

• Monitor blood pressure and pulse rate periodically throughout treatment; consider discontinuing drug if sustained increases persist.

• Monitor liver function tests.

Patient teaching

• Instruct patient to take drug with or without food but that taking with food may increase tolerability.

◀€ Advise patient (and significant other as appropriate) to monitor patient's mental status carefully and to immediately report increased depression or suicidal thoughts or behavior (especially in child or adolescent).

◀€ Instruct patient to immediately report signs and symptoms of serotonin syndrome (from shivering and diarrhea to severe symptoms such as muscle rigidity, fever, and seizures).

◀€ Instruct patient to immediately report signs and symptoms of neuroleptic malignant syndrome, such as fever, muscle rigidity, altered mental status (including catatonic signs), irregular pulse or blood pressure, rapid heartbeat, and excessive sweating.

◀€ Tell patient to immediately report signs and symptoms of liver problems (such as yellowing of skin or eyes).

◀€ Caution patient not to stop taking drug suddenly and that drug must be tapered.

• Instruct patient to report headache, difficulty concentrating, memory impairment, weakness, or unsteadiness.

• Tell patient to monitor blood pressure and pulse rate regularly and report sustained increases.

• Tell patient to report signs and symptoms of bleeding, including easy bruising.

• Advise patient to avoid alcohol use while taking drug.

• Advise patient to consult prescriber before taking other prescription or nonprescription drugs, especially aspirin or NSAIDs.

• Caution patient to avoid driving and other hazardous activities until drug's effects on concentration and alertness are known.

• As appropriate, review all other significant and life-threatening adverse reactions and interactions, especially those related to the drugs, tests, and behaviors mentioned above.

milrinone lactate
Apo-Milrinone✦

Pharmacologic class: Bipyridine phosphodiesterase inhibitor
Therapeutic class: Inotropic
Pregnancy risk category C

Action
Increases cellular levels of cyclic adenosine monophosphate, causing inotropic action that relaxes vascular smooth muscle and increases myocardial contractility

Availability
Injection: 1 mg/ml in 10-, 20-, and 50-ml vials
Injection (premixed): 200 mcg/ml in dextrose 5% in water (D_5W)

Indications and dosages
➤ Heart failure
Adults: Initially, 50 mcg/kg I.V. bolus given slowly over 10 minutes, followed by continuous I.V. infusion of 0.375 to 0.75 mcg/kg/minute. Don't exceed total daily dosage of 1.13 mg/kg.

Dosage adjustment
• Renal impairment

Contraindications
• Hypersensitivity to drug

Precautions
Use cautiously in:
• atrial flutter or fibrillation, supraventricular and ventricular arrhythmias, renal impairment, electrolyte abnormalities, decreased blood pressure, severe aortic or pulmonic valvular disease, acute phase of myocardial infarction (not recommended), electrolyte abnormalities, abnormal blood digoxin level

m

- elderly patients
- pregnant or breastfeeding patients
- children (safety and efficacy not established).

Administration

- Dilute 1 mg/ml solution with half-normal saline solution, normal saline solution, or D_5W per manufacturer's instructions.

◀፤ Don't administer through same I.V. line as furosemide or torsemide (precipitate will form).

- Deliver I.V. slowly over 10 minutes.
- Expect to titrate infusion rate depending on response.

Route	Onset	Peak	Duration
I.V.	5-15 min	1-2 hr	3-6 hr

Adverse reactions

CNS: headache
CV: hypotension, chest pain, angina, **ventricular or supraventricular arrhythmias, ventricular tachycardia or fibrillation**

Interactions

None significant

Patient monitoring

- Monitor vital signs and ECG. Watch closely for ventricular arrhythmias, sustained tachycardia, and fibrillation.
- Assess cardiovascular status closely. Stay alert for complaints of chest pain.

◀፤ Stop drug and contact prescriber immediately if patient's systolic pressure drops 30 mm Hg or more.

Patient teaching

- Instruct patient to change position slowly, to avoid light-headedness or dizziness from hypotension.
- As appropriate, review all other significant and life-threatening adverse reactions.

minocycline hydrochloride

Aknemin ⊕, Dentomycin ⊕, Dom-Minocycline❋, Dynacin, Gen-Minocycline❋, Minocin, Novo-Minocycline❋, PMS-Minocycline❋, Ratio-Minocycline❋, Riva-Minocycline❋, Sandoz Minocycline❋, Sebomin ⊕, Sebren ⊕, Solodyn

Pharmacologic class: Tetracycline
Therapeutic class: Anti-infective
Pregnancy risk category D

Action

Binds reversibly to 30S ribosome, inhibiting bacterial protein synthesis

Availability

Capsules: 50 mg, 75 mg, 100 mg
Capsules (pellet-filled): 50 mg, 100 mg
Microspheres (sustained-release): 1 mg
Suspension: 50 mg/5 ml
Tablets: 50 mg, 75 mg, 100 mg

ⓘ Indications and dosages

➤ Infections caused by susceptible organisms
Adults: Initially, 200 mg P.O. then 100 mg P.O. q 12 hours or 50 mg P.O. q 6 hours
Children ages 8 and older: 4 mg/kg P.O. followed by 2 mg/kg q 12 hours
➤ Gonorrhea in penicillin-sensitive patients
Adults: Initially, 200 mg P.O., then 100 mg q 12 hours for at least 4 days
➤ Uncomplicated gonococcal urethritis in men
Adults: 100 mg P.O. q 12 hours for 5 days
➤ Syphilis
Adults: Initially, 200 mg P.O., then 100 mg q 12 hours for 10 to 15 days
➤ Acne
Adults: 50 mg P.O. one to three times daily

Dosage adjustment
- Renal impairment

Contraindications
- Hypersensitivity to drug, its components, or tetracyclines

Precautions
Use cautiously in:
- sulfite sensitivity, renal disease, hepatic impairment, nephrogenic diabetes insipidus
- cachectic or debilitated patients
- pregnant (last half of pregnancy) or breastfeeding patients
- children younger than age 8 (not recommended).

Administration
- Ask patient about sulfite sensitivity before giving.
- Give with 8 oz. of water, with or without food.
- Know that drug is used in penicillin-sensitive patients.

Route	Onset	Peak	Duration
P.O.	Unknown	1-4 hr	Unknown

Adverse reactions
CNS: headache
CV: pericarditis
EENT: pharyngitis
GI: nausea, vomiting, diarrhea, oral candidiasis, stomatitis, mouth ulcers
GU: bladder or vaginal yeast infection
Metabolic: eosinophilia, **hemolytic anemia, thrombocytopenia**
Skin: photosensitivity, rash
Other: dental caries; dental infection; gingivitis; periodontitis; tooth disorder, pain, or discoloration; superinfection; hypersensitivity reactions including **anaphylaxis**

Interactions
Drug-drug. *Adsorbent antidiarrheals:* decreased minocycline absorption
Antacids containing aluminum, calcium, or magnesium; calcium, iron, and magnesium supplements; sodium bicarbonate: decreased minocycline absorption
Cholestyramine, colestipol: decreased oral absorption of minocycline
Hormonal contraceptives: decreased contraceptive efficacy
Methoxyflurane: nephrotoxicity
Penicillin: interference with bactericidal action of penicillin
Sucralfate: blocked absorption of minocycline
Warfarin: increased anticoagulant effect
Drug-diagnostic tests. *Alanine aminotransferase, alkaline phosphatase, amylase, aspartate aminotransferase, bilirubin, blood urea nitrogen:* increased levels
Hemoglobin, platelets, neutrophils, white blood cells: decreased levels
Urinary catecholamines: false elevation
Drug-food. *Dairy products:* decreased minocycline absorption
Drug-behaviors. *Alcohol use:* decreased antibiotic effect
Sun exposure: increased risk of photosensitivity reaction

Patient monitoring
- Assess patient's oral health closely for dental problems.
- Monitor patient for superinfection, especially oral, bladder, and vaginal yeast infections.
- Evaluate CBC and renal and liver function tests frequently.
- ◀ Watch closely for hypersensitivity reactions, including anaphylaxis.

Patient teaching
- Tell patient he may take with or without food, followed by a full glass of water. Instruct him to space doses evenly over 24 hours and to take one dose 1 hour before bedtime.
- Advise patient not to take with antacids or iron, calcium, or magnesium products.

m

Reactions in **bold** are life-threatening.　　◀ Clinical alert

🔊 Instruct patient to immediately report fever, chills, skin rash, unusual bleeding or bruising, sore throat, or mouth pain or discomfort.

• Stress importance of good oral hygiene to minimize adverse oral and dental effects.

• Tell patient to complete entire course of therapy even after symptoms improve.

🔊 Caution patient not to use outdated minocycline because it may cause serious kidney disease.

• Inform female patient that drug may make hormonal contraceptives ineffective. Urge her to use barrier contraception.

• Tell pregnant patient that drug may stain fetus' teeth if taken during last half of pregnancy.

• Advise female patient to tell prescriber if she is breastfeeding.

• As appropriate, review all other significant and life-threatening adverse reactions and interactions, especially those related to the drugs, tests, foods, and behaviors mentioned above.

minoxidil

Apo-Gain✦, Gen-Minoxidil✦, Loniten⊕✦, Minox✦, Regaine⊕, Rogaine, Rogaine Extra Strength

Pharmacologic class: Peripheral vasodilator (direct-acting)

Therapeutic class: Antihypertensive, hair growth stimulant

Pregnancy risk category C

FDA BOXED WARNING

• Drug may cause serious adverse effects (such as pericardial effusion occasionally progressing to tamponade) and may exacerbate angina pectoris. Reserve it for hypertensive patients who respond inadequately to maximum therapeutic doses of diuretic and two other antihypertensives.

• Give under close supervision, usually concurrently with therapeutic doses of beta blocker to prevent tachycardia and increased myocardial workload. Usually, drug also must be given with diuretic to prevent serious fluid accumulation. Patients with malignant hypertension and those already receiving guanethidine should be hospitalized when therapy begins so they can be monitored to avoid too rapid, or large orthostatic, blood pressure decreases.

Action

Reduces blood pressure by relaxing vascular smooth muscle, causing vasodilation. Action in hair growth stimulation unclear; vasodilatory action may enhance microcirculation around hair follicles.

Availability

Tablets: 2.5 mg, 10 mg
Topical solution: 2%, 5%

🖊 Indications and dosages

➢ Severe symptomatic hypertension; hypertension associated with end-organ damage

Adults and children ages 12 and older: 5 mg/day as a single dose, increased carefully q 3 days. Usual range is 10 to 40 mg/day in single or divided doses. For rapid blood pressure control with careful monitoring, dosage may be adjusted q 6 hr. Maximum dosage is 100 mg/day.

Children younger than age 12: 0.2 mg/kg/day P.O. as a single dose. May increase in increments of 50% to 100% until blood pressure control is optimal. Usual range is 0.25 to 1 mg/kg/day; maximum recommended dosage is 50 mg/day.

➢ Male-pattern baldness; diffuse hair loss or thinning in women; adjunct to hair transplantation

---

Adults: Apply 1 ml of 2% or 5% topical solution to affected area b.i.d. for 4 months or longer.
➤ Alopecia areata
Adults: Apply 1 ml of 2% or 5% topical solution to scalp b.i.d.

Contraindications

• Hypersensitivity to drug or its components
• Dissecting aortic aneurysm
• Pheochromocytoma

Precautions

Use cautiously in:
• recent MI, malignant hypertension, heart failure, angina pectoris, severe renal impairment
• concurrent guanethidine therapy
• pregnant or breastfeeding patients.

Administration

• Give oral form with meals to decrease GI upset.
◀€ If patient is also receiving guanethidine, discontinue that drug 1 to 3 days before starting minoxidil, to avoid severe orthostatic hypotension.
• Know that oral form is usually given with a beta-adrenergic blocker or diuretic to control hypertension.

Route	Onset	Peak	Duration
P.O.	30 min	2-3 hr	2-5 days
Topical	Unknown	Unknown	Unknown

Adverse reactions

CV: ECG changes (such as T-wave changes), tachycardia, angina, **pericardial effusion, cardiac tamponade, heart failure**
GI: nausea, vomiting
Respiratory: pulmonary edema
Skin: hypertrichosis
Other: weight gain, edema

Interactions

Drug-drug. *Antihypertensives, nitrates:* additive hypotension

Guanethidine: severe orthostatic hypotension
Nonsteroidal anti-inflammatory drugs: decreased minoxidil efficacy
Drug-diagnostic tests. *Alkaline phosphatase, blood urea nitrogen, creatinine, plasma renin activity, sodium:* increased levels
Hematocrit, hemoglobin, red blood cells: decreased levels

Patient monitoring

• Monitor vital signs and ECG.
• Assess daily weight and fluid intake and output.
◀€ Monitor cardiovascular status carefully. Stay alert for signs and symptoms of heart failure.
• Watch for hypertrichosis.
• Know that hematologic and renal values usually return to pretreatment levels with continued therapy.

Patient teaching

• Instruct patient to take oral form with meals to decrease GI upset.
• Advise patient to weigh himself daily and report sudden gains.
• Tell patient taking oral form that drug may darken, lengthen, and thicken body hair. Tell him to shave or use depilatory to reduce unwanted hair growth. Reassure him that unwanted growth will disappear 1 to 6 months after he stops taking drug.
◀€ Instruct patient to immediately report difficulty breathing (especially when lying down) or pain in chest, arm, or shoulder.
• Teach patient how to use topical form. Urge him to read package insert carefully.
• Caution patient not to use topical form on other body parts and not to let it contact mucous membranes.
• Tell patient using topical form that new scalp hair will be soft and barely visible. Caution him to use only 1 ml twice daily, regardless of amount of balding. Remind him not to stop using

m

---

drug suddenly, because new hair growth will be lost.

• As appropriate, review all other significant and life-threatening adverse reactions and interactions, especially those related to the drugs and tests mentioned above.

mirtazapine

Apo-Mirtazapine✤, Dom-Mirtazapine✤, Gen-Mirtazapine✤, Novo-Mirtazapine✤, PHL-Mirtazapine✤, PMS-Mirtazapine✤, Ratio-Mirtazapine✤, Remeron, Remeron RD✤, Remeron Soltab, Riva-Mirtazapine✤, Sandoz Mirtazapine✤, Zispin⊕

Pharmacologic class: Piperazino-azepine derivative

Therapeutic class: Tetracyclic antidepressant

Pregnancy risk category C

FDA | BOXED WARNING

• Drug may increase risk of suicidal thinking and behavior in children and adolescents with major depressive disorder and other psychiatric disorders. Risk must be balanced with clinical need, as depression itself increases suicide risk. With patient of any age, observe closely for clinical worsening, suicidality, and unusual behavior changes when therapy begins. Advise family and caregivers to observe patient closely and communicate with prescriber as needed.

• Drug isn't approved for use in pediatric patients.

Action

Potentiates effects of norepinephrine and serotonin by blocking their synaptic reuptake. Also exerts anticholinergic activity by disrupting muscarinic receptors.

Availability

Tablets: 15 mg, 30 mg, 45 mg
Tablets (orally disintegrating): 15 mg, 30 mg, 45 mg

⊘ Indications and dosages

➤ Depression

Adults: Initially, 15 mg/day as a single dose at bedtime; may increase dosage q 1 to 2 weeks up to 45 mg/day. For maintenance, 15 to 45 mg/day.

Dosage adjustment

• Renal or hepatic impairment
• Elderly patients

Contraindications

• Hypersensitivity to drug
• MAO inhibitor use within past 14 days

Precautions

Use cautiously in:
• hepatic or renal impairment
• history of seizures, cardiovascular or cerebrovascular disease, or psychiatric illness
• elderly patients
• pregnant or breastfeeding patients
• children (safety not established).

Administration

• Administer orally disintegrating tablet without water. Have patient place it on tongue until it melts. Make sure tablet isn't broken.

• Be aware that drug is usually used in conjunction with psychotherapy.

◀ Don't give within 14 days of MAO inhibitors.

Route	Onset	Peak	Duration
P.O.	1-2 wk	≥6 wk	Unknown

Adverse reactions

CNS: drowsiness, dizziness, abnormal dreams, abnormal thinking, asthenia, tremor, confusion, **suicidal behavior or ideation (especially in child or adolescent)**

CV: orthostatic hypotension, chest pain

EENT: sinusitis

GI: constipation, dry mouth

GU: urinary frequency, urinary tract infection

Hematologic: agranulocytosis

Musculoskeletal: back pain, myalgia

Respiratory: increased cough, dyspnea

Skin: photosensitivity

Other: flulike symptoms, edema, increased appetite, weight gain, increased thirst

Interactions

Drug-drug. *Benzodiazepines, other CNS depressants:* additive CNS depression

Drugs metabolized by CYP450 enzyme: altered metabolism of these drugs

MAO inhibitors: hypertension, seizures, death

Drug-diagnostic tests. *Alanine aminotransferase, cholesterol, triglycerides:* increased levels

Drug-herbs. *Chamomile, hops, kava, skullcap, valerian:* increased CNS depression

S-adenosylmethionine (SAM-e), St. John's wort: increased risk of serotonergic adverse effects (including serotonin syndrome)

Drug-behaviors. *Alcohol use:* additive CNS effects

Patient monitoring

• Monitor vital signs, especially for orthostatic hypotension.

• Assess neurologic status.

• Watch for weight gain caused by edema or increased appetite.

• Stay alert for urinary tract infection, sinusitis, and flulike symptoms.

🔊 Monitor CBC with white cell differential. Stay alert for agranulocytosis.

🔊 Watch for suicidal behavior or ideation (especially in child or adolescent).

Patient teaching

• Advise patient to take with food or milk to reduce GI upset.

• Tell patient he may crush conventional tablets if he can't swallow them whole.

• Instruct patient to take orally disintegrating tablet without water. Tell him to place it on tongue until it melts and to make sure tablet isn't broken.

• Advise patient that therapeutic effects may take 2 to 3 weeks.

🔊 Tell patient to immediately report sore throat, fever, mouth sores, or other signs or symptoms of infection.

🔊 Instruct patient (or parent) to immediately report suicidal thoughts or actions (especially in child or adolescent).

🔊 Caution patient not to discontinue drug abruptly. Dosage must be tapered.

• If drug causes oversedation, tell patient to consult prescriber about taking entire daily dose at bedtime.

• Caution patient to avoid driving and other hazardous activities until he knows how drug affects concentration and alertness.

• Tell patient to avoid alcohol and to discuss herbal use with prescriber.

• Instruct patient to avoid exposure to excessive sunlight or sun lamps.

• As appropriate, review all other significant and life-threatening adverse reactions and interactions, especially those related to the drugs, tests, herbs, and behaviors mentioned above.

m

misoprostol

Apo-Misoprostol✤, Cytotec, Novo-Misoprostol✤, PMS-Misoprostol✤

Pharmacologic class: Prostaglandin E₁ analog

Therapeutic class: Antiulcerative, cytoprotective agent

Pregnancy risk category X

FDA | BOXED WARNING

- In pregnant women, drug can cause abortion, premature birth, or birth defects. Uterine rupture has occurred when drug was given to pregnant women to induce labor or to induce abortion beyond week 8 of pregnancy.
- Don't give to pregnant women to reduce risk of nonsteroidal anti-inflammatory drug (NSAID)-induced ulcers.
- Advise patients of drug's abortifacient property and warn them not to give it to others.
- Don't use drug to reduce risk of NSAID-induced ulcers in women of childbearing potential unless patient is at high risk for complications from gastric ulcers linked to NSAIDs or at high risk for gastric ulcers. In such patients, drug may be prescribed if patient has had negative serum pregnancy test within 2 weeks before starting therapy; is able to comply with effective contraceptive measures; has received both oral and written warnings of drug's hazards, risk of possible contraception failure, and danger to other women of childbearing potential should drug be taken by mistake; and will begin drug only on second or third day of next normal menstrual period.

Action

Reduces gastric acid secretion and increases gastric mucus and bicarbonate production, creating a protective coating on gastric mucosa

Availability

Tablets: 100 mcg, 200 mcg

💊 Indications and dosages

➤ To prevent gastric ulcers caused by NSAIDs

Adults: 200 mcg q.i.d. with food, with last daily dose given at bedtime. If intolerance occurs, decrease to 100 mcg q.i.d.

Off-label uses

- Duodenal ulcer
- Pregnancy termination

Contraindications

- Prostaglandin hypersensitivity
- Pregnancy

Precautions

Use cautiously in:
- females of childbearing age
- breastfeeding patients
- children younger than age 18 (safety not established).

Administration

🔊 Before starting therapy, make sure female patient understands dangers of taking drug while pregnant or breastfeeding.
- Be aware that drug should not be used in females of childbearing age, except those who need NSAIDs and are at high risk for complications from NSAID-associated gastric ulcers.
- For antiulcer use in females, start therapy on day 2 or 3 of normal menses.

Route	Onset	Peak	Duration
P.O.	Rapid	14-20 min	3-6 hr

Adverse reactions

CNS: headache

GI: nausea, vomiting, diarrhea, constipation, abdominal pain, dyspepsia, flatulence

GU: miscarriage, menstrual disorders, postmenopausal bleeding

Interactions
Drug-drug. *Magnesium-containing antacids:* increased risk of diarrhea

Patient monitoring
• Assess GI status. Report significant adverse reactions.
• Monitor menstrual pattern or postmenopausal bleeding. Report significant problems.

Patient teaching
• Instruct patient to take with food.
• Advise patient to report diarrhea, abdominal pain, and menstrual irregularities.
◀℥ Tell patient drug may cause spontaneous abortion. Stress importance of using reliable contraception.
• Instruct female patient using drug for ulcer treatment to start therapy on second or third day of normal menses.
• Caution patient not to take magnesium-containing antacids, which may worsen diarrhea.
• As appropriate, review all other significant adverse reactions and interactions, especially those related to the drugs mentioned above.

mitomycin
Mutamycin

Pharmacologic class: Antitumor antibiotic
Therapeutic class: Antineoplastic
Pregnancy risk category C

• Give under supervision of physician experienced in cancer chemotherapy, in facility with adequate diagnostic and treatment resources.
• Most common and severe toxic effect is bone marrow suppression.
• Some patients receiving systemic drug have experienced hemolytic uremic syndrome, a serious complication consisting primarily of microangiopathic hemolytic anemia, thrombocytopenia, and irreversible renal failure. Syndrome may arise at any time during systemic therapy, but most cases occur at doses of 60 mg or higher. Blood product transfusion may exacerbate symptoms.

Action
Selectively inhibits DNA synthesis by causing cross-linking of DNA strands and suppressing RNA and protein synthesis, resulting in cell death

Availability
Injection: 5-mg, 20-mg, and 40-mg vials

⚠ Indications and dosages
➤ Disseminated adenocarcinoma of stomach or pancreas (given with other chemotherapeutic agents); palliative treatment when other therapies fail
Adults: 20 mg/m² I.V. as a single dose. Repeat cycle q 6 to 8 weeks, adjusting dosage if necessary.

Dosage adjustment
• Reduced white blood cell or platelet count

Contraindications
• Hypersensitivity to drug
• Thrombocytopenia, coagulation disorders, increased bleeding tendency

---

Reactions in **bold** are life-threatening.   ◀℥ Clinical alert

Precautions

Use cautiously in:
- active infections, decreased bone marrow reserve, impaired hepatic function
- history of pulmonary disorders
- elderly patients
- pregnant or breastfeeding patients.

Administration

◀彡 Follow facility policy for handling, administering, and disposing of mutagenic, teratogenic, and carcinogenic drugs.
- Reconstitute 5-mg vial with 10 ml of sterile water. Shake, let mixture stand, and administer by direct I.V. injection through Y-tube or three-way stopcock. Infuse over 5 to 10 minutes through line with running infusion of normal saline solution or dextrose 5% in water.

◀彡 Avoid extravasation and contact with skin, mucous membranes, and eyes.

Route	Onset	Peak	Duration
I.V.	Unknown	Unknown	Unknown

Adverse reactions

GI: nausea, vomiting, anorexia, mouth ulcers, stomatitis
GU: renal failure, hemolytic uremic syndrome
Hematologic: anemia, **leukopenia, thrombocytopenia**
Respiratory: pulmonary toxicity, interstitial pneumonitis
Skin: reversible alopecia; pruritus; desquamation; phlebitis, necrosis, and sloughing with I.V. site extravasation
Other: fever

Interactions

Drug-drug. *Live-virus vaccines:* decreased antibody response to vaccine, increased risk of adverse reactions
Other antineoplastics: additive bone marrow depression
Vinca alkaloids: respiratory toxicity

Patient monitoring

◀彡 Closely monitor CBC with white cell differential and platelet count. Stay alert for evidence of blood dyscrasias.
- Assess kidney function tests. Measure fluid intake and output and evaluate fluid balance.

◀彡 Watch for signs and symptoms of hemolytic uremic syndrome (irritability, fatigue, pallor, and decreased urinary output).

◀彡 Closely monitor I.V. site and skin integrity to prevent extravasation.

◀彡 Assess respiratory status carefully to detect severe pulmonary problems.

Patient teaching

◀彡 Teach patient to recognize and immediately report signs and symptoms of hemolytic uremic syndrome, blood dyscrasias, and renal failure.

◀彡 Instruct patient to report cough or shortness of breath, even if it occurs several months after therapy ends.
- Advise patient to limit exposure to infections and to avoid live vaccines.
- Tell patient drug may cause hair loss. Discuss options for dealing with this problem.
- As appropriate, review all other significant and life-threatening adverse reactions and interactions, especially those related to the drugs mentioned above.

mitoxantrone hydrochloride

Novantrone, Onkotrone✦

Pharmacologic class: Antibiotic antineoplastic

Therapeutic class: Antineoplastic, immune modifier

Pregnancy risk category D

- Administer slowly into free-flowing I.V. infusion. Never give I.M., subcutaneously, intra-arterially, or intrathecally; severe local tissue damage may occur with extravasation.
- Except in acute nonlymphocytic leukemia, drug generally shouldn't be given to patients with baseline neutrophil counts below 1,500/mm³. Obtain frequent peripheral blood cell counts on all patients to monitor for bone marrow depression.
- Myocardial toxicity, whose severe form manifests as potentially fatal congestive heart failure (CHF), may occur during therapy or months to years afterward. Risk increases with cumulative dose. In cancer patients, risk of symptomatic CHF is about 2.6% for those receiving up to a cumulative dose of 140 mg/m². Monitor patients for evidence of cardiotoxicity and ask about CHF symptoms before starting therapy. In multiple sclerosis (MS) patients who reach cumulative dose of 100 mg/m², monitor for evidence of cardiotoxicity before each subsequent dose; they shouldn't receive cumulative dose above 140 mg/m².
- Active or dormant cardiovascular disease, previous or concomitant radiation to mediastinal or pericardial area, previous anthracycline or anthracenedione therapy, or concurrent use of other cardiotoxic drugs may increase cardiotoxicity risk.
- Secondary acute myelogenous leukemia has occurred in cancer patients and MS patients who received drug. Refractory secondary leukemia is more common when drug is given with DNA-damaging antineoplastics, when patients have been heavily pretreated with cytotoxic drugs, or when dosages have been escalated.

Action

Selectively inhibits DNA synthesis by causing cross-linking of DNA strands and suppressing RNA and protein synthesis, resulting in cell death

Availability

Injection: 2 mg/ml in 10-ml, 12.5-ml, and 15-ml vials

❷ Indications and dosages

➣ Acute nonlymphocytic leukemia (given with other agents)
Adults: For induction—12 mg/m²/day I.V. on days 1 to 3, with 100 mg/m² of cytosine arabinoside given for 7 days as a continuous I.V. infusion (over 24 hours) on days 1 through 7. If remission doesn't occur, second course may follow, with mitoxantrone given for 2 days and cytosine arabinoside for 5 days at same daily dosages. For consolidation therapy—12 mg/m²/ day mitoxantrone I.V. on days 1 and 2 and 100 mg/m² cytosine arabinoside I.V. as a continuous infusion over 24 hours on days 1 through 5, given 6 weeks after induction therapy.
➣ Pain in patients with advanced hormone-refractory prostatic cancer (given with corticosteroids)
Adults: 12 to 14 mg/m² I.V. given over 15 to 30 minutes q 21 days
➣ Multiple sclerosis
Adults: 12 mg/m² I.V. given over 5 to 15 minutes q 3 months. Maximum cumulative lifetime dosage is 140 mg/m².

Contraindications

- Hypersensitivity to drug

Precautions

Use cautiously in:
- bone marrow depression, heart failure, chronic debilitating illness, hepatobiliary dysfunction
- elderly patients
- pregnant or breastfeeding patients
- children.

Administration

◀€ Follow facility policy for handling, administering, and disposing of mutagenic, teratogenic, and carcinogenic drugs.

• Dilute with 50 ml or more of normal saline solution or dextrose 5% in water (D_5W). Infuse I.V. over 3 to 5 minutes into running line of normal saline solution or D_5W.

• Alternatively, dilute drug further in normal saline solution or D_5W and infuse intermittently I.V. over 15 to 30 minutes.

◀€ If extravasation occurs, stop infusion immediately.

◀€ Avoid contact with skin, mucous membranes, and eyes.

• Be aware that drug isn't indicated for primary progressive multiple sclerosis.

Route	Onset	Peak	Duration
I.V.	Unknown	Unknown	Unknown

Adverse reactions

CNS: headache, **seizures**
CV: heart failure, arrhythmias, cardiotoxicity
EENT: conjunctivitis, mucositis
GI: nausea, vomiting, diarrhea, abdominal pain, stomatitis, **GI bleeding**
GU: urinary tract infection, blue-green urine, **renal failure**
Hematologic: anemia, **bone marrow depression, leukopenia, thrombocytopenia**
Hepatic: jaundice, **hepatotoxicity**
Metabolic: hyperuricemia
Respiratory: cough, dyspnea
Skin: rash, petechiae, bruising, alopecia
Other: fever, infection, hypersensitivity reaction

Interactions

Drug-drug. *Anthracycline antineoplastics (daunorubicin, doxorubicin, idarubicin):* increased risk of cardiomyopathy
Live-virus vaccines: decreased antibody response to vaccine
Other antineoplastics: additive bone marrow depression

Drug-diagnostic tests. *Alanine aminotransferase, aspartate aminotransferase, bilirubin, uric acid:* increased levels

Patient monitoring

◀€ Monitor CBC with white cell differential. Watch for evidence of blood dyscrasias.

• Assess vital signs, ECG, and respiratory and cardiovascular status.

• Monitor kidney and liver function tests. Measure fluid intake and output and evaluate fluid balance.

• Monitor temperature. Stay alert for fever and signs and symptoms of urinary tract and other infections.

Patient teaching

◀€ Advise patient to immediately report chest pain, seizure, easy bruising or bleeding, change in urination pattern, yellowing of skin or eyes, or difficulty breathing.

• Instruct patient to limit exposure to infections and to avoid live vaccines.

• Tell patient drug may turn urine blue-green.

• Advise patient to minimize GI upset by eating small, frequent servings of food and drinking plenty of fluids.

• Tell female patient to inform prescriber if she is pregnant or breastfeeding.

• As appropriate, review all other significant and life-threatening adverse reactions and interactions, especially those related to the drugs and tests mentioned above.

modafinil

Alertec✦, Apo-Mofafinil✦, Provigil

Pharmacologic class: Nonamphetamine CNS stimulant
Therapeutic class: Analeptic
Controlled substance schedule IV
Pregnancy risk category C

Action
Unknown. Thought to stimulate CNS by decreasing the release of gamma-aminobutyric acid (a CNS depressant), thereby increasing mental alertness.

Availability
Tablets: 100 mg, 200 mg

🕩 Indications and dosages
➤ Narcolepsy
Adults: 200 mg/day P.O. as a single dose in morning

Dosage adjustment
• Severe hepatic impairment

Contraindications
• Hypersensitivity to drug

Precautions
Use cautiously in:
• recent myocardial infarction, unstable angina, severe hepatic impairment, hyperthyroidism, hypertension, glaucoma, anxiety
• history of left ventricular hypertrophy, ischemic ECG changes, chest pain, arrhythmias, or mitral valve prolapse with previous CNS stimulant use
• history of psychosis
• drug abuse
• pregnant or breastfeeding patients
• children (safety and efficacy not established).

Administration
• Give without food (food delays drug absorption).

Route	Onset	Peak	Duration
P.O.	Unknown	2-4 hr	Unknown

Adverse reactions
CNS: headache, dizziness, nervousness, insomnia, depression, anxiety, amnesia, tremor, emotional lability
CV: hypertension, chest pain, vasodilation, hypotension, syncope, **arrhythmias**

EENT: abnormal vision, amblyopia, epistaxis, rhinitis, pharyngitis
GI: nausea, vomiting, diarrhea, dry mouth, anorexia
GU: abnormal urine, urinary retention, albuminuria, abnormal ejaculation
Hematologic: eosinophilia
Metabolic: hyperglycemia
Musculoskeletal: joint disorders, neck pain and rigidity
Respiratory: lung disorder, dyspnea, **asthma**
Skin: dry skin
Other: fever, chills, herpes simplex infection

Interactions
Drug-drug. *Carbamazepine, phenobarbital, rifampin, other CYP3A4 inducers:* decreased modafinil blood level
Cyclosporine, theophylline: decreased blood levels of these drugs
Diazepam, phenytoin, propranolol, tricyclic antidepressants, warfarin: increased blood levels of these drugs
Hormonal contraceptives: decreased contraceptive efficacy
Itraconazole, ketoconazole, other CYP3A4 inhibitors: increased modafinil blood level
Methylphenidate: delayed modafinil absorption
Drug-diagnostic tests. *Aspartate aminotransferase, eosinophils, gamma-glutamyl transferase, glucose:* increased levels
Hepatic enzymes: abnormal levels

Patient monitoring
• Monitor respiratory and cardiovascular status, including vital signs and ECG.
• Monitor neurologic status, including mood, motor function, cognition, and emotional lability.
• Monitor blood glucose level in diabetic patient.
• Monitor patient carefully if he is also receiving MAO inhibitors. (However, interaction studies with MAO inhibitors haven't been done.)

m

Reactions in **bold** are life-threatening. ◀️€ Clinical alert

Patient teaching
• Tell patient he may take with or without food, but that food may delay drug absorption up to 1 hour.
◀€ Advise patient to immediately report chest pain, irregular heart beats, light-headedness, or fainting.
• Caution patient to avoid driving and other hazardous activities until he knows how drug affects concentration, vision, motor function, and alertness.
• Instruct female patient to use reliable nonhormonal contraception during and for 1 month after therapy.
• Tell diabetic patient to monitor blood glucose level closely and stay alert for hyperglycemia.
• As appropriate, review all other significant and life-threatening adverse reactions and interactions, especially those related to the drugs and tests mentioned above.

moexipril hydrochloride
Perdix ⊕, Univasc

Pharmacologic class: Angiotensin-converting enzyme (ACE) inhibitor
Therapeutic class: Antihypertensive
Pregnancy risk category C (first trimester), *D* (second and third trimesters)

FDA | BOXED WARNING

• When used during second or third trimester of pregnancy, drug may cause fetal harm or death. Discontinue drug as soon as possible when pregnancy is detected.

Action
Inhibits conversion of angiotensin I to the vasoconstrictor angiotensin II, inactivates bradykinin and other vasodilatory prostaglandins, increases plasma renin levels, and reduces aldosterone levels. Net effect is systemic vasodilation.

Availability
Tablets: 7.5 mg, 15 mg

⚕ Indications and dosages
➤ Hypertension
Adults: 7.5 mg P.O. daily 1 hour before a meal; may increase if blood pressure control is inadequate. Range is 7.5 mg to 30 mg/day in one or two divided doses given 1 hour before a meal.

Dosage adjustment
• Renal impairment
• Concurrent diuretic therapy

Contraindications
• Hypersensitivity to drug
• Angioedema secondary to ACE inhibitor use

Precautions
Use cautiously in:
• renal or hepatic impairment, hypovolemia, hyponatremia, aortic stenosis or hypertrophic cardiomyopathy, cardiac or cerebrovascular insufficiency
• family history of angioedema
• concurrent diuretic therapy
• black patients
• elderly patients
• pregnant or breastfeeding patients
• children (safety not established).

Administration
• Give 1 hour before meals (food reduces drug absorption).
• Adjust dosage, as ordered, according to blood pressure response.

Route	Onset	Peak	Duration
P.O.	30 min	6 hr	Up to 24 hr

Adverse reactions
CNS: dizziness, fatigue
CV: chest pain, peripheral edema

EENT: pharyngitis, sinusitis
GI: nausea, diarrhea
GU: urinary frequency
Metabolic: hyperkalemia
Musculoskeletal: myalgia
Respiratory: upper respiratory infection, increased cough
Skin: rash, flushing, angioedema
Other: fever, flulike symptoms, hypersensitivity reaction

Interactions

Drug-drug. *Allopurinol:* increased risk of hypersensitivity reaction
Antacids: decreased moexipril absorption
Antihypertensives, general anesthetics, nitrates, phenothiazines: additive hypotension
Cyclosporine, indomethacin, potassium-sparing diuretics, potassium supplements, salt substitutes: hyperkalemia
Digoxin, lithium: increased blood levels of these drugs
Diuretics: excessive hypotension
Nonsteroidal anti-inflammatory drugs: blunted antihypertensive response
Drug-diagnostic tests. *Alanine aminotransferase, alkaline phosphatase, aspartate aminotransferase, bilirubin, blood urea nitrogen, creatinine, potassium:* increased levels
Antinuclear antibody: positive titer
Sodium: decreased level
Drug-food. *Salt substitutes containing potassium:* hyperkalemia
Drug-behaviors. *Acute alcohol ingestion:* additive hypotension

Patient monitoring

• Monitor vital signs and neurologic and cardiovascular status.
• Assess respiratory status, staying alert for persistent dry cough.
• Evaluate for allergic reactions and angioedema.
• Know that moexipril monotherapy is less effective in black patients, who may need additional concurrent antihypertensives.

Patient teaching

• Instruct patient to take 1 hour before a meal.
• Tell patient to report persistent dry cough and signs or symptoms of infection (especially upper respiratory infection).
• Advise patient to change position slowly (especially during first few days of therapy), to minimize hypotension and dizziness.
• Instruct patient to limit foods high in potassium and avoid salt substitutes containing potassium.
• As appropriate, review all other significant and life-threatening adverse reactions and interactions, especially those related to the drugs, tests, foods, and behaviors mentioned above.

montelukast sodium
Singulair

m

Pharmacologic class: Leukotriene receptor antagonist
Therapeutic class: Antiasthmatic
Pregnancy risk category B

Action

Blocks action of leukotrienes, decreasing smooth muscle contractions and edema in bronchial airways and preventing inflammation and bronchospasm

Availability

Oral granules: 4-mg base/packet
Tablets: 10 mg
Tablets (chewable): 4 mg, 5 mg

⊘ Indications and dosages

➤ Long-term asthma management
Adults and children ages 15 and older: 10-mg tablet P.O. daily in evening

---

Children ages 6 to 14: 5-mg chewable tablet P.O. daily in evening

Children ages 2 to 5: 4-mg chewable tablet or one 4-mg packet oral granules P.O. daily in evening

Children ages 12 to 23 months: 4-mg packet oral granules P.O. daily in evening

➤ Prevention of exercise-induced bronchoconstriction (EIB)

Adults and children ages 15 and older: Single-dose, 10-mg tablet P.O. at least 2 hours before exercise; additional dose shouldn't be taken within 24 hours. Patients already taking 1 tablet daily for another indication shouldn't take an additional dose.

Children ages 6 to 14: 5-mg chewable tablet P.O. at least 2 hours before exercise; additional dose shouldn't be taken within 24 hours. Patients already taking 1 tablet daily for another indication shouldn't take an additional dose.

➤ Seasonal allergic rhinitis

Adults: 10 mg P.O. daily

Children ages 2 to 5: 4 mg P.O. daily either as either chewable tablet or packet of oral granules

➤ Perennial allergic rhinitis

Adults and children ages 15 and older: 10 mg tablet P. O. daily

Children ages 6 to 14: 5 mg P.O. daily as chewable tablet

Children ages 2 to 5: 4 mg P.O. daily as either chewable tablet or one 4-mg packet of oral granules

Children ages 6 to 23 months: 1 packet (4 mg) oral granules P.O. daily

Off-label use

• Chronic urticaria

Contraindications

• Hypersensitivity to drug or its components

Precautions

Use cautiously in:

• acute asthma attack, hepatic impairment, phenylketonuria

• pregnant or breastfeeding patients

• children younger than age 6 when used for EIB prevention (safety not established)

• children younger than age 2 when used for seasonal allergy (safety not established)

• children younger than age 1 when used for asthma (safety not established)

• children younger than age 6 months when used for perennial allergy (safety not established).

Administration

• Give with or without food.

• Administer oral granules either directly in mouth, dissolved in 1 teaspoon (5 mL) cold or room temperature baby formula or breast milk, or mixed with spoonful of cold or room temperature soft foods (applesauce, carrots, rice, or ice cream only). Don't open packet until ready to use. After opening packet, administer full dose (with or without mixing with baby formula, breast milk, or food); dose must be given within 15 minutes. If granules have been mixed with baby formula, breast milk, or food, don't store for future use.

• Ensure that patient taking drug for prevention of EIB has short-acting beta-agonist available for rescue.

Route	Onset	Peak	Duration
P.O.	Unknown	3-4 hr	Unknown
P.O. (chewable)	Unknown	2-2.5 hr	Unknown
P.O. (granules)	Unknown	Unknown	Unknown

Adverse reactions

CNS: fatigue, headache, dizziness, asthenia, agitation, aggressive behavior or hostility, anxiousness, depression, disorientation, dream abnormalities, hallucinations, insomnia, irritability,

restlessness, somnambulism, tremor, **suicidal thinking and behavior (including suicide)**
EENT: nasal congestion, otitis and sinusitis (in children)
GI: abdominal pain; nausea and diarrhea (in children); dyspepsia; infectious gastroenteritis
Respiratory: cough
Skin: rash
Other: dental pain, influenza, fever

Interactions

Drug-drug. *CYP450 inducers (such as phenobarbital, rifampin):* decreased montelukast effects
Drug-diagnostic tests. *Alanine aminotransferase, aspartate aminotransferase, eosinophils:* increased levels

Patient monitoring

• Assess eosinophil count.
• Monitor temperature. Watch for fever and other signs and symptoms of infection.
◀♪ Monitor patient for change in mood or behavior, including suicidal ideation.

Patient teaching

• Advise patient (or caregiver) who has asthma or asthma and rhinitis to take drug in evening.
• Instruct patient (or caregiver) who has EIB not to take another dose within 24 hours of previous dose.
• Inform patient (or caregiver) that he may sprinkle granules onto soft foods (applesauce, carrots, rice, or ice cream only) and take immediately. Drug isn't intended to be dissolved in any liquid other than breast milk or baby formula. Don't store drug that has been mixed with food or liquids for future use.
• Instruct patient or caregiver that after opening packet of oral granules, dose must be taken within 15 minutes.
◀♪ Tell patient or caregiver that drug is for preventive use only, not for treatment of acute asthma attacks and that

appropriate rescue medication should be available.
◀♪ Instruct patient or caregiver to notify prescriber if mood or behavior changes.
• Caution patient to avoid driving and other hazardous activities, because drug causes dizziness.
• As appropriate, review all other significant adverse reactions and interactions, especially those related to the drugs and tests mentioned above.

---

morphine hydrochloride
Doloral✤, Morphitec✤

morphine sulfate, morphine sulphate⊕
Astramorph PF, Avinza, Duramorph, Filnarine⊕, Filnarine SR⊕, Infumorph, Kadian, Morcap SR⊕, Morphogesic⊕,Morphogesic SR⊕, MS Contin, MST Continus⊕, MXL⊕, Novo-Morphine✤, Oramorph SR, Oramorph SR⊕, PMS Morphine Sulfate SR✤, Ratio-Morphine Sulfate SR, Rhotard⊕, Sevredol⊕, Statex✤, Sulfate SR✤, Zomorph⊕

Pharmacologic class: Opioid agonist
Therapeutic class: Opioid analgesic
Controlled substance schedule II
Pregnancy risk category C

FDA | BOXED WARNING

• Avinza (morphine sulfate) capsules are modified-release form indicated for once-daily P.O. administration to relieve moderate to severe pain requiring continuous, around-the-clock opioids for extended time. Instruct

---

patients to swallow capsules whole or sprinkle contents on applesauce. Warn them never to chew, crush, or dissolve capsules or consume alcoholic beverages or use prescription or nonprescription drugs containing alcohol during therapy, as this may lead to rapid release and absorption of potentially fatal dose.

• Intrathecal dosage of morphine sulfate injection is usually one-tenth of epidural dosage.

Action

Interacts with opioid receptor sites, primarily in limbic system, thalamus, and spinal cord. This interaction alters neurotransmitter release, altering perception of and tolerance for pain.

Availability

morphine hydrochloride
Rectal suppositories: 20 mg, 30 mg
Syrup: 1 mg/ml, 5 mg/ml, 10 mg/ml, 20 mg/ml, 50 mg/ml
Tablets: 10 mg, 20 mg, 40 mg, 60 mg
morphine sulfate
Capsules: 15 mg, 30 mg
Capsules (extended-release): 10 mg, 20 mg, 30 mg, 50 mg, 60 mg, 80 mg, 90 mg, 100 mg, 120 mg, 200 mg
Capsules (sustained-release): 10 mg, 20 mg, 30 mg, 50 mg, 60 mg, 100 mg
Oral solution: 2 mg/ml, 4 mg/ml, 20 mg/ml (concentrate), 10 mg/5 ml, 20 mg/5 ml, 100 mg/5 ml
Rectal suppositories: 5 mg, 10 mg, 20 mg, 30 mg
Solution for epidural injection (extended-release, liposomal): 10 mg/ml, 15 mg/1.5 ml, 20 mg/2-ml vials
Solution for epidural or intrathecal use (preservative free, for continuous microinfusion device): 10 mg/ml and 25 mg/ml in 20-ml vials
Solution for epidural or I.V. injection (preservative-free): 0.5 mg/ml, 1 mg/ml
Solution for I.M., I.V., or subcutaneous injection: 1 mg/ml, 2 mg/ml, 4 mg/ml,
5 mg/ml, 8 mg/ml, 10 mg/ml, 15 mg/ml, 25 mg/ml, 50 mg/ml
Solution for I.V. injection (for patient-controlled analgesia [PCA] device):
1 mg/ml, 2 mg/ml, 3 mg/ml, 5 mg/ml
Tablets: 15 mg, 30 mg
Tablets (controlled-release, sustained-release): 15 mg, 30 mg, 60 mg, 100 mg, 200 mg
Tablets (soluble): 10 mg, 15 mg, 30 mg

💋 Indications and dosages

➤ Severe to moderate pain
Oral use—
Adults: 5 to 30 mg P.O. (immediate-release) q 4 hours p.r.n. Or 20 mg P.O. (controlled-release, Kadian) once or twice daily p.r.n. Or 200 mg P.O. (MS Contin) in opioid-tolerant patients who require daily morphine-equivalent dosages above 400 mg.
I.M. or subcutaneous use—
Adults: 5 to 20 mg/70 kg I.M. or subcutaneously q 4 hours p.r.n.
I.V. use—
Adults: 2 to 10 mg/70 kg I.V. p.r.n. given slowly over 4 to 5 minutes. As a continuous I.V. infusion, 0.1 to 1 mg/ml in dextrose 5% in water delivered by controlled-infusion device.
Rectal use—
Adults: 10 to 30 mg P.R. q 4 hours p.r.n.
Epidural use—
Adults: Initially 5 mg (Astramorph PF, Duramorph) injected in lumbar region (may relieve pain up to 24 hours). If response isn't adequate within 1 hour, carefully give incremental doses of 1 to 2 mg p.r.n., up to 10 mg/24 hours. For continuous epidural infusion, 2 to 4 mg/24 hours. For epidural injection (DepoDur) before orthopedic leg surgery, recommended dosage is 15 mg; before lower abdominal or pelvic surgery, 10 to 15 mg. For cesarean section after umbilical cord clamping, recommended dosage is 10 mg.
Intrathecal use—
Adults: Usual intrathecal dosage is one-tenth of epidural dosage; 0.2 to

1 mg as a single injection in lumbar area may relieve pain up to 24 hours.

Dosage adjustment
• Adults weighing less than 50 kg (110 lb)
• Elderly patients
• Children

Contraindications
• Hypersensitivity to drug, tartrazine, bisulfites, or alcohol
• Acute bronchial asthma
• Upper airway obstruction
• Respiratory depression
• GI obstruction, paralytic ileus

Precautions
Use cautiously in:
• head trauma; increased intracranial pressure; severe renal, hepatic, or pulmonary disease; hypothyroidism; adrenal insufficiency; prostatic hypertrophy
• elderly or debilitated patients
• pregnant or breastfeeding patients.

Administration
• For best response, give at pain onset.
• Give oral form with food or milk to minimize GI upset.
• If desired, crush immediate-release form and mix with food or fluids.
• Don't crush or break extended-release form; remind patient to swallow it whole.
• If desired, open sustained-release capsules (Kadian) and sprinkle entire contents onto small amount of food (such as applesauce). Have patient consume mixture immediately without chewing, crushing, or dissolving pellets.
• When giving by direct I.V., dilute in at least 5 ml of sterile water for injection or normal saline solution. Give 2.5 to 10 mg over 4 to 5 minutes.
• For continuous I.V. infusion, use infusion pump or PCA pump. Titrate

dosage to provide adequate pain relief.
• Don't use parenteral form if it's cloudy or contains visible particulates.

Route	Onset	Peak	Duration
P.O.	Unknown	60-120 min	4-5 hr
P.O. (extended)	Unknown	Unknown	8-24 hr
I.V.	Rapid	20 min	4-5 hr
I.M.	10-30 min	30-60 min	4-5 hr
Subcut.	20 min	50-90 min	4-5 hr
Epidural	6-30 min	Unknown	Up to 24 hr
Epidural (ext., liposomal)	Unknown	Unknown	Unknown
Intrathecal	Rapid (min)	Unknown	Up to 24 hr
P.R.	Unknown	20-60 min	4-5 hr

Adverse reactions
CNS: confusion, sedation, dizziness, dysphoria, euphoria, floating feeling, hallucinations, headache, nightmares
CV: hypotension, bradycardia
EENT: blurred vision, diplopia, miosis
GI: nausea, vomiting, constipation, dry mouth
GU: urinary retention
Respiratory: apnea, respiratory depression, respiratory arrest
Skin: flushing, itching, sweating
Other: physical or psychological drug dependence, drug tolerance

Interactions
Drug-drug. *Antihistamines, barbiturates, clomipramine, sedative-hypnotics, tricyclic antidepressants:* additive CNS depression
Buprenorphine, butorphanol, dezocine, nalbuphine, pentazocine: decreased analgesia
Cimetidine: decreased morphine metabolism and increased effects
MAO inhibitors: severe, unpredictable reactions

m

Reactions in **bold** are life-threatening. ◀€ Clinical alert

Mixed opioid agonist-antagonists: precipitation of withdrawal symptoms in physically dependent patients

Warfarin: increased anticoagulant effect

Drug-diagnostic tests. *Amylase, lipase:* increased levels

Drug-herbs. *Chamomile, hops, kava, skullcap, valerian:* increased CNS depression

Drug-behaviors. *Alcohol use:* increased CNS depression

Patient monitoring

• Monitor vital signs. Contact prescriber if respiratory rate is 10 breaths/minute or less.

• Assess pain character, location, and intensity.

• Monitor fluid intake and output. Stay alert for urinary retention.

• Monitor bowel elimination pattern. If constipation occurs, intervene as appropriate.

• Assess neurologic status. Implement safety measures as needed to prevent injury.

• Evaluate patient for signs and symptoms of physical or psychological dependence. Be watchful for drug hoarding.

Patient teaching

• Tell patient he may crush immediate-release form and mix with food or fluids.

• Advise patient not to crush or break extended-release form. Instruct him to swallow it whole.

• Tell patient he may open sustained-release capsule (Kadian), sprinkle entire contents of capsule onto a small amount of food (such as applesauce), and consume immediately. Stress importance of not chewing, crushing, or dissolving pellets.

• Advise patient to take drug at the first sign of pain, because continuous dosing is more effective than p.r.n. dosing.

🔊 Tell patient and caregiver that drug may cause respiratory depression. Instruct them to immediately report respiratory rate of 10 breaths/minute or less.

• Inform patient that drug may cause constipation or urinary retention. Encourage high-fiber diet and high fluid intake.

• Stress importance of taking drug only as prescribed. Point out that drug may cause psychological or physical dependence.

• Caution patient to avoid driving and other hazardous activities until he knows how drug affects concentration, vision, and alertness.

• Teach patient and caregiver about appropriate safety measures to prevent injury.

• Caution patient to avoid alcohol and other CNS depressants during and for 24 hours after therapy.

• Advise patient to avoid herbs, which may worsen adverse CNS effects.

• As appropriate, review all other significant and life-threatening adverse reactions and interactions, especially those related to the drugs, tests, herbs, and behaviors mentioned above.

moxifloxacin hydrochloride
Avelox, Moxeza, Vigamox

Pharmacologic class: Fluoroquinolone
Therapeutic class: Anti-infective
Pregnancy risk category C

FDA | BOXED WARNING

• Fluoroquinolones for systemic use are associated with an increased risk of tendinitis and tendon rupture in all ages. This risk is further increased in patients usually over age 60, with concomitant use of corticosteroids, and in kidney, heart, and lung transplant recipients.

• Fluoroquinolones, including Avelox, may exacerbate muscle weakness in patients with myasthenia gravis. Avoid Avelox in patients with known history of myasthenia gravis.

Action

Selectively inhibits DNA synthesis by disrupting DNA replication and transcription and suppressing protein synthesis, causing bacterial cell death

Availability

Injection (premixed): 400 mg/250-ml bag
Ophthalmic solution: 5% (3 ml in 4-ml bottle)
Tablets: 400 mg

⍟ Indications and dosages

➤ Acute bacterial sinusitis
Adults: 400 mg P.O. or I.V. q 24 hours for 10 days
➤ Acute bacterial exacerbation of chronic bronchitis
Adults: 400 mg P.O. or I.V. q 24 hours for 5 days
➤ Community-acquired pneumonia
Adults: 400 mg P.O. or I.V. q 24 hours for 7 to 14 days
➤ Uncomplicated skin and skin-structure infections
Adults: 400 mg P.O. or I.V. q 24 hours for 7 days
➤ Bacterial conjunctivitis
Adults: Instill one drop of Vigamox ophthalmic solution into affected eye t.i.d. for 7 days or one drop of Moxeza ophthalmic solution into affected eye b.i.d. for 7 days.

Contraindications

• Hypersensitivity to drug, its components, or other fluoroquinolones

Precautions

Use cautiously in:

• known or suspected CNS disorders that may predispose to seizures or lower seizure threshold, peripheral neuropathy, diarrhea, renal impairment, cirrhosis, bradycardia, acute myocardial ischemia, dialysis
• prolonged QTc interval, hypokalemia, and drugs that prolong QT interval
• history of myasthenia gravis (avoid use)
• elderly patients
• pregnant or breastfeeding patients (safety not established except in post-exposure inhalation anthrax)
• children younger than age 18 (except in post-exposure inhalation anthrax)
• children younger than age 4 months (Moxeza ophthalmic use) or age 1 (Vigamox ophthalmic use).

Administration

• Give premixed I.V. dose over 60 minutes. Avoid bolus or rapid infusion.
• Don't mix with other drugs in same I.V. line.
• Know that although milk or yogurt may impair absorption of P.O. moxifloxacin, drug may be given with other calcium products.

Route	Onset	Peak	Duration
P.O.	Within 1 hr	1-3 hr	24 hr
I.V.	Rapid	End of infusion	24 hr
Ophthalmic	Unknown	Unknown	Unknown

Adverse reactions

CNS: dizziness, drowsiness, headache, confusion, light-headedness, insomnia, agitation, hallucinations, acute psychoses, tremor, **seizures**
CV: hypertension, vasodilation, tachycardia, **prolonged QT interval, arrhythmias**
EENT: conjunctivitis; decreased visual acuity; keratitis; eye dryness, discomfort, pain, pruritus, and hyperemia; subconjunctival hemorrhage; tearing;

m

Reactions in **bold** are life-threatening.   ◀€ Clinical alert

otitis media; pharyngitis; rhinitis (all with ophthalmic solution)
GI: nausea, diarrhea, abdominal pain, **pseudomembranous colitis**
GU: vaginitis
Hematologic: eosinophilia, **thrombocytopenia, leukopenia**
Musculoskeletal: joint pain, tendinitis, tendon rupture
Respiratory: increased cough (with ophthalmic solution)
Skin: rash, photosensitivity, phototoxicity, **Stevens-Johnson syndrome**
Other: altered taste (with ophthalmic solution), phlebitis at I.V. site, superinfection, fever, exacerbation of myasthenia gravis, hypersensitivity reactions including **anaphylaxis**

Interactions

Drug-drug. *Amiodarone, bepridil, disopyramide, erythromycin, pentamidine, phenothiazines, pimozide, procainamide, quinidine, sotalol, tricyclic antidepressants:* increased risk of serious adverse cardiovascular reactions
Antacids, bismuth subsalicylate, iron salts, sucralfate, zinc salts: decreased moxifloxacin absorption
Nonsteroidal anti-inflammatory drugs: increased risks of CNS stimulation and seizures
Theophylline: increased theophylline blood level and possible toxicity
Warfarin and its derivatives: enhanced anticoagulant effect
Drug-diagnostic tests. *Alanine aminotransferase, alkaline phosphatase, aspartate aminotransferase, bilirubin, lactate dehydrogenase, platelets:* increased levels
Drug-food. *Concurrent tube feedings, milk, yogurt:* impaired absorption of P.O. moxifloxacin
Drug-herbs. *Dong quai, St. John's wort:* phototoxicity
Fennel: decreased moxifloxacin absorption
Drug-behaviors. *Sun exposure:* phototoxicity

Patient monitoring

◀€ Watch for hypersensitivity reaction (such as anaphylaxis) and other allergic reactions, which may occur after initial dose. Discontinue drug at first sign of rash, jaundice, or other signs or symptoms of hypersensitivity.
• Monitor cardiovascular and neurologic status closely.
◀€ Stay alert for tendinitis and Achilles tendon rupture. Discontinue drug if tendon pain or inflammation occurs.
• Monitor CBC and liver function tests.
• Assess GI status. Report signs or symptoms of pseudomembranous colitis. Be aware that if pseudomembranous colitis is suspected or confirmed, ongoing antibiotic use not directed against *Clostridium difficile* may need to be discontinued.
• Watch closely for superinfection.
• Discontinue drug if peripheral neuropathy or phototoxicity occurs.
• Closely monitor prothrombin time, International Normalized Ratio, or other suitable anticoagulation tests if drug is given concomitantly with warfarin or its derivatives.

Patient teaching

• Advise patient to take tablets once a day with or without food, 4 hours before or 8 hours after antacids, multivitamins, sucralfate, or preparations containing aluminum, magnesium, iron, or zinc.
◀€ Tell patient drug may cause serious allergic reactions even several days after therapy begins. Advise him to stop taking drug and report these reactions immediately.
◀€ Urge patient to stop taking drug and promptly report tendon pain, diarrhea with blood or pus, and signs and symptoms of superinfection.
• Teach patient how to use eye drops. Caution him to avoid touching

applicator tip to eye, finger, or other object.

• Instruct patient being treated for bacterial conjunctivitis not to wear contact lenses.

• Caution patient to avoid driving and other hazardous activities until he knows how drug affects concentration and alertness.

• As appropriate, review all other significant and life-threatening adverse reactions and interactions, especially those related to the drugs, tests, foods, herbs, and behaviors mentioned above.

mupirocin (pseudomonic acid, pseudomonic acid A)

Bactroban, Bactroban Nasal 2%, Taro-Mupirocin✸

Pharmacologic class: Dermatologic agent
Therapeutic class: Anti-infective, topical
Pregnancy risk category B

Action

Inhibits bacterial protein and RNA synthesis by reversibly and specifically binding to bacterial isoleucyl-transfer RNA synthetase. Bactericidal.

Availability

Intranasal ointment: 2.15%
Topical cream: 2%
Topical ointment: 2%

⟐ Indications and dosages

➤ Impetigo
Adults and children ages 2 months to 16 years: Apply a small amount of ointment topically t.i.d. for 3 to 5 days. Reevaluate if no response.
➤ Infected traumatic skin lesions

Adults and children ages 3 months to 16 years: Apply a small amount of cream topically t.i.d. for 10 days.
➤ Nasal colonization of methicillin-resistant *Streptococcus aureus*
Adults and children ages 12 and older: Apply intranasal ointment (half of single-use tube to each nostril) topically to anterior nares b.i.d. for 5 days.

Contraindications

• Hypersensitivity to drug or its components

Precautions

Use cautiously in:
• moderate or severe renal impairment (with large doses)
• breastfeeding patients
• children younger than age 12 (intranasal ointment), younger than age 3 months (cream), or younger than age 2 months (ointment).

Administration

• After intranasal application, press nares together repeatedly to distribute drug.
• Avoid contact with eyes.
• Discontinue use if sensitization or severe local irritation occurs.
• If desired, cover affected area with gauze dressing after applying cream or ointment.
• Don't use intranasal form with any other nasal spray.
• Don't use Bactroban ointment on mucosal surfaces. Use Bactroban Nasal (mupirocin calcium ointment) intranasally.
• Know that although mupirocin isn't absorbed systemically, polyethylene glycol (its water-miscible ointment base) may be absorbed from open wounds and damaged skin and may be excreted by the kidneys.

Route	Onset	Peak	Duration
Topical, intranasal	Not systemically absorbed		

m

Adverse reactions
CNS: headache (with intranasal use)
EENT: rhinitis, nasal stinging or
burning, pharyngitis (all with
intranasal use)
GI: mouth and lip sores
Skin: pruritus (with intranasal use);
dry skin, rash, redness, stinging or
pain, secondary wound infection
Other: taste disorders (with intranasal
use)

Interactions
None significant

Patient monitoring
• Monitor for drug efficacy.

Patient teaching
• Instruct patient to wash affected area
with soap and water and dry it thoroughly, then apply small amount of
drug to area and rub in gently. If
desired, tell him to apply gauze
dressing.
• Advise patient to complete entire
course of therapy, even if symptoms
disappear. Tell him to try not to miss
doses.
• If patient misses a dose, tell him to
apply dose as soon as he remembers.
However, if it's almost time for next
dose, advise him to skip missed dose
and resume regular dosing schedule.
• Advise patient to contact prescriber
if skin infection doesn't improve
within 3 to 5 days or if it worsens.
• Caution patient not to apply drug to
eye or mucous membranes (except
nasal form for intranasal use).
• As appropriate, review all other significant adverse reactions.

muromonab-CD3
Orthoclone OKT3

Pharmacologic class: Murine monoclonal antibody
Therapeutic class: Immunosuppressant
Pregnancy risk category C

FDA | BOXED WARNING

• Give under supervision of physician
experienced in immunosuppressive
therapy and management of solid-
organ transplant patients, in facility
equipped for cardiopulmonary resuscitation where patient can be monitored
closely based on health status.
• Drug may cause anaphylactic and
anaphylactoid reactions and occasionally life-threatening or lethal systemic,
cardiovascular, and CNS reactions.
Monitor patient's fluid status closely
before and during therapy. Methylprednisolone pretreatment is recommended to minimize symptoms of
cytokine release syndrome.

Action
Binds to and blocks function of T lymphocytes responsible for antigen recognition, thereby reversing graft rejection

Availability
Injection: 1 mg/1 ml in 5-ml ampules

⚡ Indications and dosages
➤ Acute allograft rejection in kidney
transplant patients; steroid-resistant
acute allograft rejection in heart and
liver transplant patients
**Adults and children weighing more
than 30 kg (66 lb):** 5 mg/day I.V. for 10
to 14 days
**Children weighing 30 kg (66 lb) or
less:** 2.5 mg/day I.V. for 10 to 14 days

Contraindications
- Hypersensitivity to drug or other murine products
- Uncompensated heart failure
- Uncontrolled hypertension
- Predisposition to or history of seizures
- Antimouse antibody titer of 1:1000 or higher
- Pregnancy or breastfeeding

Precautions
Use cautiously in:
- fever
- children younger than age 2.

Administration
- In kidney transplant patients, know that therapy should start as soon as acute kidney rejection is diagnosed. In heart and liver transplant patients, therapy should start when physician determines that steroid therapy hasn't reversed allograft rejection.
- ◀︎ Know that drug must be given in facility equipped and staffed to treat cardiopulmonary arrest.
- For I.V. bolus injection, draw solution into syringe through low-protein-binding 0.2- or 0.22-micron filter. Discard filter and attach needle-free adapter.
- Administer bolus over less than 1 minute.
- Give antipyretics to decrease fever and corticosteroids to reduce allergic response, as prescribed.

Route	Onset	Peak	Duration
I.V.	Immediate	Unknown	1 wk

Adverse reactions
CNS: fatigue, headache, weakness, tremors, hallucinations, **aseptic meningitis, cerebral edema, seizures, encephalopathy**
CV: chest pain, hypertension, hypotension, **heart failure, tachycardia, cardiac arrest, shock**
EENT: vision loss, blurred vision, conjunctivitis, photophobia, tinnitus, otitis media

GI: nausea, vomiting, diarrhea
GU: oliguria, anuria
Respiratory: dyspnea, wheezing, **severe pulmonary edema, adult respiratory distress syndrome (ARDS)**
Skin: flushing
Other: fever, chills, flulike symptoms, infection, **anaphylaxis, cytokine release syndrome**

Interactions
Drug-drug. *Indomethacin:* increased muromonab blood level, encephalopathy and other adverse CNS effects
Live-virus vaccines: increased viral replication and effects
Other immunosuppressants: increased risk of infection
Drug-diagnostic tests. *Blood urea nitrogen, creatinine:* increased levels
Drug-herbs. *Astragalus, echinacea, melatonin:* interference with immunosuppressant effect

Patient monitoring
- Evaluate vital signs and cardiovascular status. Monitor ECG closely.
- ◀︎ Stay alert for signs and symptoms of cytokine release syndrome, including fever up to 41.6 °C (107 °F), chills, rigor, nausea, vomiting, abdominal pain, diarrhea, malaise, joint and muscle pain, headache, and tremors.
- ◀︎ Be aware that most adverse reactions occur within 30 minutes to 6 hours of first dose.
- Monitor temperature closely. Stay alert for fever and other signs and symptoms of infection.
- ◀︎ Assess neurologic status and respiratory status closely. Evaluate for evidence of aseptic meningitis, encephalopathy, cerebral edema, pulmonary edema, and ARDS.

Patient teaching
- Inform patient that drug can cause serious adverse reactions. Reassure him that he will be monitored closely and will receive interventions to relieve

m

Reactions in **bold** are life-threatening.   ◀︎ Clinical alert

these reactions. Teach him which signs and symptoms to report immediately.
• Reassure patient that adverse reactions will subside as treatment progresses.
• Advise female patient to avoid becoming pregnant or breastfeeding during therapy.
• As appropriate, review all other significant and life-threatening adverse reactions and interactions, especially those related to the drugs, tests, and herbs mentioned above.

mycophenolate mofetil
CellCept

mycophenolate mofetil hydrochloride
CellCept Intravenous

mycophenolate sodium
Myfortic

Pharmacologic class: Mycophenolic acid derivative

Therapeutic class: Immunosuppressant

Pregnancy risk category D

FDA | **BOXED WARNING**

• Increased susceptibility to infection and possible lymphoma development may result from immunosuppression. Give drug under supervision of physician experienced in immunosuppressive therapy and management of renal, cardiac, or hepatic transplant patients, in facility with adequate diagnostic and treatment resources. Physician responsible for maintenance therapy should have complete information needed for patient follow-up.

• Use of CellCept during pregnancy is associated with increased risk of pregnancy loss and congenital malformations. Female patients of childbearing potential who are taking CellCept must use contraception.

Action
Inhibits binding of interleukin (IL)-1 to IL-1 receptors, preventing proliferation and differentiation of activated B and T cells. Binds to intracellular proteins to prevent T-cell activation, suppressing immune responses.

Availability
Capsules: 250 mg
Injection: 500 mg/vial
Oral suspension: 200 mg/ml (after constitution)
Tablets: 500 mg
Tablets (delayed-release): 180 mg, 360 mg

Indications and dosages
➤ To prevent organ rejection in patients receiving allogeneic kidney transplants
Adults: 1 g P.O. or I.V. b.i.d. or 720 mg P.O. b.i.d. (delayed-release), given with corticosteroids and cyclosporine
Children: 400 mg/m² P.O. b.i.d. (delayed-release), up to a maximum of 720 mg b.i.d.; or 600 mg/m² P.O. b.i.d., up to a maximum daily dosage of 2 g/10 ml (oral suspension). Given with corticosteroids and cyclosporine.
➤ To prevent organ rejection in patients receiving allogeneic heart transplants
Adults: 1.5 g P.O. or I.V. b.i.d., given with corticosteroids and cyclosporine. May start I.V. therapy less than 24 hours after transplantation; switch to P.O. dosing when tolerated.
➤ To prevent organ rejection in patients receiving allogeneic liver transplants

Adults: 1.5 g b.i.d. P.O. or 1 g I.V. b.i.d., given with corticosteroids and cyclosporine

Dosage adjustment
- Severe chronic renal impairment
- Neutropenia

Contraindications
- Hypersensitivity to drug or its components, mycophenolic acid, or polysorbate 80 (I.V. form)

Precautions
Use cautiously in:
- lymphoma, cancer, neutropenia, renal disease, or GI disorders
- elderly patients
- pregnant or breastfeeding patients
- children (indicated for kidney transplant only).

Administration
- Give P.O. form at least 1 hour before or 2 hours after meals. To enhance absorption, don't give with other drugs.
- Give delayed-released tablets whole. Don't let patient crush or chew them.
- Know that pharmacist should mix oral solution before dispensing.
- ◀𝄞 Be aware that drug is teratogenic. Avoid inhaling powder in capsules or letting powder contact skin, mucous membranes, or eyes. If contact occurs, wash skin thoroughly with soap and water or flush eyes with water.
- Know that delayed-release tablets aren't interchangeable with immediate-release tablets, capsules, or oral suspension.
- For I.V. use, reconstitute with dextrose 5% in water and dilute to 6 mg/ml. Administer over 2 hours.
- ◀𝄞 Don't give by rapid I.V. push or bolus.

Route	Onset	Peak	Duration
P.O.	Unknown	30-75 min	7.5-18 hr
P.O. (delayed, suspension)	Unknown	Unknown	Unknown
I.V.	Unknown	Unknown	10-17 hr

Adverse reactions
CNS: headache, dizziness, insomnia, asthenia, tremor
CV: chest pain, hypertension, peripheral edema
EENT: pharyngitis, oral moniliasis
GI: nausea, vomiting, diarrhea, constipation, abdominal pain, dyspepsia, **GI hemorrhage**
GU: urinary tract infection, hematuria, **renal tubular necrosis**
Hematologic: anemia, hypochromic anemia, **leukocytosis, leukopenia, thrombocytopenia**
Metabolic: hypophosphatemia, hyperglycemia, hypokalemia, **hyperkalemia**
Musculoskeletal: back pain
Respiratory: dyspnea, cough, bronchitis, pneumonia
Skin: acne, rash
Other: pain, fever, opportunistic infections, **fatal infections, sepsis, lymphoma and other cancers** (especially of skin)

Interactions
Drug-drug. *Acyclovir, ganciclovir, other drugs that undergo renal tubular secretion:* increased risk of toxicity from either drug
Antacids containing aluminum or magnesium: decreased mycophenolate absorption
Cholestyramine: reduced mycophenolate bioavailability
Hormonal contraceptives: reduced contraceptive efficacy
Phenytoin, theophylline: increased blood levels of both drugs
Probenecid, salicylates: increased mycophenolate blood level
Drug-diagnostic tests. *Cholesterol:* increased level
Drug-herbs. *Astragalus, echinacea, melatonin:* interference with immunosuppressant effect

m

Reactions in **bold** are life-threatening.   ◀𝄞 Clinical alert

Patient monitoring
- Monitor CBC with white cell differential, electrolyte levels, lipid panel, blood chemistry, and liver function tests frequently.
- Evaluate vital signs. Assess cardiovascular and respiratory status carefully. Watch for signs and symptoms of bronchitis and pneumonia.
- ◀℥ Assess all body systems carefully for signs and symptoms of infection.
- ◀℥ Monitor patient closely for bleeding tendency.

Patient teaching
- Advise patient to take oral drug at least 1 hour before or 2 hours after meals. Tell him not to crush, break, or chew tablets, not to open or chew capsules, and not to take with other drugs.
- ◀℥ If capsule breaks, tell patient not to inhale powder or let it contact skin, mucous membranes, or eyes. If contact occurs, tell him to wash skin thoroughly with soap and water or flush eyes with water.
- ◀℥ Instruct patient to take his temperature and promptly report fever or other signs or symptoms of infection. Tell him to immediately report unusual bleeding or bruising.
- Caution patient to avoid driving and other hazardous activities until he knows how drug affects concentration and alertness.
- Instruct patient to avoid crowds and people with known infections.
- Advise patient not to take herbs without consulting prescriber.
- Tell patient to avoid live-virus vaccines.
- ◀℥ Instruct patient to avoid excessive exposure to sunlight and ultraviolet light, because of increased risk of skin cancer.
- ◀℥ Tell female patient to use abstinence or two other contraceptive methods during and for 6 weeks after therapy (even if she has a history of infertility). Urge her to report suspected pregnancy immediately.
- As appropriate, review all other significant and life-threatening adverse reactions and interactions, especially those related to the drugs, tests, and herbs mentioned above.

nabilone
Cesamet

Pharmacologic class: Synthetic cannabinoid
Therapeutic class: Antiemetic
Controlled substance schedule II
Pregnancy risk category C

Action
Unclear. Drug has complex effects on CNS, including relaxation, drowsiness, and euphoria; antiemetic effect may result from interaction with cannabinoid receptor system in neural tissues.

Availability
Capsules: 1 mg

⚕ Indications and dosages
➤ Nausea and vomiting associated with cancer chemotherapy in patients who respond inadequately to conventional antiemetics
Adults: 1 to 2 mg P.O. twice daily; give initial dose 1 to 3 hours before chemotherapy. Maximum daily dose, 6 mg given in divided doses three times daily.

Contraindications
- Hypersensitivity to drug or other cannabinoids

Precautions
Use cautiously in:
- hepatic or renal impairment, hypertension, cardiac disease, QT interval prolongation, psychiatric disorders (current or previous)
- history of substance abuse
- concurrent use of sedatives, hypnotics, other psychoactive drugs, or CNS depressants
- concurrent alcohol use
- pregnant or breastfeeding patients
- elderly patients
- children (safety and efficacy not established).

Administration
- On day of chemotherapy, give 1 to 3 hours before chemotherapeutic drug is administered.
- To minimize adverse reactions, give recommended lower starting dosage and increase dosage as necessary.
- Know that drug may be given two or three times daily during entire course of each chemotherapy cycle and, if needed, for 48 hours after last dose of each chemotherapy cycle.

Route	Onset	Peak	Duration
P.O.	Unknown	2 hr	Unknown

Adverse reactions
CNS: drowsiness, euphoria, dysphoria, inebriated feeling, mood swings, irritability, fatigue, malaise, ataxia, headache, poor concentration, disorientation, anxiety, depersonalization, depersonalization syndrome, speech disorder or disturbance, insomnia, abnormal dreams, vertigo, lightheadedness, dizziness, orthostatic dizziness, twitching, depression, confusion, asthenia, sedation, hallucinations, paresthesia, memory disturbance, perception disturbance, seizures, dystonia, numbness, akathisia, tremor, incoordination, toxic psychosis, paranoia, apathy, thought disorder, panic disorder, withdrawal, nervousness, phobic neurosis, emotional disorder, hyperactivity, hypotonia, sinus headache
CV: orthostatic hypotension
EENT: visual disturbances, pharyngitis, nasal congestion, dry throat, dry nose, nosebleed, voice change, thick tongue sensation
GI: nausea, dry mouth
GU: increased or decreased urination, urinary retention, urinary frequency
Metabolic: thirst
Musculoskeletal: muscle pain, back pain, neck pain, joint pain
Respiratory: dyspnea, wheezing, cough
Skin: excessive sweating, pruritus, rash, photosensitivity
Other: taste changes, increased appetite, fever, hot flashes, chills, unspecified pain, bacterial infection, chest pain, allergic reaction

Interactions
Drug-drug. *Amitriptyline, amoxapine, desipramine, other tricyclics:* additive tachycardia, hypertension, drowsiness
Amphetamines, cocaine, other sympathomimetics: additive hypertension, tachycardia, possible cardiotoxicity
Anticholinergics, antihistamines, tricyclic antidepressants: increased tachycardia and hypertension
Antihistamines, atropine, scopolamine, other anticholinergics: additive or superadditive tachycardia, drowsiness
Antihistamines, barbiturates, benzodiazepines, buspirone, lithium, muscle relaxants, opioids, other CNS depressants: additive drowsiness and CNS depression
Antipyrine, barbiturates: decreased clearance of these drugs
Disulfiram, fluoxetine: reversible hypomanic reaction
Opioids: cross-tolerance and mutual potentiation
Naltrexone: enhanced nabilone effects
Theophylline: increased theophylline metabolism

n

Drug-behaviors. *Alcohol use:* increased positive mood effects, increased CNS depression
Sun exposure: increased risk of skin reactions

Patient monitoring

• Ensure that patient remains under supervision of responsible adult, especially during initial use and dosage adjustments.
• Monitor vital signs for orthostatic hypotension and tachycardia.
🔊 Check for adverse CNS reactions. Report significant depression, paranoid reaction, or emotional lability. Be aware that adverse psychiatric reactions can last for 48 to 72 hours after treatment ends.
• Monitor for excessive use, abuse, or misuse of drug.
• Monitor patient's nutritional and hydration status.

Patient teaching

• Instruct patient to take drug on day of chemotherapy 1 to 3 hours before chemotherapeutic drug is scheduled.
• Teach patient about significant CNS side effects (especially mood changes) and cardiovascular side effects. Stress importance of taking drug only as pre-scribed and needed.
• Inform patient that drug may cause additive CNS depression if used with alcohol or other CNS depressants (such as sleeping pills, tranquilizers, or anxiolytics).
🔊 Advise patient, family member, or caregiver to immediately report depression, suicidal thoughts, paranoid reactions, and other serious CNS reactions.
• Caution patient to avoid driving and other hazardous activities until drug effects are known.
• Instruct breastfeeding patient not to use drug while breastfeeding.

• As appropriate, review all other significant adverse reactions and interactions, especially those related to the drugs and behaviors mentioned above.

nabumetone
Gen-Nabumetone✤, Nabumetone✤, Novo-Nabumetone✤, Relifex✇, Sandoz✤

Pharmacologic class: Nonsteroidal anti-inflammatory drug (NSAID)
Therapeutic class: Antiarthritic
Pregnancy risk category C (first and second trimesters), ***D*** (third trimester)

FDA | BOXED WARNING

• Drug may increase risk of serious cardiovascular thrombotic events, myocardial infarction, and stroke. Risk may increase with duration of use. Patients with cardiovascular disease or risk factors for it may be at greater risk.
• Drug increases risk of serious GI adverse events, including bleeding, ulcers, and stomach or intestinal perforation. These events can occur at any time during use and without warning. Elderly patients are at greater risk.
• Drug is contraindicated for treatment of perioperative pain in setting of coronary artery bypass graft surgery.

Action
Unknown. Thought to stimulate anti-inflammatory response and block pain impulses by inhibiting cyclooxygenase, an enzyme needed for prostaglandin synthesis.

Availability
Tablets: 500 mg, 750 mg

⬤ Indications and dosages
➤ Rheumatoid arthritis; osteoarthritis
Adults: 1,000 mg/day P.O. as a single dose or in two divided doses; may increase up to 2,000 mg/day

Contraindications
• Hypersensitivity to drug
• Active GI bleeding or ulcer disease
• History of aspirin- or NSAID-induced asthma, urticaria, or other allergic-type reaction
• Concurrent use of other NSAIDs
• Pregnancy (third trimester)

Precautions
Use cautiously in:
• severe cardiovascular, renal, or hepatic disease
• history of ulcer disease
• pregnant (first or second trimester) or breastfeeding patients
• children (safety and efficacy not established).

Administration
• Give with food or milk to increase absorption.
• In chronic therapy, use lowest effective dosage.

Route	Onset	Peak	Duration
P.O.	1-2 hr	5 hr	12-24 hr

Adverse reactions
CNS: dizziness, drowsiness, fatigue, headache, insomnia, malaise, nervousness
CV: vasculitis
EENT: abnormal vision, tinnitus
GI: nausea, vomiting, diarrhea, constipation, abdominal pain, dyspepsia, flatulence, stomatitis, dry mouth, **GI bleeding**
Skin: pruritus, rash, **angioedema**
Other: edema, fluid retention, allergic reactions including **anaphylaxis**

Interactions
Drug-drug. *Acetaminophen:* increased risk of adverse renal reactions (with chronic nabumetone use)
Anticoagulants, cefamandole, cefoperazone, cefotetan, clopidogrel, eptifibatide, plicamycin, thrombolytics, ticlopidine, tirofiban, valproic acid: increased risk of bleeding
Antihypertensives, diuretics: decreased nabumetone efficacy
Antineoplastics: increased risk of adverse hematologic reactions
Aspirin, corticosteroids, other NSAIDs, potassium supplements: additive adverse GI effects
Cyclosporine: increased risk of renal toxicity
Insulins, oral hypoglycemics: increased hypoglycemic effect
Methotrexate: increased risk of methotrexate toxicity

Patient monitoring
◀𝄇 Watch closely for signs and symptoms of angioedema, anaphylaxis, or other hypersensitivity reactions (including hives, swelling, shortness of breath, and abdominal pain).
• Monitor GI status. Report nutritional deficiencies.
• Assess vital signs.
• Monitor fluid intake and output.

Patient teaching
• Tell patient he may crush tablet if he can't swallow it whole.
• To minimize GI upset, advise patient to take drug with food; eat small, frequent servings of healthy food; and drink plenty of fluids.
• Advise patient to continue taking drug for entire duration prescribed.
◀𝄇 Teach patient to recognize and immediately report signs and symptoms of hypersensitivity reaction and angioedema (hives, swelling, shortness of breath, abdominal pain).
• Caution patient to avoid driving and other hazardous activities until he

n

Reactions in **bold** are life-threatening.   ◀𝄇 Clinical alert knows how drug affects concentration, vision, strength, and alertness.

• Advise patient not to drink alcohol. Tell him to avoid aspirin, ibuprofen, and over-the-counter preparations (unless prescribed).

• Caution female patient not to take drug, especially during third trimester.

• As appropriate, review all other significant and life-threatening adverse reactions and interactions, especially those related to the drugs mentioned above.

nadolol

Apo-Nadolol♦, Corgard, Novo-Nadolol♦

Pharmacologic class: Beta-adrenergic blocker (nonselective)

Therapeutic class: Antianginal, antihypertensive

Pregnancy risk category C

FDA | BOXED WARNING

• Catecholamine hypersensitivity may occur after drug withdrawal. Angina exacerbation and in some cases, myocardial infarction have followed abrupt withdrawal. When discontinuing long-term nadolol, reduce dosage gradually over 1 to 2 weeks and monitor patient carefully. If angina worsens markedly or acute coronary insufficiency develops, reinstate drug promptly and take other appropriate measures to manage angina. Caution patient not to interrupt or stop therapy without physician's advice. Because coronary artery disease is common and may be unrecognized, don't discontinue drug abruptly, even in patients treated only for hypertension.

Action

Blocks stimulation of beta$_1$- and beta$_2$-adrenergic receptor sites, decreasing cardiac output and thereby slowing heart rate and reducing blood pressure

Availability

Tablets: 20 mg, 40 mg, 80 mg, 120 mg, 160 mg

⟋ Indications and dosages

➤ Angina pectoris

Adults: Initially, 40 mg P.O. daily; may increase by 40 to 80 mg q 3 to 7 days p.r.n., up to a maximum of 240 mg/day

➤ Hypertension

Adults: Initially, 40 mg P.O. daily; may increase by 40 to 80 mg q 7 days p.r.n., up to 320 mg/day

Dosage adjustment

• Renal impairment

Off-label uses

• Hyperthyroidism
• Migraine headache
• Parkinson's tremor

Contraindications

• Hypersensitivity to drug or other beta-adrenergic blockers
• Pulmonary edema or cardiogenic shock
• Sinus bradycardia or heart block
• Heart failure (unless secondary to tachyarrhythmia treatable with beta blockers)
• Bronchial asthma (including severe chronic obstructive pulmonary disease)

Precautions

Use cautiously in:

• renal or hepatic impairment, pulmonary disease, diabetes mellitus, thyrotoxicosis
• history of severe allergic reactions
• elderly patients
• pregnant or breastfeeding patients
• children (safety not established).

Administration
• Give with or without food.
• Be aware that drug may be given alone or with diuretic for hypertension.

Route	Onset	Peak	Duration
P.O.	5 days	3-4 hr	24 hr

Adverse reactions
CNS: dizziness, fatigue, paresthesia, behavior changes, sedation
CV: bradycardia, peripheral vascular insufficiency (Raynaud's phenomenon), **heart failure**
EENT: blurred vision, dry eyes, nasal congestion
GI: nausea, constipation, diarrhea, abdominal discomfort or bloating, indigestion, anorexia
Respiratory: bronchospasm
Skin: rash

Interactions
Drug-drug. *Amphetamines, ephedrine, epinephrine, norepinephrine, phenylephrine, pseudoephedrine:* severe vasoconstriction and bradycardia
Antihypertensives, nitrates: additive hypotension
Clonidine: increased hypotension and bradycardia
Digoxin: additive bradycardia
Diltiazem, general anesthetics, phenytoin (I.V.), verapamil: additive myocardial depression
Insulins, oral hypoglycemics: altered glycemic control
Nonsteroidal anti-inflammatory drugs: decreased antihypertensive action
Thyroid hormones: decreased nadolol efficacy
Drug-behaviors. *Acute alcohol ingestion:* additive hypotension
Cocaine use: severe vasoconstriction, bradycardia

Patient monitoring
• Monitor vital signs and peripheral circulation. Notify prescriber of heart rate below 55 beats/minute.

• Assess for signs and symptoms of heart failure or bronchospasm.

Patient teaching
• Advise patient to take drug with meals and a bedtime snack to minimize GI upset.
• Teach patient how to measure pulse and blood pressure; tell him when to notify prescriber.
• Instruct patient to avoid over-the-counter products containing stimulants, such as some cold and flu remedies and nasal decongestants.
• Tell diabetic patient and family that drug may mask hypoglycemia symptoms. Advise patient to monitor urine or blood glucose regularly.
• Caution patient to avoid driving and other hazardous activities until he knows how drug affects concentration and alertness.
• As appropriate, review all other significant and life-threatening adverse reactions and interactions, especially those related to the drugs and behaviors mentioned above.

nafarelin acetate
Synarel

Pharmacologic class: Gonadotropin-releasing hormone (GnRH)
Therapeutic class: Hormone
Pregnancy risk category X

Action
Inhibits secretion of gonadotropin, a luteinizing hormone (LH)-releasing hormone. Initially increases pituitary production of LH and follicle-stimulating hormone (FSH), which ultimately leads to deactivation of testicular and ovarian functions.

Reactions in **bold** are life-threatening.   ◀€ Clinical alert

Availability

Nasal spray: 2 mg/ml in 10-ml bottle
(200 mcg/spray)

💋 Indications and dosages

➤ Endometriosis
Adults: One spray (200 mcg) intranasally in one nostril in morning and one spray in other nostril in evening (400 mcg/day). May increase to one spray in each nostril in morning and evening (800 mcg/day).
➤ Central precocious puberty
Children: Two sprays in each nostril in morning and evening (1,600 mcg/day). May increase up to 1,800 mcg/day (three sprays in alternating nostrils t.i.d.).

Contraindications

• Hypersensitivity to GnRH, its analogs, or sorbitol
• Undiagnosed abnormal vaginal bleeding
• Pregnancy or breastfeeding

Precautions

Use cautiously in:
• rhinitis, ovarian cysts, major risk factors for bone density loss (such as chronic alcoholism or chronic corticosteroid use).

Administration

• Make sure patient isn't pregnant before starting therapy.
• For endometriosis, start therapy on day 2 to day 4 of menstrual period.
• If patient needs topical decongestant, wait at least 2 hours after nafarelin dose before giving.
• Know that retreatment for endometriosis isn't recommended.

Route	Onset	Peak	Duration
Intranasal	Within 4 wk	3-4 wk	3-6 mo

Adverse reactions

CNS: emotional lability, headache, depression, insomnia, **seizures**
CV: chest pain, **thromboembolism**
EENT: nasal irritation, rhinitis
GU: vaginal dryness, bleeding, or discharge; menses cessation; transient breast enlargement; decreased libido
Musculoskeletal: reduced bone density, myalgia
Respiratory: dyspnea
Skin: urticaria, rash, pruritus, acne, oily skin, hirsutism, transient pubic hair increase
Other: weight changes, hot flashes, edema, body odor, hypersensitivity reaction

Interactions

Drug-drug. *Topical nasal decongestants:* reduced nafarelin absorption

Patient monitoring

• Monitor patient for emotional lability or depression.
• Assess nasal mucosa for erosion.
• Monitor vital signs. Weigh patient regularly; report edema.
• Stay alert for adverse hormonal effects, including hot flashes, menses cessation followed by breakthrough bleeding, hirsutism, acne, decreased libido, and vaginal dryness.
🔊 Closely monitor patient for signs and symptoms of seizures and thromboembolism.

Patient teaching

• Instruct patient to complete entire course of therapy. Advise her to keep enough of drug on hand to prevent interruption.
• Inform patient that regular menstruation should cease after 4 to 6 weeks of therapy but that breakthrough bleeding may still occur.
• Tell patient ovulation may still occur. Instruct her to use barrier contraception during therapy and to report suspected pregnancy.
• Caution patient not to breastfeed.

• Teach patient about adverse hormonal effects. Identify which signs and symptoms to report.

• Inform patient that drug may cause emotional changes or depression. Advise her to report these to prescriber.

◀€ Instruct patient to immediately report signs and symptoms of seizures and thromboembolism.

• As appropriate, review all other significant adverse reactions and interactions, especially those related to the drugs mentioned above.

nalbuphine hydrochloride
Nubain

Pharmacologic class: Opioid agonist-antagonist
Therapeutic class: Analgesic, adjunct to anesthesia
Pregnancy risk category C

Action
Binds to opiate receptors in CNS, inhibiting ascending pain pathways. This inhibition alters perception of and response to painful stimuli.

Availability
Injection: 10 mg/ml, 20 mg/ml

⊘ Indications and dosages
➤ Moderate to severe pain
Adults: 10 mg/70 kg I.V., I.M., or subcutaneously q 3 to 6 hours p.r.n., up to 160 mg/day. Maximum for single dose is 20 mg.
➤ Adjunct to balanced anesthesia
Adults: 0.3 mg to 3 mg/kg I.V. over 10 to 15 minutes, followed by maintenance dose of 0.25 mg to 0.50 mg/kg I.V. in single doses p.r.n.

Contraindications
• Hypersensitivity to drug

Precautions
Use cautiously in:
• increased intracranial pressure, head trauma, myocardial infarction, severe heart disease, respiratory depression, renal or hepatic disease, impaired ventilation, hypothyroidism, adrenal insufficiency, prostatic hypertrophy, emotional instability, alcoholism
• history of substance abuse or dependence
• pregnant or breastfeeding patients
• children.

Administration
◀€ Make sure emergency resuscitation equipment and naloxone (antidote) are available before starting therapy.
• For I.M. use, inject deep into large muscle mass; rotate injection sites.
• When giving I.V. for pain, infuse undiluted over 2 to 3 minutes into vein or I.V. line with compatible solution (such as dextrose 5% in water, normal saline solution, or lactated Ringer's solution).

Route	Onset	Peak	Duration
I.V.	2-3 min	30 min	3-6 hr
I.M.	15 min	1 hr	3-6 hr
Subcut.	15 min	Unknown	3-6 hr

Adverse reactions
CNS: dizziness, sedation, headache, vertigo
CV: hypertension, hypotension, tachycardia, bradycardia
EENT: miosis
GI: nausea, vomiting, dry mouth
Respiratory: dyspnea, **respiratory depression**
Skin: sweating, clammy skin
Other: hypersensitivity reactions including **anaphylaxis**

Interactions
Drug-drug. *CNS depressants (including general anesthetics, MAO inhibitors, sedative-hypnotics, tranquilizers, tricyclic antidepressants):* additive CNS effects

n

Reactions in **bold** are life-threatening.　　　　◀€ Clinical alert

Drug-diagnostic tests. *Amylase, lipase:* increased levels

Drug-herbs. *Chamomile, hops, kava, skullcap, valerian:* increased CNS depression

Drug-behaviors. *Alcohol use:* additive CNS and respiratory depression

Patient monitoring

• Monitor vital signs. Watch for respiratory depression and heart rate changes.

• Evaluate patient for CNS changes. Institute safety measures as needed to prevent injury.

◀€ Watch for hypersensitivity reactions, including anaphylaxis.

Patient teaching

• Instruct patient to change position slowly and carefully to avoid dizziness from sudden blood pressure decrease.

• Tell patient to avoid CNS depressants (including alcohol, sedative-hypnotics, and some herbs) for at least 24 hours after taking nalbuphine.

• Advise patient to consult prescriber before taking herbs.

• Caution patient to avoid driving and other hazardous activities until he knows how drug affects concentration, vision, and alertness.

• As appropriate, review all other significant and life-threatening adverse reactions and interactions, especially those related to the drugs, tests, herbs, and behaviors mentioned above.

naproxen

Apo-Naproxen✤, EC-Naprosyn, Gen Naproxen✤, Naprosyn, Naprosyn-E✤, Naprosyn-EC⊕, Naprosyn SR✤, Novo-Naprox✤, Nu-Naprox✤, Nycopren⊕, PMS-Naproxen EC✤, Riva-Naproxen✤

naproxen sodium

Aflaxen, Aleve, Anaprox, Anaprox DS, Apo-Napro-Na✤, Apo-Napro-Na DS✤, Arthroxen⊕, Gen-Naproxen EC✤, Napratec⊕, Naprelan, Novo-Naprox Sodium✤, Novo-Naprox Sodium DS✤, Riva-Naproxen Sodium✤, Synflex✤, Synflex⊕

Pharmacologic class: Nonsteroidal anti-inflammatory drug (NSAID)

Therapeutic class: Nonopioid analgesic, antipyretic, anti-inflammatory

Pregnancy risk category B (first and second trimesters), **D** (third trimester)

FDA | BOXED WARNING

• Drug may increase risk of serious cardiovascular thrombotic events, myocardial infarction, and stroke (which can be fatal). Risk may increase with duration of use. Patients with cardiovascular disease or risk factors for it may be at greater risk.

• Drug increases risk of serious GI adverse events, including bleeding, ulcers, and stomach or intestinal perforation (which can be fatal). These events can occur at any time during use and without warning. Elderly patients are at greater risk.

• Drug is contraindicated for treatment of perioperative pain in setting of coronary artery bypass graft surgery.

Action

Unknown. Thought to inhibit prostaglandin synthesis.

Availability

naproxen
Oral suspension: 125 mg/5 ml
Tablets: 250 mg, 375 mg, 500 mg
Tablets (delayed-release): 375 mg, 500 mg

✤ Canada   ⊕ UK   ☙ Hazardous drug   ⊗ High-alert drug

naproxen sodium
Caplets, tablets: 220 mg, 275 mg, 550 mg
Tablets (controlled-release): 375 mg, 500 mg, 750 mg

Indications and dosages

➤ Pain; osteoarthritis; ankylosing spondylitis; dysmenorrhea; bursitis; acute tendinitis
Adults: 250 to 500 mg (naproxen) P.O. b.i.d. (up to 1.5 g/day); 375 to 500 mg (naproxen delayed-release) P.O. t.i.d.; 250 mg, 375 mg, or 500 mg (naproxen oral suspension) P.O. b.i.d.; 275 to 550 mg (naproxen sodium) P.O. b.i.d. (up to 1.65 g/day)
Children: 10 mg/kg P.O. daily in two divided doses (naproxen only)
➤ Mild to moderate pain; primary dysmenorrhea
Adults: Initially, 500 mg (naproxen) P.O., followed by 250 mg q 6 to 8 hours p.r.n., to a maximum of 1.25 g/day. Or initially, 550 mg (naproxen sodium) P.O., followed by 275 mg q 6 to 8 hours p.r.n., to a maximum of 1,375 mg/day.
➤ Gout
Adults: Initially, 750 mg (naproxen) P.O., followed by 250 mg q 8 hours or initially, 825 mg (naproxen sodium) P.O., followed by 275 mg q 8 hours. On day 1, 1,000 to 1,500 mg (naproxen sodium controlled-release formulation) P.O. once daily, followed by 1,000 mg once daily until attack has subsided.
➤ Management of pain, primary dysmenorrhea, acute tendinitis and bursitis
Adults: Initially, two 500-mg naproxen sodium controlled-release tablets P.O. once daily. Or, for patients requiring greater analgesic benefit, two 750-mg naproxen sodium controlled-release tablets P.O. once daily. Or, three 500-mg naproxen sodium controlled-release tablets may be used for a limited period. Thereafter, total daily dose shouldn't exceed two 500-mg tablets.

➤ Rheumatoid arthritis, osteoarthritis, ankylosing spondylitis
Adults: Initially, two 375-mg naproxen sodium controlled-release tablets P.O. once daily, one 750-mg tablet P.O. once daily, or two 500-mg tablets P.O. once daily. During long-term administration, adjust dosage up or down depending on patient's clinical response. Use lowest effective dose in all patients. (Patients already taking naproxen 250 mg, 375 mg, or 500 mg b.i.d. may have their total daily dosage replaced with naproxen sodium controlled-release tablets as a single daily dose.)

Dosage adjustment
• Renal or hepatic impairment
• Elderly patients

Contraindications
• Hypersensitivity to drug or other NSAIDs
• Asthma, urticaria, or allergic-type reactions after taking aspirin or other NSAIDs
• Perioperative pain in the setting of coronary artery bypass graft surgery

Precautions
Use cautiously in:
• severe cardiovascular, renal, or hepatic disease
• advanced renal disease (not recommended)
• history of ulcer disease or GI bleeding (use with extreme caution)
• chronic alcohol use or abuse
• elderly patients
• pregnant patients
• breastfeeding patients (avoid use)
• children (naproxen sodium controlled-release) and naproxen use in children younger than age 2 (safety not established).

n

Administration
• Give with food or milk to avoid GI upset.

Route	Onset	Peak	Duration
P.O. (analgesia)	1 hr	2-4 hr	8-12 hr
P.O. (anti-inflamm.)	14 days	2-4 wk	Unknown

Adverse reactions
CNS: dizziness, drowsiness, headache, vertigo, light-headedness
CV: palpitations, tachycardia, hypertension
GU: renal toxicity (with long-term use in patients in whom renal prostaglandins have a compensatory role in maintenance of renal perfusion), **renal papillary necrosis**
EENT: visual disturbances, tinnitus, auditory disturbances
GI: nausea, diarrhea, constipation, heartburn, abdominal pain, stomatitis, **GI bleeding**
Skin: rash, pruritus, skin eruptions, sweating, photosensitivity, **exfoliative dermatitis, Stevens-Johnson syndrome, toxic epidermal necrolysis**
Other: thirst, edema, allergic reactions including **anaphylaxis**

Interactions
Drug-drug. *Acetaminophen (chronic use), cyclosporine:* increased risk of adverse renal effects
Anticoagulants, thrombolytics: increased anticoagulant effect
Antihypertensives, cefamandole, cefoperazone, cefotetan, diuretics, eptifibatide: decreased response
Antineoplastics, methotrexate: increased risk of nephrotoxicity
Aspirin: decreased naproxen efficacy
Aspirin, corticosteroids, other NSAIDs: additive adverse GI effects
Clopidogrel, plicamycin, ticlopidine, valproic acid: increased risk of bleeding
Insulin, oral hypoglycemics: increased risk of hypoglycemia
Lithium: increased lithium blood level and risk of nephrotoxicity
Other photosensitizing agents: increased risk of photosensitivity
Probenecid: increased naproxen blood level, increased risk of toxicity
Drug-diagnostic tests. *Alanine aminotransferase, alkaline phosphatase, aspartate aminotransferase, blood urea nitrogen, creatinine, lactate dehydrogenase, potassium:* increased levels
Bleeding time: prolonged for up to 4 days after therapy ends
Creatinine clearance, glucose, hematocrit, hemoglobin, leukocytes, platelets: decreased values
Urine 5-hydroxy-indoleacetic acid, urine steroids: test interference
Drug-herbs. *Anise, arnica, chamomile, clove, dong quai, fenugreek, feverfew, garlic, ginger, ginkgo, ginseng, licorice:* increased anticoagulant effect, increased risk of bleeding

Patient monitoring
• Monitor GI status. Stay alert for signs and symptoms of GI bleeding.
◀≋ In long-term use, assess CBC with white cell differential and coagulation studies, and monitor for visual and hearing impairment and renal toxicity.
• Monitor cardiovascular status for tachycardia, palpitations, hypertension, and edema.
• Monitor blood glucose level closely in diabetic patients.
◀≋ Monitor patient for signs and symptoms of serious skin manifestations; discontinue drug at first appearance of rash or other signs of hypersensitivity.

Patient teaching
• Tell patient to take medication with food or milk followed by 8 oz of water, and to stay upright for 30 minutes afterward.
• Inform patient that he may crush or break regular tablets but must swallow delayed- or controlled-release form whole.

❦ Canada   ⊕ UK   ⚜ Hazardous drug   ⊗ High-alert drug

• Tell patient that drug's full therapeutic effect may take up to 2 weeks.
• Caution patient not to exceed recommended dosage.
◀€ Instruct patient how to recognize and immediately report signs and symptoms of renal toxicity and serious skin manifestations.
• Advise patient to use sunscreen to prevent photosensitivity reaction.
• Instruct patient not to take over-the-counter medications unless prescribed.
• Tell patient to consult prescriber before taking herbs.
• Advise female patient to tell prescriber if she is pregnant or breastfeeding before starting drug.
• As appropriate, review all other significant and life-threatening adverse reactions and interactions, especially those related to the drugs, tests, and herbs mentioned above.

naratriptan hydrochloride
Amerge, Naramig⊕

Pharmacologic class: Selective 5-hydroxytryptamine$_1$ (5-HT$_1$) agonist
Therapeutic class: Vascular headache suppressant, antimigraine drug
Pregnancy risk category C

Action
Binds with specific 5-HT$_1$ receptors in intracranial blood vessels and sensory trigeminal nerves, leading to vasoconstriction and migraine relief

Availability
Tablets: 1 mg, 2.5 mg

⦸ Indications and dosages
➤ Migraine headache
Adults: 1 or 2.5 mg P.O. as single dose; may repeat in 4 hours. Don't exceed

5 mg in 24 hours; don't use to treat more than four headaches per month.

Dosage adjustment
• Mild to moderate renal or hepatic impairment

Contraindications
• Hypersensitivity to drug or its components
• Hemiplegic or basilar headaches
• Severe renal, cardiovascular or hepatic impairment
• History of cerebrovascular or peripheral vascular conditions
• Ischemic bowel disease
• Uncontrolled hypertension
• Use of ergot-type drugs (such as dihydroergotamine) and other 5-HT$_1$ agonists within 24 hours
• MAO inhibitor use within past 14 days

Precautions
Use cautiously in:
• mild to moderate renal or hepatic impairment, cardiovascular risk factors
• elderly patients (not recommended)
• pregnant or breastfeeding patients
• children (safety not established).

Administration
• Know that drug does not prevent migraine.
• Give only if patient's cardiovascular status has been evaluated and determined to be safe, and if first dose can be given under supervision.

Route	Onset	Peak	Duration
P.O.	30-60 min	2-3 hr	Up to 24 hr

Adverse reactions
CNS: dizziness, drowsiness, malaise, fatigue, paresthesia, **cerebral hemorrhage, subarachnoid hemorrhage, stroke, other cerebrovascular events**
CV: significant blood pressure elevation including hypertensive

---

Reactions in **bold** are life-threatening.   ◀€ Clinical alert

crisis (rare), **coronary artery vasospasm, myocardial infarction, ventricular fibrillation or tachycardia**
GI: nausea, vomiting, **colonic ischemia with abdominal pain, bloody diarrhea**
Other: pain or pressure sensation in throat or neck, **peripheral vascular ischemia, serotonin syndrome,** hypersensitivity including **anaphylaxis or anaphylactoid reactions**

Interactions

Drug-drug. *Ergot-type compounds (dihydroergotamine, methysergide):* prolonged vasospastic reaction
Hormonal contraceptives: increased naratriptan blood level and effects
MAO inhibitors: increased systemic exposure to naratriptan, increased risk of adverse reactions
Selective serotonin reuptake inhibitors: weakness, hyperreflexia, incoordination
Sibutramine: serotonin syndrome
Drug-herbs. *S-adenosylmethionine (SAM-e), St. John's wort:* increased risk of adverse serotonergic effects
Drug-behaviors. *Cigarette smoking:* increased naratriptan metabolism

Patient monitoring

• Maintain especially close monitoring in patients with cardiovascular risk factors (such as hypertension, hypercholesterolemia, obesity, diabetes mellitus, cigarette smoking, strong family history), postmenopausal women, and men older than age 40.
• Assess vital signs and ECG.
• Monitor neurologic status closely. Institute safety measures as needed to prevent injury.
🔊 Discontinue drug if serotonin syndrome is suspected.

Patient teaching

• Tell patient to take at first sign of headache.
• Advise patient to take second dose (if approved) at least 4 hours after first dose if headache has not gone away completely or has returned.
• Caution patient not to take more than two tablets in a 24-hour period.
🔊 Instruct patient how to recognize and immediately report signs and symptoms of stroke and other neurologic conditions, serotonin syndrome, hypersensitivity, or bloody diarrhea.
• Advise patient to avoid driving and other hazardous activities until he knows how drug affects concentration and alertness.
• Tell patient to avoid cigarette smoking and to discuss herb use with prescriber.
• As appropriate, review all other significant and life-threatening adverse reactions and interactions, especially those related to the drugs, herbs, and behaviors mentioned above.

natalizumab
(Tysabri)

Pharmacologic class: Recombinant humanized IgG4K monoclonal antibody
Therapeutic class: Immunologic agent
Pregnancy risk category C

FDA | BOXED WARNING

• Drug increases risk of progressive multifocal leukoencephalopathy (PML), an opportunistic viral infection of the brain that usually leads to death or severe disability.
• Monitor patient and withhold drug immediately at first sign or symptom suggestive of PML.
• Drug is available only through a special restricted distribution program, TOUCH® Prescribing Program, and must be administered only to patients enrolled in this program.

Action
Binds to the α4-subunit of α4β1 and α4β7 integrins expressed on the surface of all leukocytes except neutrophils, and inhibits the α4-mediated adhesion of leukocytes to their counterreceptor(s). The receptors for the α4 family of integrins include vascular cell adhesion molecule-1 (VCAM-1), which is expressed on activated vascular endothelium, and mucosal address in cell adhesion molecule-1 (MAdCAM-1) present on vascular endothelial cells of the GI tract. Disruption of these molecular interactions prevents transmigration of leukocytes across the endothelium into inflamed parenchymal tissue. Specific mechanisms by which drug exerts its effects in multiple sclerosis (MS) and Crohn's disease haven't been fully defined.

Availability
Solution for infusion: 300 mg/15-ml vial (20 mg/ml)

ⓘ Indications and dosages
➤ Relapsing forms of MS; moderately to severely active Crohn's disease in patients with evidence of inflammation who have had inadequate response to or can't tolerate conventional therapy
Adults: 300 mg by I.V. infusion over approximately 1 hour q 4 weeks. In Crohn's disease, discontinue in patient who hasn't experienced therapeutic benefit by 12 weeks of induction therapy and in patient who can't discontinue long-term concomitant steroids within 6 months of starting natalizumab.

Contraindications
- Hypersensitivity to drug
- History of or current PML

Precautions
Use cautiously in:
- hepatic impairment

- infections, immune reconstitution inflammatory syndrome
- concurrent use of TNF*a* inhibitors, antineoplastics, prolonged immunosuppressant or immunomodulatory therapy; systemic medical condition resulting in significantly compromised immune system (avoid use)
- pregnant or breastfeeding patients
- children younger than age 18 (safety and efficacy not established).

Administration
◀﹦ Don't give as I.V. push or bolus.
- To prepare solution, withdraw 15 ml of drug concentrate from vial. Inject concentrate into 100 ml 0.9% sodium chloride injection, leading to concentration of 2.6 mg/ml. Don't use other I.V. diluents or mix with other drugs. Gently invert vial to mix completely; don't shake. Following dilution, infuse solution immediately or refrigerate at 2° to 8° C (36° to 46° F), and use within 8 hours.
- Infuse 300 mg in 100 ml 0.9% sodium chloride injection over approximately 1 hour (infusion rate approximately 5 mg/minute). After infusion is complete, flush with 0.9% sodium chloride injection.
◀﹦ Observe patient during infusion and for 1 hour after infusion is complete. Promptly discontinue infusion at first sign or symptom consistent with a hypersensitivity reaction.
◀﹦ Obtain MRI scan in MS patients before starting therapy to help differentiate subsequent MS signs and symptoms from those of PML. Withhold drug immediately at first sign or symptom suggestive of PML.
- Be aware that a baseline brain MRI in patients with Crohn's disease may help distinguish preexisting lesions from newly developed lesions.
◀﹦ For patients with Crohn's disease who start drug while taking long-term corticosteroids, start steroid withdrawal as soon as therapeutic benefit

has occurred. If patient can't discontinue systemic corticosteroids within 6 months, discontinue natalizumab.

◄€ Discontinue drug in patients with jaundice or other evidence of significant liver injury.

Route	Onset	Peak	Duration
I.V.	Unknown	Unknown	Unknown

Adverse reactions
CNS: headache, fatigue, depression, somnolence, vertigo, tremor, **PML**
EENT: tonsillitis, pharyngolaryngeal pain, sinusitis
GI: nausea, diarrhea, constipation, dyspepsia, gastroenteritis, abdominal discomfort, flatulence, aphthous stomatitis, exacerbation of Crohn's disease, **intestinal obstruction or stenosis**
GU: vaginitis; irregular menstruation; dysmenorrhea; amenorrhea; ovarian cyst; urinary tract infection; urinary incontinence, urgency, frequency
Hepatic: abnormal liver function test values
Musculoskeletal: arthralgia, extremity pain, back pain, muscle cramps, joint swelling, limb injury
Respiratory: upper and lower respiratory tract infections, cough
Skin: rash, dermatitis, pruritus, urticaria, dry skin, skin laceration, thermal burn
Other: infections, chest discomfort, seasonal allergy, weight changes, tooth infections, toothache, herpes infection, night sweats, rigors, peripheral edema, influenza-like illness, **immunosuppression, infusion reactions,** hypersensitivity reactions including **anaphylaxis**

Interactions
Drug-drug. *Corticosteroids, immunosuppressants (such as azathioprine, cyclosporine, 6-mercaptopurine, methotrexate), TNFα inhibitors:* increased risk of PML and other infections

Drug-diagnostic tests. *Circulating basophils, eosinophils, lymphocytes, monocytes, nucleated RBCs:* increased levels
Hemoglobin: decreased level

Patient monitoring
• Monitor CBC with differential and hepatic function tests.

◄€ Continue to monitor patient for hypersensitivity reactions; infection; hepatotoxicity; signs and symptoms of immune reconstitution inflammatory syndrome (including unanticipated clinical decline in patient's condition after return of immune function and in some cases after apparent clinical improvement; and PML signs and symptoms (such as progressive weakness on one side of the body, limb clumsiness, vision disturbances, and changes in thinking, memory, and orientation leading to confusion and personality changes).

Patient teaching
• Explain the TOUCH Prescribing Program to patient.

◄€ Instruct patient to immediately report hypersensitivity reactions (such as flushing, nausea, headache, dizziness, fatigue, hives, or itching); signs and symptoms of infections; signs and symptoms of hepatotoxicity (such as yellowing of skin or eyes, dark urine, or right upper abdominal pain or discomfort); unanticipated clinical decline in condition or new signs and symptoms; or signs and symptoms of PML (such as progressive weakness on one side of the body, limb clumsiness, vision disturbances, and changes in thinking, memory, and orientation leading to confusion and personality changes).

• Instruct patient to tell prescriber about all drugs he's taking, because some drugs have potential for serious drug interactions and shouldn't be taken with natalizumab.

- Advise female patient of childbearing age that drug should be used during pregnancy only if potential benefit justifies potential risk to fetus.
- Advise breastfeeding patient that she should decide whether to discontinue breastfeeding or discontinue drug, taking into account importance of drug for her treatment.
- As appropriate, review all other significant and life-threatening adverse reactions and interactions, especially those related to the drugs and tests mentioned above.

nateglinide
Starlix

Pharmacologic class: Amino acid derivative
Therapeutic class: Hypoglycemic
Pregnancy risk category C

Action
Decreases blood glucose level by stimulating insulin secretion from pancreatic beta cells; interacts with calcium and potassium channels in pancreas

Availability
Tablets: 60 mg, 120 mg

Indications and dosages
➤ To decrease glucose levels in type 2 (non-insulin-dependent) diabetes mellitus not adequately controlled by diet and exercise
Adults: 120 mg P.O. t.i.d. up to 30 minutes before meals, or 60 mg P.O. t.i.d. if patient is near glycosylated hemoglobin (HbA1c) goal

Contraindications
- Hypersensitivity to drug or its components
- Diabetic ketoacidosis
- Type 1 (insulin-dependent) diabetes mellitus

Precautions
Use cautiously in:
- renal or hepatic impairment, adrenal or pituitary insufficiency
- elderly or malnourished patients
- pregnant or breastfeeding patients.

Administration
- Give 30 minutes before meals. If meal is missed, don't give dose.
- Know that drug may be given alone or with metformin.

Route	Onset	Peak	Duration
P.O.	Rapid	Within 1 hr	4 hr

Adverse reactions
CNS: dizziness
GI: diarrhea
Metabolic: hypoglycemia
Musculoskeletal: back pain, joint pain
Respiratory: upper respiratory tract infection, bronchitis, coughing
Other: flulike symptoms, trauma

Interactions
Drug-drug. *Beta-adrenergic blockers, MAO inhibitors, nonsteroidal anti-inflammatory drugs, salicylates:* increased hypoglycemic effect
Corticosteroids, sympathomimetics, thiazides, thyroid products: reduced hypoglycemic effect
Drug-diagnostic tests. *Glucose:* decreased level

Patient monitoring
- Monitor blood glucose and HbA1c levels.
- Assess pulmonary status for bronchitis, upper respiratory infection, and flulike signs and symptoms.
- Monitor musculoskeletal status. Check for back pain and arthropathy.
- Note GI complaints, and identify nutritional deficiencies.

Patient teaching
- Instruct patient to take dose up to 30 minutes before each main meal.

- Advise patient not to skip a meal. If he does, tell him to also skip accompanying nateglinide dose, to prevent hypoglycemia.
- Teach patient how to monitor blood and urine for glucose and ketones, as prescribed.
- Instruct patient to report adverse CNS effects and signs and symptoms of respiratory infection.
- Caution patient to avoid driving and other hazardous activities until he knows how drug affects sensation and balance.
- As appropriate, review all other significant and life-threatening adverse reactions and interactions, especially those related to the drugs and tests mentioned above.

nebivolol
Bystolic

Pharmacologic class: Beta-adrenergic blocker
Therapeutic class: Antihypertensive
Pregnancy risk category C

Action
Not fully known. The following factors may be involved: decreased heart rate, reduced myocardial contractility, decreased tonic sympathetic outflow to periphery from cerebrovasomotor centers, suppressed renin activity, vasodilation, and decreased peripheral vascular resistance.

Availability
Tablets: 2.5 mg, 5 mg, 10 mg

🚫 Indications and dosages
➤ Hypertension
Adults: Individualized; 5 mg P.O. daily. If patient requires further blood pressure reduction, dosage may be increased at 2-week intervals up to 40 mg P.O. daily.

Dosage adjustment
- Moderate hepatic impairment or severe renal impairment (creatinine clearance less than 30 ml/minute)

Contraindications
- Hypersensitivity to drug or its components
- Severe bradycardia, heart block greater than first degree, cardiogenic shock, decompensated cardiac failure, sick sinus syndrome (unless permanent pacemaker is in place)
- Severe hepatic impairment

Precautions
Use cautiously in:
- moderate hepatic impairment
- severe renal impairment
- congestive heart failure (CHF)
- peripheral vascular disease
- bronchospastic disease (use not recommended)
- diabetic patients receiving hypoglycemic drugs
- known or suspected pheochromocytoma
- concurrent use of myocardial depressants, AV conduction inhibitors (such as cardiac glycosides and certain calcium antagonists), or antiarrhythmics (such as disopyramide)
- perioperative use with anesthetics that depress myocardial function (such as ether, cyclopropane, or trichloroethylene)
- pregnant patients
- breastfeeding patients (use not recommended)
- children (safety and efficacy not established).

Administration
- Give with or without food.
- Be aware that drug may be used alone or in combination with other antihypertensives.
- Know that drug shouldn't be combined with other beta blockers. Closely monitor patients receiving

---

catecholamine-depleting drugs (such as reserpine or guanethidine), because added beta blockade may decrease sympathetic activity excessively. In patients receiving nebivolol with clonidine, discontinue nebivolol for several days before gradually tapering clonidine.

◀€ Don't withdraw drug abruptly; taper over 1 to 2 weeks when possible. Drug may mask signs and symptoms of hyperthyroidism, such as tachycardia; abrupt withdrawal may exacerbate signs and symptoms of hyperthyroidism or may trigger thyroid storm.

Route	Onset	Peak	Duration
P.O.	Unknown	1.5-4 hr	Unknown

Adverse reactions

CNS: headache, fatigue, dizziness, insomnia
CV: bradycardia
GI: nausea, diarrhea
Respiratory: dyspnea
Skin: rash
Other: chest pain, peripheral edema

Interactions

Drug-drug. *Antiarrhythmics (such as disopyramide), myocardial depressants or AV conduction inhibitors (such as cardiac glycosides and certain calcium antagonists):* increased risk of slowed AV conduction and bradycardia
Cimetidine: increased d-nebivolol (active isomer) blood level
CYP2D6 inhibitors (such as fluoxetine, paroxetine, propafenone, quinidine): increased d-nebivolol blood level
Other beta-adrenergic blockers: excessive reduction of sympathetic activity
Sildenafil: decreased effect of sildenafil
Drug-diagnostic tests. *Blood urea nitrogen, triglycerides, uric acid:* increased levels
Cholesterol, high-density lipoproteins, platelet count: decreased

Patient monitoring

◀€ Be aware that beta blockade may further depress myocardial contractility and trigger more severe heart failure in patients with compensated CHF. If CHF worsens, consider discontinuing drug.

◀€ During perioperative use, closely monitor patients receiving anesthetics that depress myocardial function, such as ether, cyclopropane, or trichloroethylene. Also, know that if drug is withdrawn before major surgery, the heart's impaired ability to respond to reflex adrenergic stimuli may increase risks of general anesthesia and surgery.

• Because of significant negative inotropic and chronotropic effects in patients treated with verapamil- or diltiazem-type beta blockers or calcium channel blockers, use caution in patients treated concomitantly with these agents; monitor ECG and blood pressure.

Patient teaching

• Tell patient drug may be taken with or without food.
• Advise patient not to stop taking drug unless prescriber approves.
◀€ Instruct patient to immediately report difficulty breathing, increasing shortness of breath, excessively slow pulse, or weight gain.
• Caution patient to avoid driving and other hazardous activities until drug's effects on alertness are known.
• Advise breastfeeding patient not to breastfeed during therapy.
• As appropriate, review all other significant adverse reactions and interactions, especially those related to the drugs and tests mentioned above.

nefazodone hydrochloride

Pharmacologic class: Phenylpiperazine
Therapeutic class: Antidepressant
Pregnancy risk category C

FDA | BOXED WARNING

- Drug may increase risk of suicidal thinking and behavior in children and adolescents with major depressive disorder and other psychiatric disorders. Risk must be balanced with clinical need, as depression itself increases suicide risk. With patient of any age, observe closely for clinical worsening, suicidality, and unusual behavior changes when therapy begins. Advise family and caregivers to observe patient closely and communicate with prescriber as needed.
- Drug isn't approved for use in pediatric patients.

Action

Potentiates effects of norepinephrine and serotonin by blocking synaptic reuptake in nerve cells and disrupting alpha$_1$-adrenergic receptors

Availability

Tablets: 50 mg, 100 mg, 150 mg, 200 mg, 250 mg

⃠ Indications and dosages

➤ Major depression
Adults: Initially, 100 mg P.O. b.i.d. May increase weekly up to 600 mg/day in two divided doses.

Dosage adjustment

- Elderly patients

Contraindications

- Hypersensitivity to drug, its components, or other phenylpiperazines
- Active hepatic disease, baseline transaminase elevation, or previous drug withdrawal necessitated by hepatic damage
- MAO inhibitor use within past 14 days
- Concurrent cisapride (not available in U.S.), pimozide, carbamazepine, or triazolam therapy

Precautions

Use cautiously in:
- cardiovascular or cerebrovascular disease
- history of suicide attempt, drug abuse, or mania
- elderly patients
- pregnant or breastfeeding patients
- children younger than age 18 (safety not established).

Administration

- Give with food or milk if GI upset occurs.
- Know that tablets may be crushed.
- 🔊 Don't give concurrently with cisapride, pimozide, carbamazepine, or triazolam.
- 🔊 Don't give within 14 days of MAO inhibitors.

Route	Onset	Peak	Duration
P.O.	Days-wks	Few wks	Unknown

Adverse reactions

CNS: dizziness, asthenia, agitation, light-headedness, insomnia, drowsiness, confusion, weakness, headache, impaired memory, poor concentration, paresthesia, psychomotor retardation, tremor, **suicidal behavior or ideation (especially in child or adolescent)**
CV: hypotension, orthostatic hypotension, peripheral edema
EENT: abnormal or blurred vision, eye pain, tinnitus, pharyngitis
GI: nausea, vomiting, diarrhea, constipation, dyspepsia, dry mouth
GU: urinary frequency or retention, urinary tract infection
Hepatic: hepatotoxicity, hepatic failure
Respiratory: increased cough
Skin: rash, pruritus
Other: increased appetite, thirst, infection, chills, fever, flulike symptoms

Interactions

Drug-drug. *Alprazolam, triazolam:* increased blood level and effects of these drugs

Antihypertensives, nitrates: additive hypotension

Carbamazepine, cisapride, pimozide: increased nefazodone blood level, leading to toxicity

CNS depressants (including antihistamines, opioids, sedative-hypnotics): additive CNS depression

Digoxin: increased digoxin blood level

HMG-CoA reductase inhibitors: increased risk of myopathy

MAO inhibitors: potentially fatal reactions (hyperpyrexia, excitation, seizures, delirium, coma)

Drug-diagnostic tests. *CBC, cholesterol, glucose, hematocrit:* decreased levels

Hepatic enzymes: increased levels

Drug-herbs. *Chamomile, hops, kava, skullcap, valerian:* increased CNS depression

S-adenosylmethionine (SAM-e), St. John's wort: increased risk of adverse serotonergic effects, including serotonin syndrome

Drug-behaviors. *Acute alcohol ingestion:* additive hypotension

Alcohol use: increased CNS depression

Patient monitoring

• Monitor vital signs with patient lying down, sitting, and standing. Notify prescriber if blood pressure drops 20 mm Hg.

• Assess CBC.

◀≹ Monitor liver function tests frequently. Notify prescriber of abnormal results.

• Closely monitor neurologic status.

• Evaluate patient for withdrawal symptoms (which may occur if therapy stops abruptly).

◀≹ Monitor closely for increasing depression and suicidal ideation (especially in child or adolescent).

Patient teaching

• Advise patient to take with food or milk to minimize GI upset.

• Tell patient to crush drug if he can't swallow it whole.

• Inform patient that therapeutic response may take up to 4 weeks. Encourage him to keep taking drug as prescribed.

◀≹ Tell patient drug may cause adverse CNS effects. Advise him to report significant mood changes (especially depression or suicidal thoughts). Caution parent to report these problems in child or adolescent.

◀≹ Instruct patient to immediately report unusual tiredness, yellowing of skin or eyes, nausea, or anorexia.

• Instruct patient to rise slowly and carefully, to avoid dizziness from temporary blood pressure drop.

• Tell patient to avoid alcohol and to consult prescriber before taking herbs.

◀≹ Instruct patient not to stop taking drug abruptly. Dosage must be tapered.

• As appropriate, review all other significant and life-threatening adverse reactions and interactions, especially those related to the drugs, tests, herbs, and behaviors mentioned above.

nelarabine
Arranon, Atriance ⊕ ✤

Pharmacologic class: Antimetabolite
Therapeutic class: Antineoplastic
Pregnancy risk category D

FDA BOXED WARNING

• Administer I.V. only.

• Give under supervision of physician experienced in use of cancer chemotherapy.

• Drug has caused severe neurologic events, including severe somnolence,

---

seizures, and peripheral neuropathy. Demyelination-associated events also have occurred. Drug discontinuation doesn't always lead to full recovery from these events. Monitor patient closely for neurologic changes; discontinue drug for serious neurologic events.

Action
Inhibits DNA synthesis in leukemic blasts, leading to cell death

Availability
Solution for injection: 250 mg/50 ml

⚠ Indications and dosages
➤ T-cell acute lymphoblastic leukemia and T-cell lymphoblastic lymphoma in patients whose disease hasn't responded to at least two chemotherapy regimens or who've relapsed after such therapy
Adults: 1,500 mg/m^2 I.V. undiluted over 2 hours on days 1, 3, and 5; repeat every 21 days. Continue therapy until disease progresses, unacceptable toxicity occurs, patient becomes eligible for bone marrow transplant, or patient no longer benefits from therapy.
Children: 650 mg/m^2 I.V. undiluted over 1 hour daily for 5 consecutive days; repeat every 21 days. Continue therapy until disease progresses, unacceptable toxicity occurs, patient becomes eligible for bone marrow transplant, or patient no longer benefits from therapy.

Dosage adjustment
• Neurologic or hematologic toxicity

Contraindications
• Hypersensitivity to drug or its components

Precautions
Use cautiously in:
• renal or hepatic dysfunction

• patients undergoing concurrent intrathecal chemotherapy
• patients previously treated with intrathecal chemotherapy or craniospinal irradiation
• concurrent administration of live vaccines (immunocompromised patients)
• elderly patients
• pregnant or breastfeeding patients.

Administration
• Administer undiluted.
• Infuse over 2 hours in adults or over 1 hour in children.
• In patients at risk for tumor lysis syndrome, take measures to prevent hyperuricemia (such as hydration, urine alkalization, and allopurinol prophylaxis).
◀€ Discontinue drug if serious neurologic adverse reactions occur.

Route	Onset	Peak	Duration
I.V.	Unknown	End of infusion	Unknown

Adverse reactions
CNS: confusional state, insomnia, depression, headache, peripheral neuropathy, somnolence, paresthesia, hypoesthesia, fine motor dysfunction, neurologic disorder, tremor, ataxia, abnormal gait, dizziness, amnesia, balance disorder, sensory loss, demyelination, asthenia, fatigue, rigors, decreased level of consciousness, **seizures, cerebral hemorrhage, coma**
CV: tachycardia, chest pain, hypotension
EENT: blurred vision, epistaxis, sinusitis
GI: nausea, vomiting, diarrhea, constipation, abdominal pain, abdominal distention, stomatitis, anorexia
Hematologic: anemia, **neutropenia, thrombocytopenia, leukopenia**
Metabolic: dehydration
Musculoskeletal: myalgia, arthralgia, back pain, muscle weakness, extremity pain
Respiratory: pneumonia, cough, dyspnea, exertional dyspnea, wheezing, pleural effusion

Skin: petechiae
Other: abnormal taste, infection, fever, edema, peripheral edema, pain, non-cardiac chest pain

Interactions
Drug-drug. *Pentostatin:* decreased nelarabine efficacy
Drug-diagnostic tests. *Bilirubin, serum creatinine, transaminases:* increased
Blood albumin, CBC, calcium, glucose, magnesium, platelets, potassium: decreased

Patient monitoring
◀€ Watch closely for neurologic events, such as somnolence, confusion, seizures, ataxia, motor incoordination, and peripheral neuropathy (which may not subside even after therapy ends). Know that previous craniospinal irradiation or current or previous intrathecal chemotherapy may increase patient's risk of adverse neurologic events.
• Closely monitor patients with hepatic or renal dysfunction for adverse reactions.
• Monitor CBC regularly.

Patient teaching
• Instruct patient or caregiver to read patient information leaflet thoroughly.
◀€ Urge patient or caregiver to immediately report neurologic symptoms, such as extreme sleepiness, confusion, seizures, unsteadiness or weakness on walking, difficulty with tasks such as buttoning clothing, and numbness and tingling in fingers, hands, or feet.
◀€ Tell patient to immediately report easy bruising, bleeding, fever, or signs or symptoms of infection.
• Inform patient that he'll need to undergo frequent blood tests.
• Instruct patient to avoid live virus vaccines.
• Caution patient to avoid driving and other hazardous activities until drug effects are known.

• Urge female with childbearing potential to avoid pregnancy and breastfeeding during therapy.
• As appropriate, review all other significant and life-threatening adverse reactions and interactions, especially those related to the drugs and tests mentioned above.

nelfinavir mesylate
Viracept

Pharmacologic class: Protease inhibitor
Therapeutic class: Antiretroviral
Pregnancy risk category B

Action
Inhibits action of human immunodeficiency virus (HIV) protease and prevents cleavage of viral polyproteins, resulting in production of immature, noninfectious virus

Availability
Oral powder: 50 mg/1 g powder (1 g powder/level scoopful)
Tablets: 250 mg, 625 mg

⚕ Indications and dosages
➢ HIV infection
Adults and children older than age 13: 750 mg P.O. t.i.d. or 1,250 mg b.i.d., given with other antiretrovirals
Children ages 2 to 13: 20 to 30 mg/kg P.O. t.i.d., given with a meal or light snack

Contraindications
• Hypersensitivity to drug or its components
• Concurrent use of amiodarone, dihydroergotamine, ergonovine, ergotamine, midazolam, pimozide, quinidine, rifampin, sildenafil (when used

n

for pulmonary arterial hypertension), or triazolam

Precautions
Use cautiously in:
- moderate or severe hepatic impairment (avoid use)
- hemophilia, diabetes mellitus
- concurrent use of lovastatin, simvastatin, or St. John's wort (not recommended)
- concurrent use of other HMG-CoA reductase inhibitors also metabolized by the CYP3A pathway, proton pump inhibitors, and rifampin
- phenylketonuria (oral powder contains phenylalanine)
- breastfeeding patients.

Administration
- Give tablets with food.
- For adult who can't swallow tablets whole, crush and mix in food or dissolve in small amount of water. Have patient consume mixture immediately, or refrigerate for up to 6 hours.
- For child who can't swallow tablets, mix oral powder with small amount of water, formula, or milk. Have child consume mixture immediately, or refrigerate for up to 6 hours.
- Don't mix powder with water in its original container.
- Don't mix powder with acidic juice (combination produces bitter taste).
- ◀€ Don't give concurrently with amiodarone, astemizole, cisapride, dihydroergotamine, ergotamine, midazolam, quinidine, rifampin, terfenadine, or triazolam.

Route	Onset	Peak	Duration
P.O.	Rapid	2-4 hr	8 hr

Adverse reactions
CNS: anxiety, depression, dizziness, drowsiness, emotional lability, headache, hyperkinesia, insomnia, malaise, migraine headache, sleep disorders, weakness, myasthenia, paresthesia, **suicidal ideation, seizures**
EENT: acute iritis, rhinitis, sinusitis, pharyngitis
GI: nausea, diarrhea, abdominal pain, flatulence
GU: nephrolithiasis, sexual dysfunction
Hematologic: anemia, **leukopenia, thrombocytopenia**
Metabolic: dehydration, hyperuricemia, hyperglycemia, **hypoglycemia**
Musculoskeletal: joint pain, arthritis, back pain, myalgia, myopathy
Respiratory: dyspnea, **bronchospasm**
Skin: pruritus, rash, sweating, fungal dermatitis, folliculitis, urticaria
Other: fever, body fat redistribution, allergic reactions, **immune reconstitution syndrome**

Interactions
Drug-drug. *Amiodarone, dihydroergotamine, ergotamine, midazolam, quinidine, triazolam:* excessive sedation, vasoconstriction, serious arrhythmias
Atorvastatin, rosuvastatin: increased statin concentration
Azithromycin, bosentan, colchicine, inhaled fluticasone, salmeterol: increased concentration of these drugs
Carbamazepine, phenobarbital, phenytoin, rifampin: decreased nelfinavir blood level and efficacy
Delavirdine: increased nelfinavir concentration, decreased delavirdine concentrations
HMG-CoA reductase inhibitors: increased risk of serious reactions, such as myopathy and rhabdomyolysis
Hormonal contraceptives: decreased contraceptive blood level and efficacy
Immunosuppressants (cyclosporine, sirolimus, tacrolimus): increased immunosuppressant concentration
Indinavir, saquinavir: increased indinavir or saquinavir concentration and increased nelfinavir concentration

---

Methadone, trazodone: decreased concentration of these drugs

Nevirapine: decreased nelfinavir concentration

Rifabutin: decreased rifabutin metabolism and effects

Ritonavir: increased nelfinavir concentration

Sildenafil, tadalafil, vardenafil: increased risk of adverse events

Warfarin: affected warfarin concentration

Drug-diagnostic tests. *Alanine aminotransferase, alkaline phosphatase, amylase, aspartate aminotransferase, creatine kinase, gamma-glutamyl transpeptidase, lactic dehydrogenase lipids, uric acids:* increased levels

Blood glucose: increased or decreased level

Hemoglobin, platelets, white blood cells: decreased levels

Drug-food. *Most foods:* enhanced drug absorption

Drug-herbs. *St. John's wort:* decreased nelfinavir blood level and efficacy

Patient monitoring

◀€ Watch for signs and symptoms of depression and suicidal ideation.

• Evaluate neurologic status closely, particularly for seizures and sensorimotor dysfunction.

• Assess CBC, lipid panel, uric acid level, and HIV-specific tests.

• Watch for secondary infections, particularly fungal and EENT infections.

◀€ Be aware that immune reconstitution syndrome may occur in patients receiving combination antiretroviral therapy. During initial phase of therapy, patient whose immune system responds may develop an inflammatory response to indolent or residual opportunistic infections (such as *Mycobacterium avium* complex, cytomegalovirus, *Pneumocystis jiroveci* pneumonia, and

tuberculosis), which may necessitate further evaluation and treatment.

Patient teaching

• Advise patient to take with a meal or snack. Inform him that he may mix oral powder with nonacidic fluids.

• Tell patient he may take missed dose up to 1 hour before next scheduled dose.

◀€ Instruct patient to report depression or suicidal thoughts.

• Tell patient that drug may predispose him to other infections, especially fungal and EENT infections. Advise him to avoid crowds and to wash hands often and thoroughly.

• Tell patient with phenylketonuria (or caregiver) that powder contains phenylalanine.

◀€ Tell patient to immediately report new or worsening signs or symptoms.

◀€ Advise patient not to use St. John's wort while taking this drug.

• Advise female patient to use reliable barrier contraception.

• Advise female patient not to breastfeed, because breast milk may transfer HIV to infant.

• Caution patient to avoid driving and other hazardous activities until he knows how drug affects concentration, vision, strength, and alertness.

• As appropriate, review all other significant and life-threatening adverse reactions and interactions, especially those related to the drugs, tests, foods, and herbs mentioned above.

neomycin sulfate
Neo-Fradin, Nivemycin ✛

Pharmacologic class: Aminoglycoside
Therapeutic class: Anti-infective
Pregnancy risk category D

FDA | BOXED WARNING

• Systemic absorption follows oral use and may lead to toxic reactions. Observe patient closely for indications of toxicity. Neurotoxicity (including ototoxicity) and nephrotoxicity have occurred, even at recommended doses. Perform serial, vestibular, and audiometric tests as well as renal function tests, especially in high-risk patients. Risk of nephrotoxicity and ototoxicity is greater in patients with renal impairment. Ototoxicity may be delayed, and patients developing cochlear damage won't have symptoms during therapy; total or partial deafness may occur long after drug is stopped.

• Neuromuscular blockage and respiratory paralysis may follow oral use. Consider these risks, especially to patients receiving anesthetics or neuromuscular blockers (such as tubocurarine, succinylcholine, and decamethonium) and those receiving massive transfusions of citrated anticoagulated blood. If blockage occurs, calcium salts may reverse these phenomena, but patient may need mechanical respiratory assistance.

• Avoid concurrent or sequential systemic, oral, or topical use of other aminoglycosides or neurotoxic drugs, as toxicity may be additive.

• Advanced age and dehydration increase risk of toxicity.

• Avoid giving drug concurrently with potent diuretics, as some diuretics are ototoxic. Also, I.V. diuretics may enhance neomycin toxicity by altering its blood and tissue levels.

Action

Interferes with bacterial protein synthesis by binding to 30S ribosomal subunit, causing misreading of genetic code. Inaccurate peptide sequence then forms in protein chain, causing bacterial death.

Availability

Ointment: 0.5%
Oral solution: 125 mg/5 ml
Tablets: 500 mg

⚕ Indications and dosages

➤ Preoperative intestinal antisepsis
Adults: 1 g P.O. q hour for four doses, then 1 g q 4 hours for 24 hours or 1 g at 19 hours, 18 hours, and 9 hours before surgery
➤ Hepatic encephalopathy
Adults: 4 to 12 g/day P.O. in divided doses
➤ Superficial bacterial infections
Adults: Apply ointment topically one to five times daily.

Contraindications

• Hypersensitivity to drug or other aminoglycosides
• Intestinal obstruction

Precautions

Use cautiously in:
• renal impairment, neuromuscular diseases (such as myasthenia gravis), hearing impairment
• obese patients
• elderly patients
• pregnant or breastfeeding patients
• children under age 18 (safety not established).

Administration

• Give preoperative dose before bowel surgery, after cathartic administration, as ordered.

Route	Onset	Peak	Duration
P.O.	Variable	1-4 hr	Unknown
Topical	Unknown	Unknown	Unknown

Adverse reactions

CNS: neuromuscular blockade
EENT: ototoxicity (with prolonged, high-dose use)
GI: nausea, vomiting, diarrhea, malabsorption syndrome

🍁 Canada   ⊕ UK   ⚘ Hazardous drug   ⊗ High-alert drug

GU: nephrotoxicity (with prolonged, high-dose use)
Other: superinfection

Interactions
Drug-drug. *Acyclovir, amphotericin B, cephalosporin, cisplatin, other amino-glycosides, vancomycin:* increased risk of ototoxicity and nephrotoxicity
Digoxin: decreased digoxin absorption
Dimenhydrinate: masking of ototoxicity symptoms
Oral anticoagulants: increased anticoagulant effect
Potent loop diuretics: increased risk of ototoxicity

Patient monitoring
• Assess for neuromuscular blockade, ototoxicity, and nephrotoxicity.
• Monitor kidney function tests.

Patient teaching
• Instruct patient to drink plenty of water.
• Tell patient to complete full course of therapy.
• Inform patient that drug may cause muscle weakness.
• Instruct patient to report hearing problems and change in urination pattern.
• Caution patient to avoid driving and other hazardous activities until he knows how drug affects neuromuscular status.
• Tell patient he'll undergo frequent blood testing during therapy.
• As appropriate, review all other significant and life-threatening adverse reactions and interactions, especially those related to the drugs mentioned above.

neostigmine bromide
Prostigmin

neostigmine methylsulfate
PMS-Neostigmine Methylsulfate✤,
Prostigmin

Pharmacologic class: Anticholinesterase
Therapeutic class: Muscle stimulant
Pregnancy risk category C

Action
Inhibits enzyme acetylcholinesterase, leading to increased acetylcholine concentration at synapse and prolonged acetylcholine effects. Exerts direct cholinomimetic effect on skeletal muscle.

Availability
Injection (methylsulfate): 2 mg/ml, 1 mg/ml, 0.5 mg/ml, 0.25 mg/ml
Tablets (bromide): 15 mg

🕖 Indications and dosages
➤ Myasthenia gravis
Adults: 15 mg/day P.O.; may increase p.r.n. up to 375 mg/day; average dosage is 150 mg/day. Or 1 ml of 1:2,000 solution (0.5 mg) subcutaneously or I.M. based on response and tolerance.
➤ Postoperative abdominal distention and bladder atony
Adults: 0.5 to 1 mg I.M. or subcutaneously. If given for urinary retention and no response occurs within 1 hour, catheterize patient as ordered and repeat dose q 3 hours for five doses.
➤ Antidote for nondepolarizing neuromuscular blockers
Adults: 0.5 to 2.5 mg I.V.; repeat p.r.n. up to 5 mg. Precede initial dose with 0.6 to 1.2 mg atropine sulfate I.V., as ordered.

Contraindications
• Hypersensitivity to cholinergics or bromide
• Mechanical obstruction of GI or urinary tract
• Peritonitis

n

Reactions in **bold** are life-threatening. Clinical alert

Precautions
Use cautiously in:
• asthma, peptic ulcer, bradycardia, arrhythmias, recent coronary occlusion, vagotonia, hyperthyroidism, seizure disorder
• pregnant or breastfeeding patients.

Administration
◀€ Before giving, ensure that atropine sulfate is available to treat cholinergic crisis.
• Know that atropine may be combined with usual neostigmine dose to decrease risk of adverse reactions.
• Give oral form 1 hour before or 2 hours after a meal.
• Administer I.V. dose undiluted directly into vein or I.V. line. Give 0.5-mg dose slowly over 1 minute.
◀€ Keep resuscitation equipment nearby.

Route	Onset	Peak	Duration
P.O.	45-75 min	1-2 hr	2-4 hr
I.V.	4-8 min	1-2 hr	2-4 hr
I.M., subcut.	20-30 min	1-2 hr	2-4 hr

Adverse reactions
CNS: dizziness, headache, drowsiness, asthenia, **loss of consciousness**
CV: hypotension, tachycardia, bradycardia, **atrioventricular (AV) block, cardiac arrest**
EENT: vision changes, lacrimation, miosis
GI: nausea, vomiting, diarrhea, abdominal cramping, flatulence, increased peristalsis
GU: urinary frequency
Musculoskeletal: muscle cramps, spasms, and fasciculations; joint pain
Respiratory: dyspnea, **bronchospasm, respiratory depression, respiratory arrest, laryngospasm**
Skin: rash, urticaria, flushing
Other: **anaphylaxis**

Interactions
Drug-drug. *Aminoglycosides, anticholinergics, atropine, corticosteroids, local and general anesthetics:* reversal of anticholinergic effects
Cholinergics: additive toxicity
Kanamycin, neomycin, streptomycin: increased neuromuscular blockade
Succinylcholine: potentiation of neuromuscular blockade, prolonged respiratory depression

Patient monitoring
◀€ Monitor vital signs. Assess patient for hypotension, bradycardia or tachycardia, AV block, and evidence of impending cardiac arrest.
• Evaluate respiratory and neurologic status.

Patient teaching
• Instruct patient to take tablets 1 hour before or 2 hours after meals.
◀€ Tell patient drug may alter his respiratory and cardiac status. Teach him to recognize and immediately report warning signs.
• Caution patient to avoid driving and other hazardous activities until he knows how drug affects concentration, vision, muscle function, and alertness.
• As appropriate, review all other significant and life-threatening adverse reactions and interactions, especially those related to the drugs mentioned above.

nesiritide
Natrecor

Pharmacologic class: Human B-type natriuretic peptide
Therapeutic class: Vasodilator
Pregnancy risk category C

Action
Binds to receptors on vascular smooth muscle and endothelial cells, causing smooth muscle relaxation and vasodilation. As a result, systemic and pulmonary pressures decrease and diuresis occurs.

Availability
Injection: 1.5 mg in single-use vials

Indications and dosages
➤ Acutely decompensated heart failure in patients who have dyspnea at rest or with minimal activity
Adults: 2 mcg/kg I.V. bolus, followed by continuous I.V. infusion of 0.01 mcg/kg/minute

Contraindications
• Hypersensitivity to drug or its components
• Systolic pressure below 90 mm Hg
• Primary therapy for cardiogenic shock

Precautions
Use cautiously in:
• restrictive or obstructive cardiomyopathy, constrictive pericarditis, pericardial tamponade, renal dysfunction, hypotension
• pregnant or breastfeeding patients.

Administration
🔊 Know that nesiritide is a high-alert drug.
• For I.V. use, prime tubing before connecting to patient. Withdraw bolus and infuse over 60 seconds into I.V. port of tubing. Follow immediately with constant infusion delivering 0.01 mcg/kg/minute.
• Know that drug should be mixed and infused in dextrose 5% in water, normal saline solution, or dextrose in half-normal saline solution.
🔊 Don't mix with other drug solutions. Always administer through separate line.

• Know that nesiritide therapy beyond 48 hours has not been studied.

Route	Onset	Peak	Duration
I.V.	Immediate	15 min	Unknown

Adverse reactions
CNS: dizziness, headache, insomnia, anxiety
CV: hypotension, angina pectoris, bradycardia, ventricular extrasystole, **ventricular tachycardia**
GI: nausea, vomiting, abdominal pain
Musculoskeletal: leg cramps, back pain
Respiratory: cough, hemoptysis, **apnea**
Other: injection site reactions

Interactions
Drug-drug. *Angiotensin-converting enzyme inhibitors, nitrates:* increased hypotension
Bumetanide, enalaprilat, ethacrynate sodium, furosemide, heparin, hydralazine, insulin: physical and chemical incompatibility with nesiritide
Drug-diagnostic tests. *Hematocrit, hemoglobin:* decreased values

Patient monitoring
• Monitor vital signs and pulmonary artery wedge pressure continuously during and for several hours after infusion.
• Assess cardiovascular status closely.

Patient teaching
• Tell patient he'll be monitored closely during and for several hours after infusion.
• Inform patient that drug may cause serious adverse effects. Reassure him that he'll receive appropriate interventions to relieve symptoms.
• Instruct patient to report chest pain, dizziness, palpitations, and other uncomfortable symptoms.
• As appropriate, review all other significant and life-threatening adverse reactions and interactions, especially those related to the drugs and tests mentioned above.

n

nevirapine
Viramune, Viramune XR

Pharmacologic class: Nonnucleoside reverse transcriptase inhibitor
Therapeutic class: Antiretroviral
Pregnancy risk category C

FDA | BOXED WARNING

- Drug has caused severe, life-threatening, and in some cases fatal hepatotoxicity, particularly in first 18 weeks. In some cases, patients had nonspecific, prodromal signs or symptoms of hepatitis and progressed to hepatic failure. These events are commonly associated with rash. Women and patients with higher CD4+ cell counts at initiation of therapy are at increased risk. Women with CD4+ cell counts greater than 250/mm^3, including pregnant women receiving nevirapine in combination with other antiretrovirals for treatment of HIV-1 infection, are at greatest risk. However, hepatotoxicity associated with nevirapine use can occur in both men and women, and at any time during treatment. Hepatic failure has also been reported in patients without HIV taking nevirapine for postexposure prophylaxis (PEP). Use of nevirapine for occupational and nonoccupational PEP is contraindicated. Patients must discontinue drug and seek immediate medical help if they develop hepatitis signs or symptoms or have increased transaminase levels along with rash or other systemic symptoms.
- Severe, life-threatening skin reactions (including fatal cases) have occurred; these have included Stevens-Johnson syndrome, toxic epidermal necrolysis, and hypersensitivity reactions. Patients who develop signs or symptoms of severe skin reactions or hypersensitivity reactions must discontinue drug and seek immediate medical help.
- Monitor patients intensively during first 18 weeks of therapy. Be especially vigilant during first 6 weeks. Don't restart drug in patient who has had clinical hepatitis or transaminase elevations combined with rash or other systemic symptoms, or after severe rash, or hypersensitivity reaction.

Action
Inhibits human immunodeficiency virus (HIV) nonnucleoside reverse transcriptase by binding directly to reverse transcriptase and blocking RNA-dependent and DNA-dependent polymerase activity

Availability
Oral suspension: 50 mg/5 ml
Tablets: 200 mg
Tablets (extended-release): 400 mg

⊘ Indications and dosages
➣ Treatment of HIV-1 infection
Adults: 200 mg P.O. daily for 14 days, then 200 mg (immediate-release) P.O. b.i.d., given in combination with other antiretrovirals; 400 mg (extended-release) P.O. daily after either a 14-day 200-mg lead-in regimen or after switching from a 200-mg b.i.d. regimen.
Children ages 15 days and older: 150 mg/m^2 (immediate-release tablet or oral suspension) P.O. once daily for 14 days, followed by 150 mg/m^2 b.i.d. thereafter. Total daily dosage shouldn't exceed 400 mg for any patient.

Dosage adjustment
- Chronic hemodialysis

Off-label uses
- Prophylaxis of maternal-fetal HIV transmission

♦ Canada   ⊕ UK   ⚕ Hazardous drug   ⊗ High-alert drug

Contraindications

- Hypersensitivity to drug or its components
- Moderate or severe hepatic impairment (Child-Pugh Class B or C, respectively)
- Use as part of occupational and nonoccupational postexposure prophylaxis regimens

Precautions

Use cautiously in:
- impaired renal or hepatic function
- pregnant or breastfeeding patients
- children.

Administration

- Be aware that drug should be given alone for first 14 days to reduce incidence of rash.
- If patient experiences rash during 14-day lead-in period with immediate-release form, don't initiate extended-release form until rash has resolved.
- Don't continue immediate-release lead-in dosing regimen beyond 28 days. If immediate-release dosing is interrupted for more than 7 days, restart recommended dosing, including 14-day lead-in dosing.
- For patients who interrupt extended-release dosing for more than 7 days, restart recommended lead-in dosing with immediate-release form using one 200-mg tablet daily for first 14 days.
- Be aware that drug shouldn't be started in adult females with CD4+ cell counts greater than 250/mm^3 or in adult males with CD4+ cell counts greater than 400/mm^3 because of serious and life-threatening hepatotoxicity, unless benefit outweighs risk.
- Give with or without food.

Route	Onset	Peak	Duration
P.O.	Unknown	4 hr	Unknown

Adverse reactions

CNS: paresthesia, headache, malaise, fatigue
GI: nausea, diarrhea, abdominal pain
Hematologic: agranulocytosis
Hepatic: hepatitis, hepatotoxicity, hepatic failure
Musculoskeletal: myalgia, pain
Skin: rash, blistering, toxic epidermal necrolysis, **Stevens-Johnson syndrome**
Other: fever

Interactions

Drug-drug. *Antiarrhythmics, antifungals, calcium channel blockers, cancer chemotherapy, ergot alkaloids, immunosuppressants, motility agents, opiate agonists:* possible decreased plasma concentrations of these drugs
Anticoagulants: possible increased or decreased anticoagulant plasma concentrations
Clarithromycin, efavirenz, indinavir, ketoconazole, methadone: decreased activity of these drugs
Ethinyl estradiol, norethindrone: decreased contraceptive plasma levels
Fluconazole: increased nevirapine level
Lopinavir/ritonavir: decreased lopinavir activity
Nelfinavir: decreased nelfinavir active metabolite, minimum nelfinavir concentration
Rifabutin: increased rifabutin level
Drug-diagnostic tests. *Alanine aminotransferase, aspartate aminotransferase, bilirubin, gamma-glutamyltransferase:* increased levels
Hemoglobin, neutrophils: decreased levels
Drug-herbs. *St. John's wort:* decreased nevirapine blood level

Patient monitoring

🔊 Check closely for rash (which may be first sign of Stevens-Johnson syndrome), especially during first 6 months of therapy.
- Monitor patient's weight, temperature, and chest X-ray periodically.
- Assess patient's appetite and energy and physical activity levels.
- Monitor liver function tests and CBC with white cell differential.

Reactions in **bold** are life-threatening.

🔊 Clinical alert

Patient teaching
• Tell patient he may take with or without food.
• Tell patient or caregiver to shake suspension gently before use and that it's important to take the entire measured dose of suspension by using an oral dosing syringe or dosing cup.
• Tell patient or caregiver that the extended-release tablet must be swallowed whole and must not be chewed, crushed, or divided.
• Instruct patient to take missed dose as soon as he remembers. But if it's almost time for next dose, tell him to skip missed dose. Caution him not to double the dose.
• Inform female patient that hormonal contraceptives, implants, or shots may be ineffective during nevirapine therapy. Urge her to use alternative birth-control method.
◀€ Teach patient to recognize and immediately report rash, easy bruising or bleeding, and signs and symptoms of hepatotoxicity.
• Inform patient that nevirapine won't cure HIV or prevent its transmission.
• Caution female not to breastfeed, because breast milk may transfer HIV to infant.
• As appropriate, review all other significant and life-threatening adverse reactions and interactions, especially those related to the drugs, tests, and herbs mentioned above.

nicardipine hydrochloride
Cardene, Cardene IV, Cardene SR

Pharmacologic class: Calcium channel blocker
Therapeutic class: Antianginal, antihypertensive
Pregnancy risk category C

Action
Inhibits calcium transport into myocardial and vascular smooth muscle cells, causing cardiac output and myocardial contractions to decrease

Availability
Capsules: 20 mg, 30 mg
Capsules (sustained-release): 30 mg, 45 mg, 60 mg
Injection: 2.5 mg/ml in 10-ml ampules

🖊 Indications and dosages
➤ Chronic stable angina, given alone or with beta-adrenergic blockers
Adults: Titrate dosage individually, starting with 20 to 40 mg P.O. (immediate-release) t.i.d. Wait at least 3 days before increasing dosage.
➤ Hypertension, given alone or with other antihypertensives
Adults: Titrate dosage individually, starting with 20 mg P.O. (immediate release) t.i.d. Wait at least 3 days before increasing dosage. Dosage range is 20 to 40 mg P.O. t.i.d. Patient may be switched to sustained-release capsules at nearest equivalent daily dosage of immediate-release capsules, starting with 30 mg P.O. b.i.d. Effective range is 30 to 60 mg/day.
➤ Short-term treatment of hypertension when oral therapy isn't feasible or desirable
Adults: Continuous I.V. infusion of 0.5 mg/hour (equal to 20 mg P.O. q 8 hours), or 1.2 mg/hour (equal to 30 mg P.O. q 8 hours), or 2.2 mg/hour (equal to 40 mg P.O. q 8 hours)

Off-label uses
• Raynaud's disease
• Heart failure
• Migraine

Contraindications
• Hypersensitivity to drug
• Advanced aortic stenosis

Precautions
Use cautiously in:
- hepatic or mild renal impairment
- hypotension, heart failure, significant left ventricular dysfunction
- pheochromocytoma
- pregnant or breastfeeding patients (safety not established)
- children younger than age 18 (safety not established).

Administration
- Give immediate-release capsules without regard to meals; if GI upset occurs, give with meals. Don't give with grapefruit or grapefruit juice.
- Don't open, crush, break, or let patient chew sustained-release capsules. Give with meals, but not with high-fat meals, grapefruit, or grapefruit juice.
- For I.V. use, dilute each 25-mg ampule with 240 ml of compatible I.V. fluid (such as dextrose 5% in water, normal saline solution, dextrose 5% with normal saline solution, or half-normal saline solution) to a concentration of 0.1 mg/ml.

◄€ Don't dilute with sodium bicarbonate 5% or lactated Ringer's injection (incompatible).
- Don't mix with furosemide, heparin, or thiopental.

◄€ Give by slow I.V. infusion. Titrate dosage to blood pressure response.

Route	Onset	Peak	Duration
P.O.	20 min	0.5-2 hr	8 hr
P.O. (sustained)	Unknown	Unknown	12 hr
I.V.	Few min	45 min	Unknown

Adverse reactions
CNS: dizziness, headache, asthenia, drowsiness, paresthesia
CV: hypotension, peripheral edema, chest pain, increased angina, palpitations, tachycardia
GI: nausea, dyspepsia, dry mouth

Musculoskeletal: myalgia
Skin: flushing

Interactions
Drug-drug. *Cimetidine:* increased nifedipine blood level
Cyclosporine: increased cyclosporine blood level
Fentanyl anesthesia: increased hypotension
Drug-food. *Grapefruit, grapefruit juice:* increased drug blood level and effects
High-fat meal (sustained-release form): decreased drug blood level
Drug-herbs. *Ephedra (ma huang), yohimbine:* antagonism of drug's antihypertensive effect
St. John's wort: decreased nifedipine blood level
Drug-behaviors. *Alcohol use:* additive hypotension, increased drowsiness or dizziness

Patient monitoring
- Assess vital signs and cardiovascular status.
- Monitor fluid intake and output. Assess for signs and symptoms of heart failure.

Patient teaching
- Tell patient he may take immediate-release capsules without regard to meals. If GI upset occurs, advise him to take them with food, but not with grapefruit or grapefruit juice.
- Tell patient not to open, crush, break, or chew sustained-release capsules. Instruct him to take them with meals, but not with high-fat meals, grapefruit, or grapefruit juice.
- Tell patient to monitor blood pressure and report abnormal findings.

◄€ Advise patient to immediately report chest pain or blood pressure drop.
- Instruct patient to consult prescriber before drinking alcohol or taking herbs or over-the-counter drugs (especially cold remedies).

n

Reactions in **bold** are life-threatening. ◄€ Clinical alert

• As appropriate, review all other significant adverse reactions and interactions, especially those related to the drugs, foods, herbs, and behaviors mentioned above.

nicotine

nicotine inhaler
Nicotrol Inhaler

nicotine nasal spray
Nicotrol NS

nicotine polacrilex
Commit, Nicorette, Nicotinell⊕

nicotine transdermal system
Clear Nicoderm CQ, Nicoderm CQ, Nicopatch⊕, Nicorette Patch⊕, NiQuitin⊕, Prostep❦

Pharmacologic class: Cholinergic
Therapeutic class: Smoking deterrent
Pregnancy risk category C (gum), *D* (inhalation, nasal, transdermal)

Action
Supplies nicotine during controlled withdrawal from cigarette smoking. Binds selectively to nicotinic-cholinergic receptors in central and peripheral nervous systems, autonomic ganglia, adrenal medulla, and neuromuscular junction. At low doses, has a stimulating effect; at high doses, a reward effect.

Availability
Chewing gum: 2 mg, 4 mg
Inhalation: 42 cartridges/system, each containing 10 mg nicotine (delivers 4 mg)

Nasal spray: 10 mg/ml (0.5 mg/spray) in 10-ml bottles (100 doses)
Transdermal patch: 7 mg/day, 11 mg/day, 14 mg/day, 15 mg/day, 21 mg/day, 22 mg/day

Indications and dosages
➤ Adjunctive therapy (with behavior modification) for nicotine withdrawal
Transdermal system—
Adults: 21 mg/day transdermally (Habitrol) for 4 to 8 weeks, then 14 mg/day for 2 to 4 weeks, then 7 mg/day for 2 to 4 weeks, for a total of 8 to 16 weeks; patient must wear system 24 hours/day. Or 21 mg/day transdermally (Nicoderm CQ) for 6 weeks, then 14 mg/day for 2 weeks, then 7 mg/day for 2 weeks, for a total of 10 weeks; patient must wear system 24 hours/day. Or 15 mg/day transdermally (one Nicotrol patch) for 6 weeks; patient must wear system 16 hours/day, removing it at bedtime.
Adults, adolescents, and children weighing less than 45 kg (100 lb) who smoke fewer than 10 cigarettes daily or have underlying cardiovascular disease: 14 mg/day transdermally (Habitrol) for 4 to 8 weeks, then 7 mg/day for 2 to 4 weeks, for a total of 6 to 8 weeks; patient must wear system 24 hours/day. Or 14 mg/day transdermally (Nicoderm CQ) for 6 weeks, then 7 mg/day for 2 weeks, for a total of 8 weeks; patient must wear system 24 hours/day.
Nasal spray—
Adults: One spray intranasally in each nostril once or twice per hour, up to five times per hour or 40 times per day, for no longer than 6 months
Inhalation—
Adults: For optimal response, at least six cartridges inhaled daily for first 3 to 6 weeks, to a maximum of 16 cartridges daily for up to 12 weeks. Patient self-titrates dosage to required nicotine level (usually 6 to 16 cartridges daily),

followed by gradual withdrawal over 6 to 12 weeks.

Chewing gum—

Adults: Use as needed depending on smoking urge or chewing rate, or use on fixed schedule q 1 to 2 hours. Initial requirement may range from 18 to 48 mg/day, not to exceed 60 mg/day.

Route	Onset	Peak	Duration
Gum	Rapid	15-30 min	Unknown
Inhalation	Rapid	15 min	Unknown
Nasal spray	Rapid	4-15 min	Unknown
Transdermal (Habitrol)	Rapid	6-12 hr	Unknown
Transdermal (Nicoderm CQ)	Rapid	2-4 hr	Unknown

Contraindications

• Hypersensitivity to drug or its components or to menthol (inhaler only)
• Allergy to adhesive (transdermal forms only)

Precautions

Use cautiously in:
• cardiovascular disease, hypertension, bronchospastic disease, diabetes mellitus, pheochromocytoma, peripheral vascular disease, hyperthyroidism, peptic ulcer disease, hepatic disease
• immediately after myocardial infarction, severe arrhythmia, or severe or worsening angina (use not recommended)
• skin disorders (transdermal form)
• dental disorders, esophagitis, pharyngitis, stomatitis (gum form)
• females of childbearing age
• pregnant or breastfeeding patients.
• children under age 18 (safety and efficacy not established).

Administration

• Apply patch when patient awakens and remove patch (as prescribed) at same time each day.
• Administer nasal spray regularly during first week, to help patient get used to irritant effects.
• With inhalation use, give at least six cartridges daily for first 3 to 6 weeks.
• Encourage patient to titrate dosage to level required, followed by gradual withdrawal.

Adverse reactions

CNS: headache, dizziness, drowsiness, poor concentration, nervousness, weakness, paresthesia, insomnia, abnormal dreams

CV: chest pain, hypertension, tachycardia, **atrial fibrillation**

EENT: sinusitis; pharyngitis (with gum); mouth and throat irritation (with inhaler); nasopharyngeal irritation, rhinitis, sneezing, watering eyes, eye irritation (with nasal spray)

GI: nausea, vomiting, diarrhea, constipation, abdominal pain, dry mouth, dyspepsia; increased salivation, sore mouth (with gum)

GU: dysmenorrhea

Musculoskeletal: joint pain, back pain, myalgia; jaw ache (with gum)

Respiratory: increased cough (with nasal spray or inhaler), **bronchospasm**

Skin: burning at patch site, erythema, pruritus, cutaneous hypersensitivity, rash, sweating (all with transdermal patch)

Other: abnormal taste, increased appetite (with gum), allergy, hiccups

Interactions

Drug-drug. *Acetaminophen, adrenergic antagonists (such as prazosin, labetalol), clozapine, furosemide, imipramine, oxazepam, pentazocine, propranolol and other beta-adrenergic blockers, theophylline:* increased effects of these drugs

Bupropion: treatment-emergent hypertension

Insulin: decreased insulin requirement

n

Reactions in **bold** are life-threatening.   ◀◉ Clinical alert

Isoproterenol, phenylephrine: increased requirements for these drugs
Propoxyphene: decreased nicotine metabolism
Drug-food. *Caffeine-containing foods and beverages:* increased nicotine effects
Drug-behaviors. *Cigarette smoking:* increased nicotine metabolism and effects

Patient monitoring

• Assess for signs and symptoms of nicotine withdrawal (irritability, drowsiness, fatigue, headache).

◀≀ Watch for bronchospasm and evidence of nicotine toxicity (nausea, vomiting, diarrhea, increased salivation, headache, dizziness, visual disturbances).

Patient teaching

◀≀ Caution patient against any type of smoking during therapy. Urge him to immediately report chest tightness or difficulty breathing.

• If patient uses gum, advise him to chew one piece whenever nicotine craving occurs. Instruct him to chew it slowly until he feels a tingling sensation, then store it between cheek and gum until tingling disappears.

• Instruct patient to apply transdermal patch to clean, dry skin of upper arm or torso when he awakens; to keep it in place when showering, bathing, or swimming; and to remove it at same time each day.

• If patient uses nasal spray, instruct him to tilt head back slightly when spraying. Remind him not to sniff, swallow, or inhale through nose.

• If patient uses inhalation form, teach him to puff continuously for 20 minutes and to use at least six cartridges daily for first 3 to 6 weeks.

• As appropriate, review all significant and life-threatening adverse reactions and interactions, especially those related to the drugs, foods, and behaviors mentioned above.

nifedipine

Adalat CC, Adalat LA✚, Adalat P.A.✿, Adalat Retard✚, Adalat XL✿, Adipine✚, Afeditab CR, Angiopine✚, Apo-Nifed✿, Calchan✚, Cardilate MR✚, Coracten✚, Fortipine✚, Gen-Nifedical✿, Hypolar Retard✚, Neozipine XL✚, Nifediac CC, Nifedical XL, Nifedipress MR✚, Nifopress MR✚, Novo-Nifedin✿, Nu-Nifed, Procardia, Procardia XL, Slofedipine✚, Tensipine✚, Valni Retard✚, Valni XL✚

Pharmacologic class: Calcium channel blocker
Therapeutic class: Antianginal, antihypertensive
Pregnancy risk category C

Action

Inhibits calcium transport into myocardial and vascular smooth muscle cells, suppressing contractions. Dilates main coronary arteries and arterioles and inhibits coronary artery spasm, increasing oxygen delivery to heart and decreasing frequency and severity of angina attacks.

Availability

Capsules: 5 mg, 10 mg, 20 mg
Tablets (extended-release): 10 mg, 20 mg, 30 mg, 60 mg, 90 mg

⦿ Indications and dosages

➤ Vasospastic (Prinzmetal's) angina; chronic stable angina
Adults: Initially, 10 mg P.O. (immediate-release) t.i.d. titrated over 7 to 14 days; usual effective range is 10 to

20 mg t.i.d., not to exceed 180 mg/day. Patient may be switched to extended-release at nearest equivalent of immediate-release daily dosage (for instance, 30-mg immediate-release dose may be switched to 90-mg extended-release dose). Total extended-release dosage should not exceed 90 mg/day.

➢ Hypertension

Adults: 30 to 60 mg/day P.O. (extended-release only) titrated over 7 to 14 days to a maximum of 120 mg/day

Off-label uses

- Aortic regurgitation
- Heart failure
- Migraine
- Prevention of labor

Contraindications

- Hypersensitivity to drug

Precautions

Use cautiously in:
- chronic renal insufficiency
- hypotension, aortic stenosis, heart failure, significant left ventricular dysfunction (especially when used with beta-adrenergic blockers), peripheral edema
- elderly patients
- pregnant or breastfeeding patients (safety not established)
- children (safety not established).

Administration

- Give immediate-release form with or without food. If GI upset occurs, give with meals, but never with grapefruit or grapefruit juice.
- Don't crush or break extended-release tablet. Make sure patient swallows it whole. Give on empty stomach, and not with grapefruit or grapefruit juice.
- Know that Procardia XL and Adalat CC are not equivalent because of their pharmacokinetic differences.
- Be aware that only extended-release tablets are used to treat hypertension.

Route	Onset	Peak	Duration
P.O.	20 min	Unknown	6-8 hr
P.O. (Adalat PA)	Unknown	4 hr	12 hr
P.O. (Adalat CC, PA, XL)	Unknown	6 hr	24 hr

Adverse reactions

CNS: headache, dizziness, fatigue, asthenia, paresthesia, vertigo
CV: peripheral edema, chest pain, hypotension
EENT: epistaxis, rhinitis
GI: nausea, constipation
GU: urinary frequency, erectile dysfunction
Musculoskeletal: leg cramps
Skin: flushing, rash

Interactions

Drug-drug. *Beta-adrenergic blockers*: increased risk of heart failure, severe hypotension, or angina exacerbation
Cimetidine: increased nifedipine blood level
Coumarin anticoagulants: increased prothrombin time
Digoxin: increased risk of digoxin toxicity
Quinidine: decreased quinidine blood level
Drug-diagnostic tests. *Antinuclear antibody, direct Coombs' test:* false-positive results
Drug-food. *Grapefruit, grapefruit juice:* increased nifedipine blood level and effects
Drug-herbs. *Ephedra (ma huang), yohimbine:* antagonism of nifedipine effect
Ginkgo, ginseng: increased nifedipine blood level
St. John's wort: decreased nifedipine blood level
Drug-behaviors. *Alcohol use:* additive hypotension

n

Patient monitoring
• Monitor vital signs and cardiovascular status. Stay alert for chest pain and edema.
• Watch for rash.

Patient teaching
• Tell patient he may take immediate-release form with or without meals. If GI upset occurs, tell him to take it with meals, but never with grapefruit or grapefruit juice.
• Caution patient not to crush or break extended-release tablets. Tell him to swallow them whole. Advise him to take on empty stomach, and not with grapefruit or grapefruit juice.
• Inform patient that angina attacks may occur 30 minutes after a dose. Explain that these attacks are usually temporary and don't mean that drug should be withdrawn.
◀€ Tell patient to report rash immediately.
• Caution patient to avoid driving and other hazardous activities until he knows how drug affects concentration, balance, and alertness.
• Instruct patient to consult prescriber before taking herbs or over-the-counter drugs (especially cold remedies).
• As appropriate, review all other significant adverse reactions and interactions, especially those related to the drugs, tests, foods, herbs, and behaviors mentioned above.

nilotinib
Tasigna

Pharmacologic class: Protein-tyrosine kinase inhibitor
Therapeutic class: Antineoplastic
Pregnancy risk category D

FDA BOXED WARNING
• Drug prolongs QT interval and may lead to sudden death. Don't give to patients with hypokalemia, hypomagnesemia, or long-QT syndrome. Correct hypokalemia or hypomagnesemia before starting drug and monitor for these imbalances periodically. Avoid concomitant drugs known to prolong QT interval; also avoid strong CYP3A4 inhibitors. Instruct patient not to eat 2 hours before or 1 hour after taking dose. Obtain ECG to monitor QTc at baseline, 7 days after drug initiation, periodically thereafter, and after dosage adjustments.
• Reduce dosage in patients with hepatic impairment.

Action
Inhibits proliferation of murine leukemic cell lines mediated by BCR-ABL kinase and human cell lines derived from patients with Philadelphia chromosome–positive (Ph+) chronic myeloid leukemia (CML)

Availability
Capsules: 200 mg

⚕ Indications and dosages
➤ Chronic-phase or accelerated-phase Ph+ CML in patients resistant or intolerant to previous imatinib therapy
Adults: 400 mg P.O. q 12 hours
➤ Newly diagnosed Philadelphia chromosome positive CML
Adults: 300 mg P.O. q 12 hours

Dosage adjustment
• QTc longer than 480 msec
• Hematologic toxicity
• Moderate or severe non-hematologic toxicity
• Concomitant use of CYP3A4 inducers
• Hepatic impairment

Off-label uses

• Ph+ acute lymphoblastic leukemia (ALL)
• Systemic mastocytosis with *c-kit* receptor activation
• Hypereosinophilic syndrome

Contraindications

• Hypokalemia
• Hypomagnesemia
• Long-QT syndrome

Precautions

Use cautiously in:
• hepatic impairment
• rare hereditary problems of galactose intolerance, severe lactase deficiency, or glucose-galactose malabsorption (use not recommended)
• myelosuppression
• electrolyte abnormalities
• history of pancreatitis
• pregnant or breastfeeding patients
• children (safety and efficacy not established).

Administration

◀€ Correct hypophosphatemia and hypokalemia before starting drug.
• Don't give with food. Know that patient shouldn't consume food for at least 2 hours before or 1 hour after dose.
• Administer capsule whole with water.
• Be aware that drug may be given in combination with hematopoietic growth factors, if indicated.

Route	Onset	Peak	Duration
P.O.	Unknown	3 hr	Unknown

Adverse reactions

CNS: headache, fatigue, asthenia, insomnia, dizziness, paresthesia, vertigo, **intracranial hemorrhage**
CV: palpitations, hypertension, flushing, **QT interval prolongation and sudden death**
EENT: dysphonia, nasopharyngitis
GI: nausea, vomiting, diarrhea, constipation, abdominal pain, abdominal discomfort, dyspepsia, flatulence, anorexia
Hematologic: anemia, **neutropenia, thrombocytopenia, leukopenia, pancytopenia, febrile neutropenia**
Hepatic: hepatotoxicity
Metabolic: electrolyte abnormalities
Musculoskeletal: arthralgia, myalgia, extremity pain, bone pain, muscle spasms, back pain, chest pain
Respiratory: cough, dyspnea, exertional dyspnea, pneumonia
Skin: rash, pruritus, eczema, urticaria, alopecia, erythema, hyperhidrosis, dry skin
Other: fever, peripheral edema, night sweats, weight changes

Interactions

Drug-drug. *Drugs eliminated by CYP2B6, CYP2C8, or CYP2C9:* decreased blood levels of these drugs
Drugs eliminated by CYP3A4 (such as warfarin), CYP2C8, CYP2C9, CYP2D6, or UGT1A1: increased blood levels of these drugs
Drugs that inhibit P-glycoprotein ABCB1: increased nilotinib blood level
Midazolam: increased midazolam exposure
P-glycoprotein substrates: increased blood levels of these drugs
Strong CYP3A4 inducers (such as carbamazepine, dexamethasone, phenytoin, rifabutin, rifampin, rifapentin, phenobarbital): decreased nilotinib blood level
Strong CYP3A4 inhibitors (such as atazanavir, clarithromycin, indinavir, itraconazole, ketoconazole, nefazodone, nelfinavir, ritonavir, saquinavir, telithromycin, voriconazole): increased nilotinib blood level
Drug-diagnostic tests. *Albumin, calcium, magnesium, neutrophils, phosphorus, platelets, sodium, white blood cells:* decreased levels
ALP, ALT, AST, bilirubin, blood glucose, creatinine, serum amylase, serum lipase: increased levels
Potassium: increased or decreased level

n

Drug-food. *Grapefruit products:* increased nilotinib blood level
High-fat meal: increased nilotinib onset
Drug-herbs. *St. John's wort:* decreased nilotinib blood level

Patient monitoring

◀ɛ Closely monitor for prolonged QT interval if patient has hepatic impairment or is receiving strong CYP3A4 inhibitors.

• Obtain complete blood count every 2 weeks for first 2 months of therapy and monthly thereafter, or as indicated.

• Periodically monitor electrolyte and lipase levels and liver function tests.

Patient teaching

• Tell patient not to take drug with food and not to consume food for at least 2 hours before or 1 hour after dose.

• Advise patient to take capsules whole with water.

◀ɛ Instruct patient to avoid grapefruit products and St. John's wort.

• Tell lactose-intolerant patient that drug contains lactose.

◀ɛ Instruct patient to immediately notify prescriber if symptoms of QTc prolongation (faintness or irregular heartbeat) occur.

◀ɛ Urge patient to immediately report signs or symptoms of liver damage, such as nausea, fatigue, anorexia, yellowing of skin or eyes, dark urine, light-colored stools, itching, or abdominal tenderness.

• Advise female patient that drug may harm fetus. Caution her to avoid pregnancy.

• Advise breastfeeding patient to seek guidance to help her decide whether to discontinue breastfeeding or discontinue drug.

• As appropriate, review all other significant and life-threatening adverse reactions and interactions, especially those related to the drugs, tests, food, and herbs mentioned above.

nilutamide
Anandron✚, Nilandron

Pharmacologic class: Antiandrogen
Therapeutic class: Antineoplastic
Pregnancy risk category C

FDA | BOXED WARNING

• Drug may cause interstitial pneumonitis. Though rare, interstitial changes have led to hospitalization and death postmarketing. Most cases occurred within first 3 months of therapy and reversed after drug was stopped. Obtain routine chest X-ray before starting treatment, and be prepared to obtain baseline pulmonary function tests if ordered. Instruct patient to report new or worsening shortness of breath; this symptom warrants immediate drug withdrawal pending evaluation.

Action

Inhibits testosterone uptake in target tissue, preventing normal androgenic response and arresting tumor growth in androgen-sensitive tissue

Availability

Tablets: 50 mg, 150 mg

ⓘ Indications and dosages

➤ Metastatic prostate cancer (used with surgical castration)
Adults: 300 mg/day P.O. for 30 days, starting on day of or day after surgery; then 150 mg/day P.O.

Contraindications

• Hypersensitivity to drug or its components

• Severe hepatic or respiratory insufficiency

✚ Canada   ⊕ UK   ☣ Hazardous drug   ⊗ High-alert drug

Precautions
Use cautiously in:
- renal impairment.

Administration
- Give with or without food.
- Start therapy on same day as or day after surgical castration.

Route	Onset	Peak	Duration
P.O.	Rapid	Days	Wks

Adverse reactions
CNS: dizziness, depression, hyperesthesia, insomnia
CV: hypertension, peripheral edema, **heart failure**
EENT: abnormal vision, impaired dark and light adaptation, chromatopsia
GI: nausea, vomiting, constipation, dyspepsia, anorexia
GU: hematuria, nocturia, urinary tract infection, gynecomastia, testicular atrophy, decreased libido, erectile dysfunction
Hematologic: anemia, **aplastic anemia**
Hepatic: hepatitis
Respiratory: dyspnea, upper respiratory infection, **interstitial pneumonia**
Other: flulike symptoms, pain, fever, hot flushes, alcohol intolerance

Interactions
Drug-drug. *Phenytoin, theophylline, vitamin K:* increased risk of toxicity from these drugs
Drug-diagnostic tests. *Alanine aminotransferase, aspartate aminotransferase:* increased levels
Drug-behaviors. *Alcohol use:* disulfiram-like reaction

Patient monitoring
- Check for signs and symptoms of hepatitis. Monitor liver function tests.
- Monitor CBC.
- Assess fluid intake and output and weight. Watch for signs and symptoms of heart failure.
- Monitor respiratory status, including chest X-rays.

Patient teaching
- Advise patient he may take with or without food.
- Tell patient therapy will start on day of or day after surgical castration.
- Caution patient not to stop taking drug without consulting prescriber.
- Instruct patient to weigh himself daily and report sudden increases.
- 🔊 Advise patient to report new onset or worsening of dyspnea as well as signs and symptoms of hepatotoxicity, such as nausea, vomiting, abdominal pain, unusual tiredness, or yellowing of skin or eyes.
- Advise patient to avoid alcohol during therapy, because serious adverse reactions may occur.
- Tell patient drug may impair his adaptation to darkness and light, which may cause difficulty driving at night or through tunnels.
- As appropriate, review all other significant and life-threatening adverse reactions and interactions, especially those related to the drugs, test, and behaviors mentioned above.

nimodipine
Nimotop

Pharmacologic class: Calcium channel blocker
Therapeutic class: Cerebral vasodilator
Pregnancy risk category C

FDA | BOXED WARNING

- Don't give by I.V. or other parenteral route. Deaths and serious or life-threatening adverse events have occurred when capsule contents have been injected parenterally.

Action

Inhibits calcium transport into vascular smooth muscle cells, suppressing contractions; also dilates coronary and cerebral arteries

Availability

Capsules: 30 mg

⊘ Indications and dosages

➤ Subarachnoid hemorrhage

Adults: 60 mg P.O. q 4 hours for 21 days. Therapy should start within 96 hours of subarachnoid hemorrhage.

Dosage adjustment

• Hepatic impairment

Contraindications

None

Precautions

Use cautiously in:
• hepatic impairment, hypotension
• elderly patients
• pregnant or breastfeeding patients (safety not established)
• children (safety not established).

Administration

• Give at least 1 hour before or 2 hours after meals. Don't let patient consume grapefruit or grapefruit juice within 1 hour before or 2 hours after dose.
• If patient can't swallow capsule, puncture it with sterile needle and empty contents into syringe. Administer through nasogastric tube, then flush with normal saline solution (30 ml).

Route	Onset	Peak	Duration
P.O.	Unknown	1 hr	4 hr

Adverse reactions

CNS: headache, depression
CV: hypotension, peripheral edema, ECG abnormalities, bradycardia, tachycardia
GI: nausea, diarrhea, abdominal discomfort
Musculoskeletal: muscle cramps
Respiratory: dyspnea
Skin: acne, flushing, rash

Interactions

Drug-drug. *Other calcium channel blockers:* enhanced cardiovascular effects
Drug-diagnostic tests. *Liver function tests:* abnormal results
Drug-food. *Any food:* decreased drug blood level and effects
Grapefruit juice, grapefruit juice: increased drug blood level and effects
Drug-herbs. *Ephedra (ma huang), yohimbine:* antagonism of nimodipine effects
St. John's wort: decreased drug blood level
Drug-behaviors. *Alcohol use:* increased hypotension

Patient monitoring

• Monitor weight and fluid intake and output. Stay alert for fluid retention.
• Assess neurologic status and mood, watching for signs of depression.
• Check vital signs and ECG.

Patient teaching

• Tell patient to complete full course of therapy (21 days).
• Advise patient to take on an empty stomach 1 hour before or 2 hours after a meal. Instruct him to not to consume grapefruit or grapefruit juice within 1 hour before or 2 hours after taking drug.
• Tell patient to report irregular heartbeat, shortness of breath, rash, or swollen hands or feet.
• Instruct patient to minimize GI upset by eating small, frequent meals.
• Advise patient to weigh himself daily and report sudden weight gain.
• As appropriate, review all other significant adverse reactions and interactions, especially those related to the drugs, tests, foods, herbs, and behaviors mentioned above.

---

nisoldipine
Sular, Syscor✠

Pharmacologic class: Calcium channel blocker
Therapeutic class: Antihypertensive
Pregnancy risk category C

Action
Suppresses calcium transport into vascular smooth muscle cells. This suppression inhibits vasoconstriction and dilates coronary arteries, improving myocardial oxygen uptake.

Availability
Tablets (extended-release): 8.5 mg, 17 mg, 22.5 mg, 34 mg

⟩ Indications and dosages
➣ Hypertension
Adults: Initially, 17 mg P.O. daily; may increase by 8.5 mg per week or longer intervals to attain adequate blood pressure control. Usual maintenance dosage is 17 to 34 mg daily.

Contraindications
• Hypersensitivity to drug or dihydropyridine calcium channel blockers

Precautions
Use cautiously in:
• heart failure and left ventricular dysfunction, hepatic impairment, renal disease, coronary artery disease, hypotension
• concurrent phenytoin use
• elderly patients
• pregnant or breastfeeding patients
• children (safety not established).

Administration
• Give with meals, but not with high-fat meals, grapefruit, or grapefruit juice.

• Don't crush or break extended-release tablets. Make sure patient swallows them whole.
• Know that drug may be given alone or with other antihypertensives.

Route	Onset	Peak	Duration
P.O.	Unknown	6-12 hr	24 hr

Adverse reactions
CNS: headache, dizziness
CV: peripheral edema, chest pain, vasodilation, hypotension, palpitations
EENT: pharyngitis, sinusitis
GI: nausea
Skin: rash

Interactions
Drug-drug. *Cimetidine:* increased nisoldipine blood level
Phenytoin, other CYP3A4 inducers: decreased nisoldipine blood level and efficacy
Drug-food. *Grapefruit juice:* significantly increased drug blood level and effects
High-fat meal: decreased drug blood level
Drug-herbs. *Ephedra (ma huang), yohimbine:* antagonism of nimodipine effects
St. John's wort: decreased nimodipine blood level
Drug-behaviors. *Alcohol use:* increased hypotensive effects

Patient monitoring
• Check vital signs and ECG.
• Monitor fluid intake and output. Watch for peripheral edema.

Patient teaching
• Tell patient to swallow extended-release tablets whole and not to crush or break them.
• Advise patient to take with food, but not high-fat food. Recommend small, frequent meals.

n

Reactions in **bold** are life-threatening.   ◀◁ Clinical alert

- Instruct patient to avoid high-fat meals, alcohol, grapefruit, and grapefruit juice.
- Tell patient to immediately report irregular heart beat, shortness of breath, swelling, pronounced dizziness, rash, or chest pain.
- As appropriate, review all other significant adverse reactions and interactions, especially those related to the drugs, foods, herbs, and behaviors mentioned above.

nitazoxanide
Alinia

Pharmacologic class: Antiprotozoal
Therapeutic class: Anti-infective
Pregnancy risk category B

Action
Impedes pyruvate:ferredoxin oxido-reductase enzyme-dependent electron transfer reaction, which is essential to anaerobic energy metabolism

Availability
Oral suspension: 100 mg/5 ml
Tablets: 500 mg

🖊 Indications and dosages
➤ Diarrhea caused by *Giardia lamblia* or *Cryptosporidium parvum*
Adults and children ages 12 and older: 500 mg (tablet or 25 ml suspension) P.O. every 12 hours with food for 3 days
Children ages 4 to 11: 200 mg (10 ml suspension) P.O. every 12 hours with food for 3 days
Children ages 1 to 3: 100 mg (5 ml suspension) P.O. every 12 hours with food for 3 days

Contraindications
- Hypersensitivity to drug or its components

Precautions
Use cautiously in:
- renal, hepatic, or biliary disease or dysfunction; immunodeficiency (including human immunodeficiency virus); diabetes mellitus (suspension)
- concurrent use of warfarin or other highly plasma protein–bound drugs
- elderly patients
- pregnant or breastfeeding patients
- children younger than age 11 (tablets) or age 1 (suspension).

Administration
- Give with food.
- Because a single tablet contains more nitazoxanide than recommended for pediatric dosing, don't give tablets to children younger than age 11.
- Keep suspension container tightly closed and shake well before each use. Suspension may be stored for 7 days; after that, discard unused portion.

Route	Onset	Peak	Duration
P.O.	Unknown	1-4 hr	Unknown

Adverse reactions
CNS: headache
GI: nausea, vomiting, diarrhea, abdominal pain

Interactions
Drug-drug. *Warfarin and other highly plasma protein–bound drugs with narrow therapeutic index:* competition for binding sites, resulting in increased nitazoxanide blood level and efficacy

Patient monitoring
- Monitor renal and liver function tests frequently in patients with renal, hepatic, or biliary dysfunction.
- Monitor blood glucose levels in diabetic patients taking oral suspension.

Patient teaching
- Instruct patient to take drug with food.

• Inform diabetic patient that oral suspension contains sucrose.
• As appropriate, review all other significant adverse reactions and interactions, especially those related to the drugs mentioned above.

nitrofurantoin
Apo-Nitrofurantoin ✤, Furadantin, Novo-Furantoin ✤

nitrofurantoin macrocrystals
Macrobid, Macrodantin

Pharmacologic class: 5-nitrofuran derivative
Therapeutic class: Anti-infective, urinary tract anti-infective
Pregnancy risk category B

Action
Inhibits bacterial enzymes required for normal cell activity at low concentrations; inhibits normal cell-wall synthesis at high concentrations

Availability
Capsules: 25 mg, 50 mg, 100 mg (macrocrystals)
Capsules (extended-release): 100 mg (macrocrystals)
Oral suspension: 25 mg/5 ml
Tablets: 50 mg, 100 mg (macrocrystals)

💊 Indications and dosages
➤ Active urinary tract infections (UTIs)
Adults: 50 to 100 mg P.O. q.i.d. or 100 mg q 12 hours (extended-release), continued for 1 week, or for 3 days after urine becomes sterile
Children older than 1 month: 5 to 7 mg/kg/day P.O. in four divided doses, continued for 1 week, or for 3 days after urine becomes sterile

➤ Chronic suppression of UTIs
Adults: 50 to 100 mg P.O. at bedtime
Children: 1 mg/kg/day P.O. in one or two divided doses

Contraindications
• Hypersensitivity to drug or parabens (oral suspension)
• Oliguria, anuria, or significant renal impairment
• Pregnancy near term (38 to 42 weeks' gestation), imminent labor onset, labor and delivery
• Infants younger than 1 month

Precautions
Use cautiously in:
• diabetes mellitus, renal impairment
• blacks and patients of Mediterranean or near-Eastern descent (because of possible G6PD deficiency)
• elderly or debilitated patients
• pregnant (to week 32) or breastfeeding patients.

Administration
• As appropriate, obtain specimens for repeat urine culture and sensitivity tests before therapy.
• To avoid GI upset and increase drug bioavailability, give with food or milk.

Route	Onset	Peak	Duration
P.O.	Unknown	30 min	6-12 hr

Adverse reactions
CNS: dizziness, drowsiness, headache, asthenia, peripheral neuropathy, vertigo
CV: chest pain
EENT: nystagmus
GI: nausea, vomiting, diarrhea, abdominal pain, anorexia, parotitis, pancreatitis
Hematologic: eosinophilia, **agranulocytosis, thrombocytopenia, leukopenia, granulocytopenia, G6PD deficiency anemia, hemolytic anemia, megaloblastic anemia**
Hepatic: hepatitis, hepatic necrosis

n

Musculoskeletal: arthralgia, myalgia
Respiratory: asthma attacks, **pulmonary hypersensitivity reactions** including **diffuse interstitial pneumonitis** (with prolonged therapy)
Skin: rash, exfoliative dermatitis, alopecia, pruritus, urticaria, angioedema, photosensitivity, **Stevens-Johnson syndrome**
Other: drug fever, chills, superinfection (limited to urinary tract), hypersensitivity reactions including **anaphylaxis, lupus-like syndrome**

Interactions

Drug-drug. *Anticholinergics:* increased nitrofurantoin absorption and bioavailability
Drugs that can cause pulmonary toxicity: increased risk of pneumonitis
Hepatotoxic drugs: increased risk of hepatotoxicity
Magnesium salts: decreased nitrofurantoin absorption
Neurotoxic drugs: increased risk of neurotoxicity
Uricosurics (such as probenecid): decreased renal clearance and increased blood level of nitrofurantoin
Drug-diagnostic tests. *Alanine aminotransferase, alkaline phosphatase, aspartate aminotransferase, bilirubin, blood urea nitrogen, creatinine:* increased levels
Granulocytes, platelets, hemoglobin: decreased levels
Urine glucose tests using Benedict's reagent or Fehling's solution: false-positive results
Drug-food. *Any food:* increased drug bioavailability

Patient monitoring

• Monitor patient's response to therapy. Assess urine culture and sensitivity tests.
◄€ Watch for and immediately report peripheral neuropathy.
◄€ Assess respiratory status. Watch for signs and symptoms of serious pulmonary hypersensitivity reaction.

◄€ Monitor CBC and liver function tests closely. Stay alert for evidence of hematologic and hepatic disorders.
• Evaluate patient for rash.

Patient teaching

• Instruct patient to take with food or milk at regular intervals around the clock.
• Advise patient to complete entire course of therapy.
• Tell patient not to take magnesium-containing drugs (such as antacids) during therapy.
• Caution patient not to drive or perform other hazardous activities until he knows how drug affects vision, concentration, and alertness.
◄€ Tell patient to immediately report fever, chills, cough, chest pain, difficulty breathing, rash, bleeding or easy bruising, dark urine, yellowing of skin or eyes, numbness or tingling of fingers or toes, or intolerable GI distress.
• Advise female patient to avoid taking drug during pregnancy, especially near term.
• As appropriate, review all other significant and life-threatening adverse reactions and interactions, especially those related to the drugs, tests, and foods mentioned above.

nitroglycerin

Minitran, Nitrek, Nitro-Dur, Nitroject✣, Nitrolingual, Nitromist, Nitronal✠, Nitroquick, Nitrostat

Pharmacologic class: Nitrate
Therapeutic class: Antianginal
Pregnancy risk category C

Action

Inhibits calcium transport into myocardial and vascular smooth muscle cells,

---

suppressing contractions. Dilates main coronary arteries and arterioles, inhibits coronary artery spasm, increases oxygen delivery to heart, and reduces frequency and severity of angina attacks.

Availability

Capsules (extended-release): 2.5 mg, 6.5 mg, 9 mg
Injection: 0.5 mg/ml, 5 mg/ml
Ointment (transdermal): 2%
Solution for injection: 25 mg/250 ml, 50 mg/250 ml, 50 mg/500 ml, 100 mg/250 ml, 200 mg/500 ml
Spray (translingual): 0.4 mg/spray in 14.5-g canister (200 doses)
Tablets (buccal, extended-release): 1 mg, 2 mg, 3 mg, 5 mg
Tablets (extended-release): 2.6 mg, 6.5 mg, 9 mg
Tablets (sublingual): 0.3 mg, 0.4 mg, 0.6 mg
Transdermal system (patch): 0.1 mg/hour, 0.2 mg/hour, 0.3 mg/hour, 0.4 mg/hour, 0.6 mg/hour, 0.8 mg/hour

⏀ Indications and dosages

➢ Management and prophylaxis of angina pectoris
Adults: For acute angina attack, 0.3 to 0.6 mg S.L., repeated q 5 minutes for 15 minutes p.r.n.; or one to two translingual sprays, repeated q 5 minutes for 15 minutes p.r.n. For long-term or prophylactic use, 1-mg extended-release buccal tablet q 5 hours, with dosage and frequency increased p.r.n.; or 2.5 to 9 mg (extended-release tablets) P.O. q 8 to 12 hours; or 1.3 to 6.5 mg (extended-release capsules) P.O. q 8 to 12 hours.
➢ Hypertension during surgery; adjunct in heart failure
Adults: 5 mcg/minute I.V., increased by 5 mcg/minute q 3 to 5 minutes up to 20 mcg/minute, then increased by 10 to 20 mcg/minute q 3 to 5 minutes (dosage based on hemodynamic parameters)
➢ Heart failure associated with acute myocardial infarction (MI)

Adults: 12.5 to 25 mcg I.V., then a continuous infusion of 10 to 20 mcg/minute q 5 to 10 minutes; increase by 5 to 10 mcg/minute q 5 to 10 minutes as needed to a maximum of 200 mcg/minute.

Contraindications

• Hypersensitivity to drug, other organic nitrates, nitrites, or adhesives (transdermal form)
• Angle-closure glaucoma
• Orthostatic hypotension
• Hypotension or uncorrected hypovolemia (I.V. form)
• Early MI (S.L. form)
• Increased intracranial pressure (as from head trauma or cerebral hemorrhage)
• Severe anemia
• Pericardial tamponade or constrictive pericarditis
• Concurrent sildenafil therapy

Precautions

Use cautiously in:
• severe renal or hepatic impairment, glaucoma, hypertrophic cardiomyopathy
• hypovolemia, normal or decreased pulmonary capillary wedge pressure (with I.V. use)
• alcohol intolerance (with large I.V. doses)
• pregnant or breastfeeding patients
• children (safety not established).

Administration

• Administer tablets and capsules with water. Don't crush, break, or let patient chew them.
• For S.L. use, administer under tongue or in buccal pouch; instruct patient not to swallow tablet. For acute angina, give at pain onset. For angina prophylaxis, give before activities that may cause anginal pain.
• For translingual use, spray directly onto oral mucosa. Don't let patient inhale spray. Give at pain onset and as needed prophylactically before activities that trigger angina.

Reactions in **bold** are life-threatening.   🔊 Clinical alert

• For transdermal use, apply system to skin site with little hair and movement. Don't apply to distal extremities. Rotate application sites to avoid irritation and sensitization.

• Apply transdermal ointment to skin by spreading prescribed amount over 6" × 6" area (using an applicator, not your fingers). Cover area with plastic wrap and tape. Rotate sites to reduce risk of irritation and inflammation.

◀ Know that solution for injection is a concentrate. Dilute with dextrose 5% in water or normal saline solution before giving by I.V. infusion.

◀ Don't mix solution for injection with other drugs, and don't give by direct I.V. injection.

• Be aware that solution for injection is affected by type of infusion set used and that dosage is based on use of conventional PVC tubing. When using nonabsorbent tubing, reduce dosage.

• For I.V. use, administer with infusion pump. Increase dosage in increments of 5 mcg/minute every 3 to 5 minutes p.r.n. to achieve desired blood pressure response. Once achieved, reduce dosage and lengthen dosage adjustment intervals.

◀ Don't give concurrently with sildenafil (may cause life-threatening hypotension).

Route	Onset	Peak	Duration
P.O. (extended)	40-60 min	Unknown	8-12 hr
I.V.	Immediate	Unknown	Several min
Buccal (extended)	Unknown	Unknown	5 hr
S.L.	1-3 min	Unknown	30-60 min
Transdermal (ointment)	20-60 min	Unknown	4-8 hr
Transdermal (patch)	40-60 min	Unknown	8-24 hr
Translingual	2-4 min	Unknown	30-60 min

Adverse reactions

CNS: dizziness, headache
CV: hypotension, syncope
Hematologic: methemoglobinemia
Skin: contact dermatitis (with transdermal or ointment use), rash, exfoliative dermatitis, flushing

Interactions

Drug-drug. *Antihypertensives, beta-adrenergic blockers, calcium channel blockers, haloperidol, phenothiazines:* additive hypotension
Drugs with anticholinergic properties (antihistamines, phenothiazines, tricyclic antidepressants): decreased absorption of lingual, S.L., or buccal nitroglycerin
Sildenafil: increased risk of potentially fatal hypotension
Drug-diagnostic tests. *Cholesterol:* false elevation
Methemoglobin: significant levels (with excessive doses)
Urine catecholamines, urine vanillyl-mandelic acid: increased levels
Drug-behaviors. *Alcohol use, acute alcohol ingestion:* increased risk of potentially fatal hypotension

Patient monitoring

◀ With I.V. use, monitor blood pressure frequently. Titrate dosage to obtain desired results.

• With transdermal use, check for rash or skin irritation.

• Monitor patient for angina relief.

Patient teaching

• Instruct patient to place S.L. tablet directly under tongue and hold it there as it dissolves. Caution him not to chew or swallow tablet.

• Tell patient to use drug before physical activities that may cause angina.

• Instruct patient to take drug at pain onset and repeat every 5 minutes for three doses. If pain doesn't subside, advise him to seek medical attention.

• Tell patient not to chew or crush sustained-release tablets.
• Advise patient to apply correct amount of ointment using applicator. Caution him to avoid rubbing site. Instruct him to cover ointment with plastic wrap and tape it, to wash hands after placement, and to rotate sites.
• Advise patient to consult prescriber or pharmacist before changing brands of transdermal system. Different brands may have different drug concentrations.
• As appropriate, review all significant and life-threatening adverse reactions and interactions, especially those related to the drugs, tests, and behaviors mentioned above.

---

nitroprusside sodium
Nipride❦, Nitropress

Pharmacologic class: Vasodilator
Therapeutic class: Antihypertensive
Pregnancy risk category C

FDA BOXED WARNING

• After reconstitution with appropriate diluent, drug isn't suitable for direct injection. Dilute reconstituted solution further in sterile 5% dextrose injection before infusing.
• Drug may cause steep blood pressure decrease. In patients not properly monitored, this decrease can lead to irreversible ischemic injury or death. Give drug only when available equipment and personnel allow continuous blood pressure monitoring.
• Except when used briefly or at low infusion rates, drug gives rise to significant amount of cyanide ion, which can reach toxic, potentially lethal levels. Infusion at maximum dosage rate should never last more than 10 minutes.

If blood pressure isn't adequately controlled after 10 minutes of maximum-rate infusion, end infusion immediately. Monitor acid-base balance and venous oxygen concentration, but be aware that, although these tests may indicate cyanide toxicity, they provide imperfect guidance.
• Review these warnings thoroughly before giving drug.

Action
Interferes with calcium influx and intracellular activation of calcium, causing peripheral vasodilation and direct blood pressure decrease

Availability
Injection: 50 mg/vial in 2 ml- and 5-ml vials

Indications and dosages
➤ Hypertensive emergencies; controlled hypotension during anesthesia
Adults and children: 0.3 to 10 mcg/kg/minute I.V., titrated to response

Dosage adjustment
• Hepatic insufficiency
• Renal impairment
• Elderly patients

Contraindications
• Hypertension caused by aortic coarctation or atrioventricular shunting
• Acute heart failure caused by reduced peripheral vascular resistance
• Congenital (Leber's) optic atrophy, tobacco amblyopia
• Inadequate cerebral circulation
• Moribund patients

Precautions
Use cautiously in:
• hepatic or renal disease, fluid and electrolyte imbalances, hypothyroidism
• elderly patients
• pregnant or breastfeeding patients
• children.

Administration

◀€ Be aware that nitroprusside is a high-alert drug.

◀€ Give only in settings with trained personnel and continuous blood pressure monitoring equipment.

• Dilute 50 mg in 2 to 3 ml of dextrose 5% in water (D_5W); then dilute in 250 to 1,000 ml of D_5W.

• Administer with microdrip regulator, infusion pump, or other device that allows precise flow rate measurement.

• Wrap infusion solution in aluminum foil or other opaque material to protect it from light.

Route	Onset	Peak	Duration
I.V.	1-2 min	1-10 min	10 min

Adverse reactions

CNS: increased intracranial pressure
CV: ECG changes, bradycardia, tachycardia, **marked hypotension**
GI: ileus
Hematologic: decreased platelet aggregation, **methemoglobinemia**
Metabolic: hypothyroidism
Skin: rash, flushing
Other: pain, irritation, and venous streaking at injection site; too-rapid blood pressure decrease (causing apprehension, restlessness, palpitations, retrosternal discomfort, nausea, retching, abdominal pain, diaphoresis, headache, dizziness, muscle twitching); **thiocynate or cyanide toxicity** (initially, tinnitus, miosis, and hyperreflexia) at blood level of 60 mg/L; **severe cyanide toxicity** (air hunger, confusion, **lactic acidosis, death**) at level of 200 mg/L

Interactions

Drug-drug. *Enflurane, ganglionic blockers, halothane, negative inotropic drugs, volatile liquid anesthetics:* severe hypotension
Drug-diagnostic tests. *Creatinine:* increased level

Methemoglobin: hemoglobin sequestration as methemoglobin

Patient monitoring

◀€ Measure blood pressure frequently (preferably with continuous arterial line) to detect rapid drop.

• Monitor injection site closely to avoid extravasation. Use central line whenever possible. Ensure that infusion rate is precisely controlled to prevent too-rapid infusion.

• Obtain baseline ECG and monitor for changes.

◀€ Watch for signs and symptoms of cyanide toxicity (lactic acidosis, dyspnea, headache, vomiting, confusion, and loss of consciousness).

Patient teaching

• Tell patient he'll be closely monitored during therapy.

◀€ Instruct patient to immediately report headache, nausea, or pain at injection site.

• As appropriate, review all other significant and life-threatening adverse reactions and interactions, especially those related to the drugs and tests mentioned above.

nizatidine

Apo-Nizatidine✦, Axid, Axid AR, Dom-Nizatidine✦, Gen-Nizatidine✦, Novo-Nizatidine✦, PHL-Nizatidine✦, PMS-Nizatidine✦, Zinga⊕

Pharmacologic class: Histamine$_2$ (H_2)-receptor antagonist
Therapeutic class: Antiulcer drug
Pregnancy risk category B

Action

Inhibits histamine action at H_2-receptor sites in gastric parietal cells,

---

reducing gastric acid secretion and pepsin production

Route	Onset	Peak	Duration
P.O.	Unknown	0.5-3 hr	8-12 hr

Availability
Capsules: 150 mg, 300 mg
Oral solution: 15 mg/ml
Tablets: 75 mg

⚡ Indications and dosages
➤ Active duodenal ulcer
Adults: 300 mg P.O. daily at bedtime or 150 mg b.i.d. for up to 8 weeks
➤ Maintenance of healed duodenal ulcers
Adults and children ages 12 and older: 150 mg P.O. daily at bedtime for up to 1 year
➤ Esophagitis and associated heartburn caused by gastroesophageal reflux disease (GERD)
Adults: 150 mg P.O. b.i.d. for up to 12 weeks
➤ Active benign gastric ulcer
Adults: 150 mg P.O. b.i.d. or 300 mg P.O. once daily at bedtime
➤ Erosive esophagitis; GERD
Children ages 12 and older: 150 mg P.O. b.i.d. for up to 8 weeks

Dosage adjustment
• Moderate to severe renal impairment
• Elderly patients

Contraindications
• Hypersensitivity to drug or other H$_2$-receptor antagonists

Precautions
Use cautiously in:
• mild renal impairment
• elderly patients
• pregnant or breastfeeding patients
• children younger than age 12 (safety and efficacy not established).

Administration
• Give with or without food.
• If patient is to take drug twice daily, give one dose in morning and one at bedtime.

Adverse reactions
CNS: dizziness, drowsiness, headache, anxiety, nervousness, insomnia, abnormal dreams, asthenia
CV: chest pain
EENT: amblyopia, sinusitis, rhinitis, pharyngitis
GI: nausea, vomiting, diarrhea, constipation, dyspepsia, abdominal pain, flatulence, anorexia, dry mouth
Hematologic: anemia
Musculoskeletal: back pain, myalgia
Respiratory: cough
Skin: rash, pruritus
Other: tooth disorder, infection, fever, pain

Interactions
Drug-drug. *Salicylates (high doses):* increased salicylate blood level
Drug-diagnostic tests. *Alanine aminotransferase, alkaline phosphatase, aspartate aminotransferase:* elevated levels
Urobilinogen tests using Multistix: false-positive result
Drug-herbs. *Pennyroyal:* altered rate of herbal metabolite formation

Patient monitoring
• Monitor liver and renal function tests.
• Check temperature; watch for fever and other signs and symptoms of infection.

Patient teaching
• Advise patient to take once-daily dose at bedtime with or without food, or twice-daily doses in morning and at bedtime.
• Instruct patient to take exactly as prescribed. Caution him not to take other OTC drugs (especially aspirin).
• Tell patient to report signs and symptoms of infection.

n

Reactions in **bold** are life-threatening.   ◀€ Clinical alert

- Caution patient to avoid driving and other hazardous activities until he knows how drug affects concentration and alertness.
- As appropriate, review all other significant adverse reactions and interactions, especially those related to the drugs, tests, and herbs mentioned above.

norelgestromin/ethinyl estradiol
Evra ♦, Ortho Evra

Pharmacologic class: Estrogen
Therapeutic class: Hormone
Pregnancy risk category X

FDA | BOXED WARNING

- Cigarette smoking increases risk of serious cardiovascular adverse effects from hormonal contraceptive use. Risk increases with age and with heavy smoking (15 or more cigarettes per day) and is quite marked in women older than age 35. Strongly advise women who use hormonal contraceptives not to smoke.
- Risk of venous thromboembolism (VTE) among women ages 15 to 44 who used the transdermal patch compared to women who used oral contraceptives containing 30 to 35 mcg of ethinyl estradiol (EE) and either levonorgestrel or norgestimate was assessed in four U.S. case-control studies using electronic health care claims data. Odds ratios ranged from 1.2 to 2.2; one of the studies found a statistically significant increased risk of VTE for current patch users.
- The pharmacokinetic (PK) profile for the transdermal patch is different from the PK profile for oral

contraceptives in that it has higher steady state concentrations and lower peak concentrations. Area under the time-concentration curve and average concentration at steady state for EE are approximately 60% higher in women using the patch compared with women using an oral contraceptive containing 35 mcg of EE. In contrast, peak concentrations for EE are approximately 25% lower in women using the patch. It's unknown whether there are changes in risk of serious adverse events based on the differences in PK profiles of EE in women using the patch compared with women using oral contraceptives containing 30 to 35 mcg of EE. Increased estrogen exposure may increase risk of adverse events, including VTE.

Action
Suppresses gonadotropin and inhibits ovulation by causing changes in cervical mucus and endometrium, thereby preventing egg implantation

Availability
Transdermal patch: 6 mg norelgestromin and 0.75 mg ethinyl estradiol (releases 150 mcg norelgestromin and 20 mcg ethinyl estradiol q 24 hours)

𝆺 Indications and dosages
➢ To prevent pregnancy
Adults: Apply patch on day 1 of menstrual cycle (or first Sunday after period begins). Change patch weekly thereafter for 3 weeks (on same day each week), and then remove patch for fourth week. Repeat q month.

Contraindications
- Hypersensitivity to drug or its components
- Undiagnosed abnormal genital bleeding
- Known or suspected breast cancer or history of such cancer

- Endometrial carcinoma or other known or suspected estrogen-dependent neoplasia
- Thromboembolism, history of thromboembolic disease, known thrombophilic conditions
- Current or past cerebrovascular or coronary artery disease
- Valvular heart disease with complications
- Diabetes with vascular involvement
- Persistent blood pressure values at or above 160 mm Hg systolic or 100 mm Hg diastolic
- Headache with focal neurologic symptoms
- Cholestatic jaundice of pregnancy, jaundice with previous hormonal contraceptive use
- Acute or chronic hepatic disease with abnormal liver function
- Hepatic adenomas or carcinomas
- Major surgery with prolonged immobilization
- Known or suspected pregnancy

Precautions

Use cautiously in:
- cardiovascular disease, renal disease, asthma, bone disease, migraine, lipid disorders, fibrocystic breasts, increased risk for endometrial cancer, sexually transmitted diseases
- family history of breast or genital tract cancer
- abnormal mammogram
- elderly patients (use not indicated)
- women with body weight at or above198 lb (90 kg)
- breastfeeding patients
- children before menarche (use not indicated).

Administration

- Apply patch to clean, dry, intact skin on buttock, abdomen, upper torso, or upper outer arm.
- Change patch on same day each week (except for fourth week, when patch is removed).

Route	Onset	Peak	Duration
Transdermal	Rapid	2 days	Unknown

Adverse reactions

CNS: headache, dizziness, lethargy, depression, emotional lability, **increased risk of cerebrovascular accident**

CV: edema, hypertension, **myocardial infarction, thromboembolism**

EENT: contact lens intolerance, worsening of myopia or astigmatism

GI: nausea, vomiting, jaundice, abdominal cramps, bloating, anorexia, gallbladder disease, **pancreatitis**

GU: amenorrhea, dysmenorrhea, breakthrough bleeding, cervical erosion, vaginal candidiasis, breast tenderness, breast enlargement or secretion, menstrual cramps, libido loss, **increased risk of breast or endometrial cancer**

Hepatic: cholestatic jaundice, **hepatic adenoma**

Metabolic: hyperglycemia, hypercalcemia, sodium and water retention

Musculoskeletal: leg cramps

Respiratory: upper respiratory infection, **pulmonary embolism**

Skin: acne, oily skin, increased pigmentation, urticaria, patch site reaction

Other: increased appetite, weight changes

Interactions

Drug-drug. *Acetaminophen, ascorbic acid, atorvastatin, miconazole (vaginal capsules):* increased ethinyl estradiol blood level

Antibiotics, barbiturates, carbamazepine, fosphenytoin, phenobarbital, phenytoin, rifampin: decreased contraceptive efficacy

Corticosteroids: enhanced corticosteroid effects

Cyclosporine: increased risk of cyclosporine toxicity

n

Reactions in **bold** are life-threatening.   ◀€ Clinical alert

CYP3A4 inhibitors (such as ketoconazole, itraconazole): increased hormone level

Dantrolene, other hepatotoxic drugs: increased risk of hepatotoxicity

Insulin, oral hypoglycemics, warfarin: altered requirements for these drugs

Protease inhibitors: increased contraceptive metabolism

Tamoxifen: interference with tamoxifen effects

Drug-diagnostic tests. *Antithrombin III, folate, low-density lipoproteins, pyridoxine, total cholesterol, urine pregnanediol:* decreased levels

Cortisol; factors VII, VIII, IX, and X; glucose; high-density lipoproteins; phospholipids; prolactin; prothrombin; sodium; triglycerides: increased levels

Metyrapone test: false decrease

Thyroid function tests: false interpretation

Drug-food. *Caffeine:* increased blood caffeine level

Drug-herbs. *Black cohosh:* increased adverse drug effects

Red clover: interference with hormonal therapy

Saw palmetto: antiestrogenic effects

St. John's wort: decreased drug blood level and effects

Drug-behaviors. *Smoking (15 or more cigarettes daily):* increased risk of adverse cardiovascular reactions

Patient monitoring

• Evaluate menstrual pattern.

◀€ Monitor blood pressure. Watch for signs and symptoms of thromboembolic disease (swelling or warmth in calf, sudden chest pain, shortness of breath).

• Check blood glucose level in diabetic patient.

Patient teaching

• Instruct patient to start using patch on first day of menstrual period or on first Sunday after period starts. Advise her to use calendar to keep track of which day each week to change patch.

• Tell patient to remove patch during fourth week of each cycle. Explain that she will have bleeding that week.

• Advise patient to check daily to ensure that patch is attached firmly to skin. Explain that if patch is detached for 1 day or less, she should try to reattach it more firmly. If patch is detached for more than 1 day or for an unknown length of time, she should start with new patch and new calendar.

• Instruct patient to use alternative contraception during first week of patch use.

◀€ Inform patient that smoking while using patch increases risk of thromboembolic disease and other serious cardiovascular reactions. Stress importance of not smoking. Tell her to immediately report swelling or warmth in calf, chest pain, or shortness of breath.

• Advise breastfeeding patient to use other forms of contraception until she has completely weaned her infant.

• As appropriate, review all other significant and life-threatening adverse reactions and interactions, especially those related to the drugs, tests, foods, herbs, and behaviors mentioned above.

norepinephrine bitartrate
Levophed, Noradrenaline ⊕

Pharmacologic class: Sympathomimetic

Therapeutic class: Alpha- and beta-adrenergic agonist, cardiac stimulant, vasopressor

Pregnancy risk category C

FDA | BOXED WARNING

• If extravasation occurs, infiltrate area promptly with 10 to 15 ml of saline solution containing 5 to 10 mg phentolamine to prevent sloughing and necrosis. Use syringe with fine hypodermic needle, and infiltrate solution liberally throughout area. Give phentolamine as soon as possible; its sympathetic blockade causes immediate local hyperemic changes if area is infiltrated within 12 hours.

Action

Stimulates beta$_1$ and alpha$_1$ receptors in sympathetic nervous system, causing vasoconstriction, increased blood pressure, enhanced contractility, and decreased heart rate

Availability

Injection: 1 mg/ml

🕭 Indications and dosages

➤ Severe hypotension

Adults: 8 to 12 mcg/minute I.V.; then titrate based on blood pressure response. For maintenance, 2 to 4 mcg/minute.

Contraindications

• Concurrent cyclopropane or halothane anesthesia
• Hypotension caused by blood volume deficit (except in emergencies until blood volume replacement is completed), profound hypoxia or hypercarbia
• Mesenteric or peripheral vascular thrombosis

Precautions

Use cautiously in:
• sulfite sensitivity (some products), especially in asthmatic patients
• arterial embolism, cardiac disease, peripheral vascular disease, hypertension, hyperthyroidism
• patients receiving MAO inhibitors or tricyclic antidepressants concurrently
• elderly patients
• pregnant or breastfeeding patients
• children (safety and efficacy not established).

Administration

• Mix with dextrose 5% in water or dextrose 5% in normal saline solution.
• Inspect solution to make sure it's clear and colorless. Don't infuse if it's brown or pink.
• Administer through infusion pump. Titrate infusion rate to achieve and maintain low-normal systolic blood pressure (80 to 100 mm Hg).
• Continue infusion until adequate blood pressure and tissue perfusion persist without drug therapy.
• Gradually titrate dosage downward.
• To avoid extravasation, administer only into large vein (antecubital) or through central line. Don't use femoral vein in patients who are elderly or have occlusive vascular disorders.
🕭 To prevent delivery of large drug concentrations, avoid line stasis and flushing.

Route	Onset	Peak	Duration
I.V.	Immediate	Immediate	1-2 min after infusion ends

Adverse reactions

CNS: headache, anxiety
CV: bradycardia, **severe hypertension, arrhythmias**
Respiratory: respiratory difficulty
Skin: irritation with extravasation, necrosis
Other: ischemic injury

Interactions

Drug-drug. *Alpha-adrenergic blockers:* antagonism of norepinephrine effects
Antihistamines, ergot alkaloids, guanethidine, MAO inhibitors, oxytocin, tricyclic antidepressants: severe hypertension
Bretylium, inhalation anesthetics: increased risk of arrhythmias

Patient monitoring

🕭 Check blood pressure every 2 minutes until desired pressure is achieved. Recheck every 5 minutes for duration of infusion.

n

Reactions in **bold** are life-threatening.   🕭 Clinical alert

- Maintain continuous ECG monitoring and blood pressure monitoring.
◀◢ Be aware that headache may signal extreme hypertension and overdose.
- Monitor infusion site for extravasation.
◀◢ Watch for signs and symptoms of peripheral vascular insufficiency (decreased capillary refill, pale to cyanotic to black skin color).
◀◢ Never leave patient unattended during infusion.

Patient teaching
- When patient is alert, explain why he's receiving drug.
- Reassure patient he'll be monitored continuously until he's stable.

norethindrone acetate
Aygestin, Camila, Errin, Jolivette, Nora-BE, Nor-QD, Ortho Micronor

Pharmacologic class: Progesterone, hormone
Therapeutic class: Progestin
Pregnancy risk category X

Action
Inhibits pituitary gonadotropin secretion, suppressing follicular maturation and ovulation and stimulating mammary tissue growth

Availability
Tablets: 0.35 mg, 5 mg

🖊 Indications and dosages
➤ Endometriosis
Adults: 5 mg Aygestin P.O. daily for 2 weeks, increased in increments of 2.5 mg/day q 2 weeks until 15 mg daily is reached
➤ Amenorrhea; abnormal uterine bleeding
Adults: 2.5 to 10 mg Aygestin P.O. daily starting on day 5 of menstrual cycle

➤ Prevention of pregnancy
Adults: 1 tablet (0.35 mg) P.O. daily

Contraindications
- Hypersensitivity to drug
- Impaired liver function or liver disease
- Thromboembolic disorders
- Known or suspected breast cancer
- Undiagnosed vaginal bleeding
- Known or suspected pregnancy
- As a diagnostic test for pregnancy

Precautions
Use cautiously in:
- hypertension, blood dyscrasias, bone marrow disease, hepatic or renal disease, gallbladder disease, heart failure, diabetes mellitus, depression, migraine, asthma, seizure disorder
- family history of breast or reproductive tract cancer
- breastfeeding patients.

Administration
- Give with or without food.
- When administering for endometriosis, amenorrhea, or abnormal uterine bleeding, know that therapy may continue for 6 to 9 months or until breakthrough bleeding necessitates a temporary halt.
- When administering for prevention of pregnancy, know that drug must be given continuously every day at the same time with no interruptions between pill packs.

Route	Onset	Peak	Duration
P.O.	Variable	Unknown	24 hr

Adverse reactions
CNS: migraine, depression, insomnia, drowsiness
EENT: retinal vascular lesions, sudden partial or complete vision loss, proptosis, diplopia, **papilledema**
GI: nausea

GU: breakthrough bleeding, menstrual flow changes, amenorrhea, changes in cervical erosion and secretions, breast tenderness and secretion
Hepatic: cholestatic jaundice
Metabolic: fluid retention, decreased glucose tolerance
Skin: rash, urticaria, acne, hirsutism, chloasma
Other: edema, weight gain or loss, fever

Interactions

Drug-drug. *Hepatic enzyme-inducing drugs (such as carbamazepine, phenobarbital, phenytoin, rifampin):* decreased norethindrone efficacy
Drug-diagnostic tests. *Alkaline phosphatase; amino acids; factors VII, VIII, IX, and X; nitrogen; pregnanediol:* increased levels
Gamma-glutamyltransferase, high-density lipoproteins: decreased levels
Drug-herbs. *Cola nut, guarana, yerba maté:* increased CNS stimulation
St. John's wort: decreased contraceptive efficacy
Drug-behaviors. *Smoking:* risk of serious cardiovascular reactions

Patient monitoring

• Monitor pretreatment and annual physical exams to check blood pressure, breasts, abdomen, pelvic organs, and Pap smear results.
◀ Assess for signs and symptoms of depression, especially in patients with history of depression. Stop giving drug if significant depression recurs.
• Check blood glucose level in diabetic patients.

Patient teaching

• Instruct patient to avoid pregnancy or to discontinue drug if she gets pregnant (may cause serious fetal anomalies or fetal death).
◀ Advise patient to discontinue drug and consult prescriber if she experiences sudden partial or complete vision loss.

• If patient is receiving drug to treat amenorrhea, tell her to mark administration days on calendar.
• Instruct patient taking drug to prevent pregnancy to take drug every day at the same time without interruption between pill packs.
• Tell diabetic patient to monitor blood glucose level closely and to watch for hyperglycemia.
• Instruct patient to report breakthrough bleeding, spotting, change in menstrual flow, or amenorrhea.
• Caution patient not to smoke during therapy.
• As appropriate, review all other significant and life-threatening adverse reactions and interactions, especially those related to the drugs, tests, herbs, and behaviors mentioned above.

norfloxacin
Noroxin, Utinor⊕

n

Pharmacologic class: Fluoroquinolone
Therapeutic class: Anti-infective
Pregnancy risk category C

FDA BOXED WARNING

• Fluoroquinolones for systemic use are associated with an increased risk of tendinitis and tendon rupture in all ages. This risk is further increased in patients usually over age 60, with concomitant use of corticosteroids, and in kidney, heart, and lung transplant recipients.
• Drug may exacerbate muscle weakness in patients with myasthenia gravis. Avoid use in patients with known history of myasthenia gravis.

Action
Inhibits bacterial DNA synthesis by blocking DNA gyrase in susceptible

---

gram-negative and gram-positive aerobic and anaerobic bacteria

Route	Onset	Peak	Duration
P.O.	Rapid	2-3 hr	12 hr

Availability
Tablets: 400 mg

⚡ Indications and dosages
➤ Urinary tract infections (UTIs) caused by *Escherichia coli, Klebsiella pneumoniae,* or *Proteus mirabilis*
Adults: 400 mg P.O. q 12 hours for 3 days
➤ UTIs caused by all organisms except *E. coli, K. pneumoniae,* and *P. mirabilis*
Adults: 400 mg P.O. q 12 hours for 7 to 10 days. For complicated UTIs, may give for up to 21 days.
➤ Gonorrhea
Adults: 800 mg P.O. as a single dose
➤ Prostatitis caused by *E. coli*
Adults: 400 mg P.O. q 12 hours for 28 days

Dosage adjustment
• Renal impairment

Contraindications
• Hypersensitivity to drug
• History of tendinitis or tendon rupture with fluoroquinolone use

Precautions
Use cautiously in:
• CNS diseases or disorders, renal impairment, cirrhosis, bradycardia, acute myocardial ischemia
• known history of myasthenia gravis (avoid use)
• elderly patients
• pregnant or breastfeeding patients (safety not established except in postexposure inhalation or cutaneous anthrax).
• children younger than age 18.

Administration
• Give with glass of water 1 hour before or 2 hours after a meal.
• Don't give antacids within 2 hours of norfloxacin.

Adverse reactions
CNS: dizziness, light-headedness, drowsiness, headache, asthenia, insomnia, agitation, confusion, acute psychoses, hallucinations, tremors, **increased intracranial pressure, seizures**
CV: vasodilation, **QT prolongation, arrhythmias**
GI: nausea, diarrhea, abdominal pain, **pancreatitis, pseudomembranous colitis**
GU: interstitial cystitis, vaginitis
Hematologic: leukopenia
Hepatic: hepatitis
Metabolic: hyperglycemia, **hypoglycemia**
Musculoskeletal: tendinitis, tendon rupture
Skin: rash, hyperhidrosis, photosensitivity, phototoxicity, **Stevens-Johnson syndrome**
Other: altered taste, myasthenia gravis exacerbation, hypersensitivity reactions including **anaphylaxis**

Interactions
Drug-drug. *Antacids, bismuth, iron salts, subsalicylate, sucralfate, zinc salts:* decreased norfloxacin absorption
Antineoplastics: decreased norfloxacin blood level
Cimetidine: interference with norfloxacin elimination
Corticosteroids: increased risk of tendon rupture
Nitrofurantoin: antagonism of norfloxacin's antibacterial effects in GU tract
Other fluoroquinolones: increased risk of nephrotoxicity
Probenecid: decreased renal elimination of norfloxacin
Theophylline: increased theophylline blood level, greater risk of toxicity
Warfarin: increased anticoagulant effect

Drug-diagnostic tests. *Alanine aminotransferase, alkaline phosphatase, aspartate aminotransferase, bilirubin, eosinophils, lactate dehydrogenase, platelets:* increased levels
Hemoglobin, hematocrit: decreased values
Drug-food. *Caffeine:* decreased hepatic metabolism of caffeine
Milk or yogurt (consumed alone): impaired drug absorption
Tube feedings: impaired drug absorption
Drug-herbs. *Dong quai, St. John's wort:* phototoxicity
Fennel: decreased drug absorption
Drug-behaviors. *Sun exposure:* phototoxicity

Patient monitoring
• Monitor vital signs and cardiovascular status.
• Check fluid intake and output. Keep patient well-hydrated.
◀€ Watch for signs and symptoms of tendinitis or tendon rupture.
• Assess patient's response to therapy. Obtain specimens for repeat culture and sensitivity tests if he relapses or doesn't improve.
• Monitor renal function.

Patient teaching
• Tell patient to take on empty stomach with full glass of water, 1 hour before or 2 hours after a meal.
• If patient needs antacid for GI upset, instruct him not to take it within 2 hours of norfloxacin.
◀€ Advise patient to stop taking drug and promptly report rash; severe GI problems; tendon pain, swelling, or inflammation; or weakness.
• Caution patient to avoid driving and other hazardous activities until he knows how drug affects concentration and alertness.
• Teach patient ways to counteract photosensitivity, such as by wearing sunglasses and avoiding excessive exposure to bright light.

• As appropriate, review all other significant and life-threatening adverse reactions and interactions, especially those related to the drugs, tests, foods, herbs, and behaviors mentioned above.

nortriptyline hydrochloride
Allegron⊕, Apo-Nortriptyline✴, Aventyl, Dom-Nortriptyline✴, Gen-Nortriptyline✴, Novo-Nortriptyline✴, Norventyl✴, Nu-Nortriptyline✴, Pamelor, PMS-Nortriptyline✴, Ratio-Nortriptyline✴

Pharmacologic class: Tricyclic compound
Therapeutic class: Antidepressant
Pregnancy risk category D

FDA | BOXED WARNING
• Drug may increase risk of suicidal thinking and behavior in children and adolescents with major depressive disorder and other psychiatric disorders. Risk must be balanced with clinical need, as depression itself increases suicide risk. With patient of any age, observe closely for clinical worsening, suicidality, and unusual behavior changes when therapy begins. Advise family and caregivers to observe patient closely and communicate with prescriber as needed.
• Drug isn't approved for use in pediatric patients.

Action
Increases serotonin and norepinephrine release by blocking their reuptake by presynaptic neurons; also possesses anticholinergic properties

Availability

Capsules: 10 mg, 25 mg, 50 mg, 75 mg
Oral solution: 10 mg/5 ml

ⓘ Indications and dosages

➤ Depression
Adults: 25 mg P.O. t.i.d. or q.i.d., up to a maximum of 150 mg daily

Dosage adjustment

• Elderly patients
• Adolescents

Off-label uses

• Postherpetic neuralgia
• Neurologic pain

Contraindications

• Hypersensitivity to drug or dibenzazepines
• Acute recovery phase of myocardial infarction
• MAO inhibitor use within past 14 days

Precautions

Use cautiously in:
• asthma, cardiovascular disease, cardiac or hepatic disease, hyperthyroidism, increased intraocular pressure, angle-closure glaucoma, urinary retention, severe depression
• history of seizures
• elderly patients (especially elderly men with prostatic hyperplasia)
• pregnant or breastfeeding patients
• children (use not recommended).

Administration

• Give as prescribed, either in divided doses three or four times daily or as single dose at bedtime.
• Administer with meals or snack to minimize stomach upset.
◀€ Don't give within 14 days of MAO inhibitors.

Route	Onset	Peak	Duration
P.O.	2-3 wk	6 wk	Unknown

Adverse reactions

CNS: dizziness, drowsiness, fatigue, headache, lethargy, insomnia, agitation, confusion, extrapyramidal reactions, hallucinations, **seizures, suicidal behavior or ideation** (especially in child or adolescent)
CV: hypotension, ECG changes, palpitations, **heart block, arrhythmias, myocardial infarction, cerebrovascular accident**
EENT: blurred vision, dry eyes
GI: nausea, constipation, anorexia, dry mouth, **paralytic ileus**
GU: urinary retention, gynecomastia
Hematologic: blood dyscrasias
Hepatic: jaundice, **hepatotoxicity**
Skin: photosensitivity
Other: unpleasant taste, weight gain

Interactions

Drug-drug. *Anticholinergics, anticholinergic-like drugs (including antidepressants, antihistamines, atropine, disopyramide, haloperidol, phenothiazines, quinidine):* additive anticholinergic effects
Antihypertensives: poor therapeutic response to antihypertensives
Antithyroid drugs: increased risk of agranulocytosis
Cimetidine, fluoxetine, hormonal contraceptives: increased nortriptyline blood level and possible toxicity
Clonidine: hypertensive crisis
CNS depressants (including antihistamines, opioids, sedative-hypnotics): additive CNS depression
Decongestants, vasoconstrictors: additive adrenergic effects
MAO inhibitors: hypertension, hyperpyrexia, seizures, death
Drug-diagnostic tests. *Alkaline phosphatase, bilirubin:* increased levels
Glucose: increased or decreased level
Drug-herbs. *Angel's trumpet, belladonna, henbane, jimson weed, scopolia:* increased anticholinergic effects
Chamomile, hops, kava, skullcap, scopolia, valerian: increased CNS depression
St. John's wort: decreased drug blood level and efficacy

Drug-behaviors. *Alcohol use:* increased drowsiness, impaired motor skills

Patient monitoring
• Check vital signs and ECG.
• Monitor bladder and bowel function. Stay alert for urine retention and constipation.
• Assess neurologic status and document mood swings.
• Monitor liver function tests.
◀ Watch for suicidal tendency, especially in child or adolescent.

Patient teaching
• Explain that drug's full effect may take 4 weeks.
• Tell patient drug may cause drowsiness or dizziness, but these effects should subside within a few weeks.
◀ Advise patient (and family as appropriate) to immediately report worsening depression or suicidal ideation, especially in child or adolescent.
• Caution patient to avoid driving and other hazardous activities until he knows how drug affects him.
• Tell patient to avoid alcohol and to consult prescriber before using herbs.
• As appropriate, review all other significant and life-threatening adverse reactions and interactions, especially those related to the drugs, tests, herbs, and behaviors mentioned above.

nystatin
Bio-Statin, Candistatin✢, Dom-Nystatin✢, Mycostatin, Nadostine✢, Nilstat✢, Nyaderm✢, Nystan ⊕, Nystop, Pedi-Dri, PMS-Nystatin✢, Ratio-Nystatin✢

Pharmacologic class: Antifungal
Therapeutic class: Anti-infective
Pregnancy risk category A

Action
Interferes with fungal cell-wall synthesis, inhibiting formation of ergo sterols, increasing cell-wall permeability, and causing osmotic instability

Availability
Cream: 100,000 units/g
Ointment: 100,000 units/g
Powder: 100,000 units/g
Suspension: 100,000 units/ml
Tablets: 500,000 units
Troches: 200,000 units
Vaginal tablets: 100,000 units

⚕ Indications and dosages
➤ Candidiasis (topical use)
Adults and children: Apply cream, ointment, or powder two or three times daily until healing is complete.
➤ Oral candidiasis
Adults: 400,000 to 600,000 units (suspension) P.O. q.i.d. Have patient gargle and then swallow half of dose in each side of mouth.
Infants: 200,000 units (suspension) P.O. q.i.d. Use half of dose in each side of mouth.
Newborn and premature infants: 100,000 units (suspension) P.O. q.i.d. Use half of dose in each side of mouth.
➤ GI infections
Adults: 500,000 to 1 million units (one to two tablets) P.O. t.i.d. Continue for 48 hours after desired response occurs.
➤ Vaginal candidiasis
Adults: 100,000 units (one vaginal tablet) intravaginally daily for 2 weeks, or 100,000- to 500,000-unit applicatorful (cream) intravaginally once or twice daily for 2 weeks

Contraindications
• Hypersensitivity to drug or its components

Precautions
Use cautiously in:
• renal or hepatic disease, achlorhydria
• pregnant or breastfeeding patients
• children younger than age 2.

n

Reactions in **bold** are life-threatening. ◀ Clinical alert

Administration

- Give oral suspension by placing half of dose in each side of patient's mouth. Instruct patient to hold suspension in mouth, swish it around, or gargle for several minutes before swallowing it.
- To prepare oral solution from powder, add one-eighth teaspoon to 120 ml of water and stir well. Give immediately.
- Advise patient to let troche dissolve slowly and completely in mouth. Tell her not to chew or swallow it whole.
- Know that nystatin vaginal tablets can be given orally to treat oral candidiasis.
- To apply cream, ointment, or powder, gently and thoroughly massage preparation into skin.
- Use applicator provided for vaginal administration.

Route	Onset	Peak	Duration
P.O., topical, vaginal	Unknown	Unknown	Unknown

Adverse reactions

GI: nausea, vomiting, diarrhea, GI distress, oral irritation
GU: vulvovaginal irritation (with intravaginal form)
Skin: pruritus, rash

Interactions

Drug-drug. *Topical corticosteroids:* increased corticosteroid absorption
Drug-behaviors. *Latex contraceptive use:* damage to contraceptive (with intravaginal use)

Patient monitoring

- If patient takes oral tablets, inspect oral mucous membranes for irritation.
- With topical use, monitor affected area for increase in redness, swelling, or irritation.

Patient teaching

- Advise patient to continue taking for at least 48 hours after symptoms resolve.
- Instruct patient to let lozenge dissolve slowly in mouth. Tell her not to chew or swallow it.
- If patient misses a dose, tell her to take dose as soon as possible and then resume her regular dosing schedule.
- Inform patient that diabetes mellitus, reinfection by sexual partner, tight-fitting pantyhose, and use of antibiotics, hormonal contraceptives, or corticosteroids predispose her to vaginal infection. Urge her to wear cotton underwear.
- Tell female patient to practice careful hygiene in affected areas.
- Instruct patient using vaginal tablets to wash applicator thoroughly after each use.
- Tell patient to continue therapy during menstruation.
- As appropriate, review all significant adverse reactions and interactions, especially those related to the drugs and behaviors mentioned above.

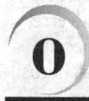

octreotide acetate
Sandostatin, Sandostatin LAR

Pharmacologic class: Somatostatin analog
Therapeutic class: Antidiarrheal
Pregnancy risk category B

Action

Suppresses secretion of serotonin, serotonin metabolites, and gastrohepatic peptides, increasing fluid and electrolyte absorption from GI tract. Also suppresses growth hormone, insulin, and glucagon.

Availability
Depot injection: 10 mg, 20 mg, 30 mg
Injection: 0.05 mg/ml, 0.1 mg/ml, and 0.5 mg/ml in 1-ml ampules; 0.2 mg/ml and 1 mg/ml in 5-ml vials

🝙 Indications and dosages
➤ Diarrhea and flushing associated with carcinoid tumors
Adults: 100 to 600 mcg (Sandostatin) subcutaneously or I.V. daily in two to four divided doses for 2 weeks. Then, depending on response, 20 mg (LAR Depot) I.M. q 4 weeks for 2 months.
➤ Diarrhea caused by vasoactive intestinal peptide tumors (VIPomas)
Adults: 200 to 300 mcg (Sandostatin) subcutaneously or I.V. daily in two to four divided doses for 2 weeks. Then, depending on response, 20 mg (LAR Depot) I.M. q 2 weeks for 2 months.
➤ Acromegaly
Adults: 50 to 100 mcg (Sandostatin) subcutaneously or I.V. two or three times daily. Then, depending on response, 20 mg (LAR Depot) I.M. q 4 weeks for 3 months. Then adjust based on growth hormone levels.

Dosage adjustment
• Renal impairment

Off-label uses
• Dumping syndrome (postprandial hypotension)
• GI and pancreatic fistulas
• Variceal bleeding

Contraindications
• Hypersensitivity to drug or its components

Precautions
Use cautiously in:
• gallbladder disease, renal impairment, hyperglycemia or hypoglycemia, fat malabsorption

• pregnant or breastfeeding patients
• children.

Administration
• When giving subcutaneously, rotate administration site with each injection.
◀≣ Don't give LAR Depot I.V.
• Mix I.M. solution and inject deep into gluteal muscle over 3 minutes. Don't use deltoid.
• For I.V. administration, dilute in 50 to 200 ml of dextrose 5% in water or normal saline solution. Infuse over 15 to 30 minutes.
• Know that octreotide suppression test and octreotide scintigraphy may be done to determine if drug will aid carcinoid tumor treatment.
• Drug may be kept at room temperature for 2 weeks. Refrigerate ampules.

Route	Onset	Peak	Duration
Subcut., I.V.	Unknown	0.4 hr	Up to 12 hr
I.M.	Unknown	2 wk	Up to 4 wk

Adverse reactions
CNS: dizziness, drowsiness, fatigue, headache, weakness
CV: edema, bradycardia, conduction abnormalities, **arrhythmias**
EENT: vision disturbances
GI: nausea, vomiting, diarrhea, abdominal pain, cholelithiasis, fat malabsorption
Skin: flushing
Metabolic: hypothyroidism, hyperglycemia, **hypoglycemia**
Other: injection site pain

Interactions
Drug-drug. *Cyclosporine:* reduced cyclosporine blood level
Insulin, oral hypoglycemics: altered requirements for these drugs
Orally administered drugs: altered absorption of these drugs
Drug-diagnostic tests. *Glucose:* increased or decreased level
Hepatic enzymes: slightly increased levels

Reactions in **bold** are life-threatening.   ◀≣ Clinical alert

Schilling's test: abnormal results
Thyroxine, vitamin B$_{12}$: decreased levels
Drug-food. *Fats:* altered octreotide absorption

Patient monitoring

- Assess bowel sounds and stool frequency and consistency.
- Monitor vital signs and fluid intake and output. Stay alert for dehydration or edema.
- Evaluate diabetic patient for hypoglycemia or hyperglycemia.
- Know that in women with active acromegaly, normalization of growth hormone and insulin-like growth factor-1 may restore fertility.

Patient teaching

- Tell patient being treated for carcinoid tumor to keep track of number of daily stools or flushing episodes.
- Instruct patient to weigh himself daily and report significant changes.
- Advise female with childbearing potential to use adequate contraception while taking drug.
- If patient will use drug at home, teach correct methods for injection, storage, and needle disposal.
- Caution patient to avoid driving and other hazardous activities until he knows how drug affects concentration, vision, and alertness.
- As appropriate, review all other significant and life-threatening adverse reactions and interactions, especially those related to the drugs, tests, and foods mentioned above.

ofloxacin
Exocin⊕, Floxin, Ocuflox, Tarivid⊕

Pharmacologic class: Fluoroquinolone
Therapeutic class: Anti-infective
Pregnancy risk category C

FDA BOXED WARNING

- Fluoroquinolones for systemic use are associated with an increased risk of tendinitis and tendon rupture in all ages. This risk is further increased in patients usually over age 60, with concomitant use of corticosteroids, and in kidney, heart, and lung transplant recipients.
- Drug may exacerbate muscle weakness in patients with myasthenia gravis. Avoid use in patients with known history of myasthenia gravis.

Action

Inhibits bacterial DNA synthesis by inhibiting DNA gyrase in susceptible bacteria

Availability

Ophthalmic solution: 3 mg/ml (0.3%)
Otic solution: 0.3%
Tablets: 200 mg, 300 mg, 400 mg

🖊 Indications and dosages

➤ Prostatitis caused by *Escherichia coli*
Adults: 300 mg P.O. q 12 hours for 6 weeks
➤ Complicated urinary tract infections caused by *E. coli, Klebsiella pneumoniae,* or *Proteus mirabilis*
Adults: 200 mg P.O. q 12 hours for 10 days
➤ Uncomplicated cystitis caused by *E. coli* or *K. pneumoniae*
Adults: 200 mg P.O. q 12 hours for 3 days
➤ Acute uncomplicated urethral and cervical gonorrhea
Adults: 400 mg P.O. as a single dose
➤ Nongonococcal cervicitis or urethritis caused by *Chlamydia trachomatis*; mixed infections of cervix or urethra caused by *C. trachomatis* or *Neisseria gonorrhoeae*
Adults: 300 mg P.O. q 12 hours for 7 days
➤ Acute bacterial exacerbation of chronic bronchitis, community-acquired pneumonia, and

uncomplicated skin and skin-structure infections caused by susceptible organisms

Adults: 400 mg P.O. q 12 hours for 10 days

➤ Acute pelvic inflammatory disease

Adults: 400 mg P.O. q 12 hours for 10 to 14 days

➤ Bacterial conjunctivitis

Adults and children ages 1 and older: One to two drops of ophthalmic solution in affected eye q 2 to 4 hours on days 1 and 2; then one to two drops q.i.d. on days 3 through 7

➤ Corneal ulcers

Adults: One to two drops of ophthalmic solution in affected eye q 30 minutes while awake on days 1 and 2, then one to two drops q hour while awake on days 3 to 7, then one to two drops q.i.d. while awake on days 7 to 9

➤ Otitis externa

Adults and children ages 13 and older: 10 drops of otic solution into affected ear daily for 7 days

➤ Chronic suppurative otitis media with perforated tympanic membrane

Adults and children ages 12 and older: 10 drops of otic solution into affected ear b.i.d. for 14 days

Dosage adjustment
• Renal impairment
• Severe hepatic impairment

Contraindications
• Hypersensitivity to drug or other fluoroquinolones

Precautions
Use cautiously in:
• underlying CNS disease, renal impairment, cirrhosis, bradycardia, acute myocardial ischemia
• known history of myasthenia gravis (avoid use)
• history of tendinitis or tendon rupture with fluoroquinolone use
• dialysis patients
• elderly patients

• pregnant or breastfeeding patients (safety not established except in postexposure inhalation or cutaneous anthrax).
• children younger than age 18 (except in postexposure inhalation or cutaneous anthrax and in ophthalmic and otic use).

Administration
• Don't give zinc- or iron-containing drugs within 2 hours of ofloxacin.

Route	Onset	Peak	Duration
P.O.	Rapid	1-2 hr	12 hr
Ophthalmic, otic	Unknown	Unknown	Unknown

Adverse reactions
CNS: dizziness, drowsiness, headache, light-headedness, insomnia, acute psychoses, agitation, confusion, tremors, hallucinations, **increased intracranial pressure, seizures**
CV: chest pain, vasodilation
GI: nausea, diarrhea, constipation, abdominal pain, **pseudomembranous colitis**
GU: interstitial cystitis, vaginitis
Hematologic: eosinophilia, **leukopenia**
Musculoskeletal: tendinitis, tendon rupture, joint pain, back pain
Skin: rash, photosensitivity, phototoxicity, **Stevens-Johnson syndrome**
Other: altered taste, superinfection, myasthenia gravis exacerbation

Interactions
Drug-drug. *Amiodarone, bepridil, disopyramide, erythromycin, pentamidine, phenothiazines, pimozide, procainamide, quinidine, sotalol, tricyclic antidepressants:* increased risk of serious adverse cardiovascular reactions
Antacids, bismuth subsalicylate, iron or zinc salts, sucralfate: decreased ofloxacin absorption
Corticosteroids: increased risk of tendon rupture
Probenecid: decreased renal elimination of ofloxacin

O

Theophylline: increased theophylline blood level and possible toxicity
Warfarin: increased warfarin effects
Drug-diagnostic tests. *Alanine aminotransferase, aspartate aminotransferase, platelets:* increased levels
Hemoglobin, hematocrit: decreased values
Drug-food. *Milk or yogurt (consumed alone), tube feedings:* impaired drug absorption
Drug-herbs. *Fennel:* decreased drug absorption
Dong quai, St. John's wort: phototoxicity
Drug-behaviors. *Sun exposure:* phototoxicity

Patient monitoring

• Assess patient for signs and symptoms of superinfection.
• Inspect for rash. Check for signs and symptoms of hypersensitivity reaction.
◀⑀ Watch for fever with diarrhea; diarrhea containing pus; or severe, persistent diarrhea; and tendinitis or tendon rupture.
• Evaluate neurologic status closely.

Patient teaching

• Encourage patient to maintain fluid intake of at least 1,500 ml daily to prevent crystalluria.
• Inform patient being treated for gonorrhea that partners must be treated.
◀⑀ Tell patient to immediately report fever and diarrhea, especially if stool contains blood, pus, mucus. Caution him not to treat diarrhea without consulting prescriber.
◀⑀ Instruct patient to stop taking drug and immediately report rash or tendon pain or inflammation.
• Instruct patient not to take iron- or zinc-containing drugs or antacids within 2 hours of ofloxacin.
• Teach patient ways to counteract photosensitivity, such as by wearing sunglasses and avoiding excessive exposure to bright light.
• Teach patient how to use eye or ear drops. Caution him not to touch dropper tip to any surface (including eye or ear).
• As appropriate, review all other significant and life-threatening adverse reactions and interactions, especially those related to the drugs, tests, foods, herbs, and behaviors mentioned above.

olanzapine
Zyprexa, Zyprexa IntraMuscular, Zyprexa, Zydis

olanzapine pamoate
Zyprexa Relprevv

Pharmacologic class: Thienobenzodiazepine
Therapeutic class: Antipsychotic
Pregnancy risk category C

FDA | BOXED WARNING

• Elderly patients with dementia-related psychosis are at increased risk for death. Drug isn't approved for patients with dementia-related psychosis.
• When using olanzapine and fluoxetine in combination, refer to boxed warning section of package insert for Symbyax (olanzapine and fluoxetine).
• Adverse events with signs and symptoms consistent with olanzapine overdose, in particular sedation, including coma and delirium (postinjection delirium-sedation syndrome), have been reported after injections of Zyprexa Relprevv. Injections must be administered in a registered health care facility with ready access to emergency response services. After each injection, patients must be observed at the health care facility by a health care professional for at least 3 hours. Because of this risk, Zyprexa Relprevv is available only through a restricted distribution

program called Zyprexa Relprevv Patient Care Program, which requires prescriber, health care facility, patient, and pharmacy enrollment.

Action
Unknown. Thought to antagonize dopamine and serotonin type 2 in CNS. Also antagonizes muscarinic receptors in respiratory tract, causing cholinergic activation.

Availability
Injection powder for suspension (extended-release): 210 mg/vial, 300 mg/vial, 405 mg/vial
Solution for injection: 10-mg vials
Tablets: 2.5 mg, 5 mg, 7.5 mg, 10 mg, 15 mg, 20 mg
Tablets (orally disintegrating): 5 mg, 10 mg, 15 mg, 20 mg

⚡ Indications and dosages
➤ Schizophrenia
Adults: Initially, 5 to 10 mg (Zyprexa, Zyprexa Zydis) P.O. daily with a target dosage of 10 mg/day within several days; may increase or decrease q week by 5 mg/day (not to exceed 20 mg/day). Periodically reevaluate long-term usefulness of drug for individual patient. Or, for Zyprexa Relprevv dosages corresponding to Zyprexa target oral dosages, see chart below:

Target dosages (Zyprexa P.O.)	Dosing first 8 weeks (Zyprexa Relprevv I.M.)	Maintenance dosage after 8 weeks (Zyprexa Relprevv I.M.)
10 mg/day	210 mg/ 2 weeks or 405 mg/ 4 weeks	150 mg/ 2 weeks or 300 mg/ 4 weeks
15 mg/day	300 mg/ 2 weeks	210 mg/ 2 weeks or 405 mg/ 4 weeks
20 mg/day	300 mg/ 2 weeks	300 mg/ 2 weeks

Adolescents: Initially, 2.5 or 5 mg (Zyprexa, Zyprexa Zydis) P.O. daily with a target dosage of 10 mg/day. When dosage adjustments are needed, increments or decrements of 2.5 or 5 mg are recommended to a maximum of 20 mg/day.
➤ Bipolar I disorder (manic or mixed episodes)
Adults: Initially, 10 or 15 mg (Zyprexa, Zyprexa Zydis) P.O. daily; may increase or decrease q 24 hours by 5 mg/day (not to exceed 20 mg/day). Or 10 mg I.M. (Zyprexa IntraMuscular); maximum dosage is three 10-mg doses I.M. 2 to 4 hours apart. Or initially, 10 mg (Zyprexa, Zyprexa Zydis) P.O. daily when administered as adjunctive treatment to lithium or valproate.
Adolescents: Initially, 2.5 or 5 mg (Zyprexa, Zyprexa Zydis) P.O. daily with a target dosage of 10 mg/day. When dosage adjustments are necessary, increments or decrements of 2.5 or 5 mg are recommended to a maximum of 20 mg/day.
➤ Agitation associated with schizophrenia and bipolar I mania
Adults: 10 mg I.M. (Zyprexa IntraMuscular) or 5 mg or 7.5 mg I.M. when clinically warranted; maximum of three doses 2 to 4 hours apart. If agitation persists after initial dose, subsequent doses up to 10 mg may be given. If ongoing olanzapine therapy is clinically indicated, 5 to 20 mg/day (Zyprexa, Zyprexa Zydis) P.O. may be initiated as soon as clinically appropriate.
➤ Depressive episodes associated with bipolar I disorder
Adults: Initially, 5 mg (Zyprexa, Zyprexa Zydis) P.O. and 20 mg fluoxetine P.O. daily in the evening. Dosage adjustments, if indicated, can be made according to efficacy and tolerability within ranges of 5 to 12.5 mg (Zyprexa or Zyprexa Zydis) and fluoxetine 20 to 50 mg.

O

➤ Treatment-resistant depression
Adults: Initially, 5 mg (Zyprexa, Zyprexa Zydis) P.O. and 20 mg fluoxetine P.O. daily in the evening. Dosage adjustments, if indicated, can be made according to efficacy and tolerability within ranges of 5 to 20 mg (Zyprexa or Zyprexa Zydis) and fluoxetine 20 to 50 mg.

Dosage adjustment
• Elderly or debilitated patients
• Patients predisposed to hypotensive reactions
• Patients who otherwise exhibit a combination of factors that may result in slower metabolism of olanzapine, or who may be more pharmacodynamically sensitive to olanzapine

Off-label uses
• Borderline personality disorder (with oral use)

Contraindications
None

Precautions
Use cautiously in:
• hepatic impairment, cardiovascular or cerebrovascular disease, diabetes mellitus, prostatic hypertrophy, angle-closure glaucoma, phenylketonuria (with orally disintegrating tablets)
• history of seizures, paralytic ileus, or suicide attempt
• elderly patients
• pregnant or breastfeeding patients
• children younger than age 18 (safety not established).

Administration
• Administer without regard to meals.
• When administering as combination therapy, give in the evening.
• To remove orally disintegrating tablet from package, peel back foil; don't push tablet through foil.

• Establish tolerability with oral olanzapine before initiating treatment with I.M. forms.
• Be aware that the two Zyprexa intramuscular formulations have different dosing schedules; Zyprexa IntraMuscular is a short-acting formulation and Zyprexa Relprevv is a long-acting formulation.
🔊 Be aware that I.M. forms are intended for deep I.M. injection into the gluteal muscle only. Don't give I.V. or subcutaneously.
• Reconstitute Zyprexa IntraMuscular for I.M. injection with 2.1 ml of sterile water for injection only, into single-packaged vial.
• After reconstituting Zyprexa IntraMuscular solution for injection, withdraw total contents of vial for 10-mg dose; 1.5 ml for 7.5-mg dose; 1 ml for 5-mg dose, or 0.5 ml for 2.5-mg dose.
• Use Zyprexa IntraMuscular solution for I.M. injection within 1 hour of reconstitution.
• Be aware that total Zyprexa daily dosages above 30 mg P.O. or 10 mg I.M. given more often than 2 hours after initial dose and 4 hours after second dose aren't recommended.
• Be aware that Zyprexa Relprevv may be irritating to the skin. Use gloves when reconstituting and flush area with water if contact is made with skin.
• Before administering Zyprexa Relprevv injection, confirm that someone will accompany patient after a 3-hour observation period. If this can't be confirmed, don't give the injection.
• Know that Zyprexa Relprevv must be suspended using only the diluent provided. After following manufacturer's directions for reconstitution, suspension concentration is 150 mg/ml. Final volume to inject is 1 ml for 150-mg dose, 1.4 ml for 210-mg dose, 2 ml for 300-mg dose, and 2.7 ml for 405-mg dose.
• Use Zyprexa Relprevv suspension immediately after removing from vial.

- Inject Zyprexa Relprevv deep into the gluteal muscle only. Don't massage injection site after injection.
- Don't combine in syringe with diazepam, lorazepam, or haloperidol.

Route	Onset	Peak	Duration
P.O.	Unknown	6 hr	Unknown
I.M. (Zyprexa IntraMuscular)	Rapid	15-45 min	Unknown
I.M. (Zyprexa Relprevv)	Unknown	1 wk	Wks-Months

Adverse reactions

CNS: dizziness, headache, weakness, fatigue, restlessness, sedation, insomnia, mood changes, agitation, personality disorder, impaired speech, tardive dyskinesia, dystonia, tremor, extrapyramidal effects, **neuroleptic malignant syndrome, coma, postinjection delirium-sedation syndrome**
CV: orthostatic hypotension, chest pain, tachycardia
EENT: amblyopia, rhinitis, pharyngitis
GI: nausea, constipation, abdominal pain, increased salivation, dry mouth
GU: urinary incontinence, urinary tract infection
Hematologic: leukopenia, neutropenia, agranulocytosis
Metabolic: goiter, increased thirst, hyperprolactinemia, hyperlipidemia, **severe hyperglycemia**
Musculoskeletal: hypertonia, joint pain
Respiratory: cough, dyspnea
Skin: ecchymosis, photosensitivity
Other: increased appetite, weight gain or loss, fever, flulike symptoms, impaired body temperature regulation, **death**

Interactions

Drug-drug. *Antihypertensives, diazepam:* additive hypotension
Carbamazepine, omeprazole, rifampin: decreased olanzapine effects
CNS depressants: additive CNS depression

Dopamine agonists, levodopa: antagonism of these drugs' effects
Fluvoxamine: decreased olanzapine clearance
Lorazepam: increased somnolence with I.M. olanzapine
Drug-diagnostic tests. *Alanine aminotransferase, alkaline phosphatase, aspartate aminotransferase, bilirubin, glucose, creatinine phosphokinase, gammaglutamyltransferase, LDL cholesterol, lipids, prolactin, serum glucose, total cholesterol, triglycerides:* elevated levels
Neutrophils, platelets: decreased count
Drug-behaviors. *Alcohol use:* additive CNS depression, potentiated orthostatic hypotension
Smoking: increased drug clearance
Sun exposure: increased risk of photosensitivity

Patient monitoring

- Assess patient's mental status during therapy.
- Monitor vital signs during dosage adjustment periods.
- Make sure patient takes drug and doesn't hoard it.
- ◀≋ Watch for signs and symptoms of neuroleptic malignant syndrome (fever, respiratory distress, tachycardia, seizures, diaphoresis, hypertension or hypotension, tiredness, severe muscle stiffness, loss of bladder control).
- Evaluate patient for onset of akathisia, tardive dyskinesia, and extrapyramidal effects.
- ◀≋ Watch for signs of increasing depression.
- ◀≋ Monitor blood glucose level closely, especially in patient with diabetes mellitus. Severe hyperglycemia, coma, and death may occur.
- Watch for orthostatic hypotension before I.M. injection. Keep patient recumbent if drowsiness or dizziness follows injection.
- Monitor baseline and periodic lipid and liver enzyme levels.

O

Reactions in **bold** are life-threatening.　　　　◀≋ Clinical alert

◀⣐ Monitor CBC frequently during first few months of therapy; consider discontinuing drug at first sign of a clinically significant decline in white blood cells (WBCs) in the absence of other causative factors. Discontinue drug in patients with severe neutropenia (absolute neutrophil count less than 1,000/mm³) and monitor WBC until recovery.

◀⣐ Monitor patient for signs and symptoms of postinjection delirium-sedation syndrome after Zyprexa Relprevv injections.

◀⣐ Be aware that the possibility of a suicide attempt is inherent in patients with schizophrenia or bipolar I disorder; close supervision of high-risk patients should accompany drug therapy.

Patient teaching

• Tell patient he may take without regard to meals.

• Instruct patient to remove orally disintegrating tablet from package by peeling back foil—not by pushing tablet through foil. Instruct him to remove tablet from foil using dry hands, and place entire tablet in mouth. Tell him tablet will disintegrate with or without liquid.

• Tell patient drug may cause extrapyramidal symptoms, akathisia, and tardive dyskinesia leading to involuntary movements, tremors, rigidity, muscle contractions, and restlessness.

◀⣐ Caution patient with diabetes mellitus to monitor blood glucose closely.

• Tell patient to move slowly when sitting up or standing to avoid dizziness. Advise him to dangle legs briefly before getting out of bed.

• Advise patient to avoid smoking, alcohol, or other CNS depressants.

• Tell patient to exercise in moderation and to avoid overly hot baths and showers, because drug impairs body temperature regulation.

• Caution patient to avoid driving and other hazardous activities until he knows how drug affects concentration and alertness.

◀⣐ Instruct patient or caregiver how to recognize and report signs and symptoms of infection and postinjection delirium-sedation syndrome.

• As appropriate, review all other significant and life-threatening adverse reactions and interactions, especially those related to the drugs, tests, and behaviors mentioned above.

olmesartan medoxomil
Benicar, Olmetec⊕

Pharmacologic class: Angiotensin II type 1-receptor antagonist

Therapeutic class: Antihypertensive

Pregnancy risk category C (first trimester), *D* (second and third trimesters)

FDA   BOXED WARNING

• When used during second or third trimester of pregnancy, drug may cause fetal harm or death. Discontinue as soon as possible when pregnancy is detected.

Action
Selectively blocks binding of angiotensin II to specific tissue receptors in vascular smooth muscle and adrenal gland. This action blocks vasoconstrictive effects of renin-angiotensin system as well as aldosterone release, thereby reducing blood pressure and possibly preventing vascular remodeling related to arteriosclerosis.

Availability
Tablets: 5 mg, 20 mg, 40 mg

🚺 Indications and dosages
➤ Hypertension
Adults and children ages 6 to 16 weighing more than 35 kg (77 lb): 20 mg P.O. once daily; may titrate to 40 mg daily after 2 weeks, if needed
Children ages 6 to 16 weighing 20 kg (44 lb) to less than 35 kg (77 lb): 10 mg P.O. daily; may titrate to 20 mg daily after 2 weeks, if needed.

Dosage adjustment
• Volume depletion

Contraindications
• Hypersensitivity to drug or its components

Precautions
Use cautiously in:
• hepatic disease, renal dysfunction, hypovolemia, sodium depletion
• elderly patients
• pregnant patients (first trimester; not recommended in second and third trimesters)
• breastfeeding patients
• children (safety and efficacy not established).

Administration
• Give with or without food.
• Know that drug may be used alone or with other antihypertensives.

Route	Onset	Peak	Duration
P.O.	Variable	1-2 hr	Unknown

Adverse reactions
CNS: fatigue, dizziness, headache, insomnia
CV: orthostatic hypotension, chest pain, peripheral edema, syncope, tachycardia
EENT: sinusitis, rhinitis, pharyngitis
GI: nausea, diarrhea, constipation, abdominal pain, dry mouth
GU: hematuria
Hematologic: hyperglycemia

Musculoskeletal: back pain, arthritis, muscle weakness
Respiratory: upper respiratory infection symptoms, bronchitis, cough
Skin: dry skin, rash, inflammation, pruritus, alopecia, angioedema
Other: dental pain, flulike symptoms

Interactions
Drug-diagnostic tests. *Triglycerides:* increased level
Drug-herbs. *Ephedra (ma huang):* antagonism of antihypertensive effect

Patient monitoring
• Monitor vital signs and cardiovascular status. Stay alert for orthostatic hypotension, syncope, and peripheral edema.
• Check temperature and watch for signs and symptoms of flu and other infections (especially respiratory and EENT infections).
• Watch for angioedema.
• In volume-depleted patient, monitor blood pressure carefully after initial dose. Transient blood pressure drop may occur.

Patient teaching
• Tell patient to take at same time each day, with or without food.
• Advise patient to promptly report signs and symptoms of infection, particularly respiratory symptoms.
• Inform patient that when he begins therapy, inadequate fluid intake, excessive perspiration, vomiting, or diarrhea may cause blood pressure to drop. Tell him to change position slowly to avoid dizziness or fainting.
• Caution patient to avoid driving and other hazardous activities until he knows how drug affects concentration and alertness.
◀ Tell female patient to notify prescriber immediately if she suspects pregnancy.
• As appropriate, review all other significant adverse reactions and interactions, especially those related to the tests and herbs mentioned above.

Reactions in **bold** are life-threatening.   ◀ Clinical alert

olsalazine sodium
Dipentum

Pharmacologic class: Salicylate
Therapeutic class: Anti-inflammatory
Pregnancy risk category C

Action
Unknown. Converts to active form, mesalamine, which blocks cyclooxygenase and inhibits prostaglandin production in colon.

Availability
Capsules: 250 mg

⚠ Indications and dosages
➤ Ulcerative colitis in patients who can't tolerate sulfasalazine
Adults: 500 mg P.O. b.i.d.

Contraindications
• Hypersensitivity to drug or other salicylates

Precautions
Use cautiously in:
• hepatic or renal impairment, severe allergy, bronchial asthma
• pregnant or breastfeeding patients
• children younger than age 14.

Administration
• Give with meals to reduce GI irritation.

Route	Onset	Peak	Duration
P.O.	Variable	60 min	Unknown

Adverse reactions
CNS: headache, fatigue, depression, vertigo
GI: nausea, vomiting, diarrhea, abdominal pain, cramps, dyspepsia, bloating, stomatitis
Musculoskeletal: joint pain
Respiratory: upper respiratory infection
Skin: rash, itching

Interactions
Drug-drug. *Anticoagulants, coumarin derivatives:* prolonged prothrombin time, increased International Normalized Ratio
Drug-food. *Any food:* decreased GI irritation

Patient monitoring
• Monitor neurologic status. Stay alert for depression.
• Assess GI symptoms. Encourage adequate fluid intake to avoid dehydration.
• Monitor urinalysis, blood urea nitrogen, and creatinine in patients with renal impairment.

Patient teaching
• Instruct patient to take with food and to continue taking drug even after symptoms improve.
• Tell patient to eat appropriate foods in small, frequent servings to minimize GI upset.
• Advise patient to contact prescriber if symptoms worsen or don't improve after 1 to 2 months of therapy.
• Tell patient he may require periodic proctoscopy and sigmoidoscopy to determine response to drug.
• Caution patient to avoid driving and other hazardous activities until he knows how drug affects mood and wakefulness.
• As appropriate, review all significant adverse reactions and interactions, especially those related to the drugs and foods mentioned above.

omalizumab
Xolair

Pharmacologic class: Recombinant DNA-derived immunoglobulin G subclass 1 (IgG1) monoclonal antibody
Therapeutic class: Monoclonal antibody
Pregnancy risk category B

• Anaphylaxis, presenting as bronchospasm, hypotension, syncope,
urticaria, or angioedema of throat or
tongue, has occurred after administration of omalizumab. Anaphylaxis has
occurred after first dose but also has
occurred beyond 1 year after beginning
treatment. Closely observe patients for
appropriate period after administration and be prepared to manage anaphylaxis that can be life-threatening.
Inform patients of signs and symptoms of anaphylaxis and have them
seek immediate medical care should
signs and symptoms occur.

Action
Inhibits binding of IgE to high-affinity
IgE receptors on surface of mast cells
and basophils

Availability
Powder for injection: 150 mg/vial

⚠ Indications and dosages
➤ Persistent asthma in patients with
positive skin tests or in vitro reactivity
to perennial allergens whose symptoms
aren't adequately controlled by inhaled
corticosteroids
**Adults and adolescents ages 12 and
older:** 150 to 375 mg subcutaneously
q 2 to 4 weeks, with dosing frequency
determined by serum IgE level and weight

Dosage adjustment
• Significant weight change

Contraindications
• Hypersensitivity to drug

Precautions
Use cautiously in:
• elderly patients
• pregnant or breastfeeding patients
• children younger than age 12.

Administration
◀€ Be aware that omalizumab isn't a
rescue drug and isn't intended for
acute asthma attacks or status
asthmaticus.
◀€ Don't discontinue abruptly.
• Don't administer more than 150 mg
per injection site.
• Prepare injection only with sterile
water for injection.

Route	Onset	Peak	Duration
Subcut.	Unknown	7-8 days	Unknown

Adverse reactions
CNS: headache, fatigue, dizziness
EENT: sinusitis, pharyngitis, earache
Musculoskeletal: arthralgia, fracture,
leg or arm pain
Respiratory: upper respiratory infection
Skin: pruritus, dermatitis
Other: injection-site reaction, viral
infection, pain, **cancer, anaphylaxis**

Interactions
Drug-diagnostic tests. *Serum IgE:* elevated level

Patient monitoring
◀€ Monitor patient for severe hypersensitivity reactions, including anaphylaxis.
◀€ Watch for signs and symptoms of
cancer (rare).

Patient teaching
◀€ Tell patient to take exactly as prescribed and not to change dosage or
stop drug abruptly (unless hypersensitivity reaction occurs).
◀€ Instruct patient to discontinue
drug and notify prescriber immediately at first sign of hypersensitivity
reaction, such as rash, hives, or itching.
• Inform patient that asthma symptoms may not improve immediately
after starting drug.
• Tell patient drug isn't intended for
acute asthma attacks.
• As appropriate, review all other significant and life-threatening adverse reactions and interactions, especially those
related to the tests mentioned above.

omega-3-acid ethyl esters
Lovaza

Pharmacologic class: Combination ethyl esters of omega-3 fatty acids, principally eicosapentaenoic acid (EPA) and docosahexaenoic acid (DHA)

Therapeutic class: Lipid-regulating agent

Pregnancy risk category C

Action
Unclear. May include inhibition of acyl-CoA:1,2-diacylglycerol acyltransferase, increased mitochondrial and peroxisomal β-oxidation in the liver, decreased lipogenesis in the liver, and increased plasma lipoprotein lipase activity; may reduce synthesis of triglycerides in the liver because EPA and DHA are poor substrates for the enzymes responsible for triglyceride synthesis, and EPA and DHA inhibit esterification of other fatty acids.

Availability
Capsules: 1 g

⚠ Indications and dosages
➤ Adjunct to diet to reduce triglyceride levels in patients with severe (500 mg/dl or greater) hypertriglyceridemia
Adults: 4 g P.O. daily as a single 4-g dose or as 2-g dose P.O. b.i.d.

Contraindications
• Hypersensitivity to drug or its components

Precautions
Use cautiously in:
• hepatic impairment
• hypersensitivity to fish or shellfish
• pregnant or breastfeeding patients
• children (safety and efficacy not established).

Administration
• Administer capsules whole with meals.
• Assess triglyceride levels carefully before starting therapy, and identify other causes (such as diabetes mellitus, hypothyroidism, or drugs) of high triglyceride levels; manage as appropriate.
• Ensure patient is on appropriate lipid-lowering diet before starting drug.

Route	Onset	Peak	Duration
P.O.	Unknown	Unknown	Unknown

Adverse reactions
GI: vomiting, constipation, GI disorder, eructation, dyspepsia
Hepatic: increased liver enzyme levels
Skin: pruritus, rash
Other: taste perversion

Interactions
Drug-drug. *Anticoagulants, other drugs affecting coagulation (such as aspirin, NSAIDs):* prolonged bleeding time
Drug-diagnostic tests. *ALT, AST, LDL-C:* increased levels

Patient monitoring
• Monitor hepatic function tests in patients with hepatic impairment.
• Monitor LDL-C and triglyceride levels periodically.

Patient teaching
• Tell patient to take capsules whole with meals and not to break open, crush, dissolve, or chew them.
• Instruct patient to tell prescriber if he's allergic to fish.
• Advise patient to maintain lipid-lowering diet.
• As appropriate, review all other significant adverse reactions and interactions, especially those related to the drugs and tests mentioned above.

omeprazole magnesium

Heartburn Relief⊕, Losec✦⊕,
Mepradec⊕, Prilosec, Prilosec OTC,
Ratio-Omeprazole✦, Sandoz
Omeprazole✦, Zanprol⊕

omeprazole and sodium bicarbonate

Zegerid, Zegerid OTC

Pharmacologic class: Proton pump
inhibitor
Therapeutic class: Antiulcer drug
Pregnancy risk category C

Action

Reduces gastric acid secretion and
increases gastric mucus and bicarbonate production, creating protective
coating on gastric mucosa and easing
discomfort from excess gastric acid

Availability

Capsules (delayed-release): 10 mg,
20 mg, 40 mg
*Powder for oral suspension (delayed-
release):* 2.5 mg, 10 mg in packets
Tablets (delayed-release): 20 mg

⦿ Indications and dosages

➤ Gastroesophageal reflux disease
Adults: 20 mg P.O. (capsules, powder)
daily for 4 weeks
➤ Erosive esophagitis
Adults: 20 mg P.O. (capsules, powder)
daily for 4 to 8 weeks
➤ Short-term treatment of active
duodenal ulcer
Adults: 20 mg P.O. (capsules, powder)
daily for 4 weeks. Some patients may
need 4 additional weeks of therapy.
➤ To reduce risk of duodenal ulcers
caused by *Helicobacter pylori*
Adults: 40 mg P.O. (capsules) daily in
morning, given with clarithromycin t.i.d.
for 2 weeks; then 20 mg daily for 2 weeks
➤ Gastric ulcers
Adults: 40 mg P.O. (capsules) daily for
4 to 8 weeks
➤ Pathologic hypersecretory conditions,
including Zollinger-Ellison syndrome
Adults: Initially, 60 mg P.O. (capsules)
daily; may increase up to 120 mg t.i.d.
Divide daily dosages above 80 mg.
➤ Frequent heartburn (two or more
episodes a week)
Adults ages 18 and older: 20 mg P.O.
(OTC tablets, capsules, or powder)
daily for 14 days

Off-label uses

• Posterior laryngitis
• To enhance pancreatin efficacy in treating steatorrhea in cystic fibrosis patients

Contraindications

• Hypersensitivity to drug or its
components

Precautions

Use cautiously in:
• hepatic disease
• hypomagnesemia
• concurrent use of clopidogrel (avoid
use)
• pregnant or breastfeeding patients
• children (safety not established).

Administration

• Give 30 to 60 minutes before a meal,
preferably in morning.
• If desired, give concurrently with
antacids.
• Know that if patient has ulcer at start
of therapy, treatment may be extended.
• When giving through nasogastric
tube, use powder for oral suspension,
or separate capsule and mix pellets
with water. Agitate syringe while
injecting. After administration, flush
with 30 to 60 ml of water.
• Don't crush capsules.

O

Reactions in **bold** are life-threatening.   ◀€ Clinical alert

- Be aware that symptomatic response doesn't rule out gastric cancer.

Route	Onset	Peak	Duration
P.O.	Within 1 hr	Within 2 hr	72-96 hr
P.O. (delayed)	Unknown	10-90 min	Unknown

Adverse reactions

CNS: dizziness, headache, asthenia
GI: nausea, vomiting, diarrhea, constipation, abdominal pain
Metabolic: hypomagnesemia
Musculoskeletal: back pain; fractures of hip, wrist, spine (with long-term daily use)
Respiratory: cough, upper respiratory tract infection
Skin: rash

Interactions

Drug-drug. *Ampicillin, cyanocobalamin, iron salts, ketoconazole:* reduced absorption of these drugs
Clarithromycin: increased omeprazole blood level
Clopidogrel: diminished antiplatelet activity
Diazepam, phenytoin, warfarin: prolonged elimination and increased effects of these drugs
Digoxin: increased digoxin absorption and blood level, possible digoxin toxicity
Drugs metabolized by CYP450 system: competitive metabolism
Methotrexate: increased methotrexate serum level
Penicillins: serious and occasionally fatal hypersensitivity reactions including anaphylaxis
Rifampin: substantially decreased omeprazole concentrations
Drug-diagnostic tests. *Alanine phosphatase, alkaline aminotransferase, aspartate aminotransferase, bilirubin:* increased levels
Gastrin: increased level during first 1 to 2 weeks of therapy
Serum chromogranin A: increased level may cause false-positive results in diagnostic investigations for neuroendocrine tumors
Serum magnesium: decreased level
Drug-herbs. *St John's wort:* substantially decreased omeprazole concentration

Patient monitoring

- Assess vital signs.
- Check for abdominal pain, emesis, diarrhea, or constipation.
- Evaluate fluid intake and output.
- Watch for elevated liver function test results (rare).
- Monitor magnesium level before starting drug and periodically thereafter in patients expected to be on long-term treatment or who take proton pump inhibitors with other drugs such as digoxin or drugs that may cause hypomagnesemia.

Patient teaching

- Tell patient to take 30 to 60 minutes before a meal, preferably in morning.
- Instruct patient to swallow capsules or tablets whole and not to chew or crush them. If he can't swallow capsule, tell him he may open it, carefully sprinkle and mix entire contents into 1 tbsp of cool applesauce, and swallow immediately with glass of water.
- Instruct patient on how to use delayed-release oral suspension: Empty contents of a 2.5-mg packet of powder into a container with 5 ml of water or 10-mg packet of powder into a container with 15 ml of water; don't use other liquids or foods. Stir and allow drug to thicken for 2 to 3 minutes. Stir well and drink within 30 minutes. If any drug remains after drinking, add more water to container, stir, and drink immediately.
- Inform patient taking OTC delayed-release tablets for heartburn that full effect may take 1 to 4 days. Advise him not to take tablets for more than 14 days without consulting health care professional.

🍁 Canada   ✠ UK   ☣ Hazardous drug   ⊗ High-alert drug

- Advise patient to avoid St John's wort while taking this drug.
- Caution patient to avoid driving and other hazardous activities until he knows how drug affects concentration and alertness.
- As appropriate, review all other significant adverse reactions and interactions, especially those related to the drugs and tests mentioned above.

onabotulinumtoxinA (Toxin type A)
Botox, Botox Cosmetic, Vistabel⊕, Xeomin⊕

abobotulinumtoxinA (Toxin type A)
Dysport

incobotulinumtoxinA (Toxin type A)
Xeomin

rimabotulinumtoxinB (Toxin type B)
Myobloc, NeuroBloc⊕

Pharmacologic class: Neurotoxin
Therapeutic class: Neuromuscular blocker
Pregnancy risk category C

FDA | BOXED WARNING

- Postmarketing reports indicate that the effects of all botulinum toxin products may spread from the area of injection to produce symptoms consistent with botulinum toxin effects, including asthenia, generalized muscle weakness, diplopia, blurred vision, ptosis, dysphagia, dysphonia, dysarthria, urinary incontinence, and breathing difficulties. These signs and symptoms have

been reported hours to weeks after injection. Swallowing and breathing difficulties can be life-threatening, and deaths have occurred.
- The risk of signs and symptoms is probably greatest in children treated for spasticity, but signs and symptoms can also occur in adults treated for spasticity and other conditions, particularly in patients who have underlying conditions that would predispose them to these symptoms.
- In unapproved uses, including spasticity in children and adults, and in approved indications, cases of spread of effect have been reported at dosages comparable to those used to treat cervical dystonia and at lower dosages.

Action
Blocks neuromuscular transmission by binding to receptor sites on motor nerve terminals and inhibiting acetylcholine release, thereby causing localized muscle denervation. As a result, local muscle paralysis occurs, which leads to muscle atrophy and reinnervation due to development of new acetylcholine receptors.

Availability
Toxin type A—(onabotulinumtoxinA)
Powder for injection: 100 units/vial
Toxin type A— abobotulinumtoxinA
Freeze-dried powder for injection: 300 units/vial, 500 units/vial
Toxin type A—(incobotulinumtoxinA)
Powder for injection, lyophilized: 50 units in single-use vials, 100 units in single-use vials
Toxin type B—(rimabotulinumtoxinB)
Solution for injection: 5,000-units/ml vial

⬤ Indications and dosages
Toxin type A (onabotulinumtoxinA)
➤ Temporary improvement in appearance of moderate to severe glabellar lines associated with corrugator or procerus muscle activity

Adults ages 65 and younger: *Botox cosmetic only*—Total of 20 units (0.5-ml solution) injected I.M. as divided doses of 0.1 ml into each of five sites: two in each corrugator muscle and one in procerus muscle. Injection usually needs to be repeated q 3 to 4 months to maintain effect. *Dysport*—50 units I.M. in five equal aliquots of 10 units each to achieve clinical effect *Xeomin*—Or, 20 units per treatment session divided into five equal I.M. injections of 4 units each.

➤ Treatment of blepharospasm in patients previously treated with onabotulinumtoxinA (Botox)
Adults: *Xeomin*—When initiating therapy, base dose, number, and location of injections on the previous dosing of onabotulinumtoxinA (Botox). If previous dose of Botox isn't known, the recommended starting dose is 1.25 to 2.5 units per injection site.

➤ Upper limb spasticity
Adults: *Botox*—75 to 360 units I.M. divided among selected muscles at a given treatment session. Dose can be repeated no sooner than 12 weeks after the previous injection.

➤ Prophylaxis of headaches in patients with chronic migraine (15 or more days per month with headache lasting 4 hours a day or longer)
Adults: *Botox*—155 units as 0.1-ml (5 units) injections per each site divided across seven head and neck muscles

➤ Severe axillary hyperhidrosis inadequately managed by topical agents
Adults: *Botox*—50 units per axilla injected into defined hyperhidrotic area

➤ Blepharospasm
Adults: 1.25 to 2.5 units injected into medial and lateral pretarsal orbicularis oculi of upper eyelid and lateral pretarsal orbicularis oculi of lower eyelid

➤ Strabismus
Adults: 1.25 to 5 units injected into eyelid (dosage varies with strabismus severity). Dose can be repeated in 7 to 14 days if patient has adequate response; with inadequate response, dosage may be doubled.

Toxin types A and B (**onabotulinumtoxinA, abobotulinumtoxinA, incobotulinumtoxinA, rimabotulinumtoxinB**)

➤ Treatment of cervical dystonia to decrease severity of abnormal head position and neck pain in both botulinum toxin-naïve and previously treated patients
Adults: *Xeomin*—120 units injected I.M. into affected muscles per treatment session.

➤ To relax skeletal muscles and reduce severity of abnormal head position and neck pain associated with cervical dystonia
Adults: *Botox*—Usual dosage is 236 units injected I.M. locally into affected muscles. Dosage ranges from 198 to 300 units. *Dysport*—500 units I.M. as a divided dose among affected muscles in patients with or without a history of prior treatment with botulinum toxin. *Myobloc*—2,500 to 5,000 units I.M. injected locally into affected muscles.

Contraindications
• Hypersensitivity to drug or its components
• Allergy to cow's-milk protein (Dysport)
• Acute urinary tract infection or acute urinary retention (Botox intradetrusor injections)
• Active infection at injection site

Precautions
Use cautiously in:
• cardiovascular disease, peripheral neuropathy, neuromuscular disorders, compromised respiratory function, dysphagia
• inflammation at injection site, injections near vulnerable anatomical structures
• pregnant or breastfeeding patient
• children younger than age 12; children younger than age 18 (*Dysport, Xeomin*)

Administration

- Be aware that only trained professional medical personnel should inject this drug.
- Be aware that botulinum toxin products aren't interchangeable.

Toxin type A (onabotulinumtoxinA) when administered for eye disorders

- Reconstitute by slowly injecting preservative-free normal saline solution into drug vial.
- Rotate vial gently to mix drug; then draw up at least 20 units (0.5-ml solution) and expel air bubbles.
- Remove needle used for reconstitution, and attach 30G needle. Then inject drug as divided doses of 0.1 ml into each of five sites (two in each corrugator muscle, one in procerus muscle).
- Prepare eye with several drops of local anesthetic and ocular decongestant, as prescribed, several minutes before injection for blepharospasm or strabismus.
- When administering for upper limb spasticity, dilute with preservative-free normal saline solution to 200 units/4 ml or 100 units/2 ml. Then, using a 25G to 30G needle for superficial muscles and a longer 22G needle for deeper musculature, inject no more than 50 units per site.

Toxin type A (abobotulinumtoxinA)

- Reconstitute each 300-unit vial with 0.6 ml preservative-free normal saline solution and each 500-unit vial with 1 ml preservative-free normal saline solution.
- Swirl vial gently to mix drug.
- Remove needle used for reconstitution. Use a 23G to 25G needle for administration. Then inject 10 units into each of five sites (two in each corrugator muscle and one in the procerus muscle).
- Use within 4 hours of reconstitution.

Toxin type B (rimabotulinumtoxinB)

- Draw up prescribed dose from preservative-free, 3.5-ml single-use vial.
- Don't shake vial.
- Divide prescribed dose and inject locally into affected muscles.

Route	Onset	Peak	Duration
I.M.	Mins-hrs	Unknown	3-4 mo
I.M. (blepharospasm)	3 days	1-2 wk	3 mo
I.M. (strabismus)	1-2 days	Unknown	1-2 wk
I.M. (cervical dystonia [Dysport])	Unknown	2-4 wk	Unknown

Adverse reactions

CNS: headache, dizziness
CV: hypertension, **arrhythmias, myocardial infarction (MI)**
EENT: blepharoptosis, conjunctivitis, keratitis, eye dryness, double vision, tearing, increased sensitivity to light, sinusitis, pharyngitis
GI: nausea, dyspepsia, difficulty swallowing
Musculoskeletal: back pain, neck pain, muscle weakness
Respiratory: pneumonia, bronchitis, upper respiratory tract infection
Skin: skin tightness, ecchymosis
Other: tooth disorder, injection site redness, edema, or pain, flulike symptoms, facial muscle paralysis, infection, **anaphylaxis**

Interactions

Drug-drug. *Aminoglycosides, anticholinesterase compounds, clindamycin, lincomycin, magnesium sulfate, other neuromuscular blockers (such as succinylcholine), polymyxin B, quinidine:* increased risk of adverse effects

Patient monitoring

- Stay alert for signs and symptoms of anaphylaxis, particularly after first dose.
- Monitor vital signs and ECG, watching for evidence of hypertension, arrhythmias, and MI.
- Assess effect of drug on affected muscles; check for paralysis.
- ◀€ Be aware that spread of toxin effects may lead to swallowing and

breathing difficulties and death. Provide immediate medical attention if respiratory, speech, or swallowing difficulties occur.

• Monitor temperature. Watch for signs and symptoms of respiratory and EENT infections as well as flulike symptoms.

Patient teaching

◀ Instruct patient to seek immediate medical attention if respiratory, speech, or swallowing difficulties occur.

• Teach patient about desired effect of injection. Advise patient to report paralysis.

• Instruct patient to report signs and symptoms of infection, particularly flulike illness and EENT and respiratory infections.

• Inform patient being treated for blepharospasm (uncontrollable blinking) that he may experience transient eyelid drooping, corneal inflammation, double vision, dry eyes, tearing, and light sensitivity.

• As appropriate, review all other significant and life-threatening adverse reactions and interactions, especially those related to the drugs mentioned above.

ondansetron hydrochloride

Apo-Ondansetron✲, Dom-Ondansetron✲, Gen-Ondansetron✲, Novo-Ondansetron✲, Ondemet⊕, PHL-Ondansetron✲, PMS-Ondansetron✲, Ratio-Ondansetron✲, Sandoz Ondansetron✲, Zofran, Zofran ODT, Zofran Preservative Free

Pharmacologic class: Serotonin type 3 (5-HT$_3$) antagonist

Therapeutic class: Antiemetic

Pregnancy risk category B

Action

Blocks serotonin at 5-HT$_3$ receptor sites in vagal nerve terminals by disrupting CNS chemoreceptor trigger zone

Availability

Injection: 2 mg/ml in 2- and 20-ml vials
Injection (premixed): 32 mg/50 ml single-dose containers
Injection USP (preservative-free): 2 mg/ml in 2-ml single-dose vials
Oral solution: 4 mg/5 ml
Tablets: 4 mg, 8 mg, 24 mg
Tablets (orally disintegrating): 4 mg, 8 mg

🖉 Indications and dosages

➤ To prevent nausea and vomiting caused by moderately emetogenic chemotherapy

Adults and children older than age 12: 8 mg (tablet) or 10 ml (oral solution) P.O. b.i.d.; give first dose 30 minutes before chemotherapy and repeat dose 8 hours later. Give 8 mg (tablet) or 10 ml (oral solution) P.O. q 12 hours for 1 to 2 days after chemotherapy ends.

Children ages 4 to 11: 4 mg (tablet) or 5 ml (oral solution) P.O. q 8 hours; give first dose 30 minutes before chemotherapy and repeat dose 4 and 8 hours later. Give 4 mg (tablet) or 5 ml (oral solution) P.O. q 8 hours for 1 to 2 days after chemotherapy ends.

➤ To prevent nausea and vomiting caused by highly emetogenic chemotherapy

Adults and children older than age 12: 32 mg I.V. as a single dose infused over 15 minutes, starting 30 minutes before chemotherapy; or three 0.15-mg/kg doses I.V., with first dose infused over 15 minutes, starting 30 minutes before chemotherapy and repeated 4 hours and 8 hours later.

➤ To prevent nausea and vomiting caused by radiation

Adults and children older than age 12: 8 mg (tablet) or 10 ml (oral solution) P.O. 1 to 2 hours before radiation and

repeated q 8 hours, depending on radiation type, location, and extent
➤ Prevention and treatment of postoperative nausea and vomiting
Adults and children older than age 12: 16 mg (tablet) or 20 ml (oral solution) P.O. 1 hour before anesthesia induction, or 4 mg I.V. or I.M. before anesthesia or postoperatively
Children ages 2 to 12 weighing more than 40 kg (88 lb): 4 mg I.V. before anesthesia or postoperatively
Children ages 2 to 12 weighing less than 40 kg (88 lb): 0.1 mg/kg I.V. before anesthesia or postoperatively

Dosage adjustment
• Hepatic impairment

Contraindications
• Hypersensitivity to drug
• Concurrent use of apomorphine

Precautions
Use cautiously in:
• hepatic disease
• congenital long QT syndrome (avoid use)
• hypersensitivity to other selective 5-HT3 receptor antagonists
• phenylketonuria (with orally disintegrating tablets)
• pregnant or breastfeeding patients
• children younger than age 12.

Administration
• Give first dose before emetogenic event.
• Remove orally disintegrating tablet by peeling back foil with dry hands; don't push tablet through foil backing. After removing, place tablet on patient's tongue, where it will dissolve within seconds. Tell patient to swallow saliva.
• Give undiluted when administering I.M. before anesthesia induction.
• Give undiluted by direct I.V. immediately before anesthesia induction, or postoperatively if nausea and vomiting occur. Administer slowly, over at least

30 seconds (preferably over 2 to 5 minutes).
• For intermittent I.V. infusion, dilute in 50 ml of dextrose 5% in water (D_5W) and normal saline solution or D_5W and half-normal saline solution. Infuse over 15 minutes.
• When giving I.V., don't use flexible plastic container in series connection.

Route	Onset	Peak	Duration
P.O., I.V.	Rapid	15-30 min	4-8 hr
I.M.	Rapid	40 min	Unknown

Adverse reactions
CNS: headache, dizziness, malaise, drowsiness, fatigue, weakness, extrapyramidal reactions
CV: chest pain, hypotension, ECG changes including **QT-interval prolongation (rare and mostly with I.V. use), torsades de pointes (postmarketing reports)**
GI: constipation, diarrhea, abdominal pain, dry mouth
GU: urinary retention
Respiratory: bronchospasm
Skin: rash
Other: pain at injection site, shivering, **anaphylaxis**

Interactions
Drug-drug. *Drugs that alter hepatic enzyme activity:* altered pharmacokinetics of ondansetron
Drug-diagnostic tests. *Alanine aminotransferase, aspartate aminotransferase, bilirubin:* transient elevations

Patient monitoring
• Monitor GI status.
• Assess for extrapyramidal reactions.
• Check vital signs. Watch for hypotension and bronchospasm.
• Monitor fluid intake and output. Stay alert for urinary retention.
🔊 Be aware that cases of torsades de pointes have been reported. Monitor ECG in patients with electrolyte abnormalities (such as hypokalemia or

O

---

hypomagnesemia), congestive heart failure, or bradyarrhythmias, and in patients taking other drugs that lead to prolonged QT interval.

◀€ Be aware that using ondansetron after abdominal surgery or with chemotherapy-induced nausea and vomiting may mask a progressive ileus or gastric distention.

Patient teaching
• Tell patient to remove orally disintegrating tablet by peeling back foil with dry hands—not by pushing tablet through foil backing. Instruct him to place tablet on tongue, where it will dissolve within seconds, and then to swallow saliva.

◀€ Instruct patient to immediately report extrapyramidal symptoms, irregular heartbeats, abdominal distention after abdominal surgery, or allergic reaction.

• Inform patient with phenylketonuria (or caregiver) that powder contains phenylalanine.

• Caution patient to avoid driving and other hazardous activities until he knows how drug affects concentration and alertness.

• As appropriate, review all other significant and life-threatening adverse reactions and interactions, especially those related to the drugs and tests mentioned above.

orlistat
Alli, Xenical

Pharmacologic class: GI lipase inhibitor
Therapeutic class: Weight control drug
Pregnancy risk category X

Action
Inhibits absorption of dietary fats in stomach and small intestine

Availability
Capsules: 60 mg (over-the-counter drug), 120 mg

🕖 Indications and dosages
➤ Obesity management (in conjunction with reduced-calorie diet); to reduce risk of regaining after weight loss
Adults: 120 mg (Xenical) P.O. t.i.d. with each main meal containing fat (during or up to 1 hour after the meal)
➤ Weight loss in overweight adults (in conjunction with reduced-calorie and low-fat diet)
Adults ages 18 and older: 60 mg (Alli) P.O. t.i.d. with each meal containing fat

Contraindications
• Hypersensitivity to drug or its components
• Chronic malabsorption syndrome or cholestasis
• Patients who have had organ transplant or are taking drugs to reduce organ rejection (such as cyclosporine), patients with known problems absorbing food (Alli)
• Pregnancy

Precautions
Use cautiously in:
• hypothyroidism, nephrolithiasis, diabetes mellitus, clinically significant GI disease, fat-soluble vitamin deficiencies
• history of bulimia or anorexia nervosa
• breastfeeding patients
• children.

Administration
• Know that organic causes of obesity should be ruled out before therapy starts.
• Give three times daily with meal containing fat (Alli) or up to 1 hour after a meal (Xenical).
• If patient misses a meal or eats a fat-free meal, omit dose.
• Know that orlistat therapy is frequently combined with psychotherapy.

Route	Onset	Peak	Duration
P.O.	Unknown	8 hr	48-72 hr

Adverse reactions

CNS: *Xenical:* dizziness, headache, fatigue, insomnia, depression, anxiety

EENT: *Xenical:* ear, nose, and throat symptoms

GI: fecal urgency, flatus with discharge, oily or increased bowel movements, oily spotting, fecal incontinence

GU: *Xenical:* urinary tract infection (UTI), vaginitis, menstrual irregularities

Hepatic: severe liver injury (rare)

Musculoskeletal: *Xenical:* back pain, arthritis, myalgia, tendinitis

Respiratory: *Xenical:* upper or lower respiratory infection

Skin: *Xenical:* dry skin, rash

Other: *Xenical:* dental pain, tooth disorder, influenza

Interactions

Drug-drug. *Beta-carotene, fat-soluble vitamins:* reduced vitamin absorption

Cyclosporine: reduced cyclosporine blood level (Xenical)

Pravastatin: increased lipid-lowering effects (Xenical)

Warfarin: altered coagulation parameters

Patient monitoring

◀ℰ Monitor hepatic function closely. If liver injury is suspected, discontinue drug immediately and continue to monitor liver function tests.

• Watch for signs and symptoms of UTI, respiratory infection, and EENT disorders.

• Monitor patient for weight loss.

• Evaluate patient's diet for appropriate caloric intake.

• Be aware that patient may develop an elevated urinary oxalate level. Monitor renal function in patients at risk for renal insufficiency.

Patient teaching

• Instruct patient to take with meals as directed. Tell him he may omit a dose if he misses a meal or eats a fat-free meal.

• Advise patient to consume reduced-calorie diet and to spread daily fat intake over three main meals.

• Inform patient that drug predisposes him to EENT, respiratory, and urinary infections. Instruct him to promptly report signs and symptoms.

◀ℰ Instruct patient to report signs or symptoms of hepatic dysfunction (anorexia, pruritus, jaundice, dark urine, light-colored stools, or right upper quadrant pain).

• Tell patient about common adverse GI reactions, including problems controlling bowel movements. If significant GI upset occurs, encourage him to consult prescriber about taking psyllium at bedtime or with each dose.

• Advise patient to ask prescriber if he should take a daily multivitamin containing vitamins A, D, E, K, and beta-carotene at least 2 hours before or after taking drug.

• As appropriate, review all other significant adverse reactions and interactions, especially those related to the drugs mentioned above.

oseltamivir phosphate   **O**
Tamiflu

Pharmacologic class: Viral neuro-aminidase inhibitor

Therapeutic class: Antiviral

Pregnancy risk category C

Action

Inhibits influenza virus neuraminidase, altering viral particle aggregation and decreasing viral release from infected cells

Availability

Capsules: 30 mg, 45 mg, 75 mg

Powder for oral suspension: 12 mg/ml

⁄ Indications and dosages

➢ To prevent influenza type A

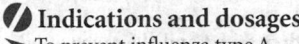

Adults and children older than age 13: 75 mg P.O. daily for 10 days, starting within 2 days of exposure; 75 mg P.O. daily during community outbreak of influenza for up to 6 weeks

Children ages 1 and older weighing more than 40 kg (88 lb): 75 mg P.O. daily for 10 days, starting within 2 days of exposure; continue dosing during community outbreak of influenza for up to 6 weeks

Children ages 1 and older weighing more than 23 kg up to 40 kg (more than 51 lb up to 88 lb): 60 mg P.O. daily for 10 days, starting within 2 days of exposure; continue dosing during community outbreak of influenza for up to 6 weeks

Children ages 1 and older weighing more than 15 kg up to 23 kg (33 lb up to 51 lb): 45 mg P.O. daily for 10 days, starting within 2 days of exposure; continue dosing during community outbreak of influenza for up to 6 weeks

Children ages 1 and older weighing 15 kg (33 lb) or less: 30 mg P.O. daily for 10 days, starting within 2 days of exposure; continue dosing during community outbreak of influenza for up to 6 weeks

➤ Treatment of influenza type A

Adults and children older than age 13: 75 mg P.O. b.i.d. for 5 days, starting within 2 days of symptom onset

Children ages 1 and older who weigh more than 40 kg (88 lb): 75 mg P.O. b.i.d. for 5 days, starting within 2 days of symptom onset

Children ages 1 and older who weigh more than 23 kg and up to 40 kg (51 to 88 lb): 60 mg P.O. b.i.d. for 5 days, starting within 2 days of symptom onset

Children ages 1 year and older who weigh more than 15 kg and up to 23 kg (33 to 51 lb): 45 mg P.O. b.i.d. for 5 days, starting within 2 days of symptom onset

Children ages 1 and older who weigh less than 15 kg (33 lb): 30 mg P.O. b.i.d. for 5 days, starting within 2 days of symptom onset

Dosage adjustment
• Renal impairment

Contraindications
• Hypersensitivity to drug or its components

Precautions
Use cautiously in:
• chronic cardiac or renal disease, respiratory disorders
• elderly patients
• pregnant or breastfeeding patients
• children younger than age 1 (safety and efficacy not established).

Administration
• For flu treatment, give first dose at onset of symptoms. For flu prevention, give within 2 days of exposure.

Route	Onset	Peak	Duration
P.O.	Variable	2.5	6 hr

Adverse reactions
CNS: headache, dizziness, fatigue, insomnia, unusual behavior, confusion
GI: nausea, vomiting, diarrhea
Respiratory: cough, bronchitis
Skin: epidermal necrolysis, erythema multiforme, Stevens-Johnson syndrome
Other: hypersensitivity reactions **(including anaphylaxis)**

Interactions
None significant

Patient monitoring
◀€ Monitor patient closely for allergic reaction or severe rash; discontinue drug immediately if these occur.
• Closely monitor patient for unusual behavior or confusion.
• Monitor respiratory status. Watch for signs and symptoms of secondary infection.

Patient teaching
- Instruct patient to take as soon as flu symptoms occur and to complete entire course of therapy.
- Advise patient to take with food or milk to minimize GI irritation.
- Tell patient to prepare oral solution by adding water to powder and shaking well.
- 🔊 Instruct patient or caregiver to discontinue drug and seek immediate medical attention if rash or swelling of lips, face, or throat occurs
- Instruct patient or caregiver to report change in behavior.
- Caution patient not to share drug with others, even if they have similar symptoms.
- Instruct patient to consult prescriber before taking other drugs.
- As appropriate, review all other significant adverse reactions.

oxaliplatin
Eloxatin

Pharmacologic class: Alkylator
Therapeutic class: Antineoplastic
Pregnancy risk category D

FDA BOXED WARNING

- Anaphylaxis may occur within minutes of administration. Epinephrine, corticosteroids, and antihistamines have been used to relieve symptoms.

Action
Unclear. Thought to form reactive platinum complexes that inhibit DNA synthesis through formation of interstrand and intrastrand cross-linking of DNA molecules. Cell-cycle-phase nonspecific.

Availability
Powder for reconstitution for injection, lyophilized: 5 mg/ml in 50-mg and 100-mg single-use vials
Solution for injection: 5 mg/ml in 10-ml, 20-ml, and 40-ml single-use vials

Indications and dosages
➤ Metastatic cancer of colon or rectum, given with 5-fluorouracil (5-FU) and leucovorin
Adults: On day 1, 85 mg/m² oxaliplatin I.V. infusion and 200 mg/m² leucovorin; give both drugs simultaneously over 2 hours, followed by 400 mg/m² I.V. bolus of 5-FU over 2 to 4 minutes, then 600 mg/m² 5-FU I.V. as 22-hour continuous infusion. On day two, 200 mg/m² leucovorin I.V. infusion over 2 hours, followed by 400 mg/m² 5-FU I.V. bolus over 2 to 4 minutes, then 600 mg/m² 5-FU I.V. as 22-hour continuous infusion.

Contraindications
- Hypersensitivity to drug or platinum products

Precautions
Use cautiously in:
- thrombocytopenia
- radiation therapy
- recent pneumococcal or smallpox vaccination
- elderly patients
- pregnant or breastfeeding patients
- children.

Administration
- 🔊 Follow facility policy for preparing, handling, and administering mutagenic, teratogenic, and carcinogenic drugs.
- Premedicate patient with antiemetics, as prescribed.
- Reconstitute with sterile water or dextrose 5% in water (D_5W)—never with normal saline solution or other solutions containing chloride.

• Further dilute reconstituted drug in 250 to 500 ml of D_5W.
• Infuse over 2 hours simultaneously with leucovorin, but in a separate I.V. bag.
• Don't use administration sets or needles that contain aluminum.
◀€ Be aware of importance of using leucovorin rescue with this drug.
◀€ Avoid extravasation, which may cause necrosis and other severe reactions.
• Know that treatment cycles are usually repeated every 2 weeks.

Route	Onset	Peak	Duration
I.V.	Unknown	Unknown	Unknown

Adverse reactions

CNS: headache, dizziness, fatigue, insomnia, peripheral neuropathy
CV: cardiac abnormalities
EENT: decreased visual acuity, hearing loss, tinnitus, rhinitis, pharyngitis
GI: severe nausea, vomiting, diarrhea, constipation, dyspepsia, gastroesophageal reflux, mucositis, flatulence, stomatitis, anorexia
GU: hematuria, dysuria
Hematologic: anemia, **thrombocytopenia, leukopenia, pancytopenia, neutropenia, hemolytic uremic syndrome**
Metabolic: hypokalemia
Respiratory: dyspnea, cough, upper respiratory infection, **pulmonary fibrosis**
Skin: alopecia, rash, flushing, extravasation, redness, swelling, angioedema
Other: weight loss, increased cold sensitivity, pain at injection site, **anaphylaxis**

Interactions

Drug-drug. *Aminoglycosides, loop diuretics:* increased risk of nephrotoxicity
Aspirin, nonsteroidal anti-inflammatory drugs: increased risk of bleeding

Live-virus vaccines: decreased antibody response to vaccine
Myelosuppressants: increased bone marrow depression
Drug-diagnostic tests. *Alanine aminotransferase, aspartate aminotransferase, bilirubin, creatinine:* increased levels
Hemoglobin, neutrophils, platelets, white blood cells: decreased levels
Drug-behaviors. *Alcohol use:* increased risk of bleeding

Patient monitoring

◀€ Monitor I.V. site frequently to avoid extravasation.
• Monitor CBC, blood chemistry, and kidney and liver function tests before each treatment cycle.
◀€ Watch closely for blood dyscrasias, hemolytic uremic syndrome, serious pulmonary problems, and anaphylaxis.
• Conduct complete neurologic exam before and after each dose.
• Monitor vital signs and ECG. Evaluate cardiovascular and respiratory status closely.
• Assess patient's comfort level. Keep him warm during infusion to minimize neurologic effects.
• Watch for signs and symptoms of toxicity (paresthesia, nausea, vomiting).

Patient teaching

• Inform patient that chemotherapy drugs can cause many adverse effects.
• Tell patient he'll receive drug from trained health care professionals in hospital setting.
◀€ Instruct patient to inform nurse immediately if drug contacts his skin, eyes, or mouth.
• Advise patient to notify nurse if pain or redness occurs at I.V. site.
• Instruct patient to stay warm and avoid iced drinks to minimize neurologic symptoms.
◀€ Tell patient to report itching, hives, swelling of hands or face, chest tightness, difficulty breathing, unsteadiness,

severe diarrhea or vomiting, or tingling sensation in hands, arms, legs, or feet.
• As appropriate, review all other significant and life-threatening adverse reactions and interactions, especially those related to the drugs, tests, and behaviors mentioned above.

oxaprozin
Apo-Oxaprozin✣, Daypro, Rhoxal-Oxaprozin✣

Pharmacologic class: Propionic acid derivative, nonsteroidal anti-inflammatory drug (NSAID)
Therapeutic class: Anti-inflammatory, analgesic
Pregnancy risk category C (first and second trimesters), *D* (third trimester)

FDA | BOXED WARNING

• Drug may increase risk of serious cardiovascular thrombotic events, myocardial infarction, and stroke. Risk may increase with duration of use. Patients with cardiovascular disease or risk factors for it may be at greater risk.
• Drug increases risk of serious GI adverse events, including bleeding, ulcers, and stomach or intestinal perforation. These events can occur at any time during use and without warning. Elderly patients are at greater risk.
• Drug is contraindicated for treatment of perioperative pain in setting of coronary artery bypass graft surgery.

Action
Unclear. Thought to inhibit prostaglandin synthesis by blocking cyclooxygenase (COX-2), thereby reducing inflammation.

Availability
Tablets: 600 mg

💊 Indications and dosages
➤ Rheumatoid arthritis; osteoarthritis
Adults: 1,200 mg daily in two to three divided doses. Maximum daily dosage is 1,800 mg (1,200 mg for potassium form).

Dosage adjustment
• Mild disease
• Renal impairment
• Low body weight

Contraindications
• Hypersensitivity to drug
• Concurrent use of other NSAIDs (including aspirin)
• Active GI bleeding or ulcer disease

Precautions
Use cautiously in:
• severe cardiovascular or hepatic disease, renal impairment
• history of ulcer disease
• pregnant or breastfeeding patients
• children (safety not established).

Administration
• Give with food or after meals if GI upset occurs.
• Use lowest effective dosage to minimize adverse reactions.

Route	Onset	Peak	Duration
P.O.	Unknown	3-5 hr	Unknown

Adverse reactions
CNS: dizziness, fatigue, headache, agitation, anxiety, confusion, depression, insomnia, malaise, paresthesia, tremor
CV: edema, vasculitis, blood pressure changes
EENT: abnormal vision, tinnitus
GI: nausea, vomiting, diarrhea, constipation, abdominal pain, gastritis, dyspepsia, duodenal ulcer, flatulence,

O

---

stomatitis, dry mouth, anorexia, **GI bleeding**
GU: albuminuria, azotemia, **interstitial nephritis, acute renal failure**
Hematologic: anemia
Hepatic: cholestatic jaundice, **hepatitis**
Respiratory: dyspnea, **hypersensitivity pneumonitis**
Skin: rash, pruritus, diaphoresis, photosensitivity, angioedema, **Stevens-Johnson syndrome**
Other: appetite and weight increases, allergic reactions including **anaphylaxis**

Interactions

Drug-drug. *Alcohol, aspirin and other NSAIDs, corticosteroids, potassium supplements:* additive adverse GI effects and toxicity
Anticoagulants, cefamandole, cefoperazone, cefotetan, clopidogrel, eptifibatide, plicamycin, thrombolytics, ticlopidine, tirofiban, vitamin A: increased risk of bleeding
Antineoplastics: increased risk of adverse hematologic reactions
Insulin, oral hypoglycemics: increased hypoglycemic effects of these drugs
Methotrexate: increased risk of methotrexate toxicity
Drug-diagnostic tests. *Alanine aminotransferase, alkaline phosphatase, aspartate aminotransferase, blood urea nitrogen, creatinine, lactate dehydrogenase, potassium:* increased levels
Bleeding time: prolonged (for up to 2 weeks after drug discontinuation)
Creatinine clearance, glucose, hemoglobin, hematocrit, platelets, white blood cells: decreased levels
Liver function tests: abnormal results
Drug-herbs. *Alfalfa, anise, arnica, astragalus, bilberry, black currant seed oil, bladderwrack, bogbean, boldo (with fenugreek), borage oil, buchu, capsaicin, cat's claw, celery, chamomile, chapparal, chincona bark, clove, clove oil, dandelion, dong quai, evening primrose oil, fenugreek, feverfew, garlic, ginger, ginkgo, ginseng, guggul, licorice,*

papaya extract, red clover, rhubarb, safflower oil, skullcap, tan-shen: increased anticoagulant effect and bleeding risk

Patient monitoring

• Monitor kidney and liver function tests, coagulation studies, and CBC.
◀€ Watch for signs and symptoms of acute renal failure, nephritis, hepatitis, bleeding tendency, and anemia.
• Monitor hearing and vision, including results of eye exams.
◀€ Watch for and promptly report rash or swelling.
• Assess respiratory status closely. Stay alert for dyspnea and pneumonitis.

Patient teaching

• Instruct patient to take with food or meal.
• Inform patient that many common over-the-counter drugs (including acetaminophen, aspirin, and other NSAIDs) and herbal preparations increase drug's adverse effects. Tell him to consult prescriber before taking these products.
◀€ Instruct patient to immediately report rash, unusual tiredness, yellowing of skin or eyes, easy bruising or bleeding, change in urination pattern, weight gain, arm or leg swelling, vision changes, and black or tarry stools.
• Advise patient to minimize GI upset by eating small, frequent servings of food and drinking plenty of fluids.
• Caution patient to avoid driving and other hazardous activities until he knows how drug affects concentration and alertness.
• Advise patient on long-term therapy to have periodic eye exams.
• As appropriate, review all other significant and life-threatening adverse reactions and interactions, especially those related to the drugs, tests, and herbs mentioned above.

oxazepam
Apo-Oxazepam✷, Bio-Oxaxepam✷, Novoxapam✷, PMS-Oxazepam✷, Riva Oxazepam✷

Pharmacologic class: Benzodiazepine
Therapeutic class: Anxiolytic, sedative-hypnotic
Controlled substance schedule IV
Pregnancy risk category D

Action
Suppresses CNS stimulation at limbic and subcortical levels by potentiating effects of gamma-aminobutyrate, an inhibitory neurotransmitter. This suppression reduces anxiety and diminishes alcohol withdrawal symptoms.

Availability
Capsules: 10 mg, 15 mg, 30 mg
Tablets: 15 mg

⦰ Indications and dosages
➤ Mild to moderate anxiety
Adults: 10 to 15 mg P.O. three to four times daily
➤ Severe anxiety; alcohol withdrawal symptoms
Adults: 15 to 30 mg P.O. three to four times daily

Dosage adjustment
• Elderly patients

Off-label uses
• Insomnia

Contraindications
• Hypersensitivity to drug or tartrazine (some products)

Precautions
Use cautiously in:
• hepatic dysfunction, severe chronic obstructive pulmonary disease, myasthenia gravis, CNS depression, uncontrolled severe pain
• history of suicide attempt or drug abuse
• concurrent use of other benzodiazepines
• elderly or debilitated patients
• pregnant or breastfeeding patients.

Administration
• Administer with or without food.
• Taper dosage after long-term therapy.

Route	Onset	Peak	Duration
P.O.	45-90 min	3 hr	6-12 hr

Adverse reactions
CNS: dizziness, drowsiness, headache, confusion, poor memory, hangover effect, slurred speech, depression, paradoxical stimulation
CV: orthostatic hypotension, hypotension, ECG changes, tachycardia
EENT: blurred vision, mydriasis, tinnitus
GI: nausea, vomiting, constipation, diarrhea
GU: urinary retention, urinary incontinence
Hematologic: leukopenia
Hepatic: jaundice, **hepatitis**
Respiratory: respiratory depression
Skin: rash, dermatitis, itching
Other: physical and psychological drug dependence, drug tolerance, withdrawal symptoms

Interactions
Drug-drug. *Azole antifungals:* increased oxazepam blood level, greater risk of toxicity
Hormonal contraceptives, phenytoin: decreased oxazepam efficacy
Levodopa: decreased levodopa efficacy
Other CNS depressants (including antidepressants, antihistamines, other benzodiazepines, sedative-hypnotics, opioids): additive CNS depression
Theophylline: decreased sedative effect of oxazepam

O

Reactions in **bold** are life-threatening. ◀€ Clinical alert

Drug-diagnostic tests. *Alanine aminotransferase, alkaline phosphatase, aspartate aminotransferase, lactate dehydrogenase:* increased levels
Hematocrit, thyroid uptake of sodium iodide 123I and 131I, white blood cells: decreased values
Drug-food. *Cabbage:* decreased drug blood level
Drug-herbs. *Chamomile, hops, kava, valerian, skullcap:* increased CNS depression
Drug-behaviors. *Alcohol use:* increased CNS depression

Patient monitoring

◀🎔 Monitor liver function tests and watch for signs and symptoms of hepatitis.
• Check vital signs. Stay alert for respiratory depression, orthostatic hypotension, and tachycardia.
• Monitor neurologic status. As needed, take measures to prevent injury.
• Watch for signs and symptoms of psychological or physical dependence.
• When tapering, watch for withdrawal symptoms.

Patient teaching

• Tell patient he may take with or without meals, but should avoid cabbage.
• Advise patient to take exactly as prescribed. Tell him drug can cause dependence, and emphasize importance of following tapering instructions to avoid withdrawal symptoms.
◀🎔 Urge patient to immediately report unusual tiredness, nausea, appetite loss, or yellowing of skin or eyes.
• Tell patient to change position slowly to avoid blood pressure decrease.
• Instruct patient to report severe dizziness, weakness, persistent drowsiness, palpitations, or visual changes.
• Advise patient not to drink alcohol.
• Caution patient to avoid driving and other hazardous activities until he knows how drug affects vision, cognition, and balance.
• As appropriate, review all other significant and life-threatening adverse reactions and interactions, especially those related to the drugs, tests, foods, herbs, and behaviors mentioned above.

oxcarbazepine

Apo-Oxcarbazepine✱, Trileptal

Pharmacologic class: Carboxamide derivative
Therapeutic class: Anticonvulsant
Pregnancy risk category C

Action

Blocks sodium channels in neural membranes, stabilizing hyperexcitable states and inhibiting neuronal firing and impulse transmission in brain

Availability

Oral suspension: 300 mg/5-ml bottle
Tablets: 150 mg, 300 mg, 600 mg

🩸 Indications and dosages

➢ Adjunctive therapy for partial seizures
Adults: 300 mg P.O. b.i.d. May increase by up to 600 mg/day q week, to a maximum of 1,200 mg/day.
Children ages 2 to 16: Initially, 8 to 10 mg/kg/day P.O. to a maximum of 600 mg/day
➢ Conversion to monotherapy for partial seizures
Adults: 300 mg P.O. b.i.d. May increase by 600 mg/day at weekly intervals over 2 to 4 weeks, to a maximum of 2,400 mg/day
Children ages 4 to 16: Initially, 8 to 10 mg/kg/day P.O. given in two divided doses, increased to a maximum of 10 mg/kg/day

➤ Initiation of monotherapy

Adults: 300 mg P.O. b.i.d., increased by 300 mg/day P.O. q 3 days up to 1,200 mg/day

Children ages 4 to 16: Initially, 8 to 10 mg/kg/day P.O. given in two divided doses; increase by 5 mg/kg q 3 days to a maximum of 1,200 mg/day

Dosage adjustment
- Renal impairment
- Children ages 2 to younger than 4 weighing less than 20 kg (44 lb)

Contraindications
- Hypersensitivity to drug or its components

Precautions
Use cautiously in:
- renal impairment
- pregnant or breastfeeding patients
- children younger than age 2 (safety not established).

Administration
- Administer twice daily with or without food.
- Shake oral suspension well. If desired, mix in small glass of water.

Route	Onset	Peak	Duration
P.O.	Unknown	Unknown	Unknown

Adverse reactions
CNS: dizziness, vertigo, drowsiness, fatigue, headache, ataxia, tremor, emotional lability
EENT: abnormal vision, diplopia, nystagmus, rhinitis
GI: nausea, vomiting, diarrhea, constipation, abdominal pain, dyspepsia
Metabolic: hyponatremia
Skin: acne, rash
Other: thirst, allergic reactions, edema, lymphadenopathy

Interactions
Drug-drug. *Carbamazepine, valproic acid, verapamil:* decreased oxcarbazepine blood level
CNS depressants (including antidepressants, antihistamines, opioids, sedative-hypnotics): additive CNS depression
Felodipine, hormonal contraceptives: decreased blood levels of these drugs
Phenobarbital: decreased oxcarbazepine and increased phenobarbital blood levels
Phenytoin: increased phenytoin blood level
Drug-diagnostic tests. *Sodium:* decreased level
Drug-behaviors. *Alcohol use:* additive CNS depression

Patient monitoring
- Monitor neurologic status closely for changes in cognition, mood, wakefulness, balance, and gait.
- Check sodium level. Watch for signs and symptoms of hyponatremia.

Patient teaching
- Instruct patient to take at same time each day, with or without food.
- Tell patient to report vision changes and significant neurologic changes.
- Advise patient to have periodic eye exams.
- Tell female patient that drug makes hormonal contraceptives less effective.
- Inform patient that he may need frequent tests to check drug blood levels.
- Tell patient not to drink alcohol.
- Caution patient to avoid driving and other hazardous activities until he knows how drug affects him.
- As appropriate, review all significant adverse reactions and interactions, especially those related to the drugs, tests, and behaviors mentioned above.

O

Reactions in **bold** are life-threatening. 🔊 Clinical alert

oxybutynin
Cystrin⊕, Kentera⊕, Oxytrol

oxybutynin chloride
Apo-Oxybutynin✣, Ditropan, Ditropan XL, Dom-Oxybutynin✣, Gelnique, Gen-Oxybutynin✣, Lyrinel XL⊕, Novo-Oxybutynin✣, Nu-Oxybutynin✣, PHL-Oxybutynin✣, PMS-Oxybutynin✣, Uromax✣

Pharmacologic class: Anticholinergic
Therapeutic class: Urinary tract antispasmodic
Pregnancy risk category B

Action
Inhibits acetylcholine action at postganglionic receptors, relaxing smooth muscle lining of GU tract and preventing bladder irritability

Availability
Syrup: 5 mg/5 ml
Tablets: 5 mg
Tablets (extended-release): 5 mg, 10 mg, 15 mg
Topical gel: 1 g in 1.14-ml sachet
Transdermal system (patch): 39 cm²/ 36 mg

⏻ Indications and dosages
➤ Frequent urination, urinary urgency or incontinence, and nocturia caused by neurogenic bladder; overactive bladder
Adults: 5 mg P.O. two to three times daily (not to exceed 5 mg q.i.d.); or 5 to 15 mg P.O. once daily (extended-release); or one 3.9 mg/day transdermal system applied twice weekly; or apply contents of one gel sachet daily.
Children older than age 5: 5 mg P.O. b.i.d., to a maximum of 5 mg t.i.d.

Dosage adjustment
• Elderly patients

Contraindications
• Hypersensitivity to drug
• Glaucoma
• Intestinal obstruction, severe colitis, atony, paralytic ileus, megacolon, or hemorrhage
• Obstructive uropathy, urinary retention
• Myasthenia gravis
• Acute hemorrhage with shock

Precautions
Use cautiously in:
• cardiovascular disease, hyperthyroidism, GI disease
• elderly patients
• pregnant or breastfeeding patients
• children younger than age 5 (safety not established).

Administration
• Give oral forms without regard to food.
• Don't crush or break tablets.
• Apply contents of one gel sachet to dry, intact skin on the abdomen, upper arms, shoulders, or thighs.

Route	Onset	Peak	Duration
P.O.	30-60 min	3-6 hr	6-10 hr
P.O. (extended)	30-60 min	3-6 hr	Up to 24 hr
Transdermal	24-48 hr	48-96 hr	96 hr after removal
Gel	Unknown	Unknown	Unknown

Adverse reactions
CNS: dizziness, drowsiness, hallucinations, insomnia, weakness, anxiety, restlessness, headache
CV: palpitations, hypotension, tachycardia
EENT: blurred vision, cycloplegia, increased intraocular pressure, mydriasis, photophobia

---

GI: nausea, vomiting, diarrhea, constipation, bloating, dry mouth

GU: urinary hesitancy, urinary retention, erectile dysfunction, suppressed lactation

Metabolic: hyperthermia

Skin: decreased sweating, urticaria, application-site reactions

Other: allergic reactions, fever, hot flashes

Interactions

Drug-drug. *Anticholinergics, anticholinergic-like drugs (including amantadine, antidepressants, disopyramide, haloperidol, phenothiazines):* additive anticholinergic effects

Atenolol: increased atenolol absorption

CNS depressants (including antidepressants, antihistamines, opioids, sedative-hypnotics): additive CNS depression

Digoxin: increased digoxin blood level (with extended-release oxybutynin)

Haloperidol: decreased haloperidol blood level, tardive dyskinesia, worsening of schizophrenia

Levodopa: decreased levodopa efficacy

Nitrofurantoin: increased nitrofurantoin blood level, greater risk of toxicity

Drug-herbs. *Angel's trumpet, jimsonweed, scopolia:* increased anticholinergic effects

Drug-behaviors. *Alcohol use:* additive CNS depression

Patient monitoring

• Monitor vital signs and temperature. Watch for hypotension, fever, and tachycardia.

• Evaluate patient's vision.

• Assess results of cystometric studies. Stay alert for urinary retention.

Patient teaching

• Tell patient he may take with or without food. Caution him not to crush, break, or chew extended-release tablets.

• Instruct patient to apply transdermal patch to dry, intact skin on abdomen, hip, or buttock. Tell him to use a new

skin area with each new system and not to reapply new patch to same site within 7 days. Caution him not to cut or puncture patch.

• Instruct patient to apply contents of one gel sachet daily to dry, intact skin on the abdomen, upper arms, shoulders, or thighs. Tell patient to use a new skin area daily. Advise patient to cover application site with clothing if skin-to-skin contact at application site is anticipated and to wash hands immediately after product application. Warn patient that gel is flammable and to avoid open fire or smoking until gel has dried.

• Tell patient to report blurred vision, fever, skin rash, nausea, or vomiting.

• Advise patient he'll need to undergo periodic bladder exams.

• Caution patient to avoid driving and other hazardous activities if drug causes drowsiness or blurred vision.

• As appropriate, review all other significant adverse reactions and interactions, especially those related to the drugs, herbs, and behaviors mentioned above.

oxycodone hydrochloride

Oxecta, OxyContin, Oxynorm ✛, Roxicodone, Supeudol ✦

Pharmacologic class: Opioid agonist

Therapeutic class: Narcotic analgesic

Controlled substance schedule II

Pregnancy risk category B

FDA   BOXED WARNING

• Drug is opioid agonist and Schedule II controlled substance, with abuse potential similar to morphine. This potential must be considered when prescribing or dispensing drug.

• Extended-release tablets are indicated for managing moderate to severe pain when continuous, around-the-clock analgesia is needed for extended period of time. Extended-release tablets aren't intended for as-needed analgesia.

• Extended-release 80-mg tablets are for use only in opioid-tolerant patients. This strength may cause fatal respiratory depression when given to patients without previous opioid exposure.

• Instruct patients to swallow extended-release tablets whole. Caution them not to break, chew, or crush them, as this causes rapid release and absorption of potentially fatal dose.

Action
Unknown. Thought to interact with opioid receptor sites primarily in limbic system, thalamus, and spinal cord, blocking transmission of pain impulses.

Availability
Capsules (immediate-release): 5 mg
Solution (oral): 5 mg/5 ml
Tablets: 5 mg, 7.5 mg, 10 mg, 15 mg, 20 mg, 30 mg
Tablets (controlled-release): 10 mg, 15 mg, 20 mg, 30 mg, 40 mg, 60 mg, 80 mg

🖉 Indications and dosages
➣ Moderate to severe pain
Adults: 5 mg P.O. q 6 hours p.r.n., increased gradually to 10 to 30 mg q 6 hours p.r.n.
➣ Moderate or severe pain when continuous around-the-clock analgesia is needed
Adults: 10 mg P.O. (controlled-release) q 12 hours. For patients already taking opioids, use total oral oxycodone daily equianalgesic dosage and then round down to closest tablet strength. For breakthrough pain, give supplemental immediate-release doses.

Dosage adjustment
• Hepatic disease
• Renal impairment
• Debilitated or opioid-naive patients

Off-label uses
• Postherpetic neuralgia (controlled-release form)

Contraindications
• Hypersensitivity to drug
• Paralytic ileus
• When opioids are contraindicated (as in respiratory depression, severe bronchial asthma, hypercarbia)

Precautions
Use cautiously in:
• head trauma; increased intracranial pressure (ICP); severe renal, hepatic, or pulmonary disease; hypothyroidism; adrenal insufficiency; urethral stricture; undiagnosed abdominal pain or prostatic hyperplasia; extensive burns; alcoholism
• history of substance abuse
• prolonged or high-dose therapy
• elderly or debilitated patients
• labor and delivery
• pregnant or breastfeeding patients
• children younger than age 18.

Administration
• Be aware that drug has high abuse potential.
• Know that controlled-release Oxy-Contin isn't indicated for p.r.n. pain control but is reserved for patients who need continuous, around-the-clock analgesia.
• Be aware that 80-mg controlled-release tablets are for opioid-tolerant patients only.
🔊 Never break, crush, or let patient chew controlled-release forms. Otherwise, rapid release and absorption of potentially fatal dose may occur.
• Give Oxecta tablets whole. Don't crush or dissolve tablets or administer by nasogastric, gastric, or other feeding

tubes, because this may cause obstruction of feeding tubes.

• When discontinuing, taper dosage gradually to prevent withdrawal symptoms.

Route	Onset	Peak	Duration
P.O.	15-30 min	1 hr	4-6 hr
P.O. (controlled)	Unknown	24-36 hr	>12 hr

Adverse reactions

CNS: dizziness, asthenia, drowsiness, euphoria, light-headedness, insomnia, confusion, anxiety, twitching, abnormal dreams and thoughts

CV: orthostatic hypotension, **circulatory depression, bradycardia, shock**

GI: nausea, vomiting, constipation, diarrhea, ileus, abdominal pain, dyspepsia, gastritis, anorexia

GU: urinary retention

Respiratory: apnea, respiratory depression, respiratory arrest

Skin: pruritus, sweating

Other: chills, fever, hiccups, physical and psychological drug dependence

Interactions

Drug-drug. *Antihistamines, sedative-hypnotics:* additive CNS depression

Barbiturates, protease inhibitors: increased respiratory and CNS depression

Opioid agonist-antagonists: precipitation of opioid withdrawal in physically dependent patients

Drug-diagnostic tests. *Amylase, lipase:* increased levels

Drug-behaviors. *Alcohol use:* additive CNS depression

Patient monitoring

◀≣ Monitor vital signs and respiratory status. Withhold drug in significant respiratory or CNS depression.

• Assess patient's pain level frequently.

• Monitor bowel and bladder function.

• Assess patient for anxiety, twitching, and other CNS symptoms.

• Closely monitor head-trauma patient. Drug may increase ICP while masking signs and symptoms.

• Carefully assess patient with acute abdominal pain. Drug may obscure diagnosis.

• Stay alert for drug hoarding, tolerance, and dependence.

Patient teaching

◀≣ Caution patient not to break, crush, chew, or dissolve controlled-release tablets. Warn him that doing so may cause rapid drug release and absorption (possibly fatal).

• Tell patient taking controlled-release form not to drive for 3 to 4 days after dosage increase, after consuming even a single alcoholic beverage, or if also taking antihistamines or other drugs that cause drowsiness.

• Tell patient to take Oxecta tablets whole.

◀≣ Instruct patient to promptly report adverse reactions, especially difficulty breathing or slow pulse.

• Advise patient not to drink alcohol.

• Tell patient not to be alarmed if controlled-release tablets appear in stools; drug has already been absorbed.

• Advise ambulatory patient to change position slowly, to avoid dizziness from orthostatic hypotension.

• Instruct patient to consult prescriber before taking other drugs.

• Caution patient to avoid driving and other hazardous activities, because drug may cause drowsiness or dizziness.

• As appropriate, review all other significant and life-threatening adverse reactions and interactions, especially those related to the drugs, tests, and behaviors mentioned above.

O

Reactions in **bold** are life-threatening.   ◀≣ Clinical alert

oxymorphone hydrochloride
Opana, Opana ER, Oxynorm ⊕

Pharmacologic class: Opioid agonist
Therapeutic class: Narcotic analgesic
Controlled substance schedule II
Pregnancy risk category C

FDA | BOXED WARNING

- Drug is morphine-like opioid agonist and Schedule II controlled substance, with abuse potential similar to other opioids. This potential must be considered when prescribing or dispensing drug.
- Drug is indicated for managing moderate to severe pain when continuous, around-the-clock opioid is needed for extended period. It isn't intended for as-needed analgesia.
- Instruct patients to swallow extended-release tablets whole. Caution them not to break, chew, dissolve, or crush them, as this causes rapid release and absorption of potentially fatal dose.
- Caution patient not to consume alcoholic beverages or take prescription or nonprescription medications containing alcohol during therapy, as this may increase drug blood levels and cause potentially fatal overdose.

Action
Unknown. Thought to interact with opioid receptor sites primarily in limbic system, thalamus, and spinal cord, blocking pain impulse transmission.

Availability
Injection: 1 mg/ml, 1.5 mg/ml
Tablets: 5 mg, 10 mg

Tablets (extended-release): 5 mg, 7.5 mg, 10 mg, 15 mg, 20 mg, 30 mg, 40 mg

🕖 Indications and dosages
➢ Moderate to severe pain
Adults: 1 to 1.5 mg I.M. or subcutaneously q 4 to 6 hours p.r.n.; or initially, 0.5 mg I.V., increased cautiously until pain relief is satisfactory
➢ To reduce labor pain
Adults: 0.5 to 1 mg I.M.
➢ Initiation of therapy for moderate to severe acute pain in opioid-naïve patients
Adults: 10 to 20 mg (Opana) P.O. q 4 to 6 hours depending on initial pain intensity. If deemed necessary to initiate therapy at lower dose, start with 5 mg. Adjust dosage based on patient's response to initial dose. Dose can then be adjusted to acceptable level of analgesia taking into account pain intensity and adverse effects experienced. For chronic around-the-clock opioid therapy, give 5 mg (Opana ER) q 12 hours; thereafter, individually adjust dosage, preferably at increments of 5 to 10 mg q 12 hours every 3 to 7 days to level that provides adequate analgesia and minimizes side effects; give under close supervision of prescribing physician.
➢ Moderate to severe acute pain when converting from parenteral to oral form in patients requiring continuous, around-the-clock opioid treatment for extended period
Adults: 10 times patient's total daily parenteral oxymorphone dose as Opana, in four or six equally divided doses (for example, approximately 10 mg Opana may be needed to provide pain relief equivalent to total daily I.M. dose of 4 mg oxymorphone); titrate dosage to optimal pain relief or combine with acetaminophen/nonsteroidal anti-inflammatories for optimal pain relief. Or 10 times patient's total daily parenteral oxymorphone dose as

Opana ER, in two equally divided doses (for example, approximately 20 mg Opana ER q 12 hours may be needed to provide pain relief equivalent to total daily parenteral dose of 4 mg oxymorphone.

➤ Moderate to severe acute pain when converting from other oral opioids to Opana or Opana ER

Adults: Refer to published relative potency information, keeping in mind that conversion ratios are only approximate. In general, it's safest to start Opana therapy by administering half of calculated total daily dose of Opana in four to six equally divided doses P.O. q 4 to 6 hours. Or, for patients requiring continuous, around-the-clock opioid treatment for extended period, give Opana ER in two divided doses P.O. q 12 hours. Gradually adjust initial dosage of Opana or Opana ER until adequate pain relief and acceptable adverse effects have been achieved.

➤ Moderate to severe acute pain in opioid-experienced patients when converting from Opana to Opana ER

Adults: Administer half patient's total daily oral Opana dose as Opana ER P.O. q 12 hours.

Dosage adjustments

• Mild hepatic impairment (Opana, Opana ER)
• Severe hepatic impairment (Numorphan)
• Moderate to severe renal impairment (Opana, Opana ER)
• Concurrent use of other CNS depressants (Opana, Opana ER)
• Elderly or debilitated patients

Contraindications

• Hypersensitivity to drug or its components, or morphine analogs
• Any situation in which opioids are contraindicated, such as respiratory depression (in absence of resuscitative equipment or in unmonitored

settings) and acute or severe bronchial asthma or hypercarbia
• Pulmonary edema secondary to chemical respiratory irritant (Numorphan)
• Suspected or existing paralytic ileus
• Moderate and severe hepatic impairment (Opana, Opana ER)

Precautions

Use cautiously in:
• head trauma, increased intracranial pressure, severe renal disease, hypothyroidism, adrenal insufficiency, urethral stricture, undiagnosed abdominal pain or prostatic hyperplasia, biliary tract disease, pancreatitis, extensive burns, alcoholism
• history of substance abuse
• prolonged or high-dose therapy
• elderly or debilitated patients
• labor and delivery
• pregnant or breastfeeding patients
• Pain in immediate postoperative period (first 12 to 24 hours), or if pain is mild or not expected to persist for extended period (Opana ER)
• Children younger than age 18.

Administration

• Give oral on empty stomach at least 1 hour before or 2 hours after eating.
• Tell patient to swallow extended-release tablets whole and not to break, chew, dissolve, or crush tablets.
• Be aware that extended-release tablets are not for p.r.n. use.
• Be aware that extended-release tablets are indicated only for postoperative use if patient had already been receiving drug before surgery or if postoperative pain is expected to be moderate or severe and persist for extended period.

◀̇ Be aware that administration from any source (such as beverages or drugs) may result in increased plasma drug levels and potentially fatal overdose of oxymorphone.

Reactions in **bold** are life-threatening.   ◀̇ Clinical alert

◀€ Keep naloxone available to reverse respiratory depression, if necessary.
• Give I.V. dose by direct injection over 2 to 3 minutes.

Route	Onset	Peak	Duration
P.O.	Unknown	Unknown	Unknown
I.V.	5-10 min	30-60 min	3-6 hr
I.M., subcut.	10-15 min	30-60 min	3-6 hr

Adverse reactions

CNS: somnolence (Opana, Opana ER), sedation, headache, drowsiness, confusion, dysphoria, euphoria, dizziness, hallucinations, lethargy, impaired mental and physical performance, depression, restlessness, insomnia, paradoxical stimulation, **seizures**
CV: hypotension, orthostatic hypotension, palpitations, **bradycardia, tachycardia**
EENT: blurred vision, miosis, diplopia, visual disturbances, tinnitus
GI: abdominal distention, flatulence (Opana), abdominal pain, dyspepsia (Opana ER), nausea, vomiting, constipation, biliary tract spasm, cramps, dry mouth, anorexia, **paralytic ileus, toxic megacolon**
GU: urinary hesitancy or retention, urethral spasm, antidiuretic effect
Respiratory: suppressed cough reflex, hypoxia (Opana), **atelectasis, respiratory depression, allergic bronchospastic reaction, allergic laryngeal edema or laryngospasm, apnea**
Skin: rash, urticaria, pruritus, facial flushing, diaphoresis
Other: pyrexia (Opana, Opana ER), physical or psychological drug dependence, drug tolerance, allergic reaction, injection site reaction (Numorphan)

Interactions

Drug-drug. *Agonist/antagonist analgesia (such as buprenorphine, butorphanol, nalbuphine, or pentazocine):* reduced oxymorphone effect; may precipitate withdrawal symptoms (Opana, Opana ER)
Anticholinergics: increased risk of urinary retention or severe constipation
Antihistamines (first-generation), antipsychotics, barbiturates, general anesthetics, MAO inhibitors, sedative-hypnotics, skeletal muscle relaxants, tricyclic antidepressants: increased risk of respiratory depression
Propofol: increased risk of bradycardia (Numorphan)
Drug-diagnostic tests. *Amylase, lipase:* increased levels
Drug-behaviors. *Alcohol use or abuse, opiate abuse:* increased risk of respiratory depression

Patient monitoring

◀€ Closely monitor respiratory status. Stay alert for respiratory depression and allergic responses affecting bronchi and larynx.
• Monitor vital signs and ECG.
• With prolonged use, watch for signs and symptoms of drug dependence.
• Assess neurologic status carefully. Institute protective measures as needed.
• Monitor patient receiving Opana or Opana ER for breakthrough pain and adverse reaction (especially severe constipation).

Patient teaching

◀€ Instruct patient to immediately report seizures or difficulty breathing.
• Tell patient to rise slowly when changing position, to avoid dizziness from blood pressure decrease.
• Instruct patient taking Opana or Opana ER to report episodes of breakthrough pain and adverse reactions (especially severe constipation that may lead to paralytic ileus).
◀€ Advise patient not to drink alcohol from any source because doing so may result in fatal overdose.

- Caution patient not to drive or perform other hazardous activities.
- Tell patient not to stop taking drug suddenly after several weeks, because withdrawal symptoms may occur.
- As appropriate, review all other significant and life-threatening adverse reactions and interactions, especially those related to the drugs, tests, and behaviors mentioned above.

oxytocin
Pitocin, Syntocinon✢⊕,
Syntometrine⊕

Pharmacologic class: Posterior pituitary hormone
Therapeutic class: Uterine-active agent
Pregnancy risk category NR

FDA | BOXED WARNING

- Drug isn't indicated for elective induction of labor (defined as initiation of labor in pregnant woman with no medical indications for induction). Available data aren't adequate to evaluate benefits versus risk.

Action
Unknown. Thought to directly stimulate smooth muscle contractions in uterus and cervix.

Availability
Injection: 10 units/ml ampule or vial

⚕ Indications and dosages
➤ To induce or stimulate labor
Adults: Initially, 1-ml ampule (10 units) in compatible I.V. solution infused at 1 to 2 milliunits/minute (0.001 to 0.002 units/minute). Increase rate in increments of 1 to 2 milliunits/minute q 15 to 30 minutes until acceptable contraction pattern is established.
➤ To control postpartum bleeding
Adults: 10 to 40 units in compatible I.V. solution infused at rate adequate to control bleeding; or 10 units I.M. after placenta delivery
➤ Incomplete abortion
Adults: 10 units in compatible I.V. solution infused at 10 to 20 milliunits/minute (0.01 to 0.02 units/minute)

Off-label uses
- Antepartal fetal heart rate testing
- Breast enlargement

Contraindications
- Hypersensitivity to drug
- Cephalopelvic disproportion
- Fetal distress when delivery is not imminent
- Prolonged use in uterine inertia or severe toxemia
- Hypertonic or hyperactive uterine pattern
- Unfavorable fetal position or presentation that's undeliverable without conversion
- Labor induction or augmentation when vaginal delivery is contraindicated (as in invasive cervical cancer, active genital herpes, or total placenta previa)

Precautions
Use cautiously in:
- previous cervical or uterine surgery, history of uterine sepsis
- breastfeeding patients.

Administration
- Reconstitute by adding 1 ml (10 units) to 1,000 ml of normal saline solution, lactated Ringer's solution, or dextrose 5% in water.
- ◀€ Don't give by I.V. bolus injection.
- Infuse I.V. using controlled-infusion device.

O

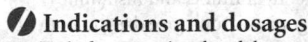

• Be aware that drug isn't routinely given I.M.
• Know that drug should be given only to inpatients at critical care facilities when prescriber is immediately available.

Route	Onset	Peak	Duration
I.V.	Immediate	40 min	1 hr
I.M.	3-5 min	40 min	2-3 hr

Adverse reactions

CNS: **seizures, coma, neonatal brain damage, subarachnoid hemorrhage**
CV: premature ventricular contractions, **arrhythmias, neonatal bradycardia**
GI: nausea, vomiting
GU: **postpartal hemorrhage; pelvic hematoma; uterine hypertonicity, spasm, or tetanic contraction; abruptio placentae; uterine rupture** (with excessive doses)
Hematologic: **afibrinogenemia**
Hepatic: **neonatal jaundice**
Other: hypersensitivity reactions including **anaphylaxis, low 5-minute Apgar score (neonate)**

Interactions

Drug-drug. *Sympathomimetics:* postpartal hypertension
Thiopental anesthetics: delayed anesthesia induction
Vasoconstrictors: severe hypertension (when given within 3 to 4 hours of oxytocin)
Drug-herbs. *Ephedra (ma huang):* increased hypertension

Patient monitoring

◀€ Continuously monitor contractions, fetal and maternal heart rate, and maternal blood pressure and ECG. Discontinue infusion if uterine hyperactivity occurs.
◀€ Monitor patient extremely closely during first and second stages of labor because of risk of cervical laceration, uterine rupture, and maternal and fetal death.
• When giving drug to control postpartal bleeding, monitor and record vaginal bleeding.
• Assess fluid intake and output. Watch for signs and symptoms of water intoxication.

Patient teaching

• Inform patient about risks and benefits of oxytocin-induced labor.
◀€ Teach patient to recognize and immediately report adverse drug effects.

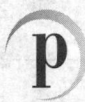

paclitaxel
Apo-Paclitaxel✤, Paxene⊕

Pharmacologic class: Antimicrotubule agent
Therapeutic class: Antineoplastic
Pregnancy risk category D

FDA | BOXED WARNING

• Give injection under supervision of physician experienced in use of cancer chemotherapy, in facility with adequate diagnostic and treatment resources.
• Anaphylaxis and severe hypersensitivity reactions may occur despite premedication. All patients should be pretreated with corticosteroids, diphenhydramine, and histamine$_2$ antagonists. Don't give drug to patients who've had previous severe reactions.
• Don't administer drug to patients with solid tumors whose baseline neutrophil counts are below 1,500 cells/mm³ or to patients with AIDS-related Kaposi's sarcoma whose

---

baseline neutrophil counts are below 1,000 cells/mm^3. To monitor for bone marrow suppression, obtain frequent peripheral blood cell counts on all patients.

• Albumin form of drug may substantially affect drug's functional properties. Don't substitute for or use with other paclitaxel forms.

Action
Stabilizes cellular microtubules to prevent depolymerization. This action inhibits microtubule network (essential for vital interphase and mitotic cellular functions) and induces abnormal microtubule arrays or bundles throughout cell cycle and during mitosis.

Availability
Concentrate for injection: 30 mg/5-ml vial, 100 mg/16.7-ml vial, 300 mg/50-ml vial

❶ Indications and dosages
➤ Advanced ovarian cancer
Adults: As first-line therapy, 175 mg/m^2 I.V. over 3 hours q 3 weeks, or 135 mg/m^2 I.V. over 24 hours q 3 weeks, followed by cisplatin. After failure of first-line therapy, 135 mg/m^2 I.V. or 175 mg/m^2 I.V. over 3 hours q 3 weeks.
➤ Breast cancer after failure of combination chemotherapy
Adults: As adjuvant treatment for node-positive breast cancer, 175 mg/m^2 I.V. over 3 hours q 3 weeks for four courses given sequentially with doxorubicin combination chemotherapy. After chemotherapy failure for metastatic disease or relapse within 6 months of adjuvant therapy, 175 mg/m^2 I.V. over 3 hours q 3 weeks.
➤ Non-small-cell lung cancer
Adults: 135 mg/m^2 I.V. over 24 hours q 3 weeks, followed by cisplatin
➤ AIDS-related Kaposi's sarcoma
Adults: 135 mg/m^2 I.V. over 3 hours q 3 weeks, or 100 mg/m^2 I.V. over 3 hours q 2 weeks

Dosage adjustment
• Advanced human immunodeficiency virus infection (when used for Kaposi's sarcoma)

Off-label uses
• Advanced head and neck cancer
• Small-cell lung cancer
• Upper GI tract adenocarcinoma
• Non-Hodgkin's lymphoma
• Pancreatic cancer
• Polycystic kidney disease

Contraindications
• Hypersensitivity to drug or castor oil
• Solid tumors when baseline neutrophil count is below 1,500 cells/mm^3
• AIDS-related Kaposi's sarcoma when baseline neutrophil count is below 1,000 cells/mm^3

Precautions
Use cautiously in:
• severe hepatic impairment, active infection, decreased bone marrow reserve, chronic debilitating illness
• patients with childbearing potential
• breastfeeding patients (not recommended)
• children (safety not established).

Administration
◀€ Follow facility protocol for handling chemotherapeutic drugs and preparing solutions.
• Dilute in dextrose 5% in water, normal saline solution, or dextrose 5% in lactated Ringer's solution per manufacturer's guidelines.
• Inspect solution for particles. Administer through polyethylene-lined administration set attached to 0.22-micron in-line filter.
• To prevent severe hypersensitivity reaction, premedicate with dexamethasone 20 mg 12 and 6 hours before infusion, as prescribed. Also give diphenhydramine 50 mg I.V., plus either cimetidine 300 mg or ranitidine 50 mg I.V. 30 to 60 minutes before paclitaxel.

◀€ Keep epinephrine available. If severe hypersensitivity reaction occurs, stop infusion immediately and give epinephrine, I.V. fluids, and additional antihistamine and corticosteroid doses, as indicated and prescribed.

Route	Onset	Peak	Duration
I.V.	Unknown	Unknown	Unknown

Adverse reactions

CNS: peripheral neuropathy
CV: hypotension, hypertension, syncope, abnormal ECG, bradycardia, **venous thrombosis**
GI: nausea, vomiting, diarrhea, stomatitis, mucositis
Hematologic: anemia, **leukopenia, neutropenia, bleeding, thrombocytopenia**
Musculoskeletal: joint pain, myalgia
Skin: alopecia, radiation reactions
Other: infection, injection site reaction, hypersensitivity reactions including **anaphylaxis**

Interactions

Drug-drug. *Carbamazepine, phenobarbital:* decreased paclitaxel blood level and efficacy
Cisplatin: increased bone marrow depression (when paclitaxel dose follows cisplatin dose)
Cyclosporine, diazepam, doxorubicin, felodipine, ketoconazole, midazolam: inhibited paclitaxel metabolism and greater risk of toxicity
Doxorubicin: increased doxorubicin blood level and toxicity
Live-virus vaccines: decreased antibody response to vaccine, increased risk of adverse reactions
Other antineoplastics: increased risk of bone marrow depression
Drug-diagnostic tests. *Liver function tests:* abnormal results
Triglycerides: increased levels

Patient monitoring

◀€ Watch closely for hypersensitivity reaction.

• Monitor heart rate and blood pressure.
• Assess infusion site for local effects and extravasation, especially during prolonged infusion.
◀€ Monitor CBC, including platelet count. If neutropenia develops, monitor patient for infection; if thrombocytopenia develops, watch for signs and symptoms of bleeding.
• If patient has preexisting cardiac conduction abnormality, maintain continuous cardiac monitoring.

Patient teaching

• Instruct neutropenic patient to minimize infection risk by avoiding crowds, plants, and fresh fruits and vegetables.
• Tell thrombocytopenic patient to avoid activities that can cause injury. Advise him to use soft toothbrush and electric razor.
◀€ Advise patient to promptly report signs and symptoms of infection, bleeding, or peripheral neuropathy (such as numbness and tingling of feet and hands).
• Tell patient to promptly report pain or burning at injection site.
• Explain that temporary hair loss may occur.
• As appropriate, review all other significant and life-threatening adverse reactions and interactions, especially those related to the drugs and tests mentioned above.

palifermin
Kepivance

Pharmacologic class: Keratinocyte growth factor (KGF) (rDNA origin)
Therapeutic class: Biologic and immunologic agent
Pregnancy risk category C

Action

Produced by recombinant DNA technology in *Escherichia coli;* binds to KGF receptor on cell surface, resulting in epithelial cell proliferation, differentiation, and migration

Availability

Powder for injection (lyophilized): 6.25 mg in single-use vials

🚫 Indications and dosages

➤ To decrease incidence and duration of severe oral mucositis in patients with hematologic malignancies who are receiving myelotoxic therapy requiring hematopoietic stem cell support
Adults: 60 mcg/kg/day I.V. bolus injection for 3 consecutive days before and 3 consecutive days after myelotoxic therapy, for a total of six doses. Give first three doses before myelotoxic therapy, with third dose given 24 to 48 hours before such therapy. Administer last three doses after myelotoxic therapy, with first of these given after (but on same day of) hematopoietic stem cell infusion and at least 4 days after most recent palifermin dose.

Contraindications

• Hypersensitivity to drug, its components, or *E. coli*–derived proteins

Precautions

Use cautiously in:
• patients with nonhematologic cancers
• use with melphalan 200 mg/m² as a conditioning regimen (not recommended)
• elderly patients
• pregnant or breastfeeding patients
• children (safety and efficacy not established).

Administration

• Reconstitute powder with 1.2 ml sterile water for injection to yield final concentration of 5 mg/ml.

🔊 Swirl vial gently during dissolution; don't shake or vigorously agitate.
• Don't filter reconstituted solution during preparation or administration.
• Use immediately (within 1 hour) after reconstituting; protect from light.
• When heparin is used to maintain I.V. line, use normal saline solution to rinse line before and after palifermin administration.
• Administer by I.V. bolus injection.
• Don't give within 24 hours before, during infusion of, or within 24 hours after myelotoxic chemotherapy.

Route	Onset	Peak	Duration
I.V.	Unknown	Unknown	Unknown

Adverse reactions

CNS: dysesthesia
CV: hypertension
EENT: tongue discoloration or thickening
Musculoskeletal: pain, arthralgias
Skin: rash, pruritus, skin toxicities, erythema
Other: altered taste, edema, fever

Interactions

Drug-drug. *Heparin:* possible binding
Drug-diagnostic tests. *Amylase, lipase:* increased

Patient monitoring

• Monitor serum amylase and lipase levels frequently.

Patient teaching

• Instruct patient to report adverse reactions, including rash, itching, skin redness, swelling, discolored tongue, and altered taste.
• As appropriate, review all other significant adverse reactions and interactions, especially those related to the drugs and tests mentioned above.

Reactions in **bold** are life-threatening.   🔊 Clinical alert

paliperidone
Invega

paliperidone palmitate
Invega Sustenna

Pharmacologic class: Benzisoxazole derivative
Therapeutic class: Antipsychotic
Pregnancy risk category C

FDA | BOXED WARNING

• Elderly patients with dementia-related psychosis are at increased risk for death. Over course of 10-week controlled trial, death rate in drug-treated patients was about 4.5%, compared to about 2.6% in placebo group. Although causes of death varied, most appeared to be cardiovascular or infectious. Don't give drug to patients with dementia-related psychosis.

Action
Unknown. In schizophrenia, therapeutic activity may be mediated through combination of central serotonin$_2$- and dopamine$_2$-receptor antagonism. Drug is a major active metabolite of risperidone.

Availability
Injection (paliperidone palmitate):
39 mg, 78 mg, 117 mg, 156 mg, 234 mg in prefilled syringes
Tablets (extended-release): 1.5 mg, 3 mg, 6 mg, 9 mg

Indications and dosages
➤ Schizophrenia
Adults: 6 mg P.O. once daily. Some patients may benefit from daily dosages as high as 12 mg or as low as 3 mg. If indicated, increase in increments of 3 mg/day at intervals of more than 5 days. Or initially, 234 mg I.M. (paliperidone palmitate) on treatment day 1 and 156 mg I.M. 1 week later. Recommended monthly maintenance dose is 117 mg; some patients may benefit from lower or higher maintenance doses within recommended range of 39 to 234 mg. Adjustment of maintenance dosage may be made monthly. When making dosage adjustments, consider paliperidone palmitate's prolonged-release characteristics, as the full effect of the dosage adjustment may not be evident for several months.
Adolescents ages 12 to 17 weighing 51 kg (112 lb) or more: 3 mg P.O. daily; increase dosage, if necessary, only after clinical reassessment at increments of 3 mg/day at intervals of more than 5 days up to a maximum of 12 mg/day.
Adolescents ages 12 to 17 weighing less than 51 kg (112 lb): 3 mg P.O. daily; increase dosage, if necessary, only after clinical reassessment at increments of 3 mg/day at intervals of more than 5 days up to a maximum of 6 mg/day.
➤ Schizoaffective disorder
Adults: 6 mg P.O. once daily. Some patients may benefit from dosages as high as 12 mg or as low as 3 mg. Maximum recommended dosage is 12 mg/day.

Dosage adjustment
• Renal impairment

Contraindications
• Hypersensitivity to drug, its components, or risperidone

Precautions
Use cautiously in:
• GI strictures (use should be avoided), cardiovascular or cerebrovascular disease, diabetes mellitus, Parkinson's disease, or conditions that raise body temperature (such as exercise,

exposure to extreme heat, and concomitant anticholinergics use)

• increased risk of hypotension (as from dehydration, hypovolemia, or antihypertensives), aspiration pneumonia, or suicide attempt

• increased risk of metabolic changes (including hyperglycemia, dyslipidemia, weight gain)

• concurrent use of other drugs that are centrally acting or prolong the QT interval (use should be avoided)

• history of seizures or breast cancer

• elderly patients with dementia-related psychosis

• pregnant or breastfeeding patients

• children younger than age 18 (safety and efficacy not established).

Administration

• Give tablets in morning with or without food.

• Administer tablets whole. Ensure that patient doesn't chew, divide, or crush them.

◄€ Administer paliperidone palmitate by deep I.M. injection only as a single injection. Don't give in divided injections. Don't administer I.V. or subcutaneously.

◄€ For first and second I.M. doses, give in the deltoid muscle using $1^1/_2$-inch 22G needle for patients 90 kg (198 lb) or more or 1-inch 23G needle for patients less than 90 kg. After the second dose, monthly maintenance doses may be given in either the deltoid or gluteal muscle. For gluteal injection, use $1^1/_2$-inch 22G needle regardless of patient weight.

Route	Onset	Peak	Duration
P.O.	Unknown	24 hr	Unknown
I.M.	1 day	13 days	126 days

Adverse reactions

CNS: dizziness, headache, akathisia, tardive dyskinesia, dystonia, extrapyramidal disorder, hypertonia, parkinsonism, sedation, somnolence, tremor, anxiety, asthenia, fatigue, **seizure, stroke (in elderly patients with dementia-related psychosis), neuroleptic malignant syndrome (NMS)**

CV: first-degree atrioventricular block, bundle-branch block, sinus arrhythmia, tachycardia, hypertension, orthostatic hypotension, prolonged QT interval, abnormal T wave, palpitations

EENT: blurred vision

GI: upper abdominal pain, dyspepsia, nausea, antiemetic effect, esophageal dysmotility, salivary hypersecretion, dry mouth

GU: hyperprolactinemia

Hematologic: leukopenia, neutropenia, agranulocytosis

Musculoskeletal: back pain, extremity pain

Respiratory: cough, dyspnea, aspiration pneumonia

Other: fever, weight gain, possible drug tolerance or dependency

Interactions

Drug-drug. *Antihypertensives:* increased risk of hypotension

Centrally acting drugs with sedative effect: increased sedation

Class IA antiarrhythmics (such as procainamide, quinidine), Class III antiarrhythmics (such as amiodarone, sotalol), anti-infectives (such as gatifloxacin, moxifloxacin), other antipsychotics (such as chlorpromazine, thioridazine), other drugs that prolong the QT interval: increased risk of prolonged QT interval

Dopamine agonists (such as levodopa): antagonized effects of these drugs

Drug-diagnostic tests. *Blood glucose, serum prolactin:* increased levels

Granulocytes, leukocytes, neutrophils: decreased counts

Drug-food. *Any food:* possibly increased paliperidone effects

Drug-behaviors. *Alcohol use:* increased sedation

P

Reactions in **bold** are life-threatening.   ◄€ Clinical alert

Patient monitoring

• Closely monitor patient at risk for suicide attempts.

• Monitor patient with diabetes regularly for signs and symptoms of worsening glycemic control.

• Stay alert for orthostatic hypotension.

◀€ Monitor patient for signs and symptoms of NMS (extremely high fever, muscle rigidity, altered mental status, irregular pulse or blood pressure, tachycardia, diaphoresis, arrhythmias). Immediately discontinue drug and take appropriate measures if NMS occurs.

◀€ Closely monitor CBC with differential, especially during first few months of therapy; discontinue drug if severe neutropenia occurs.

• Consider discontinuing drug if tardive dyskinesia occurs.

• Watch for signs and symptoms of drug tolerance, dependency, and abuse.

Patient teaching

• Inform patient he may take drug with or without food.

• Teach patient to take tablets whole and not to chew, divide, or crush them.

• Inform patient that tablet shell doesn't dissolve and may look like a complete tablet in stool.

◀€ Instruct patient to immediately discontinue drug and report signs or symptoms of NMS (such as high fever, muscle rigidity, altered mental status, irregular pulse or blood pressure, fast heart rate, or excessive sweating).

• Instruct patient to report fever or other signs and symptoms of infection.

• Tell patient drug may cause temporary blood pressure decrease if he stands or sits up suddenly. Instruct him to rise slowly and carefully.

• Advise patient to take precautions against dehydration and overheating.

• Caution patient not to consume alcohol during therapy.

• Caution patient to avoid hazardous activities until drug's effects on concentration, coordination, vision, and alertness are known.

• As appropriate, review all other significant and life-threatening adverse reactions and interactions, especially those related to the drugs, tests, foods, and behaviors mentioned above.

palivizumab
Synagis

Pharmacologic class: Monoclonal antibody
Therapeutic class: Immunologic agent
Pregnancy risk category C

Action

Neutralizes and suppresses activity of syncytial virus in respiratory tract, inhibiting respiratory syncytial virus (RSV) replication

Availability

Injection: 50 mg, 100-mg vial

⬥ Indications and dosages

➤ To prevent serious lower respiratory disease caused by RSV in high-risk children

Children: 15 mg/kg I.M. q month throughout RSV season

Contraindications

• Hypersensitivity to drug or its components

Precautions

Use cautiously in:

• thrombocytopenia, coagulation disorders, established RSV infection.

Administration

◀€ Keep epinephrine 1:1,000 available in case anaphylaxis occurs. (However, drug isn't known to cause anaphylaxis.)

• Dilute in sterile water for injection. Gently swirl for 30 seconds to avoid foaming.
• Keep reconstituted solution at room temperature for at least 20 minutes before administering. Give within 6 hours of reconstitution.
• Inject I.M. into anterolateral thigh. Avoid gluteal injection, which may damage sciatic nerve.

Route	Onset	Peak	Duration
I.M.	Unknown	Unknown	Unknown

Adverse reactions
CNS: nervousness, pain
EENT: conjunctivitis, otitis media, rhinitis, pharyngitis, sinusitis
GI: vomiting, diarrhea, gastroenteritis, oral moniliasis
Hematologic: anemia
Respiratory: upper respiratory tract infection, cough, wheezing, dyspnea, bronchiolitis, bronchitis, pneumonia, croup, **asthma, apnea**
Skin: rash, fungal dermatitis, eczema
Other: hernia, pain, fever, injection site reaction, viral infection, flulike symptoms, failure to thrive

Interactions
Drug-diagnostic tests. *Alanine aminotransferase, aspartate aminotransferase:* increased levels
Hemoglobin: decreased level
Immunological-based RSV diagnostic tests: interference, possibly leading to false-negative test results

Patient monitoring
◀≲ Watch closely for signs and symptoms of anaphylaxis immediately after dosing.
• Assess for signs and symptoms of infection, particularly EENT and respiratory infection.
• Monitor liver function tests and CBC.
• Assess patient's weight and hydration status.

Patient teaching
• Tell parent that monthly injections are necessary during RSV season (November through April).
• Inform parent that drug may cause GI symptoms and failure to thrive. Provide dietary consultation as needed.
◀≲ Caution parent that EENT and respiratory infections may follow administration. Advise parent to contact prescriber immediately if child has fever or other signs or symptoms of infection.
• As appropriate, review all other significant and life-threatening adverse reactions and interactions, especially those related to the tests mentioned above.

palonosetron hydrochloride
Aloxi

Pharmacologic class: Selective serotonin subtype 3 (5-HT$_3$) receptor antagonist
Therapeutic class: Antiemetic
Pregnancy risk category B

p

Action
Selectively binds to and antagonizes 5-HT$_3$ receptors on vagal nerve terminals and in chemoreceptor trigger zone. This action blocks serotonin release, reducing the vomiting reflex.

Availability
Solution for injection: 0.25 mg (free base) in 5-ml single-use vial

⓲ Indications and dosages
➤ To prevent nausea and vomiting caused by cancer chemotherapy
Adults: 0.25 mg I.V. as a single dose 30 minutes before chemotherapy.

Repeated doses within 7 days aren't recommended.

➤ To prevent postoperative nausea and vomiting
Adults: 0.075 mg I.V. as a single dose given over 10 seconds immediately before anesthesia induction

Contraindications
• Hypersensitivity to drug or its components

Precautions
Use cautiously in:
• hypersensitivity to other 5-HT$_3$ receptor antagonists
• diabetes mellitus, hepatic dysfunction
• pregnant or breastfeeding patients
• children.

Administration
• Flush I.V. line with normal saline solution before and after giving.
• Deliver into I.V. line over 30 seconds. Don't mix with other drugs.

Route	Onset	Peak	Duration
I.V.	Unknown	Unknown	Unknown

Adverse reactions
CNS: headache, fatigue, insomnia, dizziness, anxiety
CV: hypotension, vein discoloration and distention, nonsustained tachycardia, bradycardia
GI: constipation, diarrhea, abdominal pain, anorexia
GU: glycosuria
Metabolic: fluctuating electrolyte levels, hyperglycemia, **metabolic acidosis, hyperkalemia**
Musculoskeletal: joint pain
Other: fever, flulike symptoms

Interactions
Drug-diagnostic tests: *Alanine aminotransferase, aspartate aminotransferase, bilirubin, blood and urine glucose, potassium:* increased levels

Patient monitoring
• Monitor vital signs and ECG. Watch closely for tachycardia, bradycardia, and hypotension.
• Watch electrolyte levels for fluctuations (especially hyperkalemia and metabolic acidosis).
• Evaluate temperature. Stay alert for flulike symptoms.
• Closely monitor blood and urine glucose levels in diabetic patients. Stay alert for hyperglycemia.

Patient teaching
• Explain that drug helps prevent nausea and vomiting caused by chemotherapy.
• Teach patient to recognize and report signs and symptoms of hyperkalemia and metabolic acidosis.
• Advise patient to report flulike symptoms.
• Instruct diabetic patient to closely watch blood and urine glucose levels.
• As appropriate, review all other significant and life-threatening adverse reactions and interactions, especially those related to the tests mentioned above.

pamidronate disodium
Aredia

Pharmacologic class: Bisphosphonate, hypocalcemic

Therapeutic class: Bone resorption inhibitor

Pregnancy risk category C

Action
Inhibits normal and abnormal bone resorption and decreases calcium levels

---

Availability
Injection: 30 mg/vial, 90 mg/vial

Route	Onset	Peak	Duration
I.V.	Unknown	Unknown	Unknown

💊 Indications and dosages
➤ Hypercalcemia caused by cancer
Adults: For moderate hypercalcemia, 60 to 90 mg as a single-dose I.V. infusion over 2 to 24 hours. For severe hypercalcemia, 90 mg as a single-dose I.V. infusion over 2 to 24 hours.
➤ Osteolytic lesions caused by multiple myeloma
Adults: 90 mg I.V. as a 4-hour infusion q month
➤ Osteolytic bone metastases of breast cancer
Adults: 90 mg I.V. as a 2-hour infusion q 3 to 4 weeks
➤ Paget's disease
Adults: 30 mg I.V. daily as a 4-hour infusion for 3 days

Contraindications
• Hypersensitivity to drug, its components, or other bisphosphonates

Precautions
Use cautiously in:
• renal impairment
• pregnant or breastfeeding patients
• children (safety not established).

Administration
• Hydrate patient with saline solution as needed before starting therapy.
• Because of risk of renal failure, give no more than 90 mg in single doses.
◀≋ Reconstitute vial using 10 ml of sterile water for injection. When completely dissolved, dilute in 250 to 1,000 ml of half-normal or normal saline solution or dextrose 5% in water.
◀≋ Don't mix with solutions containing calcium, such as lactated Ringer's solution.
• Administer in I.V. line separate from all other drugs and fluids.

Adverse reactions
CNS: anxiety, headache, insomnia, psychosis, drowsiness, weakness
CV: hypertension, syncope, tachycardia, **atrial flutter, arrhythmias, heart failure**
EENT: sinusitis
GI: nausea, vomiting, diarrhea, abdominal pain, constipation, dyspepsia, stomatitis, anorexia, **GI hemorrhage**
GU: urinary tract infection
Hematologic: anemia, **neutropenia, leukopenia, granulocytopenia, thrombocytopenia**
Metabolic: hypothyroidism
Musculoskeletal: bone pain, joint pain, myalgia
Respiratory: crackles, coughing, dyspnea, upper respiratory infection, **pleural effusion**
Other: fever, generalized pain, injection site reaction

Interactions
Drug-diagnostic tests. *Creatinine:* increased level
Electrolytes, hemoglobin, magnesium, phosphorus, platelets, potassium, red blood cells, white blood cells: decreased levels

Patient monitoring
• Monitor hydration status carefully.
• Monitor vital signs and ECG. Evaluate cardiovascular and respiratory status closely.
• Assess hematologic studies and creatinine level before each treatment course.
• Assess electrolyte levels, especially calcium, magnesium, and phosphorus.
• Closely monitor fluid intake and output. Watch for signs and symptoms of urinary tract infection.

p

Reactions in **bold** are life-threatening.   ◀≋ Clinical alert

Patient teaching

- Instruct patient to weigh himself regularly and report sudden gains.
- 🔊 Advise patient to promptly report significant respiratory problems, peripheral edema, or GI bleeding.
- 🔊 Inform patient that drug lowers resistance to some infections. Tell him to immediately report fever and other signs and symptoms of infection.
- Explain importance of undergoing laboratory tests before, during, and after therapy.
- Caution patient to avoid driving and other hazardous activities until he knows how drug affects concentration, cognition, and alertness.
- Tell patient to minimize GI upset by eating small, frequent servings of food and drinking plenty of fluids.
- As appropriate, review all other significant and life-threatening adverse reactions and interactions, especially those related to the tests mentioned above.

pancrelipase

Creon, Pancreaze, Ultresa, Viokace, Zenpep

Pharmacologic class: Pancreatic enzyme
Therapeutic class: Digestant
Pregnancy risk category C

Action

Catalyzes hydrolysis of fats to monoglyceride, glycerol, and free fatty acids; proteins into peptides and amino acids; and starches into dextrins and short chain sugars, such as maltose and maltriose, in the duodenum and proximal small intestine, thereby acting like digestive enzymes physiologically secreted by the pancreas

Availability

Creon
Capsules (delayed-release): 3,000 USP units lipase, 9,500 USP units protease, 15,000 USP units amylase; 6,000 USP units lipase, 19,000 USP units protease, 30,000 USP units amylase; 12,000 USP units lipase, 38,000 USP units protease, 60,000 USP units amylase; 24,000 USP units lipase, 76,000 USP units protease, 120,000 USP units amylase

Pancreaze
Capsules (delayed-release): 4,200 USP units lipase, 10,000 USP units protease, 17,500 USP units amylase; 10,500 USP units lipase, 25,000 USP units protease, 43,750 USP units amylase; 16,800 USP units lipase, 40,000 USP units protease, 70,000 USP units amylase; 21,000 USP units lipase, 37,000 USP units protease, 61,000 USP units amylase

Ultresa
Capsules (delayed-release): 13,800 USP units lipase, 27,600 USP units protease, 27,600 USP units amylase; 20,700 USP units lipase, 41,400 USP units protease, 41,400 USP units amylase; 23,000 USP units lipase, 46,000 USP units protease, 46,000 USP units amylase

Viokace
Tablets: 10,440 USP units of lipase, 39,150 USP units of protease, 39,150 USP units of amylase; 20,880 USP units of lipase, 78,300 USP units of protease, 78,300 USP units of amylase

Zenpep
Capsules (delayed-release): 3,000 USP units lipase, 10,000 USP units protease, 16,000 USP units amylase; 5,000 USP units lipase, 17,000 USP units protease, 27,000 USP units amylase; 10,000 USP units lipase, 34,000 USP units protease, 55,000 USP units amylase; 15,000 USP units lipase, 51,000 USP units protease, 82,000 USP units amylase; 20,000 USP units lipase, 68,000 USP units protease, 109,000 USP units amylase; 25,000

USP units lipase, 85,000 USP units protease, 136,000 USP units amylase

🍴 Indications and dosages

➤ Exocrine pancreatic insufficiency due to chronic pancreatitis or pancreatectomy

Adults: Individualize dosage based on clinical symptoms, degree of steatorrhea, and fat content of diet (Viokace)

➤ Exocrine pancreatic insufficiency due to cystic fibrosis (CF), chronic pancreatitis, pancreatectomy, and other conditions

Adults and children age 4 and older: Initially, 500 lipase units/kg/meal to a maximum of 2,500 lipase units/kg/meal (or 10,000 lipase units/kg/day or less), or less than 4,000 lipase units/g fat ingested per day (Creon)

Children older than age 12 months and younger than age 4: Initially, 1,000 lipase units/kg/meal to a maximum of 2,500 lipase units/kg/meal (or 10,000 lipase units/kg/day or less), or less than 4,000 lipase units/g fat ingested per day (Creon)

Infants up to age 12 months: 3,000 lipase units/120 ml formula or per breastfeeding (Creon)

Don't exceed recommended maximum dosage set forth by the Cystic Fibrosis Foundation Consensus Conferences Guidelines.

➤ Exocrine pancreatic insufficiency due to CF and other conditions

Adults and children age 4 and older: Initially, 500 lipase units/kg/meal to a maximum of 2,500 lipase units/kg/meal (or 10,000 lipase units/kg/day or less), or less than 4,000 lipase units/g fat ingested per day (Pancreaze, Zenpep)

Adults and children age 4 and older weighing 28 kg (62 lb) or more: Initially, 500 lipase units/kg/meal to a maximum of 2,500 lipase units/kg/meal (or 10,000 lipase units/kg/day or less), or less than 4,000

lipase units/g fat ingested per day (Ultresa)

Children older than age 12 months and younger than age 4: Initially, 1,000 lipase units/kg/meal to a maximum of 2,500 lipase units/kg/meal (or 10,000 lipase units/kg/day or less), or less than 4,000 lipase units/g fat ingested per day (Pancreaze, Zenpep)

Children older than age 12 months and younger than age 4 weighing 14 kg (31 lb) or more: Initially, 1,000 lipase units/kg/meal to a maximum of 2,500 lipase units/kg/meal (or 10,000 lipase units/kg/day or less), or less than 4,000 lipase units/g fat ingested per day (Ultresa)

Infants up to age 12 months: 2,000 to 4,000 lipase units/120 ml formula or per breastfeeding (Pancreaze); 3,000 lipase units/120 ml formula or per breastfeeding (Zenpep)

Don't exceed recommended maximum dosage set forth by the Cystic Fibrosis Foundation Consensus Conferences Guidelines.

Contraindications
None

Precautions
Use cautiously in:
• proteins of porcine origin allergy
• renal impairment, gout, hyperuricemia
• fibrosing colonopathy (with high doses)
• lactose intolerance
• pregnant or breastfeeding patients
• children younger than age 12 (with high doses).

Administration
• Be aware that brands aren't interchangeable.
• Administer capsules whole with meals.
• Give to infants before each feeding but don't mix capsule contents directly into formula or breast milk.

• For infants or patients unable to swallow intact capsules, sprinkle contents on acidic soft food, such as applesauce, yogurt, or other acidic soft food with pH of 4.5 or less.

• Don't mix capsule contents with alkaline foods, such as milk, breast milk, formula, or ice cream.

• Be aware that attempting to divide capsule contents into small fractions to deliver small doses of lipase isn't recommended.

• Be aware that high-dose use (exceeding 6,000 lipase units/kg/meal) of pancreatic enzyme replacement therapy has been associated with fibrosing colonopathy and colonic strictures in children younger than age 12.

Route	Onset	Peak	Duration
P.O.	Unknown	Unknown	Unknown

Adverse reactions

CNS: dizziness, headache
EENT: nasopharyngitis
GI: nausea, vomiting, diarrhea, constipation, abdominal pain, abnormal feces, flatulence, frequent bowel movements, anal pruritus, **fibrosing colonopathy**
Hepatic: biliary tract stones
Metabolic: hyperglycemia, hypoglycemia, hyperuricemia
Respiratory: cough
Skin: pruritus, urticaria, rash
Other: viral transmission (theoretical risk), **severe allergic reactions**

Interactions

None

Patient monitoring

• Monitor patient for hyperglycemia, hypoglycemia, and hyperuricemia.

◀╎ Closely monitor patient for signs or symptoms of fibrosing colonopathy (such as abdominal pain or distention, vomiting, intermittent diarrhea, and weight loss) that may be associated with high-dose use.

Patient teaching

• Tell patient or caregiver that capsules must be swallowed whole and shouldn't be crushed or chewed.

• Advise patient or caregiver to take drug with food with a full glass of water.

• Tell patient or caregiver not to hold drug in mouth, to avoid mucosal irritation.

• Tell patient or caregiver that for infants or patients who are unable to swallow intact capsules, contents can be sprinkled on soft acidic food, such as applesauce, yogurt, or other soft acidic food.

• Tell patient or caregiver not to mix capsule contents with alkaline foods, such as milk, breast milk, formula, or ice cream.

• Inform patient or caregiver that brands aren't interchangeable.

◀╎ Tell patient or caregiver to inform prescriber of pork allergy and to immediately seek medical attention if allergic reaction occurs.

◀╎ Tell patient or caregiver to immediately report signs or symptoms of fibrosing colonopathy (such as abdominal pain or distention, vomiting, intermittent diarrhea, or difficulty passing stool).

• Instruct patient or caregiver to report signs or symptoms of high blood sugar (such as extreme thirst), low blood sugar (such as confusion, shakiness, sweating, or hunger), or high uric acid (pain or swelling around joints).

• Advise breastfeeding patient to consider risk and benefit of drug in providing adequate nutritional support for exocrine pancreatic insufficiency.

• Advise female of childbearing age to notify prescriber if she is pregnant, thinking of becoming pregnant, or is breastfeeding during therapy.

• As appropriate, review all other significant and life-threatening adverse reactions.

♣ Canada   ⊕ UK   ⚕ Hazardous drug   ⊗ High-alert drug

pantoprazole sodium
Apo-Pantoprazole✴, Co
Pantoprazole✴, Gen-Pantoprazole✴,
Novo-Pantoprazole✴, Pantoloc✴,
PMS-Pantoprazole✴, Protium⊕,
Protonix, Protonix IV, Ran-
Pantoprazole✴, Ratio-Pantoprazole✴,
Sandoz Pantoprazole✴

Pharmacologic class: Proton pump
inhibitor
Therapeutic class: GI agent
Pregnancy risk category B

Action
Reduces gastric acid secretion and
increases gastric mucus and bicarbonate production, creating protective
coating on gastric mucosa

Availability
*Granules (delayed-release oral suspen-
sion):* 40 mg
Powder for injection (freeze-dried):
40 mg/vial
Tablets (delayed-release): 20 mg, 40 mg

🖊 Indications and dosages
➤ Erosive esophagitis caused by gas-
troesophageal reflux disease (GERD)
Adults: 40 mg I.V. daily for 7 to 10
days or 40 mg P.O. daily for 8 weeks.
May repeat P.O. course for 8 addi-
tional weeks.
**Children ages 5 and older weighing
40 kg (88 lb) or more:** 40 mg P.O. daily
for up to 8 weeks
**Children ages 5 and older weighing
15 kg (33 lb) to less than 40 kg (88 lb):**
20 mg P.O. daily for up to 8 weeks
➤ Erosive esophagitis
Adults: 40 mg P.O. daily
➤ Pathologic hypersecretory conditions
Adults: Initially, 40 mg P.O. b.i.d.,
increased as needed to maximum of

240 mg P.O. daily; some patients may
need up to 2 years of therapy. Alternatively, 80 mg I.V. q 12 hours, to a
maximum of 240 mg/day (80 mg q
8 hours).

Contraindications
• Hypersensitivity to drug or any
substituted benzimidazole

Precautions
Use cautiously in:
• severe hepatic disease
• atrophic gastritis with long-term use
• increased risk of osteoporosis-related
hip, wrist, or spine fractures with long-
term use or multiple daily doses
• concurrent use of atazanavir, nelfinavir, or methotrexate
• pregnant or breastfeeding patients
• children.

Administration
• Be aware that oral granules may be
mixed with applesauce or apple juice
and given 30 minutes before a meal.
Once mixed, give drug within 10 minutes.
• Know that oral granules may be
mixed with 10 ml apple juice and
administered into nasogastric tube
using 60-ml catheter-tip syringe. Rinse
syringe with additional apple juice
so that no granules remain in
syringe.
• For I.V. administration, use in-line
filter provided. If Y-site is used, place
filter below Y-site closest to patient.
• Dilute I.V. form with 10 ml of normal saline solution; further dilute in
dextrose 5% in water, normal saline
solution, or lactated Ringer's solution,
as directed. Give over 15 minutes at a
rate no faster than 3 mg/minute.
• Don't give I.V. form with other I.V.
solutions.
• Know that I.V. form is indicated for
short-term treatment of GERD in
patients with history of erosive

P

esophagitis as alternative to P.O. therapy.

- Be aware that symptomatic response doesn't rule out gastric cancer.

Route	Onset	Peak	Duration
P.O.	Rapid	2.5 hr	>24 hr
I.V.	Rapid	Unknown	>24 hr

Adverse reactions

CNS: dizziness, headache
CV: chest pain
EENT: rhinitis
GI: vomiting, diarrhea, abdominal pain, dyspepsia
Metabolic: hyperglycemia
Musculoskeletal: hip, wrist, spine fractures (with long-term daily use)
Skin: rash, pruritus
Other: injection site reaction

Interactions

Drug-drug. *Ampicillin, cyanocobalamin, digoxin, iron salts, ketoconazole:* delayed absorption of these drugs
Atazanavir, nelfinavir: substantially decreased atazanavir or nelfinavir plasma concentration with loss of therapeutic effect and development of drug resistance
Clarithromycin, diazepam, flurazepam, phenytoin, triazolam: increased pantoprazole blood level
Sucralfate: delayed pantoprazole absorption
Warfarin: increased bleeding
Drug-diagnostic tests. *Aspartate aminotransferase, glucose:* increased levels
Tetrahydrocannabinol test: false-positive result

Patient monitoring

- Assess for symptomatic improvement.
- Monitor blood glucose level in diabetic patient.

Patient teaching

- Tell patient to swallow delayed-release tablets whole without crushing, chewing, or splitting.

- Tell patient he may take tablets with or without food.
- Explain that antacids don't affect drug absorption.
- Instruct diabetic patients to monitor blood glucose level carefully and stay alert for signs and symptoms of hyperglycemia.
- As appropriate, review all other significant adverse reactions and interactions, especially those related to the drugs and tests mentioned above.

paroxetine hydrochloride

Apo-Paroxetine❈, Co Paroxetine❈, Dom-Paroxetine❈, Gen-Paroxetine❈, Novo-Paroxetine❈, Paxil, Paxil CR, PHL-Paroxetine❈, PMS-Paroxetine❈, Riva-Paroxetine❈, Sandoz Paroxetine❈, Seroxat⊕

paroxetine mesylate

Pexeva

Pharmacologic class: Selective serotonin reuptake inhibitor (SSRI)
Therapeutic class: Antidepressant, anxiolytic
Pregnancy risk category C

FDA | BOXED WARNING

- Drug may increase risk of suicidal thinking and behavior in children and adolescents with major depressive disorder and other psychiatric disorders. Risk must be balanced with clinical need, as depression itself increases suicide risk. With patient of any age, observe closely for clinical worsening, suicidality, and unusual behavior changes when therapy begins. Advise family and caregivers to observe patient closely and communicate with prescriber as needed.

- Drug isn't approved for use in pediatric patients.

Action
Unknown. Thought to inhibit neuronal reuptake of serotonin in CNS.

Availability
paroxetine hydrochloride—
Oral suspension: 10 mg/5 ml in 250-ml bottle
Tablets: 10 mg, 20 mg, 30 mg, 40 mg
Tablets (controlled-release): 12.5 mg, 25 mg, 37.5 mg
paroxetine mesylate—
Tablets: 10 mg, 20 mg, 30 mg, 40 mg

ⓘ Indications and dosages
➤ Major depressive disorder
Adults: Initially, 20 mg/day P.O. (immediate-release) as a single dose; may increase as needed by 10 mg/day at weekly intervals (range is 20 to 50 mg); daily dosages of approximately 30 mg may maintain efficacy for up to 1 year. Or initially, 25 mg P.O. (controlled-release) daily; may increase by 12.5 mg/day at weekly intervals, up to 62.5 mg/day. Or, 20 mg/day P.O. (paroxetine mesylate) as a single dose in morning; may increase as needed by 10 mg/day at weekly intervals up to maximum of 50 mg/day; daily dosages of approximately 30 mg may maintain efficacy for up to 1 year.
➤ Obsessive-compulsive disorder
Adults: Initially, 20 mg/day P.O. (immediate-release); increase as needed by 10 mg/day at weekly intervals, up to 60 mg P.O. (range is 20 to 60 mg/day). Or, initially 20 mg P.O. (paroxetine mesylate); may increase as needed by 10 mg/day at weekly intervals up to maximum of 60 mg/day; recommended dosage is 40 mg/day.
➤ Panic disorder
Adults: Initially, 10 mg/day P.O. (immediate-release); may increase as needed by 10 mg/day at weekly intervals, up to 40 mg P.O. (range is 10 to

60 mg/day); maximum dosage is 60 mg/day, with dosage adjustments made to maintain patient on lowest effective dosage. Or initially, 12.5 mg/day P.O. (controlled-release); may increase by 12.5 mg/day at weekly intervals, to a maximum of 75 mg/day. Or, 10 mg/day P.O. (paroxetine mesylate) daily in morning; may increase as needed by 10 mg/day at weekly intervals up to maximum of 60 mg/day. Target dosage is 40 mg/day. Maintain patient on lowest effective dosage.
➤ Posttraumatic stress disorder
Adults: Initially, 20 mg/day P.O.; range is 20 to 50 mg/day. Make any dosage increases if needed in increments of 10 mg/day at intervals of at least 1 week. For maintenance, adjust to lowest effective dosage.
➤ Generalized anxiety disorder
Adults: Initially, 20 mg/day P.O.; range is 20 to 50 mg/day; however, dosages greater than 20 mg/day may not provide added benefit. Make any dosage increases if needed in increments of 10 mg/day at intervals of at least 1 week. Or, 20 mg/day P.O. (paroxetine mesylate) daily in morning.
➤ Premenstrual dysphoric disorder
Adults: 12.5 to 25 mg/day P.O. (controlled-release) daily. May give either daily throughout menstrual cycle or only during luteal phase cycle (per prescriber). Make any dosage changes if needed at intervals of at least 1 week.

Dosage adjustment
- Hepatic impairment, severe renal impairment
- Elderly or debilitated patients

Contraindications
- Hypersensitivity to drug or its components
- MAO inhibitor use within past 14 days
- Concurrent thioridazine use

P

Precautions

Use cautiously in:
- severe renal or hepatic impairment
- narrow-angle glaucoma
- diseases or conditions that may affect metabolism or hemodynamic responses
- history of seizures, mania, or suicide attempt
- increased risk of suicide attempt, hyponatremia, or abnormal bleeding
- elderly or debilitated patients
- pregnant or breastfeeding patients
- children younger than age 18 (safety not established).

Administration

- Give with or without food.
- Give controlled-release tablets whole. Make sure patient doesn't chew or crush them.

🔇 Don't give to patients receiving MAO inhibitors or thioridazine.

- Reassess patient periodically to gauge need for continued therapy.

Route	Onset	Peak	Duration
P.O.	Unknown	2-8 hr	Unknown
P.O. (controlled)	Unknown	6-10 hr	Unknown

Adverse reactions

CNS: anxiety, agitation, dizziness, drowsiness, asthenia, vascular headache, confusion, hangover, depression, paresthesia, tremor, twitching, myoclonus, amnesia, insomnia, abnormal dreams, unusual or severe mood changes, fatigue, **cerebral ischemia, suicidal behavior or ideation** (especially in child or adolescent)

CV: chest pain, hypertension, hypotension, palpitations, orthostatic hypotension, angina pectoris, ventricular or supraventricular extrasystoles, tachycardia, bradycardia, **thrombophlebitis, myocardial ischemia**

EENT: blurred vision, rhinitis, dry mouth

GI: nausea, vomiting, diarrhea, constipation, abdominal pain, dyspepsia, flatulence, anorexia

GU: urinary frequency, urinary disorders, urinary tract infection, genital disorders, ejaculatory disturbance, decreased libido

Musculoskeletal: back pain, myalgia, myasthenia, myopathy, joint pain

Respiratory: cough, bronchitis, respiratory disorders

Skin: sweating, pruritus, pallor, rash, photosensitivity, **Stevens-Johnson syndrome** (postmarketing reports)

Other: chills, edema, appetite and weight changes, accidental injury, yawning

Interactions

Drug-drug. *Cimetidine:* increased paroxetine blood level

Digoxin: decreased digoxin efficacy

Drugs metabolized by liver (such as amitriptyline, class IC antiarrhythmics, desipramine): decreased metabolism and increased effects of these drugs

5-hydroxytryptamine receptor agonists (such as frovatriptan, naratriptan, rizatriptan): weakness, hyperreflexia, incoordination

MAO inhibitors: potentially fatal reactions (hyperthermia, rigidity, myoclonus, autonomic instability, fluctuating vital signs, extreme agitation, delirium, coma)

Phenobarbital, phenytoin: decreased paroxetine efficacy

Tamoxifen: decreased tamoxifen concentration

Theophylline: increased risk of theophylline toxicity

Thioridazine: increased thioridazine blood level, serious ventricular arrhythmias, sudden death

Tryptophan: headache, nausea, sweating, dizziness

Warfarin: increased risk of bleeding (without altering prothrombin time)

Drug-diagnostic tests. *Alkaline phosphatase, bilirubin, glucose:* increased levels

5-hydroxyindole acetic acid, vanillylmandelic acid: decreased levels

Urinary catecholamines: false increases

Drug-herbs. *S-adenosylmethionine (SAM-e), St. John's wort:* increased risk of adverse serotonergic effects, including serotonin syndrome

Patient monitoring

• Check for signs and symptoms of toxicity, including drowsiness, nausea, tremor, tachycardia, confusion, and dizziness.

• Assess vital signs and cardiovascular status.

◀€ Monitor neurologic status. Watch closely for depression and suicidal behavior and ideation (especially in child or adolescent).

• Evaluate respiratory status. Stay alert for signs and symptoms of infection.

◀€ Monitor patient for signs and symptoms of Stevens-Johnson syndrome.

Patient teaching

• Tell patient to swallow controlled-release tablets whole without chewing or crushing them.

◀€ Describe signs and symptoms of drug toxicity. Tell patient to report these immediately.

◀€ Teach patient or caregiver to recognize and immediately report signs of suicidal intent or expressions of suicidal ideation (especially in child or adolescent).

◀€ Teach patient or caregiver to immediately report rash if it occurs.

• Tell patient to continue to take drug even if he feels better. Caution him not to stop therapy abruptly.

• Advise patient to consult prescriber before taking other prescription drugs or over-the-counter preparations.

• Caution patient to avoid driving and other hazardous activities until he knows how drug affects him.

• As appropriate, review all other significant and life-threatening adverse reactions and interactions, especially those related to the drugs, tests, and herbs mentioned above.

pazopanib
Votrient

Pharmacologic class: Selective multi-targeted tyrosine kinase inhibitor
Therapeutic class: Antineoplastic
Pregnancy risk category D

FDA **BOXED WARNING**

• Severe and fatal hepatotoxicity has been observed in clinical studies.
• Monitor hepatic function and interrupt, reduce, or discontinue dosing as recommended.

Action

Specifically targets growth factor receptors associated with angiogenesis and tumor-cell proliferation; also exhibits inhibition of vascular endothelial growth factor receptors, platelet-derived growth factor receptors, fibroblast growth factor receptors, stem cell factor receptor (c-Kit), interleukin-2 receptor inducible T-cell kinase, leukocyte-specific protein tyrosine kinase, and transmembrane glycoprotein receptor tyrosine kinase

Availability
Tablets: 200 mg

Indications and dosages
➤ Advanced renal cell carcinoma (RCC); advanced soft-tissue sarcoma (STS) in patients who have received prior chemotherapy
Adults: 800 mg P.O. daily. In RCC, initial dosage reduction should be 400 mg, and additional dosage decrease or increase should be in 200-mg steps based on individual tolerability. In STS, a decrease or increase should be in 200-mg steps based on individual tolerability.

p

Reactions in **bold** are life-threatening.   ◀€ Clinical alert

Dosage adjustment
- Moderate hepatic impairment
- Strong CYP3A4 inducers/inhibitors

Contraindications
None

Precautions
Use cautiously in:
- severe hepatic impairment with total bilirubin greater than three times the upper limit of normal (ULN)
- mild to moderate hepatic impairment, proteinuria
- hypothyroidism, hypertension, cardiac disease, patients at risk for developing QT-interval prolongation
- signs and symptoms of serious infection
- patients at increased risk for myocardial infarction (MI), angina, ischemic stroke, transient ischemic attack, and GI perforation or fistula
- hemoptysis; cerebral or clinically significant GI hemorrhage in past 6 months (avoid use)
- patients undergoing surgical procedures
- concurrent use of other cancer therapies (not indicated)
- concurrent use of antiarrhythmics and other drugs that may prolong QT interval
- concurrent use of strong CYP3A4 inducers or inhibitors (avoid use)
- concurrent use of CYP substrates (use not recommended)
- concurrent use of simvastatin
- elderly patients
- pregnant or breastfeeding patients
- children (safety and efficacy not established).

Administration
- Administer without food at least 1 hour before or 2 hours after a meal. Don't give with grapefruit or grapefruit juice. Don't crush tablets.

- Perform baseline ECG and LVEF evaluation, and maintain electrolytes within normal range during therapy.
- ◀≣ Perform baseline urinalysis and discontinue drug for Grade 4 proteinuria.
- Ensure patient's blood pressure is well controlled before starting drug.
- ◀≣ Before starting treatment, monitor hepatic function and interrupt, reduce, or discontinue dosing as recommended.
- ◀≣ Don't administer to patient who has had MI, angina, ischemic stroke, transient ischemic attack, hemoptysis, or clinically significant GI hemorrhage in previous 6 months.
- ◀≣ Be aware that serious infections, including some with fatal outcome, have been reported. Institute appropriate anti-infective therapy promptly and consider drug interruption or discontinuation for serious infections.
- ◀≣ Temporarily interrupt therapy in patients undergoing surgical procedures for at least 7 days before surgery. Discontinue drug in patients who develop wound dehiscence.
- ◀≣ Be aware that drug isn't indicated for use in combination with other cancer agents, because of possible increased toxicity and mortality (pulmonary hemorrhage, GI hemorrhage, and sudden death).

Route	Onset	Peak	Duration
P.O.	Unknown	2-4 hr	Unknown

Adverse reactions
CNS: fatigue, asthenia, headache
CV: hypertension, **decreased ejection fraction, congestive heart failure (CHF), QT-interval prolongation, torsades de pointes**
GI: nausea, vomiting, diarrhea, anorexia, dyspepsia, **GI perforation and fistula**
GU: proteinuria
Hematologic: leukopenia, neutropenia, thrombocytopenia, lymphocytopenia,

arterial and venous thrombotic events, hemorrhagic events
Hepatic: abnormal liver function test values, **hepatotoxicity**
Metabolic: altered electrolyte levels, hypothyroidism
Musculoskeletal: musculoskeletal pain
Respiratory: dyspnea
Skin: alopecia, rash, skin depigmentation, impaired wound healing, palmar-plantar erythrodysesthesia
Other: hair color changes, chest pain, dysgeusia, facial edema, weight loss, decreased appetite, infection, tumor pain, **reversible posterior leukoencephalopathy syndrome**

Interactions

Drug-drug. *CYP3A4 substrates (such as dextromethorphan, midazolam, paclitaxel):* inhibited metabolism of these drugs
Simvastatin: increased risk of ALT elevations
Strong CYP3A4 inducers (such as rifampin): decreased pazopanib concentration
Strong CYP3A4 inhibitors (such as clarithromycin, ketoconazole, ritonavir): increased pazopanib concentration
Drug-diagnostic tests. *ALT, AST, total bilirubin:* increased levels
Glucose: increased or decreased level
Hemoglobin, magnesium, neutrophils, phosphorus, platelets, sodium: decreased levels
Drug-food. *Any food:* increased pazopanib systemic exposure
Grapefruit juice: inhibited CYP3A4 activity and increased pazopanib plasma concentration

Patient monitoring

• Monitor CBC with differential closely.
◀ᛞ Periodically monitor urinalysis during treatment, with follow-up measurement of 24-hour urine protein as clinically indicated. Interrupt therapy and reduce dosage for 24-hour

urine protein of 3 g or more; discontinue drug for repeat episodes despite dosage reductions.
◀ᛞ Monitor serum liver function tests at least once every 4 weeks for at least first 4 months of treatment or as clinically indicated; continue periodic monitoring thereafter. If ALT levels of more than three times ULN occur concurrently with bilirubin levels of more than two times ULN, permanently discontinue drug.
◀ᛞ Closely monitor patient for QT-interval prolongation and signs or symptoms of CHF; periodically monitor ECG and maintain electrolyte levels within normal range.
• Periodically evaluate left ventricular ejection fraction in patients at risk for cardiac dysfunction, including patients who have received previous anthracycline exposure.
• Monitor patients for hypertension; treat as needed. If hypertension persists despite therapy, reduce dosage or discontinue drug as appropriate.
◀ᛞ Closely monitor patient for signs and symptoms of reversible posterior leukoencephalopathy syndrome (RPLS) (headache, seizure, lethargy, confusion, blindness, other visual and neurologic disturbances, and possibly mild to severe hypertension). Discontinue drug if RPLS develops.
◀ᛞ Closely monitor patient for signs and symptoms of infection, hemorrhage, thrombotic events, and GI perforation or fistula.
• Be aware that proactive thyroid function monitoring is recommended.
• Monitor patient for impaired wound healing after surgery.
• Closely watch for ALT elevations in patients also taking simvastatin.

Patient teaching

• Tell patient to take drug without food at least 1 hour before or 2 hours after a meal, not to crush tablets, and

p

Reactions in **bold** are life-threatening.   ◀ᛞ Clinical alert to avoid grapefruit and grapefruit juice.

🔊 Instruct patient to immediately report unusual tiredness; dizziness; numbness or weakness on one side of the body; trouble talking; shortness of breath; irregular heartbeats; high blood pressure; chest pain; bleeding; itching; yellowing of skin or eyes; dark urine; right upper abdominal pain, discomfort, or distention; wounds that don't heal; or red, painful hands and feet.

• Teach patient how to manage diarrhea and to notify prescriber if moderate to severe diarrhea occurs.

• Tell patient that drug may cause depigmentation of the hair or skin.

• Instruct patient to tell prescriber about all drugs he's taking, because some drugs have potential for serious drug interactions and shouldn't be taken with pazopanib.

• Advise female patient of childbearing age to avoid pregnancy during therapy.

• Advise breastfeeding patient that she should decide whether to discontinue breastfeeding or discontinue drug, taking into account importance of drug for her treatment.

• As appropriate, review all other significant and life-threatening adverse reactions and interactions, especially those related to the drugs, tests, and food mentioned above.

pegaptanib sodium injection
Macugen

Pharmacologic class: Selective vascular endothelial growth factor (VEGF) antagonist
Therapeutic class: Ophthalmic agent
Pregnancy risk category B

Action
Binds to extracellular VEGF, which contributes to progression of neovascular age-related macular degeneration; this action suppresses pathologic neovascularization and macular degeneration progression.

Availability
Solution for ophthalmic injection: 0.3 mg/90-microliter single-dose syringe

Indications and dosages
➤ Neovascular (wet) age-related macular degeneration
Adults: 0.3 mg by intravitreous injection into affected eye once every 6 weeks

Contraindications
• Hypersensitivity to drug or its components
• Ocular or periocular infection

Precautions
Use cautiously in:
• pregnant or breastfeeding patients
• children (safety and efficacy not established).

Administration
• Administer only by ophthalmic intravitreous injection under controlled aseptic conditions.
• Inspect drug for particulates and discoloration before administering.
• Attach threaded plastic plunger rod to rubber stopper inside syringe barrel. Don't pull back on plunger.

Route	Onset	Peak	Duration
Intravitreous	Unknown	1-4 days	Unknown

Adverse reactions
CNS: dizziness, headache, vertigo
CV: hypertension, carotid artery occlusion, chest pain, transient ischemic attack, **cerebrovascular accident**
EENT: anterior chamber inflammation, blurred vision, cataract, conjunctival

hemorrhage, corneal edema, eye discharge, eye inflammation or swelling, eye irritation or pain, increased intraocular pressure, ocular discomfort, punctate keratitis, reduced visual acuity, visual disturbance, vitreous disorder or hemorrhage, vitreous floaters or opacities, blepharitis, conjunctivitis, photopsia, allergic conjunctivitis, conjunctival edema, corneal abrasion, corneal deposits, corneal epithelial disorder, endophthalmitis, eyelid irritation, meibomianitis, mydriasis, periorbital hematoma, retinal edema, hearing loss

GI: diarrhea, nausea, vomiting, dyspepsia

GU: urinary tract infection, urinary retention

Metabolic: diabetes mellitus

Musculoskeletal: arthritis, bone spur

Respiratory: bronchitis, pleural effusion

Skin: contact dermatitis, contusion

Other: **anaphylaxis, including angioedema** (rare)

Interactions
None

Patient monitoring
• Watch for increased intraocular pressure, especially within 30 minutes of injection. Be prepared to intervene appropriately.
• Monitor patient for endophthalmitis during week after injection to promote early detection and treatment.

Patient teaching
◀€ Instruct patient to contact ophthalmologist immediately if treated eye becomes red, light-sensitive, or painful or if vision change occurs.
• As appropriate, review all other significant and life-threatening adverse reactions.

pegaspargase
(PEG-L-asparaginase)
Oncaspar

Pharmacologic class: Enzyme
Therapeutic class: Antineoplastic
Pregnancy risk category C

Action
Stimulates production of effector proteins, such as serum neopterin and 2', 5' oligodenylate synthetase; raises body temperature and reversibly lowers white blood cell and platelet counts

Availability
Injection: 750 international units/ml, 5-ml vial in phosphate-buffered saline solution

⟋ Indications and dosages
➤ Acute lymphoblastic leukemia
Adults and children with body surface area (BSA) greater than 0.6 m²: 2,500 international units/m² I.M. or I.V. q 14 days
Adults and children with BSA less than 0.6 m²: 82.5 international units/m² I.M. or I.V. q 14 days

Contraindications
• Hypersensitivity or previous serious allergic reaction (such as generalized urticaria, bronchospasm, laryngeal edema, hypotension) to drug
• Pancreatitis or history of pancreatitis
• Previous hemorrhagic events related to L-asparaginase therapy

Precautions
Use cautiously in:
• renal or hepatic disease, CNS disorders
• concurrent use of hepatotoxic agents, anticoagulants, aspirin or other

p

nonsteroidal anti-inflammatory drugs (NSAIDs)

• pregnant or breastfeeding patients.

Administration

🔊 Follow facility protocol for handling, preparing, and disposing of chemotherapeutic drugs.

🔊 Avoid inhaling vapors and contact with skin or mucous membranes.

🔊 Keep resuscitation equipment, epinephrine, oxygen, steroids, and antihistamines readily available.

• Know that I.M. route is preferred because it's less likely to cause hepatotoxicity, coagulopathy, and GI or renal disorders. For single I.M. injection, don't exceed volume of 2 ml.

• For I.V. use, dilute in 100 ml of normal saline solution or dextrose 5% in water. Infuse over 1 to 2 hours.

🔊 Don't freeze; freezing inactivates drug.

Route	Onset	Peak	Duration
I.V.	Unknown	72-96 hr	2 wk
I.M.	Unknown	Unknown	Unknown

Adverse reactions

CNS: dizziness, headache, confusion, hallucinations, emotional lability, drowsiness, neuritis, Parkinson-like syndrome, malaise, **coma, seizures**

CV: hypertension, hypotension, chest pain, peripheral edema, tachycardia, **endocarditis**

GI: nausea, vomiting, diarrhea, constipation, abdominal pain, flatulence, anorexia, **pancreatitis**

GU: glycosuria, polyuria, urinary frequency, hematuria

Hematologic: hemolytic anemia, leukopenia, pancytopenia, thrombocytopenia, disseminated intravascular coagulation

Hepatic: jaundice, fatty liver deposits, **hepatotoxicity, hepatomegaly**

Metabolic: hypoproteinemia, hyperuricemia, hyperammonemia, hyponatremia, hyperglycemia, **hypoglycemia**

Respiratory: dyspnea, cough, **bronchospasm**

Skin: rash, urticaria, pruritus, night sweats, alopecia

Other: increased appetite and thirst, weight loss, chills, fever, injection site reaction, facial or lip edema, hypersensitivity reactions including **anaphylaxis, septic shock**

Interactions

Drug-drug. *Aspirin, dipyridamole, heparin, NSAIDs, warfarin:* increased risk of bleeding or thrombosis
Methotrexate: decreased methotrexate action

Drug-diagnostic tests. *Amylase, blood urea nitrogen, creatinine, lipase, uric acid:* increased levels
Glucose: increased or decreased level
Liver function tests: abnormal results
Lymphoblasts: decreased count
Plasma proteins: altered levels

Patient monitoring

🔊 Watch for anaphylaxis and other hypersensitivity reactions, especially during first hour of therapy.

• Monitor CBC (including platelet count); fibrinogen; prothrombin and partial thromboplastin times; International Normalized Ratio; and serum amylase, lipase, and uric acid levels.

🔊 Assess neurologic status. Stay alert for decreased level of consciousness and evidence of impending seizure.

• Check for signs and symptoms of bleeding, infection, and hyperglycemia.

• Monitor heart rate, blood pressure, respiratory rate, temperature, and fluid intake and output.

Patient teaching

🔊 Teach patient to recognize and immediately report signs and symptoms of hypersensitivity reactions, bleeding, infection, and other adverse reactions.

• Tell patient drug is likely to cause reversible hair loss.

🍁 Canada   ⊕ UK   ⚕ Hazardous drug   ⊗ High-alert drug

- Stress importance of undergoing follow-up laboratory tests.
- Advise patient to avoid situations that increase risk for infection.
- Instruct patient to consult prescriber before taking other prescription drugs or over-the-counter preparations.
- As appropriate, review all other significant and life-threatening adverse reactions and interactions, especially those related to the drugs and tests mentioned above.

pegfilgrastim
Neulasta

Pharmacologic class: Granulocytic colony stimulating factor
Therapeutic class: Hematopoietic drug
Pregnancy risk category C

Action
Binds to specific cell-surface receptors on hematopoietic cells, stimulating their proliferation and differentiation in bone marrow

Availability
Injection: 6 mg/0.6 ml in prefilled syringes

Indications and dosages
➣ To reduce risk of infection in non-myeloid cancer patients who are receiving myelosuppressive drugs
Adults: 6 mg subcutaneously as a single dose once per chemotherapy cycle

Contraindications
- Hypersensitivity to drug, *Escherichia coli*-derived proteins, filgrastim, or other drug components

Precautions
Use cautiously in:
- myeloid cancers, sickle cell disease
- patients undergoing chemotherapy or radiation
- pregnant or breastfeeding patients
- children (safety and efficacy not established).

Administration
- Inspect solution for particles; discard if particles or discoloration appear.
- Don't give 14 days before to 24 hours after administration of cytotoxic chemotherapy.

Route	Onset	Peak	Duration
Subcut.	Variable	Variable	Variable

Adverse reactions
CNS: headache, weakness, fatigue, dizziness, insomnia
CV: peripheral edema
GI: nausea, vomiting, diarrhea, abdominal pain, dyspepsia, stomatitis, **splenic rupture**
Hematologic: leukocytosis, granulocytopenia
Musculoskeletal: bone pain, myalgia, joint pain
Respiratory: adult respiratory distress syndrome (ARDS) in septic patients
Skin: alopecia, mucositis
Other: taste perversion, allergic reaction, increased pain, fever, neutropenic fever, **aggravation of sickle cell disease**

Interactions
Drug-drug. *Lithium:* potentiation of neutrophil release
Drug-diagnostic tests. *Alkaline phosphatase, lactate dehydrogenase, uric acid:* increased levels

Patient monitoring
◀€ Assess for signs and symptoms of impending splenic rupture, such as left upper abdominal quadrant or shoulder pain and splenic enlargement.

p

Reactions in **bold** are life-threatening. ◀€ Clinical alert

• Monitor vital signs and temperature.
◀€ Watch for signs and symptoms of sepsis, ARDS, and neutropenic fever.
• Monitor CBC, uric acid level, and liver function tests.

Patient teaching

• Teach patient or caregiver how to administer injection and dispose of syringes at home, if appropriate.
◀€ Teach patient to recognize and immediately report respiratory distress or signs and symptoms of splenic rupture.
• Caution patient to avoid driving and other hazardous activities until he knows how drug affects concentration and alertness.
• Advise patient to minimize GI upset by eating small, frequent servings of food and drinking plenty of fluids.
• Instruct patient to have follow-up laboratory tests as needed.
• As appropriate, review all other significant and life-threatening adverse reactions and interactions, especially those related to the drugs and tests mentioned above.

peginesatide
Omontys

Pharmacologic class: Erythropoiesis-stimulating agent (ESA)
Therapeutic class: Hematologic agent
Pregnancy risk category C

FDA | BOXED WARNING

Warning: ESAs increase risk of death, myocardial infarction, stroke, venous thromboembolism, thrombosis of vascular access, and tumor progression or recurrence.
• In controlled trials, patients experienced greater risk of death, serious adverse CV reactions, and stroke when administered ESAs to target a hemoglobin level of greater than 11 g/dl.
• No trial has identified a hemoglobin target level, ESA dosage, or dosing strategy that doesn't increase these risks.
• Use the lowest dosage sufficient to reduce the need for RBC transfusions.

Action

Binds to and activates human erythropoietin receptor and stimulates erythropoiesis in human red cell precursors in vitro; increases reticulocyte count, followed by increases in hemoglobin. Rate of hemoglobin increase varies among patients and is dependent on peginesatide dosage.

Availability

Solution for injection: 2 mg/0.5 ml, 3 mg/0.5 ml, 4 mg/0.5 ml, 5 mg/0.5 ml, 6 mg/0.5 ml in single-use vials; 1 mg/0.5 ml, 2 mg/0.5 ml, 3 mg/0.5 ml, 4 mg/0.5 ml, 5 mg/0.5 ml, 6 mg/0.5 ml in prefilled syringes; 10 mg/ml, 20 mg/2 ml in multi-use vials

🚫 Indications and dosages

➢ Anemia caused by chronic kidney disease in patients on dialysis
Adults: Initially when hemoglobin level is less than 10 g/dl, 0.4 mg/kg subcutaneously or I.V. once monthly. When converting from another ESA, give once monthly based on total weekly epoetin or darbepoetin alfa dose at time of conversion.

Dosage adjustment

• Based on hemoglobin level

Contraindications

• Uncontrolled hypertension

Precautions

Use cautiously in:
• patients with chronic kidney disease and an insufficient hemoglobin response
• patients with chronic kidney disease not on dialysis

- coexistent CV disease and stroke, controlled hypertension
- anemia due to cancer chemotherapy (not indicated)
- patients undergoing coronary artery bypass graft surgery or orthopedic procedures
- pregnant or breastfeeding patients
- children (safety and efficacy not established).

Administration

- Don't dilute drug or administer with other drug solutions.
- Evaluate transferrin saturation and serum ferritin level before starting drug; administer supplemental iron therapy when serum ferritin level is less than 100 mcg/L or when serum transferrin saturation is less than 20%, as prescribed. Be aware that other causes of anemia (such as vitamin deficiency, metabolic or chronic inflammatory conditions, or bleeding) should be corrected or excluded before initiating drug.
- Monitor hemoglobin level at least every 2 weeks until stable. When adjusting therapy, consider hemoglobin rate of rise, rate of decline, ESA responsiveness, and hemoglobin variability; be aware that a single hemoglobin excursion may not require a dosing change. Don't increase dosage more frequently than once every 4 weeks.
- ◀𝄞 Be aware that for patient who doesn't respond adequately over a 12-week escalation period, increasing dosage further is unlikely to improve response and may increase risks. Drug should be used at the lowest dosage that will maintain a hemoglobin level sufficient to reduce need for RBC transfusions. Discontinue drug if responsiveness doesn't improve.
- ◀𝄞 Be aware that using ESAs to target a hemoglobin level greater than 11 g/dl increases risk of serious adverse CV reactions and hasn't been shown to provide additional benefits. Ensure that

patient's hypertension is under control before starting treatment. Reduce dosage or withhold drug if blood pressure becomes difficult to control.
- ◀𝄞 Be aware that patients with cancer receiving ESAs or patients undergoing coronary artery bypass graft surgery may be at increased risk for serious CV adverse reactions or death; patients undergoing orthopedic procedures may be at risk for deep vein thrombosis; and patients with chronic kidney disease not on dialysis may be at increased risk for CV events.
- Be aware that the presence of peginesatide-specific binding antibodies is associated with declining hemoglobin levels and may require increased drug dosages to maintain hemoglobin levels or transfusion for anemia of chronic kidney disease.
- ◀𝄞 Discontinue drug and administer appropriate therapy if a serious allergic reaction occurs.

Route	Onset	Peak	Duration
I.V.	Unknown	Unknown	Unknown
Subcutaneous	Unknown	48 hr	Unknown

Adverse reactions

CNS: headache, **seizures, stroke**
CV: procedural hypotension, hypotension, hypertension, **congestive heart failure (CHF), myocardial infarction (MI)**
GI: nausea, vomiting, diarrhea
Hematologic: thromboembolism
Metabolic: hyperkalemia
Musculoskeletal: muscle spasms, extremity pain, back pain, arthralgia
Respiratory: dyspnea, cough, upper respiratory tract infection
Other: arteriovenous fistula–site complications, pyrexia, peginesatide-specific binding antibodies, allergic reactions, **increased mortality**

Interactions

Drug-diagnostic tests. *Potassium:* increased level

Patient monitoring

• Continue to monitor hemoglobin level at least monthly provided hemoglobin level remains stable.

• Continue to evaluate transferrin saturation and serum ferritin level during treatment and to administer supplemental iron as prescribed.

◀≣ During first several months after drug initiation, closely monitor patient for neurologic symptoms; appropriately control hypertension; and watch for such CV events as stroke, MI, and CHF.

• Be aware that patient receiving peginesatide may require increased anticoagulation with heparin to prevent clotting of the extracorporeal circuit during hemodialysis.

Patient teaching

• If patient will self-administer drug, tell him to follow exact directions for injection, storage, and proper disposal of needles and syringes.

◀≣ Advise patient to immediately report allergic reactions; new-onset seizures, premonitory symptoms, or change in seizure frequency; and CV signs and symptoms.

• Advise patient of importance of having blood tests and blood pressure checks, and of compliance with antihypertensive therapy, iron supplements, and dietary restrictions.

• As appropriate, review all other significant and life-threatening adverse reactions and interactions, especially those related to the tests mentioned above.

peginterferon alfa-2a
Pegasys

Pharmacologic class: Interferon

Therapeutic class: Biological response modifier

Pregnancy risk category C

FDA BOXED WARNING

• Drug may cause or aggravate fatal or life-threatening neuropsychiatric, autoimmune, ischemic, and infectious disorders. Monitor patient closely with periodic clinical and laboratory evaluations. Withdraw drug in patients who have persistently severe or worsening signs or symptoms of these conditions. In most cases, these disorders resolve once therapy ends.

• Concurrent use with ribavirin may cause birth defects or fetal death. Use extreme care to avoid pregnancy in female patients and female partners of male patients. Also, ribavirin causes hemolytic anemia, which may result in worsening of cardiac disease. (See ribavirin package insert for additional information and other warnings.)

Action

Unclear. Thought to bind to specific cell-surface receptors, suppressing cell proliferation and viral replication. Also increases effector protein levels and reduces white blood cell (WBC) and platelet counts.

Availability

Injection: 180-mcg/ml vial, 180 mcg/0.5-ml prefilled syringe, 180 mcg/0.5-ml autoinjector for single use, 135 mcg/0.5-ml autoinjector for single use

❶ Indications and dosages

➢ Chronic hepatitis C virus infection in patients with compensated liver disease not previously treated with interferon alfa and in patients with histological evidence of cirrhosis and compensated liver disease

Adults: 180 mcg subcutaneously q week for 48 weeks. When used in combination with ribavirin, recommended ribavirin dosage and duration for peginterferon alfa-2a are based on viral genotype.

Children ages 5 and older: 180 mcg/1.73 m² × body surface area subcutaneously q week, to a maximum dose of 180 mcg in combination with ribavirin. Recommended treatment duration is based on viral genotype.

➤ Chronic HCV infection with HIV coinfection and CD4 count greater than 100 cells/mm³

Adults: 180 mcg subcutaneously q week for 48 weeks. When used in combination with ribavirin, duration for peginterferon alfa-2a is 48 weeks regardless of viral genotype.

➤ Chronic hepatitis B virus infection in patients with compensated liver disease and evidence of viral replication and liver inflammation

Adults: 180 mcg subcutaneously as monotherapy q week for 48 weeks.

Dosage adjustment
• Neutrophil count less than 750 cells/mm³ or platelet count less than 50,000 cells/mm³
• Hepatic disease
• End-stage renal disease requiring dialysis
• Serious adverse reactions

Off-label uses
• Renal cell carcinoma

Contraindications
• Hypersensitivity to drug or its components
• Autoimmune hepatitis
• Decompensated hepatic disease
• Hemoglobinopathies
• Concurrent use of didanosine (in peginterferon alfa-2a and ribavirin combination therapy)
• Infants and neonates (due to benzyl alcohol content)
• Pregnant patients, men whose female partners are pregnant

Precautions
Use cautiously in:
• thyroid disorders; bone marrow depression; hepatic, renal, or cardiac disease; pancreatitis; autoimmune disorders; pulmonary disorders; colitis; ophthalmic disorders; depression
• elderly patients
• pregnant or breastfeeding patients
• children younger than age 18.

Administration
• Keep refrigerated. Before giving, roll vial between palms for 1 minute to warm; don't shake. Protect solution from light.
• Administer undiluted in abdomen or thigh by subcutaneous injection.
• Use only one vial or prefilled syringe or disposable autoinjector per dose. Discard unused portion of single-use vials or prefilled syringes.
• Know that drug may be used alone or with ribavirin. However, monotherapy isn't recommended for treatment of chronic hepatitis C unless patient has a contraindication or significant intolerance to ribavirin.

Route	Onset	Peak	Duration
Subcut.	Gradual	72-96 hr	Unknown

Adverse reactions
CNS: dizziness, vertigo, insomnia, fatigue, rigors, poor memory and concentration, asthenia, depression, irritability, anxiety, peripheral neuropathy, mood changes, **suicidal ideation**
CV: hypertension, chest pain, **supraventricular arrhythmias, myocardial infarction**
EENT: vision loss, blurred vision, retinal artery or vein thrombosis, retinal hemorrhage, optic neuritis, retinopathy, **papilledema**
GI: nausea, vomiting, diarrhea, abdominal pain, dry mouth, anorexia, **GI tract bleeding, ulcerative and hemorrhagic colitis, pancreatitis**
Hematologic: anemia, **leukopenia, thrombocytopenia, neutropenia**
Metabolic: diabetes mellitus, aggravated hypothyroidism or hyperthyroidism

p

Musculoskeletal: myalgia, back pain, joint pain; delay in weight and height increases (children)
Respiratory: pneumonia, **interstitial pneumonitis, bronchoconstriction, respiratory failure**
Skin: alopecia, pruritus, diaphoresis, rash, dermatitis, dry skin, eczema
Other: weight loss, flulike symptoms, injection-site reaction, pain, **autoimmune phenomena, severe and possibly fatal bacterial infections, severe hypersensitivity reactions including angioedema and anaphylaxis**

Interactions
Drug-drug. *Theophylline:* increased theophylline blood level
Drug-diagnostic tests. *Absolute neutrophil count, hematocrit, hemoglobin, platelets, WBCs:* decreased values
Alanine aminotransferase: transient increase
Glucose, thyroid function tests: decreased or increased levels
Triglycerides: increased levels

Patient monitoring
◀≋ Assess cardiac and pulmonary status closely. Watch for evidence of infections and hypersensitivity reactions, including anaphylaxis.
• Before therapy begins, assess CBC (including platelet count), blood glucose level, and thyroid, kidney, and liver function tests. Continue to monitor at 1, 2, 4, 6, and 8 weeks and then every 4 weeks during therapy (more often if abnormalities occur). Monitor thyroid function tests every 12 weeks.
◀≋ Monitor for development of diabetes mellitus, hypothyroidism, and hyperthyroidism.
◀≋ If serious adverse reaction occurs, discontinue drug or adjust dosage until reaction abates, as prescribed. If reaction persists or recurs despite adequate dosage adjustment, discontinue drug.

Patient teaching
• Teach patient or caregiver how to administer injection subcutaneously in thigh or abdomen and how to dispose of equipment properly, if appropriate.
◀≋ Advise patient to promptly report rash, bleeding, bloody stools, infection symptoms (such as fever), decreased vision, chest pain, severe stomach or lower back pain, shortness of breath, depression, or suicidal thoughts.
• Instruct patient to administer drug exactly as prescribed. If he misses a dose but remembers it within 2 days, tell him to take missed dose as soon as possible; if more than 2 days have elapsed, tell him to contact prescriber.
• Caution patient not to switch brands without prescriber's approval.
• Instruct patient to have periodic eye exams.
• Advise female patient of childbearing age to avoid pregnancy and use two birth control methods before, during, and up to 6 months after therapy. Instruct male patient to use condoms.
• As appropriate, review all other significant and life-threatening adverse reactions and interactions, especially those related to the drugs and tests mentioned above.

peginterferon alfa-2b
PEG-Intron, PegIntron ⊕, Unitron Peg ✦, ViraferonPeg ⊕

Pharmacologic class: Immunomodulator
Therapeutic class: Immunologic agent
Pregnancy risk category C (monotherapy), *X* (when given with ribavirin)

FDA BOXED WARNING
• Drug may cause or aggravate fatal or life-threatening neuropsychiatric,

autoimmune, ischemic, and infectious disorders. Monitor patient closely with periodic clinical and laboratory evaluations. Withdraw drug in patients with persistently severe or worsening signs or symptoms of these conditions. In most cases, these disorders resolve once therapy ends.

• Concurrent use with ribavirin may cause birth defects or fetal death. Use extreme care to avoid pregnancy in female patients and female partners of male patients.

Action
Binds to specific cell-surface membrane receptors, causing suppression of cell proliferation, enhanced phagocytic macrophage activity, and inhibition of viral replication

Availability
Powder for injection with diluent: 50 mcg/0.5-ml vial, 80 mcg/0.5-ml vial, 120 mcg/0.5-ml vial, 150 mcg/0.5-ml vial (Redipen)

Ⰰ Indications and dosages
➤ Chronic hepatitis C virus (HCV) infection in patients with compensated liver disease
Adults ages 18 and older: For monotherapy, 1 mcg/kg/week subcutaneously for 1 year given on the same day of the week. When given with ribavirin, 1.5 mcg/kg/week subcutaneously. When used in combination with ribavirin, recommended duration in interferon alfa–naïve patients is based on viral genotype. Combination treatment duration for patients who previously failed therapy is 48 weeks, regardless of HCV genotype.
Children ages 3 to 17: 60 mcg/m^2/week subcutaneously in combination with ribavirin. Recommended treatment duration is based on viral genotype.

Dosage adjustment
• Serious adverse reactions

• Renal impairment
• Cardiac disease
• Hematologic toxicity

Contraindications
• Hypersensitivity to drug or its components
• Autoimmune hepatitis
• Decompensated hepatic damage

Precautions
Use cautiously in:
• renal insufficiency
• cardiovascular disease, patients with history of psychiatric disorders, patients with debilitating medical conditions, such as those with history of pulmonary disease
• human immunodeficiency virus, hepatitis B infection
• patients who have failed other interferon alfa therapy
• patients who develop neutralizing antibodies
• organ transplant recipients
• elderly patients
• pregnant or breastfeeding patients
• children.

Administration
• Reconstitute by holding dual-chamber glass cartridge upright with dose button down and pressing two halves of pen together until you hear an audible click. Then gently invert (don't shake) pen to mix solution.
• To administer, hold pen upright, attach supplied needle, and select appropriate dosage by pulling back on dosing button until dark bands are visible. Then turn button until dark band aligns with correct dose.
• Use reconstituted solution immediately.
• Know that drug may be used alone or with ribavirin.
• Don't use combination therapy in patients with creatinine clearance less than 50 ml/minute.

P

Reactions in **bold** are life-threatening.　　　　　◀€ Clinical alert

Route	Onset	Peak	Duration
Subcut.	Unknown	15-44 hr	Unknown

Adverse reactions

CNS: fatigue, headache, malaise, asthenia, dizziness, insomnia, depression, anxiety, emotional lability, irritability, poor concentration, agitation, nervousness, rigors, **suicidal behavior, suicidal or homicidal ideation**

CV: hypotension, tachycardia, chest pain, angina pectoris, **arrhythmias, cardiomyopathy, myocardial infarction**

EENT: vision decrease or loss, retinal artery or vein thrombosis, retinal hemorrhage, cotton-wool spots in visual field, rhinitis, sinusitis, pharyngitis

GI: nausea; vomiting; diarrhea; constipation; abdominal pain; dyspepsia; right upper abdominal quadrant pain; anorexia; dry mouth; **ulcerative, hemorrhagic, or ischemic colitis; pancreatitis**

GU: menstrual disorder

Hematologic: neutropenia, thrombocytopenia

Hepatic: hepatomegaly

Metabolic: aggravated hypothyroidism or hyperthyroidism

Musculoskeletal: myalgia, arthralgia, musculoskeletal pain

Respiratory: dyspnea, pneumonia, bronchiolitis obliterans, cough, **sarcoidosis, pulmonary infiltrates, interstitial pneumonitis, bronchoconstriction**

Skin: rash, dry skin, pruritus, sweating, flushing, alopecia

Other: exacerbation or development of autoimmune disorders, injection-site reaction, fever, viral or fungal infection, **systemic lupus erythematosus, severe hypersensitivity reactions including angioedema and anaphylaxis**

Interactions

Drug-diagnostic tests. *Bilirubin, triglycerides, uric acid:* increased levels *Glucose, thyroid function tests:* decreased or increased levels *Hemoglobin, neutrophils, platelets, white blood cells:* decreased levels

Patient monitoring

• Before therapy begins, assess CBC (including platelet count); blood glucose level, and thyroid, kidney, and liver function tests. Continue to monitor at weeks 2, 4, 8, and 12 and then every 6 weeks during therapy (more often if abnormalities occur). Monitor thyroid function tests every 12 weeks.

◀€ Assess cardiac and pulmonary status closely. Watch for signs and symptoms of infection and hypersensitivity reactions, including anaphylaxis.

◀€ Monitor neurologic status. Stay alert for such behavioral changes as irritability, anxiety, depression, and homicidal or suicidal ideation.

◀€ If serious adverse reaction occurs, know that drug will be discontinued or dosages adjusted accordingly.

• Monitor patient for development of diabetes mellitus, hypothyroidism, or hyperthyroidism.

• Be aware that if HCV level remains high after 6 months, drug should be discontinued.

Patient teaching

• Tell patient to take exactly as prescribed. If he misses a dose but remembers it within 2 days, instruct him to take it as soon as possible. However, if more than 2 days have elapsed, advise him to contact prescriber.

• Teach patient or caregiver how to administer injection subcutaneously into thigh or abdomen, if appropriate, and how to properly dispose of equipment.

◀€ Advise patient to stop drug and promptly report infection symptoms, such as high fever, easy bruising or bleeding, decreased vision, chest pain, shortness of breath, severe stomach or

---

lower back pain, depression, or suicidal or homicidal thoughts.
• Urge patient to have periodic eye exams.
• Instruct female patient of childbearing age to avoid pregnancy and to use two birth control methods before, during, and up to 6 months after therapy. Instruct male patient to use condoms.
• As appropriate, review all other significant and life-threatening adverse reactions and interactions, especially those related to the tests mentioned above.

pegvisomant
Somavert

Pharmacologic class: Growth hormone (GH) receptor antagonist
Therapeutic class: GH analog
Pregnancy risk category B

Action
Selectively binds to GH receptors on cell surfaces, where it blocks binding of endogenous GH and interferes with GH signal transduction. This action decreases blood levels of insulin-like growth factor-1 (IGF-1) and other GH-responsive serum proteins.

Availability
Solution: 10-mg, 15-mg, and 20-mg vials

Indications and dosages
➤ Acromegaly
Adults: Initial subcutaneous loading dose of 40 mg, followed by 10 mg/day subcutaneously. May adjust in 5-mg increments after serum IGF-1 measurement q 4 to 6 weeks; don't exceed maximum daily maintenance dosage of 30 mg.

Contraindications
• Hypersensitivity to drug, its components, or latex (in vial stopper)

Precautions
Use cautiously in:
• GH-excreting tumors, diabetes mellitus, hepatic dysfunction
• pregnant or breastfeeding patients
• children.

Administration
• Reconstitute in vial with 1 ml of sterile water for injection.
• Roll vial gently between palms to mix; don't shake. Withdraw prescribed dosage and administer subcutaneously.

Route	Onset	Peak	Duration
Subcut.	Unknown	Unknown	24 hr

Adverse reactions
CNS: dizziness, paresthesia
CV: chest pain, hypertension, peripheral edema
EENT: sinusitis
GI: nausea, diarrhea, abdominal pain
Musculoskeletal: back pain
Other: infection, pain, injection site reaction, accidental injury, flulike symptoms, lipohypertrophy

Interactions
Drug-drug. *Insulin, oral hypoglycemics:* decreased insulin sensitivity, reduced requirements for these drugs
Opioids: increased pegvisomant requirement
Drug-diagnostic tests. *GH assays:* interference with GH measurement
Liver function tests: abnormal results
Drug-behaviors. *Opioid addiction:* increased pegvisomant requirement

Patient monitoring
• Assess liver function tests; watch for signs and symptoms of hepatic dysfunction.

p

Reactions in **bold** are life-threatening. ◀€ Clinical alert

• Monitor serum IGF-1 level. If appropriate, discuss dosage adjustments with prescriber.
• Monitor vital signs; check for hypertension, chest pain, and peripheral edema.
• Measure temperature. Watch for signs and symptoms of infection, especially sinusitis or flulike symptoms.
• Assess blood glucose level closely in diabetic patient. Notify prescriber of significant decrease.

Patient teaching

• Teach patient proper technique for reconstituting and administering drug subcutaneously.
🔊 Instruct patient to immediately report chest pain, peripheral edema, or signs or symptoms of infection.
• Caution patient to avoid driving and other hazardous activities until he knows how drug affects him.
• Teach diabetic patient to monitor blood glucose level closely and report significant decrease.
🔊 Instruct patient to report yellowing of skin or eyes and other signs and symptoms of hepatic dysfunction. Tell him he'll undergo frequent liver function tests.
• As appropriate, review all other significant adverse reactions and interactions, especially those related to the drugs, tests, and behaviors mentioned above.

pemetrexed
Alimta

Pharmacologic class: Folic acid antagonist

Therapeutic class: Antineoplastic, antimetabolite

Pregnancy risk category D

Action
Disrupts folate-dependent metabolic processes essential for cell replication

Availability
Powder for injection: 500 mg sterile lyophilized powder in single-use vials

🚫 Indications and dosages
➤ Malignant pleural mesothelioma in patients whose disease is unresectable or who otherwise aren't eligible for curative surgery (given with cisplatin)
Adults: 500 mg/m² as an I.V. infusion over 10 minutes on day 1 of each 21-day cycle. The recommended dose of cisplatin is 75 mg/m² infused over 2 hours starting approximately 30 minutes after pemetrexed administration ends.
➤ Nonsquamous non-small-cell lung cancer
Adults: 500 mg/m² I.V. infusion over 10 minutes on day 1 of each 21-day cycle for single-agent use, or in combination with cisplatin infused over 2 hours starting approximately 30 minutes after pemetrexed administration ends

Dosage adjustment
• Hematologic toxicities, based on nadir absolute neutrophil and platelet counts
• Grade 2 to 4 neurotoxicity
• Grade 3 or higher nonhematologic toxicities (except neurotoxicity)
• Grade 3 or 4 diarrhea or any diarrhea requiring hospitalization
• Creatinine clearance below 45 ml/minute

Contraindications
• Severe hypersensitivity reaction to drug or its components

Precautions
Use cautiously in:
• hepatic or renal impairment, neurotoxicity

- pregnant or breastfeeding patients
- children (safety and efficacy not established).

Administration

- Reconstitute 500-mg vial with 20 ml preservative-free normal saline solution injection, yielding 25 mg/ml. Gently swirl vial until powder dissolves completely.
- Further dilute appropriate volume of reconstituted solution to 100 ml with preservative-free normal saline solution injection; administer I.V. over 10 minutes.
- Know that drug is physically incompatible with diluents containing calcium, including Ringer's and lactated Ringer's solutions. Administration with other drugs and diluents isn't recommended.
- Administer I.V. only.
- As ordered, pretreat with dexamethasone (or equivalent) 4 mg P.O. twice daily on day before, day of, and day after pemetrexed administration to minimize cutaneous reactions.
- When administering with cisplatin, hydrate patient with 1 to 2 L fluid infused over 8 to 12 hours before and after cisplatin administration. Maintain adequate hydration and urine output for 24 hours.
- To reduce toxicity, ensure that patient receives at least five daily doses of low-dose folic acid or multivitamin with folic acid within 7 days before first pemetrexed dose. Folic acid therapy should continue throughout course of therapy and for 21 days after final dose. Patient also must receive one I.M. injection of vitamin B_{12} during week before first pemetrexed dose and every three cycles thereafter.
- Discontinue drug if creatinine clearance is below 45 ml/minute or patient has hematologic or nonhematologic Grade 3 or 4 toxicity after two dosage reductions (except Grade 3 transaminase elevation).

- Withdraw drug immediately in patients with Grade 3 or 4 neurotoxicity.

Route	Onset	Peak	Duration
I.V.	Unknown	Unknown	Unknown

Adverse reactions

CNS: fatigue, sensory neuropathy, altered mood, depression
CV: thrombosis, embolism
EENT: pharyngitis
GI: nausea, vomiting, constipation, diarrhea without colostomy, dysphagia, esophagitis, pain on swallowing, stomatitis, anorexia
GU: renal failure
Hematologic: neutropenia, leukopenia, anemia, thrombocytopenia, febrile neutropenia
Hepatic: abnormal liver function
Musculoskeletal: myalgia, arthralgia
Respiratory: dyspnea
Skin: rash, desquamation, alopecia
Other: fever, dehydration, noncardiac chest pain, infection without neutropenia or with Grade 3 or Grade 4 neutropenia, edema, other constitutional symptoms, allergic reaction, hypersensitivity reaction

Interactions

Drug-drug. *Ibuprofen:* decreased pemetrexed clearance and increased concentration
Nephrotoxic agents: possible decrease in pemetrexed clearance
Drug-diagnostic tests. *Alanine aminotransferase, aspartate aminotransferase, serum creatinine:* increased
Creatinine clearance, hematocrit, hemoglobin, platelets, WBCs: decreased

Patient monitoring

- Monitor CBC and platelet counts frequently.
- Monitor renal and liver function tests and blood chemistry results (especially serum creatinine) periodically.

• Know that patients with mild to moderate renal insufficiency should avoid taking nonsteroidal anti-inflammatory drugs (NSAIDs) with short elimination half-lives (such as aspirin, diclofenac, and ibuprofen) for 5 days before, on day of, and for 2 days after pemetrexed administration. If concomitant NSAID use is necessary, monitor patient closely for toxicities (especially myelosuppression and renal and GI toxicity).

• Be aware that all patients should avoid NSAIDs with long half-lives (such as diflunisal, piroxicam, and sulindac) for at least 5 days before, on day of, and for 2 days after pemetrexed administration. If concomitant NSAID use is necessary, monitor patient closely for toxicities (especially myelosuppression and renal and GI toxicity).

Patient teaching

• Instruct patient to take folic acid and vitamin B_{12} before and during therapy, as prescribed.

• Advise patient to drink ten 8-oz glasses of fluid and to urinate frequently during first 24 hours after therapy that includes cisplatin.

• Teach patient to recognize signs and symptoms of anemia and to contact prescriber if temperature above 100.4 °F (38 °C) develops.

• Tell patient to consult prescriber before taking products containing ibuprofen.

• Advise female with childbearing potential to avoid pregnancy during therapy.

• Instruct breastfeeding patient to stop breastfeeding during therapy.

• As appropriate, review all other significant and life-threatening adverse reactions and interactions, especially those related to the drugs and tests mentioned above.

penicillin G benzathine
Bicillin L-A, Permapen

Pharmacologic class: Penicillin
Therapeutic class: Anti-infective
Pregnancy risk category B

Action
Inhibits biosynthesis of cell-wall mucopeptide; kills penicillin-susceptible bacteria during active multiplication stage

Availability
Suspension for I.M. injection: 600,000 units/ml in 1-, 2-, and 4-ml prefilled syringes

🖉 Indications and dosages
➤ Upper respiratory infections
Adults: 1.2 million units I.M. as a single dose
Children weighing 27 kg (60) or more: 900,000 units I.M. as a single dose
Infants and children weighing less than 27 kg (60 lb): 300,000 to 600,000 units I.M. as a single dose
➤ Early syphilis (primary, secondary, or latent)
Adults: 2.4 million units I.M. as a single dose
Children: 50,000 units/kg I.M. as a single dose, increased as needed up to adult dosage
➤ Congenital syphilis
Children younger than age 2: 50,000 units/kg I.M. as a single dose
➤ Late (tertiary) syphilis and neuro-syphilis
Adults: 2.4 million units I.M. q week for up to 3 weeks, after aqueous penicillin G or procaine penicillin therapy
➤ Gummas and cardiovascular syphilis
Adults: 2.4 million units I.M. q week for 3 weeks

➤ Yaws, bejel, and pinta
Adults: 1.2 million units I.M. as a single dose
➤ Prophylaxis of rheumatic fever and glomerulonephritis
Adults: After acute attack, 1.2 million units I.M. q month or 600,000 units q 2 weeks

Contraindications
• Hypersensitivity to penicillins, beta-lactamase inhibitors (piperacillin/tazobactam), or benzathine

Precautions
Use cautiously in:
• severe renal insufficiency, significant allergies, asthma
• pregnant or breastfeeding patients.

Administration
• Before giving, ask patient about allergy to penicillin, beta-lactamase inhibitors, and benzathine. Be aware that cross-sensitivity to cephalosporins and imipenem also may occur.
◀╠ Do not give intravenously
• Inject deep I.M. into upper outer quadrant of buttock in adult or mid-lateral thigh in infant or small child. Don't inject into gluteal muscle in child younger than age 2. Rotate injection sites with repeated doses.
◀╠ Keep epinephrine and emergency equipment at hand in case of anaphylaxis.
• Be aware that Hoigne's syndrome (transient bizarre behavior and neurologic reactions) may immediately follow I.M. injection.
• Know that in syphilis treatment, Jarisch-Hersheimer reaction (fever, chills, headache, sweating, malaise, hypotension or hypertension) may occur 2 to 12 hours after therapy begins and usually subsides within 24 hours.

Route	Onset	Peak	Duration
I.M.	Delayed	Dose dependent	Dose dependent

Adverse reactions
CNS: headache, lethargy, hallucinations, anxiety, neuropathy, fatigue, nervousness, tremors, euphoria, asthenia, Hoigne's syndrome, **cerebrovascular accident, seizures, coma**
CV: hypotension, pulmonary hypertension, vasodilation, vasovagal reaction, syncope, palpitations, tachycardia, **cardiac arrest, pulmonary embolism**
EENT: blurred vision, vision loss, laryngeal edema
GI: nausea, vomiting, diarrhea, epigastric distress, abdominal pain, colitis, blood in stool, glossitis, **pseudomembranous colitis**
GU: hematuria, proteinuria, urogenic bladder, erectile dysfunction, priapism, nephropathy, **renal failure**
Hematologic: hemolytic anemia, leukopenia, thrombocytopenia
Metabolic: hypernatremia, **hyperkalemia**
Respiratory: dyspnea, hypoxia, **apnea, pulmonary embolism**
Skin: rash, urticaria, sweating
Other: fever, superinfection, injection site reactions and pain, Jarisch-Hersheimer reaction, **anaphylaxis, serum sickness**

Interactions
Drug-drug. *Aspirin, probenecid:* increased penicillin blood level
Erythromycins, tetracyclines: decreased antimicrobial activity of penicillin
Hormonal contraceptives: decreased contraceptive efficacy
Drug-diagnostic tests. *Alanine aminotransferase, blood urea nitrogen, creatinine, eosinophils, granulocytes, hemoglobin, platelets, potassium, white blood cells:* increased levels
Direct Coombs' test: positive result
Sodium: decreased level
Urine glucose, urine protein: false-positive results

p

Reactions in **bold** are life-threatening.　　　◀╠ Clinical alert

Patient monitoring

◀€ Watch closely for anaphylaxis and serum sickness.

• In long-term therapy, monitor electrolyte levels and CBC with white cell differential; watch for electrolyte imbalances and blood dyscrasias.

• Assess neurologic status, especially for seizures and decreasing level of consciousness.

◀€ Watch for evidence of superinfection and pseudomembranous colitis.

Patient teaching

◀€ Teach patient to recognize anaphylaxis symptoms and to contact emergency medical services immediately if these occur.

◀€ Tell patient drug may cause diarrhea. Instruct him to immediately report severe, persistent diarrhea, and fever.

• Urge patient to complete entire course of therapy as prescribed, even after symptoms improve.

• Advise patient to contact prescriber if infection symptoms get worse.

• Tell female patient that drug may make hormonal contraceptives ineffective. Advise her to use barrier birth control if she wishes to avoid pregnancy.

• As appropriate, review all other significant and life-threatening adverse reactions and interactions, especially those related to the drugs and tests mentioned above.

penicillin G potassium
Pfizerpen

Pharmacologic class: Penicillin
Therapeutic class: Anti-infective
Pregnancy risk category B

Action

Inhibits biosynthesis of cell-wall mucopeptide; bactericidal against penicillin-susceptible microorganisms during active multiplication stage

Availability

Powder for injection: 1 million, 5 million, and 20 million units/vial
Premixed (frozen) solution for injection: 1 million, 2 million, and 3 million units/50 ml

⏀ Indications and dosages

➤ Meningococcal meningitis
Adults: 1 to 2 million units I.M. q 2 hours or 20 to 30 million units/day by continuous I.V. infusion for 14 days, or until afebrile for 7 days

➤ Meningitis caused by susceptible pneumococcal or meningococcal strains
Children: 250,000 units/kg/day in equally divided doses I.M. or by continuous I.V. infusion q 4 hours for 7 to 14 days (depending on causative organism)
Infants older than 7 days: 200,000 to 300,000 units/kg/day I.V. in divided doses q 6 hours
Infants less than 7 days old: 100,000 to 150,000 units/kg/day I.V. in divided doses q 12 hours

➤ Actinomycosis
Adults: 1 to 6 million units/day I.M. or I.V. for cervicofacial infections; 10 to 20 million units/day I.V. q 4 to 6 hours for 6 weeks for thoracic and abdominal infections

➤ Clostridial infections
Adults: 20 million units/day I.M. or I.V. infusion q 4 to 6 hours, given with antitoxin therapy

➤ Fusospirochetal infections
Adults: 5 to 10 million units/day I.M. or 200,000 to 500,000 units I.V. infusion q 4 to 6 hours

➤ Rat bite fever; Haverhill fever
Adults: 12 to 20 million units/day I.M. or I.V. infusion q 4 to 6 hours for 3 or 4 weeks

➤ *Pasteurella* infections
Adults: 4 to 6 million units/day I.M. or
I.V. infusion q 4 to 6 hours for 2 weeks
➤ Erysipeloid endocarditis
Adults: 12 to 20 million units/day I.M.
or I.V. infusion q 4 to 6 hours for 4 to 6
weeks
➤ Diphtheria (as adjunctive therapy
with antitoxin to prevent carrier state)
Adults: 2 to 3 million units/day I.M. or
I.V. infusion in divided doses q 4 to 6
hours for 10 to 12 days
➤ Anthrax
Adults: At least 5 million units/day
I.M. or I.V. infusion
➤ Serious streptococcal infections
Adults: 5 to 24 million units/day I.M.
or I.V. infusion in divided doses q 4 to
6 hours
➤ Neurosyphilis
Adults: 18 to 24 million units/day I.V.
(given in doses of 3 to 4 million units q
4 hours) for 10 to 14 days
➤ *Listeria* infections
Adults: 15 to 20 million units/day I.M.
or I.V. infusion q 4 to 6 hours for 2
weeks in meningitis or 4 weeks in
endocarditis
➤ Disseminated gonococcal infections
Adults: 10 million units/day I.V. (3 to
4 million units q 4 hours) for 10 to
14 days

Off-label uses
• Lyme disease
• Predental prophylaxis against bacter-
ial endocarditis

Contraindications
• Hypersensitivity to penicillins or
beta-lactamase inhibitors (piperacillin/
tazobactam)

Precautions
Use cautiously in:
• severe renal insufficiency, significant
allergies, asthma
• pregnant or breastfeeding patients.

Administration
• Before giving, ask patient about
allergy to penicillin, beta-lactamase
inhibitors, or benzathine. Know that
cross-sensitivity to imipenem and
cephalosporins also may occur.
◀€ Keep epinephrine and emergency
equipment at hand in case anaphylaxis
occurs.
• For I.V. use, dilute in sterile water for
injection, normal saline solution, or
dextrose 5% in water (D_5W). For continuous infusion, further dilute in 1 to
2 L of compatible solution and infuse
over 24 hours. For intermittent infusion, further dilute in 50 or 100 ml of
normal saline solution or D_5W;
administer over 1 to 2 hours in adults
or 15 to 30 minutes in children and
infants.
• Know that drug also may be given by
intrapleural or intrathecal route.
• Be aware that in syphilis treatment,
Jarisch-Hersheimer reaction (fever,
chills, headache, sweating, malaise,
hypotension or hypertension) may
occur 2 to 12 hours after therapy
starts and usually subsides within
24 hours.

Route	Onset	Peak	Duration
I.M.	Rapid	15-30 min	4-6 hr
I.V.	Rapid	End of infusion	4-6 hr

P

Adverse reactions
CNS: hyperreflexia, neuropathy, **coma,
seizures**
**CV: arrhythmias, cardiac arrest, heart
failure** (with high I.V. doses)
GI: nausea, vomiting, diarrhea, epigastric distress, abdominal pain, colitis,
blood in stool, glossitis, **pseudomembranous colitis**
GU: nephropathy
**Hematologic: hemolytic anemia,
leukopenia, thrombocytopenia**
Metabolic: hyperkalemia (with high-
dose, continuous I.V. infusion)

Reactions in **bold** are life-threatening.   ◀€ Clinical alert

Skin: rash, urticaria, exfoliative dermatitis

Other: pain at I.M. injection site, phlebitis at I.V. site, Jarisch-Hersheimer reaction, superinfection, **anaphylaxis, serum sickness**

Interactions

Drug-drug. *Aspirin, probenecid:* increased penicillin blood level

Erythromycins, tetracyclines: decreased antimicrobial activity of penicillin

Hormonal contraceptives: decreased contraceptive efficacy

Drug-diagnostic tests. *Alanine aminotransferase, eosinophils, granulocytes, hemoglobin, platelets, potassium, white blood cells:* increased levels

Direct Coombs' test: positive result

Sodium: decreased level

Urine glucose, urine protein: false-positive results

Patient monitoring

◀̥ Watch closely for signs and symptoms of anaphylaxis and serum sickness.

• In long-term therapy, monitor electrolyte levels and CBC with white cell differential; watch for electrolyte imbalances and blood dyscrasias.

• Closely monitor neurologic status, especially for seizures and decreasing level of consciousness.

◀̥ Stay alert for signs and symptoms of superinfection and pseudomembranous colitis.

Patient teaching

◀̥ Teach patient to recognize signs and symptoms of anaphylaxis. Tell him to contact emergency medical services immediately if these occur.

◀̥ Tell patient drug may cause diarrhea. Instruct him to immediately report severe, persistent diarrhea and fever.

• Urge patient to complete entire course of therapy as prescribed, even after symptoms improve.

• Tell patient to contact prescriber if infection symptoms worsen.

• Inform female patient that drug may make hormonal contraceptives ineffective. Advise her to use barrier birth-control method if she wishes to avoid pregnancy.

• As appropriate, review all other significant and life-threatening adverse reactions and interactions, especially those related to the drugs and tests mentioned above.

penicillin G procaine

Ayercillin✸, Crysticillin-AS✸

Pharmacologic class: Penicillin

Therapeutic class: Anti-infective

Pregnancy risk category B

Action

Inhibits biosynthesis of cell-wall mucopeptide; bactericidal against penicillin-susceptible microorganisms during active multiplication stage

Availability

Suspension for I.M. injection: 600,000 units/ml vial, 1.2 million units/2-ml vial, 2.4 million units/4-ml vial, 3 million units/10-ml vial

🖉 Indications and dosages

➤ Anthrax; bacterial endocarditis; erysipeloid and fusospirochetal infections; group A streptococcal infections; moderately severe, uncomplicated pneumococcal pneumonia and staphylococcal infections; rat-bite fever

Adults: 600,000 to 1 million units/day I.M.

➤ Diphtheria

Adults: 300,000 to 600,000 units/day I.M. given with antitoxin for 14 days.

For carrier state, 300,000 units/day I.M. for 10 days.

➤ Syphilis, yaws, bejel, pinta

Adults and children older than age 12: 600,000 units/day I.M. for 8 days; for late infections, continue for 10 to 15 days. For neurosyphilis, 2.4 million units/day I.M. for 10 to 14 days, given with probenecid.

➤ Congenital syphilis

Children: 50,000 units/kg I.M. daily for at least 10 days

➤ Uncomplicated gonorrhea

Adults: 4.8 million units/day I.M., divided into at least two doses and two sites at one visit, with P.O. probenecid given 30 minutes before injection

Off-label uses

• Lyme disease
• Predental prophylaxis against bacterial endocarditis

Contraindications

• Hypersensitivity to penicillins, beta-lactamase inhibitors (piperacillin/tazobactam), or procaine

Precautions

Use cautiously in:
• severe renal insufficiency, significant allergies, asthma
• pregnant or breastfeeding patients
• neonates.

Administration

• Before giving, ask patient about allergy to penicillin, beta-lactamase inhibitors, or benzathine. Know that cross-sensitivity to imipenem and cephalosporins may occur.

◄≀ Keep epinephrine and emergency equipment at hand in case anaphylaxis occurs.

• In adults, inject I.M. deep into upper outer aspect of buttock.

• In infants and small children, inject at a slow, steady rate into midlateral aspect of thigh.

• Be aware that Hoigne's syndrome (transient bizarre behavior and neurologic reactions) may immediately follow I.M. injection.

• Know that in syphilis treatment, Jarisch-Hersheimer reaction (fever, chills, headache, sweating, malaise, hypotension or hypertension) may occur 2 to 12 hours after therapy starts and usually subsides within 24 hours.

Route	Onset	Peak	Duration
I.M.	Delayed	1-3 hr	24 hr

Adverse reactions

CNS: lethargy, hallucinations, anxiety, depression, twitching, Hoigne's syndrome, **seizures, coma**
EENT: laryngeal edema
GI: nausea, vomiting, diarrhea, epigastric distress, abdominal pain, colitis, blood in stool, glossitis, **pseudomembranous colitis**
GU: interstitial nephritis
Hematologic: increased bleeding, hemolytic anemia, bone marrow depression, leukopenia, thrombocytopenia, granulocytopenia
Skin: rash, urticaria
Other: pain at I.M. injection site, fever, superinfection, Jarisch-Hersheimer reaction, sterile abscess, procaine toxicity, **anaphylaxis, serum sickness**

Interactions

Drug-drug. *Aspirin, probenecid:* increased penicillin blood level
Erythromycins, tetracyclines: decreased antimicrobial activity of penicillin
Hormonal contraceptives: decreased contraceptive efficacy
Drug-diagnostic tests. *Alanine aminotransferase, eosinophils, granulocytes, hemoglobin, platelets, potassium, white blood cells:* increased levels
Direct Coombs' test: positive result
Sodium: decreased level
Urine glucose, urine protein: false-positive results

P

Patient monitoring

◀€ Watch closely for signs and symptoms of anaphylaxis and serum sickness.

• In long-term therapy, monitor electrolyte levels and CBC with white cell differential. Watch for electrolyte imbalances and blood dyscrasias.

• Assess neurologic status, especially for seizures and decreasing level of consciousness.

◀€ Monitor patient for signs and symptoms of superinfection and pseudomembranous colitis.

Patient teaching

◀€ Teach patient to recognize signs and symptoms of anaphylaxis. Tell him to contact emergency medical services immediately if these occur.

◀€ Tell patient drug may cause diarrhea. Instruct him to immediately report severe, persistent diarrhea and fever.

• Stress importance of completing entire course of therapy as prescribed, even after symptoms improve.

• Advise patient to contact prescriber if infection symptoms worsen.

• Tell female patient that drug may make hormonal contraceptives ineffective. Encourage her to use barrier birth-control method if she wishes to avoid pregnancy.

• As appropriate, review all other significant and life-threatening adverse reactions and interactions, especially those related to the drugs and tests mentioned above.

penicillin V potassium

Apo-Pen VK✤, Novo-Pen-VK✤, Pen-Vee

Pharmacologic class: Penicillin
Therapeutic class: Anti-infective
Pregnancy risk category B

Action

Inhibits biosynthesis of cell-wall mucopeptide; bactericidal against penicillin-susceptible microorganisms during active multiplication stage

Availability

Oral solution: 200,000 units (125 mg)/5 ml, 400,000 units (250 mg)/5 ml
Tablets: 400,000 units (250 mg), 800,000 units (500 mg)

⊘ Indications and dosages

➤ Upper respiratory streptococcal infections, including scarlet fever and mild erysipelas
Adults and children ages 12 and older: 125 to 250 mg P.O. q 6 to 8 hours for 10 days
Children younger than age 12: 25 to 50 mg/kg/day P.O. in divided doses q 6 hours for 10 days
➤ Pneumococcal respiratory infections, including otitis media
Adults and children ages 12 and older: 250 to 500 mg P.O. q 6 hours until afebrile for at least 2 days
➤ Skin and soft-tissue staphylococcal infections; fusospirochetosis (Vincent's infection) of oropharynx
Adults and children ages 12 and older: 250 to 500 mg P.O. q 6 to 8 hours
➤ To prevent recurrence of rheumatic fever or chorea
Adults and children ages 12 and older: 125 to 250 mg P.O. b.i.d. on a continuing basis

Off-label uses

• Prophylaxis of *Streptococcus pneumoniae* septicemia in children with sickle cell anemia or splenectomy
• Early Lyme disease
• Actinomycosis
• Preexposure prophylaxis of anthrax
• Prophylaxis of bacterial endocarditis for dental procedures

---

✤ Canada   ⊕ UK   ☣ Hazardous drug   ⊗ High-alert drug

Contraindications
• Hypersensitivity to penicillins or beta-lactamase inhibitors (piperacillin/tazobactam)

Precautions
Use cautiously in:
• severe renal insufficiency
• pregnant or breastfeeding patients.

Administration
• Before giving, ask patient about allergies to penicillin, beta-lactamase inhibitors, or benzathine. Know that cross-sensitivity to imipenem and cephalosporins may occur.

◀❲ Keep epinephrine and emergency equipment at hand in case anaphylaxis occurs.

• Give with water 1 hour before or 2 hours after meals. Don't give with fruit juice or carbonated beverages.

Route	Onset	Peak	Duration
P.O.	Unknown	1 hr	6 hr

Adverse reactions
CNS: lethargy, hallucinations, anxiety, depression, twitching, **seizures, coma**
GI: nausea, vomiting, diarrhea, epigastric distress, abdominal pain, colitis, blood in stool, glossitis, **pseudomembranous colitis**
GU: interstitial nephritis
Hematologic: anemia, **hemolytic anemia, increased bleeding, leukopenia, granulocytopenia, bone marrow depression, thrombocytopenia, thrombocytopenic purpura**
Metabolic: hypokalemia, **hyperkalemia, metabolic alkalosis**
Skin: rash, urticaria
Other: fever, superinfection, **anaphylaxis, serum sickness**

Interactions
Drug-drug. *Aspirin, probenecid:* increased penicillin blood level
Erythromycins, tetracyclines: decreased antimicrobial activity of penicillin

Hormonal contraceptives: decreased contraceptive efficacy
Drug-diagnostic tests. *Alanine aminotransferase, eosinophils, granulocytes, hemoglobin, platelets:* increased levels
Albumin, lymphocytes, protein, sodium, uric acid, white blood cells: decreased levels
Direct Coombs' test: positive result
Potassium: increased or decreased level
Urine glucose, urine protein: false-positive results
Drug-herbs. *Khat:* delayed and reduced penicillin absorption

Patient monitoring
◀❲ Watch for signs and symptoms of anaphylaxis and serum sickness.
• In long-term therapy, monitor electrolyte levels and CBC with white cell differential; watch for electrolyte imbalances and blood dyscrasias.
• Assess neurologic status, especially for seizures and decreasing level of consciousness.
◀❲ Monitor patient closely for signs and symptoms of superinfection and pseudomembranous colitis.

Patient teaching
• Instruct patient to take with water 1 hour before or 2 hours after meals. Tell him not to take with fruit juice or carbonated beverages.
◀❲ Teach patient to recognize anaphylaxis symptoms. Tell him to immediately contact emergency medical services if these occur.
• Instruct patient to report signs and symptoms of superinfection.
• Advise patient to contact prescriber if infection symptoms get worse.
◀❲ Tell patient drug may cause diarrhea. Instruct him to immediately report severe, persistent diarrhea and fever.
• Instruct patient to complete entire course of therapy as prescribed, even after symptoms improve.
• Tell female patient drug may make hormonal contraceptives ineffective.

P

Reactions in **bold** are life-threatening.　　　　◀❲ Clinical alert

Advise her to use barrier birth-control method if she wishes to avoid pregnancy.
• As appropriate, review all other significant and life-threatening adverse reactions and interactions, especially those related to the drugs, tests, and herbs mentioned above.

pentamidine isethionate
NebuPent, Pentacarinat✠, Pentam 300

Pharmacologic class: Antiprotozoal
Therapeutic class: Anti-infective
Pregnancy risk category C

Action
Unknown. May interfere with nuclear metabolism and synthesis of DNA, RNA, and proteins.

Availability
Aerosol: 300 mg
Injection: 300 mg/vial

Indications and dosages
➤ *Pneumocystis jiroveci* pneumonia
Adults and children ages 5 and older: 4 mg/kg I.V. or deep I.M. daily for 14 days
➤ To prevent *P. jiroveci* pneumonia in high-risk patients with human immunodeficiency virus
Adults: 300 mg by inhalation once q 4 weeks using Respigard II nebulizer

Off-label uses
• Trypanosomiasis
• Visceral leishmaniasis

Contraindications
• History of anaphylaxis from pentamidine or diamidine compounds (inhalation only)

(*Note:* No absolute contraindications exist for patients with *P. jiroveci*.)

Precautions
Use cautiously in:
• anemia, blood dyscrasias, hepatic or renal disease, hypoglycemia, diabetes mellitus, ventricular tachycardia, hypocalcemia, hypertension, hypotension
• pregnant or breastfeeding patients
• children (safety and efficacy of inhalation solution not established).

Administration
• For I.V. infusion, dilute 300 mg-vial with sterile water for injection. Withdraw prescribed dosage, then dilute further in 50 to 250 ml of dextrose 5% in water; infuse over 60 to 120 minutes.
• For I.M. use, dilute 300 mg-vial with 3 ml of sterile water for injection. Withdraw prescribed dosage; administer deep I.M. using Z-track method.
• Keep patient supine during I.M. or I.V. administration to minimize hypotension.
• For inhalation, dilute in 6 ml of sterile water and administer through nebulizer at a flow rate of 6 L/minute from 50-psi compressed air source. Don't mix inhalation solution with other drugs.

Route	Onset	Peak	Duration
I.V.	Unknown	1 hr	Unknown
I.M., inhalation	Unknown	0.5 hr	Unknown

Adverse reactions
CNS: headache, disorientation, hallucinations, dizziness, confusion, fatigue, neuralgia
CV: chest pain, ECG abnormalities, syncope, vasodilation, vasculitis, phlebitis, hypertension, palpitations, **arrhythmias, severe hypotension**
EENT: pharyngitis

GI: nausea, vomiting, diarrhea, abdominal pain, anorexia, **acute pancreatitis**
Hematologic: anemia, **leukopenia, thrombocytopenia**
Metabolic: hypocalcemia, hyperglycemia, **hypoglycemia, hyperkalemia**
Musculoskeletal: myalgia
Respiratory: cough, dyspnea, congestion, **pneumothorax, bronchospasm**
Skin: rash, night sweats, urticaria, sterile abscess or induration at injection site
Other: metallic or bad taste, fever, chills, pain at injection site or elsewhere, edema, allergic reactions

Interactions

Drug-diagnostic tests. *Blood urea nitrogen, creatinine, liver function tests, potassium:* increased values
Calcium, hemoglobin, hematocrit, platelets, white blood cells: decreased levels
ECG: alterations
Glucose: increased or decreased level

Patient monitoring

◀€ Closely monitor blood pressure and blood glucose. Watch for arrhythmias and evidence of pulmonary infection, blood dyscrasias, and pancreatitis during and after I.M. or I.V. administration, until patient is stable. (Severe, life-threatening reactions may occur.)
• Assess I.V. site closely during and after I.V. administration. Know that sterile abscess, pain, or induration may occur at injection site.
• Evaluate neurologic status.
• Monitor CBC (including platelet count), calcium and potassium levels, and kidney and liver function tests.

Patient teaching

• Explain purpose of therapy. Stress importance of completing entire course of treatment.
◀€ Teach patient to recognize and immediately report serious cardiovascular and neurologic reactions,

abdominal pain, and easy bruising or bleeding.
• Teach patient how to use aerosol.
• Tell patient to notify prescriber if infection worsens.
• Advise patient to minimize GI upset by eating small, frequent servings of food and drinking plenty of fluids.
• Caution patient to avoid driving and other hazardous activities until he knows how drug affects concentration and alertness.
• As appropriate, review all other significant and life-threatening adverse reactions and interactions, especially those related to the tests mentioned above.

pentazocine lactate
Talwin

pentazocine hydrochloride and acetaminophen
Fortral ⊕

pentazocine hydrochloride and naloxone hydrochloride

Pharmacologic class: Opioid agonist-antagonist

Therapeutic class: Opioid analgesic, adjunct to anesthesia

Controlled substance schedule IV

Pregnancy risk category C

FDA **BOXED WARNING**

• When administering pentazocine hydrochloride and acetaminophen, be aware that acetaminophen has been associated with acute liver failure, at times resulting in liver transplant or death. Most of the cases of liver injury are associated with the use of acetaminophen at dosages that exceed

---

4,000 mg/day, and often involve more than one acetaminophen-containing product.

• Pentazocine and naloxone hydrochloride tablets are for oral use only. Severe, potentially lethal reactions may result from misuse by injection, alone or in combination with other substances.

Action
Unknown. Thought to interact with opioid receptor sites primarily in limbic system, thalamus, and spinal cord, blocking transmission of pain impulses.

Availability
Injection: 30 mg/ml (as lactate salt)
Tablets: 50 mg pentazocine and 0.5 mg naloxone (Talwin NX); 25 mg pentazocine and 650 mg acetaminophen (Talacen)

❶ Indications and dosages
➤ Moderate to severe pain; preoperative or preanesthetic medication; adjunct to surgical anesthesia
Adults: 30 mg subcutaneously, I.M., or I.V. q 3 to 4 hours (not to exceed 60 mg/dose subcutaneously or I.M., or 30 mg/dose I.V.). Maximum daily dosage is 360 mg.
➤ Moderate to severe pain
Adults: Initially, one tablet (Talwin Nx) q 3 to 4 hours, increased to two tablets p.r.n., up to a maximum of 12 tablets daily
➤ Mild to moderate pain
Adults: One tablet (Talacen) P.O. q 4 hours; up to a maximum of six tablets daily
➤ Labor
Adults: 20 mg I.V. for two or three doses at 2- to 3-hour intervals, or 30 mg I.M. as a single dose

Contraindications
• Hypersensitivity to drug, acetaminophen, or naloxone (with oral form)

Precautions
Use cautiously in:
• head trauma, increased intracranial pressure, respiratory conditions, adrenal insufficiency, seizure disorder, acute CNS manifestations, hepatic impairment, acute myocardial infarction, alcohol or narcotic use
• sulfite sensitivity (Talacen)
• history of drug abuse
• pregnant or breastfeeding patients
• children (safety not established).

Administration
• Administer each 5-mg I.V. dose by slow direct infusion over 1 minute, with patient lying supine.
• Use subcutaneous route only when necessary (may cause tissue damage).

Route	Onset	Peak	Duration
P.O. (Talwin NX)	15-30 min	1-3 hr	3 hr
P.O. (Talacen)	15-30 min	60-90 min	3 hr
I.V.	12-30 min	Unknown	3 hr
I.M., subcut.	15-20 min	15-60 min	3 hr

Adverse reactions
CNS: dizziness, drowsiness, euphoria, hallucinations, headache, sedation, dysphoria, insomnia, unusual dreams, weakness, depression, irritability, excitement, tremor, paresthesia
CV: hypertension, hypotension, syncope, tachycardia, **circulatory depression, shock**
EENT: blurred vision, diplopia, nystagmus, miosis (with high doses), tinnitus
GI: nausea, vomiting, constipation, diarrhea, dry mouth, ileus, cramps, abdominal distress, anorexia
GU: urinary retention, altered rate and strength of labor contractions

---

Hematologic: thrombocytopenia purpura (with Talacen)
Respiratory: dyspnea, transient apnea in neonates whose mothers received pentazocine during labor, **respiratory depression**
Skin: clammy skin, diaphoresis, rash, urticaria, nodules, cutaneous depression, skin and subcutaneous sclerosis, dermatitis, pruritus, flushing
Other: altered taste, chills, soft-tissue induration, stinging on injection, facial edema, physical or psychological drug dependence, drug tolerance, **anaphylaxis**

Interactions

Drug-drug. *Barbiturates, first-generation (sedating) antihistamines, other sedating drugs:* additive CNS depression
MAO inhibitors: unpredictable reactions
Opioids: decreased analgesic effects
Drug-diagnostic tests. *Amylase, lipase:* increased levels
Granulocytes, white blood cells: reduced counts
Drug-herbs. *Chamomile, hops, kava, skullcap, valerian:* increased CNS depression
Drug-behaviors. *Alcohol use:* increased CNS depression

Patient monitoring

◀⟨ Monitor vital signs. Watch closely for evidence of shock, dyspnea, and circulatory or respiratory depression.
• Monitor drug efficacy.
• In prolonged use, assess for signs and symptoms of drug dependence.

Patient teaching

◀⟨ Tell patient receiving Talacen or Talwin NX that drug is for oral use only. Life-threatening reactions may result from misusing drug by injection.
• Inform patient that withdrawal symptoms may occur if he stops taking drug suddenly after prolonged use.

• Urge patient to avoid alcohol.
• Advise patient to consult prescriber before taking other prescription drugs or over-the-counter preparations.
• Caution patient to avoid driving and other hazardous activities until he knows how drug affects him.
• Advise patient to have periodic eye exams.
• As appropriate, review all other significant and life-threatening adverse reactions and interactions, especially those related to the drugs, tests, herbs, and behaviors mentioned above.

pentobarbital sodium
Nembutal Sodium

Pharmacologic class: Barbiturate
Therapeutic class: Sedative-hypnotic, anticonvulsant
Controlled substance schedule II
Pregnancy risk category D

Action

Depresses sensory cortex, decreases motor activity, and alters cerebellar function; may interfere with nerve impulse transmission in brain

Availability

Injection: 50 mg/ml in 2-ml prefilled syringes

⟋ Indications and dosages

➤ Preoperative sedation
Adults: Initially, 150 to 200 mg I.M., or 100 mg I.V.
➤ Seizures
Adults: Initially, 100 mg. I.V.; may give additional doses after 1 minute. Maximum dosage is 500 mg.
Children: Initially, 50 mg. I.V.; may give additional doses until desired

P

Reactions in **bold** are life-threatening.   ◀⟨ Clinical alert

response occurs. Don't exceed 100 mg/dose.

Contraindications

- Hypersensitivity to drug or other barbiturates
- Nephritis (with large doses)
- Severe hepatic impairment
- Severe respiratory disease with dyspnea or obstruction
- Manifest or latent porphyria
- History of sedative-hypnotic abuse
- Subcutaneous or intra-arterial administration

Precautions

Use cautiously in:

- hepatic or renal impairment, increased risk for suicide, alcohol use
- history of drug addiction
- labor and delivery
- elderly or debilitated patients.

Administration

◀€ When giving I.V., make sure resuscitation equipment is available.
- Give I.V. by direct injection no faster than 50 mg/minute.
- Inject I.M. deep into large muscle mass.

◀€ Don't give by subcutaneous or intra-arterial routes, because severe reactions (such as tissue necrosis and gangrene) may occur.
- Know that drug is for short-term use only, losing efficacy after about 2 weeks.

Route	Onset	Peak	Duration
I.V.	Immediate	1 min	3-4 hr
I.M.	10-25 min	Unknown	3-4 hr

Adverse reactions

CNS: drowsiness, agitation, confusion, hyperkinesia, ataxia, nightmares, nervousness, hallucinations, insomnia, anxiety, abnormal thinking
CV: hypotension, syncope, **bradycardia** (all with I.V. use)

GI: nausea, vomiting, constipation
Hepatic: hepatic damage
Musculoskeletal: joint pain, myalgia, neuralgia
Respiratory: laryngospasm (with I.V. use), **bronchospasm, respiratory depression**
Skin: rash, urticaria, exfoliative dermatitis
Other: phlebitis at I.V. site, physical or psychological drug dependence, fever, hypersensitivity reactions including angioedema

Interactions

Drug-drug. *Acetaminophen:* increased risk of hepatotoxicity
Activated charcoal: decreased pentobarbital absorption
Anticoagulants, beta-adrenergic blockers (except timolol), carbamazepine, clonazepam, corticosteroids, digoxin, doxorubicin, doxycycline, felodipine, fenoprofen, griseofulvin, hormonal contraceptives, metronidazole, quinidine, theophylline, verapamil: decreased efficacy of these drugs
Antihistamines (first-generation), opioids, other sedative-hypnotics: additive CNS depression
Chloramphenicol, hydantoins, narcotics: increased or decreased effects of either drug
Divalproex, MAO inhibitors, valproic acid: decreased pentobarbital metabolism, increased sedation
Rifampin: increased pentobarbital metabolism and decreased effects
Drug-diagnostic tests. *Sulfobromophthalein:* false increase
Drug-herbs. *Chamomile, hops, kava, valerian, or skullcap:* increased CNS depression
St. John's wort: decreased pentobarbital effects
Drug-behaviors. *Alcohol use:* increased sedation, additive CNS depression

Patient monitoring
◀≶ Closely monitor blood pressure and heart and respiratory rates. Watch for evidence of respiratory depression.
• Monitor neurologic status before and during therapy.
• Assess CBC and kidney and liver function tests.
• In long-term therapy, monitor patient for signs of drug dependence.

Patient teaching
• Advise patient to avoid other CNS depressants, alcohol, and herbs.
• Caution patient to avoid driving and other hazardous activities.
• Advise patient taking hormonal contraceptives to use alternate birth-control method during therapy.
• As appropriate, review all other significant and life-threatening adverse reactions and interactions, especially those related to the drugs, tests, herbs, and behaviors mentioned above.

---

pentostatin
Nipent

Pharmacologic class: Antimetabolite
Therapeutic class: Antineoplastic
Pregnancy risk category D

FDA BOXED WARNING

• Give under supervision of physician experienced in cancer chemotherapy, in facility with adequate diagnostic and treatment resources.
• Use of higher dosages than those specified isn't recommended, as dose-limiting severe renal, liver, pulmonary, and CNS toxicities may occur.
• In study of patients with refractory chronic lymphocytic leukemia receiving drug at recommended dosage in combination with fludarabine, four of six patients had severe or fatal pulmonary toxicity. Use in combination with fludarabine isn't recommended.

Action
Unknown. Thought to inhibit adenosine deaminase, thereby increasing levels of deoxyadenosine triphosphate in cells, blocking DNA synthesis, and inhibiting ribonucleotide reductase.

Availability
Powder for injection: 10-mg vials

 Indications and dosages
➢ Hairy cell leukemia
Adults: 4 mg/m² I.V. every other week

Contraindications
• Hypersensitivity to drug

Precautions
Use cautiously in:
• renal disease, bone marrow depression
• pregnant or breastfeeding patients
• children.

Administration
• Before giving, hydrate patient with 500 to 1,000 ml of dextrose 5% and normal saline solution (or its equivalent). After administering, give 500 ml of dextrose 5% in water (D₅W) or its equivalent.
◀≶ Follow facility protocol for handling, administering, and disposing of chemotherapeutic drugs.
• Give by direct I.V. bolus injection or dilute with 25 to 50 ml of D₅W or normal saline solution; infuse over 20 to 30 minutes.

Route	Onset	Peak	Duration
I.V.	Unknown	Unknown	Unknown

Adverse reactions
CNS: headache, malaise, anxiety, confusion, depression, dizziness, insomnia,

---

nervousness, paresthesia, drowsiness, abnormal thinking, fatigue, asthenia, hallucinations, hostility, amnesia
CV: peripheral edema, cellulitis, vasculitis, hypotension, angina, tachycardia, bradycardia, phlebitis, **thrombophlebitis, cardiac arrest, heart failure, hemorrhage, ventricular asystole, pericardial effusion, sinus arrest**
EENT: abnormal vision, nonreactive pupils, photophobia, retinopathy, eye pain, conjunctivitis, dry or watery eyes, hearing loss, tinnitus, ear pain, epistaxis, pharyngitis, rhinitis
GI: nausea, vomiting, diarrhea, constipation, dyspepsia, abdominal pain, ileus, flatulence, stomatitis, glossitis, anorexia
GU: amenorrhea, breast lump, erectile dysfunction, decreased libido, renal calculi, **renal dysfunction, renal insufficiency, renal failure**
Hematologic: ecchymosis, anemia, **hemolytic anemia, agranulocytosis, aplastic anemia, leukopenia, thrombocytopenia**
Metabolic: hyperuricemia, hypercalcemia, hyponatremia
Musculoskeletal: myalgia, joint pain
Respiratory: cough, dyspnea, respiratory tract infection, **pulmonary embolism**
Skin: rash, eczema, petechiae, dry skin, pruritus, skin disorder, furunculosis, acne, alopecia, diaphoresis, photosensitivity
Other: unusual taste, gingivitis, fever, chills, pain, facial edema, lymphadenopathy, herpes simplex or herpes zoster infection, flulike symptoms, viral or bacterial infection, allergic reaction, **sepsis, neoplasm**

Interactions
Drug-drug. *Allopurinol:* hypersensitivity vasculitis
Carmustine, cyclophosphamide, etoposide: potentially fatal acute pulmonary edema and hypotension

Fludarabine: severe or fatal pulmonary toxicity
Vidarabine: increased risk and severity of adverse reactions
Drug-diagnostic tests. *Calcium, liver function tests, serum uric acid:* increased values
Granulocytes, platelets, sodium, white blood cells: decreased levels

Patient monitoring
◀€ Monitor CBC (including platelet count). Watch for evidence of blood dyscrasias.
• Assess kidney and liver function tests. Stay alert for evidence of organ dysfunction.
• Monitor temperature. Watch for signs and symptoms of bacterial and viral infection.
• Closely monitor vital signs and ECG, particularly for life-threatening arrhythmias, heart failure, and pulmonary edema.

Patient teaching
◀€ Tell patient drug lowers resistance to infection. Instruct him to avoid crowds and to immediately report fever, cough, sore throat, and other infection symptoms.
• Advise patient to minimize GI upset by eating small, frequent servings of food and drinking plenty of fluids.
• Instruct female patient of childbearing age to avoid pregnancy during drug therapy and to seek medical advice before becoming pregnant.
• Caution patient to avoid driving and other hazardous activities until he knows how drug affects concentration and alertness.
• As appropriate, review all other significant and life-threatening adverse reactions and interactions, especially those related to the drugs and tests mentioned above.

pentoxifylline

Apo-Pentoxiphylline, Neotren ✚,
Pentoxil, Pentoxiphylline ✿,
Pentoxiphylline SR ✿, Trental

Pharmacologic class: Hemorrheologic,
xanthine derivative
Therapeutic class: Hematologic agent
Pregnancy risk category C

Action

Unknown. Thought to enhance blood
flow to the circulatory system by
increasing vasoconstriction and oxygen concentrations.

Availability

*Tablets (controlled-release, extended-
release):* 400 mg

💋 Indications and dosages

➤ Intermittent claudication
Adults: 400 mg t.i.d. If adverse reactions occur, decrease to 400 mg b.i.d.

Dosage adjustment

• Renal impairment

Off-label uses

• Diabetic angiopathies and
neuropathies
• Transient ischemic attacks
• Severe idiopathic recurrent aphthous
stomatitis
• Raynaud's phenomenon

Contraindications

• Hypersensitivity to drug or methylxanthines (such as caffeine, theophylline, theobromine)
• Recent cerebral or retinal hemorrhage

Precautions

Use cautiously in:
• patients at risk for bleeding
• pregnant or breastfeeding patients
• children (safety not established).

Administration

• Give with meals to minimize GI
distress.
• Make sure patient swallows tablets
whole without crushing, breaking, or
chewing.

Route	Onset	Peak	Duration
P.O.	Variable	2-4 hr	8 hr

Adverse reactions

CNS: agitation, dizziness, drowsiness,
headache, insomnia, nervousness,
tremor, anxiety, confusion, malaise
CV: angina, edema, hypotension,
arrhythmias
EENT: blurred vision, epistaxis, laryngitis, nasal congestion, sore throat
GI: nausea, vomiting, constipation,
diarrhea, abdominal discomfort, belching, bloating, dyspepsia, flatus, cholecystitis, dry mouth, excessive salivation, anorexia
Hematologic: leukopenia
Respiratory: dyspnea
Skin: rash, urticaria, pruritus, brittle
fingernails, flushing, angioedema
Other: bad taste, weight changes,
thirst, flulike symptoms, lymphadenopathy

Interactions

Drug-drug. *Anticoagulants, nonsteroidal anti-inflammatory drugs
(NSAIDs):* increased risk of bleeding
Antihypertensives: additive hypotension
Theobromide, theophylline: increased
risk of theophylline toxicity
Drug-herbs. *Anise, arnica, asafetida,
chamomile, clove, dong quai, fenugreek, feverfew, garlic, ginger, ginkgo,
ginseng, licorice:* increased risk of
bleeding
Drug-behaviors. *Smoking:* decreased
pentoxifylline efficacy

p

Patient monitoring

- Monitor vital signs and cardiovascular status. Watch for arrhythmias, angina, edema, and hypotension.
- Frequently monitor prothrombin time and International Normalized Ratio in patients receiving warfarin concurrently.
- Assess theophylline level in patients receiving theophylline-containing drugs concurrently.

Patient teaching

- Instruct patient to take with meals and to swallow tablets whole without crushing, breaking, or chewing.
- 🔊 Inform patient that drug can cause serious adverse effects. Instruct him to immediately report chest pain, swelling, and flulike symptoms.
- Tell patient smoking may make drug less effective and that many over-the-counter preparations (including aspirin, NSAIDs, and herbs) increase risk of bleeding.
- As appropriate, review all other significant and life-threatening adverse reactions and interactions, especially those related to the drugs, herbs, and behaviors mentioned above.

perindopril erbumine
Aceon, Apo-Perindopril✦, Coversyl✛

Pharmacologic class: Angiotensin-converting enzyme (ACE) inhibitor
Therapeutic class: Antihypertensive
Pregnancy risk category D

FDA | BOXED WARNING

- Drugs that act directly on the renin-angiotensin system can cause injury to or death of a developing fetus. Discontinue drug as soon as possible when pregnancy is detected.

Action

Inhibits conversion of angiotensin I to angiotensin II (a potent vasoconstrictor). This effect leads to decreased plasma angiotensin II, reduced vasoconstriction, enhanced plasma renin activity, and decreased aldosterone activity.

Availability

Tablets: 2 mg, 4 mg, 8 mg

🚫 Indications and dosages

➤ Essential hypertension
Adults: 4 mg P.O. daily; may titrate upward to 16 mg/day, given as a single dose or in two divided doses. (Start with 2 to 4 mg/day in patients receiving diuretics.)
➤ Coronary artery disease
Adults: Initially, 4 mg P.O. daily for 2 weeks; then increase as tolerated to a maintenance dosage of 8 mg P.O. daily.

Dosage adjustment

- Renal impairment
- Elderly patients

Off-label uses

- Heart failure
- Diabetic nephropathy

Contraindications

- Hypersensitivity to drug or other ACE inhibitors
- Hereditary or idiopathic angioedema

Precautions

Use cautiously in:
- hepatic failure, renal impairment, renal artery stenosis, hyperkalemia, cough
- black patients
- pregnant or breastfeeding patients
- children (safety not established).

Administration

- Give without regard to food.
- 🔊 Know that drug (especially first dose) may cause angioedema. Keep

epinephrine and antihistamines at hand in case of airway obstruction.
• For elderly patient, titrate dosage upward very slowly.
• Know that drug may be given alone or with other drugs.

Route	Onset	Peak	Duration
P.O.	1 hr	3-7 hr	12-24 hr

Adverse reactions

CNS: dizziness, fatigue, headache, insomnia, sleep disorder, weakness, asthenia, drowsiness, vertigo, depression, paresthesia

CV: hypotension, angina pectoris, palpitations, chest pain, abnormal ECG, tachycardia

EENT: ear infection, sinusitis, rhinitis, pharyngitis

GI: nausea, vomiting, diarrhea, abdominal pain, flatulence

GU: proteinuria, urinary tract infection, erectile or other male sexual dysfunction, decreased libido, menstrual disorder

Metabolic: hyperkalemia

Musculoskeletal: back, arm, leg, neck, or joint pain; hypertonia; myalgia; arthritis

Respiratory: cough, upper respiratory infection

Skin: rash, **angioedema**

Other: fever, viral infection, edema

Interactions

Drug-drug.
Antihypertensives, general anesthetics, nitrates, phenothiazines: additive hypotension
Diuretics: excessive hypotension
Gold (sodium aurothiomalate): increased risk of rare nitritoid reactions (including facial flushing, nausea, vomiting, and hypotension)
Lithium: increased lithium toxicity
Nonsteroidal anti-inflammatory drugs: may result in deterioration of renal function, including acute renal failure

and attenuated ACE inhibitor antihypertensive effect
Potassium-sparing diuretics, potassium supplements: increased risk of hyperkalemia

Drug-diagnostic tests. *Alanine aminotransferase, aspartate aminotransferase, blood urea nitrogen, creatinine, potassium, triglycerides:* increased levels
Hematocrit, hemoglobin: decreased values

Drug-food. *Salt substitutes containing potassium:* hyperkalemia

Drug-herbs. *Capsaicin:* cough

Drug-behaviors. *Acute alcohol ingestion:* additive hypotension

Patient monitoring

• Assess blood pressure. Be aware that dosage increases or concomitant diuretic use may cause severe hypotension.

◀╪ Watch for angioedema, especially after first dose.

• Stay alert for signs and symptoms of infection, particularly EENT and respiratory infections.

• Monitor potassium level. Watch for signs and symptoms of hyperkalemia.

• Monitor liver and kidney function tests before and during therapy.

◀╪ In black patients, watch closely for angioedema and monitor drug efficacy. Monotherapy may be less effective in these patients.

Patient teaching

• Tell patient to take at same time each day, with or without food.

◀╪ Instruct patient to stop using drug and contact prescriber immediately if hoarseness or difficulty swallowing or breathing occurs.

• Tell patient to avoid excessive perspiration or decreased fluid intake, which may cause symptomatic blood pressure drop. Inform him that vomiting or diarrhea also may lower blood pressure.

• Tell patient to report signs and symptoms of infection.

p

Reactions in **bold** are life-threatening.   ◀╪ Clinical alert

• Advise patient not to use potassium-containing salt substitutes.

◀€ Caution female patient of childbearing age to contact prescriber immediately if she suspects pregnancy.

• As appropriate, review all other significant and life-threatening adverse reactions and interactions, especially those related to the drugs, tests, foods, herbs, and behaviors mentioned above.

---

perphenazine
Apo-Perphenazine✻, Fentazin⊕

Pharmacologic class: Phenothiazine, dopaminergic antagonist
Therapeutic class: Antipsychotic, antiemetic
Pregnancy risk category NR

Action
Unknown. Thought to antagonize dopamine and serotonin type 2 in CNS. Also antagonizes muscarinic receptors in respiratory tract, causing cholinergic activation.

Availability
Tablets: 2 mg, 4 mg, 8 mg, 16 mg

🚫 Indications and dosages
➣ Schizophrenia in nonhospitalized patients
Adults and children older than age 12: Initially, 4 to 8 mg P.O. t.i.d.
➣ Schizophrenia in hospitalized patients
Adults and children older than age 12: Initially, 8 to 16 mg P.O. two to four times daily, increased p.r.n.; avoid dosages greater than 64 mg daily.
➣ Severe nausea and vomiting
Adults: 8 to 16 mg P.O. daily in divided doses, to a maximum of 24 mg.

Off-label uses
• Intractable hiccups

Contraindications
• Hypersensitivity to drug, its components, or related compounds
• Blood dyscrasias
• Bone marrow depression
• Hepatic damage
• Subcortical damage
• Coma
• Concurrent use of high-dose CNS depressants

Precautions
Use cautiously in:
• respiratory disorders, hepatic or renal dysfunction, breast cancer, alcohol withdrawal symptoms, suicidal tendency, surgery
• patients taking CNS depressants or anticholinergics
• elderly patients
• pregnant or breastfeeding patients
• children younger than age 12.

Administration
• Give with food to avoid GI upset.

Route	Onset	Peak	Duration
P.O.	Variable	1-3 hours	Unknown

Adverse reactions
CNS: drowsiness, dizziness, insomnia, vertigo, headache, hyperactivity, nocturnal confusion, bizarre dreams, tremor, ataxia, slurring, exacerbation of psychotic symptoms, paranoid reactions, parkinsonism, dystonias, akathisia, tardive dyskinesia, hyperreflexia, cerebrospinal fluid abnormality, catatonic-like state, paradoxical stimulation, **seizures, neuroleptic malignant syndrome**
CV: hypotension, orthostatic hypotension, hypertension, peripheral edema, ECG changes, tachycardia, bradycardia, **cardiac arrest, heart failure**
EENT: glaucoma, blurred vision, miosis, mydriasis, corneal and lens deposits, pigmentary retinopathy, oculogyric

---

crisis, photophobia, nasal congestion, dysphagia
GI: nausea, vomiting, diarrhea, constipation, obstipation, abnormal tongue color or movement, dry mouth, anorexia, **adynamic ileus**
GU: dark urine, urinary retention, urinary frequency, urinary incontinence, bladder paralysis, galactorrhea, lactation, breast enlargement, menstrual irregularities, inhibited ejaculation, libido changes
Hematologic: hemolytic anemia, leukopenia, agranulocytosis, thrombocytopenic purpura
Hepatic: jaundice, biliary stasis
Metabolic: hyponatremia, glycosuria, hyperglycemia, **hypoglycemia, syndrome of inappropriate antidiuretic hormone secretion, pituitary tumor**
Musculoskeletal: numbness and aching of arms and legs
Respiratory: dyspnea, suppressed cough reflex, **asthma, bronchospasm, laryngospasm, laryngeal edema**
Skin: urticaria, pallor, erythema, eczema, pruritus, perspiration, pigmentation changes, photosensitivity, angioedema, exfoliative dermatitis
Other: increased appetite, weight gain, fever, systemic lupus erythematosus-like syndrome, hypersensitivity reactions including **anaphylactoid reaction**

Interactions

Drug-drug. *Anticholinergics:* increased risk of adverse anticholinergic reactions
CNS depressants: increased perphenazine effects, increased adverse CNS reactions
Tricyclic antidepressants: increased perphenazine blood level, greater risk of adverse reactions
Drug-diagnostic tests. *Eosinophils, liver function tests:* increased values
Glucose: increased or decreased level
Granulocytes, hemoglobin, platelets, sodium, white blood cells: decreased levels

Pregnancy test: false-positive result
Drug-herbs. *Kava:* dystonic reactions
St. John's wort: photosensitivity
Yohimbe: yohimbe toxicity
Drug-behaviors. *Alcohol use:* increased CNS depression
Sun exposure: increased risk of photosensitivity reaction

Patient monitoring

◀€ Watch for anaphylactoid reaction and angioedema. Monitor neurologic status; stay alert for signs and symptoms of neuroleptic malignant syndrome (high fever, unstable blood pressure, stupor, muscle rigidity, autonomic dysfunction), parkinsonian symptoms, and catatonic-like state.
• Monitor cardiovascular status and vital signs periodically.
◀€ Evaluate respiratory status, especially for dyspnea and airway spasm.
◀€ Monitor CBC, glucose level, and liver function tests. Watch for evidence of blood dyscrasias.

Patient teaching

• Explain importance of combining drug therapy with psychotherapy.
• Tell patient to take exactly as prescribed and to report adverse reactions promptly.
• Instruct patient to avoid sun exposure and to wear sunscreen outdoors to prevent photosensitivity reaction.
• Advise patient to consult prescriber before taking other prescription drugs or over-the-counter preparations.
• Caution patient to avoid driving and other hazardous activities until he knows how drug affects him.
• Instruct patient to avoid alcohol, smoking, caffeine, and herbs.
• As appropriate, review all other significant and life-threatening adverse reactions and interactions, especially those related to the drugs, tests, herbs, and behaviors mentioned above.

p

pertuzumab
Perjeta

Pharmacologic class: Recombinant humanized monoclonal antibody

Therapeutic class: Antineoplastic

Pregnancy risk category D

FDA | BOXED WARNING

• Exposure to pertuzumab can result in embryo-fetal death and birth defects. Studies in animals have resulted in oligohydramnios, delayed renal development, and death. Advise patients of these risks and the need for effective contraception.

Action
Targets the extracellular dimerization domain (Subdomain II) of the human epidermal growth factor receptor (EGRF) 2 protein (HER2) and thereby blocks ligand-dependent heterodimerization of HER2 with other HER family members, including EGRF, HER3, and HER4. As a result, pertuzumab inhibits ligand-initiated intracellular signaling through two major signal pathways, mitogen-activated protein kinase and phosphoinositide 3-kinase. Inhibition of these signaling pathways can result in cell growth arrest and apoptosis, respectively. In addition, pertuzumab mediates antibody-dependent cell-mediated cytotoxicity.

Availability
Solution for injection: 420 mg/14-ml single-use vial

🛈 Indications and dosages
➢ HER2-positive metastatic breast cancer in patients who have not received prior anti-HER2 therapy or chemotherapy for metastatic disease

Adults: Initially, 840 mg by 60-minute I.V. infusion, followed by 420 mg over 30 to 60 minutes by I.V. infusion q 3 weeks thereafter. When administered with trastuzumab, recommended initial dose of trastuzumab is 8 mg/kg by 90-minute I.V. infusion, followed by 6 mg/kg over 30 to 90 minutes by I.V. infusion q 3 weeks thereafter. When administered with docetaxel, recommended initial dose of docetaxel is 75 mg/m^2 by I.V. infusion; may escalate to 100 mg/m^2 q 3 weeks if initial dose is well tolerated.

Dosage adjustment
• Left ventricular ejection fraction (LVEF) less than 40% or LVEF of 40% to 45% with a 10% or greater absolute decrease below pretreatment values

Contraindications
None

Precautions
Use cautiously in:
• pregnant and breastfeeding patients
• children (safety and efficacy not established).

Administration
• Be aware that HER2 testing should be performed for selection of patients appropriate for treatment with this drug.
• Assess LVEF before starting drug.
• Verify pregnancy status before starting drug.
🔊 Administer as an I.V. infusion only. Don't give as an I.V. push or bolus.
• Withdraw appropriate volume of drug solution from vial(s). Dilute in a 250-ml normal saline solution-in only PVC or non-PVC polyolefin infusion bag. Mix diluted solution by gentle inversion. Don't shake and don't mix with other drugs. Don't use dextrose (5%) solution.
• Administer immediately once prepared. If diluted infusion solution isn't

---

used immediately, it can be stored at 2° C to 8° C (36° F to 46° F) for up to 24 hours.

◀€ Observe patient closely for 60 minutes after first infusion. If significant infusion-associated reaction occurs, slow or interrupt infusion and administer appropriate medical therapies. Discontinue drug immediately if patient develops a serous hypersensitivity reaction.

• Be aware that drug should be withheld or discontinued if trastuzumab treatment is withheld or discontinued. If docetaxel is discontinued, treatment with pertuzumab and trastuzumab may continue.

• Be aware that pertuzumab dosage reductions aren't recommended.

Route	Onset	Peak	Duration
I.V.	Unknown	Unknown	Unknown

Adverse reactions

CNS: headache, dizziness, fatigue, peripheral neuropathy, asthenia, insomnia
CV: left ventricular dysfunction
EENT: increased lacrimation, nasopharyngitis
GI: nausea, vomiting, diarrhea, constipation, stomatitis
Hematologic: anemia, leukopenia, neutropenia, **febrile neutropenia**
Musculoskeletal: myalgia, arthralgia
Respiratory: upper respiratory tract infection, dyspnea, **pleural effusion**
Skin: alopecia, rash, nail disorder, pruritus, dry skin, paronychia
Other: mucosal inflammation, pyrexia, dysgeusia, decreased appetite, peripheral edema, **infusion and hypersensitivity reactions including anaphylaxis**

Interactions
None

Patient monitoring
◀€ Closely monitor patient for 30 minutes after each subsequent infusion for infusion and hypersensitivity reactions. If a significant infusion-associated reaction occurs, slow or interrupt infusion and administer appropriate medical therapies. Monitor patients carefully until complete resolution of signs and symptoms. Consider permanent discontinuation in patients with severe infusion reactions.

◀€ Continue to assess LVEF at regular intervals (every 3 months) during treatment to ensure LVEF is within institution's normal limits. If LVEF is less than 40%, or is 40% to 45% with a 10% or greater absolute decrease below pretreatment value, withhold pertuzumab and trastuzumab and repeat LVEF assessment within approximately 3 weeks. Discontinue pertuzumab and trastuzumab if LVEF hasn't improved or has declined further, unless benefits to patient outweigh risks.

• Monitor women who become pregnant during pertuzumab therapy for oligohydramnios. If oligohydramnios occurs, perform fetal testing appropriate for gestational age and consistent with community standards of care.

Patient teaching
◀€ Tell patient to immediately report fever, chills, fatigue, headache, vomiting, weakness, rash, muscle pain, leg swelling, or shortness of breath.

• Advise female patient of childbearing potential to use effective contraception while receiving this drug and for 6 months after last dose.

• Advise breastfeeding patient that she should decide whether to discontinue breastfeeding or discontinue drug, taking into account importance of drug for her treatment.

• As appropriate, review all other significant and life-threatening adverse reactions mentioned above.

p

Reactions in **bold** are life-threatening.   ◀€ Clinical alert

phenazopyridine hydrochloride

AZO-Gesic, Azo-Standard, Baridium, Phenazo ✳, Prodium, Pyridium, ReAzo, UTI Relief

Pharmacologic class: Nonopioid analgesic
Therapeutic class: Urinary analgesic
Pregnancy risk category B

Action

Unknown. Thought to act locally on urinary tract mucosa to produce analgesic or anesthetic effects, relieving urinary burning, urgency, and frequency.

Availability

Tablets: 95 mg, 97.2 mg, 100 mg, 200 mg

Indications and dosages

➣ Pain caused by lower urinary tract irritation
Adults: 200 mg P.O. t.i.d.
Children: 12 mg/kg P.O. daily in three divided doses

Contraindications

• Hypersensitivity to drug
• Renal insufficiency

Precautions

Use cautiously in:
• hepatitis
• pregnant or breastfeeding patients
• children younger than age 12.

Administration

• Give with or after meals.
• Discontinue after 2 days, as prescribed, when administering with antibiotics.

Route	Onset	Peak	Duration
P.O.	Unknown	Unknown	6-8 hr

Adverse reactions

CNS: headache
EENT: contact lens staining
GI: GI disturbances
GU: bright orange urine, **renal toxicity**
Hepatic: hepatotoxicity
Hematologic: hemolytic anemia, methemoglobinemia
Skin: rash, pruritus
Other: anaphylactoid-like reaction

Interactions

Drug-diagnostic tests. *Bilirubin, glucose, ketones, protein, steroids:* interference with urine tests based on spectrophotometry or color reactions

Patient monitoring

• Monitor patient for symptomatic improvement of urinary tract infection (UTI).
• Assess follow-up urine culture after antibiotic therapy ends.
◀▌ Monitor for yellowing of skin or sclera. This change may indicate drug accumulation caused by impaired renal excretion, warranting drug withdrawal.

Patient teaching

• Explain drug therapy and measures to help prevent UTI recurrence.
• Tell patient drug may discolor urine and tears and may stain clothing and contact lenses.
◀▌ Advise patient to contact prescriber promptly if symptoms don't improve or if skin or eyes become yellow.
• As appropriate, review all other significant and life-threatening adverse reactions and interactions, especially those related to the tests mentioned above.

phenobarbital
PMS-Phenobarbital, Solfoton

phenobarbital sodium
Luminal Sodium

Pharmacologic class: Barbiturate
Therapeutic class: Anxiolytic, anticonvulsant, sedative-hypnotic
Controlled substance schedule IV
Pregnancy risk category D

Action
Interferes with gamma-aminobutyric acid receptors, blocking nerve impulse transmission in CNS, which reduces motor activity and raises seizure threshold

Availability
Capsules: 16 mg
Elixir: 15 mg/5 ml, 20 mg/5 ml
Injection: 30 mg/ml and 60 mg/ml in 1-ml prefilled syringes; 65 mg/ml in 1-ml vials; 130 mg/ml in 1-ml prefilled syringes, 1-ml vials, and 1-ml ampules
Tablets: 15 mg, 16 mg, 30 mg, 60 mg, 90 mg, 100 mg

⊘ Indications and dosages
➤ Tonic-clonic (grand mal) and partial seizures; febrile seizures in children
Adults: 60 to 100 mg/day P.O. as a single dose or in two or three divided doses; or initially, 100 to 320 mg I.V. p.r.n. (a total of 600 mg I.V. in a 24-hour period).
Infants and children: Loading dose of 15 to 20 mg/kg P.O. (produces drug blood level of 20 mcg/ml shortly after dosing). To achieve therapeutic blood level (10 to 25 mcg/ml), children usually need higher dosage/kg than adults. Follow loading dose with 3 to 6 mg/kg/day P.O. Alternatively, 4 to 6 mg/kg/day I.M. or I.V. for 7 to 10 days to achieve blood level of 10 to 15 mcg/ml.
➤ Status epilepticus
Adults: 200 to 320 mg I.M. or I.V., repeated q 6 hours p.r.n.
Children: 15 to 20 mg/kg I.V. given over 10 to 15 minutes
➤ Sedation or hypnotic effect
Adults: For sedation, 30 to 120 mg/day P.O. or 30 to 120 mg/day I.M. or I.V. in two or three divided doses. As a hypnotic, 100 to 200 mg P.O. or 100 to 320 mg I.M. or I.V. at bedtime. Don't exceed 400 mg in a 24-hour period.
➤ Preoperative sedation
Adults: 100 to 200 mg I.M. 60 to 90 minutes before surgery
Children: 1 to 3 mg/kg I.M. or I.V., as prescribed.

Dosage adjustment
• Impaired hepatic or renal function
• Elderly or debilitated patients

Off-label uses
• Prevention and treatment of hyperbilirubinemia

Contraindications
• Hypersensitivity to drug or other barbiturates
• Manifest or latent porphyria
• Nephritis (with large doses)
• Severe respiratory disease with dyspnea or obstruction
• History of sedative-hypnotic abuse
• Subcutaneous or intra-arterial administration

Precautions
Use cautiously in:
• hepatic dysfunction, renal impairment, seizure disorder, fever, hyperthyroidism, diabetes mellitus, severe anemia, pulmonary or cardiac disease
• history of suicide attempt or drug abuse
• chronic phenobarbital use
• elderly or debilitated patients

Reactions in **bold** are life-threatening. ◀€ Clinical alert

- pregnant or breastfeeding patients
- children younger than age 6.

Administration

- Inject I.M. deep into large muscle mass; limit volume to 5 ml.
- 🔊 Give I.V. no faster than 60 mg/minute. Keep resuscitation equipment at hand.
- Stop injection immediately if patient complains of pain or if circulation at injection site diminishes (indicating inadvertent intra-arterial injection).
- 🔊 Don't give by subcutaneous route; severe reactions (such as pain and tissue necrosis) may occur.
- 🔊 Know that when given I.V. for status epilepticus, drug may take 15 minutes to attain peak blood level in brain. If injected continuously until seizures stop, drug brain level would keep rising and could exceed that required to control seizures. To avoid barbiturate-induced depression, use minimal amount required and wait for anticonvulsant effect to occur before giving second dose.
- Use parenteral route only when patient can't receive drug P.O.
- Know that drug is intended only for short-term use, losing efficacy after about 2 weeks.

Route	Onset	Peak	Duration
P.O.	30-60 min	Unknown	10-16 hr
I.V.	5 min	30 min	10-16 hr
I.M.	10-30 min	Unknown	10-16 hr

Adverse reactions

CNS: headache, dizziness, anxiety, depression, drowsiness, excitation, delirium, lethargy, agitation, confusion, hyperkinesia, ataxia, vertigo, nightmares, nervousness, paradoxical stimulation, abnormal thinking, hallucinations, insomnia, CNS depression
CV: hypotension, syncope, **bradycardia** (with I.V. use)
GI: nausea, vomiting, constipation

Hematologic: megaloblastic anemia
Hepatic: hepatic damage
Musculoskeletal: joint pain, myalgia
Respiratory: hypoventilation, **laryngospasm, bronchospasm, apnea** (with I.V. use); **respiratory depression**
Skin: rash, urticaria, exfoliative dermatitis, **Stevens-Johnson syndrome**
Other: phlebitis at I.V. site, drug dependence, hypersensitivity reactions including angioedema

Interactions

Drug-drug. *Acetaminophen:* increased risk of hepatotoxicity
Activated charcoal: decreased phenobarbital absorption
Anticoagulants, beta-adrenergic blockers (except timolol), carbamazepine, clonazepam, corticosteroids, digoxin, doxorubicin, doxycycline, felodipine, fenoprofen, griseofulvin, hormonal contraceptives, metronidazole, quinidine, theophylline, verapamil: decreased efficacy of these drugs
Chloramphenicol, hydantoins, narcotics: increased or decreased effects of either drug
Cyclophosphamide: increased risk of hematologic toxicity
Divalproex, MAO inhibitors, valproic acid: decreased phenobarbital metabolism, increased sedative effect
Other CNS depressants (including first-generation antihistamines, opioids, other sedative-hypnotics): additive CNS depression
Rifampin: increased phenobarbital metabolism and decreased effects
Drug-diagnostic tests. *Bilirubin:* decreased level in neonates and patients with seizure disorders or congenital nonhemolytic unconjugated hyperbilirubinemia
Drug-herbs. *Chamomile, hops, kava, skullcap, valerian:* increased CNS depression
St. John's wort: decreased drug effects

Drug-behaviors. *Alcohol use:* additive CNS effects

Patient monitoring

• Monitor vital signs; watch for brady-cardia and hypotension.

◀≋ In patients with seizure disorders, know that drug withdrawal may cause status epilepticus.

• Assess neurologic status. Institute safety measures as needed.

◀≋ Closely monitor respiratory status, especially for respiratory depression and airway spasm.

• Monitor phenobarbital blood level, CBC, and kidney and liver function tests.

• Watch for signs of drug dependence.

Patient teaching

◀≋ Instruct patient to promptly report rash, facial and lip edema, syncope, dyspnea, or depression.

◀≋ Stress importance of taking exactly as prescribed, with or without food. Caution patient not to stop therapy abruptly, especially if he's taking drug for seizures.

• Tell patient that prolonged use may lead to dependence.

• Instruct patient to seek medical advice before taking other prescription or over-the-counter drugs.

• Caution patient to avoid driving and other hazardous activities until he knows how drug affects him.

• Advise patient to avoid herbs, alcohol, and other CNS depressants.

• Instruct patient taking hormonal contraceptives to use alternate birth-control method.

• As appropriate, review all other significant and life-threatening adverse reactions and interactions, especially those related to the drugs, tests, herbs, and behaviors mentioned above.

phentolamine mesylate
Rogitine ✦ ⊕

Pharmacologic class: Alpha-adrenergic blocker

Therapeutic class: Diagnostic agent, antihypertensive agent in pheochromocytoma

Pregnancy risk category C

Action

Competitively blocks postsynaptic (alpha$_1$) and presynaptic (alpha$_2$) adrenergic receptors. Acts on arterial tree and venous bed, reducing total peripheral resistance and lowering venous return to heart.

Availability
Powder for injection: 5 mg

🚫 Indications and dosages

➤ To prevent or control hypertensive episodes before or during pheochromocytomectomy

Adults: 5 mg I.V. or I.M. 1 to 2 hours before surgery, then 5 mg I.V. during surgery as indicated

Children: 1 mg I.V. or I.M. 1 to 2 hours before surgery, then 1 mg I.V. during surgery as indicated

➤ To aid pheochromocytoma diagnosis

Adults: 2.5 or 5 mg (in 1 ml of sterile water) by I.V. injection; record blood pressure q 30 seconds for 3 minutes, then q minute for next 7 minutes. Or 5 mg (in 1 ml sterile water) I.M.; record blood pressure q 5 minutes for 30 to 45 minutes.

➤ To prevent or treat dermal necrosis after norepinephrine extravasation

Adults: For prevention, add 10 mg to each liter of I.V. solution containing norepinephrine. For treatment, inject 5 to 10 mg in 10 ml of normal saline

p

solution into extravasated area within 12 hours.

Off-label uses
• Hypertensive crisis caused by MAO inhibitors
• Rebound hypertension caused by withdrawal of clonidine, propranolol, or other antihypertensives
• Erectile dysfunction (given with papaverine)

Contraindications
• Hypersensitivity to drug
• Coronary artery disease
• Myocardial infarction (MI) or history of MI
• Coronary insufficiency
• Angina

Precautions
Use cautiously in:
• patients receiving cardiac glycosides concurrently
• pregnant or breastfeeding patients.

Administration
• Reconstitute powder by diluting with 1 ml of sterile water for injection.
• For pheochromocytoma diagnosis, withhold sedatives, analgesics, and nonessential drugs for 24 to 72 hours before test (until hypertension returns). Keep patient supine until blood pressure stabilizes; then rapidly inject drug I.V. Maximum effect usually occurs within 2 minutes of dosing.

Route	Onset	Peak	Duration
I.V., I.M.	Immediate	Unknown	Brief

Adverse reactions
CNS: weakness, dizziness
CV: tachycardia, acute and prolonged hypotension, orthostatic hypotension, **arrhythmias**

EENT: nasal congestion
GI: nausea, vomiting, diarrhea
Skin: flushing

Interactions
Drug-drug. *Ephedrine, epinephrine:* antagonism of these drugs' effects
Drug-herbs. *Ephedra (ma huang):* antagonism of vasoconstrictive effects

Patient monitoring
• When using for norepinephrine extravasation, monitor injection site closely and assess blood pressure, heart rate, and respiratory rate.
• For pheochromocytoma diagnosis, monitor blood pressure. In pheochromocytoma, systolic and diastolic pressures drop immediately and steeply. Monitor and record blood pressure immediately after injection, at 30-second intervals for first 3 minutes, and at 1-minute intervals for next 7 minutes. Systolic decrease of 60 mmHg and diastolic decrease of 25 mmHg within 2 minutes after I.V. administration indicates a positive reaction for pheochromocytoma.

Patient teaching
• Explain drug administration procedure.
◀€ Instruct patient to promptly report adverse reactions. Assure him he'll be monitored closely.
• Tell patient to withhold other drugs (especially sedatives and analgesics) for at least 24 hours before pheochromocytoma testing, if appropriate.
• As appropriate, review all other significant and life-threatening adverse reactions and interactions, especially those related to the drugs and herbs mentioned above.

phenylephrine hydrochloride

Afrin Children's Pump Mist, AH-Chew D, Coricidin, Fenox, Minims Phenylephrine♣, Mydfrin♣, Neo-Synephrine, Preferin♣, Rhinall, Sudafed PE, Vicks Sinex Ultra Fine Mist

Pharmacologic class: Sympathomimetic, alpha-adrenergic agonist

Therapeutic class: Vasopressor, nasal decongestant, ophthalmic vasoconstrictor

Pregnancy risk category C

FDA | BOXED WARNING

• Clinicians should be completely familiar with package insert before using injection form.

Action

Stimulates alpha-adrenergic receptors, increasing blood pressure and causing pronounced vasoconstriction in skin, mucous membranes, and mucosa. Produces mydriasis by contracting pupillary dilator muscle.

Availability

Injection: 10 mg/ml
Nasal solution: 0.125%, 0.25%, 0.5%, 1%
Ophthalmic solution: 0.12%, 2.5%, 10%
Tablets (chewable): 10 mg

🩺 Indications and dosages

➤ Mild to moderate hypotension
Adults: 1 to 10 mg subcutaneously or I.M.; don't exceed an initial dosage of 5 mg.
➤ Severe hypotension and shock
Adults: 0.1 to 0.18 mg/minute I.V. infusion. For maintenance infusion, 40 to 60 mcg/minute.

➤ To prevent hypotension during spinal anesthesia
Adults: 2 to 3 mg subcutaneously or I.M. 3 to 4 minutes before spinal anesthetic is injected
➤ Hypotensive emergency during spinal anesthesia
Adults: 0.2 mg I.V., up to a maximum of 0.5 mg/dose
➤ To prolong spinal anesthesia
Adults: 2 to 5 mg added to anesthetic solution (prolongs spinal block by up to 50%)
➤ Vasoconstrictor for regional anesthesia
Adults: 1 mg of phenylephrine added to every 20 ml of local anesthetic solution
➤ Paroxysmal supraventricular tachycardia
Adults: 0.5 mg by rapid I.V. injection, not to exceed initial dosage of 0.5 mg. Subsequent dosages (determined by blood pressure) shouldn't exceed preceding dosage by more than 0.1 to 0.2 mg; maximum dosage is 1 mg.
➤ Nasal congestion
Adults: One or two sprays of 0.25% or 0.5% nasal solution in each nostril q 3 to 4 hours p.r.n.; severe congestion may warrant 1% solution. Or 10 to 20 mg P.O. (chewable tablets) q 4 hours.
➤ Vasoconstriction and pupil dilation
Adults: After topical anesthetic is applied, instill one drop of 2.5% ophthalmic solution into lacrimal sac; repeat 1 hour later.
➤ Uveitis
Adults: Instill one drop of 2.5% or 10% ophthalmic solution to upper surface of cornea. May repeat up to three times p.r.n.
➤ Open-angle glaucoma
Adults: Instill one drop of 10% ophthalmic solution to upper surface of cornea as often as necessary.
➤ For wide pupil dilation before intraocular surgery

p

Adults: Instill 2.5% or 10% ophthalmic solution, as prescribed, into lacrimal sac 30 to 60 minutes before surgery.
➤ Refraction
Adults: Before procedure, instill one drop of 2.5% ophthalmic solution combined with a rapid-acting cycloplegic into lacrimal sac, as prescribed.
Children: Before procedure, instill one drop of 2.5% ophthalmic solution into lacrimal sac 5 minutes after cycloplegic administration, as prescribed.
➤ Provocative test for angle-closure glaucoma
Adults: 2.5% ophthalmic solution applied to dilate pupil, with intraocular pressure (IOP) measured before application and after dilation. IOP rise of 3 to 5 mm Hg suggests angle block in patients with glaucoma; however, negative response doesn't rule out glaucoma from other causes.
➤ Retinoscopy (shadow test)
Adults: 2.5% ophthalmic solution
➤ Blanching test
Adults: Instill one to two drops of 2.5% ophthalmic solution into affected eye.
➤ Decongestant to relieve minor eye irritation
Adults: Instill one or two drops of 0.12% ophthalmic solution into eye(s) up to q.i.d. p.r.n.

Dosage adjustment
• Hyperthyroidism
• Cardiac disease
• Elderly patients

Contraindications
• Hypersensitivity to drug or its components
• Severe hypertension
• Ventricular tachycardia
• Angle-closure glaucoma
• Aneurysm (10% ophthalmic solution)
• During intraocular surgery when corneal epithelial barrier has been disturbed (ophthalmic solution)
• Elderly patients with severe arteriosclerotic or cerebrovascular disease
• Some low-birth-weight infants

Precautions
Use cautiously in:
• sulfite sensitivity (some products)
• hyperthyroidism, partial heart block, bradycardia, hypertension, cardiac disease, arteriosclerosis, unstable vasomotor syndrome
• type 1 (insulin-dependent) diabetes mellitus, hypertension, hyperthyroidism, arteriosclerosis or other cardiac disease (10% ophthalmic solution)
• within 21 days of MAO inhibitors (2.5% or 10% ophthalmic solution)
• elderly patients
• pregnant or breastfeeding patients.

Administration
• In emergencies, drug may be given by direct I.V. injection. Dilute 1 ml of solution containing 10 mg/ml with 9 ml of sterile water for injection.
◀ For I.V. infusion, dilute 10 mg in 500 ml of dextrose 5% in water or normal saline solution; titrate dosage until blood pressure is slightly below patient's normal level or until maximum dosage is reached. Infuse I.V. in large vein (preferably through central venous catheter) using infusion pump. After condition stabilizes, taper dosage gradually; don't withdraw abruptly. Avoid extravasation.
◀ Be aware that systemic absorption of ophthalmic solution during pupil dilation in patients with angle-closure glaucoma may trigger asthma attack.
• As ordered, apply a drop of suitable topical anesthetic before instilling ophthalmic solution, to prevent pain and drug dilution (caused by excessive lacrimation induced by pain).
◀ Compress lacrimal sac for 1 minute after instilling 10% ophthalmic solution, to avoid excessive systemic absorption (which could cause serious cardiovascular problems, especially in elderly patients).
• Be aware that patients with heavily pigmented irides may require larger

ophthalmic doses for diagnostic procedures.

Route	Onset	Peak	Duration
P.O.	Unknown	Unknown	Unknown
I.V.	Immediate	Unknown	15-20 min
I.M., subcut.	10-15 min	Unknown	0.5-2 hr
Nasal	15-20 min	Unknown	0.5-4 hr
Ophth. (0.12%)	Rapid	Unknown	30 min-4 hr
Ophth. (2.5%)	Rapid	15-60 min	3 hr
Ophth. (10%)	Rapid	10-60 min	6 hr

Adverse reactions

CNS: headache, weakness, anxiety, restlessness, tremor, light-headedness, dizziness, drowsiness, insomnia, hallucinations, nervousness, restlessness, giddiness, prolonged psychosis, orofacial dystonia
CV: hypertension, palpitations, tachycardia, bradycardia, **arrhythmias**
EENT: with ophthalmic solution—transient pigment floaters in aqueous humor; rebound miosis; rebound hyperemia (with prolonged use); light sensitivity; photophobia; blurred vision; allergic conjunctivitis; eye burning, stinging, and irritation; transient epithelial keratitis; decreased IOP; with nasal solution—rebound congestion, burning, stinging, sneezing, dryness, local irritation
GI: nausea, vomiting, gastric irritation, anorexia
GU: urinary retention (in males with prostatitis)
Hematologic: leukopenia, agranulocytosis, thrombocytopenia
Musculoskeletal: brow ache (with ophthalmic solution)
Respiratory: asthmatic episodes
Skin: sweating, rash, urticaria, contact dermatitis, necrosis and sloughing (with extravasation at I.V. site)

Interactions

Drug-drug. *Beta-adrenergic blockers:* blocked cardiostimulatory effects of phenylephrine
Bretylium, sympathomimetics: serious arrhythmias
Furazolidone: excessive hypertension
Guanethidine, methyldopa: decreased antihypertensive effects
Halogenated hydrocarbon anesthetics: serious arrhythmias
MAO inhibitors: severe headache, hypertension, hyperpyrexia
Oxytocics, tricyclic antidepressants: increased pressor response
Drug-diagnostic tests. *Tonometry:* false-normal readings (with ophthalmic form)
Drug-behaviors. *Sun exposure:* photophobia

Patient monitoring

• Monitor ECG continuously during I.V. administration; monitor blood pressure every 5 to 15 minutes until it stabilizes, then every 30 to 60 minutes.
• Monitor central venous pressure and fluid intake and output. Keep in mind that drug doesn't eliminate need for fluid resuscitation.
• Assess CBC; watch for evidence of blood dyscrasias.
• Monitor I.V. site; extravasation can cause tissue damage.
• Assess for symptomatic improvement in patients using nasal form.
🔊 Monitor for adverse reactions, particularly life-threatening asthmatic episodes.

Patient teaching

• Tell patient to take exactly as directed and not to exceed recommended dosage.
• Advise patient using nasal solution that dropper, inhaler, or spray dispenser shouldn't be used by more than one person. Teach proper instillation technique: instill nasal solution into dependent nostril with head down and in lateral position. Stay in this position

p

for 5 minutes; then instill solution in other nostril in same manner. Advise patient to rinse container tip with hot water after each use. Instruct him to discontinue use and contact prescriber if symptoms don't improve after 3 days. Tell him not to use for more than 3 days and to contact prescriber if symptoms persist.

• Teach proper technique for instilling eye drops. Stress importance of compressing lacrimal sac after instilling, to decrease systemic drug absorption. Tell patient that ophthalmic solution may cause light sensitivity lasting several hours. Inform elderly patient that he may see transient floaters 40 to 45 minutes after administration.

• As appropriate, review all other significant and life-threatening adverse reactions and interactions, especially those related to the drugs, tests, and behaviors mentioned above.

phenytoin
(diphenylhydantoin)
Dilantin-125, Dilantin Infatabs

phenytoin sodium
(diphenylhydantoin sodium)
Dilantin Kapseals, Diphenylan✢, Epanutin✤, Phenytek✢

Pharmacologic class: Hydantoin derivative
Therapeutic class: Anticonvulsant
Pregnancy risk category D

Action
Thought to limit seizure activity by promoting sodium efflux from neurons in motor cortex and reducing activity in brainstem centers responsible for tonic phase of tonic-clonic seizures

Availability
Capsules (prompt-release): 30 mg, 100 mg
Capsules (extended-release): 30 mg, 100 mg
Injection: 50 mg/ml in 2- and 5-ml ampules
Oral suspension: 30 mg/5 ml, 125 mg/5 ml
Tablets (chewable): 50 mg

⏀ Indications and dosages
➤ Status epilepticus
Adults: Loading dose of 10 to 15 mg/kg by slow I.V., then a maintenance dosage of 100 mg P.O. or I.V. q 6 to 8 hours
Neonates and children: Loading dose of 15 to 20 mg/kg I.V. in divided doses of 5 to 10 mg/kg
➤ Generalized tonic-clonic (grand mal) and complex partial (psychomotor, temporal lobe) seizures
Adults: Loading dose of 1 g P.O. (extended-release) in three divided doses (400 mg, 300 mg, and 300 mg) at 2-hour intervals in hospitalized patients requiring rapid steady-state serum levels (when I.V. route isn't desired). Maintenance dosing usually starts 24 hours after loading dose. Patients who haven't had previous treatment usually start at 100 mg (125 mg suspension) P.O. t.i.d., adjusted as needed to a maximum of 600 mg (625 mg suspension) P.O. daily. Alternatively, if divided doses control seizures, one daily dose of 300 mg P.O. (extended-release phenytoin sodium).
Children: Initially, 5 mg/kg/day P.O. in two or three equally divided doses; maintenance dosage individualized and given in two to three divided doses (not to exceed 300 mg/day).
➤ To prevent seizures during neurosurgery
Adults: 100 to 200 mg I.M. at 4-hour intervals

Off-label uses
- Arrhythmias
- Severe preeclampsia
- Trigeminal neuralgia
- Recessive dystrophic epidermolysis bullosa, junctional epidermolysis bullosa

Contraindications
- Hypersensitivity to drug
- Sinus bradycardia, sinoatrial block, second- or third-degree atrioventricular block, Adams-Stokes syndrome

Precautions
Use cautiously in:
- hepatic disease, diabetes mellitus, skin rash
- pregnant or breastfeeding patients (safety not established).

Administration
- Before I.V. use, check designated line for patency and flush with normal saline solution. Deliver no faster than 50 mg/minute for adults or 1 to 3 mg/kg/minute in children and neonates; then flush with normal saline solution. Avoid extravasation (can cause severe tissue damage).
- 🔊 Don't administer I.V. into dorsal hand veins, because purple glove syndrome may occur.
- When giving oral solution through nasogastric tube, dilute dose with sterile water or normal saline solution; after administration, flush tube with at least 20 ml of diluent.
- Withhold enteral feedings for at least 1 hour before and 1 hour after oral administration.
- Give I.M. only as last resort (may cause pain and reduce drug absorption).
- Know that patients with history of renal or hepatic disease should not receive P.O. loading dose.

Route	Onset	Peak	Duration
P.O.	Unknown	3 hr	6-12 hr
P.O. (extended)	Unknown	4-12 hr	12-36 hr
I.V.	Unknown	Rapid	12-24 hr
I.M.	Unknown	Erratic	12-24 hr

Adverse reactions
CNS: headache, fatigue, dizziness, drowsiness, weakness, depression, ataxia, slurred speech, confusion, agitation, dysarthria, dyskinesia, extrapyramidal symptoms, insomnia, irritability, twitching, nervousness, numbness, psychotic disturbances, tremor, CNS depression (with I.V. use), **coma**

CV: vasodilation, edema, chest pain, **tachycardia, hypotension** (increased with I.V. use), **cardiovascular collapse** (with I.V. use)

EENT: diplopia, amblyopia, nystagmus, visual field defect, eye pain, conjunctivitis, photophobia, mydriasis, hearing loss, tinnitus, ear pain, epistaxis, rhinitis, sinusitis, pharyngitis

GI: nausea, vomiting, diarrhea, constipation, lip enlargement, dry mouth

GU: pink, red, or reddish-brown urine; gynecomastia; Peyronie's disease

Hepatic: jaundice, **toxic hepatitis, hepatic damage**

Hematologic: macrocytosis, simple anemia, **megaloblastic anemia, monocytosis, leukocytosis, hemolytic anemia, thrombocytopenia, agranulocytosis, granulocytopenia, leukopenia, pancytopenia**

Metabolic: hypocalcemia, diabetes insipidus, hyperglycemia

Musculoskeletal: back pain, pelvic pain, osteomalacia

Respiratory: dyspnea, increased cough and sputum, pneumonia, hyperventilation, hypoxia, hemoptysis, bronchitis, **apnea, asthma, aspiration pneumonia, pulmonary fibrosis, atelectasis, pneumothorax**

p

Reactions in **bold** are life-threatening.   🔊 Clinical alert

Skin: rash, pruritus, bruising, exfoliative dermatitis, hypertrichosis, hirsutism, alopecia, **Stevens-Johnson syndrome**
Other: gingival hyperplasia, altered taste, fever, lymphadenopathy, weight gain or loss, injection site reaction, coarsened facial features, lupus erythematosus syndrome, allergic reactions

Interactions
Drug-drug. *Acetaminophen, amiodarone, carbamazepine, cardiac glycosides, corticosteroids, dicumarol, disopyramide, doxycycline, estrogens, haloperidol, hormonal contraceptives, methadone, metapyrone, mexiletine, quinidine, theophylline, valproic acid:* increased metabolism and decreased effects of these drugs
Activated charcoal, antacids, sucralfate: decreased phenytoin absorption
Allopurinol, amiodarone, benzodiazepines, chloramphenicol, chlorpheniramine, cimetidine, disulfiram, fluconazole, ibuprofen, isoniazid, metronidazole, miconazole, omeprazole, phenacemide, phenothiazines, phenylbutazone, salicylates, succinimides, sulfonamides, tricyclic antidepressants, trimethoprim, valproic acid: increased phenytoin effects
Antineoplastics, barbiturates, carbamazepine, diazoxide, folic acid, influenza vaccine, loxapine, nitrofurantoin, pyridoxine, rifampin, theophylline: decreased phenytoin effects
Cyclosporine, dopamine, furosemide, levodopa, levonorgestrel, mebendazole, muscle relaxants, nondepolarizing phenothiazines, sulfonylureas: decreased effects of these drugs
Drug-diagnostic tests. *Alkaline phosphatase, eosinophils, gamma-glutamyl-transferase, glucose:* increased levels
Dexamethasone (1-mg) suppression test, metyrapone test: interference with test results
Free thyroxine, serum thyroxine: decreased levels

Drug-food. *Enteral tube feedings:* decreased phenytoin absorption
Folic acid: decreased folic acid absorption
Drug-behaviors. *Acute alcohol ingestion:* increased phenytoin blood level
Chronic alcohol ingestion: decreased phenytoin blood level

Patient monitoring
• Assess blood pressure, ECG, and heart rate, especially during I.V. loading dose. Watch for adverse reactions.
• Monitor phenytoin blood level; therapeutic range is 10 to 20 mcg/ml.
• Evaluate CBC and kidney and liver function tests.
• Closely monitor prothrombin time and Internationalized Normal Ratio in patients receiving warfarin concurrently.
• Monitor drug efficacy.

Patient teaching
• Explain drug therapy, need for follow-up tests, and importance of taking drug exactly as prescribed.
• Caution patient not to stop therapy abruptly.
• Advise patient to avoid alcohol.
◀€ Instruct patient to report rash immediately.
• Inform patient that drug may discolor urine.
• Tell female patient drug may make hormonal contraceptives ineffective.
• Instruct patient to practice good dental hygiene to minimize gingival hyperplasia.
• Encourage patient to seek medical advice before taking over-the-counter preparations.
• As appropriate, review all other significant and life-threatening adverse reactions and interactions, especially those related to the drugs, tests, foods, and behaviors mentioned above.

pimecrolimus
Elidel

Pharmacologic class: Dermatologic agent
Therapeutic class: Immunomodulator
Pregnancy risk category C

FDA BOXED WARNING

• Drug's long-term safety hasn't been established.
• Rare cases of lymphoma and skin cancer have occurred in patients who used drug. Avoid continuous long-term use in any age-group and limit application to areas of atopic dermatitis.
• Drug isn't indicated for use in children younger than age 2.

Action
Unknown. Thought to inhibit T-cell activation by blocking transcription of early cytokines. Also blocks release of inflammatory cytokines and mediators from mast cells after stimulation by antigen/immunoglobin E.

Availability
Cream: 1%

Indications and dosages
➤ Mild to moderate atopic dermatitis
Adults and children ages 2 and older: Apply 1% cream topically b.i.d. to clean, dry, affected area.

Contraindications
• Hypersensitivity to drug or its components

Precautions
Use cautiously in:
• eczema herpeticum (Kaposi's varicelliform eruption), varicella zoster (chickenpox or shingles), herpes simplex infection, lymphadenopathy, mononucleosis, acute infectious Netherton's syndrome, skin infections or papilloma, warts, immunocompromised state
• concurrent use of CYP3A inhibitors
• pregnant or breastfeeding patients
• children younger than age 2 (safety not established).

Administration
• Apply thin layer to affected area.
• Don't use with occlusive dressing (may increase systemic absorption).

Route	Onset	Peak	Duration
Topical	Not systemically absorbed		

Adverse reactions
CNS: headache
EENT: sinus congestion, rhinorrhea
GI: nausea, vomiting, diarrhea, gastritis
Respiratory: upper respiratory tract infection
Skin: pruritus, application-site reaction or discomfort
Other: pyrexia, increased risk of viral or bacterial infections

Interactions
Drug-drug. *CYP3A inhibitors (such as calcium channel blockers, cimetidine, erythromycin):* inhibition of action by hepatic enzymes that eliminate pimecrolimus
Drug-behaviors. *Sunbathing:* possible increased risk of skin cancer

Patient monitoring
• Reevaluate at 6 weeks if lesions haven't healed.
• Discontinue therapy, as prescribed, if disease resolves.

Patient teaching
• Tell patient to apply to clean, dry skin and to wash hands afterward (unless hands are being treated).

p

◀€ Clinical alert

- Caution patient not to use occlusive dressings.
- Tell patient drug may cause local reaction, such as a feeling of warmth or burning sensation. Advise him to contact prescriber if reaction is severe or lasts more than 1 week.
- Advise patient to apply missed dose as soon as possible. If it's almost time for next dose, tell him to skip missed dose and resume regular schedule.
- Tell patient to avoid natural or artificial sunlight and to use adequate sunblock on skin and lips.
- Instruct patient to contact prescriber if no improvement occurs after 6 weeks or if condition worsens.
- As appropriate, review all other significant adverse reactions and interactions, especially those related to the drugs and behaviors mentioned above.

pioglitazone hydrochloride

Actos, Apo-Pioglitazone✹, Co Pioglitazone✹, Gen-Pioglitazone✹, Novo-Pioglitazone✹, PMS-Pioglitazone✹, Ratio-Pioglitazone✹, Sandoz Pioglitazone✹

Pharmacologic class: Thiazolidinedione
Therapeutic class: Hypoglycemic
Pregnancy risk category C

FDA | BOXED WARNING

- Drug may cause or exacerbate heart failure. After starting therapy or increasing dosage, observe patient carefully for signs and symptoms of heart failure. If these develop, manage patient according to current standards of care and consider discontinuing drug or reducing dosage.
- Drug isn't recommended in patients with symptomatic heart failure. In patients with established New York Heart Association Class III or IV heart failure, drug initiation is contraindicated.

Action

Enhances insulin sensitivity in muscle and adipose tissue; inhibits hepatic gluconeogenesis

Availability

Tablets: 15 mg, 30 mg, 45 mg

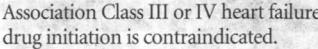 Indications and dosages

➤ Adjunct to diet and exercise to improve glycemic control in type 2 (non-insulin-dependent) diabetes mellitus
Adults: 15 to 30 mg/day; may increase to 45 mg/day if needed

Contraindications

- Hypersensitivity to drug, its components, or rosiglitazone
- Established New York Heart Association Class III or IV heart failure

Precautions

Use cautiously in:
- edema, hepatic impairment
- symptomatic heart failure (use not recommended)
- female patients of childbearing age
- pregnant or breastfeeding patients
- children (safety and efficacy not established).

Administration

- Give with or without food.
- Know that drug may be used with sulfonylureas, metformin, or insulin when combination of diet, exercise, and monotherapy doesn't achieve adequate glycemic control.

Route	Onset	Peak	Duration
P.O.	30 min	2 hr	24 hr

Adverse reactions

CNS: headache
CV: congestive heart failure (CHF) or exacerbation of CHF

EENT: sinusitis, pharyngitis
Hematologic: anemia
Metabolic: aggravation of diabetes mellitus, **hypoglycemia, hyperglycemia**
Musculoskeletal: myalgia
Respiratory: upper respiratory infection
Other: tooth disorders, pain, edema

Interactions

Drug-drug. *Hormonal contraceptives:* decreased contraceptive efficacy
Ketoconazole: increased pioglitazone effects
Drug-diagnostic tests. *Creatine kinase:* transient increase
Hematocrit, hemoglobin: decreased values (usually during first 4 to 12 weeks of therapy)
Drug-herbs. *Chromium, coenzyme Q10, fenugreek:* additive hypoglycemic effects
Glucosamine: poor glycemic control

Patient monitoring

◀€ Monitor patient carefully for signs and symptoms of heart failure (including excessive, rapid weight gain; dyspnea; and edema) after initiation and after dosage increases. Consider discontinuation or dosage reduction if these symptoms appear.

• Assess patient's weight and compliance with diet and exercise program.
• Monitor liver function tests before and during therapy.
• Monitor glycosylated hemoglobin, hemoglobin, hematocrit, and blood glucose levels.
• Assess for signs and symptoms of hypoglycemia or hyperglycemia.

Patient teaching

• Instruct patient to take exactly as prescribed. Tell him he may take drug without regard to food.
• Tell patient drug may increase his risk for EENT and respiratory infections. Instruct him to contact prescriber if symptoms occur.

◀€ Advise patient to immediately report unexplained nausea, vomiting, abdominal pain, fatigue, anorexia, dark urine, fever, trauma, infection, rapid weight gain, edema, or shortness of breath.

• Tell premenopausal anovulatory patient that drug may cause ovulation. Recommend use of reliable contraception.
• Advise female of childbearing age to contact prescriber promptly if pregnancy occurs.
• As appropriate, review all other significant and life-threatening adverse reactions and interactions, especially those related to the drugs, tests, and herbs mentioned above.

piperacillin sodium and tazobactam sodium
Tazocin ✚, Zosyn

Pharmacologic class: Penicillin (extended-spectrum), beta-lactamase inhibitor
Therapeutic class: Anti-infective
Pregnancy risk category B

Action
Piperacillin inhibits bacterial cell-wall synthesis, resulting in cell death. Tazobactam increases piperacillin efficacy.

Availability
Powder for injection: 2 g piperacillin and 0.25 g tazobactam/vial, 3 g piperacillin and 0.375 g tazobactam/vial, 4 g piperacillin and 0.5 g tazobactam/vial

⚕ Indications and dosages
➤ Community-acquired pneumonia; ruptured appendix; peritonitis; pelvic inflammatory disease; skin and skin-structure infections

---

Reactions in **bold** are life-threatening. ◀€ Clinical alert

Adults and children older than age 12:
3.375 g (3 g piperacillin and 0.375 g tazobactam) I.V. q 6 hours for 7 to 10 days
➤ Nosocomial pneumonia
Adults and children ages 12 and older:
3.375 g (3 g piperacillin and 0.375 g tazobactam) I.V. over 30 minutes q 4 hours for 7 to 14 days, given with an aminoglycoside

Dosage adjustment
• Renal impairment

Contraindications
• Hypersensitivity to penicillins, cephalosporins, imipenems, or beta-lactamase inhibitors
• Neonates

Precautions
Use cautiously in:
• heart failure, renal insufficiency (in children), seizures, bleeding disorders, uremia, hypokalemia, cystic fibrosis
• patients with sodium restrictions
• pregnant or breastfeeding patient
• children younger than age 12 (safety and efficacy not established).

Administration
• Ask patient about allergy to penicillins, cephalosporins, imipenems, or beta-lactamase inhibitors before giving.
• Dilute each gram with 5 ml of diluent, such as sterile or bacteriostatic water for injection, normal saline solution for injection, dextrose 5% in water, dextrose 5% in normal saline solution for injection, or 6% dextran in normal saline solution. Don't use lactated Ringer's solution.
• Shake vial until drug dissolves. Dilute again to a final volume of 50 ml; infuse over 30 minutes.
• Don't mix with other drugs. If possible, stop primary infusion while piperacillin infuses.
• Don't mix in same container with aminoglycosides, which are chemically incompatible with piperacillin.

Route	Onset	Peak	Duration
I.V.	Immediate	Immediate	Unknown

Adverse reactions
CNS: headache, insomnia, agitation, dizziness, anxiety, lethargy, hallucinations, depression, twitching, **coma, seizures**
CV: hypertension, chest pain, tachycardia
EENT: rhinitis, glossitis
GI: nausea, vomiting, diarrhea, constipation, dyspepsia, abdominal pain, **pseudomembranous colitis**
GU: proteinuria, hematuria, vaginal candidiasis, vaginitis, **oliguria, interstitial nephritis, glomerulonephritis**
Hematologic: anemia, **increased bleeding, bone marrow depression, leukopenia, thrombocytopenia**
Metabolic: hypokalemia, hypernatremia
Respiratory: dyspnea
Skin: rash, pruritus
Other: fever; pain, edema, inflammation, or phlebitis at I.V. site; superinfection; hypersensitivity reactions including **serum sickness and anaphylaxis**

Interactions
Drug-drug. *Aminoglycosides:* aminoglycoside inactivation
Aspirin, probenecid: increased piperacillin blood level
Hormonal contraceptives: decreased contraceptive efficacy
Methotrexate: increased risk of methotrexate toxicity
Tetracyclines: decreased piperacillin efficacy
Vecuronium: prolonged neuromuscular blockade
Drug-diagnostic tests. *Coombs' test, urine glucose tests using copper reduction method (Clinitest, Benedict's or Fehling's solution), urine protein:* false-positive results
Eosinophils: increased count
Granulocytes, hemoglobin, platelets, white blood cells: decreased levels

Patient monitoring

- Assess neurologic status, especially for seizures.
- Monitor vital signs and fluid intake and output.
- Evaluate electrolyte levels, CBC with white cell differential, and culture and sensitivity tests. Watch for evidence of hypokalemia and blood dyscrasias.
- In patients receiving high doses or prolonged therapy, monitor for signs and symptoms of bacterial or fungal superinfection and pseudomembranous colitis.
- Monitor patient's dietary sodium intake (drug has high sodium content).
🔊 Immediately report rash, hives, severe diarrhea, black tongue, sore throat, fever, or unusual bleeding or bruising.

Patient teaching

- Tell patient to monitor urinary output and report significant changes.
- Instruct patient to report unusual pain, redness, swelling, or other changes at infusion site.
- As appropriate, review all other significant and life-threatening adverse reactions and interactions, especially those related to the drugs and tests mentioned above.

piroxicam

Apo-Piroxicam✲, Brexidol⊕, Dom-Piroxicam✲, Feldene, Gen-Piroxicam✲, Novo-Pirocam✲, Nu-Pirox✲ PMS-Piroxicam✲, PRO-Piroxicam✲

Pharmacologic class: Oxicam derivative, nonsteroidal anti-inflammatory drug (NSAID)

Therapeutic class: Analgesic, anti-inflammatory, antipyretic

Pregnancy risk category C (first and second trimesters), *D* (third trimester)

FDA BOXED WARNING

- Drug may increase risk of serious cardiovascular thrombotic events, myocardial infarction, and stroke (which can be fatal). Risk may increase with duration of use. Patients with cardiovascular disease or risk factors for it may be at greater risk.
- Drug increases risk of serious GI adverse events, including bleeding, ulcers, and stomach or intestinal perforation (which can be fatal). These events can occur at any time during use and without warning. Elderly patients are at greater risk.
- Drug is contraindicated for treatment of perioperative pain in setting of coronary artery bypass graft surgery.

Action

Inhibits cyclooxygenase (an enzyme needed for prostaglandin synthesis), stimulating anti-inflammatory response and blocking pain impulses

Availability

Capsules: 10 mg, 20 mg

Indications and dosages

➤ Inflammatory disorders (such as arthritis)
Adults: 20 mg P.O. daily as a single dose or in two divided doses

Dosage adjustment

- Hepatic or renal impairment
- Elderly patients

Off-label uses

- Dysmenorrhea
- Ankylosing spondylitis
- Gout

Contraindications

- Hypersensitivity to drug or other NSAIDs (including aspirin)
- Active GI bleeding or ulcer disease
- Third trimester of pregnancy

Precautions

Use cautiously in:
- renal impairment, severe cardiovascular or hepatic disease
- history of ulcer disease
- pregnant patients in first or second trimester
- breastfeeding patients (not recommended)
- children (safety not established).

Administration

- Give with milk, antacids, or food to minimize GI upset.

Route	Onset	Peak	Duration
P.O. (analgesia)	1 hr	Unknown	48-72 hr
P.O. (anti-inflam.)	7-12 days	2-3 wk	Unknown

Adverse reactions

CNS: headache, drowsiness, dizziness
CV: edema, hypertension, vasculitis, tachycardia, **arrhythmias**
EENT: blurred vision, tinnitus
GI: nausea, vomiting, diarrhea, constipation, abdominal pain, flatulence, dyspepsia, anorexia, **severe GI bleeding**
GU: proteinuria, **renal failure**
Hematologic: anemia, **blood dyscrasias**
Hepatic: jaundice, **hepatitis**
Skin: rash
Other: allergic reactions including **anaphylaxis**

Interactions

Drug-drug. *Acetaminophen (chronic use), cyclosporine, gold compounds:* increased risk of adverse renal reactions
Anticoagulants, cefamandole, cefoperazone, cefotetan, clopidogrel, eptifibatide, heparin, plicamycin, thrombolytics, ticlopidine, tirofiban, valproic acid, vitamin A: increased risk of bleeding
Antineoplastics: increased risk of hematologic toxicity
Aspirin: decreased piroxicam blood level and efficacy
Corticosteroids, other NSAIDs: additive adverse GI reactions

Diuretics, other antihypertensives: decreased response to these drugs
Insulin, oral hypoglycemics: increased risk of hypoglycemia
Lithium: increased lithium blood level and risk of toxicity
Probenecid: increased piroxicam blood level and risk of toxicity
Drug-diagnostic tests. *Alanine aminotransferase, alkaline phosphatase, aspartate aminotransferase, blood urea nitrogen, creatinine, electrolytes, lactate dehydrogenase:* increased levels
Bleeding time: prolonged
Hematocrit, hemoglobin, platelets, white blood cells: decreased levels
Liver function tests: abnormal results
Drug-herbs. *Alfalfa, anise, arnica, astragalus, bilberry, black currant seed oil, bladderwrack, bogbean, boldo, borage oil, buchu, capsaicin, cat's claw, celery, chaparral, cinchona bark, clove oil, coenzyme Q10, dandelion, danshen, dong quai, evening primrose oil, fenugreek, feverfew, garlic, ginger, ginkgo, guggul, papaya extract, red clover, rhubarb, safflower oil, skullcap, St. John's wort:* increased anticoagulant effect, greater bleeding risk

Patient monitoring

- Monitor vital signs and cardiovascular status. Stay alert for hypertension and arrhythmias.
- Monitor kidney and liver function tests, hearing, and CBC.
- 🔊 Watch for signs and symptoms of drug-induced hepatitis and GI toxicity, including ulcers and bleeding.
- Monitor for signs and symptoms of infection, which drug may mask.

Patient teaching

- Advise patient to take with milk, antacids, or food to minimize GI upset.
- Tell patient drug may mask signs and symptoms of infection. Instruct him to contact prescriber if he suspects he has an infection.

◀≹ Teach patient to recognize and immediately report signs and symptoms of allergic reaction or GI bleeding.
• Inform patient that many herbs increase the risk of GI bleeding. Caution him not to use herbs without prescriber's approval.
• Instruct patient to drink plenty of fluids and to report decreased urination.
• Caution patient to avoid driving and other hazardous activities until he knows how drug affects concentration and alertness.
• Tell female patient to inform prescriber if she is pregnant or breastfeeding.
• As appropriate, review all other significant and life-threatening adverse reactions and interactions, especially those related to the drugs, tests, and herbs mentioned above.

pitavastatin
Livalo

Pharmacologic class: HMG-CoA reductase inhibitor
Therapeutic class: Antihyperlipidemic
Pregnancy risk category X

Action
Increases rate at which body removes cholesterol from blood and reduces production of cholesterol by inhibiting enzyme that catalyzes early rate-limiting step in cholesterol synthesis

Availability
Tablets: 1 mg, 2 mg, 4 mg

🖉 Indications and dosages
➤ Primary hyperlipidemia, mixed dyslipidemia
Adults: 2 mg P.O. daily; may increase to maximum of 4 mg daily

Dosage adjustment
• Renal impairment
• Patient with end-stage renal disease on dialysis
• Concurrent use of erythromycin or rifampin

Contraindications
• Hypersensitivity to drug or its components
• Active liver disease, unexplained persistent transaminase elevations
• Concurrent use of cyclosporine
• Women of childbearing age
• Breastfeeding

Precautions
Use cautiously in:
• patients with severe renal impairment not on dialysis (use not recommended)
• patients with predisposing factors for myopathy (such as untreated hypothyroidism)
• patients who consume substantial quantities of alcohol or have history of chronic liver disease
• concurrent use of protease inhibitors (such as lopinavir, ritonavir), erythromycin, fibric acids (such as fenofibrate, gemfibrozil), rifampin, or niacin
• elderly patients
• children (safety and efficacy not established).

Administration
• Check liver function tests before starting therapy.
• Administer with or without food.

Route	Onset	Peak	Duration
P.O.	Unknown	1 hr	12 hr

Adverse reactions
CNS: headache
EENT: nasopharyngitis
GI: diarrhea, constipation
Hepatic: liver enzyme abnormalities

Musculoskeletal: arthralgia, myalgia, back pain, extremity pain, **rhabdomyolysis**

Skin: rash, pruritus, urticaria

Other: influenza, hypersensitivity

Interactions

Drug-drug. *Cyclosporine, erythromycin, fibric acids, niacin, protease inhibitors, rifampin:* increased pitavastatin effect and risk of myopathy

Drug-diagnostic tests. *Alanine aminotransferase (ALT), alkaline phosphatase, aspartate aminotransferase (AST), bilirubin, blood glucose, creatine kinase:* increased levels

Drug-food. *Grapefruit juice:* increased drug area under the curve

Patient monitoring

◀€ Discontinue drug if markedly elevated creatine kinase level occurs or myopathy is diagnosed or suspected.

◀€ Temporarily withhold drug if an acute serious condition suggests myopathy or predisposes to development of renal failure secondary to rhabdomyolysis (such as sepsis, hypotension, dehydration, major surgery, trauma, uncontrolled seizures, or severe metabolic, endocrine, and electrolyte disorders).

• Analyze lipid levels 4 weeks after starting therapy and after dosage titration; monitor liver enzyme levels 12 weeks after starting therapy, after dosage titration, and periodically thereafter. Should an increase in ALT or AST level of more than three times the upper limit of normal persist, dosage reduction or drug withdrawal is recommended. Continue to monitor patient who develops increased transaminase levels until abnormalities resolve.

• In patient receiving warfarin concurrently, closely monitor prothrombin time and International Normalized Ratio.

Patient teaching

• Tell patient to take drug with or without food.

◀€ Instruct patient to immediately report to prescriber if unexplained muscle pain, tenderness, or weakness occurs, especially if accompanied by malaise or fever.

• Caution patient to avoid or decrease alcohol intake.

• Advise breastfeeding patient not to breastfeed while taking drug.

• Advise female patient of childbearing age to use an effective method of birth control to prevent pregnancy while using drug and if she becomes pregnant, advise her to stop taking drug and notify prescriber.

• As appropriate, review all other significant and life-threatening adverse reactions and interactions, especially those related to the drugs, tests, and food mentioned above.

posaconazole
Noxafil, Posanol ✱

Pharmacologic class: Triazole
Therapeutic class: Antifungal
Pregnancy risk category C

Action

Inhibits fungal ergosterol synthesis (key component of fungal cell membrane) by inhibiting lanosterol 14-alpha demethylase and causing methylated sterol precursors to accumulate

Availability

Oral suspension (immediate-release): 40 mg/ml in 123-ml bottle

ⓘ Indications and dosages

➤ Prophylaxis of invasive *Aspergillus* and *Candida* infections in patients at risk for these infections because of severe immunocompromise (such as hematopoietic stem-cell transplant recipients with graft-versus-host disease and those who have hematologic cancers with prolonged neutropenia from chemotherapy)

Adults and children age 13 and older: 200 mg (5 ml) P.O. three times daily for duration of therapy based on recovery from neutropenia or immunosuppression

➤ Oropharyngeal candidiasis

Adults and children age 13 and older: Loading dose of 100 mg (2.5 ml) P.O. twice daily on first day, then 100 mg P.O. once daily for 13 days

➤ Oropharyngeal candidiasis refractory to itraconazole or fluconazole

Adults and children age 13 and older: 400 mg (10 ml) P.O. twice daily for duration of therapy based on disease severity and clinical response

Off-label uses

- Esophageal candidiasis
- *Fusarium* infection
- Mycosis

Contraindications

- Hypersensitivity to drug or its components
- Concurrent use of astemizole, cisapride, ergot alkaloids, halofantrine, pimozide, quinidine, sirolimus, or terfenadine

Precautions

Use cautiously in:
- hypersensitivity to other azoles
- potentially proarrhythmic conditions, severe underlying medical conditions (such as hematologic cancers), preexisting hepatic impairment
- pregnant or breastfeeding patients
- children younger than age 13 (safety and efficacy not established).

Administration

- Before starting drug, make rigorous attempts to correct potassium, magnesium, and calcium imbalances.
- Advise patient to take each dose with full meal or liquid nutritional supplement to enhance drug absorption.
- ◀€ Don't give concurrently with astemizole, cisapride, ergot alkaloids, halofantrine, pimozide, quinidine, or terfenadine.

Route	Onset	Peak	Duration
P.O.	Unknown	3-5 hr	Unknown

Adverse reactions

CNS: seizure, insomnia, anxiety, headache, fatigue, dizziness, weakness
CV: prolonged QT interval, hypertension, hypotension, tachycardia
EENT: blurred vision, epistaxis, pharyngitis
GI: nausea, vomiting, diarrhea, constipation, abdominal pain, dyspepsia, flatulence, mucositis, dry mouth, oral candidiasis, anorexia
GU: vaginal hemorrhage
Hematologic: anemia, **neutropenia, febrile neutropenia, thrombocytopenia**
Hepatic: cholestasis, hepatic damage, **hepatic failure**
Metabolic: adrenal insufficiency (rare), dehydration
Musculoskeletal: arthralgia, back pain
Respiratory: cough, dyspnea, upper respiratory tract infection, pneumonia
Skin: rash, pruritus, petechiae
Other: unusual taste, weight loss, fever, bacteremia, herpes simplex, edema, leg edema, rigors, cytomegalovirus infection

Interactions

Drug-drug. *Astemizole, cisapride, halofantrine, pimozide, quinidine, terfenadine:* elevated blood levels of these drugs, leading to prolonged QT interval and increased risk of life-threatening arrhythmias (including torsades de pointes)

p

Reactions in **bold** are life-threatening.   ◀€ Clinical alert

Benzodiazepines metabolized through CYP3A4 (such as midazolam), phenytoin, rifabutin: increased blood levels of these drugs

Calcium channel blockers metabolized through CYP3A4 (such as amlodipine, diltiazem, felodipine): increased blood levels of these drugs, causing increased toxicity risk

Cimetidine, phenytoin, rifabutin: decreased posaconazole blood level

Cyclosporine, sirolimus, tacrolimus: elevated blood levels of these drugs, causing increased risk of nephrotoxicity and other serious adverse reactions

Ergot derivatives (dihydroergotamine, ergotamine): increased blood levels of these drugs, causing increased ergotism risk

HMG-CoA reductase inhibitors metabolized through CYP3A4 (such as atorvastatin, fluvastatin, lovastatin): increased blood levels of these drugs, causing increased risk of rhabdomyolysis

Vinca alkaloids (such as vinblastine, vincristine): increased vinca alkaloid blood levels, causing increased neurotoxicity risk

Drug-diagnostic tests. *Alanine aminotransferase, alkaline phosphatase, aspartate aminotransferase, bilirubin, gamma-glutamyltransferase, serum creatinine:* increased levels

Drug-food. *Nonfat, high-fat, or liquid nutritional supplements:* approximately three- to four-fold increase in drug mean C_{max} and area under the curve values

Patient monitoring

• Monitor serum potassium, magnesium, and calcium levels before and frequently during therapy.

• Obtain liver function tests and bilirubin level at start of therapy and periodically throughout. If liver function tests become abnormal during therapy, stay alert for signs and symptoms of more severe hepatic injury; consider withdrawing drug if these occur.

• Monitor blood drug levels frequently if patient is receiving concurrent cyclosporine, sirolimus, or tacrolimus. Consider reducing dosage as appropriate.

◀€ Monitor ECG if patient has potentially proarrhythmic condition or is receiving concurrent drugs that may prolong QT interval and are metabolized through CYP3A4. Stay alert for prolonged QT interval.

• Watch for breakthrough fungal infections in patients with severe diarrhea, vomiting, or severe renal impairment and in those receiving drugs that may decrease blood drug level or who can't eat a full meal or tolerate oral nutritional supplements.

Patient teaching

• Instruct patient to take each dose with full meal or liquid nutritional supplement.

• Advise patient to inform prescriber of all drugs he is taking because serious interactions may occur.

◀€ Urge patient to contact prescriber immediately if he develops signs or symptoms of liver impairment, such as unusual tiredness, weakness, nausea, itching, yellowing of eyes or skin, upper right abdominal tenderness, or flulike symptoms.

◀€ Tell patient to contact prescriber immediately if he develops irregular heartbeats or other cardiac symptoms.

◀€ Advise patient to notify prescriber of severe diarrhea or vomiting, because these conditions may alter blood drug level.

• Stress importance of keeping appointments for follow-up laboratory tests.

• Caution patient to avoid driving and other hazardous activities because drug may alter vision.

• As appropriate, review all other significant and life-threatening adverse reactions and interactions, especially those related to the drugs, tests, and foods mentioned above.

potassium acetate

Pharmacologic class: Mineral, electrolyte
Therapeutic class: Electrolyte replacement, nutritional supplement
Pregnancy risk category C

Action

Maintains acid-base balance, isotonicity, and electrophysiologic balance throughout body tissues; crucial to nerve impulse transmission and contraction of cardiac, skeletal, and smooth muscle. Also essential for normal renal function and carbohydrate metabolism.

Availability

Concentrate for injection: 2 mEq/ml in 20-, 50-, and 100-ml vials; 4 mEq/ml in 50-ml vials

⍟ Indications and dosages

➢ To prevent or treat potassium depletion; diabetic acidosis; metabolic alkalosis; arrhythmias; periodic paralysis attacks; hyperadrenocorticism; primary aldosteronism; healing phase of burns or scalds; overmedication with adrenocorticoids, testosterone, or corticotropin
Adults: Dosage highly individualized. For potassium level above 2.5 mEq/L, give 40 mEq/L as additive to I.V. infusion at a maximum rate of 10 mEq/hour; maximum daily dosage is 200 mEq. For potassium level less than 2 mEq/L, give 80 mEq/L as additive to I.V. infusion at a maximum rate of 40 mEq/hour (with cardiac monitoring); maximum daily dosage is 400 mEq.
Children: Dosage highly individualized; up to 3 mEq/kg or 40 mEq/m²/day as additive to I.V. infusion.

Contraindications

- Acute dehydration
- Heat cramps
- Hyperkalemia
- Hyperkalemic familial periodic paralysis
- Severe renal impairment
- Severe hemolytic reactions
- Untreated Addison's disease
- Severe tissue trauma
- Concurrent use of potassium-sparing diuretics, angiotensin-converting enzyme (ACE) inhibitors, or salt substitutes containing potassium

Precautions

Use cautiously in:
- cardiac disease, renal impairment, diabetes mellitus, hypomagnesemia
- pregnant or breastfeeding patients
- children (safety and efficacy not established).

Administration

- Make sure patient is well hydrated and urinating before starting therapy.
- ◀⁞ Give only as additive to I.V. infusion. Never give by I.V. push or I.M. route, and never give undiluted. Use peripheral line with maximum rate of 40 mEq/hour (with cardiac monitoring).
- ◀⁞ To ensure that potassium is well mixed in compatible solution, don't add potassium to I.V. bottle in hanging position.
- ◀⁞ Dilute in compatible I.V. solution. Administer slowly to reduce risk of fatal hyperkalemia.
- Know that maximum infusion rate without cardiac monitoring is 20 mEq/hour. Infusion rates above 20 mEq/hour necessitate cardiac monitoring.
- If patient complains of burning with I.V. administration, decrease flow rate.
- Be aware that potassium preparations are not interchangeable.
- Know that dosages are expressed in mEq of potassium and that potassium acetate contains 10.2 mEq/g.

p

Reactions in **bold** are life-threatening.   ◀⁞ Clinical alert

Route	Onset	Peak	Duration
I.V.	Rapid	End of infusion	Unknown

Adverse reactions

CNS: confusion, unusual fatigue, restlessness, asthenia, flaccid paralysis, paresthesia, absent reflexes

CV: ECG changes, hypotension, **arrhythmias, heart block, cardiac arrest**

GI: nausea, vomiting, diarrhea, abdominal discomfort, flatulence

Metabolic: hyperkalemia

Musculoskeletal: weakness and heaviness of legs

Respiratory: respiratory paralysis

Other: irritation at I.V. site

Interactions

Drug-drug. *ACE inhibitors, potassium-sparing diuretics, other potassium-containing preparations:* increased risk of hyperkalemia

Drug-diagnostic tests. *Potassium:* increased level

Drug-food. *Salt substitutes containing potassium:* increased risk of hyperkalemia

Drug-herbs. *Dandelion:* increased risk of hyperkalemia

Licorice: decreased response to potassium

Patient monitoring

• Monitor renal function, fluid intake and output, and potassium, creatinine, and blood urea nitrogen levels.

◀€ Know that potassium is contraindicated in severe renal impairment and must be used with extreme caution (if at all) in patients with any degree of renal impairment, because of risk of life-threatening hyperkalemia.

• Assess vital signs and ECG. Watch for arrhythmias.

• Evaluate patient's neurologic status. Stay alert for neurologic complications.

• Monitor I.V. site for irritation.

Patient teaching

• Instruct patient to report unusual pain, redness, swelling, or other reactions at infusion site.

• Advise patient to report nausea, vomiting, confusion, numbness and tingling, unusual tiredness or weakness, or heavy feeling in legs.

• Instruct patient to avoid salt substitutes.

• As appropriate, review all other significant and life-threatening adverse reactions and interactions, especially those related to the drugs, tests, foods, and herbs mentioned above.

potassium bicarbonate

Pharmacologic class: Mineral, electrolyte

Therapeutic class: Electrolyte replacement, nutritional supplement

Pregnancy risk category C

Action

Maintains acid-base balance, isotonicity, and electrophysiologic balance throughout body tissues; crucial to nerve impulse transmission and contraction of cardiac, skeletal, and smooth muscle. Also essential for normal renal function and carbohydrate metabolism.

Availability

Tablets for effervescent oral solution: 25 mEq

🚫 Indications and dosages

➣ To prevent potassium depletion

Adults: Dosage highly individualized. Usual dosage is 25 mEq/day P.O. in divided doses.

➣ To treat potassium depletion

Adults: 50 to 100 mEq/day P.O. in divided doses, not to exceed a maximum daily dosage of 150 mEq

Contraindications
- Hypersensitivity to tartrazine or alcohol (with some products)
- Acute dehydration
- Heat cramps
- Hyperkalemia
- Hyperkalemic familial periodic paralysis
- Severe renal impairment
- Severe hemolytic reaction
- Severe tissue trauma
- Untreated Addison's disease
- Concurrent use of potassium-sparing diuretics, angiotensin-converting enzyme (ACE) inhibitors, or salt substitutes containing potassium

Precautions
Use cautiously in:
- cardiac disease, renal impairment, diabetes mellitus, hypomagnesemia
- pregnant or breastfeeding patients
- children (safety and efficacy not established).

Administration
- Ensure that patient is adequately hydrated and urinating before starting therapy.
- Give with meals and a full glass of water or juice to minimize GI upset.
- Be aware that potassium preparations aren't interchangeable.
- Know that dosages are expressed in mEq of potassium and that potassium bicarbonate contains 10 mEq potassium/g.

Route	Onset	Peak	Duration
P.O.	Unknown	1-2 hr	Unknown

Adverse reactions
CNS: confusion, unusual fatigue, restlessness, asthenia, flaccid paralysis, paresthesia
CV: ECG changes, hypotension, **heart block, arrhythmias, cardiac arrest**
GI: nausea, vomiting, diarrhea, abdominal discomfort, flatulence

Metabolic: hyperkalemia
Musculoskeletal: weakness and heaviness of legs

Interactions
Drug-drug. *ACE inhibitors, potassium-sparing diuretics, other potassium-containing preparations:* increased risk of hyperkalemia
Drug-diagnostic tests. *Potassium:* increased level
Drug-food. *Salt substitutes containing potassium:* increased risk of hyperkalemia
Drug-herbs. *Dandelion:* increased risk of hyperkalemia
Licorice: decreased response to potassium

Patient monitoring
- Monitor renal function, fluid intake and output, and potassium, creatinine, and blood urea nitrogen levels.
- 🔊 Be aware that potassium is contraindicated in patients with severe renal impairment and must be used with extreme caution (if at all) in patients with any degree of renal impairment, because of risk of life-threatening hyperkalemia.
- Assess vital signs. Check ECG for arrhythmias.
- Monitor neurologic status. Stay alert for neurologic complications.

Patient teaching
- Instruct patient to dissolve tablets thoroughly in 4 to 8 oz of cold water or juice and to sip solution over 5 to 10 minutes with a meal.
- Advise patient to minimize GI upset by eating small, frequent servings of food and drinking plenty of fluids.
- Tell patient to report nausea, vomiting, confusion, numbness and tingling, unusual tiredness or weakness, or a heavy feeling in legs.
- Instruct patient to avoid salt substitutes.

P

Reactions in **bold** are life-threatening. 🔊 Clinical alert

• As appropriate, review all other significant and life-threatening adverse reactions and interactions, especially those related to the drugs, tests, foods, and herbs mentioned above.

potassium chloride

Apo-K✢, K10✢, Kaon, Kay-Cee-L⊕, K-Dur✢, K-Lor, Klor-Con, K-Lyte✢, Klotrix, K-Med✢, K-Tab, Micro-K, Riva K 20 SR✢, Slow-K✢⊕, Slow-Pot

Pharmacologic class: Mineral, electrolyte

Therapeutic class: Electrolyte replacement, nutritional supplement

Pregnancy risk category C

Action
Maintains acid-base balance, isotonicity, and electrophysiologic balance throughout body tissues; crucial to nerve impulse transmission and contraction of cardiac, skeletal, and smooth muscle. Also essential for normal renal function and carbohydrate metabolism.

Availability
Capsules (extended-release): 8 mEq, 10 mEq
Powder for oral solution: 20 mEq, 25 mEq
Parenteral injection (concentrate): 2 mEq/ml
Parenteral solution: 0.1 mEq/ml, 0.2 mEq/ml, 0.3 mEq/ml, 0.4 mEq/ml
Potassium chloride in 5% dextrose injection: 10 mEq/L, 20 mEq/L, 30 mEq/L, 40 mEq/L
Potassium chloride in 0.9% sodium chloride injection: 20 mEq/L, 40 mEq/L
Potassium chloride in dextrose and lactated Ringer's injection: various strengths
Potassium chloride in dextrose and sodium chloride injection: various strengths
Solution (oral): 6.7 mEq, 10 mEq, 13.3 mEq, 15 mEq, 20 mEq, 30 mEq, 40 mEq
Tablets: 500 mg, 595 mg
Tablets (effervescent): 25 mEq, 50 mEq
Tablets (extended-release): 8 mEq, 10 mEq, 20 mEq
Tablets (extended-release crystals): 10 mEq, 20 mEq
Tablets (extended-release, film coated): 8 mEq, 10 mEq
Tablets (film-coated): 2.5 mEq, 10 mEq

❂ Indications and dosages
➤ To prevent potassium depletion
Adults: Dosage highly individualized. Usual single dosage is 20 mEq/day P.O. in divided doses.
➤ Potassium depletion; diabetic acidosis; metabolic alkalosis; arrhythmias; periodic paralysis attacks; hyperadrenocorticism; primary aldosteronism; healing phase of scalds or burns; overmedication with adrenocorticoids, testosterone, or corticotropin
Adults: Dosage highly individualized. 40 to 100 mEq/day P.O. in divided doses, not to exceed 20 mEq in a single dose. For serum potassium level above 2.5 mEq/L, 40 mEq/L as additive to I.V. infusion at a maximum rate of 10 mEq/hour; maximum daily dosage is 200 mEq. For serum potassium level less than 2 mEq/L, 80 mEq/L as additive to I.V. infusion at a maximum rate of 40 mEq/hour (with cardiac monitoring); maximum daily dosage is 400 mEq.
Children: Dosage highly individualized; give up to 3 mEq/kg or 40 mEq/m²/day as additive to I.V. infusion.

Contraindications
• Hypersensitivity to tartrazine or alcohol (with some products)
• Acute dehydration
• Heat cramps
• Hyperkalemia

✢ Canada   ⊕ UK   ⚔ Hazardous drug   ⊗ High-alert drug

- Hyperkalemic familial periodic paralysis
- Severe renal impairment
- Severe hemolytic reactions
- Severe tissue trauma
- Untreated Addison's disease
- Esophageal compression caused by enlarged left atrium (with wax matrix forms)
- Concurrent use of potassium-sparing diuretics, angiotensin-enzyme converting (ACE) inhibitors, or salt substitutes containing potassium

Precautions
Use cautiously in:
- cardiac disease, renal impairment, diabetes mellitus, hypomagnesemia
- pregnant or breastfeeding patients
- children (safety and efficacy not established).

Administration
◀≶ Know that I.V. potassium chloride is a high-alert drug.

◀≶ Give I.V. form as additive by infusion only. Never give undiluted or by I.V. push or I.M. route. Use peripheral line and infuse at a maximum rate of 40 mEq/hour (with cardiac monitoring).

◀≶ Dilute in compatible I.V. solution per manufacturer's instructions. Administer slowly to reduce risk of fatal hyperkalemia.

◀≶ To ensure that potassium is well mixed in compatible solution, don't add potassium to I.V. bottle in hanging position.

◀≶ Be aware that maximum infusion rate without cardiac monitoring is 20 mEq/hour. Rates above 20 mEq/hour require cardiac monitoring.

- Make sure patient is well-hydrated and urinating before starting therapy.
- If patient complains of burning with I.V. administration, decrease flow rate.

- Give P.O. form with meals and a full glass of water or juice, to minimize GI upset.
- Ensure that patient swallows wax-matrix tablets completely, to avoid serious esophageal problems.
- Don't give wax matrix tablets to patients who have swallowing problems or possible esophageal compression.
- Be aware that potassium preparations aren't interchangeable.
- Know that dosages are expressed in mEq of potassium and that potassium chloride contains 13.4 mEq potassium/g.

Route	Onset	Peak	Duration
P.O.	Unknown	1-2 hr	Unknown
I.V.	Rapid	End of infusion	Unknown

Adverse reactions
CNS: confusion, unusual fatigue, restlessness, asthenia, flaccid paralysis, paresthesia, absent reflexes
CV: ECG changes, hypotension, **arrhythmias, heart block, cardiac arrest**
GI: nausea, vomiting, diarrhea, abdominal discomfort, flatulence
Metabolic: hyperkalemia
Musculoskeletal: weakness and heaviness of legs
Respiratory: respiratory paralysis
Other: irritation at I.V. site

Interactions
Drug-drug. *ACE inhibitors, potassium-sparing diuretics, other potassium-containing preparations:* increased risk of hyperkalemia
Drug-diagnostic tests. *Potassium:* increased level
Drug-food. *Salt substitutes containing potassium:* increased risk of hyperkalemia

p

Reactions in **bold** are life-threatening. ◀≶ Clinical alert

Drug-herbs. *Dandelion:* increased risk of hyperkalemia
Licorice: decreased response to potassium

Patient monitoring
• Monitor renal function, fluid intake and output, and potassium, creatinine, and blood urea nitrogen levels.
• Assess vital signs and ECG. Stay alert for arrhythmias.
• Monitor neurologic status. Watch for neurologic complications.
• Monitor I.V. site for irritation.
◀◁ Know that potassium is contraindicated in patients with severe renal impairment and must be used with extreme caution (if at all) in patients with any degree of renal impairment, because of risk of life-threatening hyperkalemia.

Patient teaching
• Instruct patient to mix and dissolve powder completely in 3 to 8 oz of water or juice.
• Tell patient to swallow extended-release capsules whole without crushing or chewing them.
• Instruct patient to take oral form with or just after a meal, with a glass of water or fruit juice.
• Tell patient to sip diluted liquid form over 5 to 10 minutes.
• Advise patient to report nausea, vomiting, confusion, numbness and tingling, unusual fatigue or weakness, or a heavy feeling in legs.
• Tell patient to minimize GI upset by eating frequent, small servings of food and drinking plenty of fluids.
• Inform patient that although wax matrix form may appear in stool, drug has already been absorbed.
• Advise patient not to use salt substitutes.
• As appropriate, review all other significant and life-threatening adverse reactions and interactions, especially those related to the drugs, tests, foods, and herbs mentioned above.

potassium iodide
Iostat, Pima, SSKI, Thyrosafe, ThyroShield

Pharmacologic class: Iodine, iodide
Therapeutic class: Antithyroid agent, expectorant
Pregnancy risk category D

Action
Rapidly inhibits thyroid hormone release, reduces thyroid vascularity, and decreases thyroid uptake of radioactive iodine after radiation emergencies or administration of radioactive iodine isotopes. As expectorant, thought to increase respiratory tract secretions, thereby decreasing mucus viscosity.

Availability
Saturated solution (SSKI): 1 g potassium iodide/ml in 30- and 240-ml bottles
Solution (strong iodine solution, Lugol's solution): 5% iodine and 10% potassium iodide in 120-ml bottle
Syrup: 325 mg potassium iodide/5 ml
Tablets: 130 mg (available only through state and federal agencies)

⏀ Indications and dosages
➤ Preparation for thyroidectomy
Adults and children: One to five drops SSKI P.O. t.i.d. or three to six drops strong iodine solution P.O. t.i.d. for 10 days before surgery
➤ Thyrotoxic crisis
Adults and children: 500 mg P.O. (approximately 10 drops SSKI) q 4 hours or 1 ml P.O. (strong iodine solution) t.i.d., at least 1 hour after initial propylthiouracil or methimazole dose
➤ Radiation protectant in emergencies
Adults older than age 40 with predicted thyroid exposure of 500

centigrays (cGy), adults ages 18 to 40 with predicted exposure of 10 cGy, pregnant or breastfeeding women with predicted exposure of 5 cGy, and adolescents weighing 70 kg (154 lb) or more with predicted exposure of 5 cGy: 130 mg P.O. (tablet)

Children ages 3 to 18 (except adolescents weighing 70 kg [154 lb] or more) with predicted thyroid exposure of 5 cGy: 65 mg P.O. (tablet)

Children ages 1 month to 3 years with predicted thyroid exposure of 5 cGy: 32 mg P.O. (tablet)

Infants from birth to age 1 month with predicted thyroid exposure of 5 cGy: 16 mg P.O. (tablet)

➤ Expectorant

Adults: 300 to 650 mg P.O. (SSKI) three or four times daily, given with at least 6 oz of fluid

Children: 60 to 250 mg P.O. (SSKI) q.i.d., given with at least 6 oz of fluid

Off-label uses
• Lymphocutaneous sporotrichosis

Contraindications
• Hypersensitivity to iodine, shellfish, or bisulfites (with some products)
• Hypothyroidism
• Renal impairment
• Acute bronchitis
• Addison's disease
• Acute dehydration
• Heat cramps
• Hyperkalemia
• Tuberculosis
• Iodism
• Concurrent use of potassium-containing drugs, potassium-sparing diuretics, or salt substitutes containing potassium

Precautions
Use cautiously in:
• cystic fibrosis, adolescent acne, hypocomplementemic vasculitis, goiter, autoimmune thyroid disease

• pregnant or breastfeeding patients
• children.

Administration
• Dilute saturated solution with at least 6 oz of water.

◀≀ Don't give concurrently with other potassium-containing drugs or potassium-sparing diuretics, because of increased risk of hyperkalemia, arrhythmias, and cardiac arrest.

• Know that U.S. government stockpiles potassium iodide 130-mg tablets for emergency use.

• When giving to very young children or patients who can't swallow tablets, crush tablet, dissolve in 20 ml of water, and add 20 ml of selected beverage (such as orange juice).

• Be aware that potassium iodide use as expectorant has been largely replaced by safer and more effective drugs.

Route	Onset	Peak	Duration
P.O.	24 hr	10-15 days	Variable

Adverse reactions
CNS: confusion; unusual fatigue; paresthesia, pain, or weakness in hands or feet

Metabolic: thyroid hyperplasia, goiter (with prolonged use), thyroid adenoma, severe hypothyroidism, **hyperkalemia, iodism** (with large doses or prolonged use)

Musculoskeletal: weakness and heaviness of legs

Other: tooth discoloration (with strong iodide solution), hypersensitivity reactions including angioedema, fever, cutaneous and mucosal hemorrhage, serum sickness-like reaction

Interactions
Drug-drug. *Lithium, other thyroid drugs:* additive hypothyroidism
Potassium-sparing diuretics, other potassium preparations: increased risk

p

Reactions in **bold** are life-threatening. ◀≀ Clinical alert of hyperkalemia, arrhythmias, and cardiac arrest

Drug-diagnostic tests. *Radionuclide thyroid imaging:* altered test results
Thyroid uptake of ^{131}I, ^{123}I, sodium pertechnetate Tc 99m: decreased uptake
Drug-food. *Salt substitutes containing potassium:* increased risk of hyperkalemia

Patient monitoring

◀€ In long-term use, check for signs and symptoms of iodism (metallic taste, sore teeth and gums, sore throat, burning of mouth and throat, coldlike symptoms, severe headache, productive cough, GI irritation, diarrhea, angioedema, rash, fever, and cutaneous or mucosal hemorrhage). Discontinue drug immediately if these occur.

• Monitor potassium level; watch for signs and symptoms of potassium toxicity.

• Assess ECG, renal function, fluid intake and output, and creatinine and blood urea nitrogen levels.

• Monitor thyroid function tests. Watch for evidence of hypothyroidism or hyperthyroidism.

Patient teaching

• Tell patient to dilute in at least 6 oz of water or juice and to take with meals.

• Advise patient to sip strong iodine solution through a straw to help prevent tooth discoloration.

◀€ Teach patient to recognize and immediately report signs and symptoms of iodism and potassium toxicity.

• Instruct patient to minimize GI upset by eating small, frequent servings of food and drinking plenty of fluids.

• Inform patient that many salt substitutes are high in potassium. Advise him not to use these without prescriber's approval.

• Caution patient not to take drug if she is pregnant or breastfeeding (except in emergency use).

• As appropriate, review all other significant and life-threatening adverse reactions and interactions, especially those related to the drugs, tests, and foods mentioned above.

pralatrexate

Folotyn

Pharmacologic class: Folic acid antagonist

Therapeutic class: Antineoplastic

Pregnancy risk category D

Action

Competitively inhibits dihydrofolate reductase and is a competitive inhibitor for polyglutamylation by the enzyme folylpolyglutamyl synthetase, resulting in depletion of thymidine and other biological molecules, the synthesis of which depends on single carbon transfer

Availability

Solution for injection: 20 mg/1 ml, 40 mg/2 ml in single-use vials

Indications and dosages

➤ Relapsed or refractory peripheral T-cell lymphoma

Adults: 30 mg/m² by I.V. push over 3 to 5 minutes weekly for 6 weeks in 7-week cycles until disease progression or unacceptable toxicity occurs. Give with supplemental oral folic acid and I.M. vitamin B_{12}.

Dosage adjustment

• Mucositis
• Hematologic toxicities
• Liver function test abnormalities of Grade 3 or greater

Contraindications

None

Precautions

Use cautiously in:
• moderate to severe renal impairment, liver function test abnormalities
• thrombocytopenia, neutropenia, anemia, mucositis, dermatologic reactions, tumor lysis syndrome
• pregnant or breastfeeding patients (avoid use)
• children (safety and efficacy not established).

Administration

• Be aware that drug should be administered under supervision of qualified physician experienced in the use of antineoplastics, with appropriate management of complications and adequate diagnostic and treatment facilities readily available.
• Obtain serum chemistry tests, including renal and hepatic function, before start of first and fourth dose of a given cycle.
• Before administering, be aware that mucositis should be Grade 1 or less, platelet count should be 100,000/mm^3 or more for first dose and 50,000/mm^3 or more for all subsequent doses, and absolute neutrophil count (ANC) should be 1,000/mm^3 or more.
• Don't dilute drug.
• Administer by I.V. push over 3 to 5 minutes through side port of a free-flowing 0.9% Sodium Chloride Injection I.V. line once weekly for 6 weeks in 7-week cycles (6 weeks on drug and 1 week off each cycle) until progressive disease or unacceptable toxicity occurs.
• Be aware that patient should take low-dose (1.0 to 1.25 mg) oral folic acid daily, initiated during 10-day period preceding first pralatrexate dose, with dosing continued during full course of therapy and for 30 days after last pralatrexate dose. In addition, patient should receive vitamin B$_{12}$ (1 mg) I.M. no more than 10 weeks before first pralatrexate dose and every 8 to 10 weeks thereafter. Subsequent vitamin B$_{12}$ injections may be given the same day as pralatrexate treatment.
• Omit or modify doses for hematologic toxicities, Grade 2 or greater mucositis, severe dermatologic reactions, or liver function test abnormalities of Grade 3 or greater. Omitted doses must not be made up at end of cycle, and once a dosage has been reduced for toxicity, it must not be reescalated.

Route	Onset	Peak	Duration
I.V.	Unknown	Unknown	Unknown

Adverse reactions

CNS: fatigue, asthenia
CV: tachycardia
EENT: epistaxis, pharyngolaryngeal pain
GI: nausea, vomiting, diarrhea, constipation, abdominal pain, anorexia, stomatitis, mucositis of GI tract
GU: mucositis of GU tract
Hematologic: anemia, neutropenia, leukopenia, thrombocytopenia, **febrile neutropenia**
Hepatic: liver function test abnormalities
Metabolic: hypokalemia
Musculoskeletal: extremity pain, back pain
Respiratory: dyspnea, cough, upper respiratory tract infection
Skin: rash, pruritus
Other: pyrexia, dehydration, edema, night sweats, **sepsis, tumor lysis syndrome**

Interactions

Drug-drug. *Probenecid, other drugs that may affect relevant transporter systems (such as NSAIDs):* delayed pralatrexate clearance resulting in increased pralatrexate exposure with subsequent increased risk of systemic toxicity

P

Reactions in **bold** are life-threatening.   ◄€ Clinical alert

Drug-diagnostic tests. *ALT, AST, transaminases:* increased levels
Platelets, potassium: decreased levels

Patient monitoring

• Monitor CBC with differential and severity of mucositis weekly.

• Continue to monitor serum chemistry tests, including renal and hepatic function.

◀€ Continue to closely monitor patient for tumor lysis syndrome (irregular heartbeat, shortness of breath, high potassium level, high uric acid level, impaired mental ability, kidney failure), and dermatologic reactions.

Patient teaching

• Inform patient about the need to take folic acid and vitamin B$_{12}$ during treatment.

◀€ Instruct patient to immediately report signs and symptoms of infection (including fever), skin reactions, mucositis, tumor lysis syndrome (irregular heartbeat, shortness of breath, impaired mental ability, urinary problems), yellowing of skin or eyes, dark urine, or right upper abdominal pain or discomfort.

• Instruct patient to tell prescriber about all drugs he's taking, including nonprescription drugs, because some drugs have potential for serious drug interactions.

• Advise female patient of childbearing age to avoid pregnancy and breastfeeding during therapy.

• As appropriate, review all other significant and life-threatening adverse reactions and interactions, especially those related to the drugs and tests mentioned above.

pramipexole dihydrochloride

Apo-Pramipexole✸, Mirapex, Mirapex ER, Mirapexin✛, Novo-Pramipexole✸, PMS-Pramipexole✸

Pharmacologic class: Non-ergot dopamine agonist
Therapeutic class: Antidyskinetic
Pregnancy risk category C

Action

Unknown. May directly stimulate postsynaptic dopamine receptors in corpus striatum (unlike levodopa, which may increase brain's dopamine concentration).

Availability

Tablets: 0.125 mg, 0.25 mg, 0.5 mg, 0.75 mg, 1 mg, 1.5 mg
Tablets (extended-release): 0.375 mg, 0.75 mg, 1.5 mg, 2.25 mg, 3 mg, 3.75 mg, 4.5 mg

🕖 Indications and dosages

➤ Idiopathic Parkinson's disease
Adults: Initially, 0.125 mg P.O. t.i.d.; may increase by 0.125 mg q 5 to 7 days over 6 to 7 weeks. Maintenance dosage ranges from 1.5 to 4.5 mg/day in three divided doses. Or, 0.375 mg (extended-release) P.O. daily; may increase no more frequently than every 5 to 7 days, first to 0.75 mg/day and then by 0.75-mg increments up to a maximum recommended dosage of 4.5 mg/day. Assess therapeutic response and tolerability at a minimal interval of 5 days or longer after each dose increment.
➤ Moderate to severe primary restless leg syndrome
Adults: Initially, 0.125 mg P.O. once daily 2 to 3 hours before bedtime. For

patients requiring additional symptomatic relief, increase dosage as needed every 4 to 7 days, up to dosage of 0.5 mg once daily.

Dosage adjustment
• Renal impairment

Contraindications
• Hypersensitivity to drug or its components

Precautions
Use cautiously in:
• renal impairment
• elderly patients
• pregnant or breastfeeding patients
• children (safety not established).

Administration
• Administer extended-release tablets whole.
• Know that patients may be switched overnight from immediate-release tablets to extended-release tablets at the same daily dose; however, dosage adjustment may be needed in some patients.
• Don't give at same time as other CNS depressants.
• Don't stop therapy abruptly. Taper dosage over 1 week.

Route	Onset	Peak	Duration
P.O.	Unknown	2 hr	8 hr

Adverse reactions
CNS: headache, dizziness, drowsiness, hallucinations, asthenia, confusion, dyskinesia, insomnia, hypertonia, unsteadiness, sleep attacks, abnormal dreams, amnesia
CV: orthostatic hypotension
EENT: retinal deterioration
GI: nausea, constipation, dyspepsia, dry mouth
GU: urinary frequency, erectile dysfunction
Musculoskeletal: leg cramps

Respiratory: fibrotic complications (such as retroperitoneal fibrosis, pulmonary infiltrates, pleural effusion or thickening)
Skin: rhabdomyolysis (immediate release tablets)
Other: accidental injury, edema

Interactions
Drug-drug. *Cimetidine:* increased pramipexole blood level
Dopamine antagonists (such as butyrophenones, metoclopramide, phenothiazines, thioxanthenes): decreased pramipexole efficacy
Levodopa: increased risk of hallucinations and dyskinesia

Patient monitoring
• Evaluate patient for therapeutic and adverse effects.
• Assess blood pressure; watch for orthostatic hypotension.
• Monitor neurologic status, especially for sleep attacks and extrapyramidal symptoms.
• Watch closely for pulmonary complications.

Patient teaching
• Instruct patient to take drug with food if it causes nausea. Tell him not to take at same time as other CNS depressants.
• Instruct patient to swallow extended-release tablets whole and not to chew, crush, or divide them.
• Advise patient to report respiratory problems, dyskinesia, hallucinations, and sleep attacks.
• Tell patient drug may cause erectile dysfunction. Encourage him to discuss this effect with prescriber.
• Inform patient and family that drug's neurologic and motor effects increase risk of sudden onset of sleep without warning and accidental injury. Teach them ways to prevent injury.
🔊 Advise patient and family to contact prescriber if vision changes or

P

Reactions in **bold** are life-threatening.   🔊 Clinical alert

unexplained muscle pain, tenderness, or weakness occurs.

• Tell patient to move slowly when sitting up or standing, to avoid dizziness from sudden blood pressure decrease.

• As appropriate, review all other significant and life-threatening adverse reactions and interactions, especially those related to the drugs mentioned above.

pramlintide acetate
Symlin

Pharmacologic class: Synthetic amylin
Therapeutic class: Hypoglycemic
Pregnancy risk category C

FDA | BOXED WARNING

• Drug is used with insulin and has been linked to increased risk of insulin-induced severe hypoglycemia, especially in patients with type 1 diabetes. When severe hypoglycemia occurs, it arises within 3 hours after injection. If it occurs while patient operates a motor vehicle or heavy machinery or performs other high-risk activities, serious injuries may occur. Careful patient selection, patient instruction, and insulin dosage adjustments are crucial to reduce risk.

Action
Mimics amylin activity to modulate gastric emptying, prevent postprandial rise in plasma glucagons, and cause feeling of satiety leading to decreased caloric intake and potential weight loss

Availability
Solution for injection: 0.6 mg/ml in 5-ml vials; 1.5-ml disposable multidose pen-injector containing 1,000 mcg/ml; 2.7-ml disposable multidose 120 pen-injector containing 1,000 mcg/ml

🕡 Indications and dosages
➤ Type 1 diabetes mellitus as adjunct treatment in patients who take insulin with meals but haven't obtained desired glycemic control despite optimal insulin therapy

Adults: Initially, 15 mcg subcutaneous injection immediately before major meals; after 3 days, increase in 15-mcg increments to maintenance dosage of 30 or 60 mcg as tolerated. Decrease preprandial rapid- or short-acting insulin dosages (including fixed-mix insulins) by 50%.

➤ Type 2 diabetes mellitus as adjunct treatment in patients who take insulin with meals but haven't obtained desired glycemic control despite optimal insulin therapy, with or without concurrent sulfonylurea, metformin, or both

Adults: Initially, 60 mcg subcutaneous injection immediately before major meals; after 3 to 7 days, increase to 120 mcg as tolerated. Decrease preprandial rapid- or short-acting insulin dosages (including fixed-mix insulins) by 50%.

Contraindications
• Hypersensitivity to drug or its components
• Confirmed gastroparesis
• Hypoglycemia unawareness

Precautions
Use cautiously in:
• patients with poor compliance to insulin therapy or hemoglobin A1c levels above 9%
• patients with recurrent or severe hypoglycemia who've required treatment during past 6 months
• concurrent insulin therapy for type 1 diabetes

🍁 Canada   ⊕ UK   ☡ Hazardous drug   ⊗ High-alert drug

- concurrent use of drugs that stimulate GI motility
- elderly patients
- pregnant or breastfeeding patients
- children (safety and efficacy not established).

Administration
- Administer immediately before major meals (at least 250 kcal or 30 g carbohydrates).
- Give pramlintide and insulin as separate injections.
- Inject pramlintide and insulin more than 2″ apart.

Route	Onset	Peak	Duration
Subcut.	Unknown	19-21 min	Unknown

Adverse reactions
CNS: headache, dizziness, fatigue
EENT: pharyngitis
GI: nausea, vomiting, abdominal pain, anorexia
Metabolic: severe hypoglycemia
Musculoskeletal: arthralgia
Respiratory: cough
Other: allergic reaction

Interactions
Drug-drug. *Angiotensin-converting enzyme inhibitors, disopyramide, fibric acid derivatives, fluoxetine, monoamine oxidase inhibitors, oral hypoglycemics, pentoxifylline, propoxyphene, salicylates, sulfonamide antibiotics:* increased hypoglycemic effect, increased risk of hypoglycemia
Beta-adrenergic blockers, clonidine, guanethidine, reserpine: blunting of early hypoglycemia symptoms
Drugs that delay gastric emptying (such as atropine) or slow food absorption (such as acarbose): exacerbated delay in gastric emptying, slow food absorption
Insulin: severe hypoglycemia (may occur within 3 hours of insulin administration)

Oral drugs for which rapid effect is desired (such as analgesics): delayed absorption of these drugs

Patient monitoring
- Monitor premeal and postmeal blood glucose levels closely; watch for hypoglycemia.

Patient teaching
- Instruct patient to take drug immediately before major meals.
- Teach patient how to self-administer injection; describe proper storage, handling, and disposal of drug and supplies.
- Instruct patient to inject pramlintide and insulin separately, more than 2″ apart. Caution patient not to mix them together.
- Teach patient to recognize and immediately report hypoglycemia symptoms; tell him these may occur within 3 hours after pramlintide injection.
- As appropriate, review all other significant and life-threatening adverse reactions and interactions, especially those related to the drugs mentioned above.

prasugrel
Effient

Pharmacologic class: Thienopyridine platelet inhibitor
Therapeutic class: Antiplatelet drug
Pregnancy risk category B

FDA BOXED WARNING
- Drug can cause significant, sometime fatal, bleeding.
- Don't use in patients with active pathological bleeding or history of

transient ischemic attack or stroke (patients age 75 and older).

• Drug is generally not recommended, because of increased risk of fatal and intracranial bleeding and uncertain benefit. In high-risk situations (such as patients with diabetes or history of prior myocardial infarction, where its effect appears to be greater), its use may be considered.

• Don't start drug in patients likely to undergo urgent coronary artery bypass graft (CABG). If possible, discontinue drug at least 7 days before any surgery.

• Additional risk factors for bleeding include body weight of less than 132 lb (60 kg), propensity for bleeding, concomitant use of medications that increase bleeding risk (such as warfarin, heparin, fibrinolytics, and nonsteroidal anti-inflammatory drugs [prolonged use]). Suspect bleeding in patient who is hypotensive and has recently undergone coronary angiography, percutaneous coronary intervention (PCI), CABG, or other surgical procedures.

• If possible, manage bleeding without discontinuing drug. Discontinuing drug, particularly in first few weeks after acute coronary syndrome, increases risk of subsequent cardiovascular events.

Action

Inhibits platelet activation and aggregation through irreversible binding of its active metabolite to the P2Y12 class of adenosine diphosphate receptors on platelets

Availability

Tablets: 5 mg, 10 mg

🕖 Indications and dosages

➤ Reduction of rate of thrombotic cardiovascular events in patients with acute coronary syndrome who are to be managed with PCI as follows: patients with unstable angina or non-ST-elevation myocardial infarction (MI) and patients with ST-elevation MI when managed with primary or delayed PCI

Adults: Initially, 60 mg P.O. as loading dose; then, 10 mg P.O. daily (with aspirin 75 to 325 mg daily)

Dosage adjustment

• Adults weighing less than 132 lb

Contraindications

• Hypersensitivity to drug or its components
• Active pathological bleeding
• History of transient ischemic attack or cerebrovascular accident

Precautions

Use cautiously in:
• CABG-related bleeding, patients at general risk for bleeding
• thrombotic thrombocytopenia purpura
• low body weight (less than 132 lb)
• elderly patients age 75 and older (use not recommended except in high-risk situations, such as diabetes and history of MI)
• pregnant or breastfeeding patients
• children (safety and efficacy not established).

Administration

• Administer with or without food.
🔊 Be aware that premature drug discontinuation increases risk of stent thrombosis, MI, and death.

Route	Onset	Peak	Duration
P.O.	Unknown	30 min	Unknown

Adverse reactions

CNS: headache, dizziness, fatigue, **intracranial hemorrhage**
CV: hypertension, hypotension, bradycardia, peripheral edema, **atrial fibrillation**

EENT: epistaxis
GI: nausea, diarrhea, **GI hemorrhage**
Hematologic: leukopenia, bleeding, **life-threatening bleeding, thrombotic thrombocytopenia purpura**
Metabolic: hypercholesterolemia, hyperlipidemia
Musculoskeletal: back pain, extremity pain
Respiratory: dyspnea, cough
Skin: rash
Other: chest pain, pyrexia, **newly diagnosed malignancies**

Interactions
Drug-drug. *Nonsteroidal anti-inflammatory drugs, warfarin:* increased risk of bleeding
Drug-diagnostic tests. *Cholesterol, lipids:* increased levels
White blood cells: decreased count

Patient monitoring
◀€ Closely monitor coagulation studies and CBC with white cell differential and watch for evidence of bleeding.
• Monitor cholesterol and lipid levels closely.

Patient teaching
• Instruct patient to take drug with or without food.
◀€ Instruct patient to immediately report to prescriber blood in stool or urine or unanticipated, prolonged, or excessive bleeding.
◀€ Instruct patient to promptly report to prescriber if fever, weakness, extreme skin paleness, purple skin patches, or neurologic changes, such as dizziness or headache, occur.
• Advise patient to notify all health care professionals that he's taking prasugrel.
• Advise patient not to take other prescription or nonprescription drugs or dietary supplements without first discussing with prescriber.
• Caution patient not to discontinue drug without first discussing with prescriber.

• As appropriate, review all other significant and life-threatening adverse reactions and interactions, especially those related to the drugs and tests mentioned above.

pravastatin sodium
Apo-Pravastatin✷, CO Pravastatin✷, Dom-Pravastatin✷, Gen-Pravastatin✷, Lipostat✦, Novo-Pravastatin✷, Nu-Pravastatin✷, PHL-Pravastatin,✷, PMS-Pravastatin✷, Pravachol, Ran-Pravastatin✷, Ratio-Pravastatin✷, Riva-Pravastatin✷, Sandoz Pravastatin✷

Pharmacologic class: HMG-CoA reductase inhibitor
Therapeutic class: Antilipemic
Pregnancy risk category X

Action
Inhibits HMG-CoA reductase, an enzyme that catalyzes cholesterol synthesis pathway. This action decreases cholesterol, triglyceride, apolipoprotein B, and low-density lipoprotein (LDL) levels and increases high-density lipoprotein levels.

Availability
Tablets: 10 mg, 20 mg, 40 mg, 80 mg

⏀ Indications and dosages
➤ Adjunct to diet to reduce risk of total mortality by reducing coronary death, myocardial infarction, revascularization, stroke or transient ischemic attack, and progression of coronary atherosclerosis in patients with clinically evident coronary heart disease; to reduce elevated total cholesterol, LDL cholesterol (LDL-C), apolipoprotein B, and triglyceride (TG) levels and increase high-density lipoprotein levels in patients with primary

hypercholesterolemia and mixed dyslipidemia; to reduce elevated serum TG
levels in patients with hypertriglyceridemia; to treat patients with primary dysbetalipoproteinemia who
aren't responding to diet

Adults: 40 mg P.O. once daily. Use 80-
mg dose only for patients not reaching
LDL-C goal with 40 mg. Adjust dosage
at 4 weeks according to patient's
response and established treatment
guidelines.

➤ Heterozygous familial hypercholesterolemia after failure of adequate trial
of diet therapy

Adolescents ages 14 to 18: 40 mg P.O.
daily

Children ages 8 to 13: 20 mg P.O. daily

Dosage adjustment

• Significant renal impairment
• Concurrent use of niacin

Contraindications

• Hypersensitivity to drug or other
HMG-CoA reductase inhibitors
• Active hepatic disease or unexplained,
persistent transaminase elevations
• Pregnancy, breastfeeding, females of
childbearing age

Precautions

Use cautiously in:
• renal impairment; severe hypotension or hypertension; severe acute
infection; severe metabolic, endocrine,
or electrolyte disorders; uncontrolled
seizures; visual disturbances; myopathy; major surgery; trauma; alcoholism
• history of hepatic disease
• concurrent use of gemfibrozil (avoid
use)
• concurrent use of colchicine, fibrates,
or lipid-modifying doses of niacin
(1 g/day or greater)
• children younger than age 8 (safety
not established).

Administration

• If patient's also receiving bile-acid
resin, give pravastatin at bedtime, at
least 4 hours after resin.

Route	Onset	Peak	Duration
P.O.	Unknown	Unknown	Unknown

Adverse reactions

CNS: headache, malaise, fatigue, dizziness, insomnia, anxiety, depression,
tremor, vertigo, memory loss, peripheral nerve palsy, paresthesia, peripheral
neuropathy, asthenia

EENT: impaired extraocular eye movements, cataract progression, ophthal-
moplegia, dry eyes

GI: nausea, vomiting, diarrhea, constipation, abdominal or biliary pain, flatulence, dyspepsia, heartburn, anorexia,
pancreatitis

GU: decreased libido, erectile dysfunction, gynecomastia

Hematologic: anemia, **thrombocytopenia, leukopenia**

Hepatic: jaundice, cholestatic jaundice,
fatty liver changes, **hepatoma, hepatic
necrosis, hepatitis**

Musculoskeletal: joint pain, myalgia,
myositis, **rhabdomyolysis**

Respiratory: dyspnea, upper respiratory tract infection

Skin: nodules, skin discoloration,
alopecia, dry skin, pruritus, rash,
urticaria, nail changes, photosensitivity

Other: altered taste, localized pain,
rare hypersensitivity reactions (including polymyalgia rheumatica, arthritis,
dermatomyositis, vasculitis, purpura,
positive antinuclear antibody,
eosinophilia, fever, chills, flushing,
**hemolytic anemia, epidermal necrol-
ysis, erythema multiforme**, Stevens-
Johnson syndrome, angioedema,
lupus erythematosus–like reaction,
and anaphylaxis**)

Interactions

Drug-drug. *Clarithromycin, colchicine,
cyclosporine, erythromycin, fibrates,*

gemfibrozil, lipid-modifying doses of niacin, other HMG-CoA reductase inhibitors: increased risk of myopathy

Drug-diagnostic tests. *Alanine aminotransferase, aspartate aminotransferase, creatine kinase, creatinine phosphokinase:* increased levels

Patient monitoring

• Watch for signs and symptoms of allergic reaction.

• Monitor vital signs and cardiovascular status.

◀€ Evaluate liver function tests before starting therapy, 6 to 12 weeks later, and at least semiannually thereafter. Also monitor lipid levels, and watch for evidence of hepatic disorders (rare).

◀€ Assess creatine kinase level if patient has muscle pain or is receiving other drugs associated with myopathy. Discontinue drug if myopathy is diagnosed or suspected. Continue to monitor for signs and symptoms of rhabdomyolysis (rare).

Patient teaching

• Caution patient not to take with antacids.

◀€ Teach patient to recognize and immediately report signs and symptoms of allergic response and other adverse reactions, especially myositis.

• Tell patient drug may cause headache and musculoskeletal pain. Encourage him to discuss activity recommendations and pain management with prescriber.

◀€ Advise patient to promptly report unusual fatigue, yellowing of skin or eyes, and unexplained muscle pain, tenderness, or weakness.

• Advise female of childbearing age to notify prescriber of suspected pregnancy. Caution her not to breastfeed during therapy.

• Tell male patient that drug may cause erectile dysfunction and abnormal ejaculation. Suggest that he discuss these issues with prescriber.

• Caution patient to avoid driving and other hazardous activities until he knows how drug affects concentration, alertness, and vision.

• As appropriate, review all other significant and life-threatening adverse reactions and interactions, especially those related to the drugs, tests, and herbs mentioned above.

prednisolone
Delacortril⊕, Deltastab⊕, Precortisyl⊕, Prelone

prednisolone acetate
Diopred✦, Omnipred, Pred Forte Ophthalmic, Pred Mild Ophthalmic

prednisolone sodium phosphate
Inflamase Mild Ophthalmic✦, Oraprad, Oraprad ODT, Pediapred, Predsol⊕

Pharmacologic class: Corticosteroid (intermediate-acting)

Therapeutic class: Anti-inflammatory, immunosuppressant

Pregnancy risk category C

Action

Exerts potent anti-inflammatory (glucocorticoid) and weak sodium-retaining (mineralocorticoid) activity. Glucocorticoid activity causes profound and varied metabolic effects.

Availability

Oral solution: 5 mg/ml
Suspension for injection (acetate): 25 mg/ml, 40 mg/ml, 50 mg/ml

p

Suspension (ophthalmic): 0.12%, 0.125%, 1%
Syrup: 5 mg/5 ml, 15 mg/5 ml
Tablets: 5 mg
Tablets (orally disintegrating, sodium phosphate): 10 mg, 15 mg, 30 mg

ⓘ Indications and dosages

➤ Severe inflammation; immunosuppression

Adults: Dosage individualized based on diagnosis, severity of condition, and response. Usual dosage ranges from 5 to 60 mg P.O. (prednisolone) daily in two to four divided doses, or 4 to 60 mg I.M. (acetate) daily in divided doses, or 5 to 50 mg P.O. (sodium phosphate) daily in divided doses.

➤ Acute exacerbation of multiple sclerosis

Adults: 200 mg P.O. daily for 1 week, followed by 80 mg every other day for 1 month

➤ Refractory bronchial asthma

Children: 1 to 2 mg/kg/day (sodium phosphate) as a single dose or in divided doses; may continue for 3 to 10 days or until symptoms resolve or patient achieves peak expiratory flow rate of 80% of personal best

➤ Nephrotic syndrome in children

Children: 60 mg/m^2 P.O. (sodium phosphate solution) daily in three divided doses for 4 weeks, then 4 weeks of alternate-day therapy at single doses of 40 mg/m^2

➤ Various allergic conditions and dermatologic, endocrine, GI, hematologic, neoplastic, nervous system, ophthalmic, respiratory, and rheumatic disorders

Adults: Variable and individualized depending on condition being treated and patient response. Initially, 10 to 60 mg (ODT) P.O. daily.

Children: Variable and individualized depending on condition being treated. Initial dosage range is 0.14 to 2 mg/kg/day P.O. in three or four divided doses.

➤ Steroid-responsive inflammatory eye conditions

Adults: In severe cases, initially one to two drops (acetate or sodium phosphate) instilled into conjunctival sac q hour during day and q 2 hours at night. In mild or moderate inflammation or in severe cases that respond favorably, one to two drops q 3 to 12 hours.

Contraindications

• Hypersensitivity to drug, other corticosteroids, alcohol, bisulfite, or tartrazine (with some products)
• Systemic fungal infections
• Active untreated infections (except in selected patients with meningitis)
• Acute superficial herpes simplex, keratitis, fungal or viral eye diseases, tuberculosis of eye, or after uncomplicated removal of superficial corneal foreign body (ophthalmic use)
• Idiopathic thrombocytopenic purpura (with I.M. use)
• Live-virus vaccines (with immunosuppressive prednisolone dosages)

Precautions

Use cautiously in:
• diabetes mellitus, glaucoma, renal or hepatic disease, hypothyroidism, cirrhosis, diverticulitis, nonspecific ulcerative colitis, recent intestinal anastomoses, inflammatory bowel disease, thromboembolic disorders, seizures, myasthenia gravis, heart failure, hypertension, osteoporosis, ocular herpes simplex, immunosuppression, emotional instability
• pregnant or breastfeeding patients
• children younger than age 6 (younger than age 2 when treated for nephrotic syndrome; younger than age 1 month when treated for aggressive lymphomas and leukemias with ODT form).

Administration

🔊 Be aware that prednisolone has many different formulations that may be given by various routes: P.O., I.M., or ophthalmic. Before administering, make sure formulation can be given by prescribed route.

• Don't break ODT tablets.

• Place ODT tablet on tongue and either swallow tablet whole or allow it to dissolve in mouth with or without water.

• Inject I.M. form deep into gluteal muscle. Rotate injection sites.

• Avoid subcutaneous injection.

🔊 In systemic therapy, don't discontinue drug abruptly, even if inhaled steroid is added.

• Know that additional corticosteroids are needed during stress or trauma.

Route	Onset	Peak	Duration
P.O. (prednisolone, sod. phos.)	Unknown	1-2 hr	1.25-1.5 days
I.M. (acetate)	Slow	Unknown	Unknown
Ophth. (acetate, sod. phos.)	Unknown	Unknown	Unknown

Adverse reactions

CNS: headache, nervousness, depression, euphoria, personality changes, psychosis, vertigo, paresthesia, insomnia, restlessness, **seizures, meningitis, increased intracranial pressure, hypertrophic cardiomyopathy in premature infants**

CV: hypotension, hypertension, vasculitis, **thrombophlebitis, thromboembolism, fat embolism, arrhythmias, heart failure, shock**

EENT: cataracts, glaucoma, visual disturbances, exacerbation of ocular infection, secondary ocular infections, globe perforation at corneal or scleral thinning site, transient stinging or burning of eyes, dry eyes, corneal ulcers, mydriasis (all with ophthalmic use); posterior subcapsular cataracts (especially in children), glaucoma, nasal irritation and congestion, rebound congestion, sneezing, epistaxis, nasopharyngeal and oropharyngeal fungal infections, perforated nasal septum, anosmia, dysphonia, hoarseness, throat irritation (with long-term use)

GI: nausea, vomiting, abdominal distention, rectal bleeding, dry mouth, esophageal candidiasis, esophageal ulcer, **pancreatitis, peptic ulcer**

GU: amenorrhea, irregular menses

Hematologic: purpura

Metabolic: sodium and fluid retention, hypokalemia, hypocalcemia, hyperglycemia, decreased carbohydrate tolerance, growth retardation (in children), diabetes mellitus, cushingoid effects (with long-term use), **hypothalamic-pituitary-adrenal suppression** (with systemic use longer than 5 days), **adrenal suppression** (with high-dose, long-term use)

Musculoskeletal: muscle weakness or atrophy, myalgia, myopathy, osteoporosis, aseptic joint necrosis, spontaneous fractures (with long-term use), osteonecrosis, tendon rupture

Respiratory: cough, wheezing, **bronchospasm**

Skin: urticaria, rash, pruritus, contact dermatitis, acne, striae, poor wound healing, thin fragile skin, bruising, hirsutism, petechiae, subcutaneous fat atrophy, urticaria, angioedema

Other: aggravation or masking of infections, increased or decreased appetite, weight gain (with long-term use), facial edema and erythema, edema, hypersensitivity reaction

Interactions

Drug-drug. *Amphotericin B, mezlocillin, piperacillin, thiazide and loop diuretics, ticarcillin:* additive hypokalemia

Anticholinesterase drugs: decreased anticholinesterase effect (when prednisolone is used for myasthenia gravis)

p

Aspirin, other nonsteroidal anti-inflammatory drugs: increased risk of GI discomfort and bleeding

Cardiac glycosides: increased risk of digitalis toxicity due to hypokalemia

Cyclosporine: therapeutic benefits in organ transplant recipients, but with increased risk of toxicity

Erythromycin, indinavir, itraconazole, ketoconazole, ritonavir, saquinavir: increased prednisolone blood level and effects

Hormonal contraceptives: impaired metabolism and increased effects of prednisolone

Isoniazid: decreased isoniazid blood level

Live-virus vaccines: decreased antibody response to vaccine, increased risk of adverse effects

Oral anticoagulants: reduced anticoagulant requirement, opposition to anticoagulant action

Phenobarbital, phenytoin, rifampin: decreased prednisolone efficacy

Salicylates: reduced salicylate blood level

Somatrem: inhibition of somatrem's growth-promoting effects

Theophylline: altered pharmacologic effects of either drug

Skin tests: suppressed results

Drug-diagnostic tests. *Calcium, potassium, thyroid ^{131}I uptake, thyroxine, triiodothyronine:* decreased levels

Cholesterol, glucose: increased levels

Nitroblue tetrazolium test for bacterial infection: false-negative result

Skin tests: suppressed results

Drug-herbs. *Alfalfa:* activation of quiescent systemic lupus erythematosus

Echinacea: increased immune-stimulating effects

Ephedra (ma huang): decreased drug blood level

Ginseng: potentiation of immunomodulating effect

Licorice: prolonged drug activity

Drug-behaviors. *Alcohol use:* increased risk of gastric irritation and GI ulcers

Patient monitoring

• Monitor weight, blood pressure, and electrolyte levels.

• Watch for cushingoid effects (moon face, central obesity, buffalo hump, hair thinning, high blood pressure, frequent infections).

🔊 Assess patient for depression and psychosis.

• Monitor blood glucose level carefully in diabetic patient.

• Evaluate for signs and symptoms of infection, which drug may mask or exacerbate.

🔊 Monitor for signs and symptoms of early adrenal insufficiency (fatigue, weakness, joint pain, fever, anorexia, shortness of breath, dizziness, syncope).

• Assess musculoskeletal status for joint, tendon, and muscle pain.

Patient teaching

• Tell patient to take oral dose with food or milk to reduce GI upset.

• Instruct patient to remove ODT tablet from blister just before taking.

• Instruct patient to place ODT tablet on tongue and either swallow tablet whole or allow it to dissolve in mouth with or without water. Caution patient not to cut, split, or break tablet.

🔊 Teach patient to recognize and immediately report cushingoid effects and signs and symptoms of early adrenal insufficiency.

🔊 Advise patient and significant other to immediately report depression or psychosis.

• Explain that drug increases risk of infection. Instruct patient to contact prescriber at first sign of infection.

🔊 Caution patient not to suddenly stop drug (including ophthalmic forms). Instruct him to discuss any changes in therapy with prescriber.

◀€ Tell patient to immediately report bleeding or joint, muscle, tendon, or abdominal pain.

• Inform patient that he may need higher dosage during periods of stress. Encourage him to wear or carry medical identification stating this.

• Tell patient to avoid vaccinations during therapy. Mention that others in household shouldn't receive oral polio vaccine because they could pass poliovirus to him.

• Caution patient not to take over-the-counter drugs or herbs during therapy.

• Teach patient how to use eye drops. Caution him not to touch dropper tip to eye or any other surface.

• As appropriate, review all other significant and life-threatening adverse reactions and interactions, especially those related to the drugs, tests, herbs, and behaviors mentioned above.

prednisone
Apo-Prednisone✦, Winpred✦

Pharmacologic class: Corticosteroid (intermediate acting)
Therapeutic class: Anti-inflammatory, immunosuppressant
Pregnancy risk category C

Action
Decreases inflammation by reversing increased cell capillary permeability and inhibiting migration of polymorphonuclear leukocytes. Suppresses immune system by reducing lymphatic activity.

Availability
Oral solution: 5 mg/ml, 5 mg/5 ml
Syrup: 5 mg/5 ml
Tablets: 1 mg, 2.5 mg, 5 mg, 10 mg, 20 mg, 50 mg

⚕ Indications and dosages
➤ Severe inflammation; immunosuppression
Adults: Dosage individualized based on diagnosis, severity of condition, and response. Usual dosage is 5 to 60 mg P.O. daily as a single dose or in divided doses.
➤ Acute exacerbation of multiple sclerosis
Adults: 200 mg P.O. daily for 1 week, then 80 mg every other day for 1 month
➤ Adjunctive therapy for *Pneumocystis jiroveci* pneumonia in AIDS patients
Adults: 40 mg P.O. b.i.d. for 5 days, then 40 mg once daily for 5 days, then 20 mg once daily for 11 days

Contraindications
• Hypersensitivity to drug, other corticosteroids, alcohol, bisulfite, or tartrazine (with some products)
• Systemic fungal infections
• Live-virus vaccines (with immunosuppressant doses)
• Active untreated infections (except in selected meningitis patients)

Precautions
Use cautiously in:
• diabetes mellitus, glaucoma, renal or hepatic disease, hypothyroidism, cirrhosis, diverticulitis, nonspecific ulcerative colitis, recent intestinal anastomoses, inflammatory bowel disease, thromboembolic disorders, seizures, myasthenia gravis, heart failure, hypertension, osteoporosis, hypothyroidism, ocular herpes simplex, immunosuppression, emotional instability
• pregnant or breastfeeding patients
• children under age 6.

Administration
• Give with food or milk to reduce GI upset.
• Administer once-daily dose early in morning.

p

Reactions in **bold** are life-threatening.   ◀€ Clinical alert

Route	Onset	Peak	Duration
P.O.	Unknown	1-2 hr	1.25-1.5 days

Adverse reactions

CNS: headache, nervousness, depression, euphoria, personality changes, psychosis, vertigo, paresthesia, insomnia, restlessness, **seizures, meningitis, increased intracranial pressure**

CV: hypotension, hypertension, vasculitis, **heart failure, thrombophlebitis, thromboembolism, fat embolism, arrhythmias, shock**

EENT: posterior subcapsular cataracts (especially in children), glaucoma, nasal irritation and congestion, rebound congestion, sneezing, epistaxis, nasopharyngeal and oropharyngeal fungal infections, perforated nasal septum, anosmia, dysphonia, hoarseness, throat irritation (all with long-term use)

GI: nausea, vomiting, abdominal distention, rectal bleeding, esophageal candidiasis, dry mouth, esophageal ulcer, **pancreatitis, peptic ulcer**

GU: amenorrhea, irregular menses

Hematologic: purpura

Metabolic: sodium and fluid retention, hypokalemia, hypocalcemia, hyperglycemia, decreased carbohydrate tolerance, diabetes mellitus, growth retardation (in children), cushingoid effects (with long-term use), **hypothalamic-pituitary-adrenal suppression** (with systemic use longer than 5 days), **adrenal suppression** (with high-dose, long-term use)

Musculoskeletal: muscle weakness or atrophy, myalgia, myopathy, osteoporosis, aseptic joint necrosis, spontaneous fractures (with long-term use), osteonecrosis, tendon rupture

Respiratory: cough, wheezing, **bronchospasm**

Skin: rash, pruritus, contact dermatitis, acne, striae, poor wound healing, hirsutism, thin fragile skin, petechiae, bruising, subcutaneous fat atrophy, urticaria, angioedema

Other: bad taste, increased or decreased appetite, weight gain (with long-term use), facial edema, aggravation or masking of infections, hypersensitivity reaction

Interactions

Drug-drug. *Amphotericin B, mezlocillin, piperacillin, thiazide and loop diuretics, ticarcillin:* additive hypokalemia

Aspirin, other nonsteroidal anti-inflammatory drugs: increased risk of GI discomfort and bleeding

Cardiac glycosides: increased risk of digitalis toxicity due to hypokalemia

Cyclosporine: therapeutic benefits in organ transplant recipients, but with increased risk of toxicity

Erythromycin, indinavir, itraconazole, ketoconazole, ritonavir, saquinavir: increased prednisone blood level and effects

Hormonal contraceptives: impaired metabolism and increased effects of prednisone

Isoniazid: decreased isoniazid blood level

Live-virus vaccines: decreased antibody response to vaccine, increase risk of adverse effects

Oral anticoagulants: reduced anticoagulant requirements, opposition to anticoagulant action

Phenobarbital, phenytoin, rifampin: decreased prednisone efficacy

Salicylates: reduced salicylate blood level

Somatrem: inhibition of somatrem's growth-promoting effects

Theophylline: altered pharmacologic effects of either drug

Drug-diagnostic tests. *Calcium, potassium, thyroid ^{131}I uptake, thyroxine, triiodothyronine:* decreased levels

Cholesterol, glucose: increased levels

Nitroblue tetrazolium test for bacterial infection: false-negative result

Drug-herbs. *Alfalfa:* activation of quiescent systemic lupus erythematosus

Echinacea: increased immune-stimulating effects

Ephedra (ma huang): decreased drug blood level

Ginseng: potentiation of immunomodulating effect

Licorice: prolonged drug activity

Drug-behaviors. *Alcohol use:* increased risk of gastric irritation and GI ulcers

Patient monitoring

• Monitor weight, blood pressure, and electrolyte levels.

• Watch for cushingoid effects (moon face, central obesity, buffalo hump, hair thinning, high blood pressure, frequent infections).

◀€ Check for signs and symptoms of depression and psychosis.

• Assess blood glucose level carefully in diabetic patient.

• Monitor patient for signs and symptoms of infection, which drug may mask or exacerbate.

◀€ Assess for early indications of adrenal insufficiency (fatigue, weakness, joint pain, fever, appetite loss, shortness of breath, dizziness, syncope).

• Monitor musculoskeletal status for joint, tendon, and muscle pain.

Patient teaching

• Tell patient to take with food or milk to reduce GI upset.

◀€ Teach patient to recognize and immediately report signs and symptoms of early adrenal insufficiency and cushingoid effects.

◀€ Inform patient that drug increases his risk of infection. Instruct him to contact prescriber at first sign of infection.

◀€ Caution patient not to stop drug suddenly. Advise him to discuss any changes in therapy with prescriber.

◀€ Tell patient to immediately report bleeding or joint, muscle, tendon, or abdominal pain.

◀€ Advise patient or significant other to immediately report depression or psychosis.

• Caution patient not to take herbs or over-the-counter drugs during therapy.

• Instruct patient to avoid vaccinations during therapy. Tell him that others in household shouldn't receive oral polio vaccine because they could pass poliovirus to him.

• Tell patient he may need higher dosage during periods of stress. Encourage him to wear or carry medical identification stating this.

• As appropriate, review all other significant and life-threatening adverse reactions and interactions, especially those related to the drugs, tests, herbs, and behaviors mentioned above.

pregabalin capsules CV
Lyrica

Pharmacologic class: Miscellaneous anticonvulsant

Therapeutic class: Anticonvulsant

Pregnancy risk category C

Action

Unclear. Binds with high affinity to CNS alpha$_2$-delta site (auxiliary subunit of voltage-gated calcium channels), possibly resulting in antinociceptive and antiseizure effects.

Availability

Capsules: 25 mg, 50 mg, 75 mg, 100 mg, 150 mg, 200 mg, 225 mg, 300 mg

⍚ Indications and dosages

➣ Adjunct for partial-onset seizures in adults

Adults: Initially, 75 mg P.O. b.i.d. or 50 mg P.O. t.i.d.; may increase to maximum of 600 mg P.O. daily given in

---

divided doses based on response and tolerance

➤ Neuropathic pain related to diabetic peripheral neuropathy

Adults: Initially, 50 mg P.O. t.i.d. in patients with creatinine clearance of at least 60 ml/minute; may increase to maximum of 100 mg P.O. t.i.d. within 1 week based on efficacy and tolerance

➤Postherpetic neuralgia

Adults: Initially, 75 mg P.O. b.i.d., or 50 mg P.O. t.i.d. in patients with creatinine clearance of at least 60 ml/minute; may increase to maximum of 300 mg P.O. daily within 1 week based on efficacy and tolerance. Tolerant patients who don't obtain sufficient pain relief after 2 to 4 weeks of 300 mg daily may receive up to 300 mg b.i.d. or 200 mg t.i.d. Reserve dosages above 300 mg daily for patients with ongoing pain who tolerate 300 mg daily.

➤ Fibromyalgia

Adults: Initially, 75 mg P.O. b.i.d. in patients with creatinine clearance of at least 60 ml/minute; may increase to 150 mg P.O. b.i.d. within 1 week based on efficacy and tolerance. If patient doesn't obtain sufficient benefit at 300 mg daily, dosage may be increased further to 225 mg b.i.d. Dosages above 450 mg daily aren't recommended.

Dosage adjustment

• Renal impairment

Contraindications

• Hypersensitivity to drug or its components

Precautions

Use cautiously in:

• abnormal creatinine clearance

• concurrent use of thiazolidinedione antidiabetics

• history of angioedema episode

• concurrent use of drugs associated with angioedema (such as angiotensin-converting enzyme inhibitors)

• elderly patients

• children (safety and efficacy not established).

Administration

• Give with or without food.

• To discontinue drug, withdraw gradually over at least 1 week to reduce risk of increased seizure frequency in patients with history of seizure disorders.

Route	Onset	Peak	Duration
P.O.	Unknown	1.5 hr	Unknown

Adverse reactions

CNS: dizziness, somnolence, euphoria, balance disorder, abnormal thinking, asthenia, neuropathy, ataxia, vertigo, confusion, incoordination, abnormal gait, tremor, amnesia, nervousness, headache, speech disorder, twitching, myoclonus, fatigue, feeling drunk, hypertonia, hypoesthesia, paresthesia, lethargy, anxiety, disorientation, depression, depersonalization, stupor

EENT: abnormal or blurred vision, diplopia, nystagmus, conjunctivitis, sinusitis, otitis media, tinnitus, pharyngolaryngeal pain

GI: vomiting, constipation, flatulence, abdominal distention, gastroenteritis, dry mouth

GU: urinary incontinence, urinary frequency, decreased libido, anorgasmia, erectile dysfunction

Metabolic: hypoglycemia, fluid retention

Musculoskeletal: back pain, myasthenia, arthralgia, muscle spasms

Respiratory: dyspnea, bronchitis

Skin: ecchymosis, pruritus

Other: increased appetite, weight gain, edema, peripheral edema, accidental injury, pain, chest pain, infection, allergic reaction, **angioedema, hypersensitivity reactions** including **anaphylactoid reactions** (rare)

Interactions
Drug-drug. *Gabapentin:* slight decrease in pregabalin rate of absorption

Lorazepam, oxycodone: exacerbated effects on cognitive and gross motor functioning

Drug-diagnostic tests. *Serum glucose:* decreased level

Drug-behaviors. *Alcohol use:* exacerbated effects on cognitive and gross motor functioning

Patient monitoring
◀ Monitor patient closely for hypersensitivity reaction and angioedema; if these effects occur, discontinue drug and begin emergency measures immediately.

• Know that patients with history of drug or alcohol abuse may be more likely to misuse or abuse drug.

Patient teaching
• Instruct patient to take drug with or without food.

◀ Teach patient to recognize signs and symptoms of angioedema and to discontinue drug and seek immediate medical care if these arise.

◀ Inform patient that drug may cause hypersensitivity reactions, such as wheezing, dyspnea, rash, hives, and blisters. Advise patient to discontinue drug and seek medical care if these reactions occur.

• Inform patient that drug may cause weight gain and edema.

• Advise patient to avoid driving and other hazardous activities until drug's effects on vision and alertness are known.

• Caution patient to avoid alcohol while taking drug.

• As appropriate, review all other significant and life-threatening adverse reactions and interactions, especially those related to the drugs, tests, and behaviors mentioned above.

primaquine phosphate

Pharmacologic class: 8-aminoquinoline compound

Therapeutic class: Antimalarial

Pregnancy risk category C

FDA | BOXED WARNING

• Familiarize yourself completely with full contents of accompanying leaflet before prescribing or administering.

Action
Unknown. Thought to disrupt parasitic mitochondria and bind to native DNA, leading to structural changes that disrupt metabolic processes and to inhibition of gametocyte and erythrocyte forms. Destroys some gametocytes and makes others incapable of undergoing maturation division.

Availability
Tablets: 26.3 mg (15 mg base)

🚫 Indications and dosages
➤ To prevent or treat relapse of malaria caused by *Plasmodium vivax*
Adults: 15 mg base P.O. daily for 14 days
Children: 0.3 mg base/kg/day P.O. for 14 days, to a maximum of 15 mg base daily

Off-label uses
• *Pneumocystis jiroveci* pneumonia

Contraindications
• Hypersensitivity to drug
• Concurrent use of quinacrine, other hemolytic drugs, or myelosuppressants
• Bone marrow depression

Reactions in **bold** are life-threatening.   ◀ Clinical alert

• Systemic disease with history of or tendency to granulocytopenia (such as lupus erythematosus or rheumatoid arthritis)

Precautions

Use cautiously in:

• porphyria, methemoglobinemia, methemoglobin reductase deficiency, hemolytic anemia in G6PD deficiency (particularly in Blacks, Asians, and persons of Mediterranean descent), iodine deficiency, anemia

• pregnant patients.

Administration

Before giving, check prescription to see if dosage is written as mg or mg base.

• Start therapy during last 2 weeks of suppression course with chloroquine or comparable drug, or after suppression course ends.

Route	Onset	Peak	Duration
P.O.	Unknown	1-3 hr	Unknown

Adverse reactions

CNS: headache, dizziness, asthenia

CV: hypertension

EENT: blurred vision, difficulty focusing

GI: nausea, vomiting, diarrhea, constipation, abdominal pain, epigastric distress

Hematologic: mild anemia, **leukocytosis, hemolytic anemia, methemoglobinemia**

Skin: pruritus, skin eruptions, pallor

Interactions

Drug-drug. *Aluminum and magnesium salts:* decreased GI absorption of primaquine

Quinacrine: increased risk of primaquine toxicity

Drug-diagnostic tests. *Hemoglobin, red blood cells:* decreased levels

White blood cells: increased or decreased count

Patient monitoring

Monitor CBC. Watch for evidence of blood dyscrasias or hemolytic reaction (dark urine, chills, fever, chest pain, bluish skin). Stop drug and notify prescriber at once if these occur.

• Monitor blood pressure.

Patient teaching

• Advise patient to take with food to minimize GI upset.

Teach patient to recognize and immediately report signs and symptoms of hemolytic reactions.

• Caution patient to avoid driving and other hazardous activities until he knows how drug affects concentration, vision, and alertness.

• Instruct patient to complete entire course of therapy as prescribed, even after symptoms improve.

• As appropriate, review all other significant and life-threatening adverse reactions and interactions, especially those related to the drugs and tests mentioned above.

primidone

Apo-Primidone*, Mysoline

Pharmacologic class: Barbiturate

Therapeutic class: Anticonvulsant

Pregnancy risk category NR

Action

Unknown. May raise seizure threshold by decreasing neuronal firing after being converted to phenobarbital.

Availability

Suspension: 250 mg/5 ml

Tablets: 50 mg, 250 mg

Indications and dosages

➤ Grand mal, psychomotor, or focal epileptic seizures

Adults and children ages 8 and older:
Initially, 100 to 125 mg P.O. at bedtime on days 1 to 3, then 100 to 125 mg P.O. b.i.d. on days 4 to 6, then 100 to 125 mg P.O. t.i.d. on days 7 to 9, followed by a maintenance dosage of 250 mg P.O. three or four times daily

Children younger than age 8: Initially, 50 mg P.O. at bedtime on days 1 to 3, then 50 mg P.O. b.i.d. on days 4 to 6, then 100 mg P.O. b.i.d. on days 7 to 9. For maintenance, 125 to 250 mg t.i.d. or 10 to 25 mg/kg/day in divided doses.

Dosage adjustment
• Renal impairment

Off-label uses
• Benign familial (essential) tremor

Contraindications
• Hypersensitivity to drug or phenobarbital
• Porphyria

Precautions
Use cautiously in:
• hepatic, renal, or chronic obstructive pulmonary disease
• pregnant or breastfeeding patients
• hyperactive children.

Administration
• Don't change brands. Bioequivalency problems have occurred.
◀€ Don't stop therapy suddenly. Dosage must be tapered.
• Know that drug may be given alone or with other anticonvulsants.

Route	Onset	Peak	Duration
P.O.	Unknown	3-4 hr	Unknown

Adverse reactions
CNS: headache, dizziness, stimulation, drowsiness, sedation, confusion, hallucinations, psychosis, ataxia, vertigo, hyperirritability, emotional disturbances, paranoid symptoms, **coma**

EENT: diplopia, nystagmus, eyelid edema
GI: nausea, vomiting, anorexia
GU: erectile dysfunction
Hematologic: megaloblastic anemia, thrombocytopenia
Skin: flushing, rash

Interactions
Drug-drug. *Acetazolamide, succinimide:* decreased primidone blood level
Carbamazepine: decreased primidone blood level, increased carbamazepine blood level
Hydantoins, isoniazid, nicotinamide: increased primidone blood level
Drug-diagnostic tests. *Hemoglobin, platelets:* decreased levels
Liver function tests: altered results

Patient monitoring
• Monitor primidone and phenobarbital blood levels.
• Monitor CBC and blood chemistry. Watch for evidence of blood dyscrasias.
• Assess neurologic status regularly. Stay alert for excessive drowsiness and emotional status changes.

Patient teaching
◀€ Caution patient not to discontinue therapy suddenly. Advise him to discuss dosage changes with prescriber.
◀€ Instruct patient to immediately report unusual bleeding, bruising, or rash.
• Tell patient drug may cause sexual dysfunction. Advise him to discuss this issue with prescriber.
• Caution patient to avoid driving and other hazardous activities until he knows how drug affects concentration, vision, and alertness.
• As appropriate, review all other significant and life-threatening adverse reactions and interactions, especially those related to the drugs and tests mentioned above.

p

Reactions in **bold** are life-threatening.　　　◀€ Clinical alert

probenecid
Benuryl✢

Pharmacologic class: Sulfonamide-derived uricosuric

Therapeutic class: Antigout drug, tubular blocking agent

Pregnancy risk category B

Action
Promotes uric acid excretion from kidney by blocking tubular reabsorption; also inhibits tubular secretion of weak organic acids (most penicillins and cephalosporins, some beta-lactams)

Availability
Tablets: 0.5 g

⏱ Indications and dosages
➤ Hyperuricemia caused by gout
Adults and children weighing more than 50 kg (110 lb): After acute gout attack subsides, 250 mg P.O. b.i.d. for 1 week, then 500 mg b.i.d.; may increase by 500 mg/day q 4 weeks (not to exceed 3 g/day)
➤ To prolong action or increase blood level of penicillins or cephalosporins
Adults: 500 mg P.O. q.i.d.
Children ages 2 to 14: Initially, 25 mg/kg or 0.7 g/m², then a maintenance dosage of 40 mg/kg/day or 1.2 g/m² in four divided doses
➤ Gonorrhea
Adults: 1 g P.O. as a single dose given with or immediately before prescribed ampicillin dose

Dosage adjustment
• Renal impairment

Off-label uses
• Hyperuricemia secondary to thiazide therapy

Contraindications
• Hypersensitivity to drug
• Acute gout attack
• Uric acid calculi
• Blood dyscrasias
• Concurrent salicylate use
• Concurrent penicillin use in patients with renal impairment
• Children younger than age 2

Precautions
Use cautiously in:
• peptic ulcer, renal impairment
• pregnant or breastfeeding patients.

Administration
◀ Don't give until acute gout attack subsides.
• Ensure high fluid intake and alkaline urine during therapy.

Route	Onset	Peak	Duration
P.O.	30 min	2-4 hr	8 hr

Adverse reactions
CNS: headache, dizziness
GI: nausea, vomiting, diarrhea, abdominal pain, anorexia
GU: urinary frequency, uric acid calculi, renal colic, **nephrotic syndrome**
Hematologic: anemia, **hemolytic anemia, aplastic anemia**
Hepatic: hepatitis, **hepatic necrosis**
Metabolic: gout exacerbation
Musculoskeletal: costovertebral pain
Skin: flushing, rash, pruritus
Other: sore gums, fever, hypersensitivity reactions including **anaphylaxis**

Interactions
Drug-drug. *Acyclovir, allopurinol, barbiturates, cephalosporins, pantothenic acid, penicillins:* increased blood levels of these drugs, enhanced uric acid–reducing effect of probenecid
Benzodiazepines: faster onset and prolonged effects of these drugs
Clofibrate: increased clofibrate blood level
Dapsone: accumulation of dapsone and its metabolites

Dyphylline: increased half-life and decreased clearance of dyphylline

Methotrexate, nonsteroidal anti-inflammatory drugs, rifampin, sulfonamides: increased blood levels, therapeutic effects, and toxicity of these drugs

Oral hypoglycemics: increased half-life and effects of these drugs

Penicillamine: increased pharmacologic effect of penicillamine

Salicylates: decreased probenecid or salicylate activity

Thiopental: extended anesthetic effect of thiopental

Zidovudine: increased risk of zidovudine toxicity

Drug-diagnostic tests. *Urine glucose tests using copper reduction method (such as Clinitest):* false-positive result

Patient monitoring

• Monitor kidney and liver function tests, CBC, and blood urea nitrogen level.

• Assess fluid intake and output to ensure good hydration and reduce urinary side effects.

• During first 6 to 12 months of therapy, monitor pattern and severity of acute gout attacks to assess need for additional anti-inflammatory drugs.

Patient teaching

• Advise patient to take with food or milk to minimize GI upset.

• Teach patient about causes of gout and proper use of drug. Stress that he must wait until acute attack subsides and then take drug regularly to prevent further attacks.

• Tell patient drug may exacerbate acute gout attacks for first 6 to 12 months, necessitating colchicine or other anti-inflammatory drug for 3 to 6 months.

• Instruct patient to drink 2 to 3 liters of fluids daily.

• Tell patient with gout to limit foods high in purine (such as anchovies, organ meats, and legumes).

• Instruct diabetic patient to test urine glucose level during therapy.

• As appropriate, review all other significant and life-threatening adverse reactions and interactions, especially those related to the drugs and tests mentioned above.

procainamide hydrochloride

Pharmacologic class: Membrane stabilizer

Therapeutic class: Antiarrhythmic (class IA)

Pregnancy risk category C

FDA | BOXED WARNING

• Prolonged use often leads to positive antinuclear antibody (ANA) test, with or without symptoms of lupus erythematosus-like syndrome. If positive ANA titer develops, weigh benefits versus risks of continued therapy.

Action

Decreases myocardial excitability by inhibiting conduction velocity. Also depresses myocardial contractility.

Availability

Injection: 100 mg/ml, 500 mg/ml

⊘ Indications and dosages

➢ Life-threatening ventricular arrhythmias

Adults: 100 mg by slow I.V. push at a rate of 50 mg/minute, repeated q 5 minutes until arrhythmia subsides, up to a maximum advisable dosage of 1 g. Alternatively, loading dose of 500 to 600 mg by I.V. infusion over 25 to 30 minutes. With either I.V. method, maximum loading dose is 1 g. When arrhythmia subsides, give continuous I.V. infusion of 2 to 6 mg/minute. Or 50 mg/kg I.M. in divided doses q 3 to 6 hours until patient can tolerate P.O. therapy.

Dosage adjustment
• Renal impairment

Contraindications
• Hypersensitivity to drug, tartrazine, procaine, or sulfites
• Complete heart block
• Torsades de pointes
• Lupus erythematosus

Precautions
Use cautiously in:
• procaine hypersensitivity, renal impairment, ischemic heart disease, heart failure, first-degree heart block, atypical ventricular tachycardia, myasthenia gravis, systemic lupus erythematosus, cytopenia
• patients receiving other antiarrhythmics concurrently
• pregnant or breastfeeding patients
• children.

Administration
◀€ Ask patient about procaine sensitivity before giving; cross-sensitivity may occur.
• For I.V. use, dilute with dextrose 5% in water.
• Administer I.V. doses with patient in supine position to avoid hypotensive effects.
• When giving by I.V. infusion, use infusion pump to ensure that drug infuses at 50 mg/minute or less.
◀€ Don't leave patient's bedside during I.V. administration.

Route	Onset	Peak	Duration
I.V.	Immediate	Immediate	Unknown
I.M.	10-30 min	15-60 min	Unknown

Adverse reactions
CNS: headache, dizziness, confusion, psychosis, restlessness, asthenia, depression, neuropathy, **seizures**

CV: hypotension, bradycardia, **atrioventricular block, ventricular fibrillation, ventricular asystole, cardiovascular collapse, cardiac arrest**
GI: nausea, vomiting, diarrhea, anorexia
Hematologic: hemolytic anemia, agranulocytosis, thrombocytopenia, neutropenia
Skin: rash, urticaria, pruritus, flushing
Other: bitter taste, lupuslike syndrome, edema

Interactions
Drug-drug. *Amiodarone:* increased procainamide blood level and risk of toxicity
Anticholinesterase drugs: decreased anticholinesterase effects
Antihypertensives: additive hypotension
Beta-adrenergic blockers, cimetidine, ranitidine, trimethoprim: increased procainamide blood level
Lidocaine: additive cardiodepressant action, conduction abnormalities
Neuromuscular blockers: increased skeletal muscle relaxation
Other antiarrhythmics: additive or antagonistic effects, additive toxicity
Trimethoprim: increased pharmacologic effect of procainamide
Drug-herbs. *Henbane:* increased anticholinergic activity
Jimsonweed: adverse cardiovascular effects
Licorice: prolonged QT interval
Drug-behaviors. *Alcohol use:* altered drug blood level

Patient monitoring
◀€ When giving I.V., stay at patient's bedside and monitor blood pressure and ECG continuously.
◀€ If ECG shows prolonged QT interval and QRS complexes, heart block, or worsening arrhythmia, stop drug therapy, run rhythm strip, and contact prescriber immediately.
• Assess blood levels of procainamide and *N*-acetylprocainamide (drug's active metabolite).
◀€ Monitor electrolyte levels, CBC, and antinuclear antibody titers. Watch

---

♣ Canada   ⊕ UK   ☣ Hazardous drug   ⊗ High-alert drug

for signs and symptoms of blood dyscrasias.
• Evaluate patient for signs and symptoms of lupuslike syndrome.

Patient teaching

◀≀ Advise patient to immediately report cardiovascular symptoms or bleeding tendency.
• Emphasize importance of taking exactly as prescribed. Advise patient to use alarm clock to help him remember to take nighttime doses.
• Advise patient to avoid alcohol.
• Instruct patient not to take herbal remedies unless prescriber approves.
• As appropriate, review all other significant and life-threatening adverse reactions and interactions, especially those related to the drugs, herbs, and behaviors mentioned above.

procarbazine hydrochloride

Matulane

Pharmacologic class: Alkylating agent
Therapeutic class: Antineoplastic
Pregnancy risk category D

FDA | BOXED WARNING

• Give under supervision of physician experienced in use of potent antineoplastics, in setting with adequate clinical and laboratory facilities to monitor patient.

Action

Thought to inhibit DNA, RNA, and protein synthesis, resulting in death of rapidly dividing cells. Also inhibits MAO.

Availability

Capsules: 50 mg

⚠ Indications and dosages

➤ Hodgkin's disease

Adults: 2 to 4 mg/kg P.O. daily as a single dose or in divided doses for 1 week, then 4 to 6 mg/kg P.O. daily until white blood cell (WBC) count is less than 4,000/mm^3 or platelet count is less than 100,000/mm^3, or until desired response occurs. With desired response, give maintenance dosage of 1 to 2 mg/ kg P.O. daily (rounded off to nearest 50 mg). As component of MOPP (mechlorethamine, vincristine, procarbazine, prednisone) regimen for advanced Hodgkin's disease, usual dosage is 100 mg/m^2 P.O. daily on days 1 to 14 of 28-day cycle.

Children: Dosage highly individualized. Usual dosage is 50 mg/m^2 P.O. daily for first week, then 100 mg/m^2 P.O. daily until leukopenia, thrombocytopenia, or desired response occurs. With desired response, maintenance dosage is 50 mg/m^2 P.O. daily.

Off-label uses

• Brain tumor
• Lymphoma

Contraindications

• Hypersensitivity to drug
• Inadequate bone marrow reserve

Precautions

Use cautiously in:
• infection, chronic debilitating illness, headache, hepatic or renal impairment, cardiovascular disease, heart failure, diarrhea, stomatitis, pheochromocytoma, psychiatric illness, alcoholism
• patients who have undergone radiation therapy or received other chemotherapy drugs within previous month
• elderly patients
• pregnant or breastfeeding patients
• females of childbearing age.

P

Administration

• Weigh patient; know that dosages are based on weight. However, use caution in patients with edema or ascites.

Route	Onset	Peak	Duration
P.O.	Rapid	1 hr	Unknown

Adverse reactions

CNS: confusion, dizziness, drowsiness, hallucinations, headache, mania, depression, nightmares, psychosis, syncope, tremor, neuropathy, paresthesia, **seizures**

CV: edema, hypotension, tachycardia

EENT: nystagmus, photophobia, retinal hemorrhage

GI: nausea, vomiting, diarrhea, dysphagia, ascites, stomatitis, dry mouth, anorexia

GU: gonadal suppression, gynecomastia

Hematologic: anemia, **leukopenia, thrombocytopenia**

Hepatic: hepatic dysfunction

Respiratory: cough, **pleural effusion**

Skin: alopecia, photosensitivity, pruritus, rash

Interactions

Drug-drug. *Digoxin:* decreased digoxin blood level

Levodopa: flushing, hypertension

Opioids: deep coma, death

Sympathomimetics (indirect-acting): abrupt, life-threatening hypertension

Tricyclic antidepressants: severe toxicity and fatal reactions (including blood pressure fluctuations, seizures, and coma)

Drug-diagnostic tests. *Hematocrit, hemoglobin, platelets, reticulocytes, WBCs:* decreased levels

Drug-food. *Caffeine-containing foods and beverages:* hypertension, arrhythmias

Tyramine-containing foods and beverages: life-threatening hypertension

Drug-behaviors. *Alcohol use:* disulfiram-like reaction

Patient monitoring

• Monitor vital signs and nutritional status.

• Assess fluid intake and output. Watch for evidence of fluid overload.

◀€ Monitor neurologic status for seizures, paresthesia, neuropathy, and confusion. Discontinue drug and notify prescriber if these occur.

◀€ Monitor CBC and platelet count. Discontinue drug and contact prescriber if WBC count falls below 4,000/mm³ or platelet count falls below 100,000/mm³.

◀€ Evaluate patient's concurrent drug use to ensure that he isn't receiving other drugs that could cause potentially fatal interactions.

◀€ Check for diarrhea. Discontinue drug and contact prescriber if patient has frequent bowel movements or watery stools.

• Monitor blood urea nitrogen level, liver and kidney function tests, and urinalysis.

◀€ Discontinue drug at first sign of hypersensitivity, stomatitis, diarrhea, or bleeding.

Patient teaching

• Instruct patient to avoid caffeine-containing foods and beverages.

◀€ Tell patient to avoid foods and beverages containing tyramine (such as cheese, Chianti wine, tea, coffee, cola, and bananas).

• Advise patient to avoid alcohol.

• Tell female of childbearing age to discuss contraception with prescriber.

• As appropriate, review all other significant and life-threatening adverse reactions and interactions, especially those related to the drugs, tests, foods, and behaviors mentioned above.

---

prochlorperazine
Compazine✤, Compro, Stemetil✤

prochlorperazine edisylate
Compazine✤

prochlorperazine maleate
Buccastem⊕, Compazine✤, Proziere⊕, Stemetil✤⊕

Pharmacologic class: Phenothiazine
Therapeutic class: Antiemetic, antipsychotic, anxiolytic
Pregnancy risk category C

Action
Exerts anticholinergic, CNS depressant, and antihistaminic effects. Depresses release of hypothalamic and hypophyseal hormones, decreases sensitivity of middle-ear labyrinth, and reduces conduction in vestibular-cerebellar pathways.

Availability
Capsules (extended-release, maleate): 10 mg, 15 mg, 30 mg
Injection (edisylate): 5 mg/ml
Oral solution (edisylate): 5 mg/5 ml
Suppositories: 2.5 mg, 5 mg, 25 mg
Tablets: 5 mg, 10 mg, 25 mg

💊 Indications and dosages
➤ Nausea
Adults: 5 to 10 mg P.O. three to four times daily or 15 mg P.O. once daily or 10 mg P.O. (extended-release) b.i.d., up to 40 mg/day. Or 2.5 to 10 mg I.V., not to exceed 40 mg/day.
Children weighing 18 to 38 kg (40 to 85 lb): 2.5 mg P.O. or P.R. t.i.d. or 5 mg P.O. or P.R. b.i.d., not to exceed 15 mg/day
Children weighing 13.6 to 17.7 kg (30 to 39 lb): 2.5 mg P.O. or P.R. two or three times daily, not to exceed 10 mg/day
Children weighing 9 to 13 kg (20 to 29 lb): 2.5 mg P.O. or P.R. daily to b.i.d., not to exceed 7.5 mg/day
➤ Nausea and vomiting related to surgery
Adults: 5 to 10 mg I.V. 15 to 30 minutes before anesthesia induction, repeated once if necessary; or 5 to 10 mg I.M. 1 to 2 hours before anesthesia induction, repeated once in 30 minutes if necessary
➤ Schizophrenia
Adults and children older than age 12: For mild symptoms, 5 to 10 mg P.O. three to four times daily; for moderate to severe symptoms in hospitalized or supervised patients, 10 mg P.O. three to four times daily, increased p.r.n. q 2 to 3 days to 50 to 75 mg P.O. daily or up to 150 mg/day as tolerated p.r.n. for more severely disturbed patients. Or 10 to 20 mg I.M.; may repeat q 2 to 4 hours for up to four doses p.r.n.
Children ages 2 to 12: Initially, 2.5 mg P.O. or P.R. two or three times daily (maximum of 10 mg on day 1); then increase based on response. Don't exceed 25 mg/day for children ages 6 to 12 or 20 mg/day for children ages 2 to 5.
➤ Anxiety
Adults and children older than age 12: 5 mg P.O. three to four times daily; or 15 mg P.O. (extended-release) once daily or 10 mg P.O. (extended-release) q 12 hours; up to 20 mg/day for a maximum of 12 weeks

Off-label uses
• Migraine

Contraindications
• Hypersensitivity to drug or other phenothiazines
• Coma
• Concurrent use of large amounts of CNS depressants
• Pediatric surgery
• Children younger than age 2 or weighing less than 9 kg (20 lb)

Reactions in **bold** are life-threatening.　◀𝄞 Clinical alert

p

Precautions

Use cautiously in:
• cardiovascular or hepatic disease, glaucoma, seizures
• anticipated exposure to extreme heat
• children with acute illness.

Administration

• For I.V. infusion, dilute 20 mg in 1 L of compatible I.V. solution, such as normal saline solution.
• Don't mix in same syringe with other drugs.
• Know that injection solution may cause contact dermatitis. Don't get it on hands or clothing.
◀€ Give I.V. by slow infusion only. Don't give as bolus.
• Know that I.M. injection is not preferred because it can cause local irritation. However, if I.M. route is prescribed, inject deep into upper outer quadrant of gluteal area.
• Don't give by subcutaneous route.
• After desired response, switch to P.O. form as prescribed.
• When infusing I.V., watch for hypotension. Keep patient supine for 30 minutes after infusion.

Route	Onset	Peak	Duration
P.O.	30-40 min	Unknown	3-4 hr
P.O. (extended)	30-40 min	Unknown	10-12 hr
I.V.	Rapid (min)	10-30 min	3-4 hr
I.M.	10-20 min	10-30 min	3-4 hr
P.R.	60 min	Unknown	3-4 hr

Adverse reactions

CNS: sedation, extrapyramidal reactions, tardive dyskinesia, **neuroleptic malignant syndrome**
CV: orthostatic hypotension, ECG changes, tachycardia
EENT: blurred vision, lens opacities, pigmentary retinopathy, dry eyes
GI: constipation, ileus, dry mouth, anorexia
GU: pink or reddish-brown urine, urinary retention, galactorrhea
Hematologic: agranulocytosis, leukopenia
Hepatic: cholestatic jaundice, **hepatitis**
Metabolic: hyperthermia
Skin: photosensitivity, pigmentation changes, rash
Other: allergic reactions

Interactions

Drug-drug. *Anticonvulsants:* reduced seizure threshold
Antineoplastics: masking of antineoplastic toxicity
CNS depressants (including antihistamines, anticholinergics, opioids, other phenothiazines, sedative-hypnotics): additive CNS depression
Guanethidine: inhibition of antihypertensive effects
Oral anticoagulants: decreased anticoagulant effect
Phenytoin: increased or decreased phenytoin blood level
Propranolol: increased blood levels of both drugs
Thiazide diuretics: increased risk of orthostatic hypotension
Drug-diagnostic tests. *Liver function tests:* abnormal results
Phenylketonuria test: false-positive result
Drug-herbs. *Betel nut:* increased risk of extrapyramidal reactions
Evening primrose oil: increased risk of seizures
Kava: increased risk of drug-related adverse reactions
Drug-behaviors. *Alcohol use:* additive CNS depression

Patient monitoring

◀€ Monitor neurologic status, especially for signs and symptoms of neuroleptic malignant syndrome (high fever, sweating, unstable blood pressure, stupor, muscle rigidity, and autonomic dysfunction).
• In long-term therapy, assess for other adverse CNS effects, including

extrapyramidal symptoms and tardive dyskinesia.

• Monitor patient closely if he's receiving drug for nausea and vomiting associated with chemotherapy, because it may mask symptoms of chemotherapy toxicity.

• Evaluate CBC and liver function tests.

Patient teaching

• Instruct patient to dilute oral solution with tomato or fruit juice, milk, coffee, soda, tea, water, or soup.

◀℣ Teach patient to recognize and immediately report signs and symptoms of an allergic reaction or neuroleptic malignant syndrome.

• Inform patient about drug's other CNS effects. Tell him to contact prescriber if these occur.

• Caution patient to avoid driving and other hazardous activities until he knows how drug affects concentration, vision, alertness, and motor skills.

• Tell patient drug may turn urine pink or reddish brown.

• As appropriate, review all other significant and life-threatening adverse reactions and interactions, especially those related to the drugs, tests, herbs, and behaviors mentioned above.

progesterone
Crinone, Endometrin, Prometrium

Pharmacologic class: Progestin
Therapeutic class: Hormone
Pregnancy risk category B (oral), *D* (injection), *NR* (vaginal)

FDA | BOXED WARNING

• Estrogen plus progestin therapy shouldn't be used for prevention of cardiovascular disease or dementia.

• The Women's Health Initiative (WHI) estrogen plus progestin substudy reported increased risk of stroke, deep vein thrombosis, pulmonary embolism, and myocardial infarction in postmenopausal women (ages 50 to 79) during 5.6 years of treatment with daily oral conjugated estrogens (0.625 mg) combined with medroxyprogesterone acetate (2.5 mg) relative to placebo.

• The substudy also demonstrated increased risk of invasive breast cancer.

• The WHI Memory Study estrogen plus progestin ancillary study of the WHI reported increased risk of dementia in postmenopausal women ages 65 and older.

Action
Suppresses ovulation by altering the vaginal epithelium, relaxing uterine smooth muscle, and promoting mammary tissue growth. Also inhibits pituitary activity and causes withdrawal bleeding in presence of estrogen.

Availability
Injection (in sesame or peanut oil with benzyl alcohol): 50 mg/ml in 10-ml vials
Micronized capsules (oral) in peanut oil: 100 mg, 200 mg
Micronized vaginal gel: 4%, 8%

❗ Indications and dosages
➤ Secondary amenorrhea
Adults: 400 mg/day P.O. in evening for 10 days, or 5 to 10 mg/day I.M. for 6 to 8 days, given 8 to 10 days before expected menstrual period. Or 45 mg (one applicatorful of 4% gel) vaginally once every other day for up to six doses; may increase to 90 mg (one applicatorful of 8% gel) once every other day for up to six doses.
➤ Dysfunctional uterine bleeding
Adults: 5 to 10 mg I.M. daily for 6 days

P

➤ To prevent postmenopausal estrogen-induced endometrial hyperplasia

Adults: 200 mg/day P.O. at bedtime for 14 days on days 8 to 21 of 28-day cycle or on days 12 to 25 of 30-day cycle. If patient currently receives estrogen 1.25 mg/day, 300 mg progesterone in two divided doses (100 mg 2 hours after breakfast and 200 mg at bedtime); further adjustment may be required.

➤ Corpus luteum insufficiency; assisted reproduction technology

Adults: For luteal-phase support, 90 mg (one applicatorful of 8% gel) vaginally once daily. For in vitro fertilization, 90 mg (one applicatorful of 8% gel) vaginally once daily, starting within 24 hours of embryo transfer and continued through day 30 after transfer; if pregnancy occurs, treatment may continue for up to 12 weeks. For partial or complete ovarian failure, 90 mg (one applicatorful of 8% gel) vaginally b.i.d. while patient undergoes donor oocyte transfer; if pregnancy occurs, treatment may last up to 12 weeks.

Contraindications

• Hypersensitivity to drug, peanuts (injection, micronized capsules), or sesame (injection)
• Thromboembolic disease
• Cerebrovascular disease
• Severe hepatic disease
• Porphyria
• Breast or reproductive system cancer
• Missed abortion
• Undiagnosed vaginal bleeding
• Diagnosis of pregnancy

Precautions

Use cautiously in:
• renal or cardiovascular disease, seizure disorders, fluid retention, diabetes mellitus, asthma, migraine, depression
• history of hepatic disease
• breastfeeding patients.

Administration

• Before first dose, make sure patient has read package insert regarding adverse effects. Reinforce written information with oral review.
🔊 Before first I.M. dose, ask if patient has allergy to peanuts or sesame. Before giving micronized capsules, ask about peanut allergy.
• Inject I.M. dose deep into muscle. Rotate injection sites.

Route	Onset	Peak	Duration
P.O.	Unknown	2-4 hr	Unknown
I.M., vaginal	Unknown	Unknown	Unknown

Adverse reactions

CNS: depression, emotional lability, **cerebrovascular accident**
CV: thrombophlebitis, thromboembolism
EENT: retinal thrombosis
GI: abdominal cramps
GU: amenorrhea, breakthrough bleeding, spotting, cervical erosions, breast tenderness, menstrual flow changes, galactorrhea
Hepatic: hepatitis
Respiratory: pulmonary embolism
Skin: melasma, rash, angioedema
Other: gingival bleeding, weight gain or loss, hypersensitivity reactions including **anaphylaxis**

Interactions

Drug-drug. *Conjugated estrogens:* increased levels of both drugs
Drug-diagnostic tests. *Alkaline phosphatase, amino acids, low-density lipoproteins:* increased levels
Chloride and sodium excretion: reduced (with high doses)
High-density lipoproteins: decreased level
Pregnanediol excretion: reduced
Thyroid function tests: altered results
Drug-herbs. *Red clover:* interference with drug effects

Drug-behaviors. *Smoking:* increased risk of thromboembolic effects

Patient monitoring

◀€ Watch for evidence of thromboembolic disorders, including cerebrovascular accident, pulmonary embolism, diplopia, proptosis, or sudden partial or complete vision loss (may signal retinal thrombosis). If these occur, discontinue drug and notify prescriber immediately.

◀€ Assess for emotional lability and depression.

Patient teaching

◀€ Teach patient to recognize and immediately report signs and symptoms of thromboembolic disorders.

◀€ Instruct patient and significant other to stay alert for and immediately report depression.

• Advise patient to monitor weight regularly and report significant changes.

• Tell female patient that drug may cause menstrual abnormalities.

• Advise female patient to discuss breastfeeding with prescriber before taking drug.

◀€ Instruct patient to immediately report possible pregnancy.

• Tell patient that smoking increases thromboembolism risk. Encourage her to stop smoking if she smokes.

• As appropriate, review all other significant and life-threatening adverse reactions and interactions, especially those related to the drugs, tests, herbs, and behaviors mentioned above.

promethazine hydrochloride

Avomine ✦, Histantil ✿, Phenergan ✿, PMS-Promethazine, Promethegan, Sominex ✦, Ziz ✦

Pharmacologic class: Phenothiazine (nonselective)

Therapeutic class: Antihistamine, antiemetic, sedative-hypnotic

Pregnancy risk category C

FDA BOXED WARNING

• Don't use promethazine in patients younger than age 2 due to potential for fatal respiratory depression. (Postmarketing cases of respiratory depression have been reported in these patients.)

• Use caution when administering to pediatric patients age 2 years and older. Preferably, use lowest effective dosage in these patients and avoid concurrent use of other drugs with respiratory depressant effects.

• Promethazine injection can cause severe chemical irritation and damage to tissue regardless of administration route. Irritation and damage can result from perivascular extravasation, unintentional intra-arterial injection, and intraneuronal or perineuronal infiltration.

• Adverse reactions to I.V. injection include burning, pain, thrombophlebitis, tissue necrosis, and gangrene. In some cases, surgical intervention, including fasciotomy, skin graft, or amputation, has been required.

• Because of risks of I.V. injection, preferred parenteral administration route is deep I.M. injection. Subcutaneous injection is contraindicated.

P

Action
Blocks effects but not release of histamine and exerts strong alpha-adrenergic effect. Also inhibits chemoreceptor trigger zone in medulla and alters dopamine effects by indirectly reducing reticular stimulation in CNS.

Availability
Injection: 25 mg/ml and 50 mg/ml in 1-ml ampules and 1- and 10-ml vials
Suppositories: 12.5 mg, 25 mg, 50 mg
Syrup: 6.25 mg/5 ml
Tablets: 12.5 mg, 25 mg, 50 mg

🕖 Indications and dosages
➤ Type 1 hypersensitivity reaction
Adults: 25 mg P.O. or P.R. at bedtime or 12.5 mg P.O. before meals and at bedtime. Or 25 mg I.M. or I.V.; may repeat in 2 hours.
Children older than age 2: 25 mg P.O. or P.R. at bedtime or 6.25 to 12.5 mg P.O. t.i.d.
➤ Motion sickness
Adults: Initially, 25 mg P.O. or P.R. 30 to 60 minutes before traveling; may repeat 8 to 12 hours later if needed. On successive travel days, 25 mg P.O. or P.R. b.i.d. (on arising and before evening meal).
Children older than age 2: 12.5 to 25 mg P.O. or P.R. b.i.d.
➤ Sedation
Adults: 25 to 50 mg P.O., I.M., I.V., or P.R. at bedtime
Children older than age 2: 12.5 to 25 mg P.O. or P.R. at bedtime
➤ Adjunct to preoperative or postoperative analgesia
Adults: 25 to 50 mg P.O., P.R., I.M., or I.V. given with appropriately reduced dosage of narcotic or barbiturate and required dosage of belladonna alkaloid
Children older than age 2: 0.5 mg/lb P.O., P.R., I.M., or I.V., given with appropriately reduced dosage of narcotic or barbiturate and required dosage of belladonna alkaloid

➤ Nausea
Adults: 25 mg P.O. or P.R.; may repeat doses of 12.5 to 25 mg P.O. or P.R. q 4 to 6 hours p.r.n. Or 12.5 to 25 mg I.M. or I.V.; may repeat q 4 hours p.r.n.
Children older than age 2: 25 mg or 0.5 mg/lb P.O. or P.R.; may repeat doses of 12.5 to 25 mg P.O. or P.R. q 4 to 6 hours p.r.n. May give I.M. or I.V. as no more than half of adult dosage. Know that drug should not be given if cause of vomiting is unknown.

Contraindications
• Hypersensitivity to drug
• Previous idiosyncratic reaction to phenothiazines
• Coma
• Intra-arterial and subcutaneous injection
• Children younger than age 2

Precautions
Use cautiously in:
• cardiovascular or hepatic disease, seizures, bone marrow depression, narrow-angle glaucoma, prostatic hypertrophy, stenosing peptic ulcer, pyloroduodenal or bladder neck obstruction
• CNS depression caused by narcotics, barbiturates, general anesthesia, tranquilizers, or alcohol
• pregnant or breastfeeding patients.

Administration
• Don't give I.V. at concentrations greater than 25 mg/ml or faster than 25 mg/minute.
• Use light-resistant covering for I.V. drug.
🔊 Inject I.M. deep into large muscle. Don't give by subcutaneous route.

Route	Onset	Peak	Duration
P.O., I.M., P.R.	20 min	Unknown	4-12 hr
I.V.	3-5 min	Unknown	4-12 hr

Adverse reactions

CNS: confusion, disorientation, fatigue, marked drowsiness, sedation, dizziness, extrapyramidal reactions, insomnia, nervousness, **neuroleptic malignant syndrome**

CV: hypertension, hypotension, bradycardia, tachycardia

EENT: blurred vision, diplopia, tinnitus

GI: constipation, dry mouth

Hematologic: blood dyscrasias

Hepatic: cholestatic jaundice

Respiratory: respiratory depression

Skin: photosensitivity, rash

Other: hypersensitivity reaction

Interactions

Drug-drug. *Anticholinergics:* additive anticholinergic effects

CNS depressants: additive CNS depression

Epinephrine: reversal of epinephrine's vasopressor effects

MAO inhibitors: increased extrapyramidal effects

Drug-diagnostic tests. *Glucose:* increased level

Granulocytes, platelets, white blood cells: decreased counts

Pregnancy test: false-positive or false-negative result

Skin tests using allergen extracts: false-negative results

Drug-herbs. *Betel nut:* increased risk of extrapyramidal reactions

Evening primrose oil: increased risk of seizures

Kava: increased risk of adverse drug effects

Drug-behaviors. *Alcohol use:* additive CNS depression

Sun exposure: increased risk of photosensitivity

Patient monitoring

◀€ Monitor neurologic status. Stay alert for signs and symptoms of neuroleptic malignant syndrome (high fever, sweating, unstable blood pressure, stupor, muscle rigidity, and autonomic dysfunction).

• In long-term therapy, assess for other adverse CNS effects, including extrapyramidal reactions.

• Monitor CBC and liver function tests.

Patient teaching

◀€ Teach patient to recognize and immediately report signs and symptoms of hypersensitivity reaction or neuroleptic malignant syndrome.

• Tell patient about drug's other significant neurologic effects. Instruct him to contact prescriber if these occur.

• Caution patient to avoid driving and other hazardous activities until he knows how drug affects concentration, vision, alertness, and motor skills.

• As appropriate, review all other significant and life-threatening adverse reactions and interactions, especially those related to the drugs, tests, herbs, and behaviors mentioned above.

propafenone hydrochloride

APO-Propafenone✦, Arythmol✢, Gen-Propafenone✦, PMS-Propafenone✦, Rythmol, Rythmol SR

p

Pharmacologic class: Direct membrane stabilizer

Therapeutic class: Antiarrhythmic (class IC)

Pregnancy risk category C

FDA | BOXED WARNING

• In study of patients with asymptomatic, non-life-threatening ventricular arrhythmias who'd had myocardial infarctions more than 6 days but less than 2 years previously, excessive mortality or nonfatal cardiac arrest rate occurred in those treated with encainide or flecainide, compared with

---

Reactions in **bold** are life-threatening.   ◀€ Clinical alert

patients in carefully matched placebo groups. Given drug's known proarrhythmic properties and lack of evidence of improved survival for any antiarrhythmic in patients without life-threatening arrhythmias, reserve drug for patients with life-threatening ventricular arrhythmias.

Action
Slows conduction velocity in atrioventricular (AV) node, decreases automaticity, and increases ratio of effective refractory period to action potential duration; also has mild beta-adrenergic blocking properties

Availability
Tablets: 150 mg, 225 mg, 300 mg
Capsules (sustained-release): 225 mg, 325 mg, 425 mg

⬮ Indications and dosages
➤ Patients without structural heart disease to treat life-threatening ventricular arrhythmias; paroxysmal atrial fibrillation or flutter and paroxysmal supraventricular tachycardia associated with disabling symptoms
Adults: Dosage highly individualized based on response and tolerance. Initially, 150 mg P.O. (prompt-release) q 8 hours (450 mg/day); may increase after 3 to 4 days to 225 mg P.O. q 8 hours (675 mg/day) or, if necessary, up to 300 mg P.O. q 8 hours (900 mg/day). Don't exceed 900 mg/day P.O.
➤ Symptomatic atrial fibrillation in patients without structural heart disease
Adults: Dosage individualized based on response and tolerance. Initially, 225 mg P.O. (extended-release) q 12 hours; may increase at 5-day intervals to 325 mg q 12 hours or, if necessary, up to 425 mg q 12 hours.

Dosage adjustment
• Hepatic disease

• Significant widening of the QRS complex or second- or third-degree AV block
• Ventricular arrhythmia with marked previous myocardial damage
• Elderly patients

Contraindications
• Hypersensitivity to drug
• Sinoatrial, AV, and intraventricular disorders of impulse generation or conduction (such as sick sinus node syndrome, AV block) unless artificial pacemaker is in place
• Cardiogenic shock
• Bradycardia
• Uncontrolled heart failure
• Marked hypotension
• Bronchospastic disorders, severe obstructive pulmonary disease
• Electrolyte imbalances

Precautions
Use cautiously in:
• hepatic or renal impairment, myasthenia gravis
• concurrent use of both a CYP2D6 inhibitor and a CYP3A4 inhibitor with extended-release propafenone (avoid use)
• concurrent use of amiodarone or quinidine (not recommended)
• pregnant or breastfeeding patients
• children.

Administration
• Give prompt-release tablets with food (but not with grapefruit juice) in three divided doses daily, once every 8 hours. Give extended-release capsules whole with or without food.

Route	Onset	Peak	Duration
P.O.	Variable	3.5 hr	Unknown
P.O. (extended)	Unknown	3-8 hr	Unknown

Adverse reactions
CNS: headache, dizziness, drowsiness, syncope, vertigo, confusion, asthenia,

speech disturbances, memory loss, ataxia, paresthesia, anxiety, abnormal dreams, insomnia, tremor

CV: palpitations, angina, chest pain, hypotension, bradycardia, premature ventricular contractions, **first-degree AV block, supraventricular or ventricular arrhythmias, heart failure, atrial fibrillation, intraventricular conduction delay**

EENT: blurred vision, tinnitus

GI: nausea, vomiting, diarrhea, constipation, dyspepsia, abdominal pain or cramps, flatulence, dry mouth, anorexia

GU: reversible disorders of spermatogenesis

Hematologic: purpura, **hemolytic anemia, leukopenia, agranulocytosis, thrombocytopenia, neutropenia**

Hepatic: cholestasis, **abnormal hepatic function**

Musculoskeletal: muscle weakness, myalgia, leg cramps, myasthenia gravis exacerbation

Respiratory: dyspnea

Skin: rash, alopecia, diaphoresis

Other: altered taste, edema

Interactions

Drug-drug. *Amiodarone:* conduction and repolarization changes

Beta-adrenergic blockers: increased blood level and effects of beta-adrenergic blockers metabolized by liver

Cimetidine: increased propafenone blood level

CYP1A2 inhibitors (such as amiodarone), CYP2D6 inhibitors (such as desipramine, paroxetine, ritonavir, sertraline), CYP3A4 inhibitors (such as erythromycin, ketoconazole, ritonavir, saquinavir): increased propafenone plasma level

Digoxin, drugs metabolized by CYP2D6 (such as desipramine, haloperidol, imipramine, venlafaxine), warfarin: increased plasma concentrations of these drugs

Lidocaine: increased CNS adverse reactions

Orlistat: reduced propafenone concentration

Quinidine: delayed propafenone metabolism

Rifampin: decreased blood level and antiarrhythmic efficacy of propafenone

Drug-diagnostic tests. *Antinuclear antibody:* positive titer

Bleeding time: prolonged

Creatine kinase, glucose: increased levels

Granulocytes, white blood cells: decreased counts

Drug-food. *Grapefruit juice:* increased propafenone plasma level

Patient monitoring

• Monitor ECG and vital signs.

• Evaluate neurologic status. Stay alert for decreasing level of consciousness.

◀€ Monitor CBC and liver function tests. Watch for evidence of blood dyscrasias and abnormal hepatic function.

• Monitor respiratory status for dyspnea.

Patient teaching

• Instruct patient to take prompt-release tablets with food.

• Tell patient to take extended-release capsules whole with or without food and not to crush or divide capsule contents.

◀€ Tell patient which cardiac, neurologic, and respiratory adverse effects to report immediately.

◀€ Instruct patient to immediately report unusual bleeding or bruising.

• Caution patient to avoid driving and other hazardous activities until he knows how drug affects concentration, vision, and alertness.

• As appropriate, review all other significant and life-threatening adverse reactions and interactions, especially those related to the drugs, tests, and herbs mentioned above.

p

---

propranolol hydrochloride

Apo-Propranolol✦, Bedranol SR⊕, Betachron E-R, Beta-Prograne⊕, Dom-Propranolol✦, Half Beta-Prograne⊕, Half Inderal LA⊕, Inderal LA, Innopran XL, Novopranol✦, Nu-Propranolol✦, PMS Propranolol✦, Rapranol SR⊕, Slo-Pro⊕, Syprol⊕

Pharmacologic class: Beta-adrenergic blocker (nonselective)

Therapeutic class: Antianginal, antiarrhythmic (class II), antihypertensive, vascular headache suppressant

Pregnancy risk category C

FDA | BOXED WARNING

• In patients with angina pectoris, exacerbations of angina and, in some cases, myocardial infarction (MI) have followed abrupt drug withdrawal. For planned withdrawal, reduce dosage gradually over at least a few weeks and caution patient not to interrupt or stop therapy without physician's advice. If therapy is interrupted and angina exacerbation occurs, consider reinstituting drug and taking other measures to manage unstable angina. As coronary artery disease may be unrecognized, it may be prudent to follow same advice in patients at risk for occult atherosclerotic heart disease who receive drug for other indications.

Action

Blocks stimulation of beta$_1$-adrenergic (myocardial) and beta$_2$-adrenergic (pulmonary, vascular, and uterine) receptor sites. This action decreases cardiac output, slows heart rate, and reduces blood pressure.

Availability

Capsules (extended-release, sustained-release): 60 mg, 80 mg, 120 mg, 160 mg
Injection: 1 mg/ml
Oral solution: 4 mg/ml, 8 mg/ml, 80 mg/ml
Tablets: 10 mg, 20 mg, 40 mg, 60 mg, 90 mg

⟋ Indications and dosages

➤ Angina pectoris

Adults: 80 to 320 mg P.O. daily in three to four divided doses or 160 mg (extended- or sustained-release) P.O. daily; maximum daily dosage is 320 mg.

➤ Hypertension

Adults: 40 mg P.O. b.i.d. or 80 mg (extended- or sustained-release) P.O. daily. Maximum daily dosage is 640 mg; usual maintenance dosage is 120 to 240 mg/day.

➤ Prophylaxis after MI

Adults: 180 to 240 mg P.O. daily in three to four divided doses; maximum daily dosage is 240 mg.

➤ Hypertrophic subaortic stenosis

Adults: 20 to 40 mg P.O. three to four times daily (before meals and at bedtime) or 80 to 160 mg (extended- or sustained-release) P.O. daily

➤ Adjunctive therapy in pheochromocytoma

Adults: 60 mg P.O. daily in divided doses for 3 days, given after primary therapy with alpha-adrenergic blocker

➤ To prevent migraine or vascular headache

Adults: 80 mg P.O. (extended- or sustained-release) daily; may increase as needed up to 240 mg/day. Effective range is 160 to 240 mg/day.

➤ Essential tremor

Adults: 40 mg P.O. b.i.d.; if necessary, 240 to 320 mg/day. Maximum daily dosage is 320 mg.

➤ Arrhythmias

Adults: 10 to 30 mg P.O. (tablets or oral solution) three or four times daily

---

➤ Life-threatening arrhythmias; arrhythmias occurring during anesthesia

Adults: 1 to 3 mg slow I.V. injection. If necessary, give second dose after 2 minutes and additional doses at intervals of no less than 4 hours until desired response occurs.

Contraindications

- Hypersensitivity to drug, its components, or other beta-adrenergic blockers
- Uncompensated heart failure
- Cardiogenic shock
- Sinus bradycardia, heart block greater than first degree
- Bronchospastic disease

Precautions

Use cautiously in:

- renal or hepatic impairment, sinus node dysfunction, pulmonary disease, diabetes mellitus, hyperthyroidism, Raynaud's syndrome, hypertensive emergencies, myasthenia gravis
- concurrent thioridazine use
- history of severe allergic reactions
- elderly patients
- pregnant or breastfeeding patients
- children (safety not established).

Administration

◀€ Take apical pulse for 1 full minute. Withhold dose and notify prescriber if patient has bradycardia or tachycardia.

◀€ Be aware that I.V. use is usually reserved for arrhythmias that are life-threatening or occur during anesthesia.

- Inject I.V. dose directly into large vein or into tubing of compatible I.V. solution (dextrose 5% in water, normal or half-normal saline solution, or lactated Ringer's solution).
- Don't give as continuous I.V. infusion.
- For intermittent I.V. infusion, dilute with normal saline solution and infuse in 0.1- to 0.2-mg increments over 10 to 15 minutes.

◀€ Keep I.V. isoproterenol, atropine, or glucagon at hand in case of emergency.

◀€ Don't stop giving drug suddenly. Dosage must be tapered.

Route	Onset	Peak	Duration
P.O.	30 min	60-90 min	6-12 hr
P.O. (extended, sustained)	Unknown	6 hr	24 hr
I.V.	Immediate	1 min	4-6 hr

Adverse reactions

CNS: fatigue, asthenia, anxiety, dizziness, drowsiness, insomnia, memory loss, depression, mental status changes, nervousness, paresthesia, nightmares

CV: peripheral vasoconstriction, orthostatic hypotension, bradycardia, **arrhythmias, heart failure, myocardial infarction and sudden death** (with abrupt withdrawal in angina therapy)

EENT: blurred vision, dry eyes, nasal congestion, rhinitis, sore throat

GI: nausea, vomiting, diarrhea, constipation, dry mouth

GU: erectile dysfunction, decreased libido

Hematologic: purpura, **thrombocytopenic purpura**

Metabolic: fluid retention, hyperglycemia, **hypoglycemia** (increased in children), **thyrotoxicosis** (with abrupt withdrawal in hypertension therapy)

Musculoskeletal: joint pain, back pain, myalgia, muscle cramps

Respiratory: wheezing, **bronchospasm, pulmonary edema**

Skin: pruritus, rash

Other: fever

Interactions

Drug-drug. *Antacids (aluminum-based):* decreased propranolol absorption

Anticholinergics, tricyclic antidepressants: antagonism of cardiac beta-adrenergic blocking effect

p

Reactions in **bold** are life-threatening.   ◀€ Clinical alert

Chlorpromazine: additive hypotension
Cimetidine: increased propranolol blood level and risk of toxicity
Digoxin: additive bradycardia
Diuretics, other antihypertensives: increased hypotensive effect
Glucagon, isoproterenol: antagonism of propranolol's effects
Insulin, oral hypoglycemics: impaired glucose tolerance, increased risk of hypoglycemia
Neuromuscular blockers: increased neuromuscular blockade (with high propranolol doses)
Nonsteroidal anti-inflammatory drugs: decreased hypotensive effect
Theophylline: decreased theophylline clearance, antagonism of theophylline's bronchodilating effect
Thioridazine: increased thioridazine blood level, leading to prolonged QT interval
Drug-diagnostic tests. *Alkaline phosphatase, blood urea nitrogen, eosinophils, lactate dehydrogenase, serum transaminases, triiodothyronine:* increased levels
Glucose: decreased or increased level
Platelets, thyroxine: decreased levels
Drug-behaviors. *Acute alcohol ingestion:* additive hypotension

Patient monitoring

• Monitor vital signs, ECG, and central venous pressure.
• Assess fluid balance. Check for signs and symptoms of heart failure.
• Monitor CBC and liver and thyroid function tests.
• Watch closely for signs and symptoms of hypoglycemia, which drug may mask.
• Monitor blood glucose level in diabetic patient, to identify need for altered insulin or oral hypoglycemic dosage. Be aware that in labile diabetes, hypoglycemia may be accompanied by steep blood pressure rise.

Patient teaching

• Advise patient to take with meals at same time every day to minimize GI upset.
◀€ Caution patient not to stop taking drug suddenly. Tell him dosage must be tapered.
• Tell patient to monitor pulse and to promptly report bradycardia or tachycardia.
• Inform patient that drug may cause muscle aches or bone pain. Advise him to discuss activity recommendations and pain management with prescriber.
• Caution patient to avoid driving and other hazardous activities until he knows how drug affects concentration, vision, and alertness.
• As appropriate, review all other significant and life-threatening adverse reactions and interactions, especially those related to the drugs, tests, and behaviors mentioned above.

propylthiouracil (PTU)
Propyl-Thyracil✶

Pharmacologic class: Thioamide derivative
Therapeutic class: Antithyroid agent
Pregnancy risk category D

FDA | **BOXED WARNING**

• Drug has caused severe liver injury and acute liver failure, in some cases fatal. These reports of hepatic reactions include cases requiring liver transplant.
• Reserve drug for patients intolerant of methimazole and in whom radioactive iodine therapy or surgery isn't appropriate for management of hyperthyroidism.
• Because of risk of fetal abnormalities associated with methimazole, propylthiouracil may be treatment of choice

when an antithyroid drug is indicated during or just before first trimester.

Action
Directly interferes with thyroid synthesis by preventing iodine from combining with thyroglobulin, leading to decreased thyroid hormone levels

Availability
Tablets: 50 mg

⚕ Indications and dosages
➤ Hyperthyroidism
Adults: Initially, 300 to 450 mg P.O. daily in equally divided doses q 8 hours; for maintenance, 100 to 150 mg P.O. daily.
➤ Thyrotoxic crisis
Adults: 200 mg P.O. q 4 to 6 hours during first 24 hours, then a maintenance dosage of 100 to 150 mg P.O. daily

Contraindications
• Hypersensitivity to drug

Precautions
Use cautiously in:
• decreased bone marrow reserve
• pregnancy and breastfeeding patients
• children.

Administration
• Give with meals to reduce GI upset.
• Be aware that drug shouldn't be used in children unless patient is allergic to or intolerant of methimazole, and there are no other treatment options available.

Route	Onset	Peak	Duration
P.O.	Unknown	1-1.5 hr	Unknown

Adverse reactions
CNS: drowsiness, headache, vertigo, neuritis, paresthesia
GI: nausea, vomiting, diarrhea, epigastric distress

Hematologic: agranulocytosis, leukopenia, thrombocytopenia
Hepatic: jaundice, **hepatic necrosis, liver failure**
Metabolic: hypothyroidism
Musculoskeletal: joint pain, myalgia
Skin: rash, urticaria, pruritus, skin discoloration, alopecia, cutaneous vasculitis
Other: taste loss, fever, lymphadenopathy, parotitis, edema

Interactions
Drug-drug. *Anticoagulants:* potentiation of anticoagulant effect
Drug-diagnostic tests. *Alanine aminotransferase, alkaline phosphatase, aspartate aminotransferase, bilirubin, lactate dehydrogenase:* increased levels
Granulocytes, platelets: decreased levels
Prothrombin time: prolonged

Patient monitoring
• Monitor CBC and liver and thyroid function tests.
• Assess for signs and symptoms of hypothyroidism (cold intolerance, nonpitting edema, fatigue, weight gain, and depression).
◀℈ Monitor for severe rash, fever, jaundice, or enlarged cervical lymph nodes. If present, stop therapy and notify prescriber.

Patient teaching
• Instruct patient to take with meals to reduce GI upset.
• Teach patient to recognize and report signs and symptoms of hypothyroidism and jaundice.
• Advise patient to discuss iodine intake (as in iodized salt and shellfish) with prescriber.
• Tell patient to avoid over-the-counter cold remedies that contain iodine.
• Caution patient to avoid driving and other hazardous activities until he knows how drug affects concentration and alertness.
• Advise female patient of childbearing age to discuss pregnancy or breastfeeding with prescriber before taking.

p

Reactions in **bold** are life-threatening.   ◀℈ Clinical alert

• As appropriate, review all other significant and life-threatening adverse reactions and interactions, especially those related to the drugs and tests mentioned above.

pseudoephedrine hydrochloride

Contac Non Drowsy⊕, Galsud⊕, Genaphed, Kidkare Decongestant, Meltus Decongestant⊕, Non-Drowsy Sudafed Decongestant⊕, Robidrine✦, Silfedrine Children's, Sudafed, Sudafed Children's Nasal Decongestant, Sudafed 12 Hour, Sudo-Tab, Sudodrin, SudoGest

pseudoephedrine sulfate

Drixoral Nasal Decongestant, Drixoral Non-Drowsy Formula

Pharmacologic class: Sympathomimetic

Therapeutic class: Decongestant (systemic)

Pregnancy risk category C

Action

Stimulates alpha-adrenergic receptors, causing vasoconstriction of respiratory tract; relaxes bronchial smooth muscle through beta$_2$-adrenergic stimulation

Availability

pseudoephedrine hydrochloride
Capsules: 60 mg
Capsules (extended-release): 120 mg, 240 mg
Capsules (soft gel): 30 mg
Oral solution: 15 mg/5 ml, 30 mg/5 ml
Syrup: 30 mg/5 ml
Tablets: 30 mg, 60 mg

Tablets (chewable): 15 mg
Tablets (extended-release): 120 mg, 240 mg
pseudoephedrine sulfate
Tablets (extended-release, film-coated): 120 mg

⬦ Indications and dosages
➤ Nasal, sinus, or eustachian tube congestion
Adults and children ages 12 and older: 60 mg P.O. q 4 to 6 hours p.r.n. (not to exceed 240 mg/day); or 120 mg (extended-release) q 12 hours or 240 mg (extended-release) q 24 hours

Contraindications
• Hypersensitivity to drug or other sympathomimetics
• Alcohol intolerance (with some liquid products)
• Hypertension
• Severe coronary artery disease
• MAO inhibitor use within past 14 days
• Children younger than age 12 (extended-release forms)

Precautions
Use cautiously in:
• hyperthyroidism, diabetes mellitus, prostatic hypertrophy, ischemic heart disease, glaucoma
• elderly patients (more sensitive to drug's CNS effects)
• pregnant or breastfeeding patients.

Administration
• Give at least 2 hours before bedtime to minimize insomnia.

Route	Onset	Peak	Duration
P.O.	30 min	Unknown	4-8 hr
P.O. (extended)	60 min	Unknown	12 hr

Adverse reactions
CNS: anxiety, nervousness, dizziness, drowsiness, excitability, fear, hallucinations, headache, insomnia, restlessness, asthenia, **seizures**

✦ Canada   ⊕ UK   ⚕ Hazardous drug   ⊗ High-alert drug

CV: palpitations, hypertension, tachycardia, **cardiovascular collapse**
GI: anorexia, dry mouth
GU: dysuria
Respiratory: respiratory difficulty

Interactions
Drug-drug. *Beta-adrenergic blockers:* increased pressor effects of pseudoephedrine
MAO inhibitors: hypertensive crisis
Mecamylamine, methyldopa, reserpine: decreased antihypertensive effect of these drugs
Other sympathomimetics: additive effects, greater risk of toxicity
Drug-food. *Foods that acidify urine:* decreased drug efficacy
Foods that alkalize urine: increased drug efficacy

Patient monitoring
• Monitor vital signs.
• Assess neurologic and cardiovascular status regularly.

Patient teaching
• Advise patient to take at least 2 hours before bedtime to reduce insomnia.
• Tell patient not to crush or break extended-release tablets or capsules.
• Advise patient to discontinue use and consult prescriber if he experiences nervousness, dizziness, or insomnia.
• Tell patient to consult prescriber before taking other over-the-counter products.
• Caution patient to avoid driving and other hazardous activities until he knows how drug affects concentration and alertness.
• As appropriate, review all other significant and life-threatening adverse reactions and interactions, especially those related to the drugs and foods mentioned above.

psyllium
Fiberall, Fibrelief⊕, Fibro-Lax, Fibro-XL, Fybogel⊕, Hydrocil Instant, Isogel⊕, Ispagel⊕, Karacil✦, Konsyl, Metamucil, Metamucil Orange Flavor, Metamucil Sugar Free, Modane Bulk, Natural Fiber Therapy, Prodiem Plain✦, Regulan⊕, Reguloid, Reguloid Sugar Free

Pharmacologic class: Psyllium colloid
Therapeutic class: Bulk-forming laxative
Pregnancy risk category B

Action
Stimulates lining of colon, increasing peristalsis and water absorption of stool and promoting evacuation

Availability
Chewable pieces: 1.7 g/piece, 3.4 g/piece
Granules: 2.5 g/tsp, 4.03 g/tsp
Powder: 3.3 g/tsp, 3.4 g/tsp, 3.5 g/tsp, 4.94 g/tsp
Powder (effervescent): 3.4 g/packet, 3.7 g/packet
Wafers: 3.4 g/2 wafers

Indications and dosages
➤ Chronic constipation; ulcerative colitis; irritable bowel syndrome
Adults and children ages 12 and older: 30 g daily in divided doses of 2.5 to 7.5 g/dose P.O. in 8 oz of water or juice

Contraindications
• Hypersensitivity to drug
• Intestinal obstruction
• Abdominal pain or other appendicitis symptoms
• Fecal impaction

Precautions
Use cautiously in:
- phenylketonuria
- pregnant patients.

Administration
- Mix powder with 8 oz of cold liquid (such as orange juice) to mask taste.
- Give diluted drug immediately after mixing, before it congeals. Follow with another glass of fluid.

Route	Onset	Peak	Duration
P.O.	12-24 hr	3 days	Variable

Adverse reactions
GI: nausea; vomiting; diarrhea (with excessive use); abdominal cramps with severe constipation; anorexia; **esophageal, gastric, small-intestine, or rectal obstruction** (with dry form)
Respiratory: asthma (rare)
Other: severe allergic reactions including **anaphylaxis**

Interactions
None significant

Patient monitoring
- Monitor patient's bowel movements.
- Check for signs and symptoms of severe (but rare) allergic reactions, such as anaphylaxis and asthma.

Patient teaching
- Tell patient to dissolve in 8 oz of cold beverage and drink immediately, followed by another glass of liquid.
- Caution patient not to take without dissolving in liquid.
- Instruct patient to take after meals if drug decreases his appetite.
- Tell patient drug usually causes bowel movement within 12 to 24 hours but may take as long as 3 days.
- ◀€ Instruct patient to immediately stop taking drug and notify prescriber if signs and symptoms of allergic reaction occur.

- Advise diabetic patient to use sugar-free drug form.
- Instruct patient with phenylketonuria to avoid forms containing phenylalanine.
- As appropriate, review all other significant and life-threatening adverse reactions.

pyrazinamide
PMS Pyrazinamide✤, Tebrazid✤

Pharmacologic class: Niacinamide derivative
Therapeutic class: Antitubercular
Pregnancy risk category C

Action
Unknown. Thought to exert bacteriostatic activity.

Availability
Tablets: 500 mg

🖊 Indications and dosages
➤ Tuberculosis
Adults and children: 15 to 30 mg/kg/day P.O., not to exceed 2 g/day; or 50 to 70 mg/kg P.O. twice weekly, up to a maximum of 4 g/dose; or 50 to 70 mg/kg/dose P.O. three times weekly, up to a maximum of 3 g/dose

Dosage adjustment
- Renal impairment

Contraindications
- Hypersensitivity to drug
- Severe hepatic disease
- Acute gout

Precautions
Use cautiously in:
- renal failure, diabetes mellitus, porphyria, chronic gout, history of gout
- pregnant or breastfeeding patients
- children younger than age 13.

Administration
- Give with other antituberculars, as prescribed, to reduce risk of resistant organisms.
- Be aware that drug therapy may last 6 months or longer.

Route	Onset	Peak	Duration
P.O.	Rapid	2 hr	Unknown

Adverse reactions
CNS: headache
GI: nausea, vomiting, diarrhea, peptic ulcer, abdominal cramps, anorexia
GU: dysuria, increased uric acid secretion
Hematologic: hemolytic anemia
Hepatic: hepatotoxicity
Metabolic: hyperuricemia, gout
Musculoskeletal: joint pain
Skin: urticaria, photosensitivity

Interactions
Drug-drug. *Ethionamide:* increased risk of hepatotoxicity
Probenecid: decreased probenecid efficacy (possibly precipitating gout)
Drug-diagnostic tests. *Acetest or Ketostix urine test:* false interpretation
Liver function tests: abnormal results
Uric acid: increased level

Patient monitoring
- Monitor CBC, uric acid level, and liver and kidney function tests.
- Assess for signs and symptoms of gout, hepatic failure, and hemolytic anemia.
- ◀€ Discontinue at first sign of hepatic impairment or hyperuricemia accompanied by acute gouty arthritis.

Patient teaching
- Advise patient to take regularly with other antituberculars, as prescribed.
- ◀€ Teach patient to recognize and immediately report signs and symptoms of gout and liver impairment.
- As appropriate, review all other significant and life-threatening adverse reactions and interactions, especially those related to the drugs and tests mentioned above.

pyridostigmine bromide
Mestinon, Mestinon-SR✲, Mestinon Timespan, Regonol

Pharmacologic class: Anticholinesterase
Therapeutic class: Muscle stimulant, antimyasthenic
Pregnancy risk category C

Action
Prevents acetylcholine destruction, resulting in stronger contractions of muscles weakened by myasthenia gravis or curare-like neuromuscular blockers

Availability
Injection: 5 mg/ml
Syrup: 60 mg/5 ml
Tablets: 60 mg
Tablets (extended-release): 180 mg

⏀ Indications and dosages
➤ Myasthenia gravis
Adults: 600 mg P.O. given over 24 hours, with doses spaced for maximum symptom relief. For myasthenic crisis, 2 mg or $\frac{1}{30}$ of oral dose I.M. or very slow I.V. q 2 to 3 hours.
➤ Postoperative reversal of nondepolarizing neuromuscular blockers
Adults: 10 to 20 mg slow I.V. injection (range is 0.1 to 0.25 mg/kg) with or immediately after 0.6 to 1.2 mg atropine sulfate I.V.

Dosage adjustment
- Renal impairment
- Seizure disorders

P

Off-label uses
- Myasthenia gravis in children
- Constipation in patients with Parkinson's disease
- Nerve agent prophylaxis

Contraindications
- Hypersensitivity to drug or bromides
- Mechanical intestinal or urinary tract obstruction

Precautions
Use cautiously in:
- seizure disorders, bronchial asthma, coronary occlusion, arrhythmias, bradycardia, hyperthyroidism, peptic ulcer, vagotonia, cholinergic crisis
- pregnant or breastfeeding patients
- children (safety and efficacy not established).

Administration
🔊 Don't exceed I.V. injection rate of 1 mg/minute.
🔊 Don't give concurrently with other anticholinesterase drugs.
- Have atropine available for use in emergencies.

Route	Onset	Peak	Duration
P.O.	20-30 min	Unknown	Unknown
P.O. (extended)	30-60 min	Unknown	6-12 hr
I.V.	2-5 min	Unknown	2-4 hr
I.M.	<15 min	Unknown	2-4 hr

Adverse reactions
CNS: headache, dysarthria, dysphoria, drowsiness, dizziness, headache, syncope, **loss of consciousness, seizures**
CV: decreased cardiac output leading to hypotension, bradycardia, nodal rhythm, **atrioventricular block, cardiac arrest, arrhythmias**
EENT: diplopia, lacrimation, miosis, spasm of accommodation, conjunctival hyperemia
GI: nausea, vomiting, diarrhea, abdominal cramps, increased peristalsis, flatulence dysphagia, increased salivation
GU: urinary frequency, urgency, or incontinence
Musculoskeletal: muscle weakness, fasciculations, and cramps; joint pain
Respiratory: increased pharyngeal and tracheobronchial secretions, dyspnea, **central respiratory paralysis, respiratory muscle paralysis, laryngospasm, bronchospasm, bronchiolar constriction**
Skin: diaphoresis, flushing, rash, urticaria
Other: thrombophlebitis at I.V. site, cholinergic crisis, anaphylaxis

Interactions
Drug-drug. *Aminoglycosides:* potentiation of neuromuscular blockade
Anesthetics (general and local), antiarrhythmics: decreased anticholinesterase effects
Atropine, belladonna derivatives: suppression of parasympathomimetic GI symptoms (leaving only fasciculations and voluntary muscle paralysis as signs of anticholinesterase overdose)
Corticosteroids: decreased anticholinesterase effects; after corticosteroid withdrawal, increased anticholinesterase effects
Ganglionic blockers (such as mecamylamine): increased anticholinesterase effects
Magnesium: antagonism of beneficial anticholinesterase effects
Nondepolarizing neuromuscular blockers (atropine, pancuronium, tubocurarine): antagonism of neuromuscular blockade and reversal of muscle relaxation after surgery (with parenteral pyridostigmine)
Other anticholinesterase drugs: in patients with myasthenia gravis, symptoms of anticholinesterase overdose that mimic underdose, causing patient's condition to worsen
Succinylcholine: increased and prolonged neuromuscular blockade (including respiratory depression)

♦ Canada   ⊕ UK   ☢ Hazardous drug   ⊗ High-alert drug

Patient monitoring

• Assess patient's response to each dose.
• Monitor vital signs, ECG, and cardiovascular and respiratory status.
◀€ Assess for signs and symptoms of overdose, which indicate cholinergic crisis.

Patient teaching

• If patient is using syrup, advise him to pour it over ice.
• Instruct patient using extended-release tablets not to crush them.
◀€ Teach patient to recognize and promptly report signs and symptoms of overdose, including muscle fasciculations, sweating, excessive salivation, and constricted pupils.
• Tell patient drug may cause headache and muscle cramps. Encourage him to discuss activity recommendations and pain management with prescriber.
• Advise patient to monitor and report his response to ongoing therapy so that optimal dosage can be determined.
• As appropriate, review all other significant and life-threatening adverse reactions and interactions, especially those related to the drugs mentioned above.

pyrimethamine

Daraprim

Pharmacologic class: Folic acid antagonist

Therapeutic class: Antiprotozoal, antimalarial

Pregnancy risk category C

Action

Inhibits reduction of dihydrofolic acid to tetrahydrofolic acid (folinic acid) by binding to and reversibly inhibiting dihydrofolate reductase

Availability

Tablets: 25 mg

Indications and dosages

➤ To control plasmodia transmission and suppress susceptible strains
Adults and children ages 10 and older: 25 mg P.O. daily for 2 days, given with a sulfonamide
➤ Toxoplasmosis
Adults: Initially, 50 to 75 mg P.O. daily for 1 to 3 weeks, given with a sulfonamide. Depending on response and tolerance, reduce dosages of both drugs by 50% and continue therapy for 4 to 5 more weeks.
Children: 1 mg/kg P.O. daily in two equally divided doses for 2 to 4 days, then reduced to 0.5 mg/kg/day for approximately 1 month. Alternatively, 2 mg/kg (up to 100 mg) P.O. daily in two equally divided doses for 3 days, then 1 mg/kg (up to 25 mg) in two equally divided doses for 4 weeks, given with sulfadiazine for 4 weeks.
➤ Prophylaxis of malaria caused by susceptible plasmodia strains
Adults and children older than age 10: 25 mg P.O. weekly
Children ages 4 to 10: 12.5 mg P.O. weekly
Infants and children younger than age 4: 6.25 mg P.O. weekly

Off-label uses

• Isosporiasis
• Prophylaxis of *Pneumocystis jiroveci* pneumonia

Contraindications

• Hypersensitivity to drug
• Megaloblastic anemia caused by folate deficiency
• Concurrent folate antagonist therapy

Precautions

Use cautiously in:
• anemia, bone marrow depression, hepatic or renal impairment, G6PD deficiency

p

- history of seizures
- patients more than 16 weeks pregnant
- breastfeeding patients.

Administration

- Administer with meals.
- When giving tablets to young children, crush them and administer as oral suspension in water, cherry syrup, or sweetened solution.
- Know that because of worldwide resistance to pyrimethamine, its use alone to prevent or treat acute malaria is no longer recommended.
- Be aware that fixed combination of pyrimethamine and sulfadoxine is available and has been used for uncomplicated mild to moderate malaria caused by chloroquine-resistant *Plasmodium falciparum* and for presumptive self-treatment by travelers.

Route	Onset	Peak	Duration
P.O.	Unknown	2-6 hr	2 wk

Adverse reactions

CNS: headache, light-headedness, insomnia, malaise, depression, **seizures**
CV: arrhythmias
EENT: dry throat
GI: nausea, vomiting, diarrhea, anorexia, atrophic glossitis
GU: hematuria
Hematologic: megaloblastic anemia, leukopenia, pancytopenia, thrombocytopenia
Metabolic: hyperphenylalaninemia
Respiratory: pulmonary eosinophilia
Skin: pigmentation changes, dermatitis, erythema multiforme, **toxic epidermal necrolysis, Stevens-Johnson syndrome**
Other: fever, **anaphylaxis**

Interactions

Drug-drug. *Lorazepam:* hepatotoxicity
Myelosuppressants (including antineoplastics): increased risk of bone marrow depression

Drug-diagnostic tests. *Platelets, white blood cells:* decreased counts

Patient monitoring

- Monitor CBC. Watch for evidence of blood dyscrasias.
- Assess for signs and symptoms of folic acid deficiency.
- Closely monitor neurologic and cardiovascular status. Stay alert for seizures and arrhythmias.
- ◀€ Watch for evidence of erythema multiforme, including sore throat, cough, mouth sores, rash, iritic lesions, and fever. Report early signs before condition can progress to Stevens-Johnson syndrome.

Patient teaching

- Advise patient to take with meals.
- ◀€ Tell patient to discontinue drug and contact prescriber at first sign of rash.
- Caution patient to avoid driving and other hazardous activities until he knows how drug affects concentration and alertness.
- As appropriate, review all other significant and life-threatening adverse reactions and interactions, especially those related to the drugs and tests mentioned above.

quetiapine fumarate
Seroquel, Seroquel XR

Pharmacologic class: Dibenzothiazepine derivative
Therapeutic class: Atypical antipsychotic
Pregnancy risk category C

FDA | BOXED WARNING

• Elderly patients with dementia-related psychosis are at increased risk for death. Over course of 10-week controlled trial, death rate in drug-treated patients was about 4.5%, compared to about 2.6% in placebo group. Although causes of death varied, most appeared to be cardiovascular or infectious. Don't give drug to patients with dementia-related psychosis.

• Drug may increase risk of suicidal thinking and behavior in children and adolescents with major depressive disorder and other psychiatric disorders. Risk must be balanced with clinical need, as depression itself increases suicide risk. With patient of any age, observe closely for clinical worsening, suicidality, and unusual behavior changes when therapy begins. Advise family and caregivers to observe patient closely and communicate with prescriber as needed.

• Drug isn't approved for use in pediatric patients.

Action

Unknown. Antipsychotic effects may occur through antagonism of dopamine D_2 and serotonin 5-HT_2 receptors. Other effects may result partly from antagonism of other receptors, such as histamine H_1 and alpha$_1$-adrenergic receptors.

Availability

Tablets: 25 mg, 50 mg, 100 mg, 200 mg, 300 mg, 400 mg
Tablets (extended-release): 50 mg, 150 mg, 200 mg, 300 mg, 400 mg

✔ Indications and dosages

➤ Schizophrenia
Adults: Initially, 25 mg P.O. b.i.d., on day 1, increased by 25 to 50 mg given two to three times daily on days 2 and 3 to range of 300 to 400 mg by day 4.

Further adjustments can be made in increments of 25 to 50 mg b.i.d. in intervals of not less than 2 days. Recommended dosage range is 150 to 750 mg/day. Or, 300 mg P.O. (extended-release tablet) once daily, preferably in evening; dosage should be titrated to 400 to 800 mg based on response and tolerability. Dosage increases may be done at 1-day intervals at increments of up to 300 mg.

Children and adolescents ages 13 to 17: Immediate-release tablets administered twice daily, with total daily dosage for initial 5 days of therapy as 50 mg P.O. on day 1, 100 mg on day 2, 200 mg on day 3, 300 mg on day 4, and 400 mg on day 5. After day 5, adjust dosage within recommended range of 400 to 800 mg/day based on response and tolerability. Make dosage adjustments in increments of no greater than 100 mg/day. Based on response and tolerability, may administer three times daily.

➤ Acute manic episodes associated with bipolar I disorder
Adults: Immediate-release tablets administered twice daily, with total daily dosages as 100 mg P.O. on day 1, 200 mg on day 2, 300 mg on day 3, and 400 mg on day 4. Increase in increments of no more than 200 mg/day up to 800 mg/day by day 6. Recommended dosage range is 400 to 800 mg/day. May be given as monotherapy or as adjunctive therapy with lithium or divalproex. Or, extended-release tablets 300 mg P.O. on day 1, 600 mg on day 2, and 400 to 800 mg on day 3. Recommended dosage range is 400 to 800 mg/day.

Children and adolescents ages 10 to 17: Immediate-release tablets administered twice daily, with total daily dosage for initial 5 days of therapy as 50 mg P.O. on day 1, 100 mg on day 2, 200 mg on day 3, 300 mg on day 4, and 400 mg on day 5. After day 5, adjust dosage within recommended range of

q

400 to 600 mg/day based on response and tolerability. Adjust dosage in increments of no more than 100 mg/day. Based on response and tolerability, may administer three times daily.

➤ Depression associated with bipolar disorder

Adults: Immediate-release or extended-release tablets administered once daily at bedtime as 50 mg P.O. on day 1, 100 mg on day 2, 200 mg on day 3, and 300 mg on day 4. Maximum dosage is 300 mg/day.

➤ Adjunctive treatment of major depressive disorder

Adults: Initially, 50 mg (extended-release) P.O once daily in the evening on days 1 and 2 and 150 mg (extended-release) P.O. once daily on days 3 and 4 as adjunct to existing antidepressive therapy. Recommended dosage is 150 to 300 mg/day.

Dosage adjustment
• Hepatic impairment
• History of hypotensive reactions
• Elderly or debilitated patients

Off-label uses
• Bipolar disorder
• Mania
• Obsessive-compulsive disorder
• Posttraumatic stress disorder
• Psychosis related to Parkinson's disease

Contraindications
• None

Precautions
Use cautiously in:
• diabetes mellitus, hepatic impairment, cardiovascular disease (including family history of QT-interval prolongation, congestive heart failure, and cardiac hypertrophy), cerebrovascular disease, dehydration, hypovolemia, Alzheimer's dementia, hypothyroidism
• history of seizures, suicide attempt, or hypotensive reactions
• history of cardiac arrhythmias such as bradycardia, hypokalemia or

hypomagnesemia, concurrent use of other drugs that prolong the QTc interval, congenital QT-interval prolongation (avoid use)
• concurrent use of drugs known to cause electrolyte imbalance
• elderly or debilitated patients
• pregnant patients
• children (safety not established).

Administration
• Monitor fasting blood lipids before treatment.
• Give immediate-release tablets with or without food; give extended-release tablets without food or with a light meal.
🔊 Don't confuse Seroquel with Serzone (an antidepressant).

Route	Onset	Peak	Duration
P.O.	Rapid	1.5 hr	8-12 hr
P.O. (extended)	Unknown	6 hr	Unknown

Adverse reactions
CNS: dizziness, sedation, cognitive impairment, extrapyramidal symptoms, tardive dyskinesia, **neuroleptic malignant syndrome, seizures, suicide**
CV: tachycardia, palpitations, peripheral edema, orthostatic hypotension, hypertension, **QT-interval prolongation**
EENT: cataracts, ear pain, rhinitis, pharyngitis
GI: constipation, dyspepsia, dry mouth, anorexia
Hematologic: leukopenia
Metabolic: hypothyroidism
Respiratory: cough, dyspnea
Skin: diaphoresis
Other: weight gain, flulike symptoms, acute withdrawal symptoms with abrupt cessation

Interactions
Drug-drug. *Antihistamines, opioids, sedative-hypnotics, other CNS depressants:* additive CNS depression

Antibiotics (such as gatifloxacin, moxifloxacin), antipsychotics (such as chlorpromazine, thioridazine, ziprasidone), Class 1A antiarrhythmics (such as procainamide, quinidine), Class III antiarrhythmics (such as amiodarone, sotalol), drugs known to prolong QTc interval (such as levomethadyl acetate, methadone, pentamidine): increased risk of prolonged QTc interval

Antihypertensives: increased risk of hypotension

Barbiturates, carbamazepine, corticosteroids, phenytoin, rifampin, thioridazine: increased clearance and decreased efficacy of quetiapine

Dopamine agonists, levodopa: antagonism of these drugs' effects

Erythromycin, fluconazole, itraconazole, ketoconazole, other CYP450-3A4 inhibitors: increased quetiapine effects

Drug-diagnostic tests. *Alanine aminotransferase, aspartate aminotransferase:* asymptomatic elevations

Total cholesterol, triglycerides: increased levels

Urine tricyclic antidepressant assay: false-positive screen

White blood cells: decreased count

Drug-behaviors. *Alcohol use:* increased CNS effects

Patient monitoring

◀€ Monitor neurologic status, especially for signs and symptoms of tardive dyskinesia, suicidal ideation, or neuroleptic malignant syndrome.

• Be aware that patient should undergo lens examination when starting treatment and at 6-month intervals during long-term treatment.

• Monitor blood pressure for orthostatic hypotension.

◀€ Monitor patient closely for prolonged QT interval.

• Monitor fasting blood lipids periodically during treatment.

◀€ Monitor CBC and differential in patients with preexisting low white blood cell (WBC) count; discontinue

drug at first sign of WBC decrease in absence of other causes.

Patient teaching

• Tell patient to take immediate-release tablets with or without food and to take extended-release form preferably in the evening, swallowed whole, without food or with a light meal.

• Instruct patient not to crush, break, or chew extended-release tablets.

◀€ Teach patient to recognize and immediately report signs and symptoms of neuroleptic malignant syndrome (such as high fever, sweating, unstable blood pressure, stupor, muscle rigidity, changes in mood or behavior and tardive dyskinesia) and prolonged QT interval.

• Instruct patient to move slowly when sitting up or standing, to avoid dizziness from sudden blood pressure decrease.

◀€ Tell patient not to stop taking drug abruptly. Tell him dosage must be tapered.

• Caution patient not to drink alcohol.

• Instruct patient to avoid driving and other hazardous activities until he knows how drug affects concentration and alertness.

• As appropriate, review all other significant and life-threatening adverse reactions and interactions, especially those related to the drugs, tests, and behaviors mentioned above.

quinapril hydrochloride
Accupril, Accupro ⊕, Quinil ⊕

Pharmacologic class: Angiotensin-converting enzyme (ACE) inhibitor
Therapeutic class: Antihypertensive
Pregnancy risk category D

Reactions in **bold** are life-threatening.   ◀€ Clinical alert

• Drugs that act directly on the renin-angiotensin system can cause injury to or death of a developing fetus. Discontinue drug as soon as possible when pregnancy is detected.

Action
Inhibits conversion of angiotensin I to angiotensin II, a potent vasoconstrictor; decreases cardiac output. Increases plasma renin levels and reduces aldosterone levels, causing systemic vasodilation.

Availability
Tablets: 5 mg, 10 mg, 20 mg, 40 mg

⚡ Indications and dosages
➤ Hypertension
Adults: Initially, 10 to 20 mg P.O. daily for patients not receiving diuretics, with subsequent dosages adjusted at 2-week intervals according to blood pressure response at peak (2 to 6 hours) and trough (predose) blood levels; for maintenance, 20 to 80 mg/day as a single dose or in two divided doses. In patients receiving diuretics, discontinue diuretic 2 to 3 days before starting quinapril; if blood pressure isn't controlled, resume diuretic. If diuretic can't be discontinued, start therapy with 5 mg/day quinapril.
➤ Adjunct in heart failure
Adults: Initially, 5 mg P.O. b.i.d., titrated weekly until effective dosage is determined. For maintenance, 20 to 40 mg/day in two evenly divided doses.

Dosage adjustment
• Renal impairment
• Elderly patients

Off-label uses
• Aortic insufficiency
• Atherosclerosis
• Postoperative hypertension
• Myocardial infarction
• Diabetic or nondiabetic neuropathy

Contraindications
• Hypersensitivity to drug or other ACE inhibitors
• Angioedema caused by other ACE inhibitors

Precautions
Use cautiously in:
• autoimmune diseases, aortic stenosis, renal artery stenosis, hypertrophic cardiomyopathy, cerebrovascular or cardiac insufficiency, collagen vascular disease, hepatic or renal impairment, hypovolemia, hyponatremia, hypotension, neutropenia, chronic cough, proteinuria, febrile illness
• family history of angioedema
• risk factors for development of hyperkalemia, including renal insufficiency, diabetes mellitus, concurrent use of potassium-sparing diuretics, potassium supplements, or potassium-containing salt substitutes
• concurrent use of nonsteroidal anti-inflammatory drugs (NSAIDs) in patients who are elderly, volume-depleted (including those on diuretics), or with compromised renal function
• concurrent immunosuppressant, lithium, or diuretic therapy
• black patients
• elderly patients
• pregnant or breastfeeding patients
• children (safety not established).

Administration
• Administer with or without food, but not with high-fat meal.
• Know that if quinapril alone doesn't adequately control blood pressure, a diuretic may be added.

Route	Onset	Peak	Duration
P.O.	0.5-1 hr	2-6 hr	Up to 24 hr

Adverse reactions

CNS: dizziness, drowsiness, fatigue, headache, insomnia, depression, vertigo, paresthesia, asthenia, malaise, nervousness, syncope
CV: hypotension, angina pectoris, palpitations, chest pain, tachycardia, **arrhythmias**
EENT: amblyopia, sinusitis, pharyngitis
GI: nausea, vomiting, diarrhea, constipation, abdominal pain, anorexia, dry mouth
GU: erectile dysfunction
Metabolic: hyperkalemia
Musculoskeletal: back pain
Respiratory: cough, dyspnea
Skin: rash, pruritus, alopecia, flushing, diaphoresis, photosensitivity
Other: taste disturbances, fever, viral infections, hypersensitivity reactions including **anaphylaxis**

Interactions

Drug-drug.
Diuretics, other antihypertensives: increased hypotension
Gold (sodium aurothiomalate): increased risk of rare nitritoid reactions (including facial flushing, nausea, vomiting, and hypotension)
Lithium: increased serum lithium level and lithium toxicity
NSAIDs: may result in deterioration of renal function, including acute renal failure and attenuated ACE inhibitor antihypertensive effect
Potassium-sparing diuretics, potassium supplements: increased risk of hyperkalemia
Tetracyclines: decreased tetracycline absorption
Drug-diagnostic tests. *Alanine aminotransferase, alkaline phosphatase, aspartate aminotransferase, bilirubin, blood urea nitrogen, creatinine, potassium:* increased levels
Drug-food. *High-fat foods:* decreased rate and extent of drug absorption
Salt substitutes containing potassium: increased risk of hyperkalemia

Patient monitoring

• Monitor vital signs and cardiovascular status. Be sure to ask patient if he's experiencing angina.
• Assess CBC and liver function tests.
• Monitor potassium level. Watch for evidence of hyperkalemia.
◀€ Watch closely for signs and symptoms of angioedema, especially in black patients after first dose.
• Assess for dry, nonproductive cough and signs and symptoms of infection.
• Monitor renal function periodically in patients receiving concurrent NSAID therapy.

Patient teaching

• Tell patient he may take with or without food, but not with high-fat meal.
◀€ Advise patient to immediately report facial or tongue swelling or difficulty breathing.
• Instruct patient to monitor and record his blood pressure.
• Tell patient to promptly report dry, nonproductive cough and signs and symptoms of infection.
• Instruct patient to move slowly when sitting up or standing, to avoid dizziness or light-headedness from sudden blood pressure decrease.
• Tell patient that excessive fluid loss (as from sweating, vomiting, or diarrhea) and inadequate fluid intake increase the risk of light-headedness (especially in hot weather).
• Caution patient to avoid driving and other hazardous activities until he knows how drug affects concentration and alertness.
• Advise patient to avoid salt substitutes containing potassium.
• Tell female patient to notify prescriber of possible pregnancy. Caution her not to breastfeed.
• As appropriate, review all other significant and life-threatening adverse reactions and interactions, especially those related to the drugs, tests, foods, herbs, and behaviors mentioned above.

q

Reactions in **bold** are life-threatening.   ◀€ Clinical alert

quinidine gluconate
Apo-Quin-G ♣

quinidine sulfate
Apo-Quinidine ♣

Pharmacologic class: Cinchona alkaloid

Therapeutic class: Antiarrhythmic (class IA), antimalarial

Pregnancy risk category C

FDA | **BOXED WARNING**

- In many trials of antiarrhythmic therapy for non-life-threatening arrhythmias, active antiarrhythmic therapy has led to increased deaths; risk of active therapy is probably greatest in patients with structural heart disease. Deaths associated with quinidine were more than three times as high as deaths in placebo group. Another analysis showed that in patients with non-life-threatening ventricular arrhythmias, quinidine-associated deaths were consistently higher than those linked to various alternative antiarrhythmics.

Action
Slows conduction and prolongs refractory period, reducing myocardial irritability and interrupting or preventing certain arrhythmias. As an antimalarial, acts primarily as intra-erythrocytic schizonticide.

Availability
quinidine gluconate
Injection: 80 mg/ml
Tablets (extended-release): 324 mg
quinidine sulfate
Tablets: 200 mg, 300 mg
Tablets (extended-release): 300 mg

ⓘ Indications and dosages
➤ Test dose
Adults: 200 mg sulfate P.O. as a single dose or 200 mg gluconate I.M. to check for idiosyncratic reaction
➤ Premature atrial and ventricular contractions
Adults: 200 to 300 mg sulfate P.O. three to four times daily, or gluconate (extended-release) given as 324 to 660 mg P.O. q 8 to 12 hours
➤ Paroxysmal supraventricular tachycardia (PSVT)
Adults: 400 to 600 mg sulfate P.O. q 2 or 3 hours until arrhythmia ends; or 324 to 660 mg (extended-release) P.O. q 8 to 12 hours. For parenteral use, 400 mg gluconate I.M., repeated q 2 hours if necessary; or 330 mg gluconate I.V. (up to 750 mg) in diluted solution, infused no faster than 1 ml/minute.
➤ To convert atrial fibrillation to sinus rhythm
Adults: 200 mg sulfate P.O. q 2 or 3 hours for five to eight doses, increased daily until sinus rhythm returns or toxic effects occur; maximum daily dosage is 4 g. Or 300 mg sulfate (extended-release) P.O. q 8 to 12 hours, increased cautiously if necessary. Or 324 to 660 mg gluconate (extended-release) P.O. q 8 to 12 hours. For parenteral use, 800 mg gluconate I.V. in diluted solution, infused no faster than 0.25 mg/kg/minute.
➤ Severe, life-threatening *Plasmodium falciparum* malaria
Adults: Loading dose of 10 mg/kg gluconate I.V. diluted in 5 ml/kg of normal saline solution (or 250 ml of normal saline solution in otherwise healthy, 50-kg [110-lb] patient) by continuous infusion over 1 to 2 hours, then a continuous maintenance infusion of 0.02 mg/kg/minute for 72 hours or until parasitemia drops to less than 1% or oral therapy can begin. Or alternative loading dose of 24 mg/kg gluconate I.V. diluted in 250 ml of

0.9% sodium chloride injection by intermittent infusion over 4 hours, followed by maintenance dosage of 12 mg/kg I.V. at 8-hour intervals, starting 8 hours after loading dose, infused over 4 hours for 7 days or until patient tolerates oral therapy.

Dosage adjustment
• Hepatic insufficiency

Off-label uses
• Myocardial infarction

Contraindications
• Hypersensitivity to drug or related cinchona derivatives
• Thrombocytopenia with previous quinidine therapy
• Myasthenia gravis
• Complete heart block
• Left bundle-branch block or other severe intraventricular conduction defects
• Aberrant ectopic impulses and abnormal rhythm
• History of prolonged QT interval or drug-induced torsades de pointes
• Digoxin toxicity

Precautions
Use cautiously in:
• potassium imbalance, renal or hepatic disease, heart failure, respiratory depression
• elderly patients
• pregnant or breastfeeding patients
• children.

Administration
◀€ Before first dose, assess apical pulse and blood pressure. If patient has bradycardia or tachycardia, withhold dose and contact prescriber.
• If patient has atrial fibrillation, expect to give digoxin, calcium channel blocker, beta-adrenergic blocker, and possibly an anticoagulant before administering quinidine.

• If sinus rhythm isn't restored after patient has received a total of 10 mg/kg quinidine gluconate, other means of cardioversion may be considered.
• Monitor blood pressure and ECG; titrate flow rate to correct arrhythmia.
• When giving large doses, monitor blood pressure and ECG continuously.
• Know that quinidine gluconate is the only parenteral cinchona alkaloid antimalarial commercially available in U.S. Because newer antiarrhythmics have replaced quinidine in many cardiac uses, it may not be readily available and prescribers may not be familiar with its use. For information about availability or use, contact manufacturer at 800-821-0538.

Route	Onset	Peak	Duration
P.O. (extended)	Unknown	3-5 hr	Unknown
P.O. (sulfate)	Unknown	1-3 hr	Unknown
I.V.	Immediate	Immediate	Unknown
I.M.	30-90 sec	Unknown	Unknown

Adverse reactions
CNS: vertigo, headache, ataxia, apprehension, excitement, delirium, syncope, confusion, depression, dementia
CV: ECG changes, hypotension, vasculitis, tachycardia, premature ventricular contractions, paradoxical tachycardia, **ventricular tachycardia, ventricular fibrillation, ventricular flutter, ventricular ectopy, torsades de pointes, complete atrioventricular (AV) block, widened QRS complex, prolonged QT interval, asystole, aggravated heart failure, arterial embolism, vascular collapse**
EENT: diplopia, blurred vision, mydriasis, abnormal color perception, scotoma, photophobia, night blindness, optic neuritis, decreased hearing, tinnitus

q

Reactions in **bold** are life-threatening.   ◀€ Clinical alert

GI: nausea, vomiting, diarrhea, abdominal pain, increased salivation, anorexia
GU: lupus nephritis
Hematologic: purpura, **hemolytic anemia, hypothrombinemia, leukocytosis, shift to left in white blood cell differential, neutropenia, thrombocytopenia, thrombocytopenic purpura, agranulocytosis**
Hepatic: hepatotoxicity
Respiratory: acute asthma attack, respiratory arrest
Skin: rash, pruritus, urticaria, photosensitivity, angioedema
Other: fever, cinchonism, lupuslike syndrome, hypersensitivity reaction

Interactions
Drug-drug. *Amiodarone:* increased quinidine blood level, causing potentially fatal arrhythmias
Antacids, cimetidine: increased quinidine blood level
Anticholinergics: additive vagolytic effect
Anticoagulants, beta-adrenergic blockers, procainamide, propafenone, tricyclic antidepressants: increased effects of these drugs
Barbiturates, hydantoins, nifedipine, rifampin, sucralfate: decreased therapeutic effect of quinidine
Cardiac glycosides: increased cardiac glycoside blood level, greater risk of toxicity
Cholinergics: decreased quinidine effect (may cause failure to terminate PSVT)
Depolarizing (decamethonium, succinylcholine) and nondepolarizing (tubocurarine, pancuronium) neuromuscular blockers: potentiation of neuromuscular blockade
Diltiazem, verapamil: decreased quinidine clearance, resulting in hypotension, bradycardia, ventricular tachycardia, AV block, or pulmonary edema
Disopyramide: increased disopyramide or decreased quinidine blood level

Potassium, urinary alkalizers: increased blood level and effects of quinidine
Drug-diagnostic tests. *Granulocytes, hemoglobin, platelets:* decreased levels
Creatine kinase, hepatic enzymes: increased levels
Renal function tests: altered results
Drug-food. *Grapefruit juice:* inhibited drug metabolism
Reduced sodium intake: increased quinidine blood level
Drug-herbs. *Jimsonweed:* adverse cardiovascular effects
Licorice: additive effects

Patient monitoring
◀≀ Monitor ECG and vital signs closely. Assess for worsening heart failure, especially with I.V. use.
• Assess CBC, kidney and liver function tests and quinidine blood level.
• Watch for signs and symptoms of blood dyscrasias.
◀≀ Closely monitor respiratory status. Stay alert for asthma attacks and impending respiratory arrest.
• Monitor for adverse GI effects, which may signify drug toxicity.

Patient teaching
• Advise patient to take with food to reduce GI upset.
• Instruct patient not to crush or chew extended-release tablets.
◀≀ Teach patient to recognize and immediately report signs and symptoms of toxicity, including tinnitus, nausea, headache, dizziness, and visual disturbances.
• Caution patient to avoid potassium supplements, licorice, and grapefruit juice. Tell him to maintain constant level of sodium intake.
• Advise patient to consult prescriber before taking herbs.
• As appropriate, review all other significant and life-threatening adverse reactions and interactions, especially those related to the drugs, tests, foods, and herbs mentioned above.

quinine sulfate
Apo-Quinine✦, Novo-Quinine✦,
Qualaquin

Pharmacologic class: Cinchona alkaloid
Therapeutic class: Antimalarial
Pregnancy risk category C

FDA | **BOXED WARNING**

• Using drug for treatment or prevention of nocturnal leg cramps may
cause serious and life-threatening
hematologic reactions, including
thrombocytopenia and hemolytic uremic syndrome/thrombotic thrombocytopenic purpura (TTP). Chronic renal
impairment associated with development of TTP has occurred. Risks associated with drug use in absence of evidence of its effectiveness in treatment
or prevention of nocturnal leg cramps
outweigh potential benefits.

Action
Unknown. Thought to interfere with
DNA synthesis by increasing pH in
intracellular organelles of susceptible
parasites.

Availability
Capsules: 324 mg

ⓘ Indications and dosages
➤ Uncomplicated *Plasmodium falciparum* malaria
Adults and children age 16 and older:
648 mg (two capsules) P.O. q 8 hours
for 7 days

Dosage adjustment
• Severe chronic renal impairment

Contraindications
• Hypersensitivity to drug (including
but not limited to thrombocytopenia,

idiopathic thrombocytopenia purpura,
thrombocytopenic purpura, hemolytic
uremic syndrome, blackwater fever),
mefloquine, quinidine
• G6PD deficiency
• Optic neuritis
• Tinnitus
• Prolonged QT interval
• Myasthenia gravis

Precautions
Use cautiously in:
• renal or hepatic impairment
• hypoglycemia
• concurrent use of digoxin and drugs
known to prolong QT interval, including Class IA antiarrhythmics (such as
disopyramide, procainamide, quinidine) and Class III antiarrhythmics
(such as amiodarone, dofetilide,
sotalol)
• concurrent use of antacids, rifampin,
ritonavir, neuromuscular blockers,
macrolide anti-infectives, CYP3A4
substrates, including astemizole, cisapride, terfenadine (not available in
U.S.), pimozide, halofantrine, quinidine (avoid use)
• pregnant or breastfeeding patients.
• children younger than age 16 (safety
and efficacy of capsules not
established).

Administration
• Give with or without food.

Route	Onset	Peak	Duration
P.O.	Unknown	1-3 hr	4-11 hr

Adverse reactions
CNS: headache, vertigo, syncope,
apprehension, restlessness, excitement,
confusion, delirium, dizziness, **seizures**
CV: angina, vasculitis, **cardiac rhythm
or conduction disturbances**
EENT: diplopia, amblyopia, blurred
vision, scotoma, abnormal color perception, photophobia, night blindness,
mydriasis, optic atrophy, hearing loss,
tinnitus

q

GI: nausea, vomiting, diarrhea, abdominal cramps, epigastric pain, dysphagia
GU: hemolytic uremic syndrome
Hematologic: hemolytic anemia, hypoprothrombinemia, acute hemolysis, thrombocytopenic purpura, agranulocytosis
Hepatic: hepatotoxicity
Metabolic: hypothermia, **hypoglycemia**
Respiratory: asthma
Skin: rash, pruritus, photosensitivity, flushing, diaphoresis
Other: cinchonism, facial edema, hypersensitivity reactions including fever and **hemolytic uremic syndrome**

Interactions

Drug-drug. *Aminophylline, theophylline:* increased quinine mean area under the curve (AUC) and C_{max}.
Antacids: delayed or decreased quinine absorption
Atorvastatin, other HMG-CoA reductase inhibitors that are CYP3A4 substrates: increased risk of myopathy
Cimetidine: decreased metabolism and increased effects of quinine
Class IA, Class III antiarrhythmics: increased risk of ECG abnormalities, including prolonged QT interval
CYP3A4 inducers (such as carbamazepine, phenobarbital, phenytoin): decreased quinine plasma concentration and increased carbamazepine, phenobarbital, and phenytoin AUC and C_{max}
CYP3A4 inducers or inhibitors, CYP3A4 and CYP2D6 substrates: decreased efficacy and increased adverse effects of these drugs
Digoxin: increased digoxin blood level
Other antimalarials including halofantrine, mefloquine: increased risk of seizures, ECG abnormalities, and cardiac arrest
Neuromuscular blockers: increased effects of these drugs, leading to respiratory difficulty
Rifampin: increased metabolism and decreased effects of quinine

Ritonavir: increased quinine mean AUC, C_{max}, and elimination half-life
Succinylcholine: delayed succinylcholine metabolism
Tetracycline: increased quinine mean plasma concentration
Urinary alkalizers (such as acetazolamide, sodium bicarbonate): increased quinine blood level and risk of toxicity
Warfarin: increased warfarin effects, increased risk of bleeding
Drug-diagnostic tests. *Urinary 17-ketogenic steroids:* elevated levels

Patient monitoring

◀€ Monitor for signs and symptoms of hypersensitivity reaction, including fever and hemolytic uremic syndrome. Discontinue drug if signs or symptoms of hypersensitivity occur.

• Stay alert for signs and symptoms of cinchonism, including tinnitus, headache, nausea, and visual disturbances.

◀€ Assess for bleeding tendency, arrhythmias, and hepatotoxicity.

• Monitor CBC, renal and liver function tests, and quinine and glucose levels.

Patient teaching

• Tell patient he may take with or without food.

◀€ Teach patient to recognize and immediately report signs and symptoms of cinchonism, cardiac arrhythmias, nephrotoxicity, and hepatotoxicity.

◀€ Instruct patient to report unusual bleeding or bruising.

• Tell female patient to discuss pregnancy or breastfeeding with prescriber before taking drug.

• As appropriate, review all other significant and life-threatening adverse reactions and interactions, especially those related to the drugs and tests mentioned above.

---

quinupristin and dalfopristin
Synercid

Pharmacologic class: Streptogramin
Therapeutic class: Anti-infective
Pregnancy risk category B

FDA **BOXED WARNING**

• Drug combination is approved for treating serious or life-threatening infections related to vancomycin-resistant *Enterococcus faecium* bacteremia under the Food and Drug Administration's accelerated approval regulations that allow marketing of products for use in life-threatening conditions when other therapies aren't available.

Action
Synergistic effects of drug combination interfere with bacterial cell-wall synthesis by disrupting DNA and RNA transcription

Availability
Injection: 500 mg/10 ml (150 mg quinupristin, 350 mg dalfopristin), 600 mg/10 ml (180 mg quinupristin, 420 mg dalfopristin)

⚕ Indications and dosages
➤ Serious or life-threatening infections caused by vancomycin-resistant *Enterococcus faecium*
Adults and adolescents ages 16 and older: 7.5 mg/kg by I.V. infusion over 1 hour q 8 hours
➤ Complicated skin and skin-structure infections caused by *Staphylococcus aureus* (methicillin-susceptible) or *Streptococcus pyogenes*

Adults and adolescents ages 16 and older: 7.5 mg/kg by I.V. infusion over 1 hour q 12 hours for at least 7 days

Dosage adjustment
• Hepatic impairment

Contraindications
• Hypersensitivity to drug or other streptogramins

Precautions
Use cautiously in:
• hepatic impairment
• breastfeeding patients
• children younger than age 16 (safety and efficacy not established).

Administration
◀€ Don't mix with other drugs or saline solution.
• For intermittent infusion through a common I.V. line, flush line with dextrose 5% in water (D_5W) before and after giving drug.
• Add 5 ml of sterile water or D_5W to powdered drug in vial, and swirl gently by hand until powder dissolves; don't shake vial. Solution should be clear.
• Within 30 minutes of first dilution, draw up prescribed dosage and dilute further in D_5W to a final concentration of 2 mg/ml or less.
• Know that if patient has a central venous catheter and is fluid-restricted, drug may be given in 100 ml of D_5W.
• Administer by infusion pump over 60 minutes.
• If significant peripheral vein irritation occurs, dilute in 500 to 750 ml of D_5W.
• Be aware that duration of therapy depends on infection site and severity.

Route	Onset	Peak	Duration
I.V.	Unknown	Unknown	Unknown

Adverse reactions
CNS: headache
CV: thrombophlebitis

Reactions in **bold** are life-threatening.　　　　◀€ Clinical alert

GI: nausea, vomiting, diarrhea
Musculoskeletal: joint pain, myalgia
Skin: rash, pruritus
Other: inflammation, pain, or edema at infusion site

Interactions

Drug-drug. *Drugs metabolized by CYP450-3A4 (antiretrovirals; antineoplastics, such as vinca alkaloids, docetaxel, and paclitaxel; astemizole; benzodiazepines; calcium channel blockers; carbamazepine; cisapride; corticosteroids; disopyramide; HMG-CoA reductase inhibitors; immunosuppressants such as cyclosporine and tacrolimus; lidocaine; quinidine; terfenadine):* increased therapeutic and adverse effects of these drugs
Drug-diagnostic tests. *Alanine aminotransferase, aspartate aminotransferase, bilirubin:* increased levels

Patient monitoring

• Monitor closely for infusion site reactions and thrombophlebitis. If these problems occur, consider increasing infusion volume, changing infusion site, or infusing through peripherally inserted central catheter or central venous catheter.
• Assess weight and fluid intake and output to help detect edema.
• Monitor bilirubin level.

Patient teaching

◀ Instruct patient to immediately report pain or redness at infusion site.
• Tell patient to report muscle aches and pains.
• As appropriate, review all other significant and life-threatening adverse reactions and interactions, especially those related to the drugs and tests mentioned above.

rabeprazole sodium

AcipHex, Novo-Rabeprazole✤, Pariet✚, PMS-Rabeprazole✤, Ran-Rabeprazole✤

Pharmacologic class: Proton pump inhibitor
Therapeutic class: Gastric antisecretory agent
Pregnancy risk category B

Action

Reduces gastric acid secretion and increases gastric mucus and bicarbonate production, creating a protective coating on gastric mucosa

Availability

Tablets (delayed-release): 20 mg

Indications and dosages

➤ Erosive or ulcerative gastroesophageal reflux disease (GERD)
Adults: 20 mg P.O. daily for 4 to 8 weeks. If healing doesn't occur within 8 weeks, another 8 weeks of therapy may be considered. Maintenance dosage is 20 mg P.O. daily.
➤ GERD
Adults: 20 mg P.O. daily for 4 weeks. If symptoms don't resolve after 4 weeks, another course of therapy may be considered.
➤ Short-term treatment of symptomatic GERD
Adolescents ages 12 and older: 20 mg P.O. daily for up to 8 weeks
➤ Hypersecretory conditions, including Zollinger-Ellison syndrome
Adults: Initially, 60 mg P.O. daily; adjust dosage as needed up to 100 mg P.O. daily as a single dose or 60 mg

P.O. b.i.d. Maximum daily dosage is 120 mg.

➤ Duodenal ulcer

Adults: 20 mg P.O. daily for up to 4 weeks

➤ *Helicobacter pylori* eradication

Adults: 20 mg P.O. b.i.d. for 7 days (given with amoxicillin and clarithromycin)

Off-label uses

• Dyspepsia
• Benign gastric ulcer

Contraindications

• Hypersensitivity to drug, its components, or benzimidazoles

Precautions

Use cautiously in:

• severe hepatic impairment
• concurrent use of atazanavir (not recommended)
• pregnant patients
• breastfeeding patients (not recommended)
• children (safety not established).

Administration

• Don't crush or split tablets.
• Give without regard to food.

Route	Onset	Peak	Duration
P.O.	Within 1 hr	Unknown	24 hr

Adverse reactions

CNS: headache
Metabolic: hypomagnesemia
Musculoskeletal: fractures of hip, wrist, spine (with long-term daily use)

Interactions

Drug-drug. *Atazanavir:* substantially decreased atazanavir plasma concentration and reduced therapeutic effect
Combined administration of rabeprazole, amoxicillin, and clarithromycin: increased rabeprazole and 14-hydroxy-clarithromycin plasma concentrations

Gastric pH-dependent drugs (such as digoxin, ketoconazole): increased or decreased absorption
Methotrexate: possibly elevated and prolonged methotrexate serum level
Warfarin: increased risk of bleeding
Drug-diagnostic tests. *Magnesium:* decreased level

Patient monitoring

• Stay alert for symptomatic response, but know that a positive response doesn't rule out gastric cancer.
• Monitor magnesium level before starting therapy and periodically thereafter in patients expected to be on prolonged therapy or who take proton pump inhibitors with drugs such as digoxin or drugs that may cause hypomagnesemia (such as diuretics).

Patient teaching

• Tell patient he may take with or without food. Instruct him not to crush, chew, or split tablets.
• Caution female patient not to breastfeed during therapy.
• As appropriate, review all significant adverse reactions and interactions, especially those related to the drugs mentioned above.

raloxifene
Evista

Pharmacologic class: Nonsteroidal benzothiophene derivative

Therapeutic class: Selective estrogen receptor modulator, bone resorption inhibitor

Pregnancy risk category X

FDA | BOXED WARNING

• An increased risk of deep vein thrombosis and pulmonary embolism is

---

Reactions in **bold** are life-threatening.   ◀€ Clinical alert

associated with raloxifene. Women with history of or active venous thromboembolism shouldn't take this drug.
• A trial in postmenopausal women with documented coronary heart disease or at increased risk for major coronary events found increased risk of death due to stroke. Consider risk-benefit ratio in women at risk for stroke.

Action
Binds to estrogen receptors, activating estrogen pathways and increasing bone mineral density. These effects decrease bone resorption and turnover.

Availability
Tablets: 60 mg

🚫 Indications and dosages
➤ Treatment and prevention of osteoporosis in postmenopausal women; reduction of invasive breast cancer risk in postmenopausal women with osteoporosis; reduction of invasive breast cancer risk in postmenopausal women at high risk for invasive breast cancer
Adults: 60 mg P.O. daily

Off-label uses
• Prophylaxis of cardiovascular disease

Contraindications
• Hypersensitivity to drug or its components
• History of thromboembolic events
• Premenopausal women
• Females of childbearing age
• Pregnancy or breastfeeding
• Children

Precautions
Use cautiously in:
• altered lipid metabolism, hepatic dysfunction
• concurrent estrogen therapy (use not recommended)

• immobilized patients and others at increased risk for thromboembolic events.

Administration
• Give with or without food.

Route	Onset	Peak	Duration
P.O.	Unknown	6 hr	Unknown

Adverse reactions
CNS: depression, insomnia, vertigo, syncope, hypoesthesia, migraine, neuralgia
CV: chest pain, peripheral edema, varicose veins, **deep-vein thrombosis, thrombophlebitis**
EENT: conjunctivitis, sinusitis, rhinitis, pharyngitis, laryngitis
GI: nausea, vomiting, diarrhea, abdominal pain dyspepsia, flatulence, gastroenteritis
GU: urinary tract infection or disorder, cystitis, vaginitis, leukorrhea, endometrial disorder, **vaginal hemorrhage**
Musculoskeletal: leg cramps, joint pain, myalgia, arthritis, tendon disorder
Respiratory: cough, pneumonia, bronchitis, **pulmonary embolism**
Skin: rash, diaphoresis
Other: weight gain, hot flashes, infection, pain, flulike symptoms

Interactions
Drug-drug. *Cholestyramine:* reduced raloxifene absorption
Highly protein-bound drugs (such as diazepam, diazoxide, lidocaine): interference with binding of these drugs
Warfarin: decreased prothrombin time
Drug-diagnostic tests. *Albumin, apolipoprotein B, calcium, fibrinogen, inorganic phosphate, low-density lipoproteins, platelets, protein, total cholesterol:* decreased levels
Apolipoprotein A1; corticosteroid-binding, sex steroid–binding, and thyroid-binding globulin: increased levels

Patient monitoring

◀€ Watch for thromboembolic events, especially during first 4 months of therapy.

• Stay alert for other adverse effects, particularly leg cramps, other musculoskeletal complaints, and respiratory disorders.

• Assess bone mineral density test results.

• Monitor for unexplained vaginal bleeding.

Patient teaching

• Tell patient she may take with or without food.

• Instruct patient to read package insert before starting drug and then periodically.

◀€ Teach patient to recognize and immediately report symptoms of blood clots.

• Instruct patient to stop taking drug 3 days before anticipated period of prolonged immobility, and to restart it only after she regains normal mobility.

• Tell patient that drug may cause hot flashes, but that these are normal effects.

• Advise patient to report unexplained vaginal bleeding or leg cramps.

• As appropriate, review all other significant and life-threatening adverse reactions and interactions, especially those related to the drugs and tests mentioned above.

raltegravir

Isentress

Pharmacologic class: Human immunodeficiency virus (HIV) integrase-strand transfer inhibitor

Therapeutic class: Antiretroviral

Pregnancy risk category C

Action

Rapidly blocks HIV integrase (enzyme needed for HIV replication), leading to viral load reduction and increased CD4+ count

Availability

Tablets (chewable): 25 mg, 100 mg
Tablets (film-coated): 400 mg

⊘ Indications and dosages

➤ HIV-1 infection in adults used in combination with other antiretrovirals

Adults and adolescents ages 12 and older: 400 mg film-coated tablet P.O. b.i.d.

Children age 6 to younger than age 12 weighing at least 25 kg (55 lb): One 400-mg film-coated tablet P.O. b.i.d. or chewable tablets, weight based to maximum of 300 mg P.O. b.i.d.

Children age 6 to younger than age 12 weighing less than 25 kg (55 lb): Chewable tablets, weight based to maximum of 300 mg P.O. b.i.d.

Children age 2 to younger than age 6 weighing at least 10 kg (22 lb): Chewable tablets, weight based to maximum of 300 mg P.O. b.i.d.

Contraindications

None

Precautions

Use cautiously in:

• treatment-naive adults (safety and efficacy not established)

• increased risk of myopathy or rhabdomyolysis (such as with concomitant use of drugs known to cause these conditions)

• elderly patients

• pregnant patients

• breastfeeding patients (use not recommended)

• children younger than age 2 (safety and efficacy not established).

r

Administration
- Administer with or without food.
- Be aware that film-coated tablets can't be substituted with chewable tablets.

Route	Onset	Peak	Duration
P.O.	Unknown	Unknown	Unknown

Adverse reactions
CNS: headache, fatigue, asthenia, dizziness, insomnia
CV: myocardial infarction
GI: nausea, vomiting, diarrhea, abdominal pain, gastritis
GU: toxic nephropathy, renal failure, renal tubular necrosis
Hematologic: anemia, **neutropenia**
Hepatic: hepatitis
Musculoskeletal: myopathy, **rhabdomyolysis**
Skin: lipodystrophy, **Stevens-Johnson syndrome, toxic epidermal necrolysis**
Other: fever, herpes simplex, immune reconstitution syndrome, hypersensitivity reaction

Interactions
Drug-drug. *Strong UGT1A1 inducers (such as rifampin):* reduced raltegravir blood level
UGT1A1 inhibitors (such as atazanavir): increased raltegravir blood level
Drug-diagnostic tests. *Absolute neutrophil count, hemoglobin, platelets:* decreased levels
ALP, ALT, AST, blood glucose, creatine kinase, lipase, pancreatic enzymes, total bilirubin: increased levels

Patient monitoring
- Monitor renal function tests.
- Be aware that immune reconstitution syndrome has occurred in patients receiving drug with combination antiretroviral therapy. During initial phase of therapy, patient whose immune system responds may develop inflammatory response to indolent or residual opportunistic infections (such as *Mycobacterium avium* complex, cytomegalovirus, *Pneumocystis jiroveci* pneumonia, or tuberculosis), which may necessitate further evaluation and treatment.
- Be aware that severe, potentially life-threatening and fatal skin reactions have been reported, including Stevens-Johnson syndrome, hypersensitivity reaction, and toxic epidermal necrolysis. Immediately discontinue drug if severe hypersensitivity, severe rash, or rash with systemic symptoms or liver aminotransferase elevations develops. Closely monitor clinical status, including liver aminotransferases.

Patient teaching
- Tell patient drug may be taken with or without food.
- Inform patient with phenylketonuria that chewable tablets contain phenylalanine.
- Inform patient that drug doesn't cure HIV infection or reduce risk of passing it to others through sexual contact, needle sharing, or blood exposure.
- 🔊 Advise patient to immediately report muscle weakness, urinary problems, new infections, rash, fever, general malaise, swelling of face or throat, or chest pain.
- Instruct female patient to notify prescriber if she is pregnant or intends to become pregnant.
- Caution breastfeeding patient to discontinue breastfeeding while taking drug, because of potential HIV transmission and adverse reactions in infants.
- As appropriate, review all other significant and life-threatening adverse reactions and interactions, especially those related to the drugs and tests mentioned above.

🍁 Canada   ⊕ UK   ☣ Hazardous drug   ⊗ High-alert drug

ramelteon
Rozerem

Pharmacologic class: Melatonin receptor agonist
Therapeutic class: Hypnotic
Pregnancy risk category C

Action
Promotes sleep through activity at melatonin MT_1 and MT_2 receptors, which are thought to be involved in maintaining circadian rhythm underlying normal sleep-wake cycle

Availability
Tablets: 8 mg

Indications and dosages
➤ Insomnia marked by difficulty with sleep onset
Adults: 8 mg P.O. within 30 minutes of going to bed

Contraindications
• Hypersensitivity to drug or its components

Precautions
Use cautiously in:
• sleep apnea, chronic obstructive pulmonary disease, hepatic impairment
• concurrent use of fluvoxamine
• pregnant or breastfeeding patients
• children (safety and efficacy not established).

Administration
• Give within 30 minutes of patient's bedtime.
• Don't give with or immediately after a high-fat meal.

Route	Onset	Peak	Duration
P.O.	Unknown	0.5-1.5 hr	Unknown

Adverse reactions
CNS: headache, somnolence, fatigue, dizziness, exacerbated insomnia, depression
GI: nausea, diarrhea
Musculoskeletal: myalgia, arthralgia
Respiratory: upper respiratory tract infection
Other: altered taste, influenza

Interactions
Drug-drug. *Fluconazole, fluvoxamine, ketoconazole:* increased ramelteon blood level
Rifampin: decreased ramelteon efficacy
Drug-diagnostic tests. *Blood cortisol:* decreased
Drug-food. *High-fat meals:* altered ramelteon absorption
Drug-herbs. *American elder, bishop's weed, cat's claw, devil's claw, eucalyptus, feverfew, ginkgo, kava, licorice, pomegranate:* increased ramelteon blood level
Valerian: additive sedation, increased ramelteon blood level
Drug-behaviors. *Alcohol use:* additive psychomotor impairment

Patient monitoring
• Monitor prolactin and testosterone levels, if ordered, in patient who develops unexplained amenorrhea, galactorrhea, decreased libido, or fertility problems.
• Evaluate patient for physical and psychiatric disorders before and during therapy. Worsening of insomnia or onset of new behavioral or cognitive symptoms could signal underlying psychiatric disorder.

Patient teaching
• Instruct patient to take drug within 30 minutes of going to bed.
• Advise patient not to take drug with or immediately after a high-fat meal.
• Caution patient to avoid driving and other hazardous activities until drug effects are known.

r

- Advise patient to contact prescriber if insomnia worsens.
- Instruct patient to report menses cessation, excessive or spontaneous lactation, decreased libido, or fertility problems.
- As appropriate, review all other significant adverse reactions and interactions, especially those related to the drugs, tests, food, herbs, and behaviors mentioned above.

ramipril
Altace, Apo-Ramipril✿, Co Ramipril✿, Lopace✿, Novo-Ramipril*, Ratio-Ramipril✿, Sandoz Ramipril✿, Tritace⊕

Pharmacologic class: Angiotensin-converting enzyme (ACE) inhibitor
Therapeutic class: Antihypertensive
Pregnancy risk category D

FDA | BOXED WARNING

- Drugs that act directly on the renin-angiotensin system can cause injury to or death of a developing fetus. Discontinue drug as soon as possible when pregnancy is detected.

Action
Inhibits conversion of angiotensin I to angiotensin II, a potent vasoconstrictor. Increases plasma renin levels and reduces aldosterone levels, causing systemic vasodilation and decreased cardiac output.

Availability
Capsules: 1.25 mg, 2.5 mg, 5 mg, 10 mg

⬮ Indications and dosages
➤ Hypertension

Adults: Initially, 2.5 mg P.O. daily in patients not receiving diuretics; may increase dosage slowly p.r.n. according to response. For maintenance, 2.5 to 20 mg/day P.O. as a single dose or in two equally divided doses. If ramipril alone doesn't control blood pressure, a diuretic may be added.
➤ To reduce the risk of myocardial infarction (MI), cerebrovascular accident, or death from cardiovascular causes
Adults: Initially, 2.5 mg P.O. daily for 1 week, followed by 5 mg P.O. daily for the next 3 weeks, then increased as tolerated to a maintenance dosage of 10 mg P.O. daily. In hypertensive patients and those who've had a recent MI, may divide maintenance dose.
➤ Heart failure after MI
Adults: Initially, 2.5 mg P.O. b.i.d.; may decrease to 1.25 mg b.i.d. if higher dosage causes hypotension. Titrate toward target dosage of 5 mg b.i.d. at 3-week intervals.

Dosage adjustment
- Renal impairment
- Concurrent diuretic use

Off-label uses
- Angina associated with syndrome X
- Atherosclerosis
- Mitral insufficiency
- Renovascular hypertension
- Diabetic or nondiabetic nephropathy
- Erythrocytosis

Contraindications
- Hypersensitivity to drug or other ACE inhibitors
- Angioedema with previous ACE inhibitor use or history of hereditary or idiopathic angioedema

Precautions
Use cautiously in:
- autoimmune diseases, aortic stenosis, hypertrophic cardiomyopathy, cerebrovascular or cardiac insufficiency, collagen vascular disease,

febrile illness, hepatic or renal impairment, hypotension, neutropenia, chronic cough, proteinuria, renal artery stenosis

• risk factors for development of hyperkalemia (including renal insufficiency, diabetes mellitus, concurrent use of potassium-sparing diuretics, potassium supplements, or potassium-containing salt substitutes)
• family history of angioedema
• concurrent immunosuppressant or diuretic therapy
• black patients
• elderly patients
• pregnant patients
• breastfeeding patients (avoid use)
• children (safety not established).

Administration
• If possible, discontinue diuretics 2 to 3 days before ramipril therapy begins to prevent severe hypotension.
• If patient can't swallow capsule, open it and mix contents in water or apple juice or sprinkle in small amount of applesauce.
• Know that drug may be used alone or with other antihypertensives.

Route	Onset	Peak	Duration
P.O.	1-2 hr	2-4 hr	24 hr

Adverse reactions
CNS: dizziness, light-headedness, fatigue, headache, vertigo, asthenia
CV: hypotension, orthostatic hypotension, angina pectoris, tachycardia, **MI, heart failure**
EENT: blurred vision, sinusitis
GI: nausea, vomiting, diarrhea
Hematologic: purpura, **agranulocytosis**
Metabolic: hyperkalemia
Musculoskeletal: muscle cramps
Respiratory: cough, asthma, upper respiratory tract infection, **bronchospasm**
Skin: rash, pruritus, urticaria, photosensitivity, **angioedema, anaphylactoid reactions**
Other: fever

Interactions
Drug-drug. *Diuretics, other antihypertensives:* increased hypotension
Gold (sodium aurothiomalate): increased risk of rare nitritoid reactions (including facial flushing, nausea, vomiting, and hypotension)
Lithium: increased lithium blood level and risk of toxicity
Nonsteroidal anti-inflammatory drugs: may result in deterioration of renal function, including acute renal failure and attenuated ACE inhibitor antihypertensive effect
Potassium-sparing diuretics, potassium supplements: increased risk of hyperkalemia
Drug-diagnostic tests. *Alanine aminotransferase, alkaline phosphatase, aspartate aminotransferase, bilirubin, blood urea nitrogen, creatinine, potassium:* increased levels
Drug-food. *Any food:* decreased rate (but not extent) of drug absorption
Salt substitutes containing potassium: increased risk of hyperkalemia

Patient monitoring
• Assess vital signs and cardiovascular status. Ask patient if he's experiencing angina.
• Monitor CBC and liver function tests.
• Closely monitor potassium level. Watch for signs and symptoms of hyperkalemia.
◀€ Stay alert for signs and symptoms of hypersensitivity reactions (including angioedema), especially in black patients after first dose
• Evaluate for dry, nonproductive cough.

Patient teaching
• Tell patient he may take with or without food.
◀€ Instruct patient to immediately report swelling of tongue or face or difficulty breathing.
• Teach patient how to monitor and record blood pressure.

r

Reactions in **bold** are life-threatening.   ◀€ Clinical alert

- Tell patient drug may cause dry, non-productive cough. Instruct him to report this problem if it becomes bothersome.
- Caution patient to avoid driving and other hazardous activities until he knows how drug affects concentration and alertness.
- Advise patient to move slowly when sitting up or standing, to avoid dizziness from sudden blood pressure decrease.
- Inform patient that excessive fluid loss (as from sweating, vomiting, or diarrhea) and inadequate fluid intake increase risk of light-headedness (especially in hot weather).
- Tell patient to avoid salt substitutes containing potassium.
- Advise female patient to tell prescriber if she is pregnant. Caution her not to take drug during third trimester or when breastfeeding.
- As appropriate, review all other significant and life-threatening adverse reactions and interactions, especially those related to the drugs, tests, foods, herbs, and behaviors mentioned above.

ranitidine hydrochloride
Acid Reducer✲, Apo-Ranitidine✲, Co Ranitidine✲, Gavilast⊕, Histac⊕, Raciran⊕, Ranitil⊕, Rantek⊕, Zantac, Zantac 75, Zantac EFFERdose

Pharmacologic class: Histamine$_2$-receptor antagonist
Therapeutic class: Antiulcer drug
Pregnancy risk category B

Action
Reduces gastric acid secretion and increases gastric mucus and bicarbonate production, creating a protective coating on gastric mucosa

Availability
Capsules (liquid-filled): 150 mg, 300 mg
Solution for injection: 25 mg/ml in 2-, 6-, and 40-ml vials
Solution for injection (pre-mixed): 50 mg/50 ml in 0.45% sodium chloride
Syrup: 15 mg/ml
Tablets: 150 mg, 300 mg
Tablets (effervescent): 150 mg

🕭 Indications and dosages
➤ Active duodenal ulcer
Adults: 150 mg or 10 ml P.O. b.i.d., or 300 mg or 20 ml P.O. daily, or 50 mg I.V. or I.M. q 6 to 8 hours
➤ To maintain healing of duodenal ulcers
Adults: 150 mg or 10 ml P.O.
➤ Benign gastric ulcer
Adults: 150 mg or 10 ml P.O. b.i.d. For maintenance, 150 mg or 10 ml P.O. or 50 mg I.V. or I.M. q 6 to 8 hours.
➤ Active duodenal and gastric ulcers
Children ages 1 month to 16 years: 2 to 4 mg/kg/day P.O., up to a maximum of 300 mg/day
➤ To maintain healing of duodenal and gastric ulcers
Children ages 1 month to 16 years: 2 to 4 mg/kg/day P.O., up to a maximum of 150 mg/day
➤ Erosive esophagitis
Adults: 150 mg or 10 ml P.O. q.i.d.
Children ages 1 month to 16 years: 5 to 10 mg/kg P.O. daily in two divided doses
➤ Gastroesophageal reflux disease
Adults: 150 mg or 10 ml P.O. b.i.d.
Children ages 1 month to 16 years: 5 to 10 mg/kg P.O. daily in two divided doses
➤ Pathologic hypersecretory conditions, including Zollinger-Ellison syndrome
Adults: 150 mg or 10 ml P.O. b.i.d., adjusted according to patient's needs. In severe cases, up to 6 g/day may be

needed. Continue therapy as long as indicated.

➤ Hospitalized patients with pathologic hypersecretory conditions, including Zollinger-Ellison syndrome; intractable duodenal ulcers; patients who can't receive oral drugs

Adults: 50 mg I.M. q 6 to 8 hours, or 50 mg intermittent I.V. bolus q 6 to 8 hours, or 50 mg intermittent I.V. infusion q 6 to 8 hours.

Children ages 1 month to 16 years: 2 to 4 mg/kg/day I.V. in divided doses q 6 to 8 hours, up to a maximum of 50 mg q 6 to 8 hours

Dosage adjustment

- Renal or hepatic impairment
- Debilitated patients

Off-label uses

- Asthma
- GI hemorrhage
- *Helicobacter pylori* infection
- Short-bowel syndrome
- Immunosuppression reversal
- Psoriasis
- Aspiration pneumonitis prophylaxis

Contraindications

- Hypersensitivity to drug or its components
- Alcohol intolerance (with some oral products)
- History of acute porphyria

Precautions

Use cautiously in:
- renal or hepatic impairment, heart rhythm disturbances, phenylketonuria (effervescent tablets)
- elderly patients
- pregnant or breastfeeding patients.

Administration

- For intermittent I.V. bolus injection, dilute in normal saline solution or other compatible solution to a concentration not exceeding 2.5 mg/ml.

Inject no faster than 4 ml/minute (5 minutes).

- For continuous I.V. infusion in patients with Zollinger-Ellison syndrome, add to dextrose 5% in water (D_5W) or other compatible solution; dilute to a concentration not exceeding 2.5 mg/ml, and start infusion at 1 mg/kg/hour. After 4 hours, if measured gastric acid output exceeds 10 mEq/hour or symptoms occur, increase dosage in increments of 0.5 mg/kg/hour, and remeasure acid output.
- Give P.O. doses with or without food. Give once-daily dose at bedtime.
- For intermittent I.V. infusion, dilute in D_5W or other compatible solution to a concentration not exceeding 0.5 mg/ml. Infuse no faster than 7 ml/minute (15 to 20 minutes).
- Be aware that premixed Zantac solution of 50 mg in half-normal saline solution (50 ml) doesn't require dilution. Infuse over 15 to 20 minutes.
- Know that I.V. form may be added to total parenteral nutrition solutions.
- Inject I.M. undiluted deep into large muscle.

Route	Onset	Peak	Duration
P.O.	Unknown	1-3 hr	8-12 hr
I.V., I.M.	Unknown	15 min	8-12 hr

Adverse reactions

CNS: headache, agitation, anxiety
GI: nausea, vomiting, diarrhea, constipation, abdominal discomfort or pain
Hematologic: reversible **granulocytopenia** and **thrombocytopenia**
Hepatic: hepatitis
Skin: rash
Other: pain at I.M. injection site, burning or itching at I.V. site, hypersensitivity reaction

Interactions

Drug-drug. *Antacids:* decreased ranitidine absorption

r

Reactions in **bold** are life-threatening.   ◀€ Clinical alert

Propantheline: delayed ranitidine absorption and increased peak blood level

Drug-diagnostic tests. *Creatinine:* slight elevation

Hepatic enzymes: increased levels

Urine protein tests using Multistix: false-negative results

Drug-herbs. *Yerba maté:* decreased drug clearance

Drug-behaviors. *Smoking:* decreased ranitidine effects

Patient monitoring

• Assess vital signs.
• Monitor CBC and liver function tests.

Patient teaching

• Tell patient he may take oral drug with or without food. Advise him to take once-daily prescription drug at bedtime.
• Instruct patient to dissolve EFFER-dose in 6 to 8 oz of water before taking.
• Caution patient to avoid driving and other hazardous activities until he knows how drug affects concentration and alertness.
• Tell patient smoking may decrease drug effects.
• As appropriate, review all other significant and life-threatening adverse reactions and interactions, especially those related to the drugs, tests, herbs, and behaviors mentioned above.

ranolazine
Ranexa

Pharmacologic class: Piperazine derivative

Therapeutic class: Antianginal

Pregnancy risk category C

Action

Unclear. Appears to modulate myocardial metabolism by partially inhibiting fatty acid oxidation, thereby increasing glucose oxidation and generating more adenosine triphosphate.

Availability

Tablets (extended-release): 500 mg, 1,000 mg

⑪ Indications and dosages

➤ Chronic angina

Adults: Initially, 500 mg P.O. twice daily, increased to maximum recommended dosage of 1,000 mg P.O. twice daily if needed

Dosage adjustment

• Concurrent use of moderate CYP3A inhibitors, such as diltiazem, verapamil, and erythromycin
• Concurrent use of P-gp inhibitors such as cyclosporine

Contraindications

• Liver cirrhosis
• Concurrent use of strong CYP3A inhibitors (such as ketoconazole, clarithromycin, nelfinavir)
• Concurrent use of CYP3A inducers (such as rifampin, phenobarbital, St. John's wort)

Precautions

Use cautiously in:
• concurrent digoxin therapy, QT-interval prolongation, drugs that prolong QT interval, moderate CYP3A inhibitors (including diltiazem, verapamil, aprepitant, erythromycin, fluconazole, grapefruit juice, or grapefruit-containing products)
• patients age 75 and older
• pregnant or breastfeeding patients
• children (safety and efficacy not established).

Administration

• Administer without regard to meals.
• Don't give with grapefruit juice.

Route	Onset	Peak	Duration
P.O.	Unknown	2-5 hr	Unknown

Adverse reactions
CNS: dizziness, headache, vertigo
CV: palpitations
EENT: tinnitus, dry mouth
GI: nausea, vomiting, constipation, abdominal pain
Respiratory: dyspnea
Other: peripheral edema

Interactions
Drug-drug. *CYP3A inducers such as carbamazepine, phenobarbital, phenytoin, rifabutin, rifampin, rifapentin:* decreased ranolazine plasma concentration
CYP3A inhibitors such as diltiazem, ketoconazole, macrolide antibiotics, paroxetine, protease inhibitors, verapamil: increased ranolazine blood level
Digoxin, simvastatin: increased blood levels of these drugs
P-gp inhibitors (such as cyclosporine): increased ranolazine exposure
Drug-food. *Grapefruit juice and grapefruit-containing products:* increased ranolazine blood level

Patient monitoring
• Obtain baseline and follow-up ECGs to evaluate drug effects on QT interval.
• Monitor blood pressure regularly in patients with severe renal impairment.

Patient teaching
• Inform patient that drug can be taken with or without food, but not with grapefruit juice or grapefruit-containing products.
• Advise patient not to chew or crush tablets.
• Instruct patient to consult prescriber before taking other prescription or over-the-counter drugs or herbal products.
• Inform patient that drug isn't intended for acute angina episodes.
• Caution patient to avoiding driving and other hazardous activities until drug effects are known.

• Advise female with childbearing potential to tell prescriber if she is pregnant or plans to become pregnant.
• Advise female not to breastfeed during therapy.
• As appropriate, review all other significant adverse reactions and interactions, especially those related to the drugs and foods mentioned above.

rasagiline
Azilect

Pharmacologic class: MAO inhibitor (type B)
Therapeutic class: Antiparkinsonian agent, antidyskinetic
Pregnancy risk category C

Action
Unknown. Thought to increase dopaminergic activity by irreversibly inhibiting MAO type B in nerve cells, increasing dopamine availability to brain cells

Availability
Tablets: 0.5 mg, 1 mg

Ⓘ Indications and dosages
➤ Initial monotherapy for idiopathic Parkinson's disease
Adults: 1 mg P.O. daily
➤ Adjunctive treatment of idiopathic Parkinson's disease in patients receiving levodopa
Adults: 0.5 mg P.O. once daily. If patient doesn't achieve sufficient clinical response, dosage may be increased to 1 mg P.O. once daily.

Dosage adjustment
• Mild hepatic impairment
• Concurrent use of ciprofloxacin and other CYP1A2 inhibitors

r

Contraindications
- Within 14 days of other MAO inhibitors or meperidine
- Concurrent use with cyclobenzaprine, dextromethorphan, methadone, propoxyphene, tramadol, and St. John's wort

Precautions
Use cautiously in:
- mild hepatic impairment (use not recommended in moderate or severe hepatic impairment), melanoma
- concurrent use of levodopa, antidepressants, or CYP1A2 inhibitors (such as ciprofloxacin)
- pregnant or breastfeeding patients
- children (safety and efficacy not established).

Administration
- Give with or without food.
- 🔇 Don't give tyramine-rich foods, beverages, dietary supplements, or over-the-counter (OTC) cough or cold medications during therapy because of possible hypertensive crisis.
- 🔇 Don't give within 14 days of other MAO inhibitors, meperidine, cyclobenzaprine, dextromethorphan, methadone, propoxyphene, tramadol, or St. John's wort.

Route	Onset	Peak	Duration
P.O.	Unknown	1 hr	Unknown

Adverse reactions
CNS: headache, vertigo, dizziness, agitation, anxiety, somnolence, amnesia, confusion, dystonia, hypertonia, abnormal gait, ataxia, dyskinesia, hyperkinesia, paresthesia, neuropathy, tremor, depression, malaise, abnormal dreams, asthenia, myasthenia, hallucinations, **stroke**
CV: orthostatic hypotension, syncope, angina, **bundle-branch block**
EENT: conjunctivitis, epistaxis, rhinitis
GI: abdominal pain, dyspepsia, indigestion, nausea, vomiting, diarrhea, constipation, dysphagia, gastroenteritis, dry mouth, gingivitis, anorexia, **GI hemorrhage**
GU: hematuria, urinary incontinence, erectile dysfunction, decreased libido
Hematologic: leukopenia, anemia, **hemorrhage**
Musculoskeletal: arthralgia, arthritis, neck pain, tenosynovitis, bursitis, leg cramps
Respiratory: asthma, dyspnea, increased cough
Skin: alopecia, skin cancer, rash, sweating, pruritus, skin ulcer, ecchymosis, photosensitivity reaction
Other: falls, accidental injury, flulike syndrome, chest pain, fever, infection, hernia, weight loss, allergic reaction

Interactions
Drug-drug. *Antidepressants (selective serotonin reuptake inhibitors, tricyclic and tetracyclic antidepressants):* severe CNS toxicity, high fever, possible death
Carbidopa-levodopa, levodopa: increased incidence of dyskinesia, hallucinations, and orthostatic hypotension
CYP1A2 inhibitors (including ciprofloxacin): increased rasagiline blood level and possible increased adverse reactions
Dextromethorphan: bizarre behavior
Meperidine, methadone, propoxyphene, tramadol: increased risk of serious and possibly fatal reactions
Other MAO inhibitors, vitamin supplements containing tyramine: increased risk of hypertensive crisis
Sympathomimetics (including amphetamines, cold remedies, nasal decongestants, and weight-loss preparations containing vasoconstrictors): severe hypertensive reactions
Drug-diagnostic tests. *Albumin:* increased value
Drug-food. *Tyramine-containing foods (aged, dried, fermented meats; pickled fish; improperly stored meats and fish; broad bean pods; aged cheeses;*

unpasteurized beers; red wines; concentrated yeast extracts; sauerkraut; soybean products): increased risk of hypertensive crisis

Drug-herbs. *St. John's wort:* bizarre behavior

Drug-behaviors. *Alcohol use:* hypertensive crisis

Patient monitoring

◀€ Stay alert for hypertensive crisis in patients using concurrent drugs that may cause this serious interaction.

• Be alert for dopaminergic adverse effects and exacerbation of preexisting dyskinesias when rasagiline is used as adjunct to levodopa. Levodopa dosage may need to be reduced.

• Monitor for orthostatic hypotension during first 2 months of therapy, especially when drug is used as adjunct to levodopa.

• Inspect patient frequently for signs of melanoma.

• In patient with hepatic insufficiency, obtain periodic liver function tests.

Patient teaching

• Tell patient he may take drug with or without food.

◀€ Stress importance of avoiding alcohol and certain foods, beverages, prescription drugs, and OTC preparations during therapy and for 14 days afterward. Ask pharmacist to give patient complete list of foods, beverages, and medications to avoid.

• Instruct patient to avoid using herbs during therapy unless prescriber approves.

◀€ Instruct patient or caregiver to immediately report occipital headache, confusion, palpitations, stiff neck, unexplained nausea or vomiting, sweating, dilated pupils, and visual disturbances (indications of hypertensive crisis).

◀€ Instruct patient to immediately report skin changes.

• Tell patient drug may cause blood pressure to drop if he stands or sits up suddenly. Advise him to rise slowly and carefully.

• Instruct patient to report hallucinations promptly.

• Caution patient to avoid hazardous activities until he knows how drug affects concentration and alertness.

• As appropriate, review all other significant and life-threatening adverse reactions and interactions, especially those related to the drugs, tests, foods, herbs, and behaviors mentioned above.

---

rasburicase
Elitek, Fasturtek

Pharmacologic class: Recombinant urate oxidase enzyme

Therapeutic class: Antimetabolite

Pregnancy risk category C

FDA **BOXED WARNING**

• Drug may cause severe hypersensitivity reactions (including anaphylaxis), severe hemolysis in patients with G6PD deficiency, and methemoglobinemia. Withdraw immediately and permanently if patient shows evidence of these problems. Before starting therapy, screen patients at higher risk for G6PD deficiency (those of African or Mediterranean ancestry).

• Drug causes spuriously low uric acid levels.

Action
Catalyzes oxidation of uric acid into an inactive soluble metabolite

Availability
Powder for injection: 1.5 mg/vial

⊘ Indications and dosages

➤ Chemotherapy-induced hyper-uricemia in patients with leukemia, lymphoma, or solid-tumor cancers
Adults and children: 0.2 mg/kg by I.V. infusion over 30 minutes as a single daily dose for 5 days. Chemotherapy should begin 4 to 24 hours after first dose.

Contraindications

• Hypersensitivity to drug or its components
• History of anaphylaxis, hemolytic anemia, or methemoglobinemia as a reaction to rasburicase
• G6PD deficiency

Precautions

Use cautiously in:
• pregnant or breastfeeding patients
• children younger than age 2.

Administration

• Know that patients at high risk for G6PD deficiency (those of African or Mediterranean descent) should be screened for this disorder before therapy starts.
• Give 4 to 24 hours before first chemotherapy dose, as ordered.
• Dilute by adding 1-ml vial of diluent provided. Swirl gently; don't shake. Dilute further by injecting diluted dose into infusion bag containing appropriate volume of normal saline solution, to achieve final volume of 50 ml.
• Administer daily by I.V. infusion over 30 minutes.
◀€ Don't give as I.V. bolus.
• Don't use I.V. filters.
• Don't mix with other drugs. Use a separate I.V. line, or flush line with 15 ml of normal saline solution before and after infusing rasburicase.
• Know that more than one course of treatment isn't recommended.

Route	Onset	Peak	Duration
I.V.	4 hr	96 hr	Unknown

Adverse reactions

CNS: headache
GI: nausea, vomiting, diarrhea, constipation, abdominal pain
Hematologic: neutropenia, methemoglobinemia, severe hemolysis (in patients with G6PD deficiency)
Respiratory: respiratory distress
Skin: rash
Other: fever, mucositis, hypersensitivity reactions including **anaphylaxis, sepsis**

Interactions

Drug-diagnostic tests. *Neutrophils:* decreased count
Uric acid: interference with measurement (if blood is at room temperature)

Patient monitoring

• Monitor for signs and symptoms of hypersensitivity reaction.
• Assess for respiratory distress and signs and symptoms of infection.
• Monitor CBC and uric acid level frequently.
◀€ Watch closely for signs and symptoms of hemolysis, especially in patients of African or Mediterranean descent.

Patient teaching

◀€ Teach parents and patient (as appropriate) to recognize and immediately report adverse effects, including hypersensitivity reaction.
◀€ Tell patient or parents (as appropriate) drug may cause sepsis. Instruct patient or parents to monitor temperature and immediately report fever and other signs and symptoms of infection.
• As appropriate, review all other significant and life-threatening adverse reactions and interactions, especially those related to the tests mentioned above.

---

repaglinide
Gluconorm, NovoNorm⊕, Prandin

Pharmacologic class: Meglitinide
Therapeutic class: Hypoglycemic
Pregnancy risk category C

Action
Inhibits alpha-glucosidases, enzymes that convert oligosaccharides and disaccharides to glucose. This inhibition lowers blood glucose level, especially in postprandial hyperglycemia.

Availability
Tablets: 0.5 mg, 1 mg, 2 mg

Indications and dosages
➤ Adjunct to diet and exercise in type 2 (non-insulin-dependent) diabetes mellitus uncontrolled by diet and exercise alone, or combined with metformin in type 2 diabetes mellitus uncontrolled by diet, exercise, and either repaglinide or metformin alone
Adults: 0.5 to 4 mg P.O. before each meal; may adjust at 1-week intervals based on blood glucose response. Maximum daily dosage is 16 mg.

Contraindications
• Hypersensitivity to drug or its components
• Diabetic ketoacidosis
• Type 1 (insulin-dependent) diabetes mellitus
• Administration with gemfibrozil

Precautions
Use cautiously in:
• renal or hepatic impairment; adrenal or pituitary insufficiency; stress caused by infection, fever, trauma, or surgery

• concurrent use of CYP2C8 inhibitors (such as trimethoprim, gemfibrozil, montelukast)
• concurrent use of CYP3A4 inhibitors (such as ketoconazole, itraconazole, erythromycin)
• concurrent use of CYP3A4 or CYP2C8 inducers (such as rifampin, barbiturates, carbamazepine)
• elderly or malnourished patients
• pregnant or breastfeeding patients
• children.

Administration
• Give 15 to 30 minutes before meals. Administer two, three, or four times daily, if needed, to adapt to patient's meal pattern.

Route	Onset	Peak	Duration
P.O.	Within 30 min	60-90 min	<4 hr

Adverse reactions
CNS: headache, paresthesia
CV: angina, chest pain
EENT: sinusitis, rhinitis
GI: nausea, vomiting, diarrhea, constipation, dyspepsia
GU: urinary tract infection
Metabolic: hyperglycemia, **hypoglycemia**
Musculoskeletal: joint pain, back pain
Respiratory: upper respiratory infection, bronchitis
Other: tooth disorder, hypersensitivity reaction

Interactions
Drug-drug. *Barbiturates, carbamazepine, rifampin:* decreased repaglinide blood level
Beta-adrenergic blockers, chloramphenicol, MAO inhibitors, nonsteroidal antiinflammatory drugs, probenecid, sulfonamides, warfarin: potentiation of repaglinide effects
Calcium channel blockers, corticosteroids, estrogens, hormonal contraceptives, isoniazid, phenothiazines, phenytoin, nicotinic acid, sympathomimetics,

r

---

thyroid preparations: loss of glycemic control
Clarithromycin: increased repaglinide area under the curve and C_{max}
Cyclosporine: increased repaglinide plasma concentration
Erythromycin, ketoconazole, miconazole: decreased repaglinide metabolism, increased risk of hypoglycemia
Gemfibrozil, itraconazole: significantly increased repaglinide exposure
Simvastatin: increased repaglinide level
Drug-food. *Any food:* decreased drug bioavailability
Drug-herbs. *Aloe gel (oral), bitter melon, chromium, coenzyme Q10, fenugreek, gymnema sylvestre, psyllium, St. John's wort:* additive hypoglycemic effects
Glucosamine: poor glycemic control

Patient monitoring

• Monitor blood glucose and glycosylated hemoglobin levels.
• Monitor patient's meal pattern. Consult prescriber about adjusting dosage if patient adds or misses a meal.
• Assess for angina, shortness of breath, or other discomforts.
• Watch for signs and symptoms of bronchitis and upper respiratory, urinary, and EENT infections.

Patient teaching

• Tell patient to take 15 to 30 minutes before each meal.
• Instruct patient to monitor blood glucose level carefully. Teach him to recognize signs and symptoms of hypoglycemia and hyperglycemia.
• Advise patient to report signs and symptoms of infection.
• As appropriate, review all other significant and life-threatening adverse reactions and interactions, especially those related to the drugs, foods, and herbs mentioned above.

reteplase, recombinant
Rapilysin ⊕, Retavase

Pharmacologic class: Tissue plasminogen activator
Therapeutic class: Thrombolytic enzyme
Pregnancy risk category C

Action
Converts plasminogen to plasmin, which in turn breaks down fibrin and fibrinogen, thereby dissolving thrombus

Availability
Injection: Retavase Half-Kit—one vial of 10.4 units (18.1 mg)/vial; Retavase Kit—two vials of 10.4 units (18.1 mg)/vial

⚕ Indications and dosages
➤ Acute myocardial infarction
Adults: 10 units by I.V. bolus over 2 minutes, repeated in 30 minutes

Off-label uses
• Pulmonary embolism

Contraindications
• Hypersensitivity to drug or alteplase
• Active internal bleeding
• Bleeding diathesis
• Recent intracranial or intraspinal surgery or trauma
• Intracranial neoplasm
• Arteriovenous malformation or aneurysm
• Severe uncontrolled hypertension
• History of cerebrovascular accident

Precautions
Use cautiously in:
• previous puncture of noncompressible vessels, major surgery, obstetric delivery, organ biopsy, trauma,

---

hypertension, conditions that may cause left-sided heart thrombus (including mitral stenosis), acute pericarditis, subacute bacterial endocarditis, hemostatic defects, diabetic hemorrhagic retinopathy, cerebrovascular disease, severe hepatic or renal dysfunction, septic thrombophlebitis or occluded AV cannula at a seriously infected site, other conditions in which bleeding poses a significant hazard

- concurrent use of oral anticoagulants (such as warfarin)
- patients older than age 75
- pregnant or breastfeeding patients.

Administration

◀€ If patient shows signs or symptoms of bleeding or anaphylaxis after first bolus dose, withhold second bolus and contact prescriber immediately.
- Use only diluent supplied (preservative-free sterile water for injection) to reconstitute drug into colorless solution of 1 unit/ml.
- If drug foams, let it sit until foam subsides.
- Don't use solution if it is discolored or contains visible precipitates.
- Don't give with other drugs in same I.V. line. Know that drug is incompatible with heparin.

Route	Onset	Peak	Duration
I.V.	Immediate	End of infusion	Variable

Adverse reactions

CNS: **intracranial hemorrhage**
CV: **arrhythmias, hemorrhage**
GI: nausea, vomiting, **GI bleeding**
GU: **hematuria**
Hematologic: anemia, **bleeding tendency**
Other: fever, bleeding at puncture sites

Interactions

Drug-drug. *Anticoagulants, indomethacin, phenylbutazone, platelet aggregation inhibitors (such as abciximab,*

aspirin, dipyridamole): increased risk of bleeding
Drug-diagnostic tests. *Hemoglobin:* decreased level
International Normalized Ratio, partial thromboplastin time, prothrombin time: increased
Drug-herbs. *Ginkgo, many other herbs:* increased risk of bleeding

Patient monitoring

◀€ Check closely for signs and symptoms of bleeding in all body systems. Monitor coagulation studies and CBC.
- Monitor ECG for arrhythmias caused by coronary thrombolysis.
- Assess neurologic status to detect early signs and symptoms of intracranial hemorrhage.

Patient teaching

- Teach patient about drug's anticoagulant effect. Review safety measures to avoid injury, which can cause uncontrolled bleeding.
◀€ Instruct patient to immediately report signs and symptoms of bleeding problems.
- Tell patient he'll undergo frequent blood testing during therapy.

ribavirin

Copegus, Rebetol, Ribasphere, Virazole

Pharmacologic class: Synthetic nucleoside analog
Therapeutic class: Antiviral
Pregnancy risk category X

FDA BOXED WARNING

- Ribavirin monotherapy isn't effective in treating chronic hepatitis C infection and shouldn't be used alone for this indication.

• Drug's main clinical toxicity is hemolytic anemia, which may worsen cardiac disease and lead to fatal and nonfatal myocardial infarctions. Don't administer to patients with history of significant or unstable cardiac disease.

• Drug is contraindicated in pregnant women and their male partners. Caution female patients and female partners of male patients receiving ribavirin to use extreme care to avoid pregnancy during therapy and for 6 months afterward.

Action
Unknown. Thought to inhibit RNA and DNA synthesis by depleting nucleotides and blocking replication and maturation of viral cells.

Availability
Capsules: 200 mg
Powder to be reconstituted for inhalation (Virazole): 6 g in 100-ml glass vial
Tablets: 200 mg

⨍ Indications and dosages
➤ Chronic hepatitis C infection
Note: Dosage calculated solely on basis of patient's weight.
Adults and children weighing 75 kg (165 lb) or more: 600 mg P.O. q morning and evening, given with interferon alfa-2b
Adults weighing less than 75 kg (165 lb) and children weighing more than 61 kg (134 lb): 400 mg P.O. q morning and 600 mg P.O. q evening, given with interferon alfa-2b
Children weighing 50 to 61 kg (110 to 134 lb): 400 mg P.O. b.i.d., given with interferon alfa-2b
Children weighing 37 to 49 kg (81 to 108 lb): 200 mg P.O. every morning and 400 mg P.O. every evening, given with interferon alfa-2b

Children weighing 25 to 36 kg (55 to 79 lb) : 200 mg P.O. b.i.d., given with interferon alfa-2b
➤ Hospitalized children with severe lower respiratory infection caused by respiratory syncytial virus
Infants and young children: 20 mg/ml by inhalation as a starting solution in Viratek Small Particle Aerosol Generator (SPAG-2) for 12 to 18 hours daily for 3 to 7 days. Give by oxygen hood from SPAG-2 unit to infant who isn't mechanically ventilated.

Dosage adjustment
• Cardiovascular disease
• Chronic obstructive pulmonary disease (COPD)
• Renal impairment
• Hemoglobin below 10 g/dl

Off-label uses
• Influenza A or B
• Pneumonia caused by adenovirus
• Severe lower respiratory tract infection in adults
• Genital herpes
• Hemorrhagic fever

Contraindications
• Hypersensitivity to drug or its components
• Autoimmune hepatitis (oral combination therapy)
• Creatinine clearance below 50 ml/minute
• Significant or unstable cardiac disease
• Hemoglobinopathy (such as sickle cell anemia, thalassemia major)
• Females of childbearing age (inhalation form)
• Pregnancy, pregnant partner of male patient (oral drug)
• Breastfeeding

Precautions
Use cautiously in:
• decompensated hepatic disease, coinfection with hepatitis B or human immunodeficiency virus, COPD

- liver or other transplant recipients
- patients who don't respond to interferon.

Administration

◀€ Be aware that oral form must be given with interferon alfa-2b injection.

- Give aerosol by Viratek SPAG-2 only. Don't use other aerosol-generating equipment.
- Dilute powder in sterile water for injection. Don't use solutions with antimicrobial ingredients.
- Know that drug may be given by oral or nasal inhalation.
- Discard solution in SPAG-2 every 24 hours before adding new solution.

◀€ Avoid prolonged contact with aerosol, which can cause headache or eye irritation.

Route	Onset	Peak	Duration
Oral	Unknown	Unknown	Unknown
Inhalation	Slow	60-90 min	Unknown

Adverse reactions

CNS: fatigue, headache, nervousness, depression, **suicidal ideation**
CV: hypotension, bradycardia (with inhalation form), **cardiac arrest**
EENT: conjunctivitis, eyelid erythema or rash
GI: nausea, dyspepsia, anorexia, **pancreatitis**
Hematologic: reticulocytosis, hemolytic anemia
Respiratory: bacterial pneumonia, pneumothorax, bronchospasm, pulmonary edema, apnea, worsening respiratory status (with inhalation form)
Skin: rash, pruritus

Interactions

Drug-drug. *Abacavir, didanosine, lamivudine, stavudine, zalcitabine, zidovudine:* potentially fatal lactic acidosis
Stavudine, zidovudine: decreased antiviral activity

Drug-diagnostic tests. *Alanine aminotransferase, aspartate aminotransferase, bilirubin:* increased levels
Hemoglobin: decreased level
Reticulocytes: increased count

Patient monitoring

◀€ Carefully monitor patient's respiratory status. Check ventilator often to ensure that drug precipitates don't impede function.

◀€ Monitor ECG and vital signs. Watch for hypotension, bradycardia, and other signs of impending cardiac arrest or worsening respiratory condition.

◀€ Assess neurologic status. Stay alert for depression and suicidal ideation.

- Monitor liver function tests and CBC with white cell differential.

Patient teaching

- Explain drug delivery system and precautions carefully to patient or to parents of children receiving inhalation form.

◀€ Tell patient or parents that drug may cause depression or suicidal thoughts, which should be reported immediately.

◀€ Instruct patient or parents to immediately report new or worsening respiratory symptoms.

- Counsel sexually active patients (both males and females) about appropriate birth control. Tell them to use extreme care to avoid pregnancy. Stress importance of using two forms of effective contraception during and for 6 months after treatment (when using oral ribavirin).
- Advise female patient not to breastfeed.
- As appropriate, review all other significant and life-threatening adverse reactions and interactions, especially those related to the drugs and tests mentioned above.

r

rifabutin
Mycobutin

Pharmacologic class: Rifamycin derivative

Therapeutic class: Antimycobacterial

Pregnancy risk category B

Action
Inhibits RNA synthesis by blocking RNA transcription in susceptible organisms (mycobacteria and some gram-positive and gram-negative bacteria)

Availability
Capsules: 150 mg

⚠ Indications and dosages
➤ To prevent disseminated *Mycobacterium avium intracellulare* complex in patients with advanced human immunodeficiency virus (HIV) infection
Adults: 300 mg P.O. daily as a single dose or in two divided doses

Off-label uses
• Tuberculosis
• Prophylaxis and treatment of *M. avium intracellulare* in children

Contraindications
• Hypersensitivity to drug
• Active tuberculosis

Precautions
Use cautiously in:
• severe hepatic disease
• pregnant or breastfeeding patients.

Administration
• Give in divided doses twice daily with food to reduce GI upset.

Route	Onset	Peak	Duration
P.O.	Unknown	2-3 hr	>24 hr

Adverse reactions
CNS: headache, asthenia, weakness
CV: pressure sensation in chest
EENT: uveitis; discolored tears, saliva, or sputum
GI: nausea, vomiting, diarrhea, dyspepsia, abdominal pain, eructation, flatulence, discolored feces, anorexia
GU: discolored urine
Hematologic: eosinophilia, **neutropenia, leukopenia, thrombocytopenia**
Musculoskeletal: joint pain, myalgia
Respiratory: dyspnea
Skin: rash, discolored skin or sweat
Other: abnormal taste, fever, flulike symptoms

Interactions
Drug-drug. *Clarithromycin, itraconazole, saquinavir:* reduced blood levels and efficacy of these drugs
Delavirdine: decreased delavirdine blood level, increased rifabutin blood level
Drugs metabolized by liver (such as zidovudine): altered blood levels of these drugs
Hormonal contraceptives: decreased contraceptive efficacy
Indinavir, nelfinavir, ritonavir: increased rifabutin blood level
Drug-diagnostic tests. *Alanine aminotransferase, aspartate aminotransferase, eosinophils:* increased levels
Neutrophils, platelets, white blood cells: decreased counts
Drug-food. *High-fat foods:* delayed drug absorption

Patient monitoring
• Monitor CBC with white cell differential. Watch for signs and symptoms of blood dyscrasias.
• Assess nutritional status.
• Closely monitor vital signs and temperature. Stay alert for dyspnea and flulike symptoms.

Patient teaching

• Advise patient to take twice daily with food (but not high-fat food) if GI upset occurs. To further minimize GI upset, teach him to eat small, frequent servings of healthy food and drink plenty of fluids.

• Instruct patient to take exactly as prescribed, even after symptoms subside.

◀€ Tell patient to immediately report easy bruising or bleeding.

• Tell patient drug may turn tears, urine, and other body fluids reddish or brownish orange. Instruct him not to wear contact lenses during therapy because drug may stain them permanently.

• Inform patient that drug occasionally causes eye inflammation. Instruct him to report symptoms promptly.

• Caution patient to avoid driving and other hazardous activities until effects of drug are known.

• As appropriate, review all other significant and life-threatening adverse reactions and interactions, especially those related to the drugs, tests, and foods mentioned above.

rifampin (rifampicin❋)

Rifadin, Rofact❋

Pharmacologic class: Rifamycin derivative
Therapeutic class: Antitubercular
Pregnancy risk category C

Action

Inhibits RNA synthesis by blocking RNA transcription in susceptible organisms (mycobacteria and some gram-positive and gram-negative bacteria)

Availability

Capsules: 150 mg, 300 mg
Powder for injection: 600 mg/vial

🖊 Indications and dosages

➤ Tuberculosis
Adults: 10 mg/kg/day (up to 600 mg/day) P.O. or I.V. infusion as a single dose
Children: 10 to 20 mg/kg/day (up to 600 mg/day) P.O. or I.V. infusion as a single dose
➤ Asymptomatic *Neisseria meningitidis* carriers
Adults: 600 mg P.O. or I.V. infusion b.i.d. for 2 days
Children ages 1 month and older: 10 mg/kg/day P.O. or I.V. infusion (up to 600 mg/day) q 12 hours for 2 days
Infants younger than 1 month old: 5 mg/kg P.O. or I.V. infusion q 12 hours for 2 days

Off-label uses

• *Mycobacterium avium intracellulare* complex infection
• Brucellosis
• *Haemophilus influenzae* type B
• Severe staphylococcal bone and joint infections
• Prosthetic valve endocarditis caused by coagulase-negative staphylococci
• Leprosy
• Prophylaxis in high-risk close contact of patients with *N. meningitidis* infections

Contraindications

• Hypersensitivity to drug or other rifamycin derivatives

Precautions

Use cautiously in:
• porphyria
• history of hepatic disease
• concurrent use of other hepatotoxic drugs
• pregnant or breastfeeding patients.

Administration

• Add 10 ml of sterile water to vial to yield a 60-mg/ml solution for I.V. infusion.
• Further dilute in 100 ml of dextrose 5% in water (D_5W) and infuse over

r

30 minutes, or add to 500 ml of D_5W and infuse over 3 hours.

• Give oral doses with a full glass of water 1 hour before or 2 hours after a meal.

• For an adult who can't swallow capsules or for a young child, mix capsule contents with syrup, shake well, and administer.

• If patient can't receive dextrose, use normal saline solution to dilute. Don't use other I.V. solutions.

Route	Onset	Peak	Duration
P.O.	Rapid	2-4 hr	12-24 hr
I.V.	Rapid	End of infusion	12-24 hr

Adverse reactions

CNS: ataxia, confusion, drowsiness, fatigue, headache, asthenia, psychosis, generalized numbness

EENT: conjunctivitis; discolored tears, saliva, and sputum

GI: nausea, vomiting, diarrhea, abdominal cramps, dyspepsia, epigastric distress, flatulence, discolored feces, anorexia, sore mouth and tongue, **pseudomembranous colitis**

GU: discolored urine

Hematologic: eosinophilia, transient **leukopenia, hemolytic anemia, hemolysis, disseminated intravascular coagulation (DIC), thrombocytopenia**

Hepatic: jaundice

Metabolic: hyperuricemia

Musculoskeletal: myalgia, joint pain

Respiratory: dyspnea, wheezing

Skin: flushing, rash, pruritus, discolored sweat, **erythema multiforme, toxic epidermal necrolysis, Stevens-Johnson syndrome**

Other: flulike symptoms, hypersensitivity reactions including vasculitis

Interactions

Drug-drug. *Barbiturates, beta-adrenergic blockers, cardiac glycosides, clarithromycin, clofibrate, cyclosporine, dapsone, diazepam, doxycycline, fluoroquinolones (such as ciprofloxacin), haloperidol, levothyroxine, methadone, progestins, quinine, tacrolimus, theophylline, tricyclic antidepressants, zidovudine:* increased metabolism of these drugs

Chloramphenicol, corticosteroids, disopyramide, efavirenz, estrogens, fluconazole, hormonal contraceptives, itraconazole, ketoconazole, nevirapine, quinidine, opioid analgesics, oral hypoglycemics, phenytoin, quinidine, ritonavir, theophylline, tocainide, verapamil, warfarin: decreased efficacy of these drugs

Delavirdine, indinavir, nelfinavir, saquinavir: decreased blood levels of these drugs

Hepatotoxic drugs (including isoniazid, ketoconazole, pyrazinamide): increased risk of hepatotoxicity

Drug-diagnostic tests. *Alanine aminotransferase, alkaline phosphatase, aspartate aminotransferase, bilirubin, blood urea nitrogen, uric acid:* increased levels

Dexamethasone suppression test: interference with results

Direct Coombs' test: false-positive result

Folate, vitamin B_{12} assay: interference with standard assays

Hemoglobin: decreased value

Liver function tests: abnormal values (transient)

Sulfobromophthalein uptake and excretion test: delayed hepatic uptake and excretion

Drug-behaviors. *Alcohol use:* increased risk of hepatotoxicity

Patient monitoring

• Monitor kidney and liver function tests, CBC, and uric acid level.

🔊 Watch for signs and symptoms of bleeding tendency, especially DIC.

• Assess for signs and symptoms of hepatic impairment.

• Monitor bowel movements for diarrhea, which may signal pseudomembranous colitis.

Patient teaching
• Advise patient to take oral dose 1 hour before or 2 hours after meals. If drug causes significant GI upset, instruct him to take it with meals. To further minimize GI upset, teach him to eat small, frequent servings of food and drink plenty of fluids.

◀€ Instruct patient to immediately report easy bruising or bleeding, fever, malaise, appetite loss, nausea, vomiting, or yellowing of skin or eyes.

• Tell patient drug may color his tears, urine, and other body fluids reddish or brownish orange. Instruct him not to wear contact lenses during therapy, because drug may stain them permanently.

• Instruct patient not to drink alcohol.

• Caution patient to avoid driving and other hazardous activities until he knows how drug affects concentration and alertness.

• As appropriate, review all other significant and life-threatening adverse reactions and interactions, especially those related to the drugs, tests, and behaviors mentioned above.

rifapentine
Priftin

Pharmacologic class: Rifamycin derivative
Therapeutic class: Antitubercular
Pregnancy risk category C

Action
Inhibits RNA synthesis by blocking RNA transcription in susceptible organisms (mycobacteria and some gram-positive and gram-negative bacteria)

Availability
Tablets: 150 mg

⚡ Indications and dosages
➤ Pulmonary tuberculosis (TB)
Adults: *Intensive-phase treatment*—600 mg P.O. twice weekly for 2 months, with doses spaced 72 hours apart; must be given with at least one other antitubercular. *Continuation-phase treatment*—600 mg P.O. once weekly for 4 months, given with another antitubercular.

Off-label uses
• *Mycobacterium avium intracellulare* complex infection

Contraindications
• Hypersensitivity to drug or other rifamycin derivatives

Precautions
Use cautiously in:
• hepatic disorders, porphyria
• concurrent protease inhibitor therapy for human immunodeficiency virus infection
• elderly patients
• pregnant or breastfeeding patients
• children younger than age 12.

Administration
• Know that drug is given with at least one other antitubercular.
• Expect to give drug with pyridoxine to adolescents, malnourished patients, and patients at risk for neuropathy.

Route	Onset	Peak	Duration
P.O.	Slow	5-6 hr	17-18 hr

Adverse reactions
CNS: headache, fatigue, anxiety, dizziness, aggressive behavior
CV: hypertension, peripheral edema
EENT: visual disturbances; discolored tears, sputum, and saliva
GI: nausea, vomiting, diarrhea, dyspepsia, esophagitis, gastritis, discolored feces, anorexia, **pancreatitis**
GU: hematuria, pyuria, proteinuria, urinary casts, discolored urine

r

◀€ Clinical alert

Hematologic: anemia, thrombocytosis, hematoma, purpura, eosinophilia, **neutropenia, leukopenia**
Hepatic: hepatitis
Metabolic: hyperuricemia, hypovolemia, **hyperkalemia**
Musculoskeletal: gout, arthritis, joint pain
Skin: rash, pruritus, acne, urticaria, discolored skin and sweat
Other: edema

Interactions

Drug-drug. *Amitriptyline, anticoagulants, barbiturates, beta-adrenergic blockers, chloramphenicol, clofibrate, corticosteroids, cyclosporine, dapsone, delavirdine, diazepam, digoxin, diltiazem, disopyramide, doxycycline, fentanyl, fluconazole, fluoroquinolones, haloperidol, hormonal contraceptives, indinavir, itraconazole, ketoconazole, methadone, mexiletine, nelfinavir, nifedipine, nortriptyline, oral hypoglycemics, phenothiazines, progestin, quinidine, quinine, ritonavir, saquinavir, sildenafil, tacrolimus, theophylline, thyroid preparations, tocainide, verapamil, warfarin, zidovudine:* decreased actions of these drugs
Antiretroviral drugs: decreased efficacy of these drugs
Drug-diagnostic tests. *Alanine aminotransferase, alkaline phosphatase, aspartate aminotransferase, bilirubin, eosinophils, lactate dehydrogenase, potassium, uric acid:* increased levels
Folate, vitamin B_{12} assays: interference with standard assays
Hemoglobin, neutrophils, platelets, white blood cells: decreased values

Patient monitoring

• Monitor CBC, uric acid level, and liver function tests. Watch for signs and symptoms of blood dyscrasias and hepatitis.
• Assess vital signs and fluid intake and output. Stay alert for hypertension and edema.
• Closely monitor nutritional status and hydration.

Patient teaching

🔈 Instruct patient to immediately report fever, malaise, appetite loss, nausea, vomiting, or yellowing of skin or eyes.
• Emphasize importance of taking with companion drugs, as prescribed, to prevent growth of resistant TB strains.
• Tell patient drug may color tears, urine, and other body fluids reddish or brownish orange. Instruct him not to wear contact lenses during therapy, because drug may stain them permanently.
• Advise patient to take with meals and to minimize GI upset by eating small, frequent servings of healthy food and drinking plenty of fluids.
• Tell patient to monitor his weight and report sudden gains. Also tell him to report swelling.
🔈 Instruct patient to immediately report rash or unusual bleeding or bruising.
🔈 Caution patient to avoid driving and other hazardous activities until he knows how drug affects concentration, vision, and alertness.
• As appropriate, review all other significant and life-threatening adverse reactions and interactions, especially those related to the drugs and tests mentioned above.

rifiximin
Xifaxan

Pharmacologic class: Rifampin-related antibiotic
Therapeutic class: Anti-infective
Pregnancy risk category C

Action
Binds to beta-subunit of bacterial DNA-dependent RNA polymerase, inhibiting bacterial RNA synthesis

Availability
Tablets: 200 mg, 550 mg

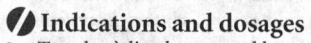 Indications and dosages
➤ Travelers' diarrhea caused by non-invasive strains of *Escherichia coli*
Adults and children age 12 and older: 200 mg P.O. three times daily for 3 days
➤ Reduction of risk of overt hepatic encephalopathy recurrence
Adults: 550 mg P.O. b.i.d.

Off-label uses
• Hepatic encephalopathy

Contraindications
• Hypersensitivity to drug, its components, or rifamycin anti-infectives

Precautions
Use cautiously in:
• elderly patients
• pregnant or breastfeeding patients
• children (safety and efficacy not established in those younger than age 12).

Administration
• Administer with or without food.
• Don't give to patients with diarrhea complicated by fever or blood in stool or to patients with suspected *Campylobacter jejuni, Shigella,* or *Salmonella* infection.

Route	Onset	Peak	Duration
P.O.	Unknown	Unknown	Unknown

Adverse reactions
CNS: headache
GI: nausea, vomiting, constipation, flatulence, abdominal pain, rectal tenesmus, defecation urgency, **pseudomembranous colitis**

Other: pyrexia, overgrowth of susceptible organisms

Interactions
None

Patient monitoring
• Monitor for fever, blood in stools, and worsening of diarrhea.
• Monitor patient's fluid and electrolyte status.
• Monitor for new infections; if needed, consider alternative therapy.

Patient teaching
• Tell patient drug can be taken with or without food.
◀ Advise patient to stop drug and notify prescriber if diarrhea symptoms worsen or last beyond 48 hours.
• As appropriate, review all other significant or life-threatening adverse reactions.

riluzole
Rilutek

Pharmacologic class: Glutamate antagonist
Therapeutic class: Amyotrophic lateral sclerosis (ALS) agent
Pregnancy risk category C

r

Action
Unknown. Thought to inhibit amino acid accumulation on motor neurons of CNS, improving nerve impulse transmission.

Availability
Tablets: 50 mg

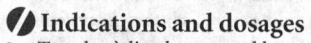 Indications and dosages
➤ ALS
Adults: 50 mg P.O. q 12 hours

Reactions in **bold** are life-threatening. ◀ Clinical alert

Off-label uses
- Cervical dystonia
- Huntington's disease

Contraindications
- Hypersensitivity to drug or its components

Precautions
Use cautiously in:
- hepatic or renal insufficiency, neutropenia, febrile illness
- elderly patients
- female patients and Japanese patients (may have decreased metabolic capacity to eliminate drug)
- pregnant or breastfeeding patients
- children.

Administration
- Give at least 1 hour before or 2 hours after a meal to maximize absorption.

Route	Onset	Peak	Duration
P.O.	Unknown	Unknown	Unknown

Adverse reactions
CNS: headache, dizziness, drowsiness, asthenia, hypertonia, depression, insomnia, malaise, vertigo, circumoral paresthesia
CV: hypertension, orthostatic hypotension, tachycardia, palpitations, peripheral edema, phlebitis, **cardiac arrest**
EENT: rhinitis, sinusitis, oral candidiasis
GI: nausea, vomiting, diarrhea, abdominal pain, dyspepsia, flatulence, stomatitis, dry mouth, anorexia
GU: urinary tract infection, dysuria
Hematologic: neutropenia
Musculoskeletal: back pain, joint pain
Respiratory: decreased lung function, increased cough, pneumonia
Skin: pruritus, eczema, alopecia, exfoliative dermatitis
Other: tooth disorders, weight loss

Interactions
Drug-drug. *Allopurinol, methyldopa, sulfasalazine:* increased risk of hepatotoxicity

CYP450-1A2 inducers (such as omeprazole, rifampin): increased riluzole elimination
CYP450-1A2 inhibitors (such as amitriptyline, phenacetin, quinolones, theophylline): decreased riluzole elimination
Drug-diagnostic tests. *Alanine aminotransferase, aspartate aminotransferase, bilirubin, gamma-glutamyltransferase:* increased levels
Drug-food. *High-fat foods:* decreased riluzole absorption
Drug-behaviors. *Alcohol use:* increased risk of hepatotoxicity

Patient monitoring
- Monitor liver function tests and CBC.
- Assess vital signs and cardiovascular status, particularly for hypertension, orthostatic hypotension, and peripheral edema.
- Closely monitor respiratory status for decreased lung function and pneumonia.
- Monitor weight, nutritional status, and hydration.
- Closely monitor females and patients of Japanese origin, who are at increased risk for adverse reactions.

Patient teaching
- Tell patient to take 1 hour before or 2 hours after a meal, at same time each day.
- Instruct patient to take his temperature regularly and report fever.
- 🔊 Teach patient to immediately report arm or leg swelling, difficulty breathing, and other signs of decreased lung function.
- Advise patient to minimize GI upset by eating small, frequent servings of food and drinking plenty of fluids.
- Caution patient to avoid high-fat foods and alcohol.
- Instruct patient to move slowly when sitting up or standing, to avoid dizziness from sudden blood pressure decrease.
- As appropriate, review all other significant and life-threatening adverse reactions and interactions, especially those related to the drugs, tests, foods, and behaviors mentioned above.

---

rimantadine hydrochloride
Flumadine

Pharmacologic class: Miscellaneous and anticholinergic-like agent
Therapeutic class: Antiviral
Pregnancy risk category C

Action
Prevents nucleic acid uncoating during viral cell replication, preventing penetration in host. Also causes dopamine release from neurons.

Availability
Syrup: 50 mg/5 ml
Tablets: 100 mg

⚕ Indications and dosages
➤ Treatment of influenza type A
Adults: 100 mg P.O. b.i.d.
➤ Prophylaxis of influenza type A
Adults and children older than age 10: 100 mg P.O. b.i.d.
Children younger than age 10: 5 mg/kg P.O. daily. Maximum dosage is 150 mg daily.

Dosage adjustment
- Renal or hepatic disease
- Seizure disorders
- Elderly patients

Off-label uses
- Parkinson's disease

Contraindications
- Hypersensitivity to drug or amantadine

Precautions
Use cautiously in:
- history of seizures or renal or hepatic disease
- pregnant or breastfeeding patients
- children younger than age 1.

Administration
- Give several hours before bedtime.
- Start therapy within 48 hours of symptom onset and continue for at least 1 week.

Route	Onset	Peak	Duration
P.O.	Slow	6 hr	Unknown

Adverse reactions
CNS: headache, dizziness, fatigue, depression, insomnia, poor concentration, asthenia, nervousness
CV: hypotension
EENT: tinnitus
GI: nausea, vomiting, diarrhea, abdominal pain, dyspepsia, dry mouth, anorexia
Respiratory: dyspnea
Skin: rash

Interactions
Drug-drug. *Acetaminophen, aspirin:* decreased rimantadine peak blood level
Cimetidine: increased rimantadine blood level

Patient monitoring
- Assess patient's flu symptoms. Notify prescriber if symptoms don't improve within 2 to 3 days.
- Monitor vital signs; watch for hypotension.
- Closely monitor nutritional status and hydration.

Patient teaching
- Advise patient to take several hours before bedtime.
- If patient's taking syrup, tell him to use specially marked oral syringe or measuring device to ensure accurate dose.
- Instruct patient to contact prescriber if symptoms don't improve within 2 to 3 days.
- Caution patient to avoid driving and other hazardous activities until he knows how drug affects concentration, motor function, and alertness.

r

• As appropriate, review all other significant adverse reactions and interactions, especially those related to the drugs mentioned above.

risedronate sodium
Actonel, Atelvia

Pharmacologic class: Bisphosphonate
Therapeutic class: Calcium regulator
Pregnancy risk category C

Action
Inhibits osteoclast-mediated bone resorption. Also exerts antiresorptive effect, probably by directly inhibiting mature osteoclast activity or indirectly inhibiting osteoblasts.

Availability
Tablets: 5 mg, 30 mg, 35 mg, 150 mg
Tablets (delayed-release): 35 mg

🕖 Indications and dosages
➤ Prevention of postmenopausal osteoporosis
Adults: 5 mg P.O. daily or 35 mg P.O. weekly (immediate-release)
➤ Treatment of postmenopausal osteoporosis
Adults: 5 mg P.O. daily, or 35 mg P.O. weekly, or 150 mg P.O. monthly (immediate-release). Or, 35 mg P.O. weekly (delayed-release).
➤ Osteoporosis in men
Adults: 35 mg (immediate-release) P.O. weekly
➤ Glucocorticoid-induced osteoporosis
Adults: 5 mg (immediate-release) P.O. daily
➤ Paget's disease
Adults: 30 mg (immediate-release) P.O. daily for 2 months. If indicated, may retreat with same dosage after post-treatment observation period of at least 2 months.

Off-label uses
• Hypercalcemia of malignancy
• Primary hyperparathyroidism

Contraindications
• Hypersensitivity to drug, its components, or other bisphosphonates
• Hypocalcemia
• Inability to stand or sit upright for at least 30 minutes
• Esophageal abnormalities that delay esophageal emptying, such as stricture or achalasia

Precautions
Use cautiously in:
• hypotension, upper GI disorders, difficulty swallowing
• severe renal impairment with creatinine clearance less than 30 ml/minute (not recommended)
• pregnant or breastfeeding patients
• children (use not indicated)

Administration
• Be aware that hypocalcemia and other disturbances of bone and mineral metabolism should be effectively treated before starting drug.
• Give immediate-release tablets with 6 to 8 oz of water 30 minutes before first food or beverage of day (other than water).
• Give delayed-release tablets in the morning immediately after breakfast with at least 4 oz of plain water.
🔊 Make sure patient stays upright for at least 30 minutes after taking.
• Be aware that patient with poor dietary intake may need calcium and vitamin D supplements.
• Give calcium, magnesium, or aluminum supplements or antacids at different time of day so they don't interfere with risedronate absorption.

Route	Onset	Peak	Duration
P.O.	Rapid	1 hr	Unknown
P.O. (delayed)	Unknown	Unknown	Unknown

Adverse reactions

CNS: headache, anxiety, depression, dizziness, vertigo, syncope, asthenia
CV: hypertension, vasodilation, angina, chest pain, cardiovascular disorder, peripheral edema
EENT: cataract, conjunctivitis, dry eyes, otitis media, rhinitis, sinusitis, pharyngitis
GI: nausea, vomiting, diarrhea, constipation, abdominal pain, dyspepsia, flatulence, gastroenteritis, colitis, esophageal irritation, dry mouth, anorexia, **esophageal stricture or perforation (rare)**
GU: urinary tract infection
Hematologic: anemia
Musculoskeletal: bone, back, or joint pain; bone fracture; bursitis; myalgia; arthritis; leg and muscle cramps; jaw osteonecrosis
Respiratory: crackles, cough, bronchitis, pneumonia
Skin: rash, pruritus, ecchymosis, **skin cancer**
Other: accidental injury, infection, neck pain, flulike symptoms, allergic reactions, **neoplasm**, hypersensitivity reactions **including angioedema** (rare)

Interactions

Drug-drug. *Antacids, aspirin, calcium- or magnesium-based supplements or laxatives, iron preparations:* decreased risedronate absorption
Nonsteroidal anti-inflammatory drugs, salicylates: increased GI irritation
Drug-diagnostic tests. *Bone-imaging diagnostic agents:* interference with test agents
Calcium, phosphorus: decreased levels
Drug-food. *Any food:* decreased drug absorption

Patient monitoring

• Watch for difficulty swallowing and signs and symptoms of esophageal irritation. Discontinue drug if new or worsening symptoms occur.
• Assess skin for unusual findings that may indicate skin cancer.
• Monitor patient for severe bone, joint, or muscle pain; consider discontinuing drug if symptoms are severe

Patient teaching

• Advise patient to read patient information insert before starting therapy.
🔊 Stress importance of taking immediate-release tablets with a full glass (6 to 8 oz) of water at least 30 minutes before first food or drink of day and delayed-release tablets in the morning immediately after breakfast with at least 4 oz of plain water. Tell patient to stay upright for at least 30 minutes afterward.
🔊 Instruct patient to stop drug and notify prescriber if difficulty or pain on swallowing, midline chest pain, or severe, persistent heartburn occurs.
• Tell patient that chewing or sucking tablet may cause mouth irritation.
• Tell patient to report signs and symptoms of colitis.
• Advise patient taking calcium-, magnesium-, or aluminum-based supplements or antacids to take them at least 2 hours after risedronate.
• Advise patient to promptly report leg cramps or bone, joint, or jaw pain.
• As appropriate, review all other significant and life-threatening adverse reactions and interactions, especially those related to the drugs, tests, and foods mentioned above.

r

---

risperidone

Novo-Risperidone✽, PHL-Risperidone✽, PMS-Risperidone✽, Ran-Risperidone✽, Ratio-Risperidone✽, Risperdal, Risperdal Consta, Risperdal M-Tab, Riva-Risperidone✽, Sandoz Risperisone✽

Pharmacologic class: Benzisoxazole derivative
Therapeutic class: Antipsychotic
Pregnancy risk category C

FDA BOXED WARNING

• Elderly patients with dementia-related psychosis are at increased risk for death. Over course of 10-week controlled trial, death rate in drug-treated patients was about 4.5%, compared to about 2.6% in placebo group. Although causes of death varied, most appeared to be cardiovascular or infectious. Don't give drug to patients with dementia-related psychosis.

Action

Antagonizes serotonin$_2$ and dopamine$_2$ receptors in CNS. Also binds to alpha$_1$- and alpha$_2$-adrenergic receptors and histamine H$_1$ receptors.

Availability

Oral solution: 1 mg/ml in 30-ml bottles
Powder for injection (extended-release microspheres): 12.5 mg, 25-mg, 37.5-mg, 50-mg vials in dose pack with diluent in prefilled syringes
Tablets: 0.25 mg, 0.5 mg, 1 mg, 2 mg, 3 mg, 4 mg
Tablets (orally disintegrating): 0.5 mg, 1 mg, 2 mg, 3 mg, 4 mg

🖊 Indications and dosages
➤ Schizophrenia

Adults: Initially, 2 mg P.O. daily (as once daily or 1 mg b.i.d.). May increase dosage at 24-hour intervals or more in increments of 1 to 2 mg per day, as tolerated, to recommended dosage of 4 to 8 mg/day. In some patients, slower titration may be appropriate. Efficacy has been demonstrated with a range of 4 to 16 mg/day. However, dosages above 6 mg/day for b.i.d. dosing weren't demonstrated to be more efficacious than with lower dosages, were associated with more extrapyramidal symptoms and other adverse effects, and generally aren't recommended. Or, 25 mg deep I.M. q 2 weeks; some patients may benefit from a higher dosage (37.5 or 50 mg). Maximum dosage is 50 mg I.M. q 2 weeks. Efficacy hasn't been evaluated for longer than 12 weeks.

Adolescents ages 13 to17: 0.5 mg P.O. as single daily dose in morning or evening. Dosage adjustments, if indicated, should occur at intervals of not less than 24 hours, in increments of 0.5 or 1 mg/day, as tolerated, to recommended dosage of 3 mg/day.

➤ Short-term management of acute manic or mixed episodes associated with bipolar 1 disorder as monotherapy or as adjunct to lithium or valproate

Adults: Initially, 2 to 3 mg/day P.O. May adjust in increments or decrements of 1 mg/day at 24-hour intervals. Range is 1 to 6 mg/day. Or, 25 mg I.M. q 2 weeks; some patients may benefit from higher dosage (37.5 or 50 mg). Make upward adjustments no more frequently than q 4 weeks. Maximum dosage is 50 mg I.M. q 2 weeks.

➤ Short-term management of bipolar 1 disorder as monotherapy

Children and adolescents ages 10 to 17: 0.5 mg P.O. daily as a single daily dose in the morning or evening. May adjust in increments or decrements of 0.5 to 1 mg/day at 24-hour intervals as tolerated, to recommended target

---

dose of 1 to 2.5 mg/day. Range is 1 to 6 mg/day.

➤ Irritability due to autistic disorder
Children and adolescents ages 5 to 17: Initially, 0.25 mg P.O. (Risperdal) daily for patients weighing less than 20 kg (44 lb) and 0.5 mg/day for patients weighing 20 kg or more. After minimum of 4 days, increase as needed to recommended dosage of 0.5 mg/day for patients weighing less than 20 kg and 1 mg/day for patients weighing 20 kg or more. Maintain this dosage for minimum of 14 days. If sufficient clinical response not achieved, consider dosage increases at 2-week or more intervals in increments of 0.25 mg/day for patients weighing less than 20 kg or 0.5 mg/day for patients weighing 20 kg or more. Effective dosage range is 0.5 to 3 mg/day. Once sufficient clinical response has been achieved and maintained, consider gradually lowering dosage to achieve optimal balance of efficacy and safety.

Dosage adjustment
• Mild to moderate hepatic or renal impairment (appropriate oral dosage titration should occur before initiation of I.M. dosing)
• Severe hepatic or renal impairment (with oral use)
• Elderly or debilitated patients
• Concurrent use of enzyme inducers (such as carbamazepine, phenobarbital, phenytoin, rifampin), fluoxetine, or paroxetine

Off-label uses
• Tourette syndrome

Contraindications
• Hypersensitivity to drug

Precautions
Use cautiously in:
• renal or hepatic impairment, cardiovascular disease, prolonged QT interval, dysphagia, hyperprolactinemia,

hypothermia or hyperthermia, Parkinson's disease, phenylketonuria, tardive dyskinesia, metabolic changes that may increase cardiovascular or cerebrovascular risk (such as hyperglycemia, dyslipidemia, weight gain), previous diagnosis of breast cancer or prolactin-dependent tumors
• history of seizures, drug abuse, or suicide attempt
• elderly or debilitated patients
• pregnant patients
• breastfeeding patients (use not recommended)
• children (safety not established for Risperdal Consta, Risperdal M-Tab, and Risperdal in children weighing less than 33 lb [15 kg]), children younger than age 5 with autistic disorder, younger than age 10 with bipolar disorder, or younger than age 13 with schizophrenia (Risperdal).

Administration
• Record baseline blood pressure before starting therapy.
◀€ Do not give powder for injection I.V.
• Be aware that oral drug tolerability should be established before starting I.M. therapy in patients who have never taken oral risperidone.
• Be aware that oral risperidone (or another antipsychotic) should be given with the first I.M. injection and continued for 3 weeks (then discontinued) to ensure that adequate therapeutic plasma concentrations are maintained before the main release phase of long-acting risperidone injection.
• When reconstituting powder for injection, use only the diluent and needle supplied.
• Shake vial vigorously for a minimum of 10 seconds to ensure homogeneous suspension. When properly mixed, the suspension appears uniform, thick, and milky with visible particles.
• If 2 minutes elapse before giving injection, shake vial vigorously before

r

administering. Give injection within 6 hours of reconstitution.

• Don't combine two different dose strengths of I.M. drug in a single administration.

• For I.M. use, inject deep into buttock; rotate injection sites between buttocks.

• Be aware that children and adolescents experiencing persistent somnolence may benefit from once-daily Risperdal dose administered at bedtime, from administering half daily dose twice daily, or from reduction of dose.

Route	Onset	Peak	Duration
P.O.	1-2 wk	Unknown	Up to 6 wk
I.M.	Unknown	Unknown	Unknown

Adverse reactions

CNS: tremor, parkinsonism, aggressive behavior, dizziness, drowsiness, extrapyramidal reactions, headache, increased dreams, longer sleep periods, insomnia, sedation, fatigue, nervousness, agitation, anxiety, tardive dyskinesia, hyperkinesia, akathisia, **transient ischemic attack (TIA), cerebrovascular accident (CVA), neuroleptic malignant syndrome, suicide**

CV: orthostatic hypotension, chest pain, tachycardia, **arrhythmias**

EENT: vision disturbances, rhinitis, sinusitis, pharyngitis

GI: nausea, vomiting, diarrhea, constipation, abdominal pain, dyspepsia, dry mouth, increased salivation, anorexia, dysphagia

GU: difficulty urinating, polyuria, galactorrhea, dysmenorrhea, menorrhagia, decreased libido

Hematologic: leukopenia, neutropenia, **agranulocytosis**

Metabolic: dyslipidemia, hyperprolactinemia, hyperglycemia, worsening of diabetes mellitus

Musculoskeletal: joint or back pain

Respiratory: cough, dyspnea, upper respiratory tract infection

Skin: pruritus, diaphoresis, rash, dry skin, seborrhea, increased pigmentation, photosensitivity

Other: toothache, fever, impaired temperature regulation, weight changes

Interactions

Drug-drug. *Antihistamines, opioids, sedative-hypnotics:* additive CNS depression

Carbamazepine: increased metabolism and decreased efficacy of risperidone

Clozapine: decreased metabolism and increased effects of risperidone

Levodopa, other dopamine agonists: decreased antiparkinsonian effects of these drugs

Drug-diagnostic tests. *Blood glucose, prolactin:* increased levels

Granulocytes, leukocytes, neutrophils: decreased counts

Drug-behaviors. *Alcohol use:* increased CNS depression

Sun exposure: increased risk of photosensitivity

Patient monitoring

◀✺ Closely monitor neurologic status, especially for mood changes or suicidal ideation, neuroleptic malignant syndrome (high fever, sweating, unstable blood pressure, stupor, muscle rigidity, and autonomic dysfunction), extrapyramidal reactions, TIA, CVA, and tardive dyskinesia.

◀✺ Closely monitor CBC with differential, especially during first few months of therapy; discontinue drug if severe neutropenia occurs.

• Monitor blood pressure, particularly for orthostatic hypotension.

• Assess body temperature. Check for fever and other signs and symptoms of infection.

• Monitor patient with diabetes mellitus for worsening of glucose control. Patients with risk factors for diabetes mellitus who are starting treatment with risperidone should undergo fasting blood glucose testing at the beginning of and periodically during treatment. Monitor all patients receiving drug for signs and symptoms of hyperglycemia, including polydipsia, polyuria, polyphagia, and weakness. Also watch for other metabolic changes such as dyslipidemia or significant weight gain.

• Reassess patients periodically to determine need for maintenance treatment.

Patient teaching

• Instruct patient to remove orally disintegrating tablet from blister pack, place on tongue immediately, and swallow as tablet dissolves.

• Tell patient to mix oral solution with water, coffee, orange juice, or low-fat milk. Tell him solution isn't compatible with cola or tea.

• Advise patient to use effective bedtime routine to avoid sleep disorders.

◀€ Teach patient to recognize and immediately report signs and symptoms of serious adverse reactions, mood changes or suicidal ideation, including tardive dyskinesia, and neuroleptic malignant syndrome.

• Instruct patient to move slowly when sitting up or standing, to avoid dizziness from sudden blood pressure decrease.

• Tell patient that excessive fluid loss (as from sweating, vomiting, or diarrhea) and inadequate fluid intake increase risk of light-headedness (especially in hot weather).

• Caution patient to avoid driving and other hazardous activities until he knows how drug affects concentration and alertness.

• Advise female patient to tell prescriber if she is or plans to become pregnant. Caution her not to breastfeed during therapy.

• Advise patient not to drink alcohol.

• As appropriate, review all other significant and life-threatening adverse reactions and interactions, especially those related to the drugs and behaviors mentioned above.

ritonavir
Norvir

Pharmacologic class: Protease inhibitor
Therapeutic class: Antiretroviral
Pregnancy risk category B

FDA | BOXED WARNING

• Coadministration with certain nonsedating antihistamines, sedative hypnotics, antiarrhythmics, or ergot alkaloids may cause potentially serious or life-threatening adverse events.

Action
Inhibits human immunodeficiency virus (HIV) nonnucleoside reverse transcriptase by binding directly to reverse transcriptase and blocking RNA-dependent and DNA-dependent polymerase activity

Availability
Capsules: 100 mg
Oral solution: 80 mg/ml
Tablets: 100 mg

Indications and dosages
➤ HIV in combination with other antiretrovirals
Adults: Initially, 300 mg P.O. b.i.d.; increase by 100 mg b.i.d. q 2 to 3 days, up to a usual maintenance dosage of 600 mg b.i.d.
Children age 1 month and older: 350 to 400 mg/m² P.O. b.i.d., not to exceed 600 mg b.i.d. Start with 250 mg/m² P.O. b.i.d.; increase by 50 mg/m² P.O. b.i.d. q 2 to 3 days, up to a usual maintenance dosage of 400 mg P.O. b.i.d. If patient doesn't tolerate 400 mg/m²

r

b.i.d. due to adverse reactions, the highest tolerated dose may be used for maintenance therapy, or alternative therapy should be considered.
Children ages 2 and older: 400 mg/m^2 b.i.d., not to exceed 600 mg b.i.d. Start with 250 mg/m^2 to minimize nausea.

Dosage adjustment
• Concurrent use of other protease inhibitors

Off-label uses
• Chronic hepatitis B

Contraindications
• Hypersensitivity to drug or its components
• Concurrent use of alfuzosin, amiodarone, cisapride, dihydroergotamine, ergonovine, ergotamine, flecainide, lovastatin, methylergonovine, oral midazolam, pimozide, propafenone, quinidine, sildenafil (Revatio, when used for pulmonary arterial hypotension), simvastatin, triazolam, voriconazole, or St. John's wort

Precautions
Use cautiously in:
• hepatic disease, diabetes mellitus, hemophilia types A and B
• underlying structural heart disease, preexisting conduction system abnormalities, ischemic heart disease, cardiomyopathies
• concurrent use with drugs that prolong PR interval (including calcium channel blockers, beta-adrenergic blockers, digoxin, atazanavir)
• concurrent use with drugs for erectile dysfunction (such as sildenafil, tadalafil, vardenafil)
• concurrent use with fluticasone, atorvastatin, lovastatin, simvastatin, and St. John's wort (use not recommended)
• pregnant or breastfeeding patients.

Administration
• Give with meals to increase absorption.
• Mix oral solution with chocolate milk or liquid nutritional supplement to mask taste.
• Know that drug is usually given with other antiretrovirals.
◀€ Don't give concurrently with amiodarone, astemizole, bepridil, cisapride, dihydroergotamine, ergonovine, ergotamine, flecainide, methylergonovine, midazolam, pimozide, propafenone, quinidine, terfenadine, or triazolam. Serious interactions may occur.

Route	Onset	Peak	Duration
P.O.	Rapid	2-4 hr	Unknown

Adverse reactions
CNS: headache, dizziness, depression, insomnia, drowsiness, asthenia, paresthesia, syncope, malaise
CV: vasodilation, **prolonged PR interval**
EENT: pharyngitis
GI: nausea, vomiting, diarrhea, constipation, dyspepsia, flatulence, abdominal pain, anorexia, **pancreatitis**
Musculoskeletal: myalgia
Skin: diaphoresis, mild skin eruptions, **Stevens-Johnson syndrome (rare)**
Respiratory: bronchospasm
Other: abnormal taste, fever, pain, allergic reactions including **anaphylaxis (rare), immune reconstitution syndrome**

Interactions
Drug-drug. *Amiodarone, bepridil, cisapride, flecainide, midazolam, pimozide, propafenone, quinidine, triazolam:* inhibited metabolism of these drugs, leading to life-threatening reactions (such as arrhythmias, prolonged sedation, and respiratory depression)
Amitriptyline, anticoagulants, atovaquone, carbamazepine, clozapine, cyclosporine, desipramine, diltiazem, disopyramide, divalproex, dofetilide,

dronabinol, ethinyl estradiol, lamotrigine, phenytoin, sulfamethoxazole, theophylline, zidovudine: increased risk of toxicity of these drugs

Amprenavir: increased amprenavir blood level

Astemizole, cisapride, encainide: increased risk of arrhythmias

Atorvastatin, cerivastatin, lovastatin, simvastatin, terfenadine: increased blood levels of these drugs, increased risk of rhabdomyolysis

Barbiturates, nevirapine, phenytoin, rifamycins: decreased ritonavir blood level

Bupropion: increased risk of seizures

Clarithromycin, efavirenz: increased blood levels of both drugs

Dihydroergotamine, ergonovine, ergotamine, methylergonovine: ergot toxicity

Fluconazole: increased ritonavir blood level

Fluticasone: increased fluticasone exposure resulting in decreased cortisol concentration

Drug-diagnostic tests. *Alanine aminotransferase, aspartate aminotransferase, cholesterol, creatine kinase, gamma-glutamyltransferase, triglycerides, uric acid:* increased levels

Hematocrit, hemoglobin, neutrophils, red blood cells, white blood cells: decreased levels

Drug-herbs. *St. John's wort:* decreased ritonavir blood level

Patient monitoring

• Monitor CBC, liver function tests, electrolyte levels, and lipid panel.

• Assess neurologic status closely. Stay alert for depression.

• Monitor bone mineral density in patients with history of pathologic fractures or who are at risk for osteopenia.

◀≋ Monitor for signs and symptoms of immune reconstitution syndrome, especially during initial phase of combination antiretroviral treatment when patients whose immune systems

respond may develop an inflammatory response to indolent or residual opportunistic infections (such as *Mycobacterium avium* infection, cytomegalovirus, *Pneumocystis jiroveci* pneumonia, or tuberculosis), which may necessitate further evaluation and treatment.

• Monitor vital signs and watch for syncope.

• Closely monitor nutritional and hydration status.

Patient teaching

• Advise patient to take with meals to increase absorption.

• Encourage patient or caregiver to mix oral solution with chocolate milk or liquid nutritional supplement to mask taste. Tell caregiver that oral solution is recommended for children older than age 1 month who can't swallow capsules or tablets and, when possible, to administer dose using a calibrated dosing syringe.

• Tell patient to swallow tablets whole and not to chew, break, or crush them.

• Tell patient drug may cause numbness, tingling, weakness, and other CNS effects that increase his injury risk. Urge him to use appropriate safety precautions.

• Instruct patient to report depression.

• Advise patient not to take nonprescription drugs or herbal products, particularly St. John's wort, without consulting prescriber.

• Tell female patient not to breastfeed because of risk of serious adverse reactions and possible HIV transmission to infant.

• As appropriate, review all other significant adverse reactions and interactions, especially those related to the drugs, tests, and herbs mentioned above.

r

rituximab
MabThera ⊕, Rituxan

Pharmacologic class: Murine/human monoclonal antibody
Therapeutic class: Antineoplastic
Pregnancy risk category C

FDA   BOXED WARNING

- Deaths from infusion reactions have occurred within 24 hours of rituximab infusion. Approximately 80% of fatal reactions were linked to first infusion. If severe infusion reaction develops, discontinue infusion and intervene appropriately.
- Acute renal failure requiring dialysis, severe mucocutaneous reactions, and progressive multifocal leukoencephalopathy have been reported.

Action
Binds to CD20 antigen on malignant B lymphocytes; recruits immune effector functions to mediate B-cell lysis (possibly through complement-dependent cytotoxicity and antibody-dependent cell-mediated cytotoxicity)

Availability
Injection: 10 mg/ml in 10-ml (100-mg) and 50-ml (500-mg) vials

⏀ Indications and dosages
➤ Non Hodgkin's lymphoma (NHL)
Adults: 375 mg/m² by I.V. infusion according to the following schedules:
Relapsed or refractory, low grade or follicular, CD20-positive B-cell NHL: Give weekly for four or eight doses.
Retreatment for relapsed or refractory, low grade or follicular, CD20-positive B-cell NHL: Give weekly for four doses.
Previously untreated, follicular, CD20-positive, B-cell NHL: Give on day 1 of each cycle of cyclophosphamide, vincristine, prednisolone (CVP) chemotherapy, for up to eight doses.
Non-progressing, low-grade, CD20-positive B-cell NHL, after first line CVP chemotherapy: Following completion of six to eight cycles of CVP chemotherapy, give weekly for four doses at 6-month intervals to a maximum of 16 doses.
Diffuse large B-cell NHL: Give on day 1 of each cycle of chemotherapy for up to eight infusions.
Dosage in combination with ibritumomab: On day 1, rituximab 250 mg/m² by I.V. infusion. Within 4 hours after rituximab infusion, give 5 mCi In-111 ibritumomab I.V. On days 7, 8, and 9, give rituximab 250 mg/m² by I.V. infusion and platelet-count-dependent dose of Y-90 ibritumomab I.V.
➤ Moderately to severely active rheumatoid arthritis in patients who have had an inadequate response to one or more tumor necrosis factor antagonist
Adults: Two 1,000 mg I.V. infusions separated by 2 weeks in combination with methotrexate. Give subsequent courses every 24 weeks or based on clinical evaluation, but not sooner than every 16 weeks.
➤ Chronic lymphocytic leukemia (CLL) in combination with fludarabine and cyclophosphamide (FC)
Adults: 375 mg/m² I.V. day before start of FC chemotherapy; then 500 mg/m² on day 1 of cycles 2 to 6 (every 28 days).

Off-label uses
- Waldenström's macroglobulinemia

Contraindications
- Hypersensitivity to drug, its components, or murine products

Precautions
Use cautiously in:
- history of drug allergy or sensitivity

- previous exposure to murine-based monoclonal antibodies
- high level of circulating malignant cells
- cardiac or pulmonary conditions
- pregnant or breastfeeding patients
- children.

Administration

- Follow facility policy regarding handling, administration, and disposal of chemotherapeutic drugs.
- Know that *Pneumocystis jiroveci* pneumonia and antiherpetic viral prophylaxis is recommended for patients with CLL during treatment and for up to 12 months following treatment, as appropriate.
- To reduce the incidence and severity of infusion reactions, premedicate patient with diphenhydramine and acetaminophen, as prescribed. In addition, for patients with rheumatoid arthritis, give I.V. methylprednisolone (or its equivalent) 30 minutes before each infusion.
- Consider withholding antihypertensive agents 12 hours before giving drug to help prevent hypotension.
- Give drug as I.V. infusion.
- ◀≋ Never give as I.V. bolus or I.V. push.
- Don't mix or dilute with other drugs.
- Dilute in dextrose 5% in water (D₅W) or normal saline solution to a concentration of 1 to 4 mg/ml. Invert bag gently to mix solution.
- Administer the first infusion at an initial rate of 50 mg/hr. If no infusion reaction occurs, increase the infusion rate in 50 mg/hr increments every 30 minutes, to a maximum of 400 mg/hr.
- If the patient tolerates the first infusion well, administer subsequent infusions at an initial rate of 100 mg/hr and increase by 100 mg/hr increments every 30 minutes to a maximum of 400 mg/hr, as tolerated.
- ◀≋ Be aware that a severe infusion reaction may occur usually after first infusion. This reaction consists of a complex of hypoxia, pulmonary infiltrates, acute respiratory distress syndrome, M.I., ventricular fibrillation, or cardiogenic shock. If such a reaction occurs, stop infusion immediately and treat appropriately.
- If hypersensitivity reaction (non-IgE-mediated) or infusion reaction that is not severe occurs, interrupt or temporarily slow infusion. When symptoms improve, infusion can continue at half of previous rate.

Route	Onset	Peak	Duration
I.V.	Variable	Variable	6-12 mo

Adverse reactions

CNS: dizziness, headache, nervousness, hypertonia, hyperesthesia, insomnia, agitation, malaise, paresthesia, asthenia, fatigue, tremor, rigors
CV: hypotension, hypertension, peripheral edema, chest pain, tachycardia, bradycardia, angina, **arrhythmias**
EENT: conjunctivitis, lacrimation disorders, rhinitis, sinusitis, pharyngitis
GI: nausea, vomiting, diarrhea, constipation, abdominal pain, dyspepsia, anorexia
GU: renal toxicity
Hematologic: anemia, **neutropenia, leukopenia, thrombocytopenia**
Metabolic: hyperglycemia, hypocalcemia
Musculoskeletal: myalgia, back pain
Respiratory: dyspnea, cough, bronchitis, **bronchospasm**
Skin: pruritus, rash, urticaria, flushing, dermatitis, angioedema, **toxic epidermal necrolysis, Stevens-Johnson syndrome**
Other: altered taste, fever, chills, pain at injection site, hypersensitivity reactions including **sepsis, severe infusion reaction**

Interactions

Drug-drug. *Cisplatin:* increased risk of renal failure

Live-virus vaccines: increased risk of infection from vaccine
Drug-diagnostic tests. *Calcium, hemoglobin, neutrophils, platelets, white blood cells:* decreased values
Glucose, lactate dehydrogenase: increased levels

Patient monitoring

• Monitor closely for signs and symptoms of hypersensitivity reaction.

◀≋ Stop drug immediately and notify prescriber if patient develops signs or symptoms of Stevens-Johnson syndrome or other severe mucocutaneous reactions (including severe rash).

◀≋ Monitor pulse and blood pressure throughout I.V. infusion. Stop infusion if hypotension, bronchospasm, or angioedema occurs. Then consult prescriber about restarting infusion at half of previous rate.

◀≋ Monitor ECG throughout infusion. Stop infusion if serious arrhythmia develops.

• Monitor CBC, blood glucose, and electrolyte levels.

• Assess for signs and symptoms of infection, including fever.

Patient teaching

◀≋ Tell patient to immediately report signs and symptoms of hypersensitivity reaction or severe skin reaction.

◀≋ Instruct patient to take his temperature daily and immediately report fever and other signs or symptoms of infection.

◀≋ Instruct patient to immediately report unusual bleeding or bruising.

• Advise patient to minimize GI upset by eating small, frequent servings of food and drinking plenty of fluids.

• As appropriate, review all other significant and life-threatening adverse reactions and interactions, especially those related to the drugs and tests mentioned above.

rivastigmine tartrate
Exelon

Pharmacologic class: Cholinesterase inhibitor

Therapeutic class: Anti-Alzheimer's drug

Pregnancy risk category B

Action

Unknown. Thought to enhance cholinergic function by elevating acetylcholine levels in brain through reversible inhibition of its hydrolysis by cholinesterase.

Availability

Capsules: 1.5 mg, 3 mg, 4.5 mg, 6 mg
Oral solution: 2 mg/ml
Transdermal patch: 4.6 mg/24 hours, 9.5 mg/24 hours

Indications and dosages

➤ Mild to moderate dementia of Alzheimer's disease

Adults: Initially, 1.5 mg P.O. b.i.d. May increase to 3 mg b.i.d. after 2 weeks; may increase further to 4.5 mg b.i.d. and 6 mg b.i.d., if tolerated, after 2 weeks at previous dosage. Typical effective range is 6 to 12 mg/day, up to a maximum of 12 mg/day. Or initially, apply one 4.6-mg patch to the skin q 24 hours. After minimum of 4 weeks, may increase to maintenance dose of one 9.5-mg patch applied to the skin q 24 hours.

➤ Mild to moderate dementia of Parkinson's disease

Adults: Initially, 1.5 mg P.O. b.i.d. May increase to 3 mg b.i.d. after 2 weeks; may increase further to 4.5 mg b.i.d. and 6 mg b.i.d. if tolerated, after 4 weeks at previous dosage. Typical effective range is 3 to 12 mg/day, up to a maximum of 12 mg/day. Or initially, apply one 4.6-mg patch to the skin q 24 hours. After minimum of 4 weeks, may increase to maintenance dose of one 9.5-mg patch applied to the skin q 24 hours.

Off-label uses
• Huntington's disease

Contraindications
• Hypersensitivity to drug, its components, or carbamate derivatives

Precautions
Use cautiously in:
• renal or hepatic impairment, diabetes mellitus, obstructive pulmonary disease, neurologic conditions that can cause seizures, peptic ulcers, GI bleeding, supraventricular conduction disorders
• patients older than age 85
• pregnant patients.

Administration
• Give with food in morning and evening.

Route	Onset	Peak	Duration
P.O.	Unknown	1 hr	12 hr

Adverse reactions
CNS: depression, dizziness, headache, confusion, insomnia, psychosis, hallucinations, anxiety, tremor, drowsiness, fatigue, syncope, asthenia
CV: chest pain, hypertension, peripheral edema
EENT: rhinitis, pharyngitis
GI: nausea, vomiting, diarrhea, constipation, abdominal pain, flatulence, eructation, dyspepsia, anorexia
GU: urinary tract infection, urinary incontinence
Musculoskeletal: back pain, joint pain, bone fractures
Respiratory: upper respiratory infection, cough, bronchitis
Skin: rash, diaphoresis
Other: weight loss, pain, flulike symptoms

Interactions
Drug-drug. *Anticholinergics:* interference with anticholinergic effects
Cholinergic agonists (such as bethanechol), succinylcholine and similar neuromuscular blockers: synergistic effects
Drug-herbs. *S-adenosylmethionine (SAM-e), St. John's wort:* increased risk of serotonin syndrome
Drug-behaviors. *Nicotine use:* increased drug clearance

Patient monitoring
• Monitor patient's nutritional and hydration status, especially at start of therapy.
• Assess vital signs and cardiovascular status. Stay alert for chest pain and peripheral edema.
• Closely monitor cognitive status, particularly memory. Report significant decline or improvement.
• Assess temperature. Watch for fever and other signs and symptoms of infection.

Patient teaching
• Instruct caregiver to give with food in morning and evening.
• Instruct caregiver to use dosing syringe provided with oral solution to withdraw prescribed amount of solution from container; patient may swallow directly from syringe. Or, drug may be mixed with a small glass of water, cold fruit juice, or soda; stir mixture and have patient drink entire amount.
• Instruct caregiver how to apply transdermal patch.
• Inform caregiver that drug initially may worsen CNS impairment. Recommend appropriate safety measures.
• Tell caregiver that memory improvement generally is subtle and that drug works by preventing further memory loss.
• Inform caregiver that drug commonly causes nausea, vomiting,

r

Reactions in **bold** are life-threatening.　　　◀€ Clinical alert

decreased appetite, and weight loss, especially at start of therapy.

• Advise caregiver to watch for and report weight loss, dehydration, and signs and symptoms of GI bleeding.

• Tell caregiver that drug interacts with many over-the-counter products and nicotine. Advise him to discuss these products with prescriber before giving to patient.

• As appropriate, review all other significant adverse reactions and interactions, especially those related to the drugs, herbs, and behaviors mentioned above.

rizatriptan benzoate
Maxalt, Maxalt-MLT, Maxalt RPD✤

Pharmacologic class: Serotonin 5-hydroxytryptamine ($5-HT_1$) receptor agonist
Therapeutic class: Antimigraine drug
Pregnancy risk category C

Action
Thought to act as agonist at specific $5-HT_1$ receptor sites in intracranial vessels, causing vasoconstriction. Also may act on sensory trigeminal nerves, reducing transmission along pain pathways.

Availability
Tablets: 5 mg, 10 mg
Tablets (orally disintegrating): 5 mg, 10 mg

🚫 Indications and dosages
➤ Acute migraine
Adults: 5 to 10 mg P.O.; may repeat in 2 hours, not to exceed 30 mg in 24 hours. For patients receiving propranolol concurrently, 5 mg P.O., up to a maximum of three doses in 24 hours.

Children ages 6 to 17 weighing 40 kg (88 lb) or more: 10 mg P.O. as a single dose. For patients receiving propranolol concurrently, 5 mg P.O., up to a maximum of three doses in 24 hours.
Children ages 6 to 17 weighing less than 40 kg (88 lb): 5 mg P.O. as a single dose. Don't prescribe drug for propranolol-treated children who weigh less than 40 kg.

Contraindications
• Hypersensitivity to drug or its components
• Ischemic heart disease or other significant cardiovascular disease
• Ischemic bowel disease
• Transient ischemic attacks
• Basilar or hemiplegic migraine
• Uncontrolled hypertension
• Use of other $5-HT_1$ agonists or ergot-type compounds (dihydroergotamine, methysergide) within 24 hours
• MAO inhibitor use within past 14 days

Precautions
Use cautiously in:
• severe renal impairment (especially in dialysis patients), moderate hepatic impairment, cardiovascular risk factors
• phenylketonuria (PKU) in patients receiving orally disintegrating tablets
• pregnant or breastfeeding patients
• children younger than age 6 (safety not established).

Administration
• Place orally disintegrating tablet on patient's tongue to dissolve. Make sure he swallows it with saliva only. Don't give with beverages.
🔊 Don't give within 14 days of MAO inhibitors (may cause serious adverse reactions).

Route	Onset	Peak	Duration
P.O.	30 min	1-1.5 hr	Unknown

Adverse reactions

CNS: headache, dizziness, drowsiness, asthenia, fatigue, paresthesia, decreased mental acuity, euphoria, tremor

CV: chest pain, tightness, heaviness, or pressure; **hypertensive crisis; arrhythmias, myocardial infarction (MI) (rare)**

GI: nausea, vomiting, diarrhea, dry mouth

Respiratory: dyspnea

Skin: flushing

Other: neck, throat, or jaw pain, tightness, or pressure; hot flashes; warm or cold sensations; **noncoronary vasospastic reactions, serotonin syndrome**

Interactions

Drug-drug. *Ergot or ergot-type compounds (such as dihydroergotamine, methysergide), other 5-HT$_1$ agonists:* additive vasoactive effects

MAO inhibitors, propranolol: increased rizatriptan blood level, greater risk of adverse effects

Selective serotonin reuptake inhibitors: weakness, hyperreflexia, incoordination

Drug-herbs. *S-adenosylmethionine (SAM-e), St. John's wort:* increased risk of adverse serotonergic effects, including serotonin syndrome

Patient monitoring

• Monitor patient's response to drug. Assess need for repeat doses.

• Assess vital signs and cardiovascular status, especially if patient has cardiovascular risk factors. Discontinue drug if arrhythmia occurs.

◀◉ Be aware that drug may cause noncoronary vasospastic reactions, such as peripheral vascular ischemia, GI vascular ischemia and infarction (abdominal pain and bloody diarrhea), splenic infarction, and Raynaud's syndrome. In patients who experience signs or symptoms suggestive of noncoronary vasospasm reaction, rule out

the suspected vasospasm reaction before giving additional doses.

◀◉ Be aware that drug may cause serotonin syndrome. Discontinue drug if serotonin syndrome is suspected.

Patient teaching

• Teach patient how to use drug. Stress that it's effective only in treating diagnosed migraine—not in preventing migraine or treating other types of headache.

• Advise patient to peel back blister pack of Maxalt-MLT with dry hands and place tablet on tongue. Tell him to swallow drug with saliva only, not beverages.

• Tell patient he may repeat dose in 2 hours if headache recurs, but should take no more than 30 mg in 24 hours.

• Inform patient with PKU that orally disintegrating tablets contain phenylalanine.

◀◉ Teach patient how to recognize and immediately report signs and symptoms of significant increases in blood pressure, arrhythmia, MI, serotonin syndrome, and vasospastic reactions.

◀◉ Instruct female patient to immediately report possible pregnancy.

• As appropriate, review all other significant adverse reactions and interactions, especially those related to the drugs and herbs mentioned above.

r

ropinirole hydrochloride

Adartrel ✦, Requip, Requip XL

Pharmacologic class: Dopamine agonist
Therapeutic class: Antidyskinetic
Pregnancy risk category C

Action
Unknown. Thought to stimulate dopamine receptors in brain.

Availability
Tablets: 0.25 mg, 0.5 mg, 1 mg, 2 mg, 3 mg, 4 mg, 5 mg
Tablets (extended-release): 2 mg, 4 mg, 6 mg, 8 mg

⦸ Indications and dosages
➤ Idiopathic Parkinson's disease
Adults: For conventional tablets, initially, 0.25 mg P.O. t.i.d. for 1 week, followed by 0.5 mg P.O. t.i.d. for 1 week, then 0.75 mg t.i.d. for 1 week, and then 1 mg t.i.d. for 1 week. After week 4, may increase by 1.5 mg/ day q week, up to 9 mg/day; then may increase further by up to 3 mg/day q week, up to 24 mg/day. For extended-release tablets, initially 2 mg P.O. once daily for 1 to 2 weeks, followed by increases of 2 mg/day at 1-week or longer intervals as appropriate, depending on therapeutic response and tolerability, up to a recommended maximum dosage of 24 mg/day.
➤ Moderate to severe primary restless leg syndrome
Adults: Initially, 0.25 mg P.O. once daily, 1 to 3 hours before bedtime. After 2 days, may increase dosage to 0.5 mg once daily and to 1 mg once daily during week 2. For weeks 3 through 6, may increase dosage by 0.5 mg/week, to a dosage of 3 mg; at week 7, dosage may be increased to 4 mg (immediate-release tablets only).

Contraindications
• Hypersensitivity to drug or its components

Precautions
Use cautiously in:
• severe hepatic impairment or cardiovascular disease, bradycardia
• elderly patients
• pregnant patients

• breastfeeding patients (use not recommended).

Administration
• Give with food if drug causes nausea.
• Assess patient for therapeutic response and tolerability at 1-week intervals (minimum) or longer after each dosage increment.
• Know that drug withdrawal should occur over 7 days, with frequency reduced to twice-daily dosing for first 4 days and then to once-daily dosing for next 3 days.

Route	Onset	Peak	Duration
P.O.	30-60 min	1-2 hr	16 hr

Adverse reactions
CNS: headache, dizziness, confusion, drowsiness, fatigue, neuralgia, amnesia, hyperesthesia, yawning, dystonia, increased dyskinesia, hyperkinesia, akathisia, hallucinations, abnormal thinking, poor concentration, syncope, vertigo, myoclonus, asthenia, malaise, sleep attacks
CV: orthostatic hypotension, hypertension, palpitations, extrasystole, peripheral edema, peripheral ischemia, chest pain, tachycardia, **atrial fibrillation**
EENT: abnormal vision, rhinitis, sinusitis, pharyngitis
GI: nausea, vomiting, flatulence, abdominal pain, dyspepsia, dry mouth, anorexia
GU: urinary tract infection, decreased libido, erectile dysfunction
Respiratory: bronchitis, dyspnea
Skin: diaphoresis, flushing
Other: viral infection, pain, edema

Interactions
Drug-drug. *Butyrophenones (such as haloperidol), metoclopramide, phenothiazines, thioxanthenes:* decreased ropinirole effects
Ciprofloxacin, estrogens: increased ropinirole effects

Drugs that alter activity of CYP450-1A2 enzyme system: altered ropinirole clearance

Levodopa: increased levodopa effects

Drug-diagnostic tests. *Alkaline phosphatase, blood urea nitrogen:* increased levels

Drug-herbs. *Kava:* decreased ropinirole efficacy

Patient monitoring

• Monitor vital signs, especially for orthostatic hypotension. Assess for peripheral edema.

• Assess neurologic status carefully. Report severe adverse reactions.

• Monitor nutritional and hydration status.

Patient teaching

• Encourage patient to take drug with food if it causes nausea.

• Instruct patient to swallow extended-release tablets whole and not to chew, crush, or divide them.

• Inform patient that hallucinations may occur during ropinirole therapy.

• Advise patient that he may experience the urge to gamble, increased sexual urges, or other intense urges and the inability to control these urges.

• Inform patient (and caregiver, as appropriate) that drug can cause serious CNS reactions; tell him which ones to report. Recommend appropriate safety measures.

• Instruct patient to move slowly when sitting up or standing, to avoid dizziness from sudden blood pressure decrease.

◀ Caution patient not to stop drug abruptly. Dosage must be tapered.

• Advise patient to report swelling of hands or feet.

• Caution patient to avoid driving and other hazardous activities until he knows how drug affects concentration, vision, and alertness.

• As appropriate, review all other significant and life-threatening adverse reactions and interactions, especially those related to the drugs, tests, and herbs mentioned above.

rosiglitazone maleate
Avandia

Pharmacologic class: Thiazolidinedione

Therapeutic class: Hypoglycemic

Pregnancy risk category C

FDA **BOXED WARNING**

• Thiazolidinediones, including rosiglitazone maleate, may cause or exacerbate heart failure in some patients. After initiating therapy or increasing dosage, observe patient carefully for heart failure signs and symptoms (including excessive, rapid weight gain; dyspnea; or edema). If these occur, manage condition per current standards of care and consider withdrawing drug or lowering dosage.

• Drug isn't recommended in patients with symptomatic heart failure and is contraindicated in those with established New York Heart Association Class III or IV heart failure.

• A meta-analysis of 52 clinical trials, most of which compared rosiglitazone maleate to placebo, showed drug to be associated with a statistically significant increased risk of myocardial infarction (MI). Three other trials, comparing rosiglitazone to other approved oral antidiabetic agents or placebo, showed a statistically nonsignificant increased risk of MI, and a statistically nonsignificant decreased risk of death. No clinical trials directly compared cardiovascular risk of rosiglitazone and pioglitazone (another thiazolidinedione), but in a separate trial, pioglitazone (when

r

---

compared to placebo) didn't show an increased risk of MI or death.

• Because of the possibly increased risk of MI, rosiglitazone is available only through a restricted distribution program called the AVANDIA-Rosiglitazone Medicines Access Program. Both prescribers and patients need to enroll in the program.

Action
Inhibits alpha-glucosidases, enzymes that convert oligosaccharides and disaccharides to glucose. This inhibition lowers blood glucose level, especially in postprandial hyperglycemia.

Availability
Tablets: 2 mg, 4 mg, 8 mg

🜛 Indications and dosages
➤ Adjunct to diet and exercise to improve glycemic control in adults with type 2 diabetes mellitus who are either already taking rosiglitazone or not already taking rosiglitazone and are unable to achieve adequate glycemic control on other antidiabetics and, in consultation with their healthcare provider, have decided not to take pioglitazone for medical reasons

Adults: 4 mg P.O. once daily or 2 mg b.i.d. After 8 to 12 weeks, may increase to 8 mg daily or 4 mg b.i.d. if needed.

Off-label uses
• Polycystic ovary syndrome

Contraindications
• Established New York Heart Association (NYHA) Class III or IV heart failure

Precautions
Use cautiously in:
• diabetic ketoacidosis, type 1 (insulin-dependent) diabetes mellitus (use not recommended)

• edema, NYHA Class I and II heart failure, elevated liver enzymes, jaundice
• concurrent use of insulin (not recommended)
• pregnant patients
• breastfeeding patients (use not recommended)
• children (safety and efficacy not established).

Administration
🔊 Obtain liver enzyme results before starting drug. Be aware that therapy shouldn't be initiated in patient with elevated baseline liver enzyme levels (alanine aminotransferase [ALT] level greater than 2.5 times the upper limit of normal) or if patient exhibits clinical evidence of active liver disease.

• Give with or without food.
• Be aware that drug is active only in presence of endogenous insulin and thus is ineffective in diabetic ketoacidosis or type 1 diabetes mellitus.

Route	Onset	Peak	Duration
P.O.	Unknown	Unknown	12-24 hr

Adverse reactions
CNS: fatigue, headache
CV: hypertension, **heart failure, increased risk of myocardial infarction**
EENT: macular edema, decreased visual acuity, nasopharyngitis
GI: diarrhea
GU: menstrual dysfunction
Hematologic: anemia
Metabolic: hyperglycemia, **hypoglycemia**
Musculoskeletal: back pain, arthralgia, increased risk of fracture
Respiratory: upper respiratory infection
Other: edema, injury, weight gain

Interactions
Drug-drug. *CYP2C8 inducers (such as rifampin):* decreased rosiglitazone area under the curve (AUC)

CYP2C8 inhibitors (such as gemfibrozil): increased rosiglitazone AUC
Drug-diagnostic tests. *Free fatty acids, high-density lipoproteins, liver enzymes, low-density lipoproteins, total cholesterol:* increased levels
Hematocrit, hemoglobin: decreased levels

Patient monitoring
• Monitor CBC, lipid panel, blood glucose, and glycosylated hemoglobin levels.
• Monitor patient's weight. Assess for fluid retention, which may lead to heart failure. Be aware that dosage increases should be accompanied by careful monitoring for adverse reactions related to fluid retention.
◀€ Closely monitor liver function tests. Be aware that patients with mildly elevated liver enzymes (ALT level 2.5 times ULN) at baseline or during therapy should be evaluated to determine cause of the liver enzyme elevation and if liver enzyme elevation resolves or worsens. If at any time ALT level increases to more than 3 times ULN, recheck liver enzyme levels as soon as possible. If ALT level remains at 3 times ULN, discontinue drug. If jaundice occurs, discontinue drug.

Patient teaching
• Tell patient he may take with or without food.
• Advise patient to monitor blood glucose level regularly and report significant changes.
◀€ Inform patient that drug may increase fluid retention, causing or exacerbating heart failure. Encourage him to weigh himself regularly and report sudden weight gain, swelling, or shortness of breath.
◀€ Teach patient to recognize and immediately report signs and symptoms of heart attack or liver problems.
• Tell patient to promptly report vision changes.

• Tell patient he'll undergo regular blood testing during therapy.
• Advise female patient that drug may result in ovulation in some premenopausal anovulatory women. Inform patient she may be at increased risk for pregnancy while taking this drug; recommend adequate contraception.
• Caution female patient not to breast-feed during therapy.
• As appropriate, review all other significant and life-threatening adverse reactions and interactions, especially those related to the tests and herbs mentioned above.

rosuvastatin calcium
Crestor

Pharmacologic class: HMG-CoA reductase inhibitor
Therapeutic class: Antilipemic
Pregnancy risk category X

Action
Selectively and competitively inhibits HMG-CoA reductase, which catalyzes its conversion to the cholesterol precursor mevalonate and thus limits cholesterol synthesis. This action increases high-density lipoprotein level and decreases low-density lipoprotein (LDL) level.

Availability
Tablets: 5 mg, 10 mg, 20 mg, 40 mg

🕭 Indications and dosages
➤ Primary prevention of cardiovascular disease; adjunct to diet for hyperlipidemia, mixed dyslipidemia, hypertriglyceridemia, primary dysbetalipoproteinemia (type III hyperlipoproteinemia); slowing of progression of atherosclerosis

---

Adults: 5 to 40 mg P.O. daily. Use 40-mg dose only for patients not reaching LDL-C goal with 20 mg.

➤ Homozygous familial hypercholesterolemia

Adults: 20 mg/day P.O. daily. (Response to therapy should be estimated from preapheresis LDL-C levels.).

➤ Heterozygous familial hypercholesterolemia after failure of an adequate trial of diet therapy

Children ages 10 to 17: 5 to 20 mg P.O. daily. Maximum recommended dosage is 20 mg/day. Individualize dosages according to recommended goal of therapy. Make adjustments at intervals of 4 weeks or more.

Dosage adjustment

• Patients with severe renal impairment (creatinine clearance less than 30 ml/minute/1.73 m^2) not on hemodialysis
• Unexplained persistent proteinuria or hematuria
• Concurrent use of cyclosporine, niacin, fenofibrate, gemfibrozil, or combination of lopinavir and ritonavir or atazanavir and ritonavir
• Asian patients

Contraindications

• Hypersensitivity to drug or its components
• Active hepatic disease or persistent, unexplained hepatic enzyme elevations
• Women who are pregnant or may become pregnant
• Breastfeeding patients

Precautions

Use cautiously in:
• predisposing factors for myopathy (such as renal impairment, advanced age, hypothyroidism)
• heavy alcohol use or history of chronic liver disease
• hypersensitivity to other HMG-CoA reductase inhibitors (such as fluvastatin, simvastatin)
• proteinuria and hematuria
• concurrent use of drugs that may decrease levels or activity of endogenous steroid hormones (such as ketoconazole, spironolactone, and cimetidine)
• concurrent use of fenofibrate, lipid-modifying doses (1 g/day or more) of niacin, coumarin anticoagulants, protease inhibitors given in combination with ritonavir
• concurrent use of gemfibrozil (avoid use or, if used, don't exceed 10 mg daily)
• elderly patients
• children younger than age 10 (safety and efficacy not established).

Administration

🔊 Check liver function tests before therapy starts.
• Give with or without food.
• Measure lipid levels within 2 to 4 weeks after therapy starts and after titration.
• Know that drug should be used as adjunct to other lipid-lowering treatments, such as diet.

Route	Onset	Peak	Duration
P.O.	Unknown	3-5 hr	Unknown

Adverse reactions

CNS: headache, dizziness, anxiety, depression, insomnia, hypertonia, paresthesia, asthenia, tremor, vertigo, neuralgia
CV: palpitations, tachycardia, chest pain, angina pectoris, hypertension, vasodilation, peripheral edema
EENT: rhinitis, sinusitis, pharyngitis
GI: nausea, vomiting, diarrhea, constipation, abdominal pain, dyspepsia, flatulence, gastritis, gastroenteritis, **pancreatitis**
GU: urinary tract infection, **myoglobinuria, acute renal failure**
Hepatic: fatal and nonfatal hepatic failure (rare)
Hematologic: anemia

♣ Canada　　✣ UK　　⚕ Hazardous drug　　⊗ High-alert drug

Metabolic: hyperglycemia, diabetes mellitus
Musculoskeletal: myalgia, myopathy, joint pain, **rhabdomyolysis**
Skin: rash, pruritus, urticaria
Other: hypersensitivity reactions (including **angioedema**)

Interactions

Drug-drug. *Antacids:* decreased rosuvastatin blood level
Cyclosporine, gemfibrozil protease inhibitor combinations lopinavir/ritonavir and atazanavir/ritonavir: increased rosuvastatin bioavailability
Hormonal contraceptives: increased contraceptive blood level
Niacin in lipid-modifying doses (1 g/day or more): increased risk of enhanced musculoskeletal effects
Warfarin: increased International Normalized Ratio
Drug-diagnostic tests. *Alanine aminotransferase (ALT), alkaline phosphatase, aspartate aminotransferase (AST), bilirubin, creatine kinase (CK), glucose:* increased levels
Thyroid function tests: altered results
Urine protein: present beyond trace

Patient monitoring

◀€ Monitor CK, creatinine, and urine protein levels closely. Also watch for signs and symptoms of rhabdomyolysis with acute renal failure: CK level above 10 times normal limits, muscle ache or weakness, creatinine elevation, and urine protein level beyond trace, accompanied by hematuria. If these findings occur, withhold drug and notify prescriber immediately.

◀€ Monitor liver function tests 12 weeks after therapy begins, after dosage increases, and at least semiannually thereafter. Reduce dosage or withdraw drug if ALT or AST persists at three times normal levels.

◀€ Temporarily withhold drug in patients with acute, serious conditions predisposing to renal failure caused by rhabdomyolysis (such as sepsis, hypotension, major surgery, trauma, uncontrolled seizures, or severe metabolic, endocrine, and electrolyte disorders).

• Monitor blood glucose, electrolyte levels, and lipid panel.

• Assess vital signs and cardiovascular status, especially for tachycardia and palpitations.

• Monitor for signs and symptoms of respiratory tract infection.

• Stay alert for tremor and asthenia.

Patient teaching

• Tell patient he may take with or without food. If he's using antacids, instruct him to take these 2 hours after rosuvastatin.

• Instruct patient to maintain a standard cholesterol-lowering diet.

◀€ Tell patient to immediately report unexplained muscle pain, tenderness, or weakness (particularly if accompanied by malaise or fever).

◀€ Caution female patient of childbearing age not to take drug if she is pregnant, plans to become pregnant, or is breastfeeding.

• Teach patient how to check blood or urine glucose level and recognize signs and symptoms of hypoglycemia and hyperglycemia.

• Tell patient that foods, beverages, and preparations containing caffeine or ephedra may increase drug's stimulant effect. Encourage him to limit caffeine intake and avoid ephedra.

• Advise patient against heavy alcohol use, which increases risk of liver disease.

• As appropriate, review all other significant and life-threatening adverse reactions and interactions, especially those related to the drugs, tests, foods, and herbs mentioned above.

r

Reactions in **bold** are life-threatening.   ◀€ Clinical alert

ruxolitinib
Jakafi

Pharmacologic class: Kinase inhibitor
Therapeutic class: Antineoplastic
Pregnancy risk category C

Action
Inhibits Janus-associated kinases
(JAKs) JAK1 and JAK2, which mediate the signaling of a number of
cytokines and growth factors important for hematopoiesis and immune
function. Myelofibrosis, a myeloproliferative neoplasm, is known to be
associated with dysregulated JAK1
and JAK2 signaling.

Availability
Tablets: 5 mg, 10 mg, 15 mg, 20 mg,
25 mg

ⓘ Indications and dosages
➤ Patients with intermediate- or
high-risk myelofibrosis (including
primary myelofibrosis, post-
polycythemia vera myelofibrosis and
post-essential thrombocythemia
myelofibrosis)
Adults: 20 mg P.O. b.i.d. for patients
with platelet count greater than
200×10^9/L, and 15 mg P.O. b.i.d for
patients with platelet count between
100×10^9/L and 200×10^9/L. Increase
dosage based on response and as recommended to maximum of 25 mg
P.O. b.i.d. Discontinue after
6 months if no spleen reduction or
symptom improvement.

Dosage adjustment
• Absolute neutrophil count (ANC)
greater than 0.75×10^9/L
• Concomitant use of strong CYP3A4
inhibitors

• Decreased platelet count and
thrombocytopenia
• Failure to achieve reduction from
pretreatment baseline in either palpable spleen length of 50% or 35%
reduction in spleen volume as measured by computed tomography scan
or magnetic resonance imaging
• Platelet count greater than 125×10^9/L at 4 weeks and platelet count
never below 100×10^9/L
• Renal and hepatic impairment

Contraindications
None

Precautions
Use cautiously in:
• renal or hepatic impairment
• end-stage renal disease (creatinine
clearance less than 15 mL/minute) not
requiring dialysis and patients with
moderate or severe renal impairment
and platelet count less than 100×10^9/L (avoid use)
• hepatic impairment in patients with
platelet count less than 100×10^9/L
(avoid use)
• patients with thrombocytopenia,
anemia, neutropenia; patients at risk
for infection
• ANC levels greater than 0.75×10^9/L
• concurrent use of strong CYP3A4
inhibitors in patients with platelet
count less than 100×10^9/L (avoid
use)
• pregnant or breastfeeding patients
• children (safety and efficacy not
established).

Administration
• Administer with or without food
but not with grapefruit juice.
• For patients unable to ingest tablets,
give through nasogastric (NG) tube
by suspending one tablet in approximately 40 ml of water, stirring for
approximately 10 minutes, and
administering within 6 hours after

---

tablet has dispersed. Rinse NG tube with approximately 75 ml of water.
• Obtain CBC before start of therapy.
• Ensure that serious infections are resolved before start of therapy.
◀€ Be aware that thrombocytopenia, anemia, and neutropenia can occur. Manage by dosage reduction, dose interruption, or transfusion. After recovery of platelet count above 50×10^9/L, restart or increase dosing after recovery of platelet count to acceptable levels.
• When discontinuing drug for reasons other than thrombocytopenia, consider gradually tapering dosage, for example, by 5 mg b.i.d. weekly.

Route	Onset	Peak	Duration
P.O.	Unknown	1-2 hr	Unknown

Adverse reactions
CNS: headache, dizziness
GI: flatulence
GU: urinary tract infections
Hematologic: anemia, **neutropenia, thrombocytopenia**
Skin: bruising
Other: weight gain, herpes zoster

Interactions
Drug-drug. *CYP3A4 inducers (such as rifampin):* decreased ruxolitinib C_{max} and area under the curve (AUC)
Mild or moderate CYP3A4 inhibitors (such as erythromycin): increased ruxolitinib C_{max} and AUC
Strong CYP3A4 inhibitors (such as boceprevir, clarithromycin, conivaptan, indinavir, itraconazole, ketoconazole, lopinavir/ritonavir, mibefradil, nefazodone, nelfinavir, posaconazole, ritonavir, saquinavir, telaprevir, telithromycin, voriconazole): increased ruxolitinib C_{max}, AUC, and half-life
Drug-diagnostic tests. *ALT, AST, cholesterol:* increased levels
Hemoglobin, neutrophils, platelets, RBCs: decreased levels

Drug-food. *Grapefruit juice:* increased ruxolitinib C_{max}, AUC, and half-life

Patient monitoring
• Monitor CBC with differential every 2 to 4 weeks until dosages are stabilized, then as clinically indicated.
• Monitor renal and hepatic function tests closely.
• Assess patient for risk of developing serious bacterial, mycobacterial, fungal, and viral infections and promptly initiate appropriate treatment.

Patient teaching
• Tell patient to take drug with or without food but not with grapefruit juice.
• For patient unable to ingest tablets, tell patient or caregiver to give through NG tube by suspending one tablet in approximately 40 ml of water, stirring for approximately 10 minutes, and administering within 6 hours after tablet has dispersed. Then rinse NG tube with approximately 75 ml of water.
• Inform patient of importance of having CBC before starting drug and regularly during teatment.
◀€ Instruct patient to immediately report signs and symptoms of low CBC (unusual bleeding, bruising, fatigue, shortness of breath) or infection (fever, chills, aches, weakness, painful rash or blisters).
• Instruct patient to tell prescriber about all drugs he's taking, because some drugs have potential for serious drug interactions and shouldn't be taken with ruxolitinib.
• Teach patient with end-stage renal disease to take drug on dialysis days after each dialysis session.
• Teach patient about early signs and symptoms of herpes zoster; advise patient to seek treatment as early as possible if these occur.

r

• Advise breastfeeding patient that she should decide whether to discontinue breastfeeding or discontinue drug, taking into account importance of drug for her treatment.

• As appropriate, review all other significant and life-threatening adverse reactions and interactions, especially those related to the drugs, tests, and food mentioned above.

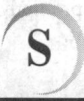

salmeterol xinafoate
Serevent ✦, Serevent Diskus

Pharmacologic class: Beta$_2$-adrenergic receptor agonist (long-acting)
Therapeutic class: Bronchodilator
Pregnancy risk category C

FDA | BOXED WARNING

• Drug may increase risk of asthma-related death. Currently available data are inadequate to determine whether concurrent use of inhaled corticosteroids or other long-term asthma control drugs mitigates the increased risk of asthma-related death from long-acting beta$_2$-adrenergic agonists. Because of this risk, use of salmeterol xinafoate for the treatment of asthma without a concomitant long-term asthma control medication such as an inhaled corticosteroid is contraindicated. When treating asthmatic patients, use only as additional therapy for those not adequately controlled on other asthma-controller medications or whose disease severity clearly warrants treatment with two maintenance therapies (including salmeterol). Once asthma control is achieved and maintained, assess patient at regular intervals and step down therapy (for example, discontinue salmeterol xinafoate), if possible, without loss of asthma control and maintain patient on a long-term asthma-control medication such as an inhaled corticosteroid. Don't use salmeterol for patients whose asthma is adequately controlled on low- or medium-dose inhaled corticosteroids

• Available data from controlled clinical trials suggest that long-acting beta$_2$-adrenergic agonists increase risk of asthma-related hospitalization in children and adolescents. For children and adolescents with asthma who require addition of a long-acting beta$_2$-adrenergic agonist to an inhaled corticosteroid, a fixed-dose combination product containing both an inhaled corticosteroid and a long-acting beta$_2$-adrenergic agonist should ordinarily be used to ensure adherence with both drugs. In cases in which use of a separate long-term asthma-control medication (for example, inhaled corticosteroid) and a long-acting beta$_2$-adrenergic agonist is clinically indicated, take appropriate steps to ensure adherence with both treatment components. If adherence can't be assured, a fixed-dose combination product containing both an inhaled corticosteroid and a long-acting beta$_2$-adrenergic agonist is recommended.

Action

Stimulates intracellular adenylate cyclase, an enzyme that catalyzes conversion of adenosine triphosphate to cyclic-3', 5'-adenosine monophosphate (cAMP). Increased cAMP levels relax bronchial smooth muscle and inhibit release of mediators of immediate hypersensitivity (especially from mast cells).

Availability
Powder for inhalation using Diskus delivery system: 50 mcg/blister (60 blisters)

⚠ Indications and dosages
➤ Maintenance treatment of asthma; prevention of bronchospasm in patients with reversible obstructive airway disease; maintenance treatment of bronchospasm in patients with chronic obstructive pulmonary disease (COPD)
Adults and children older than age 4: 50 mcg (one inhalation) b.i.d. approximately 12 hours apart
➤ Prevention of exercise-induced bronchospasm
Adults and children older than age 4: 50 mcg (one inhalation) 30 to 60 minutes before exercise. Withhold additional doses for at least 12 hours.

Off-label uses
• Cystic fibrosis
• High-altitude pulmonary edema
• Atopic asthma

Contraindications
• Hypersensitivity to drug or its components
• Acute asthma attack

Precautions
Use cautiously in:
• cardiovascular disease, diabetes mellitus, hyperthyroidism
• concurrent use of MAO inhibitors or tricyclic antidepressants (extreme caution required)
• pregnant or breastfeeding patients
• children younger than age 4.

Administration
• To use Serevent Diskus, activate device and hold in horizontal position.
• Make sure patient doesn't exhale into device.
• Preferably, give doses 12 hours apart in morning and evening.

Route	Onset	Peak	Duration
Inhalation	10-25 min	3-4 hr	12 hr

Adverse reactions
CNS: headache, nervousness, dizziness, tremor
CV: palpitations, hypertension, tachycardia, **arrhythmias**
GI: nausea, diarrhea, abdominal pain
Metabolic: hyperglycemia, **hypokalemia**
Musculoskeletal: muscle cramps and soreness
Respiratory: paradoxical bronchospasm
Skin: urticaria, angioedema, rash
Other: hypersensitivity reaction

Interactions
Drug-drug. *Beta-adrenergic blockers:* decreased salmeterol efficacy, increased risk of severe bronchospasm in patients with asthma or COPD
Diuretics (except potassium-sparing): increased risk of hypokalemia and ECG changes
MAO inhibitors, tricyclic antidepressants: potentiation of salmeterol's cardiovascular actions
Drug-diagnostic tests. *Glucose:* increased level
Potassium: decreased level
Drug-food. *Caffeine-containing foods and beverages:* increased stimulant effect
Urine-acidifying foods: increased drug blood level
Drug-herbs. *Caffeine-containing herbs (such as cola nut, yerba maté), ephedra (ma huang):* increased stimulant effect

Patient monitoring
• Assess pulmonary status and vital signs.
◀€ Stay alert for signs and symptoms of hypersensitivity reaction, particularly rash, urticaria, angioedema, and paradoxical bronchospasm.

S

Patient teaching

- Remind patient that drug isn't a rescue bronchodilator and won't give immediate relief in emergency.
- Teach patient proper technique for using inhaler or Diskus. Instruct him not to exhale into device or use a spacer with Diskus.
- Advise patient to keep Diskus dry. Tell him not to rinse, wash, or take it apart.
- Instruct patient to take regular doses 12 hours apart. Tell him to take doses for exercise-induced bronchospasm 30 to 60 minutes before exercising.
- Advise patient to take drug exactly as prescribed and not to exceed one inhalation twice daily.
- Tell patient to consult prescriber if he needs more inhalations than usual.
- Caution patient not to stop taking drug without consulting prescriber.
- As appropriate, review all other significant and life-threatening adverse reactions and interactions, especially those related to the drugs, tests, foods, and herbs mentioned above.

saquinavir mesylate
Invirase

Pharmacologic class: Protease inhibitor
Therapeutic class: Antiretroviral
Pregnancy risk category B

Action
Inhibits human immunodeficiency virus (HIV) protease, preventing cleavage of HIV polyproteins and blocking virus replication and maturation

Availability
Capsules: 200 mg
Tablets: 500 mg

⚠ Indications and dosages

➤ Advanced HIV infection in selected patients
Adults older than age 16: 1,000 mg P.O. b.i.d. given only in combination with ritonavir b.i.d.

Contraindications

- Clinically significant hypersensitivity (for example, anaphylactic reaction, Stevens-Johnson syndrome) to drug or its components and ritonavir
- When administered with ritonavir in patients with severe hepatic impairment
- Congenital or documented acquired QT-interval prolongation, refractory hypokalemia or hypomagnesemia, or concurrent therapy with other drugs that prolong QT interval
- Complete atrioventricular (AV) block without implanted pacemaker, or patient at high risk for complete AV block

Precautions
Use cautiously in:
- hepatic disease, hemophilia types A and B, diabetes mellitus
- pregnant or breastfeeding patients
- children younger than age 16.

Administration
- Give around the clock without missing doses, within 2 hours of a full meal.
- ◀€ Know that drug is given *only* in combination with ritonavir, which inhibits its metabolism. Give both drugs at same time.
- ◀€ Don't give concurrently with CYP3A substrates (such as alfuzosin, amiodarone, bepridil, cisapride, dofetilide, dihydroergotamine, ergonovine, ergotamine, flecainide, lovastatin, methylergonovine, oral midazolam, pimozide, propafenone, quinidine, rifampin, simvastatin, sildenafil when used for pulmonary arterial hypertension, systemic lidocaine,

trazodone, triazolam). Life-threatening reactions may occur.

Route	Onset	Peak	Duration
P.O.	Unknown	Unknown	Unknown

Adverse reactions

CNS: headache, dizziness, paresthesia, asthenia, depression, insomnia, anxiety, confusion, ataxia, **seizures, suicidal ideation, intracranial hemorrhage**
CV: chest pain, peripheral vasoconstriction, **thrombophlebitis**
GI: nausea, vomiting, diarrhea, constipation, abdominal pain, flatulence, dyspepsia, buccal mucosal ulcers, pancreatitis
GU: urinary retention, nephrolithiasis, **oliguria, acute renal insufficiency**
Hematologic: hemolytic anemia, pancytopenia, thrombocytopenia, acute myeloblastic leukemia
Hepatic: jaundice, **portal hypertension, exacerbation of chronic hepatic disease** (with grade 4 elevated liver function test results)
Metabolic: hyperglycemia, diabetes mellitus (exacerbation or new onset), hypercalcemia, **hyperkalemia, hypoglycemia**
Musculoskeletal: musculoskeletal pain
Respiratory: bronchitis, cough
Skin: rash, **Stevens-Johnson syndrome**
Other: altered taste, drug fever, allergic reactions, immune reconstitution syndrome

Interactions

Drug-drug. *Alfuzosin, digoxin, sildenafil when used for pulmonary arterial hypertension, tadalafil, tricyclic antidepressants, vardenafil:* increased blood levels of these drugs
Antiarrhythmics (amiodarone, bepridil, dofetilide, flecainide, propafenone, quinidine), astemizole, cisapride, pimozide, propafenone, systemic lidocaine, terfenadine: increased blood levels of these drugs, life-threatening arrhythmias

Benzodiazepines, calcium channel blockers: increased blood levels of these drugs
Carbamazepine, dexamethasone, nevirapine, phenobarbital, phenytoin, rifabutin, rifampin: reduced saquinavir steady-state level
Clarithromycin, indinavir, ketoconazole, nelfinavir, ritonavir: increased saquinavir blood level
Ergot derivatives: elevated blood level of these drugs, life-threatening reactions such as acute ergot toxicity (peripheral vasospasm and ischemia of extremities and other tissues)
HIV-1 protease inhibitors (atazanavir): possible additive effects on PR interval prolongation
HMG-CoA reductase inhibitors: increased risk of myopathy (including rhabdomyolysis)
Oral midazolam, triazolam: increased risk of life-threatening prolonged or increased sedation or respiratory depression
Nonnucleoside reverse transcriptase inhibitors (delavirdine, nevirapine): increased saquinavir blood level
Rifampin: increased risk of severe hepatocellular toxicity
Warfarin: altered International Normalized Ratio
Drug-diagnostic tests. *Alanine aminotransferase (ALT), amylase, aspartate aminotransferase (AST), bilirubin, calcium, creatinine phosphokinase, potassium:* increased levels
Blood glucose: increased or decreased level
Phosphate: decreased level
Platelets, red blood cells, white blood cells: decreased counts
Drug-food. *Any food:* increased drug absorption
Grapefruit juice: elevated drug blood level, increased pharmacologic and adverse effects
Drug-herbs. *Garlic capsules:* decreased saquinavir blood level
St. John's wort: 50% reduction in saquinavir blood level

S

◀€ Clinical alert

Patient monitoring

◀€ Be aware that immune reconstitution syndrome may occur in patients receiving combination antiretroviral therapy. During initial phase of therapy, patient whose immune system responds may develop inflammatory response to indolent or residual opportunistic infections (such as *Mycobacterium avium* complex, cytomegalovirus, *P. jiroveci* pneumonia, and tuberculosis), which may necessitate further evaluation and treatment.

• Monitor platelet count, CBC, liver function tests, electrolytes, and uric acid and bilirubin levels. Watch for evidence of life-threatening blood dyscrasias and portal hypertension.

• Assess nutritional status and hydration.

• Monitor neurologic status. Stay alert for depression, suicidal ideation, seizures, and signs or symptoms of intracranial hemorrhage.

Patient teaching

• Tell patient to take with food (but not grapefruit juice) or within 2 hours of a full meal. Stress importance of taking doses around the clock on a regular schedule.

◀€ Inform patient (and significant other as appropriate) that drug may cause depression and suicidal thoughts, which should be reported immediately.

• Advise patient to notify prescriber if rash occurs.

◀€ Teach patient to recognize and immediately report signs and symptoms of liver disorder or bleeding tendency.

• Tell patient drug interacts with many other drugs, causing serious reactions. Advise him to discuss all drug use with prescriber before therapy starts.

• Caution patient to avoid St. John's wort and garlic capsules during therapy.

• Instruct female patient not to breast-feed, because she may transmit drug effects and HIV to infant.

• As appropriate, review all other significant and life-threatening adverse reactions and interactions, especially those related to the drugs, tests, foods, and herbs mentioned above.

sargramostim (GM-CSF)
Leukine

Pharmacologic class: Granulocyte-macrophage colony stimulating factor

Therapeutic class: Hematopoietic agent

Pregnancy risk category C

Action

Stimulates proliferation and differentiation of hematopoietic cells that activate mature granulocytes and macrophages of target cells

Availability

Liquid: 500 mcg/ml
Powder for injection: 250 mcg

𝕀 Indications and dosages

➤ Post peripheral blood progenitor cell (PBPC) transplantation

Adults: 250 mcg/m^2/day I.V. over 24 hours or subcutaneously once daily, starting immediately after progenitor cell infusion

➤ Mobilization of PBPCs into peripheral blood for collection by leukapheresis

Adults: 250 mcg/m^2/day I.V. over 24 hours or subcutaneously once daily, continued throughout harvesting

➤ Neutrophil recovery after chemotherapy in acute myelogenous leukemia

Adults: 250 mcg/m^2/day I.V. over 4 hours, starting 4 days after completion of chemotherapy induction

➤ Bone-marrow transplantation failure or engraftment delay
Adults: 250 mcg/m^2/day as 2-hour I.V. infusion for 14 days. If engraftment doesn't occur, may repeat after 7 days of drug hiatus.
➤ Myeloid reconstitution after autologous or allogeneic bone-marrow transplantation
Adults: 250 mcg/m^2/day as a 2-hour I.V. infusion, starting 2 to 4 hours after autologous bone marrow infusion and at least 24 hours after last chemotherapy or radiotherapy dose

Off-label uses
• Crohn's disease
• Melanoma
• Wound healing
• Mucositis
• Stomatitis
• Vaccine adjuvant

Contraindications
• Hypersensitivity to drug, its components, or yeast products
• Excessive leukemic myeloid blasts in bone marrow or peripheral blood (10% or more)
• Within 24 hours before or after chemotherapy or radiation therapy

Precautions
Use cautiously in:
• renal or hepatic insufficiency, fluid retention, pulmonary disorders, pulmonary infiltrates, heart failure, leukocytosis, transient supraventricular arrhythmias
• cancer patients undergoing sargramostim-mobilized PBPC collection
• patients receiving purged bone marrow or previously exposed to intensive chemotherapy or radiation therapy
• pregnant or breastfeeding patients
• children.

Administration
◀€ Don't give within 24 hours of chemotherapy or radiation therapy.
• Add 1 ml of sterile water to powder for injection by directing water stream against side of vial and swirling vial gently to disperse contents.
• Avoid shaking or agitating solution.
• For a final drug concentration below 10 mcg/ml, add human albumin 0.1% to saline solution; then dilute drug in normal saline solution.
• Infuse as soon as possible after reconstitution, but no more than 6 hours after mixing.
• Don't add other drugs to infusion; don't use in-line filter.

Route	Onset	Peak	Duration
I.V.	Immediate	2 hr	3-6 hr
Subcut.	15 min	1-3 hr	6 hr

Adverse reactions
CNS: malaise, asthenia
CV: peripheral edema, tachycardia, hypotension, transient supraventricular tachycardia, **pericardial effusion**
GI: nausea, vomiting, diarrhea, anorexia, stomatitis, **GI hemorrhage**
GU: urinary tract disorder, **abnormal renal function**
Hematologic: blood dyscrasias, hemorrhage
Hepatic: hepatic damage
Musculoskeletal: joint pain, myalgia, bone pain
Respiratory: dyspnea, lung disorder
Skin: rash, alopecia
Other: fever, chills, sepsis, edema, first-dose reaction (respiratory distress, hypoxia, syncope, tachycardia, hypotension, flushing)

Interactions
Drug-drug. *Corticosteroids, lithium:* potentiation of myeloproliferative effects
Vincristine: severe peripheral neuropathy

S

Patient monitoring

• Monitor for dyspnea. Halve dosage and contact prescriber if dyspnea occurs.
• Assess CBC with white cell differential. Check for presence of blast cells, and watch for signs and symptoms of blood dyscrasias.
• Closely monitor vital signs and fluid intake and output. Stay alert for signs and symptoms of fluid overload.
• ◀≋ Monitor liver function tests, and watch for evidence of hepatic damage and bleeding (especially GI hemorrhage).

Patient teaching

◀≋ Tell patient sargramostim is a powerful drug that can cause significant adverse reactions. Teach him to recognize and report serious reactions at once.
◀≋ Instruct patient to immediately report unusual bleeding or bruising or yellowing of skin or eyes.
• Tell patient drug may cause weakness and musculoskeletal pain.
• Inform patient that he'll undergo regular blood testing during therapy.
• As appropriate, review all other significant and life-threatening adverse reactions and interactions, especially those related to the drugs mentioned above.

saxagliptin
Onglyza

Pharmacologic class: Dipeptidyl peptidase-4 (DPP-4) inhibitor
Therapeutic class: Hypoglycemic
Pregnancy risk category B

Action

Inhibits DPP-4 and slows inactivation of incretin hormones, thereby increasing blood concentrations and reducing fasting and postprandial glucose concentrations in a glucose-dependent manner in patients with type 2 diabetes mellitus

Availability

Tablets: 2.5 mg, 5 mg

◉ Indications and dosages

➤ Adjunct to diet and exercise to improve glycemic control in patients with type 2 diabetes mellitus
Adults: 2.5 to 5 mg P.O. daily

Dosage adjustment

• Moderate, severe, or end-stage renal disease
• Concurrent use of strong CYP450 inhibitors

Contraindications

• History of serious hypersensitivity to drug (such as anaphylaxis, angioedema, or exfoliative skin conditions)

Precautions

Use cautiously in:
• renal impairment, history of pancreatitis
• concurrent use of insulin secretagogues or strong CYP450 and CYP3A4/5 inhibitors
• pregnant or breastfeeding patients
• children (safety and efficacy not established).

Administration

• Assess renal function before starting therapy.
◀≋ Before starting drug, identify possible risk factors for pancreatitis, such as history of pancreatitis, alcoholism, gallstones, or hypertriglyceridemia.
• Administer without regard to meals.
• Be aware that drug shouldn't be used for the treatment of type 1 diabetes mellitus or diabetic ketoacidosis.

Route	Onset	Peak	Duration
P.O.	Unknown	2 hr	Unknown

Adverse reactions

CNS: headache
EENT: sinusitis
GI: vomiting, abdominal pain, gastroenteritis, **acute pancreatitis**
GU: urinary tract infection
Metabolic: hypoglycemia
Respiratory: upper respiratory tract infection
Skin: urticaria, **exfoliative skin conditions**
Other: peripheral edema, facial edema, hypersensitivity (including **anaphylaxis and angioedema**)

Interactions

Drug-drug. *Insulin secretagogues (such as sulfonylureas):* possible increased risk of hypoglycemia
Strong CYP3A4/5 inhibitors (such as atazanavir, clarithromycin, indinavir, itraconazole, ketoconazole, nefazodone, nelfinavir, ritonavir, saquinavir, telithromycin): significantly increased saxagliptin effect
Drug-diagnostic tests. *Lymphocytes:* decreased count
Drug-food. *Any food:* increased saxagliptin area under the curve

Patient monitoring

• Monitor blood glucose and hemoglobin A_{1C} levels and renal function tests periodically during therapy.
• Monitor CBC with differential, particularly lymphocyte count, in patients with unusual or prolonged infection.
◀€ Observe patient carefully for signs and symptoms of pancreatitis. If pancreatitis is suspected, promptly discontinue drug and initiate appropriate management.

Patient teaching

• Tell patient to take drug with or without food. Tell patient not to split or cut tablet.
• Teach patient about signs and symptoms of hypoglycemia (blurred vision, confusion, tremor, diaphoresis, excessive hunger, drowsiness, increased heart rate) and how to treat it, especially if taking saxagliptin with other drugs that may cause hypoglycemia.
◀€ Instruct patient to discontinue drug and immediately report signs and symptoms of hypersensitivity reaction (such as hives, rash, or swelling of face, lips, or throat) or pancreatitis (persistent severe abdominal pain, sometimes radiating to the back, which may or may not be accompanied by vomiting).
• Instruct patient to routinely monitor blood glucose level at home.
• As appropriate, review all other significant adverse reactions and interactions, especially those related to the drugs, tests, and food mentioned above.

scopolamine (hyoscine⊕)

Scopoderm TTS ⊕, Transderm-Scop, Transderm-V✤

scopolamine hydrobromide (hyoscine hydrobromide)

Buscopan⊕, Kwells⊕

Pharmacologic class: Antimuscarinic, belladonna alkaloid
Therapeutic class: Antiemetic, antivertigo agent, anticholinergic
Pregnancy risk category C

Action

Acts as competitive inhibitor at postganglionic muscarinic receptor sites

S

of parasympathetic nervous system and on smooth muscles that respond to acetylcholine but lack cholinergic innervation. May block cholinergic transmission from vestibular nuclei to higher CNS centers and from reticular formation to vomiting center.

Availability

Injection: 1 mg/ml in 1-ml vials, 0.4 mg/ml in 0.5-ml ampules and 1-ml vials, 0.86 mg/ml in 0.5-ml ampules
Transdermal system (Transderm-Scop): 1.5 mg/patch (releases 0.5 mg scopolamine over 3 days)

🖊 Indications and dosages

➤ Preanesthetic sedation and obstetric amnesia
Adults: 0.3 to 0.6 mg I.M., I.V., or subcutaneously 45 to 60 minutes before anesthesia, usually given with analgesics
➤ Postoperative nausea and vomiting
Adults: One transdermal patch placed behind ear on evening before surgery and kept in place for 24 hours after surgery. For cesarean section, one transdermal patch placed behind ear 1 hour before surgery.
➤ Motion sickness
Adults: One transdermal patch placed behind ear 4 hours before anticipated need, replaced q 3 days if needed

Contraindications

• Hypersensitivity to scopolamine, other belladonna alkaloids, or barbiturates
• Hypersensitivity to bromides (injection only)
• Angle-closure glaucoma
• Acute hemorrhage
• Myasthenia gravis
• Obstructive uropathy (including prostatic hypertrophy)
• Obstructive GI disease (including paralytic ileus and intestinal atony)
• Reflux esophagitis

• Ulcerative colitis or toxic megacolon
• Hepatic or renal impairment
• Chronic lung disease (with repeated doses)

Precautions

Use cautiously in:
• suspected intestinal obstruction; pulmonary or cardiac disease; tachyarrhythmia or tachycardia; open-angle glaucoma; autonomic neuropathy; hypertension; hyperthyroidism; ileostomy or colostomy
• history of seizures or psychosis
• elderly patients
• pregnant or breastfeeding patients (safety not established)
• children.

Administration

• For I.V. use, give by direct injection at prescribed rate after diluting with sterile water.
• After removing protective strip from transdermal patch, avoid finger contact with exposed adhesive layer to prevent contamination.

Route	Onset	Peak	Duration
I.M., Subcut.	30 min	1 hr	4-6 hr
I.V.	10 min	1 hr	2-4 hr
Transdermal	4 hr	Unknown	72 hr

Adverse reactions

CNS: drowsiness, dizziness, confusion, restlessness, fatigue
CV: tachycardia, palpitations, hypotension, transient heart rate changes
EENT: blurred vision, mydriasis, photophobia, conjunctivitis
GI: constipation, dry mouth
GU: urinary hesitancy or retention
Skin: decreased sweating, rash

Interactions

Drug-drug. *Antidepressants, antihistamines, disopyramide, quinidine:* additive anticholinergic effects

Antidepressants, antihistamines, opioid analgesics, sedative-hypnotics: additive CNS depression

Oral drugs: altered absorption of these drugs

Wax-matrix potassium tablets: increased GI mucosal lesions

Drug-herbs. *Angel's trumpet, jimsonweed, scopolia:* increased anticholinergic effects

Drug-behaviors. *Alcohol use:* increased CNS depression

Patient monitoring

• Assess vital signs and neurologic, cardiovascular, and respiratory status.

• Monitor patient for urinary hesitancy or retention.

Patient teaching

• Tell patient transdermal patch is most effective if applied to dry skin behind ear 4 hours before traveling.

• Caution patient to avoid touching exposed adhesive layer of transdermal patch.

• Advise patient to wash and dry hands thoroughly before and after applying patch.

• If patch becomes dislodged, instruct patient to remove it and apply new patch on a different site behind ear.

• Tell patient that using patch for more than 72 hours may cause withdrawal symptoms (headache, nausea, vomiting, dizziness). Advise him to limit use when feasible.

• Inform patient that his eyes may be markedly sensitive to light during patch use. Instruct him to wear sunglasses and use other measures to guard eyes from light.

• Caution patient to avoid alcohol because it may increase CNS depression.

• As appropriate, review all other significant adverse reactions and interactions, especially those related to the drugs, herbs, and behaviors mentioned above.

selegiline hydrochloride

Apo-Selegiline✦, Dom-Selegiline✦, Eldepryl, Emsam, Gen-Selegiline✦, Novo-Selegiline✦, Nu-Selegiline✦, PMS-Selegiline, Zelapar

Pharmacologic class: MAO inhibitor (type B)

Therapeutic class: Antidyskinetic

Pregnancy risk category C

FDA | BOXED WARNING

• Drug may increase risk of suicidal thinking and behavior in children and adolescents with major depressive disorder (MDD) and other psychiatric disorders. Anyone considering using it for MDD in a child or adolescent must balance risk with clinical need, as depression itself increases suicide risk. With patient of any age, observe closely for clinical worsening, suicidality, and unusual behavior changes when therapy begins. Advise family and caregivers to observe patient closely and communicate with prescriber as needed.

• Drug isn't approved for use in pediatric patients.

Action

Unknown. Thought to increase dopaminergic activity by inhibiting MAO type B in nerve cells, increasing dopamine availability to brain cells.

Availability

Capsules: 5 mg

Tablets: 5 mg

Tablets (orally disintegrating): 1.25 mg

S

◀€ Clinical alert

Transdermal system: 6 mg/24 hours, 9 mg/24 hours, 12 mg/24 hours

⏀ Indications and dosages

➤ Adjunctive treatment of Parkinson's disease in patients who don't respond to carbidopa-levodopa alone
Adults: 10 mg P.O. daily in divided doses. After 2 to 3 days, attempt to reduce carbidopa-levodopa dosage (typically by 10% to 30%). Or initially, 1.25 mg (orally disintegrating tablets) P.O. daily for at least 6 weeks. May increase after 6 weeks to 2.5 mg P.O. daily based on effect and tolerability.
➤ Major depressive disorder
Adults: Initially, apply 6 mg/24 hours patch; increase in dose increments of 2 mg/24 hours up to a maximum dose of 12 mg/24 hours at intervals of no less than two weeks, if needed.

Off-label uses

• Initial therapy for Parkinson's disease
• Alzheimer's disease
• Narcolepsy
• Adjunct in schizophrenia

Contraindications

• Hypersensitivity to drug or its components
• Concurrent meperidine therapy

Precautions

Use cautiously in:
• patients receiving tricyclic antidepressants (TCAs), selective serotonin reuptake inhibitors (SRRIs), or dextromethorphan, carbamazepine, and analgesics such as tramadol, methadone, and propoxyphene
• patients with pheochromocytoma
• elderly patients
• pregnant or breastfeeding patients
• children.

Administration

• Give orally disintegrating tablets in the morning before breakfast; don't give food or liquid 5 minutes before and after administration.
• Give capsules or regular tablets with breakfast and lunch, but restrict foods high in tyramine (such as aged cheese, red wine, yogurt, and smoked high-protein foods).
◀€ Don't give within 14 days of TCAs or SSRIs (5 weeks for fluoxetine because of its long half-life).
• Apply patch to dry, intact skin on the upper torso (below the neck and above the waist), upper thigh, or the outer surface of the upper arm once every 24 hours.

Route	Onset	Peak	Duration
P.O.	Unknown	0.5-2 hr	Unknown

Adverse reactions

CNS: agitation, anxiety, bradykinesia, chorea, confusion, delusions, depression, dizziness, hallucinations, headache, dyskinesias, increased akinetic involuntary movements, insomnia, lethargy, light-headedness, loss of balance, syncope, vivid dreams
CV: orthostatic hypotension, hypertension, new or increased angina, palpitations, **arrhythmias**
GI: nausea, diarrhea, abdominal pain, dry mouth, buccal mucosa irritation (with orally disintegrating tablets)
GU: urinary retention
Musculoskeletal: leg pain, low back pain
Other: generalized aches, weight loss

Interactions

Drug-drug. *Adrenergics:* increased pressor response
Buspirone: elevated blood pressure
Dextromethorphan: brief episodes of psychosis or bizarre behavior
Levodopa: increased adverse reactions to levodopa
Meperidine and analgesics such as tramadol, methadone, and propoxyphene: stupor, muscle rigidity, severe agitation, fever, death

Other MAO inhibitors: hypertensive crisis
SSRIs, TCAs: severe mental status changes, CNS toxicity (with possible hyperpyrexia and death)
Drug-food. *Tyramine-rich foods (such as aged cheese, red wine, yogurt, smoked high-protein foods):* hypertensive crisis
Drug-herbs. *Cacao:* vasopressor effects
Ginseng: headache, tremor, mania
St. John's wort: life-threatening adverse reactions

Patient monitoring
• Monitor vital signs and cardiovascular status.
• Assess neurologic status and motor function. Institute safety measures as needed to prevent injury.
• Monitor weight and fluid intake and output.
• Monitor CBC and liver and kidney function tests.

Patient teaching
• Tell patient to take capsules or regular tablets with or without food, but he should avoid foods and beverages high in tyramine. Provide a list of these foods and beverages.
• Instruct patient (and caregiver as appropriate) to take orally disintegrating tablets in the morning before breakfast and not to push these tablets through the foil backing. Tell patient to peel back the backing of one or two blisters (as prescribed) with dry hands, gently remove the tablet, then immediately place the tablet on top of the tongue where it will disintegrate in seconds. Remind patient to avoid ingesting food or liquids for 5 minutes before and after taking orally disintegrating tablets.
• Inform patient to avoid tyramine-rich foods and beverages beginning on the first day of application of 9mg/24hours- or 12mg/24hours-patch and continue to avoid these foods and beverages for two weeks after a dose reduction to the

6mg/24hours-patch or following the discontinuation of the 9mg/24hours- or 12mg/24hours-patch.
• Instruct patient (and caregiver as appropriate) to monitor neurologic status and motor function and to institute safety precautions as needed to prevent injury.
• Instruct patient to move slowly when sitting up or standing, to avoid dizziness from sudden blood pressure decrease.
• Tell patient (or caregiver) that drug may cause serious interactions with many drugs. Instruct him to tell all prescribers he's taking it.
• Tell patient not to use St. John's wort without consulting with prescriber.
• As appropriate, review all other significant and life-threatening adverse reactions and interactions, especially those related to the drugs, foods, and herbs mentioned above.

senna, sennosides
Argoral❄, Black Draught, Ex-Lax Gentle, Fleet Pedia-Lax Quick Dissolve, Fletcher's, Maximum Relief Ex-Lax, Nu-Lax❄, Perdiem, Senexon, Senna-Gen, Sennatural, Senokot, Senokot Granules, SenokotXTRA, Senolax, Sure-Lax✠

Pharmacologic class: Anthraquinone laxative
Therapeutic class: Laxative (stimulant)
Pregnancy risk category C

Action
Causes local irritation in colon, which promotes peristalsis and bowel evacuation. Softens feces by increasing water and electrolytes in large intestine.

Availability
Granules: 15 mg/tsp

Reactions in **bold** are life-threatening.   ◀€ Clinical alert

Liquid: 8.8 mg/5 ml, 25 mg/5 ml,
33.3 mg/ml (concentrate)
Tablets: 8.6 mg, 10 mg, 15 mg, 17 mg,
25 mg
Strips (orally disintegrating): 8.6 mg
Tablets (chewable): 10 mg, 15 mg

⃠ Indications and dosages
➤ Acute constipation; preparation for
bowel examination
Adults and children ages 12 and older:
For acute constipation, 12 to 50 mg
P.O. daily or b.i.d. For bowel preparation, 105 to 157.5 mg (concentrate)
12 to 14 hours before scheduled
procedure.
Children ages 6 to 11: 50% of adult
dosage. Or, two orally disintegrating
strips; don't exceed four strips in
24 hours.
Children ages 2 to 5: 33% of adult
dosage. Or, one orally disintegrating
strip; don't exceed two strips in
24 hours.

Contraindications
• Hypersensitivity to drug or its com-
ponents
• GI bleeding or obstruction
• Suspected appendicitis or undiag-
nosed abdominal pain
• Acute surgical abdomen
• Fecal impaction
• Inflammatory bowel disease (such as
Crohn's disease)

Precautions
Use cautiously in:
• pregnant or breastfeeding patients
• children.

Administration
• Give with a full glass of cold water.
• To prepare patient for bowel examination, give 12 to 14 hours before procedure, followed by a clear liquid diet.

Route	Onset	Peak	Duration
P.O.	6-24 hr	Unknown	Unknown

Adverse reactions
GI: nausea, vomiting, diarrhea, abdominal cramps, nutrient malabsorption,
yellow or yellowish-green feces, loss of
normal bowel function (with excessive
use), dark pigmentation of rectal
mucosa (with long-term use), protein-
losing enteropathy
GU: reddish-pink discoloration of
alkaline urine, yellowish-brown discoloration of acidic urine
Metabolic: electrolyte imbalances
(such as hypokalemia)
Other: laxative dependence (with long-
term or excessive use)

Interactions
Drug-diagnostic tests. *Calcium, potassium:* decreased levels

Patient monitoring
• Assess bowel movements to determine laxative efficacy.
• In long-term use, monitor fluid
balance, nutritional status, and electrolyte levels and watch for laxative
dependence.

Patient teaching
• Tell patient using drug for constipation
to take at bedtime with a glass of water.
• Instruct patient to place orally disintegrating strips on the tongue, allow strip
to dissolve, then drink plenty of water.
• In long-term use, advise patient to
watch for and report signs and symptoms of nutritional deficiencies and
fluid and electrolyte imbalance.
• If patient will undergo bowel examination, advise him to take drug 12 to
14 hours before procedure, followed by
a clear liquid diet.
• As appropriate, review all other significant adverse reactions and interactions, especially those related to the
tests mentioned above.

sertraline hydrochloride

Apo-Sertraline✱, Co Sertraline,
Dom-Sertraline, Gen-Sertraline✱,
Lustral⊕, Novo-Sertraline✱, Nu-
Sertraline✱, PHL-Sertraline✱, PMS-
Sertraline✱, Ratio-Sertraline✱, Riva-
Sertraline✱, Sandoz Sertraline✱,
Zoloft

Pharmacologic class: Selective
serotonin reuptake inhibitor (SSRI)
Therapeutic class: Antidepressant
Pregnancy risk category C

FDA BOXED WARNING

• Drug may increase risk of suicidal
thinking and behavior in children and
adolescents with major depressive disorder (MDD) and other psychiatric
disorders. Risk must be balanced with
clinical need, as depression itself
increases suicide risk. With patient of
any age, observe closely for clinical
worsening, suicidality, and unusual
behavior changes when therapy begins.
Advise family and caregivers to observe
patient closely and communicate with
prescriber as needed.
• Drug isn't approved for treating
MDD in pediatric patients.

Action

Inhibits neuronal uptake of serotonin
in CNS, potentiating serotonin activity;
has little effect on norepinephrine or
dopamine uptake

Availability

Oral concentrate: 20 mg/ml
Tablets: 25 mg, 50 mg, 100 mg

⚡ Indications and dosages

➤ Depression
Adults: Initially, 50 mg/day P.O. depending on response. May increase at weekly
intervals to a maximum of 200 mg/day.
➤ Obsessive-compulsive disorder
Adults and children ages 13 to 17: Initially, 50 mg/day P.O. May increase at
weekly intervals to a maximum of 200
mg/day.
Children ages 6 to 12: 25 mg/day P.O.
➤ Panic disorder; social anxiety disorder; posttraumatic stress disorder
Adults: Initially, 25 mg/day P.O. After 1
week, may increase to 50 mg/day;
depending on response, may then
increase at weekly intervals to a maximum of 200 mg/day.
➤ Premenstrual dysphoric disorder
Adults: Initially, 50 mg/day P.O., either
throughout entire menstrual cycle or
only during luteal phase. For maintenance, 50 to 150 mg/day.

Off-label uses

• Premature ejaculation

Contraindications

• Hypersensitivity to drug or its
components
• MAO inhibitor use within past
14 days
• Concurrent pimozide use
• Concurrent use of disulfiram (oral
concentrate)

Precautions

Use cautiously in:
• seizures disorders, severe hepatic or
renal impairment, increased risk for
suicide
• history of mania
• concurrent use of serotonergic
agents such as tryptophan (use not
recommended)
• pregnant or breastfeeding patients
• children.

S

Administration

• Give as a single dose in morning or evening.

◀€ Don't use rubber dropper when giving concentrate to patient with latex allergy.

◀€ Don't give concurrently with pimozide or within 14 days of MAO inhibitors.

Route	Onset	Peak	Duration
P.O.	Unknown	4.5-8.5 hr	Unknown

Adverse reactions

CNS: dizziness, drowsiness, fatigue, headache, insomnia, agitation, anxiety, confusion, emotional lability, poor concentration, mania, nervousness, weakness, yawning, tremor, hypertonia, hypoesthesia, paresthesia, **suicidal behavior or ideation** (especially in child or adolescent), **neuroleptic malignant syndrome–like reactions**

CV: chest pain, palpitations

EENT: vision abnormalities, tinnitus, rhinitis, pharyngitis

GI: nausea, vomiting, diarrhea, constipation, dyspepsia, flatulence, abdominal pain, dry mouth, anorexia

GU: urinary frequency, urinary disorders, sexual dysfunction, menstrual disorders

Musculoskeletal: back pain, myalgia

Skin: diaphoresis, rash

Other: altered taste, increased appetite, fever, thirst, hot flashes, **serotonin syndrome**

Interactions

Drug-drug. *Adrenergics:* increased adrenergic sensitivity, increased risk of serotonin syndrome

Cimetidine: increased sertraline blood level and effects

Clozapine, most benzodiazepines, phenytoin, tricyclic antidepressants, tolbutamide, warfarin: increased blood levels and effects of these drugs

Disulfiram: disulfiram reaction, indicated by nausea, vomiting, flushing, throbbing headache, diaphoresis, cardiovascular and respiratory reactions (with sertraline oral concentrate)

Drugs affecting serotonergic system (selective serotonin reuptake inhibitors, selective norepinephrine reuptake inhibitors), linezolid, lithium, tramadol, triptans, tryptophan: increased risk of serotonin syndrome

Drugs metabolized by CYP450-2DC or CYP450-3A4: increased blood levels of these drugs

MAO inhibitors: potentially fatal reactions (hyperthermia, rigidity, myoclonus, autonomic instability)

Pimozide: increased pimozide blood level

Sumatriptan: weakness, hyperreflexia, incoordination

Drug-diagnostic tests. *Alanine aminotransferase, aspartate aminotransferase:* increased levels

Immunoassay screening tests for benzodiazepines: false-positive results

Drug-herbs. *S-adenosylmethionine (SAM-e), St. John's wort:* increased risk of serotonergic side effects, including serotonin syndrome

Drug-behaviors. *Alcohol use:* increased CNS effects

Patient monitoring

◀€ Monitor patient's mental status carefully. Stay alert for mood changes and indications of suicidal ideation, especially in child or adolescent.

◀€ Monitor patient for development of potentially life-threatening serotonin syndrome or neuroleptic malignant syndrome–like reactions.

• Evaluate neurologic status regularly. Institute safety measures, as appropriate, to prevent injury.

• Monitor temperature. Watch for fever and other signs or symptoms of infection.

Patient teaching

• Advise patient to take once a day, either in morning or night, with or without food.

- If evening dose causes insomnia, recommend switching to morning dose.
- Instruct patient to mix oral concentrate with 4 oz of recommended liquid only. Advise him to swallow diluted drug immediately after mixing.
- Tell patient using oral concentrate that drug contains alcohol.

◀€ Caution patient not to stop taking drug suddenly. Dosage must be tapered.
- Inform patient that drug may cause serious interactions with many common drugs. Instruct him to tell all prescribers he's taking it.

◀€ Advise patient (and significant other as appropriate) to monitor his mental status carefully and to immediately report increased depression or suicidal thoughts or behavior (especially in child or adolescent).

◀€ Teach patient to recognize and immediately report signs and symptoms of serotonin syndrome or neuroleptic malignant syndrome.
- Caution patient to avoid driving and other hazardous activities until he knows how drug affects concentration and alertness.
- As appropriate, review all other significant and life-threatening adverse reactions and interactions, especially those related to the drugs, tests, herbs, and behaviors mentioned above.

sildenafil
Revatio

sildenafil citrate
Viagra

Pharmacologic class: Phosphodiesterase type 5 (PDE5) inhibitor
Therapeutic class: Anti-erectile dysfunction agent
Pregnancy risk category B

Action
Inhibits PDE5, enhancing the effects of nitric oxide released during sexual stimulation. This action inactivates cyclic guanosine monophosphate (cGMP), which then increases cGMP levels in corpus cavernosum. Resulting smooth muscle relaxation promotes increased blood flow and subsequent erection. Also relaxes pulmonary vascular smooth muscle cells and, to a lesser degree, vasodilation in systemic circulation.

Availability
Injection (Revatio): 10 mg in 12.5-ml single-use vial
Tablets: 20 mg (Revatio); 25 mg, 50 mg, 100 mg (Viagra)

🖊 Indications and dosages
➤ Erectile dysfunction
Adults: 50 mg P.O., preferably 1 hour before anticipated sexual activity. Range is 25 to 100 mg taken 30 minutes to 4 hours before sexual activity, not to exceed one dose daily.
➤ Pulmonary hypertension (Revatio only)
Adults: 20 mg P.O. t.i.d. approximately 4 to 6 hours apart, with or without food. Higher doses not recommended. Or, 10 mg by I.V. bolus t.i.d.

Dosage adjustment
- Hepatic or renal impairment (Viagra)
- Concurrent use of hepatic isoenzyme inhibitors (such as cimetidine, erythromycin, itraconazole, ketoconazole) (Viagra)
- Elderly patients (Viagra)

Contraindications
- Hypersensitivity to drug
- Concurrent use of nitrates (nitroglycerin, isosorbide mononitrate or dinitrate)

S

Precautions

Use cautiously in:

- serious cardiovascular disease (such as history of myocardial infarction, cerebrovascular accident, or serious arrhythmia within past 6 months); coronary artery disease (current or previous) with unstable angina; resting blood pressure below 90/50 mm Hg or above 170/110 mm Hg (current or previous); heart failure (current or previous); renal or hepatic impairment (current or previous); bleeding disorder; active peptic ulcer; anatomic penile deformity; retinitis pigmentosa; conditions associated with priapism (sickle cell anemia, multiple myeloma, leukemia); pulmonary veno-occlusive disease; use not recommended for any of these conditions
- history of uncontrolled hypertension or hypotension
- concurrent use of alpha blockers and antihypertensives (particularly bosentan)
- concurrent use of potent CYP3A inhibitors such as erythromycin, ketoconazole, itraconazole, ritonavir, or saquinavir (use not recommended)
- patients older than age 65
- pregnant or breastfeeding patients
- children (safety and efficacy not established).

Administration

🔇 Don't give concurrently with nitrates.
- Administer Viagra 30 minutes to 4 hours before sexual activity.
- If administering Revatio I.V., give by bolus injection only.

Route	Onset	Peak	Duration
P.O.	Within 1 hr	Unknown	Up to 4 hr
I.V.	Unknown	Unknown	Unknown

Adverse reactions

CNS: headache, dizziness, anxiety, drowsiness, vertigo, transient global amnesia, insomnia, paresthesia, seizures, cerebrovascular hemorrhage, transient ischemic attack
CV: hypertension, hypotension, myocardial infarction (MI), cardiovascular collapse, ventricular arrhythmias, sudden death
EENT: transient vision loss, blurred or color-tinged vision, increased light sensitivity, ocular redness, retinal bleeding, vitreous detachment or traction, photophobia, hearing loss, epistaxis, rhinitis, sinusitis nasal congestion
GI: diarrhea, dyspepsia, gastritis
Musculoskeletal: myalgia
Respiratory: exacerbation of dyspnea
GU: hematuria, urinary tract infection, priapism
Skin: flushing, rash, erythema, pyrexia
Other: hypersensitivity including anaphylactic reactions (rare)

Interactions

Drug-drug. *Alpha blockers, Antihypertensives, nitrates:* increased risk of hypotension
Enzyme inducers, rifampin: reduced sildenafil blood level
Hepatic isoenzyme inhibitors (such as cimetidine, erythromycin, itraconazole, ketoconazole), protease inhibitors (such as indinavir, nelfinavir, ritonavir, saquinavir): increased sildenafil blood level and effects
Drug-food. *High-fat diet:* reduced drug absorption, decreased peak level

Patient monitoring

- Monitor cardiovascular status carefully.
- Evaluate patient's vision and hearing.
- Assess for drug efficacy.

Patient teaching

- Advise patient taking drug for erectile dysfunction to take 30 minutes to 4 hours before sexual activity.

- Tell patient not to exceed prescribed dosage or take more than one dose daily.
- ◀≋ Instruct patient to stop sexual activity and contact prescriber immediately if chest pain, dizziness, or nausea occurs.
- ◀≋ Teach patient to recognize and immediately report serious cardiac and vision problems and sudden decrease in or loss of hearing.
- Inform patient that drug can cause serious interactions with many common drugs. Instruct him to tell all prescribers he's taking it.
- ◀≋ Caution patient never to take drug with nitrates, because of risk of potentially fatal hypotension.
- Instruct patient not to take other PDE5 inhibitors.
- Instruct patient to report priapism (persistent, painful erection) or erections lasting more than 4 hours.
- Tell patient that high-fat diet may interfere with drug efficacy.
- Caution patient to avoid driving and other hazardous activities until he knows how drug affects concentration and alertness.
- As appropriate, review all other significant and life-threatening adverse reactions and interactions, especially those related to the drugs and foods mentioned above.

silodosin
Rapaflo

Pharmacologic class: Alpha₁-adrenergic receptor antagonist
Therapeutic class: Benign prostatic hyperplasia (BPH) agent
Pregnancy risk category B

Action
Selectively inhibits alpha$_1$-adrenergic receptors in the lower urinary tract, relaxing smooth muscle in bladder neck and prostate

Availability
Capsules: 4 mg, 8 mg

Indications and dosages
➤ BPH
Adults: 8 mg P.O. daily

Dosage adjustment
- Moderate renal impairment

Contraindications
- Severe hepatic or renal impairment
- Concomitant administration with strong CP450 3A4 (CYP3A4) inhibitors

Precautions
Use cautiously in:
- moderate renal impairment
- orthostatic hypotension
- cataract surgery (risk of intraoperative floppy iris syndrome)
- concurrent use with other alpha blockers, antihypertensives, moderate CYP3A4 inhibitors, PDE5 inhibitors
- concurrent use with strong P-glycoprotein inhibitors (not recommended)
- females (not indicated)
- children (safety and efficacy not established).

Administration
- Administer drug with a meal.

Route	Onset	Peak	Duration
P.O.	Unknown	2-6 hr	Unknown

Adverse reactions
CNS: dizziness, headache, insomnia, asthenia
CV: orthostatic hypotension

Reactions in **bold** are life-threatening.   ◀≋ Clinical alert

EENT: nasopharyngitis, nasal congestion, rhinorrhea, sinusitis
GI: diarrhea, abdominal pain
GU: retrograde ejaculation
Hematologic: purpura

Interactions

Drug-drug. *Antihypertensives:* increased dizziness and hypotension
PDE5 inhibitors (such as tadalafil): increased risk of symptomatic hypotension
Strong CYP3A4 inhibitors (such as clarithromycin, itraconazole, ketoconazole, ritonavir, strong P-glycoprotein inhibitors (such as cyclosporine): increased silodosin plasma concentration
Drug-diagnostic tests. *Prostate-specific antigen:* increased level

Patient monitoring

• Monitor renal and hepatic function tests closely.
• Monitor blood pressure. Stay alert for orthostatic hypotension.

Patient teaching

• Instruct patient to take drug with a meal.
• Advise patient to move slowly when sitting up or standing, to avoid dizziness or light-headedness from sudden blood pressure decrease.
• Caution patient to avoid driving and other hazardous activities until drug's effects on concentration and alertness are known.
• Advise patient to tell ophthalmologist about taking silodosin before cataract surgery or other procedures involving the eyes, even if patient is no longer taking drug.
• As appropriate, review all other significant adverse reactions and interactions, especially those related to the drugs and tests mentioned above

simethicone (simeticone⊕)

Dentinox Colic Drops⊕, Equalizer Gas Relief, GasAid, Gas-X, Gas-X Extra Strength, Genasyme, Infacol♣⊕, Infantaire Gas, Maximum Strength Mylanta Gas, Mylanta Gas, Mylicon, Mylicon Infant Drops, Ovol♣, Phazyme, Wind-Eze⊕

Pharmacologic class: Methylated linear siloxane mixture
Therapeutic class: Antiflatulent, antifoam agent
Pregnancy risk category NR

Action

Causes gas bubbles to coalesce and allows gas to pass through GI tract via belching or passing of flatus. Silicone antifoam spreads on surface of aqueous liquids, forming a film of low surface tension that causes foam bubbles to collapse.

Availability

Capsules: 95 mg, 125 mg
Capsules (liquid-filled): 125 mg, 166 mg
Drops: 40 mg/0.6 ml, 40 mg/1 ml, 95 mg/1.425 ml
Suspension: 40 mg/0.6 ml, 50 mg/5 ml
Tablets: 60 mg, 62.5 mg, 80 mg, 95 mg
Tablets (chewable): 40 mg, 80 mg, 125 mg, 150 mg, 166 mg

🕭 Indications and dosages

➢ Excess gas in GI tract after surgery or from air swallowing, dyspepsia, peptic ulcer, or diverticulitis
Adults and children older than age 12: 40 to 125 mg P.O. q.i.d. after meals and at bedtime, up to 500 mg/day
Children ages 2 to 12: 40 mg P.O. q.i.d., up to 240 mg/day
Children younger than age 2: 20 mg P.O. q.i.d.

♣ Canada   ⊕ UK   ☠ Hazardous drug   ⊗ High-alert drug

Contraindications
- Hypersensitivity to drug
- Intestinal perforation or obstruction

Precautions
Use cautiously in:
- abdominal pain of unknown cause (especially when accompanied by fever).

Administration
- Give as needed after meals and at bedtime.

Route	Onset	Peak	Duration
P.O.	Immediate	Unknown	3 hr

Adverse reactions
None significant

Interactions
None significant

Patient monitoring
- Monitor GI status to assess drug efficacy.

Patient teaching
- Tell patient to take after meals and at bedtime as needed.
- Caution patient not to take dose higher than indicated on package unless prescriber approves.

simvastatin
Apo-Simvastatin✱, Co Simvastatin✱, Dom-Simvastatin✱, Gen-Simvastatin✱, Novo-Simvastatin✱, Nu-Simvastatin✱, PHL-Simvastatin*, PMS-Simvastatin✱, Ranzolont⊕, Ratio-Simvastin✱, Riva-Simvastatin✱, Sandoz Simvastatin✱, Simvador⊕, Zocor

Pharmacologic class: HMG-CoA reductase inhibitor
Therapeutic class: Antihyperlipidemic
Pregnancy risk category X

Action
Inhibits hepatic enzyme HMG-CoA reductase, interrupting cholesterol synthesis and low-density lipoprotein (LDL) consumption. Net effect is total cholesterol and serum triglyceride reductions.

Availability
Tablets: 5 mg, 10 mg, 20 mg, 40 mg, 80 mg

Indications and dosages
➤ Adjunct to diet to reduce risk of coronary heart disease (CHD) deaths, cardiovascular events, and hyperlipidemia
Adults: Initially, 10 to 20 mg P.O. daily in the evening. For patients at high risk for a CHD event due to existing CHD, diabetes, peripheral vessel disease, or history of stroke or other cerebrovascular disease, initial dosage is 40 mg/day. Range is 5 to 40 mg/day. Restrict use of 80-mg dose to patients who have been taking simvastatin 80 mg long term (for example, for 12 months or more) without evidence of muscle toxicity. Patients unable to achieve their LDL-C goal utilizing 40-mg dose should not be titrated to 80-mg dose, but should be placed on alternative LDL-C–lowering treatment that provides greater LDL-C lowering effects.
➤ Adjunct to other lipid-lowering treatments (such as LDL apheresis) or if such treatments are unavailable for patients with homozygous familial hypercholesterolemia
Adults: 40 mg/day P.O. in the evening.
➤ Heterozygous familial hypercholesterolemia after failure of an adequate trial of diet therapy
Adolescent boys and postmenarchal girls ages 10 to 17: Initially, 10 mg P.O. daily in the evening. Range is 10 to 40 mg/day; maximum dose is 40 mg/day. Adjust at intervals of 4 weeks or longer.

S

Dosage adjustment
• Severe renal impairment
• Concurrent use of amiodarone, amlodipine, diltiazem, fibrates, niacin, ranolazine, verapamil, or voriconazole
• Elderly patients

Contraindications
• Hypersensitivity to drug or its components
• Active hepatic disease or unexplained persistent serum transaminase elevations
• Concurrent use of cyclosporine, danazol, gemfibrozil, or strong CYP3A4 inhibitors
• Women who are pregnant or may become pregnant
• Breastfeeding patients

Precautions
Use cautiously in:
• severe renal impairment; severe acute infection; hypotension; severe metabolic, endocrine, or electrolyte problems; uncontrolled seizures; visual disturbances; myopathy; major surgery; trauma; alcoholism
• history of hepatic disease, liver enzyme abnormalities
• concurrent use of amiodarone, amlodipine, colchicine, digoxin, diltiazem, and lipid-modifying dosages (1 g/day or more) of niacin-containing products, other fibrates, ranolazine, verapamil, or warfarin
• concurrent use of simvastatin in dosages exceeding 20 mg/day with lipid-modifying dosages (1 g/day or more) of niacin-containing products in Chinese patients (avoid use)
• large quantities of grapefruit juice (avoid use)
• elderly patients
• children younger than age 10 (safety not established).

Administration
• Check liver function tests before starting therapy.

• Give with evening meal. Don't give with large amounts of grapefruit juice.

Route	Onset	Peak	Duration
P.O.	Unknown	Unknown	Unknown

Adverse reactions
CNS: headache, asthenia
GI: nausea, vomiting, diarrhea, constipation, abdominal pain or cramps, flatulence, dyspepsia
Musculoskeletal: myalgia, **rhabdomyolysis**
Respiratory: upper respiratory infection

Interactions
Drug-drug. *Amiodarone, calcium channel blockers (such as amlodipine, diltiazem, verapamil), colchicine, other lipid-lowering drugs (such as fibrates or lipid-modifying doses of niacin-containing products), ranolazine, voriconazole:* increased risk of myopathy including rhabdomyolysis
Cyclosporine, danazol, diltiazem, gemfibrozil, nefazodone, strong CYP3A4 inhibitors (clarithromycin, erythromycin, HIV protease inhibitors, itraconazole, ketoconazole, posaconazole, telithromycin): increased risk of severe myopathy or rhabdomyolysis
Digoxin: slightly increased digoxin blood level
Warfarin: modestly increased anticoagulant effects
Drug-diagnostic tests. *Alanine aminotransferase, aspartate aminotransferase:* increased levels
Drug-food. *Grapefruit juice (more than 1 qt daily):* increased drug blood level, greater risk of adverse reactions
Drug-behaviors. *Alcohol use:* increased risk of hepatotoxicity

Patient monitoring
◀€ Watch closely for myositis and other adverse musculoskeletal reactions. Know that drug may cause rhabdomyolysis.

- Monitor liver function tests, CBC, and lipid levels.
- In patients receiving warfarin concurrently, closely monitor prothrombin time and International Normalized Ratio.

Patient teaching

- Advise patient to take with evening meal, but not with large amounts of grapefruit juice.
- Tell patient drug may take up to 4 weeks to be effective.
- ◀€ Caution patient to stop taking drug and contact prescriber if she suspects she is pregnant.
- ◀€ Teach patient to recognize and report signs and symptoms of myopathy or hepatic disorders.
- Instruct patient to avoid alcohol use.
- As appropriate, review all other significant and life-threatening adverse reactions and interactions, especially those related to the drugs, tests, foods, herbs, and behaviors mentioned above.

sipuleucel-T
Provenge

Pharmacologic class: Autologous cellular immunotherapy
Therapeutic class: Antineoplastic
Pregnancy risk category None

Action

Not clearly understood. Induces an immune response targeted against prostatic acid phosphatase (PAP), an antigen expressed in most prostate cancers. During ex vivo culture with PAP-GM-CSF (granulocyte macrophage-colony stimulating factor), APCs (tumor suppressor genes) take up and process the recombinant target antigen into small peptides that are then displayed on the APC surface.

Availability

Suspension for injection: 50 million autologous CD54+ cells activated with PAP-GM-CSF suspended in 250 ml of lactated Ringer's injection in infusion bag

⚠ Indications and dosages

➣ Asymptomatic or minimally symptomatic metastatic castration-resistant (hormone refractory) prostate cancer
Adults: 50 million autologous CD54+ cells activated with PAP-GM-CSF in lactated Ringer's solution by I.V. infusion over approximately 60 minutes; give three complete doses at approximately 2-week intervals

Contraindications

None

Precautions

Use cautiously in:
- cardiac or pulmonary conditions
- infusion reactions
- concurrent use of chemotherapy or immunosuppressive therapy.

Administration

- Be aware that drug is for autologous use only.
- Don't infuse drug until confirmation of product release has been received from manufacturer.
- Premedicate with acetaminophen and an antihistamine such as diphenhydramine approximately 30 minutes before infusing drug, to prevent infusion reactions.
- Administer by I.V. infusion only. Don't use a cell filter.
- Gently mix and resuspend bag's contents; inspect for clumps and clots. Small clumps of cellular material should disperse with gentle manual mixing. Don't administer if bag leaks during handling or if clumps remain in bag.
- ◀€ Interrupt or slow infusion for acute infusion reactions. If infusion

S

Reactions in **bold** are life-threatening.   ◀€ Clinical alert

must be interrupted, don't resume infusion if infusion bag is held at room temperature for more than 3 hours.
• Observe patient for at least 30 minutes after each infusion.
• Be aware that if patient is unable to receive scheduled infusion for any reason, patient will need to undergo an additional leukapheresis procedure if course of treatment is to be continued.
• Be aware that drug isn't recommended for patients with visceral disease and less than 6-month life expectancy.

Route	Onset	Peak	Duration
I.V.	Unknown	Unknown	Unknown

Adverse reactions

CNS: headache, dizziness, fatigue, paresthesia, asthenia, insomnia, tremor, **cerebrovascular events**
CV: hypertension
GI: nausea, vomiting, diarrhea, constipation, anorexia, oral paresthesia
GU: hematuria, urinary tract infection
Hematologic: anemia
Musculoskeletal: back pain, joint and muscle ache, extremity pain, muscle and bone pain, neck pain, muscle spasms
Respiratory: dyspnea, upper respiratory tract infection, cough
Skin: rash
Other: chills, fever, pain, citrate toxicity, influenza-like illness, peripheral edema, hot flushes, chest pain, sweating, weight loss, **risk of transmitting infectious diseases, acute infusion reactions**

Interactions

None

Patient monitoring

◀€ Continue to observe patient for infusion reaction after each infusion.
◀€ Monitor patient for cerebrovascular events, including hemorrhagic and ischemic strokes.

Patient teaching

• Inform patient that each infusion is preceded by a leukapheresis procedure approximately 3 days before drug infusion and that it's important to maintain all scheduled appointments and arrive at each appointment on time, because the leukapheresis and infusions must be appropriately spaced and drug expiration time must not be exceeded.
• Explain importance of premedication before starting infusion.
◀€ Instruct patient to immediately report signs and symptoms of acute infusion reactions (such as fever, chills, fatigue, breathing problems, dizziness, high blood pressure, nausea, vomiting, headache, or muscle aches).
• Instruct patient to promptly notify prescriber if fever or swelling or redness around catheter site occurs, because these could indicate an infected catheter.
• Instruct patient to tell prescriber about all drugs he's taking, especially immunosuppressants.
• As appropriate, review all other significant and life-threatening adverse reactions mentioned above.

sirolimus
Rapamune

Pharmacologic class: Macrocyclic lactone
Therapeutic class: Immunosuppressant
Pregnancy risk category C

FDA BOXED WARNING

• Immunosuppression may increase patient's susceptibility to infection and lymphoma development. Give under supervision of physician experienced in immunosuppressive therapy and

---

management of renal transplant patients, in facility with adequate diagnostic and treatment resources. Physician responsible for maintenance therapy should have complete information needed for patient follow-up.

• Safety and efficacy of sirolimus as an immunosuppressant haven't been established in liver or lung transplant patients; therefore, such use isn't recommended.

• Sirolimus in combination with tacrolimus was associated with excess mortality and graft loss in a study in de novo liver transplant patients. Many of these patients had evidence of infection at or near time of death. In this and another study in de novo liver transplant patients, sirolimus in combination with cyclosporine or tacrolimus was associated with an increase in hepatic artery thrombosis (HAT); most cases of HAT occurred within 30 days after transplantation and most led to graft loss or death.

• Cases of bronchial anastomotic dehiscence, most fatal, have occurred in de novo lung transplant patients when sirolimus was used as part of an immunosuppressive regimen.

Action
Inhibits early activation and proliferation of T lymphocytes and inhibits cell cycle progression at a later stage

Availability
Oral solution: 1 mg/ml
Tablets: 1 mg, 2 mg

⚕ Indications and dosages
➤ Prevention of organ rejection in patients with kidney transplants
Adults and adolescents older than age 13 who weigh more than 40 kg (88 lb): Initially, 6 mg P.O. as a single dose as soon as possible after transplantation, then a maintenance dosage of 2 mg P.O. once daily. Usually given with cyclosporine and corticosteroids.

Dosage adjustment
• Mild to moderate hepatic failure

Contraindications
• Hypersensitivity to drug or its components

Precautions
Use cautiously in:
• renal or hepatic disease, cancer, diabetes mellitus, hyperlipidemia, infectious complications
• patients with liver or lung transplants (use not recommended)
• concurrent use of aminoglycosides, amphotericin B, and other nephrotoxic agents
• concurrent use of strong CYP3A4 inhibitors such as ketoconazole, voriconazole, itraconazole, erythromycin, telithromycin, or clarithromycin or strong CYP3A4 inducers such as rifampin or rifabutin (use not recommended)
• pregnant or breastfeeding patients
• children younger than age 13.

Administration
• Administer consistently either with or without food.
• Use syringe provided to withdraw prescribed amount. Dilute oral solution in a glass or plastic (not Styrofoam) cup containing at least 2 oz of water or orange juice. Don't use other fluids, especially grapefruit juice.
• Swirl cup to mix drug thoroughly; discard syringe. Administer diluted drug right away. Then fill cup with 4 oz of water or orange juice, and have patient drink fluid right away.
◀≋ If solution touches skin or mucous membranes, immediately wash affected area with soap and water.
• Wait 4 hours after the cyclosporine dose (if prescribed) before giving sirolimus.

S

Reactions in **bold** are life-threatening. ◀≋ Clinical alert

Route	Onset	Peak	Duration
P.O.	Unknown	1-3 hr	Unknown

Adverse reactions

CNS: headache, drowsiness, paresthesia, hypoesthesia, hypertonia, hypertonia, emotional lability, dizziness, confusion, syncope, malaise, asthenia, depression, anxiety, tremor, insomnia

CV: hypertension, hypotension, tachycardia, chest pain, edema, palpitations, vasodilation, peripheral edema, peripheral vascular disorders, **thrombophlebitis, thrombosis, heart failure, atrial fibrillation, hemorrhage, pericardial effusion**

EENT: abnormal vision, cataract, conjunctivitis, hearing loss, ear pain, otitis media, tinnitus, epistaxis, rhinitis, sinusitis, pharyngitis

GI: nausea, vomiting, diarrhea, constipation, abdominal pain, dyspepsia, hernia, enlarged abdomen, ascites, esophagitis, eructation, flatulence, gastritis, gastroenteritis, dysphagia, stomatitis, mouth ulcers, oral candidiasis, anorexia, **peritonitis**

GU: dysuria, nocturia, pyuria, urinary retention, hematuria, albuminuria, urinary frequency or incontinence, urinary tract infection, pelvic pain, kidney or bladder pain, hydronephrosis, erectile dysfunction, scrotal edema, testes disorders, **oliguria, GU tract hemorrhage, renal tubular necrosis, toxic nephropathy**

Hematologic: anemia, bruising, polycythemia, **leukocytosis, thrombocytopenia, leukopenia, thrombotic thrombocytopenia**

Metabolic: hyperlipidemia, glycosuria, hyperglycemia, diabetes mellitus, hypokalemia, hypophosphatemia, hypovolemia, hypercalcemia, dehydration, Cushing's syndrome, **acidosis**

Respiratory: dyspnea, cough, upper respiratory infection, bronchitis, hypoxia, pneumonia, **atelectasis, pleural effusion, pulmonary edema, asthma, interstitial lung disease (including pneumonitis, bronchiolitis obliterans organizing pneumonia, pulmonary fibrosis)**

Skin: skin ulcers, skin hypertrophy, pruritus, fungal dermatitis, hirsutism, rash, acne, cellulites, **non-melanoma skin cancer**

Other: gingivitis, gum hyperplasia, weight changes, neck pain, fever, abscess, chills, facial edema, flulike symptoms, infection, lymphadenopathy, abnormal healing, , lymphocele, fluid accumulation (including lymphedema, ascites), **opportunistic infections (such as tuberculosis, fatal infections, sepsis),** hypersensitivity reactions **(including anaphylactic/anaphylactoid reactions, angioedema, exfoliative dermatitis, hypersensitivity vasculitis) lymphoma**

Interactions

Drug-drug. *Aminoglycosides, amphotericin, other nephrotoxic drugs:* increased risk of nephrotoxicity

Bromocriptine, cimetidine, clarithromycin, danazol, erythromycin, fluconazole, indinavir, itraconazole, metoclopramide, nicardipine, ritonavir, verapamil, other CYP3A4 inhibitors: decreased sirolimus metabolism and increased blood level

Carbamazepine, phenobarbital, phenytoin, rifabutin, rifampin, other CYP3A4 inducers: decreased sirolimus blood level

Cyclosporine, diltiazem: increased sirolimus blood level

Live-virus vaccines: reduced vaccine efficacy

Drug-diagnostic tests. *Blood urea nitrogen, cholesterol, creatinine, hepatic enzymes, lipids, red blood cells:* increased levels

Calcium, glucose, phosphate, white blood cells: increased or decreased levels

Hemoglobin, magnesium, platelets, sodium: decreased levels

Drug-food. *Grapefruit juice:* decreased sirolimus metabolism and increased blood level

Drug-herbs. *Astragalus, echinacea, melatonin, St. John's wort:* decreased sirolimus efficacy

Patient monitoring

• Watch closely for signs and symptoms of infection and hypersensitivity reactions.

• Monitor renal function tests, lipid panel, electrolyte levels, blood chemistry studies, and sirolimus blood level.

• Evaluate all body systems carefully, especially cardiovascular, respiratory, and renal.

• Assess neurologic status closely. Implement safety precautions as needed to prevent injury.

• Be aware that cases of *Pneumocystis carinii* pneumonia have occurred in patients not receiving antimicrobial prophylaxis. Therefore, antimicrobial prophylaxis for *P. carinii* pneumonia should be administered for 1 year following transplantation. In addition, cytomegalovirus (CMV) prophylaxis is recommended for 3 months after transplantation, particularly for patients at increased risk for CMV disease.

• Watch for abnormal wound healing, especially in patients with body mass index greater than 30 kg/m^2.

Patient teaching

• Teach patient correct procedure for taking drug.

• Advise patient to take consistently either with or without food, but not with grapefruit juice.

• Instruct patient to wait 4 hours after cyclosporine dose (if prescribed) before taking sirolimus.

◀╞ Tell patient to wash affected area with soap and water immediately if drug touches his skin or mucous membranes.

• Inform patient that drug affects almost every body system. Advise him to report significant adverse reactions.

◀╞ Advise patient that drug lowers resistance to infection. Instruct him to immediately report fever, cough, breathing problems, sore throat, or other signs and symptoms of infection.

• Caution patient to avoid driving and other hazardous activities until he knows how drug affects concentration and alertness.

◀╞ Instruct patient to immediately report unusual bleeding or bruising.

◀╞ Advise female patient to use effective contraception before and during therapy and for 12 weeks after discontinuation.

◀╞ Caution patient to limit exposure to sunlight and ultraviolet light. Advise him to wear protective clothing and to use sunscreen with a high protection factor to help prevent skin cancer.

• As appropriate, review all other significant and life-threatening adverse reactions and interactions, especially those related to the drugs, tests, foods, and herbs mentioned above.

sitagliptin phosphate
Januvia

Pharmacologic class: Dipeptidyl peptidase 4 (DPP-4) inhibitor

Therapeutic class: Hypoglycemic

Pregnancy risk category B

Action

Inhibits DPP-4 and slows inactivation of incretin hormones, helping to regulate glucose homeostasis through increased insulin release and decreased glucagon levels

S

Availability
Tablets: 25 mg, 50 mg, 100 mg

🖊 Indications and dosages
➤ Adjunct to diet and exercise to improve glycemic control in type 2 diabetes mellitus
Adults: 100 mg P.O. once daily

Dosage adjustment
• Moderate to severe renal insufficiency or end-stage renal disease

Contraindications
• History of serious hypersensitivity to drug (such as anaphylaxis or angioedema)

Precautions
Use cautiously in:
• concurrent administration of drugs that cause hypoglycemia (such as sulfonylureas or insulin)
• renal impairment, history of pancreatitis
• pregnant or breastfeeding patients
• children younger than age 18 (safety and efficacy not established).

Administration
• Assess renal function before starting therapy.
◀€ Before starting drug, ask patient about possible risk factors for pancreatitis, such as history of pancreatitis, alcoholism, gallstones, or hypertriglyceridemia. However, it's unknown if these conditions make it more likely that pancreatitis will occur.
• Give with or without food.
• Be aware that drug shouldn't be used to treat type 1 diabetes mellitus or diabetic ketoacidosis.
• Know that when drug is used with a sulfonylurea, a lower dose of sulfonylurea may be required, to reduce risk of hypoglycemia.

Route	Onset	Peak	Duration
P.O.	Rapid	1-4 hr	Unknown

Adverse reactions
CNS: headache
EENT: nasopharyngitis
GI: abdominal pain, nausea, vomiting, diarrhea, **pancreatitis**
GU: acute renal failure
Respiratory: upper respiratory tract infection
Other: hypersensitivity reactions (including **anaphylaxis, angioedema, exfoliative skin conditions such as Stevens-Johnson syndrome**)

Interactions
Drug-drug. *Digoxin:* minimally increased digoxin effect and blood level
Insulin, sulfonylureas: possible increased hypoglycemia risk

Patient monitoring
• Monitor renal function periodically.
• Measure patient's weight and body mass index periodically during therapy.
• Monitor blood glucose and hemoglobin A_{1c} levels periodically during therapy.
◀€ Monitor patient for signs and symptoms of hypersensitivity reactions and immediately stop drug and institute emergency measures if such reactions occur.
• Check for diabetes signs and symptoms and disease progression routinely during therapy.
◀€ Be aware of postmarketing reports of acute pancreatitis, including fatal and nonfatal hemorrhagic or necrotizing pancreatitis. If pancreatitis is suspected, promptly discontinue drug.

Patient teaching
• Instruct patient to take drug with or without food.
• Teach patient about signs and symptoms of hypoglycemia (such as blurred vision, confusion, tremor, sweating, excessive hunger, drowsiness, and fast heart rate).

🍁 Canada   ⊕ UK   ⚗ Hazardous drug   ⊗ High-alert drug

◀፝ Teach patient about signs and symptoms of hypersensitivity reactions (such as rash, throat swelling, or difficulty breathing) and to immediately contact prescriber if these occur.

◀፝ Instruct patient to immediately discontinue drug and report if signs and symptoms of pancreatitis occur (persistent severe abdominal pain, sometimes radiating to the back, which may or may not be accompanied by vomiting).

• Instruct patient to routinely monitor blood glucose levels at home.

• As appropriate, review all other significant adverse reactions and interactions, especially those related to the drugs mentioned above.

sodium bicarbonate
Arm & Hammer Baking Soda, Bell/ans, Citrocarbonate, Naturalyte✤

Pharmacologic class: Fluid and electrolyte agent
Therapeutic class: Alkalinizer, antacid
Pregnancy risk category C

Action
Restores body's buffering capacity; neutralizes excess acid

Availability
Injection: 4% (2.4 mEq/5 ml), 4.2% (5 mEq/10 ml), 5% (297.5 mEq/500 ml), 7.5% (8.92 mEq/10 ml and 44.6 mEq/50 ml), 8.4% (10 mEq/10 ml and 50 mEq/50 ml)
Oral solution (Citrocarbonate): sodium 30.46 mEq/3.9 g and sodium citrate 1.82 g/3.9 g
Tablets: 325 mg, 650 mg

❼ Indications and dosages
➤ Metabolic acidosis

Adults and children: 2 to 5 mEq/kg by I.V. infusion over 4 to 8 hours. However, dosage highly individualized based on patient's condition and blood pH and carbon dioxide content.
➤ Urinary alkalization
Adults: Initially, 4 g P.O.; then 1 to 2 g P.O. q 4 hours
Children: 1 to 10 mEq/kg/day P.O. in divided doses given q 4 to 6 hours
➤ Renal tubular acidosis
Adults: For distal tubular acidosis, 0.5 to 2 mEq/kg P.O. daily in four to five equal doses. For proximal tubular acidosis, 4 to 10 mEq/kg P.O. daily in divided doses.
➤ Antacid
Adults: 300 mg to 2 g P.O. up to q.i.d., given with a glass of water

Contraindications
• Hypocalcemia
• Metabolic or respiratory alkalosis
• Hypernatremia
• Hypokalemia
• Severe pulmonary edema
• Seizures
• Vomiting resulting in chloride loss
• Diuretic use resulting in hypochloremic alkalosis
• Acute ingestion of mineral acids (with oral form)

Precautions
Use cautiously in:
• renal insufficiency, heart failure, hypertension, peptic ulcer, cirrhosis, toxemia
• pregnant patients.

Administration
• For I.V. use, infuse at prescribed rate using controlled infusion device.
◀፝ Don't give concurrently with calcium or catecholamines (such as norepinephrine, dobutamine, dopamine). If patient is receiving sodium bicarbonate with any of these drugs, flush I.V. line thoroughly after each dose to prevent contact between drugs.

S

Route	Onset	Peak	Duration
P.O.	Unknown	Unknown	Unknown
I.V.	Immediate	Immediate	Unknown

Adverse reactions

CNS: headache, irritability, confusion, stimulation, tremors, twitching, hyperreflexia, weakness, **seizures of alkalosis**, **tetany**

CV: irregular pulse, edema, **cardiac arrest**

GI: gastric distention, belching, flatulence, acid reflux, **paralytic ileus**

GU: renal calculi

Metabolic: hypokalemia, fluid retention, hypernatremia, **hyperosmolarity** (with overdose), **metabolic alkalosis**

Respiratory: slow and shallow respirations, **cyanosis, apnea**

Other: weight gain, pain and inflammation at I.V. site

Interactions

Drug-drug. *Anorexiants, flecainide, mecamylamine, methenamine, quinidine, sympathomimetics:* increased urinary alkalization, decreased renal clearance of these drugs

Chlorpropamide, lithium, methotrexate, salicylates, tetracycline: increased renal clearance and decreased efficacy of these drugs

Enteric-coated tablets: premature gastric release of these drugs

Drug-diagnostic tests. *Lactate, potassium, sodium:* increased levels

Drug-herbs. *Oak bark:* decreased sodium bicarbonate action

Patient monitoring

◀€ When giving I.V., closely monitor arterial blood gas results and electrolyte levels.

◀€ Stay alert for signs and symptoms of metabolic alkalosis and electrolyte imbalances.

• Monitor fluid intake and output. Assess for fluid overload.

◀€ Avoid rapid infusion, which may cause tetany.

• Watch for inflammation at I.V. site.

Patient teaching

• Tell patient using drug as antacid that too much sodium bicarbonate can cause systemic problems. Urge him to use only the amount approved by prescriber.

• Advise patient not to take oral form with milk. Caution him to avoid the herb oak bark.

• Tell patient sodium bicarbonate interferes with action of many common drugs. Instruct him to notify all prescribers if he's taking oral sodium bicarbonate on a regular basis.

• As appropriate, review all other significant and life-threatening adverse reactions and interactions, especially those related to the drugs, tests, and herbs mentioned above.

sodium chloride

Minims Sodium Chloride✦, Slo-Salt, Slow Sodium

Pharmacologic class: Electrolyte supplement

Therapeutic class: Sodium replacement

Pregnancy risk category C

Action

Replaces deficiencies of sodium and chloride and maintains these electrolytes at adequate levels

Availability

Injection: 0.45% sodium chloride—25 ml, 50 ml, 150 ml, 250 ml, 500 ml, 1,000 ml; 0.9% sodium chloride—2 ml, 3 ml, 5 ml, 10 ml, 20 ml, 25 ml, 30 ml, 50 ml, 100 ml, 150 ml, 250 ml, 500 ml, 1,000 ml; 3% sodium

chloride—500 ml; 5% sodium
chloride—500 ml; 14.6% sodium
chloride—20 ml, 40 ml, 200 ml; 23.4%
sodium chloride—30 ml, 50 ml,
100 ml, 200 ml
Tablets: 650 mg, 1 g, 2.25 g
Tablets (slow-release): 600 mg

🩺 Indications and dosages

➤ Water and sodium chloride
replacement; metabolic alkalosis; to
dilute or dissolve drugs for I.V., I.M.,
or subcutaneous use; to flush I.V. catheter; as a priming solution in hemodialysis; to initiate or end blood
transfusions
Adults: 0.9% sodium chloride
(isotonic solution) with dosage
individualized
➤ Hydrating solution; hyperosmolar
diabetes
Adults: 0.45% sodium chloride
(hypotonic solution) with dosage individualized
➤ Rapid fluid and electrolyte replacement in hyponatremia and hypochlo-
remia; severe sodium depletion; drastic
body water dilution after excessive
water intake
Adults: 3% or 5% sodium chloride
(hypertonic solution) with dosage
individualized, given by slow I.V. infusion with close monitoring of electrolyte levels
➤ Heat cramps caused by excessive
perspiration
Adults: See product label.

Contraindications

• Normal or elevated electrolyte levels
(with 3% and 5% solutions)
• Fluid retention

Precautions

Use cautiously in:
• renal impairment, heart failure,
edema or sodium retention, hypoproteinemia
• surgical patients.

Administration

◀€ Be aware that sodium chloride
injection is a high-alert drug.
• Dilute I.V. dose per product label.
Infuse slow I.V. to minimize risk of
pulmonary edema.
◀€ Don't confuse normal saline solution for injection with concentrates
meant for use in total parenteral nutrition.
• Avoid salt tablets for heat cramps;
they may pass through GI tract
undigested, causing vomiting and
potassium loss.

Route	Onset	Peak	Duration
P.O.	Unknown	Unknown	Unknown
I.V.	Immediate	Immediate	Unknown

Adverse reactions

CV: edema (when given too rapidly or
in excess), **thrombophlebitis, heart
failure exacerbation**
Metabolic: fluid and electrolyte disturbances (such as hypernatremia and
hyperphosphatemia), **aggravation of
existing metabolic acidosis** (with
excessive infusion)
Respiratory: pulmonary edema
Other: pain, swelling, local tenderness,
abscess, or tissue necrosis at I.V. site

Interactions

Drug-diagnostic tests. *Phosphate,
potassium, sodium:* increased levels

Patient monitoring

• Monitor electrolyte levels and blood
chemistry results.
◀€ Watch for signs and symptoms of
pulmonary edema or worsening heart
failure.
• Carefully monitor vital signs, fluid balance, weight, and cardiovascular status.
• Assess injection site closely to help
prevent tissue necrosis and thrombophlebitis.

S

Patient teaching

 Teach patient to recognize and immediately report serious adverse reactions, such as breathing problems or swelling.

• Instruct patient to report pain, tenderness, or swelling at injection site.

• As appropriate, review all other significant and life-threatening adverse reactions and interactions, especially those related to the tests mentioned above.

---

sodium iodide ^{131}I

Iodotope, Sodium Iodide ^{131}I
Therapeutic

Pharmacologic class: Radiopharmaceutical
Therapeutic class: Antithyroid drug
Pregnancy risk category X

Action

Incorporated into iodoamino acids in thyroid and deposited in follicular colloid, from where drug is slowly released. Destructive beta particles in follicle act on thyroidal parenchymal cells, minimizing damage to surrounding tissue.

Availability

Iodotope
Capsules: radioactivity ranging from 1 to 130 millicuries (mCi)/capsule at time of calibration
Sodium Iodide ^{131}I Therapeutic
Capsules: radioactivity ranging from 0.75 to 100 mCi/capsule at time of calibration
Oral solution: radioactivity ranging from 3.5 to 150 mCi/vial at time of calibration

Indications and dosages

➤ Thyroid cancer

Adults: Dosage highly individualized. Usual dosage for ablation of normal thyroid tissue is 50 mCi P.O., with subsequent dosages of 100 to 150 mCi P.O.
➤ Hyperthyroidism
Adults: 4 to 10 mCi P.O. (usually achieves remission without destroying thyroid). Toxic nodular goiter may require higher dosages.

Contraindications

• Vomiting and diarrhea
• Known or suspected pregnancy

Precautions

Use cautiously in:
• hypersensitivity to sulfites (with some products)
• breastfeeding
• children (safety and efficacy not established).

Administration

 Don't administer if you're pregnant.

• Make sure all antithyroid drugs and thyroid preparations are discontinued 7 days before radioactive iodine therapy begins. Otherwise, consult prescriber about giving thyroid-stimulating hormone for 3 days.

• Instruct patient to fast for 12 hours before therapy starts.

• Know that all doses must be measured by suitable radioactivity calibration system immediately before use.

• For female patient of childbearing age, give drug the week of or week after menstruation.

• Be aware that drug rarely is used to treat hyperthyroidism in patients younger than age 30.

Route	Onset	Peak	Duration
P.O.	Unknown	Unknown	Unknown

Adverse reactions

CNS: unusual fatigue
CV: chest pain, tachycardia
EENT: pain on swallowing, sore throat

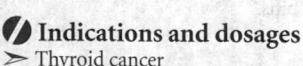

GI: nausea, vomiting, severe salivary gland inflammation

Hematologic: anemia, **leukopenia, thrombocytopenia, acute leukemia, bone marrow depression, other blood dyscrasias**

Metabolic: hypothyroidism, transient thyroiditis, **acute thyroid crisis**

Respiratory: cough

Skin: temporary hair thinning, rash, hives, urticaria

Other: chromosomal abnormalities, neck tenderness and swelling, lymphedema, increase in clinical symptoms, weight gain, **radiation sickness, death**

Interactions

Drug-drug. *Other antithyroid drugs (such as methimazole), iodine, thyroid agents:* altered uptake of sodium iodide ^{131}I

Drug-diagnostic tests. *Hemoglobin, platelets, white blood cells:* decreased levels *Procedures using contrast media:* altered sodium iodide ^{131}I uptake

Patient monitoring

◀≋ Monitor patient to make sure he's following full radiation precautions, including proper body fluid disposal.

◀≋ If you're pregnant, don't provide care to patient who has received this drug.

• If patient has received drug for thyroid cancer, limit contact with him to 30 minutes per shift on first day. Increase as required to 1 hour on second day and longer on subsequent days.

• Monitor thyroxine and thyroid-stimulating hormone blood levels, along with CBC with white cell differential.

• Assess fluid intake and output 48 hours after administration. Encourage high fluid intake.

• Watch for signs and symptoms of hypothyroidism, including fatigue, cold intolerance, depression, and sudden weight gain.

◀≋ Monitor for bleeding tendency and signs and symptoms of radiation

sickness (vomiting, dehydration, skin lesions, and fatigue).

Patient teaching

• Instruct patient to fast for 12 hours before therapy starts and to drink as much fluid as possible for 48 hours after administration.

◀≋ Teach patient and significant other how to follow full radiation exposure precautions.

◀≋ If patient is receiving drug for thyroid cancer, instruct him to avoid contact with small children. Tell him not to sleep in same room with anyone else for 7 days after receiving dose.

◀≋ Teach patient to recognize and report signs and symptoms of hypothyroidism and radiation sickness.

◀≋ Advise patient to immediately report unusual bleeding or bruising.

• Tell female patient to inform prescriber if she is pregnant or plans to become pregnant. Caution her not to breastfeed during therapy.

• As appropriate, review all other significant and life-threatening adverse reactions and interactions, especially those related to the drugs and tests mentioned above.

sodium polystyrene sulfonate

Kayexalate, K-Exit Poudre✤, Kionex, PHL-Sodium Polystyrene Sulfonate✤, PMS-Sodium Polystyrene Sulfonate✤, Resonium A✤, SPS Sodium Polystyrene Sulfonate

Pharmacologic class: Cation exchange resin

Therapeutic class: Potassium-removing resin

Pregnancy risk category C

S

Reactions in **bold** are life-threatening.   ◀≋ Clinical alert

Action

Exchanges sodium ions for potassium ions in intestine; potassium is then eliminated in feces, which decreases serum potassium level.

Availability

Oral or rectal powder for suspension: 15 g/4 level teaspoons
Suspension: 15 g/60 ml

🖊 Indications and dosages

➤ Hyperkalemia

Adults: 15 g P.O. one to four times daily in water or syrup, or 30 to 50 g P.R. q 6 hours; may instill through nasogastric tube as necessary

Contraindications

• Hypersensitivity to drug
• Hypokalemia or other electrolyte imbalances
• Obstructive bowel disease
• Neonates with reduced gut motility; oral administration in neonates

Precautions

Use cautiously in:
• renal or heart failure, severe edema, severe hypertension
• concomitant administration of sorbitol (use not recommended)
• pregnant patients
• children (efficacy not established).

Administration

• Know that drug may take hours to days to lower serum potassium level. Thus, it shouldn't be used alone to treat severe hyperkalemia.
• For rectal use, mix resin in water only; never use mineral oil. Insert #28F rubber tube 20 cm into sigmoid colon, and tape it in place. Or use indwelling urinary catheter with 30-ml balloon inflated distal to anal sphincter. Keep rectal solution at room temperature; swirl gently while administering. After giving dose, flush tubing with approximately 100 ml of sodium-free fluid;

then flush rectum to remove drug residue.
• For oral use, position patient carefully to avoid aspiration that may lead to bronchopulmonary complications.
• In elderly patients prone to fecal impaction, give cleansing enema before sodium polystyrene enema.

Route	Onset	Peak	Duration
P.O.	2-12 hr	Unknown	Unknown
P.R.	Unknown	Unknown	Unknown

Adverse reactions

GI: nausea, vomiting, constipation, fecal impaction, gastric irritation, anorexia, **intestinal necrosis, other serious GI adverse events (bleeding, ischemic colitis, perforation)**
Metabolic: sodium retention, other electrolyte abnormalities, **severe hypokalemia**

Interactions

Drug-drug. *Antacids, laxatives:* systemic alkalosis
Drug-diagnostic tests. *Calcium, magnesium, potassium:* decreased levels
Sodium: increased level

Patient monitoring

◀€ Monitor electrolyte levels. Watch for signs and symptoms of electrolyte imbalances, particularly sodium overload and hypokalemia.
◀€ Be aware that intestinal necrosis and other serious GI adverse events (bleeding, ischemic colitis, perforation) have occurred with drug use. The majority of cases occurred with concomitant use of sorbitol.
◀€ If clinically significant constipation develops, discontinue drug until normal bowel motion resumes. Be aware that magnesium-containing laxatives or sorbitol shouldn't be used to correct constipation.

Patient teaching
- Tell patient drug may cause constipation. Instruct him to report this if it becomes a problem.
- Teach patient about recommended diet (generally, low in sodium and potassium).
- For oral use, instruct patient to mix only with water, or syrup—never with orange juice.
- Advise patient to refrigerate oral solution to improve taste.
- ◀◣ Instruct patient to immediately report serious GI problems, including bleeding and abdominal pain, and early signs and symptoms of hypokalemia, including a pattern of irritable confusion and delayed thought processes.
- As appropriate, review all other significant adverse reactions and interactions, especially those related to the drugs and tests mentioned above.

solifenacin succinate
VESIcare, Vesicare ⊕

Pharmacologic class: Anticholinergic
Therapeutic class: Renal and genitourinary agent
Pregnancy risk category C

Action
Antagonizes muscarinic receptors, reducing urinary bladder smooth-muscle contractions

Availability
Tablets: 5 mg, 10 mg

✪ Indications and dosages
➤ Overactive bladder with symptoms of urge urinary incontinence, urgency, and urinary frequency

Adults: 5 mg P.O. daily initially; may increase to 10 mg P.O. daily if well tolerated

Dosage adjustment
- Moderate hepatic impairment
- Severe renal impairment
- Concurrent use of potent CYP3A4 inhibitors (such as ketoconazole)

Contraindications
- Hypersensitivity to drug or its components
- Urinary retention
- Gastric retention
- Uncontrolled angle-closure glaucoma

Precautions
Use cautiously in:
- hepatic or renal impairment, bladder outflow obstruction, decreased GI motility, GI obstructive disorder, controlled angle-closure glaucoma, congenital or acquired QT interval prolongation
- increased risk of urinary retention or heat prostration
- pregnant or breastfeeding patients
- children (safety and efficacy not established).

Administration
- Give with liquids, with or without food. Make sure patient swallows tablet whole.

Route	Onset	Peak	Duration
P.O.	Unknown	3-8 hr	Unknown

Adverse reactions
CNS: dizziness, depression, fatigue, asthenia
CV: hypertension
EENT: dry eyes, blurred vision, dry throat, pharyngitis
GI: nausea, vomiting, constipation, upper abdominal pain, dyspepsia, dry mouth
GU: urinary tract infection, urinary retention

S

Respiratory: cough
Skin: dry skin, rash, pruritus
Other: influenza, leg or foot edema

Interactions
Drug-drug. *Anticholinergics:* increased frequency or severity of adverse reactions
CYP3A4 inhibitors (such as ketoconazole): increased solifenacin blood level

Patient monitoring
• Monitor GI, renal, and hepatic function frequently.
• Monitor patient for ophthalmic disorders, especially angle-closure glaucoma. If present, stop drug until condition stabilizes.

Patient teaching
• Instruct patient to take drug with liquids, with or without food, and to swallow tablet whole.
• Advise patient to contact prescriber if severe abdominal pain or constipation lasting 3 or more days occurs.
• Caution patient to avoid driving and other hazardous activities until drug effects are known.
• Advise patient of risk for heat prostration; describe symptoms.
• Instruct patient to consult prescriber before taking over-the-counter products such as antihistamines because these may increase risk of side effects.
• As appropriate, review all other significant adverse reactions and interactions, especially those related to the drugs mentioned above.

somatropin, recombinant
Genotropin, Humatrope, Norditropin, Nutropin AQ, Nutropin AQ Pen, Nutropin Depot, Omnitrope, Saizen, Serostim, Tev-Tropin, Zomacton ✪, Zorbtive

Pharmacologic class: Posterior pituitary hormone
Therapeutic class: Growth hormone (GH)
Pregnancy risk category B (Genotropin, Saizen, Serostim), *C*

Action
Stimulates linear and skeletal growth, increases number and size of muscle cells, and influences internal organ size

Availability
Genotropin injection: 1.5 mg (about 4 international units/vial), 5.8 mg (about 15 international units/vial), 13.8 mg (about 41.4 international units/vial)
Humatrope injection: 2 mg (about 6 international units/vial), 5 mg (about 15 international units/vial), 6 mg (about 18 international units/vial), 12 mg (about 36 international units/vial), 24 mg (about 72 international units/vial)
Norditropin injection: 4 mg (12 international units/vial), 8 mg (24 international units/vial)
Norditropin injection cartridge: 5 mg/1.5 ml, 10 mg/1.5 ml, 15 mg/1.5 ml
Nutropin AQ injection: 10 mg
Nutropin AQ Pen injection cartridge: 10 mg
Nutropin Depot: 13.5-mg, 18-mg, and 22.5-mg single-use vials; 13.5-mg, 18-mg, and 22.5-mg kits
Nutropin injection: 5 mg (about 15 international units/vial), 10 mg (about 30 international units/vial)

Saizem injection: 5 g (about 15 international units/vial)
Serostim injection: 5 mg (about 15 international units/vial), 6 mg (about 18 international units/vial)
Tev-Tropin injection: 5 mg
Zorbtive injection: 8.8 mg in 10-ml vial

✔ Indications and dosages

➤ **Growth failure in children with inadequate endogenous GH**
Children: 0.16 to 0.24 mg/kg (Genotropin) subcutaneously q week in six or seven divided doses. Or 0.18 mg/kg/week (Humatrope) subcutaneously or I.M., divided equally and given on three alternate days six times weekly (or daily, if epiphyseal closure hasn't occurred). Or 0.024 to 0.034 mg/kg (Norditropin) subcutaneously six or seven times each week using NordiPen injection pen. Or 0.3 mg/kg/week (Nutropin AQ, Nutropin AQ Pen, Tev-Tropin) subcutaneously in equally divided daily doses. Or 0.06 mg/kg (Saizen) subcutaneously or I.M. three times weekly.

➤ **Endogenous GH replacement in adults with GH deficiency**
Adults: 0.04 mg/kg/week (Genotropin) subcutaneously in six or seven divided doses. Or 0.006 mg/kg/day (Humatrope) subcutaneously. Or initially, no more than 0.006 mg/kg/day (Nutropin AQ, Nutropin AQ Pen, Tev-Tropin) subcutaneously; may increase to a maximum of 0.025 mg/kg daily in patients younger than age 35 or 0.0125 mg/kg/day in patients ages 35 and older. Or 0.005 mg/kg/day (Saizen) subcutaneously; may increase to a maximum of 0.01 mg/kg/day after 4 weeks, depending on patient tolerance.

➤ **Short stature related to Turner's syndrome**
Children: 0.375 mg/kg/week (Humatrope) subcutaneously, divided into equal doses given on 3 alternate days or daily. Or up to 0.375 mg/kg/week (Nutropin AQ, Nutropin AQ Pen)

subcutaneously, divided into equal doses given three or seven times weekly.

➤ **Idiopathic short stature (non–GH-deficient) in children whose epiphyses haven't closed**
Children: Up to 0.37 mg/kg (Humatrope) subcutaneously q week. Divide dosage and give in equal doses six or seven times weekly.

➤ **Growth failure in children with Prader-Willi syndrome**
Children: 0.24 mg/kg/week (Genotropin) subcutaneously in six or seven divided doses

➤ **Infants born small for gestational age**
Children: 0.48 mg/kg/week (Genotropin) subcutaneously in six or seven divided doses

➤ **AIDS wasting or cachexia**
Adults and children weighing more than 55 kg (121 lb): 6 mg (Serostim) subcutaneously at bedtime
Adults and children weighing 45 to 55 kg (99 to 121 lb): 5 mg (Serostim) subcutaneously at bedtime
Adults and children weighing 35 to 45 kg (77 to 99 lb): 4 mg (Serostim) subcutaneously at bedtime
Adults and children weighing less than 35 kg (77 lb): 0.1 mg/kg/day (Serostim) subcutaneously at bedtime

➤ **Growth failure due to chronic renal insufficiency (up to time of kidney transplantation)**
Children: Up to 0.35 mg/kg/weekly (Nutropin AQ, Nutropin AQ Pen) subcutaneously, divided into daily doses

➤ **Short bowel syndrome in patients receiving specialized nutritional support**
Adults: 0.1 mg/kg/day subcutaneously (Zorbtive), to a maximum of 8 mg/day for no more than 4 weeks

Contraindications

• Hypersensitivity to drug, benzyl alcohol, glycerin, or metacresol (with some diluents)
• Active neoplasia

S

• Acute, critical illness after open-heart surgery, acute respiratory failure, or multiple trauma
• Children with closed epiphyses
• Neonates (Zorbtive)

Precautions
Use cautiously in:
• hypothyroidism
• diabetes mellitus.

Administration
• Reconstitute by injecting supplied diluent through rubber top of vial and aiming liquid stream at side of vial. Swirl vial gently to mix; don't shake.
• Inspect reconstituted solution. Don't use if it has visible particles or is cloudy.
• Keep diluted drug refrigerated; use within 14 days.
• When using prefilled cartridges, follow manufacturer's instructions carefully.
• Know that patients receiving Zorbtive for short bowel syndrome may receive specialized nutritional support as needed.

Route	Onset	Peak	Duration
I.M., subcut.	Unknown	1-5 hr	12-48 hr

Adverse reactions
CNS: headache, weakness
CV: mild and transient edema
GU: hypercalciuria
Hematologic: leukemia
Metabolic: fluid retention, mild hyperglycemia, hypothyroidism, **ketosis**
Musculoskeletal: localized muscle pain, tissue swelling, joint pain
Skin: rash, urticaria
Other: pain, inflammation at injection site

Interactions
Drug-drug. *Androgens, thyroid hormone:* epiphyseal closure
Corticotrophin, corticosteroids: inhibited growth response (with long-term use)

Drug-diagnostic tests. *Alkaline phosphatase, glucose, inorganic phosphorus, parathyroid hormone:* increased levels

Patient monitoring
• Monitor patient's height, X-rays, blood chemistry results, blood glucose level, and thyroid function studies.
◀€ Watch for signs and symptoms of leukemia.

Patient teaching
• Advise patient and parents that regular check-ups and blood tests are needed to detect adverse reactions.
• Teach parents how to reconstitute and administer drug. Stress importance of following manufacturer's instructions carefully when using prefilled cartridges.
• Teach parents about proper handling and disposal of syringes, needles, and cartridges.
• As appropriate, review all significant and life-threatening adverse reactions and interactions, especially those related to the drugs and tests mentioned above.

sorafenib
Nexavar

Pharmacologic class: Multikinase inhibitor
Therapeutic class: Antineoplastic
Pregnancy risk category D

Action
Decreases tumor cell proliferation in vitro and inhibits tumor growth of murine renal cell carcinoma; interacts with multiple intracellular and cell-surface kinases, several of which are involved with angiogenesis

Availability
Tablets: 200 mg

Indications and dosages
➤ Advanced renal cell carcinoma; unresectable hepatocellular carcinoma
Adults: 400 mg P.O. twice daily, continued until patient no longer benefits from therapy or experiences unacceptable toxicity

Dosage adjustment
• Bleeding event
• Cardiac ischemia or infarction
• Severe or persistent hypertension
• Skin toxicity
• Major surgery

Off-label uses
• Advanced pancreatic cancer
• Recurrent epithelial ovarian cancer
• Hepatocellular, breast, colon, colorectal, non-small-cell lung, and thyroid cancers
• Melanoma and sarcoma

Contraindications
• Hypersensitivity to drug or its components
• Combination with carboplatin and paclitaxel in patients with squamous cell lung cancer

Precautions
Use cautiously in:
• skin toxicities, hypertension, bleeding, cardiac ischemia, myocardial infarction (MI), congestive heart failure (CHF), bradyarrhythmias, or electrolyte abnormalities
• congenital long QT syndrome (avoid use)
• concurrent use of gemcitabine/cisplatin in patients with squamous cell lung cancer (not recommended)
• concurrent use of drugs known to prolong QT interval (including Class Ia and III antiarrhythmics), CYP3A4 inducers, or CYP2B6 and CYP2C8 substrates

• patients undergoing surgery
• pregnant or breastfeeding patients
• children (safety and efficacy not established).

Administration
• Administer without food (1 hour before or 2 hours after eating).

Route	Onset	Peak	Duration
P.O.	Unknown	3 hr	Unknown

Adverse reactions
CNS: fatigue, sensory neuropathy, headache, asthenia, depression
CV: hypertension, myocardial ischemia, **MI, heart failure, hypertensive crisis, prolonged QT/QTc interval**
EENT: hoarseness
GI: nausea, vomiting, diarrhea, constipation, abdominal pain, mouth pain, mucositis, stomatitis, dyspepsia, dysphagia, anorexia, **GI perforation (uncommon)**
GU: erectile dysfunction
Hepatic: drug-induced hepatitis
Hematologic: lymphopenia, anemia, **leukopenia, thrombocytopenia, neutropenia, hemorrhage**
Musculoskeletal: arthralgia, myalgia
Respiratory: cough, dyspnea
Skin: rash, desquamation, palmar-plantar erythrodysesthesia (PPE), alopecia, pruritus, dry skin, erythema, acne, flushing, exfoliative dermatitis, **Stevens-Johnson syndrome (SJS), toxic epidermal necrolysis (TEN)**
Other: decreased appetite, weight loss, flulike syndrome, fever, hypersensitivity (including **angioedema, anaphylactic reaction**)

Interactions
Drug-drug. *CYP3A4 inducers (such as carbamazepine, dexamethasone, phenytoin, phenobarbital, rifampin):* increased sorafenib metabolism and decreased blood level

S

Docetaxel: increased docetaxel area under the curve (AUC) and plasma concentration

Neomycin: decreased sorafenib mean area under the curve

Warfarin: increased risk of bleeding, elevated INR

Drug-diagnostic tests. *Amylase, bilirubin, lipase:* increased

Hemoglobin, platelets, serum phosphates, WBCs: decreased

Liver enzymes: increased

Drug-food. *High-fat meal:* reduced drug bioavailability

Drug-herbs. *St. John's wort:* decreased sorafenib blood level

Patient monitoring

• Monitor CBC with differential, platelets, serum phosphate, INR, amylase, lipase, and liver enzyme levels.

• Watch closely for PPE.

• Measure blood pressure weekly during first 6 weeks of therapy and thereafter as needed.

◀℥ Monitor for cardiac symptoms, especially prolonged QT interval, in patients with CHF, bradyarrhythmias, electrolyte abnormalities, and concurrent use of drugs known to prolong QT interval. If cardiac ischemia or infarction occurs, consider temporarily or permanently discontinuing drug.

◀℥ If GI perforation occurs, discontinue drug and initiate appropriate measures.

◀℥ Be aware that drug-induced hepatitis may result in hepatic failure and death. Discontinue drug if there is no alternative explanation for significant transaminase elevations (such as viral hepatitis or progressing, underlying malignancy).

◀℥ Monitor patient for SJS and TEN; discontinue drug if either of these conditions, which may be life-threatening, occur.

◀℥ Watch for bleeding. If bleeding necessitates medical intervention, consider discontinuing drug.

Patient teaching

• Instruct patient to take drug 1 hour before or 2 hours after eating.

◀℥ Urge patient to immediately report irregular heartbeats or signs and symptoms of liver disorder or hypersensitivity, including rash, bleeding, or chest pain.

• Advise patient to report symptoms of PPE (redness, pain, swelling, or blisters on hands and soles). Mention that these symptoms may warrant dosage decrease.

• Stress importance of weekly blood pressure checks during first 6 weeks of therapy.

• Instruct males and females to use effective birth control during therapy.

• Tell female with childbearing potential to avoid pregnancy during therapy and for at least 2 weeks after.

• Advise breastfeeding patient to stop breastfeeding during therapy.

• As appropriate, review all other significant and life-threatening adverse reactions and interactions, especially those related to the drugs, tests, foods, and herbs mentioned above.

sotalol hydrochloride

Apo-Sotalol✤, Beta-Cardone⊕, Betapace, Betapace AF, Co Sotalol✤, Dom-Sotalol✤, Gen-Sotalol✤, Med Sotalol✤, Novo-Sotalol✤, Nu-Sotalol✤, PHL-Sotalol✤, PMS-Sotalol✤, Ratio-Sotalol✤, Rhoxal-Sotalol✤, Rylosol✤, Sandoz Sotalol✤, Sorine, Sotacor✤⊕

Pharmacologic class: Beta-adrenergic blocker (nonselective)

Therapeutic class: Antiarrhythmic (classes II and III)

Pregnancy risk category B

FDA | BOXED WARNING

• To minimize risk of induced arrhythmia, patients starting or restarting drug should be placed for at least 3 days (on maintenance dosage) in facility that can provide cardiac resuscitation, continuous ECG monitoring, and creatinine clearance calculations.
• Drug also is indicated to treat documented life-threatening ventricular arrhythmias and marketed as Betapace. However, don't substitute Betapace for Betapace AF because of significant labeling differences.

Action

Blocks stimulation of cardiac beta$_1$-adrenergic and pulmonary, vascular, and uterine beta$_2$-adrenergic receptor sites. This action reduces cardiac output and blood pressure, depresses sinus heart rate, and prolongs refractory period in atria and ventricles.

Availability

Tablets: 80 mg, 120 mg, 160 mg, 240 mg
Tablets (Betapace AF): 80 mg, 120 mg, 160 mg

⬤ Indications and dosages

➤ Ventricular arrhythmias
Adults: 80 mg P.O. b.i.d. (Betapace); may increase dosage gradually. For maintenance, 160 to 320 mg/day in two to three divided doses; some patients may require 240 to 320 mg/day in divided doses. For refractory ventricular fibrillation, may increase to 480 to 640 mg/day in divided doses.
➤ Atrial fibrillation or atrial flutter
Adults: 80 mg P.O. b.i.d. (Betapace AF). With careful monitoring, may increase to 120 mg b.i.d. p.r.n., to a maximum of 160 P.O. b.i.d.

Dosage adjustment

• Renal impairment

Contraindications

• Hypersensitivity to drug
• Uncontrolled heart failure
• Bronchial asthma, chronic obstructive pulmonary disease
• Congenital or acquired long-QT syndrome
• Sinus bradycardia, second- or third-degree atrioventricular (AV) block (unless patient has pacemaker)
• Sick sinus syndrome
• Cardiogenic shock
• Hypokalemia
• Creatinine clearance below 40 ml/minute

Precautions

Use cautiously in:
• renal or hepatic impairment, diabetes mellitus, hyperthyroidism, patients undergoing major surgery
• history of severe allergic reactions
• elderly patients
• pregnant or breastfeeding patients
• children (safety not established).

Administration

• Give 1 hour before or 2 hours after meals or antacids.
• Keep in mind that Betapace and Betapace AF have different indications and are not interchangeable or therapeutically equivalent.

Route	Onset	Peak	Duration
P.O.	Unknown	2-4 hr	8-12 hr

Adverse reactions

CNS: fatigue, weakness, anxiety, dizziness, drowsiness, insomnia, memory loss, depression, mental status changes, nervousness, paresthesia, nightmares
CV: orthostatic hypotension, peripheral vasoconstriction, bradycardia, **arrhythmias, heart failure, AV block**
EENT: blurred vision, dry eyes, nasal stuffiness
GI: nausea, constipation, diarrhea
GU: erectile dysfunction, decreased libido

S

Reactions in **bold** are life-threatening.   ◀€ Clinical alert

Metabolic: hyperglycemia, **hypoglycemia**
Musculoskeletal: joint pain, back pain, muscle cramps
Respiratory: wheezing, **bronchospasm**
Skin: itching, rash
Other: lupus syndrome, hypersensitivity reaction

Interactions

Drug-drug. *Amphetamines, ephedrine, epinephrine, norepinephrine, phenylephrine, pseudoephedrine:* unopposed alpha-adrenergic stimulation, causing excessive hypotension and bradycardia
Beta-adrenergic bronchodilators, theophylline: decreased efficacy of these drugs
Calcium channel blockers: increased risk of adverse cardiovascular reactions
Class IA antiarrhythmics (such as amiodarone, quinidine): increased risk of arrhythmias
Clonidine: excessive rebound hypertension with clonidine withdrawal
Ergot alkaloids: peripheral ischemia or gangrene
General anesthetics, phenytoin (I.V.), verapamil: additive myocardial depression
Lidocaine: increased lidocaine blood level, resulting in toxicity
Sulfonylureas: increased hypoglycemic effect
Drug-diagnostic tests. *Antinuclear antibody:* increased titers
Blood urea nitrogen, glucose, lipoproteins, potassium, triglycerides, uric acid: increased levels
Drug-food. *Any food:* decreased drug absorption

Patient monitoring

• Monitor ECG, electrolyte levels, and vital signs closely for first 3 days of therapy.
• Assess patient closely for signs and symptoms of heart failure.
• In long-term use, watch for signs and symptoms of drug-induced lupus syndrome.

Patient teaching

• Tell patient drug may cause significant cardiac effects. Explain need for ECG monitoring during first few days of therapy.
🔊 Teach patient to recognize and immediately report signs and symptoms of heart failure and electrolyte imbalances.
• Inform patient that drug can cause serious interactions with many common drugs. Instruct him to tell all prescribers he's taking it.
🔊 Teach patient to recognize and promptly report signs and symptoms of drug-induced lupus syndrome.
• Advise patient that drug may cause CNS effects that increase his injury risk. Encourage him to use appropriate safety precautions.
• As appropriate, review all other significant and life-threatening adverse reactions and interactions, especially those related to the drugs, tests, and foods mentioned above.

spironolactone
Aldactone, Novo-Spiroton✶

Pharmacologic class: Aldosterone inhibitor
Therapeutic class: Potassium-sparing diuretic
Pregnancy risk category D

FDA | BOXED WARNING

• Drug induced tumors in chronic toxicity studies in rats. Use only in conditions listed under "Indications and dosages." Avoid unnecessary use.

Action

Inhibits aldosterone effects in distal renal tubule, promoting sodium and water excretion and potassium retention

Availability
Tablets: 25 mg, 50 mg, 100 mg

⚕ Indications and dosages
➤ Edema caused by heart failure, hepatic cirrhosis, or nephrotic syndrome

Adults: As sole diuretic, initially 100 mg/day P.O. (range of 25 to 200 mg) in single or divided doses, continued for 5 or more days and then adjusted to optimal therapeutic level

Children: 1 to 3 mg/kg/day P.O. as a single dose or in divided doses

➤ Essential hypertension

Adults: Initially, 50 to 100 mg/day P.O. as a single dose or in divided doses, continued for at least 2 weeks

Children: 1 to 2 mg/kg P.O. b.i.d.

➤ Hypokalemia

Adults: 25 to 100 mg/day P.O.

➤ Diagnosis and treatment of primary hyperaldosteronism

Adults: For diagnosis, 400 mg/day P.O. for 4 days in short test or for 3 to 4 weeks in long test. Resolution of hypokalemia and hypertension confirm diagnosis of primary hyperaldosteronism. Dosages of 100 to 400 mg/day P.O. may be used as a bridge to surgical therapy; in patients unsuitable for this therapy, lowest effective dosage may be used for long-term maintenance.

Off-label uses
• Acne vulgaris
• Familial male precocious puberty (given with other drugs)
• Premenstrual syndrome

Contraindications
• Anuria, acute renal insufficiency, significant impairment of renal excretory function
• Hyperkalemia

Precautions
Use cautiously in:
• hepatic dysfunction, diabetes mellitus, fluid and electrolyte imbalances, severe heart failure
• concurrent use of other potassium-sparing diuretics, such as amiloride and triamterene (avoid use)
• concurrent use of potassium supplements (avoid use with serum potassium level greater than 3.5 mEq/L)
• concurrent use of ACE inhibitors and nonsteroidal anti-inflammatory drugs (NSAIDs) (use with extreme caution)
• concurrent use of lithium (generally avoid use)
• elderly or debilitated patients
• pregnant or breastfeeding patients
• children (safety not established).

Administration
• Give single daily dose with breakfast. If two daily doses are prescribed, give second dose with food in mid-afternoon.

Route	Onset	Peak	Duration
P.O.	Unknown	1-2 hr	2-3 days

Adverse reactions
CNS: headache, drowsiness, lethargy, ataxia, confusion

GI: vomiting, diarrhea, cramping, gastritis, GI ulcers, **GI bleeding**

GU: gynecomastia, irregular menses or amenorrhea, postmenopausal bleeding, erectile dysfunction, **breast cancer**

Hematologic: agranulocytosis

Metabolic: hyponatremia, **hyperchloremic metabolic acidosis, hyperkalemia**

Skin: rash, pruritus, hirsutism, **drug rash with eosinophilia and systemic symptoms (DRESS), Stevens-Johnson Syndrome, toxic epidermal necrolysis**

Other: deepening of voice, drug fever, hypersensitivity (including **vasculitis, anaphylactic reactions**)

S

Reactions in **bold** are life-threatening. 🔊 Clinical alert

Interactions

Drug-drug. *Angiotensin-converting enzyme inhibitors, NSAIDs, potassium-sparing diuretics, potassium supplements, other potassium-containing drugs:* increased risk of hyperkalemia
Anticoagulants, heparin: reduced hypoprothrombinemic effects of these drugs
Digoxin: increased digoxin blood level
Lithium: reduced lithium renal clearance and increased risk of lithium toxicity
Salicylates: decreased diuretic effect
Drug-diagnostic tests. *Blood urea nitrogen, potassium:* increased levels
Digoxin assays: false digoxin elevation
Granulocytes: decreased count
Drug-food. *Potassium-containing salt substitutes, potassium-rich diet:* increased risk of hyperkalemia
Drug-herbs. *Licorice:* potassium loss

Patient monitoring

◀€ Monitor electrolyte levels (especially potassium), particularly in patients with severe heart failure. Watch for signs and symptoms of imbalances and metabolic acidosis. Interrupt or discontinue treatment for serum potassium level greater than 5 mEq/L or serum creatinine greater than 4 mg/dl.
• Monitor weight and fluid intake and output. Stay alert for indications of fluid imbalance.
• Monitor CBC with white cell differential.

Patient teaching

• Tell patient to take daily dose with breakfast. If two daily doses are prescribed, advise him to take second dose with food in mid-afternoon.
• Advise patient to restrict intake of high-potassium foods and to avoid licorice and salt substitutes containing potassium.
• Tell male patient drug may cause breast enlargement.

• Caution patient to avoid driving and other hazardous activities until he knows how drug affects concentration and alertness.
• As appropriate, review all other significant and life-threatening adverse reactions and interactions, especially those related to the drugs, tests, foods, and herbs mentioned above.

stavudine (d4T)
Zerit

Pharmacologic class: Nucleoside reverse transcriptase inhibitor
Therapeutic class: Antiretroviral
Pregnancy risk category C

FDA | BOXED WARNING

• Lactic acidosis and severe hepatomegaly with steatosis (including fatal cases) have occurred with use of drug alone or in combination with other nucleoside analogs. Fatal lactic acidosis has been reported in pregnant women who received stavudine–didanosine combination with other antiretrovirals. Use this combination cautiously in pregnant women and only if potential benefit clearly outweighs potential risk.
• Pancreatitis (fatal and nonfatal cases) has occurred when stavudine was used as part of combination regimen that included didanosine, in both treatment-naive and treatment-experienced patients.

Action

Inhibits replication of human immunodeficiency virus (HIV) by interfering with the enzyme reverse transcriptase, thereby terminating DNA chain

Availability
Capsules: 15 mg, 20 mg, 30 mg, 40 mg
Powder for oral solution: 1 mg/ml

ⓘ Indications and dosages
➤ HIV-1 infection
Adults weighing 60 kg (132 lb) or more: 40 mg P.O. q 12 hours
Adults and children weighing less than 60 kg (132 lb): 30 mg P.O. q 12 hours
Children weighing 30 kg (66 lb) or more: 30 mg P.O. q 12 hours
Children 14 days and older who weigh less than 30 kg (66 lb): 1 mg/kg P.O. q 12 hours
Newborns to infants 13 days old: 0.5 mg/kg P.O. q 12 hours

Dosage adjustment
• Renal impairment
• Elderly patients

Contraindications
• Hypersensitivity to drug or its components

Precautions
Use cautiously in:
• advanced HIV infection, bone marrow depression, renal failure, peripheral neuropathy, hepatic dysfunction, hyperlactatemia, lactic acidosis
• concurrent use of hydroxyurea or didanosine (avoid use)
• elderly patients (with renal impairment)
• pregnant or breastfeeding patients.

Administration
• Give with or without food.
• Know that drug is usually given with other antiretrovirals.

Route	Onset	Peak	Duration
P.O.	Variable	60-90 min	Unknown

Adverse reactions
CNS: headache, insomnia, peripheral neuropathy
GI: nausea, vomiting, diarrhea, abdominal pain, anorexia, **pancreatitis**
Hematologic: anemia, **leukopenia, thrombocytopenia**
Hepatic: hepatic steatosis, hepatitis, hepatic failure
Metabolic: increased glucose tolerance, **lactic acidosis**
Musculoskeletal: myalgia
Skin: rash
Other: body fat redistribution or accumulation, chills, fever, allergic reaction, **immune reconstitution syndrome**

Interactions
Drug-drug. *Chloramphenicol, dapsone, didanosine, ethambutol, hydralazine, hydroxyurea, lithium, phenytoin, vincristine, zalcitabine:* increased risk of peripheral neuropathy
Doxorubicin, ribavarin, zidovudine: inhibition of stavudine's absorption and metabolism
Myelosuppressants: increased bone marrow depression
Drug-diagnostic tests. *Alanine aminotransferase, amylase, aspartate aminotransferase, bilirubin, gammaglutamyl transferase, lipase:* increased levels
Neutrophils, platelets: decreased counts

Patient monitoring
◀▪ Monitor closely for signs and symptoms of lactic acidosis, hyperlactatemia, or pronounced hepatotoxicity (which may include hepatomegaly and steatosis even in the absence of marked transaminase elevations). Consult prescriber about suspending drug if these occur. Consider permanent discontinuation of drug for patients with confirmed lactic acidosis.
• Monitor patient for signs and symptoms of immune reconstitution syndrome.
• Watch for and report onset and worsening of peripheral neuropathy.
◀▪ Monitor CBC. Report evidence of bone marrow depression.

S

Reactions in **bold** are life-threatening.　　　　◀▪ Clinical alert

• Monitor liver function tests and blood chemistry results.

Patient teaching

• Tell patient he may take with or without food.

 Teach patient to recognize and promptly report signs and symptoms of lactic acidosis (such as fatigue, GI distress, and difficult or rapid breathing), hepatotoxicity, immune reconstitution syndrome, and pancreatitis.

• Instruct patient to report numbness or tingling in arms, legs, hands, or feet.

• Caution female patient not to breastfeed, because she may transmit drug effects and HIV to infant.

• As appropriate, review all other significant and life-threatening adverse reactions and interactions, especially those related to the drugs and tests mentioned above.

streptokinase
Streptase

Pharmacologic class: Group C beta-hemolytic streptococcal nonenzymatic protein
Therapeutic class: Thrombolytic
Pregnancy risk category C

Action

Converts plasminogen to plasmin, an enzyme that degrades fibrin clots and lyses thrombi and emboli

Availability

Powder for injection: 250,000, 750,000, and 1.5 million international units/vial

⏀ Indications and dosages

➤ Acute evolving transmural myocardial infarction

Adults: 1.5 million international units by I.V. infusion over 1 hour as soon as possible after symptom onset. For intracoronary infusion, 20,000 international units by I.V. bolus via coronary catheter, followed by infusion of 2,000 international units/minute over 1 hour (total of 140,000 international units).

➤ Deep-vein thrombosis (DVT)
Adults: Loading dose of 250,000 international units by I.V. infusion over 30 minutes, followed by 100,000 international units/hour I.V. for 72 hours. Begin therapy as soon as possible after thrombotic symptoms begin (preferably within 7 days).

➤ Pulmonary emboli
Adults: Loading dose of 250,000 international units by I.V. infusion over 30 minutes, then 100,000 international units/hour I.V. for 24 hours (or 72 hours if concurrent DVT is suspected). Begin therapy as soon as possible after thrombotic symptoms begin (preferably within 7 days).

➤ Arterial thrombosis or emboli
Adults: Loading dose of 250,000 international units by I.V. infusion over 30 minutes, then 100,000 international units/hour I.V. for 24 to 72 hours. Begin therapy as soon as possible after thrombotic symptoms begin (preferably within 7 days).

Contraindications

• Hypersensitivity to drug or anistreplase
• Cerebrovascular accident, intracranial or intraspinal surgery within past 2 months
• Active internal bleeding
• Intracranial neoplasm
• Severe, uncontrolled hypertension

Precautions

Use cautiously in:
• severe hepatic or renal disease, recent major surgery or trauma,

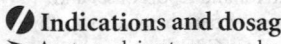

obstetric delivery, acute pericarditis, infectious endocarditis, atrioventricular malformation or aneurysm, suspected thrombus in left side of heart, septic thrombophlebitis or occluded arteriovenous cannula at seriously infected site

• conditions in which bleeding may be hard to manage (such as organ biopsy, peptic ulcer, previous puncture of noncompressible blood vessel)
• history of cerebrovascular disease
• use of drug within past 2 years
• concurrent anticoagulant use
• elderly patients
• pregnant or breastfeeding patients.

Administration

◀€ Before giving, make sure hydrocortisone is available to treat allergic reaction and aminocaproic acid is available to treat excessive bleeding.

◀€ As ordered, give test dose of 100 international units intradermally to check for hypersensitivity. Wheal-and-flare response within 20 minutes indicates probable allergy.

• To reconstitute, add 5 ml of normal saline solution or dextrose 5% in water to each vial, then dilute again to 45 ml. Roll vial gently between hands; don't shake.
• If necessary, dilute further to 50 ml in plastic container or to 500 ml in glass bottle.
• Don't mix with other drugs or give other drugs through same I.V. line.

Route	Onset	Peak	Duration
I.V.	Immediate	1 hr	4 hr
Intra-coronary	Unknown	Unknown	Unknown

Adverse reactions

CNS: headache, **intracranial hemorrhage**
CV: hypotension, **arrhythmias**
EENT: periorbital swelling
GI: nausea, vomiting, **GI hemorrhage**
GU: hematuria

Hematologic: anemia, **bleeding tendency**
Musculoskeletal: musculoskeletal pain
Respiratory: minor breathing difficulties, **bronchospasm, apnea**
Skin: urticaria, itching, flushing
Other: bleeding at puncture sites, delayed hypersensitivity reaction

Interactions

Drug-drug. *Anticoagulants, aspirin, dipyridamole, indomethacin, phenylbutazone:* increased risk of bleeding
Drug-diagnostic tests. *Hemoglobin:* decreased value
International Normalized Ratio, transaminases: increased values
Partial thromboplastin time (PTT), prothrombin time (PT): prolonged

Patient monitoring

• Monitor vital signs and neurologic status carefully after giving test dose and throughout therapy.
◀€ Watch for signs and symptoms of hypersensitivity reaction. Stop drug if these occur.
• Check for bleeding every 15 minutes for first hour, every 30 minutes for next 7 hours, then every 4 hours.
◀€ Stop therapy and contact prescriber immediately if excessive bleeding occurs.
• Assess neurologic status closely. Watch for indications of intracranial bleeding.
• Handle patient gently and sparingly. If necessary, pad bed rails to prevent injury.
• Monitor pulse rate every hour. Also monitor distal circulation.
• Monitor PTT, PT, plasma thrombin time, hemoglobin, hematocrit, and platelet count.
• Avoid giving I.M. injections during therapy.

Patient teaching

• Tell patient why he's receiving drug.
◀€ Teach patient to recognize and immediately report signs or symptoms

S

Reactions in **bold** are life-threatening.   ◀€ Clinical alert

of hypersensitivity reaction or excessive bleeding.

• Instruct patient to report unusual bruising or bleeding. Teach him safety measures to avoid bruising and bleeding.

• Advise patient that he'll undergo regular blood testing during therapy.

• As appropriate, review all other significant and life-threatening adverse reactions and interactions, especially those related to the drugs and tests mentioned above.

streptomycin sulfate

Pharmacologic class: Aminoglycoside
Therapeutic class: Anti-infective
Pregnancy risk category D

FDA | BOXED WARNING

• Risk of severe neurotoxic reactions (including vestibular and cochlear dysfunction) is markedly higher in patients with impaired renal function or prerenal azotemia. Incidence of clinically detectable, irreversible vestibular damage is particularly high.

• Neurotoxicity can lead to respiratory paralysis from neuromuscular blockade, especially when drug is given soon after anesthesia or muscle relaxants.

• Monitor renal function carefully; reduce dosage in patients with renal impairment or nitrogen retention.

• Avoid concurrent or sequential use of other neurotoxic or nephrotoxic drugs, including cephaloridine, colistin, cyclosporine, gentamicin, kanamycin, neomycin, paromomycin, polymyxin B, tobramycin, and viomycin.

• Reserve parenteral administration for settings where adequate laboratory and audiometric studies are available during therapy.

Action

Binds to 30S ribosomal subunit, inhibiting protein synthesis in bacterial cell, which causes misreading of genetic code and, ultimately, cell death

Availability

Injection: 400 mg/ml in 2.5-ml ampules, 200 mg/ml in 1-g vials

⦸ Indications and dosages

➤ Adjunct in tuberculosis and other mycobacterial infections
Adults: 15 mg/kg/day I.M., up to 1 g/day
Children: 20 to 40 mg/kg I.M. daily, up to 1 g/day
➤ Enteroccocal or streptococcal infections
Adults: 1 g I.M. b.i.d. for 1 week, then 500 mg I.M. b.i.d. for 1 week. For enterococcal endocarditis, 1 g I.M. b.i.d. given with penicillin for 1 week, then 500 mg I.M. b.i.d. for 4 weeks.
➤ Brucellosis
Adults: 1 g I.M. once or twice daily with tetracycline or doxycycline for 1 week, then once daily for at least 1 more week
➤ Tularemia
Adults: 1 to 2 g I.M. daily in divided doses for 7 to 14 days until patient is afebrile for 5 to 7 days. For tularemia caused by *Francisella tularensis*, 1 g I.M. b.i.d. for 10 days or 7.5 to 10 mg/kg I.M. b.i.d. for 10 to 14 days.
➤ Plague caused by *Yersinis pestis*
Adults: 1 g I.M. b.i.d. for 10 to 14 days

Dosage adjustment

• Renal impairment
• Elderly patients

Off-label uses

• *Mycobacterium avium-intracellulare* complex in AIDS patients

Contraindications

• Hypersensitivity to drug, other aminoglycosides, or bisulfites

Precautions

Use cautiously in:
- renal impairment, hearing impairment, neuromuscular disease (such as myasthenia gravis)
- elderly patients
- pregnant or breastfeeding patients
- infants and neonates (safety not established).

Administration

- Inject I.M. deep into upper outer quadrant of buttock.
- Alternate injection sites.
- Know that drug may be given with other antituberculars.
- Be aware that streptomycin will be withdrawn after several months or when bacteriologic smears are negative and other antituberculars are continued for 1 year.

Route	Onset	Peak	Duration
I.M.	Rapid	30-90 min	Unknown

Adverse reactions

CNS: vertigo, numbness and tingling, peripheral neuropathy, myasthenia gravis–like syndrome, **neuromuscular blockade, seizures**
CV: myocarditis
EENT: amblyopia, ototoxicity
GI: nausea, vomiting
GU: azotemia, **nephrotoxicity**
Hematologic: eosinophilia, **hemolytic anemia, pancytopenia, leukopenia, thrombocytopenia**
Hepatic: hepatic necrosis
Musculoskeletal: muscle weakness, twitching
Respiratory: apnea
Skin: rash, urticaria, exfoliative dermatitis, toxic epidermal necrolysis, angioedema
Other: fever, superinfection, **serum sickness, anaphylaxis**

Interactions

Drug-drug. *Acyclovir, amphotericin B, cephalosporin, cisplatin, potent diuretics,* *vancomycin:* increased risk of ototoxicity and nephrotoxicity
Depolarizing and nondepolarizing neuromuscular blockers, general anesthetics: potentiation of neuromuscular blockade
Dimenhydrinate: masking of ototoxicity symptoms
Indomethacin: increased streptomycin peak and trough blood levels
Parenteral penicillins (ampicillin, ticarcillin): streptomycin inactivation
Drug-diagnostic tests. *Bilirubin, blood urea nitrogen, creatinine, lactate dehydrogenase, nonprotein nitrogen:* increased levels
Granulocytes, hemoglobin, platelets, white blood cells: decreased levels

Patient monitoring

- Draw blood for peak drug level 1 hour after I.M. injection. Draw blood for trough level just before next dose.
- Monitor liver and kidney function tests. Watch for evidence of hepatotoxicity and nephrotoxicity.
- Monitor temperature. Stay alert for fever and other signs and symptoms of superinfection.
- Assess neurologic status and sensory function carefully. Watch closely for neurotoxicity, neuromuscular blockade, and seizures.
- Assess for signs and symptoms of ototoxicity.
- Monitor CBC. Watch for evidence of blood dyscrasias.

Patient teaching

- Instruct patient to report unusual bleeding or bruising.
- 🔊 Inform patient that drug can be toxic to many body systems. Teach him to recognize and immediately report serious adverse reactions.
- 🔊 Tell patient drug may promote growth of certain organisms. Advise him to immediately report signs and symptoms of superinfection.
- Inform patient that drug may impair cognitive, motor, and sensory function.

S

Reactions in **bold** are life-threatening.   🔊 Clinical alert

Advise him to use caution when driving and performing other hazardous activities.

• As appropriate, review all other significant and life-threatening adverse reactions and interactions, especially those related to the drugs and tests mentioned above.

sulfacetamide sodium
Bleph-10, Diosulf✤, Klaron, PMS-Sulfacetamide✤

Pharmacologic class: Sulfonamide
Therapeutic class: Anti-infective
Pregnancy risk category C

Action
Inhibits bacterial synthesis of folic acid by preventing condensation of pteridine with aminobenzoic acid through competitive inhibition of dihydropteroate synthetase

Availability
Lotion: 10% in 2-oz and 4-oz bottles
Ophthalmic solution: 10% in 5-ml and 15-ml dropper bottles

⍟ Indications and dosages
➣ Acne vulgaris
Adults and children ages 12 and older: Apply thin film topically to affected areas b.i.d.
➣ Superficial ocular infections (including conjunctivitis)
Adults and children ages 2 months and older: Initially, apply one to two drops of ophthalmic solution into conjunctival sac of affected eye q 2 to 3 hours. Taper by increasing dosing intervals as condition responds. Usual duration is 7 to 10 days.
➣ Adjunct in trachoma
Adults: Apply two drops of ophthalmic solution into conjunctival sac of affected eye q 2 hours; must be accompanied by systemic sulfonamide therapy.

Contraindications
• Hypersensitivity to drug or other sulfonamides

Precautions
Use cautiously in:
• sulfite allergy
• dry eye syndrome.

Administration
• To avoid contamination, don't touch container tip to eye, eyelid, or any other surface.

Route	Onset	Peak	Duration
Ophth., topical	Unknown	Unknown	Unknown

Adverse reactions
EENT: conjunctival hyperemia, eye burning, stinging, tearing (ophthalmic form)
Skin: local irritation, erythema, itching and edema (topical form), photosensitivity reaction
Other: secondary infections

Interactions
Drug-drug. *Porfimer:* increased severity of photosensitivity reaction, leading to excessive tissue damage
Silver preparations: precipitation

Patient monitoring
• Monitor patient for drug efficacy. Know that drug may be inactivated by purulent exudate.

Patient teaching
• Tell patient to apply a thin film of lotion to affected areas, as prescribed.
• Teach patient how to apply ophthalmic form. Instruct him to always wash hands first and to clean eye area of discharge by wiping from inner to outer area before applying.
• As appropriate, review all other significant adverse reactions and interactions, especially those related to the drugs mentioned above.

sulfamethoxazole-trimethoprim (co-trimoxazole⊕)

Apo-Sulfatrim❖, Apo-Sulfatrim DS❖, Bactrim, Bactrim DS, Fectrim⊕, Novo-Trimel❖, Novo-Trimel DS❖, Nu-Cotrimox❖, Nu-Cotrimox DS❖, Protrin❖, Protrin DS❖, Septra, Septra DS, Septrin⊕, Sulfatrim, Trisulfa❖, Trisulfa DS❖, Trisulfa S Suspension❖

Pharmacologic class: Sulfonamide
Therapeutic class: Anti-infective
Pregnancy risk category C

Action

Sulfamethoxazole inhibits bacterial synthesis of dihydrofolic acid by competing with para-aminobenzoic acid (PABA). Trimethoprim inhibits enzymes of folic acid pathways.

Availability

Injection: 80 mg/ml sulfamethoxazole and 16 mg/ml trimethoprim
Suspension: 200 mg sulfamethoxazole and 40 mg trimethoprim/5 ml
Tablets: 400 mg sulfamethoxazole and 80 mg trimethoprim (single strength); 800 mg sulfamethoxazole and 160 mg trimethoprim (double strength)

Indications and dosages

➤ Urinary tract infections caused by susceptible organisms
Adults: One double-strength tablet or two single-strength tablets or 20 ml suspension P.O. q 12 hours for 10 to 14 days
Children ages 2 months and older: 40 mg/kg sulfamethoxazole and 8 mg/kg trimethoprim P.O. q 12 hours for 10 days
➤ Severe urinary tract infections caused by susceptible organisms

Adults and children ages 2 months and older: 8 to 10 mg/kg (based on trimethoprim component) I.V. q 6, 8, or 12 hours for up to 14 days
➤ Shigellosis caused by susceptible strains of *Shigella flexneri* or *Shigella sonnei*
Adults: One double-strength tablet or two single-strength tablets or 20 ml suspension P.O. q 12 hours for 10 to 14 days. Alternatively, 8 to 10 mg/kg (based on trimethoprim component) I.V. q 6, 8, or 12 hours for 5 days.
Children ages 2 months and older: 40 mg/kg (sulfamethoxazole) and 8 mg/kg (trimethoprim) P.O. q 12 hours for 5 days. Alternatively, 8 to 10 mg/kg (based on trimethoprim component) I.V. q 6, 8, or 12 hours for up to 5 days.
➤ Acute exacerbation of chronic bronchitis caused by susceptible strains of *Streptococcus pneumoniae* or *Haemophilus influenzae*
Adults: One double-strength tablet or two single-strength tablets or 20 ml suspension P.O. q 12 hours for 10 to 14 days
➤ *Pneumocystis jiroveci* pneumonia
Adults and children older than 2 months: 75 to 100 mg/kg (sulfamethoxazole) and 15 to 20 mg/kg (trimethoprim) P.O. daily in equally divided doses q 6 hours for 14 to 21 days. Alternatively, 15 to 20 mg/kg (based on trimethoprim component) I.V. q 6 to 8 hours for up to 14 days.
➤ Prophylaxis of *P. jiroveci* pneumonia
Adults: One double-strength tablet P.O. daily
Children ages 2 months and older: 750 mg/m² (sulfamethoxazole) and 150 mg/m² (trimethoprim) P.O. b.i.d. in equally divided doses on 3 consecutive days each week. Total dosage should not exceed 1,600 mg sulfamethoxazole and 320 mg trimethoprim.
➤ Traveler's diarrhea caused by susceptible strains of enterotoxigenic *Escherichia coli*

S

Adults: One double-strength tablet or two single-strength tablets or 20 ml suspension q 12 hours for 5 days
➤ Acute otitis media caused by susceptible strains of *S. pneumoniae* or *H. influenzae*
Children ages 2 months and older: 40 mg/kg sulfamethoxazole and 8 mg/kg trimethoprim P.O. q 12 hours for 10 days

Off-label uses
• Granuloma inguinale
• Toxoplasmic encephalitis (as primary prophylaxis)

Dosage adjustment
• Renal impairment

Contraindications
• Hypersensitivity to sulfonamides, trimethoprim, sulfonylureas, thiazides, or loop diuretics
• Porphyria
• Marked renal or hepatic impairment
• Megaloblastic anemia caused by folate deficiency
• Pregnancy at term or when premature birth is possible
• Infants younger than 2 months (except in *P. jiroveci* pneumonia prophylaxis)

Precautions
Use cautiously in:
• urinary obstruction, renal or hepatic disease, bronchial asthma, G6PD deficiency, group A beta-hemolytic streptococcal infection, blood dyscrasias
• history of multiple allergies
• elderly patients
• pregnant (before term) or breast-feeding patients
• children.

Administration
• Dilute each 5 ml of I.V. drug in 125 ml of dextrose 5% in water.
• Infuse I.V. over 60 to 90 minutes. Avoid rapid infusion.

• Don't mix with other drugs or solutions. Don't refrigerate. Use within 6 hours after dilution.

Route	Onset	Peak	Duration
P.O.	Rapid	1-4 hr	Unknown
I.V.	Rapid	1 hr	Unknown

Adverse reactions
CNS: headache, depression, hallucinations, insomnia, drowsiness, fatigue, apathy, anxiety, ataxia, vertigo, polyneuritis, peripheral neuropathy, **seizures**
CV: allergic myocarditis or pericarditis
EENT: periorbital edema, optic neuritis, transient myopia, tinnitus
GI: nausea, vomiting, abdominal pain, stomatitis, glossitis, dry mouth, pancreatitis, anorexia, **pseudomembranous colitis**
GU: hematuria, proteinuria, **crystalluria, toxic nephrosis with oliguria and anuria, renal failure**
Hematologic: megaloblastic anemia, agranulocytosis, aplastic anemia, thrombocytopenia, leukopenia, hemolytic anemia
Hepatic: jaundice, **hepatitis, hepatocellular necrosis**
Respiratory: shortness of breath, pleuritis, **allergic pneumonitis, pulmonary infiltrates, fibrosing alveolitis**
Skin: generalized skin eruption, urticaria, pruritus, alopecia, local irritation, exfoliative dermatitis, photosensitivity reaction, **epidermal necrolysis, erythema multiforme, Stevens-Johnson syndrome**
Other: irritation at I.V. site, chills, drug fever, hypersensitivity reactions including **anaphylaxis, serum sickness, lupus-like syndrome**

Interactions
Drug-drug. *Cyclosporine:* increased nephrotoxicity
Dapsone: increased blood levels of both drugs
Hydantoins, zidovudine: increased blood levels of these drugs

---

Indomethacin, probenecid: increased sulfamethoxazole blood level
Methotrexate: increased risk of bone marrow suppression
Oral anticoagulants: increased anticoagulant effect
PABA, PABA-derived local anesthetics: inhibited sulfamethoxazole action
Sulfonylureas: increased risk of hypoglycemia
Thiazide diuretics: increased thrombocytopenic effects
Uricosuric drugs: increased uricosuric effects
Drug-diagnostic tests. *Bilirubin, blood urea nitrogen, creatinine, eosinophils, transaminases:* increased levels
Granulocytes, hemoglobin, platelets, white blood cells: decreased levels
Urine glucose tests: false-positive results
Drug-herbs. *Dong quai, St. John's wort:* increased risk of photosensitivity
Drug-behaviors. *Sun exposure:* increased risk of photosensitivity

Patient monitoring

◀≣ Monitor CBC with white cell differential. Watch for evidence of blood dyscrasias.

◀≣ Stay alert for erythema multiforme. Report early signs before condition can progress to Stevens-Johnson syndrome.

• Monitor patient for signs and symptoms of superinfection, including fever, tachycardia, and chills.

◀≣ Monitor liver function tests and assess for evidence of hepatitis.

◀≣ Check kidney function tests weekly. Evaluate patient's fluid intake, urine output, and urine pH. Report hematuria, oliguria, or anuria right away.

• Monitor neurologic status. Report seizures, hallucinations, or depression.

Patient teaching

• Advise patient to take on regular schedule as prescribed, along with a full glass of water. Tell him to drink plenty of fluids to minimize crystal formation in urine.

• If suspension is prescribed, make sure patient has a specially marked measuring spoon or other device so he can measure doses accurately.

• Instruct patient to complete full course of treatment even if he starts to feel better.

◀≣ Teach patient to recognize and immediately report signs and symptoms of hypersensitivity, especially rash.

◀≣ Inform patient that drug can cause blood disorders, GI and liver problems, serious skin reactions, and other infections. Describe key warning signs and symptoms (easy bruising or bleeding, severe diarrhea, unusual tiredness, yellowing of skin or eyes, sore throat, rash, cough, mouth sores, fever). Tell him to report these right away.

◀≣ Urge patient to promptly report scant or bloody urine or inability to urinate.

• Tell patient to contact prescriber if he develops depression.

• Teach patient effective ways to counteract photosensitivity effect. Advise him that dong quai and St. John's wort increase phototoxicity risk and should be avoided during therapy.

• Advise female patient to inform prescriber if she is pregnant. Tell her not to take drug near term.

• Caution female patient not to breastfeed, because she could pass drug effects to infant.

• As appropriate, review all other significant and life-threatening adverse reactions and interactions, especially those related to the drugs, tests, herbs, and behaviors mentioned above.

S

sulfasalazine
APO Sulfasalazine❦, Azulfidine,
Azulfidine EN-tabs, PMS-
Sulfasalazine❦, PMS-Sulfasalazine-
E.C.❦, Salazopyrin❦⊕, Salazopyrin
EN-Tabs❦, SAS Tab❦, Sulazine⊕,
Sulfazine, Sulfazine EC

Pharmacologic class: Sulfonamide
Therapeutic class: Anti-infective, GI
tract anti-inflammatory, antirheumatic
Pregnancy risk category B

Action
Unknown. Thought to inhibit prostaglandin synthesis by interfering with
secretions in colon and causing local
anti-inflammatory action.

Availability
Tablets: 500 mg
*Tablets (Azulfidine EN-tabs—delayed-
release, enteric-coated):* 500 mg

💊 Indications and dosages
➤ Ulcerative colitis
Adults: Initially, 1 to 2 g P.O. daily in
equally divided doses q 6 to 8 hours,
then 3 to 4 g P.O. daily in equally
divided doses q 6 to 8 hours. For maintenance, 500 mg q 6 hours.
Children ages 6 and older: 40 to 60
mg/kg P.O. daily in three to six divided
doses. For maintenance, 30 mg/kg P.O.
q 6 hours in four divided doses.
➤ Acute rheumatoid arthritis
Adults: Initially, 500 mg to 1 g (delayed-
release) P.O. daily for 1 week; then
increase by 500 mg/day P.O. q week up
to 2 g/day in two divided doses. If no
benefit after 12 weeks, increase to 3
g/day given in two divided doses.
➤ Polyarticular-course juvenile
rheumatoid arthritis

Children ages 6 and older: 30 to 50
mg/kg P.O. daily in two evenly divided
doses. Maximum dosage is 2 g daily.

Off-label uses
• Ankylosing spondylitis
• Crohn's disease
• Psoriatic arthritis

Contraindications
• Hypersensitivity to drug, its metabo-
lites, other sulfonamides, or salicylates
• Porphyria
• Urinary tract or intestinal
obstruction

Precautions
Use cautiously in:
• renal or hepatic disease, bronchial
asthma, G6PD deficiency, group A
beta-hemolytic streptococcal infections, blood dyscrasias
• history of multiple allergies
• pregnant or breastfeeding patients
• children younger than age 2.

Administration
• Give after meals and space doses
evenly to reduce GI effects.
• Give with a full glass of water.
• Administer delayed-release tablets
whole. Don't let patient crush or chew
them.

Route	Onset	Peak	Duration
P.O.	1.5 hr	10 hr	Unknown

Adverse reactions
CNS: headache, depression, hallucinations, insomnia, drowsiness, vertigo,
fatigue, apathy, anxiety, ataxia, polyneuritis, peripheral neuropathy,
seizures
CV: allergic myocarditis or pericarditis
EENT: periorbital edema, optic neuritis, transient myopia, tinnitus
GI: nausea, vomiting, abdominal pain,
stomatitis, glossitis, pancreatitis, dry
mouth, anorexia, **pseudomembranous
colitis**

GU: hematuria, proteinuria, orange-yellow urine, reversible oligospermia, **crystalluria, toxic nephrosis with oliguria and anuria, renal failure**
Hematologic: megaloblastic anemia, agranulocytosis, aplastic anemia, thrombocytopenia, leukopenia, hemolytic anemia
Hepatic: jaundice, **hepatitis, hepato-cellular necrosis**
Respiratory: shortness of breath, pleuritis, **cyanosis, allergic pneumonitis, pulmonary infiltrates, fibrosing alveolitis**
Skin: generalized skin eruption, urticaria, pruritus, alopecia, local irritation, orange-yellow skin discoloration, exfoliative dermatitis, photosensitivity reaction, **erythema multiforme, epidermal necrolysis, Stevens-Johnson syndrome**
Other: reversible immunoglobulin suppression, chills, drug fever, hypersensitivity reactions including **anaphylaxis, serum sickness, lupus-like syndrome**

Interactions

Drug-drug. *Digoxin, folic acid:* reduced absorption of these drugs
Drug-diagnostic tests. *Bilirubin, blood urea nitrogen, creatinine, eosinophils, transaminases:* increased levels
Granulocytes, hemoglobin, platelets, white blood cells: decreased levels
Urine glucose test: false-positive result
Drug-food. *Folic acid:* decreased folic acid absorption
Drug-herbs. *Dong quai, St. John's wort:* increased risk of photosensitivity
Drug-behaviors. *Sun exposure:* increased risk of photosensitivity

Patient monitoring

◀≣ Monitor CBC with white cell differential. Watch for evidence of blood dyscrasias.

◀≣ Stay alert for signs of erythema multiforme. Report early signs before

condition can progress to Stevens-Johnson syndrome.
• Monitor patient for signs and symptoms of superinfection, including fever, tachycardia, and chills.
◀≣ Monitor liver function tests; watch for signs and symptoms of hepatitis.
◀≣ Check kidney function tests weekly. Evaluate patient's fluid intake, urine output, and urine pH. Report hematuria, oliguria, or anuria right away.
• Monitor neurologic status. Report seizures, hallucinations, or depression.
• If patient takes drug for rheumatoid arthritis, monitor therapeutic response 4 to 12 weeks after therapy begins.

Patient teaching

• Tell patient to take on regular schedule as prescribed, along with a full glass of water. Instruct him to drink plenty of fluids to minimize crystal formation in urine.
• Urge patient to complete full course of treatment, even if he feels better after a few days.
◀≣ Instruct patient to watch for and immediately report signs and symptoms of hypersensitivity reaction, especially rash.
◀≣ Tell patient drug can cause blood disorders, GI and liver problems, serious skin reactions, and other infections. Describe key warning signs and symptoms (easy bruising or bleeding, severe diarrhea, unusual tiredness, yellowing of skin or eyes, sore throat, rash, cough, mouth sores, fever). Instruct him to report these right away.
◀≣ Advise patient to promptly report scant or bloody urine or inability to urinate.
• Instruct patient to contact prescriber if he develops depression.
• Teach patient effective ways to counteract photosensitivity effect. Tell him that dong quai and St. John's wort

S

Reactions in **bold** are life-threatening.   ◀≣ Clinical alert

increase phototoxicity risk and should be avoided during therapy.

• Inform patient that drug may discolor skin and body fluids orange-yellow and may permanently stain contact lenses.

• Advise female patient to inform prescriber if she is pregnant. Caution her not to take drug near term or when breastfeeding.

• As appropriate, review all other significant and life-threatening adverse reactions and interactions, especially those related to the drugs, tests, foods, herbs, and behaviors mentioned above.

sumatriptan succinate

Apo-Sumatriptan✤,
Co Sumatriptan✤, Dom-Sumatriptan✤, Gen-Sumatriptan✤,
Imigran⊕, Imitrex, Novo-Sumatriptan✤, PHL-Sumatriptan✤,
PMS-Sumatriptan✤, Ratio-Sumatriptan✤, Riva-Sumatriptan✤,
Sandoz Sumatriptan✤, Sumavel DosePro

Pharmacologic class: Selective 5-hydroxytryptamine$_1$ (5-HT$_1$) agonist
Therapeutic class: Vascular headache suppressant
Pregnancy risk category C

Action

Selectively activates vascular 5-HT$_1$ receptor sites, causing vasoconstriction in intracranial arteries

Availability

Injection: 6 mg/0.5-ml prefilled syringes, 0.6 mg/0.5-ml single-dose vials; 6 mg/0.5-ml prefilled, single-dose, needle-free subcutaneous delivery system; 4- and 6-mg STATdose system containing two prefilled single-dose syringe

cartridges and one STATdose Pen; 4- and 6-mg kits containing two prefilled single-dose syringe cartridges and one autoinjector pen
Nasal spray: 5 mg in 100-mcl unit dose spray device (package of six), 20 mg in 100-mcl unit dose spray device (package of six)
Tablets: 25 mg, 50 mg, 100 mg

⚡ Indications and dosages

➢ Acute migraine, cluster headaches
Adults: Initially, 25 mg P.O.; if response inadequate after 2 hours, may give up to 100 mg P.O. If migraine recurs, repeat dose q 2 hours, not to exceed 200 mg/day. Or 6 mg subcutaneously, repeated as needed after 1 hour, not to exceed 12 mg in 24 hours. If P.O. therapy will follow subcutaneous injection, additional P.O. sumatriptan may be given q 2 hours, not to exceed 100 mg/day. Or a single dose of 5, 10, or 20 mg intranasally in one nostril, repeated p.r.n. in 2 hours, not to exceed 40 mg in 24 hours.

Dosage adjustment

• Hepatic impairment

Contraindications

• Hypersensitivity to drug
• Hemiplegic or basilar migraine headache
• Ischemic cardiac, cerebrovascular, or peripheral vascular disease (such as a history of myocardial infarction, stroke, angina, or ischemic bowel)
• Uncontrolled hypertension
• Severe hepatic impairment
• MAO inhibitor use within past 14 days
• Use of other 5-HT$_1$ agonists, ergotamine-containing drugs, or ergot-type products within past 24 hours

Precautions

Use cautiously in:
• patients with cardiovascular risk factors (hypertension, hypercholesterolemia, smoking, obesity, diabetes,

family history of cardiovascular disease, men over age 40, menopausal women)
- elderly patients
- women of childbearing age
- pregnant or breastfeeding patients
- children younger than age 18 (safety not established).

Administration
- Be aware that parenteral form is for subcutaneous use only.
- Be aware that an autoinjection device is available for use with the 4- and 6-mg prefilled syringe cartridges to facilitate patient self-administration using the 4- or 6-mg dose. For patients receiving doses other than 4 or 6 mg, only the 6-mg single-dose vial dosage form should be used.
- ◀︎ If patient has risk factors for coronary artery disease, know that first dose should be given in medical setting with emergency equipment at hand.
- ◀︎ Don't give within 14 days of MAO inhibitors.
- ◀︎ Don't administer within 24 hours of other 5-HT$_1$ agonists, ergotamine-containing drugs, or ergot-type products.

Route	Onset	Peak	Duration
P.O.	Within 30 min	2-2.5 hr	Unknown
Subcut.	10-20 min	Unknown	Unknown
Intranasal	Unknown	Unknown	Unknown

Adverse reactions
CNS: headache, malaise, dizziness, drowsiness, fatigue, vertigo, anxiety, tight feeling in head, numbness
CV: angina, chest pressure or tightness, transient hypertension, ECG changes, **coronary vasospasm, myocardial infarction**
EENT: vision changes, nasal sinus discomfort, throat discomfort
GI: abdominal discomfort, dysphagia

Musculoskeletal: jaw discomfort, muscle cramps, myalgia, neck pain or stiffness
Skin: flushing; tingling; warm, cool or, burning sensation
Other: injection site reaction, feeling of heaviness or tightness

Interactions
Drug-drug. *Dihydroergotamine, ergotamine, methysergide:* increased risk of vasospastic reaction
Lithium, MAO inhibitors, selective serotonin reuptake inhibitors: weakness, hyperreflexia, incoordination
Drug-herbs. *Horehound:* enhanced serotonergic effects

Patient monitoring
- ◀︎ Monitor cardiovascular status closely. Be aware that drug may cause serious and possibly fatal cardiac disorders.
- Watch for neurologic and vision changes. Institute safety measures as needed to prevent injury.
- Monitor patient's response to drug. Assess need for repeat doses.
- Watch for injection site reaction, which should subside within 1 hour.

Patient teaching
- Instruct patient to take as soon as possible after migraine onset.
- ◀︎ Teach patient to recognize and immediately report serious cardiovascular reactions.
- Explain proper drug use. Tell patient it doesn't prevent migraine.
- With subcutaneous use, instruct patient to follow directions in the patient leaflet carefully before injecting drug and to inject dose subcutaneously using spring-loaded injector system or needle-free subcutaneous delivery system included in package. If headache recurs after dose, tell him he may take a second dose, but should wait at least 1 hour after initial dose and shouldn't exceed two 6-mg injections in a 24-hour period. Instruct

S

Reactions in **bold** are life-threatening.   ◀︎ Clinical alert

him to report injection site reaction that doesn't subside within 1 hour.

• With oral use, tell patient he may take a second dose 2 hours after first dose if migraine recurs. Tell him he may repeat oral doses every 2 hours as needed, up to 200 mg in a 24-hour period.

• With intranasal use, tell patient to spray 5, 10, or 20 mg into one nostril, as prescribed. Tell him he may repeat dose after 2 hours but shouldn't exceed 40 mg in a 24-hour period.

• Advise patient not to use drug for more than four episodes per month.

• Caution patient to avoid driving and other hazardous activities until he knows how drug affects concentration and alertness.

• As appropriate, review all other significant and life-threatening adverse reactions and interactions, especially those related to the drugs and herbs mentioned above.

sunitinib malate
Sutent

Pharmacologic class: Receptor tyrosine kinase inhibitor
Therapeutic class: Antineoplastic
Pregnancy risk category D

FDA | BOXED WARNING

• Hepatotoxicity, which has been observed in clinical trials and postmarketing experience, may be severe, and deaths have occurred.

Action
Inhibits multiple receptor tyrosine kinases, some of which are implicated in tumor growth, pathologic angiogenesis, and metastatic cancer progression

Availability
Capsules: 12.5 mg, 25 mg, 50 mg

Indications and dosages
➤ GI stromal tumor after disease progression with or intolerance to imatinib mesylate; advanced renal cell carcinoma
Adults: 50 mg P.O. daily on cycle of 4 weeks on and 2 weeks off treatment; may increase or decrease dosage in 12.5-mg increments based on safety and tolerance

Dosage adjustment
• Concurrent use of strong CYP3A4 inducers or inhibitors

Contraindications
• Hypersensitivity to drug or its components

Precautions
Use cautiously in:
• left ventricular dysfunction, hypertension, history of prolonged QT interval, concurrent use of antiarrhythmics, patients with relevant preexisting cardiac disease, bradycardia, or electrolyte disturbances
• patients who have experienced cardiac events within previous 12 months
• hepatotoxicity
• concurrent use of strong CYP3A4 inhibitors
• pregnant or breastfeeding patients
• children (safety and efficacy not established).

Administration
◀ Monitor liver function tests before start of treatment.
• Administer with or without food.
• Interrupt therapy or reduce dosage, as prescribed, in patients who lack clinical evidence of heart failure but have ejection fractions (EFs) below 50% and above 20% below baseline.

Route	Onset	Peak	Duration
P.O.	Unknown	6-12 hr	Unknown

Adverse reactions

CNS: headache, asthenia

CV: hypertension, **left ventricular dysfunction**

EENT: epistaxis, oral pain

GI: nausea, vomiting, diarrhea, constipation, abdominal pain, mucositis, stomatitis, anorexia

Hematologic: bleeding, anemia, **thrombocytopenia, neutropenia, lymphopenia, hemorrhage**

Hepatic: hepatotoxicity

Metabolic: acquired hypothyroidism, adrenal toxicity

Musculoskeletal: arthralgia, back pain, limb pain, myalgia

Respiratory: dyspnea, cough, **pulmonary embolism**

Skin: skin abnormalities, skin discoloration, rash, palmar-plantar erythrodysesthesia, alopecia, hair color changes

Other: altered taste, fatigue, fever

Interactions

Drug-drug. *Atazanavir, indinavir, itraconazole, ketoconazole, nefazodone, nelfinavir, ritonavir, saquinavir, telithromycin, voriconazole:* increased sunitinib blood level

Carbamazepine, dexamethasone, phenobarbital, phenytoin, rifabutin, rifampin, rifapentin: decreased sunitinib blood level

Drug-diagnostic tests. *Amylase, creatinine, lipase, uric acid:* increased

Liver function tests: abnormal

Serum phosphorus, potassium, sodium: decreased

Drug-food. *Grapefruit juice, pomegranate:* increased sunitinib blood level

Drug-herbs. *Alpha-lipoic acid:* decreased chemotherapeutic efficacy

American elder, bishop's weed, cat's claw, devil's claw, eucalyptus, feverfew, *Siberian ginseng, valerian:* increased sunitinib blood level

St. John's wort: unpredictable decrease in sunitinib blood level

Patient monitoring

• Obtain CBC with platelet count and blood chemistries (including phosphate) at start of each treatment cycle and frequently thereafter.

• Know that physician may order baseline and periodic evaluation of left ventricular EF in patients who experienced cardiac events within 12 months before starting drug. Watch closely for signs and symptoms of left ventricular dysfunction (especially heart failure).

• Be aware that physician may order baseline EF testing for patients without cardiac risk factors.

• Monitor for hypertension; administer standard antihypertensive therapy as ordered and needed.

• Monitor for adrenal insufficiency if patient experiences stress (as from surgery, trauma, or severe infection).

🔊 Monitor liver function tests during each cycle of treatment and as clinically indicated. Interrupt therapy for Grade 3 or 4 drug-related hepatic adverse events; discontinue drug if no resolution. Don't restart drug if severe changes in liver function tests subsequently occur or if patient has other signs and symptoms of liver failure.

Patient teaching

• Instruct patient to take drug with or without food.

🔊 Urge patient to immediately report sudden signs and symptoms of liver problems (such as yellowing of skin or eyes, unusual tiredness, loss of appetite), chest pain, swelling, or difficulty breathing.

• Tell patient drug may cause skin changes (drying, cracking, or rashes on hands or feet) and hair color changes.

S

- Advise patient to consult prescriber before taking other drugs, including over-the-counter drugs and herbs.
- Caution patient not to take St. John's wort during therapy.
- Advise female with childbearing potential to avoid pregnancy and breastfeeding during therapy.
- As appropriate, review all other significant and life-threatening adverse reactions and interactions, especially those related to the drugs, tests, foods, and herbs mentioned above.

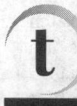

tacrolimus
Advagraf✹⊕, Prograf, Protopic

Pharmacologic class: Macrolide
Therapeutic class: Immunosuppressant
Pregnancy risk category C

FDA BOXED WARNING

- Immunosuppression may increase patient's susceptibility to infection and lymphoma development. Give under supervision of physician experienced in immunosuppressive therapy and management of organ transplant patients, in facility with adequate diagnostic and treatment resources. Physician responsible for maintenance therapy should have complete information needed for patient follow-up.
- Be aware that long-term safety of topical calcineurin inhibitors hasn't been established.
- Although a causal relationship hasn't been established, rare cases of malignancy (such as skin cancers and lymphoma) have been reported in patients treated with topical calcineurin inhibitors, including tacrolimus ointment. Therefore, continuous long-term use of tacrolimus ointment in any age-group should be avoided and application limited to areas of atopic dermatitis involvement. Tacrolimus ointment isn't indicated for use in children younger than age 2. Only 0.03% tacrolimus ointment is indicated for use in children ages 2 to 15.

Action
Unknown. Thought to inhibit T-lymphocyte activation.

Availability
Capsules: 0.5 mg, 1 mg, 5 mg
Injection: 5 mg/ml
Topical ointment: 0.03%, 0.1%

Indications and dosages
➤ Prevention of organ rejection in patients with allogeneic liver transplants
Adults: Initially, 0.1 to 0.15 mg/kg/day P.O. in two divided doses q 12 hours. Alternatively, 0.03 to 0.05 mg/kg/day by continuous I.V. infusion.
Children: 0.15 to 0.2 mg/kg/day P.O. in two divided doses q 12 hours. Alternatively, 0.03 to 0.05 mg/kg/day by continuous I.V. infusion.
➤ Prevention of organ rejection in patients with allogeneic kidney transplants
Adults: Initially, 0.2 mg/kg/day P.O. in two divided doses q 12 hours when used in combination with azathioprine, or 0.1 mg/kg/day P.O. when used in combination with mycophenolate mofetil (MMF). Alternatively, 0.03 to 0.05 mg/kg/day by continuous I.V. infusion until oral dosing can be tolerated.
➤ Prevention of heart transplant rejection
Adults: Initially, 0.075 mg/kg/day P.O. q 12 hours in two divided doses in combination with azathioprine or MMF.

➤ Moderate to severe atopic dermatitis
Adults: 0.03% or 0.1% ointment applied b.i.d. to affected area, continued 1 week after dermatitis symptoms resolve
Children ages 2 and older: 0.03% ointment applied b.i.d. to affected area, continued 1 week after dermatitis symptoms resolve

Dosage adjustment
• Hepatic or renal impairment
• Concurrent use of CYP3A inducers or inhibitors
• Black patients

Contraindications
• Hypersensitivity to drug or its components (including castor oil derivatives)

Precautions
Use cautiously in:
• severe hepatic disease, renal impairment, diabetes mellitus, hypertension, hyperkalemia, hyperuricemia, lymphoma, serious infections
• skin barrier defect with increased potential for systemic absorption of tacrolimus ointment
• premalignant and malignant skin conditions (avoid use)
• concurrent use of cyclosporine, nelfinavir, or live vaccines (avoid use)
• concurrent use of strong CYP3A4 inhibitors (such as boceprevir, clarithromycin, itraconazole, ketoconazole, ritonavir, telaprevir, voriconazole,) and strong inducers (such as rifampin, rifabutin) (not recommended)
• concurrent use of other substrates or CYP3A4 inhibitors that also have potential to prolong QT interval
• concurrent use of sirolimus (not recommended in liver and heart transplant; use with sirolimus in kidney transplant not established)
• concurrent use of other nephrotoxic drugs or drugs that cause hyperkalemia

• prolonged exposure to ultraviolet (UV) light and sunlight (avoid)
• pregnant or breastfeeding patients
• children younger than age 12 (age 2 for ointment use).

Administration
• Give oral form consistently with or without food but not with grapefruit juice.
• Give I.V. doses by infusion only. Be aware that I.V. use is reserved for patients who can't tolerate capsules orally.
• Start therapy within 24 hours of kidney transplantation and no earlier than 6 hours after liver or heart transplantation. Switch to oral dosing as soon as tolerable, starting 8 to 12 hours after I.V. dosing ends.
◀€ Before giving I.V., ensure that epinephrine 1:1,000 and oxygen are at hand in case of emergency.
• For I.V. use, dilute in normal saline solution or dextrose 5% in water to a concentration of 0.004 to 0.02 mg/ml. Give by infusion only.
• Be aware that ointment is used only as second-line therapy for the short-term and noncontinuous treatment of moderate to severe atopic dermatitis in *nonimmunocompromised* patients who have failed to respond adequately to other topical prescription treatments for atopic dermatitis.
• After applying ointment, don't place occlusive dressing or wrapping over affected area.

Route	Onset	Peak	Duration
P.O.	Unknown	1.5-3.5 hr	Unknown
I.V.	Rapid	1-2 hr	Unknown
Ointment	Unknown	Unknown	Unknown

Adverse reactions
CNS: tremor, headache, insomnia, paresthesia, delirium, asthenia, **neurotoxicities (including posterior reversible encephalopathy syndrome, delirium, seizures, and coma)**

Reactions in **bold** are life-threatening.　　　　◀€ Clinical alert

CV: hypertension, peripheral edema, **myocardial hypertrophy**
GI: nausea, vomiting, diarrhea, constipation, abdominal pain, ascites, anorexia
GU: hematuria, proteinuria, urinary tract infection, albuminuria, abnormal renal function, **oliguria, renal failure, nephrotoxicity**
Hematologic: anemia, **leukocytosis, thrombocytopenia, agranulocytosis, hemolytic anemia, pure red cell aplasia**
Metabolic: new-onset diabetes mellitus, hyperglycemia, hypomagnesemia, hypokalemia, **hyperkalemia**
Musculoskeletal: back pain
Respiratory: dyspnea, **pleural effusion, atelectasis**
Skin: burning (with ointment), rash, flushing, pruritus, alopecia
Other: pain, fever, chills, lymphadenopathy, **serious infections (including cytomegalovirus infections and polyoma virus infections), lymphoma and other malignancies, anaphylaxis**

Interactions

Drug-drug. *Bromocriptine, chloramphenicol, cimetidine, clarithromycin, clotrimazole, cyclosporine, danazol, diltiazem, erythromycin, fluconazole, itraconazole, ketoconazole, methylprednisolone, metoclopramide, metronidazole, nicardipine, omeprazole, protease inhibitors, verapamil:* increased tacrolimus blood level
Cyclosporine: increased risk of nephrotoxicity
CYP450 inducers (such as carbamazepine, phenobarbital, phenytoin, rifampin): decreased tacrolimus metabolism
Immunosuppressants (except adrenocorticoids): immunologic oversuppression
Live-virus vaccines: interference with immune response to vaccine
Mycophenolate mofetil: increased mycophenolate blood level
Nephrotoxic drugs (such as aminoglycosides, amphotericin B, cisplatin, cyclosporine): additive or synergistic effects

Drug-diagnostic tests. *Blood urea nitrogen, creatinine, glucose:* increased levels
Hemoglobin, magnesium, platelets, white blood cells: decreased levels
Liver function tests: abnormal values
Potassium: increased or decreased level
Drug-food. *Any food:* inhibited drug absorption
Grapefruit or grapefruit juice: increased drug blood level
Drug-herbs. *Astragalus, echinacea, melatonin:* decreased immunosuppression
St. John's wort: decreased tacrolimus blood level

Patient monitoring

◀€ Once I.V. infusion starts, watch closely for signs and symptoms of anaphylaxis.
• Monitor cardiac, liver, and kidney function test results. Watch for signs and symptoms of cardiovascular disorder, nephrotoxicity, and hepatic dysfunction.
◀€ Assess neurologic status for evidence of neurotoxicity (including posterior encephalopathy syndrome and seizures).
• Monitor potassium level closely. Stay alert for signs and symptoms of hyperkalemia.
• Monitor blood glucose. Watch for indications of hyperglycemia.
• Evaluate respiratory status regularly.

Patient teaching

◀€ Teach patient to recognize and immediately report serious adverse reactions.
• Tell patient to take oral doses consistently with or without food, but not with grapefruit or grapefruit juice.
• Tell diabetic patient to expect increased blood glucose level, which may warrant further antidiabetic therapy. Advise him to monitor glucose level carefully.
• Instruct patient not to place occlusive dressings or wrappings over

---

affected area after applying ointment. Tell him to use drug for 1 week after dermatitis symptoms resolve.

• Advise patient to avoid live vaccines and prolonged exposure to UV light or sunlight.

• As appropriate, review all other significant and life-threatening adverse reactions and interactions, especially those related to the drugs, tests, foods, and herbs mentioned above.

tadalafil
Cialis, Adcirca

Pharmacologic class: Phosphodiesterase type 5 (PDE5) inhibitor
Therapeutic class: Anti-erectile dysfunction agent
Pregnancy risk category B

Action
Inhibits PDE5, increasing cyclic guanosine monophosphate level and enhancing erectile function; also relaxes pulmonary vascular smooth muscle cells and vasodilation of the pulmonary vascular bed

Availability
Tablets: 2.5 mg, 5 mg, 10 mg, 20 mg, 40 mg

⏺ Indications and dosages
➤ Erectile dysfunction (for as-needed use)
Adults: Initially, 10 mg (Cialis) P.O. before anticipated sexual activity; may increase to 20 mg or decrease to 5 mg based on patient response and tolerance. For most patients, maximum recommended dosing frequency is once daily.
➤ Erectile dysfunction (for daily use)
Adults: 2.5 mg (Cialis) P.O. once daily, given at approximately the same time without regard to sexual activity; may increase to 5 mg P.O. once daily based on efficacy and tolerability
➤ Benign prostatic hyperplasia (BPH); concurrent erectile dysfunction and BPH
Adults: 5 mg (Cialis) P.O. daily at approximately the same time each day.
➤ Pulmonary hypertension
Adults: 40 mg (Adcirca) P.O. daily

Dosage adjustment
• Mild to moderate hepatic impairment or renal impairment
• Administration with alpha blockers or potent CYP3A4 inhibitors such as ketoconazole or ritonavir

Contraindications
• Hypersensitivity to drug or its components
• Concurrent use of organic nitrates (regularly or intermittently)

Precautions
Use cautiously in:
• mild to moderate hepatic or renal impairment
• severe renal impairment (avoid Adcirca use; once-daily Cialis use not recommended)
• severe hepatic impairment (Cialis use not recommended; avoid Adcirca use)
• cardiac risk that makes sexual activity inadvisable, left ventricular outflow obstruction, myocardial infarction within last 90 days, unstable angina or angina occurring during sexual intercourse, New York Heart Association Class II or greater heart failure in last 6 months, uncontrolled arrhythmias, blood pressure below 90/50 mm Hg, uncontrolled hypertension (blood pressure above 170/100 mm Hg), stroke within last 6 months, pulmonary veno-occlusive disease), erectile dysfunction whose cause hasn't been evaluated, conditions that increase risk of priapism (use not recommended)

Reactions in **bold** are life-threatening.　　　◀€ Clinical alert

• concurrent use of potent CYP450-3A4 inhibitors or inducers, or other PDE5 inhibitors (avoid use)
• concurrent use of alpha blockers (except tamsulosin 0.4 mg/day), antihypertensives, or alcohol
• pregnant or breastfeeding patients
• children (safety and efficacy not established).

Administration

• Know that patient should take drug with or without food and that patient should take Cialis before anticipated sexual activity when given on an as-needed basis.

Route	Onset	Peak	Duration
P.O.	Rapid	30 min-6 hr	Up to 36 hr

Adverse reactions

CNS: headache, fatigue, dizziness, insomnia, hyperesthesia, paresthesia, drowsiness, vertigo, asthenia, transient global amnesia
CV: angina pectoris, chest pain, hypertension, hypotension, orthostatic hypotension, palpitations, syncope, tachycardia, **myocardial infarction**
EENT: blurred vision, color vision changes, conjunctivitis, eye pain, increased lacrimation, eyelid swelling, epistaxis, nasal congestion, pharyngitis
GI: nausea, vomiting, diarrhea, dyspepsia, esophagitis, gastroesophageal reflux, gastritis, upper abdominal pain, dysphagia, dry mouth
GU: increased or spontaneous erection
Musculoskeletal: myalgia; back, neck, limb, and joint pain
Respiratory: dyspnea
Skin: pruritus, rash, sweating
Other: facial edema, pain

Interactions

Drug-drug. *Alpha-adrenergic blockers (except tamsulosin 0.4 mg/day):* marked blood pressure decrease
Angiotensin receptor blockers, enalapril, metoprolol: decreased blood pressure

CYP450-3A4 inducers (such as carbamazepine, phenobarbital, phenytoin, rifampin): decreased tadalafil blood level
CYP450-3A4 inhibitors (such as erythromycin, itraconazole, ketoconazole, ritonavir): increased tadalafil blood level
Theophylline: slight increase in heart rate
Drug-diagnostic tests. *Alanine aminotransferase, alkaline phosphatase, aspartate aminotransferase, lactate dehydrogenase, uric acid:* increased levels
Drug-food. *Grapefruit juice:* increased drug blood level
Drug-behaviors. *Alcohol use:* decreased blood pressure

Patient monitoring

• Monitor for drug efficacy.

Patient teaching

• Advise patient taking Cialis for erectile dysfunction on an as-needed basis to take before anticipated sexual activity.
• Instruct patient that when taking Cialis on a daily basis he should take tablet at approximately the same time every day, without regard to sexual activity.
• Instruct patient to take Adcirca tablets one after the other every day and not to split the dose.
◀€ Caution patient never to take concurrently with nitrates.
◀€ Instruct patient to stop sexual activity and contact prescriber immediately if chest pain, dizziness, or nausea occurs.
◀€ Advise patient to seek immediate medical attention if sudden loss of vision or sudden decrease in or loss of hearing occurs.
• Instruct patient not to take other PDE5 inhibitors.
• Instruct patient to contact prescriber if erection lasts more than 4 hours.
• Tell patient drug can cause serious interactions with many common drugs. Instruct him to tell all prescribers he is taking it.

- Caution patient to avoid driving and other hazardous activities until he knows how drug affects concentration and alertness.
- Inform patient that drug may cause temporary blood pressure drop, leading to light-headedness if he stands up suddenly. Advise him to rise slowly and carefully.
- As appropriate, review all other significant and life-threatening adverse reactions and interactions, especially those related to the drugs, tests, and foods mentioned above.

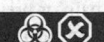

tamoxifen citrate
Apo-Tamox✶, Gen-Tamoxifen✶, Nolvadex, Nolvadex-D✶, Novo-Tamoxifen✶, PMS-Tamoxifen✶, Soltamox, Tamofen✶

Pharmacologic class: Nonsteroidal antiestrogen
Therapeutic class: Antineoplastic
Pregnancy risk category D

FDA BOXED WARNING

- For women with ductal carcinoma in situ or high risk of breast cancer, serious and life-threatening events associated with drug use in risk-reduction setting include stroke, pulmonary embolism, and uterine cancer. Some of these events were fatal. Discuss potential benefits versus potential risks of these events with these patients. In women already diagnosed with breast cancer, drug's benefits outweigh risks.

Action
Competes with estrogen receptors in tumor cells for binding to target tissues (such as breast); reduces DNA synthesis and estrogen response

Availability
Oral solution: 10 mg/5 ml
Tablets: 10 mg, 20 mg
Tablets (enteric-coated): 20 mg

⚕ Indications and dosages
➤ Adjunctive treatment of breast cancer
Adults: 20 to 40 mg P.O. daily for 5 years. Daily dosages of 20 mg may be taken as a single dose; daily dosages above 20 mg should be divided and taken b.i.d. (morning and evening).
➤ To reduce breast cancer incidence in high-risk women; treatment of ductal carcinoma in situ
Adults: 20 mg P.O. daily for 5 years

Off-label uses
- Mastalgia
- Ovulation stimulation

Contraindications
- Hypersensitivity to drug
- Concurrent warfarin use
- Women with a history of deep-vein thrombosis or pulmonary embolism
- Pregnancy or breastfeeding

Precautions
Use cautiously in:
- decreased bone marrow reserve, leukopenia, thrombocytopenia, cataracts, hyperlipidemia
- females of childbearing age.

Administration
- Don't break or crush enteric-coated tablets.
- Know that drug is indicated for reducing breast cancer risk only in high-risk women, defined as those older than age 35 who have at least a 1.67% chance of developing breast cancer over 5 years.

t

Route	Onset	Peak	Duration
P.O.	Unknown	5 hr	Unknown

Adverse reactions

CNS: confusion, depression, headache, weakness, fatigue, light-headedness

CV: chest pain, **deep-vein thrombosis**

EENT: blurred vision, ocular lesion, retinopathy, corneal opacity

GI: nausea, vomiting, abdominal cramps, anorexia

GU: vaginal bleeding, discharge, or dryness; irregular menses; amenorrhea; oligomenorrhea; ovarian cyst; pruritus vulvae; **endometrial or uterine cancer**

Hematologic: leukopenia, thrombocytopenia

Metabolic: hypercalcemia, fluid retention

Musculoskeletal: bone pain

Respiratory: cough, **pulmonary embolism**

Skin: skin changes, hair thinning or partial hair loss

Other: altered taste, weight loss, tumor flare, tumor pain, hot flashes, edema

Interactions

Drug-drug. *Aminoglutethimide, estrogens:* decreased tamoxifen effects

Antineoplastics: increased risk of thromboembolic events

Bromocriptine: increased tamoxifen blood level

Warfarin: increased anticoagulant effect

Drug-diagnostic tests. *Aspartate aminotransferase, bilirubin, calcium, creatinine, hepatic enzymes:* increased levels

Platelets, white blood cells: decreased counts

Patient monitoring

• Monitor lipid panel, calcium level, mammography results, and gynecologic exam results.

◀€ Watch for signs and symptoms of thromboembolic events, including cerebrovascular accident and pulmonary embolism.

• Monitor menstrual cycle pattern for changes that may signal endometrial or uterine cancer.

Patient teaching

• Tell patient to swallow enteric-coated tablets whole without breaking or crushing.

◀€ Instruct patient to immediately report leg or calf pain, swelling, or tenderness; unexpected shortness of breath; sudden chest pain; coughing up blood; new breast lumps; vaginal bleeding; menstrual irregularities; changes in vaginal discharge; pelvic pain or pressure; and vision changes.

• Inform patient that increase in bone or tumor pain usually means drug will be effective. Advise her to discuss pain management with prescriber.

• Stress importance of undergoing regular blood tests, mammograms, and gynecologic exams to identify early signs of serious adverse reactions.

• As appropriate, review all other significant and life-threatening adverse reactions and interactions, especially those related to the drugs and tests mentioned above.

tamsulosin hydrochloride

Bazetham⊕, Contiflo XL⊕, Flomax, Flomax CR✤, Flomaxtra⊕, Novo-Tamsulosin✤, Omnic MR⊕, Ran-Tamsulosin✤, Ratio-Tamsulosin✤, Sandoz Tamsulosin✤, Stronazon⊕, Tabphyn⊕

Pharmacologic class: Alpha-adrenergic blocker

Therapeutic class: Anti-adrenergic

Pregnancy risk category B

Action

Decreases smooth muscle contractions of prostate by binding to alpha$_1$-adrenergic receptors. This action increases urine flow and reduces symptoms of benign prostatic hyperplasia (BPH).

Availability

Capsules: 0.4 mg

ⓘ Indications and dosages

➢ BPH

Adults: 0.4 mg/day P.O. after a meal. After 2 to 4 weeks, may increase to 0.8 mg/day.

Contraindications

• Hypersensitivity to drug or its components

Precautions

Use cautiously in:
• concurrent use of other alpha-adrenergic blockers or strong CYP3A4 inhibitors (avoid use)
• concurrent use of moderate CYP3A4 inhibitors, strong or moderate CYP2D6 inhibitors, other cytochrome P450 inhibitors, warfarin, and in patients who are poor CYP2D6 metabolizers
• patients at increased risk for prostate cancer.

Administration

• Give 30 minutes after same meal each day.

Route	Onset	Peak	Duration
P.O.	Unknown	4-5 hr	9-15 hr

Adverse reactions

CNS: dizziness, headache, asthenia, insomnia, drowsiness, **syncope**, vertigo
CV: orthostatic hypotension, chest pain
EENT: rhinitis, amblyopia, pharyngitis, sinusitis
GU: retrograde or diminished ejaculation, decreased libido
Musculoskeletal: back pain
Respiratory: increased cough
Other: tooth disorder, infection

Interactions

Drug-drug. *Cimetidine:* increased tamsulosin blood level, greater risk of toxicity
Doxazosin, prazosin, terazosin: increased risk of hypotension
Ketoconazole (strong CYP3A4 inhibitor), paroxetine (strong CYP2D6 inhibitor): increased tamsulosin C_{max} and area under the curve
Drug-behaviors. *Alcohol use:* increased risk of hypotension

Patient monitoring

• Monitor blood pressure. Stay alert for orthostatic hypotension.

Patient teaching

• Tell patient to take 30 minutes after same meal each day.
• Instruct patient not to chew or open capsule. Advise him to swallow it whole.
• Tell patient to move slowly when sitting up or standing, to avoid dizziness or light-headedness from sudden blood pressure decrease.
• Caution patient to avoid hazardous activities on first day of therapy.
• Inform patient that drug may cause abnormal ejaculation. Advise him to discuss this issue with prescriber.
• As appropriate, review all other significant adverse reactions and interactions, especially those related to the drugs and behaviors mentioned above.

t

tapentadol hydrochloride

Nucynta, Nucynta ER

Pharmacologic class: Opioid agonist
Therapeutic class: Opioid analgesic
Controlled substance schedule II
Pregnancy risk category C

Reactions in **bold** are life-threatening.   ◀€ Clinical alert

FDA | BOXED WARNING

• Know that Nucynta ER is an opioid agonist and Schedule II controlled substance with an abuse liability similar to other opioid agonists, legal or illicit. Assess each patient's risk of opioid abuse or addiction before prescribing Nucynta ER. Risk of opioid abuse increases in patients with a personal or family history of substance abuse (including drug or alcohol abuse or addiction) or mental illness (such as major depressive disorder). Routinely monitor all patients receiving Nucynta ER for signs and symptoms of misuse, abuse, and addiction during treatment.

• Respiratory depression, including fatal cases, may occur with Nucynta ER, even when drug has been used as recommended and not misused or abused. Proper dosing and titration are essential; Nucynta ER should only be prescribed by health care professionals knowledgeable in the use of potent opioids for management of chronic pain. Monitor patients for respiratory depression, especially during initiation of Nucynta ER or after a dosage increase. Instruct patients to swallow tablets whole. Crushing, dissolving, or chewing extended-release tablets can cause rapid release and absorption of a potentially fatal tapentadol dose.

• Accidental ingestion of Nucynta ER, especially in children, can result in a fatal tapentadol overdose.

• Consuming alcohol with Nucynta ER may result in increased tapentadol plasma level and potentially fatal overdose. Instruct patients not to consume alcoholic beverages or use prescription or nonprescription products that contain alcohol while taking Nucynta ER.

Action
Exact mechanism unknown. Analgesic effect may be due to mu-opioid agonist activity and inhibition of norepinephrine reuptake.

Availability
Tablets: 50 mg, 75 mg, 100 mg
Tablets (extended-release): 50 mg, 100 mg, 150 mg, 200 mg, 250 mg

🕖 Indications and dosages
➤ Relief of moderate to severe acute pain
Adults ages 18 and older: 50 mg, 75 mg, or 100 mg (immediate-release) P.O. q 4 to 6 hours depending on pain intensity. On day 1, may give second dose as early as 1 hour after initial dose, if needed. Maximum daily dosage on day 1 is 700 mg and on subsequent days, 600 mg. Higher dosages not recommended.
➤ Management of moderate to severe chronic pain and neuropathic pain associated with diabetic peripheral neuropathy when continuous, around-the-clock opioid analgesic is needed for an extended period
Adult: Individualize dosing regimen according to pain severity and previous experience with similar drugs. Initially in patient not currently taking opioid analgesics, 50 mg (extended-release tablets) P.O. b.i.d. q 12 hours. Dosage range is 100 to 250 mg (extended-release tablets) P.O. b.i.d. q 12 hours. Patients receiving immediate-release form may be converted to extended-release by administering same total daily dose at half the total daily immediate-release dose q 12 hours. Maximum daily extended-release dosage is 500 mg.

Dosage adjustment
• Moderate hepatic impairment
• Elderly patients

Contraindications
- Hypersensitivity to drug or its components (extended-release form)
- Significant respiratory depression, acute or severe bronchial asthma or hypercapnia in unmonitored settings or in absence of resuscitative equipment
- Paralytic ileus
- Monoamine oxidase (MAO) inhibitor use within last 14 days

Precautions
Use cautiously in:
- severe hepatic or renal impairment (use not recommended)
- moderate hepatic impairment
- respiratory depression, hypoxia, hypercapnia, upper airway obstruction, decreased respiratory reserve (such as asthma, chronic obstructive pulmonary disease, or cor pulmonale), severe obesity, sleep apnea syndrome, myxedema, kyphoscoliosis, CNS depression, coma, hypotension
- biliary tract disease, including pancreatitis
- head injury, other intracranial injuries, increased intracranial pressure, seizures
- impaired consciousness or coma susceptible to intracranial effects of carbon dioxide retention (avoid extended-release use)
- concurrent use of other CNS depressants or serotonergic agents
- elderly or debilitated patients
- pregnant or breastfeeding patients
- children younger than age 18 (safety and efficacy not established).

Administration
- Administer with or without food. Give extended-release tablets whole.
- ◀€ Don't give concurrently or within 14 days of MAO inhibitor.
- Be aware that extended-release tablets aren't for use as an as-needed analgesic, for pain that is mild or not expected to persist for an extended time, for acute pain, or for postoperative pain unless patient is already receiving long-term opioid therapy.
- Be aware that withdrawal symptoms may occur if extended-release form is discontinued abruptly. Taper dosage to reduce withdrawal symptoms.

Route	Onset	Peak	Duration
P.O.	Unknown	Unknown	Unknown

Adverse reactions
CNS: dizziness, somnolence, headache, fatigue, tremor, lethargy, insomnia, confusion, abnormal dreams, anxiety, **seizures**
EENT: nasopharyngitis
GI: nausea, vomiting, constipation, dry mouth, dyspepsia, decreased appetite
GU: urinary tract infection
Musculoskeletal: arthralgia
Respiratory: upper respiratory tract infection, **respiratory depression**
Skin: rash, pruritus, excessive sweating
Other: hot flushing, physical or psychological drug dependence, drug tolerance, hypersensitivity

Interactions
Drug-drug. *Antidepressants, antihistamines, general anesthetics, sedative-hypnotics, other CNS depressants:* additive CNS depression leading to potentially life-threatening reactions
MAO inhibitors (such as isocarboxazid, phenelzine, tranylcypromine): increased risk of potentially fatal reactions (hyperthermia, myoclonus, autonomic instability)
Mixed agonist or antagonist opioids (such as butorphanol, nalbuphine, pentazocine): reduced analgesic effect; precipitated withdrawal symptoms
Serotonergics (such as MOA inhibitors and triptans, selective norepinephrine reuptake inhibitors, selective serotonin reuptake inhibitors, tricyclic antidepressants, other drugs that impair

---

Reactions in **bold** are life-threatening.　　　◀€ Clinical alert

t

metabolism of serotonin): risk of potentially life-threatening serotonin syndrome

Drug-behaviors. *Alcohol use:* increased CNS depression

Patient monitoring

◀€ Stay alert for overdose signs and symptoms, such as CNS and respiratory depression, GI cramping, and constipation; provide supportive measures as appropriate.

• Monitor vital signs and CNS and respiratory status.

• Assess pain level and efficacy of pain relief.

• Monitor patient for signs and symptoms of drug dependence or tolerance.

• Monitor patient for hypotension during dosage initiation and titration.

Patient teaching

• Instruct patient to take drug with or without food.

• Tell patient to take one extended-release tablet at a time with a sufficient amount of water to ensure complete swallowing immediately after placing tablet in the mouth. Tell patient that these tablets must be swallowed whole and must not be split, broken, chewed, dissolved, or crushed.

◀€ Instruct patient to stop taking drug and immediately tell prescriber if a seizure occurs.

◀€ Caution patient not to stop taking drug suddenly and that drug must be tapered.

• Advise patient to avoid alcohol use while taking drug.

• Advise patient to consult prescriber before taking other prescription or nonprescription drugs.

• Tell patient to notify prescriber if shortness of breath or difficulty breathing occurs or if nausea, vomiting, or constipation become pronounced.

• Instruct patient to move slowly when sitting up or standing to avoid dizziness or light-headedness from sudden blood pressure decrease.

• Caution patient to avoid driving and other hazardous activities until drug's effects on concentration, alertness, vision, coordination, and physical dexterity are known.

• As appropriate, review all other significant and life-threatening adverse reactions and interactions, especially those related to the drugs and behaviors mentioned above.

---

telavancin
Vibativ

Pharmacologic class: Lipoglyco-peptide
Therapeutic class: Anti-infective
Pregnancy risk category C

FDA **BOXED WARNING**

• Women of childbearing age should have serum pregnancy test before receiving telavancin.

• Avoid using telavancin during pregnancy unless potential benefit to patient outweighs potential risk to fetus.

• Adverse developmental outcomes observed in three animal species at clinically relevant doses raise concerns about potential adverse developmental outcomes in humans.

Action
Binds to bacterial membrane and disrupts membrane barrier function

Availability
Injection: 250 mg, 750 mg in single-use vials

⓪ Indications and dosages
➤ Complicated skin and skin-structure infections caused by susceptible gram-positive bacteria
Adults: 10 mg/kg I.V infusion over 60 minutes q 24 hours for 7 to 14 days

Route	Onset	Peak	Duration
P.O.	Unknown	Unknown	Unknown

Dosage adjustment
• Renal impairment

Contraindications
None

Precautions
Use cautiously in:
• renal impairment
• concurrent use of drugs known to prolong QT interval
• history of congenital long QT syndrome, known prolongation of QTc interval, uncompensated heart failure, severe left ventricular hypertrophy (avoid use)
• elderly patients
• pregnant or breastfeeding patients
• children (safety and efficacy not established).

Administration
• Obtain renal function studies before starting therapy.
• Administer slowly (over 60 minutes) to reduce risk of infusion-related reactions.
• Although drug doesn't interfere with coagulation, it does, shortly after completion of infusion, interfere with certain tests used to monitor coagulation, such as prothrombin time (PT), International Normalized Ratio (INR), activated partial thromboplastin time (aPTT), activated clotting time, and coagulation-based factor Xa tests. Don't collect blood samples for such assays immediately or shortly after infusion completion because such effects dissipate as telavancin concentration decreases.

Adverse reactions
CNS: dizziness
CV: cardiac events
GI: nausea, vomiting, diarrhea, abdominal pain, taste disturbance, *Clostridium difficile*–**associated diarrhea**
GU: foamy urine, renal events, **nephrotoxicity**
Respiratory: respiratory events
Skin: rash, pruritus, infusion-site erythema
Other: rigors, decreased appetite, infectious events, superinfection, infusion-site pain, infusion reactions

Interactions
Drug-diagnostic tests. *Activated clotting time, aPTT, coagulation-based factor Xa tests, INR, PT; urine qualitative protein assays:* interference with results

Patient monitoring
◀⟪ Be aware that new-onset or worsening renal impairment has occurred in patients taking telavancin. Monitor renal function at 48- and 72-hour intervals during treatment, or more frequently if clinically indicated, and at end of therapy.
◀⟪ Watch for *C. difficile*–associated diarrhea, which may range in severity from mild diarrhea to fatal colitis; consider discontinuing drug if *C. difficile*–associated diarrhea occurs.
• Watch for "red-man" syndrome, which can result from rapid infusion. Signs and symptoms include flushing of upper body, hypotension, pruritus, and maculopapular rash on face, neck, trunk, and limbs.

Patient teaching
◀⟪ Instruct patient to tell prescriber if severe diarrhea occurs.

t

Reactions in **bold** are life-threatening.   ◀⟪ Clinical alert

• As appropriate, review all other significant and life-threatening adverse reactions and interactions, especially those related to the tests mentioned above.

---

telithromycin
Ketek

Pharmacologic class: Ketolide antibiotic
Therapeutic class: Anti-infective
Pregnancy risk category C

FDA | BOXED WARNING

• Drug is contraindicated in myasthenia gravis because life-threatening or fatal respiratory failure has occurred in these patients.

Action
Blocks protein synthesis by binding to domains II and V of 23S rRNA of 50S ribosomal subunit. Binding at domain II enables drug to retain activity against gram-positive cocci in resistance mediated by methylases that alter domain-V binding site.

Availability
Tablets (film-coated): 300 mg, 400 mg

⚕ Indications and dosages
➣ Mild to moderate community-acquired pneumonia caused by *Streptococcus pneumoniae* (including multidrug-resistant isolates), *Haemophilus influenzae*, *Moraxella catarrhalis*, *Chlamydophila pneumoniae*, or *Mycoplasma pneumoniae*
Adults age 18 and older: 800 mg P.O. daily for 7 to 10 days

Dosage adjustment
• Severe renal impairment, with or without coexisting hepatic impairment

Contraindications
• Hypersensitivity to drug, its components, or macrolide antibiotics
• History of hepatitis or jaundice with previous use of telithromycin or macrolide antibiotics
• Concurrent use of cisapride or pimozide
• Myasthenia gravis

Precautions
Use cautiously in:
• severe renal impairment, hepatic dysfunction, congenital prolongation of QT interval, ongoing proarrhythmic conditions (such as uncorrected hypokalemia or hypomagnesemia), clinically significant bradycardia (use should be avoided)
• concurrent use of some HMG-CoA reductase inhibitors (atorvastatin, lovastatin, simvastatin), rifampin, and Class IA or Class III antiarrhythmics (use should be avoided)
• concurrent use of midazolam and other benzodiazepines metabolized by CYP3A4 that undergo high first-pass effect (such as triazolam)
• concurrent use of ergot alkaloid derivatives, metoprolol, or rifampin (use not recommended)
• pregnant or breastfeeding patients
• children younger than age 18 (safety and efficacy not established).

Administration
• Administer tablets whole with or without food.
• Give at least 1 hour before or after theophylline (if prescribed).
◀€ Don't give currently with cisapride or pimozide.

Route	Onset	Peak	Duration
P.O.	Unknown	1 hr	Unknown

Adverse reactions

CNS: headache, dizziness, fatigue, loss of consciousness

CV: prolonged QT interval with increased risk of **ventricular arrhythmias** and **torsades de pointes**

EENT: visual disturbances, poor visual accommodation

GI: nausea, vomiting, diarrhea, loose stools, light-colored stools, dysgeusia, anorexia, **pseudomembranous colitis** (possibly caused by *Clostridium difficile*)

GU: dark urine

Hepatic: abnormal hepatic function, **fulminant hepatitis, hepatic necrosis, hepatic failure**

Skin: pruritus

Other: superinfection, **hypersensitivity reactions** including **angioedema** and **anaphylaxis** (rare), **acute myasthenia gravis exacerbation**

Interactions

Drug-drug. *Atorvastatin, lovastatin, simvastatin:* increased blood levels of these drugs, increased myopathy risk

Benzodiazepines metabolized by CYP3A4 (such as midazolam, triazolam): increased blood levels of these drugs

Cisapride, pimozide: increased blood levels of these drugs, increasing risk of significantly prolonged QT interval

Class IA antiarrhythmics (such as procainamide, quinidine), Class III antiarrhythmics (such as dofetilide): interference with antiarrhythmic efficacy

Colchicine: increased serum colchicine blood level and toxicity risk

Cyclosporine, sirolimus, tacrolimus: increased blood levels of these drugs, with increased toxicity risk

CYP3A4 inducers (such as carbamazepine, phenobarbital, phenytoin, rifampin): subtherapeutic telithromycin blood level

CYP3A4 inhibitors (such as itraconazole, ketoconazole): increased telithromycin blood level

Digoxin: increased peak and trough digoxin levels

Ergot alkaloid derivatives (such as dihydroergotamine, ergotamine): acute ergot toxicity

Hexobarbital: increased hexobarbital blood level and toxicity risk

Metoprolol: increased metoprolol effect

Oral anticoagulants: possible potentiation of these drugs

Sotalol: decreased sotalol absorption

Theophylline: increased theophylline blood level, with exacerbated adverse GI reactions

Verapamil: increased verapamil blood level, causing increased risk of cardiotoxicity

Drug-diagnostic tests. *Alanine aminotransferase, aspartate aminotransferase:* increased levels

Patient monitoring

• Monitor liver function tests frequently.

🔊 Discontinue drug permanently if patient develops clinical hepatitis or transaminase elevations and other systemic symptoms.

• Monitor patient closely for adverse GI reactions, especially diarrhea.

• In patients receiving drug concurrently with anticoagulants, stay alert for potentiation of anticoagulant effects.

• In patients receiving drug concurrently with midazolam, stay alert for need to adjust midazolam dosage.

• In patients receiving drug concurrently with digoxin, monitor peak and trough digoxin levels periodically, and stay alert for adverse reactions to digoxin.

Patient teaching

• Ensure that patient has received and read medication guide that comes with drug.

• Instruct patient to take tablet whole with or without food.

• Advise patient to take drug at least 1 hour before or after theophylline (if prescribed).

• Stress importance of completing full course of therapy, even if patient feels better.

◀€ Urge patient to immediately stop taking drug and report signs and symptoms of liver damage, such as nausea, fatigue, appetite loss, yellowing of skin or eyes, dark urine, light-colored stools, itching, and tender abdomen.

◀€ Instruct patient to immediately report fainting episodes or signs of heartbeat irregularities.

◀€ Urge patient to immediately report watery or loose stools even as late as several months after taking the last dose.

◀€ Advise patient to immediately report itching, throat swelling, and other signs or symptoms of allergic reaction.

• Inform patient that drug may cause visual disturbances.

• Caution patient to avoid driving and other hazardous activities until he knows how drug affects vision and alertness.

• Advise patient to consult prescriber before taking other prescription or over-the-counter drugs or dietary supplements.

• As appropriate, review all other significant and life-threatening adverse reactions and interactions, especially those related to the drugs and tests mentioned above.

telmisartan
Micardis

Pharmacologic class: Angiotensin II receptor antagonist

Therapeutic class: Antihypertensive

Pregnancy risk category C (first trimester), **D** (second and third trimesters)

FDA   BOXED WARNING

• Drugs that act directly on the renin-angiotensin system can cause injury to or death of a developing fetus. Discontinue drug as soon as possible when pregnancy is detected.

Action
Inhibits vasoconstricting effects and blocks aldosterone-producing effects of angiotensin II at various receptor sites, including vascular smooth muscle and adrenal glands

Availability
Tablets: 20 mg, 40 mg, 80 mg

Indications and dosages
➤ Hypertension
Adults: 40 mg P.O. daily, titrated up or down within range of 20 to 80 mg daily based on response and tolerance
➤ Cardiovascular risk reduction
Adults: 80 mg P.O. daily in patients unable to take angiotensin-converting enzyme (ACE) inhibitors

Contraindications
• Hypersensitivity to drug or its components

Precautions
Use cautiously in:
• heart failure, impaired renal function secondary to primary renal disease or renal stenosis, obstructive biliary disorders, hepatic impairment, volume or sodium depletion
• patients receiving high-dose diuretics
• concomitant use of ACE inhibitors and angiotensin receptor blockers (avoid use)
• pregnant or breastfeeding patients
• children younger than age 18 (safety not established).

Administration
- Don't remove tablet from blister pack until just before giving.
- Know that drug may be used alone or with other antihypertensives.

Route	Onset	Peak	Duration
P.O.	Unknown	0.5-1 hr	24 hr

Adverse reactions
CNS: dizziness, headache, fatigue
CV: chest pain, peripheral edema, hypertension, intermittent claudication
EENT: sinusitis, pharyngitis
GI: nausea, vomiting, diarrhea, dyspepsia, abdominal pain
GU: urinary tract infection
Musculoskeletal: myalgia, back and leg pain
Respiratory: cough, upper respiratory infection
Skin: ulcer
Other: pain, flu or flulike symptoms, hypersensitivity

Interactions
Drug-drug. *Antihypertensives, diuretics:* increased risk of hypotension
Ace inhibitors (ramipril): increased ramipril steady-state C_{max} and area under the curve (AUC), decreased telmisartan C_{max} and AUC
Digoxin: increased digoxin blood level
Lithium: increased serum lithium concentration and toxicity
Nonsteroidal anti-inflammatory drugs, including selective cyclooxygenase-2 inhibitors): deterioration of renal function, including possible acute renal failure in elderly patients, volume-depleted patients (including those on diuretic therapy), or with compromised renal function; attenuated telmisartan antihypertensive effect
Drug-diagnostic tests. *Creatinine:* slight elevation

Drug-food. *Any food:* slightly reduced drug bioavailability

Patient monitoring
- Monitor blood pressure frequently and watch for signs and symptoms of hypotension.
- Closely monitor patient with impaired hepatic or renal function. Correct volume deficits as appropriate before therapy starts. Monitor fluid intake and output and creatinine level during therapy.

Patient teaching
- Tell patient to take 1 hour before or 2 hours after meals.
- Caution patient not to remove tablet from blister pack until just before taking.
- Advise patient to report swelling or chest pain.
- Teach patient to measure blood pressure regularly and report significant changes.
- Tell patient to report suspected pregnancy to prescriber. Caution her not to breastfeed.
- As appropriate, review all other significant adverse reactions and interactions, especially those related to the drugs, tests, and foods mentioned above.

temazepam
Apo-Temazepam✦, Co Temazepam✦, Dom-Temazepam✦, Gen-Temazepam✦, Novo-Temazepam✦, Nu-Temazepam✦, PHL-Temazepam✦, PMS-Temazepam✦, Ratio-Temazepam✦, Restoril

Pharmacologic class: Benzodiazepine
Therapeutic class: Sedative-hypnotic
Controlled substance schedule IV
Pregnancy risk category X

Action
Depresses CNS at limbic, thalamic, and hypothalamic levels. Enhances effects of gamma-aminobutyric acid, resulting in sedation, hypnosis, skeletal muscle relaxation, and anticonvulsant and anxiolytic activity.

Availability
Capsules: 7.5 mg, 15 mg, 22.5 mg, 30 mg

⚠ Indications and dosages
➤ Insomnia
Adults: 15 mg P.O. at bedtime p.r.n. Range is 7.5 to 30 mg.

Dosage adjustment
• Elderly or debilitated patients

Contraindications
• Hypersensitivity to drug or other benzodiazepines
• Pregnancy

Precautions
Use cautiously in:
• chronic pulmonary insufficiency, hepatic dysfunction, renal disease, psychoses, drug abuse
• history of suicide attempt or drug abuse
• elderly or debilitated patients
• breastfeeding patients
• children younger than age 15.

Administration
• Give at bedtime with or without food.

Route	Onset	Peak	Duration
P.O.	30 min	1.2-1.6 hr	Unknown

Adverse reactions
CNS: hangover, headache, dizziness, drowsiness, lethargy, fatigue, paradoxical stimulation, light-headedness, talkativeness, irritability, nervousness, confusion, euphoria, relaxed feeling, tremor, incoordination, impaired memory, nightmares, paresthesia
CV: chest pain, palpitations, tachycardia

EENT: eye irritation, pain, and swelling; photophobia; tinnitus
GI: nausea, vomiting, constipation, diarrhea, heartburn, abdominal pain, dry mouth, anorexia
Musculoskeletal: joint pain
Other: altered taste, body pain, physical or psychological drug dependence, drug tolerance

Interactions
Drug-drug. *Antidepressants, antihistamines, opioid analgesics, other sedative-hypnotics:* additive CNS depression
Digoxin: increased digoxin blood level, greater risk of toxicity
Probenecid: faster temazepam onset and prolonged effects
Theophylline: antagonism of temazepam's sedative effects
Drug-herbs. *Chamomile, hops, kava, skullcap, valerian:* increased CNS depression
Drug-behaviors. *Alcohol use:* additive CNS depression
Smoking: increased drug metabolism

Patient monitoring
• Monitor neurologic status carefully. Check for paradoxical reactions, especially in elderly patient.
• Watch for signs and symptoms of physical and psychological drug dependence. Stay alert for drug hoarding.

Patient teaching
• Advise patient to establish effective bedtime routine, to minimize insomnia.
• Inform patient (and significant other if appropriate) that drug may cause psychological and physical dependence and should be used only as prescribed and needed.
• Caution patient to avoid driving and other hazardous activities on day after taking drug, until he knows how it affects concentration and alertness.
• Instruct patient not to drink alcohol.

- Advise patient not to smoke or use herbs without consulting prescriber.
- Instruct patient to report suspected pregnancy.
- As appropriate, review all other significant adverse reactions and interactions, especially those related to the drugs, herbs, and behaviors mentioned above.

temozolomide
Temodal✦⊛, Temodar

Pharmacologic class: Alkylating agent
Therapeutic class: Antineoplastic
Pregnancy risk category D

Action
Rapidly converts to monomethyl triazeno imidazole carboxamide, an active compound that prevents DNA transcription

Availability
Capsules: 5 mg, 20 mg, 100 mg, 140 mg, 180 mg, 250 mg
Injection (powder for solution, lyophilized): 100 mg

⚠ Indications and dosages
➣ Refractory anaplastic astrocytoma
Adults: 150 mg/m² P.O. or by 90-minute I.V. infusion daily for 5 consecutive days of each 28-day treatment cycle. Adjust dosage as appropriate based on absolute neutrophil count.
➣ Newly diagnosed glioblastoma multiforme with radiotherapy
Adults: 75 mg/m² P.O. or by 90-minute I.V. infusion for 42 days with focal radiotherapy (RT), followed by initial maintenance dose of 150 mg/m² P.O. or by 90-minute I.V. infusion daily for days 1 to 5 of a 28-day cycle for six cycles. Four weeks after completing the drug plus RT phase, administer drug for an additional six cycles of maintenance treatment. Dosage in maintenance cycle 1 is 150 mg/m² P.O. or by 90-minute I.V. infusion daily for 5 days, followed by 23 days without treatment. At start of maintenance cycle 2, dosage may be escalated to 200 mg/m² based on absolute neutrophil and platelet counts. Continue dosage at 200 mg/m² daily for first 5 days of each subsequent cycle except if toxicity occurs. If dosage wasn't escalated at maintenance cycle 2, escalation shouldn't be done in subsequent cycles.

Dosage adjustment
- Neutropenia, thrombocytopenia

Contraindications
- Hypersensitivity to drug, its components, or dacarbazine

Precautions
Use cautiously in:
- severe hepatic or renal impairment, active infection, decreased bone marrow reserve, other chronic debilitating illness
- elderly patients
- pregnant or breastfeeding patients
- children (safety not established).

Administration
- Follow facility policy for handling and disposing of chemotherapeutic drugs.
- Give capsules whole daily with a full glass of water, consistently either with or without food.
- Bring powder for injection to room temperature before reconstituting with 41 ml sterile water for injection that results in a 2.5-mg/ml solution. Gently swirl but don't shake vials. Don't further dilute reconstituted solution. Use reconstituted solution within 14 hours, including infusion time. Withdraw prescribed dose and transfer into empty 250-ml infusion bag. Give reconstituted solution only by I.V.

---

infusion using infusion pump over 90 minutes. Flush lines before and after each infusion.

• Know that drug may be given in same I.V. line with normal saline solution for injection only.

• Be aware that dosages in 28-day cycle depend on nadir neutrophil and platelet counts.

Route	Onset	Peak	Duration
P.O.	Rapid	1 hr	Unknown
I.V.	Unknown	Unknown	Unknown

Adverse reactions

CNS: fatigue, headache, dysphasia, poor coordination, ataxia, anxiety, depression, dizziness, drowsiness, confusion, amnesia, insomnia, mental status changes, weakness, paresis, hemiparesis, paresthesias, **seizures**
CV: peripheral edema
EENT: abnormal vision, diplopia, pharyngitis, sinusitis
GI: nausea, vomiting, constipation, diarrhea, abdominal pain, anorexia
GU: urinary incontinence or frequency, urinary tract infection, breast pain (in women)
Hematologic: anemia, **leukopenia, thrombocytopenia**
Metabolic: adrenal hypercorticism
Musculoskeletal: abnormal gait, back pain, myalgia
Respiratory: cough, upper respiratory infection
Skin: pruritus, rash
Other: fever, viral infection, weight gain

Interactions

Drug-drug. *Antineoplastics:* additive bone marrow depression
Live-virus vaccines: decreased antibody response to vaccine, greater risk of adverse reactions
Valproic acid: decreased oral clearance of temozolomide
Drug-diagnostic tests. *Neutrophils, platelets:* decreased counts

Drug-food. *Any food:* reduced rate and extent of temozolomide absorption

Patient monitoring

🔊 Monitor CBC with white cell differential. Stay alert for evidence of bone marrow depression.

• Assess neurologic status carefully.

• Monitor fluid intake and output, and weigh patient regularly.

• Be aware that *Pneumocystis jiroveci* pneumonia prophylaxis is required during concomitant administration of RT and should be continued in patients who develop lymphocytopenia until recovery from lymphocytopenia (circulating tumor cells Grade 1 or less).

Patient teaching

• Tell patient to take capsules consistently with or without food, and with a full glass of water.

• Instruct patient to swallow capsules whole without opening or chewing them and if capsules are accidentally opened or damaged, to avoid inhalation or contact with the skin or mucous membranes.

• If drug causes nausea or vomiting, advise patient to take it 1 hour before or 2 hours after a meal.

• Inform patient that drug may cause abnormal gait and dizziness.

🔊 Instruct patient to immediately report unusual bleeding or bruising.

• Advise patient to avoid live-virus vaccines.

• Caution patient to avoid driving and other hazardous activities until he knows how drug affects concentration, alertness, and vision.

• Instruct patient to report suspected pregnancy. Caution her not to breastfeed.

• As appropriate, review all other significant and life-threatening adverse reactions and interactions, especially those related to the drugs and tests mentioned above.

tenecteplase
Metalyse ⊕, TNKase

Pharmacologic class: Tissue plasminogen activator
Therapeutic class: Thrombolytic enzyme
Pregnancy risk category C

Action
Binds to fibrin and converts plasminogen to plasmin, which breaks down fibrin clots and lyses thrombi and emboli. Causes systemic fibrinolysis.

Availability
Powder for injection: 50 mg/vial with 10-ml syringe and TwinPak Dual Cannula Device and 10-ml vial of sterile water for injection

⊘ Indications and dosages
➤ To reduce mortality associated with acute myocardial infarction
Adults weighing 90 kg (198 lb) or more: 50 mg I.V. bolus given over 5 seconds
Adults weighing 80 kg to 89 kg (176 to 197 lb): 45 mg I.V. bolus given over 5 seconds
Adults weighing 70 kg to 79 kg (154 to 175 lb): 40 mg I.V. bolus given over 5 seconds
Adults weighing 60 to 69 kg (132 to 153 lb): 35 mg I.V. bolus given over 5 seconds
Adults weighing less than 60 kg (132 lb): 30 mg I.V. bolus given over 5 seconds

Contraindications
• Hypersensitivity to drug or other tissue plasminogen activators
• Active internal bleeding
• Bleeding diathesis
• Recent intracranial or intraspinal surgery or trauma
• Severe uncontrolled hypertension
• Intracranial neoplasm
• Arteriovenous malformation or aneurysm
• History of cerebrovascular accident (CVA)

Precautions
Use cautiously in:
• previous puncture of noncompressible vessels, organ biopsy, hypertension, acute pericarditis, high risk of left ventricular thrombosis, subacute bacterial endocarditis, hemostatic defects, diabetic hemorrhagic retinopathy, septic thrombophlebitis, obstetric delivery
• patients taking warfarin concurrently
• patients older than age 75
• pregnant or breastfeeding patients.

Administration
• Reconstitute by mixing contents of prefilled syringe with 10 ml of sterile water for injection. Swirl gently; don't shake. Draw up prescribed dosage from vial, then discard remainder. Give I.V. over 5 seconds through designated line.
◀€ Don't deliver in same I.V. line with dextrose solutions. Flush I.V. line with normal saline solution before giving drug if patient has been receiving dextrose.
◀€ Give with heparin if ordered, but not through same I.V. line.

Route	Onset	Peak	Duration
I.V.	Immediate	Unknown	Unknown

Adverse reactions
CNS: intracranial hemorrhage, CVA
CV: hypotension, **arrhythmia, myocardial rupture, myocardial reinfarction, cardiogenic shock, atrioventricular block, cardiac arrest, cardiac tamponade, heart failure, pericarditis, pericardial effusion, mitral regurgitation, thrombosis, embolism, hemorrhage**

EENT: epistaxis, minor pharyngeal bleeding
GI: nausea, vomiting, **hemorrhage**
GU: hematuria
Hematologic: anemia, **bleeding tendency**
Respiratory: respiratory depression, pulmonary edema, apnea
Skin: bleeding at puncture sites, hematoma

Interactions

Drug-drug. *Anticoagulants, aspirin, dipyridamole, indomethacin, phenylbutazone:* increased bleeding risk
Drug-diagnostic tests. *Coagulation tests:* fibrinogen degradation in blood sample

Patient monitoring

◀≋ Monitor ECG. Stay alert for reperfusion arrhythmias.
◀≋ Monitor vital signs carefully. Watch for signs and symptoms of respiratory depression and reinfarction.
◀≋ Evaluate all body systems closely for signs and symptoms of bleeding. If bleeding occurs, stop drug and give antiplatelet agents, as ordered.
• Monitor CBC and coagulation studies. However, know that drug may skew coagulation results.

Patient teaching

◀≋ Inform patient that drug increases risk of bleeding. Advise him to immediately report signs and symptoms of bleeding.
• Teach patient safety measures to avoid bruising and bleeding.
• Tell patient he'll undergo regular blood tests during therapy.
• As appropriate, review all other significant and life-threatening adverse reactions and interactions, especially those related to the drugs and tests mentioned above.

tenofovir disoproxil fumarate
Viread

Pharmacologic class: Nucleoside analog reverse transcriptase inhibitor
Therapeutic class: Antiretroviral
Pregnancy risk category B

FDA | BOXED WARNING

• Severe acute exacerbations of hepatitis have been reported in patients with hepatitis B virus (HBV) infection who have discontinued anti–hepatitis B therapy. Monitor hepatic function closely with both clinical and laboratory follow-up for at least several months in patients who discontinue anti–hepatitis B therapy. If appropriate, resumption of anti–hepatitis B therapy may be warranted.
• Lactic acidosis and severe hepatomegaly with steatosis, including fatal cases, have been reported with the use of nucleoside analogs, including tenofovir.
• Drug should not be given with adefovir dipivoxil.
• Because of risk of development of human immunodeficiency virus-1 (HIV-1) resistance, drug should only be used in HIV-1 and HBV co-infected patients as part of an appropriate antiretroviral combination regimen.
• HIV-1 antibody testing should be offered to all HBV-infected patients before start of therapy. It is also recommended that all patients with HIV-1 infection be tested for presence of chronic HBV infection before start of drug therapy.
• Drug's effects on bone haven't been studied in patients with chronic HBV infection.
• In HIV-infected patients, redistribution or accumulation of body fat,

including central obesity, dorsocervical fat enlargement (buffalo hump), peripheral wasting, facial wasting, breast enlargement, and cushingoid appearance, has been observed in patients receiving combination antiretroviral therapy.

• Immune reconstitution syndrome has been reported in HIV-infected patients treated with combination antiretroviral therapy.

Action
Inhibits activity of HIV by competing with natural substrate deoxyadenosine 5'-triphosphate; disrupts cellular DNA by causing chain termination

Availability
Powder, oral: 40 mg/scoop
Tablets: 150 mg, 200 mg, 250 mg, 300 mg

Indications and dosages
➤ HIV-1 infection, chronic hepatitis B infection
Adults and adolescents age 12 and older weighing 35 kg (77 lb) or more: 300 mg P.O. daily; for patients unable to swallow tablets, give 7.5 scoops of oral powder.
➤ HIV-1 infection
Children ages 2 to younger than 12: 8 mg/kg (to maximum of 300 mg) P.O. once daily as oral powder or tablets

Dosage adjustment
• Baseline creatinine clearance less than 50 ml/minute

Contraindications
• None

Precautions
Use cautiously in:
• renal impairment
• lactic acidosis
• exacerbation of hepatitis, hepatomegaly with steatosis

• co-administration of adefovir dipivoxil or other tenofovir-containing products
• concurrent or recent use of nephrotoxic drugs.
• decreased bone marrow density
• redistribution or accumulation of body fat
• immune reconstitution syndrome
• elderly patients
• pregnant or breastfeeding patients
• children younger than age 2 with HIV-1 infection and younger than age 12 or less than 35 kg (77 lb) with chronic hepatitis B infection (safety and efficacy not established).

Administration
• Assess creatinine clearance before starting drug.
• Give tablets without regard to meals.
• Give oral powder with 2 to 4 oz of soft foods that can be swallowed without chewing (such as applesauce, baby food, or yogurt). Don't mix with liquids. Give dose immediately after mixing.
• Know that drug is usually given with other antiretrovirals for HIV infection.

Route	Onset	Peak	Duration
P.O.	Rapid	45-75 min	Unknown

Adverse reactions
CNS: headache, asthenia, depression
GI: nausea, vomiting, diarrhea, abdominal pain, flatulence, anorexia
GU: new-onset or worsening renal impairment (including acute renal failure and Fanconi syndrome)
Skin: rash
Hepatic: severe hepatomegaly with steatosis
Metabolic: hyperglycemia, **lactic acidosis**
Other: body fat redistribution, pain, **immune reconstitution syndrome**

Interactions

Drug-drug. *Acyclovir, cidofovir, didanosine, ganciclovir, indinavir, lopinavir, probenecid, ritonavir, valacyclovir, valganciclovir, other drugs eliminated by active tubular secretion (such as adefovir dipivoxil):* increased blood level of either drug

Atazanavir, lopinavir/ritonavir: increased tenofovir concentration

Drug-diagnostic tests. *Alanine aminotransferase, amylase, aspartate aminotransferase, blood and urine glucose, creatine kinase, triglycerides:* increased levels

Neutrophils: decreased count

Drug-food. *Any food:* decreased drug bioavailability and efficacy

Patient monitoring

◀€ Watch for and report signs and symptoms of lactic acidosis or hepatotoxicity.

• Monitor bone mineral density in patients with history of pathologic fractures or who are at risk for osteopenia.

◀€ Monitor for signs of immune reconstitution syndrome, especially during initial phase of combination antiretroviral treatment when patients whose immune systems respond may develop an inflammatory response to indolent or residual opportunistic infections (such as *Mycobacterium avium* infection, cytomegalovirus, *Pneumocystis jiroveci* pneumonia, or tuberculosis), which may necessitate further evaluation and treatment.

• Monitor kidney and liver function tests.

• Assess nutritional status and hydration in light of adverse GI reactions and underlying disease.

Patient teaching

• Tell patient to take tablets once daily at the same time every day with or without food and take oral powder at the same time every day with food.

• Tell patient not to mix oral powder with liquids. Tell patient to use only the dosing scoop supplied, to mix only with 2 to 4 oz of soft foods that can be swallowed without chewing (such as baby food, applesauce, or yogurt), and to take entire dose immediately after mixing.

◀€ Instruct patient to immediately report unusual tiredness or yellowing of skin or eyes.

• Tell patient drug may cause weakness and headache. Caution him to avoid driving and other hazardous activities until he knows how drug affects performance.

• Caution female patient not to breast-feed.

• As appropriate, review all other significant and life-threatening adverse reactions and interactions, especially those related to the drugs, tests, and foods mentioned above.

terazosin hydrochloride

Apo-Terazosin✿, Dom-Terazosin✿, Hytrin, Novo-Terazosin✿, Nu-Terazosin✿, PHL-Terazosin✿, PMS-Terazosin✿, Ratio-Terazosin✿

Pharmacologic class: Anti-adrenergic (peripherally acting)

Therapeutic class: Antihypertensive

Pregnancy risk category C

Action

Blocks postsynaptic alpha$_1$-adrenergic receptors, causing vasodilation and decreasing smooth muscle contractions in bladder neck and prostate

---

Availability
Capsules: 1 mg, 2 mg, 5 mg, 10 mg

Indications and dosages
➤ Hypertension
Adults: Initially, 1 mg P.O., increased slowly as needed up to 5 mg/day. Usual range is 1 to 5 mg/day, not to exceed 20 mg/day.
➤ Benign prostatic hyperplasia
Adults: 1 mg P.O. at bedtime. To achieve desired response, may increase gradually to 2 mg/day, then to 5 mg/day, and then to a maximum of 10 mg/day.

Contraindications
• Hypersensitivity to drug or other quinazoline derivatives

Precautions
Use cautiously in:
• prostate cancer, hepatic disease, dehydration, volume or sodium depletion
• pregnant or breastfeeding patients
• children (safety not established).

Administration
◀€ Don't stop therapy suddenly. Dosage must be tapered.
• Know that drug may be given as a single dose at bedtime or in two divided doses.

Route	Onset	Peak	Duration
P.O.	15 min	2-3 hr	24 hr

Adverse reactions
CNS: dizziness, headache, weakness, drowsiness, nervousness, paresthesia, vertigo, fatigue, syncope
CV: orthostatic hypotension (with first dose), rebound hypertension, chest pain, palpitations, peripheral edema, tachycardia, **arrhythmias**
EENT: blurred vision, conjunctivitis, amblyopia, nasal congestion, sinusitis
GI: nausea, vomiting, diarrhea, abdominal pain, dry mouth
GU: urinary frequency or incontinence, erectile dysfunction, priapism

Musculoskeletal: joint, back, and extremity pain; arthritis
Respiratory: dyspnea
Skin: pruritus
Other: fever, weight gain, flulike symptoms

Interactions
Drug-drug. *Estrogens, nonsteroidal anti-inflammatory drugs (NSAIDs), sympathomimetics:* decreased antihypertensive effects
Midodrine: antagonism of terazosin's action
Nitrates, other antihypertensives: additive hypotension
Drug-herbs. *Ephedra (ma huang):* antagonism of terazosin's action
Drug-behaviors. *Alcohol use:* additive hypotension

Patient monitoring
• Monitor blood pressure. Stay alert for orthostatic hypotension (first-dose effect) when therapy begins.
• Assess cardiovascular status. Report chest pain, peripheral edema, palpitations, and other significant effects.

Patient teaching
• Instruct patient to take at same time every day, with or without food.
◀€ Caution patient not to stop therapy abruptly. Dosage must be tapered.
◀€ Advise patient to immediately report swelling, breathing difficulty, palpitations, chest pain, and other cardiovascular reactions.
• Tell patient drug may cause erectile dysfunction and other sexual problems.
• Caution patient not to use NSAIDs or drink alcohol.
• Instruct patient to move slowly when sitting up or standing, to avoid dizziness from sudden blood pressure decrease.
• As appropriate, review all other significant and life-threatening adverse reactions and interactions, especially those related to the drugs, herbs, and behaviors mentioned above.

t

Reactions in **bold** are life-threatening.   ◀€ Clinical alert

terbinafine hydrochloride
Lamisil, Lamisil AT

Pharmacologic class: Synthetic allyl-amine derivative

Therapeutic class: Antifungal

Pregnancy risk category B

Action
Unclear. Thought to interfere with sterol biosynthesis of fungal cell membrane permeability by inhibiting enzymes responsible for normal fungal growth and maturation, resulting in cell death.

Availability
Cream: 1%
Gel (topical): 1%
Oral granules: 125 mg, 187.5 mg
Solution (topical): 1%
Spray (topical): 1%
Tablets: 250 mg

⚡ Indications and dosages
➤ Tinea cruris; tinea corporis; tinea pedis; tinea versicolor

Adults and children ages 12 and older: Massage cream into affected area and surrounding area once or twice daily for 7 to 14 days, not to exceed 4 weeks. Or, for tinea pedis, apply gel to affected area once daily at bedtime for 1 week. Or, for tinea cruris and tinea corporis, spray or apply gel to affected area once daily (morning or night) for 1 week. Or, for tinea pedis, spray between toes b.i.d. (morning and night) for 1 week.

➤ Onychomycosis of fingernail or toenail

Adults: For fingernail infection, 250 mg P.O. daily for 6 weeks. For toenail infection, 250 mg P.O. daily for 12 weeks.

➤ Tinea capitis

Children ages 4 and older weighing less than 25 kg (55 lb): 125 mg P.O. daily for 6 weeks

Children ages 4 and older weighing 25 to 35 kg (55 to 77 lb): 187.5 mg P.O. daily for 6 weeks

Children ages 4 and older weighing more than 35 kg (77 lb): 250 mg P.O. daily for 6 weeks

Contraindications
• Hypersensitivity to drug or its components
• Chronic active hepatic disease

Precautions
Use cautiously in:
• renal impairment (use not recommended)
• pregnant or breastfeeding patients (use not recommended)
• children younger than age 12 (safety and efficacy not established with cream, spray, or tablet use).

Administration
• Give with or without food, but not with coffee, cola, or tea.
• Know that oral granules should be sprinkled on nonacidic food, such as pudding or mashed potatoes. Fruit-based food such as applesauce shouldn't be used.
• Know that oral granules should be swallowed without being chewed.
• Don't put occlusive dressing over affected area after cream application.

Route	Onset	Peak	Duration
P.O.	Unknown	≤ 2 hr	Unknown
Topical	Unknown	Unknown	Unknown

Adverse reactions
CNS: headache, depression
EENT: visual disturbances
GI: nausea, diarrhea, dyspepsia, abdominal pain, flatulence
Hematologic: neutropenia
Hepatic: hepatic failure

Skin: burning, stinging, dryness, itching, and local irritation (with topical form); rash; pruritus; urticaria; **erythema multiforme; Stevens-Johnson syndrome**
Other: taste and smell disturbances

Interactions

Drug-drug. *Cimetidine:* decreased terbinafine clearance
Cyclosporine: increased cyclosporine clearance
Dextromethorphan: increased dextromethorphan blood level
Rifampin: increased terbinafine clearance
Warfarin: altered warfarin efficacy
Drug-diagnostic tests. *Hepatic enzymes:* increased levels
Neutrophils: decreased count
Drug-food. *Caffeine-containing foods and beverages:* decreased caffeine clearance
Drug-herbs. *Chaparral, comfrey, germander, jin bu huan, kava, pennyroyal:* increased risk of hepatotoxicity
Cola nut, guarana, yerba maté: decreased clearance of these herbs

Patient monitoring

• Monitor CBC and liver function tests.
◀€ Watch for signs and symptoms of erythema multiforme. Report early indications before they progress to Stevens-Johnson syndrome.

Patient teaching

• Tell patient he may take with or without food.
• Advise caregiver that oral granules should be sprinkled on nonacidic food, such as pudding or mashed potatoes and not to use fruit-based food such as applesauce.
• Advise caregiver that oral granules should be swallowed without being chewed.

• Instruct patient to avoid coffee, tea, and colas, which can worsen adverse drug reactions.
• Tell patient drug may take 4 weeks to be effective in fingernail infections and 10 weeks in toenail infections. Urge him to keep taking it even though symptoms don't improve right away.
◀€ Advise patient to immediately report rash, sore throat, cough, fever, or yellowing of skin or eyes.
• Instruct patient how to use topical drug, to wash affected area with soap and water and dry area completely before applying drug, and to wash hands after each use.
• Instruct patient not to place occlusive dressing over affected area after applying cream.
• Advise patient to wear well-fitting, ventilated shoes and to change shoes and socks at least once daily when receiving treatment for athlete's foot.
• Caution patient not to let topical drug contact eyes, nose, or mouth.
• As appropriate, review all other significant and life-threatening adverse reactions and interactions, especially those related to the drugs, tests, foods, and herbs mentioned above.

terbutaline sulfate
Monovent ⊕

Pharmacologic class: Selective beta₂-adrenergic receptor agonist
Therapeutic class: Bronchodilator
Pregnancy risk category B

Action

Relaxes bronchial smooth muscle by stimulating beta₂-adrenergic receptors; inhibits release of hypersensitivity mediators, especially from mast cells

Availability
Injection: 1 mg/ml
Tablets: 2.5 mg, 5 mg

🕊 Indications and dosages
➤ Bronchospasm in reversible obstructive airway disease
Adults and children older than age 12: 0.25 mg subcutaneously, repeated in 15 to 30 minutes p.r.n., up to a maximum of 0.5 mg in 4 hours. Or 2.5 to 5 mg P.O. q 6 hours t.i.d. while awake, up to a maximum of 15 mg/day in adults; 2.5 mg P.O. q 6 hours t.i.d. while awake, up to a maximum of 7.5 mg/day in children.

Dosage adjustment
• Renal impairment

Off-label uses
• Tocolytic in preterm labor

Contraindications
• Hypersensitivity to drug, its components, or sympathomimetic amines

Precautions
Use cautiously in:
• cardiovascular disorders, hypertension, arrhythmias, hyperthyroidism, diabetes mellitus, seizure disorders, glaucoma
• concurrent use of MAO inhibitors, tricyclic antidepressants, or beta-adrenergic blockers
• elderly patients
• breastfeeding patients.

Administration
• Inject subcutaneously into lateral deltoid.

Route	Onset	Peak	Duration
P.O.	30 min	2-3 hr	4-8 hr
Subcut.	15 min	30 min	1.5-4 hr

Adverse reactions
CNS: tremors, anxiety, nervousness, insomnia, headache, dizziness, drowsiness, stimulation
CV: palpitations, chest discomfort, tachycardia
GI: nausea, vomiting
Skin: diaphoresis, flushing

Interactions
Drug-drug. *Beta-adrenergic blockers:* blockage of bronchodilating effect
MAO inhibitors, tricyclic antidepressants: potentiation of terbutaline's adverse cardiovascular reactions
Other sympathomimetic amines: additive adverse cardiovascular reactions

Patient monitoring
• Monitor vital signs.
• Assess neurologic status.

Patient teaching
• Tell patient he may take with or without food.
• Advise patient or parents to establish effective bedtime routine to minimize insomnia.
• Instruct patient or parents to space doses evenly during waking hours, to avoid taking drug at bedtime.
• As appropriate, review all other significant adverse reactions and interactions, especially those related to the drugs mentioned above.

teriparatide (recombinant)
Forsteo ✦, Forteo

Pharmacologic class: Biosynthetic fragment of human parathyroid hormone
Therapeutic class: Parathyroid hormone
Pregnancy risk category C

FDA | BOXED WARNING

• In male and female rats, drug increased incidence of osteosarcoma (malignant bone tumor). Because of uncertain relevance of this finding to humans, use drug only in patients for whom potential benefits outweigh potential risk. Don't administer to patient at increased baseline risk for osteosarcoma.

Action
Stimulates new bone growth by binding to specific high-affinity cell-surface receptors

Availability
Injection: Multidose prefilled delivery device (pen) with 28 daily doses of 20 mcg/dose (600 mcg/2.4 ml)

❷ Indications and dosages
➤ Osteoporosis in patients at high risk for bone fracture
Adults: 20 mcg/day subcutaneously for up to 2 years

Contraindications
• Hypersensitivity to drug
• Conditions that increase osteosarcoma risk (such as Paget's disease, unexplained alkaline phosphatase elevation, open epiphyses, skeletal radiation therapy)
• Bone cancer metastases or history of bone cancer
• Metabolic bone disease other than osteoporosis
• Hypercalcemia

Precautions
Use cautiously in:
• urolithiasis, hypotension
• concurrent use of cardiac glycosides
• pregnant or breastfeeding patients.

Administration
• Inject subcutaneously into thigh or abdominal wall, with patient lying down.

• Know that prefilled injection pen delivers 20 mcg of drug per actuation and may be reused for up to 28 days after first injection. Discard pen in protected container after 28 days, even if it's not empty.

Route	Onset	Peak	Duration
Subcut.	Rapid	Rapid	Unknown

Adverse reactions
CNS: dizziness, headache, insomnia, depression, vertigo, asthenia
CV: hypertension, angina, syncope
EENT: rhinitis, pharyngitis
GI: nausea, vomiting, diarrhea, dyspepsia, anorexia
Metabolic: hyperuricemia
Musculoskeletal: joint pain, cramps
Respiratory: cough, dyspnea, pneumonia
Skin: rash, sweating
Other: pain

Interactions
Drug-drug. *Digoxin:* increased digoxin toxicity
Drug-diagnostic tests. *Calcium:* increased level

Patient monitoring
• Monitor respiratory and neurologic status and assess patient's mood.
• Monitor bone mineral density tests and calcium level.

Patient teaching
• Instruct patient to promptly report such adverse reactions as cough and difficulty breathing.
• Tell patient that prefilled injection pen delivers 20 mcg of drug per actuation. Inform him that he may reuse it for up to 28 days after first injection, and should then discard it in appropriate receptacle, even if it's not empty.
• Advise patient to establish effective bedtime routine to minimize insomnia.
• Caution patient to avoid driving and other hazardous activities until he

t

Reactions in **bold** are life-threatening.   ◀€ Clinical alert

knows how drug affects strength and balance.

• As appropriate, review all other significant adverse reactions and interactions, especially those related to the drugs and tests mentioned above.

testosterone

Axiron, Androderm, AndroGel, Andropatch ✛, Fortesta, Striant, Testim, Testogel ✛, Testopel Pellets, Testos ✱

testosterone cypionate

Depo-Testosterone

testosterone enanthate

Delatestryl, PMS-Testosterone Enthanate ✱

Pharmacologic class: Hormone
Therapeutic class: Androgenic and anabolic steroid, antineoplastic
Controlled substance schedule III
Pregnancy risk category X

FDA | **BOXED WARNING**

• Virilization has occurred in children secondarily exposed to testosterone gel.
• Children should avoid contact with unwashed or unclothed application sites in men using testosterone gel.
• Health care providers should advise patients to strictly adhere to recommended instructions for use.

Action

Responsible for normal growth and development of male sex organs and maintenance and maturation of secondary sex characteristics. Also decreases estrogen activity, which aids treatment of some breast cancers.

Availability

testosterone
Buccal system: 30 mg
Gel: 1% (25 mg, 50 mg), 1.62% (metered-dose pump delivers 20.25 mg/actuation), 2% (10 mg/one metered-dose pump actuation)
Injection (aqueous suspension): 100 mg/ml
Pellets (subcutaneous implant): 75 mg
Solution (topical): 30 mg/metered-dose pump actuation
Transdermal system: 2 mg/day, 4 mg/day
testosterone cypionate
Injection: 100 mg/ml, 200 mg/ml
testosterone enanthate
Injection (in oil): 200 mg/ml

🕛 Indications and dosages

➤ Male hypogonadism
Adult males: 10 to 25 mg (testosterone) I.M. two to three times weekly or 50 to 400 mg (enanthate) I.M. q 2 to 4 weeks for 3 to 4 years. Or 150 to 450 mg (pellet) implanted subcutaneously q 3 to 6 months. Or, 4 mg (transdermal system) daily, adjusted to 2 mg or 6 mg based on serum testosterone level. Or, 60 mg (one 30-mg actuation of Axiron topical solution applied to each axilla) daily at same time each morning, adjusted to 30 mg (one pump actuation) or increased from 60 to 90 mg (three pump actuations) or from 90 to 120 mg (four pump actuations) based on serum testosterone concentration from single blood draw 2 to 8 hours after applying solution and at least 14 days after starting treatment or following dosage adjustment. Or, 40 mg (four actuations of Fortesta topical gel) applied to clean, intact skin of thighs once daily in morning, adjusted to 10 mg (one pump actuation) or up to 70 mg (seven pump actuations) based on total serum testosterone level 2 hours after applying gel at approximately 14 days after starting treatment or following dosage adjustment. Or,

50 mg testosterone gel (AndroGel 1%) daily applied topically, adjusted up to 75 mg daily within 14 days, with subsequent dosages up to 100 mg daily. Or, 30 mg (buccal system) to gum region b.i.d. Or, 50 to 400 mg I.M. (cypionate) q 2 to 4 weeks.

➤ Delayed puberty

Adult males: 50 to 200 mg I.M. (enanthate only) q 2 to 4 weeks for limited duration (4 to 6 months); or 150 to 450 mg subcutaneously (pellets) q 3 to 6 months

➤ Inoperable breast cancer in women 1 to 5 years after menopause

Adults: 200 to 400 mg I.M. (enanthate) q 2 to 4 weeks

Contraindications

• Hypersensitivity to drug, its components, or tartrazine
• Males with breast cancer or suspected prostate cancer
• Females (buccal or transdermal systems or gel)
• Pregnancy or breastfeeding

Precautions

Use cautiously in:

• diabetes mellitus; edema associated with serious cardiac, hepatic, or renal disease; sleep apnea; hypercalcemia
• children younger than age 18 (safety and efficacy not established).

Administration

• Evaluate elderly patients and patients at increased risk for prostate cancer for presence of prostate cancer before starting testosterone replacement therapy.
• Inspect aqueous solution for injection. If crystals are visible, warm bottle and shake contents to dissolve crystals.
• Rotate I.M. injection sites within upper outer quadrant of gluteus maximus. Inject deeply into muscle.
• Apply gel once daily to clean, dry, intact skin on shoulder, upper arm, or abdomen.

• Place buccal system just above incisor tooth. Have patient hold it in place for 30 seconds to ensure adhesion. Rotate to other side of mouth with each application.

Route	Onset	Peak	Duration
Buccal	Slow	10-12 hr	Unknown
I.M.	Unknown	10-100 min	Unknown
Subcut.	Unknown	Unknown	3-4 mo
Topical gel	30 min	Unknown	Unknown
Transdermal	Unknown	2-4 hr	Unknown

Adverse reactions

CNS: headache, depression, emotional lability, nervousness, anxiety, asthenia, memory loss, dizziness, vertigo, **cerebrovascular accident**

CV: edema, peripheral edema, **deepvein phlebitis, heart failure**

GI: bleeding

GU: hematuria, urinary tract infection, impaired urination, scrotal cellulitis, benign prostatic hyperplasia, scrotal papilloma (with transdermal use), prostatitis, libido changes, breast pain or tenderness, gynecomastia, virilization in females, excessive hormonal effects in males

Hematologic: polycythemia, leukopenia, suppressed clotting factors

Hepatic: hepatic adenoma (with long-term enanthate use)

Metabolic: hyperphosphatemia, hypernatremia, hypercalcemia, **hypoglycemia, hyperkalemia**

Musculoskeletal: myalgia

Respiratory: sleep apnea

Skin: acne; rash, itching, burning, discomfort, irritation, burn-like blister, erythema (with transdermal use); pain, local edema, and induration at injection site (with I.M. or subcutaneous use)

Other: accidental injury, flulike symptoms, hypersensitivity reaction

t

Reactions in **bold** are life-threatening. ◀᧝ Clinical alert

Interactions

Drug-drug. *Corticosteroids:* increased risk of edema

Hepatotoxic drugs: increased risk of hepatotoxicity

Insulin, oral hypoglycemics: decreased blood glucose level

Oral anticoagulants: increased anticoagulant effect

Oxyphenbutazone: increased oxyphenbutazone blood level

Propranolol: increased propranolol clearance

Drug-diagnostic tests. *Bilirubin, liver function tests:* abnormal results

Calcium, cholesterol, hematocrit, hemoglobin, phosphate, prostate-specific antigen (with topical use), sodium: increased levels

Clotting factors, creatine excretion, glucose, serum creatinine, thyroxine, thyroxine-binding globulin: decreased levels

Urine creatine and creatinine: decreased excretion

Urine 17-ketosteroids: increased excretion

Drug-herbs. *Chaparral, comfrey, germander, jin bu huan, kava, pennyroyal:* increased risk of hepatotoxicity

Patient monitoring

• Monitor electrolyte levels, liver function tests, blood and urine calcium levels, lipid panels, CBC with white cell differential, and semen studies.

• Assess diabetic patient carefully for hypoglycemia.

• Closely monitor neurologic status. Stay alert for sleep apnea.

• Assess for early signs of excessive hormonal effects in females (virilization). If these occur, drug withdrawal may be indicated.

Patient teaching

◀€ Instruct patient to immediately report signs and symptoms of liver problems, including nausea, vomiting, yellowing of skin or eyes, and ankle swelling.

• Teach prepubertal male about signs and symptoms of excessive hormonal effects, such as acne, priapism, increased body and facial hair, and penile enlargement.

• Teach postpubertal male about signs and symptoms of excessive adverse hormonal effects, such as erectile dysfunction, gynecomastia, epididymitis, testicular atrophy, and infertility.

◀€ Tell female patient to immediately report signs of masculinization, such as excessive body or facial hair, deepening of voice, clitoral enlargement, and menstrual irregularities.

• Advise female of childbearing age to use barrier contraceptives. Caution her not to breastfeed.

• Tell patient which transdermal patches can be applied to scrotum. Instruct him to apply patch daily to clean, dry skin after removing protective liner to expose drug-containing film. To prevent irritation, instruct him to apply each patch to a different site, waiting at least 1 week before reusing same site.

• Advise patient to apply topical gel once daily to clean, dry skin on shoulder, upper arm, or abdomen. Tell him that after opening packet, he should squeeze entire contents into palm and apply immediately. Instruct him to wait until gel dries before getting dressed.

• Teach patient to place buccal system in comfortable position just above incisor tooth and hold it in place for about 30 seconds to ensure adhesion. Tell him to use opposite side of mouth with each application. Caution him not to dislodge buccal system, especially when eating, drinking, brushing teeth, or using mouthwash. If system doesn't properly adhere or falls out during 12-hour dosing interval, tell him to discard it and apply new system. If it falls out within 4 hours of next dose, tell him to apply new system and keep it in place until next regularly scheduled dose.

- Instruct patient to apply topical solution to clean, dry, intact skin of axilla area only and to allow application site to dry completely before dressing. Advise patient to wash axilla with soap and water to remove any testosterone residue if direct skin-to-skin contact with another person is anticipated.
- Tell patient drug shouldn't be used to enhance athletic performance or physique.
- As appropriate, review all other significant and life-threatening adverse reactions and interactions, especially those related to the drugs, tests, and herbs mentioned above.

tetracycline hydrochloride

Apo-Tetra🍁, Novotetra🍁,
Nu-Tetra🍁, Topicycline❋

Pharmacologic class: Tetracycline
Therapeutic class: Anti-infective
Pregnancy risk category B (topical form), ***D*** (oral form)

Action

Unknown. Thought to inhibit bacterial protein synthesis at level of 30S and 50S bacterial ribosomes and to alter cytoplasmic membrane of susceptible organisms.

Availability

Capsules: 250 mg, 500 mg

Indications and dosages

➢ Mild to moderate infections caused by susceptible organisms
Adults: 500 mg P.O. b.i.d. or 250 mg P.O. q.i.d.
➢ Severe infections caused by susceptible organisms
Adults: 500 mg P.O. q.i.d.
Children older than age 8: 25 to 50 mg/kg P.O. q.i.d.
➢ Syphilis in penicillin-allergic patients
Adults: 500 mg P.O. q.i.d. for 14 days
➢ Late syphilis (except neurosyphilis)
Adults: 500 mg P.O. q.i.d. for 28 days
➢ Leptospirosis when penicillin is contraindicated or ineffective
Adults: 1 to 2 g P.O. daily in two to four divided doses for 5 to 7 days
➢ Yaws
Adults: 1 to 2 g P.O. daily in two to four divided doses for 10 to 14 days
➢ Gonorrhea in penicillin-allergic patients
Adults: Initially, 1.5 g P.O., followed by 500 mg P.O. q 6 hours for 4 days, up to a total of 9 g
➢ Uncomplicated urethral, endocervical, or rectal infections caused by *Chlamydia trachomatis*
Adults: 500 mg P.O. q.i.d. for 7 days
➢ Rickettsial and mycoplasmal infections
Adults: 1 to 2 g P.O. daily in two to four divided doses for 7 days
➢ *Helicobacter pylori* infection
Adults: In patients with active duodenal ulcer, 500 mg P.O. q.i.d. at meals and bedtime for 14 days, given with other drugs (such as metronidazole, bismuth subsalicylate, amoxicillin, or omeprazole)
➢ Brucellosis
Adults: 500 mg P.O. q.i.d. for 3 weeks, given with streptomycin I.M. b.i.d. during week 1 and streptomycin once daily during week 2
➢ Granuloma inguinale; chancroid
Adults: 1 to 2 g P.O. daily in two to four divided doses for 2 to 4 weeks
➢ Cholera
Adults: 500 mg P.O. q 6 hours for 48 to 72 hours
➢ Plague when streptomycin is contraindicated or ineffective
Adults: 2 to 4 g P.O. q.i.d. for 10 days
Children older than age 8: 30 to 40 mg/kg P.O. q.i.d. for 10 to 14 days

➤ Tularemia as an alternative to streptomycin

Adults: 1 to 2 g P.O. daily in two to four divided doses for 1 to 2 weeks

➤ *Campylobacter* infection

Adults: 1 to 2 g P.O. daily in two to four divided doses for 10 days

➤ Relapsing fever caused by *Borrelia recurrentis*

Adults: 1 to 2 g P.O. daily in two to four divided doses for 7 days or until patient is afebrile

➤ Adjunctive treatment of inflammatory acne

Adults and adolescents: 500 mg to 1 g P.O. q.i.d. for 1 to 2 weeks, decreased gradually to 125 to 500 mg P.O. daily

Dosage adjustment

• Renal impairment

Off-label uses

• Rosacea
• Anthrax
• Arthritis
• Lyme disease
• Sclerosing agent to control pleural effusions

Contraindications

• Hypersensitivity to drug, other tetracyclines, bisulfites, or alcohol (in some products)

Precautions

Use cautiously in:

• renal disease, hepatic impairment, nephrogenic diabetes insipidus
• cachectic or debilitated patients
• pregnant or breastfeeding patients (except in anthrax treatment)
• children younger than age 8 (except in anthrax treatment).

Administration

• Give with 8 oz of water at least 1 hour before or 2 hours after a meal (especially if it includes milk or other dairy products), antacids, laxatives, or antidiarrheal drugs.

Route	Onset	Peak	Duration
P.O.	Rapid	2-3 hr	6-12 hr

Adverse reactions

CNS: paresthesia, **benign intracranial hypertension**

CV: pericarditis

EENT: abnormal conjunctival pigmentation, hoarseness, pharyngitis

GI: nausea, vomiting, diarrhea, loose bulky stools, esophageal ulcers, epigastric distress, enterocolitis, oral and anogenital candidiasis, stomatitis, black hairy tongue, glossitis, anorexia, **pancreatitis**

GU: dark yellow or brown urine, vaginal candidiasis, anogenital lesions

Hematologic: eosinophilia, **hemolytic anemia, neutropenia, thrombocytopenia, thrombocytopenia purpura**

Hepatic: fatty liver

Musculoskeletal: retarded bone growth, polyarthralgia

Respiratory: pulmonary infiltrates

Skin: photosensitivity, maculopapular or erythematous rash, increased pigmentation, urticaria, onycholysis

Other: permanent tooth discoloration (in children younger than age 8), tooth enamel defects, superinfection, hypersensitivity reactions including **anaphylaxis, serum sickness–like reaction, exacerbation of systemic lupus erythematosus**

Interactions

Drug-drug. *Adsorbent antidiarrheals, antacids, calcium, cholestyramine, cimetidine, colestipol, iron, magnesium, sodium bicarbonate:* decreased tetracycline absorption

Digoxin: increased digoxin blood level, greater risk of toxicity

Hormonal contraceptives: decreased contraceptive efficacy

Insulin: reduced insulin requirement

Lithium: increased or decreased lithium blood level

Methoxyflurane: increased risk of nephrotoxicity

Penicillin: decreased penicillin activity

Sucralfate: prevention of tetracycline absorption from GI tract

Warfarin: enhanced warfarin effects

Drug-diagnostic tests. *Alanine aminotransferase, alkaline phosphatase, amylase, aspartate aminotransferase, bilirubin, blood urea nitrogen:* increased levels

Hemoglobin, neutrophils, platelets, white blood cells: decreased levels

Urinary catecholamines: false elevation

Drug-food. *Dairy products, foods containing calcium:* decreased drug absorption

Drug-behaviors. *Alcohol use:* decreased drug efficacy

Sun exposure: increased risk of photosensitivity

Patient monitoring

• Monitor for signs and symptoms of superinfection and hypersensitivity reaction.

• With long-term use, monitor CBC, liver function tests, and (in prepubertal patients) bone growth.

• Assess neurologic status. Stay alert for benign intracranial hypertension (especially in children).

Patient teaching

• Tell patient to take oral form with 8 oz of water at least 1 hour before or 2 hours after eating a meal, consuming dairy products, or taking antacids, laxatives, or antidiarrheal drugs. Advise him to take last daily dose at least 1 hour before bedtime.

• Stress importance of completing entire course of therapy as ordered, even after symptoms improve.

◀€ Caution patient not to use outdated tetracycline, because it may cause serious kidney disease.

• Teach patient to recognize and report signs and symptoms of yeast infection and other infections.

• With long-term therapy, tell patient he'll undergo regular blood testing. Advise parents that prepubertal child should have periodic bone X-rays.

• Caution patient to avoid alcohol during therapy.

• Tell parents that tetracycline use during tooth development period (last half of pregnancy, infancy, and childhood to age 8) may cause permanent yellow, gray, or brownish tooth discoloration.

• As appropriate, review all other significant and life-threatening adverse reactions and interactions, especially those related to the drugs, tests, foods, and behaviors mentioned above.

thalidomide
Thalomid

Pharmacologic class: Synthetic glutamic acid derivative

Therapeutic class: Immunomodulator, angiogenesis inhibitor

Pregnancy risk category X

FDA | BOXED WARNING

• When taken during pregnancy, drug may cause severe, life-threatening birth defects or fetal death. Never administer to women who are pregnant or could become pregnant during therapy. Because of its toxicity and to reduce risk of fetal exposure, drug is approved for marketing only under special Food and Drug Administration–approved restricted distribution program, called System for Thalidomide Education and Prescribing Safety (S.T.E.P.S.™). Only prescribers and pharmacists registered with program are allowed to prescribe and dispense drug. Also,

---

Reactions in **bold** are life-threatening. ◀€ Clinical alert

patients must be advised of, agree to, and comply with program requirements.

• Use of thalidomide in patients with multiple myeloma results in an increased risk of venous thromboembolic events (VTEs), such as deep venous thrombosis and pulmonary embolism. Risk increases significantly when thalidomide is used in combination with standard chemotherapeutic agents, including dexamethasone. In one controlled trial, rate of VTEs was 22.5% in patients receiving thalidomide in combination with dexamethasone compared to 4.9% in patients receiving dexamethasone alone ($p = 0.002$). Patients and physicians are advised to watch for signs and symptoms of thromboembolism. Instruct patients to seek medical care if they develop signs and symptoms, such as shortness of breath, chest pain, or arm or leg swelling. Consider thromboprophylaxis based on assessment of individual patient's underlying risk factors.

Action

Suppresses excess levels of tumor necrosis factor-alpha in patients with erythema nodosum leprosum (ENL). Alters leukocyte migration by changing cell surface characteristics.

Availability

Capsules: 50 mg, 100 mg, 200 mg

⚠ Indications and dosages

➤ Cutaneous manifestations of moderate to severe ENL; to prevent and suppress recurrent ENL

Adults weighing 50 kg (110 lb) or more: 100 to 300 mg P.O. daily, or up to 400 mg P.O. daily, depending on disease severity or previous response. Continue therapy until symptoms of active reactions subside (usually after 2 weeks); then may taper in 50-mg decrements q 2 to 4 weeks.

Adults weighing less than 50 kg (110 lb): Initially, 100 mg P.O. daily, or up to 400 mg P.O. daily, depending on disease severity or previous response. Continue therapy until symptoms of active reactions subside (usually after 2 weeks); then may taper in 50-mg decrements q 2 to 4 weeks.

➤ Newly diagnosed multiple myeloma (MM)

Adults: 200 mg P.O. once daily, in combination with dexamethasone 40 mg/day P.O. on days 1 to 4, 9 to 12, and 17 to 20 every 28 days.

Dosage adjustment

• Neutropenia
• Bradycardia

Off-label uses

• Aphthous stomatitis
• Wasting syndrome associated with human immunodeficiency virus (HIV)
• Multiple myeloma
• Refractory Crohn's disease

Contraindications

• Hypersensitivity to drug or its components
• Pregnancy

Precautions

Use cautiously in:

• neutropenia, bradycardia, peripheral neuropathy, hypotension, underlying malignancy, history of seizures or risk of seizures, risk of tumor lysis syndrome

• concurrent use of drugs that slow cardiac conduction, drugs that cause peripheral neuropathy (such as alcohol, amiodarone, bortezomib, cisplatin, disulfiram, docetaxel, metronidazole, paclitaxel, phenytoin, vincristine), and hormonal contraceptives

• concurrent use of opioids, antihistamines, antipsychotics, anti-anxiety agents, or other CNS depressants (avoid use)

• breastfeeding patients (use not recommended)
• children younger than age 12 (safety not established).

Administration

◀╏ Follow all instructions provided by System for Thalidomide Education and Prescribing Safety (S.T.E.P.S.™) program, accessible at http://www.steps-info.com.

• Give with 8 oz of water just before bedtime, at least 1 hour after evening meal.

• Know that patients who need prolonged maintenance therapy to prevent cutaneous ENL recurrence and those who have flares during tapering should receive minimum effective dosage, with tapering attempted every 3 to 6 months. To taper, decrease dosage by 50 mg every 2 to 4 weeks.

Route	Onset	Peak	Duration
P.O.	48 hr	1-2 mo	Unknown

Adverse reactions

CNS: drowsiness, dizziness, vertigo, sedation, tremor, asthenia, peripheral neuropathy, fatigue, confusion, anorexia, anxiety, agitation (with MM use), headache, **seizures**
CV: bradycardia, orthostatic hypotension, peripheral edema, **deep vein thrombosis** (with MM use)
EENT: rhinitis, sinusitis, pharyngitis
GI: nausea, constipation, diarrhea, abdominal pain, oral moniliasis
GU: erectile dysfunction
Hematologic: leukopenia, **neutropenia**
Metabolic: hypocalcemia
Musculoskeletal: muscle weakness (with MM use), back pain
Respiratory: dyspnea, **pulmonary embolus** (with MM use)
Skin: dry skin, desquamation (with MM use), exfoliative, purpuric, bullous, or maculopapular rash; pruritus; fungal dermatitis; nail disorder;

photosensitivity; toxic epidermal necrolysis, **Stevens-Johnson syndrome**
Other: weight gain or loss (with MM use), fever, tooth pain, chills, accidental injury, hypersensitivity reactions, increased HIV viral load, **severe birth defects, fetal death, tumor lysis syndrome**

Interactions

Drug-drug. *Barbiturates, chlorpromazine, reserpine, sedative-hypnotics, and other CNS depressants:* increased sedation
Cardiovascular agents (such as alpha- and beta-adrenergic blockers, beta blockers, calcium channel blockers, digoxin), neuromuscular blockers (succinylcholine), lithium, noncardiovascular agents such as H$_2$ blockers (cimetidine, famotidine), tricyclic antidepressants: increased risk of bradycardia
Drugs linked to peripheral neuropathy: increased risk of peripheral neuropathy
Hormonal contraceptives: increased risk of thromboembolic disease
Drug-diagnostic tests. *Alanine aminotransferase, aspartate aminotransferase, lactate dehydrogenase, lipids, liver function tests:* increased values
Calcium, hemoglobin, neutrophils, white blood cells: decreased values
Drug-food. *High-fat meal:* interference with drug absorption
Drug-behaviors. *Alcohol use:* increased sedation, increased risk of peripheral neuropathy

Patient monitoring

◀╏ Monitor for signs and symptoms of hypersensitivity reaction. If rash occurs, discontinue drug and contact prescriber immediately. Don't restart drug if Stevens-Johnson syndrome, toxic epidermal necrolysis, or exfoliative, purpuric, or bullous rash occurs.
◀╏ Watch for and report signs and symptoms of peripheral neuropathy. If symptoms develop, discontinue drug

---

Reactions in **bold** are life-threatening.   ◀╏ Clinical alert

immediately. Usually, treatment with thalidomide should only be reinitiated if the neuropathy returns to baseline status.

• Assess CBC with white cell differential.

• Carefully monitor patient's reproductive status.

◀€ Monitor patients at risk for tumor lysis syndrome (such as those with high tumor burden before treatment) and take appropriate precautions.

◀€ Closely monitor patients with history of seizures or who are at risk for seizures for clinical changes that could precipitate acute seizure activity.

◀€ Observe patients (particularly patients being treated for MM) for signs and symptoms of thromboembolism.

• Monitor patients for bradycardia and possible syncope; dosage reduction or drug discontinuation may be required.

• Be aware that patients treated for MM who develop such adverse reactions as constipation or somnolence may benefit from temporarily discontinuing drug or continuing drug at lower dosage.

• Measure viral load after first and third months of treatment and every 3 months thereafter.

Patient teaching

• Instruct patient to take with 8 oz of water just before bedtime, at least 1 hour after dinner.

◀€ Tell patient to immediately report signs and symptoms of peripheral neuropathy, tumor lysis syndrome, seizures, thromboembolism, bradycardia, or hypersensitivity reaction, especially rash.

• Teach patient about risks of fetal exposure to drug. Carefully review relevant portions of S.T.E.P.S.™ program with patient.

• Instruct female of childbearing age to use two highly effective birth control methods simultaneously, from 1 month before first thalidomide dose until 1 month after last dose.

• Explain mandatory pregnancy testing schedule to female patient, and stress importance of compliance.

◀€ Advise female patient to contact prescriber immediately if she suspects she's pregnant.

• Caution female patient not to breast-feed.

• Instruct male patient to use latex condoms during every sexual encounter.

• Tell patient that dizziness and orthostatic hypotension may occur. Advise patient to remain upright for a few minutes before standing up from a lying position.

• Tell patient to avoid alcohol and drugs that may cause drowsiness during drug therapy.

• Advise patient not to donate blood or sperm while taking this drug and for 4 weeks after stopping drug.

• As appropriate, review all other significant and life-threatening adverse reactions and interactions, especially those related to the drugs, tests, foods, and behaviors mentioned above.

theophylline

Apo-Theo LA♣, Elixophyllin, Novo-Theophyl SR♣, Nuelin SA⊕, PMS-Theophylline♣, Pulmophyllin ELX♣, Ratio-Theo-Bronc♣, Slo-Phyllin⊕, Theo-24, Theochron, Theolair♣, Theo-Time, Uniphyl, Uniphyllin Continus⊕

Pharmacologic class: Xanthine derivative

Therapeutic class: Bronchodilator, spasmolytic

Pregnancy risk category C

Action

Relaxes bronchial smooth muscles, suppressing airway response to stimuli. Also inhibits phosphodiesterase and release of slow-reacting substance of anaphylaxis and histamine.

Availability

Capsules (immediate-release): 100 mg, 200 mg
Capsules (extended-release, 8 to 12 hours): 50 mg, 60 mg, 65 mg, 75 mg, 100 mg, 125 mg, 130 mg
Capsules (extended-release, 12 hours): 50 mg, 125 mg, 130 mg, 250 mg, 260 mg
Capsules (extended-release, 24 hours): 100 mg, 200 mg, 300 mg, 400 mg
Elixir: 80 mg/15 ml
Injection (with dextrose): 0.4 mg/ml, 0.8 mg/ml, 1.6 mg/ml, 2 mg/ml, 3.2 mg/ml, 4 mg/ml
Syrup (cherry): 80 mg/15 mg, 150 mg/15 ml
Tablets (immediate-release): 100 mg, 125 mg, 200 mg, 250 mg, 300 mg
Tablets (extended-release, 12 to 24 hours): 100 mg, 200 mg, 300 mg, 400 mg, 450 mg, 600 mg
Tablets (extended-release, 24 hours): 400 mg, 600 mg

🚺 Indications and dosages

➤ Acute bronchospasm in patients not receiving theophylline
Adults (otherwise healthy nonsmokers): Initially, 6 mg/kg P.O., followed in next 12 to 16 hours by 3 mg/kg P.O. q 6 hours for two doses, then a maintenance dosage of 3 mg/kg P.O. q 8 hours
Children ages 9 to 16; young adult smokers: Initially, 6 mg/kg P.O., followed in next 12 to 16 hours by 3 mg/kg P.O. q 4 hours for three doses, then a maintenance dosage of 3 mg/kg P.O. q 6 hours
Children ages 1 to 9: Initially, 6 mg/kg P.O., followed in next 12 to 16 hours by 4 mg/kg P.O. q 4 hours for three doses, then a maintenance dosage of 4 mg/kg P.O. q 6 hours

➤ Acute bronchospasm in patients receiving theophylline
Adults and children: Loading dose based partly on time, amount, and administration route of last dose and on expectation that each 0.5 mg/kg will produce 1 mcg/ml rise in theophylline blood level. In significant respiratory distress, loading dose may be 2.5 mg/kg P.O. or I.V. to increase theophylline level by approximately 5 mcg/ml.
➤ Chronic bronchospasm
Adults and children: *Immediate-release forms*—16 mg/kg or 400 mg P.O. daily (whichever is lower) in three to four divided doses q 6 to 8 hours. *Timed-release forms*—12 mg/kg or 400 mg P.O. daily (whichever is lower) in three to four divided doses q 8 to 12 hours. May increase dosage of either immediate- or timed-release form at 2- to 3-day intervals, to a maximum of 13 mg/kg or 900 mg daily (whichever is lower) in patients older than age 16, 18 mg/kg daily in children ages 12 to 16, 20 mg/kg daily in children ages 9 to 12, or 24 mg/kg daily in children up to age 9.

Dosage adjustment

- Cor pulmonale or heart failure
- Elderly patients
- Young adults

Off-label uses

- Essential tremor
- Apnea and bradycardia in premature infants

Contraindications

- Hypersensitivity to drug or other xanthines (such as coffee, theobromine)
- Active peptic ulcer
- Seizure disorder

Precautions

Use cautiously in:
- alcoholism; heart failure or other cardiac or circulatory impairment; hypertension; renal or hepatic disease;

COPD; hypoxemia; hyperthyroidism; diabetes mellitus; glaucoma; peptic ulcer disease
- elderly patients
- children younger than age 1.

Administration

- For I.V. delivery, use infusion solution designed for drug, or mix with dextrose 5% in water. Administer by controlled infusion pump.
- Know that for acute bronchospasm, theophylline preferably is given I.V. as 20 mg/ml of theophylline (or 25 mg/ml of aminophylline).
- Don't give timed-release form to patient with acute bronchospasm.

Route	Onset	Peak	Duration
P.O.	Rapid	1-2 hr	6 hr
P.O. (timed)	Delayed	4-8 hr	8-24 hr
I.V.	Rapid	End of infusion	6-8 hr

Adverse reactions

CNS: irritability, dizziness, nervousness, restlessness, headache, insomnia, reflex hyperexcitability, **seizures**
CV: palpitations, marked hypotension, sinus tachycardia, extrasystole, **circulatory failure, ventricular arrhythmias**
GI: nausea, vomiting, diarrhea, hematemesis, gastroesophageal reflux
GU: increased diuresis, proteinuria
Metabolic: hyperglycemia, **syndrome of inappropriate antidiuretic hormone secretion**
Musculoskeletal: muscle twitching
Respiratory: tachypnea, **respiratory arrest**
Skin: urticaria, rash, alopecia, flushing
Other: fever, hypersensitivity reaction

Interactions

Drug-drug. *Allopurinol, calcium channel blockers, cimetidine, corticosteroids, disulfiram, ephedrine, hormonal contraceptives, influenza virus vaccine, interferon, macrolides, mexiletine, nonselective beta-adrenergic blockers, quinolones, thiabendazole:* increased theophylline blood level, greater risk of toxicity
Aminoglutethimide, barbiturates, ketoconazole, rifampin, sulfinpyrazone, sympathomimetics: decreased theophylline blood level and effects
Carbamazepine, isoniazid, loop diuretics: increased or decreased theophylline blood level
Halothane: increased risk of arrhythmias
Hydantoins: decreased hydantoin blood level
Lithium: decreased therapeutic effect of lithium
Nondepolarizing muscle relaxants: reversal of neuromuscular blockade
Propofol: antagonism of propofol's sedative effects
Tetracyclines: increased risk of adverse reactions to theophylline
Drug-diagnostic tests. *Glucose:* increased level
Drug-food. *Any food:* altered bioavailability and absorption of some timed-release theophylline forms, causing rapid release and possible toxicity
Caffeine- or xanthine-containing foods and beverages: increased theophylline blood level and greater risk of adverse CNS and cardiovascular reactions
Diet high in protein and charcoal-broiled beef and low in carbohydrates: increased theophylline elimination, decreased efficacy
High-carbohydrate, low-protein diet: decreased theophylline elimination, increased risk of adverse reactions
Drug-herbs. *Caffeine-containing herbs (such as cola nut, guarana, maté):* increased theophylline blood level, greater risk of adverse CNS and cardiovascular reactions
Ephedra (ma huang): increased stimulant effect
St. John's wort: decreased theophylline blood level and efficacy

---

Drug-behaviors. *Nicotine (in cigarettes, gum, transdermal patches):* increased theophylline metabolism, decreased efficacy

Patient monitoring
• Monitor for signs and symptoms of hypersensitivity reaction, including rash and fever.
• Assess respiratory status. Monitor pulmonary function tests to gauge drug efficacy and identify adverse effects.
• Monitor cardiovascular and neurologic status carefully.
• Assess glucose level in diabetic patient.

Patient teaching
• Advise patient to take oral form with 8 oz of water 1 hour before or 2 hours after meals.
• Tell patient not to crush or chew timed-release form.
• Caution patient not to use different drug brands interchangeably.
◀▓ Instruct patient to immediately report worsening dyspnea and other respiratory problems.
• Teach patient to recognize and report adverse neurologic reactions.
• Tell patient that all nicotine forms (including cigarettes, patches, and gum) decrease drug efficacy. Discourage nicotine use.
• Advise patient that a diet high in protein and charcoal-broiled beef and low in carbohydrates makes drug less effective.
• Tell patient that a high-carbohydrate, low-protein diet increases risk of adverse reactions, as do products containing caffeine.
• Caution patient to avoid herbs, especially ephedra and St. John's wort.
• Advise patient not to take over-the-counter drugs without prescriber's approval. Tell him to inform all prescribers he's taking drug, because it interacts with many other drugs.

• As appropriate, review all other significant and life-threatening adverse reactions and interactions, especially those related to the drugs, tests, foods, herbs, and behaviors mentioned above.

thyroid, desiccated
Armour Thyroid, Nature-Throid, Westhroid

Pharmacologic class: Hormone supplement
Therapeutic class: Thyroid hormone
Pregnancy risk category A

FDA | **BOXED WARNING**

• Drug shouldn't be used alone or with other agents to treat obesity or weight loss. In euthyroid patients, doses within range of daily hormonal requirements are ineffective for weight loss. Larger doses may cause serious or life-threatening toxicity, particularly when given with sympathomimetic amines (such as those used for anorectic effects).

Action
Regulates cell growth and differentiation and increases metabolic rate of body tissues; effects mediated at cellular level

Availability
Tablets: 15 mg, 30 mg, 60 mg, 90 mg, 120 mg, 180 mg, 240 mg, 300 mg

🖊 Indications and dosages
➢ Mild hypothyroidism
Adults: Initially, 60 mg/day P.O.; may increase by 60 mg q 30 days to desired response. Usual maintenance dosage is 60 to 180 mg/day.

◀▓ Clinical alert

➤ Severe hypothyroidism
Adults: Initially, 15 mg/day P.O. daily; may increase to 30 mg/day after 2 weeks and then to 60 mg/day 2 weeks later. Assess after 1 month, and again 1 month later at 60 mg-dose. If necessary, dosage may then increase to 120 mg/day P.O. for 2 months, with assessment repeated. Subsequent assessments and dosage increases may occur up to a maximum of 180 mg/day.
➤ Congenital or severe hypothyroidism
Children: Initially, 15 mg P.O. daily; may increase to 30 mg/day after 2 weeks, with subsequent increases at 2-week intervals. Maintenance dosage may be higher in growing children than in hypothyroid adults.

Dosage adjustment
- Cardiovascular disease
- Elderly patients

Contraindications
- Hypersensitivity to drug or its components
- Adrenal insufficiency
- Thyrotoxicosis

Precautions
Use cautiously in:
- tartrazine sensitivity (some products)
- cardiovascular disease
- elderly patients
- breastfeeding patients.

Administration
- Give before breakfast each day.

Route	Onset	Peak	Duration
P.O.	Unknown	12-48 hr	Unknown

Adverse reactions
CNS: insomnia, tremors, headache
CV: palpitations, angina pectoris, hypertension, tachycardia, **arrhythmias, cardiac arrest**
GI: nausea, vomiting, diarrhea

GU: menstrual irregularities
Metabolic: heat intolerance, **thyroid storm**
Musculoskeletal: accelerated bone maturation (in children)
Skin: sweating
Other: weight loss, appetite changes, fever

Interactions
Drug-drug. *Anticoagulants, catecholamines, sympathomimetics:* increased effects of these drugs
Bile acid sequestrants: decreased thyroid hormone absorption
Digoxin, insulin, oral hypoglycemics: decreased effects of these drugs
Estrogen: decreased thyroid hormone effects
Oral anticoagulants: increased risk of bleeding
Drug-diagnostic tests. *Aspartate aminotransferase, creatine kinase, glucose, lactate dehydrogenase, protein-bound iodine:* increased levels
Thyroid function tests: decreased values
Drug-herbs. *Bugleweed, soy:* increased adverse drug reactions

Patient monitoring
◀€ Monitor for chest pain. If it occurs, withhold drug and contact prescriber.
- Assess vital signs and temperature frequently.
◀€ Monitor thyroid function tests closely. Immediately report evidence of thyroid storm.
- In diabetic patient, monitor blood glucose level closely.
- In children, monitor sleeping pulse rate and morning basal temperature.
- In female on long-term therapy, monitor bone density tests.

Patient teaching
- Tell patient to take each morning before breakfast.
◀€ Caution patient not to stop therapy abruptly. Dosage must be tapered.

◀€ Advise patient to immediately report chest pain or signs and symptoms of drug toxicity (fever, chest pain, rapid pulse, skipped heartbeats, heat intolerance, excessive sweating, nervousness, emotional instability).

• Instruct patient to tell all prescribers he's taking drug. Caution him not to use over-the-counter preparations without consulting prescriber.

• Tell diabetic patient that drug may alter blood glucose level. Encourage frequent glucose self-monitoring.

• As appropriate, review all other significant and life-threatening adverse reactions and interactions, especially those related to the drugs, tests, and herbs mentioned above.

tiagabine hydrochloride
Gabitril Filmtabs

Pharmacologic class: Nipecotic acid derivative
Therapeutic class: Anticonvulsant
Pregnancy risk category C

Action
Unknown. Thought to raise seizure threshold by enhancing activity of gamma-aminobutyric acid (a major inhibitory neurotransmitter in CNS).

Availability
Tablets: 2 mg, 4 mg, 12 mg, 16 mg, 20 mg

⏿ Indications and dosages
➤ Adjunctive treatment of partial seizures
Adults older than age 18: Initially, 4 mg P.O. once daily for 1 week; may increase as needed by 4 to 8 mg/day at weekly intervals, up to 56 mg/day in two to four divided doses

Adolescents ages 12 to 18: Initially, 4 mg P.O. once daily. May increase total daily dosage by 4 mg at start of week 2; thereafter, may increase by 4 to 8 mg q week until clinical response occurs or patient is receiving up to 32 mg/day. Give total daily dosage in two to four divided doses.

Dosage adjustment
• Hepatic impairment

Off-label uses
• Anxiety

Contraindications
• Hypersensitivity to drug or its components

Precautions
Use cautiously in:
• hepatic impairment
• pregnant or breastfeeding patients
• children younger than age 12 (safety not established).

Administration
◀€ Don't stop drug suddenly. Dosage must be tapered.
• Be aware that concomitant anticonvulsant therapy need not be modified unless indicated.

Route	Onset	Peak	Duration
P.O.	Unknown	45 min	Unknown

Adverse reactions
CNS: dizziness, insomnia, drowsiness, nervousness, asthenia, confusion, poor concentration, impaired memory, depression, emotional lability, hostility, agitation, ataxia, abnormal gait, tremors, paresthesia, speech disorder, language problems
CV: vasodilation
EENT: nystagmus, epistaxis, pharyngitis
GI: nausea, vomiting, diarrhea, abdominal pain, mouth ulcers
Musculoskeletal: myasthenia
Respiratory: increased cough
Skin: rash, pruritus

t

Reactions in **bold** are life-threatening.   ◀€ Clinical alert

Other: increased appetite, weight changes, pain, allergic reaction

Interactions
Drug-drug. *Carbamazepine, phenobarbital, phenytoin, primidone:* increased tiagabine clearance, decreased blood level

Patient monitoring
◀€ Watch for signs or symptoms of depression and suicidal ideation.
• Assess vital signs and cardiovascular status.
• Monitor closely for severe generalized weakness. If present, consult prescriber regarding possible dosage reduction.

Patient teaching
• Tell patient to take on regular schedule with food.
◀€ Caution patient not to stop therapy suddenly. Dosage must be tapered.
• Instruct patient to report signs or symptoms of depression.
◀€ Advise patient to report neurologic reactions. Tell him to contact prescriber immediately if severe overall weakness or severe depression occurs.
• Advise female patient to tell prescriber if she suspects she is pregnant.
• As appropriate, review all other significant adverse reactions and interactions, especially those related to the drugs mentioned above.

ticarcillin disodium and clavulanate potassium
Timentin

Pharmacologic class: Penicillin (extended-spectrum)
Therapeutic class: Anti-infective
Pregnancy risk category B

Action
Ticarcillin disodium inhibits bacterial cell-wall synthesis during replication; clavulanic acid extends ticarcillin's antibiotic spectrum by inactivating beta-lactamase enzymes (which otherwise would degrade ticarcillin).

Availability
Injection: 3 g ticarcillin and 100 mg clavulanic acid in 3.1-g vials

⚕ Indications and dosages
➢ Systemic and urinary tract infections caused by susceptible organisms
Adults weighing more than 60 kg (132 lb): 3.1 g (30:1 fixed-ratio combination of 3 g ticarcillin and 100 mg clavulanic acid) by I.V. infusion q 4 to 6 hours
Adults weighing less than 60 kg (132 lb): 200 to 300 mg/kg/day (based on ticarcillin content) by I.V. infusion in divided doses q 4 to 6 hours
➢ Gynecologic infections caused by susceptible organisms
Adults weighing more than 60 kg (132 lb): For moderate infections, 200 mg/kg/day (based on ticarcillin content) by I.V. infusion in divided doses q 6 hours. For severe infections, 300 mg/kg/day (based on ticarcillin content) by I.V. infusion in divided doses q 4 hours.
Adults weighing less than 60 kg (132 lb): 200 to 300 mg/kg/day by I.V. infusion q 4 to 6 hours
➢ Mild to moderate or severe infections in children caused by susceptible organisms
Children weighing more than 60 kg (132 lb): For mild to moderate infections, 3.1 g (30:1 fixed-ratio combination of 3 g ticarcillin and 100 mg clavulanic acid) by I.V. infusion q 6 hours. For severe infections, 3.1 g (30:1 fixed-ratio combination of 3 g ticarcillin and 100 mg clavulanic acid) by I.V. infusion q 4 hours.

Children ages 3 months to 16 years weighing less than 60 kg (132 lb): For mild to moderate infections, 200 mg/kg/day (based on ticarcillin content) by I.V. infusion in divided doses q 6 hours. For severe infections, 300 mg/kg/day (based on ticarcillin content) by I.V. infusion in divided doses q 4 hours.

Dosage adjustment
• Renal impairment

Contraindications
• Hypersensitivity to drug or other penicillins

Precautions
Use cautiously in:
• cystic fibrosis, renal or hepatic disease
• pregnant or breastfeeding patients.

Administration
• Ask patient about penicillin allergy before giving.
• Add 13 ml of sterile water or normal saline solution to vial; shake gently. Dilute further to 10 to 100 mg/ml of ticarcillin; infuse I.V. over 30 minutes.
• Give at least 1 hour before I.V. aminoglycosides (such as amikacin or gentamicin).

Route	Onset	Peak	Duration
I.V.	Immediate	Immediate	Unknown

Adverse reactions
CNS: headache, giddiness, dizziness, lethargy, fatigue, hyperreflexia, neuromuscular excitability, asterixis, hallucinations, stupor, **seizures**
GI: nausea, vomiting, diarrhea, flatulence, **pseudomembranous colitis**
Hematologic: eosinophilia, transient **neutropenia** and **leukopenia** (with high doses)
Skin: urticaria, rash
Other: unpleasant taste; fever; overgrowth of nonsusceptible organisms; pain, vein irritation, erythema, phlebitis, and **thrombophlebitis** at I.V. site;

hypersensitivity reactions including **anaphylaxis**

Interactions
Drug-drug. *Aminoglycosides:* physical incompatibility, causing aminoglycoside inactivation when mixed in same I.V. solution
Aminoglycosides, tetracyclines: additive activity against some bacteria
Lithium: altered lithium elimination
Probenecid: increased ticarcillin blood level
Drug-diagnostic tests. *Alanine aminotransferase, alkaline phosphatase, aspartate aminotransferase, eosinophils, lactate dehydrogenase, sodium:* increased levels
Bleeding time: prolonged
Granulocytes, hemoglobin, platelets, white blood cells: decreased levels
Liver function tests: transient increases
Urine glucose, urine protein: false-positive results

Patient monitoring
• Monitor liver function tests and CBC with white cell differential.
• Watch closely for signs and symptoms of superinfection and severe allergic reactions.
• Assess neurologic status, and stay alert for seizures.

Patient teaching
◀€ Advise patient to report skin reactions and severe diarrhea right away.
◀€ Tell patient drug may increase risk of other infections. Advise him to promptly report signs and symptoms of new infection.
• Instruct patient to limit sodium intake (drug contains sodium).
• As appropriate, review all other significant and life-threatening adverse reactions and interactions, especially those related to the drugs and tests mentioned above.

Reactions in **bold** are life-threatening.   ◀€ Clinical alert

ticlopidine hydrochloride

Apo-Ticlopidine✚, Dom-
Ticlopidine✚, Gen-Ticlopidine✚,
Novo-Ticlopidine✚, NU-
Ticlopidine✚, PMS-Ticlopidine✚,
Sandoz Ticlopidine✚, Ticlid

Pharmacologic class: Platelet aggrega-
tion inhibitor
Therapeutic class: Antiplatelet agent
Pregnancy risk category B

FDA | BOXED WARNING

• Drug may cause life-threatening
hematologic adverse reactions, including neutropenia, agranulocytosis,
thrombotic thrombocytopenic purpura (TTP), and aplastic anemia. Such
reactions may arise within several days
of starting therapy. TTP incidence
peaks after about 3 to 4 weeks; neutropenia, at approximately 4 to 6
weeks; and aplastic anemia, after about
4 to 8 weeks. Thereafter, incidence of
hematologic reactions declines.
• During first 3 months of therapy,
monitor patient hematologically and
clinically for evidence of neutropenia
or TTP. If it occurs, discontinue drug
immediately.

Action

Inhibits release of first and second
phases of adenosine diphosphate–
induced effects on platelet aggregation,
preventing thrombus formation

Availability

Tablets: 250 mg

⏱ Indications and dosages

➤ To reduce risk of thrombotic cerebrovascular accident when aspirin is
ineffective or intolerable

Adults: 250 mg P.O. b.i.d. with meals
➤ Adjunctive therapy to prevent subacute stent thrombosis in patients with
implanted coronary stents
Adults: 250 mg P.O. b.i.d. with meals,
given with antiplatelet doses of aspirin
for up to 30 days after successful stent
implantation

Dosage adjustment

• Renal impairment

Off-label uses

• Chronic arterial occlusion
• Coronary artery bypass graft
• Open-heart surgery
• Intermittent claudication
• Primary glomerulonephritis
• Sickle cell disease
• Subarachnoid hemorrhage
• Uremic patients with atrioventricular
shunts or fistulas

Contraindications

• Hypersensitivity to drug
• Hematopoietic disorders
• Hemostatic disorders or active
bleeding
• Severe hepatic disease
• History of thrombotic thrombocy-
topenia purpura (TTP) or aplastic
anemia

Precautions

Use cautiously in:
• renal or hepatic impairment
• high risk for bleeding
• elderly patients
• pregnant or breastfeeding patients
• children younger than age 18 (safety
not established).

Administration

• Give with meals.
• Don't give within 2 hours of antacids.

Route	Onset	Peak	Duration
P.O.	Within 4 days	8-11 days	2 wk

Adverse reactions

CNS: dizziness, headache, weakness, **intracerebral bleeding**

EENT: conjunctival hemorrhage, tinnitus, epistaxis

GI: nausea, vomiting, diarrhea, full sensation, GI pain, dyspepsia, flatulence, anorexia, **GI bleeding**

GU: hematuria

Hematologic: ecchymosis, eosinophilia, purpura, **TTP, thrombocytosis, neutropenia, agranulocytosis, bone marrow depression**

Skin: rashes, bruising, pruritus, urticaria

Other: pain, posttraumatic or perioperative bleeding

Interactions

Drug-drug. *Antacids:* decreased ticlopidine blood level

Aspirin: potentiation of aspirin's effect on platelets

Cimetidine (long-term use): reduced ticlopidine clearance

Digoxin: slightly decreased digoxin blood level

Phenytoin: increased phenytoin blood level, greater risk of toxicity

Theophylline: decreased theophylline clearance, greater risk of toxicity

Vitamin A: altered anticoagulant effects

Drug-diagnostic tests. *Alanine aminotransferase, alkaline phosphatase, aspartate aminotransferase:* increased levels

Granulocytes, neutrophils, platelets, white blood cells: decreased counts

Liver function tests: abnormal results

Drug-food. *Any food:* increased ticlopidine absorption

Drug-herbs. *Alfalfa, anise, arnica, astragalus, bilberry, black current seed oil, bladderwrack, bogbean, boldo, borage oil, buchu, capsacin, cat's claw, celery, chapparal, cinchona bark, clove oil, coenzyme Q10, dandelion, dong quai, evening primrose oil, fenugreek, feverfew, garlic, ginger, gingko, guggal, papaya extract, red clover, rhubarb, safflower oil, skullcap, St. John's wort, tan shen:* altered anticoagulant effects

Patient monitoring

🔊 Closely monitor coagulation studies and CBC with white cell differential. Watch for evidence of bleeding tendency and blood dyscrasias.

🔊 Assess neurologic status carefully. Stay alert for signs and symptoms of intracranial bleeding.

• Monitor liver function tests.

Patient teaching

• Tell patient to take with meals, but not within 2 hours of antacids.

🔊 Instruct patient to immediately report easy bruising or bleeding.

• Advise patient to stop taking drug 10 to 14 days before elective surgery.

• Tell patient to inform all prescribers that he is taking drug.

• Inform patient that aspirin-containing products and many herbs increase risk of bleeding. Urge him to consult prescriber before taking over-the-counter drugs or herbs.

• Caution patient to avoid activities that can cause injury. Tell him to use soft toothbrush and electric razor to avoid gum and skin injury.

• As appropriate, review all other significant and life-threatening adverse reactions and interactions, especially those related to the drugs, tests, foods, and herbs mentioned above.

tigecycline
Tygacil

Pharmacologic class: Glycylcycline antibiotic

Therapeutic class: Anti-infective

Pregnancy risk category D

Action
Inhibits protein translation in bacteria by binding to 30S ribosomal subunit and blocking entry of amino-acyl tRNA molecules into ribosomal A site, which in turn prevents incorporation of amino acid residues into elongating peptide chains

Availability
Powder for injection (lyophilized): 50 mg/5 ml in single-dose vial

⬦ Indications and dosages
➤ Treatment of skin, skin-structure infections, and complicated intra-abdominal infections caused by susceptible organisms
Adults age 18 and older: 100 mg I.V. initially, followed by 50 mg I.V. every 12 hours for 5 to 14 days, depending on infection site and severity and patient's clinical and bacteriologic process
➤ Community-acquired bacterial pneumonia caused by susceptible organisms
Adults age 18 and older: Initially, 100 mg I.V., followed by 50 mg I.V. q 12 hours for 7 to 14 days, depending on infection site and severity and patient's clinical and bacteriologic process

Dosage adjustment
• Severe hepatic impairment

Contraindications
• Hypersensitivity to drug or its components

Precautions
Use cautiously in:
• mild to moderate hepatic impairment, complicated intra-abdominal infections secondary to perforation, ventilator-associated pneumonia
• pregnant and breastfeeding patients
• children younger than age 18.

Administration
• Reconstitute with 5.3 ml of normal saline solution injection or 5% dextrose injection to yield a concentration of 10 mg/ml (50 mg).
• Swirl vial gently until drug dissolves. Immediately withdraw 5 ml of reconstituted solution from vial and add to 100-ml I.V. bag for infusion. Maximum concentration in I.V. bag should be 1 mg/ml.
• Discard reconstituted solution that isn't yellow or orange.
• Administer through dedicated I.V. line or Y-site. If same I.V. line is used for sequential infusion of several drugs, flush before and after infusion, using either normal saline solution injection or 5% dextrose injection. Use infusion solution compatible with tigecycline and other drugs given through same line.
• Administer over 30 to 60 minutes.
• Don't give amphotericin B, chlorpromazine, methylprednisolone, or voriconazole simultaneously through same Y-site.

Route	Onset	Peak	Duration
I.V.	Unknown	Unknown	Unknown

Adverse reactions
CNS: headache, dizziness, insomnia, asthenia, pseudotumor cerebri
CV: hypertension, hypotension, phlebitis
GI: nausea, vomiting, diarrhea, constipation, abdominal pain, dyspepsia, increased GI enzymes, **pseudomembranous colitis, pancreatitis**
Hematologic: anemia, leukocytosis, thrombocytopenia
Hepatic: hepatic dysfunction, hepatic failure
Metabolic: antianabolic action (with increased BUN, azotemia, acidosis, and hyperphosphatemia)
Musculoskeletal: back pain
Respiratory: increased cough, dyspnea

Skin: pruritus, rash, sweating, photosensitivity

Other: abscess, fever, infection, pain, peripheral edema, abnormal healing, superinfection, permanent tooth discoloration (during tooth development), **increase in all-cause mortality, hypersensitivity reaction (including anaphylaxis)**

Interactions

Drug-drug. *Hormonal contraceptives:* reduced contraceptive efficacy

Drug-diagnostic tests. *Alanine aminotransferase, alkaline phosphatase, amylase, aspartate aminotransferase, bilirubin, blood glucose, blood urea nitrogen:* increased

Blood protein, potassium, WBCs: decreased

Patient monitoring

• Monitor prothrombin time or other suitable anticoagulation tests if patient is receiving warfarin concomitantly.

◀ᶠ Closely monitor liver function tests; watch for signs and symptoms of hepatic impairment.

Patient teaching

◀ᶠ Instruct patient to immediately report rash and other signs or symptoms of allergic reaction.

• Tell patient to complete full course of therapy, even if he feels better.

• Advise patient taking oral hormonal contraceptives to use alternative birth control method during therapy.

• Caution female with childbearing potential to avoid pregnancy because drug may harm fetus.

• As appropriate, review all other significant and life-threatening adverse reactions and interactions, especially those related to the drugs and tests mentioned above.

timolol maleate

Apo-Timol✤, Betim⊕, Betimol, Dom-Timolol✤, Gen-Timolol✤, Istalol, Novo-Timol✤, NU-Timolol✤, PMS-Timolol✤, Rhoxal-Timolol✤, Sandoz Timolol✤, Timoptic, Timoptix-XE

Pharmacologic class: Beta-adrenergic blocker (nonselective)

Therapeutic class: Antihypertensive, vascular headache suppressant, antiglaucoma agent

Pregnancy risk category C

FDA BOXED WARNING

• Exacerbations of angina pectoris and myocardial infarction (MI) may follow abrupt withdrawal of some beta blockers. When discontinuing long-term therapy, particularly in patients with ischemic heart disease, reduce dosage gradually over 1 to 2 weeks and monitor patient carefully. If angina worsens markedly or acute coronary insufficiency develops, reinstate drug promptly (at least temporarily) and take other appropriate measures to manage unstable angina. Caution patient not to interrupt or discontinue therapy without prescriber's advice. Because coronary artery disease is common and may be unrecognized, it may be prudent not to discontinue drug abruptly even in patients treated only for hypertension.

Action

Blocks stimulation of beta₁-adrenergic (myocardial) and beta₂-adrenergic (pulmonary, vascular, uterine) receptor sites. May reduce aqueous production, which decreases intraocular pressure (IOP).

Reactions in **bold** are life-threatening. ◀ᶠ Clinical alert

Availability
Ophthalmic gel: 0.25%, 0.5%
Ophthalmic solution: 0.25%, 0.5%
Tablets: 5 mg, 10 mg, 20 mg

⏀ Indications and dosages
➤ Hypertension
Adults: Initially, 10 mg P.O. b.i.d., given alone or with a diuretic; may increase at 7-day intervals as needed. Usual maintenance dosage is 10 to 20 mg daily in two divided doses, up to 60 mg/day.
➤ Acute MI
Adults: 10 mg P.O. b.i.d. starting 1 to 4 weeks after MI
➤ To prevent vascular headaches
Adults: Initially, 10 mg P.O. b.i.d. For maintenance, 20 mg may be given as a single daily dose. Total daily dosage may be increased to a maximum of 30 mg in divided doses or decreased to 10 mg/day, depending on response and tolerance. Withdraw drug if satisfactory response doesn't occur after 6 to 8 weeks at maximum dosage.
➤ Elevated IOP in patients with ocular hypertension or open-angle glaucoma
Adults: One drop of 0.25% to 0.5% ophthalmic solution in affected eye b.i.d., or 0.25% to 0.5% ophthalmic gel in affected eye once daily

Off-label uses
• Angina pectoris
• Supraventricular arrhythmias

Contraindications
• Hypersensitivity to drug or other beta-adrenergic blockers
• Uncompensated heart failure
• Bradycardia or heart block
• Cardiogenic shock
• Bronchial asthma (current or previous), severe chronic obstructive pulmonary disease

Precautions
Use cautiously in:
• renal or hepatic impairment, diabetes mellitus, thyrotoxicosis
• elderly patients
• pregnant or breastfeeding patients
• children (safety not established).

Administration
• Measure apical pulse before giving. If patient has significant bradycardia or tachycardia, withhold dose and consult prescriber.

Route	Onset	Peak	Duration
P.O.	Unknown	1-2 hr	12-24 hr
Ophthalmic	≤ 30 min	1-2 hr	≤ 24 hr

Adverse reactions
CNS: fatigue, dizziness, asthenia, insomnia, headache, vertigo, nervousness, depression, paresthesia, hallucinations, memory loss, disorientation, emotional lability, clouded sensorium
CV: hypotension, angina pectoris exacerbation, bradycardia, **atrioventricular or sinoatrial block, arrhythmias, heart failure**
EENT: visual disturbances, dry eyes, tinnitus, nasal congestion
GI: nausea, constipation, diarrhea, abdominal discomfort
GU: erectile dysfunction, decreased libido
Metabolic: hyperuricemia, **hypoglycemia, hyperkalemia**
Musculoskeletal: joint pain
Respiratory: dyspnea, crackles, **bronchospasm, pulmonary edema**
Skin: itching, rash

Interactions
Drug-drug. *Antihypertensives, nitrates:* additive hypotension
Insulin, oral hypoglycemics: altered efficacy of these drugs
Nonsteroidal anti-inflammatory drugs: decreased antihypertensive effect of timolol

---

Quinidine: inhibited timolol metabolism, leading to increased beta-adrenergic blockade and bradycardia
Reserpine: increased risk of hypotension and bradycardia
Theophylline: reduced effects of both drugs
Drug-diagnostic tests. *Antinuclear antibodies:* increased titer
Blood urea nitrogen, liver function tests, potassium, uric acid: increased values
Glucose, high-density lipoproteins, hematocrit, hemoglobin: decreased values
Drug-herbs. *Ephedra (ma huang), St. John's wort, yohimbine:* decreased timolol efficacy

Patient monitoring
• Closely monitor vital signs, blood pressure, cardiovascular status, and ECG.
• Assess respiratory status. Check breath sounds for wheezing and bronchospasm.
• Monitor blood glucose level in patient with diabetes mellitus.

Patient teaching
• Teach patient how to measure pulse before each dose. Instruct him to contact prescriber if pulse is outside established safe range.
◀ Caution patient not to stop taking drug abruptly. Dosage must be tapered.
• Teach patient how to administer eye drops. Instruct him to use drops only as prescribed, because they are absorbed systemically. Caution him not to touch dropper tip to eye or any other surface.
◀ Teach patient to recognize and immediately report significant adverse respiratory, cardiac, and neurologic reactions.
• Inform patient that many over-the-counter drugs and herbs may decrease the efficacy of timolol. Advise him to consult prescriber before using these products.

• Advise diabetic patient that drug may lower blood glucose level. Encourage regular blood glucose monitoring.
• As appropriate, review all other significant and life-threatening adverse reactions and interactions, especially those related to the drugs, tests, and herbs mentioned above.

tinidazole
Fasigyn ✛, Tindamax

Pharmacologic class: Antiprotozoal
Therapeutic class: Anti-infective
Pregnancy risk category C

FDA BOXED WARNING

• Prolonged use of metronidazole (a structurally related drug with similar biologic effects) has caused cancer in mice and rats. Reserve tinidazole for conditions listed under "Indications and dosages."

Action
Free nitro radical (generated from tinidazole reduction by *Trichomonas* cell extracts) may explain activity against *Trichomonas* species; activity against *Giardia* and *Entamoeba* species is unknown.

Availability
Tablets: 250 mg, 500 mg

🗇 Indications and dosages
➤ Trichomoniasis caused by *Trichomonas vaginalis*
Adults: Single dose of 2 g P.O. with food, given to both sexual partners simultaneously
➤ Bacterial vaginosis in nonpregnant females

Adults: 2 g P.O. once daily with food for 2 days, or 1 g P.O. once daily with food for 5 days

➤ Giardiasis caused by *Giardia duodenalis (Giardia lamblia)*

Adults: Single dose of 2 g P.O. with food

Children older than age 3: Single dose of 50 mg/kg (up to 2 g) with food

➤ Amebiasis caused by *Entamoeba histolytica*

Adults: 2 g P.O. daily with food for 3 days

Children older than age 3: 50 mg/kg (up to 2 g) P.O. daily with food for 3 days

➤ Amebic liver abscess caused by *E. histolytica*

Adults: 2 g P.O. daily with food for 3 to 5 days

Children older than age 3: 50 mg/kg (up to 2 g) P.O. daily with food for 3 to 5 days

Dosage adjustment

• Hemodialysis patients

Contraindications

• Hypersensitivity to drug, its components, or other nitroimidazole derivatives
• First trimester of pregnancy

Precautions

Use cautiously in:
• CNS disease, hepatic dysfunction
• history of blood dyscrasias
• elderly patients
• pregnant or breastfeeding patients
• children (except to treat giardiasis and amebiasis in children older than age 3).

Administration

• Give with food to minimize GI discomfort.

Route	Onset	Peak	Duration
P.O.	Unknown	1.6 hr	Unknown

Adverse reactions

CNS: weakness, fatigue, malaise, dizziness, vertigo, ataxia, insomnia, drowsiness, giddiness, headache, transient peripheral neuropathy, **seizures**
CV: palpitations
GI: nausea, vomiting, diarrhea, constipation, dyspepsia, gastric discomfort, tongue discoloration, stomatitis, anorexia
Hematologic: transient neutropenia and leukopenia
Musculoskeletal: arthralgia, myalgia, arthritis
Other: altered taste, overgrowth of susceptible organisms, hypersensitivity reactions including **angioedema**

Interactions

Drug-drug. *Cyclosporine, lithium, tacrolimus:* possible increase in blood levels of these drugs
Cholestyramine: decreased oral bioavailability of tinidazole
CYP450 inducers (such as phenobarbital, rifampin): increased tinidazole elimination and decreased blood level
CYP450 inhibitors (such as cimetidine, ketoconazole): increased tinidazole blood level
Fluorouracil: decreased fluorouracil clearance
Fosphenytoin, phenytoin: prolonged half-life and reduced clearance of these drugs
Oxytetracycline: antagonism of therapeutic effects of tinidazole
Warfarin, other oral coumarin anticoagulants: increased effects of these drugs
Drug-diagnostic tests. *Alanine aminotransferase, aspartate aminotransferase, hexokinase glucose, lactate dehydrogenase, triglycerides:* interference with test results
Drug-behaviors. *Alcohol use:* disulfiram-like reaction during tinidazole therapy and for 3 days after

Patient monitoring

◀€ Closely monitor patient for neurologic abnormalities, such as seizures and peripheral neuropathy. If these occur, withdraw drug immediately.

• Monitor blood chemistry tests, especially liver function tests.

Patient teaching
• Advise patient to take drug with food.
• For child or other patient unable to swallow tablets, inform parent or caregiver that drug can be crushed in artificial cherry syrup and given with food.
◀€ Caution patient or caregiver to stop therapy and call prescriber immediately if seizures or numbness or tingling in extremities occurs.
• Instruct patient to avoid alcohol use during therapy.
• Advise female patient to avoid pregnancy during therapy.
• Counsel female patient to avoid breastfeeding during therapy and for 3 days after last dose.
• As appropriate, review all other significant and life-threatening adverse reactions and interactions, especially those related to the drugs, tests, and behaviors mentioned above.

---

tiotropium
Spriva ⊕, Spiriva HandiHaler

Pharmacologic class: Antimuscarinic, anticholinergic
Therapeutic class: Bronchodilator
Pregnancy risk category C

Action
Inhibits smooth-muscle muscarinic M_3-receptors, leading to bronchodilation

Availability
Capsules for inhalation: 18 mcg

⏴ Indications and dosages
➤ Long-term, once-daily maintenance treatment of bronchospasm associated with chronic obstructive pulmonary disease
Adults: Contents of one capsule inhaled orally once daily using supplied HandiHaler

Contraindications
• Hypersensitivity to atropine or its derivatives (including ipratropium) or drug components

Precautions
Use cautiously in:
• angle-closure glaucoma, prostatic hyperplasia, bladder neck obstruction, moderate to severe renal impairment, severe hypersensitivity to milk proteins
• concurrent use of other anticholinergics
• pregnant or breastfeeding patients
• children (safety and efficacy not established).

Administration
• Give contents of one capsule once daily using HandiHaler.
• Don't let patient swallow capsule.

Route	Onset	Peak	Duration
Inhalation (P.O.)	30 min	3 hr	24 hr

Adverse reactions
CNS: depression, paresthesia
CV: angina, increased heart rate
EENT: eye pain or discomfort, blurred vision, visual halos, cataract, colored images in association with red eyes (with inadvertent eye exposure), epistaxis, rhinitis, sinusitis, laryngitis, pharyngitis, dysphonia
GI: vomiting, constipation, dyspepsia, abdominal pain, gastroesophageal reflux, stomatitis, dry mouth
GU: urinary tract infection, urinary retention, urinary difficulty
Musculoskeletal: myalgia, skeletal pain, arthritis, leg pain
Respiratory: upper respiratory tract infection, coughing, **paradoxical bronchospasm**

t

Reactions in **bold** are life-threatening.   ◀€ Clinical alert

Skin: rash
Other: nonspecific chest pain, edema, infection, candidiasis, flulike symptoms, herpes zoster, **hypersensitivity reaction (including angioedema)**

Interactions
Drug-diagnostic tests. *Blood glucose, cholesterol:* increased

Patient monitoring
◀€ Closely monitor patient for allergic reaction and paradoxical bronchospasm; if these occur, discontinue drug and consider alternative therapy.
• Closely monitor patients with moderate to severe renal impairment.

Patient teaching
• Give patient information portion of package insert on HandiHaler use.
• Inform patient that drug is once-daily maintenance medicine that opens narrowed airways and helps keep them open for 24 hours. Stress that it's not for immediate (rescue) relief of breathing problems.
• Tell patient that capsules are intended for oral inhalation only and should be used only with HandiHaler device. Emphasize that HandiHaler must not be used to take any other drug.
◀€ Caution patient not to let powder get into eyes.
• Teach patient to take prescribed dose in these steps: Immediately before use, open one sealed blister foil and HandiHaler device, insert capsule, press HandiHaler button once to pierce capsule, and exhale completely before placing mouthpiece into mouth with head upright. Then breathe in slowly and deeply at a rate fast enough to hear capsule vibrate, until lungs are full. Holding breath as long as comfortable, take HandiHaler device out of mouth. Then place device back in mouth and inhale again to get full dose.

• Tell patient not to exhale into HandiHaler mouthpiece at any time.
• Caution patient not to swallow capsules.
• Tell patient not to store capsules in HandiHaler device.
• Instruct patient to clean device as shown in patient information sheet.
• Instruct patient to discard any capsules inadvertently exposed to air while preparing dose.
◀€ Tell patient to contact prescriber immediately if eye pain or discomfort, blurred vision, visual halos, or colored images occur.
◀€ Instruct patient to immediately stop drug and report signs and symptoms of hypersensitivity reaction (including itching, rash, swelling of the lips, tongue, or throat) or difficulty breathing.
◀€ Tell patient to immediately report signs and symptoms of prostatic hyperplasia or bladder-neck obstruction (such as difficulty passing urine or painful urination).
• As appropriate, review all other significant and life-threatening adverse reactions and interactions, especially those related to the tests mentioned above.

tipranavir
Aptivus

Pharmacologic class: Nonpeptidic protease inhibitor of human immunodeficiency virus type 1 (HIV-1)
Therapeutic class: Antiretroviral
Pregnancy risk category C

FDA | **BOXED WARNING**

• When given concurrently with ritonavir 200 mg, drug has been linked to reports of fatal and nonfatal intracranial hemorrhage and clinical hepatitis

---

and hepatic decompensation. Use extra vigilance in patients with chronic hepatitis B or hepatitis C co-infection.

Action
Inhibits virus-specific processing of viral Gag and Gag-Pol polyproteins in HIV-1 infected cells, preventing formation of mature virions

Availability
Capsules: 250 mg
Oral solution: 100 mg/ml

⚡ Indications and dosages
➤ Combination antiretroviral treatment of HIV-1 infected patients who are treatment-experienced and infected with HIV-1 strains resistant to more than one protease inhibitor
Adults: 500 mg P.O. twice daily given with 200 mg ritonavir
Children ages 2 to 18: 14 mg/kg P.O. with ritonavir 6 mg/kg (or 375 mg/m^2 with ritonavir 150 mg/m^2) twice daily, not to exceed maximum dosage of tipranavir 500 mg with ritonavir 200 mg twice daily. For children who develop intolerance or toxicity and can't continue with tipranavir 14 mg/kg with ritonavir 6 mg/kg, consider decreasing dosage to tipranavir 12 mg/kg with ritonavir 5 mg/kg (or tipranavir 290 mg/m^2 with ritonavir 115 mg/m^2) twice daily provided virus isn't resistant to multiple protease inhibitors.

Contraindications
• Moderate to severe hepatic impairment
• Concurrent use of amiodarone, astemizole, bepridil, cisapride, dihydroergotamine, ergonovine, ergotamine, flecainide, methylergonovine, oral midazolam, pimozide, propafenone, quinidine, terfenadine, or triazolam
• Sildenafil (Revatio) when used for pulmonary hypertension

Precautions
Use cautiously in:
• treatment-naïve patients (avoid use)
• sulfonamide allergy
• hepatic insufficiency, diabetes mellitus, hyperglycemia, hemophilia, increased risk of bleeding
• concurrent use of drugs known to increase risk of bleeding
• concurrent use of other protease inhibitors, fluticasone propionate, or salmeterol (use not recommended)
• concurrent use of calcium channel blockers, carbamazepine, itraconazole, ketoconazole, parenteral midazolam, PDE5 inhibitors (when used for erectile dysfunction), phenobarbital, phenytoin, trazodone, valproic acid
• pregnant or breastfeeding patients.

Administration
• Administer with or without food when given with ritonavir capsules or solution; must administer only with meals when given with ritonavir tablets.
• Give 2 hours before or 1 hour after antacids.

Route	Onset	Peak	Duration
P.O.	Unknown	2.9-3 hr	Unknown

Adverse reactions
CNS: fatigue, headache, depression, insomnia, asthenia, **intracranial hemorrhage**
GI: diarrhea, nausea, vomiting, abdominal pain, dyspepsia, flatulence
Hematologic: leukopenia, anemia, neutropenia, thrombocytopenia
Hepatic: hepatotoxicity
Metabolic: hyperglycemia, new-onset or exacerbations of diabetes mellitus
Respiratory: bronchitis, cough
Skin: rash
Other: pyrexia, fat accumulation or redistribution, immune reconstitution syndrome

t

Reactions in **bold** are life-threatening. ◄€ Clinical alert

Interactions

Drug-drug. *Antacids:* decreased tipranavir peak concentration

Atorvastatin, desipramine, fluticasone, itraconazole, ketoconazole, rifabutin, selective serotonin reuptake inhibitors, sildenafil, tadalafil, trazodone, vardenafil, voriconazole: increased levels of these drugs

Calcium channel blockers: possible unpredictable effects

Clarithromycin: increased levels of both drugs

Didanosine, ethinyl estradiol, methadone: decreased levels of these drugs

Disulfiram, other drugs that produce disulfiram-like reaction (such as metronidazole): increased risk of disulfiram-like reactions

Fluconazole: increased tipranavir level

Hormonal contraceptives: decreased hormonal concentration, increased risk of rash

Lovastatin, simvastatin: increased potential for serious reactions (such as myopathy and rhabdomyolysis)

Metronidazole: disulfiram-like interaction

PDE5 inhibitors: increased PDE5 inhibitor-associated adverse events, including hypotension, syncope, visual disturbances, and priapism

Rifampin: loss of virologic response, tipranavir resistance

Salmeterol: increased risk of cardiovascular adverse events including QT interval prolongation, palpitations, and sinus tachycardia

Trazodone: increased trazodone plasma concentrations

Valproic acid: decreased valproic acid effectiveness

Warfarin: altered warfarin blood level

Drug-diagnostic tests. *Alanine aminotransferase (ALT), amylase, aspartate aminotransferase (AST), cholesterol, triglycerides:* increased

Platelets, WBCs: decreased

Drug-food. *High-fat meal:* increased drug bioavailability

Drug-herbs. *St. John's wort:* loss of virologic response, tipranavir resistance

Patient monitoring

• Monitor liver function tests and watch for signs and symptoms of hepatic impairment before and during therapy. Discontinue drug if signs and symptoms of clinical hepatitis, asymptomatic increases in ALT/AST of more than 10 times upper limit of normal (ULN), or asymptomatic increases in ALT/AST of 5 to 10 times ULN with concomitant increases in total bilirubin occur.

• Monitor triglyceride and cholesterol levels before therapy starts and at periodic intervals during therapy.

• Monitor CBC, platelets, and serum amylase levels.

• Monitor INR frequently when therapy starts in patients receiving warfarin.

• Closely monitor patients with hyperglycemia or chronic hepatitis B or C.

• Because this drug interacts with many other drugs, closely monitor patient's drug regimen for possible interactions and adjust dosage, as appropriate.

• Be aware that immune reconstitution syndrome has occurred in patients treated with combination antiretroviral therapy. During initial phase of combination antiretroviral treatment, patients whose immune system responds may develop inflammatory response to indolent or residual opportunistic infections (such as *Mycobacterium avium* infection, cytomegalovirus, *Pneumocystis jiroveci* pneumonia, tuberculosis, or reactivation of herpes simplex and herpes zoster), which may necessitate further evaluation and treatment.

Patient teaching

• Instruct patient to take capsules or solution with or without food when

---

taking with ritonavir capsules or solution and to take with meals when taking with ritonavir tablets. Tell patient to swallow capsule whole, without chewing it.

• Tell patient to take drug 2 hours before or 1 hour after antacids.

◀≋ Emphasize that patient must take prescribed ritonavir dosage with this drug to achieve desired therapeutic effect.

• Instruct patient not to alter dosage or discontinue tipranavir or ritonavir without consulting prescriber.

• Advise patient to take a missed dose as soon as possible and then return to normal schedule. Caution against taking double doses.

◀≋ Instruct patient to immediately stop taking drug and contact prescriber if he develops unusual fatigue, general ill feeling, flulike symptoms, appetite loss, nausea, yellowing of skin or eyes, dark urine, pale stools, or right-sided abdominal pain.

◀≋ Tell patient to discontinue drug and promptly report severe report rash to prescriber.

• Inform patient that because drug may cause many interactions, he shouldn't take other prescription or over-the-counter drugs without consulting prescriber.

• Tell patient drug may cause body fat redistribution or accumulation.

• Instruct patient to store capsules in refrigerator and to use contents within 60 days of opening bottle.

• Advise female taking estrogen-based hormonal contraceptives to use additional or alternative birth control method during therapy.

• Instruct female not to breastfeed because of risk of transmitting HIV infection and adverse drug effects to infant.

• As appropriate, review all other significant and life-threatening adverse reactions and interactions, especially those related to the drugs, tests, foods, and herbs mentioned above.

tirofiban hydrochloride
Aggrastat

Pharmacologic class: Glycoprotein (GP IIb/IIIa)-receptor inhibitor

Therapeutic class: Platelet aggregation inhibitor

Pregnancy risk category B

Action
Inhibits reversible platelet aggregation by binding to GP IIb/IIIa receptor on platelets

Availability
Injection: 25-ml and 50-ml vials (250 mcg/ml), 100-ml and 250-ml premixed vials (50 mcg/ml)

⚡ Indications and dosages
➤ Acute coronary syndrome (given with heparin); patients undergoing percutaneous transluminal coronary angioplasty (PTCA) or atherectomy
Adults: Loading dose of 0.4 mcg/kg/minute I.V. for 30 minutes, followed by continuous I.V. infusion of 0.1 mcg/kg/minute for 48 to 108 hours in patients being managed medically. Continue infusion for 12 to 24 hours after PTCA or atherectomy.

Dosage adjustment
• Renal insufficiency

Contraindications
• Hypersensitivity to drug or its components
• Active internal bleeding or history of bleeding diathesis within past 30 days
• Cerebrovascular accident (CVA) within past 30 days, or history of hemorrhagic CVA
• History of intracranial hemorrhage, intracranial neoplasm, arteriovenous

---

malformation, aneurysm, or thrombocytopenia after previous tirofiban use
- History, symptoms, or findings that suggest aortic dissection
- Severe hypertension
- Acute pericarditis
- Major surgery or severe trauma within past 30 days
- Concurrent use of other parenteral GP IIb/IIIa inhibitors

Precautions

Use cautiously in:
- renal disease
- elderly patients
- pregnant or breastfeeding patients
- children younger than age 18 (safety not established).

Administration

◀€ Know that drug comes both in premixed vials of 50 mcg/ml and injection concentrate of 250 mcg/ml.
- Dilute injection concentrate to same concentration as premixed vial (50 mcg/ml) by withdrawing and discarding 50 ml of solution from 250-ml plastic bag of normal saline solution or dextrose 5% in water, or by withdrawing and discarding 100 ml of solution from 500-ml plastic bag of same solution and replacing with equal volume of concentrated drug form.
- Mix I.V. solution well and inspect visually before administering.
- Squeeze plastic bag and check for leaks; discard if it has leaks.
- Don't use drug in series connections with other plastic bags. Don't add other drugs to bag containing tirofiban.

Route	Onset	Peak	Duration
I.V.	Immediate	Immediate	4-6 hr

Adverse reactions

CNS: headache, dizziness, **spinal-epidural hematoma, intracranial hemorrhage**
CV: vasovagal reaction, bradycardia, **hemopericardium, coronary artery dissection**
GI: nausea, vomiting, occult bleeding, hematemesis, **retroperitoneal hemorrhage**
GU: pelvic pain, hematuria
Hematologic: bleeding, **thrombocytopenia**
Musculoskeletal: leg pain
Respiratory: pulmonary hemorrhage
Skin: diaphoresis
Other: infusion site bleeding, chills, fever, edema, allergic reactions, **anaphylaxis**

Interactions

Drug-drug. *Clopidogrel, dipyridamole, nonsteroidal anti-inflammatory drugs, oral anticoagulants (such as thrombolytics, ticlopidine, warfarin), other drugs affecting hemostasis:* increased risk of bleeding
Levothyroxine, omeprazole: increased renal clearance of tirofiban
Vitamin A: increased risk of bleeding
Drug-diagnostic tests. *Hematocrit, hemoglobin, platelets:* decreased values
Drug-herbs. *Alfalfa, anise, arnica, astragalus, bilberry, black currant seed oil, bladderwrack, bogbean, boldo (with fenugreek), borage oil, buchu, capsaicin, cat's claw, celery, chaparral, chincona bark, clove oil, dandelion, dong quai, evening primrose oil, fenugreek, feverfew, garlic, ginger, ginkgo, guggul, papaya extract, red clover, rhubarb, safflower oil, skullcap, tan-shen:* increased risk of bleeding

Patient monitoring

◀€ Monitor CBC, platelet count, and coagulation studies. Assess stool for occult blood.
- Watch for bleeding at puncture sites, especially at cardiac catheterization access site. Immobilize access site to reduce bleeding risk.
◀€ Monitor for signs and symptoms of bleeding in cranium and other body systems (especially respiratory, GI, and GU).
- Monitor vital signs and ECG.

◀╣ Assess cardiovascular status. Stay alert for signs and symptoms of coronary artery dissection or hemopericardium.

Patient teaching
◀╣ Teach patient to recognize and immediately report serious adverse reactions.
• Tell patient he will be closely monitored and undergo regular blood testing during therapy.

tizanidine hydrochloride
Apo-Tizanidine✤, Gen-Tizanidine✤, Zanaflex

Pharmacologic class: Alpha-adrenergic agonist (centrally acting)
Therapeutic class: Skeletal muscle relaxant
Pregnancy risk category C

Action
Stimulates alpha$_2$-adrenergic agonist receptor sites and reduces spasticity by inhibiting presynaptic motor neurons

Availability
Tablets: 2 mg, 4 mg

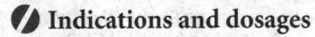 Indications and dosages
➤ Increased muscle tone associated with spasticity
Adults: Initially, 4 mg P.O. q 6 to 8 hours (no more than three doses in 24 hours). Increase in increments of 2 to 4 mg, up to 8 mg/dose or 24 mg/day (not to exceed 36 mg/day), as needed.

Contraindications
• Hypersensitivity to drug or its components

Precautions
Use cautiously in:
• renal or hepatic impairment
• elderly patients
• pregnant or breastfeeding patients
• children (safety not established).

Administration
• Give with or without food.

Route	Onset	Peak	Duration
P.O.	Unknown	1-2 hr	3-6 hr

Adverse reactions
CNS: drowsiness, asthenia, dizziness, speech disorder, dyskinesia, nervousness, anxiety, depression, hallucinations, sedation, paresthesia
CV: hypotension, bradycardia
EENT: blurred vision, pharyngitis, rhinitis
GI: vomiting, diarrhea, constipation, abdominal pain, dyspepsia, dry mouth
GU: urinary frequency, urinary tract infection
Hepatic: hepatitis
Musculoskeletal: back pain, myasthenia
Skin: rash, skin ulcers, sweating
Other: fever, infection, flulike symptoms

Interactions
Drug-drug. *Alpha$_2$-adrenergic agonist antihypertensives:* increased risk of hypotension
CNS depressants (such as antihistamines, opioids, sedative-hypnotics): additive CNS depression
Hormonal contraceptives: increased tizanidine blood level, greater risk of adverse reactions
Drug-diagnostic tests. *Alanine aminotransferase, alkaline phosphatase, aspartate aminotransferase, glucose:* increased levels
Drug-food. *Any food:* increased drug bioavailability, shorter time to peak concentration (with no effect on absorption)

t

Reactions in **bold** are life-threatening.   ◀╣ Clinical alert

Drug-behaviors. *Alcohol use:* additive CNS depression

Patient monitoring

• Monitor temperature and vital signs. Watch for orthostatic hypotension, bradycardia, and fever or other signs and symptoms of infection.
• Assess liver function tests.

Patient teaching

• Advise patient he may take with or without food.
• Tell patient to report signs or symptoms of infection or depression.
• Instruct patient to move slowly when sitting up or standing, to avoid dizziness from sudden blood pressure decrease.
◀€ Tell patient to immediately report unusual tiredness or yellowing of skin or eyes.
• Caution patient not to drink alcohol.
• Instruct patient to avoid driving and other hazardous activities until he knows how drug affects concentration and alertness.
• As appropriate, review all other significant and life-threatening adverse reactions and interactions, especially those related to the drugs, tests, foods, and behaviors mentioned above.

tobramycin

Aktob, Apo-Tobramycin✽, PMS-Tobramycin✽, TOBI, Tobrex

tobramycin sulfate

Pharmacologic class: Aminoglycoside
Therapeutic class: Anti-infective
Pregnancy risk category B (inhalation, ophthalmic), *D* (parenteral)

FDA | **BOXED WARNING**

The following boxed warnings apply to parenteral administration only:
• When giving drug by injection, observe patient closely for potential ototoxicity and nephrotoxicity. Rarely, nephrotoxicity doesn't emerge until first few days after therapy ends.
• Neurotoxicity, manifested as both auditory and vestibular ototoxicity, can occur. Auditory changes are irreversible and usually bilateral. Eighth-nerve impairment and nephrotoxicity also may develop, mainly in patients with preexisting renal damage and in those with normal renal function who receive drug for longer periods or in higher doses than those recommended. Other neurotoxicity manifestations may include numbness, skin tingling, muscle twitching, and seizures. Risk of drug-induced hearing loss increases with degree of exposure to high peak or high trough drug blood levels. Patients who develop cochlear damage may lack symptoms during therapy to warn of eighth-nerve toxicity, and partial or total irreversible bilateral deafness may continue to develop after withdrawal.
• Monitor renal and eighth-nerve function closely in patients with known or suspected renal impairment and in those whose renal functional initially is normal but who develop signs of renal dysfunction during therapy. Monitor peak and trough drug blood levels periodically during therapy; avoid levels above 12 mcg. Rising trough levels (above 2 mcg) may indicate tissue accumulation. Such accumulation, excessive peak levels, advanced age, and cumulative dose may contribute to ototoxicity and nephrotoxicity. Examine urine for decreased specific gravity and increased protein, cells, and casts. Measure blood urea nitrogen (BUN), serum creatinine, and creatinine

clearance periodically. When feasible, obtain serial audiograms. Evidence of impairment of renal, vestibular, or auditory function warrants drug withdrawal or dosage adjustment.

• Avoid concurrent or sequential use of other neurotoxic or nephrotoxic antibiotics, especially other aminoglycosides (such as amikacin, gentamicin, kanamycin, neomycin, and streptomycin), cephaloridine, cisplatin, colistin, polymyxin B, vancomycin, and viomycin. Advanced age and dehydration also increase risk.

• Don't give concurrently with potent diuretics (such as furosemide and ethacrynic acid), because these drugs are also ototoxic. Also, I.V. diuretics may increase tobramycin toxicity by altering antibiotic serum and tissue levels.

• Use drug cautiously in premature infants and neonates.

• Drug may harm fetus when given to pregnant women.

Action

Interferes with protein synthesis in bacterial cell by binding to 30S ribosomal subunit

Availability

Injection: 10 mg/ml, 40 mg/ml, 1.2-g vial
Nebulizer solution: 300 mg/5 ml in 5-ml ampule
Ophthalmic ointment: 0.3%
Ophthalmic solution: 0.3%
Pediatric solution for injection: 20 mg/2 ml
Premixed I.V. solution: 60 mg in 50 ml normal saline, 80 mg in 100 ml normal saline

⍟ Indications and dosages

➤ Serious infections caused by susceptible organisms

Adults: 3 mg/kg/day I.V. or I.M. in evenly divided doses q 8 hours. For life-threatening infections, may increase up to 5 mg/kg/day I.V. or I.M. in three or four evenly divided doses, then reduce to 3 mg/kg/day as soon as possible.

Children older than 1 week: 6 to 7.5 mg/kg/day in three or four evenly divided doses, such as 2 to 2.5 mg/kg I.V. or I.M. q 8 hours or 1.5 to 1.9 mg/kg I.V. or I.M. q 6 hours

Neonates less than 1 week old: Up to 4 mg/kg/day I.V. or I.M. in evenly divided doses q 12 hours

➤ *Pseudomonas aeruginosa* in cystic fibrosis patients

Adults and children older than age 6: 300 mg inhalation b.i.d. (preferably q 12 hours but no less than 6 hours apart) for 28 days, then off for 28 days; then repeat cycle

➤ Ocular infections caused by susceptible organisms

Adults and children: For mild to moderate infections, apply a ribbon of ophthalmic ointment (approximately 1 cm) to infected eye two or three times daily, or instill one to two drops of ophthalmic solution into infected eye q 4 hours. For severe infections, apply ophthalmic ointment q 3 to 4 hours or instill two drops of ophthalmic solution into infected eye q 30 to 60 minutes; decrease dosing frequency when improvement occurs. Therapy should continue for at least 48 hours after infection is under control.

Dosage adjustment

• Renal impairment

Contraindications

• Hypersensitivity to drug, other aminoglycosides, bisulfites (with some products), or benzyl alcohol (in neonates, with some products)

Precautions

Use cautiously in:

• renal or hearing impairment, neuromuscular diseases, obesity

• elderly patients

• pregnant or breastfeeding patients

• neonates and premature infants.

Administration

- Know that premixed I.V. solution is ready to use and requires no further dilution. Don't mix with other drugs.
- ◀€ Don't use flexible container in series connections because of risk of air embolism.
- Dilute I.V. dose from vials in 50 to 100 ml of normal saline solution or dextrose 5% in water. For child, smaller volumes are needed.
- Infuse over at least 30 minutes. Flush line after administration.
- Give cephalosporins or penicillin, if ordered, 1 hour before or after tobramycin.
- Give inhalation doses by nebulizer over 10 to 15 minutes.

Route	Onset	Peak	Duration
I.V.	Rapid	15-30 min	Unknown
I.M.	Rapid	30-90 min	Unknown
Inhalation, ophthalmic	Unknown	Unknown	Unknown

Adverse reactions

CNS: confusion, lethargy, headache, delirium, dizziness, vertigo
EENT: eye stinging (with ophthalmic form), ototoxicity, hearing loss, roaring in ears, tinnitus
GI: nausea, vomiting, diarrhea, stomatitis
GU: proteinuria, **oliguria, nephrotoxicity**
Hematologic: anemia, eosinophilia, **leukocytosis, leukopenia, thrombocytopenia, granulocytopenia**
Metabolic: hypocalcemia, hyponatremia, hypokalemia, hypomagnesemia
Musculoskeletal: muscle weakness
Respiratory: apnea
Skin: rash, urticaria, itching
Other: superinfection, fever, pain and irritation at injection site

Interactions

Drug-drug. *Cephalosporins, vancomycin:* increased risk of nephrotoxicity

Dimenhydrinate: masking of ototoxicity symptoms
General anesthetics, neuromuscular blockers: increased neuromuscular blockade and respiratory depression
Indomethacin: increased tobramycin trough and peak levels
Loop diuretics: increased risk of ototoxicity
Penicillins: physical incompatibility, tobramycin inactivation when mixed in same I.V. solution
Polypeptide anti-infectives: increased risk of respiratory paralysis and renal dysfunction
Drug-diagnostic tests. *Alanine aminotransferase, aspartate aminotransferase, bilirubin, BUN, creatinine, lactate dehydrogenase, nonprotein nitrogen, urine protein:* increased levels
Calcium, granulocytes, hemoglobin, magnesium, platelets, potassium, sodium, white blood cells: decreased levels

Patient monitoring

- Draw sample for peak drug level 1 hour after I.M. or 30 minutes after I.V. administration. Draw sample for trough level just before next dose.
- Assess liver and kidney function tests.
- Monitor CBC with white cell differential.
- Closely monitor patient's hearing.

Patient teaching

- ◀€ Tell patient drug may cause hearing impairment and other serious adverse reactions, such as unusual bleeding or bruising. Instruct him to report these reactions at once.
- Advise patient to report new signs or symptoms of infection.
- With inhalation form, teach patient how to use nebulizer. Instruct him to administer dose over 10 to 15 minutes by breathing normally through mouthpiece while sitting or standing. Remind him to use only the hand-held nebulizer and compressor originally

dispensed with drug. Advise him to use a nose clip to help him breathe through his mouth. If he uses other inhaled drugs, instruct him to take tobramycin last.

• Teach patient proper use of eye drops. Caution him not to touch dropper to eye or any other surface.

• As appropriate, review all other significant and life-threatening adverse reactions and interactions, especially those related to the drugs and tests mentioned above.

tocilizumab
Actemra

Pharmacologic class: Interleukin-6 (IL-6) receptor inhibitor
Therapeutic class: Immunomodulator
Pregnancy risk category C

FDA BOXED WARNING

• Serious infections leading to hospitalization or death, including tuberculosis (TB) and bacterial, invasive fungal, viral, and other opportunistic infections, have occurred in patients receiving tocilizumab.

• If a serious infection develops, interrupt therapy until infection is controlled.

• Perform test for latent TB; if positive, start treatment for TB before starting tocilizumab.

• Monitor all patients for active TB during treatment, even if initial latent TB test is negative.

Action

Binds specifically to both soluble and membrane-bound IL-6 receptors (sIL-6R and mIL-6R), and has been shown to inhibit IL-6–mediated signaling through these receptors; decreases levels of C-reactive protein to within normal range; decreases rheumatoid factor, erythrocyte sedimentation rate, serum amyloid A; increases hemoglobin

Availability
Solution for injection, concentrate: 80 mg/4 ml, 200 mg/10 ml, 400 mg/ 20 ml (20 mg/ml) in single-use vials

ⓘ Indications and dosages
➤ Moderate to severe active rheumatoid arthritis in patients who have had inadequate response to one or more tumor necrosis factor (TNF) antagonists
Adults: Initially (when used in combination with disease-modifying antirheumatic drugs [DMARDs] or as monotherapy), 4 mg/kg by I.V. infusion over 60 minutes q 4 weeks; may increase to 8 mg/kg by I.V. infusion over 60 minutes q 4 weeks based on clinical response. Maximum dosage, 800 mg/infusion.
➤ Active systemic juvenile idiopathic arthritis (SJIA)
Children age 2 and older weighing 30 kg (66 lb) or more: 8 mg/kg (alone or with methotrexate) by I.V. infusion over 60 minutes q 2 weeks
Children age 2 and older weighing less than 30 kg: 12 mg/kg (alone or with methotrexate) by I.V. infusion over 60 minutes q 2 weeks

Dosage adjustment
• Elevated liver enzyme levels
• Neutropenia, thrombocytopenia

Contraindications
• Hypersensitivity to drug

Precautions
Use cautiously in:
• active hepatic disease or hepatic impairment (use not recommended)
• absolute neutrophil count less than 2,000/mm^3, platelet count less than

100,000/mm³, ALT or AST more than 1.5 times the upper limit of normal (use not recommended)

- patients who may be at increased risk for GI perforation (such as patients with diverticulitis)
- patients at risk for infection
- demyelinating disorders (such as multiple sclerosis and chronic inflammatory demyelinating polyneuropathy)
- active infection (don't use)
- concurrent use of biological DMARDs such as TNF antagonists, IL-1R antagonists, anti-CD20 monoclonal antibodies, selective co-stimulation modulators, and live vaccines (avoid use)
- concurrent use of CYP3A4 substrates when decrease in effectiveness is undesirable (such as oral contraceptives, lovastatin, atorvastatin)
- concurrent use of immunosuppressants and corticosteroids
- elderly patients
- pregnant or breastfeeding patients
- children younger than age 2 and for conditions other than SJIA (safety and efficacy not established).

Administration

◀ Be aware that drug should only be administered by healthcare professional with appropriate medical support to manage anaphylaxis. If anaphylaxis or other clinically significant hypersensitivity reaction occurs, stop drug immediately and permanently.

- Evaluate patient for TB risk factors; test for latent infection before starting therapy.
- Consider risks and benefits of treatment before starting therapy in patients with chronic or recurrent infection, in those who have been exposed to TB, in those with history of serious or opportunistic infection, in those who have resided or traveled in areas of endemic TB or endemic mycoses, and in those with underlying

conditions that may predispose to infection.

- For adults and SJIA patients who weigh 30 kg or more, dilute concentrated solution to 100 ml in 0.9% sodium chloride for I.V. infusion using 100-ml infusion bag.
- For SJIA patients weighing less than 30 kg, dilute to 50 ml in 0.9% sodium chloride for I.V. infusion using 50-ml infusion bag.
- Withdraw a volume of 0.9% sodium chloride injection from infusion bag or bottle equal to volume of drug required for dose.
- Slowly add drug for I.V. infusion from each vial into infusion bag. Gently invert bag to avoid foaming to mix solution. Allow fully diluted solution to reach room temperature before infusing. Don't mix or infuse with other drugs. Discard unused product.

◀ Administer as single I.V. drip infusion over 1 hour; don't administer as bolus or push.

- Interrupt therapy if patient develops serious infection, opportunistic infection, or sepsis until infection has been controlled.

◀ Be aware that interruption or discontinuation of drug may be needed for management of dose-related laboratory abnormalities, including elevated liver enzyme levels, neutropenia, and thrombocytopenia. If appropriate, concomitant methotrexate or other drugs should be dose-modified or stopped.

- On initiation or discontinuation of tocilizumab in patients being treated with CYP450 substrates with narrow therapeutic indices, monitor therapeutic effect of drugs such as warfarin or drug concentration of drugs such as cyclosporine or theophylline.

Route	Onset	Peak	Duration
I.V.	Unknown	Unknown	Unknown

♣ Canada   ⊕ UK   ⚖ Hazardous drug   ⊗ High-alert drug

Adverse reactions

CNS: headache, dizziness

CV: hypertension

EENT: nasopharyngitis

GI: gastroenteritis, diverticulitis, mouth ulcerations, upper abdominal pain, gastritis, **GI perforation**

GU: urinary tract infection

Hematologic: neutropenia, decreased platelets

Hepatic: abnormal liver function test results, increased lipids

Musculoskeletal: bacterial arthritis

Respiratory: upper respiratory tract infection, pneumonia, bronchitis

Skin: cellulitis, rash

Other: herpes zoster exacerbation, **other serious and opportunistic infections, sepsis, malignancies, infusion reactions,** hypersensitivity reactions including **anaphylaxis**

Interactions

Drug-drug. *CYP450 substrates with narrow therapeutic indices (such as cyclosporine, theophylline, warfarin):* increased metabolism of these drugs
Omeprazole, simvastatin: decreased exposure of these drugs

Drug-diagnostic tests. *ALT, AST, HDL, LDL, total cholesterol, triglycerides:* increased levels
Neutrophils, platelets: decreased counts

Patient monitoring

• Monitor CBC with differential, particularly neutrophils and platelets, and hepatic function tests, particularly ALT and AST, every 4 to 8 weeks. Monitor ALT, AST, neutrophils, and platelets every 2 to 4 weeks in children with SJIA. Monitor lipid levels approximately 4 to 8 weeks after initiation of therapy, then at approximately 24-week intervals in adults and children.

◀€ Continue to closely watch for signs and symptoms of hypersensitivity, demyelinating disorders, serious infection, and sepsis.

• Be aware that patients who develop new infection during treatment should undergo prompt and complete diagnostic workup appropriate for immunocompromised patients, receive appropriate antimicrobial therapy, and undergo close monitoring.

• Continue to closely monitor patients for signs and symptoms of TB, including patients who tested negative for latent TB before start of therapy.

◀€ Monitor patients who may be at increased risk for GI perforation. Promptly evaluate for early identification of GI perforation in patients who present with new-onset abdominal signs and symptoms.

◀€ Be aware that treatment with immunosuppressants may increase risk of malignancies.

Patient teaching

• Instruct patient or caregiver about importance of telling prescriber about known infections before starting drug.

• Tell patient or caregiver that TB test will be done before start of therapy and tests for blood counts and liver function will be done frequently.

◀€ Instruct patient to immediately seek medical attention if hives, rash, throat swelling, or difficulty breathing occurs.

◀€ Instruct patient or caregiver of importance of immediately contacting prescriber if severe, persistent abdominal pain; change in bowel habits; infection (fever, chills, cough, or burning on urination); or other new signs and symptoms occur.

• Instruct patient or caregiver that patient shouldn't receive live vaccines during therapy.

• Advise female patient of childbearing age to inform prescriber if she becomes pregnant during therapy.

• Advise breastfeeding patient that she should decide whether to discontinue breastfeeding or discontinue drug, taking into account importance of drug for her treatment.

t

- As appropriate, review all other significant and life-threatening adverse reactions and interactions, especially those related to the drugs and tests mentioned above.

<hr>

tolcapone
Tasmar

Pharmacologic class: Catecholamine inhibitor
Therapeutic class: Antiparkinsonian
Pregnancy risk category C

FDA | BOXED WARNING

- Before prescribing or administering drug, make sure you're thoroughly familiar with prescribing information.
- Don't administer until prescriber has discussed risks with patient and patient has provided written acknowledgment that risks have been explained.
- Due to risk of hepatocellular injury (including potentially fatal, acute fulminant liver failure), drug ordinarily should be used in patients with Parkinson's disease who are receiving L-dopa/carbidopa, experiencing symptom fluctuations, and not responding satisfactorily to or not appropriate candidates for other adjunctive therapies. Withdraw therapy if patient doesn't show substantial benefit within 3 weeks of starting drug.
- Don't initiate therapy if patient has clinical evidence of hepatic disease. Don't restart therapy if patient developed hepatocellular injury while receiving drug and was withdrawn from therapy for any reason.
- Before and during therapy, obtain appropriate tests to exclude liver disease. Discontinue drug if alanine aminotransferase (ALT) or aspartate aminotransferase (AST) levels exceed two times the upper limit of normal or if clinical signs and symptoms suggest onset of hepatic dysfunction.

<hr>

Action
Unknown. When given with levodopa-carbidopa, thought to reversibly inhibit catechol *O*-methyltransferase, leading to increased levodopa bioavailability and stimulation in brain.

Availability
Tablets: 100 mg, 200 mg

⬤ Indications and dosages
➤ Adjunct to levodopa–carbidopa in idiopathic Parkinson's disease
Adults: Initially, 100 mg P.O. t.i.d. given with levodopa–carbidopa. If beneficial, may increase dosage to 200 mg P.O. t.i.d.; maximum dosage is 600 mg daily. If response inadequate after 3 weeks, stop therapy.

Contraindications
- Hypersensitivity to drug
- Nontraumatic rhabdomyolysis
- Drug-related hyperpyrexia or confusion
- Hepatic disease, alanine aminotransferase or aspartate aminotransferase elevation
- History of tolcapone-induced hepatocellular injury

Precautions
Use cautiously in:
- renal or cardiac disease, hypertension, asthma
- concurrent use of nonselective MAO inhibitor (such as phenelzine, tranylcypromine)
- pregnant or breastfeeding patients.

Administration
◀€ Before giving first dose, obtain patient's written informed consent for drug therapy.

<hr>

- Check liver function tests before starting drug.
- ◀€ Don't stop drug abruptly, because this may cause a syndrome similar to neuroleptic malignant syndrome.
- Know that levodopa–carbidopa dosage may be decreased to minimize dyskinesia.

Route	Onset	Peak	Duration
P.O.	Unknown	2 hr	Unknown

Adverse reactions

CNS: dizziness, asthenia, headache, fatigue, hypokinesia, mental deficiency, agitation, tremor, hyperactivity, paresthesia, irritability, syncope, depression, speech disorder, confusion, sleep disorder, excessive dreaming, hallucinations, drowsiness, hypertonia, imbalance, falling, hyperkinesias, dystonia, dyskinesia
CV: hypotension, chest discomfort or pain, orthostatic hypotension, palpitations
EENT: tinnitus, sinus congestion, pharyngitis
GI: nausea, vomiting, diarrhea, constipation, dyspepsia, abdominal pain, flatulence, dry mouth, anorexia
GU: hematuria, urinary tract infection (UTI), urinary incontinence, urine discoloration, urinary disorder, erectile dysfunction
Hepatic: jaundice, **severe hepatocellular injury (including fulminant hepatic failure, death)**
Musculoskeletal: neck pain, arthritis, muscle cramps, stiffness, **rhabdomyolysis**
Respiratory: upper respiratory infection, dyspnea, bronchitis
Skin: rash, dermal bleeding, diaphoresis
Other: fever, influenza

Interactions

Drug-drug. *Desipramine:* increased risk of adverse tolcapone reactions

Nonselective MAO inhibitors (such as phenelzine, tranylcypromine): inhibition of principal pathways of tolcapone metabolism
Warfarin: increased warfarin blood level
Drug-diagnostic tests. *Alanine aminotransferase, aspartate aminotransferase:* increased levels

Patient monitoring

- Monitor parkinsonian symptoms during first 3 weeks of therapy. Report improvement (or lack thereof) to help determine if therapy should continue.
- Assess neurologic status closely.
- ◀€ Monitor liver function tests. Watch closely for signs and symptoms of hepatic impairment.
- Closely monitor temperature. Stay alert for fever and other indications of infection (particularly upper respiratory infection, influenza, and UTI).

Patient teaching

- Tell patient to take drug with first levodopa–carbidopa dose of day.
- ◀€ Advise patient to immediately report signs or symptoms of liver problems (persistent nausea, fatigue, appetite loss, dark urine, itching, tenderness on right side of abdomen, and yellowing of skin or eyes).
- Instruct patient to promptly report signs and symptoms of infection.
- ◀€ Advise female patient to immediately report suspected pregnancy. Caution her not to breastfeed.
- Tell patient drug may cause involuntary movements, hallucinations, lightheadedness, and other significant reactions. Urge him to use safety measures as needed.
- Caution patient to avoid driving and other hazardous activities until he knows how drug affects concentration and alertness.
- Advise patient to move slowly when sitting up or standing, to avoid dizziness from sudden blood pressure decrease.

• As appropriate, review all other significant and life-threatening adverse reactions and interactions, especially those related to the drugs and tests mentioned above.

---

tolterodine
Detrol, Detrol LA, Detrusitol⊕, Detrusitol XL⊕

Pharmacologic class: Anticholinergic
Therapeutic class: Urinary tract antispasmodic
Pregnancy risk category C

Action
Competitively antagonizes muscarinic receptors, inhibiting bladder contractions and reducing urinary frequency

Availability
Capsules (extended-release): 2 mg, 4 mg
Tablets: 1 mg, 2 mg

⦿ Indications and dosages
➤ Overactive bladder
Adults: 2 mg (immediate-release) P.O. b.i.d.; may decrease to 1 mg P.O. b.i.d. depending on response and tolerance. Or 4 mg (extended-release) P.O. daily; may decrease to 2 mg P.O. daily, depending on response.

Dosage adjustment
• Hepatic impairment or disease
• Renal impairment
• Concurrent use of potent CYP3A4 inhibitors

Contraindications
• Hypersensitivity to drug, its components, or to fesoterodine fumarate extended-release tablets
• Urinary or gastric retention
• Uncontrolled angle-closure glaucoma

Precautions
Use cautiously in:
• GI obstruction, significant bladder outflow obstruction, controlled angle-closure glaucoma, significant hepatic impairment, renal impairment
• pregnant or breastfeeding patients
• children (safety not established).

Administration
• Give with food to increase bioavailability.

Route	Onset	Peak	Duration
P.O.	Unknown	Unknown	12 hr

Adverse reactions
CNS: headache, dizziness, vertigo, drowsiness, paresthesia, fatigue
CV: chest pain
EENT: vision abnormalities, xerophthalmia, pharyngitis
GI: diarrhea, constipation, abdominal pain, dyspepsia, dry mouth
GU: dysuria, urinary retention or frequency, urinary tract infection
Musculoskeletal: joint pain
Skin: dry skin
Other: weight gain, flulike symptoms, infection, **anaphylaxis, angioedema**

Interactions
Drug-drug. *Clarithromycin, erythromycin, itraconazole, ketoconazole, miconazole:* inhibited metabolism and increased effects of tolterodine
Drug-food. *Any food:* increased drug bioavailability

Patient monitoring
◀ Monitor patient for anaphylaxis and angioedema with first or subsequent doses. If difficulty breathing, upper airway obstruction, or fall in blood pressure occurs, discontinue drug and promptly provide appropriate treatment.
◀ Monitor patient for signs and symptoms of anticholinergic CNS effects, particularly after beginning

---

treatment or increasing dosage. Consider dosage reduction or drug discontinuation if symptoms occur.
- Monitor bladder function.
- Assess blood pressure and stay alert for chest pain.
- Monitor neurologic status. Report paresthesia or visual impairment.

Patient teaching
- Tell patient to take with food.
- If patient takes extended-release form, instruct him not to chew or crush it.
- ◀€ Instruct patient how to recognize and immediately report signs and symptoms of anaphylaxis or angioedema.
- Caution patient not to drive or operate heavy machinery until drug's effects are known.
- Advise patient to use sugarless gum or hard candy to relieve dry mouth.
- As appropriate, review all other significant adverse reactions and interactions, especially those related to the drugs and foods mentioned above.

topiramate
Apo-Topiramate✲, Co-Topiramate✲, Dom-Topiramate✲, Gen-Topiramate✲, Novo-Topiramate✲, PHL-Topiramate✲, PMS-Topiramate✲, Ratio-Topiramate✲, Sandoz-Topiramate ✲, Topamax

Pharmacologic class: Sulfamate-substituted monosaccharide derivative
Therapeutic class: Anticonvulsant
Pregnancy risk category C

Action
Blocks sodium channels, enhancing the action of gamma-amino butyrate (a neurotransmitter); also inhibits amino acid excitatory receptors

Availability
Sprinkle capsules: 15 mg, 25 mg
Tablets: 25 mg, 50 mg, 100 mg, 200 mg

🕖 Indications and dosages
➤ Adjunct in partial-onset seizures, primary generalized tonic–clonic seizures, and seizures associated with Lennox-Gastaut syndrome
Adults and children older than age 17: Initially, 25 to 50 mg P.O. daily. To achieve adequate response, may increase by 25 to 50 mg weekly, up to 200 mg b.i.d.
Children ages 2 to 16: Initially, up to 25 mg P.O. daily; increase at 1- or 2-week intervals in increments of 1 to 3 mg/kg/day given in two divided doses to achieve adequate response.
➤ Migraine prophylaxis
Adults: Dosage titrated to 100 mg P.O. daily as follows: 25 mg/day during week 1, 25 mg b.i.d. during week 2, 25 mg in morning and 50 mg in evening during week 3, and 50 mg b.i.d. during week 4
➤ Monotherapy for epilepsy
Adults and children ages 10 and older: Initially, 50 mg P.O. daily in two divided dosages. Increase dosage weekly by increments of 50 mg for first 4 weeks, then 100 mg for weeks 5 and 6. Maximum dosage is 400 mg/day in two divided doses.
Children ages 2 to younger than 10: Initially, 25 mg/day P.O. nightly for first week. Titrate dosage over 5 to 7 weeks, with total maximum daily dosage based on weight.

Dosage adjustment
- Renal impairment

Off-label uses
- Cluster headaches
- Infantile spasms
- Mood stabilization

Contraindications
None

Reactions in **bold** are life-threatening.   ◀€ Clinical alert

Precautions

Use cautiously in:
- renal or hepatic impairment, dehydration, urolithiasis, glaucoma, myopia, patients at increased risk for hyperammonemia (such as those with inborn errors of metabolism or reduced mitochondrial activity)
- concurrent use of other carbonic anhydrase inhibitors, other drugs causing metabolic acidosis, or patients on ketogenic diet (avoid use)
- concurrent use of other drugs that predispose patients to heat-related disorders (such as carbonic anhydrase inhibitors, drugs with anticholinergic activity)
- pregnant or breastfeeding patients.
- children younger than age 2 (safety and efficacy not established).

Administration

- Give without regard to meals.
- Don't break tablets, because of bitter taste.
- Administer capsules either whole or by opening capsule carefully and sprinkling entire contents into small amount of soft food. Instruct patient to swallow mixture immediately without chewing sprinkles.
- 🔊 Don't stop therapy suddenly. Dosage must be tapered.

Route	Onset	Peak	Duration
P.O.	Unknown	2 hr	12 hr

Adverse reactions

CNS: dizziness, drowsiness, fatigue, malaise, poor memory and concentration, nervousness, psychomotor slowing, speech and language problems, aggressive reaction, agitation, anxiety, confusion, depression, irritability, ataxia, paresthesia, hyperesthesia, tremor, **suicide attempt, increased seizures**

EENT: abnormal vision, diplopia, nystagmus, acute myopia, secondary angle-closure glaucoma, decreased hearing, rhinitis, sinusitis, epistaxis, pharyngitis

GI: nausea, constipation, abdominal pain, dry mouth, gastroenteritis, increased salivation (in children), anorexia

GU: renal calculi, urinary incontinence, leukorrhea

Hematologic: purpura, **leukopenia, thrombocytopenia**

Metabolic: hypocalcemia, hyperchloremia, hypernatremia, hyponatremia, hypophosphatemia, **hyperammonemia, metabolic acidosis, hypoglycemia**

Musculoskeletal: myalgia, back pain, leg pain

Respiratory: pneumonia

Skin: rash, skin disorder, alopecia, dermatitis, hypertrichosis, eczema, seborrhea, skin discoloration

Other: altered taste, weight loss, thirst, fever, flulike symptoms, hot flashes, infection, edema, hypothermia (when used in conjunction with valproic acid), hyperthermia, decreased sweating, allergic reaction

Interactions

Drug-drug. *Carbamazepine:* decreased topiramate blood level and effects

Carbonic anhydrase inhibitors (such as acetazolamide): increased risk of renal calculi

CNS depressants: increased risk of CNS depression and other adverse cognitive or neuropsychiatric reactions

Hormonal contraceptives: decreased contraceptive efficacy

Phenytoin: increased phenytoin blood level and effects, decreased topiramate blood level and effects

Valproic acid: decreased effects of both drugs

Drug-diagnostic tests. *Alanine aminotransferase, alkaline phosphatase, ammonia, aspartate aminotransferase, creatinine:* increased levels

Calcium, cholesterol, glucose, phosphate: decreased levels

🍁 Canada   ⊕ UK   ⚕ Hazardous drug   ⊗ High-alert drug

Sodium: increased or decreased level
Drug-behaviors. *Alcohol use:* increased CNS depression

Patient monitoring

◀ Monitor seizure type and pattern. Report new seizure types or worsening seizure pattern.

• Assess neurologic status closely. Report significant adverse reactions.

◀ Watch for and immediately report signs and symptoms of depression or suicidal ideation.

• Monitor fluid intake and output. Report indications of urinary tract infection, urinary incontinence, or renal calculi.

◀ Monitor vision. If patient becomes acutely nearsighted with symptoms of angle-closure glaucoma (cloudy vision, eye pain), stop drug and contact prescriber right away.

◀ Monitor patient for hyperammonemia and encephalopathy with or without concomitant valproic acid use; measure ammonia level if encephalopathic symptoms occur.

◀ Monitor patient for metabolic acidosis; obtain baseline and periodic measurements of serum bicarbonate. Consider dosage reduction or drug discontinuation if clinically appropriate.

Patient teaching

• Tell patient he may take with or without food.

• Caution patient not to crush or break tablets.

• If patient takes capsules, tell him he may open them, sprinkle contents onto small amount of soft food, and consume immediately. Tell him not to store this mixture.

◀ Caution patient not to stop drug suddenly. Dosage must be tapered.

• Instruct patient to drink plenty of fluids to reduce risk of kidney stones.

◀ Tell patient drug may cause new seizure types or worsen seizure pattern.

Instruct him to report these developments immediately.

◀ Instruct patient (and significant other as appropriate) to immediately report signs or symptoms of depression or suicidal thoughts.

◀ Instruct patient how to recognize and immediately report signs and symptoms of hyperammonemia and metabolic acidosis.

◀ Advise patient to immediately report vision changes, especially nearsightedness, cloudy vision, or eye pain.

• Caution patient not to drive or perform other hazardous activities.

• Tell patient not to drink alcohol during drug therapy.

• Advise female patient to notify prescriber of suspected pregnancy.

• As appropriate, review all other significant and life-threatening adverse reactions and interactions, especially those related to the drugs, tests, and behaviors mentioned above.

topotecan hydrochloride
Hycamtin

Pharmacologic class: DNA topoisomerase inhibitor

Therapeutic class: Antineoplastic

Pregnancy risk category D

FDA | BOXED WARNING

• Give under supervision of physician experienced in cancer chemotherapy, in facility with adequate diagnostic and treatment resources.

• Don't administer to patients with baseline neutrophil counts below 1,500 cells/mm^3. Obtain frequent peripheral blood cell counts on all patients to monitor for bone marrow depression.

Action

Regulates DNA replication and repair of broken DNA strands, relieving torsional strain; exerts cytotoxic effects during DNA synthesis

Availability

Capsules: 0.25 mg, 1 mg
Injection: 4 mg in 4-ml single-dose vials
Injection (powder for solution): 4 mg in single-dose vials

🚺 Indications and dosages

➣ Metastatic ovarian cancer or small-cell lung cancer after first-line chemotherapy fails
Adults: 1.5 mg/m² daily by I.V. infusion given over 30 minutes for 5 consecutive days, starting on day 1 of 21-day cycle
➣ Relapsed small-cell lung cancer
Adults: 2.3 mg/m² P.O. daily for 5 consecutive days; repeat every 21 days
➣ Stage IV-B, recurrent, or persistent cervical carcinoma not amenable to curative treatment with surgery or radiation therapy (in combination with cisplatin)
Adults: 0.75 mg/m² I.V. daily over 30 minutes on days 1, 2, and 3; followed by cisplatin 50 mg/m² by I.V. infusion on day 1, repeated every 21 days

Dosage adjustment

• Renal impairment
• Neutropenia
• Grade 3 or 4 diarrhea (capsules)

Contraindications

• History of severe hypersensitivity to drug or its components
• Severe bone marrow depression

Precautions

Use cautiously in:
• pregnant or breastfeeding patients
• children (safety and efficacy not established).

Administration

🔊 Before starting therapy, check blood counts. Patient must have baseline neutrophil count above 1,500 cells/mm³ and platelet count above 100,000 cells/mm³ to receive drug.
🔊 Prepare drug under vertical laminar-flow hood, wearing gloves and protective clothing. Follow facility policy for discarding used drug containers and I.V. equipment.
• If skin contacts drug, wash immediately with soap and water.
• To reconstitute, add 4 ml of sterile water to 4-mg vial. Dilute further in normal saline solution or dextrose 5% in water. Give immediately over 30 minutes using infusion pump.
• Round calculated oral daily dose to nearest 0.25 mg, and administer minimum number of 1-mg and 0.25-mg capsules. Know that the same number of capsules should be prescribed for each of the 5 dosing days.

Route	Onset	Peak	Duration
P.O.	Rapid	1-2 hr	Unknown
I.V.	Unknown	Unknown	Unknown

Adverse reactions

CNS: asthenia, fatigue, paresthesia
GI: nausea, diarrhea, constipation, abdominal pain, stomatitis, anorexia, **severe diarrhea, neutropenic colitis**
Hematologic: anemia, **leukopenia, thrombocytopenia, neutropenia**
Musculoskeletal: back pain, skeletal pain
Respiratory: coughing, dyspnea, **interstitial lung disease**
Skin: erythematous or maculopapular rash, pruritus, urticaria, dermatitis, bullous eruption, alopecia
Other: fever, body pain, **sepsis**

Interactions

Drug-drug. *Cisplatin:* severe bone marrow depression
Granulocyte colony-stimulating factor: prolonged neutropenia

Live-virus vaccines: increased risk of infection from vaccine

Drug-diagnostic tests. *Alanine aminotransferase, aspartate aminotransferase, bilirubin:* increased levels

Patient monitoring

• Closely monitor CBC with white cell differential.

◀€ Assess for signs and symptoms of bleeding tendency, severe diarrhea (with capsule use), and neutropenic colitis (fever, neutropenia, and compatible pattern of abdominal pain).

◀€ Monitor patient for signs and symptoms of interstitial lung disease (cough, fever, dyspnea, or hypoxia); discontinue drug if diagnosis is confirmed.

• Monitor closely for sepsis, other infections, and increased hepatic enzyme levels.

Patient teaching

• Tell patient to take capsules whole with or without food and not to break, divide, chew, or crush them.

◀€ Advise patient to immediately report unusual bleeding or bruising, diarrhea, abdominal pain, cough, difficulty breathing, sore throat, fever, or chills.

• Teach patient safety measures to avoid bruising and bleeding.

• Tell patient to minimize GI upset by eating small, frequent servings of food and drinking plenty of fluids.

◀€ Advise female patient to notify prescriber of suspected pregnancy. Caution her not to breastfeed during therapy.

• Inform patient that drug may cause hair loss.

• Tell patient he'll undergo regular blood testing during therapy.

• As appropriate, review all other significant and life-threatening adverse reactions and interactions, especially those related to the drugs and tests mentioned above.

torsemide (torasemide ✛)
Demadex, Torem ✛

Pharmacologic class: Loop diuretic
Therapeutic class: Diuretic, antihypertensive
Pregnancy risk category B

Action

Inhibits sodium and chloride reabsorption from ascending loop of Henle and distal renal tubule; increases renal excretion of water, sodium, chloride, magnesium, calcium, and hydrogen. Also may exert renal and peripheral vasodilatory effects. Net effect is natriuretic diuresis.

Availability

Injection: 10 mg/ml
Tablets: 5 mg, 10 mg, 20 mg, 100 mg

⏀ Indications and dosages

➤ Heart failure
Adults: 10 to 20 mg P.O. or I.V. daily. If response inadequate, double dosage until desired response occurs. Don't exceed 200 mg as a single dose.
➤ Hypertension
Adults: 5 mg P.O. daily. May increase to 10 mg daily after 4 to 6 weeks; if drug still isn't effective, additional antihypertensives may be prescribed.
➤ Chronic renal failure
Adults: 20 mg P.O. or I.V. daily. If response inadequate, double dosage until desired response occurs. Don't exceed 200 mg as a single dose.
➤ Hepatic cirrhosis
Adults: 5 or 10 mg P.O. or I.V. daily, given with aldosterone antagonist or potassium-sparing diuretic. If response inadequate, double dosage. Don't exceed 40 mg as a single dose.

t

Reactions in **bold** are life-threatening.　　　◀€ Clinical alert

Contraindications
• Hypersensitivity to drug, thiazides, or sulfonylureas
• Anuria

Precautions
Use cautiously in:
• severe hepatic disease accompanied by cirrhosis or ascites, preexisting uncorrected electrolyte imbalances, diabetes mellitus, worsening azotemia
• elderly patients
• pregnant or breastfeeding patients
• children younger than age 18.

Administration
• Give I.V. by direct injection over at least 2 minutes or by continuous I.V. infusion.
• Flush I.V. line with normal saline solution before and after administering.

Route	Onset	Peak	Duration
P.O.	Within 1 hr	1-2 hr	6-8 hr
I.V.	Within 10 min	Within 1 hr	6-8 hr

Adverse reactions
CNS: dizziness, headache, asthenia, insomnia, nervousness, syncope
CV: hypotension, ECG changes, chest pain, volume depletion, **atrial fibrillation, ventricular tachycardia, shunt thrombosis**
EENT: rhinitis, sore throat
GI: nausea, diarrhea, vomiting, constipation, dyspepsia, anorexia, rectal bleeding, **GI hemorrhage**
GU: excessive urination
Metabolic: hyperglycemia, hyperuricemia, hypokalemia
Musculoskeletal: joint pain, myalgia
Respiratory: increased cough
Skin: rash
Other: edema

Interactions
Drug-drug. *Aminoglycosides, cisplatin:* increased risk of ototoxicity

Amphotericin B, corticosteroids, mezlocillin, piperacillin, potassium-wasting diuretics, stimulant laxatives: additive hypokalemia
Antihypertensives, nitrates: additive hypotension
Lithium: increased lithium blood level and toxicity
Neuromuscular blockers: prolonged neuromuscular blockade
Nonsteroidal anti-inflammatory drugs, probenecid: inhibited diuretic response
Sulfonylureas: decreased glucose tolerance, hyperglycemia in patients with previously well-controlled diabetes
Drug-diagnostic tests. *Glucose, uric acid:* increased levels
Potassium: decreased level
Drug-herbs. *Dandelion:* interference with diuresis
Ephedra (ma huang): reduced hypotensive effect of torsemide
Geranium, ginseng: increased risk of diuretic resistance
Licorice: rapid potassium loss
Drug-behaviors. *Acute alcohol ingestion:* additive hypotension

Patient monitoring
• Monitor vital signs, especially for hypotension.
• Assess ECG for arrhythmias and other changes.
• Monitor weight and fluid intake and output to assess drug efficacy.
• Monitor electrolyte levels, particularly potassium. Stay alert for signs and symptoms of hypokalemia.
• Assess hearing for signs and symptoms of ototoxicity.
• Monitor blood glucose level carefully in diabetic patient.

Patient teaching
• Advise patient to take in morning with or without food.
• Instruct patient to move slowly when sitting up or standing, to avoid dizziness from sudden blood pressure drop.

- Tell patient to monitor weight and report sudden increases.
- Instruct diabetic patient to monitor blood glucose level carefully.
- Caution patient to avoid alcohol during drug therapy.
- Advise patient to consult prescriber before using herbs.
- As appropriate, review all other significant and life-threatening adverse reactions and interactions, especially those related to the drugs, tests, herbs, and behaviors mentioned above.

tramadol hydrochloride

ConZip, Dromadol SR⊕, Dromadol XL⊕, Larapam SR⊕, Mabron⊕, Nobligan Retard⊕, Ralivia✷, Rybix ODT, Ryzolt, Tradorec XL⊕, Tramake⊕, Tridural✷, Ultram, Ultram ER, Zamadol⊕, Zydol⊕, Zytram XL✷

Pharmacologic class: Opioid agonist
Therapeutic class: Analgesic
Pregnancy risk category C

Action

Inhibits reuptake of serotonin and norepinephrine in CNS

Availability

Tablets: 50 mg
Tablets (extended-release): 100 mg, 200 mg, 300 mg
Tablets (orally disintegrating [ODT]): 50 mg

Indications and dosages

➤ Moderate to moderately severe pain in patients who require around-the-clock treatment of pain for an extended period
Adults: In rapid titration, 50 to 100 mg (immediate-release) P.O. q 4 to 6 hours

p.r.n. (not to exceed 400 mg/day, or 300 mg/day in patients older than age 75). In gradual titration, initially 25 mg (immediate-release) P.O. daily; increase by 25 mg/day q 3 days to 100 mg/day, then increase by 50 mg/day q 3 days, up to 200 mg/day p.r.n. Alternately, 100 mg P.O (extended-release) up to a maximum of 300 mg daily. Titrate daily doses by 100-mg/day increments q 2 to 3 days (Ryzolt) or q 5 days (ConZip) to achieve a balance between adequate pain control and individual tolerability. Continue with lowest effective dose. Maximum dose is 300 mg/day. For patients on immediate-release product, calculate total 24-hour immediate-release dose and initiate at a dose rounded down to next lower 100-mg increment. Individualize dose according to patient need and tolerance, not to exceed 300 mg daily. Or, in patients not requiring rapid analgesic effect, tolerability can be improved by initiating therapy with a titration regimen. Total daily dose may be increased by 50 mg (ODT tablets) P.O. as tolerated q 3 days to reach 200 mg/day (50 mg q.i.d.). After titration, 50 to 100 mg (ODT tablets) P.O. can be administered as needed for pain relief q 4 to 6 hours, not to exceed 400 mg/day.

Dosage adjustment

- Renal or hepatic impairment

Contraindications

- Hypersensitivity to drug, its components, or opioids
- Acute intoxication with alcohol, sedative-hypnotics, centrally acting analgesics, opioid analgesics, or psychotropic agents
- Physical opioid dependence
- Significant respiratory depression, acute or severe bronchial asthma or hypercapnia in unmonitored settings or absence of resuscitative equipment

t

Precautions
Use cautiously in:
• seizure disorder or risk factors for seizures, increased intracranial pressure, head trauma, acute abdomen, patients at risk for respiratory depression, patients who use alcohol in excess, patients who suffer from emotional disturbance or depression, patients receiving CNS depressants, other opioids, anesthetics, tranquilizers, or sedative-hypnotics
• mild to severe hepatic impairment, and renal impairment with creatinine clearance less than 30 ml/minute
• history of sensitivity to phenylketones (avoid ODT use)
• history of opioid dependence or recent use of large opioid doses or patients who are suicidal or addiction-prone (use not recommended)
• concurrent use of monoamine oxidase (MAO) inhibitors (use with great caution)
• elderly patients
• pregnant or breastfeeding patients
• children younger than age 16 or 18 (ConZip) (safety not established, use not recommended).

Administration
• Give as prescribed, preferably before pain becomes severe.
🔊 Be aware that serious and rarely fatal anaphylactoid reactions have occurred, often following first dose.

Route	Onset	Peak	Duration
P.O.	1 hr	2-3 hr	4-6 hr
PO (ER)	Unknown	Unknown	Unknown

Adverse reactions
CNS: dizziness, vertigo, headache, drowsiness, anxiety, stimulation, confusion, incoordination, euphoria, nervousness, sleep disorder, asthenia, hypertonia, **seizures, suicide**
CV: vasodilation
EENT: visual disturbances

GI: nausea, vomiting, diarrhea, constipation, abdominal pain, dyspepsia, flatulence, dry mouth, anorexia
GU: urinary retention and frequency, proteinuria, menopausal symptoms
Respiratory: respiratory depression (with large doses, concomitant anesthetic use, or alcohol ingestion), **bronchospasm**
Skin: pruritus, sweating, hives, **angioedema, toxic epidermal necrolysis, Stevens-Johnson syndrome**
Other: physical or psychological drug dependence, drug tolerance, **serotonin syndrome, serious and rarely fatal anaphylactoid reactions**

Interactions
Drug-drug. *Anesthetics, antihistamines, CNS depressants, other opioids, psychotropic agents, sedative-hypnotics:* increased risk of CNS depression
Carbamazepine: increased tramadol metabolism and decreased efficacy
Serotonergic drugs (including MAO inhibitors, selective norepinephrine reuptake inhibitors, selective serotonin reuptake inhibitors, tricyclic antidepressants, triptans), drugs that impair serotonin metabolism (including MAO inhibitors), drugs that impair tramadol metabolism (such as CYP2D6 and CYP3A4 inhibitors): increased risk of serotonin syndrome and seizures
Drug-diagnostic tests. *Creatinine, hepatic enzymes:* increased levels
Hemoglobin: decreased level
Drug-herbs. *Chamomile, hops, kava, skullcap, valerian:* increased CNS depression
Drug-behaviors. *Alcohol use:* increased CNS depression

Patient monitoring
• Assess patient's response to drug 30 minutes after administration.
• Monitor respiratory status. Withhold drug and contact prescriber if respirations become shallow or slower than 12 breaths/minute.

🍁 Canada   ⊕ UK   ☣ Hazardous drug   ⊗ High-alert drug

- Monitor for physical and psychological drug dependence. Report signs to prescriber.

◀┋ Monitor patient for signs and symptoms of potentially life-threatening serotonin syndrome, which may range from shivering and diarrhea to muscle rigidity, fever, mental-status changes, and seizures.

Patient teaching

- Tell patient drug works best when taken before pain becomes severe.
- Tell patient to take extended-release tablets with or without food, to swallow them whole at same time each day with a sufficient quantity of liquid, and not to split, chew, dissolve, or crush them.
- Instruct patient to open ODT tablet blister pack and to peel back the foil on the blister; caution patient not to push tablet through foil. Instruct patient to remove a tablet and place it in the mouth, where it will dissolve in seconds and then be swallowed with saliva. Tell patient not to chew, break, or split tablet. Inform patient who has phenylketonuria that ODT tablet contains phenylalanine.
- Inform patient (and significant other as appropriate) that drug may cause respiratory depression if used with alcohol. Recommend abstinence.

◀┋ Instruct patient to immediately report seizure, suicidal behavior, or suicidal ideation.

◀┋ Instruct patient to watch for and immediately report signs and symptoms of serotonin syndrome (shivering and diarrhea, muscle rigidity, fever, and seizures).

◀┋ Tell patient to immediately report sign and symptoms of allergic reaction (such as itching, hives, difficulty breathing, or swelling of face, tongue, or throat).

- Tell patient drug interacts with many common over-the-counter drugs and herbal remedies. Instruct him to consult prescriber before taking these products.
- Inform patient that drug can cause physical and psychological dependence. Urge him to take it only as prescribed and needed.
- Caution patient to avoid driving and other hazardous activities until he knows how drug affects concentration and alertness.
- Caution patient to avoid alcohol use while taking this drug.
- As appropriate, review all other significant and life-threatening adverse reactions and interactions, especially those related to the drugs, tests, herbs, and behaviors mentioned above.

trandolapril
Goptin✚, Mavik

Pharmacologic class: Angiotensin-converting enzyme (ACE) inhibitor
Therapeutic class: Antihypertensive
Pregnancy risk category D

FDA BOXED WARNING

- Drugs that act directly on the renin-angiotensin system can cause injury to or death of a developing fetus. Discontinue drug as soon as possible when pregnancy is detected.

Action

Inhibits conversion of angiotensin I to the potent vasoconstrictor angiotensin II, promoting vasodilation. Also increases plasma renin and stimulates aldosterone secretion, inducing diuresis.

Availability

Tablets: 1 mg, 2 mg, 4 mg

⨀ Indications and dosages

➤ Hypertension

Adults: For patients not receiving diuretics, 1 mg/day P.O. in nonblack patients or 2 mg/day P.O. in black patients. If response inadequate, may increase at weekly intervals up to 4 mg/day. For patients receiving diuretics, start with 0.5 mg/day P.O.

➤ Heart failure or left ventricular dysfunction after myocardial infarction

Adults: Initially, 1 mg P.O. daily. Titrate up to 4 mg daily, if tolerated.

Dosage adjustment

- Renal impairment (creatinine clearance less than 30 ml/minute)
- Hepatic cirrhosis

Contraindications

- Hypersensitivity to drug or other ACE inhibitors
- Hereditary/idiopathic angioedema and angioedema with previous ACE inhibitor use
- Patients with diabetes mellitus taking insulin or oral hypoglycemics

Precautions

Use cautiously in:

- renal or hepatic impairment, hypovolemia, hyponatremia, aortic stenosis or hypertrophic cardiomyopathy, cerebrovascular or cardiac insufficiency, surgery and anesthesia, risk factors for hyperkalemia (including renal insufficiency, diabetes mellitus, concurrent use of potassium supplements or potassium-containing salt substitutes)
- family history of angioedema
- concurrent diuretic therapy or drugs that cause increased serum potassium level
- black patients with hypertension
- elderly patients
- pregnant patients
- breastfeeding patients (avoid use)
- children (safety not established).

Administration

- Give once or twice daily as prescribed, with or without food.

Route	Onset	Peak	Duration
P.O.	Within 1 hr	4-10 hr	Up to 24 hr

Adverse reactions

CNS: insomnia, paresthesia, dizziness, drowsiness, asthenia, syncope, **cerebrovascular accident**

CV: chest pain, palpitations, intermittent claudication, bradycardia, **first-degree atrioventricular block, cardiogenic shock**

EENT: epistaxis, sinusitis, throat inflammation

GI: vomiting, diarrhea, constipation, abdominal pain or distention, gastritis, dyspepsia, intestinal angioedema, **pancreatitis**

GU: urinary tract infection, erectile dysfunction, decreased libido

Hematologic: agranulocytosis, neutropenia

Hepatic: syndrome of cholestatic jaundice, fulminant hepatic necrosis, and death (rare)

Metabolic: hypocalcemia, gout, increased creatinine, **hyperkalemia**

Musculoskeletal: muscle cramps, myalgia, extremity pain

Respiratory: cough, dyspnea, upper respiratory infection

Skin: rash, flushing, pruritus

Other: edema, **angioedema** (face, extremities, lips, tongue, glottis, and larynx)

Interactions

Drug-drug. *Diuretics, general anesthetics, other antihypertensives:* increased risk of hypotension

Hypoglycemics (insulin, oral agents): increased risk of blood glucose–lowering effect with greater risk of hypoglycemia

Lithium: increased lithium blood level, greater risk of toxicity

Nonsteroidal anti-inflammatory drugs, including selective cyclooxygenase-2 inhibitors: increased risk of renal impairment, including acute renal failure in elderly patients, volume-depleted patients, or those with compromised renal function; loss of trandodolapril antihypertensive effect
Potassium-sparing diuretics, potassium supplements, salt substitutes containing potassium: additive hyperkalemia
Sodium aurothiomalate (gold): increased risk of nitritoid reactions (including facial flushing, nausea, vomiting, and hypotension)
Drug-diagnostic tests. *Creatinine, potassium:* increased level
Neutrophils, platelets: decreased counts
Drug-food. *Salt substitutes containing potassium:* hyperkalemia

Patient monitoring

• Monitor vital signs, especially for hypotension and bradycardia when therapy begins.
• Assess CBC with white cell differential. Watch for signs and symptoms of bleeding and infection.
• Monitor electrolyte levels, especially potassium. Stay alert for hyperkalemia.
• Assess renal function tests and fluid intake and output.
◄€ Stay alert for signs and symptoms of hypersensitivity reactions (including angioedema). Discontinue drug immediately if laryngeal stridor or angioedema of face, tongue, or glottis occurs, treat appropriately, and closely observe patient until swelling disappears.
◄€ Be aware that rarely ACE inhibitors have been associated with a syndrome of cholestatic jaundice, fulminant hepatic necrosis, and death. If patient develops jaundice, discontinue drug and provide appropriate follow-up care.

Patient teaching

• Tell patient drug may cause bleeding tendency or increase his infection risk. Teach him which warning signs to report.
◄€ Teach patient to recognize and report signs or symptoms of hyperkalemia, infection, angioedema (including intestinal angioedema that may present as abdominal pain with or without nausea), and syndrome of cholestatic jaundice.
• Instruct patient to move slowly when sitting up or standing, to avoid dizziness from sudden blood pressure drop.
• Caution patient not to exercise vigorously in hot environments.
• Advise patient not to use salt substitutes containing potassium. Tell him to avoid high-potassium foods.
• As appropriate, review all other significant and life-threatening adverse reactions and interactions, especially those related to the drugs, tests, foods, herbs, and behaviors mentioned above.

trastuzumab
Herceptin

Pharmacologic class: Recombinant DNA-derived monoclonal antibody
Therapeutic class: Antineoplastic
Pregnancy risk category B

FDA | BOXED WARNING

• Drug can result in subclinical and clinical cardiac failure manifesting as congestive heart failure and decreased left ventricular ejection fraction.
• Incidence and severity of left ventricular dysfunction were highest in patients who received trastuzumab concurrently with anthracycline-containing chemotherapy regimens.

- Discontinue trastuzumab in patients receiving adjuvant therapy and strongly consider discontinuing in patients with metastatic breast cancer who develop clinically significant decrease in left ventricular function.
- Monitor patients for decreased left ventricular function before starting trastuzumab and frequently during and after treatment. Monitor more frequently if drug is withheld in patients who develop significant left ventricular dysfunction.
- Serious infusion reactions, some fatal, and pulmonary toxicity have occurred. In most cases, signs and symptoms occurred during or within 24 hours of administration. Interrupt infusion for patients experiencing dyspnea or clinically significant hypotension.
- Discontinue drug for infusion reactions manifesting as anaphylaxis, angioedema, interstitial pneumonitis, or acute respiratory distress syndrome.
- Exacerbation of chemotherapy-induced neutropenia has also occurred.

Action

Selectively binds to human epidermal growth factor receptor 2 (HER2), inhibiting proliferation of human tumor cells that overexpress HER2

Availability

Lyophilized powder: 440-mg vial (each vial contains 20 ml bacteriostatic water for injection, 1.1% benzyl alcohol)

⊘ Indications and dosages

➤ Metastatic breast cancer in patients whose tumors overexpress HER2
Adults: As monotherapy, loading dose of 4 mg/kg I.V. infusion over 90 minutes, followed by weekly maintenance dose of 2 mg/kg I.V. infusion given over 30 minutes if loading dose was tolerated. Don't give by I.V. push.

Contraindications
None

Precautions
Use cautiously in:
- hypersensitivity to Chinese hamster ovary cell protein or to benzyl alcohol
- cardiac disease, anemia, leukopenia
- elderly patients
- pregnant or breastfeeding patients
- children younger than age 18 (safety and efficacy not established).

Administration
- Be aware that baseline left ventricular ejection fraction (LVEF) measurement should be performed immediately before starting drug.
- Follow facility policy for handling, administering, and disposal of carcinogenic, mutagenic, and teratogenic agents.
- Give antiemetic, as prescribed, before administering trastuzumab.
- 📢 Administer by I.V. infusion only. Don't give by I.V. push or bolus.
- To reconstitute, add 20 ml of bacteriostatic water for injection to vial, pointing diluent stream at lyophilized cake. Swirl vial gently; don't shake. Withdraw prescribed dose and add it to 250 ml of normal saline solution. (Don't use dextrose 5% in water.)
- Infuse loading dose I.V. over 90 minutes. Infuse weekly doses I.V. over 30 minutes.
- Immediately after reconstituting, write a date that is 28 days from reconstitution date in the space after "Do not use after" on vial label.
- If patient has benzyl alcohol hypersensitivity, reconstitute with sterile water for injection. Use immediately after reconstitution; discard unused portion.
- 📢 Never administer intrathecally; doing so causes death.

- Know that for patient who hasn't previously received chemotherapy for metastatic disease, drug is given at same dosage but in combination with paclitaxel.

Route	Onset	Peak	Duration
I.V.	Unknown	Unknown	Unknown

Adverse reactions

CNS: dizziness, headache, depression, paresthesia, insomnia, ataxia, confusion, manic reaction, **seizures**

CV: peripheral edema, hypotension, tachycardia, syncope, **arrhythmias, shock, pericardial effusion, vascular thrombosis, heart failure, cardiotoxicity, cardiac arrest, cardiomyopathy**

EENT: amblyopia, hearing loss

GI: nausea, vomiting, diarrhea, gastroenteritis, hematemesis, colitis, esophageal ulcer, stomatitis, ileus, anorexia, **intestinal obstruction, pancreatitis**

GU: urinary tract infection, hematuria, hemorrhagic cystitis, hydronephrosis, pyelonephritis, **renal failure**

Hematologic: coagulation disorder, pancytopenia, leukemia, exacerbation of chemotherapy-induced neutropenia

Hepatic: ascites, **hepatitis, hepatic failure**

Metabolic: hypothyroidism, hypercalcemia, hyponatremia

Musculoskeletal: back, bone, or joint pain; myopathy; fractures; **bone necrosis**

Respiratory: upper respiratory infection, dyspnea, **pulmonary toxicity** (dyspnea, interstitial pneumonitis, pulmonary infiltrates, pleural effusions, noncardiogenic pulmonary edema, pulmonary insufficiency and hypoxia, acute respiratory distress syndrome, pulmonary fibrosis)

Skin: cellulitis, rash, acne, herpes simplex, herpes zoster, skin ulcers

Other: weight loss, edema, infection, fever, chills, flulike syndrome, lymphangitis, hypersensitivity reactions including **anaphylaxis, infusion reaction**

Interactions

Drug-drug. *Anthracyclines, cyclophosphamide:* cardiotoxicity

Patient monitoring

◀€ Monitor closely for signs and symptoms of infusion reaction (including respiratory distress). Halt infusion if these occur.

- Monitor vital signs, especially for hypotension and bradycardia.

◀€ Use with extreme caution in patients with cardiac dysfunction. Assess cardiovascular status carefully; stay alert for heart failure, cardiomyopathy, and peripheral edema.

- Assess neurologic status for depression and paresthesia.

- Monitor respiratory status. Report increased dyspnea or flulike symptoms.

- Watch closely for signs and symptoms of infection, including herpes simplex.

- Monitor electrolyte levels and CBC with white cell differential.

- Monitor LVEF measurement every 3 months during and at completion of therapy; measure LVEF at 4-week intervals if drug is withheld for significant left ventricular cardiac dysfunction. Continue LVEF measurement every 6 months for at least 2 years after completion of therapy.

Patient teaching

◀€ Instruct patient to immediately report difficulty breathing, flulike symptoms, and fever, chills, and other signs and symptoms of infection.

◀€ Advise patient to monitor weight. Tell him to report sudden weight gain as well as swelling and other signs and symptoms of heart failure.

◀€ Instruct patient to immediately report abdominal pain, change in

t

Reactions in **bold** are life-threatening.　　　◀€ Clinical alert

bowel habits, yellowing of skin or eyes, and easy bruising or bleeding.

• Tell patient drug may cause depression. Advise him (or significant other as appropriate) to contact prescriber if this occurs.

• As appropriate, review all other significant and life-threatening adverse reactions and interactions, especially those related to the drugs mentioned above.

trazodone hydrochloride

Apo-Trazodone✤, Dom-Trazodone✤, Gen-Trazodone✤, Molipaxin⊕, Novo-Trazodone✤, Nu-Trazodone✤, Oleptro, PHL-Trazodone✤, PMS-Trazodone✤, Ratio-Trazodone✤, Trazorel✤

Pharmacologic class: Triazolopyridine derivative
Therapeutic class: Antidepressant
Pregnancy risk category C

FDA | BOXED WARNING

• Drug may increase risk of suicidal thinking and behavior in children and adolescents with major depressive disorder and other psychiatric disorders. Risk must be balanced with clinical need, as depression itself increases suicide risk. With patient of any age, observe closely for clinical worsening, suicidality, and unusual behavior changes when therapy begins. Advise family and caregivers to observe patient closely and communicate with prescriber as needed.

• Drug isn't approved for use in pediatric patients.

Action

Unclear. Thought to selectively inhibit serotonin and norepinephrine uptake in brain.

Availability

Tablets: 50 mg, 100 mg, 150 mg, 300 mg
Tablets (extended-release, bisectable): 150 mg, 300 mg

⬧ Indications and dosages

➢ Major depression
Adults: 150 mg/day P.O. (immediate-release) in three divided doses; may increase by 50 mg/day q 3 to 4 days until desired response occurs. Don't exceed 400 mg/day in outpatient or 600 mg/day in hospitalized patient. Or, 150 mg P.O. (extended-release) daily; may increase by 75 mg/day q 3 days. Don't exceed 375 mg/day.

Dosage adjustment

• Concurrent use of antihypertensives

Off-label uses

• Alcohol dependence
• Cocaine withdrawal
• Anxiety neurosis
• Insomnia

Contraindications

• Hypersensitivity to drug
• None (Oleptro)

Precautions

Use cautiously in:
• cardiovascular disease, severe hepatic or renal disease, suicidal behavior or ideation
• initial recovery period after myocardial infarction (not recommended)
• concurrent use of drugs that increase QT interval, antidopaminergic agents including antipsychotics, or nonsteroidal anti-inflammatory drugs (NSAIDs), aspirin, or other drugs that affect coagulation (avoid use)

- concurrent use or within 14 days of monoamine oxidase (MAO) inhibitors (avoid use)
- concurrent use of selective serotonin reuptake inhibitor (SSRI), selective norepinephrine reuptake inhibitor (SNRI), 5-hydroxytryptamine receptor agonist such as triptan, or serotonin precursors such as tryptophan (not recommended)
- elderly patients
- pregnant or breastfeeding patients
- children (safety not established).

Administration

- Give immediate-release tablets after meals or snacks. Give extended-release tablets whole or broken in half along score line at same time every day in late evening or at bedtime, on an empty stomach.
- Know that drug is often used in conjunction with psychotherapy.
- Be aware that when discontinuing extended-release tablets, gradual dosage reduction is recommended.
◀€ Don't administer within 14 days of MAO inhibitor use.

Route	Onset	Peak	Duration
P.O.	Unknown	1 hr	Unknown
P.O. (extended)	Unknown	9 hr	Unknown

Adverse reactions

CNS: drowsiness, confusion, dizziness, fatigue, hallucinations, headache, insomnia, nightmares, slurred speech, syncope, weakness, tremor, activation of mania or hypomania, **suicidal behavior or ideation** (especially in child or adolescent), **neuroleptic malignant syndrome-like reactions**
CV: chest pain, orthostatic hypotension, hypotension, hypertension, palpitations, tachycardia, **arrhythmias, prolonged QT interval**
EENT: blurred vision, tinnitus

GI: nausea, vomiting, diarrhea, constipation, excessive salivation, flatulence, dry mouth
GU: urinary frequency, hematuria, erectile dysfunction, priapism
Hematologic: anemia, bleeding, **leukopenia**
Metabolic: hyponatremia
Musculoskeletal: myalgia
Skin: rash
Other: serotonin syndrome

Interactions

Drug-drug. *Antihypertensives:* additive hypotension
Aspirin, NSAIDs, other drugs that affect coagulation: increased risk of bleeding
CYP3A4 inducers (such as carbamazepine): increased risk of decreased trazodone plasma concentration
CYP3A4 inhibitors (such as indinavir, itraconazole, ketoconazole): increased risk of substantial increases in trazodone plasma concentration and cardiac arrhythmias
Digoxin, phenytoin: increased blood levels of these drugs
Drugs that prolong QT interval (such as amiodarone, fluconazole, fluoxetine, imipramine): increased risk of torsades de pointes, with sudden, unexplained death
MAO inhibitors: risk of fatal reactions, including hyperthermia, rigidity, myoclonus, autonomic instability with rapid fluctuation in vital signs, and mental status changes
Other CNS depressants (such as opioid analgesics, sedative-hypnotics): additive CNS depression
Serotonergics (including SNRIs, SSRIs, triptans): increased risk of serotonin syndrome
Warfarin: risk of increased or decreased prothrombin time
Drug-diagnostic tests. *Alkaline phosphatase, bilirubin, glucose:* increased levels
Urinary catecholamines: false increases

t

Serum sodium, urinary 5-hydroxyindole acetic acid, vanillylmandelic acid: decreased levels

St. John's wort: increased risk of serotonergic effects (including serotonin syndrome)

Drug-behaviors. *Alcohol use:* additive CNS depression and hypotension

Patient monitoring

◀€ Monitor vital signs and ECG. Be aware that drug is known to prolong QT/QTc interval; some drugs that prolong QT/QTc interval can cause torsades de pointes, with sudden, unexplained death.

◀€ Monitor neurologic status. Report significant adverse reactions, particularly signs and symptoms of neuroleptic malignant syndrome-like reactions (hyperthermia, muscle rigidity, autonomic instability with possible rapid fluctuation of vital signs, and mental status changes).

• Watch for signs and symptoms of serotonin syndrome, including mental status changes (such as agitation, hallucinations, and coma), autonomic instability (such as tachycardia, labile blood pressure, and hyperthermia), neuromuscular aberrations (such as hyperreflexia, incoordination), or GI symptoms (such as nausea, vomiting, and diarrhea).

◀€ Assess patient's mood frequently. Stay alert for worsening depression and suicidal ideation.

• Watch for drug hoarding or overuse.

• When discontinuing extended-release tablets, taper dosage and watch for such symptoms as anxiety and sleep disturbance.

Patient teaching

• Tell patient to take immediate-release tablets with meals or snacks to improve drug absorption.

• Tell patient to take extended-release tablets at same time every day in late evening or at bedtime, on an empty stomach. Advise patient to swallow extended-release tablets whole or broken in half along the score line, and not to chew or crush them.

• Instruct patient to take only as prescribed. Caution him not to overuse or hoard drug.

• Advise patient (and significant other as appropriate) to monitor his mood. Explain that drug should ease depression.

◀€ Caution patient (and parent or significant other) to immediately report suicidal thoughts or behavior, especially in child or adolescent.

• Tell patient drug may cause significant adverse reactions. Instruct him to report priapism, hallucinations, fainting spells, and other serious problems.

• Instruct patient not to take over-the-counter drugs or drink alcohol during drug therapy without consulting prescriber.

• Caution patient to avoid driving and other hazardous activities until he knows how drug affects concentration, vision, and alertness. Reassure him that dizziness and drowsiness usually subside after first few weeks.

• As appropriate, review all other significant and life-threatening adverse reactions and interactions, especially those related to the drugs, tests, herbs, and behaviors mentioned above.

treprostinil sodium
Remodulin, Tyvaso

Pharmacologic class: Synthetic prostacyclin analog

Therapeutic class: Antiplatelet agent, vasodilator

Pregnancy risk category B

Action

Dilates pulmonary and systemic arterial vascular beds, reducing right and left ventricular afterload and increasing cardiac output and stroke volume. Also inhibits platelet aggregation.

Availability
Injection: 1 mg/ml, 2.5 mg/ml, 5 mg/ml, 10 mg/ml
Solution for oral inhalation: 2.9-ml ampule containing 1.74 mg treprostinil (0.6 mg/ml)

⚑ Indications and dosages
➤ To diminish exercise-induced symptoms of pulmonary artery hypertension (PAH) in patients with NYHA class II-IV symptoms
Adults: Initially, 1.25 ng/kg/minute by continuous subcutaneous infusion; if initial dose isn't tolerated, reduce infusion rate to 0.625 ng/kg/minute. For maintenance, may increase infusion rate in increments of no more than 1.25 ng/kg/minute q week for first 4 weeks, then in increments of no more than 2.5 ng/kg/minute q week, if needed. Maximum dosage is 40 ng/kg/minute.
➤ To treat pulmonary arterial hypertension (PAH) WHO Group 1 to improve exercise ability
Adults: Initially, 3 breaths (18 mcg) oral inhalation solution per treatment session q.i.d. If 3 breaths aren't tolerated, reduce to 1 or 2 breaths and subsequently increase to 3 breaths, as tolerated. For maintenance, increase dose by an additional 3 breaths at approximately 1- to 2-week intervals, if tolerated, until target dose of 9 breaths (54 mcg) is reached per treatment session q.i.d. If adverse effects preclude titration to target dose, continue at highest tolerated dose. If scheduled treatment session is missed or interrupted, resume therapy as soon as possible at usual dose. Maximum recommended dosage is 9 breaths per treatment session q.i.d.

Dosage adjustment
• Hepatic insufficiency
• Concurrent use of CYP2C8 inhibitors or inducers

Contraindications
None

Precautions
Use cautiously in:
• renal disease
• history of hepatic disease
• significant underlying lung disease such as asthma or chronic obstructive pulmonary disease (Tyvaso)
• elderly patients
• pregnant or breastfeeding patients
• children.

Administration
◀€ Give first continuous subcutaneous infusion dose in setting where resuscitation equipment is available and other health care personnel can assist if an emergency arises.
• Administer by continuous subcutaneous infusion through subcutaneous catheter with infusion pump made specifically for subcutaneous infusions.
• Expect to adjust continuous subcutaneous infusion dosage for first 6 to 12 weeks as prescriber balances symptom improvement against adverse reactions.
◀€ Don't stop infusion abruptly (may worsen PAH).
• Use oral inhalation solution only with inhalation system provided.
• Don't mix oral inhalation solution with other drugs.
• Space oral inhalation solution treatment sessions equally during waking hours, approximately 4 hours apart.

Route	Onset	Peak	Duration
Subcut.	Unknown	Unknown	Unknown
Inhal.	Unknown	Unknown	Unknown

Adverse reactions
CNS: dizziness, headache, anxiety, restlessness

CV: vasodilation, edema, hypotension, syncope
EENT: jaw pain, throat irritation, pharyngolaryngeal pain (inhalation solution)
Hematologic: bleeding
Respiratory: cough (inhalation solution)
GI: nausea, vomiting, diarrhea
Skin: rash, pruritus, flushing
Other: infusion site pain or reaction (such as erythema, rash, induration), **possible fatal bloodstream infections and sepsis** (subcutaneous infusion)

Interactions

Drug-drug. *Anticoagulants:* increased risk of bleeding
Antihypertensives, diuretics, other vasodilators: increased risk of hypotension
CYP2C8 inhibitors (such as gemfibrozil) or inducers (such as rifampin): decreased treprostinil exposure
Vitamin A: increased risk of bleeding
Drug-herbs. *Alfalfa, anise, arnica, astragalus, bilberry, black currant seed oil, bladderwrack, bogbean, boldo (with fenugreek), borage oil, buchu, capsaicin, cat's claw, celery, chaparral, chincona bark, clove oil, dandelion, dong quai, evening primrose oil, fenugreek, feverfew, garlic, ginger, ginkgo, guggul, papaya extract, red clover, rhubarb, safflower oil, skullcap, tan-shen:* increased risk of bleeding

Patient monitoring

🔊 Especially after first dose, watch closely for severe vasodilation leading to chest pain and hypotension. These signs and symptoms call for emergency measures.
🔊 Monitor vital signs. Assess carefully for indications of right ventricular failure.
• Assess neurologic status. Institute safety measures as needed to prevent injury.

🔊 Watch for infusion site reaction; be aware that route is associated with risk of bloodstream infections and sepsis, which may be fatal.

Patient teaching

• Tell patient continuous subcutaneous infusion is a long-term measure to control PAH and requires a commitment to maintain infusion system.
• Tell patient to follow instructions for operation of inhalation system and for daily cleaning of device components after last treatment session of day.
• Tell patient not to swallow and to avoid skin or eye contact with oral inhalation solution.
🔊 Instruct patient to immediately report signs and symptoms of infusion site reaction (such as redness, rash, and hardened tissue).
• Teach patient which symptoms reflect underlying disease and which may reflect adverse reactions that he should report.
• As appropriate, review all other significant adverse reactions and interactions, especially those related to the drugs and herbs mentioned above.

tretinoin
Atralin, Avita, Renova, Retin-A, Retin-A Micro, Vesanoid

Pharmacologic class: Retinoid
Therapeutic class: Antineoplastic, dermatologic agent (topical)
Pregnancy risk category C (topical), *D* (oral)

FDA | **BOXED WARNING**

• Patients with acute promyelocytic leukemia (APL) are at high risk in general and may have severe adverse reactions. Give drug under supervision of physician experienced in managing patients with acute leukemia, in facility with laboratory and supportive resources sufficient to monitor drug tolerance and protect and maintain patient compromised by drug toxicity.

• Before using drug, physician must conclude that possible benefit to patient outweighs the following known adverse effects:

• Retinoic acid-APL (RA-APL syndrome), which may be accompanied by impaired myocardial contractility, hypotension, and progressive hypoxemia. Several patients have died with multiorgan failure. Syndrome generally occurs during first month of therapy (in some cases, after first dose).

• Leukocytosis at presentation or evolving rapidly during drug therapy. Patients with high white blood cell (WBC) at diagnosis (above $5 \times 10^9/L$) have increased risk of further rapid rise in WBC counts. Rapidly evolving leukocytosis raises risk of life-threatening complications.

• Teratogenic effects. Drug therapy during pregnancy carries high risk of severe birth defects. Nonetheless, if drug is best available treatment for pregnant woman or woman of childbearing potential, ensure that she has received full information and warnings of risk to fetus and of risk of possible contraception failure, and has been taught to use two reliable contraceptive methods simultaneously during therapy and for 1 month afterward.

Action
Unknown. Thought to cause differentiation of promyelocytic leukemic blast cells, leading to apoptosis (cell shrinkage and death) and cancer remission.

Availability
Capsules: 10 mg
Topical cream: 0.02%, 0.025%, 0.05%, 0.1%
Topical gel: 0.01%, 0.025%, 0.04%, 0.1%

⚡ Indications and dosages
➤ APL when anthracycline chemotherapy fails or is contraindicated

Adults and children ages 1 and older: 45 mg/m^2/day P.O. in two evenly divided doses. Discontinue after 90 days of therapy or 30 days after complete remission occurs, whichever comes first.

➤ Acne vulgaris

Adults: Apply Avita cream, Retin-A cream gel, or Retin-A Micro gel daily before bedtime or in evening. Cover entire affected area lightly.

➤ Adjunct for mitigating fine wrinkles in patients who use comprehensive skin care and sun avoidance programs

Adults: Apply Renova 0.02% cream to face daily in evening for up to 52 weeks, using only enough to lightly cover entire affected area.

➤ Adjunct for mitigating fine wrinkles, mottled hyperpigmentation, and tactile roughness of facial skin when comprehensive skin care and sun avoidance programs alone fail

Adults ages 50 and younger: Apply Renova 0.05% cream to face daily in evening for up to 48 weeks, using only enough to lightly cover entire affected area.

Contraindications
• Hypersensitivity to drug or parabens
• Pregnancy or breastfeeding (oral use)

Precautions
Use cautiously in:
• eczema, sunburn, photosensitivity
• concurrent use of over-the-counter (OTC) acne products or abrasive soaps or cleansers with strong drying effects or high alcohol or lime content (with all topical forms)

Reactions in **bold** are life-threatening.   ◀€ Clinical alert

- concurrent use of astringents, spices, permanent wave solutions, electrolysis, hair depilatories or waxes, or photosensitizing drugs (such as fluoroquinolones, phenothiazines, tetracyclines, thiazides)
- heavily pigmented, elderly, pregnant, or breastfeeding patients (safety and efficacy not established for topical use)
- children younger than age 1 for oral use or younger than age 18 for topical use (safety and efficacy not established).

Administration

- Verify that female patient has had required pregnancy test before P.O. therapy starts.
- Know that Renova topical cream isn't indicated for acne vulgaris, and that other topical forms are indicated only for acne vulgaris. Also know that some absorption of topical products occurs.

Route	Onset	Peak	Duration
P.O.	Unknown	1-2 hr	Unknown
Topical	Unknown	Unknown	Unknown

Adverse reactions

CNS: dizziness, headache, asthenia, paresthesia, confusion, agitation, hallucinations, anxiety, aphasia, depression, agnosia, insomnia, asterixis, cerebellar edema, hypotaxia, drowsiness, slow speech, facial paralysis, hemiplegia, hyporeflexia, hypotaxia, dementia, spinal cord disorder, tremors, dysarthria, **cerebrovascular accident (CVA), coma, seizures, intracranial hypertension, cerebral hemorrhage**
CV: heart murmur, chest discomfort, peripheral edema, hypertension, hypotension, phlebitis, edema, enlarged heart, ischemia, **arrhythmias, secondary cardiomyopathy, myocarditis, myocardial infarction (MI), heart failure, pericardial**

effusion, impaired myocardial contractility, progressive hypoxemia
EENT: vision disturbances, visual acuity changes, visual field defect, absence of light reflex, hearing loss, earache, full sensation in ears
GI: nausea, vomiting, constipation, diarrhea, abdominal pain and distention, GI disorders, mucositis, dyspepsia, ulcer, anorexia, **GI hemorrhage**
GU: dysuria, urinary frequency, enlarged prostate, **renal insufficiency, renal tubular necrosis, acute renal failure**
Hematologic: leukocytosis, **disseminated intravascular coagulation (DIC), hemorrhage**
Hepatic: ascites, **hepatosplenomegaly, hepatitis**
Metabolic: fluid imbalance, **acidosis**
Musculoskeletal: bone pain or inflammation, myalgia, flank pain
Respiratory: respiratory tract disorders, dyspnea, expiratory wheezing, crackles, pneumonia, **laryngeal edema, pulmonary infiltrates, pleural effusion, bronchial asthma, pulmonary hypertension**
Skin: rash; pallor; flushing; diaphoresis; alopecia; dry skin and mucous membranes; skin changes; pruritus; cellulitis; burning, erythema, peeling, and stinging (with topical use)
Other: weight changes, fever, lymphatic disorder, hypothermia, infections, facial edema, pain, **RA-APL syndrome, multisystem failure, septicemia**

Interactions

Drug-drug. *Photosensitizing drugs (such as fluoroquinolones, phenothiazines, tetracyclines, thiazides):* increased risk of photosensitivity reaction (with topical forms)
Drug-diagnostic tests. *Cholesterol, triglycerides:* increased levels
Drug-food. *Any food:* enhanced tretinoin absorption

Drug-behaviors. *Sun exposure:* increased risk of photosensitivity

Patient monitoring

◀≸ Watch closely for septicemia, multisystem failure, and retinoic acid-APL syndrome (which causes pulmonary and pericardial effusion, fever, weight gain, and dyspnea).

◀≸ Monitor for significant adverse CNS reactions, including seizures, CVA, and cerebral hemorrhage.

◀≸ Monitor cardiovascular status. Stay alert for signs and symptoms of arrhythmias, MI, and heart failure.

◀≸ Closely monitor liver and kidney function tests. Watch for evidence of hepatitis and renal failure.

◀≸ Monitor coagulation studies. Watch closely for DIC and hemorrhage.

• Evaluate respiratory status. Stay alert for indications of pulmonary hypertension and respiratory insufficiency.

• Frequently assess lipid panel and CBC with white cell differential.

Patient teaching

• Instruct patient to take oral doses with food.

◀≸ Teach patient to recognize and immediately report serious adverse reactions.

• Tell patient he will undergo regular blood testing during oral therapy.

• Instruct patient using topical form to gently wash face with mild soap, pat skin dry, and then wait 20 to 30 minutes before applying. Advise him to apply to face in evening, using only enough to cover entire affected area lightly and only for prescribed duration.

• Caution patient to avoid OTC acne drugs and extreme weather conditions (such as wind and cold). Urge him to adhere to prescribed skin care and sunlight avoidance programs when using topical form.

• Tell patient using topical form that transient burning, erythema, peeling,

pruritus, and stinging may occur. Advise him to notify prescriber if these symptoms become severe.

• As appropriate, review all other significant and life-threatening adverse reactions and interactions, especially those related to the drugs, tests, foods, and behaviors mentioned above.

---

triamcinolone acetonide

Adcortyl◆, Kenalog, Kenalog-10, Kenalog-40, Nasacort AQ, Triaderm✦

triamcinolone hexacetonide

Aristospan Intra-Articular, Aristospan Intralesional

Pharmacologic class: Synthetic corticosteroid

Therapeutic class: Anti-inflammatory (steroidal)

Pregnancy risk category C

Action

Unknown. Thought to decrease inflammation mainly by inhibiting activities of mast cells, macrophages, and other mediators of allergic reactions. Also suppresses immune system by depressing lymphatic activity.

Availability

triamcinolone acetonide
Cream: 0.025%, 0.1%, 0.5%
Injectable suspension: 10 mg/ml, 40 mg/ml
Lotion: 0.025%, 0.1%
Ointment: 0.025%, 0.1%, 0.5%
Suspension: 55 mcg/metered spray
triamcinolone hexacetonide
Injectable suspension: 5 mg/ml, 20 mg/ml

t

ⓘ Indications and dosages

➤ Allergic rhinitis

Adults and children older than age 12: 220 mcg (two sprays of acetonide suspension) in each nostril daily. When maximum benefit has been achieved and symptoms have been controlled, reduce dosage to 110 mcg/day (one spray in each nostril daily).

Children ages 6 to 12: Initially, 110 mcg (two sprays of acetonide suspension) as one spray in each nostril once daily. Use 220 mcg (two sprays in each nostril) daily in children not responding adequately to 110 mcg daily.

Children ages 2 to 5: Recommended and maximum dosage is 110 mcg as one spray in each nostril once daily.

➤ Severe inflammation; immunosuppression

Adults and children older than age 12: 60 mg (acetonide) I.M. at 6-week intervals. For intralesional or sublesional use, 1 mg at each injection site, repeated one or more times weekly; for intra-articular, intrasynovial, or soft-tissue injection, 2.5 to 40 mg, repeated when symptoms recur. Or 0.5 mg/square inch of affected skin (hexacetonide) by intralesional or sublesional injection or 2 to 20 mg by intra-articular injection; may repeat at 3- to 4-week intervals.

Children ages 6 to 12: 0.03 to 0.2 mg/kg or 1 to 6.25 mg/m² I.M. at intervals of 1 to 7 days

➤ Corticosteroid-responsive dermatoses

Adults and children older than age 12: Apply cream, ointment, or lotion sparingly to affected area two to four times daily.

Contraindications

• Hypersensitivity to drug, tartrazine, chlorofluorocarbon propellants, alcohol, propylene glycol, or polyethylene glycol
• Systemic fungal infections (parenteral use)

• Idiopathic thrombocytopenic purpura (I.M. use)
• Administration of live-virus vaccines (with immunosuppressant doses of triamcinolone)

Precautions

Use cautiously in:
• active untreated infection, systemic infection, immunosuppression, hypertension, osteoporosis, diabetes mellitus, glaucoma, renal disease, hypothyroidism, cirrhosis, diverticulitis, nonspecific ulcerative colitis, recent intestinal anastomoses, thromboembolic disorders, seizures, myasthenia gravis, heart failure, ocular herpes simplex, emotional instability
• pregnant or breastfeeding patients
• children younger than age 2 (safety not established).

Administration

◀€ Don't withdraw systemic corticosteroids abruptly when patient begins inhalation steroid therapy.

◀€ Know that patient will need additional steroids during times of stress or trauma.

◀€ Apply cream, lotion, or ointment sparingly. Know that triamcinolone is a high-potency steroid; it can be absorbed systemically and should not be withdrawn abruptly.

◀€ Avoid intralesional injection to face or head (may cause blindness).

• Don't apply topical form near eyes.
• Know that occlusive dressing may be used with topical form when treating psoriasis or other recalcitrant conditions, but should be removed if infection occurs.

Route	Onset	Peak	Duration
I.M.	Unknown	Unknown	1-4 wk
Intra-lesional, sublesional, intra-articular	Slow	Unknown	Unknown
Topical	Unknown	Unknown	Unknown

Adverse reactions

CNS: headache, vertigo, paresthesia, syncope, personality changes, **pseudotumor cerebri, seizures**

CV: hypertension, **thrombophlebitis, arrhythmias, thromboembolism, heart failure**

EENT: cataract, glaucoma, increased intraocular pressure, exophthalmos, otitis, nasal or sinus congestion, rhinitis, epistaxis, sneezing, dry mucous membranes, pharyngitis, throat discomfort

GI: nausea, vomiting, dyspepsia, abdominal distention or pain, peptic ulcer, ulcerative esophagitis, oral candidiasis, dry mouth, **pancreatitis**

GU: cystitis, urinary tract infection, glycosuria, menstrual irregularities, vaginal candidiasis

Metabolic: fluid retention, hypernatremia, hypokalemia, hyperglycemia, hypocalcemia, decreased growth (in children), carbohydrate intolerance, exacerbation of latent diabetes mellitus, cushingoid appearance (moon face, buffalo hump), **hypokalemic alkalosis, acute adrenal insufficiency** (with abrupt withdrawal or acute stress in long-term use)

Musculoskeletal: muscle weakness; steroid myopathy; loss of muscle mass; myalgia; bursitis; tenosynovitis; osteoporosis; fractures; aseptic necrosis; with intra-articular injection—osteonecrosis, tendon rupture, post-injection flare

Respiratory: cough, wheezing, chest congestion

Skin: delayed wound healing; thin and fragile skin; petechiae; bruising; with topical use—local eruptions, pruritus, hypopigmentation or hyperpigmentation, scarring, stinging, skin maceration, secondary infection, cutaneous or subcutaneous atrophy, diaphoresis, facial erythema

Other: toothache, weight gain, fever, pain, voice alteration, hypersensitivity reaction

Interactions

Drug-drug. *Erythromycin, indinavir, itraconazole, ketoconazole, ritonavir, saquinavir:* increased triamcinolone blood level and effects

Fluoroquinolones: increased risk of tendon rupture

Live-virus vaccines: decreased antibody response to vaccine

Nonsteroidal anti-inflammatory drugs (including aspirin): increased risk of adverse GI reactions

Potassium-wasting drugs (including amphotericin B, thiazide and loop diuretics, mezlocillin, piperacillin, ticarcillin): additive hypokalemia

Drug-diagnostic tests. *Cholesterol:* increased level

Skin tests: suppressed reaction

Patient monitoring

• Monitor respiratory status. Watch for worsening signs and symptoms.

• With long-term use, assess for adverse endocrine and musculoskeletal reactions.

• Monitor carefully for signs and symptoms of infection, which drug may mask.

Patient teaching

• Teach patient correct use of drug. Make sure he has received manufacturer's patient information sheet.

• Inform patient that drug can affect many body systems. Urge him to report serious adverse effects promptly.

• Tell parents drug may make child more vulnerable to childhood infections, such as chicken pox and measles.

• As appropriate, review all other significant and life-threatening adverse reactions and interactions, especially those related to the drugs and tests mentioned above.

---

triamterene
Dyrenium, Dytac⊕

Pharmacologic class: Potassium-sparing diuretic
Therapeutic class: Diuretic
Pregnancy risk category B

FDA | BOXED WARNING

• Abnormal serum potassium elevation may occur, and is more likely in patients with renal impairment or diabetes and in elderly or severely ill patients. As uncorrected hyperkalemia may be fatal, monitor serum potassium levels frequently, especially when dosage is changed or patient has an illness that may influence renal function.

Action
Depresses sodium resorption and potassium excretion in renal distal tubule

Availability
Capsules: 50 mg, 100 mg

⟪ Indications and dosages
➤ Edema
Adults: 100 mg P.O. b.i.d. Do not exceed 300 mg/day.

Dosage adjustment
• Concurrent antihypertensive drug therapy
• Elderly patients

Off-label uses
• Diabetes insipidus

Contraindications
• Hypersensitivity to drug
• Hyperkalemia
• Severe hepatic disease
• Anuria, severe renal dysfunction (except nephrosis)
• Concurrent use of other potassium-sparing diuretics or potassium supplements

Precautions
Use cautiously in:
• hepatic dysfunction, renal insufficiency, diabetes mellitus
• history of gout or renal calculi
• elderly or debilitated patients
• pregnant or breastfeeding patients
• children (safety not established).

Administration
• Give after meals.
• Know that drug may be used alone or as adjunct to thiazide or loop diuretics.
• Make sure patient stops taking potassium supplements before starting triamterene.

Route	Onset	Peak	Duration
P.O.	2-4 hr	Unknown	12-16 hr

Adverse reactions
CNS: headache, fatigue, asthenia, dizziness
GI: nausea, vomiting, diarrhea, dry mouth
GU: azotemia, renal calculi
Hematologic: megaloblastic anemia, thrombocytopenia
Hepatic: jaundice
Metabolic: hyperglycemia, **hyperkalemia, metabolic acidosis**
Skin: rash, photosensitivity
Other: anaphylaxis

Interactions
Drug-drug. *Amantadine:* increased amantadine blood level, greater risk of toxicity
Angiotensin-converting enzyme inhibitors, cyclosporine, indomethacin, potassium-sparing diuretics, potassium supplements, other potassium-containing preparations: increased risk of hyperkalemia

---

Antihypertensives, nondepolarizing muscle relaxants, other diuretics, preanesthetic and anesthetic agents: potentiated effects of these drugs

Chlorpropamide: increased risk of hyponatremia

Cimetidine: increased bioavailability and decreased renal clearance of triamterene

Indomethacin: increased risk of acute renal failure

Lithium: decreased lithium clearance, greater risk of lithium toxicity

Drug-diagnostic tests. *Alkali reserves, hemoglobin, platelets:* decreased values

Blood urea nitrogen (BUN), creatinine, glucose, hepatic enzymes, potassium: increased levels

Liver function tests: increased values

Quinidine blood level: interference with fluorescent measurement

Drug-food. *Salt substitutes containing potassium:* increased risk of hyperkalemia

Drug-herbs. *Gossypol, licorice:* increased risk of hypokalemia

Patient monitoring

• Monitor BUN, creatinine, and electrolyte levels. Stay alert for hyperkalemia.

• Assess CBC with white cell differential.

Patient teaching

• Advise patient to take after meals to reduce nausea.

• Instruct patient to take last daily dose in early evening to avoid nocturia.

• Teach patient to recognize and report signs and symptoms of electrolyte imbalances.

• Tell patient to avoid salt substitutes. Advise him not to use herbs without consulting prescriber.

• As appropriate, review all other significant and life-threatening adverse reactions and interactions, especially those related to the drugs, tests, foods, and herbs mentioned above.

triazolam
Apo-Triazo✱, Gen-Triazolam✱, Halcion

Pharmacologic class: Benzodiazepine
Therapeutic class: Sedative-hypnotic
Controlled substance schedule IV
Pregnancy risk category X

Action
Inhibits gamma-aminobutyric acid, a neurotransmitter that activates receptors at limbic, thalamic, and hypothalamic levels of CNS

Availability
Tablets: 0.125 mg, 0.25 mg, 0.5 mg

Indications and dosages
➤ Insomnia

Adults: 0.125 to 0.5 mg P.O. at bedtime p.r.n. After 7 to 10 days, decrease dosage gradually and then discontinue.

Dosage adjustment
• Elderly or debilitated patients

Off-label uses
• Presurgical hypnotic

Contraindications
• Hypersensitivity to drug or other benzodiazepines
• Concurrent use of itraconazole, ketoconazole, or nefazodone
• Pregnancy

Precautions
Use cautiously in:
• hepatic or renal dysfunction, sleep apnea, respiratory compromise, psychosis
• history of suicide attempt or drug abuse
• elderly or debilitated patients
• breastfeeding patients

t

Reactions in **bold** are life-threatening.　　　　◀€ Clinical alert

- children younger than age 18 (safety and efficacy not established).

Administration
- Don't give with grapefruit juice.

Route	Onset	Peak	Duration
P.O.	15-30 min	2 hr	Unknown

Adverse reactions
CNS: dizziness, excessive sedation, hangover, headache, anterograde or traveler's amnesia, confusion, incoordination, lethargy, depression, paradoxical excitation, light-headedness, psychological disturbance, euphoria
GI: nausea, vomiting
Other: physical or psychological drug dependence, drug tolerance, withdrawal symptoms (tremor, abdominal and muscle cramps, vomiting, diaphoresis, dysphoria, perceptual disturbances, insomnia)

Interactions
Drug-drug. *Antidepressants, antihistamines, chloral hydrate, opioid analgesics, other psychotropic drugs:* additive CNS depression
Cimetidine, disulfiram, fluconazole, hormonal contraceptives, isoniazid, itraconazole, ketoconazole, nefazodone, rifampin, and other drugs that inhibit CYP450-3A4–mediated metabolism: decreased oxidative metabolism and increased action of triazolam
Digoxin: increased digoxin blood level, greater risk of toxicity
Macrolide anti-infectives (such as azithromycin, clarithromycin, erythromycin): increased triazolam bioavailability
Probenecid: rapid onset and prolonged effects of triazolam
Ranitidine: increased triazolam blood level
Theophylline: decreased sedative effect of triazolam
Drug-food. *Grapefruit juice:* increased triazolam blood level and effects

Drug-herbs. *Chamomile, hops, kava, skullcap, valerian:* increased CNS depression
Drug-behaviors. *Alcohol use:* increased CNS depression
Smoking: increased triazolam clearance

Patient monitoring
- Monitor neurologic status. Watch for paradoxical or rebound drug effects.
- Observe for signs of drug hoarding and drug abuse.

Patient teaching
- Tell patient to take at bedtime with a liquid other than grapefruit juice.
- Explain that drug is meant only for short-term use (7 to 10 days).
- Tell patient rebound insomnia may occur for 1 to 2 nights after he discontinues drug.
- Instruct patient to avoid alcohol use and smoking.
- Caution patient to avoid driving and other hazardous activities while under drug's influence.
- As appropriate, review all other significant adverse reactions and interactions, especially those related to the drugs, foods, herbs, and behaviors mentioned above.

trifluoperazine hydrochloride
Apo-Trifluoperazine✤, Novo-Trifluzine✤, PMS-Trifluoperazine✤, Terfluzine✤

Pharmacologic class: Piperazine phenothiazine
Therapeutic class: Antipsychotic
Pregnancy risk category C

Action
Unknown. Thought to act on subcortical levels of hypothalamic and limbic systems by producing antidopaminergic effects. Also lowers seizure threshold and exhibits some adrenergic, muscarinic, and anticholinergic activity.

Availability
Tablets: 1 mg, 2 mg, 5 mg, 10 mg

ⓘ Indications and dosages
➤ Schizophrenia
Adults: 2 to 5 mg P.O. b.i.d.; may increase gradually to obtain adequate response. Usual maintenance dosage is 15 to 20 mg/day.
Children ages 6 to 12: Initially, 1 mg P.O. once or twice daily in hospitalized patients or those under close supervision; may increase gradually up to 15 mg/day P.O. until symptoms are controlled or adverse reactions are intolerable.
➤ Nonpsychotic anxiety
Adults: 1 to 2 mg P.O. b.i.d. Do not exceed 6 mg/day or 12 weeks' duration.

Dosage adjustment
• Hepatic disease
• Elderly or debilitated patients

Contraindications
• Hypersensitivity to drug, other phenothiazines, or bisulfites
• Severe hepatic disease
• Bone marrow depression
• Blood dyscrasias
• Coma
• Concomitant use of other CNS depressants in high doses

Precautions
Use cautiously in:
• seizure disorders, cardiovascular disorders, GI obstruction, glaucoma, retinopathy
• elderly or debilitated patients
• pregnant or breastfeeding patients.

Administration
• Be aware that dosage should be adjusted to needs of individual. Lowest effective dosage should always be used.

Route	Onset	Peak	Duration
P.O.	Unknown	2-4 hr	12-24 hr

Adverse reactions
CNS: sedation, dizziness, drowsiness, insomnia, fatigue, extrapyramidal effects, tardive dyskinesia, **neuroleptic malignant syndrome (NMS)**
CV: tachycardia, hypotension, orthostatic hypotension, peripheral edema, **prolonged QT interval, torsades de pointes**
EENT: dry eyes, blurred vision, miosis, mydriasis, epithelial keratopathy, pigmentary retinopathy
GI: constipation, biliary stasis, dry mouth, anorexia, **adynamic ileus**
GU: urinary retention, glycosuria, amenorrhea, ejaculatory disorders, galactorrhea, gynecomastia
Hematologic: leukopenia, agranulocytosis
Hepatic: cholestatic jaundice
Musculoskeletal: muscle weakness
Skin: photosensitivity, altered pigmentation, erythema, rash
Other: mild fever, weight gain, allergic reaction

Interactions
Drug-drug. *Alpha-adrenergic blockers:* additive effect
Antacids containing aluminum: decreased trifluoperazine absorption
Anticholinergics, anticholinergic-like drugs (including antidepressants, antihistamines, disopyramide, other phenothiazines, quinidine): additive anticholinergic effects
Anticonvulsants: decreased seizure threshold
Antihistamines, CNS depressants, general anesthetics, opioids, sedative-hypnotics: additive CNS depression

t

Reactions in **bold** are life-threatening. ◀€ Clinical alert

Barbiturates: decreased blood levels of both drugs

Guanethidine: decreased antihypertensive effect

Lithium: increased risk of extrapyramidal reactions, disorientation, and unconsciousness

Oral anticoagulants: decreased anticoagulant effect

Phenytoin: interference with phenytoin metabolism, causing phenytoin toxicity

Propranolol: increased blood levels of both drugs

Thiazide diuretics: additive orthostatic hypotension

Drug-diagnostic tests. *Hepatic enzymes:* increased levels

Phenylketonuria test: false-positive result

Prolactin: increased level, causing interference with gonadotropin tests

Urine bilirubin: false-positive result

Drug-herbs. *St. John's wort:* increased risk of photosensitivity

Drug-behaviors. *Alcohol use:* additive CNS depression and hypotension

Sun exposure: increased risk of photosensitivity

Patient monitoring

• Monitor ECG and blood pressure. Watch closely for hypotension.

• Assess CBC (including platelet count) and liver function tests. Stay alert for signs and symptoms of hepatic damage and blood dyscrasias.

◀≋ Monitor neurologic status, especially for indications of NMS (unstable blood pressure, high fever, sweating, stupor, muscle rigidity, and autonomic dysfunction). Immediately discontinue drug if these symptoms occur.

• If signs and symptoms of tardive dyskinesia appear (repetitive, involuntary, purposeless movements, such as grimacing, tongue protrusion, lip smacking, and rapid eye blinking), consider discontinuing drug. However, some patients may require treatment despite presence of the syndrome.

Patient teaching

• Tell patient that drug's full effect usually occurs in 1 to 2 weeks.

• Instruct patient to move slowly when sitting up or standing, to avoid dizziness from sudden blood pressure drop.

◀≋ Teach patient to recognize and immediately report signs and symptoms of NMS and tardive dyskinesia.

• Caution patient to avoid driving and other hazardous activities until he knows how drug affects him.

• Tell patient to avoid alcohol and certain herbs.

• Advise patient to avoid sun exposure and to wear sunscreen and protective clothing when going outdoors.

• As appropriate, review all other significant and life-threatening adverse reactions and interactions, especially those related to the drugs, tests, herbs, and behaviors mentioned above.

trihexyphenidyl hydrochloride

Apo-Trihex✸, Broflex⊕, PMS-Trihexyphenidyl✸

Pharmacologic class: Anticholinergic
Therapeutic class: Antidyskinetic
Pregnancy risk category C

Action

Inhibits parasympathetic nervous system, relaxing smooth muscles and decreasing involuntary movements

Availability

Syrup: 2 mg/5 ml
Tablets: 2 mg, 5 mg

🖊 Indications and dosages

➢ Adjunct in idiopathic, postencephalitic, or arteriosclerotic parkinsonism

---

Adults: 1 mg P.O. on first day; may increase in 2-mg increments q 3 to 5 days, up to a maximum of 6 to 10 mg/day. In postencephalitic parkinsonism, 12 to 15 mg P.O. daily.

➤ Drug-induced extrapyramidal symptoms

Adults: Initially, 1 mg P.O. daily, increased progressively if extrapyramidal symptoms aren't controlled within several hours. Usual dosage range is 5 to 15 mg/day P.O. in divided doses.

Dosage adjustment

• Concurrent use of levodopa or other parasympathetic inhibitor
• Elderly patients

Off-label uses

• Dystonia

Contraindications

• Hypersensitivity to drug or its components
• Angle-closure glaucoma
• Pyloric or duodenal obstruction
• Stenosing peptic ulcer
• Megacolon
• Prostatic hypertrophy or bladder-neck obstruction
• Achalasia
• Myasthenia gravis

Precautions

Use cautiously in:
• chronic renal, hepatic, pulmonary, or cardiac disease; hypertension; tachycardia secondary to cardiac insufficiency; hyperthyroidism
• elderly patients
• pregnant or breastfeeding patients
• children (safety not established).

Administration

• Give with meals. However, if drug causes severe dry mouth, give before meals.
• Administer last dose at bedtime.

Route	Onset	Peak	Duration
P.O.	1 hr	2-3 hr	6-12 hr

Adverse reactions

CNS: dizziness, nervousness, drowsiness, asthenia, headache
CV: orthostatic hypotension, tachycardia
EENT: blurred vision, mydriasis, increased intraocular pressure (IOP), angle-closure glaucoma (with long-term use)
GI: nausea, vomiting, constipation, dry mouth
GU: urinary hesitancy or retention

Interactions

Drug-drug. Amantadine, other anticholinergics (including disopyramide, phenothiazines, quinidine, tricyclic antidepressants): additive anticholinergic effects
Other CNS depressants (such as antihistamines, opioids, sedative-hypnotics): additive CNS depression
Phenothiazines: decreased phenothiazine effects
Drug-herbs. Angel's trumpet, jimsonweed, scopolia: increased anticholinergic effects
Drug-behaviors. Alcohol use: additive CNS depression

Patient monitoring

• With prolonged use, monitor vision and IOP regularly.
• Assess drug efficacy to help guide dosage titration.
• Monitor vital signs. Watch for orthostatic hypotension.
• Closely monitor fluid intake and output. Stay alert for urinary retention.

Patient teaching

• Instruct patient to take with meals or, if severe dry mouth occurs, before meals.
• Tell patient drug has a bitter taste, which may be followed by numbness and tingling in mouth.

t

Reactions in **bold** are life-threatening.　◀❬ Clinical alert

- Stress importance of follow-up eye exams.
- Instruct patient to consult prescriber before taking over-the-counter preparations or herbs.
- Advise patient to avoid alcohol and hazardous activities during drug therapy.
- Tell patient to move slowly when sitting up or standing, to avoid dizziness from sudden blood pressure decrease.
- As appropriate, review all other significant adverse reactions and interactions, especially those related to the drugs, herbs, and behaviors mentioned above.

trimethobenzamide hydrochloride

Tigan

Pharmacologic class: Anticholinergic
Therapeutic class: Antiemetic
Pregnancy risk category C

Action

Unclear. Thought to block dopamine receptors and emetic impulses in chemoreceptor trigger zone, preventing nausea and vomiting.

Availability

Capsules: 300 mg
Injection: 100 mg/ml in 2-ml ampules and prefilled syringes and in 20-ml vials

⦸ Indications and dosages

➤ Nausea and vomiting
Adults: 300 mg P.O. three to four times daily or 200 mg I.M. three to four times daily

Dosage adjustment

- Renal impairment

Contraindications

- Hypersensitivity to drug
- Parenteral form in children

Precautions

Use cautiously in:
- renal impairment, arrhythmias, encephalitis, gastroenteritis, dehydration, electrolyte imbalances
- concurrent alcohol use
- elderly or debilitated patients
- pregnant or breastfeeding patients
- children with known or suspected viral illnesses.

Administration

- In I.M. use, inject deep into upper outer quadrant of gluteus maximus.
- Withhold drug in children with signs or symptoms of Reye's syndrome.

Route	Onset	Peak	Duration
P.O.	10-40 min	Unknown	3-4 hr
I.M.	15-35 min	Unknown	2-3 hr

Adverse reactions

CNS: drowsiness, dizziness, headache, depression, disorientation, parkinsonian symptoms, **coma, seizures**
CV: hypotension
EENT: blurred vision
Hematologic: blood dyscrasias
Hepatic: jaundice
Musculoskeletal: muscle cramps, opisthotonos
Skin: rash, urticaria, flushing
Other: pain and stinging at I.M. injection site, hypersensitivity reaction

Interactions

Drug-drug. *Antidepressants, antihistamines, CNS depressants, opioids, sedative-hypnotics:* additive CNS depression
Drug-behaviors. *Alcohol use:* additive CNS depression

Patient monitoring

- Monitor neurologic status, especially for parkinsonian symptoms and other serious adverse reactions.
- Assess CBC and liver function tests. Watch for blood dyscrasias and jaundice.

• Evaluate injection site for pain and stinging.
• Closely monitor patient's nutritional and hydration status. Report continuing nausea.

Patient teaching
• Advise patient to take as needed for nausea and vomiting, but only as prescribed.
• Tell patient to contact prescriber promptly if nausea persists despite therapy.
• Instruct patient to minimize nausea and vomiting by eating small, frequent servings of healthy food and drinking plenty of fluids.
• Advise patient to avoid alcohol.
• Caution patient to avoid driving and other hazardous activities until drug effects are known.
• As appropriate, review all other significant and life-threatening adverse reactions and interactions, especially those related to the drugs and behaviors mentioned above.

triptorelin pamoate
Decapeptyl SR✙,
Gonapeptyl Depot✙, Trelstar Depot, Trelstar LA

Pharmacologic class: Synthetic agonist analog of luteinizing hormone-releasing hormone (LHRH)
Therapeutic class: Antineoplastic
Pregnancy risk category X

Action
Initially causes surge in luteinizing hormone (LH), follicle-stimulating hormone (FSH), and testosterone levels. After several weeks of therapy, LH and FSH secretion decrease, causing sustained testosterone reduction equivalent to pharmacologic castration.

Availability
Microgranules for injection (lyophilized): 3.75 mg (depot), 11.25 mg (long-acting), 22.5 mg (long-acting)

❂ Indications and dosages
➤ Palliative treatment of advanced prostate cancer
Adults: 3.75 mg (depot) I.M. monthly as a single injection or 11.25 mg (long-acting) I.M. q 12 weeks as a single injection or 22.5 mg (long-acting) I.M. q 24 weeks

Off-label uses
• Infertility
• Endometriosis
• Uterine fibroids
• Precocious puberty

Contraindications
• Hypersensitivity to drug, LHRH, or other LHRH agonists
• Pregnancy
• Women of childbearing potential

Precautions
Use cautiously in:
• renal insufficiency
• prostate cancer with impending spinal cord compression or severe urinary tract disorder
• breastfeeding patients (use not recommended).

Administration
• Reconstitute with 2 ml of sterile water for injection, using accompanying syringe (don't use other diluents). Add syringe contents to vial containing particles; shake well. Withdraw vial contents and inject I.M. immediately.
• Inject deep I.M. into either buttock. Rotate injection sites.
◀ Keep epinephrine and emergency equipment at hand in case of anaphylactic reaction.

t

Reactions in **bold** are life-threatening.   ◀ Clinical alert

Route	Onset	Peak	Duration
I.M. (depot)	Slow	4 days	1 mo
I.M. (long-acting)	Slow	2-3 days	3 mo

Adverse reactions

CNS: insomnia, dizziness, headache, emotional lability, fatigue, **stroke**

CV: hypertension, **increased risk of myocardial infarction and sudden cardiac death**

GI: vomiting, diarrhea

GU: urinary retention, urinary tract infection, gynecomastia, erectile dysfunction, testicular atrophy

Hematologic: anemia

Metabolic: hyperglycemia

Musculoskeletal: skeletal or leg pain

Skin: pruritus

Other: leg edema, temporary worsening of disease, edema, hot flashes, pain at injection site, hypersensitivity reactions including **anaphylaxis**

Interactions

Drug-diagnostic tests. *Hemoglobin:* decreased value

Pituitary-gonadal function tests: misleading results (with continuous or long-term use)

Serum glucose: increased

Patient monitoring

• Monitor serum testosterone and prostate-specific antigen levels periodically to assess drug efficacy.

◀❦ Monitor patient for signs and symptoms suggestive of cardiovascular disease and manage as appropriate.

Patient teaching

• Explain drug therapy to patient. Stress need for follow-up laboratory tests.

• Tell patient prostate cancer symptoms may worsen during first few weeks of therapy.

• Instruct patient to monitor weight and report sudden weight gain or leg swelling.

• Advise female patient to tell prescriber before starting therapy if she is or plans to become pregnant. Caution her not to breastfeed during therapy.

• As appropriate, review all other significant and life-threatening adverse reactions and interactions, especially those related to the drugs and tests mentioned above.

tromethamine

Tham

Pharmacologic class: Protein substrate
Therapeutic class: Systemic alkalizer
Pregnancy risk category C

Action

Combines with hydrogen ions to form bicarbonate and a buffer, correcting acidosis. Also shows some diuretic activity.

Availability

Injection: 18 g/500 ml

💊 Indications and dosages

➤ Metabolic acidosis associated with cardiac bypass surgery

Adults: 9 ml/kg (0.32 g/kg) by slow I.V. infusion; 500 ml (18 g) is usually adequate. Maximum single dosage is 500 mg/kg infused over at least 1 hour.

➤ Metabolic acidosis associated with cardiac arrest

Adults: 3.6 to 10.8 g by I.V. injection into large peripheral vein if chest isn't open, or 2 to 6 g I.V. directly into ventricular cavity if chest is open. After reversal of cardiac arrest, patient may need additional amounts to control persistent acidosis.

➤ To correct acidity of acid-citrate-dextrose (ACD) blood in cardiac bypass surgery

Adults: 0.5 to 2.5 g added to each 500 ml of ACD blood used for priming pump-oxygenator. Usual dosage is 2 g.

Dosage adjustment
• Elderly patients

Contraindications
• Hypersensitivity to drug
• Anuria
• Uremia

Precautions
Use cautiously in:
• renal disease, severe respiratory disease, respiratory depression
• pregnant patients
• infants.

Administration
◀€ Keep intubation equipment nearby in case respiratory depression occurs.
• For metabolic acidosis associated with cardiac bypass surgery, give by slow I.V. infusion through large-bore I.V. catheter into large antecubital vein. Elevate arm after infusion.
• If extravasation occurs, discontinue drug and infiltrate affected area with 1% procaine hydrochloride (containing hyaluronidase).
• Be aware that in cardiac arrest, drug is used with standard resuscitative measures. When giving by direct I.V. injection into open chest, never inject into cardiac muscle.

Route	Onset	Peak	Duration
I.V.	Immediate	Immediate	Unknown

Adverse reactions
GU: oliguria
Hepatic: hemorrhagic hepatic necrosis
Metabolic: metabolic alkalosis, transient hypoglycemia, fluid-solute overload, hyperkalemia
Respiratory: respiratory depression
Other: fever; I.V. site infection; extravasation with venous thrombosis or phlebitis, inflammation, necrosis, and sloughing

Interactions
Drug-diagnostic tests. *Glucose:* decreased level
Potassium: increased level

Patient monitoring
• Maintain continuous cardiac monitoring.
• Monitor arterial blood gas levels. Watch for alkalosis and signs and symptoms of respiratory depression.
• Assess liver function tests. Stay alert for signs and symptoms of hepatic impairment.
• Monitor glucose and potassium levels. Watch for hypoglycemia and hyperkalemia.
• Closely monitor fluid intake and output. Check for fluid and electrolyte imbalances and oliguria related to hyperkalemia.

Patient teaching
• Explain drug therapy to patient. Assure him he will be monitored continuously.
• As appropriate, review all significant and life-threatening adverse reactions and interactions, especially those related to the tests mentioned above.

trospium chloride
Regurin ⊕, Sanctura, Sanctura XR

Pharmacologic class: Anticholinergic, antimuscarinic
Therapeutic class: Renal and genitourinary agent, antispasmodic
Pregnancy risk category C

t

Action

Antagonizes effects of acetylcholine on muscarinic receptors in cholinergically innervated organs, reducing bladder smooth muscle tone

Availability

Capsules (extended-release): 60 mg
Tablets: 20 mg

⏺ Indications and dosages

➤ Overactive bladder with symptoms of urge urinary incontinence, urgency, and urinary frequency
Adults: 20 mg P.O. twice daily 1 hour before meals or on empty stomach, or 1 60-mg capsule daily in morning with water at least 1 hour before a meal

Dosage adjustment

• Severe renal impairment
• Patients age 75 and older

Contraindications

• Hypersensitivity to drug or its components
• Preexisting or risk of urinary or gastric retention or uncontrolled angle-closure glaucoma

Precautions

Use cautiously in:
• moderate renal impairment, moderate to severe hepatic impairment, decreased GI motility, controlled angle-closure glaucoma, clinically significant bladder outflow obstruction or GI obstructive disorders
• patients at risk for heat prostration
• elderly patients
• pregnant or breastfeeding patients
• children (safety and efficacy not established).

Administration

• Give at least 1 hour before meals or on empty stomach.

Route	Onset	Peak	Duration
P.O.	Unknown	5-6 hr	Unknown

Adverse reactions

CNS: headache, fatigue, syncope, hallucinations, delirium, dizziness, drowsiness
CV: tachycardia, chest pain
EENT: dry eyes, blurred vision, dry throat
GI: vomiting, constipation (new-onset or aggravated), upper abdominal pain, dyspepsia, flatulence, abdominal distention, dry mouth
GU: urinary retention
Skin: dry skin
Other: altered taste, heat prostration, **angioedema**

Interactions

Drug-drug. *Anticholinergics:* additive anticholinergic effects
Digoxin, metformin, morphine, pancuronium, procainamide, tenofovir, vancomycin: increased blood levels of both drugs
Drug-behaviors. *Alcohol use:* increased risk of drowsiness

Patient monitoring

• Monitor renal and hepatic function tests.
• Monitor patient for decreased GI motility and urinary retention.
🔊 If patient has controlled angle-closure glaucoma, stay alert for severe eye pain accompanied by nausea, rainbows around lights, red eye, and blurred vision. Be prepared to treat immediately, as appropriate.
🔊 Be aware that angioedema associated with life-threatening upper airway swelling may occur. If involvement of the tongue, hypopharynx, or larynx occurs, promptly discontinue drug and provide appropriate treatment.

Patient teaching

• Instruct patient to take tablet 1 hour before meals on an empty stomach or to take capsule in morning with water at least 1 hour before a meal.

♣ Canada   ⊕ UK   ⚕ Hazardous drug   ⊗ High-alert drug

• Instruct patient not to consume alcohol within 2 hours of taking extended-release capsule.

• Advise patient to consult prescriber before taking over-the-counter products such as antihistamines because these may increase risk of side effects.

• Inform patient that drug increases risk of heat prostration; describe symptoms and advise him to seek prompt medical attention if these occur.

• Caution patient to avoid driving and other hazardous activities until drug effects are known.

• Advise patient to avoid alcohol use.

• As appropriate, review all other significant adverse reactions and interactions, especially those related to the drugs and behaviors mentioned above.

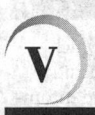

valacyclovir hydrochloride (valaciclovir⊕)
Apo-Valacyclovir✣, Valtrex

Pharmacologic class: Acyclic purine nucleoside analog
Therapeutic class: Antiviral
Pregnancy risk category B

Action
Rapidly converts to acyclovir, which interferes with viral DNA synthesis and replication

Availability
Caplets: 500 mg, 1 g

⬭ Indications and dosages
➣ Herpes zoster (shingles)
Adults: 1 g P.O. t.i.d. for 7 days. Therapy should begin at first sign or symptom of herpes zoster, within 48 hours of onset of zoster rash.

➣ Genital herpes
Adults: For initial episode, 1 g P.O. b.i.d. for 10 days. For recurrent episodes, 500 mg P.O. b.i.d. for 3 days. For chronic suppression, 1 g P.O. daily for no more than 1 year; in patients with history of fewer than nine yearly recurrences, 500 mg P.O. daily for no more than 1 year.
➣ To reduce risk of genital herpes in immunocompetent patients
Adults: 500 mg P.O. daily for source partner, along with counseling regarding safe sex practices
➣ Herpes labialis
Adults: 2 g b.i.d. for 1 day taken 12 hours apart. Begin therapy at first symptom of lesion.

Dosage adjustment
• Renal impairment

Off-label uses
• Cytomegalovirus prophylaxis

Contraindications
• Hypersensitivity to drug, its components, or acyclovir

Precautions
Use cautiously in:
• renal impairment, concurrent use of nephrotoxic drugs, inadequately hydrated patients
• elderly patients
• pregnant or breastfeeding patients
• children.

Administration
• Be aware that therapy may be ineffective if begun more than 72 hours after initial genital herpes outbreak, or more than 24 hours after symptom onset in herpes recurrence.

Route	Onset	Peak	Duration
P.O.	Unknown	1.5-2.5 hr	8-24 hr

V

Adverse reactions
CNS: headache, dizziness, depression, agitation, hallucinations, confusion, **encephalopathy**
GI: nausea, vomiting, diarrhea, abdominal pain
GU: dysmenorrhea, **acute renal failure**
Hematologic: anemia, **leukopenia, thrombocytopenia, hemolytic uremic syndrome/thrombotic thrombocytopenic purpura/ (HUS/TTP)**
Musculoskeletal: joint pain
Other: hypersensitivity reaction

Interactions
Drug-drug. *Cimetidine, probenecid:* increased valacyclovir blood level
Drug-diagnostic tests. *Alanine aminotransferase, alkaline phosphatase, aspartate aminotransferase:* increased levels

Patient monitoring
◀︎〜 Monitor CBC. Stay alert for signs and symptoms of blood dyscrasias. Discontinue drug if clinical signs and symptoms and laboratory findings consistent with HUS/TTP occur.
• Assess liver and kidney function tests.

Patient teaching
• Inform patient that herpes transmission can occur even when he is asymptomatic.
• Tell patient and significant other that no cure exists for herpes. Urge them to practice safe sex.
• Inform pregnant patient of risk of neonatal herpes infection.
• Instruct pregnant patient or female of childbearing age to tell health care provider that she has herpes. After delivery, tell her to inform neonatal care providers.
◀︎〜 Instruct patient to promptly report unusual bleeding or bruising, urinary changes, or serious adverse CNS reactions.

• As appropriate, review all other significant and life-threatening adverse reactions and interactions, especially those related to the drugs and tests mentioned above.

valganciclovir hydrochloride
Valcyte

Pharmacologic class: Synthetic guanine derivative
Therapeutic class: Antiviral
Pregnancy risk category C

FDA | BOXED WARNING

• Clinical toxicities of drug (which is metabolized to ganciclovir) include granulocytopenia, anemia, and thrombocytopenia. In animal studies, ganciclovir caused cancer, birth defects, and aspermatogenesis.

Action
Converts to its active form, inhibiting activity of cytomegalovirus (CMV)

Availability
Solution (oral): 50 mg/ml
Tablets: 450 mg

⚕ Indications and dosages
➤ Active CMV retinitis in AIDS patients
Adults: For induction therapy, 900 mg P.O. b.i.d. for 21 days. For maintenance, 900 mg P.O. daily.
➤ CMV prevention in high-risk kidney, heart, and kidney-pancreas transplant patients
Adults: 900 mg P.O. daily with food, starting within 10 days of transplantation and continuing until 100 days after transplantation

➤ CMV prevention in high-risk kidney or heart transplant patients
Children ages 4 months to 16 years: Base dosage on body surface area and creatinine clearance calculated using a modified Schwartz formula. Give oral solution P.O. daily with food, starting within 10 days of transplantation and continuing until 100 days after transplantation; round all calculated doses to the nearest 25-mg increment, with a maximum dose of 900 mg.

Dosage adjustment
• Renal impairment

Contraindications
• Hypersensitivity to drug, its components, or ganciclovir
• Absolute neutrophil count below 500 cells/mm³, platelet count below 25,000 cells/mm³, or hemoglobin below 8 g/dl

Precautions
Use cautiously in:
• cytopenia, impaired renal function
• patients receiving myelosuppressive drug therapy or radiation therapy
• elderly patients
• pregnant or breastfeeding patients.

Administration
• Avoid direct contact with broken or crushed tablet. If skin contact occurs, wash thoroughly with soap and water; if eye contact occurs, rinse eyes thoroughly with plain water.
• Know that oral solution is preferred for children but tablets may be used if the calculated doses are within 10% of available tablet strength (450 mg).

Route	Onset	Peak	Duration
P.O.	Unknown	1-3 hr	Unknown

Adverse reactions
CNS: headache, insomnia, sedation, dizziness, peripheral neuropathy, paresthesia, hallucinations, confusion, agitation, psychosis, ataxia, **seizures**

EENT: retinal detachment
GI: nausea, vomiting, diarrhea, abdominal pain
Hematologic: anemia, **bone marrow depression, aplastic anemia, pancytopenia, thrombocytopenia, neutropenia**
Other: fever, catheter-related infection, local or systemic infection, hypersensitivity reaction, **sepsis**

Interactions
Drug-drug. *Cytotoxic drugs (such as adriamycin, amphotericin B, co-trimoxazole, dapsone, doxorubicin, flucytosine, pentamidine, vinblastine, vincristine):* additive toxicity
Cilastatin, imipenem: seizures
Didanosine: decreased valganciclovir blood level, increased didanosine blood level
Nephrotoxic drugs (such as amphotericin B, cyclosporine): increased creatinine level
Probenecid: decreased renal clearance of valganciclovir
Zidovudine: increased risk of granulocytopenia and anemia
Drug-diagnostic tests. *Alanine aminotransferase, alkaline phosphatase, aspartate aminotransferase, creatinine:* increased levels
Creatinine clearance: decreased value
Granulocytes, hemoglobin, neutrophils, platelets, white blood cells: decreased levels
Drug-food. *Any food:* increased drug absorption

Patient monitoring
• Monitor CBC with white cell differential and platelet count. Watch for signs and symptoms of blood dyscrasias.
◀€ Stay alert for hypersensitivity reaction and signs and symptoms of infection.
• Closely monitor neurologic status. Observe for signs and symptoms of impending seizure.

V

Reactions in **bold** are life-threatening. ◀€ Clinical alert

- Periodically assess creatinine level and creatinine clearance.

Patient teaching
- Instruct patient to take with food.
- Instruct patient (or caregiver) how to take oral solution using oral dispenser provided.
- Explain drug therapy to patient. Stress importance of taking drug exactly as prescribed to prevent overdose.
- Tell patient to avoid direct contact with solution or broken or crushed tablets. If skin contact occurs, advise patient to wash area thoroughly with soap and water or, if eye contact occurs, to rinse eyes thoroughly with plain water.
- ◀℥ Tell patient drug can cause serious adverse reactions. Teach him which ones to report immediately.
- Advise patient to avoid driving and other hazardous activities.
- Caution female of childbearing age to avoid pregnancy and breastfeeding.
- Urge male patient to use barrier contraception during and for 90 days after therapy.
- Instruct patient to have follow-up eye exams every 4 to 6 weeks, as well as periodic laboratory tests.
- As appropriate, review all other significant and life-threatening adverse reactions and interactions, especially those related to the drugs, tests, and foods mentioned above.

valproate sodium
Apo-Divalproex✤, Apo-Valproic Syrup✤, Depacon, Dom-Divalproex✤, Dom-Valproic Acid✤, Epilem✠, Epilem Chrono✠, Episenta✠, Epival CR✠, Epival ECT✤, Gen-Divalproex✤, Gen-Valproic-Cap✤, Novo-Divalproex✤, Novo-Valproic ECC✤, Nu-Divalproex✤, Nu-Valproic✤, Orlept✠, PHL-Divalproex✤, PHL-Valproic Acid✤, PMS-Divalproex✤, PMS-Valproic Acid✤, Ratio-Valproic✤, Ratio-Valproic ECC✤, Sandoz Valproic✤

valproic acid
Convulex✠, Depakene, Stavzor

divalproex sodium
Depakote, Depakote ER, Depakote Sprinkle

Pharmacologic class: Carboxylic acid derivative
Therapeutic class: Anticonvulsant, mood stabilizer, antimigraine agent
Pregnancy risk category D

FDA | **BOXED WARNING**

- Hepatic failure resulting in death has occurred in patients receiving Depacon. Children younger than age 2 are at considerably increased risk for fatal hepatotoxicity, especially those on multiple anticonvulsants, those with congenital metabolic disorders or organic brain disease, and those with severe seizure disorders accompanied by mental retardation. In this patient group, use Depacon with extreme caution and as sole agent. Weigh benefits

---

✤ Canada   ✠ UK   ✤ Hazardous drug   ⊗ High-alert drug

of therapy against risks. Above this age-group, incidence of fatal hepatotoxicity decreases considerably in progressively older patients.

• Valproate can cause teratogenic effects, such as neural tube defects. When using it in women with childbearing potential, weigh benefits against risk of fetal injury.

• Life-threatening pancreatitis has occurred in both children and adults receiving valproate. Some cases were hemorrhagic, with rapid progression from initial symptoms to death.

Action

Increases level of gamma-aminobutyric acid in brain, reducing seizure activity

Availability

valproate sodium
Injection: 100 mg/ml in 5-ml vial
Syrup: 250 mg/5 ml
valproic acid
Capsules (delayed-release): 125 mg, 250 mg, 500 mg
Capsules (liquid-filled): 250 mg
divalproex sodium
Capsules (containing coated particles or sprinkles): 125 mg
Tablets (enteric-coated, delayed-release): 125 mg, 250 mg, 500 mg
Tablets (extended-release): 250 mg, 500 mg

⚕ Indications and dosages

➤ Complex partial seizures
Adults and children older than age 10: Initially, 10 to 15 mg/kg/day P.O. or I.V. (valproate sodium). May increase by 5 to 10 mg/kg/day q week until blood drug level is 50 to 100 mcg/ml or adverse reactions occur; don't exceed 60 mg/kg/day. If daily dosage exceeds 250 mg, give in two divided doses.
➤ Simple or complex absence seizures

Adults and children older than age 10: Initially, 15 mg/kg/day P.O. or I.V. (valproate sodium). May increase by 5 to 10 mg/kg/day at weekly intervals until therapeutic blood drug level is reached or adverse reactions occur; don't exceed 60 mg/kg/day. If daily dosage exceeds 250 mg, give in two divided doses.
➤ Mania associated with bipolar disorder
Adults: Initially, 750 mg (divalproex or valproic acid delayed-release) P.O. daily in divided doses. Titrate rapidly to desired effect or trough level of 50 to 125 mcg/ml. Don't exceed 60 mg/kg/day.
➤ To prevent migraine
Adults: 250 mg (divalproex or valproic acid delayed-release) P.O. b.i.d. Or 500 mg (divalproex extended-release) P.O. daily for 1 week (up to 1 g/day). Maximum dosage is 1 g/day.

Off-label uses

• Chorea
• Photosensitivity-related seizures
• Sedative-hypnotic withdrawal

Contraindications

• Hypersensitivity to drug or tartrazine (some products)
• Hepatic impairment
• Urea cycle disorders

Precautions

Use cautiously in:
• bleeding disorders, organic brain disease, bone marrow depression, renal impairment
• posttraumatic seizures caused by head injury (use not recommended)
• history of hepatic disease
• elderly patients
• pregnant or breastfeeding patients
• children.

Administration

• Give I.V. only when oral therapy isn't feasible.

V

- For I.V. use, dilute valproate sodium in at least 50 ml of dextrose 5% in water, lactated Ringer's solution, or normal saline solution. Infuse over 1 hour at a rate slower than 20 mg/minute.
- Know that I.V. and P.O. dosages and dosing frequencies are identical. However, patient should be switched to oral therapy as soon as possible.
- Give oral forms with food.
- Be aware that divalproex extended-release and delayed-release forms are not bioequivalent.
- Make sure patient swallows divalproex extended-release tablets and valproic acid capsules whole without chewing or crushing.
- If patient can't swallow capsule containing coated particles, sprinkle entire contents of capsule onto about 5 ml of semisolid food, such as pudding or applesauce, immediately before giving.
- Don't give syrup in carbonated beverages (may cause mouth and throat irritation).

Route	Onset	Peak	Duration
P.O. (capsules)	Rapid	1-4 hr	6-24 hr
P.O. (delayed, extended)	Unknown	Unknown	Unknown
P.O. (syrup)	Rapid	15-120 min	6-24 hr
I.V.	Rapid	End of 1-hr infusion	Unknown

Adverse reactions

CNS: confusion, dizziness, headache, sedation, ataxia, paresthesia, asthenia, tremor, drowsiness, emotional lability, abnormal thinking, amnesia, **hyperammonemic encephalopathy, suicidal behavior or ideation**
EENT: amblyopia, blurred vision, nystagmus, tinnitus, pharyngitis
GI: nausea, vomiting, diarrhea, abdominal pain, dyspepsia, anorexia, **pancreatitis**

Hematologic: leukopenia, thrombocytopenia
Hepatic: hepatotoxicity
Metabolic: hyperammonemia
Musculoskeletal: back pain
Respiratory: dyspnea
Skin: rash, alopecia, bruising
Other: abnormal taste, increased appetite, weight gain, flulike symptoms, infection, infusion site pain and reaction, **multiorgan hypersensitivity reaction**

Interactions

Drug-drug. *Activated charcoal, cholestyramine:* decreased valproate absorption
Antiplatelet agents (including abciximab, aspirin and other nonsteroidal anti-inflammatory drugs, eptifibatide, tirofiban), cefamandole, cefoperazone, cefotetan, heparin, thrombolytics, warfarin: increased risk of bleeding
Barbiturates, primidone: decreased metabolism and greater risk of toxicity of these drugs, decreased valproate efficacy
Carbamazepine: increased carbamazepine blood level, decreased valproate blood level, poor seizure control
Chlorpromazine: decreased valproate clearance and increased trough level
Cimetidine: decreased valproate clearance
Clonazepam: absence seizures in patients with history of these seizures
CNS depressants (such as antihistamines and antidepressants, MAO inhibitors, opioid analgesics, sedative-hypnotics): additive CNS depression
Diazepam: displacement of diazepam from binding site, inhibited diazepam metabolism
Erythromycin, felbamate: increased valproate blood level, greater risk of toxicity
Ethosuximide: inhibited ethosuximide metabolism
Lamotrigine: decreased valproate blood level, increased lamotrigine blood level

Phenytoin: increased phenytoin effects and risk of toxicity, decreased valproate effects

Salicylates (large doses in children): increased valproate effects

Topiramate: increased risk of hyperammonemia with and without encephalopathy and hypothermia

Tricyclic antidepressants: increased blood levels of these drugs, greater risk of adverse reactions

Zidovudine: decreased zidovudine clearance in patients with human immunodeficiency virus

Drug-diagnostic tests. *Alanine aminotransferase, alkaline phosphatase, aspartate aminotransferase, bilirubin:* increased levels

Bleeding time: prolonged

Ketone bodies: false-positive results

Platelets, white blood cells: decreased counts

Thyroid function tests: interference with results

Drug-behaviors. *Alcohol use:* additive CNS depression

Patient monitoring

◀᠁ Closely monitor neurologic status. Watch for seizures and suicidal behavior or ideation.

◀᠁ If hyperammonemia or hyperammonemic encephalopathy (unexplained lethargy and vomiting or changes in mental status) is suspected, measure ammonia level.

◀᠁ Evaluate GI status. Stay alert for signs and symptoms of pancreatitis. Consider discontinuing drug if pancreatitis is diagnosed.

◀᠁ Watch for diverse signs and symptoms of multiorgan hypersensitivity reaction, such as fever and rash associated with other organ system involvement (lymphadenopathy, hepatitis, liver function test abnormalities, hematologic abnormalities, pruritus, nephritis, oliguria, hepatorenal syndrome, arthralgia, and asthenia).

Discontinue drug if multiorgan hypersensitivity reaction occurs.

• Monitor I.V. infusion site for local reactions.

• Assess CBC (including platelet count), prothrombin time, International Normalized Ratio, and liver function tests.

• Monitor valproate blood level; therapeutic range is 50 to 100 mcg/ml.

Patient teaching

• Instruct patient to take with food to minimize GI upset.

• Tell patient taking extended-release tablets or valproic acid capsules to swallow them whole without chewing or breaking.

• Inform patient taking capsules with delayed-release pellets that he may swallow them whole or open them and sprinkle contents onto a teaspoon of semisolid food, such as pudding or applesauce.

• Tell patient (or parents) that valproate syrup shouldn't be taken with carbonated beverages.

◀᠁ Advise patient to immediately report signs and symptoms of liver dysfunction (such as malaise, weakness, lethargy, appetite loss, vomiting, or yellowing of skin or eyes), signs and symptoms of pancreatitis (such as abdominal pain, nausea, vomiting, loss of appetite), or suicidal behavior or ideation.

◀᠁ Tell patient to immediately report unexplained signs and symptoms that may reflect hypersensitivity reaction (fever, rash, hepatitis signs and symptoms, bleeding or bruising, itching, urinary problems, muscle pains, or weakness).

• If patient is taking drug for seizure control, tell him to avoid driving and other hazardous activities.

◀᠁ Caution patient not to stop therapy abruptly.

• Instruct patient to avoid alcohol.

• Stress importance of follow-up laboratory tests.

V

Reactions in **bold** are life-threatening. ◀᠁ Clinical alert

• As appropriate, review all other significant and life-threatening adverse reactions and interactions, especially those related to the drugs, tests, and behaviors mentioned above.

valsartan
Diovan

Pharmacologic class: Angiotensin II receptor antagonist

Therapeutic class: Antihypertensive

Pregnancy risk category C (first trimester), *D* (second and third trimesters)

FDA | BOXED WARNING

• Drugs that act directly on the renin-angiotensin system can cause injury to or death of a developing fetus. Discontinue drug as soon as possible when pregnancy is detected.

Action
Blocks the vasoconstrictive and aldosterone-producing effects of angiotensin II at various receptor sites, including vascular smooth muscle and adrenal glands

Availability
Tablets: 40 mg, 80 mg, 160 mg, 320 mg

⬤ Indications and dosages
➢ Hypertension
Adults: Initially, 80 to 160 mg P.O. daily. May increase as needed to a maximum of 320 mg P.O. daily, or a diuretic may be added.
Children ages 6 to 16: Initially, 1.3 mg/kg (up to 40 mg total) P.O. once daily; dosage range is 1.3 to 2.7 mg/kg (40 to 160 mg total).
➢ Heart failure
Adults: 40 mg P.O. b.i.d., titrated to 80 mg or 160 mg P.O. b.i.d., as tolerated

➢ Reduction of cardiovascular mortality in clinically stable patients with left ventricular failure or left ventricular dysfunction following myocardial infarction
Adults: 20 mg P.O. b.i.d., followed by titration to 40 mg P.O. b.i.d., with subsequent titration to a target maintenance dosage of 160 mg P.O. b.i.d., as tolerated

Dosage adjustment
• Symptomatic hypotension
• Renal dysfunction

Off-label uses
• Left ventricular hypertrophy
• Diabetic nephropathy

Contraindications
• None

Precautions
Use cautiously in:
• severe heart failure; volume or sodium depletion; hepatic or renal impairment; obstructive biliary disorders; angioedema; aortic, mitral valve, or renal artery stenosis; hyperkalemia, hypotension
• pregnant or breastfeeding patients
• children younger than age 6 (safety not established).

Administration
• Give with or without food.
• For children who can't swallow tablets or children for whom calculated dosage doesn't correspond to available tablet strength, use a suspension but be aware that exposure to the suspension is 1.6 times greater than the tablet.
• To prepare 160 ml of a 4-mg/ml suspension, add 80 ml of Ora-Plus to bottle containing eight valsartan 80-mg tablets and shake for at least 2 minutes. Allow suspension to stand for at least 1 hour. Then shake for at least 1 additional minute. Add 80 ml of Ora-Sweet to bottle and shake for at least

---

10 seconds before giving appropriate dose. May store suspension for 30 days at room temperature or up to 75 days if refrigerated.

◀€ Be aware that drug isn't recommended for children with glomerular filtration rate of less than 30 ml/minute/1.73^2.

Route	Onset	Peak	Duration
P.O.	Within 2 hr	4-6 hr	24 hr

Adverse reactions

CNS: dizziness, fatigue, headache
CV: hypotension, palpitations
EENT: sinus disorders, rhinitis, pharyngitis
GI: nausea, diarrhea, constipation, abdominal pain, dry mouth
GU: albuminuria, **renal impairment**
Hematologic: neutropenia
Metabolic: hyperkalemia
Musculoskeletal: back pain, joint pain, muscle cramps
Respiratory: cough, upper respiratory tract infection
Skin: alopecia, angioedema
Other: dental pain, fever, viral infection, edema

Interactions

Drug-drug. *Nonsteroidal anti-inflammatory drugs including selective cyclooxygenase-2 inhibitors:* increased risk of renal impairment including acute renal failure in elderly patients, volume-depleted patients, or those with compromised renal function; loss of valsartan antihypertensive effect
Other antihypertensives: increased risk of hypotension
Potassium-sparing diuretics, potassium supplements: increased risk of hyperkalemia
Drug-diagnostic tests. *Serum creatinine, serum* and *urine albumin, urine potassium:* increased levels
Drug-food. *Salt substitutes containing potassium:* increased risk of hyperkalemia

Drug-herbs. *Ephedra (ma huang):* reduced hypotensive effect of valsartan
Drug-behaviors. *Alcohol use:* increased CNS depression

Patient monitoring

• Monitor blood pressure closely, especially during initial therapy and dosage adjustments.
• Assess potassium level. Stay alert for hyperkalemia.
• Be aware that in black patients, drug may be ineffective when used alone. Additional agents may be required.

Patient teaching

• Tell patient he may take with or without food.
• For children who can't swallow tablets or children for whom calculated dosage doesn't correspond to available tablet strength, show caregiver how to prepare a suspension.
◀€ Instruct female of childbearing age to report pregnancy immediately.
• Advise breastfeeding patient to avoid breastfeeding while taking drug.
• Advise patient to avoid potassium-containing salt substitutes.
• Caution patient to avoid alcohol.
• As appropriate, review all other significant and life-threatening adverse reactions and interactions, especially those related to the drugs, tests, foods, herbs, and behaviors mentioned above.

vancomycin hydrochloride

PMS-Vancomycin✦, Vancocin

Pharmacologic class: Tricyclic glycopeptide
Therapeutic class: Anti-infective
Pregnancy risk category C (with parenteral use); B (with oral use)

Action
Binds to bacterial cell wall, inhibiting cell-wall synthesis and causing secondary damage to bacterial membrane

Availability
Capsules: 125 mg, 250 mg
Powder for injection: 500-mg vial, 1-g vial, 5-g vial, 10 g-vial

❂ Indications and dosages
➤ Severe, life-threatening infections caused by susceptible strains of methicillin-resistant staphylococci, *Staphylococcus epidermidis, Streptococcus viridans* or *Streptococcus bovis* (alone or combined with an aminoglycoside), or *Enterococcus faecalis* (combined with an aminoglycoside)
Adults: 500 mg I.V. q 6 hours or 1 g I.V. q 12 hours
Children: 10 mg/kg I.V. q 6 hours
Infants and neonates: Initially, 15 mg/kg I.V., followed by 10 mg/kg I.V. q 8 hours in infants 8 days to 1 month old, or 10 mg/kg I.V. q 12 hours in infants less than 8 days old
➤ Endocarditis prophylaxis in penicillin-allergic patients at moderate risk who are scheduled for dental and other invasive procedures
Adults: 1 g I.V. slowly over 1 to 2 hours, with infusion completed 30 minutes before invasive procedure begins
Children: 20 mg/kg I.V. over 1 to 2 hours, with infusion completed 30 minutes before invasive procedure begins
➤ Enterocolitis caused by *Staphylococcus aureus*
Adults: 500 mg to 2 g P.O. daily in three or four divided doses for 7 to 10 days
Children: 40 mg/kg P.O. daily in three or four divided doses for 7 to 10 days; total daily dose shouldn't exceed 2 g.
➤ *Clostridium difficile*–associated diarrhea
Adults: 125 mg P.O. q.i.d. for 10 days
Children: 40 mg/kg P. O. in three or four divided doses for 7 to 10 days; total daily dose shouldn't exceed 2 g.

Dosage adjustment
• Renal impairment
• Elderly patients

Off-label uses
• Peritonitis
• Meningitis
• Intraocular infections
• Febrile neutropenia

Contraindications
• Hypersensitivity to drug

Precautions
Use cautiously in:
• renal impairment, preexisting hearing loss
• concurrent use of anesthetics, immunosuppressants, or nephrotoxic or ototoxic drugs
• elderly patients
• pregnant or breastfeeding patients
• neonates.

Administration
◀€ Know that I.V. therapy is ineffective against enterocolitis and pseudomembranous diarrhea.
• For intermittent I.V. infusion, dilute by adding 10 or 20 ml of sterile water for injection to vial containing 500 mg or 1 g of drug, respectively, to yield a concentration of 50 mg/ml. Dilute further by adding at least 100 ml or 200 ml, respectively, of dextrose 5% in water or normal saline solution; infuse over at least 1 hour.
• Don't give by I.M. route.
• Be aware that capsules aren't systemically absorbed; therefore, oral therapy is ineffective in infections other than *C. difficile*–associated diarrhea and enterocolitis caused by *S. aureus.*
◀€ Keep emergency equipment and epinephrine on hand in case of anaphylaxis.

Route	Onset	Peak	Duration
P.O.	Unknown	Unknown	Unknown
I.V.	Immediate	Immediate	Unknown

Adverse reactions

CV: hypotension, **cardiac arrest, vascular collapse**
EENT: permanent hearing loss, ototoxicity, tinnitus
GI: nausea, vomiting, abdominal pain, **pseudomembranous colitis**
GU: nephrotoxicity, severe uremia
Hematologic: eosinophilia, **leukopenia, neutropenia**
Metabolic: hypokalemia
Respiratory: wheezing, dyspnea
Skin: "red man" syndrome (nonallergic histamine reaction with rapid I.V. infusion), rash, urticaria, pruritus, necrosis
Other: chills, fever, thrombophlebitis at injection site, **anaphylaxis**

Interactions

Drug-drug. *Aminoglycosides, amphotericin B, bacitracin, cephalosporins, cisplatin, colistin, nondepolarizing neuromuscular blockers, pentamidine (with parenteral use):* increased risk of nephrotoxicity and ototoxicity
Anesthetic agents (with parenteral use): erythema and histamine-like flushing
Drug-diagnostic tests. *Albumin, blood urea nitrogen (BUN), creatinine:* increased levels
Eosinophils, neutrophils: decreased counts
Potassium: decreased level

Patient monitoring

◀€ Monitor closely for signs and symptoms of hypersensitivity reactions, including anaphylaxis.
• Check drug blood level weekly. Therapeutic peak ranges from 30 to 40 g/L; therapeutic trough, 5 to 10 mg/L.
• Assess BUN and creatinine levels every 2 days, or daily in patients with unstable renal function.
• Monitor urine output daily. Weigh patient at least weekly.
• Assess hearing before and during therapy; stay alert for hearing loss.

Patient may require baseline and weekly audiograms.
• Check I.V. site often for phlebitis.
• Watch for "red-man" syndrome, which can result from rapid infusion. Signs and symptoms include hypotension, pruritus, and maculopapular rash on face, neck, trunk, and limbs.
• Monitor CBC. Watch for signs and symptoms of blood dyscrasias.
• Closely monitor respiratory status. Stay alert for wheezing and dyspnea.
◀€ Monitor vital signs and cardiovascular status, especially for vascular collapse and other signs of impending cardiac arrest.

Patient teaching

• Tell patient he may take with or without food.
• Instruct patient to take oral drug exactly as prescribed for as long as prescribed, even if symptoms improve.
• Explain importance of prophylactic I.V. therapy to patients at risk for endocarditis who are scheduled for invasive procedures.
◀€ Advise patient to promptly report rash, hearing loss, breathing problems, and signs and symptoms of "red-man" syndrome, nephrotoxicity, and blood dyscrasias.
• As appropriate, review all other significant and life-threatening adverse reactions and interactions, especially those related to the drugs and tests mentioned above.

vardenafil hydrochloride

Levitra

Pharmacologic class: Phosphodiesterase-5 (PDE5) inhibitor
Therapeutic class: Erectile dysfunction agent
Pregnancy risk category B

Action
Selectively blocks PDE5, which neutralizes cyclic guanosine monophosphate, resulting in enhanced erectile function

Availability
Tablets: 2.5 mg, 5 mg, 10 mg, 20 mg

⊘ Indications and dosages
➤ Erectile dysfunction
Adult males: 10 or 20 mg P.O. approximately 1 hour before anticipated sexual activity. Maximum dosing frequency is once daily.

Dosage adjustment
• Patients older than age 65
• Concurrent use of CYP450-3A4 inhibitors
• Concurrent HIV therapy (except highly active antiretroviral therapy)

Contraindications
• Hypersensitivity to drug
• Concurrent use of nitrates or nitrate patches to treat angina
• Concurrent use of alpha-adrenergic blockers

Precautions
Use cautiously in:
• cardiovascular disease, retinitis pigmentosa, hepatic or renal impairment, reduced hepatic blood flow
• patients at increased risk for priapism (as from sickle-cell disease, leukemia, multiple myeloma, polycythemia, or history of priapism).

Administration
• Advise patient not to take more than one tablet daily.

Route	Onset	Peak	Duration
P.O.	Unknown	1 hr	4 hr

Adverse reactions
CNS: headache
CV: hypotension
EENT: blurred vision, altered color perception, light sensitivity, rhinitis
GI: dyspepsia
Skin: flushing
Other: flulike symptoms

Interactions
Drug-drug. *Alpha-adrenergic blockers, nitrates:* hypotension
Erythromycin, itraconazole, ketoconazole, protease inhibitors: increased vardenafil blood level
Drug-diagnostic tests. *Creatine kinase:* increased level

Patient monitoring
• Monitor blood pressure and heart rate, particularly if patient has cardiovascular disease.

Patient teaching
• Tell patient he may take with or without food.
• Instruct patient to take one tablet about 1 hour before anticipated sexual activity. Caution him not to take more than one tablet daily.
• Instruct patient to promptly contact prescriber if erection lasts more than 4 hours, because irreversible damage to penis may occur.
• Caution patient not to take nitrates. Tell him to inform prescriber of other drugs he's taking.
• As appropriate, review all other significant adverse reactions and interactions, especially those related to the drugs and tests mentioned above.

varenicline
Champix✿⊕, Chantix

Pharmacologic class: Autonomic drug, miscellaneous
Therapeutic class: Smoking cessation agent
Pregnancy risk category C

FDA | BOXED WARNING

- Varenicline has caused serious neuropsychiatric events, including, but not limited to, depression, suicidal ideation, suicide attempt, and completed suicide. Some reported cases may have been complicated by signs and symptoms of nicotine withdrawal (such as depression) in patients who stopped smoking. Depression, rarely including suicidal ideation, has been reported in smokers undergoing a smoking cessation attempt without medication. However, some of these symptoms have occurred in patients taking varenicline who continued to smoke. Observe all patients taking varenicline for neuropsychiatric symptoms, such as changes in behavior, hostility, agitation, depressed mood, and suicide-related events, including ideation, behavior, and attempted suicide. These symptoms, as well as worsening of preexisting psychiatric illness and completed suicide, have occurred in some patients attempting to quit smoking while taking varenicline in postmarketing experience. These events have occurred in patients with and without preexisting psychiatric disease. Patients with serious psychiatric illness, such as schizophrenia, bipolar disorder, and major depressive disorder, didn't participate in premarketing studies of varenicline; therefore, safety and efficacy of varenicline in such patients haven't been established.
- Advise patient and caregivers that patient should stop taking varenicline and contact prescriber immediately if agitation, hostility, depressed mood, or changes in behavior or thinking not typical for patient are observed, or if patient develops suicidal ideation or suicidal behavior.
- Weigh benefits of varenicline against its risks. Varenicline has been shown to increase likelihood of abstinence from smoking for as long as 1 year compared to placebo.

Action
In smoking cessation, action presumably results from activity at nicotinic receptor subtype, where its binding produces agonist activity while simultaneously preventing nicotine binding to alpha$_4$-beta$_2$ receptors.

Availability
Tablets (film coated): 0.5 mg, 1 mg

⚡ Indications and dosages
➤ To aid smoking-cessation treatment
Adults: Begin with 1-week titration of 0.5 mg P.O. daily on days 1 to 3; then, 0.5 mg P.O. b.i.d. on days 4 to 7. Starting on day 8, give 1 mg P.O. b.i.d. till end of treatment. If patient has successfully stopped smoking at end of 12 weeks, additional course of 12 weeks is recommended to improve likelihood of long-term abstinence.

Dosage adjustment
- Severe renal impairment

Contraindications
- History of serious hypersensitivity or skin reactions to drug

Precautions
Use cautiously in:
- renal impairment
- concurrent use of drugs affected by smoking, such as insulin, theophylline, and warfarin (whose dosages may need to be adjusted)
- elderly patients
- pregnant or breastfeeding patients
- children younger than age 18 (safety and efficacy not established).

Administration
- Give with full glass of water after a meal.

Route	Onset	Peak	Duration
P.O.	Unknown	3-4 hr	Unknown

Reactions in **bold** are life-threatening.   ◀€ Clinical alert

Adverse reactions

CNS: headache, migraine, somnolence, lethargy, dizziness, syncope, attention disturbance, sensory disturbance, anxiety, depression, emotional disorder, irritability, restlessness, sleep disorders, abnormal dreams, nightmares, insomnia, fatigue, malaise, asthenia, aggression, agitation, amnesia, dissociation, mood swings, parosmia, psychomotor hyperactivity, restless leg syndrome, abnormal thinking, tremor, vertigo, **suicidal ideation suicide attempt, suicide**

CV: hot flushes, hypertension, angina pectoris, bradycardia, hypotension, palpitations, peripheral ischemia, tachycardia, **thrombosis, ventricular extrasystoles, arrhythmia, myocardial infarction**

EENT: tinnitus, epistaxis, rhinorrhea

GI: nausea, vomiting, constipation, abdominal pain, flatulence, dyspepsia, gastroesophageal reflux disease, gingivitis, anorexia, increased or decreased appetite, dysgeusia, dry mouth, **intestinal obstruction** (rare), **acute pancreatitis** (rare)

GU: polyuria, menstrual disorder, decreased libido, **acute renal failure** (rare)

Hematologic: anemia, lymphadenopathy

Musculoskeletal: arthralgia, back pain, muscle cramp, musculoskeletal pain, myalgia

Respiratory: dyspnea, upper respiratory tract disorders, **pulmonary embolism** (rare)

Skin: rash, pruritus, hyperhidrosis **Stevens-Johnson syndrome, erythema multiforme** (rare)

Other: chest pain, flulike illness, edema, thirst, increased weight, nicotine withdrawal symptoms, hypersensitivity reactions including **angioedema**

Interactions

Drug-diagnostic tests. *Liver function tests:* abnormal

Patient monitoring

◀€ Monitor patient for serious neuropsychiatric symptoms, including behavior changes, agitation, depressed mood, and suicidal ideation and behavior.

◀€ Closely monitor patient for hypersensitivity or serious skin reactions.

• Monitor patients taking drugs that may be affected by smoking; dosages of these drugs may need to be adjusted once patient quits smoking.

• Monitor liver function tests.

• Monitor renal function, especially in elderly patients.

Patient teaching

◀€ Instruct patient to discontinue drug and immediately report changes in behavior, including depression and suicidal thoughts or action; rash; or swelling of face, mouth, or throat.

• Advise patient to set date to quit smoking and to start drug 1 week before quit date. Or, patient can begin drug dosing and then quit smoking between days 8 and 35 of treatment.

• Teach patient how to titrate drug for first week of therapy.

• Instruct patient to take drug with full glass of water after eating.

• Give patient educational materials and counseling referral to support smoking-cessation attempt.

• Encourage patient who relapses after quit day to continue to try to quit smoking.

• Inform patient that nausea and insomnia are side effects and usually disappear. However, if these symptoms remain troubling, advise patient to notify prescriber, who may consider dosage reduction.

• Inform patient that some drugs may require dosage adjustment after smoking cessation.

♣ Canada   ⊕ UK   ⚕ Hazardous drug   ⊗ High-alert drug

- Caution patient to avoid driving and other hazardous activities until effects of drug and smoking cessation are known.
- As appropriate, review all other significant and life-threatening adverse reactions and interactions, especially those related to the tests mentioned above.

venlafaxine hydrochloride
Co Venlafaxine✦, Co Venlafaxine XR, Efexor⊕, Effexor, Effexor XR, Gen-Venlafaxine XR✦, Novo-Venlafaxine XR✦, PMS-Venlafaxine XR✦, Ratio-Venlafaxine XR✦, Riva-Venlafaxine XR✦, Sandoz Venlafaxine XR✦

Pharmacologic class: Phenethylamine derivative
Therapeutic class: Antidepressant, anxiolytic
Pregnancy risk category C

FDA | BOXED WARNING

- Drug may increase risk of suicidal thinking and behavior in children and adolescents with major depressive disorder and other psychiatric disorders. Risk must be balanced with clinical need, as depression itself increases suicide risk. With patient of any age, observe closely for clinical worsening, suicidality, and unusual behavior changes when therapy begins. Advise family and caregivers to observe patient closely and communicate with prescriber as needed.
- Drug isn't approved for use in pediatric patients.

Action
Inhibits neuronal serotonin and norepinephrine reuptake and slightly inhibits dopamine reuptake

Availability
Capsules (extended-release): 37.5 mg, 75 mg, 150 mg
Tablets: 25 mg, 37.5 mg, 50 mg, 75 mg, 100 mg
Tablets (extended-release): 37.5 mg, 75 mg, 150 mg, 225 mg

⍟ Indications and dosages
➤ Depression
Adults: In outpatients, 75 mg P.O. daily in two or three divided doses; may increase in increments of 75 mg/day q 4 or more days to a maximum of 225 mg/day; extended-release form can be given as a single daily dose. In hospitalized patients, 75 mg P.O. daily in two or three divided doses; may increase in increments of 75 mg/day q 4 days to a maximum of 375 mg/day given in three divided doses.
➤ Generalized anxiety disorder
Adults: Single dose of 37.5 to 75 mg (extended-release) P.O. daily; may increase in increments of 75 mg/day q 4 days to a maximum of 225 mg/day
➤ Panic disorder
Adults: 37.5 mg (extended-release) P.O. daily for 7 days; increase to 75 mg P.O. daily for 7 days; then increase by 75 mg daily at weekly intervals to a maximum of 225 mg P.O. daily
➤ Social anxiety disorder
Adults: 75 mg (extended-release capsule) P.O. daily as a single dose

Dosage adjustment
- Hepatic or renal impairment

Off-label uses
- Premenstrual dysphoric disorder

V

Contraindications
- Hypersensitivity to drug
- MAO inhibitor use within past 14 days

Precautions
Use cautiously in:
- cardiovascular disease; hypertension; heart failure, recent myocardial infarction, and other conditions in which increased heart rate poses a danger; hepatic or renal impairment; glaucoma; hyperthyroidism; hyponatremia; syndrome of inappropriate antidiuretic hormone secretion (SIADH)
- history of seizures, neurologic impairment, or drug abuse
- pregnant or breastfeeding patients
- children younger than age 18.

Administration
◀€ Don't give within 14 days of MAO inhibitors.

Route	Onset	Peak	Duration
P.O.	Within 2 wk	2-4 wk	Unknown

Adverse reactions
CNS: abnormal dreams, anxiety, dizziness, headache, insomnia, nervousness, abnormal thinking, agitation, confusion, depersonalization, drowsiness, emotional lability, worsening depression, twitching, tremor, asthenia, paresthesia, mania, hypomania, **suicidal ideation or behavior** (especially in child or adolescent)
CV: chest pain, hypertension, palpitations, tachycardia, vasodilation
EENT: visual disturbances, blurred vision, mydriasis, tinnitus, rhinitis
GI: nausea, vomiting, diarrhea, constipation, abdominal pain, dyspepsia, flatulence, dry mouth, anorexia
GU: urinary frequency or retention, sexual dysfunction, abnormal ejaculation, anorgasmia, erectile dysfunction
Metabolic: hyponatremia, **SIADH**
Skin: bruising, pruritus, rash, diaphoresis, photosensitivity

Other: altered taste, weight loss, chills, yawning

Interactions
Drug-drug. *Cimetidine:* increased venlafaxine effects
MAO inhibitors: potentially fatal reactions
Sumatriptan, trazodone: serotonin syndrome (including altered level of consciousness)
Drug-diagnostic tests. *Sodium:* decreased level
Drug-herbs. *Chamomile, hops, kava, skullcap, valerian:* increased CNS depression
S-adenosylmethionine (SAM-e), St. John's wort: increased risk of sedative or hypnotic effects

Patient monitoring
◀€ Monitor neurologic status, particularly for seizures, worsening depression, and suicidal ideation.
- Closely monitor vital signs and cardiovascular status. Stay alert for hypertension and tachycardia.
- Monitor nutritional status, hydration, and weight.

Patient teaching
- Tell patient taking extended-release capsules to swallow them whole without chewing, breaking, dividing, or dissolving.
◀€ Caution patient not to stop therapy abruptly.
◀€ Advise patient to promptly report seizures, worsening depression, or suicidal thoughts (especially in child or adolescent).
- Caution patient to avoid driving and other dangerous activities until drug effects are known.
- As appropriate, review all other significant and life-threatening adverse reactions and interactions, especially those related to the drugs, tests, and herbs mentioned above.

---

verapamil hydrochloride

Apo-Verap✳, Apo-Verap SR✳, Calan, Calan SR, Cordilox MR⊕, Covera-HS, Dom-Verapamil SR✳, Gen-Verapamil✳, Gen-Verapamil SR✳, Half Securon⊕, Isoptin, Isoptin SR, Med Verapamil✳, Novo-Veramil✳, Nu-Verap✳, Nu-Verap SR✳, PHL-Verapamil SR✳, PMS-Verapamil SR✳, Riva-Verapamil SR✳, Securon SR⊕, Univer⊕, Verapress⊕, Vera-Til SR⊕, Verelan, Verelan PM, Vertab SR⊕, Zolvera⊕

Pharmacologic class: Calcium channel blocker

Therapeutic class: Antianginal, anti-arrhythmic (class IV), antihypertensive

Pregnancy risk category C

Action

Decreases conduction of sinoatrial and atrioventricular (AV) nodes by inhibiting calcium influx into cardiac and vascular smooth muscle cells, inhibiting excitatory contraction. These effects prolong AV node refractoriness and decrease myocardial oxygen consumption.

Availability

Capsules (extended-release): 100 mg, 120 mg, 180 mg, 200 mg, 240 mg, 300 mg, 360 mg
Capsules (sustained-release): 120 mg, 180 mg, 240 mg, 360 mg
Injection: 2.5 mg/ml in 2- and 4-ml vials, ampules, and syringes
Tablets (extended-release): 120 mg, 180 mg, 240 mg
Tablets (immediate-release): 40 mg, 80 mg, 120 mg

ⓘ Indications and dosages

➤ Angina
Adults: Initially, 80 mg (immediate-release) P.O. t.i.d.; may titrate at daily or weekly intervals to 360 mg/day. Or initially, 180 mg (extended-release) P.O. once daily at bedtime, titrated up to 480 mg/day at bedtime.

➤ Supraventricular tachyarrhythmias (SVTs)
Adults: 5 to 10 mg (0.075 to 0.15 mg/kg) I.V. bolus over 2 minutes; may give additional 10 mg after 30 minutes if response inadequate. Or 240 to 480 mg (immediate-release) P.O. daily in three or four divided doses.

➤ To control ventricular rate in chronic atrial flutter or atrial fibrillation in patients receiving digoxin
Adults: 240 to 320 mg P.O. daily in three or four divided doses

➤ Hypertension
Adults: Initially, 180 mg (extended-release tablet) or 200 mg (extended-release capsule) P.O. daily at bedtime. For maintenance, may titrate up to 480 mg (extended-release tablet) or 400 mg (extended-release capsule) P.O. daily at bedtime. Or initially, 80 mg (immediate-release tablet) P.O. t.i.d.; may titrate at daily or weekly intervals up to 360 to 480 mg/day. Or initially, 240 mg (sustained-release capsule) P.O. q day in morning; for maintenance, may titrate up to 240 mg P.O. b.i.d. or 480 mg P.O. once daily in morning. Titrate based on response.

Dosage adjustment

• Renal or hepatic impairment
• Concurrent digoxin therapy

Off-label uses

• Ventricular tachycardia
• Migraine headache prophylaxis
• Neurogenic bladder
• Premature labor

V

Contraindications

- Hypersensitivity to drug or other calcium channel blockers
- Sick sinus syndrome
- Second- or third-degree AV block (except in patients with artificial pacemakers)
- Hypotension
- Heart failure, severe ventricular dysfunction, or cardiogenic shock (except when associated with SVTs)
- Atrial flutter or atrial fibrillation associated with accessory bypass tracts (such as Wolff-Parkinson-White or Lown-Ganong-Levine syndrome)

Precautions

Use cautiously in:
- renal or severe hepatic impairment; first-degree AV block; idiopathic hypertrophic cardiomyopathy; neuromuscular transmission defects (such as Duchenne's muscular dystrophy); respiratory depression; digital ulcers, ischemia, or gangrene
- elderly patients
- pregnant or breastfeeding patients.

Administration

- Give I.V. over at least 2 minutes.
- Discontinue disopyramide 48 hours before starting verapamil. Don't restart disopyramide for at least 24 hours after verapamil therapy ends.

Route	Onset	Peak	Duration
P.O. (immediate)	30 min	1-2 hr	3-7 hr
P.O. (extended)	Unknown	5-7 hr	24 hr
P.O. (sustained)	Unknown	Unknown	Unknown
I.V.	Immediate	3-5 min	2 hr

Adverse reactions

CNS: anxiety, confusion, dizziness, syncope, drowsiness, headache, jitteriness, abnormal dreams, disturbed equilibrium, psychiatric disturbances, asthenia, paresthesia, tremor, fatigue

CV: chest pain, hypotension, palpitations, peripheral edema, tachycardia, **arrhythmias, heart failure, bradycardia, AV block**

EENT: blurred vision, epistaxis, tinnitus

GI: nausea, vomiting, diarrhea, constipation, dyspepsia, dry mouth, anorexia

GU: dysuria, urinary frequency, nocturia, polyuria, sexual dysfunction, gynecomastia

Hematologic: anemia, **leukopenia, thrombocytopenia**

Metabolic: hyperglycemia

Musculoskeletal: joint stiffness, muscle cramps

Respiratory: cough, dyspnea, shortness of breath, **pulmonary edema**

Skin: dermatitis, flushing, diaphoresis, photosensitivity, pruritus, urticaria, rash, **erythema multiforme, Stevens-Johnson syndrome**

Other: gingival hyperplasia, edema, weight gain

Interactions

Drug-drug. *Antihypertensives:* additive hypotension

Aspirin: increased risk of bleeding

Beta-adrenergic blockers, other antiarrhythmics: additive adverse cardiovascular reactions

Carbamazepine, cyclosporine: increased blood levels of these drugs

CYP450-3A4 inducers (such as rifampin): decreased verapamil blood level

CYP450-3A4 inhibitors (such as erythromycin, ritonavir): increased verapamil blood level

Digoxin: increased digoxin blood level, greater risk of toxicity

Lithium: increased or decreased lithium blood level

Neuromuscular blockers (succinylcholine, tubocurarine, vecuronium): prolonged neuromuscular blockade

Theophylline: decreased verapamil clearance, increased blood level, and possible toxicity

---

Drug-diagnostic tests. *Alanine aminotransferase, alkaline phosphatase, aspartate aminotransferase, blood urea nitrogen, glucose, lactate dehydrogenase:* increased levels
Granulocytes: decreased count
Drug-food. *Coffee, tea:* increased caffeine blood level
Grapefruit juice: increased verapamil blood level and effects
Drug-herbs. *Black catechu:* increased drug effects
Cola nut, guarana: increased caffeine blood level
Ephedra (ma huang), St. John's wort: reduced hypotensive effect of verapamil
Yerba maté: decreased clearance of this herb
Drug-behaviors. *Alcohol use:* additive hypotension

Patient monitoring
• With I.V. use, monitor vital signs and ECG continuously.
• Assess blood pressure when therapy begins and when dosage is adjusted.
• Watch closely for signs and symptoms of heart failure.
◀≷ Monitor for signs and symptoms of erythema multiforme (fever, rash, sore throat, mouth sores, cough, iris lesions). Report early indications immediately, before condition can progress to Stevens-Johnson syndrome.
• Assess CBC. Watch for blood dyscrasias.
• Monitor blood glucose level. Stay alert for hyperglycemia in diabetic patients.

Patient teaching
• Instruct patient to avoid chewing, breaking, or crushing extended-release form.
◀≷ Advise patient to immediately report rash, unusual bleeding or bruising, fainting, and (in long-term use) fatigue, nausea, or yellowing of skin or eyes.

• Caution patient not to take with grapefruit juice.
• Instruct patient to limit caffeine intake and avoid alcohol.
• Advise patient to seek medical advice before using over-the-counter medications or herbs.
• Tell patient to avoid sun exposure and to wear sunscreen and protective clothing when going outdoors.
• As appropriate, review all other significant and life-threatening adverse reactions and interactions, especially those related to the drugs, tests, foods, herbs, and behaviors mentioned above.

vinblastine sulfate (VLB)

Pharmacologic class: Vinca alkaloid
Therapeutic class: Antineoplastic
Pregnancy risk category D

FDA BOXED WARNING

• Drug should be administered only by individuals experienced in giving it. *Make sure needle is positioned properly in vein before injecting drug.* Leakage into surrounding tissue during I.V. administration may cause considerable irritation. If it does, discontinue injection immediately and inject remaining portion of dose into another vein. To treat extravasation, administer local injection of hyaluronidase and apply moderate heat to affected area.
• Drug is fatal if given intrathecally. Give I.V. only.

Action
Arrests mitosis and blocks cell division, interfering with nucleic acid synthesis. Cell-cycle-phase specific.

V

Availability
Lyophilized powder for injection: 10-mg vial

⬤ Indications and dosages
➢ Hodgkin's disease; advanced testicular cancer; lymphoma; AIDS-related Kaposi's sarcoma; bladder cancer; renal cancer; non-small-cell lung cancer; melanoma; breast cancer; choriocarcinoma; histiocytosis X; mycosis fungoides

Adults: 3.7 mg/m² I.V. weekly; may increase to a maximum of 18.5 mg/m² I.V. weekly, based on response. Withhold weekly dose if white blood cell (WBC) count is less than 4,000 cells/mm³. May increase dosage in increments of 1.8 mg/m² if needed, but not after WBC count drops to approximately 3,000 cells/mm³.

Dosage adjustment
• Hepatic impairment

Contraindications
• Hypersensitivity to drug
• Significant granulocytopenia from causes other than disease being treated
• Uncontrolled bacterial infections
• Intrathecal use
• Elderly patients with cachexia or skin ulcers

Precautions
Use cautiously in:
• hepatic or pulmonary dysfunction, renal disease with hypertension, malignant-cell infiltration of bone marrow, neuromuscular disease
• females of childbearing age
• pregnant or breastfeeding patients (use not recommended).

Administration
◀⟨ Follow facility protocol for handling and preparing chemotherapeutic drugs. Take special care to avoid eye contamination.

• Know that patient is usually premedicated with antiemetic.
◀⟨ Give by I.V. route only. (Intrathecal injection is fatal.)
• Reconstitute powder in 10-mg vial with 10 ml of normal saline solution for injection, to a concentration of 1 mg/ml. Refrigerate solution and protect from light; discard after 28 days.
• Inject I.V. dose into tubing of running I.V. line, or inject directly into vein over about 1 minute.
• Avoid extravasation, which may cause tissue necrosis. If extravasation occurs, stop injection, inject hyaluronidase locally, and apply moderate heat.

Route	Onset	Peak	Duration
I.V.	Unknown	Unknown	Unknown

Adverse reactions
CNS: headache, malaise, depression, paresthesia, loss of deep tendon reflexes, peripheral neuropathy and neuritis, **cerebrovascular accident, seizures**
CV: hypertension, tachycardia, **myocardial infarction**
EENT: pharyngitis
GI: nausea, vomiting, diarrhea, constipation, bleeding ulcer, abdominal pain, stomatitis, anorexia, **paralytic ileus**
GU: aspermia
Hematologic: anemia, **thrombocytopenia, leukopenia**
Metabolic: hyperuricemia, **syndrome of inappropriate antidiuretic hormone secretion**
Musculoskeletal: bone pain, muscle pain and weakness
Respiratory: shortness of breath, **acute bronchospasm, pulmonary infiltrates**
Skin: alopecia, skin irritation
Other: weight loss; jaw pain; tumor site pain; sloughing, cellulitis, and phlebitis at I.V. site; tissue necrosis (with extravasation)

Interactions
Drug-drug. *Erythromycin, other CYP450 inhibitors:* increased vinblastine toxicity
Mitomycin: increased risk of bronchospasm and shortness of breath
Phenytoin: decreased phenytoin blood level

Patient monitoring
◄€ Assess respiratory status closely. Drug may cause acute shortness of breath and bronchospasm, especially in patients who previously received mitomycin.
• Check injection site for extravasation.
• Monitor blood pressure.
• Assess CBC. Stay alert for signs and symptoms of infection.
• Monitor closely for numbness and tingling of hands or feet and other adverse reactions.

Patient teaching
• Explain drug therapy to patient. Emphasize importance of follow-up laboratory tests.
• Tell patient to promptly report signs and symptoms of infection and to take his temperature daily.
• Inform patient that drug may cause pain over tumor site.
• Instruct female of childbearing age to avoid pregnancy. Caution her not to breastfeed during therapy.
• Encourage patient to practice good oral hygiene to help prevent infected mouth sores.
• Inform patient that hair loss is a common side effect but typically reverses after treatment ends.
• As appropriate, review all other significant and life-threatening adverse reactions and interactions, especially those related to the drugs mentioned above.

vincristine sulfate (VCR)

Pharmacologic class: Vinca alkaloid
Therapeutic class: Antineoplastic
Pregnancy risk category D

FDA BOXED WARNING

• Drug should be administered only by individuals experienced in giving it. ***Make sure needle is positioned properly in vein before injecting drug.*** Leakage into surrounding tissue during I.V. administration may cause considerable irritation. If it does, discontinue injection immediately and inject remaining portion of dose into another vein. To treat extravasation, administer local injection of hyaluronidase and apply moderate heat to affected area.
• Drug is fatal if given intrathecally. Give I.V. only.

Action
Unknown. Thought to block cell division and interfere with synthesis of nucleic acid. Cell-cycle-phase specific.

Availability
Solution for injection: 1 mg/ml in 1-, 2-, and 5-ml vials

⚡ Indications and dosages
➤ Acute leukemia
Adults: 0.4 to 1.4 mg/m^2 I.V. weekly, not to exceed 2 mg/dose. (Dosages higher than 2 mg may be used depending on patient, physician, protocol, and facility.)
Children weighing more than 10 kg (22 lb): 2 mg/m^2 I.V. weekly
Children weighing 10 kg (22 lb) or less: 0.05 mg/kg I.V. weekly

V

Dosage adjustment
- Hepatic impairment

Off-label uses
- Brain, hepatic, ovarian, testicular, and other cancers
- Neuroblastoma
- Kaposi's sarcoma
- Idiopathic thrombocytopenic purpura

Contraindications
- Hypersensitivity to drug
- Demyelinating form of Charcot-Marie-Tooth disease
- Intrathecal use

Precautions
Use cautiously in:
- infections, decreased bone marrow reserve, hepatic impairment, acute uric acid nephropathy, neuromuscular disease, pulmonary dysfunction, other chronic debilitating illnesses
- females of childbearing age
- pregnant or breastfeeding patients (use not recommended).

Administration
◀ Follow facility protocol for handling and preparing chemotherapeutic drugs. Be especially careful to avoid eye contamination.
- Be aware that patient is usually premedicated with antiemetic.
◀ Give by I.V. route only. (Intrathecal injection is fatal.)
- Inject into tubing of running I.V. line, or inject directly into vein over 1 minute.
- Avoid extravasation (may cause tissue necrosis). If extravasation occurs, stop injection, inject hyaluronidase locally, and apply moderate heat.
- Know that drug may be used with other antineoplastics in some diseases.

Route	Onset	Peak	Duration
I.V.	Unknown	4 days	7 days

Adverse reactions
CNS: agitation, insomnia, depression, mental status changes, ascending peripheral neuropathy, transient cortical blindness, **seizures, coma**
EENT: diplopia
GI: nausea, vomiting, constipation, abdominal cramps, stomatitis, anorexia, **paralytic ileus**
GU: nocturia, urinary retention, gonadal suppression, **oliguria**
Hematologic: anemia, **leukopenia, thrombocytopenia** (mild and brief)
Metabolic: hyperuricemia, **syndrome of inappropriate antidiuretic hormone secretion**
Respiratory: bronchospasm
Skin: alopecia
Other: tissue necrosis (with extravasation), phlebitis at I.V. site

Interactions
Drug-drug. *Asparaginase:* decreased hepatic metabolism of vincristine
Live-virus vaccines: decreased antibody response to vaccine, increased risk of adverse reactions
Mitomycin: increased risk of bronchospasm and shortness of breath
Drug-diagnostic tests. *Platelets:* increased or decreased count
Uric acid: increased level
White blood cells: decreased count (slight leukopenia) 4 days after therapy, resolving within 7 days

Patient monitoring
◀ Assess respiratory status. Drug may cause bronchospasm, especially in patients who previously received mitomycin.
- Monitor blood pressure.
- Evaluate neurologic status. Know that neurotoxicity is a dose-limiting adverse reaction.
- Monitor CBC with platelet count. Watch for signs and symptoms of blood dyscrasias.
- Stay alert for signs and symptoms of infection.

Patient teaching

- Explain drug therapy to patient. Emphasize importance of follow-up laboratory tests.
- Advise patient to promptly report signs and symptoms of infection and to take his temperature daily.
- Urge patient to practice good oral hygiene, to help prevent infected mouth sores.
- Instruct female of childbearing age to avoid pregnancy. Caution her not to breastfeed during therapy.
- Tell patient that hair loss is a common side effect but typically reverses once treatment ends.
- As appropriate, review all other significant and life-threatening adverse reactions and interactions, especially those related to the drugs and tests mentioned above.

vinorelbine tartrate
Navelbine

Pharmacologic class: Vinca alkaloid
Therapeutic class: Antineoplastic
Pregnancy risk category D

FDA | **BOXED WARNING**

- Give under supervision of physician experienced in use of cancer chemotherapy, in facility with adequate diagnostic and treatment resources.
- *Product is for I.V. use only.* Intrathecal administration of other vinca alkaloids has resulted in death. Syringes containing this product should be labeled "WARNING. FOR I.V. USE ONLY. FATAL IF GIVEN INTRATHECALLY."
- Severe granulocytopenia causing increased susceptibility to infection may occur. Before starting drug, patient's granulocyte count should be

at least 1,000 cells/mm³. Adjust dosage according to complete blood counts (CBCs) with differentials obtained on day of treatment.
- *Make sure I.V. needle or catheter is properly positioned before injecting drug.* Administration may lead to extravasation, causing local tissue necrosis and thrombophlebitis.

Action

Blocks cell division and interferes with nucleic acid synthesis. Cell-cycle-phase specific.

Availability

Injection: 10 mg/ml in 1- and 5-ml vials

⚡ Indications and dosages

➤ Inoperable non-small-cell lung cancer
Adults: As monotherapy, 30 mg/m² I.V. weekly given over 6 to 10 minutes. In combination therapy, 25 mg/m² weekly given with cisplatin q 4 weeks. Alternatively, in combination therapy, 30 mg/m² I.V. given with cisplatin on days 1 and 29, then q 6 weeks.

Dosage adjustment

- Hepatic impairment
- Neurotoxicity

Off-label uses

- Cervical, breast, or ovarian cancer

Contraindications

- Hypersensitivity to drug
- Pretreatment granulocyte count below 1,000 cells/mm³

Precautions

Use cautiously in:
- hepatic impairment, decreased bone marrow reserve, past or present neuropathy
- history of radiation therapy

- females of childbearing age
- pregnant or breastfeeding patients (use not recommended)
- children (safety not established).

Administration

◀€ Follow facility protocols for handling and preparing chemotherapeutic drugs. Be especially careful to avoid eye contamination.

- Know that patient is usually premedicated with antiemetic.

◀€ Give by I.V. route only. (Intrathecal injection is fatal.)

- Before use, dilute drug in syringe with dextrose 5% in water or normal saline solution to yield a concentration of 1.5 to 3 mg/ml. Or dilute in I.V. bag of compatible solution to yield a concentration of 0.5 to 2 mg/ml.
- Administer into tubing of running I.V. line or directly into vein over 6 to 10 minutes. Immediately after injection, flush line with 75 to 125 ml of compatible I.V. solution.

Route	Onset	Peak	Duration
I.V.	Unknown	7-10 days	7-15 days

Adverse reactions

CNS: fatigue, **neurotoxicity**
CV: chest pain, phlebitis
GI: nausea, vomiting, diarrhea, constipation, abdominal pain, anorexia, **pancreatitis, intestinal obstruction, paralytic ileus**
Hematologic: anemia, **bone marrow depression, severe granulocytopenia, neutropenia, thrombocytopenia**
Metabolic: hyponatremia
Musculoskeletal: joint, back, or jaw pain; myalgia
Respiratory: acute respiratory distress syndrome, acute shortness of breath, bronchospasm, interstitial pulmonary changes
Skin: alopecia, rash, skin reactions
Other: tumor site pain; irritation, pain, and phlebitis at I.V. site; **sepsis**

Interactions

Drug-drug. *Cisplatin, other antineoplastics:* increased risk and severity of bone marrow depression
Mitomycin: increased risk of acute pulmonary reaction

Drug-diagnostic tests. *Bilirubin, hepatic enzymes, liver function tests:* increased values
Granulocytes, hemoglobin, platelets, white blood cells: decreased levels

Patient monitoring

- Monitor vital signs closely.
- Assess liver function tests and CBC with platelet count.
- Watch for signs and symptoms of infection.
- Observe injection site closely for reactions and extravasation.

◀€ Closely monitor neurologic and respiratory status. Drug may lead to acute pulmonary changes, especially in patients who previously received mitomycin.

Patient teaching

- Explain drug therapy to patient. Emphasize importance of follow-up laboratory tests.
- Advise patient to promptly report signs and symptoms of infection and to take his temperature daily.
- Tell patient that hair loss is a common side effect but typically reverses once treatment ends.
- Instruct female of childbearing age to avoid pregnancy. Caution her not to breastfeed during therapy.
- Urge patient to practice good oral hygiene, to help prevent infected mouth sores.
- As appropriate, review all other significant and life-threatening adverse reactions and interactions, especially those related to the drugs and tests mentioned above.

voriconazole
Vfend

Pharmacologic class: Triazole
Therapeutic class: Antifungal
Pregnancy risk category D

Action
Inhibits fungal cytochrome P450–mediated 14-alpha-lanosterol demethylation, preventing fungal biosynthesis and inactivating fungal cell

Availability
Lyophilized powder for injection: 200 mg
Powder for oral suspension: 40 mg/ml
Tablets: 50 mg, 200 mg

ⓘ Indications and dosages
➤ Invasive aspergillosis; serious fungal infections caused by *Scedosporium apiospermum* and *Fusarium* species
Adults and children ages 12 and older: Initially, 6 mg/kg I.V. q 12 hours for two doses (each dose infused over 1 to 2 hours), followed by a maintenance dose of 4 mg/kg I.V. q 12 hours given no faster than 3 mg/kg/hour. Change to oral dosing as described below when patient can tolerate it.
Adults and children ages 12 and older weighing more than 40 kg (88 lb): 200 mg P.O. q 12 hours 1 hour before or after a meal; may increase to 300 mg P.O. q 12 hours p.r.n.
Adults and children ages 12 and older weighing less than 40 kg (88 lb): 100 mg P.O. q 12 hours at least 1 hour before or after a meal; may increase to 150 mg P.O. q 12 hours p.r.n.
➤ Esophageal candidiasis
Adults and children ages 12 and older weighing 40 kg (88 lb) or more: 200 mg P.O. q 12 hours for at least 14 days, and for at least 7 days after symptoms resolve

Adults and children ages 12 and older weighing less than 40 kg (88 lb): 100 mg P.O. q 12 hours for at least 14 days, and for at least 7 days after symptoms resolve
➤ Candidemia (in nonneutropenic patients) and other deep-tissue *Candida* infections
Adults and children ages 12 and older: 6 mg/kg I.V. q 12 hours for first 24 hours, followed by maintenance dose of 3 mg/kg I.V. q 12 hours. Or 200 mg P.O. q 12 hours for candidemia and 4 mg/kg I.V. q 12 hours or 200 mg P.O. q 12 hours for other deep-tissue *Candida* infections. Patients should be treated for at least 14 days after resolution of symptoms or after last positive culture, whichever is longer.

Dosage adjustment
• Mild to moderate hepatic impairment
• Moderate to severe renal impairment (with I.V. use)
• Adult patients weighing less than 40 kg (88 lb)
• Concurrent use of phenytoin or efavirenz

Off-label uses
• Febrile neutropenia (as empiric therapy)

Contraindications
• Hypersensitivity to drug or its components
• Concurrent use of long-acting barbiturates, ergot alkaloids, rifabutin, rifampin, CYP450-3A4 substrates (such as astemizole, cisapride, pimozide, quinidine, terfenadine), sirolimus, high-dose ritonavir, St. John's wort, or carbamazepine

Precautions
Use cautiously in:
• hypersensitivity to other azoles
• renal disease, hepatic dysfunction, risk factors for pancreatitis (such as

V

Reactions in **bold** are life-threatening.　　　　◀€ Clinical alert

recent chemotherapy, hematopoietic stem cell transplant)

• hereditary problems of galactose intolerance, Lapp lactase deficiency, or glucose-galactose malabsorption (avoid tablet use)

• concurrent use of low-dose ritonavir (avoid use unless benefit-risk to patient justifies use)

• pregnant or breastfeeding patients

• children younger than age 12 (safety and efficacy not established).

Administration

• Correct electrolyte disturbances before therapy starts.

◀€ Don't give concurrently with astemizole, cisapride, or terfenadine (no longer available in U.S.); carbamazepine; ergot alkaloids; long-acting barbiturates; pimozide; quinidine; rifabutin; rifampin; ritonavir; or sirolimus.

◀€ Don't give by I.V. bolus injection.

• Reconstitute powder with 19 ml of water for injection, to yield a volume of 20 ml. Shake vial until powder dissolves. Withdraw prescribed dose, then dilute further in compatible I.V. solution to a final concentration of 0.5 to 5 mg/ml. Give I.V. over 1 to 2 hours at a rate not exceeding 3 mg/kg/hour.

• Don't give through same I.V. line with other drugs, blood products, or electrolytes.

• To reconstitute powder for oral suspension, tap bottle to release powder. Add 46 ml of water, and shake vigorously for about 1 minute. Remove cap, push bottle adapter into neck of bottle, and replace cap. After reconstitution, suspension volume is 75 ml, providing usable volume of 70 ml (40 mg/ml). Shake bottle before each use. Use only 5-ml oral dispenser supplied. Don't mix with other drugs, and don't dilute further.

• Give oral suspension and tablets 1 hour before or after a meal.

Route	Onset	Peak	Duration
P.O.	1-2 hr	Unknown	Unknown
I.V.	Start of infusion	Unknown	Unknown

Adverse reactions

CNS: dizziness, headache, hallucinations

CV: hypotension, hypertension, tachycardia, chest pain, vasodilation, peripheral edema

EENT: photophobia, blurred vision, visual disturbances, eye hemorrhage, chromatopsia

GI: nausea, vomiting, diarrhea, abdominal pain, dry mouth, **pancreatitis**

GU: renal dysfunction, **acute renal failure**

Hematologic: anemia, **pancytopenia, leukopenia, thrombocytopenia**

Hepatic: cholestatic jaundice, **hepatic failure**

Metabolic: hypomagnesemia, hypokalemia

Musculoskeletal: fluorosis, periostitis (with long-term use)

Respiratory: respiratory disorders

Skin: pruritus, maculopapular rash, **erythema multiforme, toxic epidermal necrolysis, Stevens-Johnson syndrome**

Other: chills, fever, **sepsis, infusion-related reactions** including **anaphylaxis**

Interactions

Drug-drug. *Barbiturates (long-acting), carbamazepine, phenytoin, rifampin:* decreased voriconazole blood level

Benzodiazepines: sedation

Calcium channel blockers, HMG-CoA reductase inhibitors: increased blood levels of these drugs

Cyclosporine, sirolimus, tacrolimus: increased blood levels of these drugs, greater risk of nephrotoxicity

CYP450-3A4 substrates: increased blood levels of these drugs, causing prolonged QT interval and risk of torsades de pointes

---

Ergot alkaloids: increased blood levels of these drugs, resulting in ergotism
Non-nucleoside reverse transcriptase inhibitors, protease inhibitors: inhibited voriconazole metabolism
Rifabutin: decreased voriconazole blood level, increased rifabutin blood level
Sulfonylureas: increased sulfonylurea blood level, greater risk of hypoglycemia
Vinca alkaloids: increased risk of neurotoxicity
Warfarin, other coumarin derivatives: increased partial thromboplastin time
Drug-diagnostic tests. *Alanine aminotransferase, alkaline phosphatase, aspartate aminotransferase, bilirubin, creatinine:* increased levels
Drug-herbs. *Gossypol:* increased risk of nephrotoxicity
St. John's wort: significantly reduced voriconazole plasma exposure

Patient monitoring
• Monitor kidney and liver function tests. Watch for signs and symptoms of organ toxicity.
• Assess electrolyte levels and CBC, including platelet count.
◀€ Monitor ECG. Stay alert for prolonged QT interval.
◀€ During infusion, monitor patient for anaphylactoid-type reactions, including flushing, fever, sweating, tachycardia, chest tightness, dyspnea, faintness, nausea, pruritus, and rash; consider stopping infusion should these reactions occur.
◀€ Be aware of postmarketing reports of pancreatitis, especially in children, and monitor appropriately.
◀€ Monitor patient receiving long-term therapy for skeletal pain. Discontinue drug if radiologic findings indicate fluorosis or periostitis.
• Check for vision problems in therapy exceeding 28 days.

Patient teaching
• Explain therapy to patient. Stress importance of follow-up laboratory tests.
• Tell patient using oral form to take doses 1 hour before or after a meal.
• Emphasize importance of taking drug exactly as directed for entire duration prescribed.
• Instruct patient to promptly report adverse reactions.
• Tell female of childbearing age to immediately report pregnancy.
• Caution patient to avoid driving and other hazardous activities, because drug may cause visual disturbances.
• Advise patient to minimize GI upset by eating small, frequent servings of food and drinking plenty of fluids.
• Advise patient not to use St. John's wort without consulting prescriber.
• As appropriate, review all other significant and life-threatening adverse reactions and interactions, especially those related to the drugs, tests, and herbs mentioned above.

warfarin sodium
Apo-Warfarin✤, Coumadin, Gen-Warfarin✤, Jantoven, Marevan⊕, Novo-Warfarin✤, Taro-Warfarin✤

Pharmacologic class: Coumarin derivative
Therapeutic class: Anticoagulant
Pregnancy risk category X

W

- Drug may cause major or fatal bleeding. Bleeding is more likely during starting period and with higher dosage (resulting in higher International Normalized Ratio [INR]). Monitor INR regularly in all patients. Those at high risk for bleeding may benefit from more frequent INR monitoring, careful dosage adjustment, and shorter duration of therapy. Instruct patients about measures to minimize risk of bleeding and advise them to immediately report signs and symptoms of bleeding.

Action
Interferes with synthesis of vitamin K–dependent clotting factors (II, VII, IX, and X) and anticoagulant proteins C and S in liver

Availability
Injection: 5.4 mg/vial (2 mg/ml when reconstituted)
Tablets: 1 mg, 2 mg, 2.5 mg, 3 mg, 4 mg, 5 mg, 6 mg, 7.5 mg, 10 mg

⚱ Indications and dosages
➣ Venous thrombosis; pulmonary embolism; atrial fibrillation; myocardial infarction (MI); thromboembolic complications of cardiac valve placement
Adults: Initially, 2.5 to 10 mg P.O. or I.V. daily for 2 to 4 days, then adjusted based on prothrombin time (PT) or International Normalized Ratio (INR). Usual maintenance dosage is 2 to 10 mg P.O. daily.

Dosage adjustment
- Elderly or debilitated patients

Off-label uses
- Acute coronary syndrome
- Intracoronary stent placement
- Prevention of catheter thrombosis

Contraindications
- Hypersensitivity to drug
- Uncontrolled bleeding
- Open wounds
- Severe hepatic disease
- Hemorrhagic or bleeding tendency
- Cerebrovascular hemorrhage
- Cerebral aneurysm or dissecting aorta
- Blood dyscrasias
- Pericarditis or pericardial effusion
- Bacterial endocarditis
- Malignant hypertension
- Recent brain, eye, or spinal cord injury or surgery
- Lumbar puncture and other procedures that may cause uncontrollable bleeding
- Major regional or lumbar block anesthesia
- Threatened abortion, eclampsia, preeclampsia
- Unsupervised senile, alcoholic, or psychotic patients
- Pregnancy, females of childbearing potential

Precautions
Use cautiously in:
- cancer, heparin-induced thrombocytopenia, moderate to severe renal impairment, moderate to severe hypertension, infectious GI disease, known or suspected deficiency in protein C–mediated anticoagulant response, polycythemia vera, vasculitis, severe diabetes mellitus
- indwelling catheter use
- history of poor compliance
- elderly or debilitated patients
- breastfeeding patients
- children younger than age 18 (safety and efficacy not established).

Administration
◀≋ Be aware that warfarin is a high-alert drug.
- Know that I.V. form is reserved for patients who can't tolerate oral form. I.V. and oral dosages are identical.

- For I.V. use, reconstitute vial with 2.7 ml of sterile water for injection; administer over 1 to 2 minutes. After reconstitution, drug is stable for 4 hours at room temperature.
- Be aware that vitamin K reverses warfarin effects. If major bleeding occurs, fresh frozen plasma may be given.
- When converting to warfarin from heparin, give both drugs concomitantly for 4 to 5 days until therapeutic effect of warfarin occurs.

Route	Onset	Peak	Duration
P.O.	Several hr	0.5-3 days	2-5 days
I.V.	Unknown	Unknown	Unknown

Adverse reactions

GI: nausea, vomiting, diarrhea, abdominal cramps, stomatitis, anorexia
GU: hematuria
Hematologic: eosinophilia, **bleeding, hemorrhage, agranulocytosis, leukopenia**
Hepatic: hepatitis
Skin: rash, dermatitis, urticaria, pruritus, alopecia, dermal necrosis
Other: fever, "purple toes" syndrome (bilateral painful, purple lesions on toes and sides of feet), hypersensitivity reaction

Interactions

Drug-drug. *Abciximab, acetaminophen (chronic use), androgens, aspirin, capecitabine, cefamandole, cefoperazone, cefotetan, chloral hydrate, chloramphenicol, clopidogrel, disulfiram, eptifibatide, fluconazole, fluoroquinolones, itraconazole, metronidazole (including vaginal use), nonsteroidal anti-inflammatory drugs, plicamycin, quinidine, quinine, sulfonamides, thrombolytics, ticlopidine, tirofiban, valproic acid, zafirlukast:* increased response to warfarin, greater risk of bleeding

Barbiturates, hormonal contraceptives containing estrogen: decreased anticoagulant effect
Drug-diagnostic tests. *Alanine aminotransferase, aspartate aminotransferase, INR:* increased values
Partial thromboplastin time, PT: prolonged
Drug-food. *Vitamin K–rich foods (large amounts):* antagonism of anticoagulant effect
Drug-herbs. *Angelica:* prolonged PT
Anise, arnica, asafetida, bromelain, chamomile, clove, danshen, devil's claw, dong quai, fenugreek, feverfew, garlic, ginger, ginkgo, ginseng, horse chestnut, licorice, meadowsweet, motherwort, onion, papain, parsley, passionflower, quassia, red clover, Reishi mushroom, rue, sweet clover, turmeric, white willow, others: increased risk of bleeding
Coenzyme Q10, green tea, St. John's wort: decreased anticoagulant effect
Drug-behaviors. *Alcohol use:* enhanced warfarin activity

Patient monitoring

- Monitor PT, INR, and liver function tests.
- Watch for signs and symptoms of bleeding and hepatitis.

Patient teaching

◀€ Explain therapy to patient. Stress importance of adhering to schedule for laboratory tests.
◀€ Instruct patient to promptly report unusual bleeding or bruising.
- Caution patient to consult prescriber before taking over-the-counter preparations or herbs.
- Advise patient to inform all other health care providers (including dentist) that he is taking warfarin.
- Tell patient not to vary his intake of foods high in vitamin K (such as leafy green vegetables, fish, pork, green tea, and tomatoes), to avoid alterations in drug's anticoagulant effect.

W

🔊 Instruct females of childbearing age to report pregnancy immediately.

• Stress importance of avoiding contact sports and other activities that could cause injury and bleeding.

• Caution patient to avoid alcohol during therapy.

• As appropriate, review all other significant and life-threatening adverse reactions and interactions, especially those related to the drugs, tests, foods, herbs, and behaviors mentioned above.

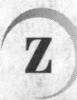

zafirlukast

Accolate

Pharmacologic class: Leukotriene receptor antagonist

Therapeutic class: Antiasthmatic, bronchodilator

Pregnancy risk category B

Action

Antagonizes activity of three leukotrienes at specific receptor sites in airway smooth muscle, inhibiting inflammation

Availability

Tablets (coated): 10 mg, 20 mg

🕊 Indications and dosages

➤ Prophylaxis and long-term treatment of asthma

Adults and children ages 12 and older: 20 mg P.O. b.i.d.

Children ages 5 to 11: 10 mg P.O. b.i.d.

Off-label uses

• Exercise-induced bronchospasm
• Chronic urticaria

Contraindications

• Hypersensitivity to drug or its components

• Hepatic impairment, including hepatic cirrhosis

Precautions

Use cautiously in:

• acute asthma attacks
• concurrent use of warfarin
• patients older than age 55
• pregnant patients
• breastfeeding patients (use not recommended)
• children younger than age 5 (safety not established).

Administration

• Give at least 1 hour before or 2 hours after a meal.

Route	Onset	Peak	Duration
P.O.	30 min	3.5 hr	12 hr

Adverse reactions

CNS: headache, dizziness, asthenia, insomnia, depression (especially in children and adolescents)

GI: nausea, vomiting, diarrhea, abdominal pain, dyspepsia

Hepatic: hepatic dysfunction including liver failure and death (rare)

Musculoskeletal: joint or back pain, myalgia

Other: fever, infection, pain

Interactions

Drug-drug. *Aspirin:* increased zafirlukast blood level

Erythromycin, theophylline: decreased zafirlukast blood level

Warfarin: increased warfarin effects, greater risk of bleeding

Drug-food. *Any food:* decreased rate and extent of zafirlukast absorption

Patient monitoring

• Assess patient's respiratory status to help evaluate drug efficacy.

◀€ Monitor liver function tests closely; watch for signs and symptoms of liver dysfunction.

Patient teaching

• Tell patient to take at least 1 hour before or 2 hours after a meal.
• Advise patient to take exactly as prescribed, even if he is symptom-free.
◀€ Tell patient to immediately report asthma attack. Advise him not to use drug for rapid relief of bronchospasm.
• Instruct patient to continue taking other asthma drugs unless prescriber directs otherwise.
◀€ Instruct patient to immediately report signs and symptoms of liver dysfunction (nausea, anorexia, fatigue, lethargy, pruritus, jaundice, flulike symptoms, or right upper quadrant abdominal pain).
• Instruct patient or caregiver to report insomnia or depression.
• Instruct female patient to consult prescriber if she plans to breastfeed.
• As appropriate, review all other significant adverse reactions and interactions, especially those related to the drugs and foods mentioned above.

zaleplon
Sonata

Pharmacologic class: Pyrazolopyrimidine, nonbenzodiazepine hypnotic
Therapeutic class: Sedative-hypnotic
Controlled substance schedule IV
Pregnancy risk category C

Action

Binds to omega-1 receptor of gamma-aminobutyric acid receptor complex, relaxing smooth muscles, reducing anxiety, and producing sedation. Also has anticonvulsant effect.

Availability

Capsules: 5 mg, 10 mg

Indications and dosages

➤ Insomnia
Adults younger than age 65: 10 mg P.O. at bedtime. Dosage above 20 mg is not recommended.

Dosage adjustment

• Mild to moderate hepatic impairment
• Elderly or debilitated patients

Contraindications

• Hypersensitivity to drug or its components

Precautions

Use cautiously in:
• tartrazine sensitivity
• severe renal impairment (use not recommended), mild to moderate hepatic impairment, respiratory impairment, depression
• history of suicide attempt
• patients weighing less than 50 kg (110 lb)
• patients older than age 65
• pregnant or breastfeeding patients (use not recommended)
• children younger than age 18 (safety not established).

Administration

• Give at bedtime.
• Don't administer with high-fat meal.

Route	Onset	Peak	Duration
P.O.	Rapid	1 hr	3-4 hr

Adverse reactions

CNS: headache, amnesia, anxiety, hallucinations, light-headedness, dizziness, drowsiness, depersonalization, transient memory or psychomotor impairment, incoordination, malaise, vertigo, asthenia, hyperesthesia, paresthesia, tremor
CV: peripheral edema

Z

EENT: abnormal vision, eye pain, ear pain, hearing sensitivity, epistaxis
GI: nausea, abdominal pain, colitis, dyspepsia, anorexia
GU: dysmenorrhea
Musculoskeletal: myalgia
Skin: photosensitivity
Other: altered sense of smell, fever

Interactions
Drug-drug. *Cimetidine:* decreased metabolism and increased effects of zaleplon
CNS depressants (including antihistamines, opioids, other sedative-hypnotics, phenothiazines, tricyclic antidepressants): additive CNS depression
CYP450-3A4 inducers (such as carbamazepine, phenobarbital, phenytoin, rifampin): decreased blood level and reduced efficacy of zaleplon
CYP450-3A4 inhibitors (such as erythromycin, ketoconazole): increased zaleplon blood level
Drug-food. *High-fat meal:* delayed drug absorption
Drug-herbs. *Chamomile, hops, kava, skullcap, valerian:* increased CNS depression
Drug-behaviors. *Alcohol use:* increased CNS depression

Patient monitoring
• Monitor drug efficacy. Insomnia persisting after 7 to 10 days warrants re-evaluation for underlying psychological or physical illness.
• Stay alert for adverse drug reactions.

Patient teaching
• Explain therapy to patient. Emphasize importance of taking drug just before bedtime or after trying to sleep—but only if he will be able to get at least 4 hours of sleep.
• Inform patient that high-fat meal slows drug absorption and delays drug effects.

• Caution patient to avoid driving and other hazardous activities while under drug's influence.
• Instruct patient to avoid alcohol during therapy.
• Tell patient rebound insomnia may occur for 1 or 2 nights after he stops taking drug.
• Advise female of childbearing age to notify prescriber if she is or plans to become pregnant or if she is breastfeeding.
• As appropriate, review all other significant adverse reactions and interactions, especially those related to the drugs, foods, herbs, and behaviors mentioned above.

zanamivir
Relenza

Pharmacologic class: Neuraminidase inhibitor
Therapeutic class: Antiviral
Pregnancy risk category C

Action
Inhibits influenza virus neuraminidase, an enzyme essential for viral replication

Availability
Powder for inhalation: 5 mg/blister

⚡ Indications and dosages
➤ Prevention of influenza
Adults and children ages 5 and older: Prophylaxis in the household setting, 2 inhalations (10 mg) once daily for 10 days. Prophylaxis during community outbreaks, 2 inhalations (10 mg) once daily for 28 days.
➤ Influenza virus A or B
Adults and children ages 7 and older: Two oral inhalations (5 mg/inhalation) b.i.d. for 5 days

Contraindications

• History of allergic reaction to components of drug, including lactose milk proteins

Precautions

Use cautiously in:
• chronic obstructive pulmonary disease, asthma, lactose intolerance
• concurrent use of live attenuated intranasal influenza vaccine (Don't administer until 48 hours after cessation of zanamivir and don't administer zanamivir until 2 weeks after administration of live attenuated influenza vaccine, unless medically indicated.)
• pregnant or breastfeeding patients
• children younger than age 7 (safety not established).

Administration

• Give two doses on day 1, spaced at least 2 hours apart. On subsequent days, space doses 12 hours apart, and give at approximately same time each day.

Route	Onset	Peak	Duration
Inhalation	Rapid	1-2 hr	12 hr

Adverse reactions

CNS: headache, dizziness
EENT: sinusitis, EENT infections
GI: nausea, vomiting, diarrhea
Respiratory: bronchitis, cough
Other: allergic reaction

Interactions

None significant

Patient monitoring

• Assess respiratory status. Watch closely for signs and symptoms of declining respiratory function.

Patient teaching

• Explain therapy to patient. Demonstrate how to use Diskhaler device.
• Tell patient to take drug exactly as prescribed for as long as directed, even if symptoms improve.

• If patient is also taking an inhaled bronchodilator, advise him to take bronchodilator before zanamivir.
• Emphasize that drug doesn't prevent spread of influenza to others.
• Instruct patient to immediately report worsening respiratory symptoms.
• As appropriate, review other significant adverse reactions.

zidovudine

Apo-Zidovudine✦, Novo-AZT✦, Retrovir

Pharmacologic class: Nucleoside reverse transcriptase inhibitor
Therapeutic class: Antiretroviral
Pregnancy risk category C

FDA BOXED WARNING

• Drug has been linked to hematologic toxicity (including neutropenia and severe anemia), particularly in patients with advanced human immunodeficiency virus (HIV) infection.
• Prolonged use is associated with symptomatic myopathy.
• Lactic acidosis and severe hepatomegaly with steatosis (including fatal cases) have occurred with use of nucleoside analogs alone or in combination, including zidovudine and other antiretrovirals.

Action

After conversion to its active metabolite, inhibits activity of HIV reverse transcriptase and terminates viral DNA growth

Availability

Capsules: 100 mg
Injection: 10 mg/ml in 20-ml vial
Syrup: 50 mg/5 ml
Tablets: 300 mg

Z

Reactions in **bold** are life-threatening.　　　　◀€ Clinical alert

⁄ Indications and dosages
➤ HIV-1 infection

Adults and children older than age 12: 600 mg P.O. total daily dosage divided into either b.i.d. or t.i.d. dosing; or 1 mg/kg I.V. five to six times daily; in combination with other antiretrovirals

Children ages 4 weeks to younger than 18 years weighing 30 kg (66 lb) or more: 600 mg P.O. total daily dosage divided into either b.i.d. or t.i.d. dosing; or 480 mg/m^2 total daily dosage divided into either b.i.d. or t.i.d. dosing. Don't exceed recommended adult dosage.

Children ages 4 weeks to younger than 18 years weighing 9 kg (20 lb) to less than 30 kg (66 lb): 18 mg/kg/day total daily dosage divided into either b.i.d. or t.i.d. dosing; or 480 mg/m^2 total daily dosage divided into either b.i.d. or t.i.d. dosing. Don't exceed recommended adult dosage.

Children ages 4 weeks to younger than 18 years weighing 4 kg (9 lb) to less than 9 kg (20 lb): 24 mg/kg/day total daily dosage divided into either b.i.d. or t.i.d. dosing; or 480 mg/m^2 total daily dosage divided into either b.i.d. or t.i.d. dosing. Don't exceed recommended adult dosage.

➤ To prevent maternal-fetal HIV transmission

Pregnant women (more than 14 weeks of pregnancy): 500 mg P.O. daily in divided doses (usually as five 100-mg doses) until labor begins; then 2 mg/kg I.V. over 1 hour followed by a continuous infusion of 1 mg/kg/hour until umbilical cord is clamped

Neonates: 2 mg/kg P.O. q 6 hours starting within 12 hours of delivery and continuing for 6 weeks. For neonates unable to receive oral dosing, 1.5 mg/kg by I.V. infusion over 30 minutes q 6 hours

Dosage adjustment
• End-stage renal disease in patients maintained on hemodialysis or peritoneal dialysis

• Hematologic toxicity
• Concurrent use of drugs (such as fluconazole or valproic acid) in patients experiencing pronounced anemia

Off-label uses
• Occupational exposure to HIV

Contraindications
• Patients who have had potentially life-threatening allergic reactions (such as anaphylaxis, Stevens-Johnson syndrome) to drug or its components

Precautions
Use cautiously in:
• renal or hepatic impairment, known risk factors for liver disease, decreased bone marrow reserve, hemoglobin less than 9.5 g/dl, granulocyte count less than 1,000 cells/mm^3
• concurrent use of Combivir or Trizivir (zidovudine-containing products) or interferon- and ribavirin-based regimens
• pregnant or breastfeeding patients.

Administration
◀€ For I.V. use, remove dose from vial and add to I.V. solution containing dextrose 5% in water, to yield a final concentration no higher than 4 mg/ml. Infuse over 1 hour. Avoid rapid infusion or bolus injection. Don't give by I.M. route.
• In adults, give by I.V. route only until patient can tolerate oral dose.
• If a child is unable to reliably swallow a capsule or tablet, give syrup formulation.

Route	Onset	Peak	Duration
P.O.	Variable	30-90 min	4 hr
I.V.	Rapid	End of infusion	4 hr

Adverse reactions
CNS: headache, paresthesia, malaise, insomnia, dizziness, drowsiness, asthenia, **seizures**

GI: nausea, vomiting, constipation, abdominal pain, dyspepsia, anorexia, **pancreatitis**
Hematologic: severe anemia (necessitating transfusions), **agranulocytopenia, severe bone marrow depression**
Hepatic: severe hepatomegaly with steatosis
Metabolic: lactic acidosis
Musculoskeletal: myalgia, back pain, myopathy
Respiratory: dyspnea
Skin: diaphoresis, rash, altered nail pigmentation
Other: abnormal taste, fever, **immune reconstitution syndrome**

Interactions

Drug-drug. *Acetaminophen, aspirin, indomethacin:* increased risk of zidovudine toxicity
Amphotericin B, dapsone, flucytosine, pentamidine: increased risk of nephrotoxicity and bone marrow depression
Cyclosporine: extreme drowsiness, lethargy
Cytotoxic drugs, myelosuppressants, nephrotoxic drugs (such as ganciclovir, interferon alfa): increased risk of hematologic toxicity
Fluconazole, methadone, probenecid, valproic acid: increased zidovudine blood level, greater risk of toxicity
Ribavirin: antagonism of zidovudine's antiviral activity
Drug-diagnostic tests. *Granulocytes, hemoglobin, platelets:* decreased levels
Drug-herbs. *St. John's wort:* decreased zidovudine efficacy

Patient monitoring

• Monitor neurologic status, especially for signs and symptoms of impending seizure.
◀╪ Periodically assess CBC and kidney and liver function tests. Be aware that drug can cause hepatotoxicity.
◀╪ Watch for signs and symptoms of pancreatitis, immune reconstitution syndrome, and lactic acidosis.

Patient teaching

• Tell patient he may take with or without food.
• Instruct patient to take capsules with at least 4 oz of fluid and to stay upright after taking.
• Explain therapy to patient. Emphasize that drug doesn't cure HIV infection.
• Urge patient to take drug exactly as prescribed.
◀╪ Teach patient to recognize and immediately report signs and symptoms of serious side effects, such as seizures.
• Stress importance of follow-up laboratory testing.
• Advise female of childbearing age to use effective contraception.
• Inform pregnant patient that drug reduces risk of, but may not prevent, HIV transmission to neonate.
• As appropriate, review all other significant and life-threatening adverse reactions and interactions, especially those related to the drugs, tests, and herbs mentioned above.

ziprasidone hydrochloride
Geodon, Zeldox❤

Pharmacologic class: Benzisoxazole derivative
Therapeutic class: Antipsychotic
Pregnancy risk category C

FDA   BOXED WARNING

• Elderly patients with dementia-related psychosis are at increased risk for death. Although causes of death varied, most appeared to be cardiovascular or infectious.
• Drug isn't approved for treatment of dementia-related psychosis.

Z

Action
Unknown. Thought to antagonize dopamine$_2$ and serotonin$_2$ receptors.

Availability
Capsules: 20 mg, 40 mg, 60 mg, 80 mg
Injection (powder, lyophilized for solution): 20 mg/ml

⚕ Indications and dosages
➤ Schizophrenia
Adults: Initially, 20 mg P.O. b.i.d. with food; may increase q 2 days up to 80 mg b.i.d. Usual maintenance dosage is 20 to 80 mg P.O. b.i.d.; maximum recommended dosage is 80 mg b.i.d. For prompt control of acute agitation, 10 to 20 mg I.M. as a single dose; depending on patient's response, may repeat 10-mg I.M. dose q 2 hours or 20-mg I.M. dose q 4 hours to a maximum daily dosage of 40 mg.
➤ Acute treatment as monotherapy of manic or mixed episodes associated with bipolar I disorder
Adults: Initially, 40 mg P.O. b.i.d. with food; may increase to 60 or 80 mg P.O. b.i.d. on second day of treatment and subsequently adjust on basis of tolerance and efficacy within range of 40 to 80 mg P.O. b.i.d. For maintenance (as an adjunct to lithium or valproate), continue treatment at same dosage on which patient was initially stabilized, within range of 40 to 80 mg P.O. b.i.d. with food; also continue periodic assessments to determine need for maintenance treatment.

Contraindications
- Hypersensitivity to drug
- History of arrhythmias, prolonged QT interval
- Recent myocardial infarction
- Uncompensated heart failure
- Concomitant use of arsenic trioxide, chlorpromazine, class IA or III antiarrhythmics, or other drugs that prolong the QT interval

Precautions
Use cautiously in:
- renal impairment, cerebrovascular disease, history of seizures or with conditions that lower seizure threshold, cardiovascular disorders, dysphagia, hyperprolactinemia
- bradycardia, hypokalemia, or hypomagnesemia (avoid use)
- adverse reactions with previous use of atypical antipsychotics (such as risperidone or clozapine)
- pregnant patients
- breastfeeding patients (use not recommended)
- children (safety and efficacy not established).

Administration
- Give with food.
- Know that P.O. therapy should replace I.M. therapy as soon as possible.
- 🔊 Don't give with drugs that prolong the QT interval.

Route	Onset	Peak	Duration
P.O.	Several hr	1-3 days	Unknown
I.M.	Unknown	1 hr	Unknown

Adverse reactions
CNS: dizziness, drowsiness, dystonia, hypertonia, asthenia, akathisia, extrapyramidal reactions, agitation, headache, insomnia, personality disorder, paresthesia, speech disorder, **neuroleptic malignant syndrome, seizures, suicide attempt**
CV: orthostatic hypotension, hypertension, tachycardia, **arrhythmias** (from prolonged QT interval)
EENT: abnormal vision, rhinitis
GI: nausea, vomiting, diarrhea, constipation, dyspepsia, dry mouth, anorexia
GU: dysmenorrhea, priapism
Metabolic: hypomagnesemia (rare), hypokalemia, hyperglycemia
Musculoskeletal: myalgia
Respiratory: cough, cold symptoms

Skin: urticaria, rash, fungal dermatitis, diaphoresis, photosensitivity
Other: accidental injury, pain at I.M. injection site

Interactions

Drug-drug. *Antihypertensives:* additive hypotension
Carbamazepine: decreased ziprasidone blood level
Centrally acting drugs: additive CNS effects
Dopamine agonists, levodopa: antagonism of these drugs' effects
Drugs that decrease potassium or magnesium level (such as diuretics) or prolong QT interval (such as dofetilide, moxifloxacin, pimozide, quinidine, sotalol, sparfloxacin, thioridazine): increased risk of arrhythmias
Ketoconazole: increased ziprasidone blood level
Drug-diagnostic tests. *Glucose, magnesium, potassium:* decreased levels
Drug-food. *Any food:* increased drug absorption
Drug-herbs. *Chamomile, hops, kava, skullcap, valerian:* increased CNS depression

Patient monitoring

◀≡ Monitor ECG before and during therapy. Stay alert for prolonged QT interval. Know that dizziness, syncope, or palpitations may signify life-threatening arrhythmias caused by prolonged QT interval.

◀≡ Obtain baseline serum potassium and magnesium levels in patients at risk for significant electrolyte disturbances. Replace potassium and magnesium as appropriate before proceeding with therapy. Periodically monitor serum potassium and magnesium levels in patients on concurrent diuretics. Discontinue drug in patients with persistent QTc measurements greater than 500 msec.

• In patients with preexisting low white blood cell count (WBC) or history of leukopenia or neutropenia, determine WBC count frequently during first few months of therapy; discontinue drug at first sign of WBC decrease in the absence of other causative factors.

• Monitor patients with risk factors for diabetes mellitus for signs and symptoms of hyperglycemia, including polydipsia, polyuria, polyphagia, and weakness, and perform glucose testing before and during treatment.

• Assess blood pressure for hypertension and orthostatic hypotension.

◀≡ Monitor neurologic status, especially for neuroleptic malignant syndrome and tardive dyskinesia. Immediately discontinue drug and provide appropriate treatment if these conditions develop. However, some patients who develop tardive dyskinesia may require this drug despite the presence of the syndrome.

◀≡ Be aware that patient with bradycardia, hypokalemia, or hypomagnesemia is at greater risk for torsades de pointes and sudden death.

◀≡ Closely supervise patients at high risk for suicide.

◀≡ Discontinue drug in patients who develop a rash without an identified cause.

Patient teaching

• Tell patient to take with food.

• Explain therapy and need for follow-up laboratory testing.

◀≡ Advise patient to promptly report suicidal thoughts or actions, extrapyramidal reactions (such as repetitive, involuntary, purposeless movements), severe thirst or other signs of hyperglycemia, rash, fainting, seizures, high fever, sweating, unstable blood pressure, stupor, muscle rigidity, or suspected infection.

• Instruct patient to consult prescriber before taking over-the-counter preparations.

Z

- Caution patient to avoid driving and other hazardous activities until drug effects are known.
- Instruct patient to move slowly when sitting up or standing, to avoid dizziness from sudden blood pressure drop.
- Advise patient to avoid sun exposure and to wear sunscreen and protective clothing when going outdoors.
- As appropriate, review all other significant and life-threatening adverse reactions and interactions, especially those related to the drugs and herbs mentioned above.

zoledronic acid
Aclasta✤❋, Reclast, Zometa

Pharmacologic class: Third-generation bisphosphonate
Therapeutic class: Calcium regulator
Pregnancy risk category D

Action
Inhibits osteoclast-mediated bone by blocking resorption of mineralized bone and cartilage, eventually causing cell death and limiting tumor growth. Also limits calcium release produced by tumor.

Availability
Concentrate for dilution for infusion (Zometa): 4 mg/5 ml single-use vial
Solution for infusion (Reclast): 5 mg/100 ml in ready-to-infuse bottles
Solution for infusion (Zometa): 4 mg/100 ml in single-use ready-to-use bottles

❶ Indications and dosages
➤ Hypercalcemia caused by cancer
Adults: 4 mg (Zometa) I.V. as a single dose infused over 15 minutes. If albumin-corrected calcium level doesn't return to normal or stay normal, retreatment with 4 mg I.V. begins no sooner than 7 days after initial treatment. For single dose, maximum recommended dosage is 4 mg.
➤ Multiple myeloma; bone metastasis from solid tumors in conjunction with standard antineoplastic therapy
Adults: 4 mg I.V. (Zometa) as a single dose infused over 15 minutes q 3 to 4 weeks for patients with creatinine clearance greater than 60 ml/minute. Optimal duration of therapy is unknown.
➤ Paget's disease of bone
Adults: 5 mg (Reclast) I.V. as single dose in 100 ml ready-to-infuse solution infused over 15 minutes with constant infusion rate by vented infusion line
➤ Treatment of osteoporosis in men and postmenopausal women
Adults: 5 mg (Reclast) I.V. as single 5-mg infusion over 15 minutes once yearly
➤ Prevention of osteoporosis in postmenopausal women
Adults: 5 mg (Reclast) I.V. as single 5-mg infusion over 15 minutes once every 2 years
➤ Treatment and prevention of glucocorticoid-induced osteoporosis
Adults: 5 mg (Reclast) I.V. as single 5-mg infusion over 15 minutes once yearly

Dosage adjustment
- Renal impairment (Zometa)

Contraindications
- Hypersensitivity to drug or its components
- Hypocalcemia (Reclast)
- Patients with creatinine clearance less than 35 ml/minute and those with evidence of acute renal impairment (Reclast)

Precautions
Use cautiously in:
- bone metastasis with severe renal impairment (use not recommended)

- asthma, renal dysfunction, hepatic insufficiency, history of hypoparathyroidism
- pregnant patients (avoid Reclast use)
- concurrent use of nephrotoxic drugs
- breastfeeding patients
- children (use not indicated)

Administration

- Before starting therapy, make sure patient is adequately hydrated.
- Don't allow drug to come in contact with calcium-containing solutions; administer as single I.V. solution.
- Reconstitute Zometa concentrate for infusion by adding 5 ml of sterile water for injection to 4-mg vial. Dilute further by adding reconstituted drug to 100 ml of normal saline solution or dextrose 5% in water.
- ◀≋ To avoid inadvertent injection of undiluted Zometa concentrate for infusion, don't store undiluted drug in a syringe.
- Be aware that Zometa ready-to-use solution for infusion (for single-use only) may be administered directly without further preparation.
- To prepare reduced Zometa dosages for patients with baseline creatinine clearance of 60 ml/minute or less, see manufacturer's directions.
- Give Reclast I.V. in 100 ml ready-to-infuse solution administered by vented infusion line. Infusion time must not be less than 15 minutes, with constant infusion rate. Following infusion, flush I.V. line with 10 ml normal saline.
- Be aware that a single Reclast dose shouldn't exceed 5 mg.
- ◀≋ Give by I.V. infusion over no less than 15 minutes. (Faster infusion may cause renal failure.)
- Be aware that all patients must be adequately supplemented with oral calcium and vitamin D daily during treatment with this drug.

Route	Onset	Peak	Duration
I.V. (Zometa)	Unknown	Unknown	7-28 days
I.V. (Reclast)	Rapid	End of infusion	Short

Adverse reactions

CNS: dizziness, lethargy, rigors, asthenia, headache, agitation, confusion, insomnia, anxiety, drowsiness, fatigue, paresthesia
CV: hypotension
EENT: conjunctivitis
GI: nausea, vomiting, diarrhea, constipation, dysphagia, anorexia
GU: urinary tract infection, **renal toxicity**
Hematologic: anemia, **neutropenia**
Metabolic: dehydration, hypomagnesemia, **hypocalcemia,** hypophosphatemia
Musculoskeletal: myalgia, joint or bone pain, osteonecrosis of jaw, atypical subtrochanteric and diaphyseal femoral fractures
Respiratory: dyspnea, cough, **pleural effusion**
Skin: rash
Other: flulike syndrome, pyrexia, pain, peripheral edema, infection, fever, chills, infusion site reactions, hypersensitivity reactions (including rare cases of **urticaria, angioedema, and anaphylactic reaction or shock**)

Interactions

Drug-drug. *Aminoglycosides, loop diuretics, other nephrotoxic agents, thalidomide:* increased risk of renal toxicity
Drug-diagnostic tests. *Calcium, hemoglobin, magnesium, phosphorus, platelets, potassium, red blood cells, white blood cells:* decreased levels
Creatinine: increased or decreased level

Patient monitoring

- Monitor electrolyte levels (especially calcium). Watch for signs and symptoms of electrolyte imbalance.

Z

• Assess vital signs. Stay alert for hypotension, dyspnea, and pleural effusion.
◀€ Closely monitor fluid intake and output and creatinine level. Check for signs and symptoms of renal toxicity.
• Monitor CBC with platelet count.
◀€ Be aware that drug may cause atypical femur fractures. Evaluate patient with thigh or groin pain and consider discontinuing or interrupting therapy based on an individual benefit-risk assessment. Also, if severe incapacitating bone, joint, or muscle pain occurs, withhold drug.

Patient teaching

• Explain therapy to patient, including associated risk of renal failure and need for follow-up laboratory tests.
• Tell patient to report shortness of breath, unusual bleeding or bruising, decreased urine output, or other significant problems.
• Instruct patient to take daily oral calcium supplement and multivitamin containing vitamin D as prescribed.
• Tell patient to avoid invasive dental procedures while taking this drug.
• Advise female of childbearing age to avoid pregnancy and breastfeeding.
• As appropriate, review all other significant and life-threatening adverse reactions and interactions, especially those related to the drugs and tests mentioned above.

zolmitriptan
Zomig Rapimelt✿❀, Zomig-ZMT

Pharmacologic class: Selective 5-hydroxytryptamine receptor agonist
Therapeutic class: Antimigraine agent
Pregnancy risk category C

Action

Blocks serotonin release, constricting inflamed and dilated cerebral and cranial blood vessels and reducing nerve transmission in trigeminal pain pathways

Availability

Nasal spray: 5-mg single-use spray device
Tablets (immediate-release): 2.5 mg, 5 mg
Tablets (orally disintegrating): 2.5 mg

⚕ Indications and dosages
➤ Acute migraine
Adults: 1.25 to 2.5 mg (immediate-release) P.O., repeated if migraine returns in 2 hours or less; maximum dosage is 10 mg in any 24-hour period. Or 2.5 mg (orally disintegrating tablet) P.O., repeated if migraine returns in 2 hours or less; maximum dosage is 10 mg in any 24-hour period. Alternatively, one dose of nasal spray (5 mg); if migraine returns, may repeat dose after 2 hours; don't exceed maximum daily dosage of 10 mg in any 24-hour period.

Dosage adjustment
• Hepatic impairment

Contraindications
• Hypersensitivity to drug
• Hemiplegic or basilar migraine
• Ischemic cardiac disease or other significant cardiac disease
• Uncontrolled hypertension
• Cerebrovascular accident or transient ischemic attack
• Peripheral vascular disease, including ischemic bowel disease
• Use of ergot-type or ergot-containing drugs or other 5-HT$_1$ agonists within past 24 hours
• MAO inhibitor use within past 14 days

Precautions
Use cautiously in:
• hepatic or renal impairment

- risk factors for coronary artery disease (such as strong family history of this disease, diabetes mellitus, obesity, cigarette smoking, high cholesterol level, men older than age 40, postmenopausal women)
- elderly patients
- pregnant or breastfeeding patients
- children.

Administration

- Place orally disintegrating tablet on patient's tongue, where it should dissolve.
- Don't break orally disintegrating tablet in half.
- Know that each nasal spray unit is intended for one use only.

Route	Onset	Peak	Duration
P.O.	Unknown	2 hr	Unknown
Nasal	15 min	2-5 hr	24 hr

Adverse reactions

CNS: paresthesia, asthenia, dizziness, insomnia, hyperesthesia, drowsiness, syncope, vertigo, agitation, depression, anxiety, emotional lability, fatigue, malaise
CV: chest pain, heaviness, or tightness; hypertension; palpitations; angina; **arrhythmias**
EENT: dry eyes, ear pain, tinnitus, epistaxis, altered sense of smell, laryngitis
GI: nausea, vomiting, dyspepsia, dysphagia, gastroenteritis, esophagitis, dry mouth
GU: urinary frequency, hematuria, polyuria, cystitis
Hepatic: hepatic dysfunction
Metabolic: hyperglycemia
Musculoskeletal: leg cramps, neck pain, tenosynovitis, myasthenia, myalgia, back pain
Respiratory: bronchitis, hiccups
Skin: pruritus, rash, diaphoresis, bruising, urticaria, photosensitivity
Other: unusual taste, flushing, sweating or redness in face (with nasal spray); fever; chills; excessive thirst; facial or tongue edema; pressure or tightness in throat or jaw; yawning; warm or cold sensation

Interactions

Drug-drug. *Cimetidine:* doubling of zolmitriptan's half-life
Ergot-containing drugs: vasospasm
Fluoxetine, fluvoxamine, paroxetine, sertraline: weakness, incoordination, hyperreflexia
MAO inhibitors: increased zolmitriptan effects
Drug-diagnostic tests. *Blood glucose:* increased level
Drug-herbs. *S-adenosylmethionine (SAM-e), St. John's wort:* serotonin syndrome
Drug-behaviors. *Smoking:* increased risk of adverse cardiovascular effects

Patient monitoring

- Assess therapeutic response to help gauge drug efficacy.
- Watch for adverse cardiovascular and respiratory reactions, particularly dyspnea and chest pain or tightness.
- Assess blood glucose level in diabetic patient.

Patient teaching

◀❰ Tell patient to immediately report shortness of breath or pain or tightness in chest or throat.
- Explain that drug is intended to treat migraine, not prevent it.
- Tell patient to remove orally disintegrating tablet from blister pack just before taking it, and then place it on his tongue and let it dissolve. Instruct him not to break it.
- Teach patient proper use of nasal spray. Tell him each unit is intended for one use only.
- Caution patient to avoid driving and other hazardous activities during severe migraine or if drug causes adverse CNS effects.

Z

Reactions in **bold** are life-threatening.   ◀❰ Clinical alert

- Inform patient that smoking may increase drug's cardiovascular risks.
- Advise female of childbearing age not to take drug if she is, might be, or plans to become pregnant.
- Advise patient to avoid sun exposure and to wear sunscreen and protective clothing when going outdoors.
- As appropriate, review all other significant and life-threatening adverse reactions and interactions, especially those related to the drugs, tests, herbs, and behaviors mentioned above.

zolpidem tartrate
Ambien, Ambien CR, Edluar, Intermezzo, Stilnoct⊕, Zolpimist

Pharmacologic class: Imidazopyridine
Therapeutic class: Sedative-hypnotic
Controlled substance schedule IV
Pregnancy risk category B

Action
Depresses CNS by binding to gamma-aminobutyric acid receptors

Availability
Oral spray: 5 mg/actuation
Tablets: 5 mg, 6.25 mg, 10 mg, 12.5 mg
Tablets (sublingual): 1.75 mg, 3.5 mg, 5 mg, 10 mg

🖊 Indications and dosages
➤ Insomnia
Adults: 10 mg P.O. (Ambien) or 12.5 mg P.O.(Ambien CR), or 10 mg (Edluar) sublingual, or 10 mg oral spray (two sprays) immediately before bedtime
➤ As-needed use for treatment of insomnia when middle-of-the-night awakening is followed by difficulty returning to sleep
Adults: 1.75 mg (Intermezzo) sublingually for women and 3.5 mg

(Intermezzo) sublingually for men, taken only once per night if needed

Dosage adjustment
- Hepatic impairment
- Concurrent use of CNS depressants
- Elderly or debilitated patients

Off-label uses
- Long-term treatment of insomnia
- Insomnia related to selective serotonin reuptake inhibitors
- Postoperative sedation

Contraindications
- Hypersensitivity to drug

Precautions
Use cautiously in:
- pulmonary disease, hepatic or severe renal impairment
- history of psychiatric illness, suicide attempt, or substance abuse
- elderly or debilitated patients
- pregnant or breastfeeding patients
- children (safety not established).

Administration
- Don't give with or immediately after a meal.

Route	Onset	Peak	Duration
P.O.	Rapid	30 min-2 hr	6-8 hr
P.O. (spray)	Unknown	0.9 hr	Unknown
S.L.	Unknown	30 min-2 hr	Unknown

Adverse reactions
CNS: amnesia, ataxia, confusion, euphoria, vertigo, daytime drowsiness, dizziness, drugged feeling
EENT: diplopia, abnormal vision
GI: nausea, vomiting, diarrhea, dry mouth
Other: hypersensitivity reaction, physical or psychological drug dependence, drug tolerance

Interactions
Drug-drug. *Antihistamines, opioid analgesics, phenothiazines, sedative-hypnotics,*

tricyclic antidepressants: increased CNS depression

Ketoconazole, ritonavir: increased blood level and enhanced effects of zolpidem

Rifampin: decreased zolpidem efficacy

Drug-herbs. *Chamomile, hops, kava, skullcap, valerian:* increased CNS depression

Drug-behaviors. *Alcohol use:* increased CNS depression

Patient monitoring
• Monitor for physical and psychological drug dependence. Watch for drug hoarding.
• Assess for adverse reactions, including confusion, ataxia, and amnesia.

Patient teaching
• Tell patient to take immediately before bedtime (and not after a meal), because it works quickly.
• Instruct patient to place sublingual tablet under the tongue, where it will disintegrate; tell patient not to swallow tablet and not to take it with water.
• Instruct patient that oral spray pump needs to be primed initially and after not using spray for 14 days. Tell patient to fully press down on pump to make sure a full dose (5 mg) of oral spray is sprayed directly into the mouth over the tongue with each spray.
• Advise patient to take only when he is able to get a full night's sleep (7 to 8 hours) before he needs to be active again. Tell patient to use oral spray only if 4 hours of bedtime remain before planned time of waking.
• Stress that drug is meant only for short-term use (7 to 10 days).
• Tell patient rebound insomnia may occur for 1 to 2 nights after he discontinues drug.
• Inform patient that drug may cause amnesia, drowsiness, and a drugged feeling the next day.

• Caution patient to avoid driving and other hazardous activities while under drug's influence.
• As appropriate, review all other significant adverse reactions and interactions, especially those related to the drugs, herbs, and behaviors mentioned above.

zonisamide
Zonegran

Pharmacologic class: Sulfonamide
Therapeutic class: Anticonvulsant
Pregnancy risk category C

Action
Raises seizure threshold and reduces seizure duration, probably by stabilizing neuronal membranes through action on sodium and calcium channels

Availability
Capsules: 25 mg, 50 mg, 100 mg

Indications and dosages
➤ Adjunctive treatment of partial seizures

Adults and children older than age 16: Initially, 100 mg P.O. daily for 2 weeks, then, if required, increased to 200 mg P.O. daily for at least 2 weeks. May increase in 100-mg increments at 2-week intervals to 300 to 400 mg daily as required. Daily dosage ranges from 100 to 600 mg.

Dosage adjustment
• Hepatic or renal impairment
• Elderly patients

Off-label uses
• Infantile spasms
• Progressive myoclonic epilepsy
• Weight loss

Z

Contraindications
• Hypersensitivity to drug or other sulfonamides

Precautions
Use cautiously in:
• hepatic or renal disease
• pregnant or breastfeeding patients
• children younger than age 16 (safety not established).

Administration
• Give with or without food.

Route	Onset	Peak	Duration
P.O.	Unknown	2-6 hr	24 hr

Adverse reactions
CNS: drowsiness, fatigue, agitation, irritability, depression, dizziness, psychomotor slowing, psychosis, asthenia, abnormal gait, incoordination, tremor, ataxia, headache, confusion, impaired memory, hyperesthesia, paresthesia, **seizures**
EENT: diplopia, amblyopia, nystagmus, tinnitus, rhinitis, pharyngitis
GI: nausea, vomiting, diarrhea, dyspepsia, dry mouth, anorexia, **pancreatitis**
GU: renal calculi
Hematologic: anemia, **leukopenia**
Respiratory: cough
Skin: rash, pruritus, bruising, **Stevens-Johnson syndrome**
Other: abnormal taste, weight loss, allergic reactions, oligohidrosis and hyperthermia (in children), flulike symptoms, accidental injury

Interactions
Drug-drug. *Carbamazepine, phenobarbital, phenytoin, valproic acid:* decreased zonisamide blood level and effects

CYP450-3A4 inducers: decreased zonisamide half-life
CYP450-3A4 inhibitors: increased zonisamide blood level
Drug-diagnostic tests. *Blood urea nitrogen, creatine kinase, creatinine:* increased levels
Platelets, white blood cells: decreased counts

Patient monitoring
• Monitor CBC with white cell differential.
• Assess neurologic status; report significant adverse reactions.
• Monitor renal function tests. Watch for signs and symptoms of renal calculi.
◀ Monitor for rash, which may be first sign of Stevens-Johnson syndrome. If rash occurs, discontinue drug and notify prescriber immediately.

Patient teaching
• Explain therapy to patient. Instruct him to keep seizure diary and show it to prescriber.
• Instruct patient to swallow capsules whole. Advise him to drink 6 to 8 glasses of water daily to help prevent kidney stones.
◀ Warn patient that stopping drug abruptly may cause status epilepticus.
• Caution patient to avoid driving and other hazardous activities until he knows how drug affects him and until seizures are well controlled.
◀ Tell patient to immediately report rash, fever, sore throat, sudden back pain, depression, speech or language problems, or painful urination.
• As appropriate, review all other significant and life-threatening adverse reactions and interactions, especially those related to the drugs and tests mentioned above.

Part 2

Drug classes
Vitamins and minerals
Herbs and supplements

Drug classes

The collective monographs below cover the most common drug classes, and provide general information for the most commonly used generic drugs in each class. The drugs listed in each class are those covered in individual monographs in this book; the list is not intended to be comprehensive.

Keep in mind that drugs in the same class may vary as to contraindications, precautions, adverse reactions, interactions, and patient monitoring. For specific information on a particular drug, see the individual monograph. Also, because pregnancy risk category and interactions may differ for the drugs in a given class, this information is not included in the monographs below.

alpha₁-adrenergic agents

Alpha₁-adrenergic blockers: alfuzosin hydrochloride, doxazosin mesylate, phentolamine mesylate, silodosin, tamsulosin hydrochloride, terazosin hydrochloride

Centrally acting alpha-adrenergic agonists: clonidine hydrochloride, methyldopa, methyldopa hydrochloride

Peripherally acting alpha-adrenergic agonists: midodrine hydrochloride

Action

Alpha₁-adrenergic blockers selectively block postsynaptic alpha₁-adrenergic receptors, causing dilation of arterioles and veins, in turn lowering supine and standing blood pressure. *Centrally acting alpha-adrenergic agonists* reduce sympathetic outflow from CNS and decrease peripheral resistance, renal vascular resistance, heart rate, and blood pressure. *Peripherally acting alpha-adrenergic agonists* activate alpha-adrenergic receptors of the arteriolar and venous vasculature, increasing vascular tone and blood pressure.

Indications

Hypertension, refractory heart failure, peripheral vascular disorders, benign prostatic hypertrophy, orthostatic hypotension (midodrine only), severe pain in cancer patients (injectable clonidine only)

Contraindications and precautions

• Contraindicated in hypersensitivity to drug and concomitant administration with strong CP450 3A4 (CYP3A4) inhibitors (silodosin)

• Use cautiously in orthostatic hypotension; cataract surgery; concurrent use of other alpha blockers; antihypertensives; moderate CYP3A4 inhibitors; PDE5 inhibitors; and strong P-glycoprotein inhibitors (not recommended) with silodosin; renal insufficiency; angina pectoris; overt heart failure; when adding diuretics to drug regimen; in pregnant or breastfeeding patients; and in children (safety not established).

Adverse reactions

CNS: dizziness, headache, asthenia, drowsiness, nervousness, paresthesia, vertigo, fatigue

CV: orthostatic hypotension (with first dose of alpha₁-adrenergic blocker), rebound hypertension, chest pain, palpitations, peripheral edema, tachycardia, **arrhythmias**

EENT: blurred vision, conjunctivitis, nasal congestion, sinusitis

---

Reactions in **bold** are life-threatening.   ◀€ Clinical alert

GI: nausea, vomiting, diarrhea, abdominal pain, dry mouth
GU: urinary frequency or incontinence, priapism, erectile dysfunction, gynecomastia (with centrally acting agonists)
Musculoskeletal: joint, back, or extremity pain
Respiratory: dyspnea
Skin: pruritus, angioedema, urticaria, alopecia (with centrally acting agonists)
Other: fever, weight gain

Patient monitoring

• Monitor electrolyte levels, ECG, and vital signs.

---

antacids

aluminum hydroxide, calcium carbonate, magnesium hydroxide, magnesium oxide, sodium bicarbonate

Action

Neutralize gastric acidity, which increases pH of stomach and duodenal bulb. Aluminum-containing antacids bind with phosphate ions in intestine to form insoluble aluminum phosphate, which is excreted in feces.

Indications

Peptic ulcer, gastric hyperacidity, upset stomach associated with hyperacidity. Magnesium oxide is indicated for magnesium deficiency or depletion caused by malnutrition, restricted diet, alcoholism, or magnesium-depleting drugs.

Contraindications and precautions

• Contraindicated in hypersensitivity to drug, renal calculi, hypercalcemia, and hypophosphatemia
• Use cautiously in renal impairment, chronic pain syndrome, recent massive GI hemorrhage, and pregnant patients.

Adverse reactions

CNS: aluminum toxicity, encephalopathy (aluminum-containing antacids)
GI: diarrhea (magnesium-containing antacids); constipation, possibly leading to intestinal obstruction (aluminum-containing antacids)
Metabolic: dose-dependent rebound hyperacidity; milk-alkali syndrome; hypermagnesemia in renal failure patients (magnesium-containing antacids); hypophosphatemia, aluminum accumulation in blood (aluminum-containing antacids)
Musculoskeletal: osteomalacia, aluminum accumulation in bone (aluminum-containing antacids)

Patient monitoring

• Assess for constipation.
• Monitor serum electrolyte levels as appropriate.

---

anti-Alzheimer's agents

donepezil hydrochloride, galantamine hydrobromide, memantine, rivastigmine tartrate

Action

Reversibly inhibit acetylcholinesterase hydrolysis in CNS, which increases acetylcholine level and promotes nerve impulse transmission. Unlike donepezil, galantamine, and rivastigmine, memantine binds preferentially to cation channels operated by *N*-methyl-D-aspartate and doesn't affect reversible acetylcholinesterase inhibition.

Indications

Mild to moderate Alzheimer's disease, moderate to severe Alzheimer's disease (memantine only)

Contraindications and precautions

• Contraindicated in hypersensitivity to drug, piperidine derivatives, or acridines; angle-closure glaucoma; undiagnosed skin lesions; and jaundice with previous use of these drugs

• Use cautiously in moderate to severe renal or hepatic dysfunction, GI bleeding, seizures, cardiovascular disease, sick sinus syndrome, asthma or chronic obstructive pulmonary disease, impaired urinary outflow, diabetes mellitus, obesity, history of ulcer, postmenopausal patients, elderly patients, pregnant or breastfeeding patients, and children.

Adverse reactions

CNS: tremor, confusion, insomnia, psychosis, hallucinations, depression, dizziness, headache, anxiety, nervousness, drowsiness, fatigue, abnormal dreams, irritability, paresthesia, aggression, vertigo, ataxia, restlessness, abnormal crying, syncope, aphasia, **seizures**

CV: chest pain, hypotension, hypertension, peripheral edema, vasodilation, **atrial fibrillation**

EENT: cataract, blurred vision, eye irritation, rhinitis, pharyngitis, sore throat

GI: nausea, vomiting, diarrhea, constipation, abdominal pain, flatulence, eructation, anorexia

GU: urinary tract infection, urinary frequency or incontinence, increased libido

Metabolic: dehydration, hot flashes

Musculoskeletal: back and joint pain, bone fracture, muscle cramps, arthritis

Respiratory: upper respiratory infection, cough, bronchitis, dyspnea, influenza

Skin: rash, pruritus, urticaria, diaphoresis, flushing

Other: toothache, weight loss, pain, accidental trauma, flulike symptoms

Patient monitoring

• Assess for severe nausea, vomiting, and diarrhea (which may lead to dehydration and weight loss).

◀◊ Watch closely for adverse reactions in patients with a history of GI bleeding, arrhythmias, seizures, pulmonary conditions, or use of nonsteroidal antiinflammatory drugs.

• Monitor alanine aminotransferase level weekly during first 18 weeks of therapy.

antiarrhythmics

adenosine, amiodarone hydrochloride, atropine sulfate, diltiazem hydrochloride, digoxin, disopyramide phosphate, dronedarone, esmolol hydrochloride, flecainide acetate, ibutilide fumarate, lidocaine hydrochloride, phenytoin, phenytoin sodium, procainamide hydrochloride, propafenone hydrochloride, propranolol hydrochloride, quinidine gluconate, quinidine sulfate, sotalol hydrochloride, verapamil hydrochloride

Action

Varies with classification and subdivision (which are based on drug's action on cardiac muscle). *Class I* antiarrhythmics decrease rate of sodium entry during depolarization, reduce rate of action potential, and lengthen effective refractory period of fast-response fibers. Class I antiarrhythmics fall into three subdivisions. *Class IA* drugs (such as disopyramide, procainamide, and quinidine) depress phase 0 and lengthen the action potential. *Class IB* drugs (such as lidocaine, phenytoin, and tocainide) somewhat depress phase 0 and shorten the action potential. *Class IC* drugs (such as flecainide and propafenone) greatly depress phase 0

Reactions in **bold** are life-threatening.   ◀◊ Clinical alert and slow conduction. Moricizine shares properties of class IA, IB, and IC antiarrhythmics.

Class II antiarrhythmics (such as propranolol) competitively block beta-adrenergic receptors and depress phase 4 depolarization.

Class III antiarrhythmics (such as amiodarone, bretylium, dofetilide, ibutilide, and sotalol) prolong duration of the action potential but don't affect polarization phase or resting membrane potential.

Class IV antiarrhythmics (calcium channel blockers such as verapamil) slow conduction velocity and increase atrioventricular (AV) node refractoriness.

Indications

Arrhythmias, premature ventricular tachycardia, atrial flutter, atrial fibrillation, AV heart block

Contraindications and precautions

• Contraindicated in hypersensitivity to drug, congenital or acquired long-QT syndrome, baseline QT or QTc interval greater than 440 msec, sick sinus syndrome, second- or third-degree AV block (unless patient has an artificial pacemaker), systolic pressure below 90 mm Hg, recent myocardial infarction or pulmonary congestion, pulmonary hypertension, aortic stenosis, severe renal impairment, digoxin toxicity, patients with NYHA Class IV heart failure or NYHA Class II to III heart failure with a recent decompensation requiring hospitalization or referral to specialized heart failure clinic (dronedarone), pregnancy, breastfeeding, and neonates

• Use cautiously in mild to moderate renal or hepatic impairment, enlarged prostate, myasthenia gravis, glaucoma, diabetes mellitus, potassium imbalance, conduction abnormalities, ventricular tachycardia, ventricular arrhythmias, history of serious ventricular arrhythmias or heart failure, elderly patients, and children (safety not established).

Adverse reactions

CNS: dizziness, light-headedness, agitation, jitteriness, anxiety, depression, fatigue, drowsiness, headache, syncope, malaise, involuntary movements, ataxia, paresthesia, peripheral neuropathy, incoordination, tremor, abnormal dreams, insomnia, confusion, acute psychosis, psychiatric disturbances

CV: chest pain, palpitations, peripheral edema, bradycardia, tachycardia, **hypotension,** development or worsening of **arrhythmias, heart failure, heart block**

EENT: blurred vision, angle-closure glaucoma, corneal microdeposits, optic neuritis or neuropathy, photophobia, dry eyes, tinnitus, disturbed equilibrium, epistaxis, dry nose, altered smell perception

GI: nausea, vomiting, diarrhea, constipation, abdominal pain, bloating, flatulence, dry mouth, anorexia

GU: dysuria, nocturia, polyuria, urinary hesitancy, urinary retention, erectile or other sexual dysfunction, decreased libido, epididymitis

Hematologic: anemia, **leukopenia, thrombocytopenia, agranulocytosis**

Hepatic: jaundice, **hepatic dysfunction**

Metabolic: hypokalemia, hypothyroidism, hyperthyroidism, **hypoglycemia**

Musculoskeletal: muscle weakness, aches, or cramps; joint stiffness

Respiratory: cough, dyspnea, pneumonia, **pulmonary fibrosis, adult respiratory distress syndrome**

Skin: bluish skin discoloration, rash, dermatosis, pruritus, alopecia, flushing, photosensitivity, toxic epidermal necrolysis, **Stevens-Johnson syndrome**

Other: gingival hyperplasia, edema, weight gain

Patient monitoring

• Monitor antiarrhythmic blood level.
• Assess blood pressure and pulse. Report heart rate below 50 or above 120 beats/minute.
• Monitor blood glucose and electrolyte levels and liver and kidney function tests.

◀€ Closely monitor extent of palpitations. Stay alert for fluttering or missed heartbeats, chest pain, and fainting episodes. Obtain ECG to document arrhythmias.

anticholinergics

atropine sulfate, atropine sulfate ophthalmic, benztropine mesylate, darifenacin hydrobromide, dicyclomine hydrochloride, dimenhydrinate, diphenoxylate hydrochloride and atropine sulfate, glycopyrrolate, hyoscyamine, hyoscyamine sulfate, meclizine hydrochloride, oxybutynin, oxybutynin chloride, scopolamine, scopolamine hydrobromide, solifenacin succinate, trihexyphenidyl hydrochloride, tiotropium, trimethobenzamide hydrochloride, trospium chloride

Action

Block acetylcholine action in CNS and on autonomic effectors; also block vagal effects on sinoatrial and atrioventricular nodes, causing heart rate to increase. Small doses decrease salivary and bronchial secretions and reduce sweating; intermediate doses dilate pupils, inhibit accommodation, and increase heart rate; large doses decrease GI and GU motility; even higher doses reduce gastric acid secretion.

Indications

Bradyarrhythmias, symptomatic bradycardia, heart block caused by vagal activity, peptic ulcer disease, pylorospasm, small-intestine hypertoxicity, colonic hypermotility, mild dysentery, diverticulitis, bronchospasm, spastic or overactive bladder, cystitis, infant colic, biliary or renal colic, pancreatitis, acute iritis, acute rhinitis, sialorrhea, hyperhidrosis, anticholinesterase poisoning, nausea, vomiting, dizziness, motion sickness, drug-induced extrapyramidal disorders, parkinsonism, adjunct for Parkinson's disease. Also used for cycloplegic refraction, to control gastric secretions and block cardiac vagal reflexes preoperatively, to promote diagnostic hypotonic duodenography, and to increase radiologic visibility of kidney.

Contraindications and precautions

• Contraindicated in hypersensitivity to drug, GI or GU tract obstruction, reflux esophagitis, severe ulcerative colitis, glaucoma, myasthenia gravis, intestinal atony, unstable cardiovascular status in acute hemorrhage, arrhythmias, tachycardia caused by cardiac insufficiency or thyrotoxicosis, toxic megacolon, GI infection, severe prostatic hypertrophy, bladder neck obstruction, bronchial asthma, chronic obstructive pulmonary disease, breastfeeding, and infants less than 6 months old
• Use cautiously in alcohol, sulfite, or tartrazine intolerance; high environmental temperatures; hepatic or renal impairment; autonomic neuropathy; mild to moderate prostatic hypertrophy; hyperthyroidism; coronary disease; heart failure; hypertension; hiatal hernia; ulcerative colitis; brain damage; Down syndrome; spasticity; phenylketonuria; elderly patients; pregnant patients (safety not established); neonates; and immature infants.

Adverse reactions

CNS: asthenia, nervousness, stimulation, insomnia, drowsiness, dizziness, headache, confusion

CV: palpitations, tachycardia

EENT: increased intraocular pressure, dilated pupils, blurred vision, photophobia

GI: nausea, vomiting, constipation, abdominal distention, epigastric distress, heartburn, gastroesophageal reflux, dry mouth, **paralytic ileus**

GU: urinary hesitancy or retention, erectile dysfunction, lactation suppression

Skin: urticaria, decreased diaphoresis

Other: taste loss, fever, irritation at I.M. injection site, allergic reaction, **anaphylaxis**

Patient monitoring

• Closely monitor vital signs and urine output.

anticoagulants

argatroban, bivalirudin, dalteparin sodium, danaparoid sodium, enoxaparin sodium, fondaparinux sodium, heparin calcium, heparin sodium, lepirudin, warfarin sodium

Action

Interfere with one or more parts of the pathways that lead to stable fibrin clot formation. May inhibit coagulation factors, bind to antithrombin, cause release of tissue factor pathway inhibitors, and prevent conversion of fibrinogen to fibrin.

Indications

Treatment or prophylaxis of venous thrombosis, pulmonary embolism, atrial fibrillation with embolization, myocardial infarction, or thromboembolic events (including deep-vein thrombosis); during cardiovascular surgery; prevention of thrombus formation and embolization after prosthetic valve placement; after abdominal surgery or total hip or knee replacement surgery

Contraindications and precautions

• Contraindicated in hypersensitivity to drug, uncontrolled or active major bleeding, or thrombocytopenia caused by antiplatelet antibodies associated with low-molecular-weight heparins

• Use cautiously in severe hepatic or renal disease; hypertensive or diabetic retinopathy; untreated or severe uncontrolled hypertension; hemorrhagic stroke; severe thrombocytopenia; active GI bleeding or ulcers or recent history of ulcer disease; cancer; bacterial endocarditis; history of congenital or acquired bleeding disorder; recent brain, spinal, or ophthalmic surgery; spinal or epidural anesthesia; patients weighing less than 45 kg (99 lb); elderly patients; pregnant or breastfeeding patients; and children (safety not established).

Adverse reactions

CNS: headache, dizziness, insomnia, confusion, **spinal hematoma, cerebral or intracranial bleeding**

CV: hypotension, hypertension, angina pectoris, tachycardia, **arrhythmias, pulmonary embolism, thromboembolism, myocardial infarction**

EENT: ocular hemorrhage, rhinitis, epistaxis

GI: nausea, vomiting, constipation, dyspepsia, hematemesis, anorectal bleeding, melena, flatulence, **retroperitoneal or intra-abdominal bleeding, GI hemorrhage**

GU: dysuria, hematuria, urinary tract infection, urinary retention, **vaginal hemorrhage**

Hematologic: purpura, anemia, **granulocytopenia, thrombocytopenia,**

agranulocytosis, pancytopenia, hemorrhage
Hepatic: hepatitis
Musculoskeletal: back pain
Respiratory: dyspnea, pneumonia, respiratory disorder
Skin: rash, pruritus, bullous eruption, skin necrosis, urticaria, cellulitis, injection site or wound hematoma, alopecia
Other: fever, pain, infection, dependent edema, impaired healing, hypersensitivity reaction, **congenital anomalies, fetal distress, fetal death**

Patient monitoring

◀€ Watch for tarry stools and unusual bleeding or bruising.

• Assess baseline coagulation tests and CBC with white cell differential.

• Monitor venipuncture sites for bleeding, hematoma, and inflammation.

anticonvulsants

carbamazepine, clonazepam, clorazepate dipotassium, diazepam, divalproex sodium, fosphenytoin sodium, gabapentin, lamotrigine, levetiracetam, magnesium sulfate, oxcarbazepine, pentobarbital, phenobarbital sodium, phenytoin, phenytoin sodium, pregabalin, primidone, tiagabine hydrochloride, topiramate, valproate sodium, valproic acid, zonisamide

Action

Selectively depress hyperactive brain areas responsible for seizures

Indications

Prophylaxis and treatment of status epilepticus and generalized tonic-clonic, mixed, petit mal, petit mal variant, akinetic, complex-partial, and myoclonic seizures; management of panic disorder, trigeminal neuralgia, migraine, anxiety, psychoneurotic reactions, and alcohol withdrawal; skeletal muscle relaxation for endoscopy or cardioversion

Contraindications and precautions

• Contraindicated in hypersensitivity to drug or intolerance of alcohol, propylene glycol, tartrazine, or tricyclic antidepressants; bone marrow depression; severe hepatic disease; and MAO inhibitor use within past 14 days

• Use cautiously in mild to moderate hepatic or renal disease, severe cardiac or respiratory disease, acute or chronic pain, fever, hyperthyroidism, diabetes mellitus, severe anemia, uremia, angle-closure glaucoma, coma, CNS depression, sinus bradycardia, sinoatrial block, second- or third-degree heart block, Stokes-Adams syndrome, obesity, history of suicide attempt or drug abuse, elderly or debilitated patients, and pregnant or breastfeeding patients.

Adverse reactions

CNS: dizziness, light-headedness, syncope, drowsiness, lethargy, sedation, depression, apathy, fatigue, disorientation, anger, hostility, mania or hypomania, restlessness, confusion, crying, delirium, headache, slurred speech, dysarthria, stupor, rigidity, tremor, dystonia, vertigo, euphoria, nervousness, poor concentration, vivid dreams, psychomotor retardation, paresthesia, extrapyramidal symptoms, mild paradoxical stimulation (first 2 weeks of therapy)
CV: hypertension, hypotension, palpitations, bradycardia, tachycardia, aggravation of coronary artery disease, **cardiovascular collapse, heart failure, arrhythmias**
EENT: blurred vision, diplopia, corneal opacities, nystagmus and other abnormal eye movements, conjunctivitis

---

Reactions in **bold** are life-threatening. ◀€ Clinical alert

GI: nausea, vomiting, diarrhea, constipation, abdominal pain, dysphagia, gastric disorders, stomatitis, glossitis, dry mouth, increased salivation, pharyngeal dryness, anorexia

GU: urinary hesitancy, retention, frequency, or incontinence; albuminuria; glycosuria; dysuria; nocturia; menstrual irregularities; libido changes; erectile dysfunction; gynecomastia

Hematologic: eosinophilia, **leukopenia, agranulocytosis, aplastic anemia, thrombocytopenia**

Hepatic: hepatitis

Metabolic: syndrome of inappropriate antidiuretic hormone secretion

Musculoskeletal: muscle rigidity

Respiratory: pneumonitis

Skin: photosensitivity, rash, urticaria, diaphoresis, **erythema multiforme, Stevens-Johnson syndrome**

Other: chills, fever, hiccups, weight changes, edema, lymphadenopathy, physical and psychological drug dependence, drug tolerance

Patient monitoring

• Monitor CBC, glucose and uric acid levels, urinalysis, and kidney and liver function tests.

◀≋ With I.V. use, watch closely for respiratory depression and cardiovascular collapse.

• Monitor for sore throat, easy bruising and bleeding, and epistaxis.

• Stay alert for oversedation.

antidepressants

amitriptyline hydrochloride, bupropion hydrochloride, citalopram hydrobromide, clomipramine hydrochloride, desipramine hydrochloride, desvenlafaxine, doxepin hydrochloride, duloxetine hydrochloride, escitalopram oxalate, fluoxetine hydrochloride, fluvoxamine maleate, imipramine hydrochloride, imipramine pamoate, milnacipran, mirtazapine, nefazodone hydrochloride, nortriptyline hydrochloride, paroxetine hydrochloride, paroxetine mesylate, sertraline hydrochloride, trazodone hydrochloride, venlafaxine hydrochloride

Action

Produce changes in serotonin or norepinephrine receptor systems; inhibit neuronal serotonin, norepinephrine, or dopamine reuptake

Indications

Endogenous or reactive depression, including depression associated with anxiety and sleep disturbances

Contraindications and precautions

• Contraindicated in hypersensitivity to drug, MAO inhibitor use within past 14 days, uncontrolled narrow-angle glaucoma (milnacipran)

• Use cautiously in cardiovascular disease; hypertension; hepatic or renal impairment; severe depression; increased intraocular pressure; angle-closure glaucoma; hyperthyroidism; prostatic hypertrophy; acute recovery phase after myocardial infarction (MI); electroshock therapy; elective surgery; suicidal tendency; history of seizures, neurologic impairment, mania, or drug abuse; concomitant use of serotonin precursors (such as tryptophan) and selective serotonin reuptake inhibitors and selective norepinephrine reuptake inhibitors (use not recommended); use of drugs that increase blood pressure or heart rate; use of I.V. digoxin; use of nonsteroidal anti-inflammatory drugs, aspirin, or other drugs that affect coagulation; significant alcohol use (avoid use);

obstructive uropathies (in males); elderly patients (milnacipran); pregnant or breastfeeding patients; and children younger than age 18.

Adverse reactions

CNS: lethargy, sedation, hallucinations, delusions, disorientation, anxiety, nervousness, EEG changes, fatigue, peripheral neuropathy, insomnia, restlessness, drowsiness, dizziness, syncope, extrapyramidal effects, **neuroleptic malignant syndrome, seizures, coma, cerebrovascular accident (CVA)**

CV: hypotension, hypertension, ECG changes, tachycardia, palpitations, chest pain, **arrhythmias, MI**

EENT: visual disturbances, blurred vision, mydriasis, increased intraocular pressure, dry eyes, tinnitus, rhinitis

GI: nausea, vomiting, diarrhea, constipation, epigastric or abdominal pain, dyspepsia, dry mouth, anorexia, **paralytic ileus**

GU: urinary frequency or retention, gynecomastia, sexual dysfunction

Hematologic: leukopenia, agranulocytosis, thrombocytopenia

Hepatic: hepatitis

Metabolic: blood glucose changes

Skin: rash, urticaria, diaphoresis, bruising, pruritus, photosensitivity

Other: altered taste, increased appetite, weight changes, edema, chills, yawning, hypersensitivity reaction

Patient monitoring

• Monitor CBC, blood glucose level, and kidney and liver function tests.

◀€ Assess ECG and heart sounds. Watch for tachycardia and more frequent angina attacks (which may precede MI or CVA).

• Evaluate neurologic function.

• Watch for sleep disturbances, lethargy, apathy, impaired thought processes, and poor therapeutic response.

• Check results of periodic eye exams. Report vision changes, perception of halos, eye pain, dilated pupils, headache, and nausea.

antidiabetic drugs (hypoglycemics)

acarbose, exenatide acetate, glimepiride, glipizide, glyburide, insulins, liraglutide, metformin hydrochloride, miglitol, nateglinide, pioglitazone hydrochloride, pramlintide acetate, repaglinide, rosiglitazone maleate, saxagliptin, sitagliptin phosphate, tolazamide

Action

Bind to plasma membrane of functional pancreatic beta cells, decreasing potassium permeability and membrane depolarization. These effects increase intracellular calcium transport and enhance release of secretory granules containing insulin.

Insulins promote glucose transport and stimulate carbohydrate metabolism, which inhibits the release of free fatty acids and stimulates protein metabolism and synthesis.

Indications

Type 1 (insulin-dependent) or type 2 (non-insulin-dependent) diabetes mellitus

Contraindications and precautions

• Contraindicated in hypersensitivity to drug; personal or family history of medullary thyroid carcinoma; in patients with multiple endocrine neoplasia syndrome type 2 (liraglutide); and in diabetes mellitus complicated by ketoacidosis

---

Reactions in **bold** are life-threatening. ◀€ Clinical alert

- Use cautiously in severe cardiovascular, hepatic, or renal disease; heart failure; intestinal disorders; thyroid, pituitary, or adrenal dysfunction; malnutrition; high fever; prolonged nausea or vomiting; dehydration; hypoxemia; excessive alcohol ingestion (acute or chronic); concurrent use of insulin secretagogue or strong CYP450 and CYP3A4/5 inhibitors (saxagliptin); pancreatitis; elderly patients; and pregnant or breastfeeding patients.

Adverse reactions

CNS: lethargy, sedation, hallucinations, delusions, disorientation, peripheral neuropathy, EEG changes, nervousness, restlessness, anxiety, fatigue, insomnia, drowsiness, dizziness, syncope, asthenia, extrapyramidal effects, **neuroleptic malignant syndrome, seizures, coma, cerebrovascular accident**

CV: hypotension, hypertension, ECG changes, tachycardia, palpitations, chest pain, **arrhythmias, myocardial infarction**

EENT: blurred vision, visual disturbances, mydriasis, dry eyes, increased intraocular pressure, tinnitus, rhinitis

GI: nausea, vomiting, diarrhea, constipation, epigastric or abdominal pain, dyspepsia, dry mouth, anorexia, **paralytic ileus**

GU: urinary frequency or retention, gynecomastia, sexual dysfunction

Hematologic: leukopenia, agranulocytosis, thrombocytopenia

Hepatic: hepatitis

Metabolic: hypokalemia, sodium retention, blood glucose changes, **hypoglycemia**

Skin: rash, urticaria, pruritus, diaphoresis, bruising, photosensitivity

Other: altered taste, increased appetite, weight changes, edema, chills, yawning, hypersensitivity reaction, injection site reaction

Patient monitoring

- Monitor blood glucose level, especially during times of increased stress (such as infection, fever, surgery, and trauma).
- Assess weight and nutritional status.
- Evaluate liver and kidney function tests.

antiemetics

5-HT$_3$ receptor antagonists: dolasetron mesylate, granisetron hydrochloride, ondansetron hydrochloride, palonosetron hydrochloride

Anticholinergics: dimenhydrinate, diphenhydramine hydrochloride, meclizine hydrochloride, trimethobenzamide hydrochloride

Antidopaminergics: chlorpromazine hydrochloride, metoclopramide hydrochloride, perphenazine, prochlorperazine, promethazine hydrochloride

Other: aprepitant, dronabinol

Action

Block activity of central neurotransmitters, dopamine in chemoreceptor trigger zone, acetylcholine in vomiting center, or 5-HT$_3$ receptors on vagal neurons in GI tract

Indications

Prevention of nausea and vomiting caused by chemotherapy or radiation therapy, prevention or treatment of postoperative nausea or vomiting

Contraindications and precautions

- 5-HT$_3$ receptor antagonists are contraindicated in hypersensitivity to drug. Antidopaminergics are contraindicated in coma and drug- or alcohol-induced CNS depression.

• Use cautiously in hepatic disease; premature infants (if drug contains benzyl alcohol); or sulfite or tartrazine sensitivity (if drug contains sulfite or tartrazine). Also use cautiously in patients who have or may develop prolonged conduction intervals, especially marked QTc prolongation.

Adverse reactions
CNS: anxiety, agitation, confusion, asthenia, dizziness, drowsiness, sedation, headache, malaise, fatigue, weakness, pain, vertigo, paresthesia, tremor, sleep disorder, depersonalization, ataxia, twitching, extrapyramidal syndrome
CV: hypertension, hypotension, angina, syncope, bradycardia, tachycardia, **arrhythmias, Mobitz I heart block**
EENT: epistaxis
GI: nausea, vomiting, diarrhea, constipation, dyspepsia, abdominal pain, dry mouth, anorexia
GU: hematuria, dysuria, polyuria, urinary retention, **oliguria**
Hematologic: anemia, purpura, hematoma, **leukopenia, thrombocytopenia**
Respiratory: hypoxia
Skin: rash, flushing, increased diaphoresis, pruritus
Other: altered taste, fever, chills, cold sensation, edema, facial or peripheral edema, injection site reaction, **anaphylaxis**

Patient monitoring
• Monitor CBC, liver function tests, and ECG changes.
◀€ Stay alert for prolonged PR interval and widened QRS complexes, especially in patients receiving concurrent antiarrhythmics.
• Watch for excessive diuresis.
• When giving antidopaminergics, monitor for signs and symptoms of neuroleptic malignant syndrome.

antifungals
amphotericin B, caspofungin acetate, fluconazole, flucytosine, griseofulvin, itraconazole, ketoconazole, micafungin sodium, miconazole, nystatin, posaconazol, terbinafine hydrochloride, voriconazole

Action
Varies with specific drug. See individual monographs.

Indications
Meningitis, visceral leishmaniasis in immunocompetent patients, invasive fungal infections, systemic fungal infections (histoplasmosis, coccidioidomycosis, blastomycosis, cryptococcosis, phycomycosis, disseminated candidiasis, zygomycosis), oral and perioral candidal infections, GI tract infections caused by *Candida albicans*

Contraindications and precautions
• Contraindicated in hypersensitivity to antifungals and concurrent use of cisapride or pimozide
• Use cautiously in renal, hepatic, or cardiac disease; achlorhydria; pregnant or breastfeeding patients; and children younger than age 2.

Adverse reactions
CNS: anxiety, confusion, headache, insomnia, asthenia, abnormal thinking, agitation, depression, dizziness, hallucinations, hypertonia, vertigo, psychosis, drowsiness, speech disorder, malaise, **stupor, seizures**
CV: chest pain, vasodilation, hypotension, orthostatic hypotension, hypertension, phlebitis, tachycardia, bradycardia, **supraventricular tachycardia, cardiac arrest, asystole, atrial fibrillation, shock**

Reactions in **bold** are life-threatening.　　◀€ Clinical alert

EENT: diplopia, amblyopia, blurred vision, eye hemorrhage, hearing loss, tinnitus, epistaxis, rhinitis, sinusitis, pharyngitis

GI: nausea, vomiting, diarrhea, abdominal pain, abdominal distention, melena, stomatitis, dry mouth, oral candidiasis, anorexia, **GI hemorrhage**

GU: dysuria, hematuria, albuminuria, glycosuria, urinary retention or incontinence, **oliguria, renal failure, abnormal renal function with hypokalemia**

Hematologic: anemia, eosinophilia, **leukocytosis, thrombocytopenia, leukopenia, agranulocytosis**

Hepatic: jaundice, **acute hepatic failure, hepatitis**

Metabolic: dehydration, hypomagnesemia, hypokalemia, hypocalcemia, hypernatremia, hyperglycemia, hypoproteinemia, hyperlipidemia, **acidosis**

Musculoskeletal: myalgia; joint, neck, or back pain

Respiratory: increased cough, wheezing, dyspnea, tachypnea, hypoxia, hyperventilation, hemoptysis, asthma, **pulmonary edema, pleural effusion, bronchospasm, respiratory failure**

Skin: pruritus, acne, alopecia, diaphoresis, skin discoloration, nodules, ulcers, urticaria, maculopapular rash

Other: gingivitis, weight changes, chills, fever, infection, peripheral or facial edema, pain or reaction at injection site, tissue damage (with extravasation), allergic reactions including **anaphylaxis, sepsis, multisystem failure**

Patient monitoring

• Monitor vital signs and fluid intake and output.

• Assess electrolyte levels, CBC, and kidney and liver function tests.

antigout agents (anti-hyperuricemia agents)

allopurinol, allopurinol sodium, colchicine, febuxostat, probenecid, rasburicase

Action

Decrease uric acid levels by inhibiting uric acid production or tubular reabsorption of urate or by catalyzing enzymatic oxidation of uric acid into allantoin (an inactive and soluble metabolite)

Indications

Primary or secondary gout, calcium oxalate calculi, management of uric acid levels during chemotherapy

Contraindications and precautions

• Contraindicated in hypersensitivity to drug, blood dyscrasias, or methemoglobinemia and G6PD deficiency, and concomitant use of azathioprine, mercaptopurine, or theophylline

• Use cautiously in acute gout attack during initiation of therapy, bone marrow depression, renal or hepatic disease, cardiac disease, idiopathic hemochromatosis, seizure disorders, peptic ulcer, and children (except those with cancer-related hyperuricemia); use not recommended in patients with greatly increased rate of urate formation, such as in malignant disease and its treatment and Lesch-Nyhan syndrome (febuxostat).

Adverse reactions

CNS: headache, somnolence, peripheral neuropathy, neuritis, paresthesia

CV: vasculitis, **necrotizing angiitis**

EENT: epistaxis

GI: nausea, vomiting, diarrhea, abdominal pain, gastritis, dyspepsia

GU: uremia, **renal failure**
Hematologic: ecchymosis, purpura, eosinophilia, **leukopenia, leukocytosis, thrombocytopenia**
Hepatic: cholestatic jaundice, **hepatomegaly, granulomatous hepatitis, hepatic necrosis**
Metabolic: acute gout attack
Musculoskeletal: arthralgia, myopathy
Skin: rash, vesicular bullous dermatitis, eczematoid dermatitis, pruritus, urticaria, onycholysis, lichen planus, alopecia, purpura, toxic epidermal necrolysis, **Stevens-Johnson syndrome**
Other: taste loss or perversion, fever, hypersensitivity reaction

Patient monitoring

• Assess fluid intake and output. Intake should be sufficient to yield daily output of at least 2 liters of slightly alkaline urine.
• Monitor uric acid level.

antihistamines

azelastine, brompheniramine, cetirizine hydrochloride, chlorpheniramine maleate, cyproheptadine hydrochloride, desloratadine, diphenhydramine hydrochloride, fexofenadine hydrochloride, hydroxyzine hydrochloride, hydroxyzine pamoate, levocetirizine, loratadine, promethazine

Action

Bind either nonselectively to central and peripheral histamine$_1$ (H$_1$) receptors or selectively to peripheral H$_1$ receptors, causing either CNS stimulation or depression

Indications

Sedation, nausea and vomiting, cough, parkinsonian symptoms, motion sickness, allergy symptoms, adjunct to pre- or postoperative analgesia

Contraindications and precautions

• Contraindicated in hypersensitivity to specific or structurally related antihistamines, angle-closure glaucoma, stenosing peptic ulcer, symptomatic prostatic hypertrophy, bladder neck obstruction, pyloroduodenal obstruction, MAO inhibitor use within past 14 days, elderly or debilitated patients (cyproheptadine), premature infants, and neonates
• Use cautiously in respiratory or cardiovascular disease, seizure disorders, ulcer disease, sleep apnea, renal or hepatic impairment, elderly patients, pregnant or breastfeeding patients, and children.

Adverse reactions

CNS: drowsiness, sedation, weakness, dizziness, syncope, incoordination, fatigue, lassitude, confusion, restlessness, excitation, euphoria, tremor, headache, insomnia, nightmares, paresthesia, catatonic-like state, hallucinations, disorientation, pseudoschizophrenia, vertigo, hysteria, tongue protrusion, neuritis, **seizures**
CV: orthostatic hypotension, hypotension, hypertension, palpitations, bradycardia, tachycardia, reflex tachycardia, extrasystoles, ECG changes, venous thrombosis at injection site (with I.V. promethazine), **cardiac arrest**
EENT: blurred vision; diplopia; oculogyric crisis; tinnitus; labyrinthitis; nasal stuffiness; dry mouth, nose, and throat; sore throat; **laryngeal edema**
GI: nausea, vomiting, diarrhea, constipation, epigastric distress, stomatitis, anorexia
GU: dysuria, glycosuria, urinary frequency, urinary retention, lactation, early menses, gynecomastia, inhibited ejaculation
Hematologic: thrombocytopenic purpura; hemolytic, hypoplastic, or aplastic anemia; thrombocytopenia;

Reactions in **bold** are life-threatening.   ◀€ Clinical alert

leukopenia; agranulocytosis; pancytopenia
Musculoskeletal: torticollis; tingling,
heaviness, and weakness of hands
Respiratory: thickened bronchial
secretions, chest tightness, wheezing,
asthma, **respiratory depression**
Skin: rash, dermatitis, erythema,
urticaria, excessive perspiration, angioedema, photosensitivity
Other: appetite increase, weight gain,
peripheral edema, chills, **lupus erythematosus–like syndrome, anaphylaxis**

Patient monitoring

• Monitor cardiovascular status, especially in patients with cardiovascular
disease.

• Use side rails as needed. Supervise
patient during ambulation.

antihyperlipidemics

Bile acid suppressants: cholestyramine, colesevelam hydrochloride,
colestipol hydrochloride

Fibric acid derivatives: fenofibrate,
fenofibric acid, gemfibrozil

HMG-CoA reductase inhibitors: atorvastatin calcium, fluvastatin sodium,
lovastatin, pitavastatin, pravastatin
sodium, rosuvastatin calcium,
simvastatin

Other: ezetimibe, omega-3-acid ethyl
esters

Action

Bile acid suppressants bind bile acids in
intestine to form an insoluble complex
that's excreted in feces; increased fecal
loss of bile acids enhances cholesterol
oxidation to bile acids, which lowers
low-density lipoprotein (LDL) and
cholesterol levels. *Fibric acid derivatives*
inhibit peripheral lipolysis and
decrease hepatic extraction of free fatty
acids, reducing hepatic triglyceride
production. They also inhibit synthesis
and increase clearance of apolipoprotein B (which carries very-low-density
lipoproteins [VLDLs]), thus lowering
VLDL production. *HMG-CoA reductase inhibitors* competitively inhibit
HMG-CoA reductase (an enzyme that
catalyzes the first step in cholesterol
synthesis pathway); this inhibition
decreases total cholesterol, LDL, VLDL,
triglyceride, and apolipoprotein B levels while increasing high-density lipoprotein levels.

Indications

Elevated LDL, total cholesterol, triglyceride, or apolipoprotein B levels in primary hypercholesterolemia or mixed
dyslipidemia (Fredrickson types IIa
and IIb); primary dysbetalipoproteinemia (Fredrickson type III); adjunct to
diet in hypertriglyceridemia (Fredrickson type IV)

Contraindications and precautions

• Contraindicated in hypersensitivity
to drug; active hepatic disease; complete biliary obstruction; persistent,
unexplained elevations in liver function tests; concurrent use of
cyclosporine; females of childbearing
age; and breastfeeding (pitavastatin)

• Use cautiously in severe metabolic,
endocrine, or electrolyte disorders;
visual disturbances; uncontrolled seizures; myopathy; cerebral arteriosclerosis; coronary artery disease; severe
hypotension or hypertension; history
of hepatic disease, alcoholism, renal
impairment, severe acute infection,
major surgery, or trauma; concurrent
use of protease inhibitors, erythromycin, fibric acids, rifampin, or niacin;
elderly patients (pitavastatin); females
of childbearing age; and children
younger than age 18 (safety not established).

Adverse reactions

CNS: amnesia, abnormal dreams, malaise, asthenia, emotional lability, facial paralysis, headache, hyperkinesia, incoordination, paresthesia, drowsiness, syncope, peripheral neuropathy
CV: orthostatic hypotension, palpitations, vasodilation, phlebitis, **arrhythmias**
EENT: eye hemorrhage, amblyopia, glaucoma, altered refraction, dry eyes, hearing loss, tinnitus, epistaxis, sinusitis, pharyngitis
GI: nausea, vomiting, diarrhea, constipation, abdominal cramps, abdominal or biliary pain, dyspepsia, gastroenteritis, colitis, flatulence, melena, tenesmus, dysphagia, esophagitis, pancreatitis, dry mouth, stomatitis, glossitis, anorexia, **GI ulcers, rectal hemorrhage**
GU: dysuria, nocturia, hematuria, urinary frequency or urgency, urinary retention, cystitis, renal calculi, nephritis, abnormal ejaculation, decreased libido, epididymitis, erectile dysfunction
Hematologic: anemia, **thrombocytopenia**
Hepatic: jaundice, **hepatic failure, hepatitis**
Metabolic: gout, hyperglycemia, **hypoglycemia**
Musculoskeletal: joint or back pain, bursitis, leg cramps, neck rigidity, torticollis, myalgia, myositis, myasthenia gravis
Respiratory: dyspnea, pneumonia, bronchitis
Skin: diaphoresis, acne, pruritus, rash, urticaria, alopecia, contact dermatitis, eczema, dry skin, skin ulcers, seborrhea, photosensitivity
Other: gingival hemorrhage, taste loss, increased appetite, weight gain, flulike symptoms, infection, fever, allergic reaction

Patient monitoring

• Monitor liver function tests and blood lipid panel.

anti-infectives

Aminoglycosides: amikacin sulfate, gentamicin sulfate, neomycin sulfate, streptomycin sulfate, tobramycin, tobramycin sulfate

Carbapenems: doripenem monohydrate, ertapenem sodium, imipenem cilastatin sodium, meropenem

Cephalosporins, first generation: cefadroxil, cefazolin sodium, cephalexin

Cephalosporins, second generation: cefaclor, cefoxitin sodium, cefprozil, cefuroxime axetil, cefuroxime sodium

Cephalosporins, third generation: cefdinir, cefepime hydrochloride, cefixime, cefoperazone sodium, cefotaxime sodium, cefpodoxime proxetil, ceftazidime, ceftibuten, ceftriaxone sodium

Cephalosporins, fourth generation: cefepime hydrochloride

Fluoroquinolones: ciprofloxacin, gemifloxacin, levofloxacin, moxifloxacin hydrochloride, norfloxacin, ofloxacin

Lincosamides: clindamycin hydrochloride, clindamycin palmitate hydrochloride, clindamycin phosphate

Lipoglycopeptide: telavancin

Macrolides: azithromycin, azithromycin dihydrate, clarithromycin, erythromycin, erythromycin ethylsuccinate, erythromycin lactobionate, erythromycin stearate, erythromycin (topical)

Monobactams: aztreonam

Penicillins: amoxicillin, amoxicillin trihydrate, amoxicillin and clavulanate potassium, ampicillin sodium, ampicillin sodium and sulbactam sodium, penicillin G benzathine, penicillin G potassium, penicillin G procaine, penicillin V potassium, piperacillin sodium and tazobactam sodium, ticarcillin disodium and clavulanate potassium

Streptogramins: quinupristin and dalfopristin

Sulfonamides: sulfacetamide sodium, sulfamethoxazole-trimethoprim, sulfasalazine

Tetracyclines: doxycycline, doxycycline calcium, doxycycline hyclate, doxycycline monohydrate, minocycline hydrochloride, tetracycline hydrochloride

Other: linezolid, metronidazole, metronidazole hydrochloride, mupirocin, nitazoxanide, nitrofurantoin, nitrofurantoin macrocrystals, pentamidine isethionate, rifaximin, telithromycin, tigecycline, tinidazole, vancomycin

Action
Bactericidal anti-infectives (aminoglycosides, cephalosporins, carbapenems, dapsone, fluoroquinolones, lincosamides, linezolid, macrolides and nitrofurantoin at high concentrations, metronidazole, monobactams, penicillins, quinupristin, and vancomycin) kill bacterial cells by inhibiting cell-wall synthesis of actively dividing bacterial cells via binding to one or more penicillin-bound proteins or 30S ribosomal subunits or via inhibition of DNA gyrase and topoisomerase IV.

Bacteriostatic anti-infectives (chloramphenicol, dapsone, linezolid [against enterococci and staphylococci only], macrolides and nitrofurantoin at low concentrations, quinupristin/dalfopristin [bacteriostatic against *Enterococcus faecium*], sulfonamides, telithromycin, and tetracyclines) inhibit bacterial cell growth or multiplication by giving the host immune system adequate time to mount a lethal response.

Indications
Vary with drug. See individual monographs.

Contraindications and precautions
• Contraindicated in hypersensitivity to drug. (For additional contraindications, see individual monographs.)
• Use cautiously in renal impairment, cirrhosis or other hepatic disease, neuromuscular disease, CNS disease, bradycardia, acute myocardial ischemia, parkinsonism, hearing impairment, concurrent use of drugs known to prolong QT interval or history of congenital long QT syndrome, known prolongation of QTc interval, uncompensated heart failure, severe left ventricular hypertrophy (avoid telavancin use), dialysis patients, obese patients, elderly patients, pregnant or breastfeeding patients, neonates, and premature infants.

Adverse reactions
CNS: dizziness, vertigo, tremor, numbness, depression, confusion, lethargy, nystagmus, headache, paresthesia, **neuromuscular blockade, seizures, neurotoxicity**
CV: hypotension, hypertension, palpitations, phlebitis, **thrombophlebitis**
EENT: visual disturbances; eye stinging, redness, itching, or dryness; photophobia; tinnitus; hearing loss;

ototoxicity; increased salivation; hoarseness (with tetracyclines)

GI: nausea, vomiting, diarrhea, abdominal cramps, stomatitis, oral candidiasis, black "hairy" tongue, anorexia, splenomegaly, **pseudomembranous colitis**

GU: polyuria, dysuria, azotemia, increased urinary cast excretion, erectile dysfunction, vaginal candidiasis, **nephrotoxicity, renal failure**

Hematologic: purpura, eosinophilia, lymphocytosis, **leukemoid reaction, hemolytic or aplastic anemia, neutropenia, agranulocytosis, leukopenia, thrombocytopenia, pancytopenia, hypoprothrombinemia, bone marrow depression**

Hepatic: hepatomegaly, hepatic necrosis

Metabolic: blood glucose changes

Musculoskeletal: joint pain, tendinitis, tendon rupture

Respiratory: dyspnea, apnea

Skin: rash, urticaria, pruritus, exfoliative dermatitis, alopecia, sterile abscess, **Stevens-Johnson syndrome**

Other: permanent tooth discoloration, tooth enamel defects, weight loss, superinfection, pain, irritation at I.M. injection site, induration, chills, fever, edema, **serum sickness, anaphylaxis**

Patient monitoring

• Monitor vital signs and fluid intake and output. Push fluids to help prevent renal tubular irritation.

• Monitor drug blood level.

• Watch for signs and symptoms of overgrowth of resistant organisms.

• Assess CBC and kidney function tests.

• Monitor International Normalized Ratio in prolonged therapy and in patients with malnutrition or high risk of renal or hepatic impairment.

• Assess for ototoxicity by comparing current and baseline audiograms.

antimalarials

chloroquine hydrochloride, chloroquine phosphate, doxycycline, hydroxychloroquine sulfate, mefloquine hydrochloride, primaquine hydrochloride, pyrimethamine, quinine sulfate

Action

Varies. See individual monographs.

Indications

Prophylaxis or treatment of malaria

Contraindications and precautions

• Contraindicated for prophylactic use in severe renal insufficiency, marked hepatic parenchymal damage, or blood dyscrasias. Also contraindicated in hypersensitivity to drug, megaloblastic anemia caused by folate deficiency, depression (current or previous), generalized anxiety disorder, psychosis, schizophrenia or other major psychiatric disorder, history of seizures, pregnancy at term, breastfeeding, and infants younger than 2 months old.

• Use cautiously in hepatic dysfunction, cardiac disease, and ocular lesions.

Adverse reactions

CNS: headache, psychic stimulation, psychotic episodes, **seizures**

CV: hypotension, ECG changes, **cardiomyopathy**

EENT: irreversible retinal damage; visual disturbances; night blindness; scotomatous vision with field defects of paracentral and pericentral ring types and typically temporal scotomas

GI: vomiting, abdominal cramps, atrophic glossitis, anorexia

GU: hematuria

Reactions in **bold** are life-threatening.   ◀╠ Clinical alert

Hematologic: hemolytic or mega-loblastic anemia, leukopenia, throm-bocytopenia, pancytopenia, methe-moglobinemia, agranulocytosis

Skin: pruritus, lichen planus–like erup-tions, skin and mucosal pigment changes, pleomorphic skin eruptions, alopecia, toxic epidermal necrolysis, **erythema multiforme, Stevens-John-son syndrome**

Other: hypersensitivity reactions including **anaphylaxis**

Patient monitoring
• Monitor liver function tests, CBC, and G6PD levels in susceptible patients before and periodically during therapy.

antimigraine drugs
Ergotamine derivatives: dihydroergo-tamine mesylate, ergotamine tartrate

Serotonin (5-hydroxytryptamine [5-HT₁]) receptor agonists: almotrip-tan malate, eletriptan, frovatriptan, naratriptan hydrochloride, rizatriptan hydrochloride, sumatriptan, topira-mate, zolmitriptan

Action
Ergotamine derivatives exert partial agonist or antagonist activity against tryptaminergic, dopaminergic, and alpha-adrenergic receptors (depending on their site), causing peripheral and cranial vasoconstriction and depres-sion of central vasomotor centers.

5-HT₁ receptor agonists activate serotonin 5-HT₁B/1D receptors, caus-ing cranial vasoconstriction, inhibition of neuropeptide release, and reduced impulse transmission in trigeminal pain pathways.

Indications
Migraine

Contraindications and precautions
• Contraindicated in hypersensitivity to drug; hemiplegic or basilar migraine; ischemic heart or bowel disease; severe renal or hepatic impairment; Prinzmetal's angina or other significant underlying cardiovascular disease; uncontrolled hypertension; use of ergo-tamine-containing preparations, ergot-type drugs, or other 5-HT₁ agonists within past 24 hours; MAO inhibitor use within past 14 days; and I.V. use
• Use cautiously in hypertension, hypercholesterolemia, diabetes melli-tus, cardiovascular disease, smoking, obesity, men older than age 40, menopausal women, pregnant or breastfeeding patients, and children younger than age 18.

Adverse reactions
CNS: dizziness, paresthesia, hypoesthe-sia, asthenia, drowsiness, somnolence, fatigue, headache, myasthenia, vertigo

CV: chest tightness, pressure, or heaviness

EENT: rhinitis, sinusitis, pharyngitis

GI: nausea; vomiting; diarrhea; abdom-inal pain or discomfort; stomach pain, cramps, or pressure; dyspepsia; dyspha-gia; dry mouth

Musculoskeletal: neck, throat, or jaw pain; stiffness

Other: altered taste, hot or cold sensa-tions, hot flushes, application site reaction

Patient monitoring
• Monitor ECG for changes.

antineoplastics
Alkylating agents: bendamustine hydrochloride, busulfan, carboplatin, carmustine, chlorambucil, cisplatin,

cyclophosphamide, dacarbazine, ifosfamide, lomustine, melphalan, melphalan hydrochloride, oxaliplatin, procarbazine hydrochloride, temozolomide

Antibiotic antineoplastics: bleomycin, sulfate, daunorubicin citrate liposome, daunorubicin hydrochloride, doxorubicin hydrochloride, doxorubicin hydrochloride liposomal, epirubicin hydrochloride, idarubicin, hydrochloride mitomycin, mitoxantrone hydrochloride

Antimetabolites: azacitidine, capecitabine, clofarabine, cytarabine, fluorouracil (5-fluorouracil, 5-FU), gemcitabine hydrochloride, hydroxyurea, mercaptopurine, methotrexate, methotrexate sodium, nelarabine, paclitaxel, pemetrexed, pentostatin

Antimitotics: cabazitaxel, docetaxel, paclitaxel, vinblastine sulfate, vincristine sulfate, vinorelbine tartrate

Biological antineoplastics: aldesleukin (interleukin-2, IL-2), cetuximab, denileukin diftitox, ibritumomab tiuxetan, interferon alfa-2b, recombinant, interferon gamma-1b, peginterferon alfa-2a, peginterferon alfa-2b, rituximab, trastuzumab

Cytoprotective agents: amifostine, leucovorin calcium (citrovorum factor, folinic acid), mesna

DNA topoisomerase inhibitors: irinotecan hydrochloride, topotecan hydrochloride

Enzyme antineoplastics: asparaginase, pegaspareginase

Epipodophyllotoxins: etoposide, (VP-16-213), etoposide phosphate

Folic acid antagonists: pralatrexate

Hormonal antineoplastics: anastrozole, bicalutamide, exemestane, flutamide, fulvestrant, goserelin acetate, letrozole, leuprolide acetate, medroxyprogesterone acetate, megestrol, nilutamide, raloxifene, tamoxifen citrate, triptorelin pamoate

Other: abiraterone acetate, alitretinoin, arsenic trioxide, axitinib, bortezomib, brentuximab vedotin, dasatinib, degarelix, erbulin, erlotinib, everolimus, ibritumomab tiuxetan, imatinib mesylate, lapatanib, lenalidomide, nilotinib, pazopanib, pertuzumab, ruxolitinib, sipuleucel-T, sorafenib, sunitinib maleate, tretinoin

Action
Varies with specific drug. Generally, antineoplastics inhibit normal substrate use in tumor cells, forming dysfunctional macromolecules by inserting themselves into abnormal cells; also intercalate between DNA strands and interfere with DNA templates. Some antineoplastics modify growth of hormone-dependent tumors.

Indications
Hodgkin's or non-Hodgkin's lymphoma, testicular teratomas, mycosis fungoides, breast cancer, ovarian cancer, prostate cancer, lung cancer, head and neck cancer, colorectal cancer, pancreatic cancer, bronchogenic carcinoma, malignant melanoma, chronic lymphatic or chronic myeloid leukemia, other cancers

Contraindications and precautions
• Contraindicated in hypersensitivity to drug or its components
• Use cautiously in heart disease, renal or hepatic impairment, decreased bone

marrow reserve, active infections, severe myocardial insufficiency, coagulation and bleeding disorders, active thrombophlebitis or thromboembolic disorders, shock, trauma, major surgery within previous month, elderly or debilitated patients, patients with childbearing potential, and pregnant or breastfeeding patients.

Adverse reactions

CNS: dizziness, fatigue, lethargy, asthenia, drowsiness, malaise, headache, sensory or motor dysfunction, impaired memory, confusion, agitation, depression, emotional lability, sleep disturbances, hallucinations, rigors, peripheral neuropathy, paresthesia, tremor, ataxia, flaccid paresis, abnormal gait, vertigo, syncope, cranial nerve dysfunction, hemiparesis, mental status changes, acute cerebellar dysfunction, **demyelinization, seizures, leukoencephalopathy, cerebrovascular accident, suicidal ideation**

CV: hypotension, hypertension, chest pain, peripheral edema, tachycardia, **cardiomegaly, prolonged QT interval, thromboembolic events, arrhythmias, cardiac tamponade, torsades de pointes, cardiac arrest, capillary leak syndrome, myocardial infarction, left-sided heart failure, pericardial effusion**

EENT: retinal thrombosis, corneal opacity, photophobia, diplopia, visual changes, nystagmus, lacrimation, lacrimal duct stenosis, stye, epistaxis, pharyngitis

GI: nausea, vomiting, diarrhea, constipation, fecal incontinence, abdominal pain, dyspepsia, GI ulcer, ascites, dry mouth, mucositis, oral candidiasis, dysphagia, anorexia, **intestinal perforation, paralytic ileus, GI bleeding**

GU: proteinuria, hematuria, dysuria, urinary hesitancy or retention, urinary obstruction, cystitis, bladder fibrosis, vaginitis, vaginal hemorrhage, breast swelling and tenderness, menstrual abnormalities, abortion, gynecomastia, sterility, libido loss, erectile dysfunction, decreased testes size, reduced sperm count, **progressive azotemia, hemolytic uremic syndrome, nephrotoxicity, oliguria or anuria, renal failure**

Hematologic: anemia, eosinophilia, **neutropenia, thrombocytopenia, leukopenia, leukocytosis, bone marrow depression, agranulocytosis, pancytopenia, coagulation disorders, hemorrhage**

Hepatic: jaundice, **hepatitis, hepatotoxicity**

Metabolic: hyperglycemia, fluid retention, **hyperkalemia**

Musculoskeletal: muscle twitching, joint or bone pain, decreased bone density, carpal tunnel syndrome

Respiratory: tachypnea, dyspnea, wheezing, pulmonary congestion, cough, chronic obstructive pulmonary disease, upper respiratory tract infection, **tracheoesophageal fistula, pleural effusion, interstitial pneumonitis, bronchospasm, pulmonary toxicity, pulmonary edema, respiratory failure, apnea, development or worsening of pulmonary fibrosis**

Skin: erythema, pruritus, rash, diaphoresis, night sweats, dry skin, urticaria, alopecia, phlebitis at I.V. site, palmar-plantar erythrodysesthesia, nail loss, bruising, petechiae, exacerbation of postradiation erythema, painful plaque erosions, epidermal necrolysis, exfoliative dermatitis, **Stevens-Johnson syndrome**

Other: increased appetite, weight gain, fever, chills, pain, flulike symptoms, herpes simplex or other infection, tumor flare, hypersensitivity reaction, **risk of second malignancy, anaphylaxis, sepsis, tumor lysis syndrome**

Patient monitoring

🔊 Watch for bleeding. If platelet count is low, avoid giving I.M. injections and taking rectal temperature.

• Stay alert for bone marrow depression, neutropenia, and anemia.

- Monitor fluid intake and output.
- Monitor for GI upset. Give antiemetics as needed and prescribed.

antiparkinsonian drugs

Anticholinergics: benztropine, trihexyphenidyl hydrochloride

Antivirals: amantadine hydrochloride

Dopaminergics: apomorphine hydrochloride, bromocriptine mesylate, carbidopa-levodopa, levodopa, pramipexole, ropinirole hydrochloride, tolcapone

MAO inhibitors: rasagiline, selegiline

Action
Block central cholinergic receptors or inhibit prolactin secretion; also may act as dopamine receptor agonists by activating postsynaptic dopamine receptors

Indications
Parkinson's disease

Contraindications and precautions
- Contraindicated in hypersensitivity to drug, angle-closure glaucoma, tardive dyskinesia, stenosing peptic ulcer, achalasia, pyloric or duodenal obstruction, prostatic hypertrophy, bladder neck obstruction, myasthenia gravis, and children younger than age 3
- Use cautiously in seizure disorders, arrhythmias, tachycardia, hypertension, hypotension, hepatic or renal dysfunction, alcoholism, exposure to hot environments, elderly patients, and pregnant or breastfeeding patients (safety not established).

Adverse reactions
CNS: confusion, headache, dizziness, fatigue, light-headedness, drowsiness, nervousness, insomnia, nightmares, mania, delusions, **seizures, cerebrovascular accident**
CV: hypotension, palpitations, extrasystole, bradycardia, **arrhythmias, acute myocardial infarction**
EENT: diplopia, blurred vision, burning sensation of eyes, nasal congestion
GI: nausea, vomiting, diarrhea, constipation, abdominal cramps, dry mouth, anorexia, **GI hemorrhage**
GU: urinary incontinence, frequency, or retention; diuresis; erectile dysfunction
Hepatic: hepatic failure
Musculoskeletal: leg cramps, numb fingers
Skin: urticaria; pale, cool fingers and toes; facial and arm rash; alopecia
Other: hyperthermia, **heat stroke**

Patient monitoring
- Monitor fluid intake and output and assess vital signs (especially blood pressure).

antiplatelet drugs
abciximab, anagrelide hydrochloride, cilostazol, clopidogrel bisulfate, dipyridamole, eptifibatide, prasugrel, ticlopidine hydrochloride, tirofiban hydrochloride, treprostinil sodium

Action
Inhibit platelet aggregation by reversibly preventing fibrinogen, von Willebrand's factor, and other adhesion ligands from binding to glycoprotein (GP) IIb/IIIa receptor or by inhibiting platelet fibrinogen induced by adenosine diphosphate

Indications
Acute coronary syndrome, cerebrovascular accident (CVA)

Reactions in **bold** are life-threatening.　　　◀€ Clinical alert

Contraindications and precautions

• Contraindicated in hypersensitivity to drug, CVA or abnormal bleeding within past 30 days, history of bleeding diathesis, history of hemorrhagic CVA, major surgery within past 6 weeks, concurrent or planned use of other parenteral GP IIb/IIIa inhibitors, dependence on renal dialysis, severe uncontrolled hypertension (systolic pressure above 200 mm Hg or diastolic pressure above 110 mm Hg), platelet count below 100,000/mm³, or serum creatinine of 4 mg/dl or more

• Use cautiously in hemorrhagic retinopathy; severe renal insufficiency; chronic hemodialysis; hepatic failure; platelet count below 150,000/mm³; hypotension, pulmonary edema, or pulmonary veno-occlusive disease (treprostinil); or concurrent use of thrombolytics or other drugs that affect hemostasis, thrombotic thrombocytopenic purpura, low body weight, patients age 75 and older (use not recommended except in high-risk situations), pregnant or breastfeeding patients, and children (safety and efficacy not established).

Adverse reactions

CNS: depression, somnolence, confusion, insomnia, nervousness, amnesia, migraine, dizziness, headache, **intracranial hemorrhage**

CV: chest pain, angina pectoris, orthostatic hypotension, hypertension, vasodilation, syncope, bradycardia, cardiovascular disease, **arrhythmias, thrombosis, aortic dissection, heart failure**

EENT: amblyopia, abnormal vision, visual field abnormality, diplopia, tinnitus, epistaxis, rhinitis, sinusitis

GI: nausea, diarrhea, constipation, gastritis, abdominal pain, dyspepsia, melena, eructation, aphthous stomatitis, **GI hemorrhage**

GU: dysuria, hematuria, urinary tract infection

Hematologic: anemia, ecchymosis, **bleeding, thrombocytopenia**

Hepatic: hemorrhage

Metabolic: dehydration

Musculoskeletal: arthralgia, myalgia, leg cramps or pain, pelvic pain

Respiratory: respiratory disease, pneumonia, bronchitis, asthma

Skin: skin disease, diaphoresis, alopecia, photosensitivity

Other: lymphadenopathy, fever, chills, edema, flulike symptoms, accidental injury

Patient monitoring

• Monitor CBC, platelet count, and coagulation studies.

• Watch for unusual bleeding or bruising.

• Assess vital signs and cardiovascular status.

antipsychotics

aripiprazole, asenapine, chlorpromazine hydrochloride, clozapine, fluphenazine decanoate, fluphenazine hydrochloride, haloperidol, haloperidol decanoate, haloperidol lactate, iloperidone, lithium carbonate, lithium citrate, loxapine succinate, olanzapine, paliperidone, perphenazine, prochlorperazine, prochlorperazine edisylate, prochlorperazine maleate, quetiapine fumarate, risperidone, trifluoperazine hydrochloride, ziprasidone

Action

Block postsynaptic mesolimbic and mesocortical dopamine receptors in brain, relieving hallucinations, delusions, and psychoses. Also thought to relieve anxiety by filtering internal arousal stimuli to reticular system in brain stem.

Indications

Acute or chronic psychosis, acute intermittent porphyria, nausea and vomiting, intractable hiccups, preoperative sedation

Contraindications and precautions

• Contraindicated in hypersensitivity to drug, phenothiazines, sulfites (when injected), or benzyl alcohol (sustained-release forms); angle-closure glaucoma; bone marrow depression; blood dyscrasias; myeloproliferative disorders; subcortical brain damage; cerebral arteriosclerosis; hepatic damage; coronary artery disease; severe hypotension or hypertension; coma; and severe depression

• Use cautiously in diabetes mellitus; respiratory, cerebrovascular, or cardiovascular disease; prostatic hypertrophy; CNS tumors; seizure disorders; intestinal obstruction; concomitant use of CYP1A2 inhibitors, drugs that are both substrates and inhibitors of CYP2D6, drugs with anticholinergic activity, other centrally acting drugs, certain antihypertensives, alcohol, and drugs known to prolong QT interval; patients who experience conditions that may contribute to core body temperature elevation; dehydration; elderly or debilitated patients; elderly patients with dementia-related psychosis; pregnant or breastfeeding patients (safety not established); and children with acute illness, infection, gastroenteritis, or dehydration.

Adverse reactions

CNS: drowsiness, sedation, extrapyramidal reactions, tardive dyskinesia, pseudoparkinsonism, **seizures, neuroleptic malignant syndrome**
CV: hypotension (increased with I.M. or I.V. use), tachycardia

EENT: blurred vision, lens opacities, dry eyes, nasal congestion
GI: constipation, anorexia, dry mouth, **paralytic ileus**
GU: urinary retention, menstrual irregularities, inhibited ejaculation, priapism, galactorrhea
Hematologic: eosinophilia, **hemolytic anemia, agranulocytosis, leukopenia, aplastic anemia, thrombocytopenia**
Hepatic: jaundice, **hepatitis**
Skin: photosensitivity, pigmentation changes, rash, sterile abscess
Other: allergic reactions, hyperthermia, pain at injection site

Patient monitoring

• Monitor vital signs (especially blood pressure), ECG, CBC, urinalysis, liver and kidney function tests, and periodic eye exams.

antirheumatic drugs

Biological response modifiers: adalimumab, anakinra, etanercept, glimumab, infliximab, tocilizumab

Disease-modifying agents: auranofin, aurothioglucose, azathioprine, cyclosporine, hydroxychloroquine sulfate, leflunomide, methotrexate, methotrexate sodium

Action

Biological response modifiers bind specifically to tumor necrosis factor (TNF) alpha or competitively inhibit binding of interleukin-1 (IL-1) to IL-1 type I receptors, thereby blocking biologic activity of TNF alpha or IL-1.

Disease-modifying agents suppress the immune system and decrease inflammation.

Indications

Rheumatoid arthritis

Reactions in **bold** are life-threatening.   ◀€ Clinical alert

Contraindications and precautions

• Contraindicated in hypersensitivity to drug, moderate to severe heart failure, demyelinating CNS disorder, hematologic abnormalities, poorly controlled or advanced diabetes mellitus, and significant exposure to varicella virus

• Use cautiously in severe myocardial, hepatic, or renal disease; decreased bone marrow reserve; active infection; hypotension; coma; history of or exposure to tuberculosis; elderly patients; pregnant or breastfeeding patients; and children.

Adverse reactions

CNS: confusion, hallucinations, headache, fatigue, insomnia, depression, EEG abnormalities, peripheral neuropathy, sensorimotor effects, **encephalitis, seizures**

CV: hypertension

EENT: iritis, corneal ulcers, gold deposits in ocular tissues, rhinitis, pharyngitis, sinusitis

GI: nausea, vomiting, diarrhea, constipation, abdominal cramps, flatulence, dyspepsia, dysphagia, ulcerative enterocolitis, melena, occult blood in stool, anorexia, **GI bleeding**

GU: hematuria, proteinuria, urinary tract infection, **nephrotic syndrome or glomerulitis, acute renal failure, acute tubular necrosis, acute nephritis, degeneration of proximal tubular epithelium**

Hematologic: eosinophilia, anemia, **thrombocytopenia, leukopenia, neutropenia, agranulocytosis, pancytopenia, hypoplastic anemia, aplastic anemia, pure red-cell aplasia, granulocytopenia, panmyelopathy, hemorrhagic diathesis**

Hepatic: jaundice, intrahepatic cholestasis, **hepatitis with jaundice, toxic hepatitis**

Musculoskeletal: arthralgia, back pain, myalgia, synovial destruction

Respiratory: upper respiratory infection, cough, dyspnea, **tuberculosis**

Skin: rash; urticaria; pruritus; erythema; papular, vesicular, or exfoliative dermatitis; abscess; alopecia; nail shedding; angioedema; photosensitivity

Other: bad taste, fever, chest pain, candidiasis, infection, chrysiasis, lupus-like syndrome, lymphoproliferative disease, hypersensitivity reaction, **cancer**

Patient monitoring

• Monitor for signs and symptoms of hypersensitivity reaction and infection.

• Monitor CBC with white cell differential and platelet count; assess liver and kidney function tests.

• Assess for heart failure in patients with history of cardiac disease.

antituberculars

ethambutol hydrochloride, isoniazid, pyrazinamide, rifabutin, rifampin, rifapentine, streptomycin sulfate

Action

Unknown. May interfere with synthesis of one or more bacterial metabolites, altering RNA synthesis during cell division.

Indications

Tuberculosis and atypical mycobacterial infections caused by *Mycobacterium tuberculosis*

Contraindications and precautions

• Contraindicated in hypersensitivity to drug (including drug-induced hepatitis)

• Use cautiously in severe renal impairment, malnutrition, diabetes mellitus, chronic alcoholism, diabetic retinopathy, cataracts, optic neuritis and other ocular defects, history of hepatic damage or chronic alcohol ingestion, patients older than age

50, Black or Hispanic females, postpartal patients, pregnant or breastfeeding patients, and children younger than age 13.

Adverse reactions

CNS: confusion, dizziness, hallucinations, headache, malaise, peripheral neuritis

EENT: optic neuritis, blurred vision, decreased visual acuity, eye pain, red-green color blindness

GI: nausea, vomiting, abdominal pain, anorexia

Hematologic: thrombocytopenia

Hepatic: hepatitis

Metabolic: hyperuricemia

Musculoskeletal: joint pain, gouty arthritis

Respiratory: bloody sputum

Skin: rash, toxic epidermal necrolysis

Other: fever, **anaphylaxis**

Patient monitoring

• Monitor vital signs (especially blood pressure), ECG, CBC, urinalysis, liver and kidney function tests, and periodic eye exams.

antiulcer drugs

Histamine$_2$ (H$_2$)-receptor antagonists: cimetidine hydrochloride, famotidine, nizatidine, ranitidine hydrochloride

Proton pump inhibitors: dexlansoprazole, esomeprazole magnesium, lansoprazole, omeprazole, pantoprazole sodium, rabeprazole sodium

Other: bismuth subsalicylate, misoprostol

Action

Reduce gastric acid level either by blocking H$_2$ receptors or by inhibiting the proton pump

Indications

Short-term treatment of active duodenal ulcer or benign gastric ulcer; prophylaxis of duodenal ulcer (at lower doses); treatment of gastroesophageal reflux disease, heartburn, acid indigestion, and gastric hypersecretory states (such as Zollinger-Ellison syndrome); prevention and treatment of stress-induced upper GI bleeding in critically ill patients

Contraindications and precautions

• Contraindicated in hypersensitivity to any antiulcer drug and in alcohol intolerance

• Use cautiously in renal impairment, elderly patients, pregnant or breastfeeding patients, and children.

Adverse reactions

CNS: confusion, dizziness, drowsiness, hallucinations, headache, peripheral neuropathy, **brain stem dysfunction**

CV: hypotension, **arrhythmias, cardiac arrest**

GI: nausea, diarrhea, constipation

GU: decreased sperm count, erectile dysfunction, gynecomastia

Hematologic: anemia, **neutropenia, thrombocytopenia, agranulocytosis, aplastic anemia**

Hepatic: hepatitis

Other: altered taste, pain at I.M. injection site, hypersensitivity reaction

Patient monitoring

• Monitor for resolution of GI symptoms.

• Assess CBC and liver function tests.

Reactions in **bold** are life-threatening.　　　　🔊 Clinical alert

antivirals and antiretrovirals

Antivirals: acyclovir, acyclovir sodium, amantadine hydrochloride, boceprevir, cidofovir, entecavir, famciclovir, foscarnet sodium, ganciclovir, interferon alfacon-1, interferon beta-1a, interferon beta-1b recombinant, oseltamivir phosphate, ribavirin, rimantadine hydrochloride, valacyclovir hydrochloride, valganciclovir hydrochloride, zanamivir

Antiretrovirals: abacavir sulfate, adefovir dipivoxil, atazanavir, darunavir, delavirdine mesylate, didanosine, efavirenz, emtricitabine, enfurvitide, etravirine, fosamprenavir calcium, indinavir sulfate, lamivudine, nelfinavir mesylate, nevirapine, raltegravir, ritonavir, saquinavir mesylate, stavudine, tenofovir disoproxil fumarate, tipranavir, zalcitabine, zidovudine

Action
Antivirals kill viral cells by inhibiting release of enzymes required for DNA synthesis; inhibiting viral nucleic acid, DNA, or protein synthesis; inhibiting viral replication; or inhibiting protease reaction.

Antiretrovirals inhibit activity of human immunodeficiency virus (HIV) protease or HIV-1 reverse transcriptase, or bind directly to reverse transcriptase and block RNA- and DNA-dependent DNA polymerase activities. These actions inhibit HIV replication.

Indications
Genital herpes, herpes simplex, varicella zoster, herpes zoster (shingles), influenza type A virus, hepatitis, cytomegalovirus, HIV

Contraindications and precautions
• Contraindicated in hypersensitivity to drug or its components, use with drugs primarily metabolized by CYP3A and UGT1A1, and with St. John's wort

• Use cautiously in renal or hepatic impairment; conduction abnormalities; concomitant use of drugs that may prolong PR interval, antiarrhythmics, antidepressants, high doses of ketoconazole and itraconazole, calcium channel blockers, hormonal contraceptives, proton pump inhibitors, antifungals, antigout agents, efavirenz, inhaled beta agonists, endothelin-receptor antagonists, inhaled nasal steroid, opioids, and drugs highly dependent on CYP2C8 with narrow indices without ritonavir (atazanavir); peripheral neuropathy; phenylketonuria; hyperuricemia; hypercholesterolemia; amylase elevation; history of mental illness, substance abuse, or hepatic impairment (including hepatitis B or C infection); sodium-restricted diet; elderly or debilitated patients; pregnant or breastfeeding patients; and children.

Adverse reactions
CNS: dizziness, asthenia, anxiety, abnormal thinking, hypoesthesia, agitation, confusion, hypertonia, **seizures, coma**

CV: hypotension, palpitations, bradycardia, weak pulse, pseudoaneurysm, **embolism, thrombophlebitis, nodal arrhythmias, atrioventricular block, ventricular tachycardia**

EENT: ocular hypotony, iritis, retinal detachment, diplopia

GI: nausea, vomiting, diarrhea, abdominal distention, dyspepsia, gastroesophageal reflux, hematemesis, dysphagia, dry mouth, **paralytic ileus**

GU: urinary retention, frequency, or incontinence; dysuria; prostatitis; **nephrotoxicity**

Hematologic: anemia, petechiae, **leukocytosis, thrombocytopenia, neutropenia, bleeding**

Hepatic: hepatomegaly

Metabolic: diabetes mellitus, **hyperkalemia**

Musculoskeletal: muscle contractions

Respiratory: bronchitis, dyspnea, wheezing, pneumonia, pleurisy, **pleural effusion, pulmonary edema, bronchospasm, pulmonary embolism**

Skin: rash, diaphoresis, urticaria, pruritus, bullous eruptions, pallor

Other: pain, peripheral coldness, edema, drug toxicity

Patient monitoring

• Monitor CBC and liver and kidney function tests.

• As indicated, monitor viral load and T-cell levels.

anxiolytics

Benzodiazepines: alprazolam, chlordiazepoxide hydrochloride, clonazepam, clorazepate, diazepam, lorazepam, oxazepam

Other: buspirone hydrochloride, doxepin, hydroxyzine hydrochloride, hydroxyzine pamoate

Action

Benzodiazepines potentiate effects of gamma-aminobutyric acid (GABA) and other inhibitory transmitters by binding to specific benzodiazepine receptor sites.

Other anxiolytics have unknown actions. They are thought to act on brain by inhibiting neuronal firing and reducing serotonin transmission.

Indications

Anxiety disorders

Contraindications and precautions

• Contraindicated in hypersensitivity to drug, psychosis, acute angle-closure glaucoma, significant hepatic disease, intra-arterial use (lorazepam injection), concurrent use of ketoconazole or itraconazole, breastfeeding (diazepam), and children younger than 6 months

• Use cautiously in hepatic disease, asthma, severe pulmonary disease, open-angle glaucoma, obesity, or concurrent use of CNS depressants.

Adverse reactions

CNS: sedation, somnolence, depression, lethargy, apathy, fatigue, hypoactivity, light-headedness, dizziness, memory impairment, disorientation, anterograde amnesia, restlessness, confusion, crying, sobbing, delirium, agitation, headache, slurred speech, aphonia, dysarthria, stupor, syncope, vertigo, euphoria, nervousness, irritability, poor concentration, inability to perform complex mental functions, rigidity, tremor, dystonia, akathisia, hemiparesis, paresthesia, hypotonia, unsteadiness, ataxia, incoordination, weakness, vivid dreams, psychomotor retardation, extrapyramidal symptoms, paradoxical reactions, behavior problems, hysteria, psychosis, **seizures, coma, suicidal tendency**

CV: bradycardia, tachycardia, hypertension, hypotension, palpitations, decreased systolic pressure, **cardiovascular collapse**

EENT: visual disturbances, diplopia, nystagmus, decreased hearing, auditory disturbances, nasal congestion

GI: nausea, vomiting, diarrhea, constipation, gastritis, coated tongue, difficulty swallowing, increased salivation, dry mouth, anorexia

---

Reactions in **bold** are life-threatening. ◀€ Clinical alert

GU: urinary incontinence or retention, menstrual irregularities, gynecomastia, galactorrhea, libido changes

Hematologic: anemia, eosinophilia, **leukopenia, agranulocytosis, thrombocytopenia**

Hepatic: hepatic dysfunction

Metabolic: dehydration

Musculoskeletal: muscle disturbances, joint pain

Respiratory: respiratory disturbances, partial airway obstruction

Skin: urticaria; pruritus; morbilliform, urticarial, or maculopapular rash; dermatitis; alopecia; hirsutism; ankle or facial edema; diaphoresis

Other: sore gums; appetite and weight changes; glassy-eyed appearance; fever; hiccups; edema; lymphadenopathy; pain, burning, and redness at I.M. injection site; phlebitis and thrombosis at I.V. site

Patient monitoring

• Monitor CBC and kidney and liver function tests.

• Taper dosage gradually to termination; do not withdraw quickly.

beta-adrenergic blockers

Alpha/beta-adrenergic blockers: carvedilol, labetalol

Beta-adrenergic blockers: atenolol, bisoprolol fumarate, carteolol hydrochloride, esmolol hydrochloride, metoprolol, nadolol, nebivolol, pindolol, propranolol hydrochloride, sotalol hydrochloride, timolol maleate

Action

Alpha/beta-adrenergic blockers combine selective competitive postsynaptic alpha$_1$-adrenergic blockade with nonselective, competitive beta-adrenergic blockade, causing blood pressure to decrease.

Beta-adrenergic blockers combine reversibly with beta-adrenergic receptors, blocking responses to sympathetic nerve impulses, catecholamines, or adrenergic drugs. Beta$_1$ blockade decreases heart rate, myocardial contractility, and cardiac output while slowing atrioventricular conduction. Beta$_2$ blockade increases bronchiolar airway resistance and enhances the inhibitory effect of catecholamines on peripheral vessels.

Indications

Hypertension; angina pectoris; myocardial infarction (MI); stable, symptomatic (class II or III) heart failure of ischemic, hypertensive, or cardiomyopathic origin; ventricular arrhythmias or tachycardia; tremors; chronic intraocular glaucoma; aggressive behavior; drug-induced akathisia; anxiety; migraine prophylaxis

Contraindications and precautions

• Contraindicated in hypersensitivity to drug, heart failure (unless secondary to tachyarrhythmia treatable with specific beta-adrenergic blocker), shock, sinus bradycardia, and heart block greater than first degree. Alpha/beta-adrenergic blockers are contraindicated in bronchial asthma and symptomatic hepatic impairment.

• Use cautiously in renal or hepatic impairment, pulmonary disease (especially asthma), pulmonary edema, diabetes mellitus, thyrotoxicosis, history of severe allergic reactions, elderly patients, pregnant or breastfeeding patients, and children (safety not established).

Adverse reactions

CNS: insomnia, headache, hyperactivity, malaise, CNS stimulation, dizziness, drowsiness, syncope, tremor, restlessness, nervousness, apprehension, anxiety, hyperkinesia, asthenia, vertigo, paresthesia

CV: hypertension, hypotension, tachycardia, angina, chest pain, palpitations, **arrhythmias**

EENT: abnormal vision, dry eyes, epistaxis, nasal congestion, sore throat (inhaled drug form), nasal dryness and irritation, hoarseness

GI: nausea, vomiting, heartburn, cholestasis, anorexia

GU: acute urinary bladder retention, difficulty voiding, ejaculation failure, erectile dysfunction, priapism, Peyronie's disease

Metabolic: hypokalemia, **hypoglycemia**

Musculoskeletal: muscle cramps

Respiratory: cough, wheezing, dyspnea, bronchitis, increased sputum, paradoxical airway resistance (with repeated, excessive use of inhaled form), **pulmonary edema, bronchospasm**

Skin: pallor; flushing; diaphoresis; generalized maculopapular, lichenoid, urticarial, or psoriaform rash; bullous lichen planus; facial erythema; reversible alopecia

Other: bad or unusual taste, increased appetite, edema, fever, antimitochondrial antibodies, hypersensitivity reaction, **systemic lupus erythematosus**

Patient monitoring

• Monitor CBC, ECG, blood glucose and electrolyte levels, and liver and kidney function tests.

• Assess vital signs, fluid intake and output, and weight.

bisphosphonates

alendronate sodium, etidronate disodium, pamidronate disodium, risendronate, zoledronic acid

Action

Inhibit normal and abnormal bone resorption

Indications

Osteoporosis in postmenopausal women and men, glucocorticoid-induced osteoporosis, Paget's disease, heterotopic ossification, hypercalcemia of malignancy, breast cancer, multiple myeloma, bone metastases of solid tumors

Contraindications and precautions

• Contraindicated in hypersensitivity to drug, hypocalcemia, esophageal abnormalities, clinically overt osteomalacia, renal impairment (class Dc and higher), inability to stand or sit upright for at least 30 minutes after dosing, and pregnancy

• Use cautiously in renal impairment less than class Dc; history of hypoparathyroidism or aspirin-sensitive asthma; or concurrent use of loop diuretics, aminoglycosides, or other nephrotoxic drugs.

Adverse reactions

CNS: agitation, anxiety, confusion, asthenia, depression, dizziness, headache, hypertonia, hypoesthesia, insomnia, neuralgia, fatigue, paresthesia, psychosis, somnolence, vertigo, **seizures**

CV: angina pectoris, cardiovascular disorder, chest pain, hypertension, hypotension, syncope, vasodilation, tachycardia, **atrial flutter or fibrillation, heart failure**

EENT: amblyopia, cataract, conjunctivitis, dry eyes, tinnitus, rhinitis, sinusitis, pharyngitis

GI: nausea, vomiting, diarrhea, constipation, abdominal pain, abdominal distention, acid reflux, belching, colitis, dyspepsia, gastritis, gastroenteritis, dysphagia, flatulence, esophageal ulcer, dry mouth, anorexia, **GI hemorrhage**

Reactions in **bold** are life-threatening.   ◀€ Clinical alert

Hematologic: anemia, ecchymosis, **granulocytopenia, leukopenia, neutropenia, thrombocytopenia**
Metabolic: dehydration, **fluid overload**
Musculoskeletal: arthralgia, arthritis, arthrosis, back or neck pain, bone disorder, bone fracture, bone or skeletal pain, bursitis, joint disorder, leg or other muscle cramps, myalgia
Respiratory: bronchitis, cough, dyspnea, pneumonia, crackles, upper respiratory infection, **pleural effusion**
Skin: alopecia, dermatitis, pruritus, rash
Other: taste perversion, weight loss, pain, edema, fever, flulike symptoms, infection, infusion-site reaction, allergic reaction

Patient monitoring

• Watch for signs and symptoms of GI irritation, including ulcers.
• Monitor blood pressure and calcium, potassium, phosphate, and creatinine levels.

bronchodilators

albuterol, albuterol sulfate, aminophylline, epinephrine, epinephrine hydrochloride, formoterol fumarate, ipratropium bromide, isoproterenol hydrochloride, levalbuterol hydrochloride, salmeterol xinafoate, terbutaline sulfate, theophylline, tiotropium

Leukotriene receptor antagonist:
montelukast sodium, zafirlukast

Action

Inhibit phosphodiesterase, an enzyme that degrades cyclic adenosine monophosphate (cAMP) by stimulating cAMP release and inhibiting release of slow-reacting substance of anaphylaxis and histamine. These actions cause bronchodilation, produce CNS and cardiac stimulation, promote diuresis, and increase gastric acid secretion.

Indications

Prevention of exercise-induced bronchospasm, prevention and treatment of bronchospasm in reversible obstructive airway disease

Contraindications and precautions

• Contraindicated in hypersensitivity to drug, angina, arrhythmias associated with tachycardia, ventricular arrhythmias that warrant inotropic therapy, cardiac dilatation or insufficiency, cerebral arteriosclerosis, organic brain damage, angle-closure glaucoma, local anesthesia of certain areas (such as toes or fingers), and labor
• Use cautiously in heart failure or other cardiac or circulatory impairment, hypertension, chronic obstructive pulmonary disease, renal or hepatic disease, hyperthyroidism, peptic ulcer, severe hypoxemia, diabetes mellitus, seizure disorders, glaucoma, elderly patients, pregnant or breastfeeding patients, young children, and infants.

Adverse reactions

CNS: insomnia, headache, hyperactivity, asthenia, malaise, dizziness, apprehension, anxiety, restlessness, CNS stimulation, nervousness, hyperkinesia, vertigo, drowsiness, tremor
CV: hypertension, hypotension, tachycardia, angina, chest pain, palpitations, **arrhythmias**
EENT: nasal congestion, nasal dryness and irritation, epistaxis, sore throat (with inhaled drug), hoarseness
GI: nausea, vomiting, heartburn, anorexia
Metabolic: hypokalemia, **hypoglycemia**
Musculoskeletal: muscle cramps

Respiratory: cough, wheezing, dyspnea, bronchitis, paradoxical airway resistance (with repeated, excessive use of inhaled drug), increased sputum, **bronchospasm, pulmonary edema**
Skin: pallor, flushing, diaphoresis
Other: unusual or bad taste, increased appetite, hypersensitivity reaction

Patient monitoring
• Monitor vital signs, ECG, and fluid intake and output.

calcium channel blockers
amlodipine, diltiazem hydrochloride, felodipine, isradipine, nicardipine hydrochloride, nifedipine, nimodipine, nisoldipine, verapamil hydrochloride

Action
Inhibit calcium influx through membranes of cardiac and smooth-muscle cells; this action depresses automaticity and conduction velocity in cardiac muscle, reducing myocardial contractility. Also decrease depolarization rate, atrial conduction, and total peripheral resistance.

Indications
Hypertension, angina pectoris, vasospastic (Prinzmetal's) angina, supraventricular tachyarrhythmias, rapid ventricular rate in atrial flutter or fibrillation

Contraindications and precautions
• Contraindicated in hypersensitivity to drug, sick sinus syndrome, second- or third-degree atrioventricular block (unless patient has artificial pacemaker in place), and systolic pressure below 90 mm Hg

• Use cautiously in severe renal or hepatic impairment, advanced aortic stenosis, cardiogenic shock (unless associated with supraventricular tachyarrhythmias), history of serious ventricular arrhythmias or heart failure, concurrent use of I.V. beta-adrenergic blockers, elderly patients, pregnant or breastfeeding patients, and children (safety not established).

Adverse reactions
CNS: headache, abnormal dreams, anxiety, confusion, dizziness, syncope, drowsiness, nervousness, paresthesia, tremor, asthenia, psychiatric disturbances
CV: peripheral edema, chest pain, hypotension, palpitations, bradycardia, tachycardia, **arrhythmias, heart failure**
EENT: blurred vision, disturbed equilibrium, tinnitus, epistaxis
GI: nausea, vomiting, diarrhea, constipation, dyspepsia, dry mouth, anorexia
GU: dysuria, nocturia, polyuria, sexual dysfunction, gynecomastia
Hematologic: anemia, **leukopenia, thrombocytopenia**
Metabolic: hyperglycemia
Musculoskeletal: joint stiffness, muscle cramps
Respiratory: cough, dyspnea
Skin: rash, dermatitis, pruritus, urticaria, flushing, diaphoresis, photosensitivity reaction, **erythema multiforme, Stevens-Johnson syndrome**
Other: gingival hyperplasia, altered taste, weight gain

Patient monitoring
• Monitor blood glucose and electrolyte levels, fluid intake and output, and liver and kidney function tests.
• Assess vital signs, ECG, weight, and blood pressure in both arms (with patient lying down, sitting, and standing).

---

cholinergics

bethanechol chloride, cevimeline hydrochloride, neostigmine, pyridostigmine bromide

Action

Stimulate cholinergic receptors, causing urinary bladder contraction, decreased bladder capacity, more frequent ureteral peristaltic waves, increased GI tone and peristalsis, increased lower esophageal sphincter pressure, and increased gastric secretions

Indications

Postpartum or postoperative nonobstructive urinary retention, urinary retention caused by neurogenic bladder, diagnosis of myasthenia gravis (Tensilon test), antidote for curare (to reverse nondepolarizing neuromuscular blockade)

Contraindications and precautions

• Contraindicated in hypersensitivity to drug or sulfites, hyperthyroidism, peptic ulcer, latent or active bronchial asthma, pronounced bradycardia or atrioventricular (AV) conduction defects, vasomotor instability, coronary artery disease, coronary occlusion, hypotension, hypertension, seizure disorders, parkinsonism, GI or GU tract obstruction, impaired GI or GU wall integrity, spastic GI disturbances, acute inflammatory GI tract lesions, peritonitis, marked vagotonia, and when GI tract or urinary bladder activity is undesirable (for instance, postoperatively)

• Use cautiously in arrhythmias, toxic megacolon, poor GI motility, and pregnant patients.

Adverse reactions

CNS: asthenia, dysarthria, dysphonia, dizziness, drowsiness, headache, syncope, **loss of consciousness, seizures**
CV: hypotension, AV block, bradycardia, **cardiac arrest, thrombophlebitis** (with I.V. use)
EENT: diplopia, miosis, conjunctival hyperemia, excessive lacrimation and salivation
GI: nausea, vomiting, diarrhea, abdominal cramps, dysphagia
GU: urinary frequency or incontinence
Musculoskeletal: muscle cramps, fasciculations
Respiratory: dyspnea, **respiratory muscle paralysis, central respiratory paralysis, laryngospasm, bronchospasm, respiratory arrest**
Skin: rash, diaphoresis, flushing
Other: anaphylaxis

Patient monitoring

• Monitor ECG, glucose and electrolyte levels, urinalysis, and liver and kidney function tests.

◀€ Assess platelet count in long-term use. Report unusual bleeding or bruising, petechiae, skin disorders, and signs and symptoms of diabetes mellitus.

CNS stimulants

amphetamine, dexmethylphenidate hydrochloride, dextroamphetamine sulfate, doxapram, lisdexamfetamine dimesylate, methylphenidate hydrochloride, modafinil, pemoline

Action

Cause norepinephrine release from central adrenergic neurons and increase central stimulation, which enhances motor activity and mental alertness, lifts mood, and suppresses appetite

---

Indications
Attention deficit hyperactivity disorder, narcolepsy

Contraindications and precautions
• Contraindicated in hypersensitivity to drug or tartrazine, advanced arteriosclerosis, cardiovascular disease, moderate to severe hypertension, agitation, hyperexcitable states (including hyperthyroidism), glaucoma, history of Tourette's syndrome or drug abuse, suicidal or homicidal tendency, concurrent MAO inhibitor use, breastfeeding, and children younger than age 6
• Use cautiously in mild hypertension, diabetes mellitus, depression, seizures, psychosis, long-term amphetamine use, elderly or debilitated patients, and pregnant patients.

Adverse reactions
CNS: nervousness, insomnia, dizziness, headache, dyskinesia, chorea, drowsiness, hyperactivity, restlessness, tremor, depression, Tourette's syndrome, **toxic psychosis**
CV: angina, palpitations, hypertension, hypotension, tachycardia, **arrhythmias**
EENT: blurred vision, poor accommodation
GI: nausea, vomiting, diarrhea, constipation, abdominal pain and cramps, anorexia, dry mouth
GU: erectile dysfunction, increased libido
Hematologic: anemia, **leukopenia, thrombocytopenia**
Hepatic: hepatic dysfunction, hepatic coma
Skin: rash, alopecia, exfoliative dermatitis
Other: metallic taste, weight loss, fever, psychological or physical drug dependence, drug tolerance, abnormal behavior (with abuse)

Patient monitoring
• Watch for and report fever, excitation, delirium, tremors, and twitching.
◀€ Monitor vital signs. Stay alert for arrhythmias, tachycardia, hypertension, and cardiovascular changes with psychotic syndrome.
• Watch for and report signs of drug abuse.

corticosteroids
beclomethasone dipropionate, betamethasone, betamethasone acetate and sodium phosphate, budesonide, dexamethasone, dexamethasone sodium sulfate, flunisolide, fluticasone propionate, fluticasone furoate, hydrocortisone, hydrocortisone acetate, hydrocortisone butyrate, hydrocortisone sodium succinate, hydrocortisone valerate, methylprednisolone, methylprednisolone acetate, methylprednisolone sodium succinate, prednisolone, prednisolone acetate, prednisolone sodium phosphate, prednisone, triamcinolone triamcinolone acetonide, triamcinolone hexacetonide

Action
Reduce the immune response by inhibiting prostaglandin synthesis, macrophage and leukocyte accumulation at inflammation site, phagocytosis, and lysosomal enzyme release. Also reduce numbers of T lymphocytes, monocytes, and eosinophils and interfere with immunoglobulin binding to cell-surface receptors. Some corticosteroids regulate metabolic pathways involving protein, carbohydrate, and fat; others regulate electrolyte and water balance.

Indications

Adrenocortical insufficiency; adrenal, inflammatory, allergic, hematologic, neoplastic, and autoimmune disorders; asthma; cerebral edema; Crohn's disease; hypercalcemia; acute spinal cord injury; nausea and vomiting caused by chemotherapy; prevention of organ rejection in transplant patients; prevention of neonatal respiratory distress in high-risk pregnancies

Contraindications and precautions

• Contraindicated in hypersensitivity to drug or intolerance of alcohol, bisulfites, or tartrazine and in active untreated infections
• Use cautiously in hypertension, osteoporosis, diabetes mellitus, glaucoma, immunosuppression, seizure disorders, renal disease, hypothyroidism, cirrhosis, diverticulitis, active or latent peptic ulcer, inflammatory bowel disease, ulcerative colitis, thromboembolic disorder or tendency, myasthenia gravis, heart failure, metastatic cancer, emotional instability, recent GI surgery, pregnant or breastfeeding patients, and children younger than age 6 (safety not established).

Adverse reactions

CNS: headache, nervousness, restlessness, depression, euphoria, personality changes, psychosis, vertigo, paresthesia, insomnia, **increased intracranial pressure, seizures**
CV: hypotension, hypertension, Churg-Strauss syndrome, **heart failure, thrombophlebitis, thromboembolism, fat embolism, arrhythmias, shock**
EENT: glaucoma (with long-term use), increased intraocular pressure, cataract, nasal congestion and irritation, perforated nasal septum, epistaxis, nasopharyngeal or oropharyngeal fungal infection, sneezing, dysphonia, hoarseness, throat irritation

GI: nausea, vomiting, abdominal distention, peptic ulcer, esophageal candidiasis or ulcer, pancreatitis, dry mouth, anorexia
GU: amenorrhea, irregular menses
Metabolic: decreased growth (in children), diabetes mellitus, cushingoid state, sodium and fluid retention, hyperglycemia, hypokalemia, hypocalcemia, hypercholesterolemia, **adrenal suppression, hypothalamic-pituitary-adrenal suppression** (with systemic use for more than 5 days)
Musculoskeletal: muscle wasting, muscle pain and weakness, myopathy, spontaneous fractures, aseptic joint necrosis, tendon rupture, osteoporosis, osteonecrosis
Respiratory: cough, wheezing, **bronchospasm**
Skin: rash, pruritus, contact dermatitis, acne, decreased wound healing, bruising, hirsutism, thin and fragile skin, petechiae, purpura, striae, subcutaneous fat atrophy, injection site atrophy, angioedema
Other: bad taste, increased appetite (with long-term use), weight gain, facial edema, increased susceptibility to infection, aggravation or masking of infection, immunosuppression, hypersensitivity reaction

Patient monitoring

• Monitor ECG, blood glucose and electrolyte levels, urinalysis, and kidney and liver function tests.
◀€ Assess platelet count in long-term therapy. Report unusual bleeding or bruising, petechiae, skin disorders, and signs and symptom of diabetes mellitus.
• Monitor appearance for changes that suggest Cushing's syndrome.

diuretics

Carbonic anhydrase inhibitor: acetazolamide

Loop diuretics: bumetanide, furosemide, torsemide

Osmotic diuretics: mannitol

Potassium-sparing diuretics: spironolactone, triamterene

Thiazide and thiazide-like diuretics: chlorthalidone, hydrochlorothiazide, indapamide, metolazone

Action

Carbonic anhydrase inhibitors inhibit carbonic anhydrase in kidneys, decreasing reabsorption of water, sodium, potassium, and bicarbonate. *Loop* diuretics inhibit reabsorption of sodium and chloride (and therefore water) in proximal and distal tubules and loop of Henle. *Osmotic* diuretics increase plasma osmolality, drawing water from body tissues into extracellular fluid and then out through the kidney. *Potassium-sparing* diuretics inhibit sodium reabsorption in distal renal tubule, causing sodium and water loss. *Thiazide and thiazide-like* diuretics decrease rate of sodium and chloride reabsorption by distal renal tubule and increase water excretion.

Indications

Hypertension or edema secondary to heart failure or other causes, cerebral edema, hemolytic transfusion reaction, drug toxicity, prevention of oliguria or acute renal failure

Contraindications and precautions

- Contraindicated in hypersensitivity to drug, alcohol intolerance (some liquid furosemide forms), anuria, renal decompensation, hepatic coma or precoma, severe electrolyte depletion, severe pulmonary congestion or edema, severe dehydration, and active intracranial bleeding (except during craniotomy)
- Use cautiously in severe hepatic disease accompanied by cirrhosis or ascites, electrolyte depletion, worsening azotemia, renal insufficiency (blood urea nitrogen above 30 mg/dl or creatinine clearance below 30 ml/minute), diabetes mellitus, elderly or debilitated patients, pregnant or breastfeeding patients, and children younger than age 18.

Adverse reactions

CNS: dizziness, headache, insomnia, nervousness, vertigo, asthenia, paresthesia, confusion, fatigue, drowsiness, **encephalopathy**
CV: hypotension, chest pain, volume depletion, **thrombophlebitis, arrhythmias**
EENT: blurred vision, nystagmus, hearing loss, tinnitus
GI: nausea, vomiting, diarrhea, constipation, dyspepsia, gastric irritation, dry mouth, anorexia, **acute pancreatitis**
GU: polyuria, nocturia, glycosuria, premature ejaculation, erectile dysfunction, nipple tenderness, **renal failure, oliguria**
Hematologic: leukopenia, other blood dyscrasias
Hepatic: jaundice
Metabolic: dehydration, hyperglycemia, hyperuricemia, hypokalemia, hypomagnesemia, **hypochloremic alkalosis**
Musculoskeletal: joint pain, muscle cramps, myalgia
Skin: rash, pruritus, urticaria, diaphoresis, photosensitivity
Other: weight gain

Patient monitoring

- Monitor fluid intake and output and weight.

Reactions in **bold** are life-threatening.   ◀€ Clinical alert

- Monitor CBC and blood glucose, blood urea nitrogen, creatinine, carbon dioxide, and electrolyte levels (especially potassium).
- Assess vital signs during rapid diuresis.

erectile dysfunction agents
Phosphodiesterase type 5 (PDE5) inhibitors: avanafil, sildenafil citrate, tadalafil, vardenafil hydrochloride

Other: alprostadil

Action
PDE5 inhibitors cause degradation of cyclic guanylic acid in smooth-muscle cells of corpus cavernosum, enhancing effects of nitric oxide released during sexual stimulation. These actions increase blood flow to penis and induce erection.

Alprostadil relaxes the trabecular smooth muscle and dilates cavernosal arteries, causing expansion of lacunar spaces and blood entrapment from compression of venules against the tunica albuginea. These effects induce erection.

Indications
Erectile dysfunction

Contraindications and precautions
- Contraindicated in hypersensitivity to drug or its components and in concurrent use of nitrates (regularly or intermittently), nitric oxide donors, or alpha-adrenergic blockers
- Use cautiously in anatomic penile deformation, conditions that predispose to priapism (such as sickle cell anemia, multiple myeloma, leukemia), bleeding disorders, active peptic ulcer, retinitis pigmentosa or other retinal abnormality, coronary ischemia, heart failure, multidrug antihypertensive regimen, or concurrent use of erythromycin, cimetidine, or other drugs that could prolong the half-life of erectile dysfunction agent.

Adverse reactions
CNS: dizziness, headache, fainting, hypoesthesia
CV: abnormal ECG, hypertension, hypotension, vasodilation, vasovagal reaction, peripheral vascular disorder, supraventricular extrasystoles
EENT: abnormal vision, mydriasis, nasal congestion, rhinitis, sinusitis
GI: nausea, diarrhea, dyspepsia, dry mouth
GU: urinary frequency and urgency, impaired urination, hematuria, urinary tract infection, inguinal hernia, prostate disorder, scrotal disorder or edema, testicular pain
Metabolic: hyperglycemia
Musculoskeletal: back or limb pain, leg cramps, myalgia
Respiratory: cough
Skin: rash, nonapplication site pruritus, diaphoresis, flushing, skin disorder or neoplasm
Other: accidental injury, flulike symptoms, infection, localized pain

Patient monitoring
- Monitor cardiovascular status and vision.
- Assess for drug efficacy. Watch for priapism or erections lasting beyond 4 hours, which may permanently damage penile tissue.

hematopoietic agents
Colony-stimulating factors: filgrastim, pegfilgrastim, sargramostim

Erythropoiesis-stimulating agent (synthetic): peginesatide

Human erythropoietins: darbepoetin alfa, epoetin alfa

Action
Varies with specific drug. See individual monographs.

Indications
Colony-stimulating factors—to reduce incidence of infection in myelosuppressive chemotherapy; to reduce time to neutrophil recovery and fever duration in patients with acute myelogenous leukemia and nonmyeloid cancer who are undergoing myeloablative chemotherapy followed by bone marrow transplant; mobilization of peripheral blood progenitor cell collection; severe chronic neutropenia
Human erythropoietins—anemia associated with chronic renal failure, zidovudine therapy in patients with human immunodeficiency virus, cancer patients on chemotherapy, reduction of allogeneic blood transfusions in surgery patients

Contraindications and precautions
• Contraindicated in hypersensitivity to drug or human albumin and in uncontrolled hypertension
• Use cautiously in cardiac disease, hypertension, seizures, and porphyria.

Adverse reactions
CNS: fatigue, headache, generalized weakness
CV: chest pain, hypertension, tachycardia
GI: nausea, vomiting, diarrhea, constipation, mucositis, stomatitis, anorexia
Metabolic: hyperkalemia
Musculoskeletal: skeletal pain, arthralgia, myalgia
Hematologic: neutropenic fever
Respiratory: dyspnea, cough, sore throat
Skin: alopecia, rash, urticaria
Other: fever, stinging at injection site, flulike symptoms, hypersensitivity reaction

Patient monitoring
• Monitor CBC before and frequently throughout therapy. Also monitor liver function tests and uric acid levels.
• Assess for signs and symptoms of splenic rupture, such as left upper quadrant abdominal pain, shoulder pain, and splenic enlargement.
• Watch for signs and symptoms of infection, sepsis, adult respiratory distress syndrome, and neutropenic fever.

immunosuppressants
azathioprine, basiliximab, cyclosporine, glatiramer acetate, lenalidomide, lymphocyte immune globulin, methotrexate, methotrexate sodium, muromonab-CD3, mycophenolate mofetil, mycophenolate mofetil hydrochloride, mycophenolate sodium, sirolimus, tacrolimus, thalidomide

Action
Inhibit binding of interleukin (IL)-1 to IL-1 receptors; prevent proliferation and differentiation of activated B and T cells; inhibit lymphokine production and IL-2 release; react with T-lymphocyte membranes, depleting blood of CD3+ T cells; and bind to intracellular proteins to prevent T-cell activation

Indications
Moderate to severely active rheumatoid arthritis, prevention of organ transplant rejection

Contraindications and precautions
• Contraindicated in hypersensitivity to drug or its components, fluid overload, uncompensated heart failure, seizure disorders, and pregnant patients with rheumatoid arthritis

---

Reactions in **bold** are life-threatening. ◀€ Clinical alert

• Use cautiously in renal or hepatic disease, cancer, diabetes mellitus, hyperkalemia, hyperuricemia, infection, hypertension, pregnant patients (except those with rheumatoid arthritis), breastfeeding patients, and children younger than age 13.

Adverse reactions

CNS: headache, insomnia, paresthesia, dizziness, tremor, drowsiness, anxiety, confusion, agitation, rigors, asthenia, **coma, seizures**

CV: hypotension, hypertension, tachycardia, palpitations, chest pain, ECG abnormalities, **torsades de pointes, prolonged QT interval**

EENT: blurred vision, painful red eye, dry and irritated eyes, eyelid edema, earache, tinnitus, nasopharyngitis, epistaxis, postnasal drip, sinusitis, sore throat

GI: nausea, vomiting, diarrhea, constipation, fecal incontinence, dyspepsia, abdominal pain, dry mouth, oral blisters, oral candidiasis, anorexia, **GI hemorrhage**

GU: urinary incontinence, breakthrough bleeding, **vaginal hemorrhage, renal impairment, oliguria, renal failure**

Hematologic: anemia, **thrombocytopenia, neutropenia, hemorrhage, disseminated intravascular coagulation**

Metabolic: hypomagnesemia, hyperglycemia, hypokalemia, **hyperkalemia, hypoglycemia, acidosis**

Musculoskeletal: myalgia; joint, bone, back, neck, or limb pain

Respiratory: dyspnea, cough, hypoxia, wheezing, tachypnea, decreased or abnormal breath sounds, hemoptysis, upper respiratory infection, **pleural effusion**

Skin: pruritus, dermatitis, bruising, dry skin, diaphoresis, night sweats, flushing, erythema, petechiae, hyperpigmentation, urticaria, skin lesions, pallor, local exfoliation

Other: weight changes, fever, lymphadenopathy, edema, facial edema, bacterial infection, herpes simplex infection, pain, hypersensitivity reaction, **sepsis**

Patient monitoring

• Assess for signs and symptoms of infection and injection site reaction.

• Monitor vital signs, CBC with platelet count, fluid intake and output, electrolyte and blood glucose levels, and liver and kidney function tests.

inotropics
digoxin, milrinone lactate

Action

Inhibit sodium- and potassium-activated adenosine triphosphatase phosphodiesterase, which raises intracellular and extracellular calcium levels. These effects increase myocardial contractility, prolong atrioventricular (AV) node refractory period, decrease conduction through sinoatrial and AV nodes, and relax and dilate vascular smooth muscle to reduce preload and afterload.

Indications

Heart failure, tachyarrhythmias, atrial fibrillation or flutter, paroxysmal atrial tachycardia

Contraindications and precautions

• Contraindicated in hypersensitivity to drug, known alcohol intolerance (elixir only), and ventricular fibrillation

• Use cautiously in electrolyte abnormalities (such as hypokalemia, hypercalcemia, hypomagnesemia), myocardial infarction, AV block, idiopathic hypertrophic subaortic stenosis, constrictive pericarditis, renal impairment, obesity, elderly patients, pregnant or breastfeeding patients, and children.

Adverse reactions
CNS: fatigue, headache, asthenia
CV: bradycardia, ECG changes, **arrhythmias**
EENT: blurred or yellow vision
GI: nausea, vomiting, diarrhea, anorexia
GU: gynecomastia
Hematologic: thrombocytopenia

Patient monitoring
• Monitor vital signs, weight, electrolyte levels, fluid intake and output, drug blood level, and kidney function tests.

---

laxatives
bisacodyl, calcium polycarbophil, docusate calcium, docusate sodium, lactulose, magnesium salts, methylcellulose, psyllium, senna, sennosides

Action
Stimulate smooth muscle of bowel, increasing intestinal contractions; increase stool bulk by causing water retention and inhibiting digestion in stomach. Also soften hard feces, promoting their passage through lower intestine.

Indications
Treatment of constipation, prevention of constipation in patients who should not strain during defecation (for example, after anorectal surgery or myocardial infarction), colonic evacuation for rectal and bowel examination

Contraindications and precautions
• Contraindicated in hypersensitivity to drug or its components, intestinal obstruction, undiagnosed abdominal pain, suspected appendicitis, and fecal impaction
• Use cautiously in severe cardiovascular disease, anal or rectal fissures, enteritis, ulcerative colitis, diverticulitis, pregnant or breastfeeding patients, and children younger than age 2.

Adverse reactions
GI: nausea; vomiting; diarrhea; esophageal, gastric, small-intestine, or rectal obstruction (with dry form of drug); abdominal cramps in severe constipation; anorexia
GU: reddish-pink discoloration of alkaline urine, yellow-brown discoloration of acidic urine
Metabolic: alkalosis, fluid and electrolyte imbalances
Musculoskeletal: tetany
Other: laxative dependence (with excessive long-term use)

Patient monitoring
• Monitor fluid and electrolyte balance.

---

neuromuscular blockers
Depolarizing blocker: succinylcholine chloride

Nondepolarizing blockers:
atracurium besylate, botulinum toxin type A, cisatracurium besylate, doxacurium chloride, mivacurium chloride, pancuronium bromide, rocuronium bromide, tubocurarine chloride, vecuronium bromide

Action
Depolarizing neuromuscular blockers initially excite skeletal muscle, then

---

prevent muscle contraction by prolonging the refractory period. *Nondepolarizing* (competitive) neuromuscular blockers bind competitively to cholinergic receptors on motor end plates, preventing muscle contraction.

Indications

Adjunct to anesthesia to facilitate endotracheal intubation; skeletal and smooth muscle relaxation; to facilitate orthopedic manipulation; reduction of muscle contractions during pharmacologically or electrically induced seizures; myasthenia gravis diagnosis

Contraindications and precautions

• Contraindicated in hypersensitivity to drug, low plasma pseudocholinesterase level, angle-closure glaucoma, myopathy with elevated creatine kinase level, penetrating eye injury, and personal or family history of malignant hyperthermia

• Use cautiously in heart disease; electrolyte imbalance; dehydration; neuromuscular, respiratory, or hepatic disease; pregnant or breastfeeding patients, and children younger than age 2.

Adverse reactions

CV: hypotension, bradycardia, **arrhythmias, cardiac arrest**
Musculoskeletal: profound and prolonged muscle relaxation, residual muscle weakness
Respiratory: cyanosis, **prolonged apnea, bronchospasm, respiratory depression**
Skin: rash, flushing, pruritus, urticaria
Other: hypersensitivity reaction

Patient monitoring

◀€ Monitor vital signs, pulmonary status, and temperature continuously.

nonopioid analgesics

acetaminophen, acetylsalicylic acid, celecoxib, diclofenac, potassium, diclofenac sodium, etodolac, ibuprofen, indomethacin, ketorolac tromethamine, meloxicam, nabumetone, naproxen, naproxen sodium, oxaprozin, oxaprozin potassium, phenazopyridine hydrochloride, piroxicam, propoxyphene hydrochloride, propoxyphene napsylate

Action

Inhibit cyclooxygenase, an enzyme needed for prostaglandin synthesis. This inhibition stimulates the antiinflammatory response and blocks pain impulses.

Indications

Inflammatory conditions (such as osteoarthritis, rheumatoid arthritis, and ankylosing spondylitis), dysmenorrhea, actinic keratoses, fever

Contraindications and precautions

• Contraindicated in hypersensitivity to drug or sulfonamides and in history of asthma, urticaria, or allergic reaction to aspirin or other nonsteroidal anti-inflammatory drugs

• Use cautiously in severe cardiovascular, renal, or hepatic disease; GI disorders; cardiac decompensation; active GI bleeding or ulcer; asthma; history of ulcer disease; and chronic alcohol use or abuse.

Adverse reactions

CNS: dizziness, headache, insomnia, fatigue, paresthesia, tremor, vertigo, syncope, anxiety, confusion, depression, nervousness, drowsiness, malaise, **seizures**

CV: palpitations, tachycardia, angina pectoris, hypertension, hypotension, **arrhythmias, heart failure, myocardial infarction**
EENT: abnormal vision, conjunctivitis, hearing loss, tinnitus, pharyngitis
GI: nausea, vomiting, diarrhea, constipation, abdominal pain, dyspepsia, flatulence, colitis, duodenal or gastric ulcer, gastritis, gastroesophageal reflux, esophagitis, dry mouth, **GI hemorrhage, pancreatitis**
GU: albuminuria, hematuria, urinary frequency, urinary tract infection, **renal failure**
Hematologic: anemia, purpura, **leukopenia, thrombocytopenia, other blood dyscrasias**
Hepatic: hepatitis
Metabolic: dehydration
Musculoskeletal: myalgia, joint or back pain
Respiratory: dyspnea, cough, asthma, upper respiratory infection, **bronchospasm**
Skin: rash, urticaria, diaphoresis, pruritus, alopecia, bullous eruption, angioedema, photosensitivity
Other: altered taste, increased appetite, weight changes, flulike symptoms, edema, accidental injury, fever, allergic reaction

Patient monitoring
• Monitor CBC and liver and kidney function tests.

opioid analgesics
buprenorphine hydrochloride, butorphanol tartrate, codeine sulfate, fentanyl citrate, fentanyl transdermal system, fentanyl transmucosal, hydrocodone bitartrate and acetaminophen, hydrocodone bitratrate and aspirin, hydrocodone bitratrate and ibuprofen, hydrocodone bitartrate and homatropine methylbromide, hydromorphone hydrochloride, levorphanol tartrate, meperidine hydrochloride, methadone hydrochloride, methylnaltrexone bromide, morphine hydrochloride, morphine sulfate, nalbuphine hydrochloride, oxycodone hydrochloride, oxymorphone hydrochloride, pentazocine lactate, pentazocine hydrochloride and acetaminophen, pentazocine hydrochloride and naloxone hydrochloride, tapentadol, tramadol hydrochloride

Action
Attach to specific CNS receptors, decreasing cell membrane permeability, slowing pain impulse transmission, and altering response to pain

Indications
Moderate to severe pain, intraoperative anesthesia, labor, cough, diarrhea

Contraindications and precautions
• Contraindicated in hypersensitivity to drug, significant respiratory depression, paralytic ileus, MAO inhibitor use within last 14 days, diarrhea caused by poisoning, acute bronchial asthma, and upper airway obstruction
• Use cautiously in severe cardiovascular, renal, or hepatic disease; cardiac decompensation; GI disorders; history of ulcer disease; chronic alcohol use or abuse; respiratory depression; severe obesity; sleep apnea syndrome; myxedema; kyphoscoliosis; CNS depression; coma; biliary tract disease, including pancreatitis; head injury, other intracranial injuries, increased intracranial pressure, seizures; concurrent use of other CNS depressants or serotonergic agents; elderly patients; pregnant or breastfeeding patients; and children younger than age 13.

Reactions in **bold** are life-threatening.　◀€ Clinical alert

Adverse reactions

CNS: drowsiness, sedation, dizziness, tremor, irritability, syncope, stimulation (in children)

CV: hypertension, hypotension, palpitations, bradycardia, tachycardia, extrasystole, **arrhythmias**

EENT: blurred vision, nasal dryness and congestion, dry or sore throat

GI: nausea, vomiting, constipation, epigastric distress, dry mouth, anorexia, **intestinal obstruction**

GU: urinary retention or hesitancy, dysuria, early menses, decreased libido, erectile dysfunction

Hematologic: hemolytic anemia, hypoplastic anemia, thrombocytopenia, agranulocytosis, leukopenia, pancytopenia

Respiratory: thickened bronchial secretions, chest tightness, wheezing

Skin: urticaria, rash, diaphoresis

Other: hypersensitivity reaction (with I.V. use), **anaphylactic shock**

Patient monitoring

• Assess vital signs and respiratory status.

• Monitor CBC, electrolyte levels, and liver and kidney function tests.

potassium channel blockers
dalfampridine

Action
Unknown. May increase conduction of action potentials in demyelinated axons through inhibition of potassium channels

Indications
To improve walking in patients with multiple sclerosis

Contraindications and precautions

• Contraindicated in history of seizures and moderate or severe renal impairment

• Use cautiously in mild renal impairment, pregnant or breastfeeding patients, and children younger than age 18 (safety and efficacy not established).

Adverse reactions

CNS: insomnia, dizziness, headache, asthenia, balance disorder, paresthesia, seizures

EENT: nasopharyngitis, pharyngolaryngeal pain

GI: nausea, constipation, dyspepsia

GU: urinary tract infection

Musculoskeletal: back pain

Other: multiple sclerosis relapse

Patient monitoring

• Monitor renal function tests regularly (especially creatinine clearance).

• Discontinue drug if seizure occurs.

renin-angiotensin system antagonists

Angiotensin-converting enzyme (ACE) inhibitors: benazepril hydrochloride, captopril, enalapril maleate, enalaprilat, fosinopril sodium, lisinopril, moexipril, perindopril erbumine, quinapril hydrochloride, ramipril, trandolapril

Angiotensin II receptor antagonists: candesartan cilexetil, eprosartan mesylate, irbesartan, losartan potassium, olmesartan medoxomil, telmisartan, valsartan

Selective aldosterone receptor antagonist: eplerenone

Action

ACE inhibitors lower blood pressure by preventing conversion of angiotensin I to angiotensin II, a potent vasoconstrictor that decreases peripheral resistance and aldosterone secretion.

Angiotensin II receptor antagonists block vasoconstrictive and aldosterone-secreting effects of angiotensin II by selectively blocking binding of angiotensin II to angiotensin I receptors in vascular smooth muscle, adrenal, and other tissues.

Selective aldosterone receptor antagonists bind to mineralocorticoid receptors and block binding of aldosterone, a component of the renin-angiotensin-aldosterone system. This effect decreases blood pressure.

Indications

Hypertension, heart failure, left ventricular dysfunction, multiple sclerosis, diabetic neuropathy

Contraindications and precautions

• Contraindicated in hypersensitivity to drug
• Use cautiously in renal or hepatic impairment, hypovolemia, hyponatremia, aortic stenosis and hypertrophic cardiomyopathy, cerebrovascular or cardiac insufficiency, surgery and anesthesia, concurrent diuretic therapy, family history of angioedema, Black patients with hypertension, elderly patients, pregnant or breastfeeding patients, and children (safety not established for most ACE inhibitors).

Adverse reactions

CNS: dizziness, fatigue, headache, insomnia, asthenia, drowsiness, vertigo
CV: hypotension, angina pectoris, tachycardia, **myocardial infarction**
EENT: sinusitis
GI: nausea, diarrhea, anorexia
GU: proteinuria, erectile dysfunction, decreased libido, **renal failure**
Hematologic: bone marrow depression, agranulocytosis
Hepatic: cholestatic jaundice progressing to **hepatic necrosis and death**
Metabolic: hyperkalemia
Respiratory: cough, bronchitis, dyspnea, asthma, **eosinophilic pneumonitis**
Skin: rash, angioedema
Other: taste disturbances, fever, **anaphylaxis**

Patient monitoring

• Monitor vital signs, including blood pressure in both arms with patient lying down, standing, and sitting.
• Assess fluid intake and output, electrolyte levels, CBC, and kidney and liver function tests.
• Evaluate urine for protein.
• Watch for microalbuminuria, especially in diabetic patients.

sedative-hypnotics

Barbiturates: pentobarbital, phenobarbital

Nonbarbiturates: dexmedetomidine hydrochloride, flurazepam hydrochloride, temazepam, triazolam, zaleplon, zolpidem tartrate

Action

Barbiturates cause drowsiness, sedation, and hypnosis by depressing the sensory cortex, decreasing motor activity, and altering cerebellar function.

Nonbarbiturates produce sedative, anxiolytic, muscle relaxant, and anticonvulsant effects by interacting with the gamma-aminobutyric acid–benzodiazepine receptor complex.

Indications

Short-term treatment of insomnia, sedation, preanesthesia

Contraindications and precautions

• Contraindicated in hypersensitivity to drug, barbiturate sensitivity, manifest or latent porphyria, marked hepatic dysfunction, severe respiratory disease, and nephritis

• Use cautiously in depression, respiratory compromise, pulmonary insufficiency, seizure disorders, hepatic or severe renal impairment, anxiety, elderly or debilitated patients, or history of drug abuse.

Adverse reactions

CNS: headache, nervousness, talkativeness, slurred speech, apprehension, irritability, anxiety, light-headedness, dizziness, euphoria, relaxed feeling, weakness, poor concentration, incoordination, confusion, memory impairment, depression, abnormal dreams, nightmares, insomnia, paresthesia, restlessness, fatigue, dysesthesia, drowsiness, somnolence, staggering, falling, ataxia, agitation, hyperkinesia, psychiatric disturbances, hallucinations, abnormal thinking, vertigo, lethargy, hangover effect

CV: palpitations, chest pain, tachycardia, hypotension, bradycardia, **circulatory collapse**, **thrombophlebitis** (with I.V. use)

EENT: blurred vision, burning eyes, difficulty focusing, visual disturbances, tinnitus

GI: nausea, vomiting, diarrhea, constipation, dyspepsia, GI pain, dry mouth, excessive salivation, glossitis, stomatitis, anorexia

Hepatic: jaundice, **hepatic failure** (in patients also receiving diuretics)

Hematologic: leukopenia, granulocytopenia

Musculoskeletal: joint pain

Respiratory: shortness of breath, hypoventilation, **respiratory depression**

Skin: dermatitis, diaphoresis, flushing, pruritus, rash, angioedema, exfoliative dermatitis

Other: altered taste, body pain, pain at I.M. injection site, fever (especially with long-term phenobarbital use)

Patient monitoring

• Monitor vital signs, respiratory status, CBC with white cell differential, liver function tests, and blood urea nitrogen, creatinine, and electrolyte levels. Stay alert for hyperkalemia.

• Assess neurologic status. Watch for signs and symptoms of drug dependence.

sex hormones

5-alpha reductase inhibitors: dutasteride, finasteride

Androgens: fluoxymesterone, nandrolone, testosterone

Estrogens: conjugated estrogens, esterified estrogens, estradiol, estrogens, etonogestrel and ethinyl estradiol vaginal ring, norelgestromin/ ethinyl estradiol, norethindrone acetate, norgestrel

Progestins: medroxyprogesterone, megestrol acetate, progesterone

Selective estrogen receptor modulator: raloxifene

Action

Varies with specific drug. See individual monographs.

Indications

Vary with specific drug. See individual monographs.

Contraindications and precautions

• Contraindicated in hypersensitivity to drug or its components; known or suspected breast cancer or estrogen-dependent neoplasia; undiagnosed abnormal genital bleeding; porphyria; active deep-vein thrombosis, pulmonary embolism, or history of these conditions; active or recent arterial thromboembolic disease; active thrombophlebitis or thromboembolic disorders; history of thrombophlebitis, thrombosis, or thromboembolic disorders associated with previous estrogen use; and pregnancy

• Use cautiously in endometrial or ovarian cancer, endometriosis, gallbladder disease, vision disturbances, hypertension, familial hyperlipoproteinemia, hypothyroidism, conditions that predispose to fluid retention, hypocalcemia, asthma, diabetes mellitus, seizure disorders, migraine, hepatic or renal disease, and elderly patients.

Adverse reactions
CNS: headache, migraine, syncope, depression, insomnia, vertigo, neuralgia, hypoesthesia
CV: chest pain, varicose veins
EENT: conjunctivitis, neuro-ocular lesions (such as retinal thrombosis, optic neuritis), steepened corneal curvature, contact lens intolerance, sinusitis, rhinitis, laryngitis, pharyngitis
GI: nausea, vomiting, diarrhea, dyspepsia, flatulence, abdominal pain, GI disorder, gastroenteritis
GU: urinary tract infection, cystitis, leukorrhea, uterine or endometrial disorder, urinary tract disorder, breast tenderness or pain, breast enlargement, decreased lactation, amenorrhea, vaginal candidiasis, vaginitis, **vaginal hemorrhage, invasive cervical cancer**
Musculoskeletal: arthralgia, myalgia, leg cramps, arthritis, tendon disorder
Respiratory: cough, bronchitis, pneumonia
Skin: rash, diaphoresis, hot flashes
Other: fever, infection, flulike symptoms

Patient monitoring
• Monitor liver function tests, fluid intake and output, and phosphatase, calcium glucose, and folic acid levels.
• Assess abdomen for liver enlargement.

• Monitor for breast tenderness and swelling.
• Assess bone density annually.

skeletal muscle relaxants
baclofen, carisoprodol, chlorzoxazone, cyclobenzaprine hydrochloride, dantrolene sodium, diazepam, methocarbamol, tizanidine hydrochloride

Action
Unknown. Thought to cause muscle relaxation through sedative properties and by inhibiting activity in descending reticular formation and spine. Also decrease muscle tone and involuntary movements.

Indications
Muscle spasms (as from trauma or inflammation), hyperreflexia and hypertonia (as in parkinsonism), tetanus, cerebral palsy, multiple sclerosis, tension headache

Contraindications and precautions
• Contraindicated in hypersensitivity to drug or polyethylene glycol (parenteral forms), renal impairment (parenteral forms), active hepatic disease, upper motor neuron disorder, and patients who use spasticity to maintain posture or balance
• Use cautiously in cardiac, hepatic, or renal dysfunction; history of allergies; seizure disorders (parenteral forms); pregnant or breastfeeding patients; and children (safety not established).

Adverse reactions
CNS: dizziness, anxiety, abnormal thinking, hyperesthesia, agitation, confusion, hypertonia, **seizures, coma**
CV: palpitations, hypotension, bradycardia, weak pulse, fistula, pseudoaneurysm, **thrombophlebitis,**

---

complete or incomplete atrioventricular block, pulmonary embolism, nodal arrhythmias, ventricular tachycardia
EENT: diplopia
GI: nausea, vomiting, diarrhea, dyspepsia, gastroesophageal reflux, hematemesis, dysphagia, **paralytic ileus, GI bleeding**
GU: urinary frequency or incontinence, dysuria, cystalgia, prostatitis, **renal dysfunction**
Hepatic: hepatitis
Musculoskeletal: muscle rigidity
Respiratory: abnormal breath sounds, dyspnea, wheezing, bronchitis, pneumonia, pleurisy, **pleural effusion, pulmonary edema, pulmonary embolism, bronchospasm**
Skin: rash, urticaria, pruritus, edema
Other: chills, fever

Patient monitoring
• Monitor vital signs and liver function tests.

thrombolytics
alteplase, anistreplase, drotrecogin alfa, reteplase, streptokinase, tenecteplase, urokinase

Action
Convert plasminogen to plasmin, an enzyme that degrades fibrin clots and lyses thrombi and emboli

Indications
Acute massive pulmonary embolism, acute ischemic cerebrovascular accident (CVA), thrombotic coronary arterial obstruction in acute myocardial infarction, deep-vein thrombosis, arterial emboli or thromboses, occlusion of venous access device

Contraindications and precautions
• Contraindicated in hypersensitivity to drug or other thrombolytics, active internal bleeding, bleeding diathesis, severe uncontrolled hypertension, intracranial neoplasm, arteriovenous malformation or aneurysm, recent CVA, or recent intracranial or intraspinal surgery or trauma
• Use cautiously in GI or GU bleeding, hypertension, left-sided cardiac thrombus (including mitral stenosis), acute pericarditis, subacute bacterial endocarditis, hemostatic defects, diabetic hemorrhagic retinopathy, septic thrombophlebitis, previous puncture of noncompressible vessels, trauma, obstetric delivery, organ biopsy, major surgery, patients older than age 75, and pregnant or breastfeeding patients.

Adverse reactions
CNS: intracranial hemorrhage
CV: hypotension, **arrhythmias, cholesterol embolization, venous thrombosis**
GI: nausea, vomiting, **GI or retroperitoneal bleeding**
GU: hematuria
Hematologic: anemia, **bone marrow depression, hemorrhage, bleeding tendency**
Respiratory: respiratory depression, apnea
Skin: bruising, urticaria
Other: fever, edema, phlebitis or hemorrhage at I.V. site, hypersensitivity reactions including **anaphylaxis, sepsis**

Patient monitoring
• Monitor vital signs and neurologic status closely.
◀€ Assess for unusual bleeding or bruising.
• Monitor International Normalized Ratio, prothrombin time, and partial thromboplastin time.

thyroid hormones
levothyroxine sodium; liothyronine sodium; liotrix; thyroid, desiccated

---

Action
Regulate growth and development by controlling protein synthesis; stimulate normal metabolism by oxygenating body tissues

Indications
Hypothyroidism, euthyroid or multinodal goiter, subacute or chronic lymphocytic thyroiditis

Contraindications and precautions
• Contraindicated in hypersensitivity to drug, recent myocardial infarction, adrenal insufficiency, and thyrotoxicosis
• Use cautiously in cardiovascular disease, severe renal insufficiency, uncorrected adrenocortical disorders, angina pectoris, ischemia, diabetes mellitus, myxedema, elderly patients, and pregnant or breastfeeding patients.

Adverse reactions
CNS: insomnia, irritability, nervousness, tremor, headache
CV: tachycardia, angina pectoris, hypotension, hypertension, increased cardiac output, palpitations, **arrhythmias, cardiovascular collapse**
GI: vomiting, diarrhea, abdominal cramps
GU: menstrual irregularities
Metabolic: hyperthyroidism
Musculoskeletal: accelerated bone maturation in children
Skin: alopecia (in children), diaphoresis
Other: weight loss, appetite changes, heat intolerance

Patient monitoring
• Monitor vital signs, weight, ECG, and thyroid function tests.

thyroid hormone antagonists
methimazole, potassium iodide, propylthiouracil, sodium iodide ^{131}I

Action
Rapidly inhibit iodine release and synthesis in thyroid gland, decreasing thyroid vascularity and preventing iodine uptake

Indications
Hyperthyroidism, thyroid cancer, thyrotoxicosis, to control hyperthyroidism before thyroidectomy or radioactive iodine therapy

Contraindications and precautions
• Contraindicated in hypersensitivity to thyroid hormone antagonists and in breastfeeding
• Use cautiously in bone marrow depression, tuberculosis, bronchitis, hyperkalemia, renal impairment, recent myocardial infarction, large nodular goiter, vomiting and diarrhea, patients younger than age 30, and pregnant patients.

Adverse reactions
CNS: headache, vertigo, paresthesia, neuritis, neuropathy, CNS stimulation, depression, drowsiness
CV: chest pain, tachycardia
EENT: pain on swallowing, sore throat
GI: nausea, vomiting, diarrhea, constipation, epigastric distress, GI irritation, dry mouth, salivary gland enlargement, anorexia, **paralytic ileus**
GU: nephritis
Hematologic: anemia, eosinophilia, **bone marrow depression, leukopenia, thrombocytopenia, leukemia, agranulocytosis**
Hepatic: jaundice, **hepatic dysfunction, hepatitis**
Metabolic: hypothyroidism, thyroid hyperplasia, **hyperkalemia**
Musculoskeletal: joint pain, myalgia
Respiratory: cough
Skin: rash, urticaria, skin discoloration, pruritus, erythema nodosum, exfoliative dermatitis, alopecia, acneiform eruption

---

Reactions in **bold** are life-threatening.   ◀€ Clinical alert

Other: taste loss, fullness in neck, fever, lupuslike syndrome, lymphadenopathy, lymphedema, **radiation sickness** (with sodium iodide ^{131}I)

Patient monitoring
• Monitor CBC and thyroid function tests.

---

vasodilators
bosentan, hydralazine hydrochloride, isosorbide dinitrate, isosorbide mononitrate, minoxidil, nesiritide, nitroglycerin, nitroprusside sodium

Action
Relax vascular smooth muscle by stimulating intracellular production of cyclic guanosine monophosphate

Indications
Acute angina, prophylaxis and long-term management of recurrent angina, heart failure associated with acute myocardial infarction (MI), to control blood pressure in perioperative hypertension associated with surgery

Contraindications and precautions
• Contraindicated in hypersensitivity to drug, severe anemia, angle-closure glaucoma, orthostatic hypotension, early MI, head trauma, cerebral hemorrhage, and as primary therapy in cardiogenic shock or systolic pressure below 90 mm Hg
• Use cautiously in acute MI (associated with hypertension, tachycardia, or congestive heart failure), cerebral hemorrhage, gastric hypermotility or malabsorption syndrome (with sustained-release forms), head trauma, hyperthyroidism, hypertrophic cardiomyopathy, increased intraocular pressure, orthostatic hypotension, volume depletion, and alcohol use.

Adverse reactions
CNS: headache, apprehension, malaise, rigors, restlessness, weakness, asthenia, vertigo, dizziness, agitation, anxiety, confusion, insomnia, nervousness, nightmares, incoordination, hypoesthesia, hypokinesia
CV: tachycardia, retrosternal discomfort, palpitations, orthostatic hypotension, rebound hypertension, hypotension, syncope, crescendo angina, premature ventricular contractions, **arrhythmias, atrial fibrillation**
EENT: blurred vision, diplopia
GI: nausea, vomiting, diarrhea, dyspepsia, abdominal pain, tenesmus, fecal incontinence
GU: dysuria, urinary frequency, urinary incontinence, erectile dysfunction
Hematologic: methemoglobinemia, hemolytic anemia
Musculoskeletal: arthralgia, muscle twitching, stiff neck
Respiratory: bronchitis, pneumonia, upper respiratory infection
Skin: pallor; cold sweats; increased perspiration; rash; contact or exfoliative dermatitis; cutaneous vasodilation with flushing; crusty skin lesions; pruritus; topical allergic reaction; erythematous, vesicular, or pruritic lesions; local burning or tingling sensation in oral cavity (with sublingual forms); **anaphylactoid reactions** with oral mucosal and conjunctival edema
Other: tooth disorder, increased appetite, edema

Patient monitoring
• Closely monitor ECG and vital signs (especially blood pressure).
• In suspected overdose, assess for signs and symptoms of increased intracranial pressure.
• Check arterial blood gas values and methemoglobin levels.

Vitamins and minerals

ascorbic acid (vitamin C)
Cecon, Cevi-Bid, Dull-C, Vita-C

Action
Water-soluble vitamin with antioxidant properties; stimulates collagen formation and enhances tissue repair

Availability
Capsules: 500 mg
Crystals: 1,000 mg/½ tsp
Injection: 250 mg/ml, 500 mg/ml
Liquid: 50 mg/ml, 500 mg/5 ml
Powder: 60 mg/½ tsp, 1,060 mg/½ tsp
Solution: 100 mg/ml
Tablets: 25 mg, 50 mg, 100 mg, 125 mg, 250 mg, 500 mg, 1,000 mg, 1,500 mg
Tablets (chewable): 60 mg, 100 mg, 250 mg, 500 mg, 1,000 mg
Tablets (timed-release): 500 mg, 1,000 mg, 1,500 mg

✒ Indications and dosages
➤ Recommended dietary allowance
Adults: 60 mg daily
➤ Scurvy
Adults: 300 mg to 1 g P.O., subcutaneously, I.M., or I.V. daily
Children: 100 to 300 mg P.O., subcutaneously, I.M., or I.V. daily depending on severity

Contraindications and precautions
• Prolonged use of excessive doses contraindicated in diabetes mellitus, sodium-restricted diet, concurrent anticoagulant use, and history of recurrent renal calculi
• Use cautiously in hypersensitivity to tartrazine or sulfites (if product contains these compounds), before tests for occult blood in stool, and in breast-feeding patients. Don't exceed recommended amount in pregnant patients.
• Avoid rapid I.V. infusion.

Adverse reactions
Transient mild soreness at I.M. or subcutaneous injection site; transient light-headedness or dizziness (with rapid I.V. administration)

cholecalciferol (vitamin D$_3$)
Delta-D

Action
Biologically active vitamin D metabolite; controls intestinal absorption of dietary calcium, tubular reabsorption of calcium by kidney, and (in conjunction with parathyroid hormone [PTH]), calcium mobilization from skeleton. Acts directly on bone cells to stimulate skeletal growth and on parathyroid glands to suppress PTH synthesis and secretion.

Availability
Tablets: 400 international units, 1,000 international units

✒ Indications and dosages
➤ Recommended dietary allowance (RDA)
Adults: 400 to 1,000 international units/day
Children: 400 international units/day

Contraindications and precautions
• Contraindicated in hypercalcemia, vitamin D toxicity, malabsorption

---

syndrome, and abnormal sensitivity to vitamin D effects

• Don't exceed RDA during normal pregnancy. Use cautiously in breast-feeding patients. Safety and efficacy of dosages exceeding RDA have not been established for children.

Adverse reactions

Nausea, vomiting, constipation, pancreatitis, weakness, headache, irritability, drowsiness, overt psychosis, dry mouth, metallic taste, muscle or bone pain, hypertension, hypotension, polyuria, polydipsia, anorexia, weight loss, hypercalciuria, reversible azotemia, nephrocalcinosis, conjunctivitis, photophobia, pruritus, albuminuria, elevated liver function tests results, **arrhythmias**

chromium (chromic chloride)
Chroma-Pak

Action

Serves as a component of glucose tolerance factor, which activates insulin-mediated reactions; helps maintain normal glucose metabolism and peripheral nerve function

Availability

Injection: 4 mcg/ml (as 20.5 mcg chromic chloride hexahydrate), 20 mcg/ml (as 102.5 mcg chromic chloride hexahydrate)

Indications and dosages

➤ Supplement to I.V. solutions used in total parenteral nutrition
Adults: 10 to 15 mcg/day. For metabolically stable adults with intestinal fluid loss, 20 mcg/day.
Children: 0.14 to 0.2 mcg/kg/day

Contraindications and precautions

• Preparations containing benzyl alcohol contraindicated in premature infants (may cause fatal gasping syndrome)
• Avoid use or adjust dosage in patients with renal or GI dysfunction.
• Use cautiously in pregnant patients.
• Multiple trace element solutions may cause overdose if patient's requirement for one element in formulation exceeds that for others. Chromium may need to be given separately.

Adverse reactions

Toxicity is rare at recommended dosages; hypersensitivity reaction to iodide may occur.

copper
Cupric Sulfate

Action

Serves as cofactor for ceruloplasmin, an oxidase needed for proper formation of transferrin (an iron carrier protein); helps maintain normal rate of red and white blood cell formation

Availability

Injection: 0.4 mg/ml, 2 mg/ml

Indications and dosages

➤ Supplement to I.V. solutions used in total parenteral nutrition
Adults: 0.5 to 1.5 mg/day to prevent deficiency; 3 mg/day to treat deficiency
Children: 20 mcg/kg/day to prevent deficiency; 20 to 30 mcg/kg/day to treat deficiency

Contraindications and precautions

• Multidose preparations contraindicated in patients with sensitivity to benzyl alcohol (such as premature infants, who may experience fatal gasping syndrome)

• Use cautiously in renal or GI dysfunction, Wilson's disease, and pregnant patients.

• Be aware that giving copper without zinc (or vice versa) may decrease blood level of the other mineral. Monitor levels before giving subsequent doses.

• Multiple trace element solutions may cause overdose if patient's requirement for one element in formulation exceeds that for others. Copper may need to be given separately.

Adverse reactions
None known

cyanocobalamin (vitamin B$_{12}$)
Big Shot B-12, Cyanoject, Rubramin

hydroxocobalamin, crystalline (vitamin B$_{12}$)
Hydro-Crysti-12, LA-12

Action
Essential to growth, cell reproduction, hematopoiesis, and nucleoprotein and myelin synthesis; also participates in nucleic acid synthesis. Plays a role in red blood cell formation through activation of folic acid coenzymes.

Availability
cyanocobalamin
Injection: 100 mcg/ml, 1,000 mcg/ml
Intranasal gel: 500 mcg/0.1 ml
Tablets: 25 mcg, 50 mcg, 100 mcg, 200 mcg, 250 mcg, 500 mcg, 1,000 mcg, 1,500 mcg
Tablets (extended-release): 100 mcg, 200 mcg, 500 mcg, 1,000 mcg
hydroxocobalamin
Injection: 1,000 mcg/ml

◢ Indications and dosages
➤ Recommended dietary allowance
Adults and children older than age 11: 2 mcg cyanocobalamin daily
Children ages 9 to 11: 1.8 mcg daily
Children ages 4 to 8: 1.2 mcg daily
Children ages 1 to 3: 0.9 mcg daily
➤ Vitamin B$_{12}$ deficiency
Adults: 30 mcg hydroxocobalamin I.M. daily for 5 to 10 days, depending on cause and severity; for maintenance, 100 to 200 mcg I.M. monthly
Children: Total dosage of 1 to 5 mg hydroxocobalamin I.M. given over 2 or more weeks in divided doses of 100 mcg; then a maintenance dosage of 30 to 50 mcg I.M. q 4 weeks
➤ Pernicious anemia
Adults: 100 mcg cyanocobalamin subcutaneously or I.M. daily for 7 days; then 100 mcg subcutaneously or I.M. every other day for 14 days; then 100 mcg subcutaneously or I.M. q 3 to 4 days for 2 to 3 weeks or until remission; then 100 mcg I.M. monthly or 1,000 to 2,000 mcg P.O. daily
➤ Vitamin B$_{12}$ deficiency and malabsorption in patients in remission
Adults: 500 mcg nasal gel intranasally once weekly

Contraindications and precautions
• Contraindicated in hypersensitivity to vitamin B$_{12}$, cobalt, or product components

Adverse reactions
Mild transient diarrhea, nausea, vomiting, dyspepsia, headache, anxiety, dizziness, nervousness, hypoesthesia, sore throat, severe and rapid optic nerve atrophy, back pain, myalgia, arthritis, paresthesia, abnormal gait, dyspnea, rhinitis, itching, rash, polycythemia vera; with parenteral forms—injection site pain, **pulmonary edema, heart failure, peripheral vascular thrombosis, anaphylactic shock**

Reactions in **bold** are life-threatening.

doxercalciferol
Hectorol

Action
Synthetic vitamin D analogue; acts directly on parathyroid gland to stimulate and suppress parathyroid hormone (PTH) synthesis and secretion

Availability
Capsules: 0.5 mcg, 2.5 mcg
Injection: 2 mcg/vial

Indications and dosages
➤ Elevated intact PTH levels (iPTH) in secondary hyperparathyroidism caused by chronic renal dialysis
Adults: Dosage individualized. Recommended initial dosage is 10 mcg P.O. three times weekly at dialysis (approximately every other day). Adjust as needed to lower blood iPTH level to 150 to 300 pg/ml. Maximum dosage is 20 mcg P.O. three times weekly.

Contraindications and precautions
• Contraindicated in hypersensitivity to product components, hypercalcemia, and evidence of vitamin D toxicity
• Use cautiously in elderly patients with coronary disease, renal impairment, or arteriosclerosis.

Adverse reactions
Nausea, vomiting, constipation, dyspepsia, headache, malaise, dizziness, sleep disorder, weight gain, anorexia, edema, arthralgia, abscess, dyspnea, pruritus, bradycardia

folic acid
Folvite

Action
Stimulates production of red and white blood cells and platelets in some megaloblastic anemias

Availability
Injection: 5 mg/ml
Tablets: 0.4 mg, 0.8 mg, 1 mg

Indications and dosages
➤ Recommended dietary allowance
Adults and children older than age 11: 150 to 400 mcg
Children younger than age 11: 25 to 100 mcg
➤ Megaloblastic anemia related to folic acid deficiency in sprue, nutritional deficiency, pregnancy, childhood, or infancy
Adults: Up to 1 mg/day P.O., I.M., I.V., or subcutaneously (given P.O. except in severe disease or severely impaired GI absorption). Higher dosages may be needed in severe cases, with a maintenance dosage of 0.4 mg/day. In pregnant or breastfeeding patients, 0.8 mg/day.
Children older than age 4: Maintenance dosage of 0.4 mg/day P.O., I.M., or subcutaneously (given P.O. except in severe disease or severely impaired GI absorption)
Children younger than age 4: Maintenance dosage of up to 0.3 mg/day P.O., I.M., or subcutaneously (given P.O. except in severe disease or severely impaired GI absorption)

Contraindications and precautions
• Contraindicated in pernicious, aplastic, or normocytic anemia
• Use cautiously in breastfeeding patients.

Reactions in **bold** are life-threatening.

Adverse reactions
Altered sleep pattern, malaise, poor concentration, impaired judgment, hyperactivity, anorexia, nausea, flatulence, bitter taste, allergic reaction (including rash, pruritus, erythema), **bronchospasm**

manganese, chelated

manganese chloride

Action
Serves as a cofactor in various enzyme systems; stimulates hepatic cholesterol and fatty acid synthesis and influences mucopolysaccharide synthesis

Availability
Injection: 0.1 mg/ml (as 0.36 mg manganese chloride)
Tablets: 20 mg and 50 mg of chelated manganese

⚫ Indications and dosages
➤ Recommended dietary allowance
Adults: 1.9 to 2.3 mg/day in males; 1.6 to 1.8 mg/day in females
➤ Supplement to I.V. solutions used for total parenteral nutrition
Adults: 0.15 to 0.8 mg/day
Children: 2 to 10 mcg/kg/day

Contraindications and precautions
• Use cautiously in pregnant patients and premature infants (may reach toxic levels in kidney).
• Reduce dosage in renal or GI dysfunction.
• Multiple trace element solutions may cause overdose if patient's requirement for one element in formulation exceeds that for others. Manganese may need to be given separately.

Adverse reactions
None known

niacin (nicotinic acid, vitamin B₃)
Slo-Niacin

niacinamide (nicotinamide)

Action
Serves as a component of two coenzymes essential to oxidation-reduction reactions

Availability
Capsules (extended-release): 100 mg, 250 mg, 400 mg, 500 mg
Capsules (sustained-release): 125 mg, 500 mg
Capsules (timed-release): 250 mg, 500 mg
Tablets: 25 mg, 50 mg, 100 mg, 125 mg, 250 mg, 400 mg, 500 mg
Tablets (extended-release): 250 mg, 500 mg, 750 mg, 1,000 mg
Tablets (sustained-release): 500 mg
Tablets (timed-release): 250 mg, 500 mg

⚫ Indications and dosages
➤ Recommended dietary allowance (RDA)
Adults: 15 to 20 mg P.O. daily in males; 13 to 15 mg P.O. daily in females
➤ Pellagra
Adults: Up to 500 mg daily P.O. given in divided doses
➤ Niacin deficiency
Adults: Up to 100 mg P.O. daily
➤ Hyperlipidemia
Adults: Initially, 250 mg P.O. daily; increase up to 1 or 2 g/day (given in divided doses) at 4- to 7-day intervals. Don't exceed 6 g/day.

Reactions in **bold** are life-threatening.

Contraindications and precautions

• Contraindicated in hypersensitivity to niacin, hepatic dysfunction, active peptic ulcer, severe hypotension, and arterial bleeding
• Use cautiously in heart disease (give only under doctor's supervision), gout, regular consumption of large amounts of alcohol, history of hepatic disease, and pregnant or breastfeeding patients. Don't exceed RDA in children (safety and efficacy not established).

Adverse reactions

Flushing, pruritus, urticaria, rash, dry skin, tingling, acanthosis nigricans, hyperpigmentation, diaphoresis, nausea, vomiting, diarrhea, dyspepsia, GI distress, abdominal pain, peptic ulcer, hyperuricemia, gout, decreased glucose tolerance, chills, dizziness, insomnia, migraine, transient headache, toxic amblyopia, cystoid macular edema, orthostasis, edema, hypotension, palpitations, syncope, dyspnea, abnormal liver function tests, **fulminant hepatic necrosis, hepatotoxicity, atrial fibrillation, other arrhythmias**

paricalcitol
Zemplar

Action

Synthetic vitamin D analog; suppresses parathyroid hormone in patients with chronic renal failure

Availability

Injection: 2 mcg/ml, 5 mcg/ml

⃠ Indications and dosages

➢ Hyperparathyroidism associated with chronic renal failure
Adults: 0.04 to 0.1 mcg/kg (2.8 to 7 mcg) as a single I.V. bolus dose given no more often than every other day

during dialysis. Dosage may be increased by 2 to 4 mcg at 2- to 4-week intervals.

Contraindications and precautions

• Contraindicated in hypersensitivity to components of formulation, hypercalcemia, and vitamin D toxicity
• Use cautiously in breastfeeding patients.

Adverse reactions

Nausea, vomiting, dry mouth, pruritus, allergic reaction, rash, urticaria, edema, light-headedness, chills, fever, flulike symptoms, malaise, palpitations, pneumonia, **GI bleeding, sepsis**

phytonadione (vitamin K₁)
AquaMEPHYTON, Mephyton

Action

Promotes hepatic synthesis of active prothrombin, proconvertin, plasma thromboplastin component, and Stuart factor

Availability

Aqueous colloidal solution for injection: 2 mg/ml
Tablets: 5 mg

⃠ Indications and dosages

➢ Hypoprothrombinemia caused by anticoagulant therapy
Adults: Initially, 2.5 to 10 mg P.O., I.M., subcutaneously, or I.V. (at doses not exceeding 1 mg/minute); repeat if needed within 12 to 48 hours after P.O. dose or within 6 to 8 hours of I.M., subcutaneous, or I.V. dose. Subsequent dosages determined by prothrombin time or clinical condition.
➢ Hypoprothrombinemia secondary to other causes

Reactions in **bold** are life-threatening.

Adults: 2.5 to 25 mg (rarely, up to 50 mg); dosage and administration route depend on severity and response.
Children: 5 to 10 mg; dosage and administration route depend on severity and response.

➤ Prevention and treatment of hemorrhagic disease of newborn
Neonates: For prevention, 0.5 to 1 mg I.M. as a single dose within 1 hour of birth. For treatment, 1 mg I.M. or subcutaneously if mother received oral anticoagulants.

Contraindications and precautions

• Contraindicated in hypersensitivity to drug or its components. (Life-threatening reactions resembling hypersensitivity or anaphylaxis have occurred during and immediately after I.V. injection.)
• Use cautiously in pregnant or breastfeeding patients, children, and neonates (if product contains benzyl alcohol).
• Avoid P.O. use in disorders that may prevent adequate absorption.

Adverse reactions

Hyperbilirubinemia (in infants); with parenteral administration—pain, swelling, tenderness at injection site; itchy rash after repeated injections; transient flushing sensations; peculiar taste; **anaphylactoid reactions**

pyridoxine hydrochloride (vitamin B$_6$)

Beesix, Doxine, Nestrex, Rodex

Action

Converts to physiologically active forms of vitamin B$_6$ (pyridoxal phosphate and pyridoxamine phosphate), which promote metabolic functions affecting carbohydrate, protein, and lipid use

Availability

Capsules (extended-release): 150 mg
Injection: 100 mg/ml
Tablets: 10 mg, 25 mg, 50 mg, 100 mg, 200 mg, 250 mg, 500 mg
Tablets (enteric-coated): 20 mg
*Tablets (extended-release):*100 mg, 200 mg, 500 mg

🕭 Indications and dosages

➤ Recommended dietary allowance (RDA)
Adults: 1.7 to 2 mg daily in males; 1.4 to 1.6 mg daily in females
➤ Prophylaxis or treatment of pyridoxine deficiency, including drug-induced deficiency (as from isoniazid, hydralazine, or hormonal contraceptives)
Adults: For prophylaxis, 25 to 100 mg daily P.O., I.V., or I.M. For established neuropathy, 200 mg daily.

Contraindications and precautions

• Contraindicated in hypersensitivity to pyridoxine or components of formulation
• Don't exceed RDA in children (safety and efficacy not established).
• Use cautiously in breastfeeding patients.
• Be aware that drug abuse and dependence have occurred after withdrawal from dosage of 200 mg/day.

Adverse reactions

Sensory neuropathic syndrome (including unstable gait, ataxia, clumsiness of hands, pedal and perioral numbness, paresthesia, and decreased sensation to touch, temperature, and vibration), photoallergic reaction, nausea, headache, decreased folic acid level, aspartate aminotransferase elevation, **seizures**

Reactions in **bold** are life-threatening.

retinol (vitamin A)
Aquasol A, Palmitate-A 5000

Action
Stimulates and supports retinal function, reproduction, bone growth, epithelial tissue differentiation, and embryonic development

Availability
Capsules: 10,000 international units, 15,000 international units, 25,000 international units
Injection: 50,000 international units/ml
Tablets: 5,000 international units

⏀ Indications and dosages
➤ Recommended dietary allowance (RDA)
Adults: 1,000 mcg retinol equivalents (RE) daily in males; 800 mcg RE daily in females
➤ Severe vitamin A deficiency with corneal changes
Adults and children older than age 8: 100,000 international units I.M. daily for first 3 days, followed by 50,000 international units I.M. daily for 2 weeks. Or 500,000 international units P.O. for 3 days, followed by 50,000 international units P.O. daily for 14 days, then 10,000 to 20,000 international units P.O. daily for 60 days. Or 50,000 to 100,000 international units P.O. daily for 1 to 7 days, followed by 5,000 to 75,000 international units daily for several weeks.
➤ Vitamin A deficiency with xerophthalmia
Children: 5,000 to 15,000 international units (1,500 to 4,500 RE) I.M. for 10 days or 5,000 international units/kg P.O. for 5 days or until recovery

Contraindications and precautions
• Hypersensitivity to vitamin A or components of formulation, hypervitaminosis A

• Don't exceed RDA during normal pregnancy.
• Use cautiously in patients with renal failure and in I.V. use.

Adverse reactions
Headache, irritability, vertigo, lethargy, malaise, fever, headache, hypercalcemia, weight loss, vision changes, anorexia, sticky skin, hypervitaminosis A, **increased intracranial pressure, anaphylactic shock and death** (with I.V. use)

riboflavin (lactoflavin, vitamin B₂)

Action
Serves as two coenzymes that catalyze oxidation-reduction reactions, such as glucose oxidation, amino acid deamination, and fatty acid breakdown

Availability
Tablets: 10 mg, 25 mg, 50 mg, 100 mg, 250 mg

⏀ Indications and dosages
➤ Recommended dietary allowance (RDA)
Adults: 1.4 to 1.8 mg in males; 1.2 to 1.3 mg in females
➤ Riboflavin deficiency
Adults: 5 to 30 mg P.O. daily in divided doses

Contraindications and precautions
• Use cautiously when giving more than RDA to pregnant or breastfeeding women.

Adverse reactions
None known

Reactions in **bold** are life-threatening.

selenium
Sele-Pak, Selepen

Action
Guards cell components against oxidative damage caused by peroxides generated during cellular metabolism

Availability
Injection: 40 mcg/ml

🚱 Indications and dosages
➤ Recommended dietary allowance
Adults: 40 to 70 mcg in males; 45 to 55 mcg in females
➤ Supplement to I.V. solutions used in total parenteral nutrition for prophylaxis and treatment of selenium deficiency
Adults and adolescents: 20 to 40 mcg daily for prophylaxis; 100 mcg daily for 24 to 31 days for treatment
Children: 3 mcg/kg daily (for prophylaxis or treatment)

Contraindications and precautions
• Use cautiously in renal or GI dysfunction, pregnant patients, or premature infants (if product contains benzyl alcohol, which is associated with fatal gasping syndrome). May need to decrease dosage in renal or GI dysfunction.
• Multiple trace element solutions may cause overdose if patient's requirement for one element in formulation exceeds that for others. Selenium may need to be given separately.

Adverse reactions
Lethargy, alopecia, hair discoloration, vomiting, abdominal pain, garlic breath, tremor, diaphoresis

thiamine (vitamin B₁)
Biamine, Thiamilate, Thiamine Hydrochloride

Action
Water-soluble vitamin; combines with adenosine triphosphate and thiamine diphosphokinase to form thiamine pyrophosphate, a coenzyme essential for normal growth and aerobic metabolism, nerve impulse transmission, and acetylcholine synthesis

Availability
Injection: 100 mg/ml
Tablets: 5 mg, 10 mg, 25 mg, 50 mg, 100 mg, 250 mg, 500 mg
Tablets (enteric-coated): 20 mg

🚱 Indications and dosages
➤ Recommended dietary allowance
Adults: 1.2 to 1.5 mg/day in males; 1 to 1.1 mg/day in females
➤ Thiamine deficiency (beriberi)
Adults: 10 to 20 mg I.M. t.i.d. for 2 weeks, then 5 to 30 mg P.O. daily for 1 month
➤ Wernicke's encephalopathy
Adults: Initially, 100 mg I.V., followed by 50 to 100 mg daily I.M. until patient can consume a regular balanced diet

Contraindications and precautions
• Contraindicated in thiamine hypersensitivity
• Use cautiously in pregnant or breastfeeding patients.

Adverse reactions
Warm sensation, pruritus, urticaria, weakness, diaphoresis, tenderness and induration (with I.M. use), hypersensitivity reaction, **cyanosis, pulmonary edema, GI tract hemorrhage, cardiovascular collapse, angioedema, anaphylactic shock, death**

Reactions in **bold** are life-threatening.

tocopherols (alpha tocopherols, vitamin E)
Aquavit E, d'Apha E, Nutr-E-Sol, Vita-Plus E

Action
Protects cellular components from oxidation, prevents formation of toxic oxidation products, maintains integrity of red blood cell (RBC) wall, protects RBCs against hemolysis, stimulates steroid metabolism, suppresses prostaglandin production, and inhibits platelet aggregation

Availability
Capsules: 100, 200, 400, 600, and 1,000 international units
Drops: 15 international units/0.3 ml
Liquid: 15 international units/30 ml
Solution (water-miscible): 50 international units/ml
Tablets: 100, 200, 400, 500, 600, 800, and 1,000 international units

⚕ Indications and dosages
➤ Recommended dietary allowance
Adults: 15 international units in males; 12 international units in females
➤ To prevent or treat vitamin E deficiency
Adults: 60 to 75 international units P.O. daily, to a maximum of 1,000 international units daily

Contraindications and precautions
None

Adverse reactions
Hypervitaminosis E, nausea, vomiting, diarrhea, fatigue, weakness, blurred vision, headache, rash, gonadal dysfunction, **bleeding, necrotizing enterocolitis** (in infants)

zinc chloride
zinc gluconate
zinc sulfate
Zinca-Pak

Action
Serves as cofactor for more than 70 enzymes; promotes wound healing and helps maintain normal growth rate, normal skin hydration, and taste and smell sensations

Availability
Capsules: 220 mg
Injection: 1 mg/ml (as 2.09 mg chloride)
Tablets (gluconate): 10 mg, 15 mg, 50 mg
Tablets (sulfate): 66 mg, 110 mg

⚕ Indications and dosages
➤ Recommended dietary allowance
Adults: 12 to 15 mg
➤ Dietary supplement
Adults: 25 to 50 mg P.O. daily
➤ Supplement to I.V. solution used in total parenteral nutrition (TPN)
Metabolically stable adults: 2.5 to 4 mg/day; may give additional 2 mg/day in acute catabolic states. In patients with fluid loss from small bowel, give additional 12.2 mg/L of TPN solution.

Contraindications and precautions
• Use cautiously in renal or GI dysfunction, pregnant patients, and premature infants (if product contains benzyl alcohol, which is associated with fatal gasping syndrome).
• Dosage may need to be decreased in renal or GI dysfunction.

Reactions in **bold** are life-threatening.

• Multiple trace element solutions may cause overdose if patient's requirement for one element in formulation exceeds that for others. Zinc may need to be given separately.

Adverse reactions

Restlessness, dizziness, nausea, vomiting, diarrhea, gastric ulcer

Herbs and supplements

The information provided in these monographs reflects commonly held beliefs about the actions and uses of common herbs and nutritional supplements. However, not all of these beliefs have been confirmed by clinical trials. Although herbal remedies have been used for thousands of years, few have undergone well-designed scientific studies to determine how they work, if they're safe, and whether they're effective in treating the medical conditions for which they're commonly used. Advise patients to consult a health care practitioner before using herbs or supplements to help determine if such use may be safe.

aloe

Purported action
With topical use, exerts a moisturizing effect on burns and wounds, which prevents air from drying the wound and increases blood flow to stimulate healing. With internal use, may exert a laxative effect by stimulating the large intestine and increasing peristalsis.

Reported uses
Used topically (as a gel) to inhibit infection and promote healing of minor burns, abrasions, wounds, and frostbite and to treat certain skin diseases (such as psoriasis and seborrheic dermatitis). Used internally (as liquid extract concentrate, capsules, or dried aloe latex) as a strong laxative.

Contraindications and precautions
Internal use is contraindicated in inflammatory bowel disease, elderly patients with suspected intestinal obstruction, pregnant or breastfeeding patients, and children younger than age 12.

Adverse reactions
• With topical use: redness, itching, and burning sensation in dermabraded skin
• With P.O. use: edema, cramps, diarrhea, weight loss, electrolyte abnormalities, **arrhythmias**

Interactions
Antiarrhythmics, corticosteroids, licorice, stimulant laxatives, thiazide diuretics: hypokalemia
Cardiac glycosides: increased effects of these drugs

bilberry

Purported action
Relieves mild GI tract inflammation, easing diarrhea; reduces oral mucous membrane irritation; increases microcirculation by redistributing new capillary formation; strengthens capillary walls; promotes overall health of circulatory system; and exerts a protective effect on stomach and liver (possibly through increased prostaglandin production)

Reported uses
Nonspecific diarrhea, mouth and throat irritation, to improve visual acuity and accommodation. Further studies are needed to confirm that

---

Reactions in **bold** are life-threatening.

bilberry promotes circulatory, GI, or hepatic health.

Contraindications and precautions
Contraindicated in bleeding disorders, pregnancy, and breastfeeding

Adverse reactions
- At typical dosages: GI distress, rash, drowsiness
- At higher dosages: unknown

Interactions
Anticoagulants, antiplatelet drugs, salicylates: potentiated effects, causing increased prothrombin time
Hypoglycemics: reduced blood glucose level

black cohosh

Purported action
Binds to estrogen receptors, directly or indirectly influencing luteinizing hormone release. Studies show black cohosh increases bone mineral density in rats but not in humans.

Reported uses
Menopause symptoms (as alternative to hormone replacement therapy), premenstrual syndrome, dysmenorrhea, arthritis, renal problems, malaria, sore throat

Contraindications and precautions
Contraindicated in pregnancy (may cause premature birth or miscarriage)

Adverse reactions
Headache, dizziness, CNS and visual disturbances, GI distress, nausea, vomiting, reduced heart rate, increased perspiration, weight gain

Interactions
Antihypertensives: additive hypotension
Docetaxel: increased docetaxel blood level
Hepatotoxic drugs: increased risk of hepatotoxicity

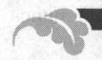

cat's claw

Purported action
Stimulates the immune system, enhances phagocytosis, dilates peripheral vessels, inhibits sympathetic nervous system activity, slows heart rate, decreases cholesterol levels, promotes diuresis, inhibits urinary bladder contraction, relaxes smooth muscle, and exerts local anesthetic effects. Studies show cat's claw has some anticancer and immunostimulant properties.

Reported uses
AIDS; inflammation; GI disorders (including colitis, inflammatory bowel disease, Crohn's disease); as an astringent, antiviral, anti-infective, and general tonic

Contraindications and precautions
Contraindicated in multiple sclerosis, tuberculosis, autoimmune disease, pregnancy, and breastfeeding. Use cautiously in GI disease (increases stomach acid secretion).

Adverse reactions
- Hypotension
- With decoction: few known risks

Interactions
Anticoagulants, antiplatelets: inhibited platelet aggregation, prolonged bleeding time
Antihypertensives: potentiated antihypertensive effects

Reactions in **bold** are life-threatening.

Benzodiazepines: increased CNS depression
CYP450-3A4 substrates (such as amiodarone, amlodipine, fentanyl, flutamide, imipramine): increased levels of these drugs
Food: enhanced cat's claw absorption
Immunosuppressants: negated immunosuppressant effects

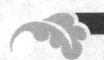

chamomile

Purported action
Reduces inflammation and fever, promotes healing of burns, and prevents ulcer formation. May also exert antispasmodic, anxiolytic, and sedative effects through action on CNS receptors.

Reported uses
Vomiting, flatulence, colic, fever, cystitis, parasitic worm infections, spasms, inflammation, anxiety; as an antibacterial, astringent, deodorant, or skin wash (to increase sloughing of necrotic tissue and promote granulation and epithelialization)

Contraindications and precautions
Contraindicated in ragweed allergy, hepatic or renal disease, pregnancy, and breastfeeding. Use cautiously in patients receiving anticoagulants.

Adverse reactions
Contact dermatitis in patients allergic to ragweed, asters, chrysanthemums, or other members of the Compositae family (such as arnica, feverfew, tansy, and yarrow), **anaphylaxis, other severe hypersensitivity reactions**

Interactions
Anticoagulants: increased anticoagulant effect

Concurrently administered drugs: delayed drug absorption
Sedatives (such as benzodiazepines): enhanced sedative effects

chondroitin

Purported action
A glycosaminoglycan (complex polysaccharide) found in extracellular matrix of connective tissue, including cornea and cartilage; thought to have protective properties (as for corneal endothelial cells and other ocular structures) without interfering with epithelialization and healing

Reported uses
Osteoarthritis, hyperlipidemia, ischemic heart disease, dry eyes, surgical aid in cataract extraction or lens implantation

Contraindications and precautions
Contraindicated in clotting disorders, prostate cancer, risk factors for prostate cancer, and patients receiving anticoagulants. Use cautiously in asthma.

Adverse reactions
Allergic reactions, alopecia, nausea, diarrhea, constipation, epigastric pain, extrasystoles, edema

Interactions
Warfarin: increased warfarin effects (with high chondroitin doses)

coenzyme Q10

Purported action
Fat-soluble, vitamin-like compound present in cells (especially concentrated

---

Reactions in **bold** are life-threatening.

in heart, liver, kidney, and pancreas). Exerts antioxidant activity, stabilizes membranes, and serves as cofactor in many metabolic pathways, especially adenosine triphosphate production in oxidative respiration.

Reported uses
Mitochondrial cytopathies (FDA-approved claim), cardiac risk reduction, heart failure, hypertension, prophylaxis of doxorubicin-induced cardiotoxicity, diabetes mellitus, immunostimulation, muscular dystrophy, statin-induced myopathy, chronic fatigue syndrome, breast cancer, Huntington's disease, Parkinson's disease, periodontal disease

Contraindications and precautions
Use cautiously in biliary obstruction, hepatic insufficiency, hypertension, diabetes mellitus, patients receiving antihypertensives, and patients undergoing chemotherapy or radiation therapy.

Adverse reactions
Anxiety, nausea, vomiting, diarrhea, flatulence, headache, **mania** or hypomania

Interactions
Antihypertensives: additive blood pressure reduction
Chemotherapy: possible cancer-cell protection
Warfarin: reduced warfarin effects

dong quai

Purported action
Exerts antispasmodic effect on smooth muscles, including those of airway and uterus. Forms containing coumarin have anticoagulant effects.

Reported uses
Asthma, allergies, menstrual disorders, menopausal symptoms, rheumatic pain, anemia, constipation, hypertension, psoriasis, skin depigmentation, ulcers; as an antispasmodic, anti-inflammatory, and anticoagulant

Contraindications and precautions
Contraindicated in patients receiving warfarin concurrently and in pregnant or breastfeeding patients (may influence uterine contractions or cause unknown effects in fetus)

Adverse reactions
- With authentic dong quai: no known reactions
- With other dong quai forms: increased risk of phototoxicity, **abortion**, uterine stimulation, and altered menstrual cycle

Interactions
Anticoagulants: increased anticoagulant effect

echinacea

Purported action
Stimulates immune system; with topical use, may have mild antibacterial and antiviral properties

Reported uses
Urinary tract and yeast infections, promotion of wound healing, prevention and treatment of upper respiratory infections (including colds and flu), allergic rhinitis, psoriasis, herpes simplex infection (topical form)

Reactions in **bold** are life-threatening.

Contraindications and precautions

Contraindicated in patients receiving immunosuppressant therapy (because of immune-stimulating properties)

Adverse reactions

Nausea, mild GI upset, allergic reactions, **anaphylaxis**

Note: Adverse reactions may be more common in patients with allergies to daisy-type plants.

Interactions

Corticosteroids: interference with chemotherapeutic effects of these drugs

CYP450-3A4 substrates (such as amiodarone, amlodipine, fentanyl, flutamide, imipramine): increased levels of these drugs

Immunosuppressants: interference with immunosuppressant effects

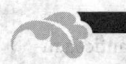

evening primrose oil

Purported action

Contains essential fatty acids (EFAs) that may improve cellular structural elements and serve as precursors to prostaglandins, which help regulate metabolic functions (including cervical ripening)

Reported uses

Disorders thought to stem from EFA deficiency or disturbed EFA metabolism, including cardiovascular disease, premenstrual syndrome, mastalgia and other breast disorders, rheumatoid arthritis, multiple sclerosis, atopic dermatitis and other dermatologic disorders, Raynaud's disease, Sjögren's syndrome, Alzheimer's disease, schizophrenia, and attention deficit hyperactivity disorder

Contraindications and precautions

Contraindicated in pregnancy, breastfeeding, and history of seizures or allergy to evening primrose oil

Adverse reactions

Headache, nausea, vomiting, diarrhea, abdominal pain, indigestion, flatulence, allergic reaction

Interactions

Anesthetics, phenothiazines: lowered seizure threshold

Anticoagulants: bleeding, bruising

Anticonvulsants: lowered seizure threshold, decreased anticonvulsant efficacy

feverfew

Purported action

Inhibits prostaglandin synthesis and serotonin release from platelets and polymorphonuclear leukocyte granules; extract may inhibit phagocytosis and platelet deposition on collagen surfaces. Exhibits antithrombotic potential and in vitro antibacterial activity, inhibits mast cell release of histamine, exerts cytotoxic activity, and suppresses enzyme release from white blood cells in inflamed joints and skin. May promote contraction and relaxation of vascular smooth muscle.

Reported uses

Menstrual pain, allergies, tinnitus, vertigo, asthma, dermatitis, psoriasis, arthritis, fever, migraine prophylaxis

Contraindications and precautions

Contraindicated in pregnancy, breastfeeding, and children younger than age 2

Reactions in **bold** are life-threatening.

Adverse reactions

- Hypersensitivity reaction, increased heart rate, oral mucosa and tongue inflammation
- After withdrawal: cluster of CNS reactions (rebound migraine, anxiety, disturbed sleep pattern), muscle and joint stiffness

Interactions

Anticoagulants, aspirin: increased antithrombotic effect of these drugs

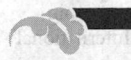

fish oils

Purported action

Contain omega-3 fatty acids, which exert anti-inflammatory and antithrombotic effects by competing with arachidonic acid in cyclooxygenase and lipoxygenase pathways and which also may suppress cyclooxygenase-2, interleukin-1 alpha, and tumor necrosis factor-alpha. Also inhibit arachidonic acid synthesis of thromboxane A_2, which causes platelet aggregation and vasoconstriction; and increase production of prostacyclin, a prostaglandin that causes vasoconstriction and reduces platelet aggregation.

Reported uses

Coronary heart disease, cardiovascular disease, cerebrovascular accident, hypertension, asthma, Crohn's disease, type 2 (non-insulin-dependent) diabetes mellitus, dysmenorrhea, fatigue, headache, herpes simplex virus type 2, hypercholesterolemia, hypertriglyceridemia, multiple sclerosis, rheumatoid arthritis, acne, rosacea, eczema, psoriasis, scleroderma, immune support; to improve circulation; to enhance cognitive performance and memory

Contraindications and precautions

Avoid large doses (more than 3 g/day) in diabetes mellitus and immunodeficiency. Use cautiously in aspirin sensitivity, bleeding disorders, cirrhosis, familial adenomatous polyposis, major depressive disorders, bipolar disorder, and concurrent antihypertensive use.

Adverse reactions

- Belching, halitosis, heartburn, increased low-density lipoprotein level, weight gain
- With large doses: **bleeding, hemorrhagic stroke,** immunosuppression, loose stools, nausea, hyperglycemia

Interactions

Anticoagulants, antiplatelet drugs, salicylates: increased risk of bleeding
Antihypertensives: additive hypotension
Hormonal contraceptives: interference with triglyceride-lowering effects of fish oils

flaxseed oil

Purported action

Contains linolenic, linoleic, and alphalinolenic acid. Linoleic acid and alphalinolenic acid are required for structural integrity of cell membranes. Alphalinolenic acid increases blood levels of omega-3 polyunsaturated fatty acids, including eicosapentaenoic acid and docosahexaenoic acid.

Reported uses

Atherosclerosis, hyperlipidemia, benign prostatic hypertrophy, constipation, diverticulitis, enteritis, gastritis, irritable bowel syndrome, menopausal symptoms, skin inflammation, systemic lupus erythematosus, nephritis, cancer prevention

---

Contraindications and precautions

Contraindicated in bowel obstruction, breast cancer, endometriosis, esophageal stricture, intestinal inflammation, ovarian cancer, uterine cancer, and uterine fibroids. Avoid medicinal doses in pregnant patients. Use cautiously in bleeding disorders or diabetes mellitus.

Adverse reactions

Diarrhea, allergic reactions, **anaphylactoid reactions, intestinal obstruction**

Interactions

Anticoagulants, antiplatelet drugs, salicylates: increased risk of bleeding
Hypoglycemics, insulins: increased risk of hypoglycemia

garlic

Purported action

Inactivates thiol enzymes (such as coenzyme A and HMG-CoA reductase) and oxidizes glutamate synthase complex, both of which are required for lipid synthesis. Also may exert mild antibacterial, antifungal, and hypotensive activity.

Reported uses

To reduce blood lipid levels (transient effect); as an antibacterial, antiseptic, or antithrombotic. Insufficient data exist regarding effects of garlic on clinical cardiovascular conditions, such as claudication and myocardial infarction.

Contraindications and precautions

Pregnant and breastfeeding patients should avoid large amounts. Use cautiously in severe renal or hepatic disease and in children.

Adverse reactions

Headache, insomnia, fatigue, vertigo, GI distress, shortness of breath, facial flushing, contact dermatitis, allergic reaction

Interactions

Anticoagulants, antiplatelet drugs, nonsteroidal anti-inflammatory drugs, other drugs and herbs with anticoagulant effects: increased prothrombin time, bleeding time, and International Normalized Ratio
Cyclosporine: decreased cyclosporine efficacy
Hormonal contraceptives: decreased contraceptive efficacy
Nonnucleoside reverse-transcriptase inhibitors, protease inhibitors: decreased efficacy of these drugs

ginger

Purported action

Inhibits prostaglandin and thromboxane biosynthesis and promotes platelet aggregation. Also possesses antiemetic, antithrombotic, antibacterial, antioxidant, antihepatotoxic, anti-inflammatory, antimutagenic, stimulant, cardiotonic, immunostimulant, diuretic, and spasmolytic properties.

Reported uses

Dyspepsia, colic, anorexia, bronchitis, and rheumatism; to stimulate digestion, increase intestinal peristalsis, promote gastric secretions, reduce cholesterol level, raise blood glucose level, and stimulate peripheral circulation; to treat nausea and vomiting associated with motion sickness, hyperemesis gravidarum, and migraine

---

Reactions in **bold** are life-threatening.

Contraindications and precautions

Large amounts are controversial in pregnant patients. Avoid use in gallstones, bleeding disorders, hypertension, hypotension, and diabetes mellitus.

Adverse reactions

CNS depression, interference with cardiac function or anticoagulant activity

Interactions

Anticoagulants: increased bleeding time

Antacids, histamine₂ blockers, hypoglycemics, insulin, proton pump inhibitors: interference with actions of these drugs

Barbiturates: enhanced barbiturate effects

ginkgo

Purported action

Exerts antioxidant and neuroprotective activity, including arteriolar vasodilation, increased tissue perfusion and cerebral blood flow, decreased arterial spasms, and reduced platelet aggregation

Reported uses

Raynaud's disease, cerebral insufficiency, anxiety, stress, tinnitus, dementia, circulatory disorders, asthma, memory impairment, headache, depression, impotence; as an adjunct in schizophrenia treatment

Contraindications and precautions

Pregnant or breastfeeding patients should avoid ginkgo. Use cautiously in diabetes mellitus, hypertension, and in patients receiving antiplatelet drugs or anticoagulants.

Adverse reactions

• Headache, dizziness, palpitations, GI and skin disorders

• With excessive use: **seizures, subdural hematoma**

• Ginkgo pollen can be strongly allergenic; contact with fleshy fruit pulp causes allergic dermatitis similar to that from poison ivy.

Interactions

Anticonvulsants: decreased efficacy of these drugs, increased risk of seizures

Buspirone, fluoxetine: hypomania

Drugs that lower seizure threshold: increased risk of seizures

Insulin: altered insulin metabolism and excretion

Thiazide diuretics: increased blood pressure

Trazodone: possible coma

ginseng

Purported action

Increases natural "killer" cell activity, stimulates interferon production, accelerates nuclear RNA synthesis, decreases blood glucose level, and increases high-density lipoprotein level; also possesses depressant, anticonvulsant, and analgesic properties

Reported uses

Fatigue, poor concentration, nervousness, hypertension or hypotension, erectile dysfunction, gastritis, cancer, some CNS and endocrine conditions

Contraindications and precautions

Contraindicated in pregnant or breastfeeding patients. Patients taking MAO inhibitors should avoid ginseng. Use cautiously in hypertension or diabetes mellitus.

Reactions in **bold** are life-threatening.

Adverse reactions

Nervousness, stimulation, hypoglycemia, diffuse mammary nodules, vaginal bleeding, ginseng abuse

Interactions

Alcohol: increased alcohol clearance
Antipsychotics, MAO inhibitors: inhibition of antipsychotic effect
Caffeine-containing preparations, stimulants: stimulant potentiation
Hypoglycemics, insulin: increased hypoglycemic effect
Immunosuppressants: decreased immunosuppressant activity
Loop diuretics: poor diuretic response
Warfarin: decreased warfarin efficacy

glucosamine

Purported action

Serves as a building block for cartilage glycosaminoglycans (GAG), aiding treatment of osteoarthritis (marked by progressive GAG degeneration). Also may possess chondroprotective, antireactive, and antiarthritic properties.

Reported uses

Osteoarthritis, joint pain and inflammation, temporomandibular joint syndrome, glaucoma; to aid weight loss

Contraindications and precautions

Diabetic patients should consult health care professional before using glucosamine because it may increase blood glucose level.

Adverse reactions

Gastric discomfort (such as nausea, vomiting, diarrhea, heartburn), headache, drowsiness, insomnia, tachycardia, pruritus

Interactions

Acetaminophen: interference with glucosamine activity
Antimitotic therapy: resistance to chemotherapeutic effects of these drugs
Diuretics: decreased glucosamine effects

goldenseal

Purported action

Contains alkaloids (hydrastine and berberine) that exert modest antimicrobial activity. May have cardiostimulatory, anti-inflammatory, peripheral vasoconstrictive, antihemorrhagic, and muscle relaxant effects.

Reported uses

Topical infections (such as wounds and herpes labialis lesions), conjunctivitis, inflamed mucous membranes (as an ingredient in cold and flu preparations), postpartum hemorrhage; as a diuretic or laxative

Contraindications and precautions

Contraindicated in hypertension, heart disease (especially arrhythmias), heart failure, and pregnancy

Adverse reactions

Rash, headache, insomnia, nausea, vomiting, abdominal pain, tachycardia, bradycardia, **seizures, respiratory depression** (with high doses)

Interactions

Antacids, histamine$_2$ antagonists, proton pump inhibitors: decreased effects of these drugs
Antihypertensives: decreased antihypertensive effect
CNS depressants: additive sedation

Reactions in **bold** are life-threatening.

grapeseed

Purported action
Exerts antioxidant, anticarcinogenic, cytoprotective, and vascular activity; also inhibits proteolytic enzymes, causing collagen stabilization

Reported uses
Prevention of cancer, cardiovascular disease, and dental caries; treatment of venous insufficiency, edema, and allergic rhinitis

Contraindications and precautions
Contraindicated in known hypersensitivity to grapeseed. Use cautiously in hepatic disease. Safety during pregnancy has not been established.

Adverse reactions
Hepatotoxicity

Interactions
Warfarin: increased risk of bleeding

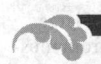

green tea

Purported action
Maintains significant blood levels of catechin, which may exert antioxidant activity against lipoproteins. Delays lipid peroxidation, exerts antimicrobial effects against oral bacteria and diarrhea-causing bacteria, and contributes antimutagenic potential against dietary carcinogens.

Reported uses
Atherosclerosis, headache, diarrhea, stomach disorders, cancer, elevated lipid levels, wounds, dental caries prophylaxis

Contraindications and precautions
Because of caffeine content, green tea should be avoided by pregnant or breastfeeding patients and by females who may become pregnant. Use cautiously in cardiac disease, renal disease, and hyperthyroidism.

Adverse reactions
Nervousness, insomnia, tachycardia, constipation, diarrhea, increased blood glucose and cholesterol levels, impaired iron metabolism, **asthma, esophageal cancer** (with heavy use)

Interactions
Hypoglycemics, insulin: interference with blood glucose control
Stimulants: increased stimulant effect
Warfarin: increased risk of bleeding

hawthorn

Purported action
Increases coronary blood flow and heart rate; exerts antiarrhythmic and positive inotropic effects

Reported uses
Atherosclerosis, angina pectoris; to regulate blood pressure and heart rhythm; as an antispasmodic or sedative

Contraindications and precautions
Contraindicated in severe renal or hepatic disease and in pregnancy and breastfeeding

Adverse reactions
Agitation, dizziness, hypotension, sedation, nausea, sweating, **toxicity** (with high doses)

Reactions in **bold** are life-threatening.

Interactions

Antiarrhythmics: enhanced antiarrhythmic action
Antihypertensives, nitrates: increased effects of these drugs
Cardiac glycosides: increased risk of cardiac glycoside toxicity
CNS depressants: increased CNS effects

kava

Purported action

Produces mild anxiolytic and anticonvulsant effects; also may exert antithrombotic effect on platelets

Reported uses

Anxiety, stress, restlessness, seizure disorders, headache, infection, local anesthesia

Contraindications and precautions

Contraindicated in history of hepatic problems. Pregnant or breastfeeding patients should avoid kava. Use cautiously in neutropenia, renal disease, and thrombocytopenia.

Adverse reactions

Morning fatigue, headache, drowsiness, mydriasis, mild GI disturbances, diarrhea, hematuria, hypertension, shortness of breath, visual disturbances, scaly rash (with heavy use)

Interactions

CNS depressants: potentiation of CNS effects
Hepatotoxic drugs: increased hepatotoxicity
Levodopa: reduced levodopa efficacy

licorice

Purported action

Licorice root derivative (carbenoxolone) soothes inflamed mucous membranes, increases life span of gastric epithelial cells by stimulating secretin release, and inhibits peptic and prostaglandin activity

Reported uses

GI complaints, cough, asthma, gastric and duodenal ulcers; used investigationally in lupus and inflammation

Contraindications and precautions

Contraindicated in renal, hepatic, and cardiovascular disease. Pregnant or breastfeeding patients should avoid licorice.

Adverse reactions

- Headache, lethargy, water retention, hypokalemia, hypernatremia, visual disturbances, hypertension, **pulmonary edema**
- With prolonged, daily use of large amounts: reactions ranging from muscle weakness to quadriplegia

Interactions

Antihypertensives, corticosteroids, diuretics: increased blood pressure
Corticosteroids, furosemide, thiazide diuretics: increased potassium loss
Digoxin: increased risk of digoxin toxicity
Estrogen: interference with estrogen therapy
Ethacrynic acid: increased mineralocorticoid activity
Insulin: hypokalemia, sodium retention

Reactions in **bold** are life-threatening.

lutein

Purported action
Serves as antioxidant and blue light filter, protecting underlying ocular tissues from photodamage. Evidence links high dietary lutein intake with reduced risk of age-related macular degeneration and cataracts. Also, serum lutein level may be inversely related to breast cancer risk.

Reported uses
Cataracts, macular degeneration, colorectal cancer

Contraindications and precautions
Use with caution in bleeding disorders and diabetes mellitus.

Adverse reactions
None reported

Interactions
Beta carotene: interference with lutein availability

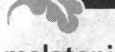

melatonin

Purported action
Endogenous melatonin plays a role in circadian rhythms: light inhibits melatonin synthesis and darkness stimulates it. Exogenous melatonin increases melatonin blood levels without affecting endogenous melatonin production; also affects body temperature regulation, cardiovascular function, and reproduction.

Reported uses
Short-term sleep pattern regulation, jet lag, tinnitus, depression, cluster headaches, cancer, thrombocytopenia caused by chemotherapy

Contraindications and precautions
Contraindicated in hepatic insufficiency, cerebrovascular disease, depression, and neurologic disorders

Adverse reactions
Headache, depression, confusion, tachycardia, pruritus

Interactions
Anticoagulants, antiplatelet drugs: increased risk of bleeding
Benzodiazepines: decreased endogenous melatonin
CNS depressants: additive sedation
Flumazenil: inhibition of melatonin effects
Fluvoxamine: increased melatonin blood level and effects
Hormonal contraceptives: increased melatonin effects
Hypoglycemics, insulin: increased insulin resistance, impaired glucose use
Immunosuppressants: interference with immunosuppressant effects
Nifedipine: interference with antihypertensive effect, increased heart rate
Verapamil: increased melatonin excretion

milk thistle

Purported action
Exerts a hepatoprotective effect, possibly by stimulating RNA and DNA synthesis. Thought to scavenge prooxidant free radicals and increase intracellular concentrations of glutathione (a substance needed to detoxify hepatic cell reactions). Also alters the outer membrane of hepatic cells and may produce an anti-inflammatory effect on platelets.

Reactions in **bold** are life-threatening.

Reported uses

Hepatic dysfunction (including damage caused by acute viral hepatitis and long-term phenothiazine or butyrophenone use), dyspepsia, gallbladder and spleen disorders; antidote for Amanita mushroom poisoning; to reduce increased total cholesterol and low-density lipoprotein levels

Contraindications and precautions

Contraindicated in pregnancy and breastfeeding

Adverse reactions

Brief GI disturbances, diarrhea, cramping, mild allergic reactions, urticaria

Interactions

Estrogens, glucuronidated drugs: increased clearance of these drugs

red yeast rice

Purported action

Contains mevinic acids (including lovastatin), which competitively inhibit HMG-CoA reductase, thereby blocking cholesterol biosynthesis

Reported uses

Diarrhea, indigestion, hyperlipidemia, poor blood circulation; to improve spleen and stomach health

Contraindications and precautions

Contraindicated in pregnancy and breastfeeding. Use cautiously in hepatic dysfunction, abnormal liver function tests, concurrent use of hepatotoxic drugs, and in persons who consume more than two alcoholic drinks daily.

Adverse reactions

Gastritis, abdominal discomfort, heartburn, flatulence, dizziness, hepatic enzyme and creatine kinase elevations, **anaphylaxis**

Interactions

Cyclosporine: increased risk of myopathy
CYP450-3A4 inhibitors: increased red yeast blood level, increased adverse reactions
Gemfibrozil, niacin: increased risk of myopathy
Grapefruit juice, HMG-CoA inhibitors (statins): increased risk of adverse reactions
Levothyroxine: abnormal thyroid function

S-adenosylmethionine (SAM-e)

Purported action

Naturally occurring molecule; plays an essential role in biochemical reactions involving enzymatic transmethylation. Contributes to synthesis, activation, and metabolism of hormones, neurotransmitters, nucleic acids, proteins, phospholipids, and some drugs.

Reported uses

Cardiovascular disease, fibromyalgia, headache, insomnia, hepatic disease, osteoarthritis, rheumatoid arthritis, depression

Contraindications and precautions

Contraindicated in concurrent use of MAO inhibitors. Use cautiously in bleeding disorders and diabetes mellitus.

Adverse reactions

Anxiety, nausea, vomiting, diarrhea, flatulence, headache, mania or hypomania

Reactions in **bold** are life-threatening.

Interactions
Antidepressants: additive effects (including additive serotonergic effects)

saw palmetto

Purported action
Reduces enlarged prostate by inhibiting testosterone 5-alpha reductase (an enzyme that converts testosterone to 5-alpha-testosterone in prostate). Inhibits cell proliferation induced by prolactin and growth factor; also may exert anti-inflammatory, immunostimulant, antiandrogenic, antiestrogenic, and astringent activity.

Reported uses
Symptomatic treatment of benign prostatic hypertrophy, including urinary frequency, reduced urinary flow, and nocturia; bronchitis; asthma

Contraindications and precautions
Contraindicated in pregnancy and in patients receiving concurrent hormone therapy (including hormonal contraceptives and hormone replacement therapy). Use cautiously in patients receiving drugs that may alter immunostimulant or anti-inflammatory activity.

Adverse reactions
Headache, hypertension, nausea, diarrhea, constipation, abdominal pain, GI upset, urinary retention

Interactions
Anticoagulants, antiplatelet drugs: increased risk of bleeding
Estrogens: interference with estrogen activity
Hormonal contraceptives: interference with contraceptive activity

shark cartilage

Purported action
Helps control cancer by inhibiting new blood vessel formation (angiogenesis) in tumors; also may have anti-inflammatory effects

Reported uses
Prostate cancer, AIDS-associated Kaposi's sarcoma, arthritis, eczema

Contraindications and precautions
Contraindicated in pregnancy or breastfeeding and in children. Use cautiously in hepatic disease.

Adverse reactions
Hepatitis

Interactions
None known

soy

Purported action
Isoflavones (phytoestrogens found in soybean) produce effects similar to those of estradiol (a female hormone). They also limit cholesterol absorption in intestine by binding to cholesterol and may enhance immune function, produce antioxidant effects, and exert beneficial effects on GI function.

Reported uses
Menopausal symptoms, osteoporosis, minor GI problems; to reduce total cholesterol and low-density lipoprotein levels. Also serves as source of fiber, protein, and minerals.

Reactions in **bold** are life-threatening.

Contraindications and precautions

Contraindicated in estrogen-dependent tumors and peanut allergy (cross-sensitivity may occur)

Adverse reactions

Some experts are concerned that phytoestrogens in soy-based infant formulas may influence CNS and psychomotor development.

Interactions

Antibiotics: decreased action of isoflavones
Estrogens: interference with hormone replacement therapy
Tamoxifen: antagonism of tamoxifen
Warfarin: decreased International Normalized Ratio, inhibited platelet aggregation

St. John's wort

Purported action

Inhibits postsynaptic serotonin reuptake or antagonizes MAO

Reported uses

Depression, wounds, muscle pain, burns; used investigationally to treat human immunodeficiency virus and certain other viruses

Contraindications and precautions

Contraindicated in concurrent use of antidepressants, in pregnant patients, and in patients planning pregnancy

Adverse reactions

Abdominal pain, constipation, other GI symptoms, dry mouth, dizziness, confusion, fatigue, mania, photosensitivity

Interactions

Bexarotene: decreased effects of St. John's wort and bexarotene
Cyclosporine, digoxin, paclitaxel, protease inhibitors, telithromycin, theophylline, tricyclic antidepressants, vinca alkaloids, warfarin: decreased efficacy of these drugs
Hormonal contraceptives: breakthrough bleeding
MAO inhibitors, selective serotonin reuptake inhibitors, serotonin agonists: increased risk of serotonin syndrome

valerian

Purported action

Binds to gamma-aminobutyric acid (GABA) and benzodiazepine receptors, stimulating release of these substances. Glutamine, a free amino acid in valerian extract, can cross the blood-brain barrier and may be metabolized to GABA, causing sedation.

Reported uses

Anxiety, nervousness, attention deficit hyperactivity disorder, depression, seizures, menopausal symptoms, menstrual cramps, tremors, restlessness, sleep disorders; as an antispasmodic

Contraindications and precautions

Avoid use in hepatic dysfunction and in pregnant or breastfeeding patients.

Adverse reactions

With overdose or prolonged use: excitability, headache, insomnia, nausea, blurred vision, **cardiac dysfunction, hepatotoxicity**

Interactions

Alcohol, antihistamines, CNS depressants: additive sedation

Reactions in **bold** are life-threatening.

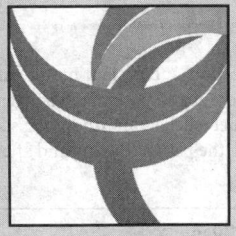

Part 3

Appendices
Selected references
Index

Common anesthetic drugs

This chart describes the indications, dosages, administration, and patient monitoring for commonly used anesthetic drugs. Although these potent and potentially dangerous drugs are usually given by specially trained personnel (such as anesthesiologists or anesthetists), the nurse is responsible for monitoring the patient during and after administration.

Drug	Indications and dosages
atracurium besylate Tracrium	➤ Adjunct to general anesthesia to promote endotracheal intubation and relax skeletal muscles during surgery **Adults and children ages 2 and older:** Initially, 0.4 to 0.5 mg/kg by I.V. bolus. For prolonged surgery, give maintenance dosage of 0.08 to 0.1 mg/kg within 20 to 45 minutes of initial dose; may repeat q 15 to 25 minutes p.r.n. During prolonged procedures, give an initial infusion of 9 to 10 mcg/kg/minute to rapidly counteract spontaneous recovery of neuromuscular function, as required; thereafter, administer at a rate of 5 to 9 mcg/kg/minute by I.V. infusion. **Children ages 1 month to 2 years:** 0.3 to 0.4 mg/kg I.V. Repeat if needed.
etomidate Amidate	➤ To induce general anesthesia **Adults and children older than age 10:** Individualized, 0.2 to 0.6 mg/kg I.V. Usual dosage is 0.3 mg/kg I.V. ➤ Adjunct to anesthesia with subpotent anesthetics, such as nitrous oxide in oxygen, during maintenance of anesthesia for short operative procedures **Adults:** Individualized in smaller increments than induction dosage.

Administration and patient monitoring

🔊 Before giving, make sure emergency respiratory equipment is at hand and that patient receives a sedative or general anesthetic.

- Give by I.V. route only (bolus, intermittent infusion, or continuous infusion). Never give I.M.
- Know that patient can hear while drug is in effect. Explain events as they occur and provide ongoing reassurance.
- Be ready to reverse drug's effects with anticholinesterase drug once spontaneous recovery begins.

🔊 Watch for anaphylaxis and injection site reaction.

- Check vital signs and airway patency until patient recovers completely from drug effects.
- Assess for pain; give analgesics p.r.n. Be aware that patient may be unable to verbalize pain while drug is in effect.
- Be aware that effect of this drug is potentiated by inhalation anesthesia; consider reduction of atracurium besylate infusion rate.
- Evaluate patient's recovery with muscle strength tests, nerve stimulation, and train-of-four monitoring.

- Before giving, ask patient about other drug usage.
- Administer slowly over 30 to 60 seconds.
- Know that solution may cause venous pain; more frequently when smaller, more distal, hand or wrist veins are used.
- Know that drug may cause cardiac depression in elderly patients, particularly those with hypertension.
- Know that drug may cause a brief period of apnea.
- Monitor respiratory status (for conscious sedation, including pulse oximetry), cardiovascular status, and CNS status.
- Know that drug isn't intended for prolonged infusion due to hazards associated with prolonged suppression of endogenous cortisol and aldosterone.

(continued)

Common anesthetic drugs (continued)

Drug	Indications and dosages
fentanyl citrate Sublimaze **fentanyl transmucosal** Actiq, Fentanyl Oralet	➤ Short-term analgesia during anesthesia and immediate preoperative and postoperative periods **Adults:** 0.05 to 0.1 mg I.M. 30 to 60 minutes before surgery as adjunct to general anesthesia. **Low dose:** 0.002 mg/kg for minor, but painful surgical procedures; maintenance dosages are rarely needed. **Moderate dose:** 0.002 to 0.02 mg/kg, when surgery becomes major; 0.025 to 0.1 mg may be administered I.V. or I.M. as maintenance dosage. **High dose:** 0.02 to 0.05 mg/kg during open heart surgery and certain more complicated neurosurgical and orthopedic procedures where surgery is more prolonged; 0.025 mg to one half the initial loading dose as maintenance dosage. **Children ages 2 to 12:** 2 to 3 mcg/kg I.V., depending on vital signs; or 5 to 15 mcg/kg transmucosally ➤ Adjunct to regional anesthesia **Adults:** 0.05 to 0.1 mg I.M. or slow I.V. over 1 to 2 minutes
ketamine	➤ To induce anesthesia **Adults:** Individualized, with initial dosage range of 1 to 4.5 mg/kg I.V. (average amount needed to produce 5 to 10 minutes of surgical anesthesia is usually 2 mg/kg). Or, 1 to 2 mg/kg I.V. at rate of 0.5 mg/kg/minute may be used. Or, initial dosage may range from 6.5 to 13 mg/kg I.M. Dose of 10 mg/kg will usually produce 12 to 25 minutes of surgical anesthesia. ➤ To maintain anesthesia **Adults:** Maintenance dosage should be adjusted according to patient's anesthetic needs and whether an additional anesthetic is used. Increments of one-half to full induction dose may be repeated as needed for anesthesia maintenance. For patients receiving I.V. diazepam–augmented anesthesia: 0.1 to 0.5 mg/minute by slow I.V. microdrip infusion augmented with diazepam 2 to 5 mg I.V. as needed.

Administration and patient monitoring

- Know that I.V. dose is given slowly over 1 to 2 minutes.
- 🔊 Keep narcotic antagonist (naloxone) and emergency equipment at hand when giving I.V.
- Know that drug is not recommended for control of mild or intermittent pain.
- 🔊 Assess for muscle rigidity in patients receiving high doses. Discuss need for neuromuscular blocker with prescriber. If blocker is given, patient will require ventilator.
- Monitor respiratory and cardiovascular functions and urinary output.
- If patient develops fever, assess for signs and symptoms of opioid toxicity, because more drug is absorbed at higher body temperatures.
- Carefully monitor hematologic studies and hepatic enzyme levels.

- Be aware that atropine, scopolamine, or another drying agent should be given at an appropriate interval before induction.
- Be aware that the 100-mg/ml concentration shouldn't be given I.V. without proper dilution.
- Dilute with an equal volume of sterile water for injection, normal saline for injection, or D_5W.
- Administer slowly over 60 seconds. Know that more rapid administration may result in respiratory depression and enhanced pressor response.
- Continually monitor cardiac function during procedure in patients with hypertension or cardiac decompensation.
- Know that if ketamine is augmented with diazepam, the two drugs must be given separately. Don't mix ketamine and diazepam in syringe or infusion bag.
- To prepare a dilute solution containing 1 mg ketamine/ml, transfer 10 ml (50-mg/ml vial) or 5 ml (100-mg/ml vial) to 500 ml of D_5W or normal saline for injection to obtain a 1-mg/ml solution.
- Know that during ketamine administration, resuscitative equipment should be present and ready for use.
- Use with caution in patient with chronic alcoholism and the acutely alcohol-intoxicated patient.
- An increase in cerebrospinal fluid pressure has occurred after ketamine administration. Use with extreme caution in patients with preanesthesia elevated cerebrospinal fluid pressure.

(continued)

Common anesthetic drugs (continued)

Drug	Indications and dosages
midazolam hydrochloride Apo-Midazolam✦, Versed	➤ To induce general anesthesia **Adults younger than age 55:** 0.3 to 0.35 mg/kg I.V. over 20 to 30 seconds if patient is not premedicated, or 0.15 to 0.35 mg/kg (usual dosage of 0.25 mg/kg) I.V. over 20 to 30 seconds if patient is premedicated. Wait 2 minutes to evaluate effect. Additional increments of 25% of initial dosage may be needed to complete induction. **Adults older than age 55 who have not been premedicated:** Initially, 300 mcg/kg I.V. for induction ➤ Continuous infusion to initiate sedation **Adults:** For rapid sedation, loading dose of 0.01 to 0.05 mg/kg by slow I.V.; repeat dose q 10 to 15 minutes until adequate sedation occurs. To maintain sedation, infuse at initial rate of 0.02 to 0.10 mg/kg/hour (1 to 7 mg/hour); adjust rate as needed.
nalbuphine hydrochloride Nubain	➤ Adjunct to balanced anesthesia **Adults:** 0.3 mg to 3 mg/kg I.V. over 10 to 15 minutes, followed by a maintenance dosage of 0.25 mg to 0.50 mg/kg I.V. in single doses p.r.n.
pancuronium bromide Pavulon	➤ Adjunct to balanced anesthesia to relax skeletal muscles for intubation **Adults and children ages 1 month and older:** Initially, 0.04 to 0.1 mg/kg I.V.; may follow with 0.01 mg/kg q 25 to 60 minutes if needed. (Dosage and infusion rates are based on type of anesthesia used and patient needs and response. Dosages listed here are typical.)
pentazocine lactate Talwin lactate	➤ Preoperative or preanesthetic medication; adjunct to surgical anesthesia **Adults:** 30 mg subcutaneously, I.M., or I.V. q 3 to 4 hours (not to exceed 30 mg I.V. or 60 mg I.M. or subcutaneously) **Children ages 1 year and older:** 0.5 mg/kg I.M. ➤ Labor **Adults:** 20 mg I.V. for two or three doses at 2- to 3-hour intervals, or 30 mg I.M. as a single dose

Administration and patient monitoring

🔊 Keep oxygen and resuscitation equipment at hand in case severe respiratory depression occurs.

- Inject I.M. deep into large muscle mass.
- Know that drug may be mixed in same syringe as atropine, meperidine, morphine, or scopolamine.
- Dilute concentrate for I.V. infusion to 0.5 mg/ml using dextrose 5% in water or normal saline solution. Infuse over at least 2 minutes; wait at least 2 minutes before giving second dose. Be aware that excessive dose or rapid I.V. delivery may cause severe respiratory depression.
- Monitor vital signs, ECG, respiratory status, and oxygen saturation.
- Assess neurologic status closely, especially in children.
- Monitor for nausea and vomiting.

🔊 Make sure emergency resuscitation equipment and naloxone (antidote) are at hand before administration begins.

- Monitor vital signs. Watch for respiratory depression and heart rate changes.
- Evaluate patient for CNS changes. Institute safety measures as needed to prevent injury.
- Watch for hypersensitivity reactions, such as anaphylaxis.
- In patients receiving morphine, meperidine, codeine, or other opiate agonists with a similar duration of action, reduce to 25% of usual initial dose.

🔊 Know that drug should be given only by specially trained personnel in settings where respiratory support is available.

- Administer through established I.V. line containing normal saline solution, lactated Ringer's solution, or dextrose 5% in water.
- Know that neostigmine can reverse drug's effects.

🔊 Make sure patient's analgesic and sedative needs are met; drug doesn't relieve pain or provide sedation.

- Monitor heart rhythm, vital signs, and pulse oximetry during and after administration.
- Evaluate fluid intake and output and potassium level.
- Assess muscle recovery using peripheral nerve stimulator and train-of-four monitoring.

- Inject each 5-mg dose over 1 minute by slow, direct I.V. infusion, with patient lying supine.
- Use subcutaneous route only when necessary (may cause tissue damage).
- Don't mix in the same syringe with barbiturates because precipitation may occur.

🔊 Monitor vital signs. Stay alert for shock, dyspnea, and circulatory or respiratory depression.

- Monitor drug efficacy.

(continued)

Common anesthetic drugs (continued)

Drug	Indications and dosages
procaine hydrochloride Novocain	➤ Infiltration anesthesia **Adults:** 350 to 600 mg of 0.25% to 0.5% of diluted solution injected as a single dose into area to be anesthetized ➤ Peripheral nerve block **Adults:** 100 ml of 1% diluted solution or 50 ml of 2% solution injected into area where peripheral nerve block is needed, or up to 200 ml of 0.5% diluted solution ➤ Spinal anesthesia **Adults:** 0.5, 1, or 2 ml of 10% solution injected into spinal area to be anesthetized, diluted in 0.5, 1, or 2 ml (respectively) of normal saline solution, sterile distilled water, or spinal fluid. Administer at 1 ml/5 seconds.
remifentanil hydrochloride Ultiva	➤ To induce anesthesia through intubation **Adults:** 0.5 to 1 mcg/kg/minute I.V., given with a hypnotic or volatile drug. May administer 1 mcg/kg I.V. over 30 to 60 seconds if endotracheal intubation will occur less than 8 minutes after drug infusion starts. ➤ To maintain anesthesia **Adults:** 0.25 to 0.4 mcg/kg/minute I.V. Increase dosage by 25% to 100% or decrease by 25% to 50% q 2 to 5 minutes p.r.n. If rate exceeds 1 mcg/kg/minute, consider increasing dosage of concomitant anesthetics to increase the depth of anesthesia. Supplemental I.V. bolus of remifentanil 1 mcg/kg may be given. **Children ages 1 to 12:** 0.25 mcg/kg/min I.V. in conjunction with halothane, sevoflurane, or isoflurane; may administer supplemental bolus of 1 mcg/kg. **Infants birth to 2 months:** 0.4 mcg/kg/minute with nitrous oxide; may administer supplemental bolus of 1 mcg/kg. ➤ To continue analgesic effect during immediate postoperative period **Adults:** Initially, 0.1 mcg/kg/minute I.V. Adjust in increments of 0.025 mcg/kg/minute q 5 minutes p.r.n. ➤ Analgesic component of monitored anesthesia care **Adults:** 0.5 to 1 mcg/kg I.V. over 30 to 60 seconds, given 90 seconds before anesthetic. As a continuous infusion, 0.05 to 0.1 mcg/kg/minute I.V. 5 minutes before anesthetic. After anesthetic is given, titrate rate to 0.025 to 0.05 mcg/kg/minute, then adjust by 0.025 mcg/kg/minute q 5 minutes p.r.n.

Administration and patient monitoring

- ◀≋ Know that drug should be given only by specially trained personnel with expertise in avoiding intravascular injections and in assessing and managing dose-related toxicities and other acute emergencies that may arise.
- ◀≋ Make sure emergency resuscitation equipment is at hand before drug is given.
- Follow label directions to reconstitute drug for selected route.
- Be aware that if necessary, epinephrine may be added to slow procaine absorption, prolong its action, or maintain hemostasis.
- ◀≋ Monitor vital signs and ECG closely, especially when drug is used for spinal anesthesia. Stay alert for evidence of impending cardiac arrest.
- ◀≋ Watch for signs and symptoms of status asthmaticus and anaphylaxis.
- ◀≋ Monitor patient's position carefully, especially after spinal anesthesia, to help prevent damage to nerves and other body tissues.
- Inspect infusion site for extravasation.

- ◀≋ Keep emergency resuscitation equipment and naloxone at hand in case of respiratory arrest.
- Add 1 ml of diluent/mg of drug. Shake well to produce a clear, colorless solution of 1 mg/ml.
- Dilute drug further in normal or half-normal saline solution, dextrose 5% in water, dextrose 5% in normal saline solution, or dextrose 5% in lactated Ringer's solution.
- Drug is for I.V. use only.
- Use infusion control pump for continuous infusion. Choose site close to venous cannula. After administering, flush I.V. tubing to clear.
- Know that delivery rates above 0.2 mcg/kg/minute may cause respiratory depression.
- ◀≋ When giving high doses, assess for muscle rigidity. Be prepared to stop therapy.
- Continuously monitor respiratory and cardiovascular function, oxygenation, and vital signs.
- Assess fluid intake and output. Watch for urinary retention.

(continued)

Common anesthetic drugs (continued)

Drug	Indications and dosages
rocuronium bromide Zemuron (P/F)	➤ Adjunct to general anesthesia to allow endotracheal intubation and relax skeletal muscles during mechanical ventilation or surgery **Adults:** Initially, I.V. bolus of 0.6 to 1.2 mg/kg (usually allows endotracheal intubation within 2 minutes and paralyzes muscles for 30 minutes). Boluses of 0.1 to 0.2 mg/kg may be given at 25% recovery for maintenance. For continuous I.V. infusion, 0.01 to 0.012 mg/kg/minute only after early evidence of recovery from intubating dose.
ropivacaine hydrochloride Naropin	➤ Lumbar epidural block **Adults:** 15 to 30 ml (75 to 150 mg) I.V. of 0.5% solution, or 15 to 25 ml (113 to 188 mg) I.V. of 0.75% solution, or 15 to 20 ml (150 to 200 mg) of a 1% solution ➤ Lumbar epidural block during labor **Adults:** 10 to 20 ml (20 to 40 mg) of 0.2% solution, then 6 to 14 ml/hour (12 to 28 mg/hour) as a continuous I.V. infusion; or 10 to 15 ml/hour (20 to 30 mg/hour) of 0.2% solution as an incremental "top-up" injection ➤ Lumbar epidural block for cesarean section **Adults:** 20 to 30 ml (100 to 150 mg) I.V. of 0.5% solution, or 15 to 20 ml (113 to 150 mg) of 0.75% solution
succinylcholine chloride Anectine, Quelicin	➤ Adjunct to anesthesia to relax skeletal muscles during short surgical procedures; endotracheal intubation with mechanical ventilation; electrically induced convulsive therapy **Adults:** 0.6 mg/kg I.V. over 10 to 30 seconds, or a continuous I.V. infusion at 0.5 to 10 mg/minute, or 0.04 to 0.07 mg/kg I.V. intermittently p.r.n. **Older children and adolescents:** 1 mg/kg I.V. over 10 to 30 seconds **Infants and young children:** 2 mg/kg I.V. over 10 to 30 second

Administration and patient monitoring

- ◀⧦ Keep emergency resuscitation equipment at hand when giving.
- ◀⧦ Be aware that drug should be given only by personnel who are specially trained in administering anesthesia and neuromuscular blockers.
- Verify that patient has received a sedative or general anesthetic before therapy begins.
- Give by rapid I.V. injection or continuous I.V. infusion in compatible solution (dextrose 5% in water or normal saline solution, normal saline solution, sterile water for injection, or lactated Ringer's solution).
- Know that maintenance dose of 0.1 mg/kg provides an extra 12 minutes of muscle relaxation; 0.15 mg/kg, an extra 17 minutes; and 0.2 mg/kg, an extra 24 minutes.
- Assess respiratory status frequently.
- Monitor vital signs and ECG continuously until patient recovers fully from neuromuscular blockade. Closely monitor recovery with nerve stimulator and train-of-four monitoring.

- ◀⧦ Know that drug should be given only by personnel specially trained in use of epidural blocks.
- Be aware that test dose (containing epinephrine) should be given.
- Use small, incremental doses for titration. Avoid rapid I.V. infusion.
- Monitor vital signs, ECG, and cardiovascular status continuously.
- Assess neurologic status. Stay alert for signs and symptoms of impending seizure.
- ◀⧦ Watch carefully for warning signs of allergic reaction and respiratory distress.

- ◀⧦ Make sure patient has received a sedative or general anesthetic before administering.
- ◀⧦ Verify that emergency resuscitation equipment is at hand before giving.
- As ordered, give test dose of 5 to 10 mg I.V. after anesthesia administration. Drug may be given if test dose does not cause respiratory depression or if such depression lasts no longer than 5 minutes.
- For I.V. use, reconstitute with dextrose 5% in water or normal saline solution; administer via intermittent or continuous I.V. infusion. Don't mix with alkaline solution, such as sodium bicarbonate, barbiturates, or thiopental sodium.
- Be aware that continuous I.V. infusion isn't recommended for children or adolescents.
- ◀⧦ Watch for life-threatening adverse reactions, including anaphylaxis, malignant hyperthermia, and hypersensitivity reaction.
- Monitor ECG and vital signs (especially respirations) until patient recovers fully.
- Assess recovery by checking hand grip, head lift, and voluntary cough response.

(continued)

Common anesthetic drugs (continued)

Drug	Indications and dosages
sufentanil Sufenta	➤ As a primary anesthetic to induce and maintain anesthesia **Adults:** Initially, 8 to 30 mcg/kg I.V., given with oxygen and a muscle relaxant. Maintenance dosage is 0.5 to 10 mcg/kg p.r.n. ➤ Analgesic adjunct to maintain balanced general anesthesia **Adults:** 1 to 8 mcg/kg I.V., with 75% of dose given immediately before intubation. Remainder can be given as 10- to 50-mcg bolus doses to maintain analgesia. ➤ Epidural analgesia during labor and delivery **Adults:** 10 to 15 mcg epidurally with bupivacaine, with or without epinephrine. May repeat twice at intervals of less than 1 hour, for a total of three doses.
vecuronium bromide Norcuron	➤ Adjunct to anesthesia to facilitate endotracheal intubation and relax skeletal muscles during surgery or mechanical ventilation **Adults and children older than age 9:** Initially, 0.08 to 0.1 mg/kg by I.V. bolus. During prolonged surgery, maintenance dose of 0.01 to 0.015 mg/kg is given by continuous I.V. infusion within 25 to 40 minutes of initial dose. In patients receiving balanced anesthesia, maintenance dose may be given q 12 to 15 minutes.

Administration and patient monitoring

- ◀≾ Know that drug should be given only by personnel who are specially trained in using I.V. and epidural anesthetics and in managing respiratory effects of potent opioids.
- ◀≾ Keep oxygen and resuscitation and intubation equipment at hand.
- Be aware that dosage is based on mean body weight.
- ◀≾ Monitor ECG and vital signs. Stay alert for signs and symptoms of shock and impending cardiac arrest.
- Assess airway patency closely. Watch for respiratory depression and airway spasms.
- Monitor neurologic status during and after administration. Institute safety measures as needed to prevent injury.
- Monitor fluid intake and output. Check for oliguria or urinary retention.

- ◀≾ Know that drug should be given by specially trained personnel and only when respiratory support is available.
- When giving by I.V. bolus, administer over 1 to 2 minutes.
- When giving by continuous I.V. infusion, reconstitute by adding bacteriostatic water for injection to yield a concentration of 1 mg/ml. Dilute further with dextrose 5% in water, normal saline solution, or lactated Ringer's solution. Administer with infusion-control device.
- Monitor heart rhythm, blood pressure, and pulse oximetry during and after administration.
- Monitor fluid intake and output and measure temperature.
- Assess muscle recovery using peripheral nerve stimulator and train-of-four monitoring.
- ◀≾ Make sure patient's analgesic and sedative needs are met. (Drug doesn't relieve pain or provide sedation.)

Common combination drug products

Many drugs (especially over-the-counter preparations) are combination products that contain several active ingredients and are sold under a discrete trade name. The combination products below are listed by trade name, followed by active ingredients and therapeutic class.

Acanya
benzoyl peroxide, clindamycin phosphate
Therapeutic class: Anti-infective, keratologic agent

Accuretic
hydrochlorothiazide, quinapril hydrochloride
Therapeutic class: Antihypertensive

Actifed
codeine phosphate, pseudoephedrine hydrochloride, triprolidine hydrochloride
Therapeutic class: Adrenergic, antihistamine, antitussive

Activella Tablets
estradiol, norethindrone acetate
Therapeutic class: Estrogen, progestin

Actonel with Calcium
risedronate sodium tablets with calcium carbonate tablets
Therapeutic class: Bone resorption inhibitor

Actoplus Met
metformin hydrochloride, pioglitazone hydrochloride
Therapeutic class: Antidiabetic agent

Adderall
amphetamine aspartate, amphetamine sulfate, dextroamphetamine saccharate, dextroamphetamine sulfate
Therapeutic class: CNS stimulant

Advair HFA
fluticasone propionate, salmeterol xinafoate
Therapeutic class: Corticosteroid, bronchodilator

Advicor
lovastatin, niacin
Therapeutic class: Antihyperlipidemic

Aggrenox
aspirin, dipyridamole
Therapeutic class: Antiplatelet drug

Aldactazide
hydrochlorothiazide, spironolactone
Therapeutic class: Diuretic

Aldoril
hydrochlorothiazide, methyldopa
Therapeutic class: Antihypertensive

Allegra-D
fexofenadine hydrochloride, pseudoephedrine hydrochloride
Therapeutic class: Antihistamine, adrenergic

Apri
desogrestrel, ethinyl estradiol
Therapeutic class: Estrogen, progestin

Arthrotec
diclofenac sodium, misoprostol
Therapeutic class: Anti-inflammatory, gastric protectant

Atacand HCT
candesartan cilexetil, hydrochlorothiazide
Therapeutic class: Antihypertensive

Atripla
efavirenz, emtricitabine, tenofovir disoproxil fumarate
Therapeutic class: Antiviral

Augmentin
amoxicillin, clavulanate potassium
Therapeutic class: Anti-infective

Avalide
hydrochlorothiazide, irbesartan
Therapeutic class: Antihypertensive

Avandamet
rosiglitazone maleate, metformin
   hydrochloride
Therapeutic class: Hypoglycemic

Avandaryl
rosiglitazone maleate and glimepiride
Therapeutic class: Hypoglycemic

Azor
amlodipine, olmesartan medoxomil
Therapeutic class: Antihypertensive

Bactrim
sulfamethoxazole, trimethoprim
Therapeutic class: Anti-infective

Caduet
amlodipine besylate, atorvastatin calcium
Therapeutic class: Antihypertensive,
   antihyperlipidemic

Capozide
captopril, hydrochlorothiazide
Therapeutic class: Antihypertensive

Ciprodex
ciprofloxacin, dexamethasone
Therapeutic class: Anti-infective, anti-
   inflammatory drug

Clarinex-D 12 hour
desloratadine and pseudoephedrine
Therapeutic class: Antihistamine and
   vasoconstrictor

Claritin-D
loratadine, pseudoephedrine sulfate
Therapeutic class: Antihistamine,
   adrenergic

Coartem
artemether, lumefantrine
Therapeutic class: Antimalarial

CombiPatch
estradiol, norethindrone acetate
Therapeutic class: Estrogen, progestin

Combivent
albuterol sulfate, ipratropium bromide
Therapeutic class: Bronchodilator

Combivir
lamivudine, zidovudine
Therapeutic class: Antiviral

Combunox
ibuprofen, oxycodone hydrochloride
Therapeutic class: Opioid analgesic

Corzide
bendroflumethiazide, nadolol
Therapeutic class: Antihypertensive

Cosopt
dorzolamide, timolol maleate
Therapeutic class: Antihypertensive,
   carbonic anhydrase inhibitor

Darvocet N-100
acetaminophen, propoxyphene
Therapeutic class: Opioid analgesic

Duetact
glimepiride, pioglitazone
Therapeutic class: Antihyperglycemic

Dyazide
hydrochlorothiazide, triamterene
Therapeutic class: Diuretic

EMLA Cream
lidocaine, prilocaine
Therapeutic class: Anesthetic

Endocet
acetaminophen, oxycodone
   hydrochloride
Therapeutic class: Opioid analgesic

Epzicom
abacavir sulfate, lamivudine
Therapeutic class: Antiviral

Exforge
amlodipine, valsartan
Therapeutic class: Antihypertensive

Exforge HCT
amlodipine, valsartan,
   hydrochlorothiazide
Therapeutic class: Antihypertensive

Femhrt
ethinyl estradiol, norethindrone acetate
Therapeutic class: Estrogen, progestin

Fioricet
acetaminophen, butalbital, caffeine
Therapeutic class: Barbiturate analgesic

Fiorinal
aspirin, butalbital, caffeine
Therapeutic class: Barbiturate analgesic

(continued)

Common combination drug products (continued)

Fosamax Plus D
alendronate sodium, cholecalciferol
Therapeutic class: Bone resorption
   inhibitor

Glucovance
glyburide, metformin hydrochloride
Therapeutic class: Hypoglycemic

Helidac
bismuth subsalicylate, metronidazole,
   tetracycline hydrochloride
Therapeutic class: Anti-infective

Humulin 70/30
insulin, recombinant human;
   insulin suspension, isophane
Therapeutic class: Hypoglycemic

Hycodan
homatropine methylbromide,
   hydrocodone bitartrate
Therapeutic class: Opioid analgesic

Hydrocet
acetaminophen, hydrocodone bitartrate
Therapeutic class: Opioid analgesic

Hyzaar
hydrochlorothiazide, losartan
   potassium
Therapeutic class: Antihypertensive

Inderide
hydrochlorothiazide, propranolol
   hydrochloride
Therapeutic class: Antihypertensive

Janumet
metformin hydrochloride, sitagliptin
Therapeutic class: Antihyperglycemic

Kaletra
lopinavir, ritonavir
Therapeutic class: Antiviral

Librax
chlordiazepoxide hydrochloride,
   clidinium bromide
Therapeutic class: Anxiolytic

Loestrin 24 FE
norethindrone acetate/ethinyl estradiol
   and ferrous fumarate
Therapeutic class: Hormonal
   contraceptive with iron

Lomotil
atropine sulfate, diphenoxylate
   hydrochloride
Therapeutic class: Antidiarrheal,
   anticholinergic

Lopressor HCT
hydrochlorothiazide, metoprolol
   tartrate
Therapeutic class: Antihypertensive

Lortab
acetaminophen, hydrocodone bitartrate
Therapeutic class: Opioid analgesic

Lotensin HCT
benazepril hydrochloride,
   hydrochlorothiazide
Therapeutic class: Antihypertensive

Lotrel
amlodipine besylate, benazepril
   hydrochloride
Therapeutic class: Antihypertensive

Maxzide
hydrochlorothiazide, triamterene
Therapeutic class: Antihypertensive,
   diuretic

Moduretic
amiloride hydrochloride, hydrochlorothiazide
Therapeutic class: Diuretic

NovoLog Mix 70/30
insulin aspart (recombinant), insulin
   aspart protamine
Therapeutic class: Hypoglycemic

NuLYTELY
polyethylene glycol, potassium chloride, sodium bicarbonate, sodium
   chloride
Therapeutic class: Laxative

Ortho-Cyclen
ethinyl estradiol, norgestimate
Therapeutic class: Contraceptive

Pediazole
erythromycin ethylsuccinate,
   sulfisoxazole acetyl
Therapeutic class: Anti-infective

Percocet
acetaminophen, oxycodone hydrochloride
Therapeutic class: Opioid analgesic

Percodan
aspirin, oxycodone hydrochloride,
oxycodone terephthalate
Therapeutic class: Opioid analgesic

Premphase
conjugated estrogens, medroxyprogesterone acetate
Therapeutic class: Contraceptive

Primaxin
cilastatin sodium, imipenem
Therapeutic class: Anti-infective

Qsymia
phentermine and topiramate extended-
release
Therapeutic class: Adjunct for weight
management

Rifamate
isoniazid, rifampin
Therapeutic class: Antitubercular

Rifater
isoniazid, pyrazinamide, rifampin
Therapeutic class: Antitubercular

Roxicet
acetaminophen, oxycodone hydrochloride
Therapeutic class: Opioid analgesic

Septra
sulfamethoxazole, trimethoprim
Therapeutic class: Anti-infective

Sinemet
carbidopa, levodopa
Therapeutic class: Antiparkinsonian

Solage
mequinol, tretinoin
Therapeutic class: Antineoplastic

Stalevo
carbidopa, entacapone, levodopa
Therapeutic class: Antiparkinsonian

Stribild
elvitegravir, cobicistat, emtricitabine,
tenofovir disoproxil fumarate
Therapeutic class: Antiviral

Symbicort
budesonide, formoterol
Therapeutic class: Antiasthmatic,
bronchodilator

Symbyax
fluoxetine hydrochloride, olanzapine
Therapeutic class: Mood stabilizer

Taclonex
calcipotriene and betamethasone
Therapeutic class: Topical agent for psoriasis vulgaris

Tarka
trandolapril, verapamil hydrochloride
Therapeutic class: Antihypertensive

Tenoretic
atenolol, chlorthalidone
Therapeutic class: Antihypertensive

Trizivir
abacavir sulfate, lamivudine, zidovudine
Therapeutic class: Antiviral

Truvada
emtricitabine, tenofovir disoproxil
fumarate
Therapeutic class: Antiviral

Tussionex
chlorpheniramine polistirex, hydrocodone polistirex
Therapeutic class: Antitussive, antihistamine

Twynsta
telmisartan, amlodipine
Therapeutic class: Antihypertensive

Tylox
acetaminophen, oxycodone hydrochloride
Therapeutic class: Opioid analgesic

Ultracet
acetaminophen, tramadol hydrochloride
Therapeutic class: Nonopioid analgesic

Ultrase
amylase, lipase, protease
Therapeutic class: Digestive enzyme

Unasyn
ampicillin sodium, sulbactam sodium
Therapeutic class: Anti-infective

Common combination drug products (continued)

Valturna
aliskiren, valsartan
Therapeutic class: Antihypertensive

Vaseretic
enalapril maleate, hydrochlorothiazide
Therapeutic class: Antihypertensive,
    diuretic

Vicodin
acetaminophen, hydrocodone bitartrate
Therapeutic class: Opioid analgesic

Vimovo
naproxen, esomeprazole magnesium
Therapeutic class: Nonsteroidal anti-
inflammatory drug, antiulcer drug

Vusion
miconazole, sodium bicarbonate
Therapeutic class: Steroid-free agent for
    diaper dermatitis

Vytorin
ezetimibe, simvastatin
Therapeutic class: Antihyperlipidemic

Zestoretic
hydrochlorothiazide, lisinopril
Therapeutic class: Antihypertensive

Ziac
bisoprolol fumarate, hydrochloro-
    thiazide
Therapeutic class: Antihypertensive

Ziana Gel
clindamycin phosphate, tretinoin
Therapeutic class: Antibiotic, retinoid

Zyrtec-D
cetirizine hydrochloride, pseudo-
    ephedrine hydrochloride
Therapeutic class: Antihistamine/
    decongestant

Adult immunization schedule by age group

This 2012 schedule shows the recommended age groups for routine administration of vaccines for adults ages 19 and older. A person may receive a combination vaccine if any components of the combination are indicated (unless the vaccine's other components are contraindicated). Consult the package insert for detailed recommendations.

For more information about recommended vaccines and contraindications for immunization, visit www.cdc.gov/vaccines or call the CDC-INFO Contact Center at 800-232-4636.

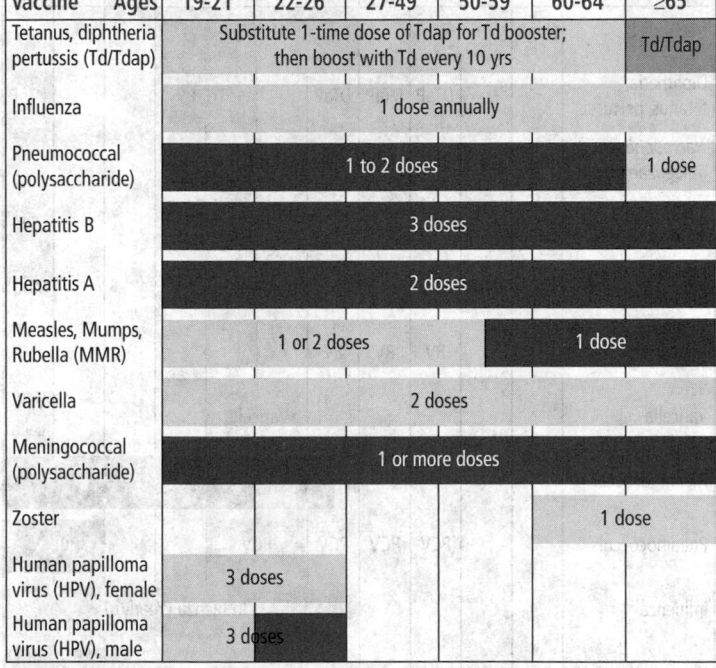

Vaccine Ages	19-21	22-26	27-49	50-59	60-64	≥65
Tetanus, diphtheria pertussis (Td/Tdap)	Substitute 1-time dose of Tdap for Td booster; then boost with Td every 10 yrs					Td/Tdap
Influenza	1 dose annually					
Pneumococcal (polysaccharide)	1 to 2 doses					1 dose
Hepatitis B	3 doses					
Hepatitis A	2 doses					
Measles, Mumps, Rubella (MMR)	1 or 2 doses			1 dose		
Varicella	2 doses					
Meningococcal (polysaccharide)	1 or more doses					
Zoster					1 dose	
Human papilloma virus (HPV), female	3 doses					
Human papilloma virus (HPV), male	3 doses					

KEY

For all persons in this age group and who lack documentation of vaccination or have no evidence of previous infection

For those with some other risk factor (medical, occupational, lifestyle, or other indications)

For patients age 65 and older if in contact with child age 12 months or younger. Td or Tdap if no infant contact.

The Adult, Childhood, and Adolescent immunization schedules (Appendices C, D, and E) have been approved by the Centers for Disease Control and Prevention's Advisory Committee on Immunization Practices, the American Academy of Family Physicians, the American College of Obstetricians and Gynecologists, the American College of Physicians, and the American College of Nurse–Midwives. Recommended adult immunization schedule-United States, 2012. MMWR 2012;61(04).

Childhood immunization schedule by age group

This 2012 schedule shows recommended ages for routine administration of childhood vaccines for children from birth through 6 years of age. A child who doesn't receive a given dose at the recommended age should receive it at a subsequent visit. Consult the package insert for detailed recommendations.

For more information about recommended vaccines, visit www.cdc.gov/vaccines or call the CDC-INFO Contact Center at 800-232-4636.

Vaccine	Birth	Age 1 mo	2 mo	4 mo	6 mo	12 mo	15 mo	18 mo	19-23 mo	2-3 yr	4-6 yr
Hepatitis B	HepB	HepB				HepB					
Diphtheria, tetanus, pertussis			DTaP	DTaP	DTaP		DTaP				DTaP
Haemophilus influenzae type b			Hib	Hib	Hib	Hib					
Inactivated poliovirus			IPV	IPV		IPV					IPV
Measles, Mumps, Rubella						MMR					MMR
Rotavirus			RV	RV	RV						
Varicella						Varicella					Varicella
Meningococcal						MCV4					
Pneumococcal			PCV	PCV	PCV	PCV					PPSV
Influenza					Influenza (Yearly)						
Hepatitis A						Dose 1					HepA series

KEY

For all persons in this age group and who lack documentation of vaccination or have no evidence of previous infection

For those with some other risk factor (medical, occupational, lifestyle, or other indications)

DTaP: Diphtheria, tetanus, pertussis
HepA: Hepatitis A vaccine
HepB: Hepatitis B vaccine
Hib: *Haemophilus influenzae* type b conjugate vaccine
IPV: Inactivated poliovirus
MMR: Measles, Mumps, Rubella
MCV4: Meningococcal conjugate vaccines, quadrivalent
PCV: Pneumococcal conjugate vaccine
PPSV: Pneumococcal polysaccharide vaccine

Adolescent immunization schedule by age group

This 2012 schedule shows recommended ages for routine administration of currently licensed vaccines to adolescent children ages 7 to 18. An adolescent who doesn't receive a given dose at the recommended age should receive it at a subsequent visit. Consult the package insert for detailed recommendations.

For more information about recommended vaccines (including precautions and contraindications for immunization and vaccine shortages), visit www.cdc.gov/vaccines or call the CDC-INFO Contact Center at 800-232-4636.

Vaccine	Ages 7-10	11-12	13-18
Tetanus, diphtheria pertussis	1 dose (if indicated)	1 dose	1 dose (if indicated)
Human papilloma virus		3 doses	Complete 3-dose series
Hepatitis B	Complete 3-dose series		
Inactivated poliovirus	Complete 3-dose series		
Measles, Mumps, Rubella	Complete 2-dose series		
Varicella	Complete 2-dose series		
Meningococcal		Dose 1	Booster at age 16
Pneumococcal			
Influenza	Influenza (yearly)		
Hepatitis A	Complete 2-dose series		

KEY

For all persons in this age group and who lack documentation of vaccination or have no evidence of previous infection

Catch-up immunization

For patients age 65 and older if in contact with child age 12 months or younger. Td or Tdap if no infant contact.

DTaP: Diphtheria, Tetanus, Pertussis
HepA: Hepatitis A vaccine
HepB: Hepatitis B vaccine
HPV: Human papillomavirus
IPV: Inactivated poliovirus
MCV4: Meningococcal conjugate vaccine
MMR: Measles, Mumps, Rubella
MPSV4: Meningococcal polysaccharide vaccine
PPV: Pneumococcal polysaccharide vaccine

Normal laboratory values for blood tests

The table below shows normal laboratory values for commonly ordered blood tests. Results may vary slightly among laboratories. Many of these values are monitored regularly to assess patient response and drug efficacy.

Hematology

White blood cell count
4,100 to 10,900/mm³

Red blood cell count
Men: 4.5 to 6.2 million/mm³
Women: 4.2 to 5.4 million/mm³

Hemoglobin
Men: 14 to 18 g/dl
Women: 12 to 16 g/dl

Hematocrit
Men: 42% to 54%
Women: 38% to 46%

Platelet count
140,000 to 400,000/mm³

Red blood cell indices
MCH: 26 to 32 pg
MCHC: 32 to 36 g/dl
MCV: 80 to 95 μm³

Reticulocyte count
0.5% to 2% of total red blood cell count

White blood cell differential
Basophils: 0.3% to 2%
Eosinophils: 0.3% to 7%
Lymphocytes: 16.2% to 43%
Monocytes: 4% to 10%
Neutrophils: 47.6% to 76.8%

Coagulation studies

Partial thromboplastin time
60 to 70 seconds

Prothrombin time
10 to 14 seconds

International Normalized Ratio
2.0 to 3.0 in patients receiving warfarin

Bleeding time
3 to 6 minutes (template and Ivy methods)
1 to 3 minutes (Duke method)

D-Dimer
< 250 μg/L

Fibrinogen
215 to 519 mg/dl

Fibrinogen degradation products
< 1:10

Chemistry

Glucose
70 to 100 mg/dl

Blood urea nitrogen (BUN)
8 to 20 mg/dl

Creatinine
Men: 0.8 to 1.2 mg/dl
Women: 0.6 to 1.1 mg/dl

BUN/creatinine ratio
6 to 22 (calculated)

Chemistry (continued)

Globulin
2.3 to 3.5 g/dl

Sodium
135 to 145 mEq/L

Potassium
3.5 to 5.0 mEq/L

Anion gap
8 to 16 mEq/L

Chloride
100 to 108 mEq/L

Carbon dioxide
22 to 34 mEq/L

Albumin
3.3 to 4.5 g/dl

Calcium
9 to 10.5 mg/dl

Magnesium
1.5 to 2.5 mEq/L

Phosphorus
2.5 to 4.5 mg/dl

Amylase
60 to 180 units/L

Lipase
0 to 110 units/L

Lactate dehydrogenase
48 to 115 IU/L

Lactic acid
3 to 12 mg/dl

Protein
6.0 to 8.5 g/dl

Uric acid
Men: 4.0 to 8.5 mg/dl
Women: 2.5 to 7.5 mg/dl

KEY MCH: Mean corpuscular hemoglobin
MCHC: Mean corpuscular hemoglobin concentration
MCV: Mean corpuscular volume

(continued)

Chemistry (continued)

Erythrocyte sedimentation rate
Men: 0 to 15 mm/hour
Women: 0 to 20 mm/hour

Glucose-6-phosphate dehydrogenase
5 to 13 units/g hemoglobin

Hemoglobin A1c
< 6.0% of total hemoglobin

B-Type natriuretic peptide
< 100 pg/ml

Zinc
60 to 130 mcg/dl

Serotonin
Men: 21 to 321 ng/ml
Women: 0 to 420 ng/ml

Arterial blood gases

pH
7.35 to 7.45 mmHg

$Paco_2$
35 to 45 mmHg

Pao_2
75 to 100 mmHg

HCO_3^-
22 to 26 mEq/L

Sao_2
94% to 100%

Lipid studies

Low-density lipoproteins
Optimal: < 100 mg/dl
Near optimal: 100 to 129 mg/dl

High-density lipoproteins
Desirable: ≥ 60 mg/dl

Total cholesterol
Desirable: < 200 mg/dl

Triglycerides
Desirable: < 200 mg/dl

Liver function studies

Alanine aminotransferase
Men: 10 to 35 units/L
Women: 9 to 24 units/L

Alkaline phosphatase
39 to 117 units/L

Aspartate aminotransferase
Men: 8 to 20 units/L
Women: 5 to 40 units/L

Serum bilirubin
Direct: ≤ 0.4 mg/dl
Indirect: ≤ 1.3 mg/dl
Total: ≤ 1.3 mg/dl

Cardiac studies

Cardiac troponin I
< 1.0 µg/ml

Creatine kinase (CK)
Total CK—
  Men: 54 to 186 IU/L
  Women: 41 to 117 IU/L
Isoenzymes—
  CK-MM: 96% to 100% of total
  CK-MB: 0% to 4% of total
  CK-BB: 0% of total

High sensitivity C-reactive protein
Low cardiovascular risk: < 1.0 mg/L
Average cardiovascular risk: 1.0 to 3.0 mg/L

Tumor-related marker studies

Carbohydrate antigen (CA) 15.3
> 25 U/ml

CA 19-9 (Siemens Chemiluminescent Method)
< 37 U/ml

CA 125 (Siemens Chemiluminescent Method)
< 21 U/ml

Carcinoembryonic antigen
< 3 ng/ml, individualized and variable (non-smokers)
< 5 ng/ml, individualized and variable (smokers)

Prostate-specific antigen
≤ 4 ng/ml

Prostatic acid phosphatase
< 0 to 2.7 ng/ml

Lymphocyte surface markers

CD3
Absolute: 840 to 3,060 cells/µL
Percentage: 57% to 85%

CD4
Absolute: 490 to 1,740 cells/µL
Percentage: 30% to 61%

CD8
Absolute: 180 to 1,170 cells/µL
Percentage: 12% to 42%

Helper: suppressor (CD4: CD8) ratio
0.86 to 5

Normal laboratory values for blood tests (continued)

Iron studies

Serum iron
40 to 180 mcg/dl

Ferritin
Men: 18 to 270 µg/ml
Women: 18 to 160 µg/ml

Iron-binding capacity
200 to 450 mcg/dl

Transferrin
88 to 341 mg/dl

Transferrin saturation
12% to 57%

Hormone studies

Cortisol, free

8:00 to 10:00 A.M.	0.07 to 0.93 mcg/dl
4:00 to 6:00 P.M.	0.04 to 0.45 mcg/dl
10:00 to 10:00 P.M.	0.04 to 0.35 mcg/dl

Cortisol, total

8:00 to 10:00 A.M.	4.6 to 20.6 mcg/dl
4:00 to 6:00 P.M.	1.8 to 13.6 mcg/dl

Estradiol
Men: < 50 pg/ml
Women: Menstruating (day of
  cycle relative to LH peak) —
  Follicular (−12): 19 to 83 pg/ml
  Follicular (−4): 64 to 183 pg/ml
  Midcycle (−1): 150 to 528 pg/ml
  Luteal (+2): 58 to 157 pg/ml
  Luteal (+6): 60 to 211 pg/ml
  Luteal (+12): 55 to 150 pg/ml
Postmenopausal (no treatment):
  0 to 31 pg/ml

Free thyroxine
0.7 to 1.9 ng/dl

Free thyroxine fraction
0.03% to 0.005%

Growth hormone
Age 1 day: 5 to 53 ng/ml
Age 1 week: 5 to 27 ng/ml
Age 1 to 12 months: 2 to 10 ng/ml
Age 1 year and older: < 5 ng/ml

Hormone studies (continued)

17-Hydroxyprogesterone
Men: 0.06 to 3.0 mg/L
Women (follicular phase): 0.2 to
  1.0 mg/L

**Parathyroid hormone,
intact**
Ages 2 to 20 years: 9 to
  52 pg/ml
Older than age 20: 8 to
  97 pg/ml

Radioactive iodine uptake
10% to 30%

Testosterone
Males > age 18: 241 to 827 ng/dl
Females > age 18: 14 to 76 ng/dl

Triiodothyronine (T$_3$)
60 to 181 ng/dl

Thyroxine (T$_4$)
4.5 to 12.5 mcg/dl

Thyroid hormone binding ratio
0.9 to 1.1

Thyroid-stimulating hormone
0.5 to 4.70 microIU/ml

Drug infusion rates

SAFETY
GUIDELINES

The tables below show infusion rates for common drug infusions. Before using these tables as your administration guide, make sure the concentration of the prescribed infusion matches the concentration shown in the table.

Adenosine (Adenoscan) infusion rates

Using this table, you can determine that the appropriate infusion rate is corrected for total body weight.

Patient's weight		
kg	lb	Infusion rate (ml/minute)
45	99	2.1
50	110	2.3
55	121	2.6
60	132	2.8
65	143	3
70	154	3.3
75	165	3.5
80	176	3.8
85	187	4.0
90	198	4.2

Aminophylline infusion rates

Although aminophylline infusion rates are highly individualized, this table can help you determine the infusion rate for an infusion containing aminophylline 500 mg (= 400 mg theophylline) in 500 ml D_5W that must be controlled by an automated infusion control device.

Dosage (mg/hour)	Dosage (mg/hour)	
Aminophylline	Theophylline	Rate (ml/hour)
10	8	10
15	12	15
20	16	20
25	20	25
30	24	30
35	28	35
40	32	40
45	36	45
50	40	50
55	44	55
60	48	60
65	52	65
70	56	70
75	60	75
80	64	80

Drug infusion rates (continued)

Argatroban infusion rates

Using this table, you can determine the infusion rate for argatroban (for a 2-mcg/kg/minute dose) that has been diluted in normal saline solution, D_5W, or lactated Ringer's solution to a concentration of 1 mg/ml.

Patient's weight (kg)	Dosage (mcg/minute)	Infusion rate (ml/hour)
50	100	6
60	120	7
70	140	8
80	160	10
90	180	11
100	200	12
110	220	13
120	240	14
130	260	16
140	280	17

Clindamycin phosphate infusion rates

Using this table, you can determine dilution and infusion rates after diluting I.V. solution to a concentration of not more than 18 mg/ml using normal saline solution, D_5W, or lactated Ringer's solution.

	Dilution and infusion rates	
Dosage (mg)	Diluent (ml)	Infusion rate (minutes)
300	50	10
600	50	20
900	50 to 100	30
1,200	100	40

Dobutamine infusion rates

Using this table, you can determine the infusion rate for an infusion containing dobutamine 250 mg mixed in 250 ml of dextrose 5% in water (1,000 mcg/ml).

Dosage (mcg/kg/ minute)	Patient's weight (kg)														
	40	45	50	55	60	65	70	75	80	85	90	95	100	105	110
	Infusion rate (ml/hour)														
0.5	1	1	2	2	2	2	2	2	2	3	3	3	3	3	3
1.5	4	4	5	5	5	6	6	7	7	8	8	9	9	9	10
2.5	6	7	8	8	9	10	11	11	12	13	14	14	15	16	17
5.0	12	14	15	17	18	20	21	23	24	26	27	29	30	32	33
7.5	18	20	23	25	27	29	32	34	36	38	41	43	45	47	50
10.0	24	27	30	33	36	39	42	45	48	51	54	57	60	63	66
12.5	30	34	38	41	45	49	53	56	60	64	68	71	75	79	83
15.0	36	41	45	50	54	59	63	68	72	77	81	86	90	95	99
20.0	48	54	60	66	72	78	84	90	96	102	108	114	120	126	132
25.0	60	68	75	83	90	98	105	113	120	128	135	143	150	158	165
30.0	72	81	90	99	108	117	126	135	144	153	162	171	180	189	198
35.0	84	95	105	116	126	137	147	158	168	179	189	200	210	221	231
40.0	96	108	120	132	144	156	168	180	192	204	216	228	240	252	264

(continued)

Dopamine infusion rates

Using this table, you can determine the infusion rate for an infusion containing dopamine 400 mg in 250 ml of dextrose 5% in water (1,600 mcg/ml).

Dosage (mcg/kg/minute)	Patient's weight (kg)													
	40	45	50	55	60	65	70	75	80	85	90	95	100	105
	Infusion rate (ml/hour)													
0.5	1	1	1	1	1	1	1	1	2	2	2	2	2	2
1.5	2	3	3	3	3	4	4	4	5	5	5	6	6	6
2.5	4	4	5	5	6	6	7	7	8	8	8	9	9	10
5.0	8	8	9	10	11	12	13	14	15	16	17	18	19	20
7.5	11	13	14	15	17	18	20	21	23	24	25	27	28	30
10.0	15	17	19	21	23	24	26	28	30	32	34	36	38	39
12.5	19	21	23	26	28	30	33	35	38	40	42	45	47	49
15.0	23	25	28	31	34	37	39	42	45	48	51	53	56	59
20.0	30	34	38	41	45	49	53	56	60	64	68	71	75	79
25.0	38	42	47	52	56	61	66	70	75	80	84	89	94	98
30.0	45	51	56	62	67	73	79	84	90	96	101	107	113	118
35.0	53	59	66	72	79	85	92	98	105	112	118	125	131	138
40.0	60	68	75	83	90	98	105	113	120	128	135	143	150	158
45.0	68	76	84	93	101	110	118	127	135	143	152	160	169	177
50.0	75	84	94	103	113	122	131	141	150	159	169	178	188	197

Epinephrine infusion rates

Use this table to determine the rate at which to infuse epinephrine 1 mg in 250 ml of dextrose 5% in water (4 mcg/ml).

Dosage (mcg/minute)	Infusion rate (ml/hour)
1	15
2	30
3	45
4	60
5	75
6	90
7	105
8	120
9	135
10	150
15	225

Drug infusion rates (continued)

Nitroglycerin infusion rates

When infusing nitroglycerin, first find the prescribed concentration and then determine the infusion rate in ml/hour.

Dosage (mcg/minute)	Nitroglycerin 25 mg/250 ml D₅W (100 mcg/ml) Infusion rate (ml/hour)	Nitroglycerin 50 mg/250 ml D₅W (200 mcg/ml) Infusion rate (ml/hour)
5	3	2
10	6	3
15	9	5
20	12	6
25	15	8
30	18	9
40	24	12
50	30	15
60	36	18
70	42	21
80	48	24
90	54	27
100	60	30

KEY   D₅W: dextrose 5% in water

Nitroprusside infusion rates

Using this table, you can determine the infusion rate for an infusion containing nitroprusside 50 mg in 250 ml of dextrose 5% in water (200 mcg/ml).

Dosage (mcg/kg/minute)	40	45	50	55	60	65	70	75	80	85	90	95	100	105	110
	Infusion rate (ml/hour)														
0.3	4	4	5	5	5	6	6	7	7	8	8	9	9	9	10
0.5	6	7	8	8	9	10	11	11	12	13	14	14	15	16	17
1.0	12	14	15	17	18	20	21	23	24	26	27	29	30	32	33
1.5	18	20	23	25	27	29	32	34	36	38	41	43	45	47	50
2.0	24	27	30	33	36	39	42	45	48	51	54	57	60	63	66
3.0	36	41	45	50	54	59	63	68	72	77	81	86	90	95	99
4.0	48	54	60	66	72	78	84	90	96	102	108	114	120	126	132
5.0	60	68	75	83	90	98	105	113	120	128	135	143	150	158	165
6.0	72	81	90	99	108	117	126	135	144	153	162	171	180	189	198
7.0	84	95	105	116	126	137	147	158	168	179	189	200	210	221	231
8.0	96	108	120	132	144	156	168	180	192	204	216	228	240	252	264
9.0	108	122	135	149	162	176	189	203	216	230	243	257	270	284	297
10.0	120	135	150	165	180	195	210	225	240	255	270	285	300	315	330

Patient's weight (kg)

(continued)

Phenylephrine infusion rates

Using this table, you can determine the infusion rate for an infusion containing phenylephrine 20 mg in 250 ml of dextrose 5% in water or normal saline solution (80 mcg/ml).

Dosage (mcg/minute)	Rate (ml/hour)	Dosage (mcg/minute)	Rate (ml/hour)
9	7	25	19
11	8	27	20
12	9	29	22
13	10	32	24
15	11	35	26
16	12	37	28
17	13	40	30
19	14	43	32
20	15	45	34
21	16	48	36
23	17	51	38
24	18	53	40

Identifying life-threatening adverse reactions

Early recognition of a life-threatening adverse drug reaction is a crucial aspect of patient care and safety. This appendix helps you identify life-threatening adverse reactions that are relatively rare or cause symptoms you may not be readily familiar with. Some reactions are potentially lethal from the onset; others can become lethal if they progress.

Acute pancreatitis
Inflammation of the pancreas
Signs and symptoms: sudden onset of epigastric pain, nausea, and vomiting

Acute respiratory distress syndrome (ARDS)
Respiratory insufficiency in which abnormal permeability of the alveolar-capillary membrane causes fluid to fill the alveoli, disrupting gas exchange
Signs and symptoms: dyspnea, tachypnea, and progressive hypoxemia despite oxygen therapy; pulmonary edema

Adrenal suppression
Condition marked by inhibition of one or more of the enzymes essential to adrenocortical hormone production
Signs and symptoms: weakness, fatigue, abdominal pain, appetite and weight loss, dizziness, orthostatic hypotension, increased skin pigmentation

Adynamic ileus
Intestinal obstruction caused by a reduction in intestinal motility
Signs and symptoms: nausea, vomiting, decreased or absent bowel sounds, abdominal distention

Agranulocytopenia
Acute condition caused by deficiencies of neutrophils, basophils, and eosinophils in the blood
Signs and symptoms: chills, fever, headache, malaise, weakness, fatigue

Alkalosis
Increase in blood alkalinity caused by buildup of alkalis or reduction of acids
Signs and symptoms: in metabolic alkalosis—apathy, confusion, stupor (when severe); in respiratory alkalosis—air hunger, muscle twitching, numbness or tingling of extremities or circumoral area

Amyloidosis
Metabolic disorder caused by deposition of protein-containing fibrils in tissues, which may attack the heart and blood vessels, brain, kidneys, liver, spleen, intestines, or endocrine glands
Signs and symptoms: vary with area of invasion

Anaphylactoid shock
Hypersensitivity reaction marked by acute airway obstruction and vascular collapse within minutes of exposure to an antigen
Signs and symptoms: edema, rash, tachycardia, hypotension, respiratory distress, seizures, unconsciousness

Anaphylaxis
Hypersensitivity reaction to an antigen to which the patient has been previously sensitized, causing sudden release of immunologic mediators either locally or throughout the body
Signs and symptoms: urticaria, angioedema, flushing, wheezing, dyspnea, increased mucus production, nausea, vomiting

(continued)

Angioedema

Vascular reaction involving deep dermal, submucosal, or subcutaneous tissues in which capillaries become dilated and more permeable; also called angioneurotic edema

Signs and symptoms: edema of skin, mucous membranes, and internal organs; urticaria; giant wheals; respiratory distress

Autoimmune phenomena

Immunologic responses, such as serum sickness, lupus, vasculitis, and hepatitis, associated with development of antibodies (as to a particular drug)

Signs and symptoms: possibly none; or signs and symptoms specific to the particular autoimmune condition

Bone marrow depression

Disruption of healthy blood cell development in the bone marrow (including red and white blood cells and platelets), which impairs or weakens the body's defense against pathogenic organisms, toxins, and irritants

Signs and symptoms: increased susceptibility to infection, fever, weakness

Cardiac tamponade

Condition marked by increased cardiac pressure, which inhibits filling of the heart chambers during diastole

Signs and symptoms: chest pain, weak peripheral pulses, distended neck veins, dyspnea, orthopnea, diaphoresis, anxiety, restlessness, pallor

Cardiomyopathy

Any disease or disorder of the heart that impairs normal cardiac performance

Signs and symptoms: shortness of breath, orthopnea, fatigue, chest pain, syncope

Cardiotoxicity

The quality of being poisonous or harmful to the heart (as with certain drugs)

Signs and symptoms: variable cardiac-related symptoms

Cardiovascular collapse

Sudden loss of effective blood flow to body tissues

Signs and symptoms: hypotension, vasovagal syncope, cardiogenic shock, cardiac arrest

Cerebral ischemia

Temporary lack of arterial or circulatory blood flow to the brain, possibly causing localized tissue death

Signs and symptoms: persistent focal neurologic deficit in the area of distribution of the involved cerebral artery

Chemical arachnoiditis

Inflammation of the arachnoid (middle) layer of the meninges of the brain and spinal cord in response to exposure to a toxic substance

Signs and symptoms: mild nausea or vomiting, headache, fever, neck or back pain and stiffness

Cholesterol embolism

Sudden obstruction of a blood vessel by cholesterol-containing plaques

Signs and symptoms: hypotension, sudden shortness of breath, weak pulse, cyanosis, chest pain, decreased level of consciousness

Clostridium difficile–associated diarrhea

Antibiotic-associated diarrhea caused by *Clostridium difficile,* a spore-forming, gram-positive, anaerobic bacillus that produces two exotoxins: toxin A and toxin B

Signs and symptoms: watery diarrhea, fever, loss of appetite, nausea, abdominal pain, abdominal tenderness, colon perforation, sepsis, and death (rarely)

Identifying life-threatening adverse reactions (continued)

Disseminated intravascular coagulation ·
Disorder marked by abnormal activation of coagulation factors in the blood, causing hemostasis, thrombosis, and possibly, organ damage
Signs and symptoms: bleeding (possibly from multiple sites), hematomas, thrombosis, petechiae, ecchymosis, cutaneous oozing

Disulfiram-like reaction
Acute, unpleasant reaction to alcohol ingestion in a patient taking disulfiram (Antabuse) for alcohol aversion therapy
Signs and symptoms: flushing, dyspnea, headache, nausea, copious vomiting, blood pressure fluctuations

Drug rash with eosinophilia and systemic symptoms (DRESS)
Rare, severe adverse reaction presenting as generalized rash, marked eosinophilia, fever, and dysfunction of one or more organ systems, including liver failure
Signs and symptoms: generalized rash, fever, and internal organ involvement weeks to months, reportedly, after starting such drugs as sulfonamides, phenobarbital, sulfasalazine, carbamazepine, phenytoin, and possibly celecoxib and ethambutol

Encephalopathy
Generalized dysfunction of the brain
Signs and symptoms: impaired speech, orientation, or cognition; sluggish reaction to stimuli

Eosinophilic pneumonitis
Infiltration of pulmonary alveoli by large numbers of eosinophils and mononuclear cells, causing inflammation
Signs and symptoms: dyspnea, cough, fever, night sweats, pulmonary edema, weight loss

Epileptiform seizures
Sudden, uncontrolled electrical discharge from the cerebral cortex caused by epilepsy
Signs and symptoms: variable; may include a cry, a fall, unconsciousness, overt seizure, amnesia, or incontinence

Erythema multiforme
Hypersensitivity reaction of the skin and mucous membranes; may take a severe multisystemic form
Signs and symptoms: rash, macules, papules, or blisters on the face, palms, and extremities

Fanconi syndrome
Congenital form of anemia caused by excessive amino acids in the blood secondary to renal tubular failure
Signs and symptoms: polyuria; growth impairment; soft, flexible, brittle bones

Granulocytopenia
Abnormal reduction in the number of granulocytes in the blood
Signs and symptoms: increased susceptibility to infection

Heart block
Interference with the normal electrical impulses of the heart, classified by the level of impairment that results (first-, second-, or third-degree block)
Signs and symptoms: prolonged PR interval, widened QRS interval, and delayed or dropped beats on ECG; other symptoms vary with the degree of heart block and may include dizziness, syncope, shortness of breath, fatigue, and orthostatic hypotension

Hepatomegaly
Liver enlargement
Signs and symptoms: possibly none; or abdominal distention, abdominal pain, and constipation

(continued)

Hepatotoxicity

Liver inflammation caused by exposure to a toxin or a toxic amount of a substance in the body
Signs and symptoms: jaundice, fatigue, weakness, altered mental status

Hyperkalemia

A condition marked by an excessive amount of potassium in the blood
Signs and symptoms: possibly none; with severe hyperkalemia—muscle weakness, arrhythmias

Hypertensive crisis

Severe blood pressure elevation, usually defined as diastolic pressure higher than 130 mmHg
Signs and symptoms: severe headache, dizziness, light-headedness

Hypertonia

Excessive tension or pressure within a muscle or an artery
Signs and symptoms: muscle pain and spasms

Hypervolemia

Abnormal increase in volume of circulating body fluid
Signs and symptoms: weight gain, peripheral edema, ascites, dyspnea, pulmonary edema, paroxysmal nocturnal dyspnea

Immune reconstitution syndrome

Enhanced immunologic response, especially during the initial phase of combination antiretroviral treatment, when patients whose immune systems respond may develop an inflammatory response to indolent or residual opportunistic infections (such as *Mycobacterium avium* infection, cytomegalovirus, *Pneumocystis jiroveci* pneumonia, or tuberculosis).

Signs and symptoms: possibly nonspecific, including new or worsening fever, persistent or cyclic fever, new pleural effusions, new or worsening lymphadenopathy, fatigue, weakness, night sweats, anorexia, weight loss, chronic diarrhea, abdominal pain, and vulnerability to infection

Impaired myocardial contractility

Decreased contractile ability of the middle layer of the heart muscle wall
Signs and symptoms: shortness of breath, chest pain, edema

Increased intracranial pressure

Increased pressure within the brain, as from increased cerebrospinal fluid pressure or a brain lesion or swelling; also called intracranial hypertension
Signs and symptoms: in infants—bulging fontanel, separated sutures, lethargy, vomiting; in older children and adults—lethargy, vomiting, headache, behavior changes, seizures, neurologic deficits, progressive decrease in level of consciousness

Interstitial pneumonia

Chronic, noninfectious inflammation of the pulmonary alveolar walls
Signs and symptoms: shortness of breath, either with activity or at rest

Ischemic colitis

Inflammation of the colon caused by lack of blood supply to mesenteric arteries of the small intestine
Signs and symptoms: abdominal pain, weight loss

Lactic acidosis

Accumulation of lactic acid in the blood caused by reduced oxygenation and perfusion to tissues, muscles, and major organs
Signs and symptoms: muscle pain, fatigue, hyperventilation, nausea, vomiting, dizziness, light-headedness

Identifying life-threatening adverse reactions (continued)

Leukocytosis
Abnormal increase in the number of white blood cells (leukocytes) in the blood
Signs and symptoms: fever, hemorrhage

Leukopenia
Abnormal reduction (below 5,000 cells/mm³) in circulating white blood cells, as from drug-induced impairment of blood cell production
Signs and symptoms: infection, fever, stomatitis, sinusitis

Lupuslike syndrome
A syndrome similar to systemic lupus erythematosus that occurs in response to drug therapy and resolves when the drug is withdrawn
Signs and symptoms: fever; red, scaly, macular skin rash; joint inflammation

Lupus nephritis
Kidney inflammation associated with systemic lupus erythematosus (SLE), marked by deposition of antigen-antibody complexes in the mesangium and basement membrane
Signs and symptoms: hypertension, peripheral edema, proteinuria, renal failure, cardiac decompensation, other symptoms of active SLE (such as fatigue, fever, rash, arthritis, CNS disease)

Megaloblastic anemia
Anemia marked by production and proliferation of megaloblasts (large immature red blood cells) in the bone marrow or circulation
Signs and symptoms: weakness, fatigue, light-headedness, headache, rapid pulse, breathlessness

Metabolic acidosis
Increase in blood acidity caused by buildup of acids or loss of bicarbonate
Signs and symptoms: lethargy, drowsiness, headache, diminished muscle tone and reflexes, hyperventilation, arrhythmias, nausea, vomiting, diarrhea, abdominal pain

Methemoglobinemia
Condition in which a portion of the iron component of hemoglobin has been oxidized to the ferric state, making it incapable of transporting oxygen
Signs and symptoms: cyanosis, dizziness, drowsiness, headache

Neoplasm
Abnormal growth of new tissue, such as a tumor
Signs and symptoms: vary with tumor site

Nephrotoxicity
The quality of causing damage to the kidney (as from a drug); usually leads to increased permeability to proteins, which results in edema and hypoalbuminemia
Signs and symptoms: proteinuria, hematuria, fluid retention

Neuroleptic malignant syndrome
Reaction to a drug that alters the brain's dopamine level or to withdrawal of a drug that increases the dopamine level
Signs and symptoms: sweating, altered mental status, seizures, renal failure

Neutropenia
Abnormal decrease in the level of neutrophils in the blood (usually below 1,500 per µL)
Signs and symptoms: infection, fever, mouth and throat sores

Osmotic nephrosis
Disruption of osmotic pressure in the kidney's renal tubule
Signs and symptoms: fluid retention, edema

Pancytopenia
Deficiency of all cellular elements of the blood, including red blood cells, white blood cells, and platelets
Signs and symptoms: bleeding from the nose and gums, easy bruising, fatigue, shortness of breath

(continued)

Papilledema

Swelling and inflammation of the optic nerve
Signs and symptoms: severe headache, visual disturbances, blindness

Pericardial effusion

Escape of fluid from blood vessels into the pericardium
Signs and symptoms: hypotension, tachycardia, muffled heart sounds, decreased breath sounds, distended jugular vein, pulsus paradoxus, widened pulse pressure, weak peripheral pulses, pericardial friction rub, tachypnea, edema, cyanosis

Pseudomembranous colitis

Condition in which an inflammatory exudate forms on epithelial tissues of the colon
Signs and symptoms: diarrhea with blood and mucus, abdominal cramps

Pseudotumor cerebri

Benign intracranial hypertension without evidence of a brain tumor
Signs and symptoms: headache, papilledema, elevated cerebrospinal fluid pressure

Pulmonary toxicity

The quality of causing damage to the lungs and alveoli (as from certain drugs)
Signs and symptoms: any respiratory sign or symptom

Renal acidosis

Acidosis caused by accumulation of phosphoric and sulfuric acids in the body, which the kidneys fail to excrete
Signs and symptoms: appetite loss, altered level of consciousness, altered respiratory rate or effort

Renal failure

Condition marked by a serum creatinine increase of 25% or more, which impairs the kidney's ability to excrete wastes, concentrate urine, and conserve electrolytes
Signs and symptoms: dehydration, fluid overload, altered neurologic status, appetite loss, weight gain, bleeding

Respiratory acidosis

Acidosis resulting from accumulation and retention of carbon dioxide in the lungs
Signs and symptoms: dyspnea, diaphoresis, tremors, decreased reflexes, decreased level of consciousness

Rhabdomyolysis

Acute disorder in which byproducts of skeletal muscle destruction accumulate in the renal tubules, causing renal failure
Signs and symptoms: See "Hyperkalemia" and "Metabolic acidosis."

Salicylate toxicity

Toxic condition caused by overdose of a salicylate, such as aspirin or an aspirin derivative
Signs and symptoms: rapid breathing, irritability, headache, vomiting, and (if extreme) seizures and respiratory failure

Sarcoidosis

Multisystemic disease that causes granulomatous lesions of organs or tissues throughout the body
Signs and symptoms: fatigue, weight loss, shortness of breath, anorexia, skin lesions, cough, skeletal changes (in later stages)

Sepsis

Systemic inflammatory response caused by pathogenic microorganisms or their toxins
Signs and symptoms: tachycardia, fever, rapid breathing, hypothermia, evidence of reduced blood flow to major organs

Serum sickness

Hypersensitivity reaction to administration of a nonprotein drug
Signs and symptoms: fever, rash, joint pain, edema, lymphadenopathy

Steatosis

Fatty liver degeneration
Signs and symptoms: possibly none; or right upper abdominal quadrant pain, abdominal discomfort, fatigue, malaise

Identifying life-threatening adverse reactions (continued)

Stevens-Johnson syndrome

Severe allergic reaction marked by severe skin and mucous membrane lesions, most often in response to a drug

Signs and symptoms: respiratory tract infection, fever, sore throat, chills, headache, malaise, vomiting, diarrhea, tachycardia, hypotension, corneal ulcers, conjunctivitis, epistaxis, dysuria, erosive vulvovaginitis, balanitis, seizures, altered level of consciousness, coma

Syndrome of inappropriate anti-diuretic hormone secretion

Metabolic disturbance marked by an increase in antidiuretic hormone, which causes a decrease in serum sodium concentration

Signs and symptoms: weakness, fatigue, malaise, headache, altered mental status, lethargy, irritability, delirium, psychosis, personality changes, anorexia, nausea, vomiting, thirst, abdominal and muscle cramps

Tardive dyskinesia

Disorder marked by slow, rhythmic involuntary movements of the face, limbs, and torso in patients who have received long-term dopaminergic antagonist therapy

Signs and symptoms: involuntary, repetitive facial grimacing and twisting; tongue protrusion; lip puckering and smacking; chewing or sucking motions; involuntary, snakelike writhing movements (such as wiggling or twisting); excessive blinking; involuntary flexion and extension movements of the fingers and hands

Tetany

Hyperexcitability of nerves and muscles caused by a decrease in extracellular calcium

Signs and symptoms: muscle twitching, cramps, sharp flexion of wrist and ankle joints, seizures

Thrombocytopenia

Abnormal decrease in the number of platelets caused by destruction of erythroid tissue in the bone marrow

Signs and symptoms: purpura, ecchymosis, petechiae, internal hemorrhage, hematuria, abdominal distention, melena

Torsade de pointes

Rapid form of ventricular tachycardia that appears as twisting or shifting QRS complexes on the ECG

Signs and symptoms: pallor, diaphoresis, rapid pulse, low or normal blood pressure, transient or prolonged loss of consciousness

Toxic epidermal necrolysis

Exfoliative skin condition that represents a severe cutaneous reaction (as to a drug, infection, or chemical exposure)

Signs and symptoms: scalded appearance of the skin, skin erosion and redness

Tumor lysis syndrome

Complication that usually follows chemotherapy treatment of myelo-lymphoproliferative diseases in which a metabolic derangement produced by rapid tumor breakdown is a consequence of therapy

Signs and symptoms: possibly no symptoms in early stages, but progression of the syndrome may lead to cardiac arrhythmias, shortness of breath, hyperkalemia, hyperuricemia, hyperphosphatemia, hypocalcemia, impaired mental ability, and renal failure

Potentially inappropriate drugs for elderly patients

Drug-drug interactions can have potentially life-threatening consequences in older adults, who often take several drugs at once for multiple diseases. Elderly patients are more susceptible to drug interactions than younger patients because of the physiologic changes associated with aging and the sheer number of drugs older patients are taking. Beers criteria, developed by Dr. Mark Beers, originally published in the *Archives of Internal Medicine* in 1991, with updated articles in 1997, 2003, 2007, and again in 2012, identified several drugs that adults ages 65 and older should avoid. This list (although not inclusive) is based on those criteria. Also refer to the manufacturer's complete package insert.

Generic drug or class	Brand names
alprazolam	Niravam, Xanax, Xanax X
amiodarone hydrochloride	Cordarone, Pacerone
amitriptyline hydrochloride	
aripiprazole	Abilify
asenapine	Saphris
aspirin > 325 mg/day	
barbiturates (except phenobarbital for seizure control)	Butisol Sodium, Luminal Sodium, Mebaral, Nembutal Sodium, Seconal Sodium
benztropine (oral)	Cogentin
brompheniramine	Bromfenac, Dimetapp Allergy, Lodrane 24, LoHist 12, Nasahist B, ND-Stat, TanaCof-XR, Vazol
carisoprodol	Soma
chlordiazepoxide hydrochloride	
chlorpheniramine maleate	Ahist, Aller-Chlor, Chlorphen, Chlor-Trimeton, CPM-12, Diabetic Tussin Allergy Relief, QDALL AR, Teldrin HBP
chlorpromazine	
chlorpropamide	Diabenese
chlorzoxazone	Parafon Forte DSC
clonazepam	Klonopin
clomipramine	
clonidine	Catapres-TTS
clonidine hydrochloride	Catapres
clorazepate	Tranxene

Potentially inappropriate drugs for elderly patients
(continued)

clozapine	Clozaril
cyclobenzaprine hydrochloride	Amrix, Fexmid, Flexeril
cyproheptadine hydrochloride	
dexchlorpheniramine	
diazepam	Valium
diclofenac potassium	Cambia, Cataflam, Zipsor
diclofenac sodium	Pennsaid, Voltaren, Voltaren XR
dicyclomine	Bentyl
diflunisal	
digoxin	Digitek, Lanoxin (> 0.125 mg/day)
diphenhydramine hydrochloride (oral)	Aler-Cap, Aler-Dryl, Aler-Tab, AllerMax, Altaryl, Banophen, Benadryl, Compoz, Diphen, Diphenhist, Genahist, Hydramine, Nytol, Siladryl, Silphen, Simply Sleep, Sleep-ettes D, Sleepinal, Sominex, Twilite, Unisom
dipyridamole (oral, short-acting)	Persantine
disopyramide	Norpace, Norpace CR
dofetilide	
doxazosin mesylate	Cardura, Cardura XR
doxepin hydrochloride (> 6 mg/day)	
dronedarone	Multaq
ergot mesyloids	
estrogens (with or without progestins)	Premarin, Premarin Intravenous
eszopiclone	Lunesta
etodolac	
ferrous sulfate (> 325 mg/day)	Feosol, Feratab, Fer-Gen-Sol, Fer-In-Sol, Fer-Iron, Slow FE
flecainide	Tambocor
fluphenazine	
fluoxetine hydrochloride (daily)	Prozac, Sarafem, Selfemra
glyburide	DiaBeta, Glynase PresTab
growth hormone	
haloperidol	

(continued)

hydroxyzine	Atarax, Vistaril
hyoscyamine sulfate	Levsin
ibuprofen	Advil, Advil Migraine, Advil Pediatric Drops, Caldolor, Children's Advil, Children's Motrin, Junior Strength Advil, Junior Strength Motrin, Motrin, Motrin IB, Motrin Infant
ibutilide	Corvert
iloperidone	Fanapt
imipramine	Tofranil
indomethacin	Indocin, Indocin SR
insulin, sliding scale	
isoxsuprine	
ketoprofen	
ketorolac tromethamine (includes parenteral)	
lorazepam	Ativan
loxapine succinate	
megestrol	Megace, Megace ES
meloxicam	
meperidine hydrochloride	Demerol
metaxalone	Skelaxin
methocarbamol	Robaxin
methyldopa	
metoclopramide hydrochloride	Reglan
mineral oil	
nabumetone	
nifidepine (short-acting)	Procardia
nitrofurantion	Furadantin, Macrobid, Macrodantin
non–COX-selective NSAIDs (long-term use of full dose): naproxen oxaprozin piroxicam	 Aleve, Anaprox, Naprosyn Daypro Feldene
olanzapine	Zyprexa
oxaprozin	Daypro
oxazepram	
paliperidone	Invega
pentazocine	Talwin

(continued)

Potentially inappropriate drugs for elderly patients
(continued)

perphenazine	
procainamide hydrochloride	
promethazine hydrochloride	Phenadoz, Phenergan, Promethagan
propafenone hydrochloride	Rythmol
quetiapine	Seroquel, Seroquel XR
quinidine	
risperidone	Risperdal, Risperdal Consta, Risperdal M-Tab
scopolamine	
sotalol hydrochloride	Betapace, Sorine
spironolactone (> 25 mg/ day)	Aldactone
temazepam	Restoril
terazosin	Hytrin
thyroid, dessicated	Armour Thyroid, Nature-Throid, Westhroid
ticlopidine hydrochloride	Ticlid
triazolam	Halcion
trifluoperazine	
trihexyphenidyl hydrochloride	
trimethobenzamide hydrochloride	Tigan
zaleplon	Sonata
ziprasidone	Geodon
zolpidem	Ambien, Ambien CR

Source: Potentially inappropriate drugs for the elderly (Beers List). *MPR*. www.empr.com/
potentially-inappropriate-drugs-for-the-elderly-beers-list/article/125908/.

Hazardous drugs

The drugs listed below have been designated as hazardous by the National Institute for Occupational Safety and Health, Centers for Disease Control and Prevention, and/or the American Society of Health-System Pharmacists. The list doesn't include all hazardous drugs. The agents listed here meet one or more of the following criteria: carcinogenicity, teratogenicity or other developmental toxicity, reproductive toxicity, organ toxicity at low doses, genotoxicity, or structure and toxicity profiles that mimic existing drugs determined to be hazardous by the above criteria. All health care workers handling these drugs must follow appropriate precautions along with recommendations included in the manufacturer's complete package insert.

acitretin
aldesleukin
alitretinoin
altretamine
amsacrine
anastrozole
arsenic trioxide
asparaginase
azacitidine
azathioprine
bacillus Calmette-Guerin vaccine
bendamustine hydrochloride
bexarotene
bicalutamide
bleomycin
bortezomib
bosentan
busulfan
capecitabine
carbamazepine
carboplatin
carmustine
cetrorelix acetate
chlorambucil
chloramphenicol
choriogonadotropin alfa
cidofovir
cisplatin
cladribine
clofarabine
clonazepam
colchicine
cyclophosphamide
cyclosporine
cytarabine

dacarbazine
dactinomycin
dasatinib
daunorubicin HCl
degarelix
denileukin
diethylstilbestrol
dinoprostone
docetaxel
doxorubicin
dronedarone HCl
dutasteride
entecavir
epirubicin
ergonovine/methylergonovine
estradiol
estramustine phosphate sodium
estrogen-progestin combinations
estrogens, conjugated
estrogens, esterified
estrone
estropipate
etoposide
everolimus
exemestane
finasteride
floxuridine
fludarabine
fluorouracil
fluoxymesterone
flutamide
fulvestrant
ganciclovir
ganirelix acetate
gemcitabine

(continued)

gemtuzumab ozogamicin
gonadotropin, chorionic
goserelin
hydroxyurea
idarubicin
ifosfamide
imatinib mesylate
irinotecan HCl
leflunomide
lenalidomide
letrozole
leuprolide acetate
lomustine
mechlorethamine
medroxyprogesterone
megestrol
melphalan
menotropins
mercaptopurine
methotrexate
methyltestosterone
mifepristone
mitomycin
mitotane
mitoxantrone HCl
mycophenolate mofetil
nafarelin
nelarabine
nilotinib
nilutamide
oxaliplatin
oxcarbazepine
oxytocin
paclitaxel
palifermin
paroxetine
pegaspargase
pemetrexed
pentamidine isethionate
pentostatin
pipobroman
piritrexim isethionate

podofilox
podophyllum resin
procarbazine
progesterone
progestins
raloxifene
rasagiline mesylate
ribavirin
risperidone
sirolimus
sorafenib
streptozocin
sunitinib malate
tacrolimus
tamoxifen
televancin
temozolomide
teniposide
testolactone
testosterone
tetracycline HCl
thalidomide
thioguanine
thiotepa
topotecan
toremifene citrate
tretinoin
trifluridine
triptorelin
uracil mustard
valganciclovir
valproic acid/divalproex sodium
valrubicin
vidarabine
vinblastine sulfate
vincristine sulfate
vindesine
vinorelbine tartrate
zidovudine
ziprasidone HCl
zoledronic acid
zonisamide

Drugs that prolong the QT interval

The drugs listed below are known to possibly cause QT-interval prolongation; and there is some evidence to show that when used as directed in labeling, these drugs can cause torsades de pointes. Other drugs or substances not listed here may also cause this problem, and the list doesn't include several drugs that have been withdrawn from the market in the United States. Monitor patients closely when administering drugs associated (some more than others) with QT-interval prolongation.

Generic name	Brand name
alfuzosin	–
amantadine hydrochloride	–
atazanavir	Reyataz
clozapine	Clozaril
dolasetron mesylate	Anzemet
dronedarone	Multaq
eribulin	Halaven
escitalopram	Lexapro
famotidine	Pepcid
fingolimod	Gilenya
flecainide acetate	Tambocor
foscarnet	–
fosphenytoin sodium	Cerebyx
gemifloxacin mesylate	Factive
granisetron hydrochloride	Granisol, Kytril, Sancuso
iloperidone	Fanapt
indapamide	Lozol
isradipine	DynaCirc CR
lapatinib	Tykerb
levofloxacin	Iquix, Levaquin, Quixin
lithium carbonate	Lithane, Lithobid
lithium citrate	–
mirtazapine	Remeron
moexipril and hydrochlorothiazide	Uniretic
nicardipine hydrochloride	Cardene, Cardene IV, Cardene SR
nilotinib	Tasigna
octreotide acetate	Sandostatin, Sandostatin LAR

(continued)

Generic name	Brand name
ofloxacin	Floxin, Ocuflox
ondansetron hydrochloride	Zofran, Zofran ODT, Zofran Preservative Free
oxytocin	Pitocin
paliperidone	Invega
pentamidine isethionate	NebuPent, Pentam
quetiapine fumarate	Seroquel, Seroquel XR
ranolazine	Ranexa
risperidone	Risperdal, Risperdal Consta, Risperdal M-Tab
sunitinib maleate	Sutent
tacrolimus	Prograf, Protopic
tamoxifen citrate	Nolvadex, Soltamox, Tamofen
telithromycin	Ketek
vardenafil hydrochloride	Levitra
venlafaxine hydrochloride	Effexor, Effexor XR
voriconazole	Vfend
ziprasidone hydrochloride	Geodon

Source: CredibleMeds. www.azcert.org/medical-pros/drug-lists/drug-lists.cfm.

Most commonly used drugs in nursing specialties

Nurses are often required to float to units in which they're not accustomed to working, where they might have to administer unfamiliar drugs. If you know ahead of time which drugs are most commonly used in the various nursing specialties, you'll be able to increase your confidence—and reduce the chance of making a drug error. The table below shows the 10 most commonly used drugs in nine nursing specialties.

Specialty	Top 10 drugs
Critical care nursing	amiodarone hydrochloride diltiazem hydrochloride dopamine hydrochloride epinephrine hydrochloride furosemide insulin lorazepam morphine sulfate nitroglycerin propofol
Emergency care nursing	acetaminophen aspirin diltiazem hydrochloride diphtheria and tetanus toxoids famotidine ibuprofen ketorolac levofloxacin metoclopramide nitroglycerin
Home care nursing	acetaminophen acetaminophen/oxycodone acetaminophen/propoxyphene napsylate digoxin diltiazem hydrochloride docusate sodium furosemide metformin hydrochloride potassium chloride warfarin
Long-term care nursing	carbidopa/levodopa digoxin docusate sodium donepezil hydrochloride enalapril maleate furosemide metoprolol tartrate mirtazapine pantoprazole sodium potassium chloride
Medical-surgical nursing	diltiazem hydrochloride furosemide

(continued)

Specialty	Top 10 drugs
Medical-surgical nursing (continued)	heparin sodium insulin levofloxacin lisinopril metformin metoprolol tartrate morphine sulfate simvastatin
Obstetric nursing	acetaminophen/codeine acetaminophen/oxycodone dinoprostone ibuprofen magnesium sulfate nalbuphine hydrochloride oxytocin penicillin promethazine hydrochloride terbutaline sulfate
Pediatric nursing	albuterol amoxicillin/clavulanate potassium amoxicillin trihydrate azithromycin co-trimoxazole fluticasone propionate gentamicin sulfate ibuprofen methylphenidate hydrochloride montelukast sodium
Post-anesthesia care nursing	bupivacaine hydrochloride fentanyl citrate hydromorphone hydrochloride lidocaine hydrochloride lorazepam meperidine hydrochloride metoclopramide hydrochloride midazolam hydrochloride morphine sulfate ondansetron hydrochloride
Psychiatric nursing	bupropion hydrochloride carbamazepine divalproex sodium escitalopram oxalate fluoxetine hydrochloride lithium carbonate olanzapine risperidone sertraline hydrochloride venlafaxine hydrochloride

Top 200 most commonly prescribed drugs

The table below lists the top 200 drugs ranked by the number of prescriptions sold in the United States in 2011.

1. Lipitor
2. Plavix
3. Nexium
4. Abilify
5. Advair Diskus
6. Seroquel
7. Singulair
8. Crestor
9. Cymbalta
10. Humira
11. Enbrel
12. Remicade
13. Actos
14. Neulasta
15. Rituxan
16. Zyprexa
17. Copaxone
18. Lexapro
19. OxyContin
20. Epogen
21. Avastin
22. Atripla
23. Spiriva Handihaler
24. Januvia
25. Lantus
26. Truvada
27. Diovan
28. Lyrica
29. Celebrex
30. Lucentis
31. Herceptin
32. Diovan HCT
33. Avonex
34. Lantus Solostar
35. Gleevec
36. Namenda
37. Enoxaparin
38. Geodon
39. Zetia
40. Tricor
41. Vyvanse
42. Suboxone
43. Lidoderm
44. Procrit
45. Eloxatin
46. Niaspan
47. Provigil
48. Aranesp
49. Androgel
50. Combivent
51. Lovenox
52. Rebif
53. Vytorin
54. Nasonex
55. Viagra
56. Symbicort
57. Seroquel XR
58. Alimta
59. Novolog
60. Lovaza
61. Humalog
62. Adderall XR
63. Neupogen
64. Flovent HFA
65. Proair HFA
66. Reyataz
67. Aciphex
68. Concerta
69. Budesonide
70. Levemir
71. Incivek
72. Varivax

(continued)

Top 200 most commonly prescribed drugs (continued)

73. Prevnar
74. Lunesta
75. Cialis
76. Solodyn
77. Novolog Flexpen
78. Isentress
79. Levaquin
80. Janumet
81. Methylphenidate ER
82. Synagis
83. Venlafaxine
84. Restasis
85. Zyvox
86. Betaseron
87. Evista
88. Erbitux
89. Benicar
90. Velcade
91. Zometa
92. Synthroid
93. Vesicare
94. Xeloda
95. Detrol LA
96. Opana ER
97. Orencia
98. Prezista
99. Ventolin HFA
100. Benicar HCT
101. Cubicin
102. Boniva
103. Sandostatin LAR
104. Actonel
105. Sensipar
106. Amphetamine Salts ER
107. Asacol
108. Loestrin 24 FE
109. Tarceva
110. Pradaxa
111. Renvela
112. Gamunex-C
113. Pristiq
114. Dexilant
115. Trilipix
116. Focalin XR
117. Avodart
118. Xolair
119. Strattera
120. Byetta
121. Humalog Kwikpen
122. Pegasys Convenience Pack
123. Gammagard Liquid
124. Prograf
125. Treanda
126. Risperdal Consta
127. Colcrys
128. Norvir
129. Premarin
130. Nuvaring
131. Xopenex
132. Travatan
133. Epzicom
134. Aloxi
135. Amphetamine Salts ER
136. Fentanyl
137. Actos Plus Met
138. Aggrenox
139. Viread
140. Metroprolol succinate
141. Forteo
142. Avapro
143. Mirena
144. Victoza 3-Pak
145. Zosyn
146. Exelon
147. Privigen
148. Revlimid
149. Lexiscan
150. Stelara
151. Adacel
152. Ortho-Tri-Cyclen Lo 28
153. Welchol
154. Angiomax

155. Gardasil
156. Lumigan
157. Pulmozyme
158. Invega
159. Reclast
160. Temodar
161. Xifaxan
162. Atorvastatin Calcium
163. NovoSeven RT
164. Bystolic
165. Invega
166. Lialda
167. Gilenya
168. Pneumovax
169. Effexor
170. Kaletra
171. Zostavax
172. Metoprolol Succinate
173. Taxotere
174. Tysabri
175. Donepezil HCL
176. Chantix
177. Xgeva
178. Nutropin AQ
179. Fluticasone Propionate
180. Avelox
181. Yervoy
182. Exforge
183. Onglyza
184. Abraxane
185. Hydrocodone/APAP
186. Synvisc-One
187. Zyprexa Zydis
188. Bupropion HCL XL
189. QVAR
190. NovoLog Flexpen Mix
191. Maxalt MLT
192. Zemplar
193. Docetaxel
194. Vancocin
195. Lamictal
196. Menactra
197. Vidaza
198. Valcyte
199. Omnipaque
200. Ranexa

Source: Top 200 products of 2011 by total dollars. *Pharmacy Times.*
www.pharmacytimes.com

Current drug shortages

In recent years, drug shortages in the United States have reached critical levels, adversely affecting drug therapy, delaying medical procedures and treatment, and contributing to medication errors. Shortages primarily affect older, sterile, injectable drugs, such as analgesics, sedatives and chemotherapeutics.

Despite the U.S. Food and Drug Administration's (FDA) efforts, drug shortages continue for a number of reasons, including a lack of raw materials, patent expirations, manufacturing costs, and manufacturing capacity. When shortages occur, the FDA provides information and helps restore availability.

Nurses should keep informed about current drug shortages and, when appropriate, take an active role in developing their facility's contingency plans. By knowing which drugs are expected to be in short supply and discussing workable alternatives with physicians and pharmacists, nurses can ease the adverse effects of ongoing drug shortages.

This list was last updated December 12, 2012. For more recent information, go to www.fda.gov/Drugs/DrugSafety/DrugShortages/default.htm.

A

Acetylcysteine Inhalation Solution
Acyclovir Sodium Injection
Alfentanil (Alfenta) Injection
Amikacin Injection
Amino Acid Products
Ammonium Chloride Injection
Atracurium besylate
Atropine Sulfate Injection

B

Bacteriostatic 0.9% Sodium Chloride
Barium Sulfate for Suspension
Bismuth subsalicylate/tetracycline hydrochloride/metronidazole (Helidac)
Bumetanide Injection
Bupivacaine Hydrochloride (Marcaine, Sensorcaine) Injection
Buprenorphine hydrochloride (Buprenex) Injection
Butorphanol (Stadol) Injection

C

Caffeine, anhydrous (125 mg/ml) and Sodium benzoate (125 mg/ml)
Caffeine and Ergotamine Tartrate Tablet
Cetrorelix Acetate for Injection (Cetrotide)
Chloroprocaine (Nesacaine) Injection
Chromic Chloride Injection
Citric Acid; Gluconolactone; Magnesium Carbonate Solution (Renacidin); Irrigation
Corticorelin Ovine Triflutate

D

Daunorubicin Hydrochloride Solution for Injection
Denileukin diftitox (Ontak) Injection
Desmopressin Injection (DDAVP)
Dexrazoxane (Zinecard) Injection
Dextroamphetamine (Dexedrine) Tablets
Dextrose Injection
Diazepam Injection
Dipyridamole Injection
Doxorubicin (Adriamycin) lyophilized powder
Doxorubicin Liposomal (Doxil) Injection

E

Edetate Calcium Disodium (Calcium Disodium Versenate) Injection
Epinephrine Injection
Epinephrine 1 mg/ml (Preservative Free)
Erythromycin Lactobionate Injection
Ethiodol (ETHIODIZED OIL) ampules
Etomidate (Amidate) Injection

F

Fentanyl Citrate (Sublimaze) Injection
Fluticasone Propionate and Salmeterol (Advair HFA) Inhalation Powder
Foscarnet Sodium (Foscavir) Injection
Fosphenytoin Sodium (Cerebyx) Injection
Fospropofol disodium (Lusedra) Injection
Furosemide Injection

G

Gallium Nitrate (Ganite) Injection

H

Heparin Sodium Premixes
Hydromorphone Hydrochloride (Dilaudid) Injection

I

Ibandronate sodium (Boniva) Injection
Intravenous Fat Emulsion
Isoniazid Tablets

K

Ketorolac Tromethamine Injection

L

Leucovorin Calcium Lyophilized Powder for Injection
Leuprolide Acetate Injection
Lidocaine (Xylocaine) Hydrochloride Injection
Lidocaine Hydrochloride, 4% Topical Solution (Laryng-O-Jet, LTA kit)
Liotrix (Thyrolar) Tablets
Lorazepam (Ativan) Injection

M

Magnesium Sulfate Injection
Mannitol (Osmitrol, Resectisol) Injection
Methadone Injection
Methazolamide (Glauctabs, Neptazane) Tablets
Methotrexate Injection
Methoxsalen (Oxsoralen) 1% topical lotion
Methyldopate Hydrochloride Injection
Metoclopramide (Reglan) Injection
Midazolam Hydrochloride (Versed) Injection
Mitomycin Powder for Injection
Morphine Sulfate Injection
Morphine Sulfate (Astramorph PF, Duramorph, Infumorph) Injection (Preservative Free)
Multi-Vitamin Infusion (Adult and pediatric)

N

Nalbuphine Hydrochloride (Nubain) Injection
Naloxone (Narcan) Injection
Naltrexone (Revia) Oral Tablets
Nefazodone (Serzone) Tablets
Nitroglycerin Ointment USP, 2% (Nitro-Bid)
Norethindrone and Ethinyl Estradiol Tablets, USP (Ovcon 50 Tablets)

O

Ondansetron (Zofran) Injection 2 mg/ml
Ondansetron Injection 32 mg/50 ml premixed
Oxymorphone Hydrochloride (Opana) Tablet

P

Pancuronium Bromide Injection

Peginterferon Alfa-2a (Pegasys) Injection, Pre-filled Syringes
Pentamidine isethionate inhalant (NebuPent)
Pentamidine isethionate for injection (Pentam 300)
Pentostatin for Injection (Nipent)
Perflutren Lipid Microsphere (DEFINITY) Injection
Phentolamine Mesylate (Regitine) Injection
Pilocarpine Hydrochloride Ophthalmic Gel 4% (Pilopine HS)
Potassium Chloride Injection 2 mEq/ml
Potassium Phosphate Injection
Procainamide Hydrochloride Injection
Prochlorperazine Injection
Promethazine Injection
Propofol (Diprivan) Injection

S

Secretin Synthetic Human (ChiRhoStim) Injection
Selenium Injection
Sodium Acetate Injection
Sodium benzoate and Sodium phenylacetate (Ammonul) Injection
Sodium Bicarbonate Injection
Sodium Chloride 0.9% (5.8 ml and 20 ml)
Sodium Chloride 23.4%
Succinylcholine (Anectine, Quelicin) Injection
Sufentanil Citrate (Sufenta) Injection
Sulfamethoxazole 80 mg/trimethoprim 160 mg/ml Injection (SMX/TMP) (Bactrim)

T

Technetium Tc 99m Bicisate for Injection
Technetium Tc 99m Sestamibi Kit for Injection
Telavancin (Vibativ) Injection
Tetracycline Capsules
Thiotepa (Thioplex) for Injection
Thyrotropin alfa (Thyrogen) Injection
Ticarcillin disodium/Clavulanic Potassium Injection (Timentin)
Ticlopidine (Ticlid) Tablets
Tobramycin Solution for Injection
Tromethamine (Tham) Injection

V

Viaspan Cold Storage Solution 1000 ml Bag
Vinblastine Sulfate Injection
Vitamin A Palmitate (Aquasol A) Injection
Vitamin K1 (Phytonadione) Injectable Emulsion

Z

Zinc Chloride Injection

Source: U.S. Food and Drug Administration. Drug shortages. www.fda.gov/Drugs/DrugSafety/DrugShortages/default.htm.

Selected references

Publications

AHFS Drug Information 2012. Bethesda, MD: American Society of Health-System Pharmacists, 2012.

American Heart Association. 2010 American Heart Association Guidelines for Cardiopulmonary Resuscitation and Emergency Cardiovascular Care. www.heart.org/idc/groups/heart-public/@wcm/@ecc/documents/downloadable/ucm_318152.pdf.

American Society of Health-System Pharmacists. ASHP guidelines on handling hazardous drugs 2005. *Am J Health-Syst Pharm.* 2006;63:1172-1193.

Bailie GR, Mason NA. *2012 Dialysis of Drugs.* Saline, MI: Renal Pharmacy Consultants, 2012.

Blumenthal M, et al. *The Complete German Commission E Monographs: Therapeutic Guide to Herbal Medicines.* Newton, MA: Integrative Medicine Communication, 1998.

Blumenthal M, et al, eds. *Herbal Medicine: Expanded Commission E Monographs.* Newton, Mass.: Integrative Medicine Communication, 2000.

Brunton L, Chabner BA, Knollman B. *Goodman & Gilman's The Pharmacological Basis of Therapeutics.* 12th ed. New York, NY: McGraw-Hill Professional, 2011.

Chameides L, Samson RA, Schnexnayder SM, et al, eds. *Pediatric Advanced Life Support Provider Manual.* Dallas, TX: American Heart Association, 2011.

Drug Facts and Comparisons 2012. Philadelphia, PA: Lippincott Williams & Wilkins, 2012.

The Elsevier Guide to Oncology Drugs & Regimens. Huntington, NY: Elsevier Oncology, 2006.

Hansten ED, Horn JR. *Drug Interactions Analysis and Management 2012.* Philadelphia, PA: Lippincott Williams & Wilkins, 2012.

Hansten ED, Horn JR. *The Top 100 Drug Interactions: A Guide to Patient Management. 2012 Edition.* Edmonds, WA: H & H Publications, 2012.

Hazinski MF, Samson R, Schexnayder S, eds. *2010 Handbook of Emergency Cardiovascular Care for Healthcare Providers.* Dallas, TX: American Heart Association, 2010.

Health Research & Educational Trust, Institute for Safe Medication Practices, & Medical Group Management Association. Patient safety tools for physician practices. www.mgma.com/pppsa/.

Institute of Medicine. *Preventing Medication Errors.* Washington, DC: National Academies Press, 2007.

Institute of Medicine. *To Err is Human: Building a Safer Health System.* Washington, DC: National Academies Press, 2000.

The Joint Commission. 2012 National patient safety goals. www. jointcommission.org/standards_information/npsgs.aspx.

King Guide to Parenteral Admixtures. Napa, CA: King Guide Publications, Inc, 2012. www.kingguide.com/.

National Institute for Occupational Safety and Health. NIOSH list of antineoplastic and other hazardous drugs in healthcare settings 2012. http://www.cdc.gov/niosh/docs/2012-150/pdfs/2012-150.pdf.

National Institute for Occupational Safety and Health. Preventing occupational exposure to antineoplastic and other hazardous drugs in health care settings. www.cdc.gov/niosh/docs/2004-165/.

PDR for Herbal Medicines, 4th ed. Montvale, NJ: Thomson Healthcare, 2007.

Physicians' Desk Reference 2013. 67th ed. Montvale, NJ: PDR Network, LLC, 2013.

Pickar GD, Abernethy AP. *Dosage Calculations.* 9th ed. Clifton Park, NY: Delmar Cengage Learning, 2012.

Polovich M. *Safe Handling of Hazardous Drugs.* 2nd ed. Pittsburgh, PA: Oncology Nursing Society, 2011.

Shargel L, Wu-Pong S, Yu A. *Applied Biopharmaceutics & Pharmacokinetics.* 6th ed. New York, NY: McGraw-Hill Medical, 2012.

Sweetman SC, ed. *Martindale: The Complete Drug Reference.* 37th ed. London: Pharmaceutical Press, 2011.

Tatro DS. *Drug Interaction Facts 2013.* Philadelphia, PA: Lippincott Williams & Wilkins, 2012.

U.S. Food and Drug Administration. MedWatch: The FDA Safety Information and Adverse Event Reporting Program. www.fda.gov/Safety/MedWatch/default.htm.

Websites

American Society of Health-System Pharmacists (drug information): www.ahfsdruginformation.com/

Centers for Disease Control and Prevention (immunization schedules): www.cdc.gov/vaccines/schedules/hcp

DailyMed (drug information): http://dailymed.nlm.nih.gov/dailymed/about.cfm

Druginfonet.com (drug information): www.druginfonet.com/index.php?pageID=official.htm

Drugs.com (drug information): www.drugs.com

Drugs@FDA (catalog of FDA-approved drugs): www.accessdata.fda.gov/scripts/cder/drugsatfda

Health Canada (Canadian drug product database): www.hc-sc.gc.ca/dhp-mps/index-eng.php

Institute for Safe Medication Practices: www.ismp.org

MedlinePlus (drug information): www.nlm.nih.gov/medlineplus/druginformation.html

U.S. Food and Drug Administration (drug information): www.fda.gov/Drugs/default.htm

U.S. Pharmacopeia (drug information): www.usp.org

Index

t: table   **Boldface:** Color section

---

t: table   **Boldface:** Color section

Boldface: Color section

Boldface: Color section

Boldface: Color section

Boldface: Color section

Boldface: Color section

     Boldface: Color section

---

t: table   **Boldface:** Color section

Boldface: Color section

Boldface: Color section

Boldface: Color section

t: table

Boldface: Color section